Haemostasis and Thrombosis

VOLUME 2

Edited by

Arthur L. Bloom

Late Professor of Haematology, University of Wales College of Medicine,
Cardiff, UK

Charles D. Forbes

Professor of Medicine, Ninewells Hospital and Medical School,
Dundee, UK

Duncan P. Thomas

Formerly Head of the Division of Haematology,
National Institute for Biological Standards and Control,
South Mimms, UK

Edward G. D. Tuddenham

Clinical Scientific Staff, Medical Research Council; Director of the Haemostasis Research Group,
Clinical Research Centre, Harrow, UK

THIRD EDITION

CHURCHILL LIVINGSTONE
EDINBURGH LONDON MADRID MELBOURNE NEW YORK AND TOKYO 1994

CHURCHILL LIVINGSTONE
Medical Division of Longman Group UK Limited

Distributed in the United States of America by Churchill Livingstone Inc., 650 Avenue of the Americas, New York, NY 10011, and by associated companies, branches and representatives throughout the world.

First edition 1981
Second edition 1987
Third edition 1994
Reprinted 1994

ISBN 0-443-04521-6

British Library of Cataloguing in Publication Data
A catalogue record for this book is available from the British Library.

Library of Congress Cataloging in Publication Data
A catalog record for this book is available from the Library of Congress.

The publisher's policy is to use **paper manufactured from sustainable forests**

Produced by Longman Singapore Publishers (Pte) Ltd
Printed in Singapore

Haemostasis and Thrombosis

VOLUME 2

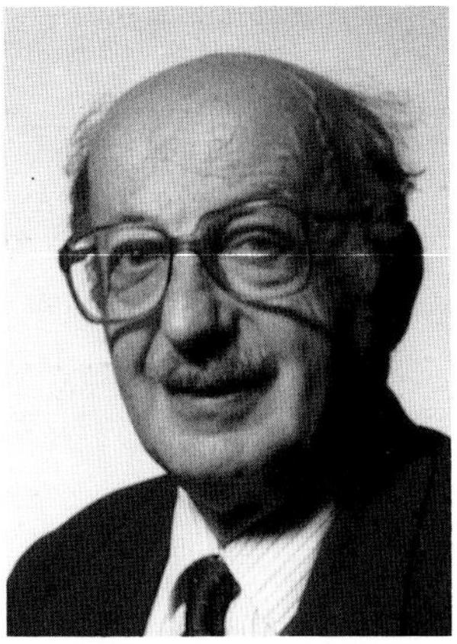

Arthur Leslie Bloom 1930–1992

In Memoriam

This third edition of Haemostasis and Thrombosis is dedicated to the memory of Professor Arthur Bloom, who died on 12 November, 1992. At the time of his death, he was Professor in Haematology at the University of Wales College of Medicine and Honorary Director of the Haemophilia Reference Centre in Cardiff.

This book was originally his idea, and reflected his deep knowledge of the field to which he had contributed so much. It is primarily due to his inspiration, enthusiasm and commitment that the book is now entering upon its second decade of life.

In common with his family, friends and patients, his fellow editors mourn the untimely death of a gentle physician, an imaginative scientist and a wise counsellor.

SI MONUMENTUM REQUIRIS, CIRCUMSPICE

For Churchill Livingstone:

Publisher: Michael Parkinson
Project Editor: Dilys Jones
Copy Editor: Jane Ward
Indexer: Monica Trigg
Production Controller: Debra Barrie
Sales Promotion Executive: Douglas McNaughton

Contents

SECTION 10
Venous thrombosis

SECTION 11
Antithrombotic therapy

Contributors

C. F. Allaart MD
Clinical Researcher, Department of Haematology, University Hospital, Leiden, The Netherlands

Maureen Andrew MD FRCP(C)
Professor, Departments of Pediatrics and Pathology, McMaster University, Hamilton, Ontario

Fedor Bachmann MD FACP
Professor Emeritus and Past Head of the Division of Haematology, Department of Medicine, University of Lausanne Medical Center, Lausanne, Switzerland

Trevor W. Barrowcliffe MA PhD
Head of Division of Haematology, National Institute for Biological Standards and Control, South Mimms, UK

Kenneth A. Bauer MD
Associate Professor of Medicine, Harvard Medical School; Chief, Hematology-Oncology Section, Brockton-West Roxbury Department of Veterans Affairs Medical Center; Associate Physician, Hematology-Oncology Division, Beth Israel Hospital, Boston, USA

Jill J. F. Belch MD FRCP
Reader in Medicine, University Department of Medicine, University of Dundee; Consultant Physician, Ninewells Hospital, Dundee, UK

Peter R. F. Bell MD FRCS
Professor, Department of Surgery, Clinical Sciences Building, Leicester Royal Infirmary, Leicester, UK

Vittorio Bertele MD
Chief of the Unit of Vascular Medicine, Istituto di Ricerche, Farmacologiche 'Mario Negri', Consorzio Mario Negri Sud, Santa Maria Imbaro, Italy

Arthur L. Bloom MD FRCP FRCPath (Deceased)
Formerly Professor in Haematology, University of Wales College of Medicine, Cardiff, UK

Nuala A. Booth PhD
Lecturer, Department of Molecular and Cell Biology, University of Aberdeen, Marischal College, Aberdeen, UK

Ernest Briët MD
Professor of Medicine, Director, Hematology Laboratories, University Hospital Leiden, The Netherlands

George J. Broze Jr MD
Professor of Medicine and Cell Biology and Physiology, Washington University School of Medicine, St Louis, USA

Robin W. Carrell PhD FRCP FRCPath
Professor of Haematology, MRC Centre Clinical School of Medicine, University of Cambridge, Cambridge, UK

Chiara Cerletti PhD
Head, Giulio Bizzozero Laboratory of Platelet and Leukocyte Pharmacology, Instituto di Ricerche, Consorzio 'Mario Negri' Sud, Santa Maria Imbaro, Italy

Desirée Collen MD PhD
Professor of Medicine, Center for Thrombosis and Vascular Research, University of Leuven, Leuven, Belgium

Barry S. Coller MD
Professor of Medicine and Pathology; Head, Division of Hematology, State University of New York at Stony Brook, New York, USA

James M. Courtney PhD Dr Sc Nat
Professor, Bioengineering Unit, University of Strathclyde, Glasgow, UK

Neville Crawford PhD
Distinguished Visiting Professor, Department of Biochemistry, Royal Free Hospital School of Medicine, London, UK

Björn Dahlbäck MD PhD
Professor of Blood Coagulation Research, Department of Clinical Chemistry, University of Lund, Malmö General Hospital, Malmö, Sweden

John F. Davidson MB FRCPEd FRCPath
Consultant Haematologist, Glasgow Royal Infirmary, Glasgow; Honorary Clinical Senior Lecturer, Glasgow University, Glasgow, UK

Earl W. Davie PhD
Professor of Biochemistry, University of Washington, Seattle, USA

David de Bono MA MD FRCP
British Heart Foundation Professor of Cardiology, University of Leicester; Consultant Cardiologist, Groby Road Hospital, Leicester, UK

Giovanni de Gaetano MD PhD
Director, Centro di Ricerche Biomediche e Farmacologiche, Consorzio 'Mario Negri Sud', Santa Maria Imbaro, Italy

Russell F. Doolittle PhD
Professor of Biology and Chemistry, Center for Molecular Genetics, University of California, San Diego, California, USA

Charles D. Forbes DSc MD FRCP(Glas Edin Lond) FRS(E) FRSA
Professor of Medicine, Ninewells Hospital and Medical School, Dundee, UK

Yoshihiro Fujimura MD
Associate Professor, Department of Blood Transfusion, Nara Medical College, Nara, Japan

Patrick J. Gaffney PhD FRCPath DSc
Scientist, Special Appointment, National Institute for Biological Standards and Control, South Mimms, UK

Allan Gaw MB ChB PhD
Research Fellow, Department of Molecular Genetics, University of Texas, Southwestern Medical Center, Dallas, Texas, USA

Paul L. F. Giangrande BSc MD MRCP MRCPath
Consultant Haematologist, Oxford Haemophilia Centre, Churchill Hospital, Oxford, UK

Francesco Giannelli MD MRCP DSc
Professor of Molecular Genetics, Division of Medical and Molecular Genetics, Guy's Hospital, London, UK

Alan R. Giles MB BS FRCP(C)
Professor, Departments of Pathology and Medicine, Queen's University, Kingston, Ontario; Director, Hemostasis Laboratory and Clinic, Kingston General Hospital, Kingston, Ontario, Canada

Samuel Z. Goldhaber MD
Associate Professor of Medicine, Harvard Medical School; Physician, Brigham and Women's Hospital, Boston, USA

Peter J. Grant MD MRCP
Senior Lecturer and Honorary Consultant, Academic Unit of Medicine, Leeds General Infirmary, Leeds, UK

Ian A. Greer MD MRCP(UK) MRCOG
Muirhead Professor and Head, Department of Obstetrics and Gynaecology, University of Glasgow; Honorary Consultant Obstetrician and Gynaecologist, Glasgow Royal Maternity Hospital and Glasgow Royal Infirmary, Glasgow, UK

Laurence A. Harker MD
Blomeyer Professor of Medicine, Emory University School of Medicine, Atlanta, Georgia; Director, Division of Hematology and Oncology, Emory University School of Medicine, Atlanta, Georgia, USA

Paul L. Harper MD MRCP MRCPath
Consultant Haematologist, West Suffolk Hospital, Bury St Edmunds, UK

Dorian O. Haskard DM MRCP
Senior Lecturer and Honorary Consultant Physician, Royal Postgraduate Medical School, Hammersmith Hospital, London, UK

Frits Haverkate PhD
Senior Research Associate, Gaubius Laboratory, IVVO-TNO, Leiden, The Netherlands

H. C. Hemker MD PhD
Professor and Chairman, Department of Biochemistry, Cardiovascular Research Institute, Maastricht and Rijles, Limburg University, Maastricht, The Netherlands

A. H. Henderson FRCP FESC
Professor of Cardiology, British Heart Foundation Sir Thomas Lewis Chair, University of Wales College of Medicine, Cardiff, UK

Anthon du P. Heyns MD DSc FFPath(SA)
Medical Director, The South African Blood Transfusion Service; Professor, Department of Haematology, School of Pathology, University of the Witwatersrand, Johannesburg, Republic of South Africa

Akitada Ichinose MD PhD
Research Associate Professor of Biochemistry, University of Washington, Department of Biochemistry, Seattle, USA

Sara Joan Israels MD
Associate Professor, Department of Pediatrics, University of Manitoba, Winnipeg, Manitoba, Canada

Craig M. Jackson PhD
President, Reagents Applications Inc., San Diego, California, USA

Harold L. James PhD
Associate Professor, Department of Biochemistry, University of Texas Health Center at Tyler, USA

Richard J. Jenny PhD
Scientific Director, Haematologic Technologies Inc., Essex Junction, Vermont, USA

Vijay V. Kakkar FRCS FRCSE
Professor of Surgical Science, Director, Thrombosis Research Institute, University of London, UK; Consultant Surgeon, Royal Brompton and Kings College Hospitals, London, UK

Raelene L. Kinlough-Rathbone MD BS PhD
Professor of Pathology, McMaster University, Hamilton, Ontario, Canada

John G. Kelton MD
Professor of Medicine and Pathology, McMaster University Medical Center, Hamilton, Ontario, Canada

Jaap Koopman PhD
Research Associate, Department of Fibrinolysis, Gaubius Laboratory, Leiden and Department of Hematology, University Hospital, Leiden, The Netherlands

David A. Lane BA PhD
Professor of Molecular Haematology, Charing Cross and Westminster Medical School, London, UK

H. Roger Lijnen PhD
Associate Professor, Center for Thrombosis and Vascular Research, University of Leuven, Leuven, Belgium

Richard I. Lindley MB BS MRCP(UK)
Research Fellow, Neurosciences Trials Unit, Department of Clinical Neurosciences, University of Edinburgh, Western General Hospital, Edinburgh, UK

Colin Longstaff PhD
Scientist, National Institute for Biological Standards and Control, South Mimms, UK

Gordon D. O. Lowe MD FRCP (Edin, Glas, Lond)
Professor, Department of Medicine, University of Glasgow; Consultant Physician and Co-Director, Haemophilia Unit, Royal Infirmary, Glasgow, UK

Christopher A. Ludlam BSc PhD FRCPath
Director, Haemophilia and Haemostasis Centre; Consultant Haematologist, Royal Infirmary, Edinburgh, UK

Mike Makris MA MB BS MRCP MRCPath
Lecturer in Haematology, University of Sheffield; Senior Lecturer in Haematology, Royal Hallamshire Hospital, Sheffield, UK

Kenneth G. Mann PhD
Professor and Chair, Department of Biochemistry, University of Vermont College of Medicine, Vermont, USA

Pier Mannuccio Mannucci MD
Professor of Internal Medicine, IRCCS Maggiore Hospital and University of Milano, Italy

Tom W. Meade DM FRCP
Director, MRC Epidemiology and Medical Care Unit; Professor of Epidemiology, Wolfson Institute of Preventive Medicine, Medical College of St Bartholomew's Hospital, London, UK

Stefan Niewiarowski MD PhD
Professor of Physiology, Department of Physiology and Sol Sherry Thrombosis Research Center, Philadelphia, USA

Alan T. Nurden PhD
Director, URA 1464 CNRS, Hopital Cardiologique, Pessac, France

Donogh Paul O'Brien PhD CBiol MIBiol
Senior Scientist, Haemostasis Research Group, Clinical Research Centre, Harrow, UK

Robin J. Olds MB ChB PhD FRCPA
Research Fellow, Institute of Molecular Medicine, John Radcliffe Hospital, Oxford, UK

Chris J. Packard BSc PhD MRCPath
Top Grade Biochemist, Institute of Biochemistry, Glasgow Royal Infirmary, Glasgow, UK

Marian A. Packham PhD
University Professor, Department of Biochemistry, University of Toronto, Toronto, Canada

Ian Peake PhD MRCPath
Professor of Molecular Medicine, Section of Molecular Genetics, Department of Medicine, University of Sheffield, Sheffield, UK

Jeremy D. Pearson MA PhD
Professor of Vascular Biology, Vascular Biology Research Centre, Biomedical Sciences Division, King's College, London, UK

Colin R. M. Prentice MD FRCP DTM&H
Professor of Medicine, University of Leeds, The General Infirmary, Leeds, UK

F. Eric Preston MD FRCP FRCPath
Professor of Haematology, Royal Hallamshire Hospital, Sheffield, UK

Martin H. Prins MD
Lecturer in Clinical Epidemiology and Internal Medicine, Academic Medical Center, Amsterdam, The Netherlands

Michael D. Randall PhD
Research Fellow, Department of Diagnostic Radiology, Cardiovascular Research Group, University of Wales College of Medicine, Cardiff, UK

Oscar Ratnoff MD LLD
Professor of Medicine, Case Western Reserve University; Physician, University Hospitals of Cleveland, Cleveland, USA

Alexander P. Reiner MD
Senior Fellow, Division of Hematology, Department of Medicine, University of Washington School of Medicine, Seattle, USA

Charles R. Rizza MD FRCPE
Consultant Physician and Director, Oxford Haemophilia Centre, Churchill Hospital, Oxford; Clinical Lecturer in Haematology, University of Oxford, UK

J. Evan Sadler MD PhD
Associate Investigator, Howard Hughes Medical Institute; Associate Professor, Department of Medicine and Department of Biochemistry and Molecular Biophysics, Washington University School of Medicine, St Louis, USA

Hidehiko Saito MD FACP
Chairman and Professor, First Department of Medicine, Nagoya University School of Medicine, Nagoya, Japan

Derek D. Sandeman BSc MRCP
Senior Registrar, Endocrinology and Diabetes, University Hospital of Wales, Cardiff, UK

Michael C. Scrutton MA DPhil DSc
Professor of Biochemistry, Division of Life Sciences, King's College, London, UK

James Shepherd MB PhD MRCPath
Professor of Pathological Biochemistry, University of Glasgow, Glasgow, UK

Jan J. Sixma MD PhD
Professor of Haematology, University Hospital Utrecht, Utrecht, The Netherlands

Jerry A. Smith BSc PhD
Postdoctoral Research Fellow, Department of Cardiology, University of Wales College of Medicine, Cardiff, UK

Johan P. Stenflo MD PhD
Professor of Clinical Chemistry, Lund University, Malmö General Hospital, Malmö, Sweden

S. L. Thein MB BS MRCP MRCPath
Clinical Scientific Staff, Medical Research Council, Molecular Haematology Unit, Institute of Molecular Medicine, John Radcliffe Hospital, Oxford, UK

Duncan P. Thomas MD MSc DPhil FRCPath
Formerly Head of the Division of Haematology, National Institute for Biological Standards and Control, South Mimms, UK

Koiti Titani PhD
Professor, Division of Biomedical Polymer Science, Institute for Comprehensive Medical Science, Fujita Health University School of Medicine, Toyoake, Aichi, Japan

John E. Tooke MA MSc DM MRCP
Consultant Physician and Senior Lecturer in Medicine, Diabetes Research Laboratories, Postgraduate Medical School, University of Exeter, Exeter, UK

Paula B. Tracy PhD
Associate Professor, Biochemistry and Medicine, University of Vermont College of Medicine, Burlington, USA

Edward G. D. Tuddenham MD FRCP(Lond) FRCPath
Clinical Scientific Staff, Medical Research Council; Director of the Haemostasis Research Group, Clinical Research Centre, Harrow, UK

A. Graham G. Turpie MB FRCP(Lond, Glasg) FACP FACC FRCPC
Professor of Medicine, McMaster University; Internist, Hamilton General Hospital, Hamilton, Ontario, Canada

A. M. H. P. van den Besselaar PhD
Biochemist, Haemostasis and Thrombosis Research Unit, Department of Haematology, Leiden University Hospital, Leiden, The Netherlands

Marc Verstraete MD PhD
Professor of Medicine, Center for Thrombosis and Vascular Research, Katholieke Universiteit Leuven, Leuven, Belgium

Isobel D. Walker MD FRCP FRCPath
Consultant Haematologist, Glasgow Royal Infirmary and Glasgow Royal Maternity Hospital; Honorary Clinical Senior Lecturer, University of Glasgow, Glasgow, UK

Theodore E. Warkentin MD
Assistant Professor of Pathology and Medicine, McMaster University; Hematologist, Department of Laboratory Medicine and Service of Clinical Hematology, Civics Hospital (General Division), Hamilton, Ontario, Canada

Charles Warlow MD FRCP
Professor of Medical Neurology, University of Edinburgh, Edinburgh, UK

James G. White MD
Regents' Professor, Laboratory Medicine – Pathology, Pediatrics; Associate Dean for Research, University of Minnesota School of Medicine, Minnesota, USA

Josiah N. Wilcox PhD
Department of Medicine, Division of Hematology, Emory University, Atlanta, USA

Preface to the Third Edition

Since the second edition of this book in 1987, knowledge of the clinical and laboratory aspects of haemostasis and thrombosis has continued to grow rapidly. This growth is reflected in the increased number of pages and chapters, especially in those dealing with biochemical and molecular mechanisms in health and disease. In a volume of this size, and with so many authors, it is inevitable that there may be overlap in some presentations. This is not necessarily detrimental and we have made no attempt to edit these out, as some repetition often gives a more rounded view of a topic.

To keep the size of the book within manageable proportions, some of the contents of the two earlier editions have been discarded to make room for new work. With the expanding scope and inevitable increasing specialisation in the field, the number of editors was increased to four. The list of contributors reflects the international nature of contemporary medicine and science, and although the editors are all based in the United Kingdom, over half the contributors are from other countries.

Sadly, the senior editor did not live to see the publication of this edition. Professor Arthur Bloom died in late 1992, to the great dismay of his many friends and colleagues around the world.

We would like to thank the many past and present contributors for their help and encouragement in producing this volume. In addition, we would like to express our gratitude to Dilys Jones, Janice Urquhart and the staff of Churchill Livingstone for their expert editorial assistance.

It is our hope that this volume will enhance development of both the clinical and the laboratory aspects of haemostasis and thrombosis.

C.D.F
D.P.T.
1993 E.G.D.T.

Preface to the First Edition

Haemostasis and thrombosis are increasingly recognised as distinct areas of special study, both in the laboratory and in the clinic. However, few texts are available that span the whole field, linking structure, biochemistry and physiology with pathology, clinical diagnosis, pharmacology and treatment, and also considering thrombosis as well as the haemorrhagic disorders. While no textbook can compete in detail with specialised monographs dealing with selected topics, in our view there is a need for a medium-sized, reasonably comprehensive textbook that covers haemostasis and its disorders and thrombosis. Many of the physiological processes involved in normal haemostasis are relevant to the development of thrombosis and to the pathogenesis of atherosclerosis, and it is illogical to divide these subjects one from the other. We hope that this book will provide information and guidance to all those interested in these areas and, if not solving their particular problems, will at least point them in the right direction. It may also serve a more mundane purpose by helping those studying for postgraduate diplomas or preparing for higher degrees. We have included chapters on the principles of laboratory and other techniques, but detailed descriptions of methods are not included – these are available in several excellent volumes. Nor have we attempted to cover in detail all the various clinical conditions where thrombosis plays an important role (such as in heart attacks and strokes), as these topics are well covered in standard textbooks.

All contributors to this volume are acknowledged experts in their field. Inevitably, in a multi-author book there is some repetition and unevenness in depth of presentation. We have attempted to reduce this, but repetition is not always a bad thing and may help to give new perspectives to difficult topics. In addtion, we have tried to integrate the contents to produce an up-to-date account of the whole field.

We would like to thank the contributors for their cooperation and the staff of Churchill Livingstone for their help and enthusiasm during preparation of this book. We would like especially to record our thanks to Miss Olive Harrison for expert editorial assistance and to our secretaries who cheerfully carried the additional burden that this volume has imposed. We hope that the final product is worthy of the efforts and hard work of all those concerned.

Cardiff and London — A. L. B.
1981 — D. P. T.

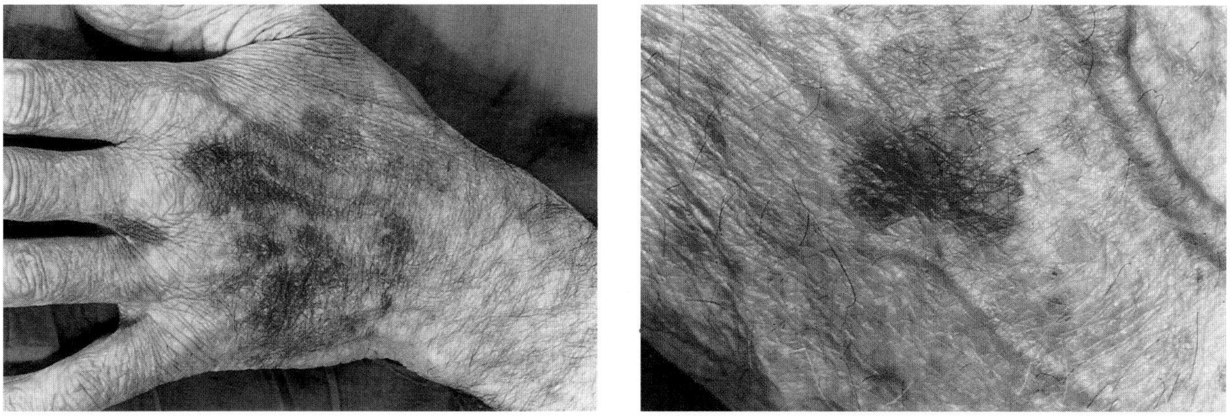

Plate 46.1 Typical appearances of senile purpura on the back of the hand in an elderly lady. Note the thin atrophied skin which has lost its elasticity and subcutaneous fat and in which the veins become extremely prominent. Lesions may be at different stages of development and resolve slowly to leave areas of brown haemosiderin ('age spots').

A

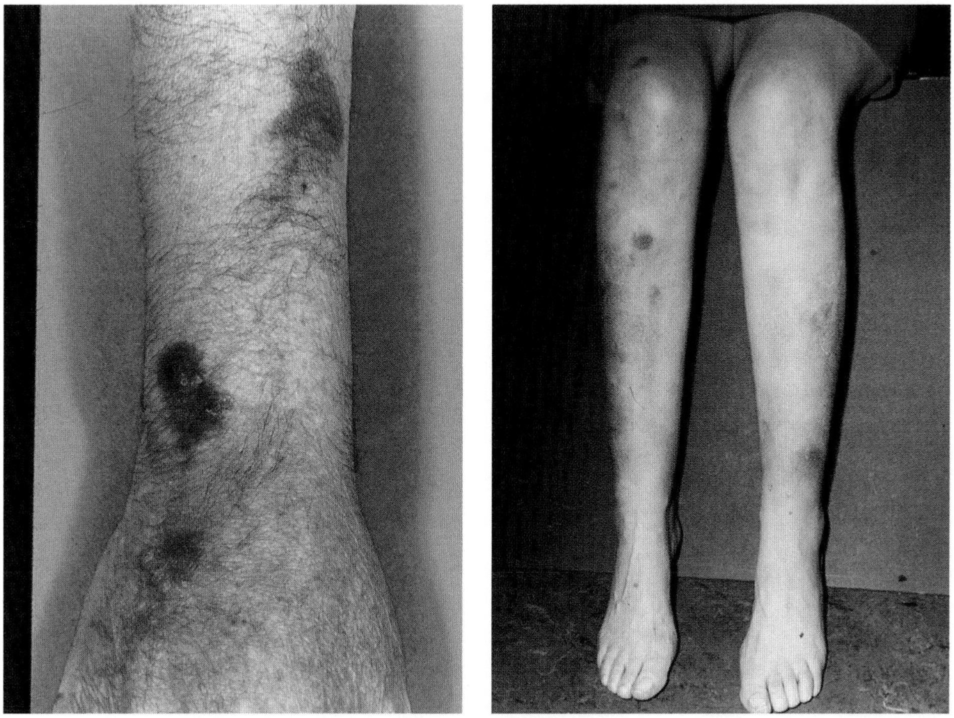

B

Plate 46.2 Typical appearances of purpura in patients taking long-term steroids. **A**, a male with rheumatoid arthritis and **B**, a young woman with systemic lupus erythematosus. The lesions are particularly noticeable on the shins and forearms and are often associated with minor trauma. The skin is thin and atrophic (as are the muscles).

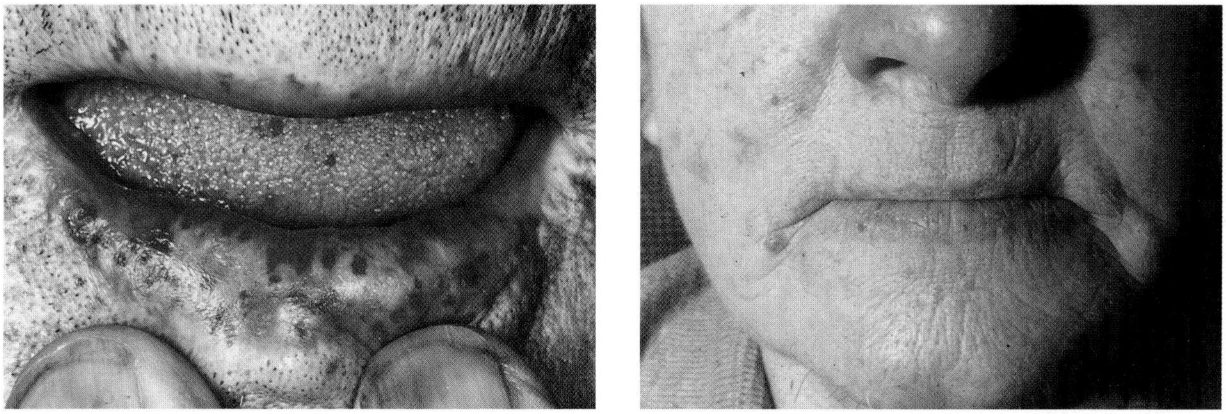

A B

Plate 46.3 Hereditary haemorrhagic telangiectasis. **A**, multiple telangiectatic spots on the lips and tongue. These blanch on pressure with a glass slide. **B**, often they are not as marked but despite this, this patient had had lifelong epistaxis and severe iron-deficient anaemia.

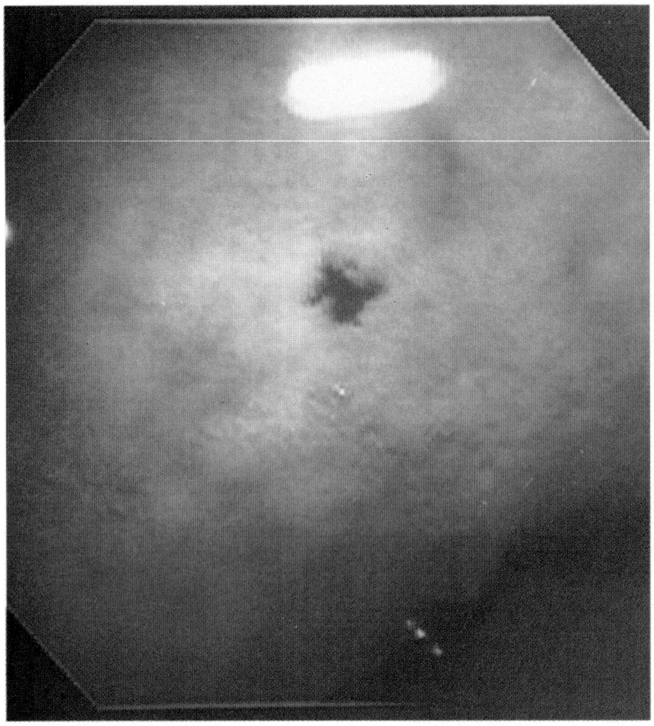

Plate 46.4 Multiple telangiectatic lesions may be found in the alimentary, respiratory and uro-genital tract. This lesion is in the duodenum.

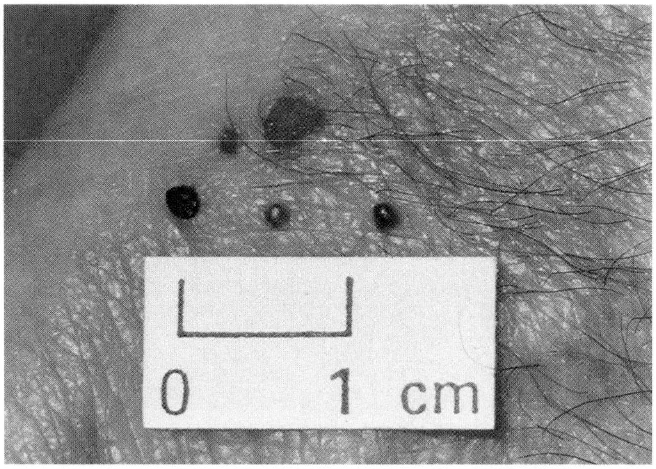

Plate 46.5 Blood blisters in the skin, self induced by mechanical trauma. Often these are found in disturbed or mentally retarded patients.

A

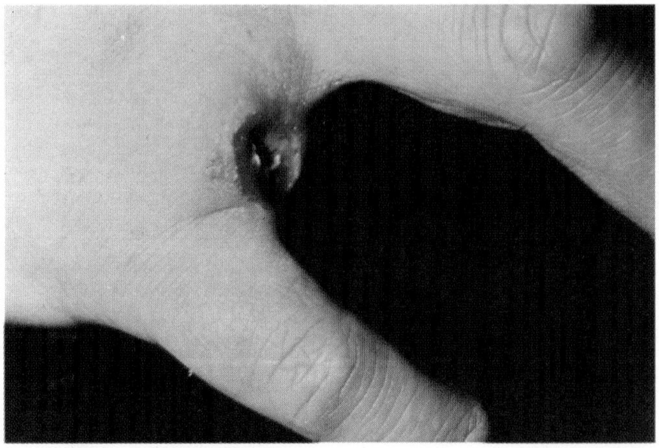

B

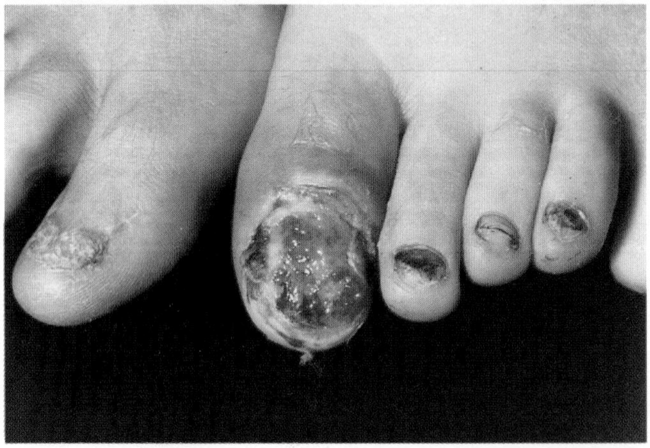

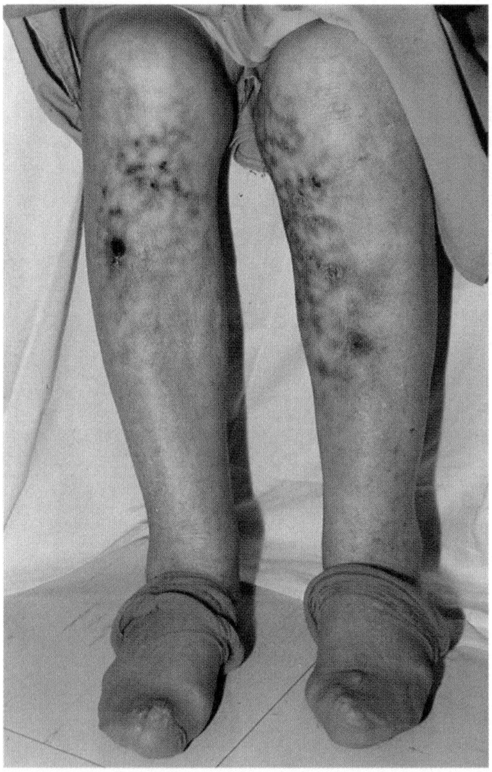

C

Plate 46.6 Separate types of deliberate self injury. **A**, this patient complained of multiple episodes of bruising followed by ulceration at the base of fingers and toes which was associated with recurrent bleeding. All tests of haemostasis were normal. The ulcers did not heal and she eventually had several amputations of digits because of superadded infection. A plaster of Paris dressing over the affected area resulted in rapid and complete healing. The presumption was that the lesions were self induced with a corrosive. **B**, this patient was investigated because of recurrent episodes of 'bleeding under the nails' which resulted in the nail sloughing off. The patient was in a psychiatric institution. No abnormality of haemostasis was found. It was eventually considered that the lesions were self induced. **C**, this lady developed multiple areas of bleeding from the skin of her shins and thighs and was referred as a case of purpura. It appeared that she had an extreme area of erythema ab igne which she excoriated to cause the bleeding.

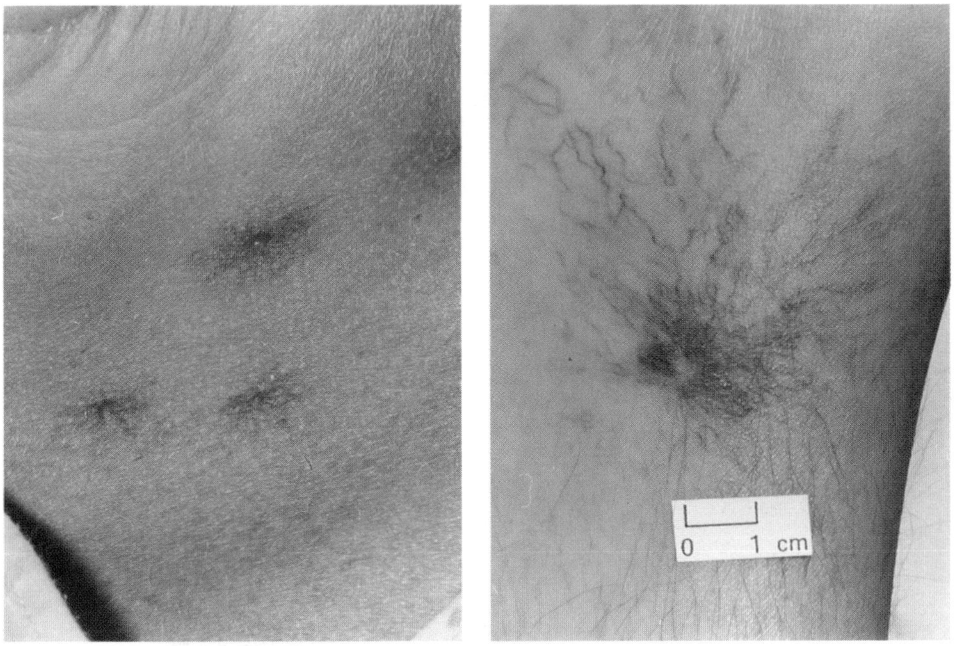

A

Plate 46.7 Vascular spiders. **A**, typical appearance of multiple spider naevi in the 'V' of the neck in a patient who has chronic liver disease – note the icteric skin. **B**, close up of a large spider naevus in the same patient. The raised central punctum where the spiral artery comes to the surface is clearly visible. Compression of this central point leads to blanching of the spiders' 'legs'.

B

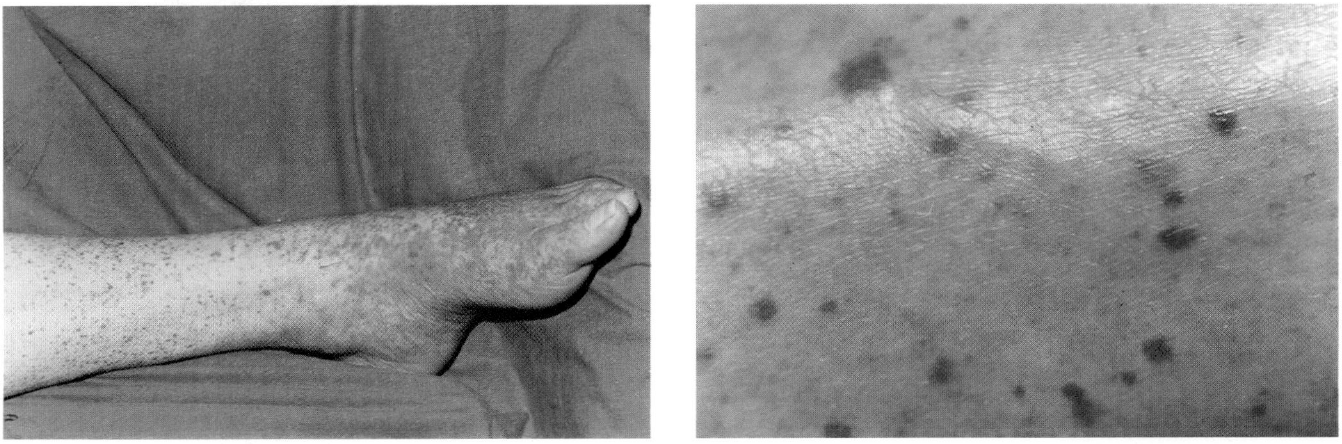

A B

Plate 46.8 Allergic or anaphylactoid purpura. **A**, this patient presented with abdominal pain and a diffuse purpuric rash of the buttocks, thighs and lower legs. There was evidence of glomerulonephritis. **B**, a close-up of the purpura to show that the lesions are raised and may be palpable.

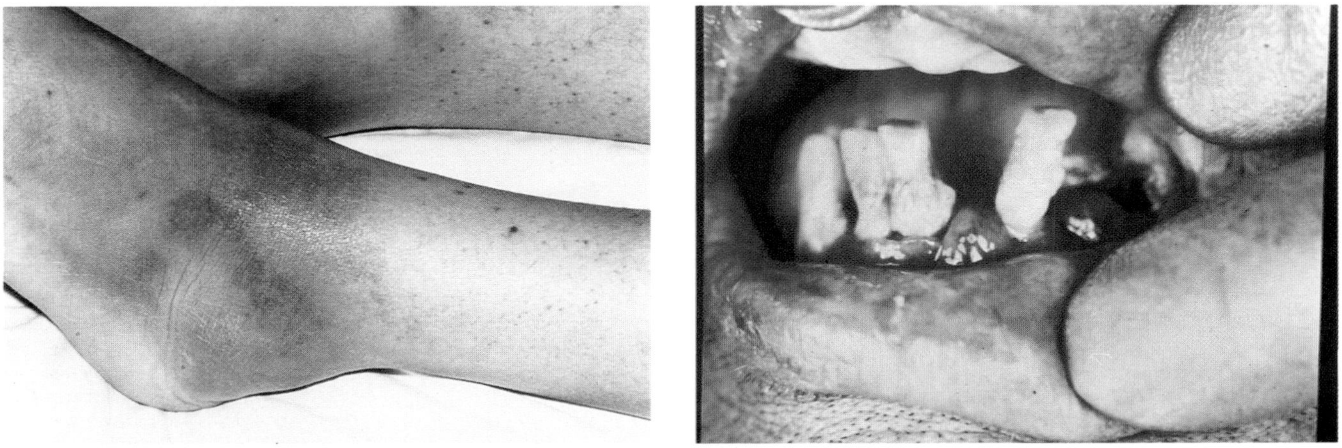

A B

Plate 46.9 Metabolic purpuras. **A**, this elderly lady lived alone and after her husband died became a recluse. She was seen in a severely neglected state with multiple sheet haemorrhages and a fine purpuric rash which was perifollicular. **B**, This patient was seen in a dental clinic with severe dental caries and spongy gums which oozed blood. He had other skin purpura. No other abnormality was present in his blood. Both patients responded to the administration of vitamin C, indeed the first patient had started to improve with the standard hospital diet even before being seen.

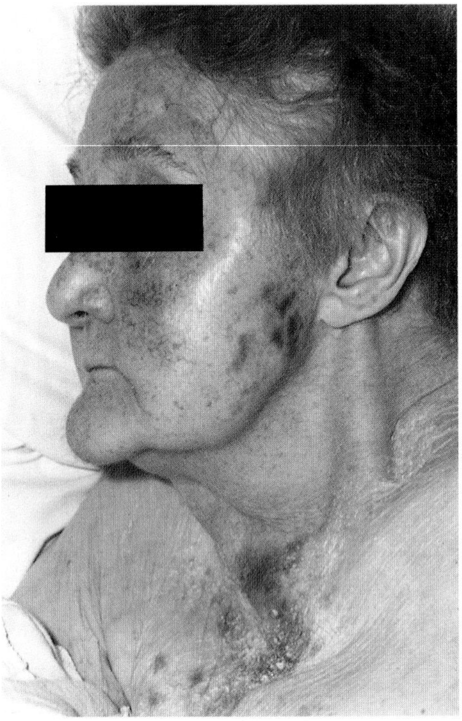

Plate 46.10 Dysproteinaemias. This old lady had multiple myeloma and multiple areas of bruising and purpura.

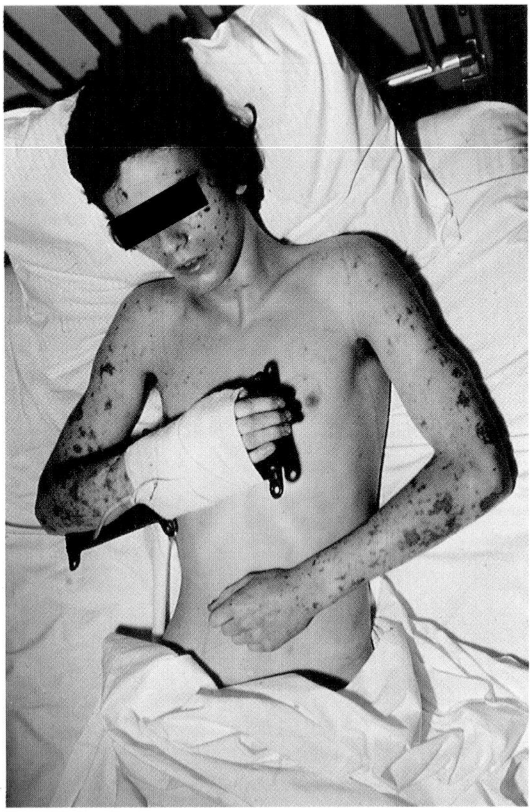

A

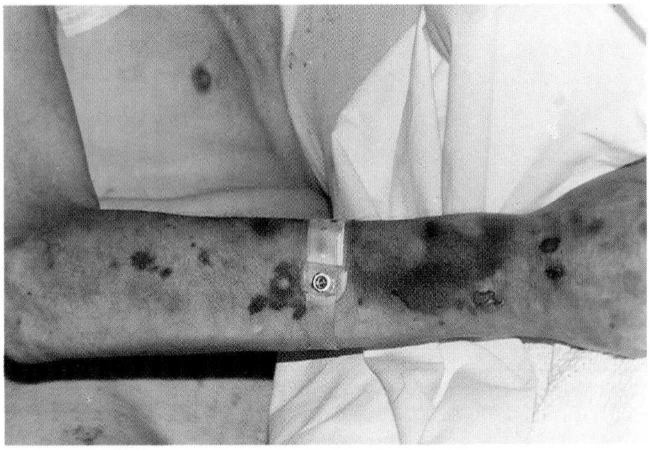

B

Plate 46.11 Purpura associated with infectious diseases. **A**, this boy rapidly deteriorated with high fever, clouding of conscious level and signs of meningism. He had a widespread purpuric rash on the skin with subconjunctival and retinal haemorrhages. **B**, this elderly man was admitted with a diagnosis of intra-abdominal sepsis probably due to rupture of a colonic diverticulum. He developed a disseminated purpuric rash associated with his Gram-negative septicaemia.

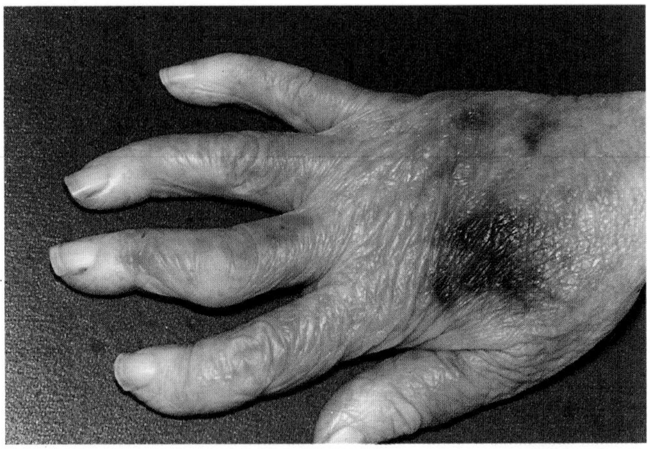

Plate 46.12 This patient with long-standing osteo-arthritis developed a diffuse purpuric rash which in areas became confluent and necrotic. No cause was determined. There was no DIC or alteration of the haemostatic profile.

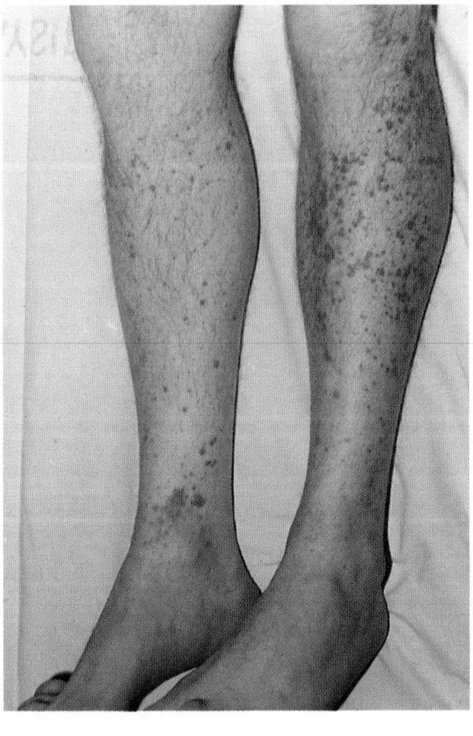

Plate 46.13 Drug-induced vessel disease. This patient was being treated for left ventricular failure with frusemide when he developed this extensive purpuric rash over the shins. There was no renal involvement. Stopping the drug resulted in gradual disappearance of the rash.

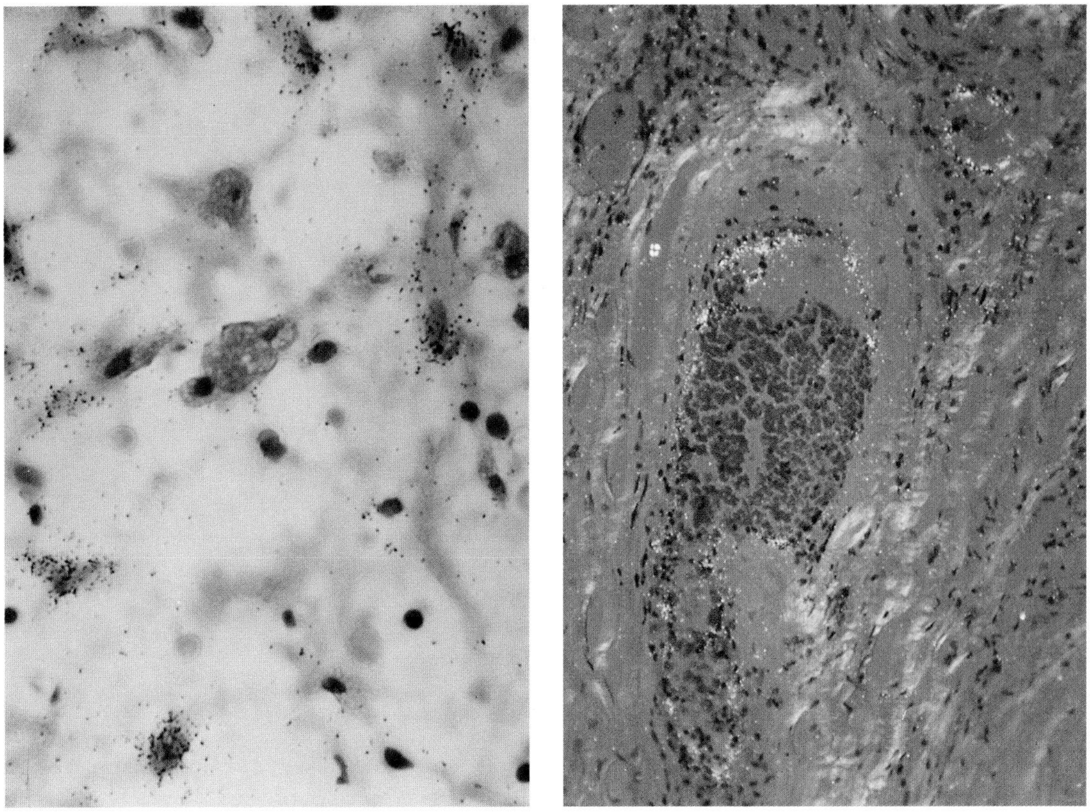

A B

Plate 49.1 PDGF expression in human atherosclerotic plaques analyzed by in situ hybridization. **A**. Mesenchymal-appearing intimal cells in a carotid plaque expressing PDGF-A chain mRNA. Frozen sections of a human carotid endarterectomy specimen were hybridized in situ with a ^{35}S-labelled riboprobe specific for PDGF-A chain mRNA. The dark spots indicate the localization of silver grains indicating presence of PDGF mRNA. **B**. Dysfunctional endothelial cells lining the vasa vasorum in the atherosclerotic plaque intima express PDGF-B chain mRNA. Positive hybridization is indicated by the silver grains appearing as white spots. Reprinted from Wilcox et al 1988 with permission.

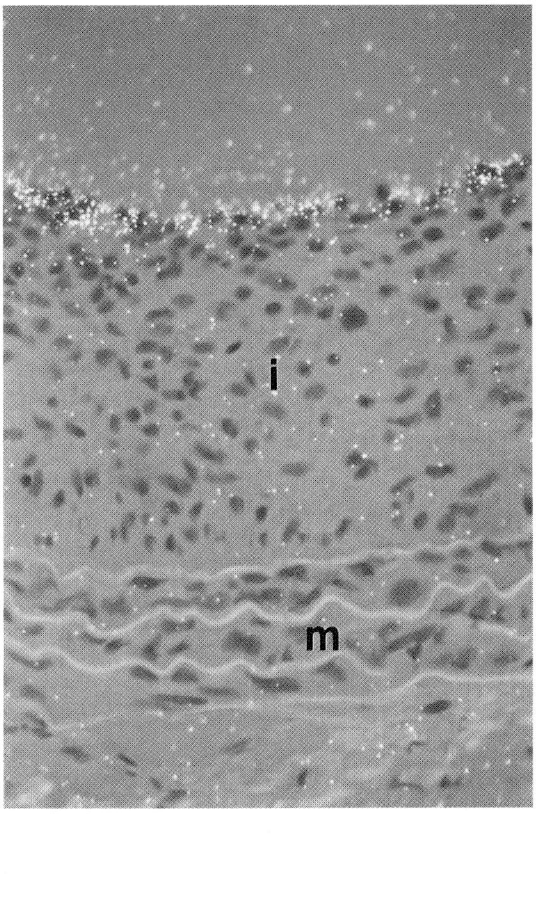

Plate 49.2 Localization of PDGF-A mRNA-containing cells in the neointima of the rat carotid artery by in situ hybridization 2 weeks after balloon catheter denudation of the endothelium. PDGF-A chain mRNA was confined to a lumenal band of proliferating smooth muscle cells at this time. Note the significant neointima generated after balloon injury. m, media; i, intima. Reproduced from Majesky et al 1990 with permission.

A 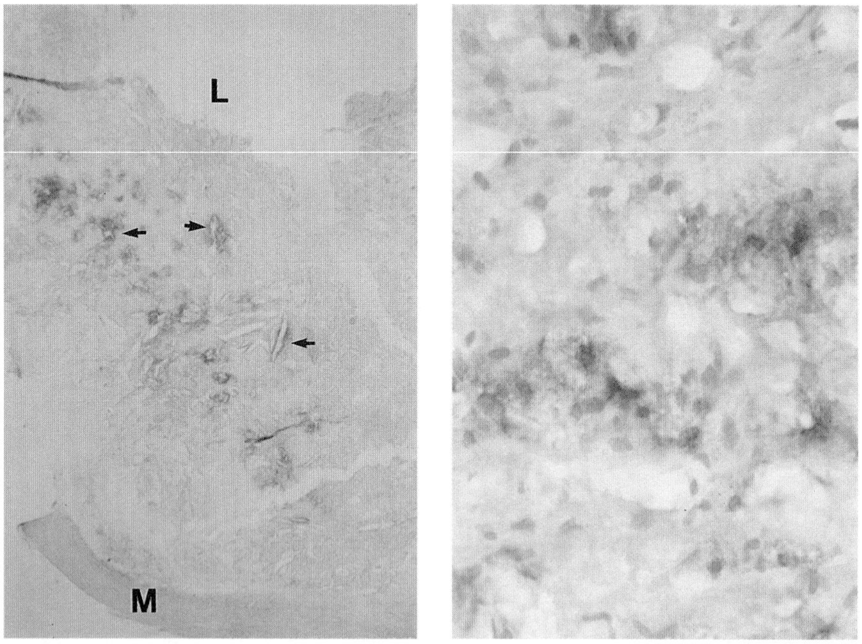

B

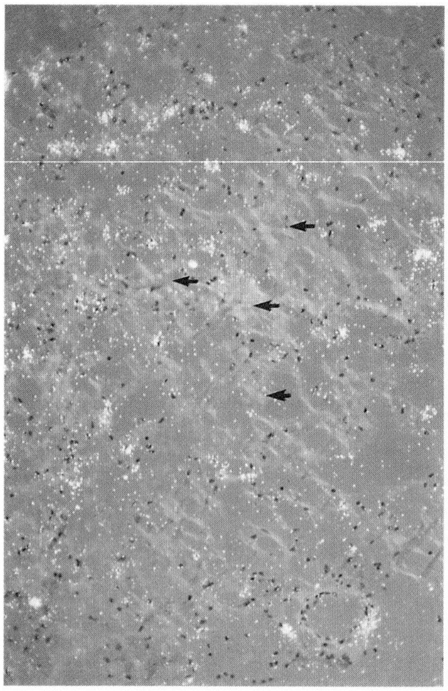

Plate 49.3 Localization of tissue factor (TF) in human atherosclerotic plaque by immunohistochemistry. **A**. Overview of TF localization in human carotid endarterectomy specimen. TF staining was heaviest in the necrotic core concentrated around the cholesterol clefts (arrows). **B**. TF protein localized to foamy macrophages in human carotid plaque. TF mRNA and protein was also found in mesenchymal-appearing intimal cells in the fibrous cap and areas of organizing thrombi but never seen in normal vessels (not shown). Reproduced from Wilcox et al 1989 with permission.

Plate 49.4 Localization of mesenchymal-appearing intimal cells in human atherosclerotic plaque expressing PDGF-A chain mRNA in areas of organizing thrombi identified by in situ hybridization. Some residual thrombus is indicated by the arrows.

A 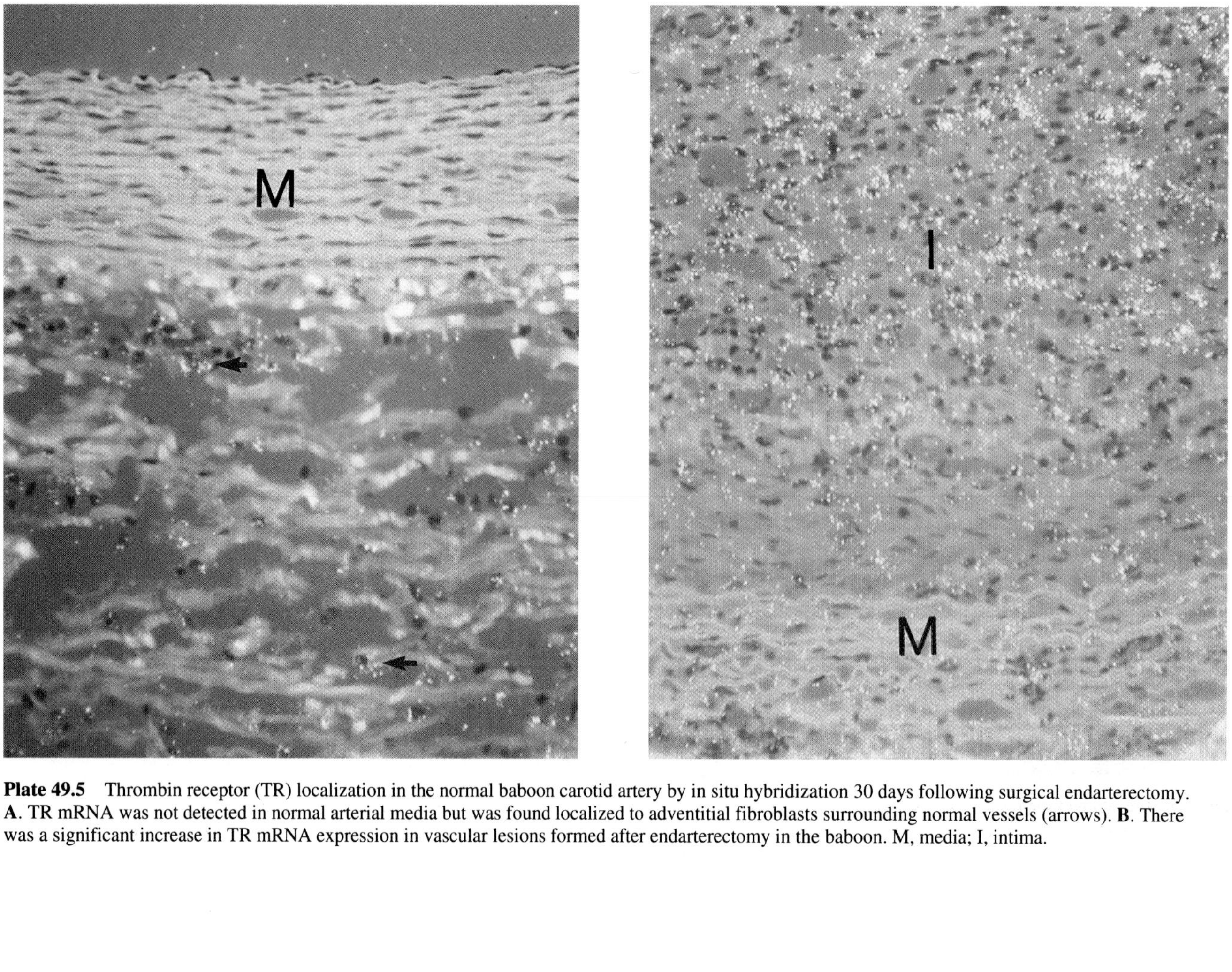

B

Plate 49.5 Thrombin receptor (TR) localization in the normal baboon carotid artery by in situ hybridization 30 days following surgical endarterectomy. **A**. TR mRNA was not detected in normal arterial media but was found localized to adventitial fibroblasts surrounding normal vessels (arrows). **B**. There was a significant increase in TR mRNA expression in vascular lesions formed after endarterectomy in the baboon. M, media; I, intima.

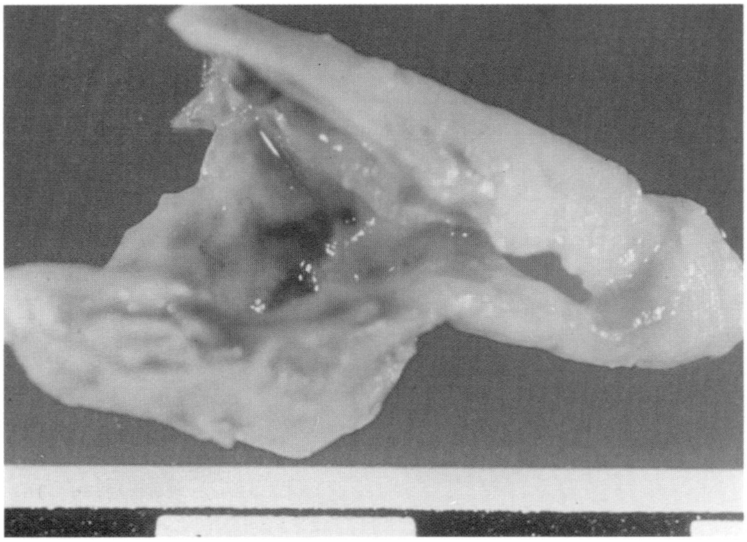

Plate 56.1 A typical partially calcified plaque removed at carotid endarterectomy.

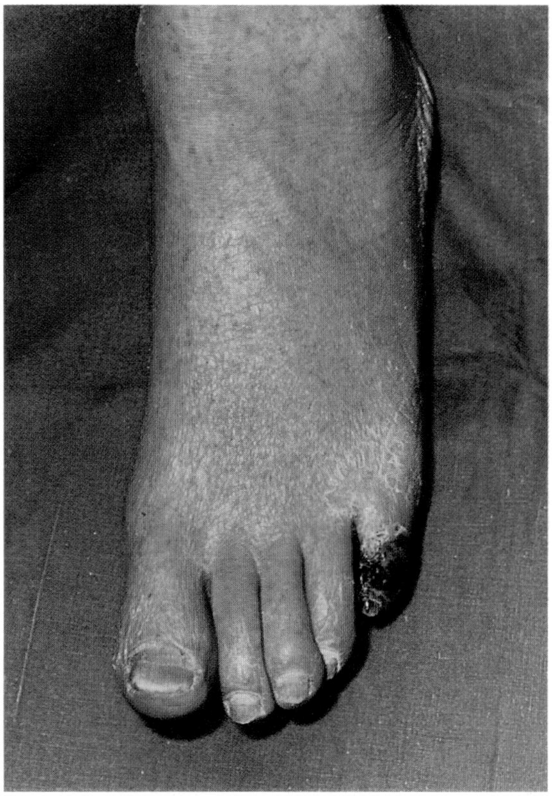

Plate 56.2 Gangrene of the little toe due to critical ischaemia.

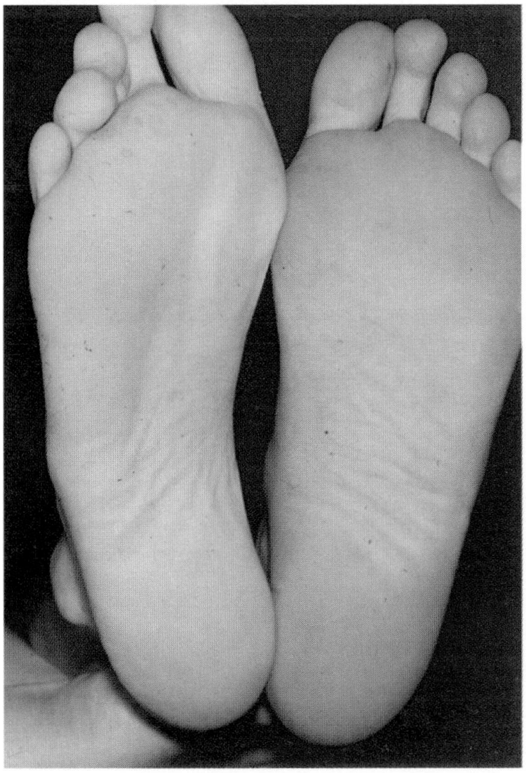

Plate 56.3 Elevation of the foot causes pallor of the affected (right) side.

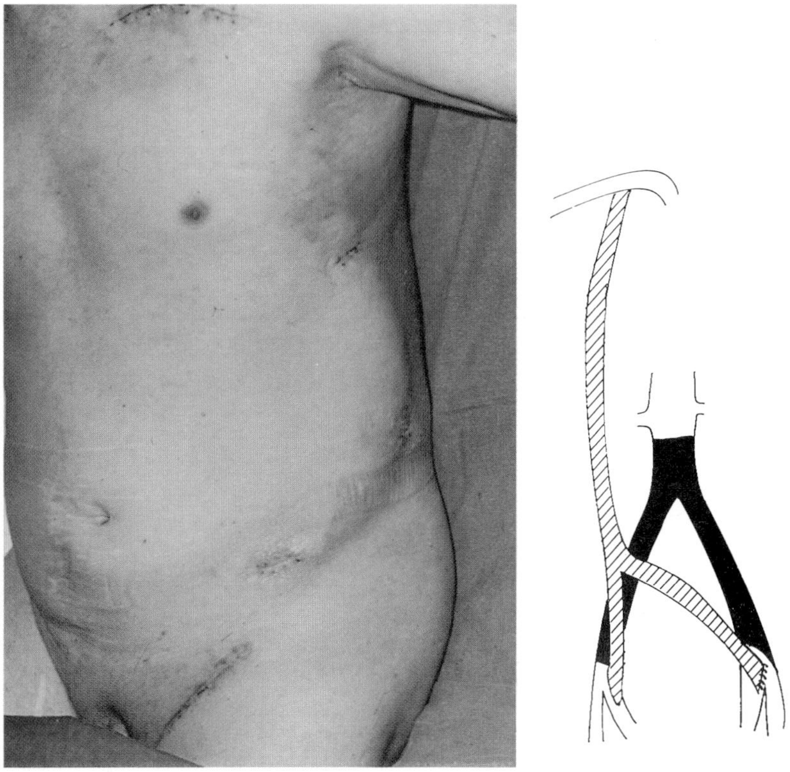

Plate 56.4 A long dacron graft can be sutured to the axillary artery above and tunnelled subcutaneously to supply both legs.

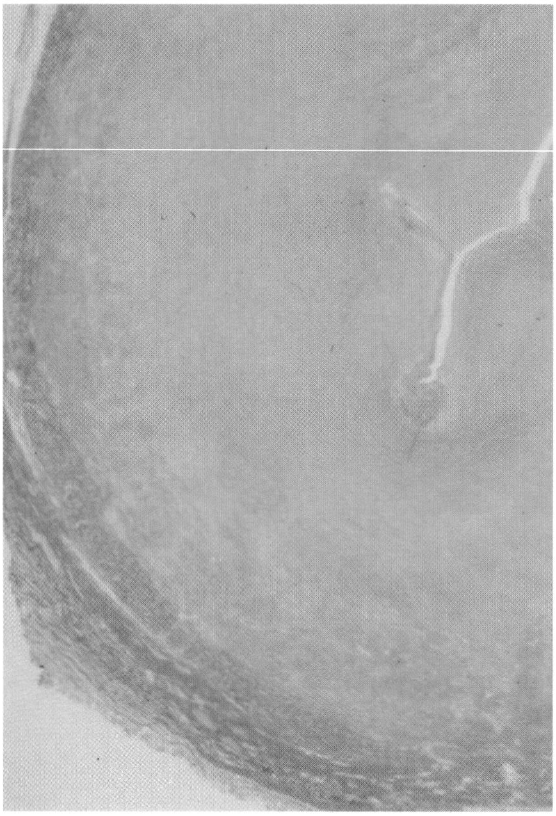

Plate 56.5 Severe intimal hyperplasia and luminal narrowing in a segment of excised vein graft.

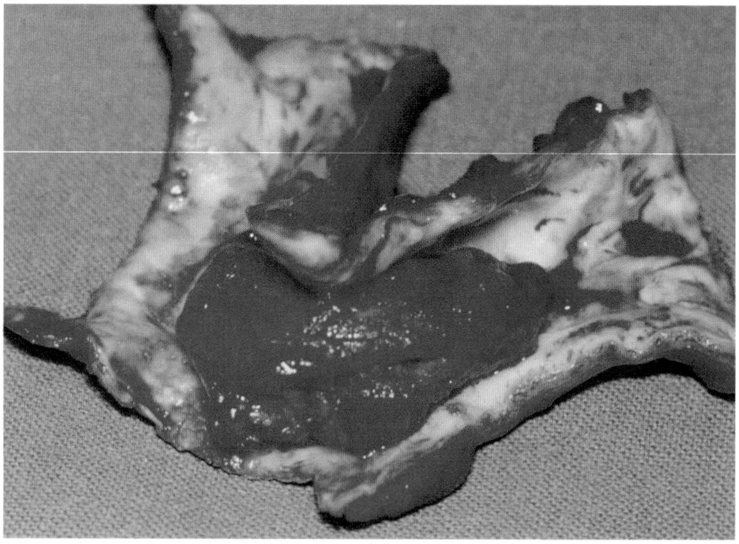

Plate 56.6 Postmortem specimen showing an embolus lodged at the aortic bifurcation.

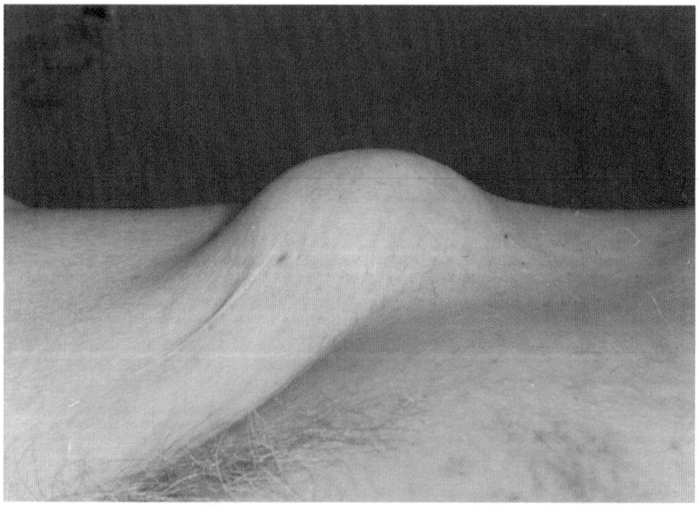

Plate 56.7 A femoral artery aneurysm.

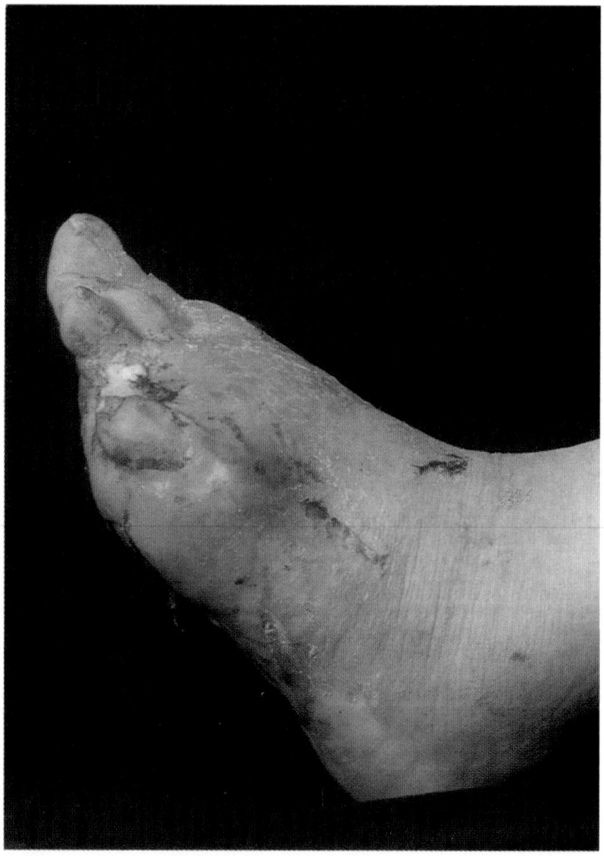

Plate 56.8 A neuropathic diabetic foot with a deep infection.

SECTION 7

Abnormalities of platelets

32. Inherited disorders of platelet function

B. S. Coller

DIAGNOSTIC APPROACH

The platelet's major homeostatic functions are to prevent and arrest haemorrhage and so abnormal bleeding is a symptom that brings individuals with platelet disorders to medical attention (Fig. 32.1). Therefore it is vital that a careful history of bleeding be obtained (Coller & Schneiderman, 1991). The mucocutaneous pattern of bleeding with platelet disorders is relatively distinctive with epistaxis, gum bleeding, easy bruising and menorrhagia the most common manifestations. Especial attention in the history should be directed at identifying the effects of previous haemostatic challenges, such as pregnancies, surgical operations, tooth extractions, and lacerating traumas, since this historical information is the best predictor of future responses to comparable insults.

Table 32.1 contains a listing of the major categories of inherited disorders of platelets organized by pathogenetic mechanism, and Figure 32.1 contains an outline of the actual steps a clinician is likely to take in trying to establish a diagnosis based upon the usual sequence of tests ordered. A logical sequence of evaluation will rapidly narrow the range of possibilities, with more specialized tests required to confirm the diagnosis. The details of performing the more specialized assays will be described with each disease; this section provides an overview.

A low platelet count will identify patients with inherited and acquired quantitative platelet disorders as well as inherited disorders of platelet function that are associated with thrombocytopenia. A review of the peripheral smear and assessment of the mean platelet volume add important information. Patients with acquired quantitative platelet disorders tend to have somewhat enlarged platelets if their thrombocytopenia is due to increased platelet destruction (e.g. autoimmune thrombocytopenia), whereas patients with acquired thrombocytopenia due to decreased platelet production (e.g. after chemotherapy) tend to have somewhat smaller than normal platelets (Paulus & Aster 1990). Several inherited thrombocytopenias, including the thrombocytopenia with absent radii (TAR) syndrome and cyclic thrombocytopenia also have near normal-sized platelets. In contrast to the modest platelet size abnormalities noted in the above disorders, there is a group of autosomal dominant giant platelet syndromes with leukocyte inclusions in which the large size of the platelets is quite dramatic (White 1987, Greinacher & Müller-Eckhardt 1990); these include the May–Hegglin anomaly (thrombocytopenia, giant platelets, and inclusions in leukocytes; Coller & Zarrabi 1981, Ricci et al 1985), Fechtner syndrome (a variant of the Alport syndrome; interstitial nephritis, congenital cataract, neurosensorial deafness, thrombocytopenia, giant platelets, and inclusions in leukocytes; White 1987, Greinacher & Müeller-Eckhardt 1990), and the Sebastion syndrome (haematological abnormalities like those in the Fechtner syndrome but without the renal, eye and ear defects; Greinacher & Müeller-Eckhardt 1990). Giant platelets are also observed in other inherited thrombocytopenias (Lecompte 1988), including Mediterranean macrothrombocytopenia (von Behrens 1975), Montreal platelet syndrome (White 1987), Epstein syndrome (White 1987), Eckstein syndrome (White 1987), Enyeart anomaly (White 1987), and Medich disorder (White 1987).

Platelet size and morphology also help to categorize patients with inherited platelet disorders that produce both quantitative and qualitative abnormalities. Thus, unusually small platelets suggests the diagnosis of Wiskott–Aldrich syndrome. Large platelets that do not have purple granules with conventional Wright blood smear stains are characteristic of the grey platelet syndrome (α-storage pool deficiency), but one needs to be certain that the stain is functioning properly on control smears and that the patient does not have a plasma factor that produces degranulation of platelets in vitro when blood is collected into EDTA (Cockbill et al 1988). The diagnosis of the grey platelet syndrome is established by assessing platelet function and α granule contents. Some patients with platelet-type (pseudo-) von Willebrand disease have mild to moderate thrombocytopenia and large platelets; their characteristic GPIb-mediated functional and biochemical

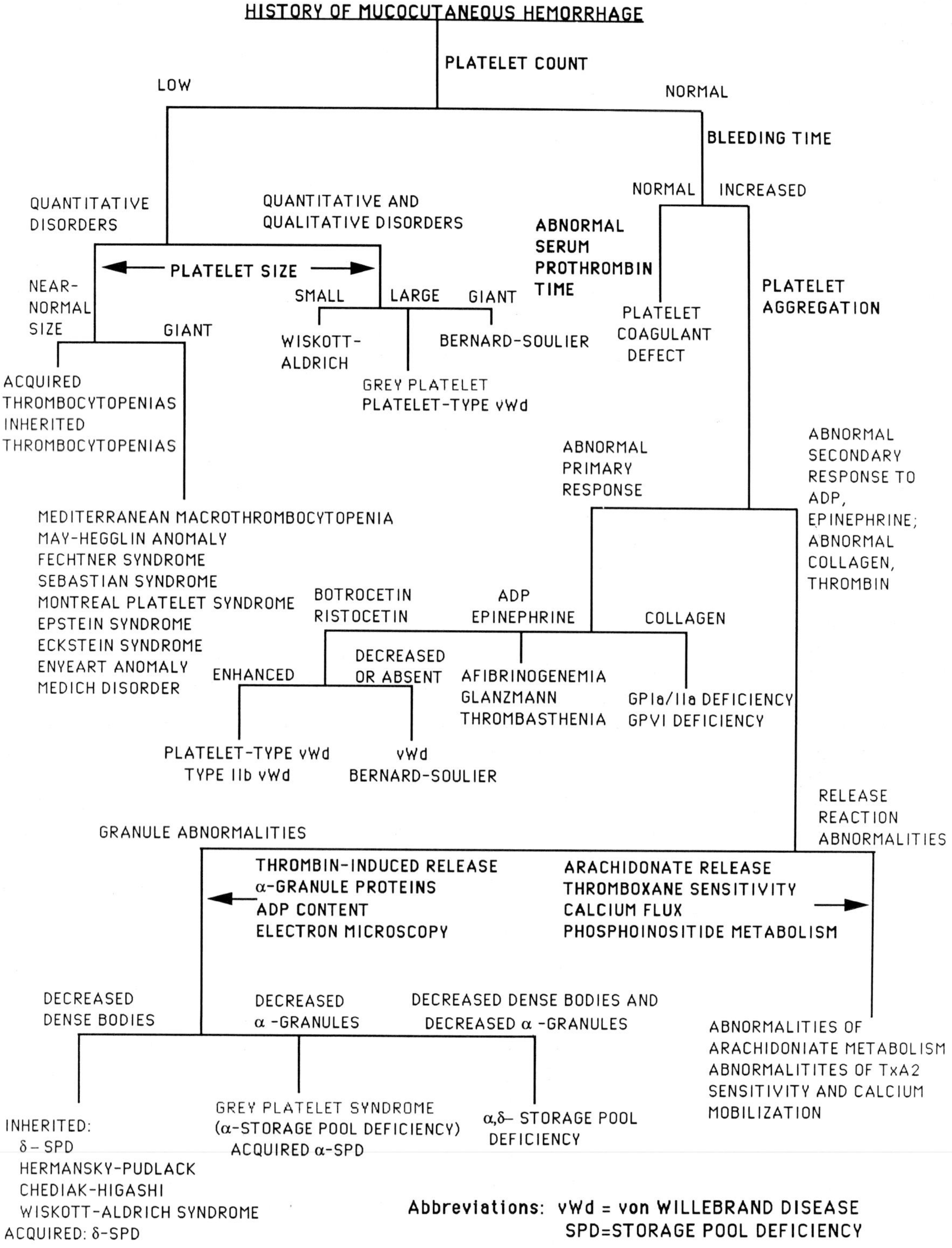

Fig. 32.1 Evaluation of patients with mucocutaneous haemorrhage for abnormalities is platelet number or function.

abnormalities confirm the diagnosis. Patients with Bernard–Soulier syndrome have giant platelets and the diagnosis is established by showing functional and biochemical abnormalities in the GPIb/IX complex and GPV.

Patients with a history of mucocutaneous bleeding but normal numbers of platelets are usually then evaluated with a bleeding time. The bleeding time is usually normal in patients with a defect in platelet coagulant activity and if this type of disorder is suspected, the serum prothrombin time is a useful screening assay. Additional tests of platelet coagulant activity can be used to confirm the diagnosis. Platelet aggregation studies can differentiate those patients

Table 32.1 Inherited disorders of platelet function

- I. Glycoprotein abnormalities
  - A. Glycoprotein IIb/IIIa — Glanzmann thrombasthenia
  - B. Glycoproteins Ib, IX, and V — Bernard–Soulier syndrome
  - C. Glycoprotein Ib — platelet-type (pseudo-) von Willebrand disease
  - D. Glycoprotein Ia/IIa (VLA-2)
  - E. Glycoprotein IV
  - F. Glycoprotein VI
  - G. CD43 — Wiskott-Aldrich syndrome
- II. Abnormalities of platelet granules
  - A. δ-storage pool deficiency
  - B. α, δ-storage pool deficiency
  - C. Grey platelet syndrome – α-storage pool deficiency
- III. Abnormalities of platelet coagulant activity
- IV. Abnormalities of signal transduction and secretion
  - A. Defects in arachidonic acid metabolism
  - B. Defects in thromboxane A_2 sensitivity and calcium mobilization

with defects in the von Willebrand factor-dependent primary wave of aggregation from those with defects in the fibrinogen-dependent primary wave of aggregation and those with defects in the secondary wave of aggregation. Two groups of patients have been described who have enhanced platelet aggregation in response to ristocetin, that is, their platelets aggregate more readily than normal platelets to low doses of ristocetin. The first is patients with platelet-type von Willebrand disease who have an abnormality in the platelet GPIb receptor that facilitates the binding of von Willebrand factor. The second is type IIb von Willebrand disease in which an abnormality in the von Willebrand factor itself leads to enhanced platelet aggregation (see Ch. 16). These disorders can be differentiated by the ability of the patient's plasma von Willebrand factor to bind to normal platelets and, in selected cases, by direct analysis of GPIb.

Platelets fail to respond to ristocetin (or the snake venom protein botrocetin) if the plasma lacks functional von Willebrand factor, as is the case in most forms of von Willebrand disease, or if the platelets lack functional GPIb receptors (Bernard–Soulier syndrome). Adding normal plasma corrects the defect in von Willebrand disease, but not in Bernard–Soulier syndrome. Further direct assessment of plasma von Willebrand factor and GPIb will establish the diagnosis. Bernard–Soulier syndrome platelets may also have a defect in thrombin-induced aggregation.

Patients with no plasma fibrinogen (afibrinogenaemia) (see Ch. 21) or with platelets that cannot bind fibrinogen because they lack a functional GPIIb/IIIa receptor (Glanzmann thrombasthenia) will not respond to ADP or adrenalin; plasma fibrinogen determinations and biochemical and functional studies of GPIIb/IIIa, which may include polyacrylamide gel electrophoresis and monoclonal antibody binding, will establish the diagnosis. An isolated defect in the primary response to collagen has been identified in patients with defects in either the GPIa/IIa receptor or GPVI. Biochemical and immunochemical studies are required to differentiate these syndromes.

A variety of platelet defects can result in abnormal secondary responses to ADP, adrenalin, collagen and thrombin, and these are broadly classified as granule abnormalities and abnormalities of the platelet release reaction. Since virtually all of the defects in the release re-action can be overcome by stimulating platelets with high doses of thrombin, one can exclude a dense granule abnormality if the release of ATP (measured using a luminescence aggregometer) in response to a high dose of thrombin is normal. Immunological or biochemical assays for α granule proteins establish the presence or absence of normal α granule contents. Electron microscopy can confirm the granule deficiencies. The loci of the defects in the platelet release reaction abnormalities can be further defined by attempting to initiate aggregation with arachidonate or a thromboxane A_2 analogue; further localization can be achieved by measuring arachidonate release, thromboxane sensitivity, calcium fluxes and phosphoinositide metabolism.

GLYCOPROTEIN ABNORMALITIES

GLYCOPROTEIN IIb/IIIa ABNORMALITIES — GLANZMANN THROMBASTHENIA

In 1918, Glanzmann, a Swiss paediatrician, described a heterogeneous group of patients with hereditary haemorrhagic diatheses and abnormal clot retraction. Since he believed the disorders were due to platelet 'weakness', he chose the evocative term thrombasthenia. Although it has been argued that Glanzmann did not intend to define a new entity, but rather to indicate the presence of haemorrhagic symptoms in relatives of patients with thrombocytopenic purpura (Hardisty et al 1964), his name has continued to be applied to a qualitative platelet abnormality syndrome that has continually been more precisely defined. Early investigators identified as hallmarks of the disorder a prolonged bleeding time and failure of platelets to clump spontaneously in shed blood or to spread on glass slides (George & Nurden 1987). Pioneering studies in the early 1960s on platelet interactions with glass beads and the identification of a heat stable factor that aggregated platelets, later identified as ADP (Gaarder et al 1961), led to the recognition that thrombasthenic platelets do not aggregate when stimulated with ADP, adrenaline, serotonin, collagen and thrombin; platelet adhesion to connective tissue, however, is normal (Hardisty et al 1964, Caen et al 1966, Zucker et al 1966, Weiss & Kochwa 1968). A reduction in platelet fibrinogen in patients with thrombasthenia was identified in the mid 1960s (Caen et al 1966, Zucker et al 1966, Weiss & Kochwa 1968, George et al 1990). At approximately the same time, the heterogeneity of patients with Glanzmann thrombasthenia was better appreciated. Caen proposed a classification into type I and type II disease based on the severity of the defects in clot retraction, platelet fibrinogen, adhesion to fibrin, and other biochemical criteria (Caen 1972).

A major improvement in understanding Glanzmann thrombasthenia came from the studies of Nurden et al (Nurden & Caen 1974, Nurden 1989) and Phillips et al (1975) in the mid 1970s who identified marked deficiencies in platelet glycoproteins IIb and IIIa in some patients with the disorder. Subsequent studies employing crossed immunoelectrophoresis and non-denaturing detergents allowed for the identification of the complex that forms between GPIIb and GPIIIa and its calcium dependence (Kunicki et al 1981, Hagen et al 1982, Pidard 1989). The technique of immunoblotting after polyacrylamide gel electrophoresis provided a much more sensitive method of detecting trace amounts of GPIIb and GPIIIa (Nurden et al 1985, Coller et al 1987, Seligsohn et al 1989). The availability of monoclonal antibodies directed against different regions of the GPIIb/IIIa complex allowed for direct evaluation of surface expression of the glycoproteins, enhanced the specificity of the immunoblot studies, and facilitated diagnosis, carrier detection, and prenatal diagnosis (McEver et al 1980, Coller et al 1983c, 1986, Seligsohn et al 1985, 1989, Ginsberg et al 1986). Collectively, all of these advanced biochemical and immunological techniques led to the recognition that, except for populations with a high rate of consanguinity, Glanzmann thrombasthenia is very heterogeneous in its glycoprotein profile, with some patients having total glycoprotein deficiencies, others having partial deficiencies, and still others with no quantitative deficiency at all (George et al 1990).

Complementing the glycoprotein investigations were simultaneous functional studies conducted in the late 1970s and early 1980s identifying a defect in the ability of thrombasthenic platelets to interact with fibrinogen, either in the absence or presence of platelet stimulation (Bennett & Vilaire 1979, Mustard et al 1979, Coller 1980). The recognition that ex vivo platelet aggregation depends on binding fibrinogen to the platelet surface (Bennett & Vilaire 1979, Peerschke 1985) and that adhesion to glass is in actuality adhesion to the fibrinogen that rapidly deposits on glass (Zucker & Vroman 1969, Zucker & McPherson 1977), provided ready explanations for the observed abnormalities in Glanzmann thrombasthenia platelet function. The fibrinogen binding abnormality also offered several potential explanations for the platelet fibrinogen deficiency, although the precise mechanism still remains somewhat uncertain (Coller et al 1991c). Although it was logical to conclude that GPIIb/IIIa was the receptor responsible for fibrinogen binding, doubts remained until the early 1980s when monoclonal antibodies were developed that both blocked fibrinogen binding to platelets and recognized the GPIIb/IIIa complex. These antibodies could reproduce the Glanzmann thrombasthenia abnormalities both in vitro and in vivo (Bennett et al 1983, Coller et al 1983c, 1991b, McEver et al 1983, Pidard et al 1983).

Ligand binding studies beginning in the mid 1980s indicated that in addition to fibrinogen, GPIIb/IIIa could also bind von Willebrand factor, fibronectin, vitronectin, and perhaps thrombospondin (Ruggeri et al 1982, 1983, Plow et al 1984, 1985a, Gralnick et al 1984, Lawler & Hynes 1989, Asch & Podack 1990). The basis for the promiscuous nature of the GPIIb/IIIa receptor became apparent when: 1) studies of related receptors in the integrin receptor family demonstrated that the peptide sequence Arg-Gly-Asp (RGD) in the ligand was crucial for binding to these integrin receptors (Ruoslahti & Pierschbacher 1987, Phillips et al 1988), and 2) all of the ligands that bound to GPIIb/IIIa contained RGD sequences in the regions of the molecule that are thought to mediate the binding (Phillips et al 1988). Moreover, small peptides containing the RGD sequence could inhibit the binding of all of the ligands to GPIIb/IIIa (Gartner & Bennett 1985, Haverstick et al 1985, Plow et al 1985b). Thus, a crucial RGD binding site exists in the GPIIb/IIIa complex. The C-terminus of the fibrinogen γ-chain also can bind to GPIIb/IIIa and the dodecapeptide made from this sequence can also inhibit the binding of all of the ligands to GPIIb/IIIa (Kloczewiak et al 1984, Plow et al 1984, Timmons et al 1984). The precise contributions of the γ-chain dodecapeptide and the two RGD sequences in fibrinogen to platelet binding are still being investigated (Savage & Ruggeri 1991, Abrams et al 1992). Evidence continues to emerge, moreover, about interactions between the ligands and GPIIb/IIIa that are distinct from both the RGD and dodecapeptide sequences (Parise et al 1992).

One of the major enigmas about Glanzmann thrombasthenia has been why a presumably single genetic defect leads to the loss of two separate proteins. Studies in the late 1980s led to the cloning of the cDNAs and genes for both GPIIb and GPIIIa (Fitzgerald et al 1987b, Poncz et al 1987), which in turn led to the identification of significant homologies with the α and β subunits, respectively, of other integrin family receptors (Phillips et al 1988). Further studies localized both genes to a very small region on chromosome 17 (Sosnoski et al 1988). Analysis of the biosynthesis of integrin receptors led to the realization that GPIIb and GPIIIa must form a complex soon after synthesis in order for correct post-translational processing and transport to the surface membrane of the platelet to occur (Cheresh & Spiro 1987, Duperray et al 1987, Bodary et al 1989, O'Toole et al 1989). If complex formation does not occur because one of the proteins is not synthesized, the uncomplexed subunit is degraded. Thus, a defect in either GPIIb or GPIIIa could lead to a loss of both subunits.

Additional studies of platelet integrins identified trace amounts of the $\alpha_v\beta_3$, vitronectin receptor on the surface of normal platelets (Lam et al 1989, Lawler & Hynes 1989, Coller et al 1991a). Since GPIIIa and β_3 have the same primary structure and are presumed to be the products of the same gene, surface expression of α_v β_3 vitronectin receptors (Pytela et al 1986, Cheresh 1987) was used to distinguish Glanzmann thrombasthenia patients whose genetic abnormality is in GPIIb from those whose defect is in GPIIIa (Burk et al 1991, Coller et al 1991a, Newman et al 1991). Thus thrombasthenic patients could be subcategorized into those who lacked $\alpha_v\beta_3$ and those who had normal to increased amounts. The $\alpha_v\beta_3$ vitronectin receptor is also promiscuous, binding fibrinogen, von Willebrand factor and probably thrombospondin, in addition to vitronectin (Cheresh et al 1989, Lawler & Hynes 1989). It also recognizes the RGD sequence (Cheresh 1987, Smith & Cheresh 1988), but it appears to differ from GPIIb/IIIa in not being able to recognize the γ-chain dodecapeptide sequence (Cheresh et al 1989).

The application of molecular biological techniques in the 1990s has led to the identification of the primary DNA defects in a small number of patients with Glanzmann thrombasthenia (Bray & Shuman 1990, Burk et al 1991, Chen et al 1991, Djaffar et al 1991, Lanza et al 1991, Newman et al 1991, Bajt et al 1992, Rifat et al 1992) and many others will certainly be identified in the near future. This information has already been used to develop DNA-based assays that improve carrier detection and prenatal diagnosis in selected groups (Peretz et al 1991). In addition, insights obtained from the qualitative GPIIb/IIIa defects present in the subset of Glanzmann thrombasthenia patients who have significant amounts of platelet GPIIb/IIIa (Nurden et al 1987, Jung et al 1988, Loftus et al 1990, Chen et al 1991, Bajt et al 1992), offer vital insights into the structure–function relationships of ligand binding.

The evolution in our understanding of Glanzmann and improved knowledge of platelet physiology permit us to define the disorder more precisely. Figure 32.2 is a schematic diagram of platelet aggregation in which either a chemical agonist or shear stress alters the platelet membrane and initiates signals that ultimately lead to more GPIIb/IIIa receptors adopting a conformation that has a high affinity for its ligands. After the binding of one or more of the ligands, other poorly-defined events occur (Peerschke 1985) that ultimately result in platelet aggregation. Positive feedback loops involved in GPIIb/IIIa activation include new synthesis by activated platelets of the important agonist thromboxane A_2 and release from platelets of preformed agonists contained in granules. This scheme of platelet aggregation indicates that failure of platelet aggregation in response to the agonists that stimulate the GPIIb/IIIa receptor, which has traditionally

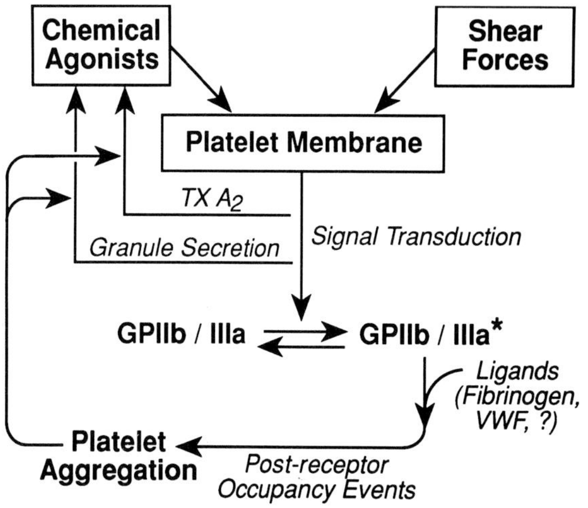

Fig. 32.2 Platelet aggregation. The sequence of events in platelet aggregation, with the recognized positive feedback loops identified.

been the functional hallmark of Glanzmann thrombasthenia, can potentially be caused by defects in the transducing mechanisms or in the GPIIb/IIIa receptor itself. In order to avoid confusion, the Platelet Subcommittee of the Scientific and Standardization Committee of the International Society on Thrombosis and Haemostasis decided in 1990 to define Glanzmann thrombasthenia as 'a congenital, hereditary reduction or absence of platelet aggregation in response to multiple physiologic agonists (e.g. ADP, thrombin, collagen) due to abnormalities of genes coding for GPIIb or GPIIIa . . .' Recognizing the potential for other defects leading to the same functional consequences, the Committee defined 'thrombasthenic state' as a 'reduction or absence of primary platelet aggregation in response to multiple agonists without abnormality of the genes coding for GPIIb/IIIa'. These definitions help to focus attention on the central role of GPIIb/IIIa in Glanzmann thrombasthenia. From a practical standpoint, since defects in the GPIIb/IIIa proteins are usually easily identified, whereas localization of the defect to the GPIIb or GPIIIa gene may take a long time, the combination of the functional abnormalities and abnormalities of the GPIIb and/or GPIIIa proteins is usually considered sufficient to establish the diagnosis.

Epidemiology

Glanzmann thrombasthenia is a rare disorder in regions of the world where consanguineous matings are unusual. For example, George et al in 1990 could only identify 12 reported cases from the United States. In contrast, in groups where consanguineous matings are common, Glanzmann thrombasthenia may be as prevalent as haemophilia. Included among the high frequency populations are 42 patients from a region in South India (Khanduri et al 1981); 39 patients from the Iraqi-Jewish population living in Israel (Reichert et al 1975, Seligsohn & Rososhansky 1982, Seligsohn et al 1991); 37 Arab patients from Israel, Jordan, and Saudi Arabia (Reichert et al 1975, Awidi 1983, Mirghani et al 1988, Seligsohn et al 1991) and a smaller number of patients from three Gypsy families (George et al 1990). The actual gene frequencies in these populations have been difficult to estimate because of problems in defining the limits of the population at risk and being certain that all affected patients have been identified. The Iraql-Jewish population in Israel, however, is well defined since it is believed to be derived from the Jews who were taken to Babylonia soon after the destruction of the Temple in Jerusalem in 586 BCE. This population remained as a distinct group within this region, which is now Iraq, with a high rate of consanguineous marriage. In 1950 and 1951 nearly the entire population moved to Israel, and by 1984, 35 Iraqi-Jewish patients with Glanzmann thrombasthenia were identified among an estimated 270 000 Iraqi-Jews living in Israel (Seligsohn & Rososhansky 1984). Thus, the homozygote frequency is one in 7714 individuals, and, assuming that the population follows the Hardy–Weinberg formula, the frequency of the carrier state (2pq) is one in 44 or 2.3%. The carrier state among the Arab population studied by Seligsohn & Rososhansky (1984) calculates to ≈0.5%. With the advent of unequivocal carrier detection by molecular biological techniques, the carrier frequency can now be directly assessed (Peretz et al 1991).

The importance of inquiring about parental consanguinity in sporadic cases of Glanzmann thrombasthenia is emphasized by George et al's (1990) identification of consanguinity in at least 39% of the 64 cases from 51 sibships that were reviewed. In groups that have intermarried over generations, however, knowledge of consanguinity may be limited. In the Iraqi-Jewish population, for example, even though all of the affected individuals appear to have the same defect, the parents of only 15 of the 28 affected sibships knew of consanguinity (Seligsohn et al 1991). In cases where there is no consanguinity, it is probably more likely that the affected patient is doubly heterozygous for two different recessive defects carried by the parents. Although thrombasthenia affects both sexes, consistent with its recessive inheritance, a slight female predominance (58% of 177 patients) was observed by George et al (1990). They ascribed this to better ascertainment in females because abnormal menstrual bleeding is likely to bring them to medical attention.

Clinical symptoms

Several major reviews of the clinical symptoms of patients with Glanzmann thrombasthenia have been reported, including those by George et al (1990) on 177 patients (123 from the literature and 64 patients from 51 sibships studied in Paris over a 33-year-period) and Seligsohn & coworkers (1991) on 55 living and four dead patients from Israel. The frequency of bleeding symptoms identified by George et al (1990) is given in Table 32.2.

Excessive ecchymoses and petechiae, presumably reflecting an exaggeration of the normal purpura and petechiae that often result from trauma at the time of delivery, are sometimes, but not usually, appreciated at birth. Circumcision without platelet transfusion support led to excessive bleeding in ten out of 12 patients, but none of five patients bled when pretreated with platelets (Seligsohn & Rososhansky, 1982). Excessive purpura in response to minimal trauma is found in virtually all affected patients throughout their lives.

Severe epistaxis is one of the cardinal manifestations of Glanzmann thrombasthenia (Seligsohn & Rososhansky 1982, George et al 1990). On occasion, the recurrent bleeding can be life-threatening and incapacitating. Guarisco et al (1987), for example, reported on a 3-year-old boy who had 18 separate hospital admissions over a 19 month period for uncontrollable epistaxis, resulting in 121 days of hospitalization; on one occasion the bleeding was brisk enough to produce hypovolemic shock. During childhood, epistaxis is common among normal individuals but rarely is it severe enough to merit the extensive medical care that is commonly required for Glanzmann thrombasthenia patients. Just as normal individuals have a decrease in epistaxis as they reach adulthood, so do patients with Glanzmann thrombasthenia, although this is not invariably the case.

Spontaneous gingival bleeding is also found in the majority of patients and can result in severe iron deficiency and the need for blood transfusions. With careful tooth and gum care, gingival bleeding can be dramatically reduced. Unfortunately, patients are often reluctant to have proper dental care because it initially causes bleeding, and inexperienced dentists are often reluctant to provide even routine care.

Table 32.2 Bleeding in patients with Glanzmann's thrombasthenia

	No. of affected patients	Frequency (%)
Symptoms		
Menorrhagia	54/55	98
Easy bruising, purpura	152/177	86
Epistaxis	129/177	73
Gingival bleeding	97/177	55
Gastrointestinal haemorrhage	22/177	12
Haematuria	10/177	6
Haemarthrosis	5/177	3
Intracranial haemorrhage	3/177	2
Visceral haematoma	1/177	1
Severity: requirements for red cell transfusions		
Patients from literature*	32/48	67
Paris patients	54/64	84

*Data are from 177 patients reviewed by George et al 1990, of whom 113 were from the literature and 64 were studied in Paris.

Menorrhagia, especially at menarche, is nearly a universal manifestation of Glanzmann thrombasthenia, and one of the potentially life-threatening complications of the disease. To account for the unusual severity of bleeding at menarche, George et al (1990) cite evidence that the early anovulatory cycles result in prolonged, and unopposed, oestrogen stimulation of proliferative endometrium.

Gastrointestinal bleeding occurred in only 12% of the patients reviewed by George et al (1990), but it was reported in 49% of the subset of patients from Israel (Seligsohn & Rososhansky 1982). The search for a bleeding site can be particularly difficult and frustrating. Haemarthroses are decidedly uncommon, and spontaneous haemarthrosis even rarer, although they do occur, emphasizing how different the pattern of bleeding is in Glanzmann thrombasthenia compared to haemophilia. Although central nervous system bleeding as a result of trauma may be more extensive in patients with Glanzmann thrombasthenia than in normals, the lack of spontaneous central nervous system bleeding is quite remarkable (George et al 1990), indicting only a minor role for platelet function mediated by GPIIb/IIIa in maintaining normal haemostasis in this vital area.

Pregnancy is tolerated well by patients with Glanzmann thrombasthenia prior to delivery, with bleeding only rarely requiring blood transfusions (George et al 1990). Excessive bleeding is common in the immediate postpartum period if platelets are not administered, but rare if platelet transfusions are administered (George et al 1990). Even after several days or weeks of successful control of haemorrhage, however, excessive bleeding can occur, necessitating repeat blood and platelet transfusions. George et al (1990) made the interesting observation that patients delivered by caesarean section did not experience delayed postpartum haemorrhage, perhaps because the products of conception and haematomas were more effectively removed. The use of low doses of PGE_2, lactate Ringer's solution by continuous intrauterine irrigation via a Foley catheter has been reported to be very effective in stopping severe postpartum haemorrhage (Peyser & Kupfermine 1990) and has been used successfully in patients with haemorrhagic disorders (Seligsohn 1992).

Surgical procedures are generally not well tolerated unless prophylactic platelet transfusions are administered. Seligsohn & Rososhansky (1984) reported that seven out of 11 patients undergoing tooth extraction without platelet transfusion bled excessively whereas only one out of 12 treated with platelets had excessive bleeding. Similarly, all nine patients undergoing major surgery with platelet transfusions had uncomplicated courses. With special precautions, however, including careful suturing, the use of resolvable, oxidized, regenerated cellulose (Surgical) and custom-designed splints made from soft acrylic, it may be possible to perform tooth extractions without platelet transfusions (Jasmin et al 1987). Another recent approach that has permitted tooth extractions without a platelet transfusion combines systemic tranexamic acid with local use of a fibrin 'glue' (Tisseal) and gel-foam (Seligsohn 1992).

The haemorrhagic diathesis in Glanzmann thrombasthenia is characterized by its variability, with some patients severely affected and others only minimally affected (George et al 1990). Since Glanzmann thrombasthenia is also a heterogeneous disorder at the molecular level, it might be expected that the clinical symptoms would echo this molecular heterogeneity. There are, however, no data at present to support this hypothesis. In particular, although there is a discrete difference in platelet $\alpha_v\beta_3$ vitronectin receptor expression between patients from the Arab population in Israel (who have normal or increased numbers of platelet $\alpha_v\beta_3$ receptors) and Iraqi-Jews (who have virtually no platelet $\alpha_v\beta_3$ receptors), the haemorrhagic diatheses within each population extend across a considerable range of severity (Coller et al 1991a). Similarly, George et al (1990) found no clear correlation between the amount of residual platelet GPIIb/IIIa and clinical severity in the patients he reviewed. Finally, as also pointed out by George et al (1990), there can be dramatic differences in severity even between siblings who are likely to share the same defect. In fact, the one patient whose disease was severe enough to justify bone marrow transplantation at age 5 had a 10-year old sister whose disease was very mild.

Therapy and management

Preventive dental care is crucial in minimizing gingival haemorrhage. Supplemental oral iron should be given continually to patients with chronic, excessive blood loss to minimize the need for transfusions or parenteral iron therapy. Consideration should also be given to supplemental folic acid for patients whose haematopoiesis is under constant stimulation to make up for chronic blood loss.

George et al (1990) reviewed the use of hormonal therapy to control menorrhagia. For severe haemorrhage, they recommended a 19-norprogesterone (e.g. norethindrone acetate), 5 mg every 4 hours until bleeding comes under control, and then 3 weeks of additional therapy with 5 mg twice a day. Therapy with a birth control pill should then begin, titrating the dose to prevent breakthrough bleeding. The endometrium is expected to atrophy with repeat cycles, leading to decreased risk of excessive bleeding. The gonadotropin-releasing hormone agonist, nasal nafarelin, is another agent that reliably prevents menses (Barbieri 1992). The nearly uniform severity of excessive bleeding with menarche has led some experts to recommend instituting birth control pills before menarche (George et al 1990). Although this may be justified, questions related to premature cessation of bone growth need to be considered as well.

Gingival haemorrhage can usually be controlled with local measures such as gel foam soaked in topical thrombin. Topical bovine thrombin, however, has been associated with the development of antibodies to bovine thrombin, factor XI, and factor V (which contaminate the thrombin preparations) in patients undergoing open heart surgery, and at least one such antibody to factor V has cross-reacted sufficiently with human factor V to cause severe haemorrhage (Nichols et al 1991, Spero et al 1991). Bovine thrombin is also a component of fibrin 'glues'.

Antifibrinolytic therapy has been used as adjunctive therapy for gingival haemorrhage and tooth extractions. Based on studies in haemophiliacs, a dose of 40 mg/kg of ε-aminocaproic acid given four times daily by mouth has been recommended (George et al 1990). Gastrointestinal side-effects frequently cause patients to discontinue the medication. Tranexamic acid is also an effective systemic antifibrinolytic agent and usually is better tolerated than ε-aminocaproic acid. It has been used successfully in preventing haemorrhage in patients with factor VIII or factor XI deficiency undergoing tooth extractions who take oral doses ranging from 0.5 g every eight hours to 1 g four times daily (Ratnoff 1987, Berliner et al 1992). As an alternative to systemic therapy, a mouthwash composed of tranexamic acid has been found effective in controlling gingival haemorrhage in haemophiliacs and patients on oral anticoagulants (Sindet-Pedersen et al 1989). Systemic treatment with antifibrinolytic agents is contraindicated in the presence of disseminated intravascular coagulation and can produce numerous side-effects (Ratnoff, 1987).

Desmopressin (1-deamino-8-D-arginine vasopressin; DDAVP) has been tested in several patients with Glanzmann thrombasthenia. Although no effect on the bleeding time was observed in five patients (Mannucci et al 1986, Mannucci 1988, George et al 1990), one patient had a decrease in bleeding time from ≈20 minutes to 14.5 minutes (DiMichele & Hathaway 1990). This last patient underwent minor dental surgery without bleeding using desmopressin therapy as an alternative to platelet transfusions (the patient was refractory to platelet transfusions). Although it seems reasonable to use bleeding time correction as an index of likely beneficial clinical effect, in truth there is little to support the assumption that there is a good correlation between the bleeding time and haemostasis at the time of surgery (Rodgers & Levin 1990). Moreover, complete correction of the Ivy bleeding time does not appear necessary for surgical haemostasis in von Willebrand disease (Borchgrevink et al 1963, Nilsson et al 1963). Thus, based on existing data, it may be inappropriate to exclude a potential benefit of desmopressin in Glanzmann thrombasthenia.

Management of recurrent epistaxis can be particularly frustrating. One approach has been described in detail by Guarisco et al (1987). Those nose bleeds that do not respond to the simple measures of elevating the patient's head and applying local pressure require medical intervention. Topical vasoconstriction and local anaesthesia are used to prepare the nose for the installation of cottonoid pledgets soaked in 0.25% oxymetazoline, which are then pressed against the septum by external compression for 5 minutes. The cottonoids are left in place and oxymetazoline applied every 8 hours until the bleeding stops. Platelet transfusions are instituted at the same time. If this is inadequate to control the bleeding, cauterization of Kiesselbach's plexus with silver nitrate sticks or trichloroacetic acid is used. If bleeding is still uncontrolled, anterior packing, posterior packing, arterial ligation, or embolic occlusion of the internal maxillary artery have been used successfully, but all of these procedures have potentially serious consequences. Even when the acute episode is well controlled, the problem of frequent recurrences remains.

Platelet transfusion therapy is the major modality for arresting haemorrhage in patients with Glanzmann thrombasthenia. Although there is abundant evidence of efficacy in preventing and treating haemorrhage (Brown et al 1975, Seligsohn & Rososhansky 1982, George et al 1990), a recent study suggests that Glanzmann thrombasthenic platelets can interfere with normal platelet function and so greater than expected platelet numbers need to be infused (Jennings et al 1991); a previous report did not find a significant inhibiting effect (Brown et al 1975). Since platelet transfusions are so important, it is useful to consider some of the recent advances in our use of this therapy (Slichter 1991). Alloimmunization can lead to a refractory state in which platelet increments do not occur, and so efforts should be made to reduce the risk of developing such antibodies. Recent evidence indicates that depleting platelet concentrates of white blood cells by selective filtration decreases the likelihood of developing alloimmunization (Sniecinski et al 1988) although there is still some controversy on this point (Slichter 1991, Schiffer 1991). Since erythrocyte transfusions also contain contaminating white blood cells and platelets, leukocyte depletion of packed red blood cell transfusions may also be useful. Moreover, even in patients who are already refractory to platelet transfusions, leukocyte depletion of platelets for transfusion may improve the recovery of circulating platelets (Saarinen et al 1990). Two additional advantages of filtration are reductions in febrile transfusion reactions and cytomegalovirus sero-conversion (Andreu 1991); the latter may be especially important if bone marrow transplantation is ever considered. Thus, at present it would seem prudent to filter all erythrocyte and platelet transfusions.

The improved recoveries of platelets matched for ABO antigens argues in favour of using type-specific platelets if available (Slichter 1991). In fact, preliminary data indicate that it may be most desirable to use ABO identical platelets rather than ABO compatible platelets to achieve the best results (Heal et al 1991). Female patients who are Rh negative and of child-bearing potential should receive Rh negative platelets if possible to avoid Rh sensitization. HLA matching improves platelet recovery in many alloimmunized patients (Slichter 1991). Although in patients with haematologic malignancies, who are immunocompromised, random donor platelets are generally used until alloimmunization occurs (Schiffer 1991), the need for long-term, intensive platelet support in Glanzmann thrombasthenia patients, who are immunocompetent, probably justifies using HLA-matched platelets from the beginning. The increased use of single donor platelets obtained by plateletpheresis using continuous flow centrifuges might even make it possible to identify a small number of HLA-matched donors who might be available to donate when needed. Platelets from family members may be useful for this purpose, but this approach jeopardizes the ability to use that relative as a bone marrow donor should the need arise. The role, if any, for intravenous gammaglobulin in improving the platelet response in alloimmunized patients remains unclear (Slichter 1991).

Prognosis

Glanzmann thrombasthenia is a severe disorder that can have life-threatening complications, but with modern therapy, the prognosis is good. George et al (1990) noted that only two of the 64 patients he analyzed in Paris died of haemorrhage. One patient died after drainage of an intrahepatic haematoma that may have been a complication of oral contraceptive therapy. The nature of the haemorrhagic death in the other patient was not identified. Six of the patients, however, had siblings that died in early childhood from haemorrhage; at least some of these deaths may have been preventable with modern therapy. Among the patients described by Seligsohn et al (1991) in Israel, two of 40 patients from the Iraqi-Jewish population died from haemorrhage and a third died of adult respiratory distress syndrome; one of 13 Arab patients died of bleeding.

The GPIIb/IIIa complex and its function

GPIIb is a 1008 amino acid glycoprotein composed of two chains: a large α chain of M_r 125 000 and a smaller β chain of M_r 25 000 held together by a single disulphide bond (Poncz et al 1987, Phillips et al 1988) (Fig. 32.3). The α- and β-chains are synthesized as a single protein that undergoes cleavage, most likely after Arg^{859} (Kolodziej et al 1991), during the maturation of the GPIIb/IIIa complex. There may be additional cleavages in the same region, resulting in minor differences in size (Charo et al 1986, Loftus et al 1988). The β-subunit contains a transmembrane domain but the α-chain does not. GPIIb shares several features common to α-subunits in the integrin receptor superfamily, most importantly the presence of divalent cation-binding domains near the N-terminus that have been implicated in ligand binding (Phillips et al 1988). The gene for GPIIb is on the long arm of chromosome 17 and consists of 30 exons spread across ≈17 kilobases (Sosnoski et al 1988, Heidenreich et al 1990). An alternatively spliced form of GPIIb has been identified (Bray et al 1990).

GPIIIa is a single chain protein of 762 amino acids with one transmembrane domain (Fitzgerald et al 1987, Zimrin et al 1988). It is identical in sequence to the β_3-integrin subunit and homologous to other integrin receptor β-subunits, sharing cysteine-rich repeats near the transmembrane region and a complex disulphide bonding pattern in the N-terminal region (Phillips et al 1988). The GPIIIa gene is within 250 kilobases of the GPIIb gene on chromosome 17 and it consists of 14 exons spanning ≈46 kilobases (Sosnoski et al 1988, Zimrin et al 1990). An alternatively processed version of GPIIIa has also been identified resulting from nonsplicing of the final exon (van Kuppevelt et al 1989). GPIIIa can also complex with the α_v-subunit to give rise to the $\alpha_v\beta_3$ vitronectin receptor (Suzuki et al 1986, Fitzgerald et al 1987a). The GPIIb/IIIa receptor is highly specific for platelets and megakaryocytes in normal tissue, whereas the $\alpha_v\beta_3$ receptor is distributed widely, including endothelial cells and osteoclasts (Beckstead et al 1986, Lawler & Hynes 1989, Lam et al 1989).

The GPIIb/IIIa receptor is the dominant platelet receptor, with at least ≈40–50 000 complexes on the surface of platelets and another ≈25 000 complexes in internal platelet pools, including the α granule membrane (Coller et al 1983, Ruggeri & Hodson 1989, Wencel-Drake 1990). In contrast, there are only ≈50–100 $\alpha_v\beta_3$ vitronectin receptors on the surface of each platelet (Coller et al 1991a). The surface and internal GPIIb/IIIa receptors appear to be in dynamic equilibrium, at least when antibodies or other ligands bind to the receptors (Wencel-Drake 1990).

The biosynthesis of GPIIb/IIIa is schematically depicted in Figure 32.4. DNA control elements that are specific for megakaryocytes initiate the synthesis of each polypeptide resulting in their appearance in the endoplasmic reticulum (Uzan et al 1991). Perhaps assisted by chaperone proteins that control protein folding (Bennett et al 1991), GPIIb and GPIIIa form a complex and undergo additional processing in the endoplasmic reticulum and Golgi apparatus, including glycosylation and GPIIb cleavage (Duperray et al 1987, O'Toole et al 1989, Kolodziej et al 1991). The complex is then transported to the plasma membrane and α granule membrane. If complex formation does not occur, proteases digest the uncomplexed protein. The α_v polypeptide can also combine

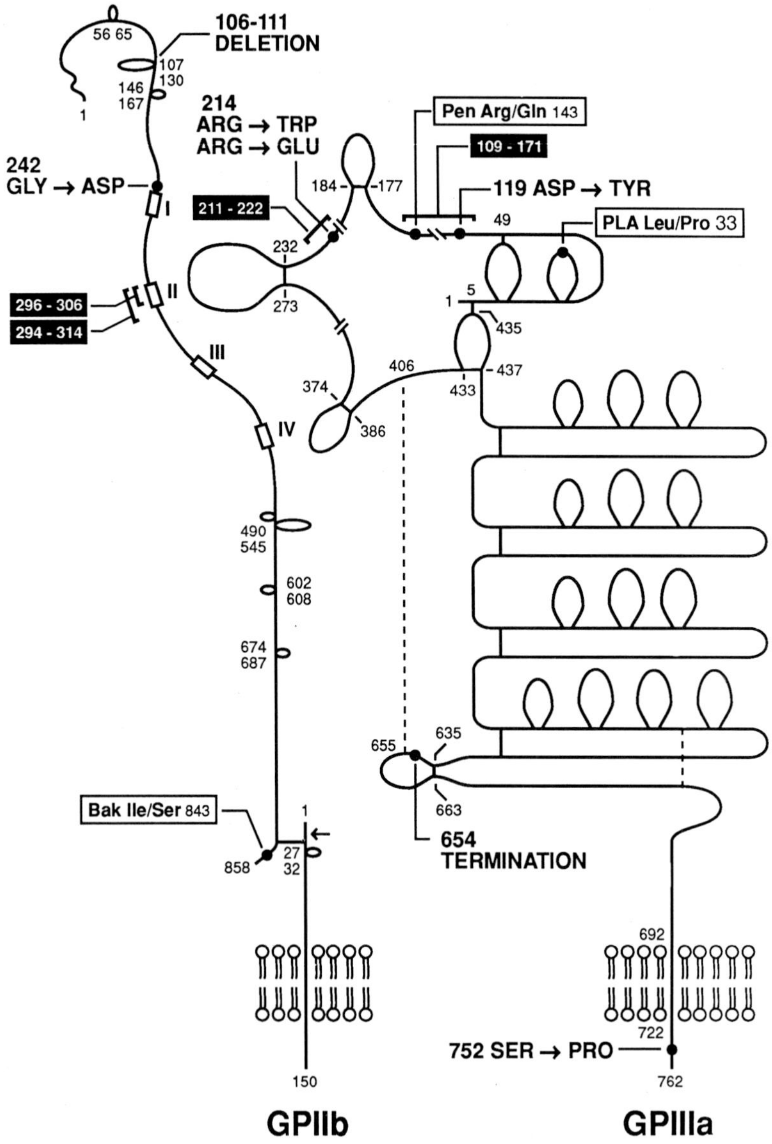

Fig. 32.3 Schematic diagram of platelet glycoproteins IIb and IIIa, including identification of documented abnormalities in Glanzmann thrombasthenia, sites of alloantigenic diversity, and regions implicated in ligand binding. Disulphide bonds have been assigned as suggested by Calvete et al (1989, 1991). The arrow near the N-terminus of GPIIbβ indicates variations in the cleavage site (Kolodzeij et al 1991). The Pen and PLA alloantigens on GPIIIa and the Bak alloantigen on GPIIb are identified in open boxes (Newman 1991, Wang et al 1991). The amino acid 294–314 region in GPIIb is implicated in ligand binding based on studies of γ-chain dodecapeptide cross-linking (amino acids 294–314) and inhibition of ligand binding by a synthetic peptide (amino acids 296–306) (D'Souza et al 1990, 1991). The region of amino acids 109–171 in GPIIIa is implicated in ligand binding based on studies of RGD-peptide cross-linking (D'Souza et al 1988) and the region of amino acids 211–222 is implicated in ligand binding based on synthetic peptide data (Charo et al 1991). The defects producing Glanzmann thrombasthenia include a deletion in GPIIb at amino acids 106–111 (Newman et al 1991), a point mutation in GPIIb at amino acid 242 (Rifat et al 1992), point mutations at amino acids 119, 214 and 752 in GPIIIa (Loftus et al 1990, Lanza et al 1991, Chen et al 1991, Bajt et al 1992) and a deletion leading to chain termination at amino acid 654 (Newman et al 1991).

with GPIIIa, producing the $\alpha_v\beta_3$ vitronectin receptor that presumably undergoes similar processing and membrane expression (Newman et al 1986, Polack et al 1989).

The GPIIb/IIIa receptor has a low affinity for its ligands when in the unactivated state, but shifts to high affinity when activated by any one of several different agonists

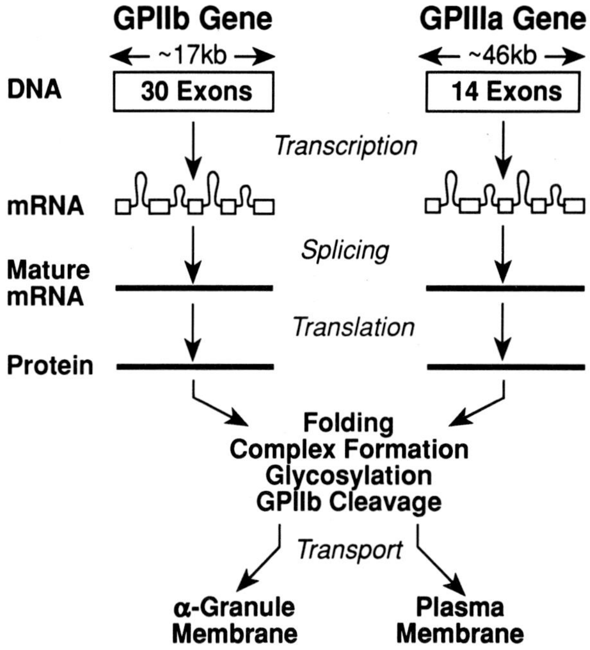

Fig. 32.4 Biosynthesis of the GPIIb/IIIa complex.

that are thought to be of potential physiological or pathological significance; these include collagen, thrombin, ADP, adrenalin, serotonin, vasopressin and perhaps, shear forces (Plow & Ginsberg 1989, Coller 1989). The mechanism by which this transformation occurs is unknown, but the result is presumed to be a comformational change in the GPIIb/IIIa receptor itself (O'Toole et al 1990). Recently, phosphatidic acid and Iysophosphatidic acid have been shown to increase the affinity of purified GPIIb/IIIa for fibrinogen, raising the possibility that one or both of these lipids are involved in the intact platelet (Smyth et al 1991, 1992). Studies of a patient with Glanzmann thrombasthenia suggest an important role for the cytoplasmic domain of GPIIIa (Chen et al 1991) and studies with deletion mutants of recombinant GPIIb/IIIa suggest an important role for the cytoplasmic domain of GPIIb (O'Toole et al 1991). The cytoplasmic domain of GPIIIa can undergo low level phosphorylation, but it is not clear if this reaction is related to receptor activation (Parise et al 1990, Hillery et al 1991).

The binding site(s) for adhesive ligands on GPIIb/IIIa has been studied extensively by a variety of techniques. Cross-linking studies of RGD peptides implicate a region near the N-terminus of GPIIIa (D'Souza et al 1988) (Fig. 32.3), whereas cross-linking studies of the γ-chain and synthetic peptide experiments implicate a region near the second calcium binding domain of GPIIb (Santoro & Lawing 1987, D'Souza et al 1990, 1991). The importance of the RGD cross-linking region of GPIIIa is supported by the finding that a patient with Glanzmann thrombasthenia and dysfunctional GPIIb/IIIa has a point mutation ($Asp^{119} \rightarrow$ Tyr) in that region. An adjacent area of GPIIIa also appears to be crucial to function, based on data from synthetic peptides (Charo et al 1991) and the identification of two other patients with Glanzmann thrombasthenia and dysfunctional GPIIb/IIIa receptors with two different mutations involving the same amino acid ($Arg^{214} \rightarrow$ Glu and $Arg^{214} \rightarrow$ Trp)(Lanza et al 1991, Bajt et al 1992). Further support for the importance of the calcium-binding domains of GPIIb comes from one patient with Glanzmann thrombasthenia and a point mutation adjacent to the first calcium binding domain ($Gly^{242} \rightarrow$ Asp) (Rifat et al 1992).

Plasminogen can bind to unstimulated platelets and the binding is increased five-fold when platelets are stimulated with thrombin. Much less plasminogen binds to both unstimulated and stimulated thrombasthenic platelets, implicating GPIIb/IIIa as the major binding site (Miles et al 1986). This is of particular note because abnormal platelet-supported fibrinolytic activity and abnormally loose platelet adsorption of plasminogen was noted by early investigators of Glanzmann thrombasthenia (Caen et al 1966).

Electron microscopical evaluation of GPIIb/IIIa, and inferences derived from studies of other integrin receptors, indicate that it is composed of a head region of ≈ 80 Å × 120 Å, containing segments from the N-termini of both GPIIb and GPIIIa, and two extended, thin, rods with hydrophobic regions near the tips, presumably representing the C-terminal regions of each glycoprotein, including the transmembrane segments (Carrell et al 1985, Kelly et al 1987, Nermut et al 1988, Weisel et al 1991). Fibrinogen has been visualized binding to isolated GPIIb/IIIa molecules primarily through its γ-chain C-terminal region, and when two different GPIIb/IIIa molecules were identified binding to a single fibrinogen molecule, the tails of the GPIIb/IIIa receptors were extended in opposite directions (Weisel et al 1991). The geometry of fibrinogen binding to GPIIb/IIIa on intact platelets (RGD- or dodecapeptide-mediated; univalent or bivalent) still remains to be defined. After fibrinogen binds to platelets it undergoes a transformation such that the binding becomes irreversible (Peerschke 1985, 1988, 1989) and new receptor-induced binding sites (RIBS) appear on the fibrinogen (Zamarron et al 1991). The GPIIb/IIIa receptor itself also undergoes changes with ligand binding that can be identified by monoclonal antibodies (Plow & Ginsberg 1989). One or more post-fibrinogen binding events appear necessary for platelet aggregation to occur (Coller 1989).

Diagnostic evaluation for Glanzmann thrombasthenia

There are three major components to the evaluation for Glanzmann thrombasthenia: global tests of platelet function, analysis of GPIIb/IIIa and $\alpha_v\beta_3$ vitronectin receptor quantity and functional integrity, and molecular genetic analysis of GPIIb and GPIIIa. Extensive study of Glanzmann thrombasthenia platelets indicate that they have essentially normal morphology; electrophoretic mobility; lifespan; adhesion to connective tissue, collagen, and von Willebrand factor; and content of calcium, magnesium, ATP, ADP, and serotonin (Caen et al 1966, Zucker et al 1966). The GPIIb/IIIa complex has, however, been implicated in platelet-calcium interactions. Brass & Shattil (1984) demonstrated abnormal high affinity and low affinity calcium-binding sites in thrombasthenic platelets and Brass (1985) implicated GPIIb/IIIa in calcium transport. Ryback (1988) found that GPIIb/IIIa incorporated into liposomes could function as a calcium channel. Powling and Hardisty (1985), however, found normal calcium uptake by stimulated thrombasthenic platelets. Platelet enzyme abnormalities have been reported in isolated patients with Glanzmann thrombasthenia, including decreases in Mg-ATPase, pyruvate kinase, glyceraldehyde 3 phosphate dehydrogenase, glutathione reductase and glutathione peroxidase, but the significance of these observations is unclear (Caen et al 1966, Moser 1968, Karpatkin & Weiss 1972).

Tests of platelet function

Platelet aggregation

When conducted with appropriate attention to the variables that may affect the results (Coller 1979), including platelet count, platelet-rich plasma pH, stirring mechanism, and elapsed time from blood drawing and platelet-rich plasma preparation, this technique provides important information on the overall ability of platelets to be activated by various agonists, undergo shape change, bind fibrinogen, and enter into aggregates. In Glanzmann thrombasthenia, the results are usually dramatic (Caen et al 1966, 1971, Zucker et al 1966, Weiss & Kochwa 1968, Cronberg 1971):

1. Adrenalin produces no observable response.
2. ADP and thrombin produce shape change but no aggregation.
3. Collagen produces shape change followed by a variable increase in light transmission that may be due to slight aggregation, but more likely is progressive platelet adhesion to the collagen fibres producing 'pseudoaggregation' (Hughes et al 1971, Coller et al 1983c).
4. Ristocetin produces a complex, dose-dependent pattern:
   a. regardless of dose; a normal or slightly reduced initial slope of 'aggregation' (which depends primarily on von Willebrand factor binding to platelet GPIb and is really an agglutination reaction)
   b. at low doses of ristocetin; when the normal response involves an identifiable second wave of aggregation, dependent upon the release reaction, studies with a monoclonal antibody to GPIIb/IIIa suggest that thrombasthenic platelets will not have the second wave (Coller et al 1983c)
   c. at high ristocetin doses; an interesting pattern of aggregation followed by disaggregation (Cohen et al 1975, Chediak et al 1979), occurring in repeating cycles, presumably reflecting GPIb-von Willebrand factor mediated agglutination followed by release of ADP (which is known to inhibit GPIb-von Willebrand factor agglutination) (Grant et al 1976), ATP and other granule contents that may also affect aggregation, followed by ADP and ATP breakdown, followed by increasing GPIb-von Willebrand factor interactions, etc.

Although the aggregometer provides quantifiable and reproducible data, it is also possible to assess platelet aggregation microscopically. In fact, the easiest, and surely most cost effective way to test for Glanzmann thrombasthenia even with very small amounts of blood is simply to make a smear from unanticoagulated blood. Normally, platelet aggregates are seen whereas none are present with thrombasthenic blood (Reichert et al 1975). This test is particularly useful for prenatal diagnosis when only very small amounts of blood are available (Champeix et al 1988), but it is very important to have confirmatory evidence if clinical decisions depend upon the diagnosis.

The aggregometer cannot detect very small platelet aggregates and techniques employing microscopic analysis or particle counters that size and count single platelets are much more sensitive. Some patients with Glanzmann thrombasthenia and detectable levels of platelet GPIIb/IIIa (type II) have given positive results with these techniques even when aggregometer tracings were considered negative (Lee et al 1981, Burgess-Wilson et al 1987).

Platelet release reaction

Release of dense body contents can be measured either by preloading platelets with radiolabelled serotonin or by monitoring release of platelet ATP by the light emitted from the reaction between luciferin and luciferase in the presence of ATP (Feinman et al 1977). The latter technique has the advantages of being able to be performed in platelet-rich plasma (avoiding the alterations that may accompany gel-filtration or washing) and permitting monitoring of release simultaneously with platelet aggregation. It does, however, require a special instrument. Release of α granule contents can be assessed by measuring the plasma content of platelet factor 4 (PF-4) or β-thromboglobulin after the platelets are stimulated and then removed by centrifugation. With adrenaline at any dose, or low doses of ADP, collagen or thrombin, release of granule contents from thrombasthenic platelets or normal platelets treated with antibodies to GPIIb/IIIa is less than from normal platelets because the aggregation process enhances release under these circumstances (Caen et al 1966, 1971, Charo et al 1977, Heptinstall & Taylor 1979, Coller et al 1983c). In contrast, with high doses of collagen and thrombin, the release reaction does not depend on platelet aggregation (Coller et al 1983c) and so thrombasthenic platelets behave in the same way as normal platelets (Caen et al 1966, Zucker et al 1966, Weiss & Kochwa 1968, Cronberg 1971, Malmsten et al 1977).

Clot retraction

Although abnormal clot retraction was the original functional assay used to define Glanzmann thrombasthenia (Glanzmann 1918), the results are variable between different patients. In fact, Caen (1972) proposed a subdivision of Glanzmann thrombasthenia into cases with absent (type 1) and subnormal (type 2) clot retraction. He also noted that $MgCl_2$ partially corrected the abnormality, but to varying extents. In general the type 2 patients have more residual GPIIb/IIIa (10–20%) than the type 1 patients (0–5%), but there is great heterogeneity at the molecular level in each group (Lee et al 1981, George et al 1990). Although the defect in clot retraction presumably reflects the abnormal interaction between platelet GPIIb/IIIa with fibrinogen/fibrin (Hantgan 1987, Gartner & Ogilvie 1988), the precise mechanism of clot retraction still remains poorly defined (Cohen et al 1982).

Interaction with glass surfaces

Normal platelets in whole blood or platelet-rich plasma adhere and spread on glass surfaces whereas Glanzmann thrombasthenic platelets do not (Caen et al 1966, Zucker et al 1966, Weiss & Kochwa 1968, Zucker & Vroman 1969, Stanford et al 1983). Evidence indicates that fibrinogen rapidly deposits on glass surfaces and so adhesion of platelets to these surfaces is probably mediated through the immobilized fibrinogen (Zucker & Vroman 1969, Stanford et al 1983). A similar process occurs during the glass bead retention test, accounting for the profound abnormality in Glanzmann thrombasthenia (Zucker et al 1966, Zucker & McPherson 1977).

Platelet coagulant activity

Both normal (Bevers et al 1986) and abnormal (Hardisty et al 1964, Caen et al 1966, Zucker et al 1966, Weiss & Kochwa 1968) results have been described, again probably reflecting whether stimulation is with doses of agonists that rely on platelet aggregation to achieve a maximal release reaction response. Variations in the assays for measuring platelet coagulant activity also may contribute to the reported differences. With maximal stimulation, however, thrombasthenic platelets appear quite capable of supporting coagulation normally (Bevers et al 1986).

Ex vivo interaction with deendothelialized blood vessels in flow chambers

This technique assesses the ability of platelets in whole blood to adhere to the subendothelium of a blood vessel, spread on the surface, and form platelet thrombi as a result of platelet aggregation. The effects of different anticoagulants and shear forces can also be tested. The most striking abnormality with Glanzmann thrombasthenia platelets is the absence of platelet thrombi. A defect in platelet spreading is also apparent, but results of platelet adhesion are normal or variably abnormal, depending upon the anticoagulant and shear rate (Tschopp et al 1975, Sakariassen et al 1986, Weiss et al 1986, Lawrence & Gralnick 1987).

Tests of platelet GPIIb/IIIa and $\alpha_v\beta_3$ receptor number and functional integrity

Techniques are based on polyacrylamide gel electrophoresis (Phillips & Agin 1977a, Clemetson 1985, Meyer & Herrmann 1985, Nurden 1985, Kehrel et al 1988). The original studies that identified the GPIIb/IIIa defects in Glanzmann thrombasthenia patients employed this technique (Nurden & Caen 1974, Phillips et al 1975, Jamieson et al 1979). Since platelet samples are solubilized in sodium dodecyl-sulphate, both surface and internal GPIIb/IIIa complexes are analyzed unless intact platelets are surface-labelled before solubilization. To avoid the overlapping mobilities of GPIIb and GPIIIa with other glycoproteins, samples can be electrophoresed both nonreduced and reduced (either separately, or sequentially on a nonreduced-reduced gel), or nondenatured proteins can be first separated by isoelectric focusing and then electrophoresed in a sodium dodecyl-sulphate polyacrylamide gel. The inter-chain and intra-chain disulphide bonds of GPIIb/IIIa result in a distinctive pattern in which the major GPIIb band decreases in M_r from 140 000 to 120 000 (since the GPIIb β chain has been lost) and the major GPIIIa band increases in M_r from 90 000 to 110 000 (since the molecule is less compact after breaking disulphide bands). Detection of all the electrophoresed proteins can be achieved with Coomassie blue staining (GPIIb can be readily detected but GPIIIa usually cannot), whereas identification of glycoproteins can be achieved with the periodic acid-Schiff stain or by reacting the gel with carbohydrate-specific lectins. To obtain increased sensitivity and to assess only the surface glycoproteins, the intact platelets can be prelabelled with protein-specific reagents (^{125}I using either lactoperoxidase or Iodogen for tyrosine groups, or biotinylation for free amino groups) or carbohydrate-specific reagents (Na^3HBH_4 reduction after periodate oxidation for vicinal hydroxyls). The gels can then be analyzed for total protein by staining and for surface glycoproteins by radioautography (^{125}I), avidin-enzyme binding, or fluorography

(^{3}H). Quantitation of the results is difficult because of the need to precisely control the amount of protein added to the gel, but comparison with dilutions of normal platelet proteins permits some estimate.

The introduction of the immunoblotting technique, in which proteins separated by polyacrylamide gel electrophoresis are blotted onto a membrane support and then the membrane is reacted with antibodies specific for certain proteins, dramatically increased the sensitivity for detecting small amounts of GPIIb/IIIa (down to ≈1% of normal) and profoundly influenced our understanding of the disorder. Patients were identified who lacked GPIIIa alone, lacked GPIIb alone, or in only a few cases, lacked both (Nurden 1985, Coller et al 1987, Jung et al 1988, Seligsohn et al 1989, Bray & Shuman 1990, Burk et al 1991). Moreover, the distribution of the residual GPIIb between the uncleaved and cleaved form, deduced from changes in M_r with disulphide bond reduction, permits some estimate of the extent to which the GPIIb precursor undergoes normal processing after synthesis (Jung et al 1988, Seligsohn et al 1989). Finally, immunoblotting permits the detection of unusual fragments or forms of GPIIb and GPIIIa that would otherwise not be detectable. Immunoblotting cannot, however, distinguish between surface and internal molecules.

Crossed immunoelectrophoresis

This technique involves platelet solubilization in the non-denaturing detergent Triton X-100, which retains GPIIb/IIIa in a complex (Hagen et al 1980, Shulman & Karpatkin 1980, Pidard 1989). Proteins are first separated according to charge in the first dimension and then they are detected by reaction with precipitating polyclonal antibodies in the second dimension. Radiolabelled monoclonal antibodies can also be incorporated to aid identification of GPIIb/IIIa, and radiolabelled fibrinogen can be layered over the gel to assess the ability of the GPIIb/IIIa complex to bind this ligand. Quantitation is imprecise but gross differences can be observed. This technique has been most helpful in identifying variants of Glanzmann thrombasthenia in which platelets contain an abnormal GPIIb/IIIa complex that is unusually sensitive to dissociation by divalent cation chelation with EDTA (Nurden et al 1987, Modderman et al 1989, George et al 1990).

Monoclonal antibody binding

Antibodies directed against either GPIIb alone, GPIIIa alone, or the GPIIb/IIIa complex can be used to assess the number of receptors on the platelet surface (Ruggeri & Hodson 1989). In addition, the antibodies can determine the number of receptors that join the platelet surface after the platelets are stimulated to undergo the release reaction. Studies using radiolabelled antibodies permit precise quantitation, with most studies, using antibodies directed against any part of the complex, finding ≈40 000–50 000 antibody molecules binding to unactivated platelets (McEver et al 1980, 1983, Bennett et al 1983, Coller et al 1983c, 1986b, Pidard et al 1983, Thiagarajan et al 1983, Newman et al 1985, Niiya et al 1987, Jordan et al 1991) and ≈75 000 molecules binding to platelets that have undergone the release reaction. What is unclear, however, is whether the antibodies are binding bivalently (to two different GPIIb/IIIa receptors) or univalently. Studies with univalent fragments of antibodies to GPIIb/IIIa suggest that the binding of intact antibody may be bivalent (Coller 1986, Niiya et al 1987, Jordan et al 1991), in which case the number of GPIIb/IIIa receptors on the platelet surface is more likely around 80 000 per platelet. This makes GPIIb/IIIa one of, if not the, densest receptor on any cell, with an average of less than 150 Å between receptors. Flow cytometry can also be used to assess the binding of monoclonal or polyclonal antibodies to platelets if the antibodies are labelled with a fluorescent molecule or if a fluorescent secondary reagent is used; although with this technique it is difficult to determine the precise number of molecules that bind per platelet, studies can be performed with very small samples, even in whole blood, offering significant advantages (Shattil et al 1985, Jennings et al 1986, Michelson 1987, Marti et al 1988).

In addition to providing quantitative information on the GPIIb/IIIa receptor number, the availability of murine monoclonal antibodies that bind near to, or at, crucial functional sites in the receptor permit the assessment of the functional integrity of the receptor. PAC1, the best studied antibody, is an IgM with a RYD sequence in one of its hypervariable regions; it is thought to bind to the same site on GPIIb/IIIa that binds RGD. Very little PAC1 binds to unactivated platelets, but activated platelets bind ≈10 000–15 000 molecules per platelet (Shattil et al 1985, Taub et al 1989). Thus, platelets from some patients with qualitative variants of Glanzmann thrombasthenia can bind significant numbers of antibody molecules directed at sites on GPIIb or GPIIIa, showing the presence of the receptor, but cannot bind antibodies that bind to critical functional sites (Lanza et al 1991, Bajt et al 1992). The binding of ligand to the GPIIb/IIIa receptor induces changes in the structure of the receptor that can be identified by the binding of antibodies such as PMI-1, which is directed against a site on the GPIIbα subunit (Ginsberg 1986, Plow & Ginsberg 1989).

The recognition that normal platelets contain trace amounts of the $\alpha_v\beta_3$ vitronectin receptor (Lam et al 1989, Lawler & Hynes 1989) permitted subcategorization of patients with Glanzmann thrombasthenia on the basis of the expression of this integrin. Monoclonal antibodies to different regions of the receptor have been used. Normal platelets only have ≈50–100 $\alpha_v\beta_3$ receptors on their surface and so technical adjustments have to be made to measure these small numbers (Coller et al 1991a). High specific activity radiolabelled antibodies are required since flow cytometry is not sensitive enough to detect this small number. It was presumed that patients with defects in GPIIIa would be deficient in $\alpha_v\beta_3$ receptors because GPIIIa is the β subunit common to both receptors (Zimrin et al 1988), and this was verified in studies on patients from the Iraqi-Jewish population (Coller et al 1991a, Newman et al 1991). Several patients with defects in GPIIb have also been studied for $\alpha_v\beta_3$ vitronectin receptor expression and their platelets appear to have increased $\alpha_v\beta_3$ receptors (Burk et al 1991, Coller et al 1991a, Rifat et al 1992), presumably because there is little or no GPIIb to compete for the pool of GPIIIa. Thus far there has been a perfect correlation between $\alpha_v\beta_3$ vitronectin receptor expression and the predicted GPIIb/IIIa receptor subunit containing the genetic abnormality, and so $\alpha_v\beta_3$ receptor expression seems to be a reliable method for determining which subunit is likely to be affected. Other thrombasthenic patients have been identified with a deficiency of $\alpha_v\beta_3$ receptors (Krissansen et al 1990) or at least trace amounts of $\alpha_v\beta_3$ (Lam et al 1989, Lawler & Hynes 1989) but their defects remain to be defined.

Ligand binding

The essential function of GPIIb/IIIa is to bind adhesive glycoprotein ligands when platelets are stimulated and so direct ligand-binding studies using radiolabelled fibrinogen, von Willebrand factor, and other ligands are useful in assessing the receptor's integrity. The major drawback of such studies is the requirement for separating platelets from plasma proteins before adding the radiolabelled ligand in order to remove the relatively large amounts of the unlabelled ligand proteins present in plasma that would reduce the specific activity. Unfortunately, all of the washing and gel filtration methods that accomplish this produce some alterations in the platelet.

^{125}I-labelled fibrinogen binding has been most extensively studied using several different agonists (Lee et al 1981, Bennett 1985, Peerschke 1985, Plow & Ginsberg 1989). High doses of ADP and thrombin result in the binding of $\approx$40 000 fibrinogen molecules per platelet. Since there are four RGD sequences and two λ-chain dodecapeptide sequences per fibrinogen molecule, there is a theoretical possibility that a single fibrinogen molecule could bind to six different GPIIb/IIIa receptors. Steric and geometric considerations make it unlikely that the RGD sequence in the coiled coil region are important in fibrinogen binding to activated platelets; the relative roles of the other RGD sequence and the γ-chain dodecapeptide are still uncertain, but both probably contribute (Harfenist et al 1984, Peerschke et al 1986, Amrani et al 1988, Shattil et al 1992). The interaction between platelets and immobilized fibrinogen appears to be even more complex, depending upon the state of platelet activation (Coller 1980, Savage & Ruggeri 1991, Parise et al 1992). Even though the $\alpha_v\beta_3$ vitronectin receptor can bind fibrinogen, the very small number of receptors makes it unlikely that this receptor contributes significantly to fibrinogen binding. There is some suggestive evidence, however, that the $\alpha_v\beta_3$ vitronectin receptor makes a minor contribution to platelet fibrinogen (Coller et al 1991c).

The platelets of patients with severe Glanzmann thrombasthenia do not bind any fibrinogen (Bennett & Vilaire 1979, Mustard et al 1979), but patients with significant amounts of residual GPIIb/IIIa usually bind some fibrinogen, and rare patients have been noted to bind considerable amounts (Lee et al 1981). Patients with variants of Glanzmann thrombasthenia usually do not bind any fibrinogen. Glanzmann thrombasthenic platelets also fail to adhere to immobilized fibrinogen (Coller 1980).

Platelet fibrinogen and vitronectin

One of the hallmarks of Glanzmann thrombasthenia is a marked reduction in platelet fibrinogen to levels that are $\leq$ 10% of normal (Zucker et al 1966, Caen et al 1966, Weiss & Kochwa 1968, Disdier et al 1989, Coller et al 1991c). Although early studies suggested that megakaryocytes can synthesize fibrinogen, the weight of more recent evidence indicates that platelet fibrinogen is taken up from plasma fibrinogen (Handagama et al 1989, 1990, Harrison et al 1989). GPIIb/IIIa appears to be the dominant receptor responsible for the uptake, but the $\alpha_v\beta_3$ receptor, which can also bind fibrinogen, may play a very minor role (Coller et al 1991c). Platelet fibrinogen can be assessed by Coomassie blue staining of platelet proteins separated by polyacrylamide gel electrophoresis, by immunoblotting studies using antifibrinogen antibodies, or by sensitive immunological assays of platelet proteins solubilized in non-denaturing detergents. To avoid contamination with plasma fibrinogen it is important that the platelets are washed well before solubilization. For reasons that remain unexplained, some patients with Glanzmann thrombasthenia have nearly normal levels of platelet fibrinogen (Karpatkin et al 1984).

Vitronectin is also contained in platelets and can be analyzed by immunoblotting or immunoassay of platelet proteins solubilized in non-denaturing detergents (Coller 1991c). Since vitronectin can bind to both GPIIb/IIIa and the $\alpha_v\beta_3$ vitronectin receptor, if its platelet content also relied on uptake from plasma in a manner similar to fibrinogen, one would anticipate a deficiency in thrombasthenic platelets, especially those lacking $\alpha_v\beta_3$ in addition to GPIIb/IIIa. The only study reported to date found a paradoxical result, with normal platelet vitronectin in patients with no GPIIb/IIIa but increased $\alpha_v\beta_3$ receptors, and increased platelet vitronectin ($\approx$4–5 fold) in patients lacking both GPIIb/IIIa and $\alpha_v\beta_3$ receptors (Coller et al

1991c). One possible explanation for these findings is that vitronectin is made in megakaryocytes and $\alpha_v\beta_3$ is required for transport out of the platelet. Vitronectin production by megakaryocytes has not, however, been demonstrated as yet.

Genetic analysis of GPIIb and GPIIIa

Defining the primary defect responsible for Glanzmann thrombasthenia in a given patient requires analysis of the patient's genetic material. The logical first step is to obtain genomic DNA from peripheral blood lymphocytes and perform Southern blot analysis with GPIIb- and GPIIIa-specific probes after enzymatic digestion of the DNA with restriction endonucleases. This should identify any major deletions or insertions in the gene. If this is normal, analysis of the cDNA for small deletions or point mutations is the next logical step. Since megakaryocyte mRNA is not easily obtained, platelet mRNA has been most commonly analyzed. Although platelets contain only small amounts of mRNA, the remarkable amplification produced by the polymerase chain reaction has made it practicable to obtain sufficient amounts of mRNA to perform a complete study from as little as 30 ml of peripheral blood (Newman et al 1991). The first step after mRNA extraction is to reverse transcribe the mRNA into cDNA, and then the cDNA can be amplified. The products can then be sequenced and compared to the published reports of the authentic sequences (Fitzgerald et al 1987b, Poncz et al 1987). An alternative strategy based on using genomic DNA is also possible since the nucleotide sequences of both the GPIIb and GPIIIa genes have been published (Heidenreich et al 1990, Zimrin et al 1990). Thus, primers based on these sequences can be used to search for the defect, to confirm a defect found in the cDNA, or to better define an abnormality identified in the cDNA if it involves an intron-exon boundary (Burk et al 1991, Newman et al 1991). In patients without family histories of consanguinity, special attention needs to be paid to the possibility that the patient is a double heterozygote with two separate abnormalities. Distinguishing between functionally unimportant polymorphisms and significant abnormalities can be difficult and so confirmatory evidence utilizing site-directed mutagenesis to produce the same abnormality in a cell line expressing recombinant GPIIb/IIIa is extremely important.

Carrier detection and prenatal diagnosis

Carriers of Glanzmann thrombasthenia have almost always been described as asymptomatic and their platelet function studies are usually normal (George et al 1990). Despite this, they have only approximately 50–60% of the normal number of GPIIb/IIIa receptors on their platelets, allowing for their identification using a variety of techniques, including complement fixation with alloimmune antisera, polyacrylamide gel electrophoresis with periodic acid-Schiff staining, crossed immunoelectrophoresis and electroimmunoassay using heterologous antisera, and monoclonal antibody binding assays (McEver et al 1980, Kunicki et al 1981a, Hermann et al 1982, Stormorken et al 1982, Zonneveld et al 1983, Coller et al 1986). Each assay measures slightly different aspects of platelet GPIIb/IIIa as described above. Even under optimal conditions, however, these assays are not definitive since some overlap between controls and carriers occurs. For example, in one study using monoclonal antibody binding that involved 37 obligate carriers and 20 controls, the assay was 92% sensitive and 92% specific (Coller et al 1986b). Since genetic counselling decisions are so vital, even this degree of accuracy leaves much to be desired. When the genetic defect in the involved kindred has been identified, carrier detection can become unequivocal. Many alternative techniques are available, including the use of unique DNA probes that are specific for the abnormal DNA sequence, and the use of direct size analysis of polymerase chain reaction products when detectable deletions are present (Newman et al 1991, Peretz et al 1991). The latter technique can actually be performed on the DNA recovered from the cells present in routine urine samples, facilitating collection of samples for analysis (Peretz et al 1991).

Platelet GPIIb/IIIa appears early in fetal development and so by 18 weeks of age it is present at the same levels as on adult platelets (Seligsohn et al 1985, Gruel et al 1986). This permits fetal blood samples to be analyzed by the techniques indicated above for expression of GPIIb/IIIa and its functional integrity. The earliest studies utilized fetoscopy in order to obtain samples of pure fetal blood (Seligsohn et al 1985, 1988), but subsequent technical advances have led to the adoption of percutaneous umbilical blood vessel sampling under ultrasound guidance (Kaplan et al 1985, Champeix et al 1988, Wautier & Gruel 1989, Seligsohn et al 1991). When the genetic abnormality is known, carrier detection can be performed at 8–10 weeks of gestation using chorionic villus biopsy as the source of DNA (Seligsohn, 1992b). Alternatively, DNA from cells obtained from amniotic fluid later in the pregnancy can also be tested (Seligsohn, 1992b). Technical advances continue to occur with enormous rapidity and so it is difficult to provide definitive estimates for the risks to the fetus and mother of each of these procedures. Of particular note, however, is the observation that several, but not all, fetuses affected with Glanzmann thrombasthenia died from exsanguination soon after fetal blood sampling (Champeix et al 1988, Seligsohn et al 1991). This contrasts with the rarity of this complication after fetal blood sampling of haemophiliacs, emphasizing the differences in bleeding patterns in these disorders.

Frequency of Glanzmann thrombasthenia subtypes

Based on clot retraction, and where available, platelet fibrinogen content and GPIIb/IIIa content, George et al (1990) categorized the 64 patients studied in Paris as type I (78%), type II (14%), or variants (8%); since 26 of the 64 patients were not tested for GPIIb/IIIa content directly, it is possible that some variants were misassigned into the other categories. Type I patients had no or minimal clot retraction, absent or severely deficient fibrinogen, less than 5% of normal GPIIb/IIIa, and absent fibrinogen binding. Type II patients had normal or moderately reduced clot retraction, substantial amounts of platelet fibrinogen, and 10–20% of normal platelet GPIIb/IIIa; their platelets bound fibrinogen in proportion to their residual GPIIb/IIIa content (Lee et al 1981). Patients were considered variants if they had the characteristic platelet function abnormalities, but had ≈50% or more of the normal amounts of GPIIb/IIIa. It is important to emphasize, however, that this categorization does not predict clinical symptoms, with both severely affected and minimally affected patients present in each group (George et al 1990). Moreover, there is significant molecular heterogeneity within each group; immunoblot studies of type I patients demonstrated that 15 of 18 had detectable GPIIIa but only seven had detectable GPIIb (George et al 1990). Iraqi-Jewish and Arab type I patients were also found to differ in immunoblot patterns and in their molecular biological defect (Coller et al 1987, Seligsohn et al 1989, Newman et al 1991).

The variants of Glanzmann thrombasthenia with 50% or more GPIIb/IIIa are of particular interest because their defects can provide important information on the mechanism by which GPIIb/IIIa becomes activated and on the structure of the ligand-binding regions. George et al (1990) reviewed five variants studied in Paris. Two of the patients (CM and MS) had GPIIb/IIIa complexes that were unstable in the presence of the calcium chelating agent EDTA, indicating an abnormality in GPIIb/IIIa complex formation (Nurden et al 1987). Neither patient had platelet fibrinogen. Patient CM never required platelet transfusions whereas patient MS required transfusion for bleeding at menarche and suffered a traumatic intracerebral haematoma at age 6. Two other patients, AP and CG, had variable clinical and molecular manifestations of the disease. The molecular biological defects in the last of these variants (*RP*, patient P) and in two other variants (*Cam* and *ET*) have recently been reported and so they will be discussed below.

Jung et al (1988) described a 21-year-old patient (SS) with mild haemorrhagic symptoms, a long bleeding time, ≈35% of normal GPIIb/IIIa on her platelets, ≈25% of normal fibrinogen binding to her activated platelets, normal platelet fibrinogen, and no aggregation in response to ADP. Immunoblot studies identified two GPIIb bands, one of which migrated abnormally. The abnormal band appeared to be an uncleaved version of GPIIb. The patient's parents were consanguineous, but the father showed the abnormal GPIIb whereas the mother did not. The father was asymptomatic and had only slightly reduced platelet aggregation; his platelets were estimated to contain 56% of the normal platelet GPIIb whereas the patient had only 20–30%.

Tanoue et al (1987) reported a 15-year-old female patient (MY) with mild purpura who had mild thrombocytopenia (70 000–110 000 platelets/μL), a prolonged bleeding time, reduced clot retraction and platelet retention, and absence of platelet aggregation in response to ADP, adrenalin and collagen. Thrombin-induced aggregation of washed platelets, however, was nearly normal. In addition, her platelets contained substantial amounts of fibrinogen. The patient had significant amounts of GPIIb/IIIa, but the proteins failed to react with the PAS stain or with concanavalin A, suggesting abnormal glycosylation.

Modderman et al (1989) described a 30-year-old female patient with a moderately-severe haemorrhagic diathesis, prolonged bleeding time and a failure of her platelets to aggregate, bind fibrinogen or retract clots when stimulated. The patient had only a partial deficiency of GPIIb/IIIa and a partial deficiency of platelet fibrinogen. The GPIIb/IIIa complex was unusually sensitive to dissociation with calcium chelation and the GPIIb appeared to be present in both the uncleaved and cleaved forms.

Molecular biological defects in Glanzmann thrombasthenia

In the recent past, the molecular biological basis of Glanzmann thrombasthenia has been identified in several affected groups and individual patients, providing important information on the biogenesis of the GPIIb/IIIa receptor and its function. Table 32.3 summarizes the data.

Glanzmann thrombasthenia III. Two siblings with type I Glanzmann thrombasthenia from a family designated GT III were studied by Bray & Shuman (1990). Neither GPIIb nor GPIIIa could be detected by immunoblotting in either patient. No platelet GPIIIa mRNA could be identified and analysis of genomic DNA revealed a mutant GPIIIa allele inherited from the father with an insertion of at least 7.2 kb in the 5′ region of the gene. The patients were presumed to have inherited an abnormal GPIIIa gene from the mother as well, but the nature of the abnormality was not defined.

Cam variant. Three members of a single Guamanian family (two males and one female) were identified by Ginsberg et al (1986) as having an unusual variant of Glanzmann thrombasthenia. Clinically, the patients had moderately severe disease requiring intermittent therapy with platelets. Their laboratory values reflected a pro-

Table 32.3 Molecular biological defects in Glanzmann's thrombasthenia

Patient or group	Category	Platelet fibrinogen	GPIIb/IIIa content	$\alpha_v\beta_3$ (% of normal)	Affected subunit	Molecular biological defect
GT III	Type I	–	No GPIIb or GPIIIa by immunoblot	–	GPIIIa	Doubly heterozygous GPIIIa defects; 1) Insertion ≥7.2 kb in 5' portion of GPIIIa, and 2) unidentified mutation leading to loss of expression
KW	Type I	–	No GPIIb and trace GPIIIa by immunoblot	190	GPIIb	Homozygous 4 kb deletion encompassing exons 2–9 of GPIIb with a pseudoexon composed of portions of introns 1 and 9
Iraqi-Jews	Type I	Trace	Trace GPIIb and no GPIIIa by immunoblot	0	GPIIIa	Homozygous 11 bp GPIIIa deletion in exon 12 leading to frameshift and premature termination at amino acid 654
Israeli Arabs	Type I	Trace	Trace GPIIb and GPIIIa by immunoblot	200	GPIIb	Homozygous 13 bp deletion at juncture of intron 3–exon 4 leading to alternative splicing, loss of 18 bp in cDNA and 6 amino acid deletion (106–111) including 1 cysteine
Paris patient	Type I	0	No GPIIIa	–	GPIIIa	Homozygous 5 kb insertion between exons 8 and 10; no GPIIIa mRNA
JF	Type I	Trace	Trace GPIIb and GPIIIa by immunoblot	201	GPIIb	G→A in GPIIb, Gly^{242}→Asp
Guamanian family	Variant	Trace	Normal GPIIb/IIIa by SDS-PAGE	–	GPIIIa	G→T in GPIIIa, Asp^{119}→Tyr
ET	Variant	Trace	Normal GPIIb/IIIa	–	GPIIIa	G→A in GPIIIa, Arg^{214}→Glu
Strasbourg variant	Variant	20%	Normal to subnormal GPIIb/IIIa	–	GPIIIa	C→T in GPIIIa, Arg^{214}→Trp
Patient P, Paris I	Variant	50%	50–60% GPIIb/IIIa by SDS-PAGE	–	GPIIIa	1. T→C in GPIIIa, Ser^{752}→Pro 2. Unidentified GPIIIA null mutation

found functional abnormality in GPIIb/IIIa as judged by platelet aggregation, fibrinogen binding, and platelet fibrinogen studies. An abnormality in GPIIb/IIIa structure involving divalent cations was inferred from the ability of a monoclonal antibody to GPIIbα (PMI-1), which only binds to normal platelets in the presence of the calcium chelator EDTA, to bind to patient platelets even in the absence of EDTA. In a subsequent study (Loftus et al 1990), these investigations identified a homozygous G to T point mutation in GPIIIa leading to a change at amino acid 119, converting an Asp into a Tyr. Confirmation was obtained by site-directed mutagenesis in an expression system. It is of note that Asp^{119} is highly conserved among integrin β-subunits and this region has previously been implicated as being near the RGD binding site (D'Souza et al 1988), making this discovery particularly exciting.

Iraqi-Jewish patients. Patients from this large population who have the classical laboratory findings of type I Glanzmann thrombasthenia and variably severe clinical disease (Reichert et al 1975, Seligsohn & Rososhansky 1984, Seligsohn et al 1991) were found to have trace amounts of immunodetectable platelet GPIIb (Seligsohn et al 1989), but no GPIIIa (Coller et al 1987). Subsequent analysis of $\alpha_v\beta_3$ vitronectin receptors supported a GPIIIa defect since the patient's platelets were also deficient in $\alpha_v\beta_3$ receptors (Coller 1991a). There were no major structural changes in their genomic DNA (Russell et al 1988), but studies of their platelet mRNA and genomic DNA revealed a homozygous 11 bp deletion in exon 12 of GPIIIa leading to a frame shift; the new sequence codes for several additional abnormal amino acids and then a termination codon after amino acid 654 (Newman et al 1991). Thus, a truncated GPIIIa molecule lacking a transmembrane domain is predicted. Two features of the disorder in these patients are particularly notable: 1) the homozygous genomic DNA GPIIIa abnormality predicts a deficiency of $\alpha_v\beta_3$ vitronectin receptors in tissues other than platelets and yet these patients appear to have their clinical abnormalities confined to the haemostatic system, and 2) there is very little processing of the residual pro-GPIIb to GPIIbα + GPIIbβ (Seligsohn et al 1989) indicating a requirement for complex formation with a more normal GPIIIa in order for GPIIb cleavage to occur.

Israeli-Arab patients. Five unrelated type I patients from this population (Reichert et al 1975, Seligsohn & Rosohansky 1984, Seligsohn et al 1991) with variably severe clinical disease share the same abnormality. Immunoblotting identified trace amounts of both GPIIb and GPIIIa (Coller et al 1987, Seligsohn et al 1989). The patients' platelets had normal to increased amounts of $\alpha_v\beta_3$ vitronectin receptors (Coller et al 1991a), suggesting the presence of a normal GPIIIa protein, and thus a presumably abnormal GPIIb protein. There were no major structural abnormalities of their genomic DNA (Russell et al 1988). Analysis of platelet mRNA and genomic DNA revealed a 13 bp deletion at the junction between intron 3 and exon 4, including the splice acceptor signal, leading to forced alternative splicing and loss of six amino acids in the protein (Newman et al 1991). One of the six amino acids is a Cys and so it is likely that this abnormal GPIIb cannot fold properly. Some of the pro-GPIIb is cleaved to GPIIbα and GPIIbβ, but less than normal (Seligsohn et al 1989). Although these patients have a marked deficiency of platelet fibrinogen, direct comparison with Iraqi-Jewish patients' platelets indicated the presence of slightly more platelet fibrinogen in the Arab patients, suggesting perhaps a minor role for $\alpha_v\beta_3$ in uptake of fibrinogen from plasma (Coller et al 1991c).

Summary and prospects for the future

The study of Glanzmann thrombasthenia has provided vital data on platelet physiology. Analysis of the GPIIb/IIIa receptor in Glanzmann patients has uncovered crucial information regarding integrin receptor biogenesis and structure–function relationships. These studies have led to advances in protein-based and DNA-based diagnosis, improving the accuracy of carrier detection and prenatal diagnosis. Moreover, insights derived from analysis of Glanzmann thrombasthenia patients have led to attempts to inhibit platelet thrombus formation in pathological conditions by blocking GPIIb/IIIa receptors (Coller et al 1991b).

The future looks even brighter, with additional molecular biological defects in patients certain to be uncovered, providing even more detailed data. Studies of acute and chronic vascular disease in large numbers of carriers of Glanzmann thrombasthenia with decreased numbers of GPIIb/IIIa receptors may allow us to ascertain whether a 40–50% decrease in GPIIb/IIIa surface receptors offers any protection from these disorders. This information will be particularly important if orally active agents that can block GPIIb/IIIa on a chronic basis become available.

Therapy for haemorrhagic episodes in Glanzmann thrombasthenia remains difficult, but advances in platelet transfusion are likely to continue to make this therapy more effective. Bone marrow transplantation is becoming safer and more likely to succeed, but the risks are so considerable that it would only be justified in the most refractory of cases. The growing enthusiasm about the prospects for gene replacement therapy also auger well, but it is impossible at present to predict when this will become safe and effective enough to be justified in Glanzmann thrombasthenia.

The history of Glanzmann thrombasthenia demonstrates the synergistic interrelationship that exists between basic and clinical research, with each new clinical insight leading to more basic studies, and each new basic insight leading to more sophisticated clinical analysis. The end is still not in sight.

GLYCOPROTEIN Ib, IX, AND V ABNORMALITIES: BERNARD–SOULIER SYNDROME

History

In 1948 the French haematologists Bernard and Soulier described a consanguineous family with two children affected with a severe bleeding disorder involving epistaxis, ecchymosis, gingival bleeding and haematemesis (Bernard & Soulier 1948, Bernard 1983). One child died at 31 months from gastrointestinal bleeding and was only incompletely evaluated, but it appeared that both children suffered from the same disorder, characterized by variable thrombocytopenia, giant platelets on the blood smear, prolonged bleeding time, and normal clot retraction. The younger sibling had a decrease in spontaneous mucocutaneous haemorrhage with age, but still had multiple episodes of trauma-related haemorrhage requiring platelet transfusions. Multiple antibodies to platelets developed in the patient, including an agglutinating antibody ('antibody P') that helped to characterize the biochemical abnormality (Degos et al 1977). His platelet count fell steadily from 1964 (80 000/μL) to 1973 (20 000/μL) for unknown reasons. In 1976 the patient died from a cerebral haemorrhage several hours after suffering head trauma as a result of a barroom brawl.

Epidemiology and inheritance

In a review published in 1983, Bernard identified 70 cases of Bernard–Soulier syndrome reported in the literature, of which 59 were considered complete descriptions. A number of cases have been reported subsequently (Berndt et al 1983b, McGill et al 1984, Michelas et al 1984, de Marco et al 1986, 1990, Heslop et al 1986, Sheffer et al 1986, Shinmyozu et al 1986, Suhasini et al 1986, de Moerloose et al 1987, Ingerslev et al 1987, Oki et al 1987, Cuthbert et al 1988, Drouin et al 1988a,b, Mant 1988, Stevens et al 1988, Nichols et al 1989, Peaceman et al 1989, Shimamoto et al 1989, Finch et al 1990, Poulsen & Taaning 1990, Ware et al 1990, Waldenstrom et al 1991). Cases have been reported from at least 15 different countries throughout Europe, Asia, Africa and North America. Consanguinity is common, occurring in 14 of the 37 families responsible for the 59 cases reported by Bernard (1983).

Clinical manifestations

The haemorrhagic manifestations in 54 patients was

also reviewed by Bernard (1983). Epistaxis was the most common symptom, occurring in 70% of the patients; ecchymoses (58%), menometrorrhagia (44%), gingival bleeding (42%), and gastrointestinal bleeding (22%) also occurred with considerable frequency. Severe post-traumatic bleeding (13%), haematuria (7%), cerebral haemorrhage (4%), and retinal haemorrhage (2%) were much rarer complications. George & Nurden (1987) emphasized the variability of bleeding manifestations in Bernard–Soulier syndrome even within families, citing a Kuwaiti patient (George et al 1981) who required platelet transfusions every 2–4 weeks for more than 12 years to control bleeding episodes whereas her sister received only two transfusions over a comparable time period.

Therapy and management

As in Glanzmann thrombasthenia, attention needs to be focused on good dental prophylaxis, hormonal control of menstruation, and iron replacement for those losing significant amounts of blood. Drugs that interfere with platelet function should be avoided. Epistaxis can be particularly difficult to control and in the most severe cases may require ligation of the arteries supplying the nose (Rodeghiero et al 1987). Several patients have had successful pregnancies and deliveries, but the course can be very difficult, with delayed bleeding and the need for emergency hysterectomy (Michelas et al 1984, Heslop et al 1986, Peaceman et al 1989).

Desmopressin was reported to decrease the bleeding time in four patients without improving ristocetin-induced aggregation in the two it was tested in (Cuthbert et al 1987, DiMichele & Hathaway 1990, Waldenstrom et al 1991); little or no effect on bleeding time was observed, however, in other patients (Heslop et al 1986, Mant 1988). Serious bleeding episodes require platelet transfusions and a description of the recent advances in platelet transfusion therapy is included in the section on Glanzmann thrombasthenia (p. 728). Plasmapheresis and intravenous gammaglobulin have been used to help increase the response to transfused platelets in patients who have become refractory to platelet transfusions (Peaceman et al 1989), but the efficacy of these manoeuvres remains uncertain. Since patients may lack GPIb, GPV and/or GPIX, they are at risk of developing antibodies to these glycoproteins, some of which may interfere with GPIb function (Degos et al 1977). In fact, the first patient described with the syndrome developed this complication and the antibody ('antibody P') reacted with GPIb and inhibited GPIb function (Degos et al 1977).

The functional and glycoprotein abnormalities in Bernard–Soulier syndrome

Since the prolongation of the bleeding time in patients with Bernard–Soulier syndrome appeared to be greater than would be expected on the basis of the decreased platelet count, a qualitative disorder in platelet function was suspected (Bernard 1983, George and Nurden 1987). This presumed defect was easily differentiated from the defect in Glanzmann thrombasthenia by the normal clot retraction and the normal or supernormal (Bithell et al 1972, Waldenstrom 1991) aggregation induced by ADP, collagen, and adrenaline. Platelet shape change, thromboxane production, and release of dense granule contents are also normal when Bernard–Soulier syndrome platelets are activated by these agonists (George & Nurden 1987).

A series of observations focused attention on the possibility that a platelet membrane receptor for von Willebrand factor was deficient in Bernard–Soulier platelets:

1. Normal platelets are agglutinated by bovine von Willebrand factor (a contaminant in early bovine fibrinogen preparations), but Bithell et al in 1972 noted that Bernard–Soulier platelets could not be agglutinated by this agent.
2. Normal platelets are agglutinated by human von Willebrand factor when the antibiotic ristocetin is added, but in 1973 Howard et al demonstrated that Bernard–Soulier platelets do not respond. Although this defect was similar to that observed when von Willebrand disease platelets were tested, it differed in that it could not be corrected by adding normal plasma. Moreover, direct measurement of von Willebrand factor binding to platelets in the presence of ristocetin confirmed the failure of von Willebrand factor to bind to Bernard–Soulier platelets in the presence of ristocetin (Zucker et al 1977, Moake et al 1980).
3. Bernard–Soulier platelets do not adhere to de-endothelialized blood vessels in flow chamber studies (Weiss et al 1974a), an abnormality very similar to that observed in patients lacking von Willebrand factor.
4. The snake venom protein botrocetin causes von Willebrand factor to bind to normal platelets, leading to agglutination, whereas agglutination of Bernard–Soulier platelets is markedly reduced or absent (Howard et al 1984, Nishio et al 1990).

Paralleling the functional studies were a series of biochemical and biophysical studies that defined the membrane abnormalities.

1. A deficiency in Bernard–Soulier platelet surface sialic acid resulting in a decrease in platelet electrophoretic mobility was discovered by Grottum and Solum in 1969.
2. A decreased amount of platelet GPIb in Bernard–Soulier platelets was identified by Nurden & Caen in 1975 using ^{125}I-labelled-platelets, a result that was rapidly confirmed using immunological techniques (Hagen et al 1980, Nurden et al 1981).

3. The alloimmune antibody (antibody P) from a patient with Bernard–Soulier syndrome reacted with GPIb, failed to react with Bernard–Soulier platelets and caused normal platelets to function like Bernard–Soulier platelets (Degos et al 1977).

4. Murine monoclonal antibodies directed against GPIb failed to react with Bernard–Soulier platelets and also produced a Bernard–Soulier-like defect in normal platelets (McMichael 1981, Ruan et al 1981, 1987, Berndt et al 1983b, Coller et al 1983b, Montgomery et al 1983).

5. Studies employing ^{3}H to label the carbohydrate component of membrane glycoproteins identified additional abnormalities in GPV (M_r 82 000) and GPIX (M_r 20 000) in patients with Bernard–Soulier syndrome (Clemetson et al 1982, Berndt 1983b).

6. Studies with monoclonal antibodies demonstrated that GPIb and GPIX form a noncovalent complex (Berndt et al 1983b, Coller et al 1983b).

The primary sequences of GPIbα, GPIbβ and GPIX have been deduced from their cDNAs, and portions of the sequence of GPV have been determined from the purified protein (Lopez et al 1987, 1988, Hickey et al 1989, Clemetson et al 1990, Roth et al 1990, Shimomura et al 1990). The gene for GPIbα is on the short arm of chromosome 17 and the gene for GPIX is probably on chromosome 3 (Wenger et al 1989, Roth 1991). The GPIbα gene is unusual in that it does not contain exons in the coding region and this may also be true of GPIX (Wenger et al 1988, Hickey et al 1990).

The most striking observation is that all four proteins have one or more leucine-rich regions that are homologous to regions in leucine-rich α_2-glycoprotein, a human serum protein of unknown function (Roth et al 1991, Ruggeri 1991) (Fig. 32.5). Glycoprotein Ibα (M_r 143 000) is composed of 610 amino acids and has seven tandem leucine-rich repeats in the N-terminal region (residues 36–200); conserved flanking sequences of 22 amino acids are present on both sides of these repeats. The segment between amino acids 220–310 has been designated a hinge region and within this region there is a span of negatively charged amino acids (269–287) and positively charged amino acids (288–301) that have been implicated in the binding of von Willebrand factor to GPIb (Roth 1991, Ruggeri 1991). Other data derived from peptides also support the importance of this region in ligand binding (Katagiri et al 1990, Vicente et al 1990, Ruggeri 1991). A five segment tandem repeat of about nine amino acids between amino acids 363 and 414 is rich in *O*-linked carbohydrate attachment sites, accounting for the heavy glycosylation in this region (Roth 1991). There are also four *N*-linked glycosylation sites in the molecule. GPIbα contains a transmembrane domain near the C-terminus. One or more disulphide bonds connect GPIbα to GPIbβ,

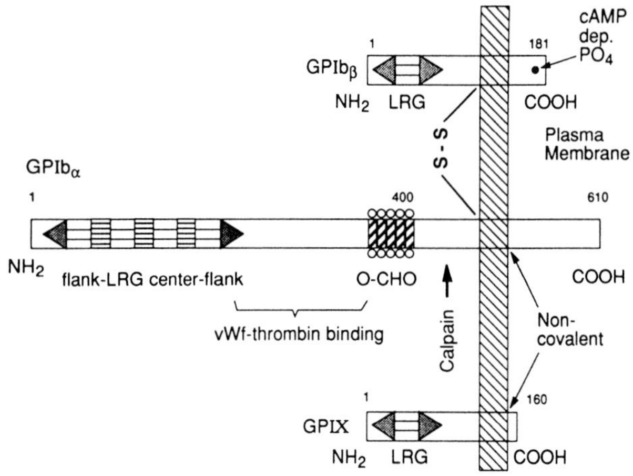

Fig. 32.5 The GPIb/IX complex. Proteins are depicted as open bars with superscripts referring to amino acid number and subscripts to N- and C-termini. Transmembrane domains demarcate larger extracellular from smaller intracellular regions extending on either side of the plasma membrane. Disulphide bonds, S–S, link the GP Ib α and β chains while GPIX is noncovalently associated with Ib. Flank-LRG centre-flank structures include conserved, 22-amino acid flanking sequences (◀▶) on either side of central, 24-amino acid LRG sequences present as one segment (Ibβ and IX) or as seven tandem repeats (Ibα). Calpain releases the extracellular portion of GPIbα, glycocalicin, with its macroglycopeptide domain marked by five, 9-amino acid tandem repeats and associated *O*-linked carbohydrate (O–CHO). The hinge region between the LRG structure and the *O*-carbohydrate region of Ibα mediates binding to vWF and thrombin. GPIbβ contains a cAMP-dependent phosphorylation (PO_4) site. (Reprinted with permission from Roth 1991.)

a protein of 181 amino acids and M_r 20 000 (Roth et al 1991). GPIbβ has only a single leucine-rich repeat surrounded by flanking sequences. It is also a transmembrane molecule and its intracytoplasmic tail has a phosphorylation site (Fox et al 1987, 1989) and a free sulphydryl group (Kalomiris & Coller 1985). GPIX (M_r 20 000) is composed of 160 amino acids, has one leucine-rich repeat with flanking sequences, and also spans the bilayer (Roth 1991). Both GPIbβ and GPIX are acylated with palmitic acid (Muszbek & Laposata 1989). GPV (M_r 82 000) is probably also a transmembrane protein with one or more leucine-rich repeats (Roth 1991).

GPIb contains several polymorphic areas. Polymorphic variations in the M_r of GPIbα have been detected in the Japanese and American populations and attributed to variations in repeat elements (Moroi et al 1984, Jung et al 1986, Lopez & Ludwig 1991, Ware et al 1991). In addition, the alloantigen Pl^{E} has been localized to GPIbα (Furihata et al 1988), and the alloantigen HPA-2 (Ko) has been identified as a $Thr^{145} \rightarrow$ Met polymorphism (Kuijpers et al 1992). The biogenesis of the GPIb complex has not been fully characterized. The absence of GPIbα, GPIbβ, GPIX, and GPV from the surface of Bernard–Soulier platelets raises the possibility that intracellular interactions between the glycoproteins is required for surface expression, and if these interactions do not occur the proteins are degraded (Roth 1991). Thus, potentially a defect in just one of the proteins could result in the absence of all four. Since GPIbα and GPIbβ are covalently coupled and GPIX is noncovalently associated with GPIb, this hypothesis is plausible and preliminary data from transfection studies lend additional support (Murata et al 1991). It is less clear, however, how GPV is involved in the interactions.

Laboratory features

Platelet morphology and deformability

The large size of Bernard–Soulier platelets on peripheral smear is one of the most striking features of the disorder. Usually more than one third of the platelets have diameters $\geqslant 3.5$ μ, with some platelets as large as 20–30 μ. The platelets in the original description of the disorder were said to resemble lymphocytes because the chromophore was gathered in the centre (Bernard & Soulier 1948). Although one study suggested that Bernard–Soulier platelets are normal in size when in suspension and only appear increased in size because of unusual spreading (Frojmovic et al 1978), the overwhelming evidence indicates that Bernard–Soulier platelets have significantly more volume and protein, as well as increased numbers of organelles (McGill et al 1984, White 1987). There is, however, considerable variability in platelet size between patients as well as in the size of platelets from a single patient. Bernard–Soulier platelets do not have distinctive abnormalities by electron microscopy, although there usually is an increase in vacuolar structures and there may be somewhat of a decrease in the open-canalicular system (White 1987). A freeze-fracture analysis of the platelets of one patient with Bernard–Soulier syndrome identified larger intramembranous particles and an abnormal distribution of particles between the fractured surfaces (Chevalier et al 1979), but a subsequent study failed to identify such abnormalities (White 1987). White et al (1984) studied the membrane rheologic properties of Bernard–Soulier platelets with micropipette elastimetry and found the plasma membranes to be considerably more deformable than normal. This abnormality was proposed to explain the apparently enhanced spreading of Bernard–Soulier platelets.

There is no clear explanation for the abnormal size and deformability of Bernard–Soulier platelets. One possible factor, however, is the recognized interaction between GPIb and actin-binding protein, linking GPIb to the platelet's cytoskeleton (Fox 1985). A deficiency in the interactions might therefore affect platelet development and the deformability of the membrane. Studies of megakaryocytes have identified vacuolar changes and irregularities in the demarcation membranes but no other specific abnormalities (Bernard 1983). Immunofluorescent studies of megakaryocytes in one patient were of note because an antibody to GPIb gave a negative result whereas an antibody to GPIX gave a weakly positive result, consistent with the hypothesis that GPIX may have been synthesized, but then been degraded when it could not complex with GPIb (Hourdille' et al 1990). Studies of this patient's platelets, however, indicated that at least some of the GPIX became associated with the plasma membrane.

Platelet aggregation

The platelets of patients with Bernard–Soulier syndrome fail to aggregate in response to the antibiotic ristocetin (Howard et al 1973) or the snake venom botrocetin (Howard et al 1984, Nishio et al 1990, Eaton et al 1991). Although a similar abnormality is seen in von Willebrand disease, the hallmark of Bernard–Soulier syndrome is that the defect is not corrected by adding back normal plasma or normal von Willebrand factor. Platelet aggregation in response to ADP, adrenalin or collagen is either normal or enhanced (Bithell et al 1972, Evensen et al 1974, Waldenstrom 1991). Thrombin-induced aggregation is usually characterized by a prolonged lag phase and diminished response at low thrombin concentrations (Jamieson & Okumura 1978). Higher thrombin concentrations can overcome the defect (Nurden et al 1986), however, and several patients have been reported to have normal thrombin-induced aggregation, although with unspecified thrombin doses (Evensen et al 1974, George et al 1981). There are serious technical problems in performing platelet aggregation studies in patients with Bernard–Soulier syndrome because the thrombocytopenia and the large size of the platelets make it difficult to obtain platelet-rich plasma at an adequate platelet count. The use of the whole blood aggregometer may circumvent these problems (Ingerman-Wojenski et al 1987, Nichols et al 1989). Similarly, monoclonal antibody studies to assess platelet GPIb can also be performed on whole blood (Montgomery et al 1983, Nichols et al 1989).

Prothrombin consumption and platelet coagulant activity

A paradoxical series of observations have been made concerning the ability of Bernard–Soulier platelets to support coagulation. When prothrombin consumption is used as the end-point of a clotting assay employing Bernard–Soulier platelets, a marked decrease in prothrombin consumption is identified (Caen & Bellucci 1983). This abnormality is also found when normal whole blood is allowed to clot in the presence of a monoclonal antibody to the von Willebrand factor binding site on GPIb (Coller et al 1983b). However, when tests of platelets' ability to enhance coagulation as judged by thrombin generation are employed ('platelet factor 3' assays), Bernard–Soulier platelets behave as if they are more active than normal, a result consistent with their increased size (Walsh et al 1975, Bevers et al 1986). Other abnormalities of Bernard–Soulier platelets include decreased collagen-induced coagulant activity, and reduced platelet-associated factors V, VIII, and XI (as judged by platelet washing) (Walsh et al 1975). It is not easy to reconcile these observations. Abnormal phospholipid content of Bernard–Soulier platelets has also been reported, with an increase in outer surface phosphatidylethanolamine and phosphatidylserine; it is possible that this contributes to the observed increase in platelet factor 3 activity (Perret et al 1983). Since von Willebrand factor circulates with factor VIII, it is possible that a defect in GPIb might translate into defective factor VIII binding to platelets, but attempts to demonstrate a functional contribution of factor VIII/von Willebrand factor binding to GPIb during coagulation have not been successful (Soberano et al 1986). Finally, it might be proposed that the decreased binding of thrombin to Bernard–Soulier platelets (see below) may facilitate thrombin-related end points by eliminating a competing binding site.

Platelet-thrombin interactions

In contrast to their brisk response to ADP, adrenalin, and collagen, Bernard–Soulier platelets aggregate more slowly than normal in the presence of low concentrations of thrombin; this defect can be completely overcome, however, by increasing the thrombin concentration (Jamieson & Okumura 1978, Nurden et al 1986, Jandrot-Perrus et al 1990). Several different hypotheses have been proposed to explain these observations. GPV is cleaved by thrombin into an M_r 69 000 fragment and early studies suggested that this cleavage may be responsible for thrombin activation of platelets (Phillips & Agin 1977b, Berndt & Phillips 1981). Since Bernard–Soulier platelets are deficient in GPV, this would furnish a logical explanation for the observed abnormality in thrombin-induced aggregation. More detailed studies, however, demonstrated that platelet activation does not correlate with GPV cleavage and thus a role for GPV in signal transduction is problematic (McGowan et al 1983, White & Krupp 1985, Bienz et al 1986). Bernard–Soulier platelets were found to have fewer thrombin binding sites than normal; this is due to the GPIb deficiency since GPIb can bind thrombin (Hagen et al 1981, Larsen & Simons 1981, Harmon & Jamieson 1986, Takamatsu et al 1986). GPIb appears to be responsible for high affinity thrombin binding to platelets, but since there are many more GPIb sites ($\approx$25 000) than high affinity thrombin-binding sites ($\approx$50), perhaps only a subpopulation of GPIb sites are involved (Ruggeri 1991). Current evidence indicates that von Willebrand factor and thrombin bind to different sites on GPIb as judged by the ability of a monoclonal antibody to block ristocetin-induced platelet agglutination without inhibiting thrombin-induced aggregation (Coller et al 1983b). Moreover, one patient with a variant form of Bernard–Soulier syndrome with an abnormal GPIb molecule had no von Willebrand factor binding but had normal high affinity thrombin binding (de Marco 1991, Ruggeri et al 1991). The recent identification of a functional thrombin receptor as a seven transmembrane domain protein unrelated to GPIb with a thrombin cleavage site may help to resolve some of the complexity (Vu et al 1991). One hypothesis that appears to be consistent with the current data is that binding to GPIb may bring thrombin in proximity to this other receptor and thus facilitate cleavage.

Platelet survival

Several early studies indicated that autologous platelet survival in Bernard–Soulier syndrome is very short whereas compatible homologous platelets survive much longer (Grottum & Solum 1969). This furnished a likely explanation for the thrombocytopenia found in the disorder. The shortened platelet survival was proposed to be a result of the reduced platelet sialic acid (Grottum & Solum 1969) since in studies where sialic acid is enzymatically removed from the platelet surface, platelet survival decreases dramatically (Greenberg et al 1979). A more recent study of four patients with Bernard–Soulier syndrome, three of whom had undergone splenectomy, using ^{111}I-labelled oxine to label the platelets, found decreased platelet recovery but nearly normal or normal platelet survival in the splenectomized patients (Heyns et al 1985). The unsplenectomized patient also had a decrease in recovery and had only about a 40% decrease in platelet survival. Platelet survival studies in Bernard–Soulier patients are technically difficult to perform because of the low counts and large platelets. Moreover, thrombocytopenia itself is a cause for shortened platelet survival. Thus, it is unclear how common a reduced platelet survival is and whether decreased survival is sufficient to explain the thrombocytopenia. It is also appropriate to note that from the standpoint of platelet clearance, there may be a substantial difference between removing sialic acid by neuraminidase treatment as opposed to having reduced sialic acid due to a membrane glycoprotein deficiency; in the first case a penultimate galactose residue will be exposed and may specifically enhance removal, whereas in the latter case no galactose will be exposed.

Ex vivo interaction with subendothelial surfaces and shear-induced platelet aggregation

Platelets from patients with Bernard–Soulier syndrome and normal platelets treated with monoclonal antibodies to GPIb fail to adhere normally to subendothelial surfaces, especially when tested at shear rates greater than 650 s^{-1} (Weiss et al 1974, 1978, 1986, Caen et al 1976,

Baumgartner et al 1976, Sakariassen et al 1986). The shear-dependence of the defect is remarkable and is also found in von Willebrand disease, presumably because the interaction is between GPIb and von Willebrand factor (Weiss et al 1978). It is not yet clear, however, whether the shear effect operates on platelet GPIb, plasma von Willebrand factor, or von Willebrand factor in the subendothelium (Roth 1991). In addition, the role of platelet von Willebrand factor remains unclear. It appears, however, as if each of the separate pools of von Willebrand factor makes a contribution to optimal adhesion (Coller 1985). Roth (1991) has reviewed the two likely mechanisms:

1. Platelet GPIb binding of von Willebrand factor, followed by the binding of this platelet-bound von Willebrand factor to the extracellular matrix
2. binding of von Willebrand factor to the extracellular matrix followed by the binding of platelet GPIb to the bound von Willebrand factor.

High shear forces can also make normal platelets aggregate directly and this process appears to be mediated by the initial binding of von Willebrand factor to GPIb, followed by platelet activation (mediated by an increase in cytosolic calcium), activation of GPIIb/IIIa receptors, binding of fibrinogen to GPIIb/IIIa, and platelet aggregation. Bernard–Soulier platelets are not aggregated by these high shear rates, reflecting the failure to bind von Willebrand factor to their surface (Peterson et al 1987, Ikeda et al 1991).

Molecular basis of Bernard–Soulier syndrome

A variety of biochemical and immunological techniques have been applied to evaluating the GPIb complex associated with Bernard–Soulier syndrome platelets. These include radiolabelling of surface glycoproteins followed by polyacrylamide gel electrophoresis, crossed-immunoelectrophoresis, direct monoclonal antibody binding studies, whole platelet ELISA studies, and immunoblotting studies using polyclonal and monoclonal antibodies against the different components. A description of these techniques and their limitations is included in the section on Glanzmann thrombasthenia (p. 733).

Given the size and multiplicity of the genes involved in forming the GPIb, GPIX and GPV proteins, a variety of different defects would be expected to be responsible for Bernard–Soulier syndrome. This is supported by the variable biochemical results in different patients, with some completely deficient in GPIb and others having considerable amounts of GPIb, up to 50% of normal (Clemetson et al 1982, Coller et al 1983b, Nurden et al 1983, De Marco et al 1986, Drouin et al 1988, Stevens et al 1988, Poulsen & Taaning 1990). There is controversy as to whether there is a concordance or discordance in glycoprotein reduction among GPIbα, GPIbβ, GPIX, and GPV in Bernard–Soulier patients, with subtle technical factors still to be standardized (Nurden et al 1989).

The Bolzano variant of Bernard–Soulier syndrome has been well characterized and permits some important insights. The patient was originally described as having classical Bernard–Soulier syndrome based on a characteristic history, platelet function abnormalities, and the complete failure of a monoclonal antibody to GPIb (AP-1) to bind to the patient's platelets (de Marco et al 1986). When later studied with a monoclonal antibody to another site on GPIb, however, the patient's platelets were seen to have about 50% of the normal amount of GPIb (de Marco et al 1990). Immunoblot studies revealed an abnormal prominence of an M_r 105 000 GPIb-related band in addition to the normal GPIb 145 000 band. The patient's platelets failed to bind ^{125}I-labelled-von Willebrand factor in the presence of ristocetin, but bound ^{125}I-α-thrombin normally, indicating a functional difference in the von Willebrand factor and thrombin binding regions. Preliminary molecular biological studies indicate that the patient is homozygous for an $Ala^{156} \rightarrow Val$ substitution in the leucine-rich repeat area of GPIbα (Ware et al 1991). A mammalian cell expression system confirmed that the $Ala^{156} \rightarrow Val$ change was sufficient to account for the changes in monoclonal antibody binding and the ability to bind von Willebrand factor.

Another Bernard–Soulier variant is a 36-year-old patient with the classic findings of Bernard–Soulier syndrome who was found to have no normal GPIbα as judged by monoclonal antibody binding and immunoblot studies; his platelets, however, did contain an M_r 40 000 protein that reacted with an antibody to GPIbα (Ware et al 1990). GPIX could not be detected at all. The patient's mother and two children had both normal GPIbα and the abnormal GPIbα in their platelets; all three were clinically normal but had reduced von Willebrand factor binding. Molecular biological studies indicated the presence of one allele with a G→A transition leading to a $Trp^{343} \rightarrow$nonsense codon and thus a GPIbα of only 342 amino acids instead of 610 amino acids. The size of the abnormal GPIbα observed in the immunoblot studies was consistent with this finding. The presumed abnormality in the other allele, which allowed full expression of only the abnormal allele, was not identified.

Finch et al (1990) reported on a family with two siblings affected by Bernard–Soulier syndrome. Immunoblot analysis revealed trace amounts of GPIbα and GPIX, but no GPV. Genetic analysis was consistent with autosomal recessive inheritance. Restriction fragment length polymorphism studies indicated that the inheritance of the disease was not linked to the inheritance of the GPIbα gene, making it likely that the defect was in one of the other proteins in the GPIb, GPIX, GPV group, or a protein important in their proper maturation.

Miller et al (1992) described three members of a family with a variant of Bernard–Soulier syndrome characterized by autosomal dominant transmission, moderate clinical bleeding, reduced, but not absent, ristocetin-induced aggregation, variably prolonged bleeding time, moderate thrombocytopenia, giant platelets, and reduced platelet affinity for binding von Willebrand factor at low ristocetin concentrations. The patient's platelets had GPIb and GPIX, but a portion of the GPIb appeared to be unusually susceptible to proteolytic digestion. The only identifiable genetic abnormality was a heterozygous base substitution at nucleotide 259 (C→T), leading to a Leu^{57}→Phe change. Since the alteration is in one of the leucine-rich repeats of GPIbα that may be important in protein–protein interactions, the authors postulate that it induces changes in the structure of GPIb leading to enhanced proteolysis and inefficient platelet agglutination. The results in this family are particularly intriguing because despite the presence of considerable amounts of GPIb and the substantial ability of platelets to bind von Willebrand factor, both thrombocytopenia and giant platelets were observed.

Summary and conclusions

Studies of patients with Bernard–Soulier syndrome have provided important information on platelet function mediated by GPIb, GPIX, and/or GPV. The defect in GPIb–von Willebrand factor interactions has served as a useful model for investigating the primary events in platelet interactions with subendothelial surfaces. It is clear, however, that our insight into this disorder is still primitive since we do not understand the basis for the morphological changes, thrombocytopenia, or inconsistent findings in platelet coagulant activity. Even the well-characterized abnormality in thrombin responsiveness remains clouded in mystery. In addition, the biogenesis of the complex is still poorly understood, especially the enigmatic role of GPV. The identification of the leucine-rich regions in each of the proteins involved is fascinating, but it is not clear where this clue will lead. The role of shear and its primary site of action also has escaped definitive analysis. The most promising opportunities for the immediate future lie in the molecular genetic analysis of affected patients and their glycoprotein expression systems since these studies will predictably lead to a much firmer knowledge of the structure–function relationships and the biogenesis of the membrane complex.

GPIb ABNORMALITIES: PLATELET-TYPE (PSEUDO-) VON WILLEBRAND DISEASE

Several different families have been reported whose platelets bind von Willebrand factor more avidly than normal platelets at low doses of ristocetin, leading to enhanced ristocetin-induced platelet aggregation (Takahashi 1980, Gralnick et al 1982, Miller & Castella 1982, Weiss et al 1982). Botrocetin-induced aggregation has also been reported to be enhanced in the patients in which it was studied (Miller & Castella 1982, Takahashi et al 1984, 1985). The plasma of these patients is deficient in the high molecular weight von Willebrand factor multimers, presumably because the patients' platelets are continually binding these multimers. Thrombocytopenia and somewhat enlarged platelets have been observed in some, but not all, cases. The patients' bleeding disorder is generally mild to moderate in severity and the bleeding time is usually, but not always, prolonged.

It is important to distinguish this syndrome from type IIb von Willebrand disease because both disorders can produce similar clinical syndromes, with enhanced ristocetin-induced platelet aggregation and plasma von Willebrand factor lacking the high molecular weight multimers. Several measurements can be helpful in the differential diagnosis (Gralnick 1982, Miller et al 1983, Weiss et al 1982):

1. Normal cryoprecipitate or purified von Willebrand factor aggregates platelets from some, but perhaps not all, patients with platelet-type von Willebrand disease but not platelets from patients with type IIb von Willebrand disease.
2. Isolated platelets from patients with platelet-type von Willebrand disease will bind normal von Willebrand factor at lower concentrations of ristocetin than will normal platelets or platelets from patients with type IIb von Willebrand disease.
3. The von Willebrand factor in the plasma of patients with type IIb von Willebrand disease will bind to normal platelets at lower than normal concentrations of ristocetin, whereas the von Willebrand factor in the plasma of patients with platelet-type von Willebrand disease will only bind at higher than normal ristocetin concentrations (White & Montgomery 1991).

Abnormalities in GPIb are thought to be responsible for the platelet-function defects in platelet-type von Willebrand disease. Abnormal electrophoretic mobility of GPIb was identified in two families with no normal GPIb and two abnormal bands, one lower than normal in M_r and the other higher than normal in M_r (Takahashi et al 1984). Molecular biological studies have identified two different heterozygous point mutations in the GPIbα DNA in two different families (Gly^{233}→Val and Met^{239}→Val) (Miller et al 1991, Russel and Roth 1991); of note, both mutations are in the GPIbα region implicated in binding von Willebrand factor (Ruggeri 1991).

Therapy of patients with platelet-type von Willebrand disease is complicated by the potential for both desmopressin and cryoprecipitate to induce thrombocytopenia, presumably as a result of excessive binding of von Willebrand factor to platelets leading to rapid platelet clearance (Miller et al 1983, Takahashi et al 1985). The in vitro response to cryoprecipitate may help to identify the patients at highest risk because one patient whose platelets failed to respond to cryoprecipitate in vitro did not become thrombocytopenic when treated with cryoprecipitate in vivo (Krizek et al 1982). For those at greatest risk, low doses of cryoprecipitate may be able to support haemostasis without inducing thrombocytopenia (Miller 1984, Takahashi 1984, 1985).

GLYCOPROTEIN Ia/IIa ABNORMALITIES

A female patient with a history of easy bruising following minor trauma beginning in her teenage years was reported by Nieuwenhuis et al in 1985 and 1986. The patient also suffered from menorrhagia (controlled with oral contraceptives and tranexamic acid) and a massive post-traumatic leg haematoma. The patient did not have epistaxis, gingival bleeding or excessive haemorrhage after either a tonsillectomy or appendectomy. Tooth extractions and a caesarean section were performed with cryoprecipitate prophylaxis, without incident. The patient's mother also had easy bruising and her maternal grandfather had episodes of severe epistaxis.

Laboratory analysis revealed a prolonged bleeding (>30 min) time, normal platelet count, and normal platelet aggregation in response to ADP, ionophore A23187, adrenalin, arachidonic acid, platelet-aggregating factor, thrombin, and ristocetin. In contrast, the patient's platelets failed to aggregate or undergo shape change in response to a variety of collagens even at very high doses. The patients' platelets also failed to undergo phospholipid metabolism in response to collagen, to adhere to collagen in the presence of EDTA in a static system, or to adhere to collagen in flow chamber studies using citrated blood. A similar adhesion abnormality was found using an arterial subendothelial surface, and spreading of adherent platelets was also impaired. Much of the residual adhesion at high shear rates, but not low shear rates, could be eliminated by an antibody to von Willebrand factor.

Analysis of radiolabelled platelet glycoproteins demonstrated a 75–85% reduction in GPIa (Nieuwenhuis et al 1985). Although not discussed by the authors, the published radioautographs also suggested a less severe deficiency in GPIIa as well. Preliminary studies with a monoclonal antibody to GPIa confirmed the abnormality (Beer et al. 1987). That the GPIIa defect is less severe than the GPIa defect is expected because GPIIa can also complex with GPIc and GPIc*, forming the VLA-5 and VLA-6 receptors (Hemler et al 1988, Piotrowicz et al 1988, Sonnenberg et al 1988). Studies from several laboratories have identified GPIa/IIa as being able to mediate platelet adhesion to collagen in the presence of magnesium (Santoro 1986, Kunicki et al 1988, Santoro et al 1988, Coller et al 1989) and so this patient's abnormality appears to support a functional role for this receptor. It is possible, however, that the GPIa/IIa defect is not the only abnormality this patient has because GPIa/IIa does not mediate platelet–collagen interactions in vitro in the presence of EDTA (Santoro 1986, Coller et al 1989) and yet the patient's platelets displayed an abnormality in collagen adhesion in the presence of EDTA. Moreover, the inhibition of collagen-induced platelet aggregation in platelet-rich plasma produced by a monoclonal antibody to GPIa/IIa is considerably less than the defect observed with the patient's platelets (Coller et al 1989).

Another patient with GPIa deficiency has been described (Kehrel et al 1988). She had a life-long bleeding tendency characterized by spontaneous petechial bleeding, menorrhagia, and postoperative haemorrhage. Laboratory data included a prolonged bleeding time and normal platelet aggregation in response to ADP, ionophore A23187, adrenalin, thrombin, arachidonic acid, and ristocetin. Platelet aggregation to collagen was reduced but not absent, and the defect could be partially overcome by increasing the collagen concentration. Unlike the first patient, this patient's platelets adhered normally to collagen in the presence of EDTA. Platelet protein analysis identified a profound abnormality in GPIa and virtually no intact thrombospondin; thrombospondin fragments were, however, detectable. The addition of purified thrombospondin to the patient's platelet-rich plasma normalized collagen-induced aggregation. At the time of menopause, the patient's haemorrhagic symptoms and platelet abnormalities mysteriously disappeared.

GPIV ABNORMALITIES

Asymptomatic individuals have been found to lack GPIV (CD36), an M_r 88 000 protein that has been implicated in mediating platelet interactions with collagen (Tandon et al 1989) and thrombospondin (Asch et al 1987), and the interactions of a variety of cells with *Plasmodium falciparum*-infected erythrocytes (Oquendo et al 1989). GPIV has also been implicated in mediating platelet–monocyte and monocyte–macrophage interactions (Silverstein et al 1989). Patients lacking GPIV can make antibodies against GPIV when exposed to platelet GPIV through pregnancy or platelet transfusions and this can lead to platelet refractoriness and neonatal isoimmune thrombocytopenia. GPIV deficiency was first identified in a patient suffering from platelet refractoriness, which is usually due to alloantigens, and so it was originally thought that the patient had an antigenic protein variant (Nak^{a-}) (Ikeda et al 1989); subsequent studies, however, indicated that the individuals lacked all immunodetectable GPIV (Yamamoto et al 1990). The incidence of GPIV deficiency varies significantly among different groups, being approximately 0.3% in the population of the United States, but 3%–11% in the Japanese population.

Platelets lacking GPIV show only a minimal defect in the rate of adhesion to collagen in the presence of calcium chelators, and virtually no defect in collagen adhesion in the presence of divalent cations (Tandon et al 1991). They have a severe abnormality, however, in interacting with malaria-infected erythrocytes. No abnormality in thrombospondin binding can be detected.

GLYCOPROTEIN VI ABNORMALITIES

A female patient with a life-long history of easy bruisability, intermittent menorrhagia and nosebleeds was reported by Moroi et al (1989) to have a slightly prolonged bleeding time and an isolated defect in collagen-induced platelet aggregation. The patient's platelets also failed to adhere to collagen fibrils in the presence of EDTA regardless of the source or type of collagen. Studies of radiolabelled platelets demonstrated a marked deficiency of GPVI, a M_r 62 000 glycoprotein, in the patient and partial deficiencies in each of her parents. The parents, however, denied consanguinity. Additional support for the role of GPVI in platelet adhesion to collagen came from studies of another patient who had idiopathic thrombocytopenic purpura and a defect in collagen-induced aggregation (Sugiyama et al 1987). The antibody from this patient reacted with a M_r 62 000 glycoprotein on normal platelets, but it failed to react with the platelets from the patient with the GPVI deficiency.

A second patient with a deficiency in GPVI was reported by Ryo et al (1992). This 26-year-old man had a very mild history of mucocutaneous bleeding. There was no parental consanguinity. He had mild thrombocytopenia, a prolonged bleeding time, decreased platelet adhesion to collagen in the presence of EDTA, and absent collagen-induced platelet aggregation. Collagen did, however, induce shape change, suggesting some interaction between platelets and collagen. Immunoblot studies identified the deficiency in GPVI.

CD43 ABNORMALITIES: WISKOTT–ALDRICH SYNDROME

Small platelets, thrombocytopenia, recurrent infections and eczema are the major characteristics of the X chromosome-linked Wiskott–Aldrich syndrome (Omerod 1985). A multiplicity of immunological abnormalities, including defects in T lymphocyte function, result in abnormal immunoglobulin levels, unresponsiveness to polysaccharide antigens, and impaired cellular immunity. The immunodeficiency is thought to be responsible for the failure of immune surveillance, which results in a dramatic increase in lymphoreticular malignancies, and the recurrent infections. Death commonly occurs before the teenage years as a result of haemorrhage, infection, or malignancy.

Platelets are remarkably small in this disorder and splenectomy consistently results in an increase in platelet size, although not necessarily to normal (Murphy et al 1972, Lum et al 1980). This suggests that the platelets become smaller after they leave the bone marrow as a result of alterations that occur in the spleen. Thrombocytopenia is variable, but can be severe. Shortened platelet survival accounts for the thrombocytopenia in most cases (Grottum et al 1969, Baldini 1972, Murphy et al 1972) and it, too, can be alleviated to some extent by splenectomy (Lum et al 1980). The defect leading to the shortened survival is intrinsic to the platelet since the survival of homologous platelets is normal. In one study, however, platelet survival in four patients was found to be only slightly decreased, and the thrombocytopenia was ascribed to ineffective thrombopoiesis (Ochs et al 1980). Although splenectomy carries with it an increased risk of sepsis, prophylactic antibiotics and pneumococcal and perhaps meningococcal vaccines, can reduce the risk (Lum et al 1980, Nathan 1980).

Although a variety of ultrastructural abnormalities have been described in Wiskott–Aldrich syndrome, the most recent studies have indicated essentially normal platelet morphology (White 1987). Platelet function abnormalities have been reported in most patients, with abnormalities in the storage pool of adenine nucleotides most common (Grottum et al 1969, Baldini 1972, Stormorken et al 1991). Several abnormalities in energy metabolism have also been described (Baldini 1972, Verhoeven et al 1989). In general, bleeding times are longer than predicted on the basis of the thrombocytopenia, but perhaps not when the platelet mass is considered.

In 1981, Parkman et al reported that Wiskott–Aldrich syndrome is associated with abnormalities in lymphocyte sialophorin (CD43, gp115, leukosialin), a membrane glycoprotein present in one form (M_r 115 000) on T lymphocytes, thymocytes, B cells, and monocytes, and in another form (M_r 135 000) on neutrophils and platelets (Remold-O'Donnell et al 1987, Shelley et al 1989, Remold-O'Donnell & Rosen 1990). Most recently, sialophorin was found to bind to ICAM-1, a ligand implicated in immunofunction (Rosenstein et al 1991); sialophorin also enhances T cell activation (Park et al 1991). The defect in sialophorin is unlikely to be the primary abnormality since the gene for sialophorin is on chromosome 16 whereas Wiskott–Aldrich syndrome is inherited as an X-linked trait. Parkman et al (1981) also identified deficiencies in platelet GPIb, another protein rich in *O*-linked carbohydrate, and GPIa in two patients. Subsequently, Higgins et al (1991) found aberrant *O*-linked oligosaccharide biosynthesis in lymphocytes and platelets from Wiskott–Aldrich syndrome patients. Pidard et al (1988), however, failed to identify either a GPIb or GPIa defect in two patients with Wiskott–Aldrich syndrome but a slight reduction in these two glycoproteins was identified in the platelets of a third patient. Stormorken et al (1991) studied a patient with a variant of Wiskott-Aldrich syndrome and also found normal GPIb.

Bone marrow transplantation can cure this disorder and thus it should be seriously considered (Nathan 1980). Splenectomy can reduce the risk of haemorrhage by increasing the platelet count and platelet volume, and may even improve platelet function.

There have been several reports of X-linked thrombocytopenia with varying manifestations of Wiskott–Aldrich syndrome (Stormorken et al 1991). In addition, although female carriers of Wiskott–Aldrich syndrome are generally asymptomatic and without platelet abnormalities, exceptions have been reported (Tornai et al 1989). These intermediately-affected individuals provide important insights into the pathophysiology, suggesting that multiple dissociable abnormalities may be responsible for the full syndrome.

OTHER PLATELET ABNORMALITIES

ABNORMALITIES OF PLATELET GRANULES

The platelet contains at least four different granules: dense bodies or δ granules, α granules, peroxisomes, and lysosomes (White 1987). A heterogeneous group of disorders affecting dense bodies and α granules have been described. Patients whose platelets only lack dense bodies are classified as having δ-storage pool deficiency (Weiss 1987, Nieuwenhuis et al 1987, Rao 1990). Included in this category are patients who have the defect as an isolated platelet abnormality and patients who have the platelet defect as part of an inherited disorder that also affects other tissues, including Hermansky–Pudlak syndrome (tyrosinase-positive oculocutaneous albinism, excessive accumulation of ceroid-like material in reticuloendothelial cells in bone marrow and other tissues, and a haemorrhagic diathesis), the Chediak–Higashi syndrome (partial oculocutaneous albinism, giant lysosomal granules, and frequent pyogenic infections) (Bell et al 1976, Rendu et al 1983, Apitz-Castro et al 1985, Weiss 1987, White 1987), and the Wiskott–Aldrich syndrome (Grottum et al 1969, Kuramoto et al 1970). Although reports of δ-storage pool deficiency in association with Ehlers–Danlos syndrome (Onel et al 1973), osteogenesis imperfecta (Hathaway et al 1972), and thrombocytopenia with absent radii (Day & Holmsen 1972) have appeared, the consistency of the relationship between these disorders and δ-storage pool deficiency remains unclear.

A heterogeneous group of patients have deficiencies affecting both the dense bodies and α granules and these patients are classified as having α,δ-storage pool disease (Weiss et al 1979, Rao 1986, Weiss 1987, White 1987). Finally, a group of patients have their defect confined to the α granules and these patients are classified as having the grey platelet syndrome (based on the lack of granule staining on peripheral smear) or α-storage pool disease (White 1987).

Granule biochemistry

Dense bodies or δ granules get their name from their appearance in electron micrographs as a result of their calcium content (White 1987). They are also rich in serotonin, which platelets take up from plasma by a transporter mechanism and then sequester in dense bodies with the aid of a proton pump in the dense granule membrane that creates a more acidic environment within the dense body (Holmsen 1990a). Approximately two thirds of the platelet's adenine nucleotides are also sequestered at high concentrations in dense bodies and the ratio of ATP/ADP within these granules is 2/3. This 'storage pool' of adenine nucleotides is not in rapid equilibrium with the cytosolic 'metabolic pool' of adenine nucleotides and the latter is characterized by a much higher ratio of ATP/ADP (8–10/1). Pyrophosphate and orthophosphate are present in dense bodies, as is adrenalin.

Platelet α granules contain a variety of proteins, some of which are synthesized by megakaryocytes while others are taken up from the surrounding plasma (Niewiarowski & Holt 1987, Holmsen 1990a). Several platelet-specific proteins are present in α granules, including platelet factor 4 (PF-4) and β-thromboglobulin. A group of cationic proteins with diverse functions have also been identified. Fibrinogen appears to be taken up into α granules from plasma by a mechanism that requires GPIIb/IIIa (Coller et al 1991c). Thrombospondin and von Willebrand factor are probably derived from megakaryocyte synthesis. Albumin and immunoglobulin G, in contrast, appear to be nonspecifically taken up into platelet α granules (George 1991). Many other proteins have been found in platelets in small amounts, but the mechanisms leading to their presence in α granules is uncertain.

δ-Storage pool deficiency

The clinical manifestations of this group of disorders are usually moderate, with variable mucocutaneous haemorrhage involving easy bruising and epistaxis, as well as bleeding after delivery, tooth extractions, and surgical procedures. Haemorrhage is rarely severe, except when patients are also taking aspirin or other antiplatelet agents (Weiss 1987, Nieuwenhuis 1987). Lethal haemorrhage has, however, been reported in the Hermansky–Pudlak syndrome (Hardisty et al 1972, Witkop 1974), especially in the perinatal and peripartum periods. In fact, in one series, haemorrhage accounted for 16% of the deaths in Hermansky–Pudlak syndrome, second only to fibrotic lung disease as a cause of death (White 1987). The inheritance of primary storage pool disease is often unclear and it is likely that a variety of different genetic abnormalities lead to the development of this disorder (Weiss 1987). There have, however, been families in which an autosomal dominant mechanism seemed responsible. When δ-storage pool deficiency is associated with another disorder, the mode of inheritance of the other disorder is the deciding factor.

Laboratory evaluation with routine platelet-function studies produces quite variable results from patient to patient, and even in the same patient over time, making it difficult to provide precise criteria (Weiss 1969, Holmsen & Weiss 1970, 1972, White et al 1971, Pareti et al 1974, Nieuwenhuis 1987, White 1987). Thus, although the bleeding time is usually somewhat prolonged, and a correlation between granule ADP content and bleeding time has been reported (Akkerman et al 1988), some patients have normal bleeding times. Since release of dense body contents, and perhaps α granule contents, are mechanisms for enhancing platelet aggregation, granule deficiencies result in abnormal aggregation patterns. The primary wave of platelet aggregation induced by ADP or adrenalin is usually normal; the abnormalities in the second wave are variable, ranging from an absent or markedly decreased response, to only a modest reduction in the response. The response to collagen-induced aggregation depends on the dose of collagen used, with low doses accentuating the abnormalities and high doses obscuring them. A useful guide recommended by Weiss (1987) to establish the correct collagen dose is to assess whether normal platelets treated with aspirin aggregate less well than untreated platelets. High doses of thrombin cause maximal release of δ granule contents even when patients have ingested aspirin or have defects in the release reaction. Therefore, one simple method to exclude δ-storage pool disease is to assess the release of ATP from platelets in response to high doses of thrombin using the bioluminescent technique incorporated into some aggregometers. A normal release excludes δ-storage pool disease but the luciferin-luciferase reagent is highly labile so spurious results can occur if care is not taken to control this variable (Soslau & Parker 1992).

Special biochemical studies have more precisely defined the platelet abnormalities in δ granule deficiency. The loss of the storage pool of adenine nucleotides results in a decrease in total platelet content of adenine nucleotides and shifts the ATP/ADP ratio to a value more closely reflecting that in the metabolic pool (8–10/1) than that in the normal storage pool (2/3) (Weiss et al 1972, 1974, 1979, Pareti et al 1974, Akkerman et al 1983, Weiss 1987, Holmsen 1990b). Platelet serotonin content is variably decreased, with some of the lowest levels recorded in patients with Hermansky–Pudlak syndrome. Kinetic studies indicate that the platelets in δ-storage pool disease have a normal initial rate of serotonin uptake from plasma, but saturation is rapidly achieved and the serotonin fails to get incorporated into δ granules; instead, it is rapidly metabolized to 5-hydroxyindoleacetic acid (Weiss et al 1974). Calcium and pyrophosphate are also deficient in the patient's platelets (Lages et al 1975). Variable abnormalities in platelet secretion and the arachidonic acid pathway have been identified, but it is not clear whether these are secondary to the aggregation abnormalities (Willis & Weiss 1973, Weiss et al 1974, Holmsen et al 1975, Weiss & Lages 1981). Recently the platelets from a patient with Hermansky–Pudlak syndrome were found to be deficient in a dense granule protein of M_r 40 000, having only 15% of the normal level (Gervard et al 1991). This protein appears to share some of the properties of synaptophysin, a synaptic vesicle protein, but with some significant differences.

Morphological studies show the platelets to be normal except for the decrease or absence of dense bodies, with patients with Hermansky–Pudlak syndrome again demonstrating the most profound deficiencies (White 1987). The defects can be detected by electron microscopy of whole mounts and thin sections of platelets fixed in the presence of calcium. Although δ granules can be identified in unstained specimens, staining with uranaffin, which specifically stains amine-containing organelles, or osmium may accentuate the abnormalities. The decrease or absence of dense bodies can also be detected using mepacrine, a fluorescent amine taken up by δ granules (Lorez et al 1979).

The management and therapy of patients with δ-storage pool disease is similar to that for Glanzmann thrombasthenia, although the need for platelet transfusions is much less common. Avoidance of aspirin and other antiplatelet agents is most important. Suppression of menses is of benefit in patients with menorrhagia. Desmopressin has been reported to normalize the bleeding time in a number of patients with storage pool disease (Nieuwenhuis & Sixma 1988, Wijermans & van Dorp 1989), but it has not been uniformly successful (Kobrinsky et al 1984, Mannucci et al 1986, Van Dorp 1990). Gerritsen et al (1978) made the interesting observation that cryoprecipitate could correct the bleeding time abnormality in patients with δ-storage pool disease. Although a mechanism involving an increase in von Willebrand factor has some plausibility, it is perhaps more likely that platelet fragments and microparticles contained in cryoprecipitate are responsible for the correction (Coller et al 1975, George et al 1986).

A reported association between δ-storage pool disease and primary pulmonary hypertension (Herve et al 1990) is of particular interest, since the authors speculate that the elevated levels of plasma serotonin and its metabolites may have been responsible for the pulmonary vascular abnormalities. Moreover, fibrotic lung disease is also associated with the Hermansky–Pudlak syndrome (White 1987).

α,δ-Storage pool deficiency

This heterogeneous group of disorders includes patients with variable deficiencies in both dense bodies and α granules; the decrease in δ granule contents is usually severe, whereas the deficiency in α granule contents ranges from mild to severe (Weiss et al 1979b, Weiss 1987). Clinically, these patients resemble the patients with δ-storage pool disease. Laboratory evaluation of platelet function also yields results similar to those in δ-storage pool disease with variable abnormalities in bleeding time and platelet aggregation.

Biochemical analysis reflects the defect in δ bodies, with low levels of serotonin and adenine nucleotides, and the characteristic increase in the ATP/ADP ratio (Weiss et al 1979b, Weiss 1987). In addition, the contents of α granules are also variably decreased. Analysis of the α granule membrane protein GMP-140 (P-selectin) in three patients from one family with partial α,δ granule deficiency and one patient with severe α,δ granule deficiency demonstrated normal platelet GMP-140 content in the three family members, but a marked reduction in GMP-140 in the patient with the severe disorder (Lages et al 1991).

Therapy and management of patients with α,δ-storage pool disease is essentially the same as for patients with δ-storage pool disease. Data on the effectiveness of desmopressin are meagre.

Grey platelet syndrome (α-storage pool deficiency)

In 1971 Raccuglia reported on an 11-year-old female with a life-long bleeding tendency, a long bleeding time, variable thrombocytopenia, and large agranular platelets that appeared grey on peripheral smear. A series of similar patients appeared subsequently, each of whom had an absence or marked deficiency of α granule proteins and morphologically identifiable α granules (Gootenberg et al 1976, Gerrard et al 1980, Levy-Toledano 1981, Berrebi et al 1981, Nurden et al 1982, Berndt et al 1983a, Coller et al 1983a, Kohler et al 1985, Srivastava et al 1987, Wills 1989, Facon et al 1990). One patient with the grey platelet syndrome also had the congenital abnormalities of Goldenhar's syndrome (Gerrard et al 1980). 24 patients from a single Japanese family have also been reported to have the grey platelet syndrome (Mori et al 1984), but the abnormalities in these patients appear to differ from the remainder of the group in that the PF-4 levels were only reduced by 50%, the platelets were not uniformly agranular, and the plasma von Willebrand antigen and ristocetin cofactor activities were significantly reduced.

Morphological analysis of grey platelets demonstrates their large size, increase in vacuolar structures, and absence of α granules (White 1987). Variable abnormalities of the dense tubular system and the open canalicular system have been described. Immunohistochemical studies indicate that the vacuolar structures are composed of α granule membranes since they react with antibodies to the α granule membrane protein GMP-140 (P-selectin) (Rosa et al 1987) and GPIIb/IIIa (Cramer et al 1990). The GMP-140 molecules can redistribute to the plasma membrane surface when platelets are stimulated with thrombin in a manner that is indistinguishable from normal. Studies using antibodies to the α granule proteins, fibrinogen, and von Willebrand factor identified small amounts of these proteins in partially filled vacuoles and in small, abortive α granules in grey platelets, further supporting the notion that the granules are present but not appropriately filled with α granule proteins (Cramer et al 1985). There is no evidence for the failure to synthesize the proteins since plasma levels of the platelet-specific proteins β-thromboglobulin and PF-4 are normal or increased (Gerrard et al 1980). Immunoelectron microscopy of megakaryocytes from patients also identified von Willebrand factor in small granules (Cramer et al 1985). Since studies in normal megakaryocytes found a progression of von Willebrand factor from the Golgi to the α granules with megakaryocyte maturation, it was concluded that the von Willebrand factor is synthesized but then not properly retained in α granules. Similar observations with cultured megakaryocytes using antibodies to PF-4 and platelet-derived growth factor (PDGF) showed localized staining early in megakaryocyte development that failed to progress normally to granular staining in later megakaryocytes (Caen et al 1987).

Collectively, the above studies have been interpreted as demonstrating that the defect in the grey platelet syndrome lies in targeting the synthesized proteins to the α granules, with the secondary phenomenon of leakage of these proteins into the surrounding milieu. Since several patients with the grey platelet syndrome have had reticulin fibrosis of their bone marrow (Berndt et al 1983a, Coller et al 1983a, Caen et al 1987), it has been postulated that leakage of platelet α granule contents into the bone marrow is responsible for this phenomenon (Caen et al 1987). PDGF has been implicated because it has the capacity to induce cells to grow and synthesize collagen. Alternatively or additionally, platelet α granules are thought to have an inhibitor of collagenase that may also contribute to the finding. Unlike the bone marrow changes in classical myelofibrosis, however, the reticulin fibrosis in patients with grey platelet syndrome does not appear to progress to bone marrow compromise.

Pulmonary fibrosis has also been reported in association with the grey platelet syndrome (Facon et al 1990), raising the intriguing possibility that leakage of α granule contents from megakaryocytes within the pulmonary circulation may occur when megakaryocytes travel to the lung just before fragmentation into platelets. It is of interest, however, that this patient did not have evidence of bone marrow fibrosis.

Platelet aggregation abnormalities have been described in the grey platelet syndrome but the defects have not been consistent. In general, aggregation by ADP and adrenalin has been normal or near normal. Aggregation in response to collagen and thrombin has shown more severe abnormalities but even these findings are inconsistent. The initial platelet-depolarization response to thrombin was normal in two patients (Greenberg-Sepersky 1985), but delayed morphological changes in response to thrombin and a delay in the release reaction have been identified (Srivastava et al 1987). In addition, abnormalities in platelet factor Va formation, phosphoinositide metabolism, protein phosphorylation and calcium mobilization have been detected (Baruch et al 1987, Enouf et al 1987, Rendu et al 1987). Thus, there is reason to think that in addition to loss of α granule contents, there is a defect in signal transduction in the grey platelet syndrome (Pfueller & David 1988). It is unclear, therefore, which of these abnormalities is responsible for the abnormal aggregation responses. Attempts to correct the aggregation abnormalities by adding back α granule proteins have not been very successful (Srivastava et al 1987), perhaps supporting a more important role for the signal-transduction abnormalities.

Therapy for patients with the grey platelet syndrome includes avoidance of drugs that interfere with platelet function and hormonal control of menses if necessary. The response to desmopressin has been inconsistent with regard to bleeding time correction (Kohler et al 1985, 1988, Pfueller et al 1987). It is uncertain, however, whether bleeding time correction is a prerequisite for a good clinical response since haemostasis after tooth extraction has been achieved with desmopressin in at least one patient even without bleeding time correction (Kohler et al 1985). Antifibrinolytic therapy with ε-aminocaproic acid or tranexamic acid may also be useful (Gootenberg et al 1986). Although bleeding in the grey platelet syndrome is usually mild, severe bleeding has been reported in association with head trauma (Gootenberg et al 1986). Under such circumstances, platelet transfusion is the most rapid and reliable method to insure an adequate number of functionally normal platelets. Raccuglia (1971) reported that, in his patient, steroids partially corrected the thrombocytopenia, and splenectomy fully corrected it, with the platelet count increasing from under 50 000/μL to almost 300 000/μL. Subsequently, however, this patient's platelet count decreased again (Gerrard et al 1980). Others have not found steroids or splenectomy to significantly affect the platelet count (Kohler et al 1985). The mechanism of thrombocytopenia has not been fully elucidated, but a modest reduction in platelet survival was found in one study (Kohler et al 1985).

Pathogenesis of granule defects

The biogenesis of membrane-bound organelles has been the subject of intense investigation, but many of the steps in forming, packing, and budding off these organelles remain poorly understood. The mechanisms by which newly synthesized proteins are targeted selectively to these organelles and the mechanisms by which plasma proteins are taken up from plasma, either nonspecifically or aided by receptors such as GPIIb/IIIa, are still incompletely defined. Several different potential abnormalities could conceivably lead to impaired granule content, including impaired production of the membranes needed for the organelles, impaired targeting of proteins to the membranes making up the nascent organelles, abnormal granule formation, or unstable granule retention of its contents. Recent advances have been made in understanding vesicle transport and the role of chaperone proteins in protein folding and targeting (Gething & Sambrook 1992, Rothman & Orci 1992). The possibility that α granules are in a constant state of recycling (Wencel-Drake 1990) adds another dimension of complexity; in fact, a reduction in platelet fibrinogen can be detected within 1 day of blocking GPIIb/IIIa receptors in vivo (Harrison et al 1990), demonstrating the extraordinarily dynamic nature of this granule.

ABNORMALITIES OF PLATELET COAGULANT ACTIVITY

Platelets facilitate thrombin generation by accelerating several reactions in the coagulation cascade, including activation of factor X and prothrombin (Walsh & Schmaier 1987, Bennett 1990). Platelet activation by many different agonists can dramatically increase the total platelet coagulant activity. This platelet attribute was initially characterized as platelet factor 3 (PF3). Subsequent studies have identified multiple potential factors that may contribute to the platelet coagulant effects, including specific interactions with the contact factors, exposure of phosphatidylserine on the surface of platelets, availability of specific receptors for activated clotting factors, release and activation of factor V in platelets, and generation of platelet microparticles that are particularly active in supporting coagulation (Walsh & Schmaier 1987, Bennett 1990).

Several patients with isolated defects in platelet coagulant activity have been reported (Girolami et al 1973, Weiss et al 1979a, Minkoff et al 1980, Sultan et al 1986). In two patients, the defect may have been acquired since the patients had coexisting Ehlers–Danlos syndrome and Hashimoto's thyroiditis in one case and chronic myelogenous leukaemia in the other. In four others, all of whom had histories of excessive bleeding, the defect appeared to be primary. The best-studied patient (Weiss et al 1979a) had an appendectomy at age three without incident, but then developed excessive bleeding after tooth extractions, tonsillectomy, parturition, and hysterectomy. She also developed a spontaneous retroperitoneal haemorrhage.

The most consistent laboratory abnormality is a shortened serum prothrombin time, which is thought to reflect decreased prothrombin consumption during coagulation (Weiss et al 1979a). Abnormalities in 'PF3 availability', that is the ability of activated platelets to accelerate coagulation, are also present. Assays of this abnormality vary considerably in design and have significant problems with reproducibility since they require preparing and maintaining platelets in an unactivated state (Weiss 1967). Thus, the relatively easy serum prothrombin time assay can be used as a screening test for the disorder. With one exception, the bleeding time was not increased in patients with this disorder, in keeping with the abnormality being localized to the clotting mechanism rather than the primary arrest of haemorrhage.

The one patient who has been studied in detail was found to have normal platelet phospholipids, but marked reductions in: binding sites for factors Va and VIIIa, the ability to support the activation of factors X and prothrombin, surface exposure of plasma membrane phosphatidylserine, and generation of platelet microparticles when platelets were activated with various agonists (Miletich et al 1979, Rosing et al 1985, Ahmad et al 1989, Sims et al 1989). Most recently, the patient's erythrocytes were also shown to share the abnormality in microparticle formation when stimulated with ionophore A23187 (Bevers et al 1992). No abnormalities in platelet calpain or aminophospholipid translocase were identified. It is most likely that this patient's platelets have a defect affecting the platelet cytoskeleton or its associated regulatory proteins.

Platelet transfusions have appeared to be effective in preventing and treating haemorrhages in the few reported cases. One patient appeared to respond to prothrombin complex concentrates, raising the possibility that some activated factors may have been able to bypass the defect.

ABNORMALITIES OF SIGNAL TRANSDUCTION AND SECRETION

The platelet has the capacity to amplify a stimulus to aggregation by:

1. Synthesizing platelet-aggregating agents, including the cyclic endoperoxides PGG_2 and PGH_2 and thromboxane A_2
2. Releasing platelet-aggregating agents from dense bodies such as ADP, adrenalin and serotonin
3. Releasing adhesive glycoproteins such as fibrinogen, von Willebrand factor, fibronectin, and vitronectin from α granules.

A complex series of reactions involving several different pathways are involved in these phenomena (Figs 32.6, 7). The major features of these reactions are:

1. Agonist binding to receptors on the platelet surface
2. Signal transduction, mediated at least in part by the heterotrimeric G proteins (Brass 1991) that activate phospholipase C
3. Phosphoinositol metabolism wherein phosphatidylinositol 4,5-biphosphate is converted by phospholipase C into inositol 1,4,5-triphosphate (which can mobilize calcium from storage sites into the cytoplasm leading to calmodulin-dependent phosphorylation of proteins, including myosin light chain kinase) and Sn-1,2-diacylglycerol (which can enhance the action of protein kinase C, leading to phosphorylation of proteins thought to be responsible for secretion) (Krolls and Schafer 1989, Holmsen 1990b, Brass 1991)
4. Arachidonic acid metabolism involving release of arachidonic acid by either phospholipase A_2 or the combination of phospholipase C and glyceride lipase, followed by sequential metabolism by the enzymes cyclo-oxygenase (forming the cyclic endoperoxides PGG_2 and PGH_2) and thromboxane synthetase, producing thromboxane A_2.

The thromboxane formed can exit from the platelet and interact with receptors on the same or other platelets to stimulate platelet aggregation (Brass 1991). With the large number of potential sites in the activation pathways for abnormalities to occur, it is not surprising that a heterogeneous group of patients have been identified with presumed defects (Wu 1982, Rao 1990). Most patients have had only mild histories of excessive bleeding and moderate prolongations of the bleeding time. The evaluation of these abnormalities has tended to rely on inferences deduced from responses to certain agonists and inhibitors rather than direct biochemical analyses and so the conclusions are considerably more tentative than in the glycoprotein disorders. Also contributing to the difficulty in localizing the defects are the multiple feedback loops that control the process, in particular the role of calcium, which serves to activate several of the key enzymes and probably also serves as a fusogen to achieve release.

Defects in arachidonic acid metabolism

Defects in arachidonic acid release from phospholipids

Rao (1984) described four patients with impaired platelet aggregation and secretion to ADP, adrenalin and collagen, but normal aggregation in response to arachidonic acid. Further studies demonstrated impaired release of arachidonic acid from platelet phospholipids in response to thrombin and normal thromboxane A_2 production in response to arachidonic acid, leading to the tentative conclusion that the abnormality in arachidonic acid release

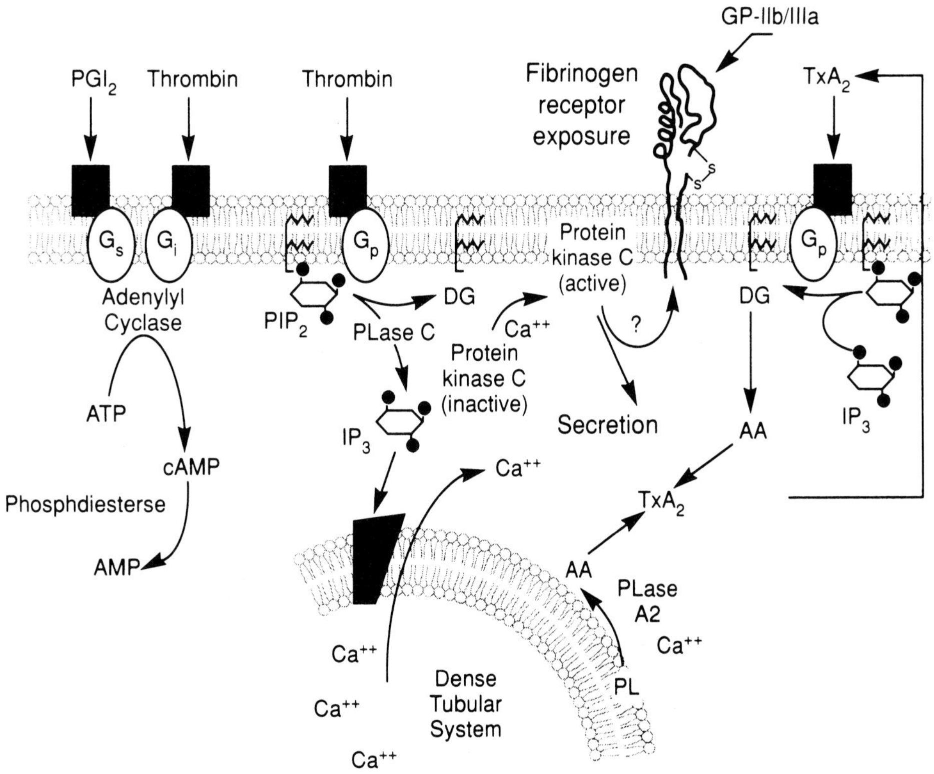

Fig. 32.6 Signal transduction during platelet activation. At the molecular level, platelet activation begins when an agonist, such as thrombin, binds to receptors on the platelet surface. This initiates a cascade of intracellular second messengers, including inositol 1,4,5-triphosphate (IP_3) and diacylglycerol (DG). IP_3 releases Ca^{2+} from the platelet dense tubular system, raising cytosolic free Ca^{2+} concentration. Diacylglycerol activates protein kinase C, shifting it to the plasma membrane and triggering granule secretion and fibrinogen receptor exposure on the glycoprotein IIb-IIIa complex. At the same time, the rising cytosolic free Ca^{2+} concentration facilitates arachidonate (AA) formation by phospholipase A_2 (PLase A_2), a process that probably occurs at both the plasma membrane and the dense tubular system membrane. Arachidonate is metabolized to thromboxane A_2 (TxA_2), which diffuses out of the cell, interacts with receptors on the platelet surface and causes further platelet activation. In many cases, the interaction between agonists and the enzymes responsible for second messenger generation is mediated by a guanine nucleotide-binding regulatory protein (G protein). In platelets, G proteins have been shown to regulate phosphoinositide hydrolysis and cAMP formation. Phospholipase C is activated by an as yet unidentified G protein referred to as G_p. Adenylyl cyclase is stimulated by the G protein, G_s, and inhibited by the G protein, G_i. (Reproduced with permission from Brass L, 1991 In: Hoffman R, Benz E J Jr, Shattil S J, Furie B, Cohn J J (eds) Haematology: basic principles and practice. Churchill Livingstone, New York.)

was primary. Subsequent studies (Rao 1990) indicated normal phospholipase A_2 but defective calcium mobilization in these patients' platelets, raising the possibility that the calcium defect is the true primary abnormality since phospholipase A_2 is a calcium-dependent enzyme. Rendu et al (1978) reported a severe defect in phospholipase activity in a patient with δ-storage pool deficiency and Hermansky–Pudlak syndrome. Holmsen et al (1987) reported on another patient with a presumed defect in arachidonic acid liberation.

Cyclo-oxygenase deficiency

Several patients have been described with deficiencies in platelet cyclo-oxygenase resulting in impaired platelet aggregation responses and diminished thromboxane synthesis (Malmsten et al 1975, Lagarde et al 1978, Pareti et al 1980, Rak and Boda 1980, Roth and Machuga 1982, Horrellou et al 1983, Rao et al 1985). The platelets of such patients do not make thromboxane from arachidonic acid, but can make it from cyclic endoperoxides. The patient described by Pareti et al (1980) also had a documented deficiency in PGI_2 production. It is of note, therefore, that this patient had a mild haemorrhagic disorder rather than a thrombotic disorder, indicating that on balance cyclo-oxygenase products are more pro-haemostatic than antithrombotic. The patient described by Rak & Boda (1980) had evidence of thrombotic vascular disease, including transient ischaemic attacks.

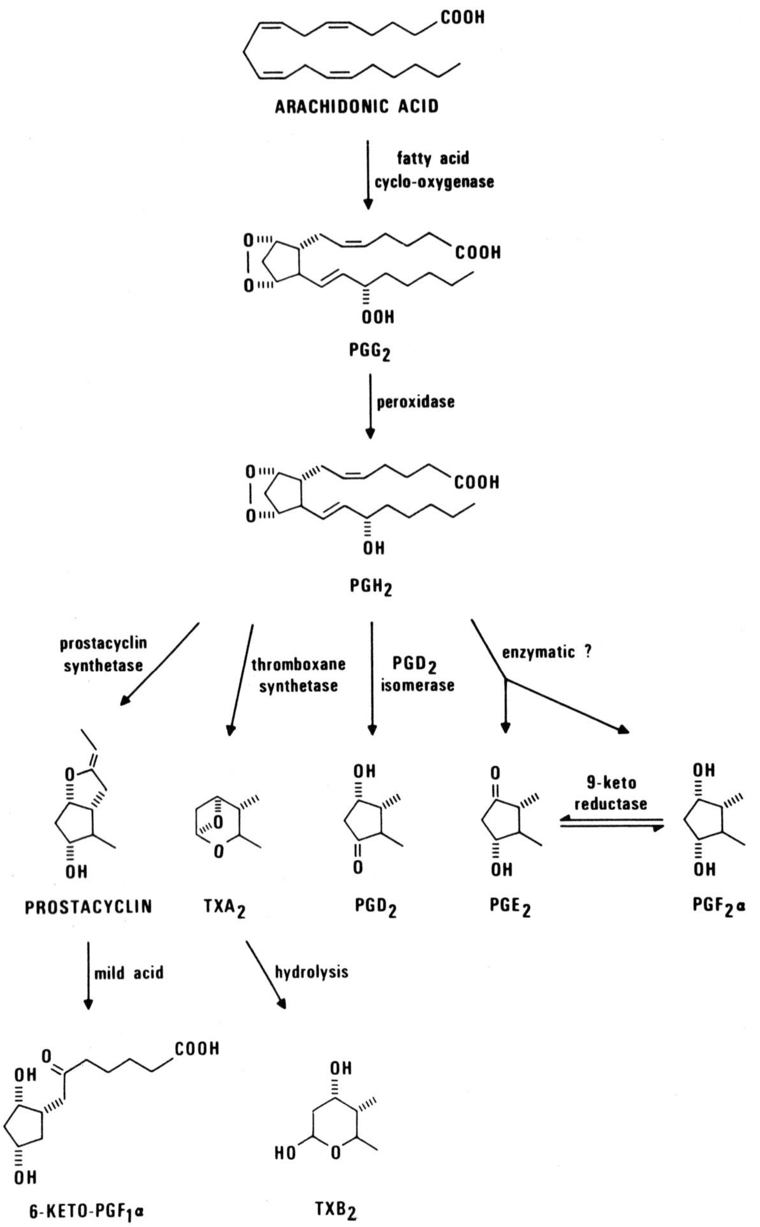

Fig. 32.7 Eicosanoid metbolism. Summary of biosynthetic pathways of prostacyclin, thromboxane A_2, and classic prostaglandins as they originate from arachidonic acid. Pathway to PGH_2 is common to all tissues that transform arachidonic acid. Subsequent fate of PGH_2 depends on the particular enzyme(s) present in each tissue. (Courtesy of Dr Robert R Gorman and reproduced from Marcus 1987 with permission.)

Thromboxane synthetase deficiency

Patients from two families have been described with putative thromboxane synthetase deficiencies based on a failure of cyclic endoperoxides to be converted into thromboxane (Mestel et al 1980, Defryn et al 1981). The patient described by Mestel et al (1980) had a variably prolonged bleeding time and a modest history of bleeding, except for a single, life-threatening gastrointestinal haemorrhage.

Defects in thromboxane A_2 sensitivity and calcium mobilization

One of the most common platelet-function abnormalities encountered is a failure of platelets to undergo secondary aggregation in response to weak agonists, but not to strong agonists. Since many of these patients' platelets have the capacity to make thromboxane, it has been inferred that their defect lies in an abnormal thromboxane A_2 receptor or a failure of thromboxane A_2 to appropriately mobilize calcium. Other defects in calcium mobilization may also be involved, and, further complicating the investigation of these patients, is the observation that ADP acts synergistically with thromboxane A_2 and so variable secretion of ADP may affect the results (Rao 1990).

A sizable number of patients with impaired thromboxane A_2 sensitivity and/or abnormal calcium mobilization have been described (Lages et al 1981, Samama et al 1981, Takahashi 1981, Wu et al 1981a,b, Koike 1984, Lages & Weiss 1988a, 1988b, Rao et al 1989). The precise abnormalities in these patients' platelets remain to be identified

REFERENCES

Abrams C S, Ruggeri Z M, Taub R, Hoxie J A, Nagaswami C, Weisel J W, Shattil S J 1992 Anti-idiotypic antibodies against an antibody to the platelet glycoprotein (GP) IIb-IIIa complex mimic GP IIb-IIIa by recognizing fibrinogen. Journal of Biological Chemistry 267: 2775–2785

Ahmad S S, Rawala-Sheikh R, Ashby B, Walsh P N 1989 Platelet receptor-mediated factor X activation by factor IXa. High-affinity IXa induced by factor VIII are deficient on platelets in Scott syndrome. Journal of Clinical Investigation 84: 824

Akkerman J-W N, Nieuwenhuis H K, Mommersteeg-Leautaud M E, Gorter G, Sixma J J 1983 ATP-ADP compartmentation in storage pool deficient platelets: correlation between granule-bound ADP and the bleeding time. British Journal of Haematology 55: 135–143

Amrani D L, Newman P J, Meh D, Mosesson M W 1988 The role of fibrinogen Aαchains in ATP, induced platelet aggregation in the presence of fibrinogen molecules containing γ′ chains. Blood 72: 919

Andreu G 1991 Role of leukocyte depletion in the prevention of transfusion-induced cytomegalovirus infection. Seminars in Hematology 28: 26–31

Apitz-Castro R, Cruz M R, Ledezma E et al 1985 The storage pool deficiency in platelets from humans with the Chediak–Higashi syndrome: study of six patients. British Journal of Haematology 59: 471–483

Asch E, Podack E 1990 Vitronectin binds to activated human platelets and plays a role in platelet aggregation. Journal of Clinical Investigation 85: 1372

Asch A S, Barnwell J, Silverstein R L, Nachman R L 1987 Isolation of the thrombospondin membrane receptor. Journal of Clinical Investigation 79: 1054–1061

Awidi A S 1983 Increased incidence of Glanzmann's thrombasthenia in Jordan as compared with Scandinavia. Scandinavian Journal of Haematology 30: 218–222

Bajt M L, Ginsberg M H, Frelinger A L, III, Berndt M C, Loftus J C 1992 A spontaneous mutation of integrin $\alpha_{IIb}\beta_3$ (platelet glycoprotein IIb-IIIa), helps define a ligand binding site. Journal of Biological Chemistry 267: 3784–3794

Baldini M G 1992 Nature of the platelet defect in the Wiskott–Aldrich syndrome. Annals of the New York Academy of Sciences 437–444

Barbieri R L 1992 Endocrinology of the female. In: Kelly W N (ed) Textbook of internal medicine. Lippincott, Philadelphia, p 2011–2013

Baruch D, Lindhout T, Dupuy E, Caen J P 1987 Thrombin-induced platelet factor Va formation in patients with a gray platelet syndrome. Thrombosis and Haemostasis 58: 768–771

Baumgartner H R, Muggli R, Tschopp T B, Turitto V T 1976 Platelet adhesion, release and aggregation in flowing blood: Effects of surface properties and platelet function. Thrombosis and Haemostasis (Stuttgart) 35: 124–138

Beckstead J H, Stenberg P E, McEver R P, Shuman M A, Bainton D F 1986 Immunohistochemical localization of membrane and alpha-granule proteins in human megakaryocytes: Application to plastic-embedded bone marrow biopsy specimens. Blood 67: 285

Beer J H, Nieuwenhuis K, Sixma J J, Coller B S 1988 Deficiency of antibody 6F1 binding to the platelets of a patient with an isolated defect in platelet-collagen interaction. Circulation 78: II-308 Abstract

Bell T G, Meyers K M, Prieur D J, Fauci A S, Wolff S M, Padgett G A 1976 Decreased nucleotide and serotonin storage associated with defective function in Chediak–Higashi syndrome cattle and human platelets. Blood 48: 175–184

Bellucci S, Devergie A, Gluckman E et al 1985 Complete correction of Glanzmann's thrombasthenia by allogeneic bone marrow transplantation. British Journal of Haematology 59: 635–641

Bennett J S 1985 The platelet-fibrinogen interaction. In: George J N, Nurden A T, Phillips D R (eds) Platelet membrane glycoproteins. Plenum Press, New York, p193

Bennett J, Shattil S J 1990 Platelet function. In: Williams W J, Beutler E, Erslev A J, Lichtman M A (eds) Hematology, 4th edn. McGraw-Hill, New York, p 1250

Bennett J S, Vilaire G 1979 Exposure of platelet fibrinogen receptors by ADP and epinephrine. Journal of Clinical Investigation 64: 1393–1401

Bennett J S, Hoxie J A, Leitman S F, Vilaire G, Cines D B 1983 Inhibition of fibrinogen binding to stimulated human platelets by a monoclonal antibody. Proceedings of the National Academy of Sciences, USA 80: 2417

Bennett J S, Kolodziel M A, Vilaire G, Gonder D, Poncz M 1991 The intracellular fate of truncated forms of the platelet glycoproteins IIb and IIIa. Blood 78(suppl 1): 719–182a (abstract)

Berliner S, Horowitz I, Martinowitz U, Brenner B, Seligsohn U 1992 Dental surgery in patients with severe factor XI deficiency without plasma replacement. Submitted

Bernard J 1983 History of congenital hemorrhagic thrombocytopathic dystrophy. Blood Cells 9: 179

Bernard J, Soulier J-P 1948 Sur une nouvelle varieté de dystrophie thrombocytaire-hemorragipare congenitale. Semaine Des Hopitaux De Paris 24: 3217

Berndt M C, Castaldi P A, Gordon S, Halley H, McPherson J J 1983a Morphological and biochemical confirmation of gray platelet syndrome in two siblings. Australian New Zealand Journal of Medicine 13: 387

Berndt M C, Gregory C, Chong B H, Zola H, Castaldi P A 1983b Additional glycoprotein defects in Bernard–Soulier's syndrome: Confirmation of genetic basis by parental analysis. Blood 62: 800–807

Berrebi A, Klepfish A, Varon D et al 1988 Gray platelet syndrome in the elderly. American Journal of Haematology 28: 270–272

Bevers E M, Comfurius P, Nieuwenhuis H K et al 1986 Platelet prothrombin converting activity in hereditary disorders of platelet function. British Journal of Haematology 63: 335–345

Bevers E M, Wiedmer T, Comfurius P et al 1992 Defective Ca^{2+}-induced microvesiculation and deficient expression of procoagulant activity in erythrocytes from a patient with a bleeding disorder: A study of the red blood cells of Scott syndrome. Blood 79: 380–388

Bienz D, Schnippering W, Clemetson K J 1986 Glycoprotein V is not the thrombin activation receptor on human platelets. Blood 68: 720

Bierling P, Fromont P, Elbez A, Duedari N, Kieffer N 1988 Early immunization against platelet glycoprotein IIIa in a newborn Glanzmann type I patient. Vox Sanguinis 55: 109–113

Bithell T C, Parekh S J, Strong R R 1972 Platelet-function studies in the Bernard–Soulier syndrome. Annals of the New York Academy of Sciences 201: 145–160

Bodary S C, Napier M A, McLean J W 1989 Expression of recombinant platelet glycoprotein IIbIIIa results in a functional fibrinogen-binding complex. Journal of Biological Chemistry 264: 18859–18862

Borchgrevink C F, Egeberg O, Godal H C et al 1963 The effect of plasma and Cohn's fraction I on the Duke and Ivy bleeding times in von Willebrand's disease. Acta Medica Scandinavica 173: 235

Brass L F 1985 Ca^{++}transport across the platelet plasma membrane: A

role for membrane glycoprotein IIb and IIIa. Journal of Biological Chemistry 260: 2231
Brass L F 1991 The biochemistry of platelet activation. In: Hoffman R, Benz Jr E J, Shattil S J, Furie B, Cohen J J (eds) Hematology: basic principles and practice. Churchill Livingstone, New York, p 1176
Brass L F, Shattil S J 1984 Identification and function of the high affinity binding sites for Ca^{2+} on the surface of platelets. Journal of Clinical Investigation 73: 626
Bray P F, Shuman M A 1990 Identification of an abnormal gene for the GPIIIa subunit of the platelet fibrinogen receptor resulting in Glanzmann's thrombasthenia. Blood 75: 881–888
Bray P F, Leung C S -I, Shuman M A 1990 Human platelets and megakaryocytes contain alternately spliced glycoprotein IIb mRNAs. Journal of Biological Chemistry 265: 9587–9590
Brown C H, III, Weisberg R J, Natelson E A, Alfrey C P Jr 1975 Glanzmann's thrombasthenia: Assessment of the response to platelet transfusions. Transfusion 15: 124
Burgess-Wilson M E, Cockbill S R, Johnston G I, Heptinstall S 1987 Platelet aggregation in whole blood from patients with Glanzmann's thrombasthenia. Blood 69: 38–42
Burk C D, Newman P J, Lyman S, Gill J, Coller B S, Poncz M 1991 A deletion in the gene for glycoprotein IIb associated with Glanzmann's thrombasthenia. Journal of Clinical Investigation 87: 270–276
Caen J P 1972 Glanzmann's thrombasthenia. Clinics in Haematology 1: 383–392
Caen J, Bellucci S 1983 The defective prothrombin consumption in Bernard–Soulier syndrome. Blood Cells 9: 389–399
Caen J P, Castaldi P A, Leclerc J C et al 1966 Congenital bleeding disorders with long bleeding time and normal platelet count. I. Glanzmann's thrombasthenia. American Journal of Medicine 41: 4
Caen J P, Cronberg S, Levy-Toledano S, Kubisz P, Pinkhas J P 1971 New data on Glanzmann's thrombasthenia. Proceedings of the Society for Experimental Biology and Medicine 136: 1082–1086
Caen J P, Nurden A T, Jeanneau C et al 1976 Bernard–Soulier syndrome: a new platelet glycoprotein abnormality. Its relationship with platelet adhesion to subendothelium and with the factor VIII von Willebrand protein. Journal of Laboratory and Clinical Medicine 87: 586–596
Caen J P, Rosa J P, Boizard B, Nurden A T 1983 Thrombasthenia Paris I variant, a model for the study of the platelet glycoprotein IIb-IIIa complex. Blood 62(suppl 1): 251a (abstract)
Caen J P, Deschamps J F, Bodevin E, Bryckaert M C, Dupuy E, Wasteson A 1987 Megakaryocytes and myelofibrosis in gray platelet syndrome. Nouvelle Revue Francaise D Hematologie 29: 109–114
Calvete J J, Henschen A, Gonzalez-Rodrigues J 1989 Complete localization of the intrachain disulphide bonds and the N-glycosylation points in the α-subunit of human platelet glycoprotein IIb. Biochemical Journal 261: 561–568
Calvete J J, Henschen A, Gonzalez-Rodriguez J 1991 Assignment of disulphide bonds in human platelet GPIIIa. Biochemical Journal 274: 63–71
Carrell N A, Fitzgerald L A, Steiner B, Erickson H P, Phillips D R 1985 Structure of human platelet membrane glycoproteins IIb and IIIa as determined by electron microscopy. Journal of Biological Chemistry 260: 1743
Champeix P, Forestier F, Daffos F, Kaplan C, Xe T I 1988 Prenatal diagnosis of a molecular variant of Glanzmann's thrombasthenia. Current Studies in Hematology and Blood Transfusions 174–179
Charo I F, Feinman R D, Detwiler T C 1977 Interrelations of platelet aggregation and sectetion. Journal of Clinical Investigation 60: 866–873
Charo I F, Fitzgerald L A, Steiner B, Rall Jr, S C, Bekeart L S, Phillips D R 1986 Platelet glycoproteins IIb and IIIa: Evidence for a family of immunologically and structurally related glycoproteins in mammalian cells. Proceedings of the National Academy of Sciences, USA 83: 8351–8356
Charo I F, Nannizzi L, Phillips D R, Hsu M A, Scarborough R M 1991 Inhibition of fibrinogen binding to GPIIb-IIIa by a GPIIIa peptide. Journal of Biological Chemistry 266: 1415–1421
Chediak J, Telfer M C, Vander Laan B, Maxey B, Cohen I 1979 Cycles of agglutination-disagglutination induced by ristocetin in thrombasthenic platelets. British Journal of Haematology 43: 113–126
Chen Y, Djaffar I, Pidard D et al 1991 The absence of activation of platelet GPIIb-IIIa, the integrin $\alpha_{IIb}\beta_3$, is associated with a point mutation of the cytoplasmic domain of GPIIIa (β_3) in a variant type of Glanzmann's thrombasthenia. Blood (Suppl 1) 78: 279a (abstract)
Cheresh D A 1987 Human endothelial cells synthesize and express an Arg-Gly-Asp-directed adhesion receptor involved in attachment to fibrinogen and von Willebrand factor. Proceedings of the National Academy of Sciences, USA 84: 6471
Cheresh D A, Spiro R C 1987 Biosynthetic and functional properties of an Arg-Gly-Asp-directed receptor involved in human melanoma cell attachment to vitronectin, fibrinogen, and von Willebrand factor. Journal of Biological Chemistry 262: 17703
Cheresh D A, Berliner S A, Vincente V, Ruggeri Z M 1989 Recognition of distinct adhesive sites on fibrinogen by related integrins on platelets and endothelial cells. Cell 58: 945
Chevalier J, Caen J P, Pinto da Silva P 1986 Freeze-fracture cytochemistry of wheat germ agglutinin and concanavalin A receptors on the plasma membrane of normal, Bernard–Soulier, and thrombasthenic platelets. American Journal of Pathology 122: 292–301
Clemetson K J 1985 Glycoproteins of the platelet plasma membrane. In: George J N, Nurden A T Philips D R (eds) Platelet membrane glycoproteins. Plenum Press, New York, p 51–85
Clemetson K J, McGregor J L, James E, Dechavanne M, Lusher E F 1982 Characterization of the platelet membrane glycoprotein abnormalities in Bernard–Soulier syndrome and comparison with normal by surface-labeling techniques and high-resolution two-dimensional gel electrophoresis. Journal of Clinical Investigation 70: 304–311
Clemetson K J, Wenger R H, Wicki A N, Clemetson J M, Kieffer N, Drouin J 1990 Molecular biology of human platelet membrane glycoprotein Ib. Progress in Clinical and Biological Research 356: 77–88
Cockbill S R, Burmester H B, Heptinstall S 1988 Pseudo grey platelet syndrome — grey platelets due to degranulation in blood collected into EDTA. European Journal of Hematology 41: 326–333
Cohen I, Gerrard J M, White J G 1982 Ultrastructure of clots during isometric contraction. Journal of Cell Biology 93: 775
Coller B S 1979 Platelet aggregation by ADP, collagen and ristocetin: A clinical review of methodology and analysis. In: Schmidt R M (ed) CRC handbook series in clinical laboratory science, section 1: hematology. CRC Press, Boca Raton, p 381
Coller B S 1980 Interaction of normal, thrombasthenia, and Bernard–Soulier platelets with immobilized fibrinogen: Defective platelet-fibrinogen interaction in thrombasthenia. Blood 55: 169–178
Coller B S 1985 Platelet-von Willebrand factor interactions. In: George J, Phillips D, Nurden A (eds) Platelet glycoproteins. Plenum, New York, p 215–244
Coller B S 1986 Activation affects access to the platelet receptor for adhesive glycoproteins. Journal of Cell Biology 103: 451–456
Coller B S 1989 Activation-dependent platelet antigens. In: Kunicki T, George J (eds) Platelet immunobiology. Lippincott, Philadelphia, p 166–189
Coller B S, Schneiderman P 1991 Clinical evaluation of hemorrhagic disorders: The bleeding history and differential diagnosis of purpura. In: Hoffman R, Benz E J, Shattil S J, Furie B, Cohen H J (eds) Hematology: basic principles and practice. Churchill Livingstone, New York, p 1176–1197
Coller B S, Zarrabi M H 1981 Platelet membrane studies in the May–Hegglin anomaly. Blood 58: 279–284
Coller B S, Hirschman R J, Gralnick H R 1975a Studies of the factor VIII/von Willebrand factor antigen on human platelets. Thrombosis Research 6: 469–480
Coller I, Glaser T, Seligsohn U 1975b Effects of ADP and ATP on bovine fibrinogen and ristocetin-induced platelet aggregation in Glauzmann's thrombasthenia. British Journal of Haematology 31: 343–347
Coller B S, Hultin M B, Nurden A T, Rosa J P, Lane B P 1983a Isolated alpha-granule deficiency (grey platelet syndrome) with slight increase in bone marrow reticulin and possible glycoprotein and/or protease defect. Thrombosis Haemostasis 50: 211 (abstract)
Coller B S, Peerschke E I, Scuder L E, Sullivan C A 1983b A murine monoclonal antibody that completely blocks the binding of

fibrinogen to platelets produces a thrombasthenic-like state in normal platelets and binds to glycoproteins IIb and/or IIIa. Journal of Clinical Investigation 72: 325–338
Coller B S, Peerschke E I, Scudder L E, Sullivan C A 1983c Studies with a murine monoclonal antibody that abolishes ristocetin-induced binding of von Willebrand factor to platelets: Additional evidence in support of GPIb as a platelet receptor for von Willebrand factor. Blood 61: 99–110
Coller B S, Peerschke E I, Seligsohn U, Scudder L E, Nurden A T, Rosa J P 1986a Studies on the binding of an alloimmune and two murine monoclonal antibodies to the platelet glycoprotein IIb-IIIba complex receptor. Journal of Laboratory and Clinical Medicine 107: 384–392
Coller B S, Seligsohn U, Zivelin A, Zwang E, Lusky A, Modan M 1986b Immunologic and biochemical characterization of homozygous and heterozygous Glanzmann thrombasthenia in the Iraqi-Jewish and Arab populations of Israel: comparison of techniques for carrier detection. British Journal of Haematology 62: 723–735
Coller B S, Seligsohn U, Little P A 1987 'Type I' Glanzmann thrombasthenia patients from the Iraqi-Jewish and Arab populations in Israel can be differentiated by platelet glycoprotein IIIa immunoblot analysis. Blood 69: 1696–1703
Coller B S, Beer J H, Scudder L E, Steinberg M H 1989 Evidence for a direct interaction of collagen with platelet GPIa/IIa and an indirect interaction with GPIIb/IIIa mediated by adhesive proteins. Blood 74: 182–192
Coller B S, Cheresh D A, Asch E, Seligsohn U 1991a Platelet vitronectin receptor expression differentiates Iraqi-Jewish from Arab patients with Glanzmann thrombasthenia in Israel. Blood 77: 75–83
Coller B S, Scudder L E, Beer J et al 1991b Monoclonal antibodies to platelet glycoprotein IIB/IIIa as antithrombotic agents. Annals of the New York Academy of Sciences 614: 193–213
Coller B S, Seligsohn U, West S M, Scudder L E, Norton K J 1991c Platelet fibrinogen and vitronection in Glanzmann thrombasthenia: Evidence consistent with specific roles for glycoprotein IIb/IIIa and $\alpha_v\beta_3$ integrins in platelet protein trafficking. Blood 78: 2603–2610
Cramer E M, Vainchenker W, Vinci G, Guichard J, Breton Gorius J 1985 Gray platelet syndrome: immunoelectron microscopic localization of fibrinogen and von Willebrand factor in platelets and megakaryocytes. Blood 66: 1309–1316
Cramer E M, Savidge G F, Vainchenker W et al 1990 Alpha-granule pool of glycoprotein IIb-IIIa in normal and pathologic platelets and megakaryocytes. Blood 75: 1220–1227
Cronberg S 1971 Abnormal behavior of platelets. In: Caen J P (ed) Platelet aggregation. Masson, Paris, p 185–191
Cuthbert R J, Watson H H, Handa S I, Abbott I, Ludlam C A 1988 DDAVP shortens the bleeding time in Bernard–Soulier syndrome. Thrombosis Research 49: 649–650
Day H J, Holmsen H 1972 Platelet adenine nucleotide 'storage pool deficiency' in thrombocytopenic absent radii syndrome. Journal of American Medical Association 221: 1053
Defreyn G, Machin S J, Carreras L O, Dauden M V, Chamone D A F, Vermylen J 1981 Familial bleeding tendency with partial platelet thromboxane synthetase deficiency: Reorientation of cyclic endoperoxide metabolism. British Journal of Haematology 49: 29–41
Degos L, Dautigny A, Brouet J C et al 1975 A molecular defect in thrombasthenic platelets. Journal of Clinical Investigation 56: 236
Degos L, Tobelem G, Lethielleux P, Levy-Toledano S, Caen J, Colombani J 1977 Molecular defect in platelet from patients with Bernard–Soulier syndrome. Blood 50: 899–903
De Marco L, Fabris F, Casonato A et al 1986 Bernard–Soulier syndrome: diagnosis by an ELISA method using monoclonal antibodies in 2 new unrelated patients. Acta Haematology 75: 203–208
De Marco L, Mazzucato M, Fabris F et al 1990 Variant Bernard–Soulier syndrome type Bolzano. A congenital bleeding disorder due to a structural and functional abnormality of the platelet glycoprotein Ib-IX complex. Journal of Clinical Investigation 86: 25–31
De Marco L, Mazzucato M, Masotti A, Fenton J W, Ruggeri Z M 1991 Function of glycoprotein Ib alpha in platelet activation induced by alpha-thrombin. Journal of Biological Chemistry 266: 35
de Moerloose P, Vogel J J, Clemetson K J, Petite J, Bienz D, Bouvier C A 1987 Bernard–Soulier syndrome in a Swiss family. Schweizerische Medizinische Wochenschrift. Journal Suisse De Medecine 117: 1817–1821
DiMichele D M, Hathaway W E 1990 Use of DDAVP in inherited and acquired platelet dysfunction. American Journal of Haematology 33: 39–45
Disdier M, Legrand C, Bouillot C, Dubernard V, Pidard D, Nurden A T 1989 Quantitation of platelet fibrinogen and thrombospondin in Glanzmann's thrombasthenia by electroimmunoassay. Thrombosis Research 53: 521–533
Djaffar I, Pidard D, Caen J, Rosa J-P 1991 An homozygous mutation in the gene coding for GPIIIa associated with Glanzmann's thrombasthenia. Blood 78(suppl 1): 1571 (abstract)
Drouin J, McGregor J L, Parmentier S, Izaguirre C A, Clemetson K J 1988 Residual amounts of glycoprotein Ib concomitant with near-absence of glycoprotein IX in platelets of Bernard–Soulier patients. Blood 72: 1086–1088
D'Souza S E, Ginsberg M H, Burke T A, Lam S C-T, Plow E F 1988 Localization of an arg-gly-asp recognition site within an integrin adhesion receptor. Science 242: 91–93
D'Souza S E, Ginsberg M H, Burke T A, Plow E F 1990 The ligand binding site of the platelet integrin receptor GPIIb-IIIa is proximal to the second calcium binding domain of its alpha subunit. Journal of Biological Chemistry 6: 3440–3446
D'Souza S E, Ginsberg M H, Matsueda G R, Plow E F 1991 A discrete sequence in a platelet integrin is involved in ligand recognition. Nature 350: 66–71
Duperray A, Berthier R, Chagnon E et al 1987 Biosynthesis and processing of platelet GPIIb-IIIa in human megakaryocytes. Journal of Cell Biology 104: 1665
Dutcher J P, Schiffer C A, Aisner J, Wiernik P H 1981 Long-term follow-up of patients with leukemia receiving platelet transfusions: identification of a large group of patients who do not become alloimmunized. Blood 58: 1007–1011
Eaton Jr. L A, Read M S, Brinkhous K M 1991 Glycoprotein Ib bioassays. Activity levels in Bernard–Soulier syndrome and in stored blood bank platelets. Archives of Pathology and Laboratory Medicine 115: 488–493
Enouf J, Lebret M, Bredoux R, Levy Toledano S, Caen J P 1987 Abnormal calcium transport into microsomes of grey platelet syndrome. British Journal of Haematology 65: 437–440
Evensen S A, Solum N O, Grottum K A, Hovig T 1974 Familial bleeding disorder with a moderate thrombocytopenia and giant blood platelets. Scandanavian Journal of Haematology 13: 203–214
Facon T, Goudemand J, Caron C et al 1990 Simultaneous occurrence of grey platelet syndrome and idiopathic pulmonary fibrosis: a role for abnormal megakaryocytes in the pathogenesis of pulmonary fibrosis? British Journal of Haematology 74: 542–543
Feinman R D, Lubowsky J, Charo I, Zabinski M 1977 The lumi-aggregometer: A new instrument for simultaneous measurement of secretion and aggregation. Journal of Laboratory and Clinical Medicine 90: 125
Finch C N, Miller J L, Lyle V A, Handin R I 1990 Evidence that an abnormality in the glycoprotein Ib alpha gene is not the cause of abnormal platelet function in a family with classic Bernard–Soulier disease. Blood 75: 2357–2362
Fitzgerald L A, Poncz M, Steiner B, Rall Jr S C, Bennett J S, Phillips D R 1987a Comparison of cDNA-derived protein sequences of the human fibronectin and vitronectin receptor alpha-subunits and platelet glycoprotein IIb. Biochemistry 26: 158
Fitzgerald L A, Steiner B, Rall Jr S C, Lo S-S, Phillips D R 1987b Protein sequence of endothelial glycoprotein IIIa derived from a cDNA clone. Journal of Biological Chemistry 262: 3936–3939
Fournier D J, Kabral A, Castaldi P A, Berndt M C 1989 A variant of Glanzmann's thrombasthenia characterized by abnormal glycoprotein IIb/IIIa complex formation. Thrombosis and Haemostasis 62: 977–983
Fox J E B 1985 Linkage of a membrane skeleton to integral membrane glycoproteins in human platelets. Identification of one of the glycoproteins as glycoprotein Ib. Journal of Clinical Investigation 76: 1673–1683
Fox J E, Berndt M C 1989 Cyclic AMP-dependent phosphorylation of glycoprotein Ib inhibits collagen-induced polymerization of actin in platelets. Journal of Biological Chemistry 264: 9520–9526

Fox J E, Reynolds C C, Johnson M M 1987 Identification of glycoprotein Ib beta as one of the major proteins phosphorylated during exposure of intact platelets to agents that activate cyclic AMP-dependent protein kinase. Journal of Biological Chemistry 262: 12627–12631

Frojmovic M M, Milton J G, Caen J P, Tobelem G 1978 Platelets from 'giant platelet syndrome (BSS)' are discocytes and normal sized. Journal of Laboratory and Clinical Medicine 91: 109–116

Furihata K, Hunter J, Aster R H, Koewing G R, Shulman N P, Kunicki T J 1988 Human anti-P1E1 antibody recognizes epitopes associated with the alpha subunit of platelet glycoprotein Ib. British Journal of Haematology 68: 103–110

Gaarder A, Jonsen J, Laland S, Hellem A, Owren P A 1961 Adenosine diphosphate in red cells as a factor in the adhesiveness of human blood platelets. Nature 192: 531

Gartner T K, Bennett J S 1985 The tetrapeptide analogue of the cell attachment site of fibronectin inhibits platelet aggregation and fibrinogen binding to activated platelets. Journal of Biological Chemistry 260: 11891

Gartner T K, Ogilvie M L 1988 Peptides and monoclonal antibodies which bind to platelet glycoproteins IIb and/or IIIa inhibit clot retraction. Thrombosis Research 49: 43

George J N 1991 Platelet IgG: Measurement, interpretation, and clinical significance. Progress in Hemostasis and Thrombosis 10: 97–126

George J, Nurden A T 1987 Inherited disorders of the platelet membrane: Glanzmann's thrombasthenia and Bernard–Soulier syndrome: In: Colman R W, Hirsh J, Marder V J, Salzman E W (eds) Hemostasis and thrombosis: basic principles and clinical practice. Lippincott, Philadelphia, p 726

George J N, Reimann T A, Moake J L, Morgan R K, Cimo P L, Sears D A 1981 Bernard–Soulier disease: A study of four patients and their parents. British Journal of Haematology 48: 459–467

George J N, Pickett E B, Heinz R 1986 Platelet membrane microparticles in blood bank fresh frozen plasma and cryoprecipitate. Blood 68: 397–309

George J N, Caen J P, Nurden A T 1990 Glanzmann's thrombasthenia: the spectrum of clinical disease. Blood 75: 1383–1395

Gerrard J M, Phillips D R, Rao G H et al 1980 Biochemical studies of two patients with the gray platelet syndrome. Journal of Clinical Investigation 66: 102–109

Gerritsen S W, Akkerman J-W N, Sixma J J 1978 Correction of the bleeding time in patients with storage pool deficiency by infusion of cryoprecipitate. British Journal of Haematology 40: 153–160

Gething M-J, Sambrook J 1992 Protein folding in the cell. Nature 355: 33–44

Ginsberg M H, Lightsey A, Kunicki T J, Kaufmann A, Marguerie G, Plow E F 1986 Divalent cation regulation of the surface orientation of platelet membrane glycoprotein IIb. Correlation with fibrinogen binding function and definition of a novel variant of Glanzmann's thrombasthenia. Journal of Clinical Investigation 78: 1103–1111

Girolami A, Brunetti A, Fioretti D et al 1973 Congenital thrombocytopathy (platelet factor 3 defect) with prolonged bleeding but normal platelet adhesiveness and aggregation. Acta Haematology 50: 116

Glanzmann E 1918 Hereditare hamorrhagische thrombasthenie. Ein Beitrag Zur Pathologie der Bluplattchen Journal Kinderkt 88: 113–141

Gerrard J M, Lint D, Sims P L et al 1991 Identification of a platelet dense granule membrane protein that is deficient in a patient with Hermansky–Pudlak syndrome. Blood 77: 101–112

Gootenberg J E, Buchanan G R, Holtkamp C A, Casey C S 1986 Severe hemorrhage in a patient with gray platelet syndrome. Journal of Pediatrics 109: 1017–1019

Gralnick H R, Williams S B, Shafer B C, Corash L 1982 Factor VIII/von Willebrand factor binding to von Willebrand's disease platelets. Blood: 328–332

Gralnick H R, Williams S B, Coller B S 1984 Fibrinogen competes with von Willebrand factor for binding to the glycoprotein IIb/IIIa complex when platelets are stimulated with thrombin. Blood 64: 797–800

Grant R A, Zucker M B, McPherson J 1976 ADP-induced inhibition of von Willebrand factor-mediated platelet agglutination. American Journal of Physiology 230: 1406

Greenberg J P, Packham M A, Guccione M A, Rand M L, Reimers H-J, Mustard J F 1979 Survival of rabbit platelets treated in vitro with chymotrypsin, plasmin, trypsin or neuraminidase. Blood 53: 916

Greenberg-Sepersky S M, Simons E R, White J G 1985 Studies of platelets from patients with the grey platelet syndrome. British Journal of Haematology 59: 603–609

Greinacher A, Müller-Eckhardt C 1990 Hereditary types of thrombocytopenia with giant platelets and inclusion bodies in the leukocytes. Blut 60: 53–60

Grottum K A, Solum N O 1969 Congenital thrombocytopenia with giant platelets: a defect in the platelet membrane. British Journal of Haematology 16: 277–290

Grottum K A, Hovig T, Holmsen H, Abrahamsen A F, Jeremic M, Seys M 1969 Wiskott-Aldrich syndrome: Qualitative platelet defects in short platelet survival. British Journal of Haematology 17: 373–387

Gruel Y, Boizard B, Daffos F, Forestier F, Caen J, Wautier J L 1986 Determination of platelet antigens and glycoproteins in the human fetus. Blood 68: 488–492

Guarisco J L, Cheney M L, Ohene-Frempong K, LeJeune F E, Blair P A 1987 Limited septoplasty as treatment for recurrent epistaxis in a child with Glanzmann's thrombasthenia. Laryngoscope 97: 336–338

Hagen I, Nurden A T, Bjerrum O J, Solum N O, Caen J 1980 Immunochemical evidence for protein abnormalities in platelets from patients with Glanzmann's thrombasthenia and Bernard–Soulier syndrome. Journal of Clinical Investigation 65: 722–731

Hagen I, Brosstad F, Solum N O, Korsmo R 1981 Crossed immunoelectrophoresis using immobilized thrombin in intermediate gel. Journal of Laboratory and Clinical Medicine 97: 213–220

Hagen I, Bjerrum O J, Gogstad G, Korsmo R, Solum N O 1982 Involvement of divalent cations in the complex between platelet glycoproteins IIb and IIIa. Biochemical et Biophysical Acta 701: 1–6

Handagama P J, Shuman M A, Bainton D F 1989 Incorporation of intravenously injected albumin, immunoglobulin G, and fibrinogen in guinea pig megakaryocyte granules. Journal of Clinical Investigation 84: 73–82

Handagama P J, Rappolee D A, Werb Z, Levin J, Bainton D F 1990 Platelet alpha-granule fibrinogen, albumin, and immunoglobulin G are not synthesized by rat and mouse megakaryocytes. Journal of Clinical Investigation 86: 1364–1368

Hantgan R R 1987 An investigation of fibrin-platelet adhesive interactions by microfluorimetry. Biochemical et Biophysical Acta 927: 5

Hardisty R M, Dormandy K M, Hutton R A 1964 Thrombasthenia: Studies on three cases. British Journal of Haematology 10: 371

Hardisty R M, Mills D C B, Ketsa-Ard K 1972 The platelet defect associated with albinism. British Journal of Haematology 23: 679–692

Hardisty R M, Machin S J, Nokes T J C et al 1983 A new congenital defect of platelet secretion: Impaired responsiveness of the platelets to cytoplasmic free calcium. British Journal of Haematology 53: 543

Harfenist E J, Packham M A, Mustard J F 1984 Effect of variant gamma chains and sialic acid content of fibrinogen upon its interactions with ADP-stimulated human and rabbit platelets. Blood 64: 1163

Harmon J T, Jamieson G A 1986 The glycocalicin portion of platelet glycoprotein Ib expresses both high and moderate affinity receptor sites for thrombin. Journal of Biological Chemistry 28: 13224–13229

Harrison P, Wilbourn B R, Debili N et al 1989 Uptake of plasma fibrinogen into the alpha granules of human megakaryocytes and platelets. Journal of Clinical Investigation 84: 1320–1324

Harrison P, Cramer E M, Wilbourn B R et al 1990 The influence of therapeutic blockage of GPIIb/IIIa on platelet alpha-granule fibrinogen. Blood 76(suppl 1): 458a (abstract)

Hathaway W E, Solomons C C, Ott J E 1972 Platelet function and pyrophosphates in osteogenesis imperfecta. Blood 39: 500

Haverstick D M, Cowan J F, Yamada K M, Santoro S A 1985 Inhibition of platelet adhesion to fibronectin, fibrinogen and von Willebrand factor substrates by a synthetic tetrapeptide derived from the cell-binding domain of fibronectin. Blood 66: 946

Heal J Rowe J, Blumberg N 1991 The importance of ABO identical platelet transfusions. Blood 78(suppl 1): 348a (abstract)

Heidenreich R, Eisman R, Surrey S et al 1990 Organization of the gene for platelet glycoprotein IIb. Biochemistry 29: 1232–1244

Heptinstall S, Taylor P M 1979 The effects of citrate and extracellular calcium ions on the platelet release reaction induced by adenosine diphosphate and collagen. Thrombosis Haemostasis 42: 778–793

Hermann F H, Meyer M, Gogstad G O, Solum N O 1982 Glycoprotein IIb-IIIa complex in platelets of patients and the heterozygotes of Glanzmann's thrombasthenia. Thrombosis Research 32: 615–621

Herve P, Drouet L, Dosquet C et al 1990 Primary pulmonary hypertension in a patient with a familial platelet storage pool disease: Role of serotonin. American Journal of Medicine 89: 117–120

Heslop H E, Hickton C M, Laird E, Tait J D, Doig J R, Beard E J 1986 Twin pregnancy and parturition in a patient with the Bernard–Soulier syndrome. Scandanavian Journal of Haematology 37: 71–73

Heyns A P, Badenhorst P N, Wessels P, Pieters H, Lotter M G 1985 Kinetics, in vivo redistribution and sites of sequestration of indium-111-labelled platelets in giant platelet syndromes. British Journal of Haematology 60: 323–330

Hickey M J, Williams S A, Roth G J 1989 Human platelet glycoprotein IX: An adhesive prototype of leucine-rich glycoproteins with flank-center-flank structures. Proceedings of the National Academy of Sciences, USA 86: 6773

Hickey M J, Deaven L L, Roth G J 1990 Human platelet glycoprotein IX: Characterization of 'full-length' cDNA and localization to chromosome 3. FEBS Letter 274: 189–192

Higgins E A, Siminovitch K A, Zhuang D L, Brockhausen I, Dennis J W 1991 Aberrant O-linked oligosaccharide biosynthesis in lymphocytes and platelets from patients with the Wiskott–Aldrich syndrome. Journal of Biological Chemistry 266: 6280–6290

Hillery C A, Smyth S S, Parise L V 1991 Phosphorylation of human platelet glycoprotein IIIa (GPIIIa). Journal of Biological Chemistry 266: 14663–14669

Holmsen H 1990a Metabolism of platelets. In: Williams W J, Beutler E, Erslev A J, Lichtman M A (eds) Hematology, 4th edn. McGraw-Hill, New York, p 1182–1200

Holmsen H 1990b Composition of platelets. In: Williams W J, Beutler E, Erslev A J, Lichtman M A (eds) Hematology, 4th edn. McGraw-Hill, New York, p 1200–1232

Holmsen H, Weiss H J 1970 Hereditary defect in the platelet release reaction caused by a deficiency in the storage pool of platelet adenine nucleotides. British Journal of Haematology 19: 643–649

Holmsen H, Weiss H J 1972 Further evidence for a deficient storage pool of adenine nucleotides on platelets from some patients with thrombocytopathia-storage pool disease. Blood 39: 197–209

Holmsen H, Setkowsky C A, Lages B, Day H J, Weiss H J, Scrutton M C 1975 Content and thrombin-induced release of acid hydrolases in gel-filtered platelets from patients with storage pool disease. Blood 46: 131–142

Holmsen H, Walsh P N, Koike K et al 1987 Familial bleeding disorder associated with deficiencies in platelet signal processing and glycoproteins. British Journal of Haematology 67: 335

Horrelou M H, Lecompte T, Lecrubier C et al 1983 Familial and constitutional bleeding disorder due to platelet cyclooxygenase deficiency. American Journal of Hematology 14: 1

Hourdille' P, Pico M, Jandrot-Perrus M, Lacaze D, Lozano M, Nurden A T 1990 Studies on the megakaryocytes of a patient with the Bernard–Soulier syndrome. British Journal of Haematology 76: 521–530

Howard M A, Hutton R A, Hardisty R M 1973 Hereditary giant platelet syndrome: A disorder of a new aspect of platelet function. British Medical Journal 586–588

Howard M A, Perkin J, Salem H H, Firkin B G 1984 The agglutination of human platelets by botrocetin: Evidence that botrocetin and ristocetin act at different sites on the factor VIII molecule and platelet membrane. British Journal of Haematology 57: 25–35

Hughes J, Caen J P, Hardisty R M, O'Brien J R 1971 Discussion in round-the-table conference on normal and modified platelet aggregation. Acta Medica Scandinavica 525(suppl): 204–205

Ikeda H, Mitani T, Ohnuma M et al 1989 A new platelet-specific antigen, Nak(a), involved in the refractoriness of HLA-matched platelet transfusion. Vox Sanguinis 57: 213

Ikeda Y, Handa M, Kawano K et al 1991 The role of von Willebrand factor and fibrinogen in platelet aggregation under varying shear stress. Journal of Clinical Investigation 87: 1234–1240

Ingerman-Wojenski C M, Smith J B, Silver M J 1982 Use of the whole-blood aggregometer to study the aggregation of 'giant' platelets. Thrombosis Research 27: 371–376

Ingerslev J, Stenbjerg S, Taaning E 1987 A case of Bernard–Soulier syndrome: study of platelet glycoprotein Ib in a kindred. European Journal of Hematology 39: 182–184

Jamieson G A, Okumura T 1978 Reduced thrombin binding and aggregation in Bernard–Soulier platelets. Journal of Clinical Investigation 61: 1861

Jamieson G A, Okumura T, Fishback B, Johnson M M, Egan J J, Weiss H J 1979 Platelet membrane glycoproteins in thrombasthenia, Bernard–Soulier syndrome, and storage pool disease. Journal of Laboratory and Clinical Medicine 93: 652–660

Jandrot-Perrus M, Rendu F, Caen J P, Levy Toledano S, Guillin M C 1990 The common pathway for alpha- and gamma-thrombin-induced platelet activation is independent of GPIb: a study of Bernard–Soulier platelets. British Journal of Haematology 75: 385–392

Jasmin J R, Dupont D, Velin P 1987 Multiple dental extractions in a child with Glanzmann's thrombasthenia: report of case. Journal of Dentistry for Children 54: 208–210

Jennings L K, Ashmun R A, Wang W C, Dockter M E 1986 Analysis of human platelet glycoproteins IIb-IIIa in Glanzmann's thrombasthenia in whole blood by flow cytometry. Blood 68: 173–179

Jennings L K, Wang W C, Jackson C W, Fox C F, Bell A 1991 Hemostasis in Glanzmann's thrombasthenia (GT): GT platelets interfere with the aggregation of normal platelets. American Journal of Pediatric Hematology and Oncology 13: 84–90

Jordan R, Wagner C, Mattis J, Weisman H, Coller B S 1991 Evidence that anti-GPIIb/IIIa monoclonal antibodies bind bivalently to platelets and that the actual GPIIb/IIIa copy numbers is ≈80 000, not ≈40 000. Thrombosis Haemostasis 65: 828(abstract)

Jung S M, Plow E F, Moroi M 1986 Polymorphism of platelet glycoprotein Ib in the United States. Thrombosis Research 42: 83

Jung S M, Yoshida N, Aoki N, Tanoue K, Yamazaki H, Moroi M 1988 Thrombasthenia with an abnormal platelet membrane glycoprotein IIb of different molecular weight. Blood 71: 915–922

Kalomiris E L, Coller B S 1985 Thiol-specific probes indicate that the beta-chain of platelet glycoprotein Ib is a transmembrane protein with a reactive endofacial sulfhydryl group. Biochemistry 24: 5430

Kaplan C, Patereau C, Reznikoff-Etievant M F, Muller J Y, Dumez Y, Kesseler A 1985 Antenatal $P1^{A1}$ typing and detection of GPIIb-IIIa complex. British Journal of Haematology 60: 586–587

Karpatkin S, Weiss H J 1972 Deficiency of glutathione peroxidase associated with high levels of reduced glutathione in Glanzmann's thrombasthenia. New England Journal of Medicine 287: 1062

Karpatkin M, Howard L, Karpatkin S 1984 Studies of the origin of platelet-associated fibrinogen. Journal of Laboratory and Clinical Medicine 104: 223–237

Katagiri Y, Hayashi Y, Yamamoto K, Tanoue K, Kosaki G, Yamazaki H 1990 Localization of von Willebrand factor and thrombin-interactive domains on human platelet glycoprotein Ibβ. Thrombosis and Haemostasis 63: 122

Kehrel B, Balleisen L, Kokott R et al 1988 Deficiency of intact thrombospondin and membrane glycoprotein Ia in platelets with defective collagen-induced aggregation and spontaneous loss of disorder. Blood 71: 1074–1078

Kehrel B, Kokott R, Stenzinger W, Balleisen L 1988 Analysis of platelet glycoproteins in thrombocytopathias using the lectin-avidin-biotin-peroxidase (LABP) technique. Folia Haematologie (Leipzig) 115: 425–429

Kelly T, Molony L, Burridge K 1987 Purification of two smooth muscle glycoproteins related to integrin: Distribution in cultured chicken embryo fibroblasts. Journal of Biological Chemistry 262: 17189

Khanduri W, Pulimood R, Sudarsanam A, Corman R H, Jadhav M, Pereira S 1981 Glanzmann's thrombasthenia: a review and report of 42 cases from South India. Thrombosis Haemostasis 46: 717–721

Kloczewiak M, Timmons S, Lukas T J, Hawiger J 1984 Platelet receptor recognition site on human fibrinogen. Synthesis and structure–function relationship of peptides corresponding to the carboxy-terminal segment of the gamma chain. Biochemistry 23: 1767

Kobrinsky N L, Israels E D, Gerrard J M et al 1984 Shortening of bleeding time by 1-deamino-8-D-arginine vasopressin in various bleeding disorders. Lancet 1: 1145

Kohler M 1988 Treatment of gray platelet syndrome. Thrombosis and Haemostasis 60: 123–124

Kohler M, Hellstern P, Morgenstern E et al 1985 Gray platelet syndrome: Selective alpha-granule deficiency and thrombocytopenia due to increased platelet turnover. Blut 50: 331–340

Koike K, Rao A K, Holmsen H et al 1984 Platelet secretion defect in patients with the attention deficit disorder and easy bruising. Blood 63: 427

Kolodziej M A, Vilaire G, Gonder D, Poncz M, Bennett J S 1991 Study of the endoproteolytic cleavage of platelet glycoprotein IIb using oligonucleotide-mediated mutagenesis. Journal of Biological Chemistry 266: 23499–23504

Krissansen G W, Elliott M J, Lucas C M et al 1990 Identification of a novel integrin beta subunit expressed on cultured monocytes (macrophages). Journal of Biological Chemistry 265: 823–830

Krizek D M, Rick M E, Williams S B, Gralnick H R 1982 Cryoprecipitate transfusion in variant von Willebrand's disease and thrombocytopenia. Annals of Internal Medicine 98: 484

Krolls M H, Schafer A I 1989 Biochemical mechanisms of platelet activation. Blood 74: 1181–1195

Kuijpers R W A M, Faber N M, Cuypers H Th M, Ouwehand W H, von dem Borne A E G Kr 1992 NH_2-terminal globular domain of human platelet glycoprotein Ib-alpha has a methionine^{145}/threonine^{145} amino acid polymorphism, which is associated with the HPA-2 (Ko) alloantigens. Journal of Clinical Investigation 89: 381–384

Kunicki T J, Pidard D, Cazenave J P, Nurden A T, Caen J P 1981a Inheritance of the human platelet alloantigen $P1^{A1}$, in type I Glanzmann's thrombasthenia. Journal of Clinical Investigation 67: 717

Kunicki T J, Pidard D, Rosa J P, Nurden A T 1981b The formation of calcium-dependent complexes of platelet membrane glycoproteins IIb and IIIa in solution as determined by crossed immunoelectrophoresis. Blood 58: 268

Kunicki T J, Nugent D J, Staats S J, Orchekowski R P, Wayner E A, Carter W G 1988 The human fibroblast class II extracellular matrix receptor mediates platelet adhesion to collagen and is identical to the platelet glycoprotein Ia-IIa complex. Journal of Biological Chemistry 263: 4516

Kuramoto A, Steiner M, Baldini M G 1970 Lack of platelet response to stimulation in the Wiskott–Aldrich syndrome. New England Journal of Medicine 282: 475

Lagarde M, Byron P A, Vargaftig B B et al 1978 Impairment of platelet thromboxane A_2 generation and of the platelet release reaction in two patients with congenital deficiency of platelet cyclooxygenase. British Journal of Haematology 38: 251

Lages B, Weiss H J 1988a Impairment of phosphatidylinositol metabolism in a patient with a bleeding disorder associated with defects of initial platelet responses. Thrombosis Haemostasis 59: 175

Lages B, Weiss H J 1988b Heterogeneous defects of platelet secretion and responses to weak agonists in patients with bleeding disorders. British Journal of Haematology 68: 53

Lages B, Scrutton M C, Holmsen H, Day H J, Weiss H J 1975 Metal ion contents of gel-filtered platelets from patients with storage pool disease. Blood 46: 119–130

Lages B, Malmstein C, Weiss H J et al 1981 Impaired platelet response to thromboxane-A_2 and defective calcium mobilization in a patient with a bleeding disorder. Blood 57: 545

Lages B, Shattil S J, Bainton D F, Weiss H J 1991 Decreased content and surface expression of alpha-granule membrane protein GMP-140 in one of two types of platelet alpha delta storage pool deficiency. Journal of Clinical Investigation 87: 919–929

Lam S C T, Plow E F, D'Souza S E, Cheresh D A, Frelinger A L, III, Ginsberg M H 1989 Isolation and characterization of a platelet membrane protein related to the vitronectin receptor. Journal of Biological Chemistry 264: 3742

Lanza E, Stierle A, Fournier D et al 1991 A new variant of Glanzmann's thrombasthenia: platelets with functionally defective GPIIb-IIIa complexes and a GPIIIa $ARG^{214} \rightarrow TRP^{214}$ mutation. Blood 78(suppl 1): 1570 (abstract)

Larsen N E, Simons E R 1981 Preparation and application of a photoreactive thrombin analogue: Binding to human platelets. Biochemistry 20: 4141–4147

Lawler J, Hynes R O 1989 An integrin receptor on normal and thrombasthenic platelets which binds thrombospondin. Blood 74: 2022

Lawrence J B, Gralnick H R 1987 Monoclonal antibodies to the glycoprotein IIb-IIIa epitopes involved in adhesive protein binding: effects on platelet spreading and ultrastructure on human arterial subendothelium. Journal of Laboratory and Clinical Medicine 109: 495–503

Lecompte T 1988 Hereditary thrombocytopenias. Current Studies in Hematology Blood Transfusions 55: 162–173

Lee H, Nurden A T, Thomaidis A, Caen J P 1981 Relationship between fibrinogen binding and platelet glycoprotein deficiencies in Glanzmann's thrombasthenia type I and type II. British Journal of Haematology 48: 47

Levy-Toledano S, Tobelem G, Legrand C et al 1978 Acquired IgG antibody occurring in a thrombasthenic patient: Its effect on human platelet function. Blood 51: 1065

Levy-Toledano S, Caen J P, Breton-Gorius J et al 1981 Gray platelet syndrome: alpha granule deficiency. Journal of Laboratory and Clinical Medicine 98: 831

Loftus J C, Plow E F, Jennings L K, Ginsberg M H 1988 Alternative proteolytic processing of platelet membrane glycoprotein IIb. Journal of Biological Chemistry 263: 11025–11028

Loftus J C, O'Toole T E, Plow E F, Glass A, Frelinger III A L, Ginsberg M H 1990 A β_3 integrin mutation abolishes ligand binding and alters divalent cation-dependent conformation. Science 249: 915–918

Lopez J A, Ludwig E H 1991 Molecular basis of platelet glycoprotein Ib polymorphism. Clinical Research 39: 327A (Abstract)

Lopez J A, Chung D W, Fujikawa K, Hagen F S, Papayannopoulou T, Roth G J 1987 Cloning of the alpha chain of human platelet glycoprotein Ib: A transmembrane protein with homology to leucine-rich $alpha_2$ glycoprotein. Proceedings of the National Academy of Sciences, USA 84: 5616

Lopez J A, Chung D W, Fujikawa K, Hagen F S, Davie E W, Roth G J 1988 The alpha and beta chains of human platelet glycoprotein Ib are both transmembrane proteins containing a leucine-rich amino acid sequence. Proceedings of the National Academy of Sciences, USA 85: 2135

Lorez H P, Richards J G, Da Prada M et al 1979 Storage pool disease: Comparative fluorescence microscopical, cytochemical and biochemical studies on amine-storing organelles of human blood platelets. British Journal of Haematology 43: 297–305

Lum L G, Tubergen D G, Corash L, Blaese R M 1980 Splenectomy in the management of the thrombocytopenia of the Wiskott–Aldrich syndrome. New England Journal of Medicine 302: 892–896

McEver R P, Baenziger N L, Majerus P W 1980 Isolation and quantitation of the platelet membrane glycoprotein deficient in thrombasthenia using a monoclonal hybridoma antibody. Journal of Clinical Investigation 66: 1311–1318

McEver R P, Bennett E M, Martin M N 1983 Identification of two structurally and functionally distinct sites on human platelet membrane glycoprotein IIb-IIIa using monoclonal antibodies. Journal of Biological Chemistry 258: 5269–5275

McGill M, Jamieson G A, Drouin J, Cho M S, Rock G A 1984 Morphometric analysis of platelets in Bernard–Soulier syndrome: size and configuration in patients and carriers. Thrombosis Haemostasis 52: 37–41

McGowan E B, Ding A, Detwiler T C 1983 Correlation of thrombin-induced glycoprotein V hydrolysis and platelet activation. Journal of Biological Chemistry 258: 11243

McMichael A J, Rust N A, Pilch J R et al 1981 Monoclonal antibody to human platelet glycoprotein I. I. Immunological studies. British Journal of Haematology 49: 501

Malmsten C, Hamberg M, Svensson J et al 1975 Physiological role of an endoperoxide in human platelets: Hemostatic defect due to platelet cyclooxygenase deficiency. Proceedings of the National Academy of Sciences, USA 72: 1446

Malmsten C, Kindahl H, Samuelsson B, Levy-Toledano S, Tobelem G, Caen J P 1977 Thromboxane synthesis and the platelet release reaction in Bernard–Soulier syndrome, thrombasthenia Glanzmann and Hermansky-Pudlak syndrome. British Journal of Haematology 35: 511–520

Mannucci P M 1986 Desmopressin (DDAVP) for treatment of disorders of hemostasis. Progress in Hemostasis and Thrombosis 8: 19

Mannucci P M 1988 Desmopressin: A nontransfusional form of treatment for congenital and acquired bleeding disorders. Blood 72: 1449

Mannucci P M, Vianello V V, Cattaneo M et al 1986 Controlled trial of desmopressin in liver cirrhosis and other conditions associated with a prolonged bleeding time. Blood 67: 1148

Mant M J 1988 DDAVP in Bernard–Soulier syndrome. Thrombosis Research 52: 77–78

Marcus A J 1987 Platelet eicosanoid metabolism. In: Colman R W, Hirsh J, Marder V J, Salzman E W (eds) Hemostasis and thrombosis: basic principles and clinical practice. Lippincott, Philadelphia, p 676–688

Marti G E, Magruder L, Schuette W E, Gralnick H R 1988 Flow cytometric analysis of platelet surface antigens. Cytometry 9: 448–455

Mestel F, Oetliker O, Beck E et al 1980 Severe bleeding associated with defective thromboxane synthetase. Lancet 1: 157

Meyer M, Herrmann F H 1985 Diversity of glycoprotein deficiencies in Glanzmann's thrombasthenia. Thrombosis and Haemostasis 54: 626–629

Michalas S, Malamitsi-Puchner A, Tsevrenis H 1984 Pregnancy and delivery in Bernard–Soulier syndrome. Acta Obstetrics and Gynecology Scandanavia 63: 185–186

Michelson A D 1987 Flow cytometric analysis of platelet surface glycoproteins: phenotypically distinct subpopulations of platelets in children with chronic myeloid leukemia. Journal of Laboratory and Clinical Medicine 110: 346–354

Miles L A, Ginsberg M H, White J G, Plow E F 1986 Plasminogen interacts with human platelets through two distinct mechanisms. Journal of Clinical Investigation 77: 2001–2009

Miletich J P, Kane W H, Hofmann S L, Stanford N, Majerus P W 1979 Deficiency of factor Xa-factor Va binding sites on the platelets of a patient with a bleeding disorder. Blood 54: 1015

Miller J L 1984 Platelet-type von Willebrand's disease. Clinical Laboratory Medicine 4: 319

Miller J L, Castella A 1982 Platelet-type von Willebrand's disease: Characterization of a new bleeding disorder. Blood 60: 790–794

Miller J L, Kupinski J M, Castella A, Ruggeri Z M 1983 Von Willebrand factor binds to platelets and induces aggregation in platelet-type but not type IIb von Willebrand disease. Journal of Clinical Investigation 72: 1532

Miller J L, Cunningham D, Lyle V A, Finch C N 1991 Mutation in the gene encoding the alpha chain of platelet glycoprotein Ib in platelet-type von Willebrand disease. Proceedings of the National Academy of Sciences USA 88: 4761–4765

Miller J L, Lyle V A, Cunningham D 1992 Mutation of Leucine-57 phenylalanine in a platelet glycoprotein Ib α-leucine tandem repeat occurring in patients with an autosomal dominant variant of Bernard–Soulier disease. Blood 79: 439–446

Minkoff I M, Wu K K, Walasek J et al 1980 Bleeding disorder due to an isolated platelet factor 3 deficiency. Annals of Internal Medicine 140: 366

Mirghani A M, Ahmed M O, Al-Sohaibani S A et al 1988 Inherited bleeding disorders in the eastern province of Saudi Arabia. Acta Haematology 79: 202–206

Moake J L, Olson J D, Troll J H, Tang S S, Funicella T, Peterson D M 1980 Binding of radioiodinated human von Willebrand factor to Bernard–Soulier, thrombasthenic and von Willebrand's disease platelets. Thrombosis Research 19: 21–27

Modderman P W, van Mourik J A, van Berkel W et al 1989 Decreased stability and structural heterogeneity of the residual platelet glycoprotein IIb/IIIa complex in a variant of Glanzmann's thrombasthenia. British Journal of Haematology 73: 514–521

Montgomery R R, Kunicki T J, Taves C et al 1983 Diagnosis of Bernard–Soulier syndrome and Glanzmann's thrombasthenia with a monoclonal assay on whole blood. Journal of Clinical Investigation 71: 385

Mori K, Suzuki S, Sugai K 1984 Electron microscopic and functional studies on platelets in gray platelet syndrome. Tohoku Journal of Experimental Medicine 143: 261–287

Moroi M, Jung S M, Yoshida N 1984 Genetic polymorphism of platelet glycoprotein Ib. Blood 64: 622

Moroi M, Jung S M, Okuma M, Shinmyozu K 1989 A patient with platelets deficient in glycoprotein VI that lack both collagen-induced aggregation and adhesion. Journal of Clinical Investigation 84: 1440–1445

Moser K 1968 A hitherto not described enzyme defect in thrombasthenia: glutathione reductase deficiency. Thrombosis Haemostasis 19: 46

Murata M, Ware J, Ruggeri Z M 1991 Expression of a soluble domain of GPIbα with structural and functional properties of the intact platelet receptor. Thrombosis Haemostasis 65: 771 (abstract)

Murphy S, Oski F A, Naiman J L, Lusch C J, Goldberg S, Gardner F H 1972 Platelet size and kinetics in hereditary and acquired thrombocytopenia. New England Journal of Medicine 286: 499–504

Mustard J F, Kinlough-Rathbone R L, Packham M A, Perry D W, Harfenist E J, Pai KRM 1979 Comparison of fibrinogen association with normal and thrombasthenia platelets on exposure to ADP or chymotrypsin. Blood 54: 987–993

Muszbek L, Laposata M 1989 Glycoprotein Ib and glycoprotein IX in human platelets are acylated with palmitic acid through thioester linkages. Journal of Biological Chemistry 264: 9716

Nathan D G 1980 Splenectomy in the Wiskott–Aldrich syndrome. New England Journal of Medicine 302: 916–917

Nermut M V, Green N M, Eason P, Yamada S S, Yamada K M 1988 Electron microscopy and structural model of human fibronectin receptor. European Molecular Biology Organisation Journal 7: 4093

Newman P J 1991 Platelet GPIIb-IIIa: Molecular variations and alloantigens. Thrombosis and Haemostasis 66: 111–118

Newman P J, Allen R W, Kahn R A, Kunicki T J 1985 Quantitation of membrane glycoprotein IIIa on intact human platelets using the monoclonal antibody, AP-3. Blood 65: 227

Newman P J, Kawai Y, Montgomery R R, Kunicki T J 1986 Synthesis by cultured human umbilical vein endothelial cells of two proteins structurally and immunologically related to platelet membrane glycoproteins IIb and IIIa. Journal of Cell Biology 103: 81

Newman P J, Seligsohn U, Lyman S, Coller B S 1991 The molecular genetic basis of Glanzmann thrombasthenia in the Iraqi-Jewish and Arab populations in Israel. Proceedings of the National Academy of Sciences, USA 88: 3160–3164

Nichols W L, Kaese S E, Gastineau D A, Otteman L A, Bowie E J 1989 Bernard–Soulier syndrome: whole blood diagnostic assays of platelets. Mayo Clinical Proceedings 64: 522–530

Nichols W L, Daniels T M, Fisher P K, Owen W G, Figueroa P I, Pineda A A 1991 Inhibitors of coagulation factor V and thrombin associated with surgical use of topical bovine thrombin or fibrin 'glue'. Blood 78(suppl 1): 63A (abstract)

Nieuwenhuis H K, Sixma J J 1988 1-Desamino 8 D-arginine vasopressin (Desmopressin) shortens the bleeding time in storage pool deficiency. Annals of Internal Medicine 108: 65

Nieuwenhuis H K, Akkerman J W N, Houdijk W P M, Sixma J J 1985 Human blood platelets showing no response to collagen fail to express surface glycoprotein Ia. Nature 318: 470–472

Nieuwenhuis H K, Sakariassen K S, Houdijk W P M, Nievelstein P F E M, Sixma J J 1986 Deficiency of platelet membrane glycoprotein Ia associated with a decreased platelet adhesion to subendothelium: A defect in platelet spreading. Blood 68: 692–695

Nieuwenhuis H K, Akkerman J W, Sixma J J 1987 Patients with a prolonged bleeding time and normal aggregation tests may have storage pool deficiency: Studies on one hundred and six patients. Blood 70: 620

Niewiarowski S, Holt J C 1987 Biochemistry and physiology of secreted platelet proteins. In: Colman R W, Hirsh J, Marder V J Salzman E W (eds) Hemostasis and thrombosis: basic principles and clinical practice, 2nd edn. Lippincott, Philadelphia, p 618–630

Niiya K, Hodson E, Bader R et al 1987 Increased surface expression of the membrane glycoprotein IIb/IIIa complex induced by platelet activation. Relationship to the binding of fibrinogen and platelet aggregation. Blood 70: 475

Nilsson I M, Magnusson S, Borchgrevink C 1963 The Duke and Ivy methods for determination of bleeding time. Thrombosis Diathesis et Haemorrhagica 10: 223

Nishio K, Fujimura Y, Niinomi K et al 1990 Enhanced botrocetin-induced type IIB von Willebrand factor binding to platelet glycoprotein Ib initiates hyperagglutination of normal platelets. American Journal of Haematology 33: 261–266

Nurden A T 1985 Glycoprotein defects responsible for abnormal platelet function in inherited platelet disorders. In: George J N, Nuerden A T, Phillips D R (eds) Platelet membrane glycoproteins. Plenum, New York, p 357

Nurden A T 1989 Congenital abnormalities of platelet membrane glycoproteins. In: Kunicki T J, George J N (eds) Platelet immunobiology, molecular and clinical aspects. Lippincott, Philadelphia, 95

Nurden A T, Caen J P 1974 An abnormal platelet glycoprotein pattern in three cases of Glanzmann's thrombasthenia. British Journal of Haematology 28: 253

Nurden A T, Caen J P 1975 Specific roles for platelet surface glycoproteins in platelet function. Nature 255: 720

Nurden A T, Dupuis D, Kunicki T J, Caen J P 1981 Analysis of the glycoprotein and protein composition of Bernard–Soulier platelets by single and two-dimensional sodium dodecyl sulfate-polyacrylamide gel electrophoresis. Journal of Clinical Investigation 67: 1431

Nurden A T, Kunicki T J, Dupuis D, Soria C, Caen J P 1982 Specific protein and glycoprotein deficiencies in platelets isolated from two patients with the grey platelet syndrome. Blood 59: 709–718

Nurden A T, Didry D, Rosa J P 1983 Molecular defects of platelets in Bernard–Soulier syndrome. Blood Cells 9: 333–358

Nurden A T, Didry D, Kieffer N, McEver R P 1985 Residual amounts of glycoproteins IIb and IIIa may be present in the platelets of most patients with Glanzmann's thrombasthenia. Blood 65: 1021

Nurden A T, George J N, Phillips D R 1986 Human platelet membrane glycoproteins. In: Shuman M, Phillips D R (eds) Biochemistry of the platelet. Academic Press, New York, p 159–224

Nurden A T, Rosa J P, Fournier D et al 1987 A variant of Glanzmann's thrombasthenia with abnormal glycoprotein IIb-IIIa complexes in the platelet membrane. Journal of Clinical Investigation 79: 962–969

Nurden A T, Rosa J P, Fournier D et al 1987 A variant of Glanzmann's thrombasthenia with abnormal GPIIb-IIIa complexes in the platelet membrane. Journal of Clinical Investigation 79: 962–969

Nurden A T, Jallu V, Hourdille' P 1989 GP Ib and Bernard–Soulier platelets. Blood 73: 2225–2227

O'Toole T E, Loftus J C, Plow E F, Glass A A, Harper J R, Ginsberg M H 1989 Efficient surface expression of platelet GPIIb-IIIa requires both subunits. Blood 74: 14–18

O'Toole T E, Loftus J C, Du X et al 1990 Affinity modulation of the alpha IIb-beta$_3$ integrin (platelet GPIIb-IIIa) is an intrinsic property of the receptor. Cell Regulation 1: 883–893

O'Toole T E, Mandelman D, Forsyth J, Shattil S J, Plow E F, Ginsberg M H 1991 Modulation of the affinity of integrin $^{\alpha}{}_{IIb}{}^{\beta}{}_{3}$ (GPIIb-IIIa) by the cytoplasmic domain of α_{IIb}. Science 845: 847

Ochs H D, Slichter S J, Harker L A, Von Behrens W E, Clark R A, Wedgwood R J 1980 The Wiskott-Aldrich syndrome: Studies of lymphocytes, granulocytes, and platelets. Blood 55: 243–252

Oki Y, Yoshioka K, Konishi M et al 1987 A case of Bernard–Soulier syndrome. Nippon Naika Gakkai Zasshi 76: 1414–1418

Onel D, Ulutin S B, Ulutin O N 1973 Platelet defect in a case of Ehlers–Danlos syndrome. Acta Haematology 50: 238

Oquendo P, Hundt E, Lawler J, Seed B 1989 CD36 directly mediates cytoadherence of Plasmodium falciparum infected erythrocytes. Cell 58: 95

Ormerod A D 1985 The Wiskott-Aldrich syndrome. Inernational Journal of Dermatology 24: 77–80

Pareti F I, Day H J, Mills D C B 1974 Nucleotide and serotonin metabolism in platelets with defective secondary aggregation. Blood 44: 789–800

Pareti F I, Mannucci P M, D'Angelo A et al 1980 Congenital deficiency of thromboxane and prostacyclin. Lancet 1: 898

Parise L V, Criss A B, Nanizzi L, Wardell M R 1990 Glycoprotein IIIa is phosphorylated in intact human platelets. Blood 75: 2363–2368

Parise L V, Steiner B, Nannizzi L, Phillips D R 1992 Evidence for novel binding sites on the platelet glycoprotein IIb and IIIa subunits for fibrinogen. Biochemical Journal 289: 445–451

Park J K, Rosenstein Y J, Remold-O'Donnell E, Bierer B E, Rosen F S, Burakoff S J 1991 Enhancement of T-cell activation by the CD43 molecule whose expression is defective in Wiskott-Aldrich syndrome. Nature 350: 706–709

Parkman R, Remold-O'Donnell E, Kenney D M, Perrine S, Rosen F S 1981 Surface protein abnormalities in lymphocytes and platelets from patients with Wiskott-Aldrich syndrome. Lancet 1387–1389

Paulus J M, Aster R H 1990 Clinical evaluation of thrombokinetics. In: Williams W J, Beutler E, Erslev A J, Lichtman M A (eds) Hematology 4th edn. McGraw-Hill, New York, p 1260–1266

Peaceman A M, Katz A R, Laville M 1989 Bernard–Soulier syndrome complicating pregnancy: a case report. Obstetrics and Gynecology 73: 457–459

Peerschke E I 1985 Platelet fibrinogen receptors. Seminars in Hematology 22: 241–259

Peerschke E I B, Francis C W, Marder V J 1986 Fibrinogen binding to human blood platelets: Effect of gamma chain carboxyterminal structure and length. Blood 67: 385

Peerschke E I B 1988 Irreversible platelet fibrinogen interactions occur independently of fibrinogen alpha chain degradation and are not mediated by intact platelet membrane glycoprotein IIb-IIIa complexes. Journal of Laboratory and Clinical Medicine 111: 84–92

Peerschke E I B 1989 Decreased accessibility of platelet-bound fibrinogen to antibody and enzyme probes. Blood 74: 682–689

Peretz H, Seligsohn U, Zwang E, Coller B S, Newman P J 1991 Detection of the Glanzmann's thrombasthenia mutations in Arab and Iraqi-Jewish patients by polymerase chain reaction and restriction analysis of blood or urine samples. Thrombosis and Haemostasis 66: 500–504

Perret B, Levy-Toledano S, Plantavid M et al 1983 Abnormal phospholipid organization in Bernard–Soulier platelets. Thrombosis Research 31: 529–537

Peterson D M, Stathopoulos N A, Giorgio T D, Hellums J D, Moake J L 1987 Shear-induced platelet aggregation requires von Willebrand factor and platelet membrane glycoproteins Ib and IIb-IIIa. Blood 69: 625–628

Peyser H R, Kupfermine M J 1990 Management of severe postpartum hemorrhage by intrauterine irrigation with prostaglandin E_1. American Journal of Obstetrics and Gynecology 162: 694–696

Pfueller S L, David R 1988 Platelet-associated immunoglobulins G, A and M are secreted during platelet activation: normal levels but defective secretion in grey platelet syndrome. British Journal of Haematology 68: 235–241

Pfueller S L, Howard M A, White J G, Menon C, Berry E W 1987 Shortening of bleeding time by 1-deamino-8-arginine vasopressin (DDAVP) in the absence of platelet von Willebrand factor in Gray platelet syndrome. Thrombosis and Haemostasis 58: 1060–1063

Phillips D R, Agin P P 1977 Platelet plasma membrane glycoproteins. Evidence for the presence of nonequivalent disulfide bonds using nonreduced-reduced two dimensional gel electrophoresis. Journal of Biological Chemistry 252: 2121

Phillips D R, Agin P P 1977 Platelet plasma membrane glycoproteins: Identification of a proteolytic substrate for thrombin. Biochemica et Biophysical Acta 75: 940

Phillips D R, Charo I F, Parise L V, Fitzgerald L A 1988 The platelet membrane glycoprotein IIb-IIIa complex. Blood 71: 831

Phillips D R, Jenkins C S P, Luscher E F, Larrieu M-J 1975 Molecular differences of exposed surface proteins on thrombasthenic platelet plasma membranes. Nature (Lond.) 257: 599–600

Pidard D 1989 The application of crossed-immunoelectrophoresis and related immunoassays to the characterization of glycoprotein structure and function. In: Kunicki T J, George J N (eds) Platelet immunobiology: molecular and clinical aspects. Lippincott, Philadelphia, p 193–234

Pidard D, Montgomery R R, Bennett J S, Kunicki T J 1983 Interaction of AP-2, a monoclonal antibody specific for the human platelet glycoprotein IIb-IIIa complex, with intact platelets. Journal of Biological Chemistry 258: 12582

Pidard D, Didry D, Le Deist F et al 1988 Analysis of the membrane glycoproteins of platelets in the Wiskott-Aldrich syndrome. British Journal of Haematology 69: 529–535

Piotrowicz R S, Orchekowski R P, Nugent D J, Yamada K Y, Kunicki T J 1988 Glycoprotein Ic-IIa functions as an activation-independent fibronectin receptor on human platelets. Journals of Cell Biology 106: 1359

Plow E F, Ginsberg M H 1989 Cellular adhesion: GPIIb-IIIa as a prototypic adhesion receptor. Progress in Hemostasis and Thrombosis 9: 117–156

Plow E F, Srouji A H, Meyer D, Marguerie G, Ginsberg M H 1984 Evidence that three adhesive proteins interact with a common recognition site on activated platelets. Journal of Biological Chemistry 259: 5388

Plow E F, McEver R P, Coller B S, Woods Jr V L, Marguerie G A, Ginsberg M H 1985a Related binding mechanisms for fibrinogen, fibronectin, von Willebrand factor and thrombospondin on thrombin-stimulated human platelets. Blood 66: 724–727

Plow E F, Pierschbacher M D, Ruoslahti E, Marguerie G, Ginsberg M H 1985b The effect of Arg-Gly-Asp-containing peptides on fibrinogen and von Willebrand factor binding to platelets. Proceedings of the National Academy of Sciences, USA 82: 8057

Plow E F, Pierschbacher M D, Ruoslahti E, Marguerie G, Ginsberg M H 1987 Arginyl-Glycyl-Aspartic acid sequences and fibrinogen binding to platelets. Blood 70: 110–115

Polack B, Duperray A, Troesch A, Berthier R, Marguerie G 1989 Biogenesis of the vitronectin receptor in human endothelial cell: Evidence that the vitronectin receptor and GPIIb-IIIa are synthesized by a common mechanism. Blood 73: 1519

Poncz M, Eisman R, Heidenreich R et al 1987 Structure of the platelet membrane glycoprotein IIb. Journal of Biological Chemistry 262: 8476–8482

Poulsen L O, Taaning E 1990 Variation in surface platelet glycoprotein Ib expression in Bernard–Soulier syndrome. Haemostasis 20: 155–161

Powling M J, Hardisty R M 1985 Glycoprotein IIb-IIIa complex and Ca^{2+} influx into stimulated platelets. Blood 66: 731

Pytela R, Pierschbacher M D, Ginsberg M H, Plow E F, Ruoslahti E 1986 Platelet membrane glycoprotein IIb/IIIa: Member of a family of Arg-Gly-Asp-specific adhesion receptors. Science 231: 1559

Raccuglia G 1971 Grey platelet syndrome: a variety of qualitative platelet disorder. American Journal of Medicine 51: 818–828

Rak K, Boda Z 1980 Hemostatic balance in congenital deficiency of platelet cyclooxygenase. Lancet 2: 44

Rao A K 1990 Congenital disorders of platelet function. Hematology and Oncology Clinics of North America 4: 65–86

Rao A K, Holmsen H 1986 Congenital disorders of platelet function. Seminars in Hematology 23: 102–118

Rao A K, Koike K, Willis J et al 1984 Platelet secretion defect associated with impaired liberation of arachidonic acid and normal myosin light chain phosphorylation. Blood 104: 116

Rao A K, Koike K, Day H J et al 1985 Bleeding disorder associated with albumin-dependent partial deficiency in platelet thromboxane production. American Journal of Clinical Pathology 83: 687

Rao A K, Kowalska M A, Disa J 1989 Impaired cytoplasmic ionized calcium mobilization in inherited platelet secretion defects. Blood 74: 664

Ratnoff O D 1987 Some therapeutic agents influencing hemostasis. In Colman R W, Hirsh J, Marder V J, Salzman E W (eds) Hemostasis and thrombosis: basis principles and clinical practice. Lippincott, Philadelphia, p 1026–1047

Reichert N, Seligsohn U, Ramot B 1975 Clinical and genetic studies of Glanzmann's thrombasthenia in Israel. Thrombosis Diathesis et Haemorrhagica 34: 806

Remold-O'Donnell E, Zimmerman C, Kenny D, Rosen F S 1987 Expression on blood cells of sialophorin, the surface glycoprotein that is defective in Wiskott–Aldrich syndrome. Blood 70: 104–109

Remold-O'Donnell E, Rosen F S 1990 Sialophorin (CD43) and the Wiskott–Aldrich syndrome. Immunodeficiency Reviews 2: 151–174

Rendu F, Breton-Gorius J, Trugnan G 1978 Studies on a new variant of Hermansky–Pudlak syndrome: Qualitative, ultrastructural, and functional abnormalities of the platelet-dense bodies associated with a phospholipase A defect. American Journal of Hematology 4: 387

Rendu F, Breton-Gorius J, Lebret M et al 1983 Evidence that abnormal platelet functions in human Chediak–Higashi syndrome are the result of a lack of dense bodies. American Journal of Pathology 11: 307–314

Rendu F, Marche P, Hovig T et al 1987 Abnormal phosphoinositide metabolism and protein phosphorylation in platelets from a patient with the grey platelet syndrome. British Journal of Haematology 67: 199–206

Ricci G, Manservigi R, Albonici L, Zavagli G, Cassai E 1985 Evidence for glycoprotein abnormality in platelets from patients with May–Hegglin anomaly. Thrombosis Haemostasis 54: 862–865

Rifat S, Coller B, Newman P et al 1992 Glanzmann thrombasthenia secondary to a $Gly^{273} \rightarrow Asp$ mutation in the 1st calcium-binding domain of platelet glycoprotein IIb. Clinical Research 40: 210A

Rodeghiero F, Castaman G, Pesavento G, Bonato F, Muleo G, Consarino C 1987 Recurrent life-threatening epistaxis in a child with Bernard–Soulier syndrome controlled by bilateral ligation of external carotids and ethmoidal arteries. Acta Haematology 77: 183–185

Rodgers R P C, Levin J 1990 A critical reappraisal of the bleeding time. Seminars in Thrombosis and Hemostasis 16: 1–20

Rosa J-P, Kieffer N, Didry D, Pidard D, Kunicki T J, Nurden A T 1984 The human platelet membrane glycoprotein complex GPIIb-IIIa expresses antigenic sites not exposed on the dissociated glycoproteins. Blood 64: 1246

Rosa J P, George J N, Bainton D F, Nurden A T, Caen J P, McEver R P 1987 Gray platelet syndrome. Demonstration of alpha granule membranes that can fuse with the cell surface. Journal of Clinical Investigation 80: 1138–1146

Rosenstein Y, Park J K, Hahn W C, Burakoff S J 1991 CD43, a molecule defective in Wiskott–Aldrich syndrome, binds ICAM-1. Nature 354: 233–235

Rosing E M, Bevers P, Confurius P et al 1985 Impaired factor X and prothrombin activation associated with decreased phospholipid exposure in platelets from a patient with a bleeding disorder. Blood 65: 1557

Roth G J 1991 Developing relationships: Arterial platelet adhesion, glycoprotein Ib, and leucine-rich glycoproteins. Blood 77: 5–19

Roth G J, Machuga R 1982 Rodioimmune assay of human platelet prostaglandin synthetase. Journal of Laboratory and Clinical Medicine 99: 187

Roth G J, Church T A, McMullen B A, Williams S A 1990 Human platelet glycoprotein V: a surface leucine-rich glycoprotein related to adhesion. Biochemical and Biophysical Research Communications 170: 153–161

Rothman J E, Orci L 1992 Molecular dissection of the secretory pathway. Nature 355: 409–415

Ruan C, Tobelem G, McMichael A J et al 1981 Monoclonal antibody to human platelet glycoprotein I. II. Effects on human platelet function. British Journal of Haematology 49: 511

Ruan C G, Du X P, Xi X D, Castaldi P A, Berndt M C 1987 A murine antiglycoprotein Ib complex monoclonal antibody, SZ 2, inhibits platelet aggregation induced by both ristocetin and collagen. Blood 69: 570–577

Ruggeri Z M 1991 The platelet glycoprotein Ib-IX complex. Progress Hemostasis and Thrombosis 10: 35–68

Ruggeri Z M, Hodson E M 1989 Use of murine monoclonal antibodies to determine platelet membrane glycoprotein structure and function. In: Kunicki T J, George J N (eds) Platelet immunobiology: molecular and clinical aspects. Lippincott, Philadelphia, p 235–254

Ruggeri Z M, Bader R, De Marco L 1982 Glanzmann thrombasthenia: Deficient binding of von Willebrand factor to thrombin-stimulated platelets. Proceedings of the National Academy of Sciences, USA 79: 6038

Ruggeri Z M, DeMarco L, Gatti L, Bader R, Montgomery R R 1983 Platelets have more than one binding site for von Willebrand factor. Journal of Clinical Investigation 72: 1

Ruoslahti E, Pierschbacher M D 1987 New perspectives in cell adhesion: RGD and integrins. Science 238: 491

Russell S D, Roth G J 1991 A mutation in the platelet glycoprotein

(GP) Ibα gene associated with pseudo-von Willebrand disease. Blood 78(Suppl 1): 131a Abstract
Russell, M E, Seligsohn U, Coller B S, Ginsberg M D, Skoglund P, Quertermous T 1988 Structural integrity of the glycoprotein IIb and IIIa genes in Glanzmann thrombasthenia patients from Israel. Blood 72: 635–638
Rybak M E, Renzulli L A, Bruns M J, Cahaly D P 1988 Platelet glycoproteins IIb and IIIa as a calcium channel in liposomes. Blood 72: 714–720
Ryo R, Yoshida A, Sugano W et al 1992 Deficiency of P62, a putative collagen receptor, in platelets from a patient with defective collagen-induced platelet aggregation. American Journal of Haematology 39: 25–31
Saarinen U M, Kekomaki R, Siimes M A, Myllyla G 1990 Effective prophylaxis against platelet refractoriness in multitransfused patients by use of leukocyte-free blood components. Blood 75: 517
Sakariassen K S, Nievelstein P F E M, Coller B S, Sixma J J 1986 The role of platelet membrane glycoproteins Ib and IIb-IIIa in platelet adherence to human artery subendothelium. British Journal of Haematology 63: 681–691
Samama M, Lecrubier C, Conard J et al 1981 Constitutional thrombocytopathy with subnormal response to thromboxane A_2. British Journal of Haematology 48: 293
Santoro S A 1986 Identification of a 160 000 dalton platelet membrane protein that mediates the initial divalent cation-dependent adhesion of platelets to collagen. Cell 46: 913
Santoro S A, Lawing Jr W J 1987 Competition for related but nonidentical binding sites on the glycoprotein IIb-IIIa complex by peptides derived from platelet adhesive proteins. Cell 48: 867–873
Santoro S A, Rajpara S M, Staatz W D, Woods Jr V L 1988 Isolation and characterization of a platelet surface collagen binding complex related to VLA-2. Biochemica et Biophysical Acta 153: 217
Savage B, Ruggeri Z M 1991 Selective recognition of adhesive sites in surface-bound fibrinogen by glycoprotein IIb-IIIa on nonactivated platelets. Journal of Biological Chemistry 266: 11227–11233
Schiffer C A 1991 Editorial: Prevention of alloimmunization against platelets. Blood 77: 1–4
Seligsohn U 1992 Private Communication
Seligsohn U, Rososhansky S 1984 A Glanzmann's thrombasthenia cluster among Iraqi Jews in Israel. Thrombosis Haemostasis 52: 230–231
Seligsohn U, Mibashan R S, Rodeck C H, Nicolaides K H, Millar D S, Coller B S 1985 Prenatal diagnosis of Glanzmann's thrombasthenia. Lancet 2: 1419
Seligsohn U, Mibashan R S, Rodeck C H, Nicolaides K H, Millar D S, Coller B S 1988 Prevention program of type I Glanzmann thrombasthenia in Israel: prenatal diagnosis. Current Studies in Hematology and Blood Transfusions 174–179
Seligsohn U, Coller B S, Zivelin A, Plow E F, Ginsberg M H 1989 Immunoblot analysis of platelet glycoprotein IIb in patients with Glanzmann thrombasthenia in Israel. British Journal of Haematology 72: 415–423
Seligsohn U, Peretz H, Newman P J, Coller B S 1992 Glanzmann thrombasthenia in Israel: Clinical, biochemical and molecular genetic characterization. In: Hereditary disorders among Jews. Oxford University Press, pp 275–282
Shattil S J, Hoxie J A, Cunningham M, Brass L F 1985 Changes in the platelet membrane protein IIb-IIIa compex during platelet activation. Journal of Biological Chemistry 260: 1107
Sheffer R, Ilan Y, Eldor A 1986 Bernard–Soulier syndrome. Harefuah 111: 119–120
Shelley C S, Remold-O'Donnell E, Davis A, III et al 1989 Molecular characterization of sialophorin (CD43), the lymphocyte surface sialoglycoprotein defective in Wiskott–Aldrich syndrome. Proceedings of the National Academy of Sciences, USA 86: 2819–2823
Shimamoto Y, Kaneoka H, Matsuzaki M et al 1989 Genetic markers and thrombin reaction in a family of Bernard–Soulier syndrome. Nippon Ketsueki Gakkai Zasshi 52: 1155–1158
Shimomura T, Fujimura K, Maehama S et al 1990 Rapid purification and characterization of human platelet glycoprotein V: The amino acid sequence contains leucine-rich repetitive modules as in glycoprotein Ib. Blood 75: 2349
Shinmyozu K, Maruyama Y, Maruyama I, Osame M, Igata A 1986 Bernard–Soulier syndrome with special reference to platelet-membrane glycoprotein abnormalities. Rinsho Ketsueki. Japanese Journal of Clinical Hematology 27: 553–559
Shulman N R, Jordan Jr, J V 1987 Platelet kinetics. In: Colman R W, Hirsh J, Marder V J, Salzman E W (eds) Hemostasis and thrombosis: basic principles and clinical practice, 2nd edn. Lippincott, Philadelphia, p 431–451
Shulman S, Karpatkin S 1980 Crossed immunoelectrophoresis of human platelet membranes. Diminished major antigen in Glanzmann's thrombasthenia and Bernard–Soulier syndrome. Journal of Biological Chemistry 255: 4320
Silverstein R L, Asch A S, Nachmann R L 1989 Glycoprotein IV mediates thrombospondin-dependent platelet-monocyte and platelet-U937 cell adhesion. Journal of Clinical Investigation 84: 546
Sims P J, Weidmer T, Esmon C T, Weiss H J, Shattil S J 1989 Assembly of the platelet prothrombinase complex is linked to vesiculation of the platelet plasma membrane. Studies in Scott syndrome: An isolated defect in platelet procoagulant activity. Journal of Biological Chemistry 264: 17049
Sindet-Pedersen S, Stenbjerg S 1986 Effect of local antifibrinolytic treatment with tranexamic acid in hemophiliacs undergoing oral surgery. Journal of Oral Maxillofactory Surgery 44: 703–707
Sindet-Pedersen S, Ramstrom G, Bernvii S, Blomback M 1989 Hemostatic effect of tranexamic acid mouthwash in anticoagulant-treated patients undergoing oral surgery. New England Journal of Medicine 320: 840–843
Slichter S J 1991 Platelet transfusions a constantly evolving therapy. Thrombosis Haemostasis 66: 178–188
Smith J W, Cheresh D A 1988 The Arg-Gly-Asp binding domain of the vitronection receptor. Journal of Biological Chemistry 263: 18726
Smyth S S, Hillery C A, Parise L V 1991 Phosphatidic and lysophosphatidic acid modulate the fibrinogen binding activity of purified platelet glycoprotein IIb-IIIa. Blood 78(Suppl 1): 278a (Abstract)
Smyth S S, Hillery C A, Parise L V 1992 The fibrinogen binding activity of platelet glucoprotein IIa-IIIa (integrin alpha-IIb beta$_3$) is modulated by lipids. Submitted
Sniecinski I, O'Donnell M R, Nowicki B, Hill L R 1988 Prevention of refractoriness and HLA-alloimmunization using filtered blood products. Blood 71: 1402–1407
Soberano M E, Clarke D, Zucker M B 1986 Binding of thrombin-activated human factor VIII to platelets. British Journal of Haematology 64: 571–585
Sonnenberg A, Modderman P W, Hogervorst F 1988 Laminin receptor on platelets is the integrin VLA-6. Nature 336: 487
Soslan G, Parker J 1992 The bioluminescent detection of platelet-released ATP: collagen-induced release and potential errors. Thrombosis Research 66: 15–21
Sosnoski D M, Emanuel B S, Hawkins A L et al 1988 Chromosomal localization of the genes for the vitronectin and fibronectin receptors alpha-subunits and for platelet glycoproteins IIb and IIIa. Journal of Clinical Investigation 81: 1993–1998
Spero J A, Triplett D A, Cmolik B L, Reid C, Clark R E 1991 A family of clotting factor inhibitors primarily involving FV and FXI occurring after cardiovascular and neurosurgical procedures. Blood 78(Suppl 1): 63a (Abstract)
Srivastava P C, Powling M J, Nokes T J, Patrick A D, Dawes J, Hardisty R M 1987 Grey platelet syndrome: studies on platelet alpha-granules, lysosomes and defective response to thrombin. British Journal of Haematology 65: 441–446
Stanford M F, Munoz P C, Vroman L 1983 Platelets adhere where flow has left fibrinogen on glass. Annals of the New York Academy of Sciences 416: 504–512
Stevens M C, Blanchette V S, Freedman M H, Sparling C, Kunicki T J 1988 A variant form of Bernard–Soulier syndrome: mild haemostatic defect associated with partial platelet GPIb deficiency. Clinical Laboratory Haematology 10: 443–451
Stormorken H, Gogstad G O, Solum N O, Pande H 1982 Diagnosis of heterozygotes in Glanzmann's thrombasthenia. Thrombosis and Haemostasis 48: 217–221
Stormorken H, Hellum B, Egeland T, Abrahamsen T G, Hovig T 1991 X-linked thrombocytopenia and thrombocytopathia: attenuated

Wiskott–Aldrich syndrome. Functional and morphological studies of platelets and lymphocytes. Thrombosis and Haemostasis 65: 300–305

Sugiyama T, Okuma M, Ushikubi F, Sensaki S, Kanaji K, Uchino H 1987 A novel platelet aggregating factor found in a patient with defective collagen-induced platelet aggregation and autoimmune thrombocytopenia. Blood 69: 1712–1720

Suhasini G, Nanivadekar S A, Sawant P D, Agarwal M B, Bichile L S, Bavdankar P Y 1986 Benard–Soulier syndrome presenting as recurrent exsanguinating haematemesis. Indian Journal of Gastroenterology 5: 137–138

Sultan Y, Brouet J C, Divergie 1976 Isolated platelet factor 3 deficiency. New England Journal of Medicine 294: 121

Suzuki S, Argaves W S, Pytela R et al 1986 cDNA and amino acid sequences of the cell adhesion protein receptor recognizing vitronectin reveal a transmembrane domain and homologies with other adhesion protein receptors. Proceedings of the National Academy of Sciences, USA 83: 8614

Takahashi H 1980 Studies of the pathophysiology and treatment of von Willebrand's disease. IV. Mechanism of increased ristocetin-induced platelet aggregation in von Willebrand's disease. Thrombosis Research 19: 857–867

Takahashi H 1985 Replacement therapy in platelet-type von Willebrand disease. American Journal of Hematology 18: 351

Takahashi H, Hattori A, Ihzumi T et al 1981 A family of platelet release mechanism abnormality with normal arachidonate metabolism and defective response to ionophore A23187. Blood Vessel 12: 223

Takahashi H, Handa M, Watanabe K et al 1984 Further characterization of platelet-type von Willebrand's disease in Japan. Blood 64: 1254–1262

Takahashi H, Nagayama R, Hattori A, Chibata A 1985 Botrocetin- and polybrene-induced platelet aggregation in platelet-type von Willebrand disease. American Journal of Hematology 18: 179

Takamatsu J, Horne M, III, Gralnick H R 1986 Identification of the thrombin receptor on human platelets by chemical crosslinking. Journal of Clinical Investigation 77: 362–368

Tandon N N, Kralisz U, Jamieson G A 1989 Identification of glycoprotein IV (CD36) as a primary receptor for platelet-collagen adhesion. Journal of Biological Chemistry 264: 7576–7583

Tandon N N, Ockenhouse C F, Greco N J, Jamieson G A 1991 Adhesive functions of platelets lacking glycoprotein IV (CD36). Blood 78: 2809–2813

Tanoue K, Hasegawa S, Yamaguchi A, Yamamoto N, Yamazaki H 1987 A new variant of thrombasthenia with abnormally glycosylated GPIIb/IIIa. Thrombosis Research 47: 323–333

Taub R, Gould R J, Garsky V M et al 1989 A monoclonal antibody against the platelet fibrinogen receptor contains a sequence that mimics a receptor recognition domain in fibrinogen. Journal of Biological Chemistry 264: 259

Thiagarajan P, Perussia B, De Marco L, Wells K, Trinchieri G 1983 Membrane proteins on human megakaryocytes and platelets identified by monoclonal antibodies. American Journal of Hematology 14: 255

Timmons S, Kloczewiak M, Hawiger J 1984 ADP-dependent common receptor mechanism for binding of von Willebrand factor and fibrinogen to human platelets. Proceedings of the National Academy of Sciences, USA 81: 4935

Tornai I, Kiss A, Laczko J 1989 Wiskott–Aldrich syndrome in a heterozygous carrier woman. European Journal of Hematology 42: 501–502

Tornai I, Kiss A, Laczko J, Nagy P M 1989 Wiskott–Aldrich syndrome in a heterozygous woman. Orvosi Hetilap 130: 679–682

Tschopp T B, Weiss H J, Baumgartner H R 1975 Interaction of thrombasthenic platelets with subendothelium: normal adhesion, absent aggregation. Experientia 31: 13

Uzan G, Prandini M H, Thevenon D, Marguerie G 1991 A negative promoter element regulates the lineage specificity of the GPIIb gene expression. Blood 78(suppl 1): 720–182a (abstract)

Van Dorp D B, Wijermans P W, Meire F, Vrensen G 1990 The Hermansky–Pudlak syndrome. Variable reaction to 1-desamino-D-arginine vasopressin for correction of the bleeding time. Ophthalmic Paediatric Genetics 11: 237–244

Van Kuppevelt T H, Languino L R, Gailit J O, Ruoslaktuki S 1989 An alternative cystoplasmic domain of the integrin P_3 subunit. Proceedings of the National Academy of Sciences, USA 86: 5415–5410

Verhoeven A J, van Oostrum I E, van Haarlem H, Akkerman J W 1989 Impaired energy metabolism in platelets from patients with Wiskott–Aldrich syndrome. Thrombosis and Haemostasis 61: 10–14

Vicente V, Houghton R A, Rugger Z M 1990 Identification of a site in the alpha chain of platelet glycoprotein Ib that participates in von Willebrand factor binding. Journal of Biological Chemistry 265: 274

Von Behrens W E 1985 Mediterranean macrothrombocytopenia. Blood 46: 199–208

Vu T-K H, Hung D T, Wheaton V I, Coughlin S R 1991 Molecular cloning of a functional thrombin receptor reveals a novel proteolytic mechanism of receptor activation. Cell 64: 1057–1068

Waldenstrom E, Holmberg L, Axelsson U, Winqvist I, Nilsson I M 1991 Bernard–Soulier syndrome in two Swedish families: effect of DDAVP on bleeding time. European Journal of Hematology 46: 182–187

Walsh P N, Schmaier A H 1992 Platelet-coagulant protein interactions. In: Colman R W, Hirsh J, Marder V J, Salzman E W (eds) Hemostasis and thrombosis: basic principles and clinical practice, 2nd edn. Lippincott, Philadelphia, p 689–709

Walsh P N, Mills D C B, Pareti F I et al 1975 Hereditary giant platelet syndrome. British Journal of Haematology 29: 639–655

Wang R G, McFarland J, Furihata K, Friedman K, Newman P J 1991 An amino acid polymorphism within the RGD binding domain of GPIIIa is associated with the PEN^A/PEN^B alloantigen. Blood 78(suppl 1): 281a (abstract)

Ware J, Russell S R, Vicente V et al 1990 Nonsense mutation in the glycoprotein Ib alpha coding sequence associated with Bernard–Soulier syndrome. Proceedings of the National Academy of Sciences, USA 87: 2026–2030

Ware J, Russell S, Murata M, Mazzucato M, DeMarco L, Ruggeri Z M 1991 Ala^{156}–Val. Substitution in platelet glycoprotein Ibalpha impairs von Willebrand factor binding and is the molecular basis of Bernard–Soulier syndrome type Bolzano. Blood 78(suppl 1): 278a (abstract)

Ware J, Russell S, Ruggeri Z M 1991 Genetic basis for the molecular polymorphisms of platelet glycoprotein Ibα. Thrombosis Haemostasis 65: 770 (abstract)

Wautier J L, Gruel Y 1989 Prenatal diagnosis of platelet disorders. Baillieres Clinical Haematology 2: 569–583

Weisel J W, Nagaswami C, Vilaire G, Bennett J S 1991 Examination of the interaction of the platelet membrane glycoprotein IIb/IIIa complex with fibrinogen by electron microscopy. Blood 78(suppl 1): 183a (abstract)

Weiss H J 1967 Platelet aggregation, adhesion and adenosine diphosphate release in thrombopathia (platelet factor 3 deficiency). American Journal of Medicine 43: 570–578

Weiss H J 1987 Inherited disorders of platelet secretion. In: Colman R W, Hirsh J, Marder V J, Salzman E W (eds) Hemostasis and thrombosis: basic principles and clinical practice, 2nd edn. Lippincott, Philadelphia, 741–747

Weiss H J, Kochwa S 1968 Studies of platelet function and proteins in 3 patients with Glanzmann thrombasthenia. Journal of Laboratory and Clinical Medicine 7: 153–165

Weiss H J, Lages B 1981 Platelet malondialdehyde production and aggregation responses induced by arachidonate, prostaglandin-G_2, collagen, and epinephrine in 12 patients with storage pool deficiency. Blood 58: 27–33

Weiss H J, Chervenick P A, Zalusky R, Factor A 1969 A familial defect in platelet function associated with impaired release of adenosine diphosphate. New England Journal of Medicine 281: 1264–1270

Weiss H J, Tschopp T B, Baumgartner H R, Sussman II, Johnson M M, Egan J J 1974 Decreased adhesion of giant (Bernard–Soulier) platelets to subendothelium. American Journal of Medicine 57: 920–925

Weiss H J, Tschopp T B, Rogers J, Brand H 1974 Studies of platelet 5-hydroxytryptamine (serotonin) in storage pool disease and albinism. Journal of Clinical Investigation 54: 421–432

Weiss H J, Turitto V T, Baumgartner H R 1978 Effect of shear rate on platelet interaction with subendothelium in citrated and native blood. Journal of Laboratory and Clinical Medicine 92: 750–764

Weiss H J, Vicic W J, Lages B A et al 1979a Isolated deficiency of platelet procoagulant activity. American Journal of Medicine 67: 206
Weiss H J, Witte L D, Kaplan K L et al 1979b Heterogeneity in storage pool deficiency: Studies on granule-bound substances in 18 patients including variants deficient in alpha-granules, platelet factor 4, beta-thromboglobulin, and platelet-derived growth factor. Blood 54: 1296–1319
Weiss H J, Meyer D, Rabinowitz R, Grima J-P, Vicic W J, Rogers J 1982 Pseudo-von Willebrand's disease. An intrinsic platelet defect with aggregation by unmodified human factor VII/von Willebrand factor and enhanced adsorption of its high-molecular-weight multimers. New England Journal of Medicine 306: 326
Weiss H J, Turitto V T, Baumgartner H R 1986 Platelet adhesion and thrombus formation on subendothelium in platelets deficient in glycoproteins IIb-IIIa, Ib, and storage granules. Blood 67: 322–330
Wencel-Drake J D 1990 Plasma membrane GPIIb/IIIa: Evidence for a cycling receptor pool. American Journal of Pathology 136: 61–70
Wenger R H, Kieffer N, Wicki A N, Clemetson K J 1988 Structure of the human blood platelet membrane glycoprotein Ib-alpha gene. Biochemical et Biophysical Acta 156: 389
Wenger R H, Wicki A N, Kieffer N, Adolph S, Hameister H, Clemetson K J 1989 The 5′ flanking region and chromosomal localization of the gene encoding human platelet membrane glycoprotein Ib-alpha. Gene 85: 517
White J G 1987 Inherited abnormalities of the platelet membrane and secretory granules. Human Pathology 18: 123–139
White J G 1990 Structural defects in inherited and giant platelet disorders. Advances in Human Genetics 19: 133–234
White G C, Krupp C L 1985 Glycoprotein V hydrolysis by thrombin. Lack of correlation with secretion. Thrombosis Research 38: 641
White J G, Edson J R, Desnick S J, Witkop Jr C J 1971 Studies of platelets in a variant of the Hermansky–Pudlak syndrome. American Journal of Pathology 63: 319–332
White J G, Burris S M, Hasegawa D, Johnson M 1984 Micropipette aspiration of human blood platelets: A defect in the Bernard–Soulier's syndrome. Blood 63: 1249–1252
White G C II, Montgomery R R 1991 Clinical aspects and therapy for von Willebrand disease. In: Hoffman R, Benz E J, Shattil S J, Furie B, Cohen H J (eds) Hematology: basic principles and practice. Churchill Livingstone, New York, p 1362–1371
Wijermans P W, Van Dorp D B 1989 Hermansky-Pudlak syndrome: correction of bleeding time by 1-desamino-8D-arginine vasopressin. American Journal of Hematology 30: 154–157
Willis A L, Weiss H J 1973 A congenital defect in platelet prostaglandin production assocated with impaired hemostasis in storage pool disease. Prostaglandins 4: 783
Wills E J 1989 Grey platelet syndrome. Ultrastructural Pathology 13: 451–455
Witkop Jr, C J, White J G, King R A 1974 Oculocutaneous albinism. In: Nyhan W L (ed) Heritable disorders of amino acid metabolism. Pattern of clinical expression and genetic variation. Wiley, New York, p 177–261
Wu K K, Le Breton G C, Tai H-H, Chen Y-C 1981 Abnormal platelet response to thromboxane A_2. Journal of Clinical Investigation 67: 1801–1804
Wu K K, Minkoff I M, Rossi E C, Chen Y-C 1981 Hereditary bleeding disorder due to a primary defect in platelet release reaction. British Journal of Haematology 47: 241–249
Wu K K 1982 Bleeding disorders due to abnormalities in platelet prostaglandins. In: Wu K K, Rossi E C (eds) Prostaglandins in clinical medicine. Year book, Chicago, p 81–92
Yamamoto N, Ikeda H, Tandon N N, et al 1990 A platelet membrane glycoprotein (GP) deficiency in healthy blood donors: Nak^{a-} platelets lack detectable GPIV (CD36). Blood 76: 1698–1703
Zaffar N, Saleem M, Ahmed S A 1987 Functional platelet defects: a clinicopathological study of 10 cases. JPMA 37: 223–228
Zamarron C, Ginsberg M H, Plow E F 1991 A receptor-induced binding site in fibrinogen elicited by its interaction with platelet membrane glycoprotein IIb-IIIa. Journal of Biological Chemistry 266: 16193–16199
Zimrin A B, Eisman R, Vilaire G, Schwartz E, Bennett J S, Poncz M 1988 Structure of platelet glycoprotein IIIa: A common subunit for two different membrane receptors. Journal of Clinical Investigation 81: 1470–1475
Zimrin A B, Gidwitz S, Lord S et al 1990 The genomic organization of platelet glycoprotein IIIa. Journal of Biological Chemistry 265: 8590–8595
Zonneveld G T E, Van Leeuwen E F, Sturk A, ten Cate J W 1983 Detection of carriers in Glanzmann's thrombasthenia. Thrombosis and Haemostasis 49: 182–186
Zucker M B, McPherson J 1977 Reactions of platelets near surfaces in vitro: lessons from the platelet retention test. Annals of the New York Academy of Sciences 283: 128–137
Zucker M B, Vroman L 1969 Platelet adhesion induced by fibrinogen adsorbed onto glass. Proceedings of the Society for Experimental Biology and Medicine 131: 318–320
Zucker M B, Pert J H, Hilgartner M W 1966 Platelet function in a patient with thrombasthenia. Blood 28: 524
Zucker M B, Kim S-J, McPherson J, Grant R A 1977 Binding of factor VIII to platelets in the presence of ristocetin. British Journal of Haematology 35: 535

33. Acquired platelet disorders

T. E. Warkentin J. G. Kelton

APPROACH TO ACQUIRED PLATELET DISORDERS

Acquired qualitative and quantitative disorders occur commonly in clinical medicine. Two important clinical decisions are needed when evaluating these patients. (1) What is the bleeding risk and (2) what is the cause of the platelet disorder?

The approach to thrombocytopenia is usually based on a consideration of the mechanism of thrombocytopenia, which can be classified as: (1) increased platelet destruction, (2) decreased platelet production, (3) platelet sequestration (hypersplenism), or (4) dilution. Usually, the mechanism of thrombocytopenia is inferred by indirect means, but sometimes a radionuclide platelet survival study is required to determine the mechanism of the thrombocytopenia. Thrombocytopenia caused by increased platelet destruction is usually classified further according to whether the pathogenesis is immune or nonimmune.

In most cases, the probable cause of platelet dysfunction is obvious from the clinical situation, e.g. uraemia, advanced liver disease, aspirin use, myeloma, myelodysplasia, myeloproliferative disorders. Less often, the responsible disorder is not obvious and requires specialized investigations, e.g. monoclonal gammopathy of undetermined significance, IgG-mediated platelet dysfunction in the absence of thrombocytopenia, antiphospholipid antibody syndrome. Spontaneous bleeding is uncommon in these disorders, and the most frequent problem faced by clinicians is whether special interventions are needed when these patients undergo invasive procedures.

EVALUATION OF THROMBOCYTOPENIA

History and physical examination

The majority of patients with thrombocytopenia or platelet dysfunction are asymptomatic. When bleeding occurs, it is mucocutaneous and can include petechiae, easy bruising, nosebleeds, and menorrhagia. The characteristic sign of severe thrombocytopenia is the presence of petechiae, which are pinpoint haemorrhages most frequently seen in dependent areas such as the feet or buttocks. Larger purpuric lesions, or ecchymoses, may also occur, often at sites of injury or venipuncture. Mucosal purpuric lesions, often forming haemorrhagic bullae, can be seen in the oral mucous membranes in patients with very severe thrombocytopenia, and indicate that urgent treatment for the thrombocytopenia should be instituted.

Sometimes, temporal characteristics are helpful diagnostic clues. For example, insidious onset of bleeding symptoms is characteristic of chronic ITP. However, the abrupt onset of severe bleeding symptoms suggests acute post-viral or drug-induced immune thrombocytopenia.

The differential diagnosis of thrombocytopenia is diverse. History should include a multiple systems review. The use of prescription and non-prescription drugs and alcohol should be recorded. Potential exposure to quinine should be considered in patients with severe thrombocytopenia. Certain physical findings may help in the diagnosis of the thrombocytopenia, including the presence of fever, lymphadenopathy, and splenomegaly.

Laboratory investigations

Peripheral blood film

The most important investigations are the complete blood count and the examination of the peripheral blood film. In general, isolated thrombocytopenia is caused by increased platelet destruction, whereas thrombocytopenia accompanied by anaemia and leukopenia is usually caused by decreased platelet production, hypersplenism, or haemodilution.

In most instances, the platelet count is quickly and accurately determined by electronic particle counters that quantify platelets based on their relative size characteristics. However, various artefacts such as ex vivo platelet clumping can lead to falsely low platelet count values (pseudothrombocytopenia, p. 768). Less commonly, spurious thrombocytosis can result if the particle counter erroneously counts as platelets such abnormal particles as red cell schistocytes, microspherocytes, leukaemic cell fragments, Pappenheimer bodies, or bacteria (Stass et al 1979, Morton et al 1980, Akwari et al 1982, Gloster et al 1985). Detecting these potential artefacts is an important reason to review the blood film in patients with thrombocytopenia or thrombocytosis.

Abnormal red and white cell morphology can be helpful in the diagnosis of quantitative and qualitative platelet disorders. For example, red cell fragments suggest that thrombocytopenia is part of a syndrome of thrombotic microangiopathy such as thrombotic thrombocytopenic purpura, haemolytic-uraemic syndrome, disseminated intravascular coagulation, or preeclampsia. 'Tear drop' and circulating nucleated red cells suggest marrow infiltration by tumour, fibrosis, or granulomata. Viral infections are suggested by the appearance of atypical lymphocytes. Bacterial or fungal infections are suggested by toxic changes in the neutrophils and monocytes such as cytoplasmic vacuolation, increased granularity, pale blue inclusions termed Döhle bodies, or protoplasmic extensions. Protozoal infections such as malaria can be confirmed by the characteristic parasitic red cell inclusions. Sometimes, rare causes of thrombocytopenia can be suggested by the peripheral blood film, including the Bernard–Soulier syndrome (thrombocytopenia, giant platelets) and May–Hegglin anomaly (thrombocytopenia, large platelets, large neutrophil Döhle bodies).

Pseudothrombocytopenia

Pseudothrombocytopenia is a relatively common laboratory artefact that occurs in up to 0.1% of all complete blood counts (Payne & Pierre 1984, Berkman et al 1991). In most cases, it is caused by platelet-reactive antibodies that bind to the GPIIb/IIIa complex at low calcium concentrations. Thus, pseudothrombocytopenia is usually EDTA-dependent, and most commonly manifests as ex vivo platelet clumping. The correct platelet count usually can be determined by collecting another blood sample into sodium citrate or heparin anticoagulants (Berkman et al 1991). Many EDTA-dependent platelet agglutinins react optimally at room temperature, and therefore maintaining the blood sample at 37°C prior to measurement may yield the correct platelet count. Other causes of pseudothrombocytopenia are listed in Table 33.1.

There are no diagnostic implications for EDTA-dependent pseudothrombocytopenia, other than the potential to result in erroneous diagnosis and treatment. For this reason, laboratories should not report an unexpectedly low platelet count unless it is confirmed by morphologic examination. Some patients have been subjected to unnecessary interventions such as splenectomy for this laboratory artefact (Onder et al 1980).

Table 33.1 Causes of pseudothrombocytopenia

Common causes
Poor blood collecting technique (thrombin generation)
EDTA-induced pseudothrombocytopenia* (Onder et al 1980, Payne & Pierre 1984, Berkman et al 1991)
Less common causes
Platelet satellitism (Bizzaro 1991)
Platelet cold agglutinins (Watkins & Shulman 1970, Cunningham & Brandt 1992)
Overfilling of vacutainer tubes (Pewarchuk et al 1992)
Platelet agglutination by rheumatoid factor immune complexes (Poskitt & Poskitt 1985a)

* Some EDTA-dependent antibodies react optimally below 37°C

Marrow examination

Megakaryocytes are normal or increased in number in patients with increased platelet destruction, hypersplenism, or haemodilution. Consequently, with rare exceptions, the marrow aspirate or biopsy is not diagnostic for these disorders. However, when thrombocytopenia is caused by poor platelet production, the marrow aspirate and biopsy may establish the diagnosis (e.g. neoplastic infiltration of the marrow, myelodysplasia, megaloblastic anaemia, aplastic anaemia, etc.). Particularly in myelodysplasia, certain dysmegakaryocytic morphologic abnormalities can be seen, including micromegakaryocytes, large mononuclear megakaryocytes and megakaryocytes with multiple but separate nuclei (Bennett 1986). Markedly reduced or absent megakaryocytes are seen in acquired or congenital amegakaryocytic thrombocytopenic disorders.

Mean platelet volume

Evaluation of the platelet size, known as mean platelet volume (MPV), can help in the classification of the thrombocytopenia (Bessman 1986). The platelet size varies inversely with the platelet count. Thus, the normal MPV range for a platelet count of 150×10^9/l is approximately 9–12 fl, whereas it is 7.5–10 fl for a platelet count of 400×10^9/l. In general, the MPV is at or above this upper normal range in destructive thrombocytopenic disorders, and reduced or at the lower end of the normal range in thrombocytopenic disorders caused by decreased marrow production or hypersplenism. This general pattern is believed to be the result of megakaryocytes responding to the thrombocytopenia by producing larger sized platelets (Corash et al 1987). A very small MPV of less than 6 fl is a clue to the diagnosis of the Wiskott–Aldrich syndrome (hereditary X-linked thrombocytopenia, atopy, immunodeficiency) and its variants (Ochs et al 1980, Standen et al 1986, Donner et al 1988).

Radionuclide platelet lifespan studies

Radionuclide platelet survival studies can be helpful in

patients in whom the cause of the thrombocytopenia is obscure. Indium-111 (^{111}In) is the optimal platelet label because of its short half life and its high platelet labelling efficiency (Snyder et al 1986). Not only can platelet survival studies determine the mechanism of thrombocytopenia, but also they can be used to identify residual splenic tissue in patients with persisting or recurrent thrombocytopenia following splenectomy for ITP. A platelet survival study should be performed when the patient's presentation, laboratory results, or response to treatment is unexpected.

Plasma glycocalicin and platelet RNA measurements

Two investigational methods that have been used to estimate platelet turnover include measurement of plasma glycocalicin (Steinberg et al 1987) and platelet RNA (Kienast & Schmitz 1990). Glycocalicin is a proteolytic fragment derived from platelet glycoprotein Ib, and is increased in disorders of increased platelet turnover. Platelet RNA can be measured in a flow cytometry using the stain thiazole orange.

Bleeding time

The bleeding time is a test of primary haemostasis, i.e. von Willebrand factor-mediated adhesion of platelets to the injured microvascular subendothelium. The most widely used assay is the Ivy technique, which involves use of a sphygmomanometer to maintain a constant venous pressure at 40 mmHg, and puncture of the forearm skin, usually using a commercially available disposable template device. The bleeding time test is widely used as a screening test for platelet dysfunction and von Willebrand's disease, and is also used to judge response to therapy (e.g. trial of desmopressin for mild von Willebrand's disease). We also use the test to help judge whether treatment should be used for mildly symptomatic thrombocytopenic patients. However, several investigators have questioned the role of the bleeding time in making clinical decisions (Rodgers & Levin 1990, Lind 1991).

Platelet aggregation studies

The develop of a simple optical method to study aggregation of platelets in response to various agonists ex vivo (Born 1962) has resulted in the widespread use of this assay in the evaluation of qualitative platelet abnormalities. Several acquired disorders of platelet function (aspirin use, acquired storage pool disorder) can be suggested by the lack of a secondary wave in response to ADP and adrenaline and by reduced aggregation to collagen. Commercially available instruments known as lumi-aggregometers utilize the luciferin/luciferase reaction to measure release of ATP from platelet dense granules and permit simultaneous investigations of platelet aggregation and granule release. Flow cytometry also has been used to assess disorders of platelet aggregation (Ginsberg et al 1990).

Overview of platelet-antibody testing

Platelet-antibody tests are often used in the evaluation of thrombocytopenic patients because immune platelet destruction is an important cause of thrombocytopenia. Literally hundreds of different assays have been described. It is useful to categorize platelet-antibody tests as direct or indirect, respectively, depending on whether antibody is measured on the patient's platelets or whether the presence of antibody in patient serum or plasma is detected. Further, platelet-antibody tests can be grouped by the general method used to detect platelet-antibody interaction (Murphy & Kelton 1990a):

1. Phase I assays measure the effect of platelet-reactive antibodies indirectly, such as by using a platelet-activation endpoint (e.g. platelet aggregation, [^{14}C]-serotonin release, platelet factor 3 activity). These assays are no longer used, except in unusual instances such as diagnostic testing for heparin-induced thrombocytopenia (Sheridan et al 1986, Warkentin et al 1992a).
2. Phase II assays employ anti-immunoglobulin probes to measure platelet-bound IgG directly or indirectly (consumption assay). Although these continue to be the most widely used assays, doubts about the validity of these assays has been raised (George 1990, Sinha & Kelton 1990, Han et al 1990, Leissinger & Stuckey 1992). These assays have a high sensitivity, but low specificity, for idiopathic thrombocytopenic purpura (Mueller-Eckhardt et al 1980, Kelton et al 1982, 1989).
3. Phase III assays have become available in recent years. These assays use techniques that indicate specific antibody/platelet membrane protein binding. For example, detection of patient serum IgG that has reacted with electrophoretically separated platelet membrane proteins on nitrocellulose (immunoblotting) is one method that was developed during the 1980s. Other methods that have been developed include immunoprecipitation (Woods et al 1987a,b), immunobead assay (McMillan et al 1987), and monoclonal antibody immobilization of platelet antigens (MAIPA) (Kiefel et al 1987). It is possible that these newer assays may be more specific tests for autoimmune thrombocytopenia (McMillan et al 1987).

Management of thrombocytopenic patients: an overview

The clinician must decide whether any treatment is required at all. For most patients, thrombocytopenia does not result in bleeding. Unfortunately, there are no definite guides to predict the risk of bleeding. The severity of the thrombocytopenia does not precisely correlate with the risk of haemorrhage, possibly because the presence of other complex clinical factors (recent surgery or trauma, coagulation defects, underlying disease that has caused the thrombocytopenia, etc.) can obscure the relationship. Measures to prevent bleeding complications should be taken, including the avoidance of trauma (intramuscular injections, arterial punctures) and avoidance of drugs that may interfere with platelet function (alcohol, aspirin).

Treatment guidelines should take into account three factors: (1) the risk of serious bleeding; (2) the cause of the thrombocytopenia; and (3) the natural history of the thrombocytopenia.

1. *Risk of bleeding.* Patients with life-threatening bleeding (intracranial haemorrhage) should immediately receive platelet transfusions. For patients without active bleeding, the clinician should estimate the risk of bleeding. Severe thrombocytopenia (platelet count less than 10×10^9/l), and the presence of mucosal blood blisters ('wet purpura'), indicates a high risk of serious bleeding, and warrants urgent treatment. For patients with less severe thrombocytopenia and minimal symptoms, obtaining the bleeding time helps to judge the haemostatic risk.

2. *Cause of the thrombocytopenia.* Disorders characterized by platelet-mediated thrombosis, such as heparin-induced thrombocytopenia and thrombotic microangiopathy, rarely have serious bleeding, but often are complicated by thrombosis. We believe that prophylactic platelet transfusions are contraindicated for these disorders. Overall, platelet function is better at the same platelet count for destructive thrombocytopenic disorders, compared with disorders of platelet production (Harker & Slichter 1972b). Presumably, this is because larger, 'hyperfunctional' platelets are produced by the normal marrow in response to peripheral platelet destruction (Corash et al 1987, Thompson & Jakubowski 1988). Prophylactic platelet transfusions should be avoided in patients with destructive thrombocytopenia, unless there is a high risk of bleeding. In contrast, prophylactic platelet transfusions are usually given to patients with leukaemia who have a platelet count below 20×10^9/l (Editorial 1987). Recent data, however, suggests that a less aggressive prophylactic approach to platelet transfusions may be acceptable (Aderka et al 1986, Gmür et al 1991).

3. *Natural history of the thrombocytopenia.* Certain disorders are characterized by short-lived, but severe, thrombocytopenia, such as alcohol-induced thrombocytopenia, septicaemia-associated thrombocytopenia, certain drug-induced thrombocytopenias and acute leukaemia. Clinicians should consider administering platelets to these patients if they are at high risk of bleeding. In contrast, when the thrombocytopenia is chronic (e.g. idiopathic thrombocytopenic purpura, amegakaryocytic thrombocytopenia, myelodysplasia), the risks of repeated prophylactic platelet transfusions are higher than the likely benefit.

Pharmacologic treatment of the thrombocytopenic patient

The adjunctive use of drug therapy to reduce the risk of thrombocytopenic bleeding is controversial.

Antifibrinolytic therapy. Orally effective antifibrinolytic drugs such as ε-aminocaproic acid and tranexamic acid have been reported to reduce bleeding in severely thrombocytopenic patients (Gardner & Helmer 1980, Garewal & Durie 1985, Bartholomew et al 1989, Ben-Bassat et al 1990). However, a small, randomized, controlled trial did not demonstrate benefit using tranexamic acid in one group of thrombocytopenic patients (Fricke et al 1991).

DDAVP (desmopressin). Desmopressin can shorten the bleeding time in some patients with moderate thrombocytopenia (Kobrinsky & Tulloch 1988, DiMichele & Hathaway 1990), although its effectiveness remains unestablished. It is unlikely to benefit patients with severe thrombocytopenia (Mannucci et al 1986).

THROMBOCYTOPENIA CAUSED BY INCREASED PLATELET DESTRUCTION

IDIOPATHIC THROMBOCYTOPENIC PURPURA (ITP)

ITP is a common autoimmune disorder of unknown etiology that is characterized by the premature destruction of IgG-coated platelets by the reticuloendothelial system (Kelton & Gibbons 1982, Karpatkin 1985).

Clinical features

For many patients with chronic ITP, the onset is insidious, and patients report bleeding symptoms over many months or years. Often, the patients are asymptomatic and are recognized when a blood count is obtained for unrelated purposes. The abrupt onset of severe, symptomatic thrombocytopenia often indicates secondary immune thrombocytopenia in adults (infectious mononucleosis-induced ITP, drug-induced thrombocytopenia).

The severity of mucocutaneous haemorrhagic symptoms and signs usually parallels the severity of the thrombocytopenia. Physical findings are limited to purpura or pallor secondary to acute or chronic bleeding. The presence of fever, lymphadenopathy, hepatomegaly, or splenomegaly suggests other diagnoses (systemic lupus erythematosus, lymphoma, HIV-associated thrombocytopenia).

Pathogenesis

The first direct evidence that ITP is the result of a humoral factor that causes premature platelet destruction was provided approximately 40 years ago when Harrington and colleagues (1951) produced thrombocytopenia in healthy volunteers who were given plasma from ITP patients. The development of new technologies to quantitate immunoglobulin on the platelet surface showed that platelet-associated immunoglobulin was elevated in most patients with ITP (Dixon et al 1975, Hegde et al 1985a). However, elevated platelet-associated IgG is not direct evidence for an immune humoral pathogenesis and is observed in other thrombocytopenic disorders (Mueller-Eckhardt et al 1980, Kelton et al 1982, 1989, Donnér et al 1990).

Direct evidence that IgG bound to platelet membrane antigens via their Fab termini (Mason & McMillan 1984) was provided during the 1980s, when new technologies such as immunoblotting (Beardsley et al 1984), immunoprecipitation (Woods et al 1984a,b, Tomiyama et al 1990a), and use of monoclonal antibodies to immobilize platelet protein antigens (Kiefel et al 1987) confirmed that IgG that specifically reacts with platelet membrane glycoproteins can be observed in most patients with ITP. Most studies have shown that GPIIb/IIIa and GPIb/IX are the most frequent target antigens in ITP (McMillan et al 1987, Kiefel et al 1991a, Kunicki & Newman 1992). Antibodies against platelet glycolipids (Van Vliet et al 1987), phospholipids (Harris et al 1985b, Font et al 1989), and vinculin (Tomiyama et al 1992) also can be detected in patients with chronic ITP, but their role in causing platelet destruction is uncertain.

Splenic lymphocytes contribute to the synthesis of platelet autoantibodies (McMillan et al 1972). The spleen also is the dominant organ of clearance of the IgG-sensitized platelets, although hepatic clearance predominates in some patients (Siegel et al 1989). Platelet lifespan studies generally show decreased platelet survival and increased turnover (Harker 1970, Branehög et al 1974). Less commonly, the platelet survival is only mildly reduced, with platelet turnover decreased (Ballem et al 1987b, Siegel et al 1989). It is uncertain whether this observation indicates megakaryocyte injury by autoantibodies (McMillan et al 1978) or intramedullary platelet destruction by marrow phagocytic cells.

The fundamental disturbance leading to autoantibody formation in ITP is not known. Lymphocytes obtained from normal spleens are capable of generating platelet-reactive antibodies (Denomme et al 1992), but the trigger of an aberrant immune reaction is not known. Some lymphocyte subclass distribution abnormalities have been reported in chronic ITP, including decreased T4-positive/T8-positive ratios (Mylvaganam et al 1985), increased numbers of $T4^{+}/T8^{+}$ lymphocytes (Mizutani et al 1985), and increased Ia-positive T lymphocyte numbers (Mizutani et al 1987).

Treatment of ITP

Emergency treatment

Emergency treatment for ITP should be instituted when patients have life-threatening haemorrhage. Immediate transfusion of platelets should be followed by high-dose intravenous IgG, followed by additional platelet transfusions (Baumann et al 1986, Murphy & Kelton 1990b). Although the transfused platelets will be destroyed by the platelet-reactive autoantibodies, transient increases in the platelet counts can be demonstrated (Carr et al 1986b).

Urgent treatment of ITP

Patients at very high risk of bleeding (severe thrombocytopenia and 'wet' purpura), as well as those who must undergo operative or other invasive procedures, should have their platelet count raised quickly to safe levels. Three approaches are used: high-dose intravenous (iv) IgG, anti-Rhesus(D) globulin, and high-dose methylprednisolone therapy.

High-dose intravenous IgG. High-dose iv IgG will raise the platelet count to safe levels ($>50 \times 10^9$/l) in approximately 80% of patients, and is the treatment of choice. The usual dosage is 1 g/kg infused over 6–8 hours, given on 2 consecutive days (Boshkov & Kelton 1989). The benefit is usually transient, lasting from 1–4 weeks. Although iv IgG is obtained from many blood donors, commercial iv IgG preparations do not transmit HIV or viral hepatitis (Imbach et al 1991). The common side-effects of headache, fever, or flushing usually respond to reduction in the rate of infusion and symptomatic therapy. Uncommon side-effects include chest pain, hypertension, hypotension, bronchospasm, and laryngeal oedema (Lederman et al 1986). Very rare adverse effects include haemolysis due to ABO haemolysins contained within the iv IgG (Kim et al 1988), acute cryoglobulinaemic nephropathy in rheumatoid factor-positive recipients (Barton et al 1987), and fatal thrombotic events in elderly patients (Woodruff et al 1986).

Anti-Rhesus(D) globulin (Anti-D). Anti-Rhesus globulin was first used by Salama and coworkers (1983, 1984). Anti-D is effective only in Rh(D)-positive patients and works by a competitive inhibition of reticuloendothelial cells by the anti-D-sensitized autologous red cells. One regimen is to administer 25 µg/kg of anti-D intravenously and repeat the dose 2 days later if no response is evident (Bussel et al 1991). Approximately 80% of patients will exhibit a significant increase in the platelet count that can last for a few weeks (Bussel et al 1991, Salama & Mueller-Eckhardt 1992). Splenectomized

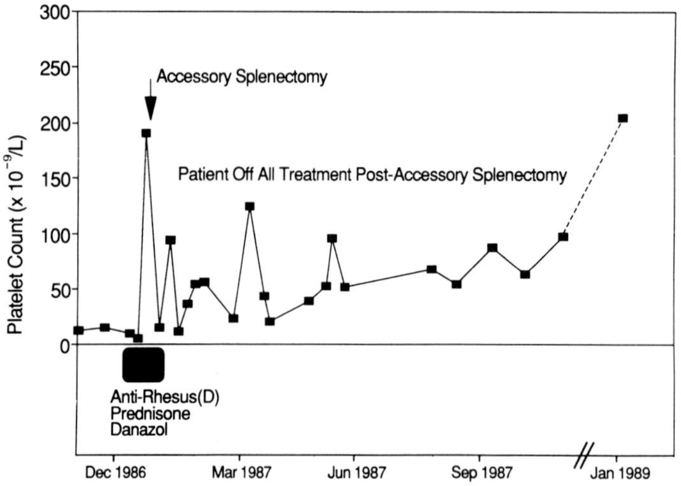

Fig. 33.1 Twenty-one year old male with refractory idiopathic thrombocytopenic purpura (ITP) for six months. His severe ITP was diagnosed in July 1986, and was refractory to corticosteroids, splenectomy (August 1986), high-dose intravenous gammaglobulin (transient response only), vincristine, danazol, plasma exchange, and cyclophosphamide. A radionuclide ^{111}Indium platelet survival study in December 1986 demonstrated a small accessory spleen, despite a peripheral blood film appearance consistent with post-splenectomy changes. The platelet count was raised pre-operatively using anti-Rhesus (D), prednisone, and danazol. Following removal of the accessory spleen, the patient had persisting but less severe thrombocytopenia, with marked improvement in bleeding symptoms. The platelet count rose slowly over the next year. This patient illustrates several principles in the management of ITP: (a) the investigation for accessory spleen(s) in patients who have refractory or relapsed ITP following splenectomy; (b) role of intermittent multiple modality treatment for high-risk bleeding periods (e.g. perioperative management); (c) avoidance of potentially toxic treatment for ITP when patients have mild-to-moderate thrombocytopenia with few or no bleeding symptoms; and, (d) late complete remission can occur in some patients with chronic ITP. (Modified, with permission from CME Publishing Ltd, Montreal, Quebec, Canada, and taken from Warkentin T E & Kelton J G. Immune thrombocytopenia. Medicine (N Am) 1989; 3rd series 30: 5495–5503.)

patients have a lower probability of response to anti-D. Anti-D may be less useful for the emergency treatment of bleeding ITP patients; however, its relatively low cost and high probability of benefit makes it an ideal treatment for patients who require a short-term increase in the platelet count (e.g. preparation for surgery) (see Fig. 33.1).

High-dose intravenous corticosteroids. High-dose methylprednisolone, 1 g daily for 3 days via the intravenous route, was as effective as iv IgG in one non-randomized study of adult ITP patients (von dem Borne et al 1988). This treatment has been used to raise the platelet count before splenectomy (Yoshida et al 1987).

Long-term therapy for ITP

Corticosteroids

Corticosteroids are frequently used in the treatment of chronic ITP. Approximately 60–70% of patients will have a clinically important increase in the platelet count in response to prednisone therapy; however, the platelet count usually decreases to baseline during tapering or following discontinuation (Berchtold & McMillan 1989, Warkentin & Kelton 1990a). Occasionally, long-term complete or partial remissions occur. In other patients, significant benefit can be achieved with small doses (prednisone 7.5 mg or less, given on alternate days). Studies have shown that smaller doses of prednisone (0.25–0.50 mg/kg/day) are just as likely to produce benefit at 6 month follow-up as conventional doses (1 mg/kg/day), although the rate in rise of the platelet count may be slower (Mazzucconi et al 1985, Bellucci et al 1988).

There are numerous side-effects of corticosteroid therapy, including hypertension, diabetes, mood changes and psychosis, fluid retention, peptic ulcer, cushingoid facies, osteoporosis, and increased risk of infection. Osteonecrosis, usually affecting the hips or shoulders, has been estimated to occur in about 5% of patients receiving corticosteroids for a prolonged period, but can also occur following intensive short-term treatment (Mankin 1992).

Splenectomy

Splenectomy is the most effective treatment for ITP. It should be considered early for patients with severe thrombocytopenia or symptomatic patients who do not have a long-term remission following a course of prednisone. Splenectomy produces a complete remission in about 70% of patients. An additional 10–20% of patients have a partial response to splenectomy. For patients with severe thrombocytopenia, the platelet count should be raised preoperatively using either corticosteroids, iv IgG, or anti-Rhesus(D). Bleeding complications are relatively uncommon even for severely thrombocytopenic patients (Jacobs et al 1986), and prophylactic platelet transfusions seldom are indicated. Perioperative corticosteroid therapy is usually given to prevent adrenal insufficiency in patients who have previously received corticosteroids.

Perioperative mortality is less than 1%, and is most frequently caused by pulmonary thromboembolism (Warkentin & Kelton 1990a). The major risk to the patient is the long-term risk of post-splenectomy sepsis. Current recommendations are that patients should be vaccinated with polyvalent pneumococcal and meningococcal vaccines at least 2 weeks before splenectomy (Centers for Disease Control 1991). *Haemophilus influenzae* type b vaccine should also be given to children, and some physicians would also administer this vaccine to adults because of the risk of *H. influenzae* bacteraemia in post-splenectomy patients (Farley et al 1992).

Refractory patients

Accessory spleens

A relapse of the ITP following an initial good response may indicate the presence of residual splenic material (accessory spleens) (Akwari et al 1987). Different approaches can be used to identify an accessory spleen, including radioisotope scanning following ^{111}In-labelled platelet survival study and CT scanning of the abdomen. The intraoperative use of a hand-held isotope detector probe has been used to locate the residual splenic material (Akwari et al 1987). The presence of Howell–Jolly bodies on the peripheral blood film does not rule out the presence of an accessory spleen as the cause of post-splenectomy relapse of ITP. Approximately 50% of patients will have a remission following removal of an accessory spleen (Berchtold & McMillan 1989).

Danazol

Danazol is a weak androgen that is effective in some adult ITP patients (Ahn et al 1983, 1987, 1989). Danazol appears to reduce platelet destruction by decreasing the number of phagocytic cell Fc receptors (Schreiber et al 1987). Usually, 400–800 mg are administered daily, although low doses (50 mg) can also be effective (Ahn et al 1987, 1989). Response is usually seen within 2 months, although a longer interval may be needed when low doses are used.

As many as 40% of patients develop subclinical elevation of liver enzymes at some time during therapy, which responds to dose reduction or discontinuation of the drug. Other side-effects include fluid retention, lethargy, myalgia, skin rash, nausea, amenorrhoea, headache, and mild virilizing effects. Rarely, peliosis of the liver and spleen (Nesher et al 1985) and idiosyncratic thrombocytopenia (Arrowsmith & Dreis 1986, Rabinowe & Miller 1987) have been observed. Danazol is contraindicated during pregnancy (Wentz 1982).

Other treatments

Other drug treatments that are effective in some refractory ITP patients include azathioprine (Quiquandon et al 1990), cyclophosphamide (Caplan & Berkman 1976, Pizzuto & Ambriz 1984), and vinca alkaloids (Manohran 1991). Still considered experimental are interferon (Proctor et al 1989), cyclosporine (Kelsey et al 1985, Matsumura et al 1988).

Alternate treatment approaches for elderly and high-risk patients

Elderly ITP patients may have a lower probability of benefit from splenectomy (Akwari et al 1987, Fenaux et al 1989) and may have a higher risk of complications. We have used splenic irradiation rather than splenectomy for these high-risk patients (Calverley et al 1992). Danazol may be more effective in older compared with younger female patients (Ahn et al 1989) and some physicians try danazol before splenectomy in these patients. Dapsone is a potent trigger of oxidant haemolysis, and has been used in some elderly, non-splenectomized patients with ITP, where it may work by blocking reticulo-endothelial function non-immunologically (Durand et al 1991b).

Diseases associated with ITP

A large number of illnesses, many of immune pathogenesis, have been associated with ITP (Table 33.2). In some cases, treatment of the associated disorder leads to a dramatic remission of the ITP (Jansen et al 1987, von dem Borne et al 1990). Otherwise, the treatment of secondary chronic ITP is similar to primary ITP, i.e. corticosteroids followed by splenectomy.

Table 33.2 Diseases associated with idiopathic thrombocytopenic purpura

Collagen vascular diseases	
	Systemic lupus erythematosus (Hegde et al 1985b, Berchtold et al 1989a)
	Rheumatoid arthritis (Hegde et al 1985b, Berchtold et al 1989a)
	Dermatomyositis (Cooper et al 1986)
	Scleroderma (Neucks et al 1980)
	Sjögren's syndrome (Berchtold et al 1989a, Sugai et al 1989)
	Mixed connective tissue disease (Berchtold et al 1989a)
Autoimmune endocrine disorders	
	Hashimoto's thyroiditis (Segal & Weintraub 1976, Herman 1980)
	Grave's disease (Pinals et al 1977, Herman 1980, Bellucci et al 1991)
	Diabetes mellitus (Hegde et al 1985b)
	Autoimmune hyperchylomicronaemia (Kihara et al 1989)
Neoplasia	
	Hodgkin's disease (Rudders et al 1972, Hegde et al 1985b, Xiros et al 1988, Berchtold et al 1989a)
	Non-Hodgkin's lymphoma (Hegde et al 1985b, Berchtold et al 1989a, Kubota et al 1989)
	Chronic lymphocytic leukaemia (Hegde et al 1985b, Berchtold et al 1989a)
	Multiple myeloma (Hegde et al 1985b, Verdirame et al 1985)
	Acute lymphoid leukaemia (Rao & Pang 1979)
	Acute myeloid leukaemia (Amylon et al 1984)
	Carcinomas (Kim & Boggs 1979, Schwartz et al 1982)
	Benign or malignant ovarian tumour (von dem Borne et al 1990, Bellucci et al 1991)
	Primary extragonadal germ cell tumour (Garnick & Griffin 1983)
Gastrointestinal disorders	
	Crohn's disease (Kosmo et al 1986)
	Ulcerative colitis (Gupta et al 1986)
	Primary biliary cirrhosis (Chalmers et al 1987, Berchtold et al 1989a)
	Coeliac disease (Stenhammar & Ljunggren 1988)
	Pernicious anaemia (Hegde et al 1985b)
Other disorders	
	Sarcoidosis (Field & Poon 1987)
	Idiopathic pulmonary fibrosis (Berchtold et al 1989a)
	Myasthenia gravis (Segal & Weintraub 1976, Pinals et al 1977, Anderson et al 1984, Jansen et al 1987)
	Retroperitoneal fibrosis (Wallach et al 1991)
	Autoimmune haemolysis (Evan's syndrome) (Hegde et al 1985b, Wang 1988, Berchtold et al 1989a)

IDIOPATHIC THROMBOCYTOPENIC PURPURA IN CHILDREN

Acute ITP in children

Acute ITP is a common disorder in young children that may be caused by transient production of platelet-reactive autoantibodies (Berchtold et al 1989b, Winiarski 1989). Typically, the child has a viral infection 1 or 2 weeks before the abrupt onset of severe thrombocytopenia (platelet count often less than 20×10^9/l). For approximately 80% of the children, the thrombocytopenia will resolve, although this may take months (Hoyle et al 1986). Rarely (less than 1%), severe sequelae such as lethal intracranial haemorrhage occur. High-dose iv IgG is a rapid way to raise the platelet count to safe levels (Imbach et al 1985, Blanchette et al 1991) and is used by most physicians. A rapid response has also been reported using high-dose methylprednisolone in acute childhood ITP (Jayabose et al 1987, van Hoff & Ritchey 1988), but this treatment has not been directly compared with iv IgG. Controlled studies indicate that oral corticosteroids also will raise the platelet count faster than no treatment (Dunn & Maurer 1984, Sartorius 1984) and some physicians would use prednisone, 4 mg/kg/day (Suarez et al 1986, Blanchette et al 1991) for symptomatic children without severe thrombocytopenia.

Chronic idiopathic thrombocytopenic purpura in children

Chronic ITP in children is usually defined as thrombocytopenia persisting for greater than 6 months. However, late remissions can occur in some children even after this interval. Serum autoantibodies reactive with GPIIb/IIIa and GPIb/IX are found in similar frequencies as seen in adults with chronic ITP (Berchtold et al 1989b), suggesting a similar pathogenesis. Phase II (platelet-associated IgG) assays are sensitive but not specific for ITP in children (Donnér et al 1990).

There is more reluctance to use long-term corticosteroid therapy (growth inhibition) or splenectomy (risk of post-splenectomy septicaemia) in children compared with adults. Symptomatic thrombocytopenia can be controlled in many of these children using repeated treatments with anti-Rhesus(D) globulin (Becker et al 1986, Andrew et al 1992) or high-dose iv IgG (Hollenberg et al 1988). Intermittent high-dose corticosteroids can also be used to treat symptomatic episodes of severe thromboctyopenia (Menichelli et al 1984).

HIV-ASSOCIATED THROMBOCYTOPENIA

There are certain differences between HIV-associated thrombocytopenia and ITP with respect to clinical features, pathogenesis, and treatment.

Clinical features

A syndrome that resembles ITP has been described in many otherwise asymptomatic HIV-infected patients (Morris et al 1982, Abrams et al 1986, Walsh & Karpatkin 1990). Prospective studies indicate that as many as 18% of asymptomatic HIV patients who are followed for several months will develop mild transient thrombocytopenia (Boyar & Beall 1991, Peltier et al 1991). However, in approximately 1–2% of patients, platelet counts are persistently below 50×10^9/l (Boyar & Beall 1991, Peltier et al 1991). Primary HIV infection is characterized by an acute infectious mononucleosis-like illness often associated with mild and transient thrombocytopenia (Cooper et al 1985).

Pathogenesis

There is evidence that at least three mechanisms contribute to the thrombocytopenia of HIV infections. These include increased platelet destruction by antibodies (Walsh et al 1984), impaired platelet production by HIV-infected megakaryocytes (Zucker-Franklin & Cao 1989), and impaired CD34 stem/progenitor cell activity resulting from an abnormal bone marrow microenvironment (Zauli et al 1992). Two types of platelet antibody have been described: immune complexes of anti-HIV antibodies and anti-F(ab′)$_2$ components (Walsh et al 1984, Karpatkin et al 1988) and platelet-reactive autoantibodies (van der Lelie et al 1987, Bettaieb et al 1989). A recent report suggests an explanation for these differing observations: some anti-HIV antibodies cross-react with an epitope on platelet GPIIb/IIIa (Bettaieb et al 1992).

In patients with advanced HIV infection, pancytopenia can occur, often with dysplastic morphologic features (Spivak et al 1984, Schneider & Picker 1985). In addition to stem/progenitor cell dysfunction, the clinician should consider marrow infections (e.g. *Mycobacterium avium/intracellulare*), HIV-associated neoplasms with marrow involvement, and drug-induced myelosuppression.

Treatment

Most patients with HIV-ITP are asymptomatic and do not require specific treatment. The following considerations apply to patients with severe thrombocytopenia.

Zidovudine

The anti-retroviral agent, zidovudine, will raise the platelet count in as many as 70% of patients (Richman et al 1987, Swiss Group 1988, Rarick et al 1991). However, the actual elevation in the platelet count tends to be modest, and seldom will zidovudine alone raise the platelet count in severely thrombocytopenic individuals to acceptable levels. Platelet lifespan studies using ^{111}In-labelled platelets demonstrate increased platelet survival in patients treated with zidovudine (Ballem et al 1989, Panzer et al 1989).

Prednisone/splenectomy

Corticosteroids are as effective as they are in ITP (and just as unlikely to produce a long-term remission) (Walsh et al 1985, Abrams et al 1986, Oksenhendler et al 1987). However, reports of worsening of oral candidiasis means that most physicians try to avoid corticosteroid therapy in HIV-infected patients. Approximately two-thirds of patients have a long-term remission following splenectomy (Walsh et al 1985, Abrams et al 1986, Oksenhendler et al 1987, Schneider et al 1987, Tyler et al 1990) and to date there does not appear to be a dramatic increase in post-splenectomy sepsis in HIV-infected patients (Tyler et al 1990).

Intravenous IgG/anti-rhesus(D) globulin

Patients with HIV-induced thrombocytopenia usually respond transiently to high-dose iv IgG or anti-D (Oksenhendler et al 1987, 1988, Pollak et al 1988) and some physicians have used repeated injections of iv IgG (Bussel & Haimi 1988) or anti-D (Rossi et al 1987, Oksenhendler et al 1988) to maintain safe platelet counts in patients with chronic, severe HIV-ITP.

Other treatments

Other treatments include danazol (Oksenhendler et al 1987), extracorporeal immunoadsorption (Snyder et al 1991), recombinant interferon (Ellis et al 1987, Northfelt et al 1991), dapsone (Durand et al 1991a), and low-dose splenic irradiation (Needleman et al 1992). There are no comparative data to recommend any of these treatments over another, and several including immunoadsorption and interferon, must be considered experimental.

Human T cell leukaemia virus type I (HTLV-I)

Recently, chronic thrombocytopenia has been described in patients that are carriers of the retrovirus HTLV-I (Matsuoka et al 1988, Takahashi et al 1991).

SYSTEMIC LUPUS ERYTHEMATOSUS AND THROMBOCYTOPENIA

Thrombocytopenia occurs in at least 10–20% of patients with systemic lupus erythematosus (SLE) (Tan et al 1982, Jonsson et al 1989). The cause of the thrombocytopenia in SLE patients is probably more complex than in ITP. Increased platelet destruction can be caused by the binding of IgG autoantibodies to platelet glycoproteins (Howe & Lynch 1987, Kaplan et al 1987), platelet-reactive immune complexes (Pfueller et al 1987) and anti-phospholipid antibodies reactive with platelet phospholipids and sulphatides (Khamashta et al 1988, Murakami et al 1991). Morphologic marrow abnormalities can include dyserythropoiesis, hypoplasia, gelatinous transformation, lymphocytosis, and plasmacytosis (Feng et al 1991), suggesting a role for impaired platelet production. Hypersplenism can explain pancytopenia in some patients. A syndrome of fever, pancytopenia, and haemophagocytosis that responds to high doses of corticosteroids has been described recently in some patients with lupus (Wong et al 1991). Some SLE patients with mild to moderate thrombocytopenia (platelet count 50–150 × 10^9/l) have a platelet function defect, with easy bruising and a prolonged bleeding time (Weiss et al 1980). Other potential contributors to the thrombocytopenia include the multisystem 'flares' of SLE, complicating infections, and side-effects of immunosuppressive medications.

If treatment is required, we try to avoid long-term corticosteroid treatment unless required for other manifestations of SLE. Danazol therapy (Agnello et al 1983, Marino & Cook 1985, West & Johnson 1988) is possibly more effective than in ITP patients. In contrast, splenectomy may be less effective (approximately 50% response rate). Intermittent cyclophosphamide has been used in patients with severe disease (Boumpas et al 1990).

ANTIPHOSPHOLIPID ANTIBODY SYNDROME

The antiphospholipid antibody syndrome consists of recurrent miscarriages, venous and arterial thrombosis (especially deep vein thrombosis, pulmonary embolism, cerebrovascular accidents), thrombocytopenia, and a variety of dermatologic findings. The spectrum of skin abnormalities includes livedo reticularis, leg ulcers, symmetric gangrene of the fingers and toes, and 'unfading acral microlivedo' (nonblanching erythematous or cyanotic macules located on the palms, soles, fingertips, or toes) (Grob & Bonerandi 1986, 1989, Grob et al 1991). Dermatopathology shows microvascular thrombosis without vasculitis (Grob et al 1991).

The thrombocytopenia tends to be intermittent and mild. Consequently, the reported incidence varies markedly in different patient series (Gastineau et al 1985, Glueck et al 1985, Harris et al 1985a). It remains unproven whether the antiphospholipid antibodies are responsible for the thrombocytopenia observed in some patients.

No laboratory features of the antiphospholipid antibodies have been identified to predict patients at highest risk for thrombosis. Long-term antiplatelet or anticoagulant therapy is thus used only in patients who have already developed an arterial or venous thrombotic event, respectively. There is anecdotal evidence that corticosteroid therapy could worsen symptoms in some patients (Davies & Triplett 1990).

IMMUNE THROMBOCYTOPENIA IN BONE MARROW TRANSPLANT RECIPIENTS

A number of factors, including infections and drug effects, can be responsible for the delayed platelet recovery in patients who have undergone bone marrow transplantation (First et al 1985). There is evidence, however, that immune platelet destruction occurs in many of these patients (Minchinton et al 1984, Anasetti et al 1989). As yet, phase III platelet-antibody assays have not been reported to confirm an autoimmune pathogenesis in these patients.

IMMUNE DRUG-INDUCED THROMBOCYTOPENIA

Heparin-induced thrombocytopenia

Heparin-induced thrombocytopenia is one of the most important adverse drug reactions in clinical medicine. Exposure to heparin is common in hospitalized patients, and clinicians should always consider this diagnosis in thrombocytopenic hospitalized patients. Heparin-induced thrombocytopenia can occur in as many as 5% of patients treated with therapeutic doses of porcine mucosal heparin. The risk is even higher when bovine heparin is used (Warkentin & Kelton 1991). Most significantly, some patients with this complication develop associated venous or arterial thrombosis. It is likely that these thrombotic complications are causally related to the heparin-induced thrombocytopenia, because (1) heparin-induced thrombocytopenia is caused by a platelet-activating IgG (Sheridan et al 1986, Kelton et al 1988); (2) the platelet activation stimulus causes platelets to produce procoagulant microparticles (Warkentin et al 1991); (3) patient serum can activate endothelial cells to cause them to produce tissue factor (Cines et al 1987) and (4) a characteristic 'white clot' consisting of platelet-rich thrombi adherent to endothelium can be demonstrated in some patients.

Heparin-induced thrombocytopenia can be difficult to distinguish from other causes of thrombocytopenia in hospitalized patients. This is because the severity of the thrombocytopenia is typically between 25–150 × 10^9/l and similar to thrombocytopenia caused by septicaemia and dilution. Sometimes, very small amounts of heparin, such as found on pulmonary artery catheters, can produce thrombocytopenia (Laster et al 1989, Moberg et al 1990).

Arterial or venous lower limb thrombosis, as well as cerebrovascular accidents and myocardial infarctions, are the most frequent thrombotic complications (Weismann & Tobin 1958, Warkentin & Kelton 1990b, 1991). Lower limb gangrene can be caused either by arterial or venous (phlegmasia cerulea dolens) thrombosis. Acute and chronic adrenal insufficiency can be caused by adrenal failure resulting from adrenal vein thrombosis, with consequent adrenal infarction and haemorrhage (Ernest & Fisher 1991). A syndrome consisting of chills, fever, and other systemic symptoms, together with abrupt thrombocytopenia, has been recently recognized in patients with heparin-induced thrombocytopenia who receive an intravenous bolus of heparin (Warkentin et al 1992d).

Most cases of heparin-induced thrombocytopenia and thrombosis go unrecognized. For example, although current data suggests that heparin-induced thrombosis occurs in as many as one in 200 patients receiving intravenous therapeutic doses of heparin for at least 7 days, the general recognition of this syndrome has only come in recent years.

Laboratory testing for heparin-induced thrombocytopenia is crucial to distinguish heparin-induced thrombocytopenia from other causes of thrombocytopenia (Sheridan et al 1986, Warkentin et al 1992a). Many centres use platelet aggregation studies in the diagnosis. However, this technique is relatively insensitive for diagnosing heparin-induced thrombocytopenia (Kelton et al 1984b, Greinacher et al 1991). To enhance sensitivity, optimally reactive donor platelets should be washed and resuspended in calcium-containing buffer and weakly positive control samples should be assayed to confirm that the test platelets can detect positive sera (Warkentin et al 1992a).

Heparin should be discontinued in suspected cases of heparin-induced thrombocytopenia. If the patient requires ongoing antithrombotic treatment, options include the defibrinogenating venom ancrod (Demers et al 1991) or the antithrombotic heparinoid, Lomoparin (Org 10172) (Chong et al 1989, Ortel et al 1992). Low molecular weight heparins should not be used because they may result in persistent thrombocytopenia and thrombosis (Warkentin & Kelton 1991). Certain types of thrombi may benefit from thrombolytic therapy (Mehta et al 1991). Platelet transfusions are contraindicated because of the risk of precipitating thrombotic complications.

Quinine- and quinidine-induced thrombocytopenia

Quinine and quinidine are relatively common causes of acute, severe thrombocytopenia (Danielson et al 1984, Nieminen & Kekomäki 1992). Quinine can be present in some cocktail mixers such as 'tonic water' and 'bitter lemon' (Belkin 1967), and in some illicit drugs (Christie et al 1983). Often, quinine is prescribed for muscle cramps (Powell et al 1988, Freiman 1990). The thrombocytopenia is usually severe (platelet counts less than 20×10^9/l) and complicated by bleeding (contrast heparin-induced thrombocytopenia). Fatal haemorrhages can occur (Freiman 1990). Treatment involves discontinuing the drug, blocking the reticuloendothelial system with high-dose iv IgG (Ray et al 1990), and transfusing platelets if the patient is judged to be at high risk of bleeding.

Quinine-induced haemolytic-uraemic syndrome

Rarely, quinine-induced thrombocytopenia is accompanied by renal failure and schistocytic haemolysis, suggesting quinine-induced haemolytic-uraemic syndrome (Spearing et al 1990, Gottschall et al 1991). It is unknown why a subset of patients with quinine-dependent IgG develop this syndrome.

Other drugs that cause severe immune thrombocytopenia

Many other drugs have been implicated as using severe idiosyncratic thrombocytopenia (platelet count $<20 \times 10^9$/l) (Table 33.3). However, confirmatory laboratory testing has only been established with relatively few agents, including some antibiotics (e.g. sulfa drugs, penicillins, cephalosporins, vancomycin, rifampin), gold, H_2-blockers (cimetidine, ranitidine), thiazide diuretics, digoxin, and benzodiazepines. In some instances, the drug-dependent

Table 33.3 Drugs implicated in immune thrombocytopenia

Drug-dependent platelet-activating IgG (Fc receptor-dependent)
Unfractionated heparin (reviewed in Warkentin & Kelton 1990), low molecular weight heparin (Eichinger et al 1991), pentosan polysulphate (Jacquin et al 1988), Arteparon (chondroitin sulphate) (Greinacher et al 1992)
Drug-dependent increase in platelet-associated IgG (Fab-dependent, Fc-independent, binding to glycoproteins IIb/IIIa or Ib/IX or both)
*Quinine (Christie et al 1985, Visentin et al 1991), *quinidine (Christie et al 1985, Visentin et al 1991), *vancomycin (Christie et al 1990, Zenon et al 1991)
Drug-dependent increase in platelet-associated IgG (glycoprotein localization is unknown)
*Ampicillin (Kelton et al 1981), *cefotetan (Christie et al 1988), *cephamandole (Lown & Barr 1987), chlorpheniramine, *cimetidine (Kelton et al 1981), *diazepam (Conti & Gandolfo 1983), digoxin, *gold (Kosty et al 1989), *hydrochlorthiazide, *mianserin (Stricker et al 1985), *'sulfa' antibiotics (Kelton et al 1981), *penicillin (Kelton et al 1981), ranitidine, *rifampin (Kakaiya et al 1989)
Probable drug-induced thrombocytopenia (established by drug rechallenge or drug-dependent phase I assay)
*Acetaminophen (Eisner & Shahidi 1972), acetazolamide, actinomycin D (Hodder et al 1985), allyl-isopropyl-acetyl-carbamide (sedormid), alprenolol, aminoglutethimide (Ardman & Rudders 1982), amiodarone (Weinberger et al 1987), antazoline, aspirin (Garg & Sarker 1974), *carbamazepine (Tohen et al 1991), cephalexin, cephalothin, chlorthalidone, *chlorthiazide, danazol (Arrowsmith & Dreis 1986, Rabinowe & Miller 1987), desferrioxamine (Walker et al 1985), desipramine, difluoromethylornithine, digitoxin, diflunisal, *diphenylhydantoin, ethchlorvynol, furosemide, gentamicin, imipramine, iopanoic acid, levamisole, *α-interferon (McLaughlin et al 1985), β-interferon, isotretinoin (Johnson & Rapini 1987), lidocaine, meprobamate, methicillin, minoxidil, morphine, methyldopa, nomifensine, novobiocin, paraaminosalicylic acid, phenylbutazone, oxprenolol, nalidixic acid (Meyboom 1984), pirenzepine, *procainamide (Meisner et al 1985), spironolactone, stibophen
Possible drug-induced thrombocytopenia (no rechallenge or in vitro testing)
Apalcillin, butobarbitone, *captopril, chlordiazopoxide/clidinium bromide, chlorpropamide, clinoril, clonazepam, diatrizoate, diazoxide, etretinate, fenoprofen, glibenclamide (Israeli et al 1988), heroin, *indomethacin, isoniazid, levodopa, lincomycin, nitroprusside, oxyphenbutazone, oxytetracycline, pentamidine, piroxicam, primidone, sulindac, ticlopidine (Takishita et al 1990), tobramycin, tolbutamide, tolmetin, toluene
Drugs with high incidence of mild thrombocytopenia and positive direct platelet-associated IgG
Valproic acid (Barr et al 1982), amrinone (Ansell et al 1984)
Drug-induced lupus anticoagulant syndrome and thromboembolism
Procainamide (Asherson et al 1989)
Drug-induced haemolytic-uraemic syndrome
Quinine (Gottschall et al 1991, Stroncek et al 1992), proguanil (Gon & Reid 1975), penicillin, ampicillin (Parker et al 1971)
Drug-induced immune haemolytic anaemia with thrombocytopenia
Note that in some cases drug-dependent thrombocytopenia has been shown (Salama & Mueller-Eckhardt 1985) and in others thrombocytopenia has been attributed to sequelae of severe intravascular haemolysis and renal failure
Diclofenac (Kramer et al 1986), doxepin (Wolf et al 1989), glafenine (Roodnat et al 1987), nomifensine (Salama & Mueller-Eckhardt 1985)

Other references are found in Hackett et al (1982). The asterisk (*) indicates that very severe thrombocytopenia (platelet count $<20 \times 10^9$/l has been documented

IgG reacts with a metabolite rather than the parent drug itself (Eisner & Shahidi 1972, Salama & Mueller-Eckhardt 1985).

Although most of these drugs produce isolated thrombocytopenia, some can produce concomitant neutropenia (e.g. quinine) or pancytopenia (e.g. gold- or carbamazepine-induced aplastic anaemia) (Williame et al 1987, Gram & Jensen 1989).

Recently, severe thrombocytopenia (platelet count $<10 \times 10^9$/l) and mucosal bleeding has been described in HIV-negative individuals following use of intravenous or intranasal cocaine (Koury 1990, Leissinger 1990, Burday & Martin 1991). This disorder appears to be caused by immune mechanisms, and responds to high-dose iv IgG therapy.

Drugs that cause mild thrombocytopenia: valproic acid and amrinone

Both valproic acid and amrinone have been described as causing a mild thrombocytopenia in a large percentage of patients shortly after commencing the drugs (Barr et al 1982, Kinney et al 1983, Ansell et al 1984). Bleeding is uncommon and some physicians choose to continue the drug. An immune pathogenesis for valproic acid-induced thrombocytopenia was suggested by elevated levels of platelet-associated IgG in affected patients in one study (Barr et al 1982).

Non-immune drug-induced thrombocytopenia

By far the most common causes of non-immune drug-induced thrombocytopenia are the anticancer drugs, which cause dose-dependent pancytopenia by direct toxic inhibition of the stem and progenitor cell populations. An important exception is the drug anagrelide that selectively suppresses platelet production (Abe Andes et al 1984). This drug has been used to treat thrombocythaemic disorders (Silverstein et al 1988, Anagrelide Study Group 1992).

Some drugs cause thrombocytopenia by non-immune mechanisms. For example, ristocetin and porcine factor VIII can cause thrombocytopenia by producing in vivo platelet agglutination (Gangarosa et al 1969, Green & Tuite 1989). Recognition of the platelet-agglutinating effect of ristocetin led to its removal from the market as an antibiotic, and resulted in the discovery of its role in promoting platelet/von Willebrand factor interactions. Hematin (used to treat attacks of porphyria) has been shown to cause platelet activation (Neely et al 1984). Protamine injections cause transient thrombocytopenia via reticuloendothelial sequestration (Heyns et al 1980).

Some drugs produce thrombocytopenia through indirect means. For example, drugs such as α-methyldopa and methotrexate can cause liver disease and hypersplenism. Thrombocytopenia due to hypersplenism was part of a scleroderma-like illness recognized during the 1970s in industrial workers exposed to vinyl chloride (Heuserman & Stutte 1977). Thrombocytopenia has been described in many patients treated with histamine$_2$-inhibiting anti-ulcer drugs such as cimetidine and ranitidine (Isaacs 1980, Spychal & Wickham 1985, Yue et al 1987). Inhibition of megakaryocyte progenitor cells by cimetidine has been described (Gross et al 1984), suggesting that marrow suppression may play a role in the pathogenesis of the thrombocytopenia.

Dose-dependent thrombocytopenia also has been reported in patients treated with various cytokines, including interleukin-2 (IL-2), granulocyte colony-stimulating factor (G-CSF), and α-interferon, which can be severe enough to cause fatal haemorrhage (McLaughlin et al 1985, Israel et al 1989, Yoshida et al 1991). For interleukin-2, data has been presented indicating both increased platelet destruction (Paciucci et al 1990) as well as megakaryocyte suppression mediated by tumour necrosis factor alpha produced by IL-2 generated lymphokine activated killer (LAK) cells (Guarini et al 1991).

INFECTIONS AND THROMBOCYTOPENIA

Thrombocytopenia is commonly seen in infected patients. Although increased platelet destruction is the most frequent mechanism for the thrombocytopenia, decreased platelet production or hypersplenism can contribute to the thrombocytopenia in some patients.

Septicaemia and thrombocytopenia: the role of DIC

Thrombocytopenia is a common feature of the infected patient, especially when microbial invasion of the bloodstream has occurred. The frequency of thrombocytopenia varies from 45–75% in bacteraemic patients (Riedler et al 1971, Corrigan 1974, Kelton et al 1979, Kreger et al 1980, Neame et al 1980), and approaches 100% for patients with septic shock or disseminated intravascular coagulation (DIC) (Corrigan & Jordan 1970, Milligan et al 1974, Oppenheimer et al 1976). Thrombin is a potent platelet agonist that could contribute to increased platelet clearance in some septic patients. Studies employing dual radiolabels found parallel increases in fibrinogen and platelet turnover in septic patients (Harker & Slichter 1972a). Elevated levels of thrombin-antithrombin complexes and soluble fibrin monomer complexes (Okajima et al 1991), as well as elevation in cross-linked D-dimer levels (Voss et al 1990), indicate that thrombin generation is a common event in septic patients. However, most patients with mild to moderate thrombocytopenia and bacteraemia have little evidence of thrombin activation indicating that other factors trigger thrombocytopenia in these patients (Neame et al 1980).

Septicaemia and thrombocytopenia: the role of immune mechanisms

Investigators have also observed high levels of platelet-associated IgG in thrombocytopenic septic patients, suggesting that humoral immune mechanisms can result in thrombocytopenia (Kelton et al 1979, Neame et al 1980). Increased levels of circulating immune complexes have also been reported in patients with septicaemia (Poskitt & Poskitt 1985b).

Thrombocytopenia occurs in almost all patients with active malaria. Immune-mediated thrombocytopenia has been shown by investigators who demonstrated that IgG from these patients bind to malarial antigens that are adsorbed to the platelet surface (Kelton et al 1983). Studies using a murine malaria model also implicate IgG-mediated platelet destruction under T lymphocyte control (Grau et al 1988).

The possible role of immune-mediated platelet destruction in sepsis led to a randomized placebo-controlled, double-blind trial of high-dose iv IgG (0.4 g/kg daily for 3 days) for septic, thrombocytopenic patients (Burns et al 1991). There was no difference in the rise in platelet count over the first 5 days following commencement of treatment; thereafter, the platelet count rose higher in the group receiving iv IgG. No clinical benefit to this treatment was observed.

Septicaemia and thrombocytopenia: the role of bacterial toxins

Some bacterial toxins such as endotoxin (Csako et al 1988, Grabarek et al 1988) and *Staphylococcus aureus* α-toxin (Bhakdi et al 1988, Arvand et al 1990) directly activate platelets and could cause thrombocytopenia. Furthermore, endogenous mediators of inflammation (e.g. platelet-activating factor) also activate platelets (Diez et al 1989).

Infections and hypersplenism

Some infections may cause thrombocytopenia by producing hypersplenism. For example, subacute bacterial endocarditis, infectious mononucleosis, and cytomegalovirus can cause reactive hyperplasia of the spleen. *Leishmania donovani* protozoa invade splenic macrophages as part of a syndrome that includes fever, weight loss, liver and spleen enlargement, lymphadenopathy, IgG hypergammaglobulinaemia, and pancytopenia (kala-azar). In contrast, hypersplenism is caused by presinusoidal portal hypertension in patients with chronic schistosomiasis.

Infections and reticuloendothelial hyperactivity (haemophagocytic syndrome)

Rarely, infections initiate an aggressively hyperphagocytic response by macrophages, resulting in phagocytosis of red cells, granulocytes, and platelets. The outcome is often fatal, even when the microbial infection is treated. Initiating infections have ranged from *Escherischia coli* cystitis (de la Serna et al 1989) and childhood roseola infection (herpesvirus-6) (Huang et al 1990), to unusual infections such as histoplasmosis (Reiner & Spivak 1988) or the zoonosis Ehrlichiosis (Abbott et al 1991). The pathophysiologic basis of the exuberant macrophage activity is unknown.

The differential diagnosis of haemophagocytosis also includes systemic lupus erythematosus (Wong et al 1991), HIV infection (Rule et al 1991), and lymphocytic neoplasms (Jaffe et al 1983, Falini et al 1990). Haemophagocytosis is also the major pathologic feature of a rare disorder known as histiocytic medullary reticulosis (Scott & Robb-Smith 1939), although many patients previously recognized as having this disorder appear to have had lymphoma (Jaffe et al 1983, Falini et al 1990).

Viral infections and thrombocytopenia

Thrombocytopenia occurs in many patients with acute viral infections, including infectious mononucleosis, cytomegalovirus, infection by human immunodeficiency virus, varicella, rubeola, rubella, herpes simplex, Kawasaki disease, and dengue (Baranski & Young 1987, Kinney et al 1992). The thrombocytopenia is usually mild and probably caused by immune mechanisms. In children, severe immune-mediated thrombocytopenia can occur 7–10 days after the onset of an otherwise unremarkable viral illness (discussed in section on childhood acute ITP, p. 774).

DIC can rarely complicate certain viral infections, including varicella, rubeola, and rubella (Baranski & Young 1987). However, DIC is a more characteristic feature of certain other viral infections, such as haemorrhagic fever with renal syndrome (Korean haemorrhagic fever) (Bruno et al 1990). The severity of bleeding often exceeds that expected for the degree of thrombocytopenia, and is caused by DIC triggered by endothelial invasion by virus.

DISSEMINATED INTRAVASCULAR COAGULATION (DIC)

Disseminated intravascular coagulation (DIC) is defined as excess thrombin generation within the vasculature that overwhelms regulatory mechanisms and results in generalized derangement of the haemostatic mechanism. The excess thrombin results in increased consumption of platelets and coagulation factors, especially fibrinogen, factors V and VIII. Consumption of inhibitors of coagulation (antithrombin III, protein C and S) can occur, which can exacerbate DIC by progressive worsening of the regulation of haemostasis. Usually there is parallel generation of plasmin, leading to increased levels of fibrin/fibrinogen degradation products (Müller-Berghaus 1989).

The clinical spectrum of DIC is wide, and ranges from laboratory abnormalities without clinical sequellae to severe bleeding caused by depletion of coagulation factors and platelets. Some patients have evidence of organ ischaemia and infarction resulting from microvascular thrombosis. For example, acute fulminant DIC in some children with meningococcal septicaemia leads to necrosis of acral tissues such as limbs and nose. Haemorrhagic adrenal necrosis can also occur.

DIC also can be chronic and compensated, with increased platelet and coagulation factor production. This type of DIC is most likely to occur in patients with underlying malignancies. Chronic DIC should be considered in patients with mild-to-moderate thrombocytopenia. Such patients often have near normal screening coagulation assays (PT and aPTT). Paracoagulation assays (e.g. protamine sulphate test) and measurement of fibrinogen/fibrin degradation products or D-dimer can confirm the diagnosis in these patients. Many of these patients develop thrombotic problems such as deep vein thrombosis, stroke, or thrombotic nonbacterial endocarditis. Some patients are benefited by heparin therapy.

The wide-ranging pathogenesis of DIC is illustrated well by an important cause of DIC in some parts of the world — snake envenomation. At least ten different platelet effects can be produced by different snake venoms, including direct platelet activation (e.g. thrombin-like, phospholipase A_2 enzymes, and other platelet-activating venoms), indirect platelet activation (e.g. procoagulant venoms that result in thrombin generation), and lectin-like peptides that agglutinate platelets (Teng & Huang 1991)

In western societies, DIC is most frequently caused by trauma (release of procoagulant tissues into the blood), septicaemia (tissue damage resulting from shock, as well as increased expression of procoagulant factors on endothelial and inflammatory cells), and malignancy (elaboration of procoagulant factors by tumour cells). Potentially life-threatening DIC also can occur in pregnant patients (e.g. amniotic fluid embolism, abruptio placentae, missed abortion, severe preeclampsia or eclampsia).

DIC is most frequently caused by systemic factors. However, in some instances, localized excess thrombin generation results in systemic depletion of coagulation factors and their inhibitors. Examples include cavernous haemangiomas that occur in childhood (Kasabach & Merritt 1940, Shim 1968) and some aortic aneurysms in adults (Micallef-Eynaud & Ludlam 1991).

A more detailed discussion of DIC is presented in Chapter 42.

THROMBOTIC MICROANGIOPATHY

Thrombotic microangiopathy is characterized by microangiopathic haemolysis, destructive thrombocytopenia, and microvascular platelet thrombi. Examination of the blood film shows red cell fragments (particularly 'helmet' and triangular forms) and thrombocytopenia. Often, there is organ dysfunction caused by microvascular thrombosis. Microscopic examination of affected organs reveals platelet-rich microthrombi in the arterioles (intraluminal hyalin microthrombi) (Neame et al 1973). Two prototypic thrombotic microangiopathic disorders have been described: thrombotic thrombocytopenic purpura (TTP) and haemolytic-ureamic syndrome (HUS).

Thrombotic thrombocytopenic purpura (TTP)

Clinical and laboratory features

TTP is rare (annual incidence approximately one in one million). Affected patients are most often young or middle-aged adults, although all ages can be affected. There is a slight female preponderance (3:2) (Petitt 1980, Kwaan 1987).

Organ dysfunction most frequently involves the central nervous system (e.g. altered level of consciousness, focal deficits, seizures), kidneys (oliguric renal failure), heart (heart failure, dysrrhythmias), lungs (respiratory distress syndrome), and pancreas (abdominal pain). Fever occurs in many patients.

Laboratory evidence of moderate-to-severe fragmentation haemolysis (anaemia, red cell fragments, polychromasia, reticulocytosis, hyperbilirubinaemia, elevated lactate dehydrogenase, absent haptoglobin) and thrombocytopenia are found in virtually all patients. Laboratory evidence of renal failure, including elevated urea and creatinine, are found in most patients. Elevated CPK and amylase levels are commonly found.

Untreated, the mortality rate exceeds 90% (Amorosi & Ultmann 1966), although it can be reduced to approximately 10–20% with treatment (Bell et al 1991, Rock et al 1991).

Pathogenesis

The acute destructive thrombocytopenia and disseminated intravascular platelet thrombi have long been interpreted to indicate a circulating platelet aggregating factor. Currently, at least two different platelet-aggregating factors have been identified. Lian and associates have described a 37 kDa protein that aggregates platelets via platelet GPIV (Lian et al 1979, 1991, Siddiqui & Lian 1985). Our group has identified a calcium-dependent cysteine protease (calpain) in the serum of TTP patients (Murphy et al 1987). Calpain is a normal constituent of blood cells that is inhibited by kininogens (Muller-Esterl 1987). Calpain can proteolyze von Willebrand factor, making it very reactive with platelets (Moore et al 1990). Previous work had suggested a role for von Willebrand factor in the pathogenesis of TTP (Moake et al 1982, Kelton et al 1984a). The calpain is carried on platelet microparticles, which make it resistant to inhibition by its natural inhibitors (Kelton et al 1992). Recently, other investigators have confirmed cysteine protease activity in TTP patients (Falanga et al 1991). It remains unknown how the calpain and platelet microparticles are generated in TTP.

Treatment

Optimal treatment for TTP is plasma given by plasma exchange (Shepard & Bukowski 1987, Rock et al 1991). The patient should receive stored plasma by infusion (75–100 ml/hour) pending arrangement of apheresis therapy. Some patients who respond incompletely, or are refractory, may respond to more intensive exchange (Brady et al 1991) or substitution of cryosupernatant (which lacks the large multimers of von Willebrand factor) for fresh frozen plasma (Byrnes et al 1990, Naumovski & Pillsbury 1991). Early relapse in responding patients is common, and therefore plasma exchange should be continued for several days or a few weeks following recovery. Patients who have recovered from an episode of TTP may develop one or more recurrences months or years following the initial episode (Rose and Eldor 1987, Onundarson et al 1992). Some physicians use high-dose corticosteroids (prednisone 200 mg/day) as initial treatment for all patients with TTP, and reserve plasma exchange for those with renal or neurologic involvement or who fail to respond to prednisone (Bell et al 1991). Anecdotal reports indicate possible benefit from splenectomy, vinca alkaloids (O'Connor et al 1992), antiplatelet agents, high-dose iv IgG (Staszewski et al 1989), and extracorporeal protein A immunoadsorption (Mittelman et al 1992). Because of the role of platelet activation in TTP, we administer aspirin to patients who are not severely thrombocytopenic.

Haemolytic-uraemic syndrome (HUS)

Clinical features

Haemolytic-uraemic syndrome can be considered a nephrotropic variant of TTP that predominantly occurs in young children. The clinical triad of HUS is fragmentation haemolysis, thrombocytopenia, and renal dysfunction. The typical presentation is oliguric renal failure in young children following a prodromal illness consisting of profuse bloody diarrhoea. However, some children with otherwise typical HUS can develop CNS, cardiac, and other organ dysfunction and clinically resemble TTP. Furthermore, the histopathologic appearance of the lesions (platelet-rich microthrombi) is identical in both disorders. HUS characteristically occurs at the extremes of age: young children and the elderly. The mortality due to HUS is estimated to be approximately 5% (Loirat et al 1988). However, this may underestimate the true severity of the illness, since children with severe illness could be classified as TTP. Approximately 4% of paediatric renal transplants in North American children were performed for HUS (Alexander et al 1990).

Pathogenesis

There is a strong association between HUS and a prodromal diarrhoeal illness characterized by infection with an organism synthesizing a shigatoxin or shiga-like toxin. In western societies, the infection is typically of a verocytotoxin (shiga-like toxin)-producing *Esch. coli* 0157 (Karmali et al 1983, Chart et al 1991). In third world countries, shigatoxin-producing *Shigella dysenteriae* type I is an important cause of HUS (Raghupathy et al 1978, Srivastava et al 1991). The pathogenetic link between these toxins and HUS is unknown.

Treatment

Clinical trials have not shown benefit using heparin (Vitacco et al 1990), urokinase plus heparin (Loirat et al 1984), or dipyridamole (Proesmans et al 1984). Two studies of plasma infusion did not show either a patient or renal survival benefit, compared with supportive treatment alone (Loirat et al 1988, Rizzoni et al 1988). However, the larger trial demonstrated lower follow-up blood creatinine levels and proteinuria, as well as less cortical necrosis in the group that received plasma infusion (Loirat et al 1988). Based on the proven efficacy of plasmapheresis in TTP, we recommend this treatment for children with severe HUS. One report describes eight children with HUS treated with high-dose iv IgG who had a more rapid recovery than historical controls (Sheth et al 1990). Gammaglobulin preparations contain IgG capable of neutralizing the shiga and shiga-like toxins (Ashkenazi et al 1988).

Other microangiopathic disorders

Illness that resemble TTP or HUS can be seen in relations with neoplasia, pregnancy, human immunodeficiency virus infection, collagen vascular diseases, certain drugs, and in transplant recipients.

Neoplasia and anticancer chemotherapy

Microangiopathic haemolysis and thrombocytopenia can occur in patients with disseminated carcinoma, particularly gastric adenocarcinoma (Brain et al 1970, Carr et al 1986a). Sometimes there is accompanying consumptive coagulopathy (Carr et al 1986a), a feature seen less frequently with typical TTP. In some cases, tumour emboli can be demonstrated pathologically (Hales & Mark 1987). A procoagulant cysteine protease material has been isolated from some of these patients (Falanga & Gordon 1985, Falanga et al 1989) that may be related to the serum platelet-activating activity that has been identified in patients with typical TTP (Falanga et al 1991). The haematologic abnormalities can respond to plasma exchange (Carr et al 1986a), but the prognosis depends on the patient's response to anticancer treatment.

In some patients, microangiopathic syndromes, including both TTP and HUS, appear to be related to the treatment of the malignancy (Antman et al 1979, Kressel et al 1981, Jackson et al 1984, Licciardello et al 1985, Fields & Lindley 1989). Mitomycin C has been implicated most frequently in causing this syndrome (D'Elia et al 1987, Lesesne et al 1989).

A recent study (Rabinowe et al 1991) found that 10% of patients develop HUS 3–12 months after bone marrow transplantation, often complicated by hypertension, oedema, and heart failure. Although the haematologic abnormalities remitted within a few weeks to months, azotaemia and hypertension usually persisted. Plasma exchange was used in the more severely affected patients, and improved the haematologic abnormalities. There was no relation with graft-versus-host disease. A similar syndrome has also been described in many children following bone marrow transplantation, in whom renal biopsy findings suggested a diagnosis of radiation-induced nephritis (Guinan et al 1988).

Drug-induced haemolytic-uraemic syndrome

HUS occurs in a subgroup of patients who develop quinine-induced thrombocytopenia (Spearing et al 1990, Gottschall et al 1991, Stroncek et al 1992). Other drugs implicated in some patients with HUS include cyclosporine (van Buren et al 1985, Keusch et al 1986), conjugated oestrogens (Ashouri et al 1982), and oral contraceptives (Hauglustaine et al 1981).

Pregnancy-associated thrombotic microangiopathy

HUS and TTP can occur in late pregnancy or during the early postpartum period (Segonds et al 1979).

Other disorders

Microangiopathic haemolysis and thrombocytopenia can sometimes occur in patients with collagen vascular diseases (Magil et al 1986, Noda et al 1990), primary pulmonary hypertension (Stuard et al 1972), and infection by HIV (Rarick et al 1992).

ALLOIMMUNE THROMBOCYTOPENIC DISORDERS

Alloantigens are genetically determined molecular variations of proteins or carbohydrates that can be recognized immunologically by some individuals after they are exposed during pregnancy or transfusion to the antigens they lack. The resulting IgG alloantibodies result in the premature destruction of the cells carrying the alloantigens. Five thrombocytopenic syndromes have been attributed to platelet-reactive alloantibodies: neonatal alloimmune thrombocytopenia, post-transfusion purpura, passive alloimmune thrombocytopenia, alloimmune platelet transfusion refractoriness, and transplantation-associated alloimmune thrombocytopenia. Table 33.4 lists the platelet alloantigens described.

NEONATAL ALLOIMMUNE THROMBOCYTOPENIA (NAT)

This is discussed subsequently in the section 'Thrombocytopenia in fetomaternal medicine' (p. 786).

Post-transfusion purpura (PTP)

Clinical features

This rare syndrome is characterized by the abrupt onset of severe thrombocytopenia and bleeding 5–10 days following receipt of a blood product, usually packed red cells. In more than 90% of instances, the thrombocytopenia remits within 60 days, but it can persist for as long as 1 year (Kunicki & Beardsley 1989). Approximately 95% of affected patients are women, usually between the ages of 40 and 80, who presumably were sensitized during a previous pregnancy. Rarely, sensitization has occurred via a previous transfusion. The thrombocytopenia is typically severe, with mucocutaneous and wound bleeding. Fatalities have been reported.

Pathogenesis

PTP is caused by platelet-reactive alloantibodies, usually anti-HPA-1a (Zw^a, Pl^{A1}), produced by the blood product recipient (Shulman et al 1961) Although invariably associated with the presence of detectable platelet alloantibodies, it remains a mystery why severe destruction of autologous platelets occurs. The first hypothesis (Shulman et al 1961) suggested that platelet alloantigens present in the blood product produced immune complexes with the alloantibodies, resulting in platelet destruction. Another suggestion was that soluble alloantigens become adsorbed onto the autologous platelets, converting them to target platelets (Kickler et al 1986). Mueller-Eckhardt (1986) has suggested that pathogenic alloantibodies cross-react with the native alloantigen in these patients (pseudospecificity). Finally, an aberrant transient autoimmune process that is somehow triggered by the alloantigen stimulus could occur (Morrison & Mollison 1966, Minchinton et al 1990).

Table 33.4 Platelet alloantigen and isoantigen systems

New HPA nomen-clature	Original designations	Caucasian genotype frequency	Caucasian phenotype frequency	Japanese genotype frequency	Japanese phenotype frequency	Clinical alloimmune syndromes described	GP localization and identification of amino acid polymorphism	Comments
HPA-1a	Zw^a, Pl^{A1}	0.85	0.98	0.98	>0.999	NAT, PTP, PTR, PAT, TAT,	IIIa (CD61) Leu^{33}/Pro^{33} amino acid polymorphism	Anti-HPA-1a is most frequent cause of severe alloimmune syndromes in Caucasians; alloimmunization associated with HLA-DRw52a (HLA-DR3 locus)
-1b	Zw^b, Pl^{A2}	0.15	0.27	0.02	0.04	NAT, PTP, PTR		
HPA-2a	Ko^b	0.911	0.992	0.864	0.982		Ib_{α} (CD42b) Met^{145}/Thr^{145} amino acid polymorphism	Usually IgM antibodies; only a single report of NAT caused by IgG anti-HPA-2b — this patient has transient amegakaryocytosis; anti-2b has been reported to cause PTR in Japan
-2b	Ko^a, Sib^a	0.089	0.169	0.136	0.254	NAT, PTR		
HPA-3a	Bak^a, Lek^a	0.61	0.85	0.54	0.79	NAT, PTP	IIb_{α} (CD41) Ile^{843}/Ser^{843} amino acid polymorphism	Although alloantigenic determinant due to amino acid polymorphism, serologic studies indicate that sialic acid residues could contribute to epitopic heterogeneity
-3b	Bak^b, Lek^b	0.39	0.66	0.46	0.71	NAT, PTP, PTR		
HPA-4a	Pen^a, Yuk^b	>0.99	>0.999	0.9917	>0.999	NAT, PTP	IIIa (CD61) Gln^{143}/Arg^{143} amino acid polymorphism	More frequent alloimmune syndromes in Japanese than Caucasians because of higher frequency of homozygous HPA-4b phenotype
-4b	Pen^b, Yuk^a	<0.01	<0.0001	0.0083	0.017	NAT		
HPA-5a	Br^b, Zav^b	0.89	0.99	–	–	NAT	Ia (CDw49b)	Can only be detected by sensitive methods; alloimmunization associated with HLA-DRw6; first and second most common cause of NAT in Japanese and Caucasian populations, respectively
-5b	Br^a, Zav^a, Hc^a	0.11	0.21	–	–	NAT, PTP, PTR, PAT		
	Pl^{E1}	0.975	0.999	–	–	–	$Ib\alpha$ (CD42b)	Alloantigen system not well established, since only one example of each alloantiserum has been identified in past 25 years; it is possible that anti-Pl^{E1} represented an isoantibody
	Pl^{E2}	0.025	0.05	–	–	NAT		
	Gov^a	0.53	0.81	–	–	PTP?	p175	Can only be identified using sensitive techniques; no clinical effects of the alloantibodies have been established
	Gov^b	0.47	0.74	–	–			
	Sr^a	<0.003	<0.01	–	–	NAT	IIIa (CD61)	'private' alloantigen system, since Sr^a antigen so far only identified in proband's family
	Va^a	<0.002	<0.004	–	–	NAT	IIb/IIIa	'private' alloantigen system, since Va^a antigen so far only identified in proband's family
	Tu^a	~0.003	~0.007	–	–	NAT	IIIa (CD61)	
	Mo^a	~0.001	~0.002	–	–	NAT	IIIa (CD61) Pro^{407}/Ala^{407}	

Table 33.4 *Cont'd*

New HPA nomenclature	Original designations	Caucasian genotype frequency	Caucasian phenotype frequency	Japanese genotype frequency	Japanese phenotype frequency	Clinical alloimmune syndromes described	GP localization and identification of amino acid polymorphism	Comments
	HLA	highly polymorphic		highly polymorphic		PTR	45 kDa heavy chain	Class I HLA antigens are present on platelets, and are the most important alloantigen target contributing to platelet transfusion refractoriness
	ABO antigens:					PTR, NAT?		Platelet recovery is less when ABO incompatible platelets are transfused.
	A	0.26	0.44					
	B	0.06	0.085					
	O	0.68	0.46					
	GP Ib isoantibody					PTR	Ib/IX complex	Anti-GPIb/IX isoantibodies can form in polytransfused Bernard–Soulier patients
	GP IIb/IIIa isoantibody					PTR	IIb/IIIa complex	Anti-GPIIb/IIIa isoantibodies can form in polytransfused Glanzmann's thrombasthenic patients
	Nak[a] GPIV isoantibody	0.94	0.9966	0.70	0.96	PTR	IV (CD36)	Anti-Nak[a] isoantibodies can form in polytransfused GPIV-deficient patients; *Nak*[a−] phenotype is common in Japan (3–4%)

Platelet alloantigen and isoantigen systems implicated in platelet alloimmune and isoimmune syndromes. The human platelet antigen (HPA) system was recently proposed to systemize platelet alloantigen nomenclature (Borne & Decary 1990). NAT, neonatal alloimmune thrombocytopenia; PTP, posttransfusion purpura; PTR, platelet transfusion refractoriness; PAT, passive alloimmune thrombocytopenia; TAT, transplantation-associated alloimmune thrombocytopenia.
Note that platelet transfusion refractoriness can be caused by either alloimmune (common) or isoimmune (rare) mechanisms.

References
HPA-1 Loghem et al 1959, Shulman et al 1964, Mueller-Eckhardt et al 1981, 1986, 1989, Newman et al 1989, Kickler et al 1990b
HPA-2 Grenet et al 1965, Marcelli-Barge et al 1973, Bizzaro & Dianese 1988, Saji et al 1989, Ishida et al 1991, Kuijpers et al 1992, Murata et al 1992
HPA-3 von dem Borne et al 1980, Boizard & Wautier 1984, Kickler et al 1988, 1990b, Kiefel et al 1989a, McGrath et al 1989, Mueller-Eckhardt et al 1989, Lyman et al 1990, Take et al 1990
HPA-4 Friedman & Aster 1985, Shibata et al 1986a,b, Furihata et al 1987, Santoso et al 1987, Simon et al 1988, Wang et al 1991
HPA-5 Kiefel et al 1988, Bierling et al 1989, Mueller-Eckhardt et al 1989, Santoso et al 1989, Smith et al 1989, Woods et al 1989, Bettaieb et al 1991, Christie et al 1991, Warkentin et al 1992c
PL[E] Shulman et al 1964, Shulman & Jordan 1982, Furihata et al 1988
Gov Kelton et al 1990
Sr[a] Kroll et al 1990
Va[a] Kekomäki et al 1992
Tu[a] Kekomäki et al 1993
Mo[a] Kuijpers et al 1993
HLA Bishop et al 1988
ABO Mueller-Eckhardt et al 1981, 1989, Lee & Schiffer 1989
GPIb/IX Degos et al 1977
GPIIb/IIIa Levy-Toledano 1978
Nak Ikeda et al 1989, Tomiyama et al 1990b, Yamamoto et al 1991

Although HPA-1a is the most frequently implicated alloantigen, HPA-1b (Taaning et al 1985), HPA-4a (Simon et al 1988) as well as both alleles of the HPA-3 system (Boizard & Wautier 1984, Kiemowitz et al 1986, Kickler et al 1988) have been implicated. All three of these alloantigen systems are located on the GPIIb/IIIa complex, and since there are approximately 50 000 copies of this complex on the platelet surface, there is the potential for severe alloimmune thrombocytopenia. In contrast, the GPIa/IIa complex (approximately 2000 copies per platelet), which has been implicated in one PTP patient, was associated with relatively mild thrombocytopenia (Christie et al 1991).

Treatment

More than 90% of patients will respond to high-dose iv IgG (1–2 g/kg), and this is the treatment of choice for PTP (Mueller-Eckhardt et al 1983, Mueller-Eckhardt 1988, Walker et al 1988). Exchange transfusion or apheresis therapy is an effective but more cumbersome treatment. Corticosteroids are often given, but their efficacy is uncertain, and are not recommended as primary therapy. Random platelet transfusions are ineffective, and can cause severe febrile and anaphylactoid reactions (Walker et al 1988). Pl^{A1}-negative platelets may give benefit to some patients (Lippman et al 1988). Red cell products should be washed before administration to remove contaminating platelet antigens. Splenectomy can be successful in some patients refractory to iv IgG and plasmapheresis (Cunningham & Lind 1989).

Future precautions

It is possible that future episodes can be prevented by administering washed or alloantigen-compatible blood products. However, not all at-risk patients will have a recurrence of PTP (Lau et al 1980), perhaps because of 'protection' by high-titre alloantibodies that immediately destroy the transfused incompatible alloantigen. Patients who have recovered from PTP should not donate blood in the future.

Passive alloimmune thrombocytopenia

Transient thrombocytopenia immediately following the infusion of a blood product containing platelet-specific alloantibodies (either anti-HPA-1a or anti-HPA-5b) has been reported (Ballem et al 1987a, Nijjar et al 1987, Scott et al 1988, Warkentin et al 1992c). The most severe episodes are caused by anti-HPA-1a alloantibodies. The duration of thrombocytopenia is usually less than 1 week (contrast post-transfusion purpura). It is important to confirm the diagnosis since the implicated blood donor should not give further donations.

Alloimmune platelet transfusion refractoriness

This is discussed in the section on platelet transfusion support of leukaemic patients (p. 789).

Transplantation-associated alloimmune thrombocytopenia

Panzer and associates (1989) described a bone marrow transplant recipient who developed late-onset alloimmune thrombocytopenia caused by residual recipient lymphoid cells that produced anti-HPA-1a alloantibodies against donor-marrow derived platelets.

THROMBOCYTOPENIA IN FETOMATERNAL MEDICINE

Incidental thrombocytopenia of pregnancy

Thrombocytopenia is a common problem in pregnancy, occurring in 5–10% of pregnant patients. The results of an ongoing prospective study in Hamilton (Burrows & Kelton 1990b) have helped to define the various causes of thrombocytopenia and have identified implications for both mother and infant. About two-thirds of thrombocytopenic women will be healthy, have no history of ITP, and have mild thrombocytopenia (platelet count 70–150 × 10^9/l): this is known as **incidental thrombocytopenia of pregnancy** (Burrows & Kelton 1988, 1990b). Incidental thrombocytopenia of pregnancy has in the past been confused with idiopathic thrombocytopenic purpura, and consequently some physicians were inappropriately aggressive in the management of these patients. In Hamilton, we have now followed over 500 of these patients, and demonstrated that this syndrome is benign. These mothers do not bleed, nor does severe thrombocytopenia occur in their infants. The frequency of thrombocytopenia in the neonates is the same as the frequency of thrombocytopenia in infants born to mothers who are healthy and who are not thrombocytopenic (2–4%). Infants with severe thrombocytopenia who are born to mothers with incidental thrombocytopenia should be investigated for the possibility of coexisting neonatal alloimmune thrombocytopenia.

Preeclampsia/eclampsia/HELLP

Thrombocytopenia (platelet count less than 150 × 10^9/l) occurs in approximately 15–20% and 50% of patients who develop preeclampsia and eclampsia, respectively (Gibson et al 1982, Schindler et al 1990). A minority of thrombocytopenic patients also have concomitant fragmentation haemolysis (schistocytes, hyperbilirubinaemia, elevated lactate dehydrogenase) and elevated liver enzymes (Pritchard et al 1954, Weinstein et al 1982, Romero et al 1989). This constellation of **h**aemolysis, **e**levated **l**iver enzymes, and **l**ow **p**latelets has been termed HELLP (Weinstein 1982), and is believed to indicate severe preeclampsia, since it is associated with a higher risk of maternal and fetal complications (Sibai et al 1986, Romero et al 1989). In some patients, the presence of HELLP predates the onset of hypertension and proteinuria (Aarnoudse et al 1986, Romero et al 1989). However, the clinical course is variable, and some patients with HELLP will respond to conservative measures alone (bed rest, antihypertensive therapy). All preeclamptic patients warrant careful repeated clinical assessment for potential serious complications, e.g. DIC, thrombotic thrombocytopenic purpura, or fatty liver of pregnancy (Goodlin 1991).

Increased platelet destruction is the mechanism of thrombocytopenia in preeclampsia (Rákóczi et al 1979, Stubbs et al 1986). In vivo platelet activation is indicated by elevated plasma β-thromboglobulin levels (Redman et al 1977) and increased urinary thromboxane metabolite levels (Van Geet et al 1990). Thrombin-induced platelet activation may occur in some patients, as suggested by elevated levels of thrombin/antithrombin complexes (Kobayashi & Terao 1987, Weiner 1988) and D-dimers (Kobayashi & Terao 1987), together with reduced antithrombin levels (Kobayashi & Terao 1987, Weiner 1988, Ho & Yang 1992). However, overt DIC is uncommon in preeclampsia (Gordon et al 1976, Leduc et al 1992), and fibrinopeptide A levels (another marker of in vivo thrombin generation) usually are not increased in preeclamptic women (Burrows et al 1987). Decreased endothelial prostacyclin synthesis due to endothelial damage could be the cause of the increased platelet turnover in these patients (Goodman et al 1982, Stubbs et al 1984). The possible role of platelet activation in the pathogenesis of preeclampsia is suggested by several studies indicating that low-dose aspirin prevents preeclampsia in high-risk patients (Wallenburg et al 1986, Schiff et al 1989).

A mild platelet function defect has been described in patients with preeclampsia, including some patients with normal platelet counts (Kelton et al 1985). To minimize the risk of the rare complication of epidural haematoma, some physicians recommend that platelet counts be obtained in all preeclamptic women, and a normal bleeding time documented before proceeding to epidural anaesthesia in those with a platelet count between 50 and 100×10^9/l (Schindler et al 1990).

Idiopathic thrombocytopenic purpura complicating pregnancy

ITP is a relatively common condition that physicians must manage during pregnancy, given the high frequency of ITP among young women. Over the past decade our concepts concerning the impact of ITP on both mother and infant have changed dramatically, and we now recognize that it is a far less dangerous condition for both mother and infant than previously thought.

For the mother with ITP, the treatment is relatively simple, with the focus being on the maternal platelet count and the interventions, if any, needed to maintain the platelet count at safe levels (above 20–50 $\times 10^9$/l). We use high-dose iv IgG because we believe it is the least dangerous agent to be used during pregnancy. An analysis of the recent larger studies (Burrows & Kelton 1990, Kaplan et al 1990, Moutet et al 1990, Samuels et al 1990) investigating ITP in pregnancy indicates that the risk of severe fetal thrombocytopenia (cord platelet count less than 50×10^9/l) is approximately 10%. Most importantly, the neonatal morbidity and mortality were generally low (intracranial bleeding <1%). Moreover, it is not possible to predict the fetal cord platelet count at delivery using either maternal clinical or laboratory features, and attempts to obtain fetal platelet counts during labour using scalp sampling are more likely to generate an erroneous result than a correct value. We believe that cordocentesis is not justified in this setting (because the intervention is more dangerous than the natural history of the disorder itself). It is our opinion that these patients can be managed by treating the mother simply for her degree of thrombocytopenia (iv IgG as needed, otherwise no treatment). Delivery is a routine vaginal delivery unless there are obstetrical indications for more aggressive intervention. However, it is important to remember that in the majority of thrombocytopenic infants born to mothers with ITP, the platelet count falls after delivery (Kelton 1983), and therefore all thrombocytopenic infants should be monitored closely after birth, as many will require treatment (iv IgG with or without platelet transfusions) to prevent the platelet count from falling to dangerous levels.

Neonatal alloimmune thrombocytopenia (NAT)

The most important alloimmune thrombocytopenic disorder is neonatal alloimmune thrombocytopenia, which causes a transient but potentially life-threatening thrombocytopenia during fetal and neonatal life. It is caused by the maternal production of IgG alloantibodies that cross the placenta and result in premature destruction of fetal platelets bearing paternally-derived platelet alloantigens (analogous to haemolytic disease of the newborn).

The frequency of the syndrome is approximately one in 1000–2000 newborn babies in western populations. In the largest investigative series, anti-HPA-1a (-Zw^a, Pl^{A1}) was found in approximately 75% of serologically-confirmed cases, and anti-HPA-5b (-Zav^a, -Br^a) was identified in 20% of cases (Mueller-Eckhardt et al 1989). However, homozygosity for HPA-5b is rare in Japanese, and anti-HPA-5b and anti-HPA-3 alloantibodies are most often implicated in this population.

Clinical features

The typical clinical picture is that of unexpected, severe thrombocytopenia in an otherwise healthy newborn. The platelet count usually continues to fall over the first few days of life, before there is a gradual recovery over days to a few weeks. It is important to emphasize that neonatal alloimmune thrombocytopenia can be severe when the implicated alloantigen system involves the GPIIb/IIIa systems. This is because the high copy number of this GP (approximately 50 000 per platelet) usually results in severe thrombocytopenia. Thrombocytopenia can occur as early as 20 weeks gestation, and generally worsens during the pregnancy (Bussel et al 1988, Kaplan et al 1988).

The risk of severe fetal or neonatal bleeding is estimated to be approximately 10–20%. Affected infants may have intracranial haemorrhage with acute and chronic sequelae. Porencephalic cysts attributable to fetal intracranial bleeds have been described. There are only about 2000 molecules of GPIa/IIa on the platelet, which may explain why neonatal alloimmune thrombocytopenia caused by anti-HPA-5 is usually milder, without bleeding symptoms. In contrast to neonatal alloimmune haemolysis, which usually occurs in second and later pregnancies, approximately half of the cases of neonatal alloimmune thrombocytopenia are found in firstborn infants.

Investigations

In suspected cases, laboratory studies are used to establish whether: (1) the mother lacks one or more platelet alloantigens, and is at risk for forming alloantibodies, and (2) serum platelet-specific alloantibodies are present. For unknown reasons, no alloantibodies can be detected in at least 20% of HPA-1a-negative mothers who have given birth to infants with suspected neonatal alloimmune thrombocytopenia (Kaplan et al 1988). A presumptive diagnosis can be made on the basis of the clinical picture and by demonstrating that the mother is homozygous for a particular alloantigen. Although many techniques (whole platelet enzyme-linked immunoassay, immunofluorescence, etc.) can be used to demonstrate alloantibodies directed against GPIIb/IIIa and GPIb, more sensitive techniques such as radioimmunoprecipitation are required to demonstrate alloantibodies against alloantigens present on low copy number platelet molecules (HPA-5, Gov systems).

Several of the platelet alloantigen systems have been characterized at the molecular level (Table 33.4). This has permitted the use of allele-specific oligonucleotide probes to type fetal platelets, using small amounts of fetal tissue (whole blood obtained by cordocentesis, or amniocytes obtained by amniocentesis) (McFarland et al 1991).

Treatment

When neonatal alloimmune thrombocytopenia is suspected during pregnancy (usually because of a history of a previously affected sibling), measures to reduce intrauterine bleeding should be undertaken. Serial ultrasound studies beginning at 20 weeks gestation should be performed to look for evidence of intracranial bleeding. If available, percutaneous umbilical blood sampling (PUBS) can be used to determine fetal platelet counts and to administer platelet transfusions in utero (Kaplan et al 1988). However, PUBS is not generally available, and serious fetal complications can occur with this procedure. At many centres, weekly injections of high-dose iv IgG, 1 g/kg, sometimes combined with dexamethasone, are given to the mother, usually beginning at 20 weeks gestation (Bussel et al 1988, Lynch et al 1992). Experimental evidence suggests that iv IgG blocks transplacental transfer of the IgG alloantibodies (Morgan et al 1991). With this treatment, the fetal platelet usually remains greater than 30×10^9/l and intracranial bleeding is usually prevented.

Delivery of the infant by Caesarian section should be performed as soon as fetal maturity has been confirmed. The advantages of Caesarian delivery are twofold: earlier delivery (which may prevent late gestation bleeding complications) and coordination of postnatal treatment. The cornerstone of postnatal treatment is the administration of washed, irradiated maternal platelets to the affected neonate (Adner et al 1969). At many centres, platelets lacking the incriminated antigen are given, but maternal platelets are preferred, since they are: (1) readily available, (2) certain to be compatible with circulating alloantibodies, and (3) less likely to cause viral infection. In an emergency, random donor platelets may be of benefit to a bleeding infant. High-dose iv IgG should also be given to the neonate to raise the platelet count (Sidiropoulos & Straume 1984, Massey et al 1987). It is important to closely monitor the platelet counts during the first days of life in all affected neonates, since the platelet count can fall further after delivery.

Table 33.5 Differential diagnosis of neonatal thrombocytopenia

Destructive thrombocytopenia
The 'sick' neonate
Septicaemia
Complications of prematurity (e.g. respiratory distress syndrome, necrotizing enterocolitis)
Birth asphyxia
Neonatal thrombosis
Parenteral fatty acid administration
Genetic disorders
Upshaw–Shulman syndrome (congenital recurrent HUS)
Homozygous protein C deficiency (causes DIC)
Aminoacidopathies
Passive immune thrombocytopenia
Neonatal alloimmune thrombocytopenia
Passive autoimmune thrombocytopenia
Maternal ITP
Maternal SLE
Maternal drug-induced immune thrombocytopenia (rare)
Aregenerative thrombocytopenia
Hereditary amegakaryocytic disorders
Isolated amegakaryocytic, e.g. thrombocytopenia/absent radii syndrome (TAR)
Generalized stem cell disorder, e.g. Fanconi's anaemia
Hereditary ineffective thrombopoiesis
Megathrombocytic, e.g. Epstein's syndrome
Normothrombocytic, usually non-syndromic
Microthrombocytic, e.g. Wiscott–Aldrich syndrome
Congenital marrow infiltration
Leukaemia, Neuroblastoma, Histiocytosis X, etc.
Congenital infections
Viral infections, e.g. congenital rubella syndrome
Other infections, e.g. congenital syphilis
Miscellaneous
Severe rhesus haemolytic anaemia
Congenital infiltrative marrow disorders
Dilutional thrombocytopenia
Blood and fluid administration (especially exchange transfusions)

Neonatal and infantal thrombocytopenia

The differential diagnosis of thrombocytopenia in the neonate comprises certain disorders that are unique to this age group (Table 33.5). Congenital thrombocytopenic disorders are discussed elsewhere in this textbook (Ch. 32).

THROMBOCYTOPENIA CAUSED BY DECREASED PLATELET PRODUCTION

Thrombocytopenia can be caused by reduced production of platelets by the megakaryocytes of the bone marrow. Megakaryocytes come from the same common stem cell as myeloid and erythroid precursor cells, and consequently, it is unusual for isolated thrombocytopenia to be caused by underproduction. Marrow disorders that generally produce pancytopenia are discussed first followed by a summary of two disorders of platelet production that are exceptions to this rule, and that are characterized by isolated thrombocytopenia: alcohol-induced thrombocytopenia and amegakaryocytic thrombocytopenia.

MARROW DISORDERS THAT USUALLY PRODUCE PANCYTOPENIA

Clonal myeloid disorders

Thrombocytopenia is an important problem in the majority of patients with one of the clonal myeloid disorders.

Acute myeloid leukaemia

Thrombocytopenia occurs in almost all patients with acute myeloid leukaemia. However, intensive platelet transfusion therapy has made bleeding an uncommon cause of death in these patients. Bleeding complications, particularly after the initiation of chemotherapy, are disproportionately greater in the promyelocytic (M3) and monocytic (M4, M5) subtypes of acute myeloid leukaemia, in which DIC can be triggered by release of procoagulant substances from the neoplastic cells (Tallman & Kwaan 1992).

Myelodysplasia

Thrombocytopenia can occur in patients with myelodysplasia. In addition many patients have marked platelet dysfunction. Moreover, the chronicity of myelodysplasia, and the lack of effective antineoplastic chemotherapy, means that many of these patients develop alloimmune refractoriness to platelet transfusions. Thus, bleeding morbidity and mortality are relatively common in this patient population. A clinically significant improvement in the platelet count will occur in some myelodysplastic patients who receive danazol (Cines et al 1985, Buzaid et al 1987). Benefit following GM-CSF may occur in some patients with myelodysplasia (Vadhan-Raj et al 1987).

Aplastic anaemia

Thrombocytopenia is an important problem in patients with aplastic anaemia. Further, the risk of alloimmune platelet transfusion refractoriness is high in aplastic anaemia patients, probably because chemotherapy with its immunosuppressive effects is not used. When aplastic anaemia patients are potential marrow transplant recipients, blood product use should be minimized and leukocyte-depleted to reduce the risk of engraftment failure (Gordon-Smith 1989).

Paroxysmal nocturnal haemoglobinuria

Paroxysmal nocturnal haemoglobinuria (PNH) is a clonal myeloid disorder that is associated with an increased frequency of unusual thromboses (e.g. portal vein thrombosis). PNH sometimes progresses to acute myeloid leukaemia or aplastic anaemia. The procoagulant tendency may be related to the absence of phosphoinositol-linked complement inhibitor proteins on PNH platelets, which causes these platelets to form procoagulant microparticles following complement activation (Wiedmer et al 1991).

Mast cell disease

In this rare group of diseases, the presence of thrombocytopenia indicates a greater likelihood of systemic involvement or of associated myelodysplasia (Travis et al 1988, Lawrence et al 1991).

Myeloproliferative disorders

Normal or increased platelet counts are usually seen in the myeloproliferative disorders. However, thrombocytopenia can occur when marrow failure results from progressive marrow fibrosis (e.g. agnogenic myeloid metaplasia, end-stage polycythaemia rubra vera) or transformation to acute leukaemia.

Coexisting platelet dysfunction in the myeloid disorders

Coexisting platelet dysfunction is particularly common in patients with myelodysplasia or myeloproliferative syndromes (Rasi & Lintula 1986, Baker & Manoharan 1988, Berndt et al 1988). Decreased GP IIb/IIIa numbers have been described in some patients with myeloproliferative disorders (Mazzucato et al 1989). Morphologic abnormalities in megakaryocytes and platelets are commonly seen (Bennett 1986). In vitro evidence of platelet *hyper*function, such as the requirement for higher aspirin concentrations to inhibit arachidonate-induced platelet aggregation, can be seen in some patients hypoaggregable to platelet agonists (Baker & Manoharan 1988).

Transfusion support of leukaemic patients

Platelet transfusions are generally given to leukaemic patients when the platelet count is less than 20×10^9/l (Editorial 1987). This recommendation is based on data in leukaemic children that indicates that serious bleeding risk increases when the platelet count falls below this level (Roy et al 1973). However, recent evidence suggests that a lower platelet count threshold can be used to guide prophylactic platelet transfusion therapy (Soloman et al 1978, Aderka et al 1986, Gmür et al 1991). Gmür and colleagues used a platelet transfusion protocol in which the platelet count threshold of less than 5×10^9/l platelets triggered prophylactic platelet transfusions for clinically stable patients without fever or bleeding. Higher platelet count thresholds were used for febrile or bleeding patients or those in whom invasive procedures were planned (Gmür et al 1991). Other investigators have also used lower platelet count thresholds together with prophylactic antifibrinolytic therapy (tranexamic acid) (Ben-Bassat et al 1990). Randomized trials comparing these new approaches with the older thresholds are needed.

Alloimmune platelet transfusion refractoriness

The platelet count response to transfusions is often suboptimal in leukaemic patients. In many cases, alloantibodies, usually against HLA antigens (Bishop et al 1988), but sometimes against platelet-specific antigens (Kickler et al 1990b), are reponsible for the poor platelet recovery. However, often other clinical factors, such as septicaemia, disseminated intravascular coagulation, splenomegaly, drugs, or poorly defined factors are related to the platelet refractoriness (Bishop et al 1988).

Management of the patient refractory to platelet transfusions

There are two major therapeutic manoeuvres used to treat patients with proven or suspected alloimmune platelet transfusion refractoriness. One is to administer HLA-matched platelets, usually obtained by pheresis of single matched donors. The other approach is to perform an in vitro crossmatch using patient serum and platelets obtained from potential donor units. Neither approach is entirely effective, probably because of the high frequency of non-alloimmune explanations for poor platelet count responses in this patient population. The benefit of iv IgG for alloimmunized patients is too small and transient to justify its use (Kickler et al 1990a).

Platelets bear variable amounts of ABO blood group antigens, and ABO incompatibility can reduce the platelet transfusion response (Lee & Schiffer 1989). Randomized trials indicate that prophylactic filtration of all blood products to reduce contaminating leukocytes will prevent many cases of alloimmunization (Lane et al 1992). However, it remains to be proven that clinically relevant platelet count improvements would result in this patient population.

Lymphoproliferative disorders

Both B and T cell lymphoproliferative disorders can be associated with thrombocytopenia. Pancytopenia is common in patients with advanced acute or chronic lymphoid malignancy that results in marrow infiltration. However, thrombocytopenia can occur by immune mechanisms in many patients with clonal lymphoproliferative disorders.

Chronic lymphocytic leukaemia, lymphoma

Immune thrombocytopenia can occur in some patients with CLL and lymphoma. In one large series, associated lymphoproliferative disorders were identified in 15% of patients with immune thrombocytopenia (Hegde et al 1985b). The incidence of immune thrombocytopenia is approximately 1–2% in patients with Hodgkin's disease (Rudders et al 1972, Xiros et al 1988). An autoimmune pathogenesis has been established by the demonstration of specific platelet glycoprotein/IgG interactions in some patients (Berchtold et al 1989a; Kubota et al 1989).

Sometimes, the thrombocytopenia responds to treatment directed at the associated neoplasm. Otherwise, the treatment of immune thrombocytopenia complicating lymphoproliferative disorders is as in ITP, with corticosteroids followed by splenectomy constituting first-line therapy. One review of immune thrombocytopenia complicating Hodgkin's disease concluded that about 30% of patients respond to corticosteroids, whereas 75% are benefited by splenectomy (Sonnenblick et al 1986). Thrombocytopenia occurring after treatment for Hodgkin's disease does not indicate a relapse of the disease, as both disorders are not necessarily causally associated.

Multiple myeloma and monoclonal gammopathies

Immune thrombocytopenia has also been described in a few patients with multiple myeloma (Verdirame et al 1985). A more frequent problem is platelet dysfunction caused by large amounts of paraprotein (p. 790).

T-lymphoproliferative disorders

Combinations of neutropenia, thrombocytopenia, and anaemia are observed in many patients with expanded populations of large lymphoid cells containing azurophilic cytoplasmic granules (Loughran et al 1985, Loughran &

Starkebaum 1987, Oshimi 1988, van Oostveen et al 1992). Some patients have associated immune disorders such as rheumatoid arthritis (Barton et al 1986). In approximately 80% of these patients with large granular lymphocytic proliferative disease, there is expansion of $CD3^+$ T cells, usually expressing TcR-$\alpha\beta$. The remainder of patients have a natural killer cell phenotype. The term T_γ-lymphoproliferative disease is used to describe those patients in whom the lymphoid cells express $Fc_\gamma III$ receptors. Both clonal and nonclonal lymphoid proliferations have been noted.

Lymphoproliferative disorders and platelet dysfunction

Platelet dysfunction is less common in the lymphoproliferative disorders compared with the clonal myeloid disorders. However, platelet dysfunction can be seen in some patients, particularly when a monoclonal gammopathy is present (multiple myeloma, Waldenstrom's macroglobulinaemia, or monoclonal gammopathy of undetermined significance). Bleeding symptoms and a prolonged bleeding time can be observed despite a normal or near-normal platelet count. Platelet dysfunction can be caused by interference of platelet surface glycoprotein function by the paraprotein (DiMinno et al 1986). It remains unexplained why some patients with hairy cell leukaemia exhibit bleeding abnormalities, including a prolonged bleeding time and defective platelet aggregation. These defects usually correct following splenectomy (Nenci et al 1981).

Purpura can be seen in patients with polyclonal hypergammaglobulinaemic disorders such as hyperglobulinaemic purpura of Waldenstrom and cryoglobulinaemia (Gorevic et al 1980). However, the bleeding time is generally normal in these patients, and the purpura are believed to be caused by perivascular deposition of immune complexes rather than platelet dysfunction.

Non-haematologic neoplastic disease

Thrombocytopenia can occur in patients with non-haematologic ('solid') malignancies. It can be caused by many factors including marrow replacement by tumour and chemotherapy-induced myelosuppression; DIC or thrombotic microangiopathy could be caused by procoagulant tumour factors in some patients (Falanga & Gordon 1985, 1989). Autoimmune thrombocytopenia can also occur in these patients (Schwartz et al 1982), but is much less common that seen with the lymphoproliferative disorders.

Megaloblastic anaemia

Thrombocytopenia can occur in patients with megaloblastic anaemia caused by folic acid or vitamin B12 deficiency. Defective DNA synthesis results in megakaryocytes of low ploidy which synthesize small platelets (Bessman 1984). Thus, the combination of small platelets (low MPV) and large, variably-sized red cells (high MCV, high RDW) suggests megaloblastic anaemia.

Iron depletion and repletion

Although iron deficiency is usually associated with a normal or elevated platelet count, thrombocytopenia can occur in some patients with severe iron-deficiency anaemia (Lopas & Rabiner 1966, Beard & Johnson 1978, Berger & Brass 1987). Occasionally, the platelet count falls to thrombocytopenic levels a few days following initiation of iron replacement therapy, then rises again (Soff & Levin 1988). The cause of thrombocytopenia in iron depletion or following repletion is unknown, although impaired platelet production has been postulated.

MARROW DISORDERS THAT USUALLY PRODUCE ISOLATED THROMBOCYTOPENIA

Alcohol-induced thrombocytopenia

Alcohol toxicity represents the most common cause of isolated thrombocytopenia caused by decreased platelet production. In one study, approximately 25% of alcoholic patients admitted to hospital were thrombocytopenic (Cowan 1980). Alcohol-induced thrombocytopenia can occur in the absence of liver disease or nutrient deficiency (Lindenbaum & Lieber 1969) and platelet counts as low as $10 \times 10^9/l$ have been described (Post & Desforges 1968). The platelet count begins to rise 2–3 days after stopping the alcohol consumption, and reaches normal values within a week or two. Occasionally the thrombocytopenia persists for weeks. Rebound thrombocytosis is common, usually occurring 10 to 17 days after stopping alcohol. Bleeding complications are uncommon and should suggest other factors, such as oesophageal varices, gastritis, peptic ulcers, coagulopathy and platelet dysfunction secondary to cirrhosis. Other causes of thrombocytopenia, including hypersplenism and folate deficiency, should be considered in these patients. Platelet dysfunction secondary to alcohol has also been described (Haut & Cowan 1974, Rand et al 1988).

Marrow examination reveals that the megakaryocytes usually appear normal, although their numbers may be decreased (Gewirtz & Hoffman 1986). Vacuolations of normoblasts and promyelocytes are typically seen (Lindenbaum & Lieber 1969). Reduced megakaryocyte numbers can occur, and may be associated with slower recovery of platelet counts (Gewirtz & Hoffman 1986). Several lines of evidence, including platelet kinetic studies (Cowan 1973), effect of alcohol consumption on pattern of platelet count recovery following plateletpheresis (Sullivan et al 1977), reduced mean platelet volumes

(Sahud 1972), and marrow culture studies (Gewirtz & Hoffman 1986, Levine et al 1986), indicate that alcohol impairs platelet production with only a minimal reduction in platelet lifespan (Cowan 1973). It appears that alcohol predominantly damages megakaryocyte maturation, rather than suppressing the progenitor CFU-meg cells (Gewirtz & Hoffman 1986, Levine et al 1986).

Amegakaryocytic thrombocytopenia

The term amegakaryocytic thrombocytopenia, also known as acquired pure amegakaryocytic thrombocytopenic purpura, describes the uncommon clinical problem of isolated thrombocytopenia with markedly decreased or absent megakaryocytes (Hoffman 1991). Amegakaryocytic thrombocytopenia can be caused by immune mechanisms, including lymphocyte-mediated damage to megakaryocyte progenitor cells (Gewirtz et al 1986) or IgG-mediated clearance of the cytokines controlling megakaryocytopoiesis (Hoffman et al 1989). Amegakaryocytic thrombocytopenia caused by presumed autoimmune mechanisms has responded in some instances to immunosuppressive therapy, including corticosteroids (Smeets & Hillen 1988), antilymphocyte or antithymocyte globulin (Faldt 1986, Manoharan et al 1989, Trimble et al 1991), and cyclosporine (Telek et al 1989).

Often, amegakaryocytic thrombocytopenia is the first manifestation of a generalized stem cell disorder (Stoll et al 1981, Hoffman et al 1982, Tricot et al 1982, Hallett et al 1989, Ridell et al 1992). Chromosome abnormalities of marrow myeloid cells may be helpful in establishing this diagnosis. Often, pancytopenia eventually ensues, and repeat marrow examination indicates myelodysplasia, acute myeloid leukaemia, or aplastic anaemia.

THROMBOCYTOPENIA CAUSED BY HYPERSPLENISM OR HAEMODILUTION

HYPERSPLENISM

The typical clinical picture of hypersplenism is mild to moderate reduction in all three cell lines together with a palpably enlarged spleen. The platelet count is usually between 50 and 150 × 10^9/l. Bleeding complications are often related to coexisting anatomic (e.g. oesophageal varices) or haemostatic (e.g. coagulopathy secondary to liver disease) problems. Only under very unusual circumstances is a splenectomy required to raise the platelet count in these patients.

HAEMODILUTION

Transfusion of large amounts of crystalloid, colloid, or packed cells can result in dilutional thrombocytopenia. Dilution is the major reason why the platelet count falls by approximately 50% in most patients undergoing cardiopulmonary bypass surgery (Harker et al 1980). Massive resuscitation for trauma patients is the major clinical situation in which dilution can coexist with more dangerous causes for thrombocytopenia, such as disseminated intravascular coagulation resulting from tissue injury or shock. Accordingly, platelet count monitoring should be done frequently in these patients, since a disproportionate fall in the platelet count may indicate DIC rather than dilution (Ciavarella et al 1987). Formerly, prophylactic platelet transfusions were often given for anticipated dilutional thrombocytopenia, but the current recommendations are to restrict platelet transfusions to patients in whom a platelet count below 50 × 10^9/l is documented or suspected, or in whom diffuse microvascular bleeding is encountered (Ciavarella et al 1987, Consensus conference 1987).

ACQUIRED QUALITATIVE PLATELET DISORDERS

Our understanding of normal and abnormal platelet/vessel wall interactions remains incomplete. Perhaps this is best exemplified by the poor correlation of in vitro tests with clinical problems. For example, the two tests used most often to assess qualitative platelet dysfunction are the bleeding time test and platelet aggregation studies. Both tests suffer from major limitations. A prolonged bleeding time is not very sensitive nor specific for identifying qualitative platelet dysfunction, or for predicting bleeding (Rodgers & Levin 1990, Lind 1991). Patients with platelet storage pool disorders often demonstrate normal platelet aggregation (Nieuwenhuis et al 1987, Israels et al 1990).

Platelet aggregation studies are flawed by numerous technical factors including: (1) the artefact of low calcium concentrations from blood chelation (which is related to the haematocrit variability among different subjects); (2) few widely accepted criteria for performance or interpretation of these assays exist (British Society Task Force 1988); (3) the considerable variation among normal individuals; (4) platelet aggregation assays are 'non-physiologic' in that plasma fibrinogen, which is essential for platelet aggregation under the conditions of platelet aggregation studies, is probably of minimal importance in physiologic platelet adhesion/aggregation, which occurs at high shear conditions.

ANTIPLATELET EFFECTS OF DRUGS

We will focus our discussion on aspirin, as clinically relevant anti-thrombotic and pro-haemorrhagic effects of this agent have been well-documented in large studies. Although many drugs have been reported to have inhibitory

Table 33.6 Drugs implicated in platelet dysfunction

Anti-platelet agents
Aspirin, dipyridamole, epoprostenol, n-3 fatty acids, iloprost, sulfinpyrazone, ticlopidine

Anti-inflammatory drugs
Non-steroidal agents (aspirin, colchicine, diclofenac, diflunisal, fenoprofen, ibuprofen, indomethacin, meclofenamic acid, mefenamic acid, naproxen, phenylbutazone, piroxicam, sulfinpyrazone, sulindac, tolmetin, zompirac). Corticosteroids (hydrocortisone, methylprednisolone)

Anti-microbial drugs
Penicillins (ampicillin, apalcillin, azlocillin, carbenicillin, methicillin, mezlocillin, nafcillin, penicillin G, piperacillin, sulbenicillin, ticarcillin). Cephalosporins (cefoperazone, cefotaxime, cephalothin, moxalactam). Other antibiotics (chlortetracycline, gentamicin, hydroxychloroquine, nitrofurantoin, quinacrine)

Diuretics
Acetazolamine, ethacrynic acid, furosemide

Cardiac, anti-hypertensive, or vasodilating drugs
Diltiazem, hydralazine, isoproterenol, isosorbide dinitrate, isosorbide mononitrate, nifedipine, nimodipine, nitroglycerin, nitroprusside, quinidine, papaverine, phenoxybenzamine, phentolamine, propranolol, reserpine, verapamil

Anaesthetic agents
Benoxinate, benzocaine, butacaine, cocaine, cyclaine, dibucaine, halothane, lidocaine, piperocaine, procaine, proparacaine, tetracaine

Bronchodilator drugs
Aminophylline, theophylline

Psychiatric drugs
Amitriptyline, chlorpromazine, desipramine, doxepin, fluphenazine, haloperidol, imipramine, nortryiptyline, promazine, promethazine, trifluoperazine

Volume expanders
Dextran, hydroxyethyl starch

Anticancer chemotherapy
Asparaginase, carmustine, daunorubicin, plicamycin, vinblastine, vincristine

Antihistamines
Chlorpheniramine, diphenhydramine, pyrilamine

Radiographic contrast agents
Iopamidol, iothalamate, ioxaglate, meglumine diatrizoate, sodium diatrizoate

Foods
Alcohol, Chinese black tree fungus (mo-er), cloves, cumin, n-3 fatty acids, garlic, ginger, onion, turmeric, vitamin C, vitamin E

Miscellaneous
Acetaminophen, aminocaproic acid, caffeine, clofibrate, cyclosporine, cyproheptadine, dicumarol, dihydroergotamine, guaifenesin, heparin, heroin, ketanserin, protamine sulphate, methysergide maleate, tissue-plasminogen activator (rt-PA), tocopherol (vitamin E)

References for this table are from Bick (1992) and George & Shattil (1991)

effects on platelet function (Table 33.6), clinical relevance has been proved in only a few instances.

Aspirin

The platelet inhibitory effect of aspirin was described 25 years ago (Weiss & Aledort 1967). Aspirin is unique among the nonsteroidal anti-inflammatory agents because it irreversibly inactivates the enzyme cyclo-oxygenase (Roth & Siok 1978, Packham 1982). Platelet cyclo-oxygenase converts arachidonate that has been liberated by phospholipases from platelet membranes during platelet activation to intermediate compounds (the cyclic endoperoxides prostaglandin PGG_2 and PGH_2). These endoperoxides are converted to thromboxane A_2 by the enzyme thromboxane synthetase. Thromboxane A_2 is a potent platelet activator that has a short half life (approximately 30 seconds). It is degraded into the stable but inactive metabolite, thromboxane B_2.

Aspirin also inhibits endothelial cell cyclo-oxygenase, where arachidonate is also converted to the identical cyclic endoperoxides. However, a different enzyme known as prostacyclin synthase converts prostaglandin H_2 to prostacyclin, which has potent vasodilatory and platelet antagonistic effects.

Aspirin inhibits both platelet and endothelial cyclo-oxygenase. Hence, it theoretically can both inhibit or enhance the haemostatic mechanism. Experimental and clinical evidence indicates that aspirin has considerable antithrombotic activity, possibly because: (1) smaller doses of aspirin may be required to inhibit platelet, compared with endothelial, cyclo-oxygenase (Baenziger et al 1977); (2) unlike the endothelial cell, the platelet is anucleate, and unable to regenerate cyclo-oxygenase; and (3) hepatic degradation of ingested aspirin localizes inhibition of platelets to their flow through the presystemic (portal) circulation, whereas endothelial cells are subsequently exposed to much smaller concentrations of aspirin (Pedersen & Fitzgerald 1984).

Effect on the bleeding time

The bleeding time increases modestly following the ingestion of aspirin. In one study (Fiore et al 1990), the peak increase occurred 4–12 hours following ingestion, and measured about 2 minutes greater than baseline (mean increase plus two standard deviations is 6 minutes). Return to baseline occurs by 48 hours. Approximately 15% of the normal population are 'hyperresponders' to aspirin (Fiore et al 1990). In some cases, a marked increase in the bleeding time after aspirin ingestion indicates the presence of a platelet or von Willebrand factor defect (Czapek et al 1978, Stuart et al 1979).

Bleeding complications of aspirin use

Theoretically, aspirin use mimics the situation in those patients with congenital cyclo-oxygenase deficiency, which is associated with a mild-to-moderate haemorrhagic tendency (Malmsten et al 1975, Lagarde et al 1978). Aspirin treatment results in increased postoperative haemorrhage following heart surgery. A large prospective, randomized study of heart surgery patients found greater chest-tube drainage (1035 against 805 ml per patient) and a higher frequency of reoperation (6.5% against 1.3%) in patients who received aspirin (Goldman et al 1988). However, it is controversial whether aspirin increases bleeding significantly during or after other surgical procedures (George & Shattil 1991).

Large prospective studies of the antithrombotic effects of aspirin also indicate that bleeding complications occur in some patients. For example, intracranial haemorrhages were significantly more common in subjects taking aspirin (Steering Committee of the Physicians' Health Study Research Group 1988).

Antithrombotic effects of aspirin

A meta-analysis of secondary prevention trials indicated that aspirin overall reduces major cardiovascular or cerebrovascular events by 23% (Antiplatelet Trialists' Collaboration 1988). A similar reduction of major vascular events was also seen in a primary prevention study of American male physicians (Steering Committee of the Physicians' Health Study Research Group 1988).

Other anti-platelet drugs with antithrombotic benefit

We summarize here a partial list of antiplatelet drugs that have been used for their antithrombotic effects.

Ticlopidine

Ticlopidine is a novel antiplatelet agent that inhibits ADP-induced platelet aggregation to a greater extent than other agonists (Thebault et al 1975, Hardisty et al 1990, McTavish et al 1990). Although it may be more effective than aspirin for the secondary prevention of cerebrovascular disease, it does not have a higher risk of bleeding complications (Hass et al 1989).

Prostacyclin and prostacyclin analogues

Prostacyclin is a potent vasodilator and anti-platelet eicosanoid synthesized by endothelial cells. Prostacyclin infusion has been shown to prolong the bleeding time in experimental animals and man (Rodgers 1990). The stable prostacyclin analogue, iloprost, has been used to inhibit platelet activation in patients with heparin-induced thrombocytopenia who require heparin during heart surgery (Kappa et al 1990).

Sulfinpyrazone

Sulfinpyrazone has little or no effect on the bleeding time (Weston et al 1977), and has been shown to interact synergistically with aspirin in the treatment of cerebrovascular disease (Canadian Cooperative Study Group 1978).

Dipyridamole

Dipyridamole, which inhibits platelet phosphodiesterase and increases inhibitory cyclic AMP levels in platelets, has little or no effect on the bleeding time (Weston et al 1977). Although one prospective blinded study of peripheral vascular disease progression indicated a superior effect of the combination of aspirin and dipyridamole compared with aspirin or placebo alone (Hess et al 1985), the consensus is that dipyridamole has little antithrombotic effect (FitzGerald 1987).

OTHER DRUGS WITH CLINICALLY SIGNIFICANT ANTI-PLATELET EFFECTS

In the following section we discuss drugs that are not used primarily for their antiplatelet effect, but which have been implicated in bleeding complications in some patients.

Antibiotics

High doses of β-lactam antibiotics will increase the bleeding times in a dose- and time-dependent fashion, sometimes markedly, and this effect can last for several days (Brown et al 1974, 1976). In one study, antibiotics were the most common explanation for prolonged bleeding times in hospitalized patients (Wisløff & Godal 1981). Clinical bleeding has been implicated for carbenicillin, mezlocillin, piperacillin, ticarcillin, cefotaxime, and moxalactam (George & Shattil 1992). Bleeding due to moxolactam can also be caused by drug-induced inhibition of vitamin K-dependent coagulation factor synthesis (Lipsky 1988).

Studies have implicated three mechanisms for the platelet dysfunction caused by penicillin: inhibition of agonist binding to platelet membrane receptors (Shattil et al 1980, Burroughs & Johnson 1990); impairment of thromboxane synthesis; and postreceptor impairment of signal transduction (Burroughs & Johnson 1990).

For patients with antibiotic-induced platelet dysfunction who require surgery (e.g. bacterial endocarditis requiring valve replacement), platelet transfusions are usually given for bleeding rather than for prophylaxis of bleeding, particularly since there is time-dependent inhibition of platelet function.

Non-steroidal anti-inflammatory drugs

Non-steroidal anti-inflammatory agents (e.g. indomethacin, naproxen) inhibit cyclo-oxygenase in a reversible, dose-dependent fashion. These drugs can cause bleeding in some circumstances.

Heparin and low molecular weight heparins

Although heparin is used because of its effects in promoting antithrombin activity, it also binds to the platelet membrane, and can result in bleeding time prolongation (Warkentin & Kelton 1990b). The binding of low molecular weight heparins to platelets is less than standard heparin, and this could be a factor in the lower incidence of bleeding complications seen in some studies with low molecular weight compared with unfractionated heparin (Levine et al 1991).

Thrombolytic therapy

At least 5% of patients develop major bleeding episodes during thrombolytic therapy. Approximately 0.5% of patients will have an intracranial haemorrhage when receiving thrombolysis for acute myocardial infarction (Erlemeier et al 1989, Sane et al 1989). Prolongation of the bleeding time following thrombolytic therapy correlated with bleeding events in one study (Gimple et al 1989). The bleeding complications are multifactorial, and related to clinical factors (use of invasive vascular catheters, hypertension), plasmin proteolysis (hypofibrinogenaemia, decreased factors V, VIII levels, von Willebrand factor degradation, anticoagulant effects of fibrinogen/fibrin degradation products), and alterations of platelet function (Sane et al 1989, Federici et al 1992, Penny & Ware 1992). Platelet transfusions should be considered in patients bleeding during thrombolytic therapy (Sane et al 1989).

Plasma expanders

Plasma expanders such as dextran and hydroxyethyl starch can prolong the bleeding time by direct inhibition of platelet function (Weiss 1967) and interference with von Willebrand factor (Sanfelippo et al 1987). These agents appear to have caused bleeding complications in some patients (Kline et al 1975, Sanfelipo et al 1987).

Ethanol

High concentrations of alcohol can decrease platelet aggregation (Haut & Cowan 1974) and thromboxane synthesis (Stuart 1979), and will potentiate the bleeding time increase caused by aspirin (Deykin et al 1982). It is unknown to what extent alcohol-induced platelet dysfunction contributes to the observations that alcohol abuse is an important risk factor for serious bleeding complications such as intracranial haemorrhage (Monforte et al 1990).

Other drugs

No clinical significance has been established for the majority of drugs shown to have in vitro or ex vivo antiplatelet effects. One example — acetaminophen — is widely regarded as a safe analgesic and antipyretic agent for patients with severe thrombocytopenia and platelet dysfunction (e.g. leukaemic patients). Yet, two studies have shown in vitro inhibition of platelet function by this drug (Shorr et al 1985, Lages & Weiss 1989).

URAEMIA

Uraemic patients have an increased incidence of haemorrhagic and thrombotic complications. Bleeding times are often elevated even in azotaemic patients who do not require dialysis (Mannucci et al 1983).

Clinical features

In one large autopsy series, approximately 5% of deaths in patients with acute renal failure were caused by bleeding (Maher & Schreiner 1962). Improved dialysis and transfusion therapy have reduced the frequency of bleeding problems in severe uraemia (Remuzzi 1988). Mucocutaneous bleeding, particularly from the upper and lower gastrointestinal tracts, is most characteristic (Lewis et al 1956, Kleinknecht et al 1972, Zuckerman et al 1985). Angiodysplasia of the stomach and duodenum is a particularly common site of bleeding in these patients (Zuckerman et al 1985). In addition, life-threatening pleural, pericardial, intracranial (particularly subdural haemorrhage), and retroperitoneal bleeding have been described (Guild et al 1957, Alfrey et al 1968, Stein et al 1970, Galen et al 1975, Milutinovich et al 1977, Janson et al 1980). The occurrence of some of these events during dialysis suggests that heparin anticoagulation could have contributed to the bleeding. Uraemic patients are also at increased risk of bleeding during surgical and other invasive procedures.

Modest decreases in platelet count during haemodialysis are frequent, and are related to platelet activation and loss via passage through the extracorporeal circuit (Hakim & Schafer 1985, Schmitt et al 1987). Moderate thrombocytopenia and thrombotic complications, particularly clot formation in the extracorporeal circuit, should suggest heparin-induced thrombocytopenia (Janson et al 1983, Leehey et al 1987, Matsuo et al 1988).

Laboratory abnormalities

The most consistently observed haemostatic abnormality in azotaemic patients is a prolonged bleeding time. The exact cause of the bleeding defect remains uncertain. Laboratory investigation is complicated by the markedly reduced haematocrit in most uraemic patients. The low haematocrits lead to lower platelet count and higher ionized calcium concentrations in chelated platelet-rich plasma samples (Ballard & Marcus 1972, Bloom et al 1986).

Abnormal platelet function

A defect in primary haemostasis was reported by Salzman & Neri (1966), who observed decreased adhesion of uraemic platelets to glass beads. More recent studies employing collagen-coated perfusion chambers (Zwaginga et al 1990, 1991a,b) and de-endothelialized rabbit segments (Escolar et al 1990) have shown defective platelet adhesion, aggregation, and spreading. Several factors interact to produce these abnormalities:

1. A normal haematocrit is essential for optimal platelet/vessel wall interaction (Escolar et al 1988, Sakariassen et al 1980); uraemic patients often have a moderate to severe anaemia (haemoglobin 70–100 g/l).
2. Decreased levels of platelet GPIb (Sloand et al 1991), as well as the largest multimers of von Willebrand factor (Gralnick et al 1988), have been reported.
3. Defective platelet activation and aggregation processes have been observed by many investigators, including impaired platelet aggregation and cytoplasmic calcium elevation to collagen, ADP, and thrombin (Di Minno et al 1985, Bloom et al 1986, Ware et al 1989, Fabris et al 1991), impaired thromboxane generation (Remuzzi et al 1983, Di Minno et al 1985, Fabris et al 1991), decreased generation of platelet procoagulant activity (platelet factor 3) (Cahalane et al 1958, Bonnin & Cheney 1961), and abnormal clot retraction (Castaldi et al 1966, Jørgensen & Ingeberg 1979).
4. Decreased platelet ADP and serotonin levels (storage pool defect) have also been reported (Eknoyan & Brown 1981, Di Minno et al 1985).

Role of uraemic toxins

Many reports indicate that uraemic 'toxins' can inhibit platelet function in vitro (Eknoyan et al 1969, Horowitz et al 1970, Rabiner & Molinas 1970, Bazylinski et al 1985, Palés et al 1987). Washed uraemic platelets demonstrate normal adhesion and aggregation when resuspended in normal plasma; in contrast, normal platelets demonstrate reduced adhesion and aggregation in the presence of uraemic plasma (Castillo et al 1986, Zwaginga et al 1991a,b).

Role of endothelium in platelet inhibition

Endothelium-derived nitric oxide is a potent antiplatelet agent (Ignarro 1989) that has recently been implicated in the pathogenesis of uraemic platelet dysfunction. Remuzzi and colleagues (1990) have developed a uraemic rat model, in which inhibition of nitric oxide generation by *N*-monomethyl-L-arginine corrects the prolonged bleeding time. A study of blood emerging from bleeding time wounds in uraemic patients showed increased 6-keto-$PGF_{1\alpha}$ levels, indicating increased microvascular prostacyclin generation (Kyrle et al 1988). These endogenous antiplatelet agents could produce the high adenylate cyclase activity and cyclic AMP levels observed in uraemic platelets (Vlachoyannis & Schoeppe 1982, Jacobsson et al 1985).

Megakaryocyte dysfunction

The circulating platelet mass, as determined by the platelet count and mean platelet volume, is reduced in patients with renal failure (Gafter et al 1987, Michalak et al 1991). Erythropoietin treatment increased the platelet counts in some studies of uraemic patients (Eschbach et al 1989, Fabris et al 1991) and can produce improved platelet function (Zwaginga et al 1991b).

Treatment

Several approaches have been used to control or prevent uraemic bleeding (Couch & Stumpf 1990). Correction of the prolonged bleeding time is the most frequent method that has been used to judge the efficacy of the treatments used.

Dialysis

The uraemic platelet function defect can be improved by aggressive dialysis. It is possible that peritoneal dialysis is more effective than haemodialysis in improving platelet function, possibly because of a more effective removal of toxic 'middle molecules' (molecular weight 300–2000) (Schoots et al 1984).

Raising the haematocrit

Raising the haematocrit by transfusion (Livio et al 1982, Fernandez et al 1985) or erythropoietin (Moia et al 1987, Gordge et al 1990, Fabris et al 1991, Zwaginga et al 1991b) can improve or correct the bleeding time by optimizing platelet/vessel wall interactions. In addition, a higher haematocrit reduces the inhibitory effects of the plasma toxins (Zwaginga et al 1991b).

Desmopressin (DDAVP)

Transient partial or complete correction of the prolonged bleeding time can be achieved by intravenous, subcutaneous, or intranasal administration of the vasopressin analogue, desmopressin (1-desamino-8-D-arginine vasopressin, DDAVP) (Mannucci et al 1983, Mannucci 1988). Benefit observed within 1 hour following use, and lasts from 4–12 hours. Repeated treatment with DDAVP produces progressively less benefit (tachyphylaxis).

Cryoprecipitate

Ten or more units of cryoprecipitate corrects or significantly improves the bleeding time in some uraemic patients, and has been used to treat bleeding episodes and prepare patients for invasive procedures (Gerritsen et al 1978, Janson et al 1980). Improvement in the bleeding time is seen at 1 to 4 hours, with peak effect between 6 and 12 hours following infusion, and a return to baseline by 24 hours. However, some investigators have not observed an improvement of the bleeding time using cryoprecipitate (Liu et al 1984).

Conjugated oestrogens

Conjugated oestrogens are effective in reducing the bleeding time in uraemic patients (Liu et al 1984, Livio et al 1986, Viganò et al 1988, Shemin et al 1990) (see Fig. 33.2). Oestrogens can be given either by the intravenous or oral route, usually for a minimum of 5 days. Maximal reduction in bleeding time occurs 3 to 7 days following start of treatment, and can persist for several days after stopping the oestrogens. The active component is 17β-oestradiol (Viganó et al 1990). Oestrogens appear to work by reducing endothelial synthesis of nitric oxide (Zoja et al 1988, 1991, Remuzzi et al 1990).

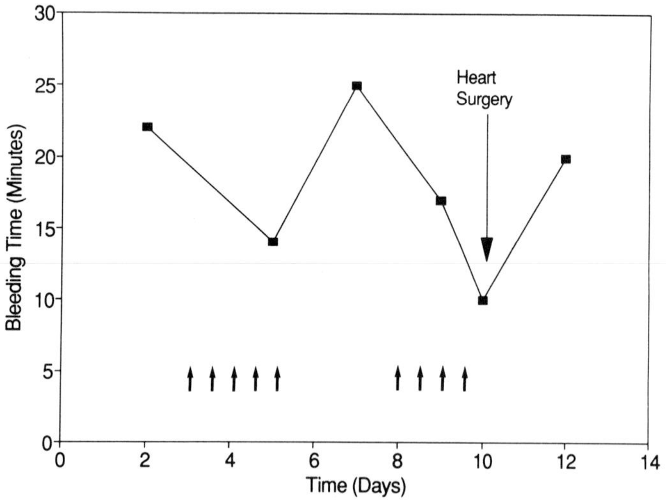

Fig. 33.2 Perioperative reduction of prolonged bleeding time in a uraemic patient using conjugated oestrogens. A 49 year old woman with moderate renal failure required open heart surgery for coronary artery disease. Conjugated oestrogens, given as 25 mg twice daily by mouth, reduced the bleeding time in preparation for open heart surgery.

MONOCLONAL AND POLYCLONAL GAMMOPATHIES

Multiple myeloma and Waldenström's macroglobulinaemia

Both coagulation and platelet function defects can occur in patients with multiple myeloma and Waldenström's macroglobulinaemia (Lackner 1973). Coagulation abnormalities usually result from the inhibition of function or less commonly by increased destruction of coagulation factors mediated by the monoclonal paraprotein. For example, a prolonged thrombin clotting time can be caused by inhibition of fibrinogen polymerization by the paraprotein, although bleeding complications are infrequent (Vigliano & Horowitz 1967, Perkins et al 1970, Lackner et al 1970). Less common coagulation abnormalities that can be complicated by serious bleeding include acquired von Willebrand's disease (Mannucci et al 1984, Takahashi et al 1986, Mohri et al 1987), primary fibrinolysis (Meyer & Williams 1985), and circulating heparin-like anticoagulants (Khoory et al 1980, Chapman et al 1984, Kaufman et al 1989).

Malignant plasma cell disorders also can be associated with defects in platelet number and function. Thrombocytopenia is common, and is usually caused by marrow suppression secondary to tumour infiltration or chemotherapy. Rarely, secondary immune thrombocytopenia can occur that responds to treatment for ITP (Verdirame et al 1985).

Platelet function abnormalities commonly are observed in patients with malignant plasma cell disorders (Cohen et al 1970, Perkins et al 1970, Lackner 1973). The coating of the platelet surface by the paraprotein has been implicated in the pathogenesis of platelet function abnormalities (Pachter et al 1959). In some patients, a specific interaction of the paraprotein with a specific platelet membrane glycoprotein, such as GPIIIa, has been described (DiMinno et al 1986). In general, the platelet inhibition correlates with the concentration of the monoclonal paraprotein (Perkins et al 1970). Accordingly, plasma exchange which reduces the paraprotein levels has been used to control serious bleeding in these patients (Cohen et al 1970, Perkins et al 1970, Mohri et al 1987). Uraemic platelet dysfunction also can occur secondary to 'myeloma kidney'.

Benign monoclonal gammopathy

Coagulation and platelet defects are less common in patients with benign monoclonal gammopathy, probably because paraprotein levels tend to be lower than in patients with malignant plasma cell disease (Perkins et al 1970). However, benign monoclonal gammopathy has been found in many patients with acquired von Willebrand's disease (Rosborough & Swaim 1978, Cass et al 1980,

Mannucci et al 1984, Stewart & Glynn 1990). If a monoclonal immunoglobulin is detected in a patient with unexplained acquired bleeding, von Willebrand factor studies should be performed. Such studies should include multimer analysis, since deficiency of predominantly the largest multimers has been reported.

Polyclonal gammopathies

Purpura can be observed in some patients with polyclonal gammopathies. Benign hyperglobulinaemic purpura of Waldenström, which occurs predominantly in young women, is characterized by recurrent, symmetric purpura in dependent areas, and polyclonal hypergammaglobulinaemia (usually with rheumatoid factor activity) Waldenström 1951, Kyle et al 1971). Perivascular infiltration by polymorphonuclear leukocytes is found in some patients. There is an increased incidence of associated sicca syndrome or systemic lupus erythematosus. Recurrent purpura and polyclonal hypergammaglobulinaemia (often with a monoclonal IgM component with rheumatoid factor activity) is also found in patients with mixed cryoglobulinaemia (Gorevic et al 1980). Cutaneous vasculitis is the cause of the purpura in these patients, who have a high incidence of concomitant arthralgias, renal, and other organ disease. The bleeding time is usually normal in patients with purpura and hypergammaglobulinaemia, consistent with the role of vascular, rather than platelet dysfunction in the pathogenesis of the purpura.

LIVER DISEASE

Moderate to severe hepatic dysfunction is associated with numerous haemostatic abnormalities, including reduction of procoagulant and anticoagulant proteins, dysfibrinogenaemia, and enhanced fibrinolysis. Thrombocytopenia also is common, usually due to hypersplenism or alcohol toxicity. In addition, some patients have platelet dysfunction, with a prolongation of the bleeding time disproportionate to the degree of thrombocytopenia. Defects in platelet aggregation and platelet factor 3 generation have been reported (Weiss & Eichelberger 1963, Ballard & Marcus 1976). Desmopressin shortened the prolonged bleeding times in two randomized, double-blind trials in cirrhotic patients (Burroughs et al 1985, Mannucci et al 1986).

CARDIOPULMONARY BYPASS SURGERY

Platelet count changes

Heart surgery requiring cardiopulmonary bypass (extracorporeal circulation) is associated with significant intraoperative and postoperative thrombocytopenia. Typically, there is a 50% reduction in the platelet count, primarily caused by dilution during 'priming' and by the loss of platelets to the bypass apparatus (Harker et al 1980, Hope et al 1981). Following surgery, the platelet count remains reduced and stable for 2–4 days, following which there is recovery to normal or elevated values. The bleeding time characteristically rises to very high levels during heart surgery (greater than 20–30 minutes), but typically shortens to below 15 minutes half an hour after protamine reversal of heparin, and corrects to normal 2–4 hours later (Harker et al 1980). Deviations from this pattern can be caused by ongoing postoperative bleeding (dilutional thrombocytopenia); heparin-induced thrombocytopenia (Walls et al 1992); disseminated intravascular coagulation (usually related to shock following heart surgery); septicaemia; and other perioperative events (Warkentin et al 1992c). Most postoperative bleeding is caused by defective surgical haemostasis, transient platelet dysfunction (Woodman & Harker 1990), and, possibly, excess fibrinolysis.

Platelet dysfunction

The cause of the platelet dysfunction after heart surgery remains incompletely understood. Platelet activation and granule release occurs when blood is exposed to the bypass apparatus (Abrams et al 1990), leading to acquired α granule deficiency (Harker et al 1980). Progressive activation of coagulation (including the contact system) and inflammation (including complement activation and release of neutrophil proteases) occurs during heart surgery, suggesting that proteolysis of platelet and coagulation proteins could cause bleeding in some patients. Protamine reversal of heparin following heart surgery can produce further decrease in the platelet count and can produce platelet and complement activation and complement activation (Hobbhahn et al 1991).

Hyperfibrinolysis

The role of excess fibrinolysis in heart surgery bleeding is controversial. Laboratory diagnosis of fibrinolysis is complicated by the marked haemodilution and progressive thrombin generation that occur during cardiopulmonary bypass surgery. The reduction of bleeding by prophylactic use of high-dose aprotinin is indirect evidence for excess fibrinolysis. However, aprotinin inhibits kallikrein as well as plasmin, and its benefits could be related to inhibition of the contact and complement systems.

Prevention of bleeding after heart surgery

Many heart surgery centres are evaluating different preventative manoeuvres to reduce bleeding after heart surgery. No consensus has emerged as to the ideal preventative approach.

Discontinue aspirin

Bleeding is increased significantly in patients who receive aspirin prior to heart surgery (Goldman et al 1988) and aspirin should be discontinued at least 5 days prior to heart surgery (Woodman & Harker 1990).

Prophylactic antifibrinolytic therapy

Blood loss was reduced approximately 40–50% in the largest randomized, double-blind trials of prophylactic high-dose aprotinin given for heart surgery (Bidstrup et al 1989, Fraedrich et al 1989, Harder et al 1991). Reduction in bleeding was also observed using ε-aminocaproic acid (Vander Salm et al 1988, DelRossi et al 1989).

Normothermic heart surgery

A recent study indicated that bleeding is reduced when normothermic surgery is performed (Yau et al 1992). This could relate to platelet dysfunction caused by cool temperatures.

Desmopressin (DDAVP)

Desmopressin given post-protamine reduced bleeding in one study (Salzman et al 1986). However, bleeding reduction was absent or marginal in two other controlled studies (Rocha et al 1988, Hackman et al 1989), and the routine use of this drug is not recommended (Woodman & Harker 1990).

Evaluation and treatment of bleeding post-cardiac surgery

There is no single, widely accepted definition for excess bleeding following heart surgery. However, in general, postoperative chest tube losses exceeding 100 ml/h is excessive (Woodman & Harker 1990). Approximately 5% of patients undergo exploratory reoperation for excess bleeding. One guideline for reoperation is bleeding that exceeds 10 ml/kg in the first postoperative hour, or an average of 5 ml/kg for the first 3 hours, or significant sudden late bleeding (Woodman & Harker 1990).

Routine laboratory testing (PT, aPTT, thrombin times, platelet count) is not helpful in guiding therapy, unless evidence for inadequate heparin neutralization (including heparin 'rebound') or severe thrombocytopenia is documented. This is because these tests do not assess the likely explanations for bleeding (platelet dysfunction, fibrinolysis, 'surgical' bleeding). In theory, bleeding time prolongation should suggest haemostatic dysfunction rather than surgical bleeding, but this has not been established.

Packed red cells are the most frequently used blood product. Patients with excess postoperative bleeding may respond to therapeutic platelet transfusions. Fresh frozen plasma and cryoprecipitate are seldom needed, unless the patient has been refractory to other treatments or there are significant abnormalities in the coagulation tests. Desmopressin (Czer et al 1987) and ε-aminocaproic acid (Lambert et al 1979) may be effective in some patients who have excess postoperative bleeding.

Platelet dysfunction caused by platelet-reactive antibodies

Some patients with normal platelet counts can have platelet dysfunction caused by antibodies that interfere with platelet function (Karpatkin & Lackner 1975). In some patients, autoantibodies that are reactive against GPIIb/IIIa (Niessner et al 1986, Meyer et al 1991) or GPIb/IX (Devine et al 1987) have been implicated. Patients with apparent ITP who are 'cured' by splenectomy, but who have persistent platelet dysfunction caused by autoantibodies have also been described (Meyer et al 1991). Further evidence that platelet-reactive antibodies could cause platelet dysfunction are observations that isoantibodies formed by Glanzmann's thrombasthenic patients lacking GPIIb/IIIa interfere with platelet function in vitro (Levy-Toledano et al 1978).

Acquired storage pool disorder

Acquired storage pool disorders include a group of acquired platelet disorders characterized by prolonged bleeding time, aggregation abnormalities (e.g. absent secondary wave to ADP, reduced aggregation to collagen and arachidonic acid), decreased ADP and ATP levels with increased ATP/ADP ratio, and granule deficiency by electron microscopy. There are two general causes of this syndrome: (1) clonal myeloid disorders, and (2) 'exhausted' platelet syndromes. For example, in some patients with myelodysplasia, myeloproliferative syndromes, and myeloid leukaemia, bleeding symptoms disproportionate to the platelet count level may be seen together with these abnormalities (Cowan et al 1975, Gerrard et al 1978, Russell et al 1981, Malpass et al 1984). Disorders that may be associated with in vivo platelet activation (e.g. cardiopulmonary bypass, systemic lupus erythematosus, other immune thrombocytopenic disorders, disseminated intravascular coagulation, thrombotic microangiopathy, renal transplant rejection, hairy cell leukaemia) also can demonstrate these abnormalities (Zahavi & Marder 1975, Pareti et al 1976, 1980, Beurling-Harbury & Galvan 1978, Harker et al 1980, Weiss et al 1980, Nenci et al 1981). It is believed that these acquired abnormalities are related to in vivo platelet activation and release of the storage granule constituents.

ACQUIRED VON WILLEBRAND DISEASE (aVWD)

Acquired von Willebrand disease can mimick acquired platelet dysfunction (mucocutaneous bleeding, normal platelet count, prolonged bleeding time). However, plasma von Willebrand factor levels and activity are reduced. Acquired inhibitors, particularly associated with monoclonal antibodies, are most commonly associated with this syndrome (Ball et al 1987, Stewart & Glynn 1990, Bloom 1991). In many of these patients, bleeding from gastrointestinal angiodysplasia occurs. Valvular heart disease can also cause deficiency of the largest multimers of von Willebrand factor (Gill et al 1986), possibly because of increased von Willebrand factor clearance at high shear rates (Chow et al 1992). The long-recognized association between aortic stenosis and gastrointestinal bleeding (Heyde 1958, Williams 1961, Schoenfeld et al 1980) could therefore be caused by acquired von Willebrand's disease (Warkentin et al 1992b).

REFERENCES

Aarnoudse J G, Houthoff H J, Weits J, Vellenga E, Huisjes H J 1986 A syndrome of liver damage and intravascular coagulation in the last trimester of normotensive pregnancy. A clinical and histopathological study. British Journal of Obstetrics and Gynaecology 93: 145–155

Abbott K C, Vukelja S J, Smith C E et al 1991 Hemophagocytic syndrome: A cause of pancytopenia in human Ehrlichiosis. American Journal of Hematology 38: 230–234

Abe Andes W, Noveck R J, Fleming J S 1984 Inhibition of platelet production induced by an antiplatelet drug, anagrelide, in normal volunteers. Thrombosis and Haemostasis 52: 325–328

Abrams D I, Kiprov D D, Goedert J J, Sarngadharan M G, Gallo R C, Volberding P A 1986 Antibodies to human T-lymphotropic virus type III and development of the acquired immunodeficiency syndrome in homosexual men presenting with immune thrombocytopenia. Annals of Internal Medicine 104: 47–50

Abrams C S, Ellison N, Budzynski A Z, Shattil S J 1990 Direct detection of activated platelets and platelet-derived microparticles in humans. Blood 75: 128–138

Aderka D, Praff G, Santo M, Weinberger A, Pinkhas J 1986 Bleeding due to thrombocytopenia in acute leukaemias and reevaluation of the prophylactic transfusion policy. American Journal of Medical Sciences 291: 147–151

Adner M M, Fisch G R, Starobin S G, Aster R H 1969 Use of 'compatible' platelet transfusions in treatment of congenital isoimmune thrombocytopenic purpura. New England Journal of Medicine 280: 244–247

Agnello V, Pariser K, Gell J, Gelfand J, Turksoy R N 1983 Preliminary observations on danazol therapy of systemic lupus erythematosus: Effects on DNA antibodies, thrombocytopenia and complement. Journal of Rheumatology 10: 682–687

Ahn Y S, Harrington W J, Simon S R, Mylvaganam R, Pall L M, So A G 1983 Danazol for the treatment of idiopathic thrombocytopenic purpura. New England Journal of Medicine 308: 1396–1399

Ahn Y S, Mylvaganam R, Garcia R O, Kim C I, Palow D, Harrington W J 1987 Low-dose danazol therapy in idiopathic thrombocytopenic purpura. Annals of Internal Medicine 107: 177–181

Ahn Y S, Rocha R, Mylvaganam R, Garcia R, Duncan R, Harrington W J 1989 Long-term danazol therapy in autoimmune thrombocytopenia: Unmaintained remission and age-dependent response in women. Annals of Internal Medicine 111: 723–729

Akwari A M, Ross D W, Stass S A 1982 Spuriously elevated platelet counts due to microspherocytosis. American Journal of Clinical Pathology 77: 220–223

Akwari O E, Itani K M, Coleman R E, Rosse W F 1987 Splenectomy for primary and recurrent immune thrombocytopenic purpura (ITP): Current criteria for patient selection and results. Annals of Surgery 206: 529–541

Alexander S R, Arbus G S, Butt K M H et al 1990 The 1989 report of the North American Pediatric Renal Transplant Cooperative Study. Pediatric Nephrology 4: 542–553

Alfrey A C, Goss J E, Ogden D A, Vogel J H K, Holmes J H 1968 Uremic hemopericardium. American Journal of Medicine 45: 391–400

Amorosi E L, Ultmann J E 1966 Thrombotic thrombocytopenic purpura: Report of 16 cases and review of the literature. Medicine (Baltimore) 45: 139–159

Amylon M D, Link M P, Glader B E 1984 Immune thrombocytopenia associated with acute nonlymphocytic leukemia. Journal of Pediatrics 105: 776–778

Anagrelide Study Group 1992 Anagrelide, a therapy for thrombocythemic states: Experience in 577 patients. American Journal of Medicine 92: 69–76

Anasetti C, Rybka W, Sullivan K M, Banaji M, Slichter S J 1989 Graft-v-host disease is associated with autoimmune-like thrombocytopenia. Blood 73: 1054–1058

Anderson M J, Woods V L Jr, Tani P, Lindstrom J M, Schmidt D, McMillan R 1984 Autoantibodies to platelet glycoprotein IIb/IIIa and to the acetylcholine receptor in a patient with chronic idiopathic thrombocytopenic purpura and myasthenia gravis. Annals of Internal Medicine 100: 829–831

Andrew M, Blanchette V S, Adams M et al 1992 A multicenter study of the treatment of childhood chronic idiopathic thrombocytopenic purpura with anti-D. Journal of Pediatrics 120: 522–527

Ansell J, Tiarks C, McCue J, Parrilla N, Benotti J R 1984 Amrinone-induced thrombocytopenia. Archives of Internal Medicine 144: 949–952

Antiplatelet Trialists' Collaboration 1988 Secondary prevention of vascular disease by prolonged antiplatelet treatment. British Medical Journal 296: 320–331

Antman K H, Skarin A T, Mayer R J, Hargreaves H K, Canellos G P 1979 Microangiopathic hemolytic anemia and cancer. A review. Medicine 58: 377–384

Ardman B, Rudders R 1982 Aminoglutethimide-induced thrombocytopenia (letter). Cancer Treatment Reports 66: 1785–1786

Arrowsmith J B, Dreis M 1986 Thrombocytopenia after treatment with danazol (letter). New England Journal of Medicine 315: 585

Arvand M, Bhakdi S, Dahlbäck B, Preissner K T 1990 Staphylococcus aureus α-toxin attack on human platelets promotes assembly of the prothrombinase complex. Journal of Biological Chemistry 265: 14377–14381

Asherson R A, Zulman J, Hughes G R V 1989 Pulmonary thromboembolism associated with procainamide induced lupus syndrome and anticardiolipin antibodies. Annals of the Rheumatic Diseases 48: 232–235

Ashkenazi S, Cleary T G, Lopez E, Pickering L K 1988 Anticytotoxin-neutralizing antibodies in immune globulin preparations: Potential use in hemolytic-uremic syndrome. Journal of Pediatrics 113: 1008–1014

Ashouri O S, Marbury T C, Fuller T J, Gaffney E, Grubb W G, Cade J R 1982 Hemolytic uremic syndrome in two postmenopausal women taking a conjugated estrogen preparation. Clinical Nephrology 17: 212–215

Baenziger N L, Dillender M J, Majerus P W 1977 Cultured human skin fibroblasts and arterial cells produce a labile platelet-inhibitory prostaglandin. Biochemical and Biophysical Research Communications 78: 294–301

Baker R I, Manoharan A 1988 Platelet function in myeloproliferative disorders: Characterization and sequential studies show multiple platelet abnormalities, and change with time. European Journal of Haematology 40: 267–272

Ball J, Malia R G, Greaves M, Preston F E 1987 Demonstration of abnormal factor VIII multimers in acquired von Willebrand's disease associated with a circulating inhibitor. British Journal of Haematology 65: 95–100

Ballard H S, Marcus A J 1972 Primary and secondary platelet aggregation in uraemia. Scandinavian Journal of Haematology 9: 198–203

Ballard H S, Marcus A J 1976 Platelet aggregation in portal cirrhosis. Archives of Internal Medicine 136: 316–319

Ballem P J, Buskard N A, Decary F, Doubroff P 1987a Post-transfusion purpura secondary to passive transfusion of anti-Pl^{A1} by blood transfusion. British Journal of Haematology 66: 113–114

Ballem P J, Segal G M, Stratton J R, Gernsheimer T, Adamson J W, Slichter S J 1987b Mechanisms of thrombocytopenia in chronic autoimmune thrombocytopenic purpura. Evidence of both impaired platelet production and increased platelet clearance. Journal of Clinical Investigation 80: 33–40

Ballem P J, Belzberg A, Devine D et al 1989 Pathophysiology of thrombocytopenia associated with HIV infection in homosexual men. A preliminary report. Blut 59: 111–114

Baranski B, Young N 1987 Hematologic consequences of viral infections. Hematology/Oncology Clinics of North America 1: 167–183

Barr R D, Copeland S A, Stockwell M L, Morris N, Kelton J G 1982 Valproic acid and immune thrombocytopenia. Archives of Disease in Childhood 57: 681–684

Bartholomew J R, Salgia R, Bell W R 1989 Control of bleeding in patients with immune and nonimmune thrombocytopenia with aminocaproic acid. Archives of Internal Medicine 149: 1959–1961

Barton J C, Prasthofer E F, Egan M L et al 1986 Rheumatoid arthritis associated with expanded populations of granular lymphocytes. Annals of Internal Medicin 104: 314–323

Barton J C, Herrera G A, Galla J H, Bertoli L F, Work J, Koopman W J 1987 Acute cryoglobulinemic renal failure after intravenous infusion of gamma globulin. American Journal of Medicine 82(3): 624–629

Baumann M A, Menitove J E, Aster R H, Anderson T 1986 Urgent treatment of idiopathic thrombocytopenic purpura with single-dose gammaglobulin infusion followed by platelet transfusion. Annals of Internal Medicine 104: 808–809

Bazylinski N, Shaykh M, Dunea G et al 1985 Inhibition of platelet function by uremic middle molecules. Nephron 40: 423–428

Beard M E J, Johnson S A N 1978 Thrombocytopenia and iron deficiency anaemia in a patient with α_1-thalassaemia trait: Response to iron therapy. Acta Haematologica 59: 114–118

Beardsley D S, Spiegel J E, Jacobs M M, Handin R I 1984 Platelet membrane glycoprotein IIIa contains target antigens that bind anti-platelet antibodies in immune thrombocytopenias. Journal of Clinical Investigation 74: 1701–1707

Becker T, Küenzlen E, Salama A et al 1986 Treatment of childhood idiopathic thrombocytopenic purpura with Rhesus antibodies (anti-D). European Journal of Pediatrics 145: 166–169

Belkin G A 1967 Cocktail purpura. An unusual case of quinine sensitivity. Annals of Internal Medicine 66: 583–586

Bell W R, Braine H G, Ness P M, Kickler T S 1991 Improved survival in thrombotic thrombocytopenic purpura-hemolytic uremic syndrome. Clinical experience in 108 patients. New England Journal of Medicine 325: 398–403

Bellucci S, Charpak Y, Chastang C, Tobelem G, and the Cooperative Group on Immune Thrombocytopenic Purpura 1988 Low doses v conventional doses of corticoids in immune thrombocytopenic purpura (ITP): Results of a randomized clinical trial in 160 children, 223 adults. Blood 71: 1165–1169

Bellucci S, Dosquet C, Boval B, Wautier J L, Caen J 1991 Association of autoimmune thrombocytopenic purpura (AITP), Graves' disease and ovarian carcinoma. Nouvelle Revue Française d'Hématologie 33: 307–309

Ben-Bassat I, Douer D, Ramot B 1990 Tranexamic acid therapy in acute myeloid leukemia: Possible reduction of platelet transfusions. European Journal of Haematology 45: 86–89

Bennett J M 1986 Classification of the myelodysplastic syndromes. Clinics in Haematology 15: 909–923

Berchtold P, McMillan R 1989 Therapy of chronic idiopathic thrombocytopenic purpura in adults. Blood 74: 2309–2317

Berchtold P, Harris J P, Tani P, Piro L, McMillan R 1989a Autoantibodies to platelet glycoproteins in patients with disease-related immune thrombocytopenia. British Journal of Haematology 73: 365–368

Berchtold P, McMillan R, Tani P, Sommerville-Nielsen S, Blanchette V S 1989b Autoantibodies against platelet membrane glycoproteins in children with acute and chronic immune thrombocytopenic purpura. Blood 74: 1600–1602

Berger M, Brass L F 1987 Severe thrombocytopenia in iron deficiency anemia. American Journal of Hematology 24: 425–428

Berkman N, Michaeli Y, Or R, Eldor A 1991 EDTA-dependent pseudothrombocytopenia: A clinical study of 18 patients and a review of the literature. American Journal of Hematology 36: 195

Berndt M C, Kabral A, Grimsley P, Watson N, Robertson T I, Bradstock K F 1988 An acquired Bernard–Soulier-like platelet defect associated with juvenile myelodysplastic syndrome. British Journal of Haematology 68: 97–101

Bessman J D 1984 The relation of megakaryocyte ploidy to platelet volume. American Journal of Hematology 16: 161–170

Bessman J D 1986 Platelets. In: Bessman J D Automated blood counts and differentials. A practical guide. Johns Hopkins University Press, Baltimore, p 57–83

Bettaieb A, Oksenhendler E, Fromont P, Duedari N, Bierling P 1989 Immunochemical analysis of platelet autoantibodies in HIV-related thrombocytopenic purpura: A study of 68 patients. Blood 73: 241–247

Bettaieb A, Fromont P, Rodet M, Godeau B, Duédari N, Bierling P 1991 Br^b, a platelet alloantigen involved in neonatal alloimmune thrombocytopenia. Vox Sanguinis 60: 230–234

Bettaieb A, Fromont P, Louache F, Oksenhendler E, Vainchenker W, Duédari N, Bierling P 1992 Presence of cross-reactive antibody between human immunodeficiency virus (HIV) and platelet glycoproteins in HIV-related immune thrombocytopenic purpura. Blood 80: 162–169

Beurling-Harbury C, Galvan C A 1978 Acquired decrease in platelet secretory ADP associated with increased postoperative bleeding in post-cardiopulmonary bypass patients and in patients with severe valvular heart disease. Blood 52: 13–23

Bhakdi S, Muhly M, Mannhardt U, Hugo F, Klapettek K, Mueller-Eckhardt C, Roka L 1988 Staphylococcal α toxin promotes blood coagulation via attack on human platelets. Journal of Experimental Medicine 168: 527–542

Bick R L 1992 Platelet function defects: A clinical review. Seminars in Thrombosis and Hemostasis 18: 167–185

Bidstrup B P, Royston D, Sapsford R N, Taylor K M 1989 Reduction in blood loss and blood use after cardiopulmonary bypass with high dose aprotinin (trasylol). Journal of Thoracic and Cardiovascular Surgery 97: 364–372

Bierling P, Fromont P, Bettaieb A, Duedari N 1989 Anti-Br^a antibodies in the French population (letter). British Journal of Haematology 73: 428–429

Bishop J F, McGrath K, Wolf M M et al 1988 Clinical factors influencing the efficacy of pooled platelet transfusions. Blood 71: 383–387

Bizzaro N 1991 Platelet satellitosis to polymorphonuclears: cytochemical, immunological, and ultrastructural characterization of eight cases. American Journal of Hematology 36: 235–242

Bizzaro N, Dianese G 1988 Neonatal alloimmune amegakaryocytosis. Case report. Vox Sanguinis 54: 112–114

Blanchette V, Adams M, MacMillan J, Wang E 1991 Initial therapy of childhood acute ITP: Results of a randomized study comparing iv IgG, oral prednisone and iv anti-D (abstract). Blood 78 (suppl 1): 345a

Bloom A L 1991 Von Willebrand factor: Clinical features of inherited and acquired disorders. Mayo Clinic Proceedings 66: 743–751

Bloom A, Greaves M, Preston F E, Brown C B 1986 Evidence against a platelet cyclooxygenase defect in uraemic subjects on chronic haemodialysis. British Journal of Haematology 62: 143–149

Boizard B, Wautier J L 1984 Lek^a, a new platelet antigen absent in Glanzmann's thrombasthenia. Vox Sanguinis 46: 47–54

Bonnin J A, Cheney K 1961 The PTF test: An improved method for

the estimation of platelet thromboplastic function. British Journal of Haematology 7: 512–522
Born G V R 1962 Aggregation of blood platelets by adenosine diphosphate and its reversal. Nature 215: 1027–1029
Boshkov L K, Kelton J G 1989 Use of intravenous gammaglobulin as an immune replacement and an immune suppressant. Transfusion Medicine Reviews 3: 82–120
Boumpas D T, Barez S, Klippel J H, Balow J E 1990 Intermittent cyclophosphamide for the treatment of autoimmune thrombocytopenia in systemic lupus erythematosus. Annals of Internal Medicine 112: 674–677
Boyar A, Beall G 1991 HIV-seropositive thrombocytopenia: The action of zidovudine. AIDS 5: 1351–1356
Brady J, Nelson J C, Lerner R G, Wuest D, Ciavarella D 1991 Intense plasma exchange as therapy for refractory thrombotic-thrombocytopenia purpura (TTP) (abstract). Blood 78 (suppl 1): 487a
Brain M C, Azzopardi J G, Baker L R I, Pineo G F, Roberts P D, Dacie J V 1970 Microangiopathic hemolytic anemia and mucin forming adenocarcinoma. British Journal of Haematology 18: 183–193
Branehög I, Kutti J, Weinfeld A 1974 Platelet survival and platelet production in idiopathic thrombocytopenic purpura (ITP). British Journal of Haematology 1974; 27: 127–143
British Society for Haematology Haemostasis and Thrombosis Task Force 1988 Guidelines on platelet function testing. Journal of Clinical Pathology 41: 1322–1330
Brown C H III, Natelson E A, Bradshaw M W, Williams T W Jr, Alfrey C P 1974 The hemostatic defect produced by carbenicillin. New England Journal of Medicine 291: 265–270
Brown C H III, Bradshaw M W, Natelson E A, Alfrey C P, Williams T W Jr, 1976 Defective platelet function following the administration of penicillin compounds. Blood 47: 949–956
Bruno P, Hassell L H, Brown J, Tanner W, Lau A 1990 The protean manifestations of hemorrhagic fever with renal syndrome. A retrospective review of 26 cases from Korea. Annals of Internal Medicine 113: 385–391
Burday M J, Martin S E 1991 Cocaine-associated thrombocytopenia. American Journal of Medicine 91: 656–660
Burns E R, Lee V, Rubinstein A 1991 Treatment of septic thrombocytopenia with immune globulin. Journal of Clinical Immunology 11: 363–368
Burroughs S F, Johnson G J 1990 β-Lactam antibiotic-induced platelet dysfunction: Evidence for irreversible inhibition of platelet activation in vitro and in vivo after prolonged exposure to penicillin. Blood 75: 1473–1480
Burrows R F, Kelton J G 1988 Incidentally detected thrombocytopenia in healthy mothers and their infants. New England Journal of Medicine 319: 142–145
Burrows R F, Kelton J G 1990a Low fetal risks in pregnancies associated with idiopathic thrombocytopenic purpura. American Journal of Obstetrics and Gynecology 163: 1147–1150
Burrows R F, Kelton J G 1990b Thrombocytopenia at delivery: A prospective survey of 6715 deliveries. American Journal of Obstetrics and Gynecology 162: 731–734
Burroughs A K, Matthews K, Qadiri M et al 1985 Desmopressin and bleeding time in patients with cirrhosis. British Medical Journal 291: 1377–1381
Burrows R F, Hunter D J S, Andrew M, Kelton J G 1987 A prospective study investigating the mechanism of thrombocytopenia in preeclampsia. Obstetrics and Gynecology 70: 334–338
Bussel J B, Haimi J S 1988 Isolated thrombocytopenia in patients infected with HIV: Treatment with intravenous gammaglobulin. American Journal of Hematology 28: 79–84
Bussel J P, Berkowitz R L, McFarland J G, Lynch L, Chitkara U 1988 Antenatal treatment of neonatal alloimmune thrombocytopenia. New England Journal of Medicine 319: 1374–1378
Bussel J B, Graziano J N, Kimberly R P, Pahwa S, Aledort L M 1991 Intravenous anti-D treatment of immune thrombocytopenic purpura: Analysis of efficacy, toxicity, and mechanism of effect. Blood 77: 1884–1893
Buzaid A C, Garewal H S, Lippman S M, Durie B G M, Katakkar S B, Greenberg B R 1987 Danazol in the treatment of myelodysplastic syndromes. European Journal of Haematology 39: 346–348
Byrnes J J, Moake J L, Klug P, Periman P 1990 Effectiveness of the cryosupernatant fraction of plasma in the treatment of refractory thrombotic thrombocytopenic purpura. American Journal of Hematology 34: 169–174
Cahalane S F, Johnson S A, Monto R W, Caldwell M J 1958 Acquired thrombocytopathy. Observations on the coagulation defect in uremia. American Journal of Clinical Pathology 30: 507–513
Calverley D G, Jones G W, Kelton J G 1992 Splenic radiation as a potential treatment for corticosteroid resistant immune thrombocytopenia. Annals of Internal Medicine 116: 977–981
Canadian Cooperative Study Group 1978 A randomized trial of aspirin and sulfinpyrazone in threatened stroke. New England Journal of Medicine 299: 53–59
Caplan S N, Berkman E M 1976 Immunosuppressive therapy of idiopathic thrombocytopenic purpura. Medical Clinics of North America 60: 971–986
Carr D J, Kramer B S, Dragonetti D E 1986a Thrombotic thrombocytopenic purpura associated with metastatic gastric adenocarcinoma. Southern Medical Journal 79: 476–479
Carr J M, Kruskall M S, Kaye J A, Robinson S H 1986b Efficacy of platelet transfusions in immune thrombocytopenia. American Journal of Medicine 80: 1051–1054
Cass A J, Bliss B P, Bolton R P, Cooper B T 1980 Gastrointestinal bleeding, angiodysplasia of the colon and acquired von Willebrand's disease. British Journal of Surgery 67: 639–641
Castaldi P A, Rozenberg M C, Stewart J H 1966 The bleeding disorder of uraemia. A qualitative platelet defect. Lancet 2: 66–69
Castillo R, Lozano T, Escolar G, Revert L, Lopez J, Ordinas A 1986 Defective platelet adhesion on vessel subendothelium in uremic patients. Blood 68: 337–342
Chapman G S, George C B, Donley D L 1984 Heparin-like anticoagulant associated with plasma cell myeloma. American Journal of Clinical Pathology 83: 764–766
Centers for Disease Control 1991 Update on adult immunization: Recommendations of the Immunization Practices Advisory Committee (ACIP). Morbidity and Mortality Weekly Report. Recommendation and Report 40 (No. RR–12): 1–94
Chalmers E A, Chan Lam D, Holden R J, Fitzimons E J 1987 Familial primary biliary cirrhosis and autoimmune thrombocytopenia. Scottish Medical Journal 32: 152
Chart H, Smith H R, Scotland S M, Rowe B, Milford D V, Taylor C M 1991 Serological identification of Escherichia coli 0157:H7 infection in haemolytic uraemic syndrome. Lancet 337: 138–140
Chong B H, Ismail F, Cade J, Gallus A S, Gordon S, Chesterman C N 1989 Heparin-induced thrombocytopenia: Studies with a low molecular weight heparinoid, Org 10172. Blood 73: 1592–1596
Chow T W, Hellums J D, Moake J L, Kroll M H 1992 Shear stress-induced von Willebrand factor binding to platelet glycoprotein Ib initiates calcium influx associated with aggregation. Blood 80: 113–120
Christie D J, Walker R H, Kolins M D, Wilner F M, Aster R H 1983 Quinine-induced thrombocytopenia following intravenous use of heroin. Archives of Internal Medicine 143: 1174
Christie D J, Mullen P C, Aster R H 1985 Fab-mediated binding of drug-dependent antibodies to platelets in quinidine- and quinine-induced thrombocytopenia. Journal of Clinical Investigation 75: 310–314
Christie D J, Lennon S S, Drew R L, Swinehart C D 1988 Cefotetan-induced immunologic thrombocytopenia. British Journal of Haematology 70: 423–426
Christie D J, van Buren N, Lennon S S, Putnam J L 1990 Vancomycin-dependent antibodies associated with thrombocytopenia and refractoriness to platelet transfusion in patients with leukemia. Blood 75: 518–523
Christie D J, Pulkrabek S, Putnam J L, Slatkoff M L, Pischel K D 1991 Posttransfusion purpura due to an alloantibody reactive with glycoprotein Ia/IIa (anti-HPA-5b). Blood 77: 2785–2789
Ciavarella D, Reed R L, Counts R B et al 1987 Clotting factor levels and the risk of diffuse microvascular bleeding in the massively transfused patient. British Journal of Haematology 67: 365–368
Cines D B, Cassileth P A, Kiss J E 1985 Danazol therapy in myelodysplasia. Annals of Internal Medicine 103: 58–60
Cines D B, Tomaski A, Tannenbaum S 1987 Immune endothelial-cell

injury in heparin-associated thrombocytopenia. New England Journal of Medicine 316: 581–589
Cohen I, Amir J, Ben-Shaul Y, Pick A, De Vries A 1970 Plasma cell myeloma associated with an unusual myeloma protein causing impairment of fibrin aggregation and platelet function in a patient with multiple malignancy. American Journal of Medicine 48: 766–776
Consensus conference 1987 Platelet transfusion therapy. Journal of the American Medical Association 257: 1777–1780
Conti L, Gandolfo G M 1983 Benzodiazepine-induced thrombocytopenia. Demonstration of drug-dependent platelet antibodies in two cases. Acta Haematologica 70: 386–388
Cooper D A, Gold J, Maclean P et al 1985 Acute AIDS retrovirus infection. Definition of a clinical illness associated with seroconversion. Lancet 1: 537–540
Cooper C, Fairris G, Cotton D W K, Steart P, Barth J H 1986 Dermatomyositis associated with idiopathic thrombocytopenia. Dermatologica 172: 173–176
Corash L, Chen H Y, Levin J, Baker G, Lu H, Mok Y 1987 Regulation of thrombopoiesis: Effects of the degree of thrombocytopenia on megakaryocyte ploidy and platelet volume. Blood 70: 177–185
Corrigan J J Jr 1974 Thrombocytopenia: A laboratory sign of septicemia in infants and children. Journal of Pediatrics 85: 219–221
Corrigan J J Jr, Jordan C M 1970 Heparin therapy in septicemia with disseminated intravascular coagulation: Effect on mortality and on correction of hemostatic defects. New England Journal of Medicine 283: 778–782
Couch P, Stumpf J L 1990 Management of uremic bleeding. Clinical Pharmacy 9: 673–681
Cowan D H 1973 Thrombokinetic studies in alcohol-related thrombocytopenia. Journal of Laboratory and Clinical Medicine 81: 64–76
Cowan D H 1980 Effect of alcoholism on hemostasis. Seminars in Hematology 17: 137–147
Cowan D H, Graham R C Jr, Baunach D 1975 The platelet defect in leukemia: Platelet ultrastructure, adenine nucleotide metabolism, and the release reaction. Journal of Clinical Investigation 56: 188–200
Csako G, Suba E A, Elin R J 1988 Endotoxin-induced platelet activation in human whole blood in vitro. Thrombosis and Haemostasis 59: 378–382
Cunningham C C, Lind S E 1989 Apparent response of refractory post-transfusion purpura to splenectomy. American Journal of Hematology 30: 112
Cunningham V L, Brandt J T 1992 Spurious thrombocytopenia due to EDTA-independent cold-reactive agglutinins. American Journal of Clinical Pathology 97: 359–362
Czapek E E, Deykin D, Salzman E W, Lian E C, Hellerstein L J, Rosoff C B 1978 Intermediate syndrome of platelet dysfunction. Blood 52: 103–113
Czer L S C, Bateman T M, Gray R J et al 1987 Treatment of severe platelet dysfunction and hemorrhage after cardiopulmonary bypass: Reduction in blood product usage with desmopressin. Journal of the American College of Cardiology 9: 1139–1147
Danielson D A, Douglas S W III, Herzog P, Jick H, Porter J B 1984 Drug-induced blood disorders. Journal of the American Medical Association 252: 3257–3260
Davies G E, Triplett D A 1990 Corticosteroid-associated blue toe syndrome: Role of antiphospholipid antibodies. Annals of Internal Medicine 113: 893–895
Degos L, Tobelem G, Lethielleux P, Levy-Toledano S, Caen J, Colombani J 1977 Molecular defect in platelets from patients with Bernard–Soulier syndrome. Blood 50: 899–903
De la Serna F J, Lopez J I, Garcia-Marcilla A, Ortiz-Conde M C, Mestre M J 1989 Hemophagocytic syndrome causing complete bone marrow failure. Report of an extreme case of a reactive histiocytic disorder. Acta Haematologica 82: 197–200
D'Elia J A, Aslani M, Schermer S, Cloud L, Bothe A, Dzik W 1987 Haemolytic-uremic syndrome and acute renal failure in metastatic adenocarcinoma treated with mitomycin: Case report and a literature review. Renal Failure 10: 107–113
DelRossi A J, Cernaianu A C, Botros S, Lemole G M, Moore R 1989 Prophylactic treatment of postperfusion bleeding using EACA. Chest 96: 27–30
Demers C, Ginsberg J S, Brill-Edwards P et al 1991 Rapid anticoagulation using ancrod for heparin-induced thrombocytopenia. Blood 78: 2194–2197
Denomme G A, Smith J W, Kelton J G, Bell D A 1992 A human monoclonal autoantibody to platelet glycoprotein IIb derived from normal human lymphocytes. Blood 79: 447–451
Devine D V, Currie M S, Rosse W F, Greenberg C S 1987 Pseudo-Bernard–Soulier syndrome: Thrombocytopenia caused by autoantibody to platelet glycoprotein Ib. Blood 70: 428–431
Deykin D, Janson P, McMahon L 1982 Ethanol potentiation of aspirin-induced prolongation of the bleeding time. New England Journal of Medicine 306: 852–854
Diez F L, Nieto M L, Fernandes-Gallardo S, Gijon M A, Crespo M S 1989 Occupancy of platelet receptors for platelet-activating factor in patients with septicemia. Journal of Clinical Investigation 83: 1733–1740
DiMichele D M, Hathaway W E 1990 Use of DDVAP in inherited and acquired platelet dysfunction. American Journal of Hematology 33: 39–45
DiMinno G, Martinez J, McKean M L, de La Rosa J, Burke J F, Murphy S 1985 Platelet dysfunction in uremia: Multifaceted defect partially corrected by dialysis. American Journal of Medicine 79: 552–559
DiMinno G, Coraggio F, Cerbone A M et al 1986 A myeloma paraprotein with specificity for platelet glycoprotein IIIa in a patient with a fatal bleeding disorder. Journal of Clinical Investigation 77: 157–164
Dixon R, Rosse W, Ebbert L 1975 Quantitative determination of antibody in idiopathic thrombocytopenic purpura: Correlation of serum and platelet-bound antibody in clinical response. New England Journal of Medicine 1975; 292: 230–236
Donnér M, Schwartz M, Carlsson K U, Holmberg L 1988 Hereditary X-linked thrombocytopenia maps to the same chromosomal region as the Wiskott–Aldrich syndrome. Blood 72: 1849–1853
Donnér M, Békássy N A, Heldrup J, Wiebe T, Garwicz S, Holmberg L 1990 Platelet surface-bound IgG and platelet-specific IgG in plasma in childhood thrombocytopenia. Acta Paediatrica Scandinavica 79: 328–334
Dunn N L, Maurer H M 1984 Prednisone treatment of acute idiopathic thrombocytopenic purpura of childhood. American Journal of Pediatric Hematology/Oncology 6: 159–164
Durand J M, Lefevre P, Hovette P, Issifi S, Mongin M 1991a Dapsone for thrombocytopenic purpura related to human immunodeficiency virus infection. American Journal of Medicine 90: 675–677
Durand J M, Lefevre P, Hovette P, Mongin M, Soubeyrand J 1991b Dapsone for idiopathic autoimmune thrombocytopenic purpura in elderly patients. British Journal of Haematology 78: 459–460
Editorial 1987 Platelet transfusion therapy. Lancet 2: 490
Eichinger S, Kyrle P A, Brenner B et al 1991 Thrombocytopenia associated with low-molecular-weight heparin (letters). Lancet 337: 1425–1426
Eisner E V, Shahidi N T 1972 Immune thrombocytopenia due to a drug metabolite. New England Journal of Medicine 287: 376–381
Eknoyan G, Brown C H 1981 Biochemical abnormalities of platelets in renal failure. Evidence for decreased platelet serotonin, adenosine diphosphate and Mg-dependent adenosine triphosphatase. American Journal of Nephrology 1: 17–32
Eknoyan G, Wachsman S J, Glueck H I, Will J J 1969 Platelet function in renal failure. New England Journal of Medicine 280: 677–681
Ellis M, Neal K, Leen C et al 1987 Alfa-2a recombinant interferon in HIV-associated thrombocytopenia. British Medical Journal 295: 1519–1520
Erlemeier H H, Zangemeister W, Burmester L, Schofer J, Mathey D G, Bleifeld W 1989 Bleeding after thrombolysis in acute myocardial infarction. European Heart Journal 10: 16–23
Ernest D, Fisher M M 1991 Heparin-induced thrombocytopaenia complicated by bilateral adrenal haemorrhage. Intensive Care Medicine 17: 238–240
Eschbach J W, Abdulhadi M H, Browne J K et al 1989 Recombinant human erythropoietin in anemic patients with end-stage renal disease. Results of a phase III multicenter clinical trial. Annals of Internal Medicine 111: 992–1000
Escolar G, Garrido M, Mazzara R, Castillo R, Ordinas A 1988

Experimental basis for the use of red cell transfusion in the management of anemic-thrombocytopenic patients. Transfusion 28: 406–411
Escolar G, Cases A, Bastida E et al 1990 Uremic platelets have a functional defect affecting the interaction of von Willebrand factor with glycoprotein IIb-IIIa. Blood 76: 1336–1340
Fabris F, Cordiano I, Randi M L et al 1991 Effect of human recombinant erythropoietin on bleeding time, platelet number and function in children with end-stage renal disease maintained by haemodialysis. Pediatric Nephrology 5: 225–228
Falanga A, Gordon S G 1985 Isolation and characterization of cancer procoagulant: A cysteine proteinase from malignant tissue. Biochemistry 24: 5558–5567
Falanga A, Shaw E, Donati M B, Consonni R, Barbui T, Gordon S G 1989 Inhibition of cancer procoagulant by peptidyl diazomethyl ketones and peptidyl sulfonium salts. Thrombosis Research 54: 389–398
Falanga A, Consonni R, Ruggenenti P, Barbui T 1991 A cathepsin-like cysteine proteinase proaggregating activity in thrombotic thrombocytopenic purpura. British Journal of Haematology 79: 474–480
Faldt R 1986 Remission of amegakaryocytic thrombocytopenia induced by antilymphocyte globulin (ALG). British Journal of Haematology 63: 205–207
Falini B, Pileri S, De Solas I et al 1990 Peripheral T-cell lymphoma associated with hemophagocytic syndrome. Blood 75: 434–444
Farley M M, Stephens D S, Brachman P S Jr, Harvey R C, Smith J D, Wenger J D, and the CDC Meningitis Surveillance Group 1992 Invasive Haemophilus influenzae disease in adults. A prospective, population-based surveillance. Annals of Internal Medicine 116: 806–812
Federici A B, Berkowitz S D, Zimmerman T S, Mannucci P M 1992 Proteolysis of von Willebrand factor after thrombolytic therapy in patients with acute myocardial infarction. Blood 79: 38–44
Fenaux P, Caulier M T, Hirschauer M C, Beuscart R, Goudemand J, Bauters F 1989 Reevaluation of the prognostic factors for splenectomy in chronic idiopathic thrombocytopenic purpura (ITP): A report on 181 cases. European Journal of Haematology 42: 259–264
Feng C S, Ng M H L, Szeto R S C, Li E K 1991 Bone marrow findings in lupus patients with pancytopenia. Pathology 23: 5–7
Fernandez F, Goudable C, Sie P et al 1985 Low haematocrit and prolonged bleeding time in uraemic patients: Effect of red cell transfusions. British Journal of Haematology 59: 139–148
Fields S M, Lindley C M 1989 Thrombotic microangiopathy with chemotherapy: Case report and review of the literature. DICP. The Annals of Pharmacotherapy 23: 582–588
Field S K, Poon M C 1987 Sarcoidosis presenting as chronic thrombocytopenia. Western Journal of Medicine 146: 481–482
Fiore L D, Brophy M T, Lopez A, Janson P, Deykin D 1990 The bleeding time response to aspirin. Identifying the hyperresponder. American Journal of Clinical Pathology 94: 292–296
First L R, Smith B R, Lipton J, Nathan D G, Parkman R, Rappeport J M 1985 Isolated thrombocytopenia after allogeneic bone marrow transplantation: Existence of transient and chronic thrombocytopenic syndromes. Blood 65: 368–374
FitzGerald G A 1987 Dipyridamole. New England Journal of Medicine 316: 1247–1257
Font J, Cervera R, Lopez-Soto A et al 1989 Anticardiolipin antibodies in patients with autoimmune diseases: Isotype distribution and clinical associations. Clinical Rheumatology 8: 475–483
Fraedrich G, Weber C, Bernard C, Hettwer A, Schlosser V 1989 Reduction of blood transfusion requirement in open heart surgery by administration of high doses of aprotinin — preliminary results. Thoracic and Cardiovascular Surgery 37: 89–91
Freiman J P 1990 Fatal quinine-induced thrombocytopenia (letter). Annals of Internal Medicine 112: 308–309
Fricke W, Alling D, Kimball J 1991 Lack of efficacy of tranexamic acid in thrombocytopenic bleeding. Transfusion 31: 345–348
Friedman J M, Aster R H 1985 Neonatal alloimmune thrombocytopenic purpura and congenital porencephaly in two siblings associated with a 'new' maternal antiplatelet antibody. Blood 65: 1412–1415
Furihata K, Nugent D J, Bissonette A, Aster R H, Kunicki T J 1987 On the association of the platelet-specific alloantigen, Pen[a], with glycoprotein IIIa. Evidence for heterogeneity of glycoprotein IIIa. Journal of Clinical Investigation 80: 1624–1630
Furihata K, Hunter J, Aster R H, Koewing G R, Shulman N R, Kunicki T J 1988 Human anti-Pl^{E1} antibody recognizes epitopes associated with the alpha subunit of platelet glycoprotein Ib. British Journal of Haematology 68: 103–110
Gafter U, Bessler H, Malachi T, Zevin D, Djaldetti M, Levi J 1987 Platelet count and thrombopoietic activity in patients with chronic renal failure. Nephron 45: 207–210
Galen M A, Steinberg S M, Lowrie E G, Lazarus J M, Hampers C L, Merrill J P 1975 Hemorrhagic pleural effusion in patients undergoing chronic hemodialysis. Annals of Internal Medicine 82: 359–361
Gangarosa E J, Johnson T R, Ramos H S 1960 Ristocetin-induced thrombocytopenia: Site and mechanism of action. Archives of Internal Medicine 105: 83–89
Gardner F H, Helmer R E III 1980 Aminocaproic acid. Use in control of hemorrhage in patients with amegakaryocytic thrombocytopenia. Journal of the American Medical Association 243: 35–37
Garewal H S, Durie B G M 1985 Anti-fibrinolytic therapy with aminocaproic acid for the control of bleeding in thrombocytopenic patients. Scandinavian Journal of Haematology 35: 497–500
Garg S K, Sarker C R 1974 Aspirin-induced thrombocytopenia on an immune basis. American Journal of the Medical Sciences 267: 129–132
Garnick M B, Griffin J D 1983 Idiopathic thrombocytopenia in association with extragonadal germ cell cancer. Annals of Internal Medicine 98: 926–927
Gastineau D A, Kazmier F J, Nicholas W L, Bowie E J 1985 Lupus anticoagulant: An analysis of the clinical and laboratory features of 219 cases. American Journal of Hematology 19: 265–275
George J N 1990 Platelet immunoglobulin G: Its significance for the evaluation of thrombocytopenia and for understanding the origin of α-granule proteins. Blood 76: 859–870
George J N, Shattil S J 1991 The clinical importance of acquired abnormalities of platelet function. New England Journal of Medicine 324: 27–39
Gerrard J M, Stoddard S F, Shapiro R S et al 1978 Platelet storage pool deficiency and prostaglandin synthesis in chronic granulocytic leukaemia. British Journal of Haematology 40: 597–607
Gerritsen S W, Akkerman J N, Sixma J J 1978 Correction of the bleeding time in patients with storage pool deficiency by infusion of cryoprecipitate. British Journal of Haematology 40: 153–160
Gewirtz A M, Hoffman R 1986 Transitory hypomegakaryocytic thrombocytopenia: aetiological association with ethanol abuse and implications regarding regulation of human megakaryocytopoiesis. British Journal of Haematology 62: 333
Gewirtz A M, Sacchetti M K, Bien R, Barry W E 1986 Cell mediated suppression of megakaryocytopoiesis in acquired amegakaryocytic thrombocytopenic purpura. Blood 68: 619–626
Gibson B, Hunter D, Neame P B, Kelton J G 1982 Thrombocytopenia in preeclampsia and eclampsia. Seminars in Thrombosis and Hemostasis 8: 234–247
Gill J C, Wilson A D, Endres-Brooks J, Montgomery R R 1986 Loss of the largest von Willebrand factor multimers from the plasma of patients with congenital cardiac defects. Blood 67: 758–761
Gimple L W, Gold H K, Leinbach R C et al 1989 Correlation between template bleeding times and spontaneous bleeding during treatment of acute myocardial infarction with recombinant tissue-type plasminogen activator. Circulation 80: 581–588
Ginsberg M H, Frelinger A L, Lam S C-T et al 1990 Analysis of platelet aggregation disorders based on flow cytometric analysis of membrane glycoprotein IIb-IIIa with conformation-specific monoclonal antibodies. Blood 76: 2017–2023
Gloster E S, Strauss R A, Jiminez J F et al 1985 Spurious elevated platelet counts associated with bacteremia. American Journal of Hematology 18: 329
Glueck H I, Kant K S, Weiss M A, Pollak V E, Miller M A, Coots M 1985 Thrombosis in systemic lupus erythematosus: Relation to the presence of circulating anticoagulants. Archives of Internal Medicine 145: 1389–1395

Gmür J, Burger J, Schanz U, Fehr J, Schaffner A 1991 Safety of stringent prophylactic platelet transfusion policy for patients with acute leukaemia. Lancet 338: 1223–1226

Goldman S, Copeland J, Moritz T et al 1988 Improvement in early saphenous vein graft patency after coronary artery bypass surgery with antiplatelet therapy: Results of a Veterans Administration Cooperative Study. Circulation 77: 1324–1332

Gon F, Reid F P 1975 A case of recurrent subacute disseminated intravascular coagulation associated with malarial prophylaxis. South African Medical Journal 49: 120–122

Goodlin R C 1991 Preeclampsia as the great impostor. American Journal of Obstetrics and Gynecology 164: 1577–1581

Goodman R P, Killam A P, Brash A R, Branch R A 1982 Prostacyclin production during pregnancy: Comparison of production during normal pregnancy and pregnancy complicated by hypertension. American Journal of Obstetrics and Gynecology 142: 817–822

Gordge M P, Leaker B, Patel A, Oviasu E, Cameron J S, Neild G H Y 1990 Recombinant human erythropoietin shortens the uraemic bleeding time without causing intravascular haemostatic activation. Thrombosis Research 57: 171–182

Gordon Y B, Ratky S M, Baker L R I, Letchworth A T, Leighton P C, Chard T 1976 Circulating levels of fibrin/fibrinogen degradation fragment E measured by radioimmunoassay in preeclampsia. British Journal of Obstetrics and Gynaecology 83: 287–291

Gordon-Smith E C 1989 Aplastic anaemia — aetiology and clinical features. Baillière's Clinics in Haematology 2 (1): 1–18

Gorevic P D, Kassab H J, Levo Y, Kohn R, Meltzer M, Prose P, Franklin E C 1980 Mixed cryoglobulinemia: Clinical aspects and long-term follow-up of 40 patients. American Journal of Medicine 69: 287–308

Gottschall J L, Elliot W, Lianos E, McFarland J G, Wolfmeyer K, Aster R H 1991 Quinine-induced immune thrombocytopenia associated with hemolytic uremic syndrome: A new clinical entity. Blood 77: 306–310

Grabarek J, Timmons S, Hawiger J 1988 Modulation of human platelet protein kinase C by endotoxic lipid A. Journal of Clinical Investigation 82: 964–971

Gralnick H R, McKeown L P, Willliams S B, Shafer B C, Pierce L 1988 Plasma and platelet von Willebrand factor defects in uremia. American Journal of Medicine 85: 806–810

Gram I, Jensen P K 1989 Carbamazepine: toxicity. In: Levy R H, Dreifuss F E, Mattson R H, Meldrum B S, Penry J K (eds) Antiepileptic drugs, 3rd edn. Raven Press, New York, p 555–565

Grau G E, Piguet P F, Gretener D, Vesin C, Lambert P H 1988 Immunopathology of thrombocytopenia in experimental malaria. Immunology 65: 501–506

Green D, Tuite G F Jr 1989 Declining platelet counts and platelet aggregation during porcine VIII:C infusions. American Journal of Medicine 86: 222–224

Greinacher A, Michels I, Kiefel V, Mueller-Eckhardt C 1991 A rapid and sensitive test for diagnosing heparin-associated thrombocytopenia. Thrombosis and Haemostasis 66: 734

Greinacher A, Michels I, Schafer M, Kiefel V, Mueller-Eckhardt C 1992 Heparin-associated thrombocytopenia in a patient treated with polysulphated chondroitin sulphate: Evidence for immunological crossreactivity between heparin and polysulphated glycosaminoglycans. British Journal of Haematology 81: 252–254

Grenet P, Dausset J, Dugas M, Petit J, Badoual J, Tangun Y 1965 Purpura thrombopenique neonatal avec isoimmunisation foeto-maternelle anti-Ko^{a}. Archives Françaises de Pédiatrie 22: 1165–1174

Grob J J, Bonerandi J J 1986 Cutaneous manifestations associated with the presence of the lupus anticoagulant. A report of two cases and a review of the literature. Journal of the American Academy of Dermatology 15: 211–219

Grob J J, Bonerandi J J 1989 Thrombotic skin disease as a marker of the anticardiolipin syndrome. Livedo vasculitis and distal gangrene associated with abnormal serum antiphospholipid activity. Journal of the American Academy of Dermatology 20: 1063–1069

Grob J J, San Marco M, Aillaud M F et al 1991 Unfading acral microlivedo. A discrete marker of thrombotic skin disease associated with antiphospholipid antibody syndrome. Journal of the American Academy of Dermatology 24: 53–58

Gross S, Worthington-White D A 1984 Cimetidine suppression of CFU-C in males. American Journal of Hematology 17: 279–286

Guarini A, Sanavio F, Novarino A, Tos A G, Aglietta M, Foa R 1991 Thrombocytopenia in acute leukemia patients treated with IL2: Cytolytic effect of LAK cells on megakaryocytic progenitors. British Journal of Haematology 79: 451–456

Guild W R, Bray G, Merrill J P 1957 Hemopericardium with cardiac tamponade in chronic uremia. New England Journal of Medicine 257: 230–231

Guinan E C, Tarbell N J, Niemeyer C M, Sallan S E, Weinstein H J 1988 Blood 72: 451–455

Gupta S, Saverymuttu S H, Marsh J C W, Hodgson H J, Chadwick V S 1986 Immune thrombocytopenic purpura, neutropenia and sclerosing cholangitis associated with ulcerative colitis in an adult. Clinical and Laboratory Haematology 8: 67–69

Hackett T, Kelton J G, Powers P 1982 Drug-induced platelet destruction. Seminars in Thrombosis and Hemostasis 8: 116–137

Hackmann T, Gascoyne R D, Naiman S C et al 1989 A trial of desmopressin (1-desamino-8-D-arginine vasopressin) to reduce blood loss in uncomplicated cardiac surgery. New England Journal of Medicine 321: 1437–1443

Hakim R M, Schafer A I 1985 Hemodialysis-associated platelet activation and thrombocytopenia. American Journal of Medicine 78: 575–580

Hales C A, Mark E J 1987 A 43-year-old woman with breast cancer and the abrupt onset of respiratory failure. New England Journal of Medicine 317: 225–235

Hallett J M, Martell R W, Sher C, Jacobs P 1989 Amegakaryocytic thrombocytopenia with duplication of part of the long arm of chromosome 3. British Journal of Haematology 71: 291–292

Han P, Kiruba R, Ho Y C 1990 Platelet-associated immunoproteins (PAIg): Specificity of measurement. Clinical and Laboratory Haematology 12: 49–56

Harder M P, Eijsman L, Roozendaal K J, van Oeveren W, Wildevuur C R H 1991 Aprotinin reduces intraoperative and postoperative blood loss in membrane oxygenator cardiopulmonary bypass. Annals of Thoracic Surgery 51: 936–941

Hardisty R M, Powling M J, Nokes T J C 1990 The action of ticlopidine on human platelets. Studies on aggregation, secretion, calcium mobilization and membrane glycoproteins. Thrombosis and Haemostasis 64: 150–155

Harker L A 1970 Thrombokinetics in idiopathic thrombocytopenic purpura. British Journal of Haematology 19: 95–104

Harker L A, Slichter S J 1972a Platelet and fibrinogen consumption in man. New England Journal of Medicine 287: 999–1005

Harker L A, Slichter S J 1972b The bleeding time as a screening test for evaluation of platelet function. New English Journal of Medicine 287: 155–159

Harker L, Malpass T W, Branson H E, Hessel II E A, Slichter S A 1980 Mechanism of abnormal bleeding in patients undergoing cardiopulmonary bypass: Acquired transient platelet dysfunction associated with selective α-granule release. Blood 56: 824–834

Harrington W J, Minnich V, Hollingsworth J W, Moore C V 1951 Demonstration of a thrombocytopenic factor in the blood of patients with thrombocytopenic purpura. Journal of Laboratory and Clinical Medicine 38: 1–10

Harris E N, Asherson R A, Gharavi A E, Morgan S H, Derue G, Hughes G R 1985a Thrombocytopenia in SLE and related autoimmune disorders: Association with anticardiolipin antibody. British Journal of Haematology 59: 227–230

Harris E N, Gharavi A E, Hegde U et al 1985b Anticardiolipin antibodies in autoimmune thrombocytopenic purpura. British Journal of Haematology 59: 231–234

Hass W K, Easton J D, Adams H P Jr et al 1989 A randomized trial comparing ticlopidine hydrochloride with aspirin for the prevention of stroke in high-risk patients. New England Journal of Medicine 321: 501–507

Hauglustaine D, van Damme B, Vanrenteghem Y, Michielsen P 1981 Recurrent hemolytic uremic syndrome during oral contraception. Clinical Nephrology 15: 148–153

Haut M J, Cowan D H 1974 The effect of ethanol on hemostatic properties of human blood platelets. Americal Journal of Medicine 56: 22–33

Hegde U M, Ball S, Zuiable A, Roter B L T 1985a Platelet associated immunoglobulins (PAIgG and PAIgM) in autoimmune thrombocytopenia. British Journal of Haematology 59: 221–226
Hegde U M, Zuiable A, Ball S, Roter B L T 1985b The relative incidence of idiopathic and secondary autoimmune thrombocytopenia: A clinical and serological evaluation in 508 patients. Clinical and Laboratory Haematology 7: 7–16
Herman J 1980 Thrombocytopenic purpura and thyroid disease (letter). Annals of Internal Medicine 93: 934
Hess H, Mietaschk A, Deichsel G 1985 Drug-induced inhibition of platelet function delays progression of peripheral occlusive arterial disease. A prospective double-blind arteriographically controlled trial. Lancet 1: 415–418
Heusermann U, Stutte H-J 1977 Zur Ätiologie der Thrombozytopenie bei der Vinylchlorid-Krankheit. Blut 35: 317–322
Heyde E C 1958 Gastrointestinal bleeding in aortic stenosis (letter). New England Journal of Medicine 259: 196
Heyns A duP, Lötter M G, Badenhorst P N et al 1980 Kinetics and in vivo redistribution of ^{111}Indium-labelled human platelets after intravenous protamine sulphate. Thrombosis and Haemostasis 44: 65–68
Ho C-H, Yang Z-L 1992 The predictive value of the hemostasis parameters in the development of preeclampsia. Thrombosis and Haemostasis 67: 214–218
Hobbhahn J, Conzen P F, Habazettl H, Gutmann R, Kellermann W, Peter K 1991 Heparin reversal by protamine in humans — complement, prostaglandins, blood cells, and hemodynamics. Journal of Applied Physiology 71: 1415–1421
Hodder F S, Kempert P, McCormack S, Bennetts G A, Katz J, Cairo M S 1985 Immune thrombocytopenia following actinomycin-D therapy. Journal of Pediatrics 107: 611–614
Hoffman R 1991 Acquired pure amegakaryocytic thrombocytopenic purpura. Seminars in Hematology 28: 303–312
Hoffman R, Bruno E, Elwell J et al 1982 Acquired amegakaryocytic thrombocytopenic purpura: A syndrome of diverse etiologies. Blood 60: 1173–1178
Hoffman R, Briddell R A, Van Besien K et al 1989 Acquired cyclic amegakaryocytic thrombocytopenia associated with an immunoglobulin blocking the action of granulocyte-macrophage colony-stimulating factor. New England Journal of Medicine 321: 97–102
Hollenberg J P, Subak L L, Ferry J J Jr, Bussel J B 1988 Cost-effectiveness of splenectomy versus intravenous gamma globulin in treatment of chronic immune thrombocytopenic purpura in childhood. Journal of Pediatrics 112: 530–539
Hope A F, Heyns A duP, Lötter M G et al 1981 Kinetics and sites of sequestration of indium 111-labeled human platelets during cardiopulmonary bypass. Journal of Thoracic and Cardiovascular Surgery 81: 880–886
Horowitz H I, Stein I M, Cohen B D 1970 Further studies on platelet inhibitory effect of guanidinosuccinic acid and its role in uremia bleeding. American Journal of Medicine 49: 336–345
Howe S E, Lynch D M 1987 Platelet antibody binding in systemic lupus erythematosus. Journal of Rheumatology 14: 482–486
Hoyle C, Darbyshire P, Eden O B 1986 Idiopathic thrombocytopenia in childhood. Edinburgh experience 1962–82. Scottish Medical Journal 31: 174–179
Huang L M, Lee C Y, Lin K H et al 1990 Human herpesvirus-6 associated with fatal haemophagocytic syndrome (letter). Lancet 336: 60–61
Ignarro L J 1989 Endothelium-derived nitric oxide: Actions and properties. Federation of American Societies for Experimental Biology Journal 3: 31–36
Ikeda H, Mitani T, Ohnuma M et al 1989 A new platelet specific antigen Nak[a] involved in the refractoriness of HLA-matched platelet transfusion. Vox Sanguinis 57: 213–217
Imbach P, Wagner H P, Berchtold W et al 1985 Intravenous immunoglobulin versus oral corticosteroids in acute immune thrombocytopenic purpura in childhood. Lancet 2: 464–468
Imbach P, Perret B A, Babington R, Kaminski K, Morell A, Heiniger H J 1991 Safety of intravenous immunoglobulin preparation: A prospective multicenter study to exclude the risk of non-A, non-B hepatitis. Vox Sanguinis 61: 240–243
Isaacs A J 1980 Cimetidine and thrombocytopenia. British Medical Journal 280: 294
Ishida F, Saji H, Maruya E, Furihata K 1991 Human platelet-specific antigen, Sib[a], is associated with the molecular weight polymorphism of glycoprotein Ibα. Blood 78: 1722–1729
Israel L, Cour V, Pihan I et al 1989 Some theoretical and practical limitations of interleukin-2. Ten cases of advanced breast cancer treated with continuous infusion of IL-2. Cancer Treatment Reviews 16: 169–171
Israeli A, Matzner Y, Or R, Raz I 1988 Glibenclamide causing thrombocytopenia and bleeding tendency: Case reports and a review of the literature. Klinische Wochenschrift 66: 223–224
Israels S J, McNicol A, Robertson C, Gerrard J M 1990 Platelet storage pool deficiency: diagnosis in patients with prolonged bleeding times and normal platelet aggregation. British Journal of Haematology 75: 118–121
Jackson A M, Rose B D, Graf L G et al 1984 Thrombotic microangiopathy and renal failure associated with antineoplastic chemotherapy. Annals of Internal Medicine 101: 41–44
Jacobs P, Wood L, Dent D M 1986 Results of treatment in immune thrombocytopenia. Quarterly Journal of Medicine 58: 153–165
Jacobsson B, Rasnas L, Nyberg G, Bregh C H, Magnusson Y, Hjalmarson A 1985 Abnormality of adenylate cyclase regulation in human platelet membranes in renal failure. European Journal of Clinical Investigation 15: 75–81
Jacquin V, Salama J, Le Roux G, Delaporte P 1988 Thromboses veineuses cérébrales et des membres supérieurs associées à une thrombopénie, induites par le polysulfate de Pentosane. Annales de Médecine Interne 139: 194–197
Jaffe E S, Costa J, Fauci A S, Cossman J, Tsokos M 1983 Malignant lymphoma and erythrophagocytosis simulating malignant histiocytosis. American Journal of Medicine 75: 741–749
Jansen P H P, Renier W O, De Vaan G, Reekers P, Vingerhoets D M, Gabreëls F J M 1987 Effect of thymectomy on myasthenia gravis and autoimmune thrombocytopenic purpura in a 13-year-old girl. European Journal of Pediatrics 146: 587–589
Janson P A, Jubelirer S J, Weinstein M J, Deykin D 1980 Treatment of the bleeding tendency in uremia with cryoprecipitate. New England Journal of Medicine 303: 1318–1322
Janson P A, Moake J C, Carpinito G 1983 Aspirin prevents heparin-induced platelet aggregation in vivo. British Journal of Haematology 53: 166–168
Jayabose S, Patel P, Inamdar S, Brilliant R, Mamtani R 1987 Use of intravenous methylprednisolone in acute idiopathic thrombocytopenic purpura. American Journal of Pediatric Hematology/Oncology 9: 133–135
Johnson T M, Rapini R P 1987 Isotretinoin-induced thrombocytopenia (letter). Journal of the American Academy of Dermatology 17: 838–839
Jonsson H, Nived O, Sturfelt G 1989 Outcome in systemic lupus erythematosus: A prospective study of patients from a defined population. Medicine 68: 141–150
Jørgensen K A, Ingeberg S 1979 Platelets and platelet function in patients with chronic uremia on maintenance hemodialysis. Nephron 23: 233–236
Kakaiya R M, Dehertogh D, Walker F J, Cummings E, Uzdejczyk M 1989 Rifampin-induced immune thrombocytopenia. A case report. Vox Sanguinis 57: 185–187
Kaplan C, Champeix P, Blanchard D et al 1987 Platelet antibodies in systemic lupus erythematosus. British Journal of Haematology 67: 89–93
Kaplan C, Daffos F, Forestier F et al 1988 Management of alloimmune thrombocytopenia: Antenatal diagnosis and in utero transfusion of maternal platelets. Blood 72: 340–343
Kaplan C, Daffos F, Forestier F et al 1990 Fetal platelet counts in thrombocytopenic pregancy. Lancet 336: 979–982
Kappa J R, Fisher C A, Todd B et al 1990 Intraoperative management of patients with heparin-induced thrombocytopenia. Annals of Thoracic Surgery 49: 714–723
Karmali A M, Steele B T, Petric M, Lim C 1983 Sporadic cases of haemolytic-uraemic syndrome associated with faecal cytotoxin and cytotoxin-producing Escherichia coli in stools. Lancet 1: 619

Karpatkin S 1985 Autoimmune thrombocytopenic purpura. Seminars in Hematology 22: 260–288
Karpatkin S, Lackner H L 1975 Association of antiplatelet antibody with functional platelet disorders. Autoimmune thrombocytopenic purpura, systemic lupus erythematosus and thrombocytopathia. American Journal of Medicine 59: 599–604
Karpatkin S, Nardi M, Lennette E, Byrne B, Poiesz B 1988 Anti HIV-1 antibody complexes on platelets of seropositive thrombocytopenic homosexuals and narcotic addicts. Proceedings of the National Academy of Sciences, USA 85: 9763–9767
Kasabach H H, Merritt K K 1940 Hemangioma with extensive purpura. American Journal of Diseases of Children 59: 1063–1070
Kaufman P A, Gockerman J P, Greenberg C S 1989 Production of a novel anticoagulant by neoplastic plasma cells: Report of a case and review of the literature. American Journal of Medicine 86: 612–616
Kekomäki R, Raivio P, Kero P 1992 A new low-frequency platelet alloantigen, Va[a], on glycoprotein IIbIIIa associated with neonatal alloimmune thrombocytopenia. Transfusion Medicine 2: 27–33
Kekomäki R, Jouhikainen T, Ollikainen J, Westman P, Laes M 1993 A new platelet alloantigen, Tu[a], on glyoprotein IIIa associated with neonatal alloimmune thrombocytopenia in two families. British Journal of Haematology 83: 306–310
Kelsey P R, Schofield K P, Geary C G 1985 Refractory idiopathic thrombocytopenic purpura (ITP) treated with cyclosporine (letter). British Journal of Haematology 60: 197–198
Kelton J G 1983 Management of the pregnant patient with idiopathic thrombocytopenic purpura. Annals of Internal Medicine 99: 796–800
Kelton J G, Gibbons S 1982 Autoimmune platelet destruction: Idiopathic thrombocytopenic purpura. 8: 83–104
Kelton J G, Neame P B, Gauldie J, Hirsh J 1979 Elevated platelet-associated IgG in the thrombocytopenia of septicemia. New England Journal of Medicine 300: 760–764
Kelton J G, Meltzer D, Moore J et al 1981 Drug-induced thrombocytopenia is associated with increased binding of IgG to platelets both in vivo and in vitro. Blood 58: 524–529
Kelton J G, Keystone J, Moore J et al 1983 Immune-mediated thrombocytopenia of malaria. Journal of Clinical Investigation 71: 832–836
Kelton J G, Powers P J, Carter C J 1982 A prospective study of the usefulness of the measurement of platelet-associated IgG for the diagnosis of idiopathic thrombocytopenic purpura. Blood 60: 1050–1053
Kelton J G, Moore J, Santos A, Sheridan D 1984a Detection of a platelet-agglutinating factor in thrombotic thrombocytopenic purpura. Annals of Internal Medicine 101: 589–593
Kelton J G, Sheridan D, Brain H, Powers P J, Turpie A G, Carter C J 1984b Clinical usefulness of testing for a heparin-dependent platelet-aggregating factor in patients with suspected heparin-associated thrombocytopenia. Journal of Laboratory and Clinical Medicine 103: 606–612
Kelton J G, Sheridan D, Santos A et al 1988 Heparin-induced thrombocytopenia: Laboratory studies. Blood 72: 925–930
Kelton J G, Murphy W G, Lucarelli A et al 1989 A prospective comparison of four techniques for measuring platelet-associated IgG. British Journal of Haematology 71: 97–105
Kelton J G, Smith J W Horsewood P, Humbert J, Hayward C P M, Warkentin T E 1990 The Gov[a/b] alloantigen system on human platelets. Blood 75: 2172–2176
Kelton J G, Warkentin T E, Hayward C P M, Murphy W G, Moore J C 1992 The calpain activity in patients with thrombotic thrombocytopenic purpura is associated with platelet microparticles. Blood: in press
Keusch G, Gmur J, Baumgartner D, Burger H R, Largiader F, Binswanger U 1986 De novo haemolytic-uraemic syndrome in two renal allograft recipients treated with cyclosporin: Successful therapy with plasma pheresis. Kidney International 30: 456
Khamashta M A, Harris E N, Gharavi A E et al 1988 Immune mediated mechanism for thrombosis: Antiphospholipid antibody binding to platelet membranes. Annals of the Rheumatic Diseases 47: 849–854
Khoory M S, Nesheim M E, Bowie E J W, Mann K G 1980 Circulating heparan sulfate proteoglycan anticoagulant from a patient with a plasma cell disorder. Journal of Clinical Investigation 65: 666–674
Kickler T S, Ness P M, Herman J H, Bell W R 1986 Studies on the pathophysiology of posttransfusion purpura. Blood 68: 347–350
Kickler T S, Herman J H, Furihata K, Kunicki T J, Aster R H 1988 Identification of Bak[b], a new platelet-specific antigen associated with posttransfusion purpura. Blood 71: 894–898
Kickler T, Braine H G, Piantadosi S, Ness P M, Herman J H, Rothko K 1990a A randomized, placebo-controlled trial of intravenous gammaglobulin in alloimmunized thrombocytopenic patients. Blood 75: 313–316
Kickler T, Kennedy S D, Braine H G 1990b Alloimmunization to platelet-specific antigens on glycoproteins IIb-IIIa and Ib/IX in multiply transfused thrombocytopenic patients. Transfusion 30: 622–625
Kiefel V, Santoso S, Weisheit M, Mueller-Eckhardt C 1987 Monoclonal antibody-specific immobilization of platelet antigens (MAIPA): A new tool for the identification of platelet-reactive antibodies. Blood 70: 1722–1726
Kiefel V, Santoso S, Katzmann B, Mueller-Eckhardt C 1988 A new platelet-specific alloantigen Br[a]. Report of 4 cases with neonatal alloimmune thrombocytopenia. Vox Sanguinis 54: 101–106
Kiefel V, Santoso S, Glockner W M, Katzmann B, Mayr W R, Mueller-Eckhardt C 1989a Posttransfusion purpura associated with an anti-Bak[b]. Vox Sanguinis 56: 93–97
Kiefel V, Santoso S, Katzmann B, Mueller-Eckhardt C 1989b The Br[a]/Br[b] system on human platelets. Blood 73: 2219–2223
Kiefel V, Santoso S, Kaufmann E, Mueller-Eckhardt C 1991a Autoantibodies against platelet glycoprotein Ib/IX: A frequent finding in autoimmune thrombocytopenic purpura. British Journal of Haematology 79: 256–262
Kiefel V, Shechter Y, Atias D, Kroll H, Santoso S, Mueller-Eckhardt C 1991b Neonatal alloimmune thrombocytopenia due to anti-Br[b] (HPA-5a). Report of three cases in two families. Vox Sanguinis 60: 244–245
Kiemowitz R M, Collins J, Davis K, Aster R H 1986 Posttransfusion purpura associated with alloimmunization against the platelet-specific antigen, Bak[a]. American Journal of Hematology 21: 79–88
Kienast J, Schmitz G 1990 Flow cytometric analysis of thiazole orange uptake by platelets: A diagnostic aid in the evaluation of thrombocytopenic disorders. Blood 75: 116–121
Kihara S, Matsuzawa Y, Kubo M et al 1989 Autoimmune hyperchylomicronemia. New England Journal of Medicine 320: 1255–1259
Kim H D, Boggs D R 1979 A syndrome resembling idiopathic thrombocytopenic purpura in 10 patients with diverse forms of cancer. American Journal of Medicine 67: 371–377
Kim H C, Park C L, Cowan J H III, Fattori F D, August C S 1988 Massive intravascular hemolysis associated with intravenous immunoglobulin in bone marrow transplant recipients. American Journal of Pediatric Hematology/Oncology 10: 69–74
Kinney E L, Ballard J O, Carlin B, Zelis R 1983 Amrinone-mediated thrombocytopenia. Scandinavian Journal of Haematology 31: 376–380
Kinney J B Jr, Albano E, Krober M S, Stevenson J G 1992 Atypical Kawasaki disease: Coronary aneurysms and thrombocytopenia. Southern Medical Journal 85: 40–42
Kleinknecht D, Jungers P, Chanard J, Barbanel C, Ganeval D 1972 Uremic and non-uremic complications in acute renal failure: Evaluation of early and frequent dialysis on prognosis. Kidney International 1: 190–196
Kline A, Hughes L E, Campbell H, Williams A, Zlosnick J, Leach K G 1975 Dextran 70 in prophylaxis of thromboembolic disease after surgery: A clinically oriented randomized double-blind trial. British Medical Journal 2: 109–112
Kobayashi T, Terao T 1987 Preeclampsia as chronic disseminated intravascular coagulation. Study of two parameters: Thrombin-antithrombin III complex and D-dimers. Gynecologic and Obstetric Investigation 24: 170–178
Kobrinsky N L, Tulloh H 1988 Treatment of refractory thrombocytopenic bleeding with 1-desamino-8-D-arginine vasopressin (desmopressin). Journal of Pediatrics 112: 993–996
Kosmo M A, Bordin G, Tani P, McMillan R 1986 Immune

thrombocytopenia and Crohn's disease (letter). Annals of Internal Medicine 104: 136
Kosty M P, Hench K, Tani P, McMillan R 1989 Thrombocytopenia associated with auranofin therapy: Evidence for a gold-dependent immunologic mechanism. American Journal of Hematology 30: 236–239
Koury M J, 1990 Thrombocytopenic purpura in HIV-seronegative users of intravenous cocaine. American Journal of Hematology 35: 134–135
Kramer M R, Levene C, Hershko C 1986 Severe reversible autoimmune haemolytic anaemia and thrombocytopenia associated with diclofenac therapy. Scandinavian Journal of Haematology 36: 118–120
Kreger B E, Craven D E, McCabe W R 1980 Gram-negative bacteremia. IV. Re-evaluation of clinical features and treatment in 612 patients. American Journal of Medicine 68: 344–355
Kressel B R, Ryan K P, Duong A T, Berengberg J, Schein P S 1981 Microangiopathic hemolytic anemia, thrombocytopenia, and renal failure in patients treated for adenocarcinoma. Cancer 48: 1738–1745
Kroll H, Kiefel V, Santoso S, Mueller-Eckhardt C 1990 Sr^a, a private platelet antigen on glycoprotein IIIa associated with neonatal alloimmune thrombocytopenia. Blood 76: 2296–2302
Kubota T, Tanoue K, Murohashi I et al 1989 Autoantibody against platelet glycoprotein IIb/IIIa in a patient with non-Hodgkin's lymphoma. Thrombosis Research 53: 379–386
Kuijpers R W A M, Ouwehand W H, Bleeker P M M, Christie D, von dem Borne A E G K 1992 Localization of the platelet-specific HPA-2 (Ko) alloantigens on the N-terminal globular fragment of platelet glycoprotein Ibα. Blood 79: 283–288
Kuijpers R W A M, Simsek S, Faber N M, Goldschmeding R, van Wermerkerken, von dem Borne A E G K 1993 Single point mutation in human glycoprotein IIIa is associated with a new platelet-specific alloantigen (Mo) involved in neonatal alloimmune thrombocytopenia. Blood 81: 70–76
Kunicki T J, Beardsley D S 1989 The alloimmune thrombocytopenias: Neonatal alloimmune thrombocytopenic purpura and post-transfusion purpura. Progress in Hemostasis and Thrombosis 9: 203–232
Kunicki T J, Newman P J 1992 The molecular immunology of human platelet proteins. Blood 80: 1386–1404
Kwaan H C 1987 Clinicopathologic features of thrombotic thrombocytopenic purpura. Seminars in Hematology 24: 71–81
Kyle R A, Gleich G J, Bayrd E D, Vaughan J H 1971 Benign hypergammaglobulinemic purpura of Waldenström. Medicine 50: 113–123
Kyrle P A, Stockenhuber F, Brenner B et al 1988 Evidence for an increased generation of prostacyclin in the microvasculature and an impairment of the platelet α-granule release in chronic renal failure. Thrombosis and Haemostasis 60: 205–208
Lackner H, Hunt V, Zucker M B, Pearson J 1970 Abnormal fibrin ultrastructure, polymerization, and clot retraction in multiple myeloma. British Journal of Haematology 18: 625–636
Lackner H 1973 Hemostatic abnormalities associated with dysproteinemias. Seminars in Hematology 10: 125–133
Lagarde M, Byron P A, Vargaftig B B, Dechavanne M 1978 Impairment of platelet thromboxane A_2 generation and of the platelet release reaction in two patients with congenital deficiency of platelet cyclo-oxygenase. British Journal of Haematology 38: 251–266
Lages B, Weiss H J 1989 Inhibition of human platelet function in vitro and ex vivo by acetaminophen. Thrombosis Research 53: 603–613
Lambert C J, Marengo-Rowe A J, Leveson J E et al 1979 The treatment of postperfusion bleeding using ε-aminocaproic acid, cryoprecipitate, fresh-frozen plasma, and protamine sulfate. Annals of Thoracic Surgery 28: 440–444
Lane T A, Anderson K C, Goodnough L T et al 1992 Leukocyte reduction in blood component therapy. Annals of Internal Medicine 117: 151–162
Laster J L, Nichols W K, Silver D 1989 Thrombocytopenia associated with heparin-coated catheters in patients with heparin-associated antiplatelet antibodies. Archives of Internal Medicine 149: 2285–2287
Lau P, Sholtis C M, Aster R H 1980 Post-transfusion purpura: An enigma of alloimmunization. American Journal of Hematology 9: 331–336
Lawrence J B, Friedman B S, Travis W D, Chinchilli V M, Metcalfe D D, Gralnick H R 1991 Hematologic manifestations of systemic mast cell disease: A prospective study of laboratory and morphologic features and their relation to prognosis. American Journal of Medicine 91: 612–624
Lederman H M, Roifman C M, Lavi S, Gelfand E W 1986 Corticosteroids for prevention of adverse reactions to intravenous immune serum globulin infusions in hypogammaglobulinemic patients. American Journal of Medicine 81: 443–446
Leduc L, Wheeler J M, Kirshon B, Mitchell P, Cotton D B 1992 Coagulation profile in severe preeclampsia. Obstetrics and Gynecology 79: 14–18
Lee E J, Schiffer C A 1989 ABO compatibility can influence the results of platelet transfusion. Results of a randomized trial. Transfusion 29: 384–389
Leehey D J, Kanak R J, Messmore H L, Nawab Z M, Popli S, Ing T S 1987 Heparin-associated thrombocytopenia in maintenance hemodialysis patients. International Journal of Artificial Organs 10: 390–392
Leissinger C A 1990 Severe thrombocytopenia associated with cocaine use. Annals of Internal Medicine 102: 737–741
Leissinger C A, Stuckey W J 1992 Unbound immunoglobulins are a major source of error in the quantitation of platelet surface-bound immunoglobulin levels. Transfusion 32: 157–161
Lesesne J B, Rothschild N, Erickson B et al 1989 Cancer-associated haemolytic-uraemic syndrome: Analysis of 85 cases from a national registry. Journal of Clinical Oncology 7: 781–789
Levine R F, Spivak J L, Meagher R C, Sieber F 1986 Effect of ethanol on thrombopoiesis. British Journal of Haematology 62: 345–354
Levine M N, Hirsh J, Gent M et al 1991 Prevention of deep vein thrombosis after elective hip surgery. A randomized trial comparing low molecular weight heparin with standard unfractionated heparin. Annals of Internal Medicine 114: 545–551
Levy-Toledano S, Tobelem G, Legrand C et al 1978 Acquired IgG antibody occurring in a thrombasthenic patient: Its effect on human platelet function. Blood 51: 1065–1071
Lewis J H, Zucker M B, Ferguson J H 1956 Bleeding tendency in uremia. Blood 11: 1073–1076
Lian E C Y, Harkness D R, Byrnes J J, Wallach H, Nunez R 1979 Presence of a platelet aggregating factor in the plasma of patients with thrombotic thrombocytopenic purpura and its inhibition by normal plasma. Blood 53: 333–338
Lian E C Y, Siddiqui F A, Jamieson G A, Tandon N N 1991 Platelet agglutinating protein p37 causes platelet agglutination through its binding to membrane glycoprotein IV. Thrombosis and Haemostasis 65: 102–106
Licciardello J T W, Moake J L, Rudy C K, Karp D D, Hong W K 1985 Elevated plasma von Willebrand factor levels and arterial occlusive complications associated with cisplatin-based chemotherapy. Oncology 42: 296–300
Lind S E 1991 The bleeding time does not predict surgical bleeding. Blood 77: 2547–2552
Lindenbaum J, Lieber C S 1969 Hematologic effects of alcohol in man in the absence of nutritional deficiency. New England Journal of Medicine 281: 333–338
Lippman S M, Lizak G E, Foung S K H, Grumet F C 1988 The efficacy of Pl^{A1}-negative platelet transfusion therapy in posttransfusion purpura. Western Journal of Medicine 148: 86–88
Lipsky J J 1988 Antibiotic-associated hypoprothrombinaemia. Journal of Antimicrobial Chemotherapy 21: 281–300
Liu Y K, Kosfeld R E, Marcum S G 1984 Treatment of uraemic bleeding with conjugated oestrogen. Lancet 2: 887–890
Livio M, Gotti E, Marchesi D, Remuzzi G, Mecca G, de Gaetano G 1982 Uraemic bleeding: Role of anaemia and beneficial effect of red cell transfusions. Lancet 2: 1013–1015
Livio M, Mannucci P M, Viganò G et al 1986 Conjugated estrogens for the management of bleeding associated with renal failure. New England Journal of Medicine 315: 731–735
Loghem J J van, Dorfmeijer H, Hart M van der, Schreur F 1959 Serological and genetical studies on a platelet antigen (Zw). Vox Sanguinis 4: 161

Loirat C, Beaufils F, Sonsino E et al 1984 Traitement du syndrome hémolytique et urémique de l'enfant par l'urokinase: Essai contrôlé coopératif. Archives Françaises de Pédiatrie 41: 15–19
Loirat C, Sonsino E, Hinglais N, Jais J P, Landais P, Fermainian J 1988 Treatment of the childhood haemolytic uraemic syndrome with plasma. A multicentre randomized controlled trial. Pediatric Nephrology 2: 279–285
Lopas H, Rabiner S F 1966 Thrombocytopenia associated with iron deficiency anemia: A report of five cases. Clinical Pediatrics 5: 609–616
Loughran T P Jr, Starkebaum G 1987 Large granular lymphocyte leukemia. Medicine 66: 397–405
Loughran T P Jr, Kadin M E, Starkebaum G et al 1985 Leukemia of large granular lymphocytes: Association with clonal chromosomal abnormalities and autoimmune neutropenia, thrombocytopenia, and hemolytic anemia. Annals of Internal Medicine 102: 169–175
Lown J, Barr A 1987 Immune thrombocytopenia induced by cephalosporins specific for thiomethyltetrazole side chain (letter). Journal of Clinical Pathology 40: 700–701
Lyman S, Aster R H, Visentin G P, Newman P J 1990 Polymorphism of human platelet membrane glycoprotein IIb associated with the Bak^a/Bak^b alloantigen system. Blood 75: 2343–2348
Lynch L, Bussel J B, McFarland J G, Chitkara U, Berkowitz R L 1992 Antenatal treatment of alloimmune thrombocytopenia. Obstetrics and Gynecology 80: 67–71
McFarland J G, Aster R H, Bussel J B, Gianopoulos J G, Derbes R S, Newman P J 1991 Prenatal diagnosis of neonatal alloimmune thrombocytopenia using allele-specific oligonucleotide probes. Blood 78: 2276–2282
McGrath K, Minchinton R, Cunningham I, Ayberk H 1989 Platelet anti-Bak^b antibody associated with neonatal alloimmune thrombocytopenia. Vox Sanguinis 57: 182
McLaughlin P, Talpaz M, Quesada J R, Saleem A, Barlogie B, Gutterman J U 1985 Journal of the American Medical Association 254: 1353–1354
McMillan R, Longmire R L, Yelenosky R, Smith R S, Craddock C G 1972 Immunoglobulin synthesis in vitro by splenic tissue in idiopathic thrombocytopenic purpura. New England Journal of Medicine 286: 681–684
McMillan R, Luiken G A, Levy R, Yelenosky R, Longmire R L 1978 Antibody against megakaryocytes in idiopathic thrombocytopenic purpura. Journal of the American Medical Association 239: 2460–2462
McMillan R, Tani P, Millard F, Berchtold P, Renshaw L, Woods V L 1987 Platelet-associated and plasma anti-glycoprotein autoantibodies in chronic ITP. Blood 70: 1040–1045
McTavish D, Faulds D, Goa K L 1990 Ticlopidine. An updated review of its pharmacology and therapeutic use in platelet-dependent disorders. Drugs 40: 238–259
Magil A B, McFadden D, Rae A 1986 Lupus glomerulonephritis with thrombotic microangiopathy. Human Pathology 17: 192–194
Maher J F, Schreiner G E 1962 Cause of death in acute renal failure. Archives of Internal Medicine 110: 493–504
Malmsten C, Hamber M, Svensson J, Samuelsson B 1975 Physiological role of an endoperoxide in human platelets: Haemostatic defect due to platelet cyclooxygenase deficiency. Proceedings of the National Academy of Sciences, USA 72: 1446–1450
Malpass T W, Savage B, Hanson S R, Slichter S J, Harker L A 1984 Correlation between prolonged bleeding time and depletion of platelet dense granule ADP in patients with myelodysplastic and myeloproliferative disorders. Journal of Laboratory and Clinical Medicine 103: 894–904
Mankin H J 1992 Nontraumatic necrosis of bone (osteonecrosis). New England Journal of Medicine 326: 1473–1479
Mannucci P M 1988 Desmopressin: A nontransfusional form of treatment for congenital and acquired bleeding disorders. Blood 72: 1449–1455
Mannucci P M, Remuzzi G, Pusineri F et al 1983 Deamino-8-D-arginine vasopressin shortens the bleeding time in uremia. New England Journal of Medicine 308: 8–12
Mannucci P M, Lombardi R, Bader R et al 1984 Studies of the pathophysiology of acquired von Willebrand's disease in seven patients with lymphoproliferative disorders or benign monoclonal gammopathies. Blood 64: 614–621
Mannucci P M, Vicente V, Vianello L et al 1986 Controlled trial of desmopressin in liver cirrhosis and other conditions associated with a prolonged bleeding time. Blood 67: 1148–1153
Manoharan A, Williams N T, Sparrow R 1989 Acquired amegakaryocytic thrombocytopenia: Report of a case and review of literature. Quarterly Journal of Medicine 70: 243–252
Manoharan A 1991 Treatment of refractory idiopathic thrombocytopenic purpura in adults. British Journal of Haematology 79: 143–147
Marcelli-Barge A, Poirier J C, Dausset J 1973 Allo-antigens and allo-antibodies of the Ko system, serological and genetic study. Vox Sanguinis 24: 1–11
Marino C, Cook P 1985 Danazol for lupus thrombocytopenia. Archives of Internal Medicine 145: 2251–2252
Mason D, McMillan R 1984 Platelet antigens in chronic idiopathic thrombocytopenic purpura. British Journal of Haematology 56: 529–534
Massey G V, McWilliams N B, Mueller D G, Napolitano A, Maurer H M 1987 Intravenous immunoglobulin in treatment of neonatal alloimmune thrombocytopenia. Journal of Pediatrics 111: 133–135
Matsumura O, Kawashima Y, Kato S et al 1988 Therapeutic effect of cyclosporine in thrombocytopenia associated with autoimmune disease. Transplantation Proceedings 20 (suppl 4): 317–322
Matsuoka T, Chikahira Y, Yamada T, Nakao K, Ueshima S, Matsuo O 1988 Effect of synthetic thrombin inhibitor (MD805) as an alternative drug on heparin induced thrombocytopenia during hemodialysis. Thrombosis Research 52: 165–171
Matsuoka T, Tamura H, Fujishita M, Kubonishi I, Taguchi H, Miyoshi I 1988 Thrombocytopenic purpura in a carrier of human T-cell leukemia virus type I. American Journal of Hematology 27: 142–143
Mazzucato M, de Marco L, de Angelis V, de Roia D, Bizzaro N, Casonato A 1989 Platelet membrane abnormalities in myeloproliferative disorders: Decrease in glycoproteins Ib and IIb/IIIa complex is associated with deficient receptor function. British Journal of Haematology 73: 369–374
Mazzucconi M G, Francesconi M, Fidani P et al 1985 Treatment of idiopathic thrombocytopenic purpura (ITP): Results of a multicentric protocol. Haematologica 70: 329–336
Mehta D P, Yoder E L, Appel J, Bergsman K L 1991 Heparin-induced thrombocytopenia and thrombosis: Reversal with streptokinase. A case report and review of literature. American Journal of Hematology 36: 275–279
Meisner D J, Carlson R J, Gottlieb A J 1985 Thrombocytopenia following sustained-release procainamide. Archives of Internal Medicine 145: 700–702
Menichelli A, Del Principe D, Rezza E 1984 Intravenous pulse methylprednisolone in chronic idiopathic thrombocytopenia. Archives of Disease in Childhood 59: 777–779
Meyboom R H B 1984 Thrombocytopenia induced by nalidixic acid. British Medical Journal 289: 962
Meyer K, Williams E C 1985 Fibrinolysis and acquired alpha-2 plasmin inhibitor deficiency in amyloidosis. American Journal of Medicine 79: 394–396
Meyer M, Kirchmaier C M, Schirmer A, Spangenberg P, Ströhl C, Breddin K 1991 Acquired disorder of platelet function associated with autoantibodies against membrane glycoprotein IIb-IIIa complex. 1. Glycoprotein analysis. Thrombosis and Haemostasis 65: 491–496
Micallef-Eynaud P D, Ludlam C A 1991 Aortic aneurysms and consumptive coagulopathy. Blood Coagulation and Fibrinolysis 2: 477–481
Michalak E, Walkowiak B, Paradowski M, Cierniewski C S 1991 The decreased circulating platelet mass and its relation to bleeding time in chronic renal failure. Thrombosis and Haemostasis 65: 11–14
Milligan G F, MacDonald J A E, Mellon A, Ledingham I M 1974 Pulmonary and hematologic disturbances during septic shock. Surgery Gynecology and Obstetrics 138: 43–49
Milutinovich J, Follette W C, Scribner B H 1977 Spontaneous retroperitoneal bleeding in patients on chronic hemodialysis. Annals of Internal Medicine 86: 189–192
Minchinton R M, Waters A H, Malpas J S, Starke I, Kendra J R,

Barrett A J 1984 Platelet- and granulocyte-specific antibodies after allogeneic and autologous bone marrow grafts. Vox Sanguinis 46 125–135

Minchinton R M, Cunningham I, Cole-Sinclair M, van der Weyden M, Vaughan S, McGrath K M 1990 Autoreactive platelet antibody in post transfusion purpura. Australian and New Zealand Journal of Medicine 20: 111–115

Mittelman A, Puccio C, Ahmed T et al 1992 Response of refractory thrombotic thrombocytopenic purpura to extracorporeal immunoadsorption (letter). New England Journal of Medicine 326: 711–712

Mizutani H, Katagiri S, Uejima K et al 1985 T-cell abnormalities in patients with idiopathic thrombocytopenic purpura: The presence of $OKT4^{+}8^{+}$ cells. Scandinavian Journal of Haematology 35: 233–239

Mizutani H, Tsubakio T, Tomiyama Y et al 1987 Increased circulating Ia-positive T cells in patients with idiopathic thrombocytopenic purpura. Clinical and Experimental Immunology 67: 191–197

Moake J L, Rudy C K, Troll J H et al 1982 Unusually large plasma factor VIII: von Willebrand factor multimers in chronic relapsing thrombotic thrombocytopenic purpura. New England Journal of Medicine 307: 1432–1435

Moberg P Q, Geary V M, Sheikh F M 1990 Heparin-induced thrombocytopenia: A possible complication of heparin-coated pulmonary artery catheters. Journal of Cardiothoracic Anesthesia 4: 226–228

Mohri H, Noguchi T, Kodama F, Itoh A, Ohkubo T 1987 Acquired von Willebrand disease due to inhibitor of human myeloma protein specific for von Willebrand factor. American Journal of Clinical Pathology 87: 663–668

Moia M, Mannucci P M, Vizzotto L, Casati S, Cattaneo M, Ponticelli C 1987 Improvement in the haemostatic defect of uraemia after treatment with recombinant human erythropoietin. Lancet 2: 1227–1229

Monforte R, Estruch R, Graus F, Nicolas J M, Urbano-Marquez A 1990 High ethanol consumption as risk factor for intracerebral hemorrhage in young and middle-aged people. Stroke 21: 1529–1532

Moore J C, Murphy W G, Kelton J G 1990 Calpain proteolysis of von Willebrand factor enhances its binding to platelet membrane glycoprotein IIb/IIIa: An explanation for platelet aggregation in thrombotic thrombocytopenic purpura. British Journal of Haematology 74: 457–464

Morgan C L, Cannell G R, Addison R S, Minchinton R M 1991 The effect of intravenous immunoglobulin on placental transfer of a platelet-specific antibody: Anti-Pl^{A1}. Transfusion Medicine 1: 209–216

Morris L, Distenfeld A, Amorosi E, Karpatkin S 1982 Autoimmune thrombocytopenic purpura in homosexual men. Annals of Internal Medicine 96: 714–717

Morrison F S, Mollison P L 1966 Post-transfusion purpura. New England Journal of Medicine 275: 243–248

Morton B D, Orringer E P, Lattart L A, Stass S A 1980 Pappenheimer bodies. An additional cause for a spurious platelet count. American Journal of Clinical Pathology 74: 310–311

Moutet A, Fromont P, Farcet J P et al 1990 Pregnancy in women with immune thrombocytopenic purpura. Archives of Internal Medicine 150: 2141–2145

Mueller-Eckhardt C 1986 Post-transfusion purpura. British Journal of Haematology 64: 419–424

Mueller-Eckhardt C, Kayser W, Mersch-Baumert K et al 1980 The clinical significance of platelet associated IgG: A study on 298 patients with various disorders. British Journal of Haematology 46: 123–131

Mueller-Eckhardt C, Kayser W, Förster C, Mueller-Eckhardt G, Ringenberg C 1981 Improved assay for the detection of platelet-specific Pl^{A1} antibodies in neonatal alloimmune thrombocytopenia. Vox Sanguinis 43: 76–81

Mueller-Eckhardt C, Küenzlen E, Thilo-Körner D, Pralle H 1983 High-dose intravenous immunoglobulin for post-transfusion purpura. New England Journal of Medicine 308: 287

Mueller-Eckhardt C, Becker T, Weisheit M, Witz C, Santoso S 1986 Neonatal alloimmune thrombocytopenia due to fetomaternal Zw^{b} incompatibility. Vox Sanguinis 50: 94

Mueller-Eckhardt C, Kiefel V, Grubert A, Kroll H, Weisheit M, Schmidt S, Mueller-Eckhardt G, Santoso S 1989 348 cases of suspected neonatal alloimmune thrombocytopenia. Lancet 1: 363–366

Müller-Berghaus G 1989 Pathophysiologic and biochemical events in disseminated intravascular coagulation: Dysregulation of procoagulant and anticoagulant pathways. Seminars in Thrombosis and Hemostasis 15: 58–87

Müller-Esterl W 1987 Novel functions of the kininogens. Seminars in Thrombosis and Hemostasis 13: 115–126

Murakami H, Lam Z, Furie B C, Reinhold V N, Asano T, Furie B 1991 Sulfated glycolipids are the platelet autoantigens for human platelet-binding monoclonal anti-DNA autoantibodies. Journal of Biological Chemistry 266: 15414–15419

Murata M, Furihata K, Ishida F, Russell S R, Ware J, Ruggeri Z M 1992 Genetic and structural characterization of an amino acid dimorphism in glycoprotein Ibα involved in platelet transfusion refractoriness. Blood 79: 3086–3090

Murphy W G, Kelton J G 1990a Techniques used to measure immunoglobulins on platelets. In: Dutcher J P (ed) Modern transfusion therapy. CRC Press, Boca Raton, vol 2: 97–124

Murphy W G, Kelton J G 1990b Platelet transfusions in idiopathic thrombocytopenic purpura. In: Dutcher J P (ed) Modern transfusion therapy. CRC Press, Boca Raton, vol 2: 125–131

Murphy W G, Moore J C, Kelton J G 1987 Calcium-dependent cysteine protease activity in the sera of patients with thrombotic thrombocytopenic purpura. Blood 70: 1683–1687

Mylvaganam R, Ahn Y S, Harrington W J, Kim C I, Gratzner H G 1985 Differences in T cell subsets between men and women with idiopathic thrombocytopenic purpura. Blood 66: 967–972

Naumovski L, Pillsbury H E 1991 Treatment of thrombotic thrombocytopenic purpura with cryosupernatant (letter). American Journal of Hematology 38: 250–251

Neame P B, Lechago J, Ling E T, Koval A 1973 Thrombotic thrombocytopenic purpura: Report of a case with disseminated intravascular platelet aggregation. Blood 42: 805–814

Neame P B, Kelton J G, Walker I R, Stewart I O, Nossel H L, Hirsh J 1980 Thrombocytopenia in septicemia: The role of disseminated intravascular coagulation. Blood 56: 88–92

Needleman S W, Sorace J, Poussin-Rosillo H 1992 Low-dose splenic irradiation in the treatment of autoimmune thrombocytopenia in HIV-infected patients. Annals of Internal Medicine 116: 310–311

Neely S M, Gardner D V, Reynolds N, Green D, Ts'Ao C-H 1984 Mechanism and characteristics of platelet activation by haematin. British Journal of Haematology 58: 305–316

Nenci G G, Gresele P, Agnelli G, Parise P 1981 Intrinsically defective or exhausted platelets in hairy cell leukaemia? (letter) Thrombosis and Haemostasis 46: 572

Nesher G, Dollberg L, Zimran A, Hershko C 1985 Hepatosplenic peliosis after danazol and glucocorticoids for ITP (letter). New England Journal of Medicine 312: 242

Neucks S H, Moore T L, Lichtenstein J R, Baldassare A R, Weiss T D, Zuckner J 1980 Localised scleroderma and idiopathic thrombocytopenia. Journal of Rheumatology 7: 741–744

Newman P J, Derbes R S, Aster R H 1989 The human platelet alloantigens, Pl^{A1} and Pl^{A2}, are associated with a $leucine^{33}/proline^{33}$ amino acid polymorphism in membrane glycoprotein IIIa, and are distinguishable by DNA typing. Journal of Clinical Investigation 83: 1778–1781

Nieminen U, Kekomäki R 1992 Quinidine-induced thrombocytopenic purpura: Clinical presentation in relation to drug-dependent and drug-independent platelet antibodies. British Journal of Haematology 80: 77–82

Niessner H, Clemetson K J, Panzer S, Mueller-Eckhardt C, Santoso S, Bettelheim P 1986 Acquired thrombosthenia due to GP IIb/IIIa-specific platelet autoantibodies. Blood 68: 571–576

Nieuwenhuis H K, Akkerman J W N, Sixma J J 1987 Patients with a prolonged bleeding time and normal aggregation tests may have storage pool deficiency: Studies on one hundred and six patients. Blood 70: 620–623

Nijjar T S, Bonacosa I A, Israels L G 1987 Severe acute thrombocytopenia following infusion of plasma containing anti-Pl^{A1}. American Journal of Hematology 25: 219–221

Noda M, Kitagawa M, Tomoda F, Iida H 1990 Thrombotic thrombocytopenic purpura as a complicating factor in a case of polymyositis and Sjögren's syndrome. American Journal of Clinical Pathology 94: 217–221

Northfelt D W, Kaplan L D, Abrams D I 1991 continuous, low-dose therapy with interferon-α for human immunodeficiency virus (HIV)-related immune thrombocytopenic purpura. American Journal of Hematology 38: 238–239

Ochs H D, Slichter S J, Harker L A, Von Behrens W E, Clark R A, Wedgwood R J 1980 The Wiskott–Aldrich syndrome: Studies of lymphocytes, granulocytes, and platelets. Blood 55: 243–252

O'Connor N T, Bruce-Jones P, Hill L F 1992 Vincristine therapy for thrombotic thrombocytopenic purpura. American Journal of Hematology 39: 234–236

Okajima K, Yang W P, Okabe H, Inoue M, Takatsuki K 1991 Role of leukocytes in the activation of intravascular coagulation in patients with septicemia. American Journal of Hematology 36: 265–271

Oksenhendler E, Bierling P, Farcet J-P, Rabian C, Seligmann M, Clauvel J-P 1987 Response to therapy in 37 patients with HIV-related thrombocytopenic purpura. British Journal of Haematology 66: 491–495

Oksenhendler E, Bierling P, Brossard Y et al 1988 Anti-RH immunoglobulin therapy for human immunodeficiency virus-related immune thrombocytopenic purpura. Blood 71: 1499–1502

Onder O, Weinstein A, Hoyer L W 1980 Pseudothrombocytopenia caused by platelet agglutinins that are reactive in blood anticoagulated with chelating agents. Blood 56: 177–182

Onundarson P T, Rowe J M, Heal J M, Francis C W 1992 Response to plasma exchange and splenectomy in thrombotic thrombocytopenic purpura. A 10-year experience at a single institution. Archives of Internal Medicine 152: 791–796

Oppenheimer L, Hryniuk W M, Bishop A J 1976 Thrombocytopenia in severe bacterial infections. Journal of Surgical Research 20: 211–214

Ortel T L, Gockerman J P, Califf R M et al 1992 Parenteral anticoagulation with the heparinoid Lomoparan (Org 10172) in patients with heparin induced thrombocytopenia and thrombosis. Thrombosis and Haemostasis 67: 292–296

Oshimi K 1988 Granular lymphocyte proliferative disorders: Report of 12 cases and review of the literature. Leukemia 2: 617–627

Pachter M R, Johnson S A, Neblett T R, Truant J P 1959 Bleeding, platelets, and marcoglobulinemia. American Journal of Clinical Pathology 31: 467–482

Paciucci P A, Mandeli J, Oleksowiz L, Ameglio F, Holland J F 1990 Thrombocytopenia during immunotherapy with interleukin-2 by constant infusion. American Journal of Medicine 89: 308–312

Packham M A 1982 Mode of action of acetylsalicylic acid. In: Barnett H J M, Hirsh J, Mustard J F (eds) Acetylsalicylic acid: New uses for an old drug. Raven Press, New York, p 63–82

Palés J L, López A, Asensio A et al 1987 Inhibitory effect of peak 2–4 of uremic middle molecules on platelet aggregation. European Journal of Haematology 39: 197–202

Panzer S, Stain C, Benda H et al 1989 Effects of 3-azidothymidine on platelet counts, indium-111-labelled platelet kinetics, and antiplatelet antibodies. Vox Sanguinis 57: 120–126

Pareti F E, Capitanio A, Mannucci P M 1976 Acquired storage pool disease in platelets during disseminated intravascular coagulation. Blood 48: 511–515

Pareti F E, Capitanio A, Mannucci L, Ponticelli C, Mannucci P M 1980 Acquired dysfunction due to the circulation of 'exhausted' platelets. American Journal of Medicine 69: 235–240

Parker J C, Barrett D A II, Hill C 1971 Mircoangiopathic hemolysis and thrombocytopenia related to penicillin drugs. Archives of Internal Medicine 127: 474–477

Payne B A, Pierre R V 1984 Pseudothrombocytopenia: A laboratory artifact with potentially serious complications consequences. Mayo Clinic Proceedings 59: 123–125

Pedersen A K, FitzGerald G A 1984 Dose-related kinetics of aspirin: Presystemic acetylation of platelet cyclooxygenase. New England Journal of Medicine 311: 1206–1211

Peltier J Y, Lambin P, Doinel C et al 1991 Frequency and prognostic importance of thrombocytopenia in symptom-free HIV-infected individuals: A 5-year prospective study. AIDS 5: 381

Penny W F, Ware J A 1992 Platelet activation and subsequent inhibition by plasmin and recombinant tissue-type plasminogen activator. Blood 79: 91–98

Perkins H A, MacKenzie M R, Fudenberg H H 1970 Hemostatic defects in dysproteinemias. Blood 35: 695–707

Petitt R M 1980 Thrombotic thrombocytopenic purpura: A thirty year review. Seminars in Thrombosis and Hemostasis 6: 350–355

Pewarchuk W, VanderBoom J, Blajchman M A 1992 Pseudopolycythemia, pseudothrombocytopenia, and pseudoleukopenia due to overfilling of blood collection vacuum tubes. Archives of Pathology and Laboratory Medicine 116: 90–92

Pfueller S L, Firkin B G, McGrath K M, Logan D 1987 Analysis of immunoglobulins that bind to platelets from serum of patients with immune thrombocytopenia: Molecular weight distribution. Thrombosis Research 47: 305–314

Pinals R S, Tomar R H, Haas D C, Farah F 1977 Graves' disease, myasthenia gravis and purpura. Annals of Internal Medicine 87: 250

Pizzuto J, Ambriz R 1984 Therapeutic experience on 934 adults with idiopathic thrombocytopenic purpura: Multicentric trial of the Cooperative Latin American Group on Hemostasis and Thrombosis. Blood 64: 1179–1183

Pollak A N, Janinis J, Green D 1988 Successful intravenous immune globulin therapy for human immunodeficiency virus-associated thrombocytopenia. Archives of Internal Medicine 148: 695–697

Poskitt T R, Poskitt P K F 1985a Spurious thrombocytopenia produced by the interaction of rheumatoid factor with antiplatelet antibody. American Journal of Hematology 18: 207–211

Poskitt T R, Poskitt P K F 1985b Thrombocytopenia of sepsis. The role of circulating IgG-containing immune complexes. Archives of Internal Medicine 145: 891–894

Post R M, Desforges J F 1968 Thrombocytopenia and alcoholism. Annals of Internal Medicine 68: 1230–1236

Powell H R, Davison P M, McCredie D A, Phair P, Walker R G 1988a Haemolytic-uraemic syndrome after treatment with metronidazole. Medical Journal of Australia 149: 222–223

Powell S E, O'Brien S J, Barnes R, Warren R F, Wickiewicz T L 1988b Quinine-induced thrombocytopenia. A case report. Journal of Bone and Joint Surgery 70A: 1097–1099

Pritchard J A, Weisman R Jr, Ratnoff O D, Vosburgh G J 1954 Intravascular hemolysis, thrombocytopenia and other hematologic abnormalities associated with severe toxemia of pregnancy. New England Journal of Medicine 250: 89–98

Proctor S J, Jackson G, Carey P et al 1989 Improvement of platelet counts in steroid-unresponsive idiopathic immune thrombocytopenic purpura after short-course therapy with recombinant α 2b interferon. Blood 74: 1894–1897

Proesmans W, Eeckels R, van Damme B et al 1984 Antithrombotic therapy in childhood hemolytic uremic syndrome: A randomized prospective study. In: Brodehl J, Ehrich J H H (eds) Paediatric nephrology. Proceedings of the Sixth International Symposium of Paediatric Nephrology, Hanover, 1983. Springer-Verlag, Berlin, p 285–288

Quiquandon I, Fenaux P, Caulier M T, Pagniez D 1990 Re-evaluation of the role of azathioprine in the treatment of adult chronic idiopathic thrombocytopenic purpura: A report on 53 cases. British Journal of Haematology 74: 223–228

Rabiner S F, Molinas F 1970 The role of phenol and phenolic acids on the thrombocytopathy and defective platelet aggregation of patients with renal failure. American Journal of Medicine 49: 346–351

Rabinowe S N, Miller K B 1987 Danazol-induced thrombocytopenia (letter). British Journal of Haematology 65: 383–384

Rabinowe S N, Soiffer R J, Tarbell N J et al 1991 Hemolytic-uremic syndrome following bone marrow transplantation in adults for hematologic malignancies. Blood 77: 1837–1844

Raghupathy P, Date A, Shastry J C M, Sudarsanam A, Jadhav M 1978 Haemolytic-uraemic syndrome complicating shigella dysentery in south Indian children. British Medical Journal 1: 1518–1521

Rákóczi I, Tallián F, Bagdány S, Gáti I 1979 Platelet life-span in normal pregnancy and pre-eclampsia as determined by a non-radioisotope technique. Thrombosis Research 15: 553–556

Rand M L, Packham M A, Kinlough-Rathbone R L, Mustard J F 1988 Effects of ethanol on pathways of platelet aggregation in vitro. Thrombosis and Haemostasis 59: 383–387

Rao S, Pang E J M 1979 Idiopathic thrombocytopenic purpura in acute lymphoblastic leukemia. Journal of Pediatrics 94: 408–409

Rarick M U, Espina B, Montgomery T et al 1991 The long-term use of zidovudine in patients with severe immune-mediated thrombocytopenia secondary to infection with HIV. AIDS 5: 1357–1361

Rarick M U, Espina B, Mochrnuk R, Trilling Y, Levine A M 1992 Thrombotic thrombocytopenic purpura in patients with human immunodeficiency virus infection: A report of three cases and review of the literature. American Journal of Hematology 40: 103–109

Rasi V, Lintula R 1986 Platelet function in the myelodysplastic syndromes. Scandinavian Journal of Haematology 36 (suppl 45): 71–73

Ray J B, Brereton W F, Nullet F R 1990 Intravenous immune globulin for the treatment of presumed quinidine-induced thrombocytopenia, DICP. The Annals of Pharmacotherapy 24: 693–695

Redman C W G, Allington M J, Bolton F G, Stirrat G M 1977 Plasma-β-thromboglobulin in pre-eclampsia. Lancet 2: 248

Reiner A P, Spivak J L 1988 Hemophagocytic histiocytosis: A report of 23 new patients and a review of the literature. Medicine 67: 369–388

Remuzzi G 1988 Bleeding in renal failure. Lancet 1: 1205–1208

Remuzzi G, Benigni A, Dodesini P et al 1983 Reduced platelet thromboxane formation in uremia. Evidence for a functional cyclooxygenase defect. Journal of Clinical Investigation 71: 762–768

Remuzzi G, Perico N, Zoja C, Corna D, Macconi D, Viganò 1990 Role of endothelium-derived nitric oxide in the bleeding tendency of uremia. Journal of Clinical Investigation 86: 1768–1771

Richman D D, Fischl M A, Grieco M H et al 1987 The toxicity of azidothymidine (AZT) in the treatment of patients with AIDS and AIDS-related complex. A double-blind, placebo-controlled trial. New England Journal of Medicine 317: 192–197

Ridell B, Kutti J, Swolin B, Wadenvik H 1992 Dysplastic megakaryopoiesis with thrombocytopenia and chromosomal aberration. American Journal of Clinical Pathology 98: 227–230

Riedler G F, Straub P W, Frick P G 1971 Thrombocytopenia in septicemia: A clinical study for the evaluation of its incidence and diagnostic value. Helvetica Medica Acta 36: 23–38

Rizzoni G, Claris-Appiani A, Edefonti A et al 1988 Plasma infusion for hemolytic-uremic syndrome in children: Results of a multicenter controlled trial. Journal of Pediatrics 112: 284–290

Rocha E, Llorens R, Paramo J A, Arcas R, Cuesta B, Trenor A M 1988 Does desmopressin acetate reduce blood loss after surgery in patients on cardiopulmonary bypass? Circulation 77: 1319–1323

Rock G A, Shumak K H, Buskard N A et al 1991 Comparison of plasma exchange with plasma infusion in the treatment of thrombotic thrombocytopenic purpura. New England Journal of Medicine 325: 393–397

Rodgers R P C 1990 Bleeding time tables. A tabular summary of pertinent literature. Seminars in Thrombosis and Hemostasis 16: 21–144

Rodgers R P C, Levin J 1990 A critical reappraisal of the bleeding time. Seminars in Thrombosis and Hemostasis 16: 1–20

Romero R, Mazor M, Lockwood C J et al 1989 Clinical significance, prevalence, and natural history of thrombocytopenia in pregnancy-induced hypertension. American Journal of Perinatology 6: 32–38

Roodnat J I, Kauffmann R H, Gerrits W B J, van Zijl A M 1987 Door glafenine veroorzaakte intravasculaire hemolyse met acute nierinsufficiëntie als gevolg van IgG-anti-glafenine-antilichamen. Nederlands Tijdschrift Geneeskunde 131: 2316–2320

Rosborough T K, Swaim W R 1978 Acquired von Willebrand's disease, platelet-release defect, and angiodysplasia. American Journal of Medicine 65: 96–100

Rose M, Eldor A 1987 High incidence of relapses in thrombotic thrombocytopenic purpura. Clinical Study of 38 patients. American Journal of Medicine 83: 437–444

Rossi E, Vimercati A R, Damasio E E et al 1987 Treatment of idiopathic thrombocytopenic purpura in HIV-positive patients with Rhesus antibodies (anti-D). Haematologica 72: 529–532

Roth G J, Siok C J 1978 Acetylation of the NH_2-terminal serine of prostaglandin synthetase by aspirin. Journal of Biological Chemistry 253: 3782–3784

Roy A J, Jaffe N, Djerassi I 1973 Prophylactic platelet transfusions in children with acute leukemia. A dose response study. Transfusion 13: 283–290

Rudders R A, Aisenberg A C, Schiller A L 1972 Hodgkin's disease presenting as 'idiopathic' thrombocytopenic purpura. Cancer 30: 220–230

Rule S, Reed C, Costello C 1991 Fatal haemophagocytic syndromes in HIV-antibody positive patient. British Journal of Haematology 79: 127

Russell N H, Salmon J, Keenan J P, Bellingham A J 1981 Platelet adenine nucleotides and arachidonic acid metabolism in the myeloproliferative disorders. Thrombosis Research 22: 389–397

Sahud M A 1972 Platelet size and number in alcoholic thrombocytopenia. New England Journal of Medicine 286: 355–356

Saji H, Maruya E, Fujii H, Maekawa T, Akiyama Y, Matsuura T 1989 New platelet antigen, Sib^a, involved in platelet transfusion refractoriness in a Japanese man. Vox Sanguinis 56: 283–287

Sakariassen K S, Bolhuis P A, Sixma J J 1980 Platelet adherence to subendothelium of human arteries in pulsatile and steady flow. Thrombosis Research 19: 547–559

Salama A, Mueller-Eckhardt C, Kiefel V 1983 Effect of intravenous immunoglobulin in immune thrombocytopenia. Competitive inhibition of reticuloendothelial system. Function by sequestration of autologous red blood cells? Lancet 2: 193–195

Salama A, Kiefel V, Amberg R, Mueller-Eckhardt C 1984 Treatment of autoimmune thrombocytopenic purpura with Rhesus antibodies (anti-Rh_0[D]). Blut 49: 29–35

Salama A, Mueller-Eckhardt C 1985 The role of metabolite-specific antibodies in nomifensine-dependent immune hemolytic anemia. New England Journal of Medicine 313: 469–474

Salama A, Mueller-Eckhardt C 1992 Use of Rh antibodies in the treatment of autoimmune thrombocytopenia. Transfusion Medicine Reviews 6: 17–25

Salzman E W, Neri L L 1966 Adhesiveness of blood platelets in uremia. Thrombosis et Diathesis Haemorrhagic 5: 84–91

Salzman E W, Weinstein M J, Weintraub R M et al 1986 Treatment with desmopressin acetate to reduce blood loss after cardiac surgery. A double-blind randomized trial. New England Journal of Medicine 314: 1402–1406

Samuels P, Bussel J B, Braitman L E et al 1990 Estimation of the risk of thrombocytopenia in the offspring of pregnant women with presumed immune thrombocytopenic purpura. New England Journal of Medicine 323: 229–235

Sane D C, Califf R M, Topol E J, Stump D C, Mark D B, Greenberg C S 1989 Bleeding after thrombolytic therapy for acute myocardial infarction: Mechanisms and management. Annals of Internal Medicine 111: 1010–1022

Sanfelippo M J, Suberviola P D, Geimer N F 1987 Development of a von Willebrand-like syndrome after prolonged use of hydroxyethyl starch. American Journal of Clinical Pathology 88: 653–655

Santoso S, Shibata Y, Kiefel V, Mueller-Eckhardt C 1987 Identification of the Yuk^b allo-antigen on platelet glycoprotein IIIa. Vox Sanguinis 53: 48–51

Santoso S, Kiefel V, Mueller-Eckhardt C 1989 Immunochemical characterization of the new platelet alloantigen system Br^a/Br^b. British Journal of Haematology 72: 191–198

Sartorius J A 1984 Steroid treatment of idopathic thrombocytopenic purpura in children. Preliminary results of a randomized cooperative study. American Journal of Pediatric Hematology/Oncology 6: 165–169

Savona S, Nardi M, Lennett E T, Karpatkin S 1985 Thrombocytopenic purpura in narcotics addicts. Annals of Internal Medicine 102: 737–741

Schiff E, Peleg E, Goldenberg M et al 1989 The use of aspirin to prevent pregnancy-induced hypertension and lower the ratio of thromboxane A_2 to prostacyclin in relatively high risk pregnancies. New England Journal of Medicine 321: 351–356

Schindler M, Gatt S, Isert P, Morgans D, Cheung A 1990 Thrombocytopenia and platelet functional defects in pre-eclampsia: Implications for regional anaesthesia. Anaesthesia and Intensive Care 18: 169–174

Schmitt G W, Moake J L, Rudy C K, Vicks S L, Hamburger R J 1987 Alterations in hemostatic parameters during hemodialysis with dialyzers of different membrane composition and flow design.

Platelet activation and factor VIII-related von Willebrand factor during hemodialysis. American Journal of Medicine 83: 411–418
Schneider D R, Picker L J 1985 Myelodysplasia in the acquired immunodeficiency syndrome. American Journal of Clinical Pathology 84: 144–152
Schneider P A, Abrams D I, Rayner A A, Hohn D C 1987 Immunodeficiency-associated thrombocytopenic purpura (IDTP). Response to splenectomy. Archives of Surgery 122: 1175–1178
Schoenfeld Y, Eldar M, Bedazovsky B, Levy M J, Pinkhas J 1980 Aortic stenosis associated with gastrointestinal bleeding. A survey of 612 patients. American Heart Journal 100: 179–182
Schoots A, Mikkers F, Cramers C, De Smet R, Ringoir S 1984 Uremic toxins and the elusive middle molecules. Nephron 38: 1–8
Schreiber A D, Chien P, Tomaski A, Cines D B 1987 Effect of danazol in immune thrombocytopenic purpura. New England Journal of Medicine 316: 503–508
Schwartz K A, Slichter S J, Harker L A 1982 Immune-mediated platelet destruction and thrombocytopenia in patients with solid tumors. British Journal of Haematology 51: 17–24
Scott R B, Robb-Smith A H T 1939 Histiocytic medullary reticulosis. Lancet 2: 194–198
Scott E P, Moilan-Bergeland J, Dalmasso A P 1988 Posttransfusion thrombocytopenia associated with passive transfusion of a platelet-specific antibody. Transfusion 28: 73–76
Segal B M, Weintraub M I 1976 Hashimoto's thyroiditis, myasthenia gravis, idiopathic thrombocytopenic purpura (letter). Annals of Internal Medicine 85: 761
Segonds A, Louradour N, Suc J M, Orfila C 1979 Postpartum hemolytic uremic syndrome: A study of three cases with a review of the literature. Clinical Nephrology 12: 229–242
Shattil S J, Bennett J S, McDonough M, Turnbull J 1980 Carbenicillin and penicillin G inhibit platelet function in vitro by impairing the interaction of agonists with the platelet surface. Journal of Clinical Investigation 65: 329–337
Shemin D, Elnour M, Amarantes B, Abuelo J G, Chazan J A 1990 Oral estrogens decrease bleeding time and improve clinical bleeding in patients with renal failure. American Journal of Medicine 89: 436–440
Shepard K V, Bukowski R M 1987 The treatment of thrombotic thrombocytopenic purpura with exchange transfusions, plasma infusions, and plasma exchange. Seminars in Hematology 24: 178–193
Sheridan D, Carter C, Kelton J G 1986 A diagnostic test for heparin-induced thrombocytopenia. Blood 67: 27–30
Sheth K J, Gill J C, Leichter H E 1990 High-dose intravenous gamma globulin infusions in hemolytic-uremic syndrome: A preliminary report (letter). American Journal of Diseases of Children 144: 268–270
Shibata Y, Matsuda I, Miyaji T, Ichikawa Y 1986a Yuk[a], a new platelet antigen involved in two cases of neonatal alloimmune thrombocytopenia. Vox Sanguinis 50: 177–180
Shibata Y, Miyaji T, Ichikawa Y, Matsuda I 1986b A new platelet antigen system, Yuk[a]/Yuk[b]. Vox Sanguinis 51: 334–336
Shim W K T 1968 Hemangiomas of infancy complicated by thrombocytopenia. American Journal of Surgery 116: 896–906
Shorr R I, Kao K-J, Pizzo S V, Rauckman E J, Rosen G M 1985 In vitro effects of acetaminophen and its analogues on human platelet aggregation and thromboxane B_2 synthesis. Thrombosis Research 38: 33–43
Shulman N R, Jordan J V Jr 1982 Platelet immunology. In: Colman R W, Hirsh J, Marder V H, Salzman E W (eds) Hemostasis and thrombosis: basic principles and clinical practice. Lippincott, Philadelphia, p 274–342
Shulman N R, Aster R H, Leitner A, Hiller M C 1961 Immunoreactions involving platelets. V. Post-transfusion purpura due to a complement-fixing antibody against a genetically controlled platelet antigen. A proposed mechanism for thrombocytopenia and its relevance in 'autoimmunity'. Journal of Clinical Investigation 40: 1597–1620
Shulman N R, Marder V J, Hiller M C, Collier E M 1964 Platelet and leukocyte isoantigens and their antibodies: Serologic, physiologic and clinical studies. Progress in Hematology 4: 222–304
Sibai B M, Taslimi M M, El-Nazer A, Amon E, Mabie B C, Ryan G M 1986 Maternal-perinatal outcome associated with the syndrome of hemolysis, elevated lever enzymes, and low platelets in severe preeclampsia-eclampsia. American Journal of Obstetrics and Gynecology 155: 501–509
Siddiqui F A, Lian E C Y 1985 Novel platelet-agglutinating protein from a thrombotic thrombocytopenic purpura plasma. Journal of Clinical Investigation 76: 1330–1337
Sidiropoulos D, Straume B 1984 The treatment of neonatal isoimmune thrombocytopenia with intravenous immunoglobulin (IgG i.v.). Blut 48: 383–386
Siegel R S, Rae J L, Barth S et al 1989 Platelet survival and turnover: Important factors in predicting response to splenectomy in immune thrombocytopenic purpura. American Journal of Hematology 30: 206–212
Silverstein M N, Petitt R M, Solberg L A Jr, Fleming J S, Knight R C, Schacter L P 1988 Anagrelide: A new drug for treating thrombocytosis. New England Journal of Medicine 318: 1292–1294
Simon T L, Collins J, Kunicki T J, Furihata K, Smith K J, Aster R H 1988 Posttransfusion purpura associated with alloantibody specific for the platelet antigen, Pen[a]. American Journal of Hematology 29: 38–40
Sinha R K, Kelton J G 1990 Current controversies concerning the measurement of platelet-associated IgG. Transfusion Medicine Reviews 4: 121–135
Sloand E M, Sloand J A, Prodouz K et al 1991 Reduction of platelet glycoprotein Ib in uraemia. British Journal of Haematology 77: 375–381
Smeets R E H, Hillen H F P 1988 Acquired amegakaryocytic thrombocytopenic purpura. Treatment with high-dose dexamethasone pulse therapy and review of the literature. Netherlands Journal of Medicine 32: 27–33
Smith J W, Kelton J G, Horsewood P et al 1989 Platelet specific alloantigens on the platelet glycoprotein Ia/IIa complex. British Journal of Haematology 72: 534
Snyder E L, Moroff G, Simon T, Heaton A, and Members of the Ad Hoc Platelet Radiolabeling Study Group 1986 Recommended methods for conducting radiolabeled platelet survival studies. Transfusion 26: 37–42
Snyder H W Jr, Bertram J H, Henry D H et al 1991 Use of protein A immunoadsorption as a treatment for thrombocytopenia in HIV-infected homosexual men: A retrospective evaluation of 37 cases. AIDS 5: 1257–1260
Soff G A, Levin J 1988 Thrombocytopenia associated with repletion of iron in iron-deficiency anemia. American Journal of the Medical Sciences 295: 35–39
Soloman J, Bofenkamp T, Fahey J L, Chillar R K, Beutler E 1978 Platelet prophylaxis in acute non-lymphoblastic leukaemia (letter). Lancet 1: 267
Sonnenblick M, Kramer M R, Hershko C 1986 Corticosteroid responsive immune thrombocytopenia in Hodgkin's disease. Oncology 43: 349–353
Spearing R L, Hickton C M, Sizeland P, Hannah A, Bailey R R 1990 Quinine-induced disseminated intravascular coagulation. Lancet 336: 1535–1537
Spivak J L, Bender B S, Quinn T C 1984 Hematological abnormalities in AIDS. American Journal of Medicine 77: 224–228
Spychal R T, Wickham N W R 1985 Thrombocytopenia associated with ranitidine. British Medical Journal 291: 1687
Srivastava R N, Moudgil A, Bagga A, Vasudev A S 1991 Hemolytic uremic syndrome in children in northern India. Pediatric Nephrology 5: 284–288
Standen G R, Lillicrap D P, Matthews N, Bloom A L 1986 Inherited thrombocytopenia, elevated serum IgA and renal disease: Identification as a variant of the Wiskott–Aldrich syndrome. Quarterly Journal of Medicine 59: 401–408
Stass S A, Holloway M L, Peterson V, Creegan W J, Gallivan M, Schumacher H R 1979 Cytoplasmic fragments causing spurious platelet counts in the leukemic phase of poorly differentiated lymphocytic leukemia. American Journal of Clinical Pathology 71: 125–128
Staszewski H, Colbourn D, Donovan V, Ludman H 1989 Thrombotic thrombocytopenic purpura: Report of a case with a possible response to high-dose intravenous gamma globulin. Acta Haematologica 82: 201–204

Steering Committee of the Physicians' Health Study Research Group 1988 Preliminary report: Findings from the aspirin component of the ongoing Physicians' Health Study. New England Journal of Medicine 318: 262–264
Stein M F, Cimino J E, Brescia M J 1970 Subdural hematoma during hemodialysis. New York State Journal of Medicine 70: 2022–2024
Steinberg M H, Kelton J G, Coller B S 1987 Plasma glycocalicin. An aid in the classification of thrombocytopenic disorders. New England Journal of Medicine 317: 1037–1042
Stenhammar L, Ljunggren C G 1988 Thrombocytopenic purpura and coeliac disease. Acta Paediatrica Scandinavica 77: 764–766
Stewart A K, Glynn M F X 1990 Acquired von Willebrand disease associated with free lambda light chain monoclonal gammopathy, normal bleeding time and response to prednisone. Postgraduate Medical Journal 66: 560–562
Stoll D B, Blum S, Pasquale D, Murphy S 1981 Thrombocytopenia with decreased megakaryocytes. Evaluation and prognosis. Annals of Internal Medicine 94: 170–175
Stricker B H C, Barendregt J N M, Claas F H J 1985 Thrombocytopenia and leucopenia with mianserin-dependent antibodies. British Journal of Clinical Pharmacology 19: 102–104
Stroncek D F, Vercellotti G M, Hammerschmidt D E, Christie D J, Shankar R A, Jacob H S 1992 Characterization of multiple quinine-dependent antibodies in a patient with episodic hemolytic uremic syndrome and immune granulocytosis. Blood 80: 241–248
Stuard I D, Heusinkveld R S, Moss A J 1972 Microangiopathic hemolytic anemia and thrombocytopenia in primary pulmonary hypertension. New England Journal of Medicine 287: 869–870
Stuart M J 1979 Ethanol-inhibited platelet prostaglandin synthesis in vitro. Journal of Studies in Alcoholism 40: 1–6
Stuart M J, Miller M L, Davey F R, Wolk J A 1979 The post-aspirin bleeding time: A screening test for evaluating hemostatic disorders. British Journal of Haematology 43: 649–659
Stubbs T M, Lazarchick J, Horger E O III 1984 Plasma fibronectin levels in preeclampsia: A possible biochemical marker for vascular endothelial damage. American Journal of Obstetrics and Gynecology 150: 885–887
Stubbs T M, Lazarchick J, van Dorsten J P, Cox J, Loadholt C B 1986 Evidence of accelerated platelet production and consumption in nonthrombocytopenic preeclampsia. American Journal of Obstetrics and Gynecology 155: 263–265
Suarez C R, Rademaker D, Hasson A, Mangogna L 1986 High-dose steroids in childhood acute idiopathic thrombocytopenia purpura. American Journal of Pediatric Hematology/Oncology 8: 111–115
Sugai S, Tachibana J, Shimizu S, Konda S 1989 Thrombocytopenia in patients with Sjogren's syndrome (letter). Arthritis and Rheumatism 32: 234
Sullivan L W, Adams W H, Liu Y K 1977 Induction of thrombocytopenia by thrombopheresis in man: Patterns of recovery in normal subjects during ethanol ingestion and abstinence. Blood 49: 197–207
Swiss Group for Clinical Studies on the Acquired Immunodeficiency Syndrome (AIDS) 1988 Zidovudine for the treatment of thrombocytopenia associated with human immunodeficiency virus (HIV): A prospective study. Annals of Internal Medicine 109: 718–721
Taaning E, Morling N, Ovesen H, Svejgaard A 1985 Posttransfusion purpura and anti-Zw^b (-Pl^{A2}). Tissue Antigens 26: 143
Takahashi H, Nagayama R, Tanabe Y, Satoh K, Hanano M, Mito M, Shibata A 1986 DDAVP in acquired von Willebrand syndrome associated with multiple myeloma. American Journal of Hematology 22: 421–429
Takahashi I, Sano M, Okamoto H et al 1991 A human T cell leukemia virus type-I carrier with recurrent thrombocytopenia and various autoantibodies. Acta Medica Okayama 45: 445–449
Take H, Tomiyama Y, Shibata Y et al 1990 Demonstration of the heterogeneity of epitopes of the platelet-specific alloantigen, Bak^a. British Journal of Haematology 76: 395–400
Takishita S, Kawazoe N, Yoshida T, Fukiyama K 1990 Ticlopidine and thrombocytopenia (letter). New England Journal of Medicine 323: 1487
Tallman M S, Kwaan H C 1992 Reassessing the hemostatic disorder associated with acute promyelocytic leukemia. Blood 79: 543–553
Tan E M, Cohen A S, Fries J F et al 1982 The 1982 revised criteria for the classification of systemic lupus erythematosus. Arthritis and Rheumatism 25: 1271–1277
Telek B, Kiss A, Pecze K, Ujhelyi P, Rak K 1989 Cyclic idiopathic pure acquired amegakaryocytic thrombocytopenic purpura: A patient treatment with cyclosporin A. British Journal of Haematology 73: 128–129
Teng C-M, Huang T-F 1991 Snake venom constituents that affect platelet function. Platelets 2: 77–87
Thebault J J, Blatrix C E, Blanchard J F, Panak E A 1975 Effects of ticlopidine, a new platelet aggregation inhibitor in man. Clinical Pharmacology and Therapeutics 18: 485–490
Thompson C B, Jakubowski J A 1988 The pathophysiology and clinical relevance of platelet heterogeneity. Blood 72: 1–8
Tohen M, Castillo J, Cole J O, Miller M G, de los Heros R, Farrer R J 1991 Thrombocytopenia associated with carbamazepine: a case series. Journal of Clinical Psychiatry 52: 496–498
Tomiyama Y, Take H, Honda S et al 1990a Demonstration of platelet antigens that bind platelet-associated autoantibodies in chronic ITP by direct immunoprecipitation procedure. British Journal of Haematology 75: 92–98
Tomiyama Y, Take H, Ikeda H et al 1990b Identification of the platelet-specific alloantigen, Nak^a, on platelet membrane glycoprotein IV. Blood 75: 684–687
Tomiyama Y, Kekomaki R, McFarland J, Kunicki T J 1992 Antivinculin antibodies in sera of patients with immune thrombocytopenia and in sera of normal subjects. Blood 79: 161–168
Travis W D, Li C-Y, Bergstralh E J, Yam L T, Swee R G 1988 Systemic mast cell disease. Analysis of 58 cases and literature review. Medicine 67: 345–368
Tricot G, Criel A, Verwilghen R L 1982 Thrombocytopenia as presenting symptom of preleukaemia in 3 patients. Scandinavian Journal of Haematology 28: 243–250
Trimble M S, Glynn M F X, Brain M C 1991 Amegakaryocytic thrombocytopenia of 4 years duration: Successful treatment with antithymocyte globulin. American Journal of Hematology 37: 126–127
Tyler D S, Shaunak S, Bartlett J A, Iglehart J D 1990 HIV-1-associated thrombocytopenia. The role of splenectomy. Annals of Surgery 211: 211–217
Vadhan-Raj S, Keating M, LeMaistre A et al 1987 Effects of recombinant human granulocyte-marcophage colony-stimulating factor in patients with myelodysplastic syndromes. New England Journal of Medicine 317: 1545–1552
van Buren D, van Buren C T, Flechner S M, Maddox A M, Verani R, Kahan B D 1985 De novo hemolytic uremic syndrome in renal transplant recipients immunosuppressed with cyclosporine. Surgery 98: 54–62
van der Lelie J, Lange J M A, Vos J J E, van Dalen C M, Danner S A, van dem Borne A E G K 1987 Autoimmunity against blood cells in human immunodeficiency-virus (HIV) infection. British Journal of Haematology 67: 109–114
Vander Salm T J, Ansell J E, Okike O N et al 1988 The role of epsilon-aminocaproic acid in reducing bleeding after cardiac operation: A double-blind randomized study. Journal of Thoracic and Cardiovascular Surgery 95: 538–540
van Geet C, Spitz B, Vermylen J, van Assche F A 1990 Urinary thromboxane metabolites in pre-eclampsia. Lancet 335: 1168–1169
van Hoff J, Ritchey A K 1988 Pulse methylprednisolone therapy for acute childhood idiopathic thrombocytopenic purpura. Journal of Pediatrics 113: 563–566
van Oostveen J W, Breit T M, de Wolf J T M et al 1992 Polyclonal expansion of T-cell receptor-$\gamma\delta^+$ T lymphocytes associated with neutropenia and thrombocytopenia. Leukemia 6: 410–418
van Vliet H H D M, Kappers-Klunne M C, van der Hel J W B, Abels J 1987 Antibodies against glycosphingolipids in sera of patients with idiopathic thrombocytopenic purpura. British Journal of Haematology 67: 103–108
Verdirame J D, Feagler J R, Commers J R 1985 Multiple myeloma associated with immune thrombocytopenic purpura. Cancer 56: 1199–1200
Viganò G, Gaspari F, Locatelli M, Pusineri F, Bonati M, Remuzzi G

1988 Dose-effect and pharmacokinetics of estrogens given to correct bleeding time in uremia. Kidney International 34: 853–858
Viganò G, Zoja C, Corna D et al 1990 17β Estradiol is the most active component of the conjugated estrogen mixture active on uremic bleeding by a receptor mechanism. Journal of Pharmacology and Experimental Therapeutics 252: 344–348
Vigliano E M, Horowitz H I 1967 Bleeding syndrome in a patient with IgA myeloma: Interaction of protein and connective tissue. Blood 29: 823–836
Visentin G P, Newman P J, Aster R H 1991 Characteristics of quinine- and quinidine-induced antibodies specific for platelet glycoproteins IIb and IIIa. Blood 77: 2668–2676
Vitacco M, Sanchez Avalos J, Gianantonio C A 1973 Heparin therapy in the hemolytic-uremic syndrome. Journal of Pediatrics 83: 271–275
Vlachoyannis J, Schoeppe W 1982 Adenylate cyclase activity and cAMP content of human platelets in uraemia. European Journal of Clinical Investigation 12: 379–381
von dem Borne A E G Kr, Decary F 1990 Nomenclature of platelet specific antigens. British Journal of Haematology 74: 239–240
von dem Borne A E G Kr, von Riesz E, Verheugt F W A et al 1980 Bak[a], a new platelet-specific antigen involved in neonatal alloimmune thrombocytopenia. Vox Sanguinis 39: 113–120
von dem Borne A E G K, Vos J J E, Pegels J G, Thomas L L M, van der Lelie H 1988 High dose intravenous methylprednisolone or high dose intravenous gammaglobulin for autoimmune thrombocytopenia. British Medical Journal 296: 249–250
von dem Borne A E G, van Oers R H J, Wiersinga W M, van der Tweel J G 1990 Complete remission of autoimmune thrombocytopenia after extirpation of a benign adenofibroma of the ovary. British Journal of Haematology 74: 119–120
Voss R, Matthias F R, Borkowski G, Reitz D 1990 Activation and inhibition of fibrinolysis in septic patients in an internal intensive care unit. British Journal of Haematology 75: 99–105
Waldenström J 1951 Three new cases of purpura hyperglobulinemia. A study in long-lasting benign increase in serum globulin. Acta Medica Scandinavica Suppl. 266: 931–946
Walker J A, Sherman R A, Eisinger R P 1985 Thrombocytopenia associated with intravenous desferrioxamine. American Journal of Kidney Diseases 6: 254–256
Walker W S, Yap P L, Kilpatrick D C, Boulton F E, Crawford R J, Sang C T M 1988 Post-transfusion purpura following open heart surgery: Management by high dose intravenous immunoglobulin infusion. Blut 57: 323–325
Wallach P M, Flannery M T, Adelman H M et al 1991 Retroperitoneal fibrosis accompanying immune thrombocytopenia. American Journal of Hematology 37: 204–205
Wallenburg H C S, Dekker G A, Makovitz J W, Rotmans P 1986 Low-dose aspirin prevents pregnancy-induced hypertension and pre-eclampsia in angiotensin-sensitive primigravidae. Lancet 1: 1
Walls J T, Curtis J J, Silver D, Boley T M, Schmaltz R A, Nawarawong W 1992 Heparin-induced thrombocytopenia in open heart surgical patients: Sequelae of late recognition. Annals of Thoracic Surgery 53: 787–791
Walsh C M, Karpatkin S 1990 Thrombocytopenia and human Immunodeficiency virus-1 infection. Seminars in Oncology 17: 367–374
Walsh C M, Nardi M A, Karpatkin S 1984 On the mechanism of thrombocytopenic purpura in sexually active homosexual men. New England Journal of Medicine 311: 635–639
Walsh C, Krigel R, Lennette E, Karpatkin S 1985 Thrombocytopenia in homosexual patients. Prognosis, response to therapy, and prevalence of antibody to the retrovirus associated with the acquired immunodeficiency syndrome. Annals of Internal Medicine 103: 542–545
Wang W C 1988 Evans syndrome in childhood: Pathophysiology, clinical course, and treatment. American Journal of Pediatric Hematology/Oncology 10: 330–338
Wang L, Juji T, Shibata Y, Kuwata S, Tokunaga K 1991 Sequence variation of human platelet membrane glycoprotein IIIa associated with the Yuk[a]/Yuk[b] alloantigen system. Proceedings of the Japanese Academy 67(B): 102–106
Ware J A, Clark B A, Smith M, Salzman E W 1989 Abnormalities of cytoplasmic Ca^{2+} in platelets from patients with uremia. Blood 73: 172–176
Warkentin T E, Kelton J G 1990a Current concepts in the management of immune thrombocytopenia. Drugs 40: 531–542
Warkentin T E, Kelton J G 1990b Heparin and platelets. Hematology/Oncology Clinics of North America 4: 243–264
Warkentin T E, Kelton J G 1991 Heparin-induced thrombocytopenia. Progress in Hemostasis and Thrombosis 10: 1–34
Warkentin T E, Santos A V, Hayward C P M, Horsewood P, Kelton J G 1991 Platelet-derived microparticles are produced by heparin-induced thrombocytopenia sera and other platelet Fc receptor stimuli (abstract). Blood 78 (suppl 1): 343a
Warkentin T E, Hayward C P M, Smith C M, Kelly P M, Kelton J G 1992a Determinants of donor platelet variability when testing for heparin-induced thrombocytopenia. Journal of Laboratory and Clinical Medicine 120: 371–379
Warkentin T E, Moore J C, Morgan D G 1992b Aortic stenosis and bleeding gastrointestinal angiodysplasia: Is acquired von Willebrand's disease the link? Lancet 340: 35–37
Warkentin T E, Smith J W, Hayward C P M, Ali A M, Kelton J G 1992c Thrombocytopenia caused by passive transfusion of anti-glycoprotein Ia/IIa alloantibody (anti-HPA-5b). Blood 79: 2480–2484
Warkentin T E, Soutar R L, Panju A, Ginsberg J S 1992d Acute systemic reactions to intravenous heparin bolus therapy: Relationship to heparin-induced thrombocytopenia (abstract). Blood 80 (suppl 1): 160a
Watkins S P Jr, Shulman N R 1970 Platelet cold agglutinins. Blood 36: 153–158
Weinberger I, Rotenberg Z, Fuchs J, Ben-Sasson E, Agmon J 1987 Amiodarone-induced thrombocytopenia. Archives of Internal Medicine 147: 735–736
Weiner C P 1988 The mechanism of reduced antithrombin III activity in women with preeclampsia. Obstetrics and Gynecology 72: 847–849
Weinstein L 1982 Syndrome of hemolysis, elevated liver enzymes, and low platelet count: A severe consequence of hypertension in pregnancy. American Journal of Obstetrics and Gynecology 142: 159–167
Weismann R E, Tobin R W 1958 Arterial embolism occurring during systemic heparin therapy. Archives of Surgery 76: 219–227
Weiss H J 1967 The effect of clinical dextran on platelet aggregation, adhesion and ADP release in man: In vivo and in vitro studies. Journal of Laboratory and Clinical Medicine 69: 37–46
Weiss H J, Aledort L M 1967 Impaired platelet/connective-tissue reaction in man after aspirin ingestion. Lancet 2: 495–497
Weiss H J, Eichelberger J W 1963 Secondary thrombocytopathia: Platelet factor 3 in various disease states. Archives of Internal Medicine 112: 827–834
Weiss H J, Rosove M H, Lages B A, Kaplan K L 1980 Acquired storage pool deficiency with increased platelet-associated IgG. Report of five cases. American Journal of Medicine 69: 711–717
Wentz A C 1982 Adverse effects of danazol in pregnancy. Annals of Internal Medicine 96: 672–673
West S G, Johnson S C 1988 Danazol for the treatment of refractory autoimmune thrombocytopenia in systemic lupus erythematosus. Annals of Internal Medicine 108: 703–706
Weston M J, Rubin M H, Langley P G, Westaby S, Williams R 1977 Effects of sulphinpyrazone and dipyridamole on capillary bleeding time in man. Thrombosis Research 10: 833–840
Wiedmer T, Hall S E, Ortel T L, Kane W H, Rosse W F, Sims P J 1991 Complement-induced vesiculation and exposure of membrane prothrombinase sites in PNH platelets (abstract). Blood 78 (suppl 1): 387a
Williame L M, Joos R, Proot F, Immesoete C 1987 Gold-induced aplastic anemia. Clinical Rheumatology 6: 600–605
Williams R C 1961 Aortic stenosis and unexplained gastrointestinal bleeding. Archives of Internal Medicine 108: 859–864
Winiarski J 1989 IgG and IgM antibodies to platelet membrane glycoprotein antigens in acute childhood idiopathic thrombocytopenic purpura. British Journal of Haematology 73: 88–92
Wisløff F, Godal H C 1981 Prolonged bleeding time with adequate

platelet count in hospital patients. Scandinavian Journal of Haematology 27: 45–50
Wolf B, Conradty M, Grohmann R, Rüther E, Witzgall H, Londong V 1989 A case of immune complex hemolytic anemia, thrombocytopenia, and acute renal failure associated with doxepin use. Journal of Clinical Psychiatry 50: 99–100
Wong K F, Hui P K, Chan J K C, Chan Y W, Ha S Y 1991 The acute lupus hemophagocytic syndrome. Annals of Internal Medicine 114: 387–390
Woodman R C, Harker L A 1990 Bleeding complications associated with cardiopulmonary bypass. Blood 76: 1680–1697
Woodruff R K, Grigg A P, Firkin F C, Smith I L 1986 Fatal thrombotic events during treatment of autoimmune thrombocytopenia with intravenous immunoglobulin in elderly patients. Lancet 2: 217–218
Woods V L Jr, Oh E H, Mason D, McMillan R 1984a Autoantibodies against the platelet glycoprotein IIb/IIIa complex in patients with chronic ITP. Blood 63: 368–375
Woods V L Jr, Kurata Y, Montgomery R R, Tani P, Mason D, Oh E H, McMillan R 1984b Autoantibodies against platelet glycoprotein Ib in patients with chronic immune thrombocytopenic purpura. Blood 64: 156–160
Woods V L Jr, Pischel K D, Avery E D, Bluestein H G 1989 Antigenic polymorphism of human very later activation protein-2 (platelet glycoprotein Ia-IIa). Platelet alloantigen Hc^a. Journal of Clinical Investigation 83: 978–985
Xiros N, Binder T, Anger B, Böhlke J, Heimpel H 1988 Idiopathic thrombocytopenic purpura and autoimmune hemolytic anemia in Hodgkin's disease. European Journal of Haematology 40: 437–441
Yamamoto N, Ikeda H, Tandon N N et al 1990 A platelet membrane glycoprotein (GP) deficiency in healthy blood donors: Nak^{a-} platelets lack detectable GPIV (CD36). Blood 76: 1698–1703
Yau T M, Carson S, Weisel R D et al 1992 The effect of warm heart surgery on postoperative bleeding. Journal of Thoracic and Cardiovascular Surgery 103: 1155–1163
Yoshida K, Wakui H, Mamiya S, Yamaguchi A, Miura A B 1987 Bolus methylprednisolone therapy in adult idiopathic thrombocytopenic purpura. Japanese Journal of Medicine 26: 172–175
Yoshida Y, Hirashima K, Asano S, Takaku F 1991 A phase II trial of recombinant human granulocyte colony-stimulating factor in the myelodysplastic syndromes. British Journal of Haematology 78: 378–384
Yue C P, Mann K S, Chan K W 1987 Severe thrombocytopenia due to combined cimetidine and phenytoin therapy. Neurosurgery 20: 963–965
Zahavi J, Marder V J 1975 Acquired 'storage pool disease' of platelets associated with circulating antiplatelet antibodies. American Journal of Medicine 56: 883–890
Zauli G, Re M C, Davis B et al 1992 Impaired in vitro growth of purified ($CD34^+$) hematopoietic progenitors in human immunodeficiency virus-1 seropositive thrombocytopenic individuals. Blood 79: 2680–2687
Zenon G J, Cadle R M, Hamill R J 1991 Vancomycin-induced thrombocytopenia. Archives of Internal Medicine 151: 995–996
Zoja C, Viganò G, Bergamelli A, Benigni A, De Gaetano G, Remuzzi G 1988 Prolonged bleeding time and increased vascular prostacyclin in rats with chronic renal failure: Effects of conjugated estrogens. Journal on Laboratory and Clinical Medicine 112: 380–386
Zoja C, Noris M, Corna D et al 1991 L-Arginine, the precursor of nitric oxide, abolishes the effect of estrogens on bleeding time in experimental uremia. Laboratory Investigation 65: 479–483
Zucker-Franklin D, Cao Y 1989 Megakaryocytes of human immunodeficiency virus-infected individuals express viral RNA. Proceedings of the National Academy of Sciences, USA 86: 5595–5599
Zuckerman G R, Cornette G L, Clouse R E, Harter H R 1985 Upper gastrointestinal bleeding in patients with chronic renal failure. Annals of Internal Medicine 102: 588–592
Zwaginga J J, IJsseldijk M J W, Beeser-Visser N, De Groot P G, Vos J, Sixma J J 1990 High von Willebrand factor concentration compensates for a primary adhesion defect in uremic blood. Blood 75: 1498–1508
Zwaginga J J, IJsseldijk M J W, de Groot P G, Vos J, de Bos Kuil R L J, Sixma J J 1991a Defects in platelets adhesion and aggregate formation in uremic bleeding disorder can be attributed to factors in plasma. Arteriosclerosis and Thrombosis 11: 733–744
Zwaginga J J, IJsseldijk M J W, de Groot P G et al 1991b Treatment of uremic anemia with recombinant erythropoietin also reduces the defects in platelet adhesion and aggregation caused by uremic plasma. Thrombosis and Haemostasis 66: 638–647

SECTION 8

Abnormalities of coagulation

34. Haemophilia and related inherited coagulation defects

C. R. Rizza

The mechanism of haemostasis following injury may be considered to consist of three apparently separate but closely interlinked stages. The first stage follows within a few seconds of injury, and consists of vasoconstriction in the damaged capillary. This is followed in a very short time by the adhesion of platelets to the damaged endothelium, by platelet aggregation to one another and their fusion to form a haemostatic plug. These two stages together are commonly considered to be the primary phase of haemostasis and are responsible for the initial cessation of bleeding from the damaged vessel. The next phase, the secondary phase, consists of activation of the blood coagulation mechanism with formation of fibrin strands which consolidate the platelet plug. The description above may suggest a distinct sequence of events with vascular, platelet and blood coagulation mechanisms acting at different times. This almost certainly is not the case and it is more likely that the different components act in concert from the moment of injury.

The importance of these different processes relative to each other and the order in which they act is to some extent determined by the nature and severity of the injury. In small blood vessels and capillaries, vasoconstriction and platelet adhesion are probably sufficient by themselves to achieve and maintain haemostasis with fibrin formation playing little part. This view is supported by the well-known observation that severely affected haemophiliacs, who have marked impairment of fibrin formation but normal platelet function, do not bleed excessively from skin punctures and superficial scratches whereas patients with quantitative or qualitative platelet defects bleed excessively from such wounds.

In more severe wounds with more tissue damage and involvement of larger blood vessels, normal clotting and fibrin deposition seems to be necessary for cessation of bleeding. In the case of large arteries containing blood at high pressure, contraction of the vessel is an important part of the haemostatic process and if contraction does not occur the blood components of the haemostatic process are unlikely by themselves to control bleeding. Detailed accounts of the part played in haemostasis by the vessel wall, platelets and the blood coagulation mechanism are given in previous Chapters.

The most severe bleeding disorders are associated with failure of the blood clotting mechanism due to a deficiency of one or more of the blood clotting factors. The deficiency may be congenital or acquired. Acquired deficiencies usually involve several factors whereas congenital deficiencies, apart from some rare instances, are single factor deficiencies. Some properties of the blood coagulation factors are shown in Table 34.1.

HAEMOPHILIA A AND HAEMOPHILIA B

Haemophilia A (classical haemophilia) and haemophilia B (Christmas disease) are the most severe and most important of the inherited bleeding disorders and will now be discussed in some detail.

The haemorrhagic features of haemophilia A and haemophilia B (Christmas disease) are identical and much of the detailed discussion of haemophilia which follows applies also to Christmas disease. The type of bleeding seen in some of the other bleeding disorders is different from that seen in haemophilia and will be described later (p. 830).

Classical haemophilia (haemophilia A) and Christmas disease (haemophilia B) are inherited life-long bleeding disorders. Both are inherited as sex-linked recessive conditions and are limited almost exclusively to males. The bleeding manifestations of the two conditions are identical and it is not possible to distinguish one from the other clinically.

HAEMOPHILIA A

Haemophilia A is the commonest of the severe inherited bleeding disorders and has been described in most human races and in several animal species including the dog (Graham et al 1975), the cat (Cotter et al 1978) and the horse (Archer 1961). Bleeding is due to a deficiency of factor VIII coagulant activity and the severity of bleeding

Table 34.1 Some properties of factors involved in blood coagulation and haemostasis

Factor	Common name	Molecular weight	Approximate amount normal plasma (μg/ml)	In vivo half life
I	Fibrinogen	340 000	3000–4000	3–4 day
II	Prothrombin	72 000	200	72 h
III	Tissue factor	220 000–300 000	0	
IV	Calcium ion	–	50	
V	Proaccelerin	300 000	10	15 h
VII	Proconvertin	63 000	1	4 h
VIII	Antihaemophilic factor	280 000	0.05	8–12 h
IX	Christmas factor	55 000	4	12–24 h
X	Stuart–Prower factor	55 000	6–8	50 h
XI	Plasma thromboplastin antecedent	160 000	8	60 h
XII	Hageman factor	90 000	40	50 h
XIII	Fibrin-stabilizing factor	320 000	30	4–7 days
Pre kallikrein	Fletcher factor	80 000	30–40	
High molecular weight Kininogen	HMWK; Fitzgerald, Flaujeac, or Williams factor	120 000	80	
	Protein C	62 000	5	
	von Willebrand's factor	>1.5 million 220 000 subunits	8	24 h

Table 34.2 Relationship of plasma factor VIII level to the severity of bleeding in haemophilia

Plasma level of factor VIII (iu/dl)	Bleeding manifestations
>40	None
20–40	Tendency to bleed after major injury, often not diagnosed
5–20	Bleeding after minor injury and surgery
1–5	Severe bleeding after minor injury. Ocasional haemarthroses and 'spontaneous' bleeding
<1	Severe haemophilia, spontaneous haemarthroses and muscle haemorrhages, joint ankylosis and crippling

Table 34.3 Haemophilia A patients registered at Haemophilia Centres in UK (1990) showing the severity of the coagulation defect and age

Age	Number of patients at factor VIII levels (%) <2% AN	2–10% AN	>10% AN	Not known	Total
<5	135	83	44	1	263
5–9	173	103	78	3	357
10–14	147	114	93	5	359
15–19	164	128	113	11	416
20–29	482	315	271	26	1094
30–39	409	269	221	27	926
40–49	275	226	176	19	696
50–59	137	149	142	11	439
60–69	66	110	136	11	323
70+	39	72	93	8	212
Not known	21	16	10	207	254
Total	2048	1585	1377	329	5339

is related to the concentration of factor VIII in the blood. Patients with low levels of factor VIII (<1–2 iu/dl) tend to bleed frequently and to bleed spontaneously into joints and muscles (Table 34. 2).

Prevalence figures for humans show considerable variation. This may be due to true differences in incidence, failure to diagnose the condition because of poor diagnostic facilities, or early death of sufferers because of environmental conditions. Statistics collected by the UK Haemophilia Centre Directors (1990) show prevalence of approximately 90 per million of population. Similar figures have been published from other European countries (Brackmann et al 1976, Mannucci & Ruggeri 1976, Nilsson 1976) and from the United States (US Department of Health Education and Welfare 1980). 39% of the 5 300 haemophilia A patients registered in the United Kingdom in the 1990 survey were severely affected with factor VIII levels of <2% of normal (Table 34.3).

Inheritance

Haemophilia A is transmitted as a sex-linked disorder. The gene for factor VIII production is situated near the end of the long arm of the X chromosome (Xq28). It is a large and complex gene (186 kb containing 26 exons) and codes for a large protein (2332 amino acids) arranged into six domains; three of these domains (A_1 A_2 A_3) are homologous to caeruloplasmin; two (C_1 C_2) are homologous to discoidin; and one domain, designated B, seems to play little part in the clotting process and is lost during the activation of factor VIII by thrombin. Interestingly domains A and C are also homologous to domains found in factor V. A large number of gene defects causing haemophilia have been identified. Most of these mutations are single nucleotide substitutions and only about 5% are insertions or deletions. The molecular biology of haemophilia is discussed in more detail in Chapters 36 and 37.

The mode of inheritance of haemophilia is illustrated in Figure 34.1. From this it can be seen that all of the sons of a haemophiliac are normal but all of his daughters are carriers. The children of a female carrier have an equal

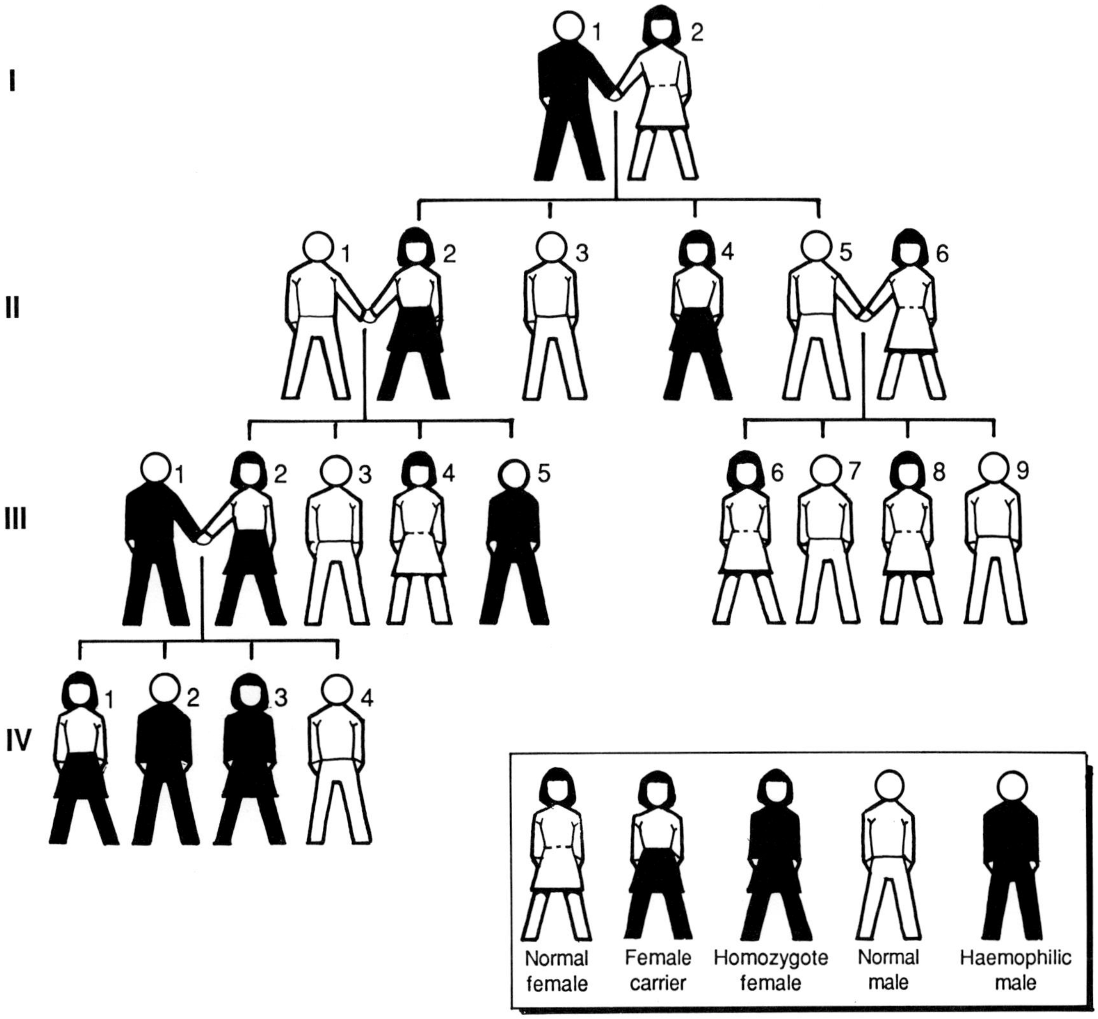

Fig. 34.1 Mode of transmission of haemophilia A and Christmas disease (haemophilia B) showing: transmission of gene by affected male — I 1; transmission of gene by carrier female — II 2; transmission of gene by affected male marrying carrier female — III 1 and III 2.

chance of being normal or affected if they are male and an equal chance of being normal or carriers if they are female. On rare occasions marriage between an affected male and a carrier female has occurred and has produced affected (homozygous) females. One such family in which there was a first cousin marriage was described by Treves (1886) and studied further in later years by Handley & Nussbrecher (1935), Merskey (1951) and Kernoff & Rizza (1973).

From epidemiological studies it appears that 30–40% of haemophiliacs have no previous family history of the disorder (Kerr 1965). This may be due to the abnormal gene passing down through several generations of carrier females without an affected male being born, so that when an affected male is eventually born the event is thought to be due to mutation. The mutation rate in man has been estimated to lie between 2 and 4 × 10^{-5} per generation (Andreassen 1943, Haldane 1947, Ikkala 1960). Calculations carried out before 1955 would unwittingly have included Christmas disease along with haemophilia. The severity of the factor VIII deficiency and bleeding symptoms run true in a particular family so that haemophilic relatives of a severely affected patient are severely affected whereas mildly affected patients tend to have mildly affected relatives. This point is of considerable importance when advising families about transmission of the condition and when prenatal diagnosis and possible termination of pregnancy is being discussed.

Clinical features

The first manifestation of haemophilia appears in early childhood but not during the neonatal period unless the child sustains some injury or undergoes surgery such as circumcision. For the first 6–9 months the child may appear to be normal without evidence of external bleeding or bruising. It has been speculated that the factor VIII from the mother may have crossed the placenta into the child but there is no evidence for this and samples of cord blood obtained from severely-affected boys immediately after birth are usually severely deficient in factor VIII. Moreover with a half life of approximately 12 hours it is extremely unlikely that any factor VIII which had crossed from mother to child could afford protection to the child for more than a few days. A more likely explanation of the absence of bleeding in early life is that the child in his cradle is protected sufficiently to avoid trauma and consequent bleeding. The picture changes however with the eruption of the child's incisor teeth and when he begins to crawl. Bleeding from the mouth is a common early manifestation of haemophilia and is usually caused by the child biting his tongue or lip. The bleeding tends to be intermittent, usually starting again when the child eats or cries, and may persist for many days or weeks resulting in severe anaemia. As the child progresses to crawling and then to walking he begins to suffer the inevitable twists and knocks associated with these activities and experiences skin bruising and haemorrhages into muscles and joints. Skin bruising is usually lumpy and often tender and commonly follows a direct blow. They are rarely a cause for concern unless very large. In a child with no previous family history of haemophilia the appearance of frequent bruising may lead to the parents being accused of 'baby battering'.

Bleeding into joints

Bleeding into joints is the most characteristic feature of severe haemophilia and is seen in the great majority of patients with factor VIII levels of <2% of normal (Fig. 34.2). Mildly affected haemophiliacs rarely have haemarthroses and are not prone to the long-term crippling effects of joint bleeding. Swelling of the joints was well recognised in the early clinical reports but it was not then recognised that the swelling was due to accumulation of blood in the joint. This was suggested by Dubois in 1838 but not until Konig's detailed report in 1892 of joint pathology in eight patients seen at his Gottingen clinic was it was generally accepted that the swelling and joint changes were due to bleeding. From his observations he recognised three stages in the pathological process.

1. An initial bleeding into the joint (haemarthrosis)
2. An inflammatory stage affecting cartilage and bone (panarthritis)
3. A final stage with permanent joint changes with erosion and destruction of cartilage and bone (regression).

In the severely affected patient joint bleeding usually starts at 2 or 3 years of age and continues throughout the patient's life. In many instances there is a history of preceding injury but in a significant number of episodes the patient cannot recall any twist or knock and bleeding seems to be spontaneous. The knees, ankles, elbows, wrists, shoulders and hips are most commonly affected. The joints of the hands are rarely affected.

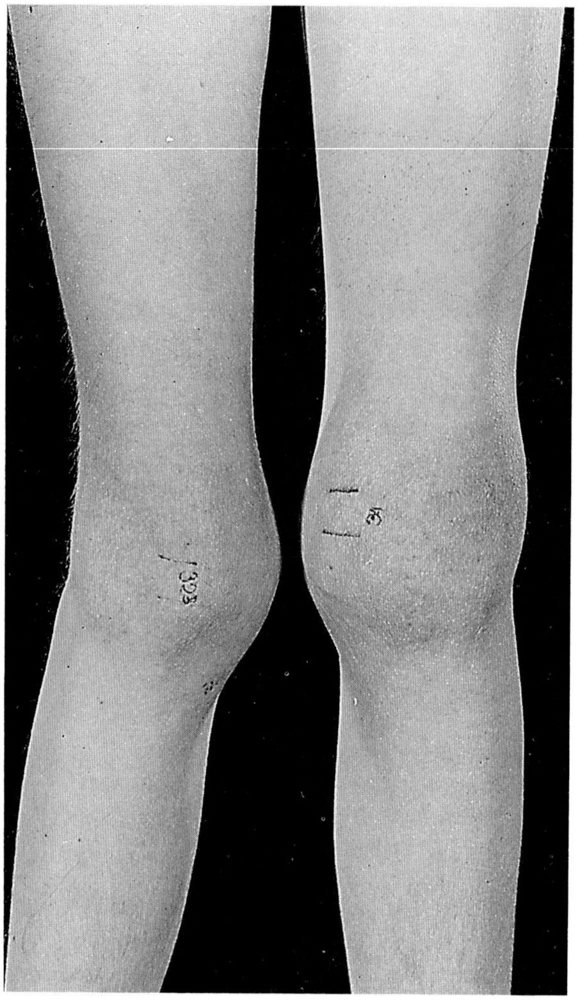

Fig. 34.2 Acute haemarthrosis of left knee. Note deformity of right knee and marked wasting of quadriceps muscles in both thighs.

Acute haemarthrosis

Bleeding into joints is the most prominent feature of severe haemophilia and it is unusual for a severely affected patient to reach adult life without having experienced haemarthrosis. The absence of a history of joint bleeding in an adult haemophiliac strongly suggests that the disease is present in a mild form. The preponderance of bleeding into knees, elbows and ankles over other joints is difficult to explain (Duthie & Rizza 1975, Houghton & Dickson 1978). It may be significant that the 'target' joints are hinge joints whereas the hip and shoulder joints are 'ball and socket' joints. Mild rotational stresses may be accommodated easily by the hip and shoulder whereas in hinge joints such stresses even although mild may cause sufficient injury to initiate bleeding. Once a joint has suffered several episodes of bleeding it often becomes the 'target' for further bleeding probably because of the chronic changes of hyperaemia and hyperplasia of the synovial membrane and joint instability resulting from the wasting of surrounding muscles. Inhibition and wasting of the quadriceps femoris muscles is a frequent and important consequence of bleeding in the knee and predisposes to further bleeding into the joint. Bleeding into one joint especially a knee or an ankle may be followed by bleeding into other joints. This has often been ascribed to the patient being in a 'bad spell'. A more likely explanation is that the original haemorrhage causes the patient to walk abnormally in an attempt to spare the bleeding joint and thereby places stress on other joints causing them to bleed. The use of walking sticks or crutches to spare the lower limbs may cause bleeding into elbows and shoulders.

Clinical features of acute haemarthrosis

Many patients say that before the onset of pain and swelling of acute haemarthrosis they are aware of premonitory abnormal sensations in the joint. They often find it difficult to describe these sensations which may include a pricking sensation, a feeling of warmth in the joint, slight stiffness or weakness. Patients soon come to recognise the significance of their particular premonitory symptoms and use them as an indication for prompt transfusion therapy.

Pain is the main disabling complaint in acute joint bleeding. This has been attributed in part to the irritating effect of blood in the synovial cavity but probably of greater importance is the rapid distension of the joint capsule which takes place. It has been shown by de Andrade et al (1965) that rapid distension of the knee joint with saline causes severe pain as well as inhibition of quadriceps femoris function. Further evidence for joint distension being the cause of the pain comes from the observation that the severe pain in haemarthrosis often diminishes dramatically with the aspiration of only a few ml of blood from the joint. In addition to pain, joint bleeding is accompanied by swelling, tenderness and heat in the joint. There is also limitation of movement with the joint held some way between full extension and flexion in a position in which the volume of the joint space is maximal and the intra-articular pressure minimal. Older patients with a badly damaged and fibrosed synovium may show very little joint swelling when they bleed but the pain may be very severe.

Before the appearance of HIV infection and AIDS in haemophiliacs, pain, swelling and heat in the joint could be confidently diagnosed as being due to haemarthrosis. Now however the possibility of pyoarthrosis must be kept in mind especially if the pain and swelling persists in spite of adequate factor replacement and if the patient is pyrexial and generally unwell. Blood culture and joint aspiration will usually reveal the diagnosis.

Aetiology and histopathology of haemarthrosis

Very little is known about the exact site of haemorrhage in joint bleeding and much of the information available has been obtained from studies in haemophilic dogs. In autopsy examinations of 33 dogs (Swanton & Wysocki 1957, Swanton 1957) it was noted that the earliest evidence of bleeding consisted of small synovial and subsynovial haemorrhages. These appeared to rupture into the joint cavity before becoming large. In joints which had suffered repeated bleeding the synovial villi were larger than normal with hyperplastic surface cells, and increased fibrous tissue and showed infiltration with lymphocytes and plasma cells. Occasionally small clots were sticking to the synovial membrane. Adhesions between adjacent villi were noted and these reduced the volume of the joint cavity and decreased the mobility of the joint capsule. Mild to moderate haemosiderosis was seen in synovial villi and this was often associated with orange-brown pigmentation of articular cartilage and tendons.

In joints which had repeated episodes of bleeding, more severe changes were seen. The tissue pigmentation was more marked and there was fibrous thickening of the synovium and widespread scarring and new fibrous tissue formation. All of these changes contributed to limitation of joint mobility. The articular cartilage showed foci of fibrillary degeneration, pitting and erosion, and irregular growth of cartilage and bone altered the shape of the surfaces. Areas of rarefaction or bone cysts may be seen in the bone adjacent to the joint which are thought to be due to degeneration of cartilage and bone rather than bone haemorrhage. Hoagland (1967) has been able to reproduce the changes characteristic of haemophilic arthropathy by injecting 1–4 ml of autologous blood six times a week into the knees of puppies.

Chronic haemophilic arthropathy

Joints which have been the target of repeated bleeding over many years show chronic degeneration changes. These changes have been well described and affect mainly the knees, ankles, elbows and hips (Ahlberg 1965, Duthie et al 1972, Arnold & Hilgartner 1977). The severity of the changes are usually directly related to the number of haemarthroses in the joint although occasionally a single severe joint haemorrhage may result in extensive joint damage.

Clinical features of chronic arthropathy. The most striking features of chronic haemophilic arthritis are loss of joint movement, fixed flexion contractures, and severe muscle wasting as a consequence of disuse. Imbalance in the action of major muscle groups especially in the thigh may lead to valgus deformities of the lower leg, and rotational deformities and posterior subluxation of the tibia on the femur (Fig. 34.3). In the very severe and advanced

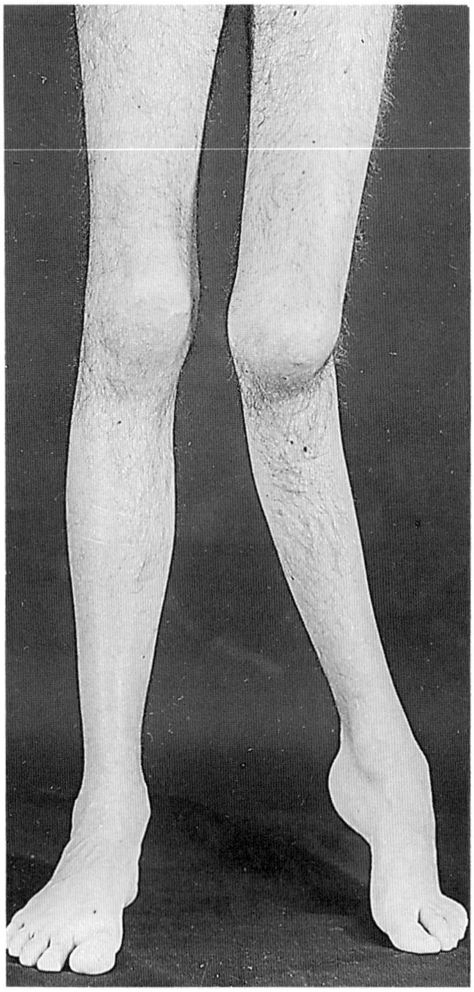

Fig. 34.3 Gross joint deformity resulting from recurrent joint haemorrhage with joint destruction.

cases, the joint may be ankylosed with complete loss of movement. Where there is still some movement in the joint, chronic pain is a common feature requiring potent analgesic drugs for its relief. Acute bleeding tends to be less frequent but when it does occur, may be extremely painful because of the tight fibrosed and contracted joint space. As a consequence of these changes the patient is severely crippled and may be confined to a wheelchair. The severe changes described above are found mainly in patients who have received no treatment or inadequate treatment with coagulation factors. During the past 20 years large amounts of potent blood coagulation factor concentrates have become available and severe crippling deformities are now less common in younger haemophiliacs who have had access to treatment with concentrates for most of their lives.

Radiology. There have been several detailed studies of the radiological changes found in haemophilic arthropathy (Ahlberg 1965, Boldero & Kemp 1966, Pettersson et al 1980). Boldero and Kemp (1966) stressed that the radiological changes seen are not diagnostic of haemophilia and may be seen in other kinds of joint disease. The radiological features of haemophilic arthropathy include epiphyseal overgrowth with enlargement of bone ends, squaring of the patella and widening of the intercondylar notch. As the joint damage progresses there is a loss of cartilage space with gross irregularity of the articular surfaces, subchondral collapse, the appearance of subchondral cysts and the development of osteophytes (Fig. 34.4). Osteoporosis is commonly seen in radiographs of joints which have been targets of repeated bleeding. Changes in joint alignment can be clearly shown on radiography with posterior subluxation of the tibia on the femur and lateral shift of the tibia on the femur being not uncommon.

Bleeding into muscles

Bleeding into muscles is the second most common type of bleeding seen in severely affected haemophiliacs. Usually this occurs after trauma but on many occasions appears to be spontaneous (Hartmann & Diamond 1957, Wilkinson et al 1961, Duthie et al 1972). Intramuscular injection of drugs is a well-known avoidable cause of muscle haematomas and should be strictly forbidden.

The muscles most frequently affected in the upper limbs are the flexor group while in the lower limbs there is a predominance of bleeding into the gastrocnemius and soleus muscles. The iliacus muscle is a particularly important site of bleeding. This muscle is closely confined behind by the pelvis and in front by the strong iliacus fascia and has the femoral nerve running across its anterior surface. Because of this, even quite small haematomas can cause severe pain with flexion and adduction of the hip as well as rapid impairment of femoral nerve function. Haemorrhages into the psoas muscles or into the retroperitoneal space may be of sufficient volume to cause severe hypovolaemia and hypotension and may endanger life.

The presence of a large volume of blood under pressure causes death of muscle fibres which can be seen on microscopy as anuclear structures within the haematoma. Within a few hours of the onset of bleeding a cellular reaction to the presence of blood becomes apparent; polymorphonuclear leukocytes appear followed by phagocytic mononuclear cells and immature connective tissue cells. The dead muscle and blood clots are slowly absorbed and healing by fibrosis takes place.

Haemophilic pseudo-tumours (blood cysts)

Sometimes if the volume of blood in a muscle haematoma is large, the resorption process is incomplete and the haematoma may persist as an encapsulated cystic lesion containing dead muscle and inspissated blood clot (Fraenkel et al 1959). Valderrama & Matthews (1965) described three types of cyst.

1. Simple cysts within the muscle fascial envelope and

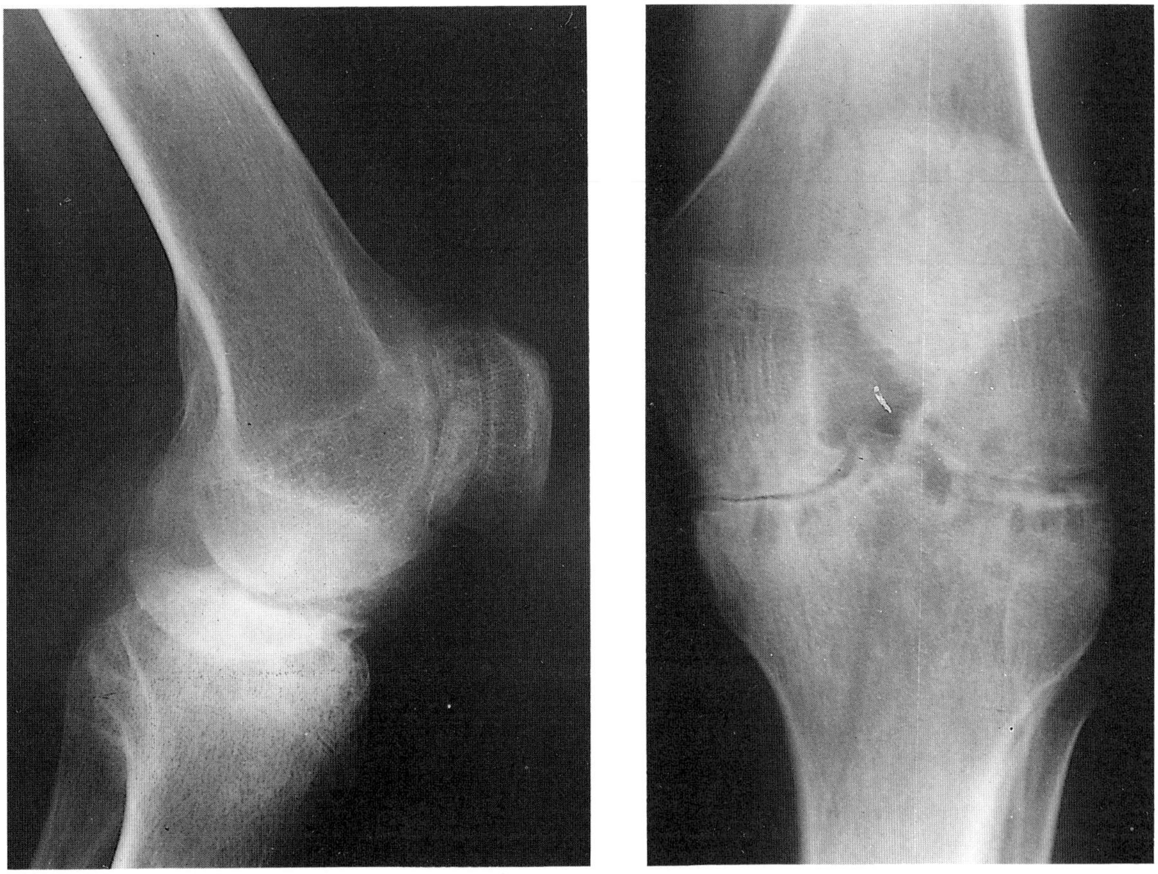

Fig. 34.4 Radiological changes in chronic haemophilic arthropathy of knee. Note loss of joint space, widening of intercondylar notch of femur, subchondral cysts and squaring of lower end of patella.

confined by tendinous attachments. This type of cyst may remain localized or may point through the skin. Bone is not usually involved.

2. Cysts arising in muscles with wide periosteal attachments (Fig. 34.5). These may enlarge to cause cortical erosion and fracture of bone.

3. Cysts arising from periosteal haemorrhage which strips and elevates the periosteum causing destruction of overlying muscle and underlying bone. Occasionally pseudo-tumours seem to arise from bone itself possibly as the result of intraosseous haemorrhage (Fig. 34.6).

Blood cysts were often thought in the past to be sarcomatous hence the name 'pseudo-tumour'. In many cases biopsy was undertaken with serious consequences including death as a result of haemorrhage or infection.

Clinical features of blood cysts. A muscle cyst usually presents as a painful mass which has grown large over months or years. There is often a history of an early injury resulting in a haematoma which never completely resolved and which enlarged and diminished over the years but became generally larger. The most common anatomical sites are the thigh and the pelvis but a number of cases have been reported in feet, hands and arms. X-ray shows

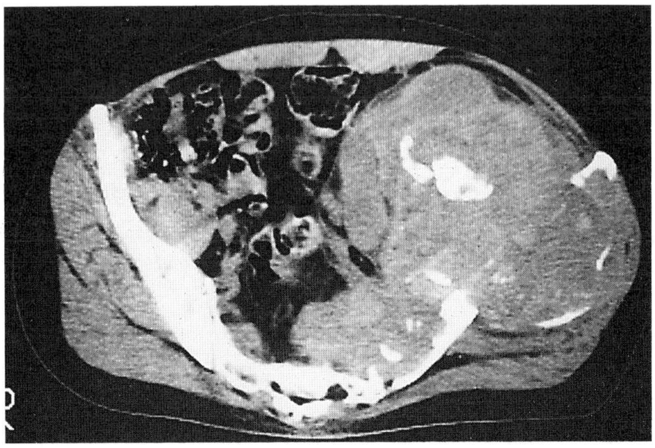

Fig. 34.5 CT scan showing haemophilic pseudo-tumour destroying ileum on left side and invading anterior aspect of sacrum.

the large soft tissue mass sometimes with destruction of adjacent bone and new irregular bone formations. Pseudo-tumours in bone may show gross destruction of the normal architecture of bone with large cyst spaces and greatly thinned bone cortex. Additional information may be obtained from ultrasonic scanning or CT scanning (Fig. 34.5).

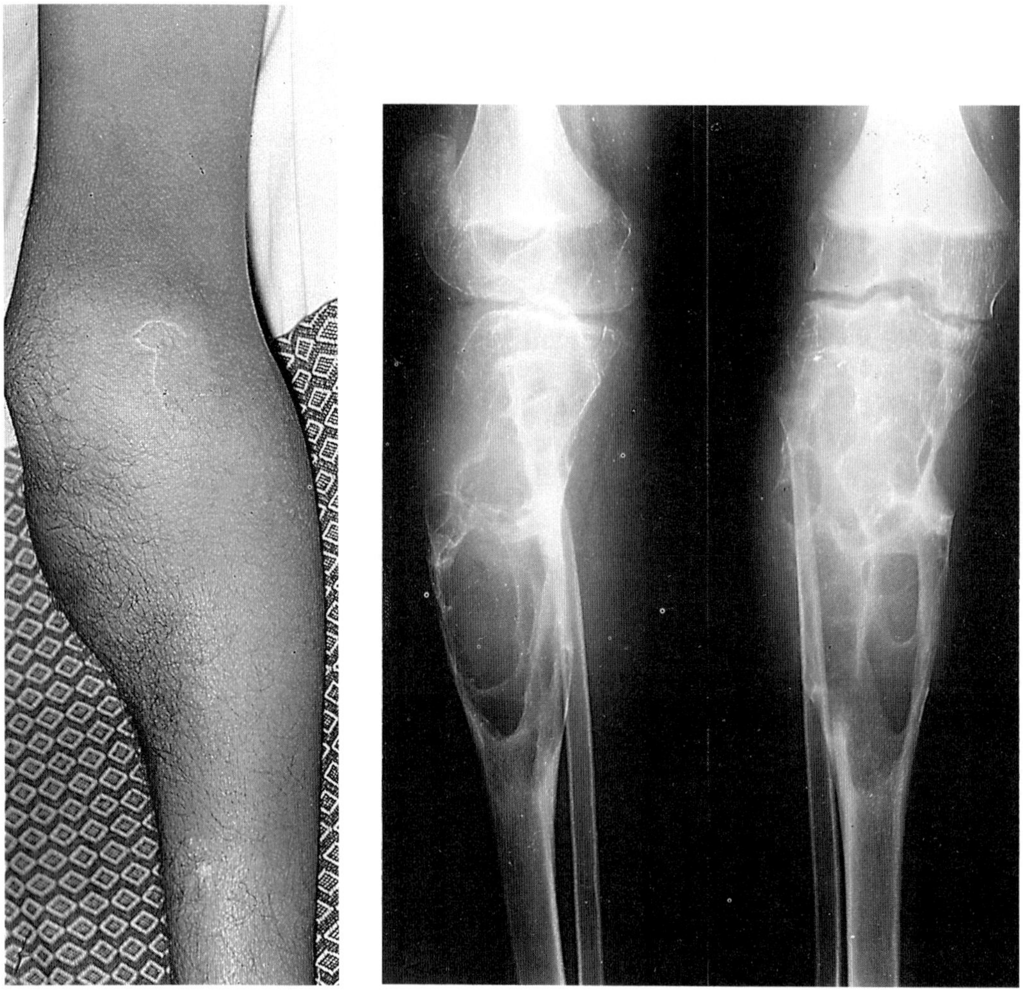

A B

Fig. 34.6 **A**, Haemophilia pseudo-tumour of bone involving upper end of tibia causing pain and swelling and **B**, lateral and anterior radiograph ic view showing gross destruction of bone and formation of numerous cysts.

Gastrointestinal bleeding

Bleeding from the gut is not uncommon in haemophiliacs (Wilkinson et al 1961, Stuart et al 1966) and, in one study, proven peptic ulceration was found in 13% of the adult haemophilic population (Forbes et al 1973). Thanks to effective treatment with factor VIII concentrate gastrointestinal bleeding is now an uncommon cause of death. These episodes should be investigated in the same way as in the non-haemophiliac. In view of the high incidence of chronic hepatitis seen in haemophilia as a consequence of infection with hepatitis C virus the possibility of bleeding oesophageal varices must be kept in mind.

Bleeding into the bowel wall is uncommon and may involve the stomach or the small or large intestine. Patients usually present with signs of symptoms of bowel obstruction. An important cause of gastrointestinal bleeding in the past was the ingestion of aspirin (Kaneshiro et al 1969, Mielke & Britten 1970). Patients with blood coagulation factor defects should never take aspirin in any form.

Intracranial haemorrhage

Until the appearance of AIDS, intracranial bleeding was the commonest cause of death in haemophiliacs in the United Kingdom and accounted for approximately 25% of all deaths (Rizza & Spooner 1983). Bleeding may be subdural, subarachnoid or into the brain substance (Potter 1965, Davies et al 1966, van Trostenburg 1975). Many haemorrhages seem to occur after apparently trivial injuries to the head but a significant number appear to be spontaneous. It is therefore essential to treat all but the most minor head injuries with factor replacement and to observe closely for 24–48 hours. CT scanning is invaluable in diagnosis and allows early neurosurgical treatment if necessary.

Haematuria

Bleeding from the renal tract is a relatively common feature of haemophilia. It is said to be rare before the age of 12 years and over 90% of severely affected patients will have had at least one episode in their lifetime (Davidson et al 1949). Bleeding usually occurs without warning and without any obvious cause and may continue for many days or weeks in spite of treatment with factor VIII. Usually however it is self-limiting and even in the days when treatment was not available was rarely a cause of death (Legg 1872). The amount of blood lost is rarely sufficient to cause anaemia. Blood loss may be so slight as to only lightly discolour the urine or may be heavy with the passage of clots. In the latter case, pain in the loin and abdomen is common, may be very severe and may require treatment with opiate analgesics. If clots obstruct the ureter, haematuria may cease for a time only to recur when the clot passes down into the bladder and the obstruction is relieved. The long-term effects of repeated haematuria and renal obstruction have been investigated by several workers (Prentice et al 1971, Wright et al 1971, Beck & Evans 1972). Prentice et al (1971), found filling defects in the renal tract in nearly 40% of patients. In addition there was evidence of dilatation of the ureter, renal pelvis or calyx in 10% of those studied. They also found abnormal renal function as measured by creatinine clearance in 30% of patients who had suffered haematuria. Two other studies however (Small et al 1982, Roberts et al 1983) found that renal function was not significantly impaired.

Haemophiliacs with haematuria should be investigated to exclude the presence of renal infection, renal stones and neoplasms. Intravenous pyelography is useful in this respect. Biochemical tests of renal function should also be carried out.

Other types of bleeding

Bleeding from the nose is common in haemophiliacs and usually follows some local injury. Upper respiratory tract infection with congestion of the nasal mucosa seems to predispose to epistaxis. Blood loss may be severe and difficult to control. If packing of the nose is found to be necessary this should be done gently so as not to cause further damage to the mucosa and packs should not be left in place too long for fear of causing local inflammation and further bleeding.

Bleeding from the mucous membranes of the mouth is a common early manifestation of haemophilia. Bleeding from the bitten tongue especially in babies may persist for days or weeks if not treated adequately. The frenulum of the upper lip is a common site for bleeding as it is frequently injured by the child pushing toys into his mouth or by trauma from the bars of his cot. Bleeding into the tongue is less common but it is potentially life-threatening as the tongue may swell rapidly making speech, swallowing and eventually breathing very difficult. Bleeding into the floor of the mouth with respiratory obstruction is a potential hazard when inferior dental nerve block is used during dental treatment without adequate factor replacement. The eruption and dehiscence of the deciduous teeth usually take place without excessive bleeding although a very loose tooth 'rocking' in the gum may cause local trauma and persistent bleeding. Removal of this tooth usually brings about cessation of haemorrhage.

Superficial cuts and needle punctures usually stop bleeding in the normal time. Deeper and more extensive laceration may stop bleeding normally but tend to bleed some hours or days later if the wound is disturbed or becomes infected and factor replacement is not given. Suturing such wounds without giving factor replacement is usually of little benefit as the wound continues to bleed under the stitches, pressure builds up and the wound breaks down. It is an old observation that suturing and application of external pressure does not control haemophilic bleeding from large wounds unless factor VIII replacement is given at the same time.

Bleeding in carriers of haemophilia

It is well known that carriers of haemophilia have factor VIII levels which are on average 50% of those found in normal women. This is due to the fact that one or other of the two X chromosomes in the somatic cells of women undergoes random inactivation (Lyonization) in early development. In the case of carriers of haemophilia, one of the X chromosomes is non-functioning with regard to factor VIII production so that random inactivation results in a factor VIII level of 50% of normal. Occasionally inactivation of the X chromosome is non-random, the normal X chromosome may be over-suppressed so that the factor VIII level may be low enough to cause bleeding symptoms. Besides easy bruising and heavy menstruation such women may bleed after surgery, childbirth and injury. The severity of bleeding symptoms, as in haemophiliacs, is inversely related to the factor VIII level. Management of the pregnant carrier of haemophilia requires close collaboration between the haematologist and the obstetrician. The level of factor VIII should be monitored during pregnancy to confirm that the expected 2–3 fold increase of factor VIII brought about by pregnancy takes place. If the factor VIII level is in the normal range at delivery there would seem to be little risk of excessive bleeding. Over the next 5–6 days however the factor VIII level returns to the pre-pregnancy level and, if this is sufficiently low, late postpartum haemorrhage may occur. It is therefore important to observe these women for 7–10 days after delivery. All obligatory or potential carriers of haemophilia should have their factor VIII level assayed before any form of surgery and, depending on the level, treated with DDAVP or factor VIII concentrate if this seems necessary. All that has been said above applies to carriers of Christmas disease with the important difference that pregnancy causes only a slight increase in the level of factor IX in the blood.

Very rarely females may suffer from severe haemophilia-like bleeding with low levels of factor VIII. The most common cause is marriage of a carrier female to an affected male which may result in a female child receiving an abnormal X chromosome from both parents. A condition like haemophilia has been reported also in women in association with partial deletion of the X chromosome, 45xx/45x mosaicism (Gilchrist et al 1965) and in a 'girl' with a male sex chromatin pattern (Nilsson et al 1959). Occasionally extreme 'Lyonisation' of the normal X chromosome may result in levels of factor VIII sufficiently low to cause severe bleeding into joints and muscles.

Diagnosis of haemophilia

Diagnosis of haemophilia is based on the clinical history, clinical examination and laboratory studies.

Clinical assessment

Severe haemophilia usually causes no problems in diagnosis. The history in a male of prolonged bleeding from injuries to the mouth or tongue in childhood followed later by bleeding into joints and muscles and excessive bleeding following dental extraction and other surgery should alert a doctor to the possibility of severe haemophilia A or B. The more mild forms of these conditions can cause problems in diagnosis, especially if the patient has not been exposed to any surgical intervention or accidental injury.

Enquiry should be made about easy or excessive bruising and some attempt should be made to assess the size of the bruises and whether or not they are accompanied by painful induration which tends to persist. The patient should be questioned about prolonged bleeding after injury and should be asked whether bleeding lasted for hours or days and whether it was intermittent. Intermittent bleeding over several days is a feature of untreated haemophilia. Special attention should be paid to the effects of surgery including dental extraction and tonsillectomy. Absence of bleeding following tonsillectomy makes it unlikely that the patient is suffering from haemophilia, severe or mild, or indeed from any inherited bleeding disorder. The possibility of a recently acquired bleeding disorder of course must always be borne in mind. A detailed family pedigree should be drawn paying particular attention to male members of the patient's maternal side of the family. It is often possible to get some indication of the severity of the condition in the patient by carefully enquiring about an affected male relative. This is of importance when dealing with a young child who has not sustained any injury to date.

Laboratory tests

As haemophilia represents a defect in the intrinsic pathway of blood coagulation only tests dependent on the intrinsic pathway may be abnormal. Hence the prothrombin time is normal as is the bleeding time and platelet count. However the whole blood clotting time, prothrombin consumption test and activated partial thromboplastin time (APTT) are abnormal in severely affected patients although they may be normal in mild haemophilia. The definitive diagnosis of haemophilia requires an assay of factor VIII to be carried out on the patient's plasma. The assay most commonly used is the one-stage assay which is based on the ability of the plasma under study to correct the defect in known haemophilic plasma in the APTT test. This assay depends on the availability of plasma from severely affected HIV-negative haemophiliacs for use as a substrate. Artificial factor VIII-deficient substrates prepared from normal plasma by immuno-absorption are now available (Takase et al 1987). The other assay method used is the two-stage method based on the thromboplastin generation test (TGT).

When carrying out factor VIII assays on plasma, appropriate standards calibrated against National or International standards must be used. Many countries now prepare freeze-dried normal plasma standards which are available as working standards. These may be obtained from the appropriate national organisations. The statistics of bioassay of blood coagulation factors and the importance of standards and controls in these assays have been discussed in detail by Kirkwood & Snape (1984) and Barrowcliffe (1984).

Psychological and socioeconomic problems in haemophiliacs and their families

Severe haemophilia produces considerable psychological strain on the patient and his family. This has increased in recent years with the advent of AIDS. When the diagnosis of haemophilia is first made the parents may experience a whole range of emotions including shock, anger, guilt, bitterness and sadness. The marriage may come under strain with the father blaming the mother, further adding to her sense of guilt. The unpredictability of the haemophilic boy's bleeding episodes causes disruption of his life routine and that of other family members. Normal children in the family may feel neglected as the haemophilic child understandably attracts the attention and concern of parents, relatives and friends and the non-haemophilic children may be the ones to have psychological problems. The provision of home treatment may help alleviate these difficulties as it enables the haemophilic boy and his family to take control of their lives.

Overprotection of the child by the parents, in particular the mother, is a natural reaction and may lead to persisting dependency on the part of the child and damaging emotional interactions and anxieties. On the other hand some adolescent haemophiliacs attempt to 'kick over the traces' and 'be normal', by pursuing dangerous hobbies and pastimes thereby exposing themselves to serious injury. Repeated episodes of bleeding may disrupt education and prevent the boy achieving his full potential. This damages his employment prospects and further adds to his problems. Most haemophiliacs however adapt well to their disorder and live full and productive lives without too many psychological problems along the way. The psychological effect of HIV infection on the haemophiliac and his family are still being assessed. There is no doubt that the psycho-sexual problems in the young haemophiliac are considerable and require great tact and understanding in their handling.

HAEMOPHILIA B (CHRISTMAS DISEASE)

Haemophilia B like haemophilia A is a life-long bleeding disorder which affects males. It is clinically indistinguishable from haemophilia A and is transmitted as a sex-linked recessive disorder. Bleeding is due to a deficiency of factor IX, a vitamin-K dependent liver factor and the severity of bleeding is related to the concentration of factor IX in the blood. During the blood coagulation process factor IX is converted by activated factor XI into an active serine protease (factor IXa) which interacts with thrombin-activated factor VIII (factor VIIIa), phospholipid and calcium ions to activate factor X.

It is now known that there are several variants of haemophilia B. Fantl et al (1956) found that the the plasma of one of their patients contained material which neutralized a factor IX antibody which had developed in another patient. This suggested that the plasma of the first patient contained a factor IX molecule that was biologically inactive. Similar results were obtained in other patients by other workers using a variety of techniques including inhibitor neutralization tests (Roberts et al 1968) counter immunoelectrophoresis (Yang 1978a) Laurell's electroimmunoassay (Orstavik et al 1978) radioimmunoassay and immunoradiometric assays (Thompson 1977, Yang 1977b, Holmberg et al 1980).

A detailed account of the different factor IX variants is given in Chapter 37. From the clinical point of view the severity of bleeding does not seem to be related to the type of variant but to the concentration of factor IX activity in the blood.

An unusual variant of haemophilia B (haemophilia B Leyden) has been described in which there is factor IX deficiency in childhood but after puberty the level of factor IX progressively rises to normal levels at an average rate of 4–5% per year (Veltkamp et al 1970, Briet et al 1982). Study of the DNA of those patients revealed mutations in the factor IX promoter region (Reitsma et al 1988, 1989, Crossley et al 1989).

Incidence

Haemophilia B is less common than haemophilia A (Ratnoff & Margolius 1957) and in the UK the prevalence is approximately 18 per million of population compared with 90 per million for haemophilia A. Occasionally a higher incidence is seen in certain areas because of geographical isolation, as in the Tenna valley in Switzerland (Duckert & Koller 1975) or for religious reasons as in the Amish community in certain parts of the United States (Wall et al 1967).

Diagnosis

The diagnosis is made from the patient's clinical history, family history and specific assay for factor IX. In severely affected patients with factor IX levels of <1% of normal the whole blood clotting time and activated partial thromboplastin time are prolonged and the prothrombin consumption test is abnormal. The prothrombin time is normal (except in patients with haemophilia Bm when tested with bovine thromboplastin) as are the bleeding time, platelet count and levels of all other coagulation factors.

The gene for factor IX has been cloned (Choo et al 1982, Kurachi & Davie 1982) and this has allowed the development of methods for carrier detection and antenatal diagnosis and for the detection of point mutations, deletions or short additions to the factor IX gene which cause haemophilia B. This exciting field is discussed in Chapter 37.

VON WILLEBRAND'S DISEASE

This inherited bleeding disorder was first described by von Willebrand in 1926 in a large family from Foglo, an island in the Aaland archipelago in the Gulf of Bothnia off the coast of Finland. After an extensive study von Willebrand concluded that this new bleeding disorder which he called 'pseudo-haemophilia' differed from classical haemophilia in three important respects:

1. The inheritance was autosomal dominant not sex-linked recessive and affected males and females equally.
2. Those affected bled from mucous membranes and skin. Haemarthroses and deep tissue haemorrhages were uncommon.
3. The skin bleeding time was prolonged which contrasted with the normal bleeding time in haemophiliacs. From this he concluded that the haemostatic defect was due to a qualitative platelet disorder. Later studies have shown that platelets behave abnormally in von Willebrand's disease but that this is due, not to an intrinsic defect in the platelets, but to a defect in their plasma environment.

In 1953 Alexander et al observed that patients with von

Willebrand's disease were deficient in factor VIII (Alexander et al 1951, Alexander & Goldstein 1953). Moreover several studies in patients with von Willebrand's disease showed that infusions of plasma, plasma fractions, normal serum or haemophilic plasma brought about a prolonged rise of factor VIII in the patient's blood (Nilsson et al 1957, Biggs et al 1963, Cornu et al 1963). Also it was shown by Salzman (1963) that the platelets of patients with von Willebrand's disease showed diminished retention when their blood was passed down a column of glass beads. In vivo studies showed diminished platelet adhesion in wounds (Borchgrevink 1960). In 1971 Howard & Firkin observed that ristocetin, an antibiotic similar in structure to vancomycin, caused aggregation of platelets in normal platelet-rich plasma but failed to do so in platelet-rich plasma from patients with von Willebrand's disease. At the same time Zimmerman et al (1971) using precipitating antisera prepared by injecting factor VIII preparations into rabbits showed, in a Laurell electro-immunoassay, that the plasma of patients with von Willebrand's disease lacked a 'factor VIII-related' antigen, now known as von Willebrand's factor antigen (vWFAg) and that this material was present in normal plasma and serum and in haemophilic plasma. In the light of new information the concept of factor VIII relatedness was replaced by the view that factor VIII and vWFAg are distinct molecules with different functions, the vWFAg acting as a carrier and stabilizer for factor VIII.

The biochemical nature and functions of vWFAg and factor VIII have been extensively studied in the past 15 years and the genes for the factors which are located on chromosome 12 and the X chromosome respectively, have been cloned. These details are presented in Chapters 16 and 35 but a brief account is given here to help in understanding the nature of the haemostatic defect in von Willebrand's disease.

von Willebrand's factor antigen is composed of a series of macromolecules of very high molecular weight ($1–15 \times 10^6$). These are built up from basic subunits with a molecular weight of approximately 250 000 which form multimers by disulphide linkage. von Willebrand's factor acts in haemostasis by promoting adhesion of platelets to subendothelium in a reaction between subendothelium components (collagen microfibrils) and a platelet membrane receptor (glycoprotein I). The large multimeric forms of vWFAg seems to be most active in promoting platelet adhesion and aggregation. vWFAg has been demonstrated on the vascular intima of many organs (Bloom et al 1973, de los Santos & Hoyer 1973) and both endothelial cells and megakaryocytes have been shown to synthesize it (Jaffe et al 1973, Nachman et al 1977). It has been suggested that vWFAg, having been secreted into the plasma by the endothelial cells, circulates to another site where it becomes linked to factor VIII. The stability of the vWFAg-VIII complex is calcium dependent.

Varieties of von Willebrand's disease

The use of techniques such as vWF (ristocetin cofactor) assay, two-dimensional immunoelectrophoresis and in particular multimer analysis by means of SDS agarose electrophoresis has made it possible to classify the disease into several types based on the structural and functional abnormalities of vWFAg (Ruggeri et al 1982a). With advances in knowledge this classification no doubt will need to be revised.

Broadly speaking there are three types of von Willebrand's disease (type I, II and III). Types I and II have been subdivided into numerous subgroups (Table 34.4).

Type I von Willebrand's disease

Type I is the commonest form of von Willebrand's disease and accounted for approximately 70% of cases in one study of 116 patients in 47 families (Hoyer et al 1983). Factor VIII, vWFAg and vWF (ristocetin cofactor) are all reduced to roughly the same extent. The bleeding time is prolonged in severely affected patients. If there is sufficient vWFAg to be detected it shows normal mobility on two-dimensional electrophoresis. Multimer analysis shows a normal multimer pattern but with reduced levels (Ruggeri et al 1982).

Several sub-types of type I von Willebrand's disease

Table 34.4 Classification of von Willebrand's disease

Type	Bleeding time	Factor VIII	vWFAg	vWF	Multimer pattern
I	Normal or prolonged	Reduced	Reduced	Reduced	All present but reduced in amount
IIa	Prolonged	Normal or reduced	Normal or reduced	Reduced	Large and intermediate forms absent
IIb	Prolonged	Normal or reduced	Normal or reduced	Normal* or reduced	Large multimers absent
IIc	Prolonged	Normal or reduced	Normal or reduced	Normal or reduced	Large multimers absent but prominent smaller forms or larger and intermediate present with prominent small forms
III	Prolonged	Reduced	None detected	None detected	None detected

* Platelets in platelet-rich plasma aggregated by low concentrations of ristocetin.

have been described based on the relative levels of vWFAg in platelets and plasma and also on the haemostatic response to infusion of DDAVP.

Type II von Willebrand's disease

Type II von Willebrand's disease is characterized by a discordant reduction of factor VIII, vWFAg and vWF (ristocetin cofactor) with vWF being more reduced than factor VIII and vWFAg. Several types of type II von Willebrand's disease have been described. In type IIa the inheritance seems to be autosomal dominant and the bleeding symptoms can be mild or severe. vWF is reduced much more than vWFAg and multimer analysis shows an abnormal pattern with loss of large and intermediate forms. Aggregation of platelets in the patient's platelet-rich plasma on addition of ristocetin is reduced. Two-dimensional immunoelectrophoresis shows increased electrophoretic mobility of vWFAg (Kernoff et al 1974, Peake et al 1974) (Fig. 34.7). vWFAg levels may be found to be higher by Laurell electroimmunoassay than by immunoradiometric assay. In type IIb von Willebrand's disease vWFAg and vWF (ristocetin cofactor) may be variable or may be normal. The large multimers of vWFAg are absent and platelets in the patient's platelet-rich plasma are aggregated by low concentrations of ristocetin which have no effect on normal platelet-rich plasma. This is an important characteristic of type IIb vWD. Some patients in this group show persistent or transient thrombocytopenia. Thrombocytopenia may follow exercise or pregnancy which bring about an increase in the level of vWF. Thrombocytopenia has also been described following administration of DDAVP. These patients apparently synthesize an abnormal vWF which is capable of binding directly to platelets thereby causing aggregation and removal of the platelet from the circulation along with the large vWF multimers attached to them.

Another similar condition, known as 'pseudo von Willebrand's disease' or 'platelet von Willebrand's disease' has been described (Takahashi 1980, Weiss et al 1982). Patients with this condition have clinical and laboratory features similar to type IIb von Willebrand's disease. The pathology here is thought to be an intrinsic defect in the platelets which react with the large multimers of normal vWF, undergo aggregation and are removed from the circulation along with the large multimers attached to them. Administration of DDAVP or cryoprecipitate may cause thrombocytopenia.

A further sub-group of type II known as type IIc has been described. Families with this condition show a double peak on two-dimensional immunoelectrophoresis in some members and a single fast running peak in others

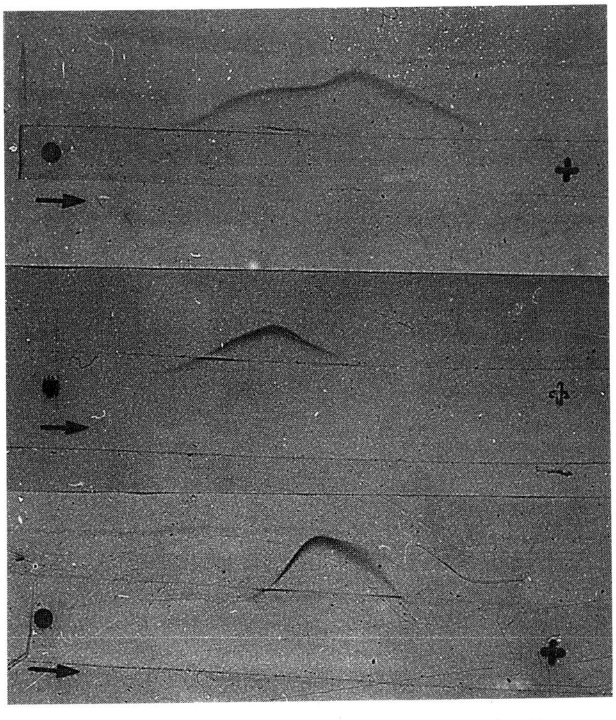

Fig. 34.7 Crossed immunoelectrophoresis of vWFAg showing increased mobility of vWFAg in type II von Willebrand's disease. **A**, patient's plasma; **B**, normal plasma; **C**, mixture of patient's plasma and normal plasma.

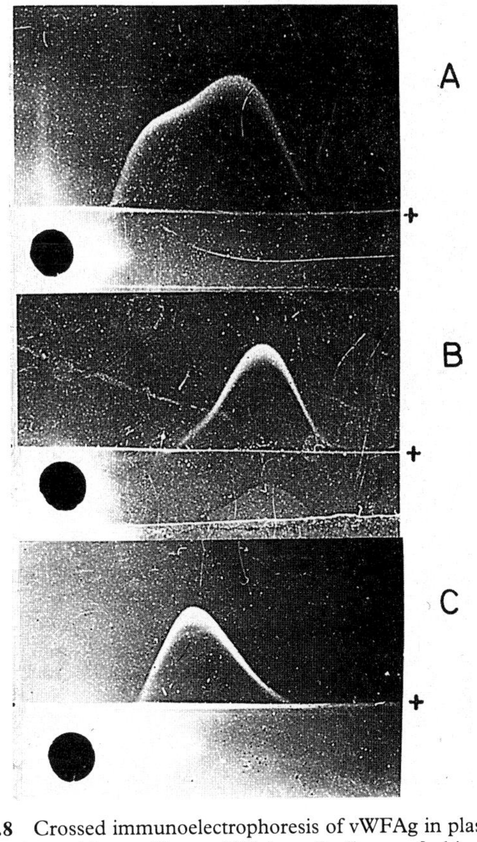

Fig. 34.8 Crossed immunoelectrophoresis of vWFAg in plasma. **B**, from a patient with type IIc von Willebrand's disease; **A**, his mother and **C**, normal plasma.

(Armitage & Rizza 1979, Ruggeri et al 1982b, Mannucci et al 1983) (Fig. 34.8). These results are interpreted as being due to a heterozygous condition (type IIc/normal) in the former subjects and a double heterozygous condition (type IIc/type I) in the latter. Multimer analysis in the heterozygous subject shows large and intermediated forms present but with a marked increase of the smallest multimers. In the double heterozygote, the large and intermediate multimers are absent but the smallest multimers are very prominent (Hoyer et al 1983). Clinically the condition seems very mild.

Type III von Willebrand's disease

In type III von Willebrand's disease, severe bleeding symptoms usually occur with haemophilia-like bleeding such as haemarthrosis and intramuscular bleeding. The skin bleeding time is greatly prolonged, the levels of vWF (ristocetin cofactor) are very low or undetectable (Shoa'i et al 1977, Zimmerman et al 1979) and the level of factor VIII procoagulant activity is low but usually measurable between 2–10% of normal. In addition these patients lack the ability to release tissue plasminogen activator in response to venous occlusion or administration of DDAVP (Ludlam et al 1980, Nilsson et al 1980). The condition is autosomal recessive and the parents of such patients are usually asymptomatic with normal or only a slight reduction in their level of vWFAg. In many cases there is no family history (Italian Working Group 1977). The incidence of parental consanguinity may be high (Shoa'i et al 1977).

Prevalence of von Willebrand's disease

von Willebrand's disease is more common than originally thought although it is difficult to obtain accurate prevalence figures because of the variability of the clinical and laboratory manifestations. Estimations of 30–40 per million and 70 per million have been made for the United Kingdom (Bloom 1980) and Switzerland (Bachman 1980) respectively. In Sweden the reported prevalence is 125 per million with most of these being relatively mild (Holmberg & Nilsson 1985). The prevalence of the severe homozygous form of the disease in Sweden was three per million and even less in other countries (Mannucci et al 1984).

Clinical features

Patients suffering the commoner heterozygous form of von Willebrand's disease, bruise easily and bleed excessively from cuts and scratches. Bleeding from the mucous membranes of the mouth, nose and gastrointestinal tract is common and in women menorrhagia may be very troublesome. Intermenstrual bleeding from the corpus luteum may occur causing abdominal pain and occasionally bleeding may be sufficient to cause a fall in haemoglobin, shock and presentation as an abdominal emergency. Postpartum haemorrhage may occur 7–10 days after delivery by which time the level of the factor VIII complex, raised during pregnancy will have returned to its basal level. Excessive bleeding may occur after dental extraction and all forms of surgery and tends to occur immediately after the injury unlike the bleeding seen in haemophiliacs which may be delayed for many hours after trauma.

Patients with homozygous von Willebrand's disease are severely affected and may have bleeding symptoms similar to those seen in haemophiliacs with recurrent haemarthroses and muscle bleeding in addition to mucous membrane bleeding.

Diagnosis

In the majority of patients, especially those with severe symptoms, the diagnosis can be made on the basis of the clinical picture, the pattern of inheritance and from the bleeding time test and assays of components of the factor VIII complex. In a typical case of von Willebrand's disease the skin bleeding time measured by the template method or by the Ivy method is prolonged and the levels of factor VIII procoagulant activity and von Willebrand's factor antigen are reduced. The ability of the patient's plasma to promote aggregation of washed fixed normal platelets in the presence of ristocetin is also reduced. This activity (ristocetin cofactor activity) is thought to reflect the platelet-related biological function of the larger multimers of von Willebrand's factor antigen. Two dimensional immunoelectrophoresis of vWFAg may give useful information showing increased mobility or selective loss of slow-moving multimers. More information about the multimeric forms of vWFAg can be obtained by SDS agarose electrophoresis of plasma, overlaying the gel with a radiolabelled antibody to vWFAg and then carrying out autoradiography. This technique however is complex and carried out at only a few centres.

The clinical and laboratory features of von Willebrand's disease may vary from member to member in the same family and from time to time in the same individual so that repeated testing may be required to reach a firm diagnosis.

FACTOR V DEFICIENCY (PARAHAEMOPHILIA)

Factor V deficiency was first described by Owren in 1947 in a 29-year-old woman. The condition is very rare and only about 65 families have been described. From the limited information available it seems to be inherited as an autosomal recessive condition although in some families it appears to be partially dominant. Consanguinity in the parents has been reported in several cases. Heterozygotes are usually asymptomatic. Occasionally the parents of a severely affected patient have reduced levels of factor V and are presumably heterozygous for the condition (Rush & Ellis 1965, Seeler 1972). Attempts to demonstrate cross-reacting material in the plasma of factor V-deficient patients using inhibitor neutralization tests have met with little success (Feinstein et al 1970, Fratantoni et al 1972, Giddings et al 1975). However Chin et al (1983) have developed an enzyme-linked immunosorbent assay using a specific factor V antibody raised in a rabbit and were able to demonstrate heterogeneity in four out of 14 patients studied.

Bleeding in factor V-deficient patients is usually relatively mild and includes easy bruising, epistaxis, prolonged bleeding from cuts, menorrhagia and bleeding following surgery. Bleeding into muscles and joints is rare and usually follows injury. In a proportion of cases the skin bleeding time is prolonged. Congenital abnormalities involving the cardiovascular and renal sytems have been described in association with factor V deficiency. Manotti et al (1989) described a family in which several members suffered thromboembolism at a young age. The factor V level was 12% of normal and bleeding after surgery did not seem to be a problem.

The most characteristic laboratory finding is a prolongation of the one-stage prothrombin time and activated partial thromboplastin time which can be corrected by the addition of adsorbed normal plasma but not by aged serum. The diagnosis is confirmed by specific assay for factor V using factor V-deficient plasma as substrate. Since deficient plasma from a severely affected patient is so difficult to obtain it is often necessary to use a factor V-deficient substrate, artificially prepared by prolonged incubation of normal oxalated plasma at 37°C.

FACTOR VII DEFICIENCY

Congenital deficiency of factor VII was first described in 1951 by Alexander and his colleagues. The condition is rare and approximately 100 cases have been described.

The inheritance pattern is probably autosomal recessive. Several different genetic variants of factor VII deficiency have been described. These have been demonstrated using inhibitor (antibody) neutralization tests to detect the presence of cross-reacting material (Goodnight et al 1971, Denson et al 1972, Briet et al 1976, Mazzucconi et al 1977). Additional information has been obtained by studying the reaction of the patient's plasma when tissue thromboplastin from different animals are used in the factor VII assay (Girolami et al 1977, 1978b, 1979, Triplett et al 1985).

The bleeding symptoms of factor VII deficiency are variable. Some patients suffer life-long bleeding whereas others seem to have very little trouble. It is not known if this variability in clinical symptoms reflects variant forms of the factor VII protein. Easy bruising, epistaxis, gastrointestinal bleeding, menorrhagia and haemarthroses are relatively common. Postoperative bleeding may occur but is not a constant feature (Ratnoff 1960, Marder & Shulman 1964).

Laboratory investigations show a prolonged one-stage prothrombin time but a normal whole blood clotting time, activated partial thromboplastin time and Russell's viper (Stypven) time. Specific assay for factor VII using a factor VII-deficient substrate plasma confirms the diagnosis.

FACTOR X (STUART–PROWER FACTOR) DEFICIENCY

Factor X deficiency which is relatively rare, was first described by Telfer et al (1956) and by Hougie et al (1957) in the two families which provided the eponym for the factor. Inheritance is autosomal and consanguinity has been reported in the parents of some affected individuals. A large number of variants of the factor have been defined using antibody neutralization techniques and tests of factor X activation via the extrinsic and intrinsic systems (Fair & Edgington 1985). Denson et al (1970) described six patients with a factor X defect and were able to demonstrate at least five different abnormalities of factor X.

Girolami et al (1970) described a large group of factor X-deficient patients in northern Italy in whom the defect (factor X Friuli) was characterized by a prolonged one-stage prothrombin time when tissue thromboplastin was used but a normal result when Russell's viper venom was used as the activating agent. The patients' plasma contained normal amounts of factor X-like cross-reacting material which showed a line of identity with normal factor X in immunodiffusion studies. They analysed the patients' plasma by one-stage assays for factor X activation by the extrinsic system and the intrinsic system, and with Russell's viper venom. They also assayed factor X by means of a specific radioimmunoassay. From their studies they found a broad spectrum of molecular variants and were able to classify the patients into at least eight groups.

Patients deficient in factor X tend to bleed severely if they are homozygous for the condition and less severely, if at all, if they are heterozygous. Bleeding after dental extraction and other forms of surgery has been described as has menorrhagia in women. Severely affected patients may suffer from haemarthroses and intramuscular haemorrhages. Occasionally the bleeding time is prolonged.

Laboratory findings include a prolonged activated partial thromboplastin time and a prolonged one-stage prothrombin time when tissue thromboplastin is used. As mentioned above, the Russell's viper venom time may be normal in certain variants of factor X deficiency. The thromboplastin generation test is abnormal when the patient's serum is used in the test. The above abnormal tests can be corrected by the addition of normal plasma or normal serum but not by alumina-adsorbed normal plasma.

PROTHROMBIN DEFICIENCY

Congenital deficiency of prothrombin is extremely rare and is probably autosomal in inheritance. Impaired synthesis of prothrombin falls into two broad groups, the hypoprothrombinaemias and dysprothrombinaemias; in the former there is a reduced concentration of the protein as measured by clotting assays and a concordant reduction in protein detectable by immunological assays; in the latter group normal or near normal amounts of the protein are detectable by immunological methods but the biological activity is greatly reduced. Shapiro and his colleagues (1969) described the first cases of dysprothrombinaemia in a family with 11 members affected. They called the prothrombin variant, prothrombin Cardeza. To date there have been about 15 reports of variant prothrombin (Shapiro et al 1969, Girolami et al 1974a, 1978a,b, Owen et al 1978, Bezeaud et al 1979, Guillin et al 1981, Inomoto et al 1987).

Patients with hypoprothrombinaemia and dysprothrombinaemia may bruise easily, bleed excessively after surgery and suffer menorrhagia. Haemarthroses seem to be very rare.

Laboratory studies in hypoprothrombinaemia show a prolongation, often slight, of the one-stage prothrombin time and occasionally a prolongation of the activated partial thromboplastin time. There is a reduction in prothrombin by one-stage or two-stage assays and a comparable reduction of cross-reacting material in immunological assays.

In the dysprothrombinaemias there is a reduced biological activity measured by coagulation tests using tissue extract but normal amounts of cross-reacting material detected by immunological assays. The use of other prothrombin activating agents such as staphylcoagulase and certain snake venoms such as *Echis carinatus* (Saw-scaled viper) *Oxyuranus scutellatus scutellatus* (Taipan), *Dispholidus typus* (Boomslang) and *Notechis scutatus* (Tiger snake) allows more detailed classification of the dysprothrombinaemias.

FIBRINOGEN DEFICIENCY

Inherited deficiency of fibrinogen is extremely rare and may be due to lack of production of the normal molecule (afibrinogenaemia, hypofibrinogenaemia) or to production of a structurally abnormal molecule (dysfibrinogenaemia).

Afibrinogenaemia

Congenital afibrinogenaemia was first described by Rabe & Salomon (1920) and further cases were described by Macfarlane (1938), Pinniger & Prunty (1946), Prentice (1951) and Hardisty & Pinninger (1956). Bleeding problems may occur at birth with bleeding from the umbilical cord. Easy bruising and excessive bleeding from cuts and following surgery has been described. Bleeding may occur from the nose and from the gastrointestinal tract and menorrhagia and postpartum haemorrhage may be troublesome. Cerebral haemorrhage has been noted as a common cause of death. In general the bleeding symptoms are milder than those seen in severe haemophilia and bleeding into muscles and joints with consequent crippling is rare.

Laboratory studies in afibrinogenaemia reveal an infinitely prolonged whole blood clotting time, activated partial thromboplastin time and one-stage prothrombin time. Addition of strong thrombin, ancrod (Arvin) or batroxobin (Reptilase) to the patient's blood or plasma fails to produce a clot and immunological tests reveal that fibrinogen is greatly reduced or absent. The levels of the other clotting factors are normal.

Inherited dysfibrinogenaemia

The first detailed account of an inherited abnormal form of fibrinogen was that of Menaché (1964) although previous reports (Fanconi 1941, Ingram 1955, Imperato & Dettori 1958) had made similar suggestions.

The abnormal fibrinogen molecule is thought to form fibrin clots in a slow and disorderly manner because of (a) slow rate of fibrinopeptide release or (b) slow polymerization of fibrin monomer. A more detailed account of the different fibrinogen variants is given in chapter 22.

Dysfibrinogenaemia seems to be autosomally inherited. The majority of those affected are heterozygous for the abnormality but a number of cases have been shown to be homozygous. A small proportion of patients have symptoms and may bleed from the mucous membranes of mouth, nose, gastrointestinal tract and uterus. Bleeding is thought to be more common in those with defective fibrinopeptide release. In some patients there is a tendency for wounds to break down and for healing to be delayed. Abortion has also been described and a number of patients have suffered repeated episodes of thrombosis. In as many as 50% of patients the condition is not associated with any clinical problems and is usually discovered by chance during routine laboratory investigations. The most consistent laboratory findings, apart from a few exceptions, is a prolonged clotting time of blood or plasma on the addition of thrombin or the snake venoms ancrod or batroxin. The one-stage prothrombin time and the activated partial thromboplastin time are usually variably prolonged. Fibrinogen estimations based on clotting with thrombin show a reduced level but estimations made by salt precipitation methods or by immunological methods usually show normal levels of fibrinogen.

FACTOR XIII (FIBRIN STABLIZING FACTOR) DEFICIENCY

Factor XIII is the precursor of a transglutaminase (transamidase) which covalently bonds and cross-links fibrin monomer thereby rendering the fibrin clot more stable and more resistant to lysis. Factor XIII has a molecular weight of 320 000 and is made up of two subunits a and b which form a tetramer a_2b_2 (Schwartz et al 1973, Israels et al 1973). During clotting, inactive factor XIII is converted to the active form by the action of thrombin in the presence of Ca^{2+}. Calcium ions are required for the dissociation of the a_2b_2 subunits. Most of the transamidase activity is formed in the activated a subunits. The b subunits may act in a regulatory or protective capacity. The first deficient patient was described by Duckert and his colleagues in 1960 although earlier studies had demonstrated the presence of a fibrin-stabilizing factor in normal blood (Robbins 1944, Laki & Lorand 1948). More than 100 cases have now been described. Inheritance is thought to be autosomal recessive and there is often a history of consanguinity in the parents. Biochemical and immunological studies have revealed considerable heterogeneity in the disorder (Lorand et al 1980, Berliner et al 1984).

Clinical features

Homozygotes present with a life-long tendency to bleed which may be severe and result in early death. Prolonged bleeding from the umbilical stump is common as is excessive bruising, bleeding into muscles and post-traumatic bleeding. Bleeding after injury is characteristically delayed several hours and wound healing may be delayed with abnormal scar formation (Duckert et al 1960). This may be due to instability of the clots in the presence of the normal fibrinolytic process, along with an abnormal fibroblast response in the absence of factor XIII (Beck et al 1961). Joint bleeding has also been described. Bleeding from mucous membranes seems to be rare. A significant number of patients suffer intracranial haemorrhage often following some minor injury. This feature alone is good reason for giving prophylactic treatment to severely affected patients. Repeated spontaneous abortion has been described in affected females.

Laboratory diagnosis

All the blood coagulation tests based on fibrin formation as the end point are normal as are the bleeding time, platelet count and tests of platelet function. A simple screening test for severe factor XIII deficiency can be made by observing the solubility of the patient's fibrin clot in 5 M urea solution or 1% monochloracetic acid. In the absence of factor XIII the clot will dissolve within a few hours. This method however is relatively insensitive because as little as 2 or 3% of the normal level of factor XIII will result in an insoluble clot. More sensitive assays may be carried out using covalent incorporation of fluorescent dansylcadaverine or radioactive putrescine into an added protein such as casein (Board 1979). Immunological assays are also available (Barbui et al 1974, Board et al 1980).

CONTACT FACTOR DEFICIENCIES

At least four plasma proteins, factor XI, factor XII, prekallikrein and high molecular weight kininogen (HMWK) are known to be involved in the contact phase of blood coagulation. As a group these have some unique properties which distinguish them from other blood coagulation factors. For example they are strongly adsorbed to negatively-charged surfaces where they can interact more easily; calcium ions are not required for their interaction; the factors take part not only in the early phase of blood coagulation but also in other important parts of the body's defence mechanism such as fibrinolysis, kinin generation and pain production in the acute inflammatory response. In spite of this most people deficient in these factors are asymptomatic apart from factor XI patients who tend to bleed.

Factor XI (plasma thromboplastin antecedent PTA) deficiency

This condition was first described by Rosenthal et al (1953) and occurs mainly in those of Ashkenazi Jewish stock (Biggs et al 1958, Rapaport et al 1961, Leiba et al 1965, Seligsohn 1978). It has been estimated that more than one in a 1000 Jews in Israel are homozygous for the condition (Seligsohn 1978). In the majority of cases which have been studied in detail there is a concordant reduction of factor XI protein and biological activity. Only two or three cases have been described where the protein is present in normal amounts and biological activity reduced.

Three point mutations have recently been described in the factor XI gene in Ashkenazi Jews (Asakai et al 1991). These have been designated type I, type II and type III mutations. In type I there is a fault in the splicing of messenger RNA. This seems to be the least common type of mutation. In type II mutation, the change results in a stop codon leading to premature termination of translation. In type III, a factor XI mutant is produced which undergoes faulty secretion from the cell. The disease is inherited as an autosomal trait. Bleeding tends to be mild and usually follows injury or some surgical procedure. There may be easy bruising and epistaxis and menorrhagia may be troublesome. The severity of bleeding may not correlate well with the degree of the factor deficiency as assessed by laboratory tests (Rimon et al 1976, Edson et al 1967). This makes it difficult to define the level of the factor required for haemostasis or to monitor treatment by means of laboratory tests. Laboratory investigation shows a normal platelet count and prothrombin time. The bleeding time is usually normal although exceptions have been described (Nossel et al 1964). The whole blood clotting time and activated partial thromboplastin time are prolonged. The diagnosis is confirmed by specific assay of factor XI using plasma from a severely deficient patient as a substrate or an artificially prepared substrate (Giddings 1971). If such substrates are not available the celite eluate test of Nossel (1964) is useful.

Factor XII (Hageman factor) deficiency

This conditon was first described by Ratnoff & Colopy (1955) and named after the patient they studied. Individuals with this deficiency have a prolonged whole blood clotting time and activated partial thromboplastin time but, despite this, rarely bleed excessively. Indeed several deficient patients including Mr Hageman himself have died from thrombotic disease (Ratnoff et al 1968, Dyerberg & Stoffersen 1980, Hellstern et al 1983, Lammle et al 1991). A few cases in which bleeding has been a feature have been described (Haanen et al 1961, Didisheim 1962, Ikkala et al 1971). A more detailed account of the biochemical nature of the defect in factor XII deficiency is given in Chapter 12.

Fletcher factor (pre-kallikrein) deficiency

Fletcher factor deficiency was first reported by Hathaway and colleagues (1965) in four siblings of a consanguineous marriage. The deficiency is not associated with bleeding and affected individuals have a prolonged activated partial thromboplastin time which shortens on prolonged exposure to the contact activating agent. Fletcher factor has been identified as plasma pre-kallikrein (Wuepper 1973, Weiss et al 1974). In a study of 18 individuals from 15 affected families Saito et al (1981) found molecular heterogeneity of the pre-kallikrein deficiency; in some there was a true deficiency of pre-kallikrein in others cross-reacting material was demonstrated using immunological methods. Interestingly all the CRM^+ samples in the above study were obtained from people of Mediterranean extraction whereas all the CRM^- samples were from black Americans.

Fitzgerald factor (Flaujeac factor, Williams factor) deficiency: Reid trait

Fitzgerald factor deficiency was first reported by Waldman & Abraham (1974) and in more detail by Saito et al (1975). The condition is characterized by prolongation of the whole blood clotting time and activated partial thromboplastin time. In this case the activated partial thromboplastin time does not shorten on prolonged incubation. In spite of what seems to be a significant defect in the early stages of the intrinsic blood coagulation pathway, people with this defect do not bleed excessively. Similar defects were reported by Lacombe et al (1975) and Coleman (1975) who named the condition, Flaujeac and Williams factor deficiency respectively after the affected families studied by them. A closely-related condition, Reid trait, was described by Lutcher (1976). In the case of Fitzgerald factor deficiency and Reid trait the plasma lacks high molecular weight kininogen. In Flaujeac and Williams deficiency there is a lack of both high and low molecular weight kininogen.

INHERITED COMBINED COAGULATION FACTOR DEFICIENCIES

Several families have been described in which a variety of combinations of coagulation factors are deficient. These conditions are relatively rare apart from factor V/VIII deficiency which has been described in about 60 families (Fischer et al 1988).

Combined deficiency of factor V and factor VIII

Combined deficiency of factor V and factor VIII was first described by Oeri et al (1954) in two brothers. Since then several similar families have been studied (Iversen & Bastrup-Madsen 1956, Jones et al 1962, Smit Sibinga et al 1972, Seligsohn et al 1982). The bleeding symptoms are usually mild or moderate in severity. Symptoms consist of easy bruising and prolonged bleeding after surgery including dental extraction. Postpartum bleeding and menorrhagia have also been described. In some cases the bleeding time has been prolonged and features of von Willebrand's disease have been noted (Ciaverella et al 1977, Akutsu et al 1987, Fischer et al 1988). In one or two families there is evidence suggesting that factor V deficiency has coincidentally occurred in a family with haemophilia A (Gobbi et al 1967, Girolami et al 1974b). In the majority of cases however the repeated autosomal transmission suggests that the combined defect exists as a distinct entity due to a single gene defect. Factor V and factor VIII both act as cofactors in the blood coagulation process and there is known to be a considerable homology in their amino acid sequences. It may well be that an abnormality in a gene necessary for post-translational modification of both factors is the cause of the combined defect.

Combined deficiencies of factors other than V and VIII are extremely uncommon and have been extensively reviewed by Soff (1981).

Deficiency of prothrombin along with one or more of the other vitamin K-dependent clotting factors has been described. Chung et al (1979) described a patient deficient in factor II, VII, IX and X in whom they postulated a defect in the γ-carboxylation mechanism or a fault in vitamin K transport. A similar case was described by Johnson et al (1980). Goldsmith et al (1982) described a mother and sister in whom prothrombin and factor X were slightly deficient, factor IX less so and factor VII was normal. The deficiencies were temporarily corrected by oral or parenteral administration of vitamin K_1.

REFERENCES

Ahlberg A 1965 Haemophilia in Sweden VII. Incidence, treatment and prophylaxis of arthropathy and other musculo-skeletal manifestations of haemophilia A and B. Acta Orthopaedica Scandinavica 77 (suppl): 3–132

Akutsu Y, Mori K, Suzuki S, Ishikawa M, Sakai H, Hiwatashi K, Fujimoto H, Endo E, Yasuda H 1987 A new disorder characterised by factor V deficiency and molecular abnormality of von Willebrand factor antigen. Thrombosis and Haemostasis 58: 133 (abstract)

Alexander B, Goldstein R 1953 Dual hemostatic defect in pseudo-hemophilia. Journal of Clinical Investigation 32: 551

Alexander B, Goldstein R, Landwehr G, Cook C D 1951 Congenital SPCA deficiency: A new hitherto unrecognised defect with hemorrhage rectified by serum and serum fractions. Journal of Clinical Investigation 30: 596–608

Andreassen M 1943 Haemofili i Danmark. (Copenhagan: E Munksgaard 1943). Opera Ex domo biologiae hereditariae humanae. Universitatis Hafniensis 6: 1–168

Archer R K 1961 True haemophilia (haemophilia A) in a thoroughbred foal. Veterinary Record 73: 338–340

Armitage H, Rizza C R 1979 Two populations of factor VIII related antigen in a family with von Willebrand's disease. British Journal of Haematology 41: 279–289

Arnold W D, Hilgartner M W 1977 Hemophilic arthropathy. Journal of Bone and Joint Surgery 59a: 287–305

Asakai R, Chung D W, Davie E W, Seligsohn U 1991 Factor X deficiency in Ashkenazi Jews in Israel. New England Journal of Medicine 325: 153–158

Bachman F 1980 Diagnostic approach to mild bleeding disorders. Seminars in Hematology 17: 292–305

Barbui T, Cartei G, Chisesi T, Dini E 1974 Electro immunoassay of plasma subunits -A and -S in a case of congenital fibrin stabilising factor deficiency. Thrombosis et Diathesis Haemorrhagica 32: 124–131

Barrowcliffe T W 1984 Standards and controls in assays of blood coagulation factors. In: Biggs R, Rizza C R (eds) Human blood coagulation, haemostasis and thrombosis. Blackwell Scientific, Oxford

Beck P, Evans K T 1972 Renal abnormalities in patients with haemophilia and Christmas disease. Clinical Radiology 23: 349–354

Beck E A, Duckert F, Ernst M 1961 The influence of fibrin stabilising factor on the growth of fibroblasts in vitro and wound healing. Thrombosis et Diathesis Haemorrhagica 6: 485–491

Berliner S L, Lusky A, Zivelin A, Modan M, Seligsohn U 1984 Hereditary factor XIII deficiency: a report of four families and definition of the carrier state. British Journal of Haematology 56: 495–505

Bezeaud A, Guillin M-C, Olmeda F, Quintana M, Gomez M 1979 Prothrombin Madrid: a new familial abnormality of prothrombin. Thrombosis Research 16: 47–58

Biggs R, Matthews J M 1963 The treatment of haemorrhage in von Willebrand's disease and the blood level of factor VIII (AHF). British Journal of Haematology 9: 203–214

Biggs R, Sharp A A, Margolis J, Hardisty R M, Stewart J, Davidson W M 1958 Defects in the early stages of blood coagulation: A report of four cases. British Journal of Haematology 4: 177–191

Bloom A L 1980 The von Willebrand Syndrome. Seminars in Hematology 17: 215–227

Bloom A L, Giddings J C, Wilks C J 1973 Factor VIII on the vascular intima: possible importance in haemostasis and thrombosis. Nature New Biology 241: 217–219

Board P G 1979 Genetic polymorphism of the A subunits of human coagulation factor XIII. American Journal of Human Genetics 31: 116–124

Board P G, Coggan M, Hamer J W 1980 An electrophoretic and quantitative analysis of coagulation factor XIII in normal and deficient subjects. British Journal of Haematology 45: 633–640

Boldero J L, Kemp H S 1966 The early bone and joint changes in haemophilia and similar blood dyscrasias. British Journal of Radiology 39: 172–180

Borchgrevink C F 1960 A method for measuring platelet adhesiveness in vivo. Acta Medica Scandinavica 168: 157–164

Brackmann H-H, Hofmann P, Etzel F, Egli H 1976 Home care of haemophilia in West Germany. Thrombosis and Haemostasis 35: 544–552

Briet E, Loeliger E A, van Tilburg N H, Veltkamp J J 1976 Molecular variant of factor VII. Thrombosis and Haemostasis 35: 289–294

Chin H C, Whitaker E, Colman R W 1983 Heterogeneity of human factor V deficiency. Evidence for the existence of antigen positive variants. Journal of Clinical Investigation 72: 493–503

Choo K H, Gould K G, Rees D J G, Brownlee G G 1982 Molecular cloning of the gene for human antihaemophilic factor IX. Nature 299: 178–180

Chung K-S, Bezeaud A, Goldsmith J C, McMillan C W, Menaché D, Roberts H R 1979 Congenital deficiency of blood clotting factors II, VII, IX and X. Blood 53: 776–787

Ciavarella N, Scaraggi F A, Petronelli M, Coviello M, Orieste A, De Mitrio V, Schiavoni M, Bonomo L 1977 von Willebrand's disease combined with factor V deficiency: variant Bario Thrombosis and Haemostasis 38: 380 (abstract)

Colman R W, Bagdasarian A, Talamo R C, Scott C F, Seavey M, Guimaraes J A, Pierce J V, Kaplan A P, Weinstein L 1975 Williams trait: human kininogen deficiency with diminished levels of plasminogen proactivator and pre-kallikrein associated with abnormalities of the Hageman factor-dependent pathways. Journal of Clinical Investigation 56: 1650–1662

Cornu P, Larrieu M J, Caen J, Bernard J 1963 Transfusion studies in von Willebrand's disease; effect on bleeding time and factor VIII assay. British Journal of Haematology 9: 189–203

Cotter S M, Brenner R M, Dodds W J 1978 Haemophilia A in three unrelated cats. Journal of American Veterinary Association 172: 166–168

Crossley P M, Winship P R, Black A, Rizza C R, Brownlee G G 1989 Unusual case of haemophilia B (letter). Lancet 1: 960

Davidson C S, Epstein R D, Miller G F, Taylor F H L 1949 Hemophilia. A clinical study of forty patients. Blood 4: 97–119

Davies S H, Turner J W, Cumming R A, Gillingham F J, Girdwood R H, Darg A 1966 Management of intracranial haemorrhage in haemophilia. British Medical Journal 2: 1627–1630

de Andrade J R, Grant C, Dixon A St J 1965 Joint distension and reflex muscle inhibition in the knee. Journal of Bone and Joint Surgery 47a: 313

de los Santos R P, Hoyer L W 1972 Antihemophilic factor in tissues: localisation by immunofluorescence. Federation Proceedings 31: 262 (abstract)

Denson K W E, Lurie A, De Cataldo F, Mannucci P M 1970 The factor X defect: recognition of abnormal forms of factor X. British Journal of Haematology 18: 317–327

Denson K W E, Conard J, Samama M 1972 Genetic variants of factor VII (letter) Lancet. 1: 1234

Didisheim P 1962 Hageman factor deficiency (Hageman trait). Archives of Internal Medicine 110: 170–177

Dubois E 1838 Observation remarquable d'hemorrhophile. Gazette Medicale de Paris 6: 43–47

Duckert F, Jung E, Schmerling D H 1960 Hitherto undescribed congenital haemorrhagic diathesis probably due to fibrin stabilising factor deficiency. Thrombosis et Diathesis Haemorrhagica 5: 179–186

Duckert F, Koller F 1975 The old Swiss hemophilia families of Tenna and Wald. In: Duckert F, Koller F. Brinkhous K M, Hemker H C (eds) Handbook of hemophilia. Excerpta Medica, Amsterdam, p 21–29

Duthie R B, Rizza C R 1975 Rheumatological manifestations of the haemophilias. Clinics in Rheumatic Diseases 1: 53–93

Duthie R B, Matthews J M, Rizza C R, Steel W M 1972 The management of musculo-skeletal problems in the haemophilias. Blackwell Scientific, Oxford

Dyerberg J, Stoffersen E 1980 Recurrent thrombosis in a patient with factor XII deficiency. Acta Haematologica 63: 278–282

Edson J R, White J G, Krivit W 1967 The enigma of severe factor XII deficiency without haemorrhagic symptoms. Distinction from Hageman factor and Fletcher factor deficiency: family study and

problems of diagnosis. Thrombosis et Diathesis Haematologica 18: 342–348
Fair D S, Edgington T S 1985 Heterogeneity of hereditary and acquired factor X deficiencies by combined immunochemical and functional analyses. British Journal of Haematology 59: 235–248
Fanconi G 1941 'Fibrinasthenie' als urasche einer schiveren haemorrhagischen. Diathese bei lues congenita. Schweizerische Medizinische Wochenschrift 71: 255–258
Fantl P, Sawers R J, Marr A G 1956 Investigation of a haemorrhagic disease due to betaprothromboplastin deficiency complicated by a specific inhibitor of thromboplastin formation. Australasian Annals of Medicine 5: 163–176
Feinstein D I, Rapaport S I, McGehee W G, Patch M J 1970 Factor V anticoagulant: clinical, biochemical, and immunological observations. Journal of Clinical Investigation 49: 1578–1588
Fischer R R, Giddings J C, Roisenberg I 1988 Hereditary combined deficiency of clotting factors V and VIII with involvement of von Willebrand factor. Clinical and Laboratory Haematology 10: 53–62
Forbes C D, Barr R D, Prentice C R M, Douglas A S 1973 Gastrointestinal bleeding in haemophilia. Quarterly Journal of Medicine (NS) 42: 503–511
Fraenkel G J, Taylor K B, Richards W C D 1959 Haemophilic blood cysts. British Journal of Surgery 46: 383–392
Fratantoni J W, Hilgartner M, Nachman R L 1972 Nature of the defect in congenital factor V deficiency: study in a patient with acquired circulating anticoagulant. Blood 39: 751–758
Giddings J C 1971 Preparation and use of a new artificial system for factor XI assay. Medical Laboratory Technology 28: 284–299
Giddings J C, Shearn S A M, Bloom A L 1975 The immunological localisation of factor V in human tissue. British Journal of Haematology 29: 57–65
Gilchrist G S, Hammond D, Melnyk J 1965 Hemophilia A in a phenotypically normal female with XX/XO mosaicism. New England Journal of Medicine 273: 1402–1406
Girolami A, Molaro G, Lazzarin M, Scarpa R, Brunetti A 1970 A 'new' congenital haemorrhagic condition due to the presence of an abnormal factor X (factor X Friuli): a study of a large kindred. British Journal of Haematology 19: 179–192
Girolami A, Bareggi G, Brunetti A, Sticchi A 1974a Prothrombin 'Padua': a new congenital dysprothrombinemia. Journal of Laboratory and Clinical Medicine 84: 654–666
Girolami A, Brunetti A, de Marco L 1974b Congenital combined factor V and factor VIII deficiency in a male born from a brother — sister incest. Blut 28: 33–42
Girolami A, Falezza G, Patrassi G, Stenico M, Vettore L 1977 Factor VII Verona coagulation disorder: double heterozygosis with an abnormal factor VII and heterzygous factor VII deficiency. Blood 50: 603–610
Girolami A, Fabris F, Dal B O, Zanon R, Ghiotto G, Burul A 1978a Factor VII Padua: a congenital coagulation disorder due to an abnormal factor VII with a peculiar activation pattern. Journal of Laboratory and Clinical Medicine 91: 387–395
Girolami A, Coccheri A, Palareti G, Poggi I, Burul A, Cappellato G 1978b Prothrombin Molise: a 'new' congenital dysprothrombinemia, double heterozygosis with an abnormal prothrombin and 'true' prothrombin deficiency. Blood 52: 115–125
Girolami A, Cattarozzi G, Dal B O, Zanon R, Cella G, Toffanin F 1979 Factor VII Padue 2: another factor VII abnormality with defective oxbrain thromboplastin activation and a complex hereditary pattern. Blood 54: 46–53
Gobbi F, Ascari E, Barbieri U 1967 Congenital combined deficiency of factor VIII (antihaemophilic globulin) and factor V (proaccelerin) in two siblings. Thrombosis et Diathesis Haemorrhagica 17: 194–204
Goldsmith G H Jr, Pence R E, Ratnoff O D, Adelstein D J, Furie B 1982 Studies on a family with combined functional deficiencies of vitamin K-dependent coagulation factors. Journal of Clinical Investigation 69: 1253–1260
Goodnight S H, Feinstein J I, Osterud B, Rapaport S I 1971 Factor VII antibody — neutralising material in hereditary and acquired factor VII deficiency. Blood 38: 1–8
Graham J B, Brinkhous K M, Dodds W J 1975 Canine and equine hemophilia. In: Brinkhous K M, Hemker H C (eds) Handbook of hemophilia. Excerpta Medica, Amersterdam, p 119–139
Guillin M C, Bezeaud A 1981 Characterisation of a variant of human prothrombin: prothrombin Madrid. Annals of the New York Academy of Sciences 370: 414
Haanen C, Hommes F, Benraad H, Morselt G 1961 A case of Hageman factor deficiency and a method to purify the factor. Thrombosis et Diathesis Haemorrhagica 5: 201–217
Haldane J B S 1947 The mutation rate of the gene for haemophilia and its segregation ratios in males and females. Annals of Eugenics 13: 262–271
Handley R S, Nussbrecher A M 1935 Hereditary Pseudo-Haemophilia. Quarterly Journal of Medicine 4: 165–178
Hardisty R M, Pinniger J L 1956 Congenital afibrinogenaemia: further observations on the blood coagulation mechanism. British Journal of Haematology 2: 139–152
Hartmann J R, Diamond L K 1957 Haemophilia and related haemorrhagic disorders. Practitioner 178: 179–190
Hathaway W E, Belhasen L P, Hathaway H S 1965 Evidence for a new plasma thromboplastin factor. I. Case report, coagulation studies and physico chemical properties. Blood 26: 521–532
Hellstern P, Kohler M, Schmengler K, Doenecke P, Wenzel E 1983 Arterial and venous thrombosis and normal response to streptokinase treatment in a young patient with severe Hageman factor deficiency. Acta Haematologica 69: 123–126
Hoagland F T 1967 Experimental hemarthrosis. The response of canine knees to injections of autologous blood. Journal of Bone and Joint Surgery 49-A: 285
Holmberg L, Gustavii B, Cordesius E, Kristofferson A C, Ljung R, Lofberg L, Stromberg P, Nilsson I M 1980 Prenatal diagnosis of hemophilia B by an immunoradiometric assay of factor IX. Blood 56: 397–401
Holmberg L, Nilsson I M 1985 von Willebrand's disease. In: Ruggeri Z M (ed) Clinics in haematology. p 467
Houghton G R, Dickson R A 1978 Lower limb arthrodeses in haemophilia. Journal of Bone and Joint Surgery 60b: 387–389
Hougie C, Barrow E M, Graham J B 1957 Stuart clotting defect. I. Segregation of an hereditary hemorrhagic state from the heterogeneous group heretofore called 'stable factor' (SPCA, proconvertin, factor VII) deficiency. Journal of Clinical Investigation 36: 485–496
Howard M A, Firkin B G 1971 Ristocetin – a new tool in the investigation of platelet aggregation. Thrombosis et Diathesis Haemorrhagica 26: 362–369
Hoyer L W, Rizza C R, Tuddenham E G D, Carta C A, Armitage H, Rotblat F 1983 von Willebrand factor multimer patterns in von Willebrand's disease. British Journal of Haematology 55: 493–507
Ikkala E 1960 Haemophilia. A study of its laboratory, clinical, genetic and social aspects based on known haemophiliacs in Finland. Scandinavian Journal of Clinical and Laboratory Investigation. 12 (suppl): 46
Ikkala E, Myllyla G, Nevanlinna H R 1971 Rare congenital coagulation factor defects in Finland. Scandinavian Journal of Haematology 8: 210–215
Imperato di C, Dettori A G 1958 Ipofibrinogenemia congenita con fibrinoastenia. Helvetica Paediatrica Acta 13: 380–399
Ingram G I C 1955 Variations in the reaction between thrombin and fibrinogen and their effects on the prothrombin time. Journal of Clinical Pathology 8: 318–323
Inomoto T, Shirakami A, Kawauchi S, Shigekiyo T, Saito S, Miyoshi K, Morita T, Iwanaga S 1987 Prothrombin Tokushima: characterisation of dysfunctional thrombin derived from a variant of human prothrombin. Blood 69: 565–569
Israels E D, Paraskevas F, Israels G L 1973 Immunological studies of coagulation factor XIII. Journal of Clinical Investigation 52: 2398–2403
Italian Working Group 1977 Spectrum of von Willebrand's disease: a study of 100 cases. British Journal of Haematology 35: 101–112
Iversen T, Bastrup-Madsen P 1956 Congenital familial deficiency of factor V (parahaemophilia) combined with deficiency of antihaemophilic globulin. British Journal of Haematology 2: 265–275
Jaffe E A, Hoyer L W, Nachman R S 1973 Synthesis of antihemophilic factor antigen by cultured human endothelial cells. Journal of Clinical Investigation 52: 2757–2764
Johnson C A, Chung K-S, McGrath K M, Bean P E, Roberts H R

1980 Characterisation of variant prothrombin in a patient deficient in factors II, VII, IX and X. British Journal of Haematology 44: 461–469
Jones J H, Rizza C R, Hardisty R M, Dormandy K M, Macpherson J C 1962 Combined deficiency of factor V and factor VIII (anti haemophilic globulin), A report of three cases. British Journal of Haematology 8: 120–128
Kaneshiro M M, Mielke C H Jr, Kasper C K, Rapaport S I 1969 Bleeding time after aspirin in disorders of intrinsic clotting. New England Journal of Medicine 281: 1039–1042
Kernoff P B A, Rizza C R 1973 Factor VIII-related antigen in female haemophilia (Letter). Lancet 2: 734
Kernoff P B A, Gruson R, Rizza C R 1974 A variant of factor VIII-related antigen. British Journal of Haematology 26: 435–439
Kerr C B 1965 Genetics of human blood coagulation. Journal of Medical Genetics 2: 221–308
Kirkwood T B L, Snape T J 1984 Statistics of bioassay of blood coagulation factors. In: Biggs R, Rizza C R (eds) Human blood coagulation, haemostasis and thrombosis. Blackwell Scientific Publications, Oxford
Konig F 1892 Die Gelenkerkrankungen bei Blutern mit besonderer Berucksichtigung der Diagnose. Samml Klinischer Vortrage Volkman, NF Chirurgie nr 11: 233–242
Kurachi K, Davie E W 1982 Isolation and characterisation of a cDNA coding for human factor IX. Proceedings of the National Academy of Sciences USA, 79: 6461–6464
Lacombe M, Varet B, Levy J 1975 A hitherto undescribed plasma factor acting at the contact phase of blood coagulation (Flaujeac factor): case report and coagulation studies. Blood 46: 761–768
Laki K, Lorand L 1948 On the solubility of fibrin clots. Science 108: 280
Lammle B, Wuillemin W A, Huber I, Krauskopf M, Zurcher C, Plugshaupt R, Furlan M 1991 Thrombo embolism and bleeding tendency in congenital factor XII deficiency — a study on 74 subjects from 14 Swiss families. Thrombosis and Haemostasis 65: 117–121
Larrieu M J, Soulier J P 1953 Deficit en facteur antihemophilique A chez une fille associe a un trouble du saignement. Revue d'Hematologie 8: 361–370
Legg J W 1872 A treatise on haemophilia, sometimes called the hereditary haemorrhagic diathesis. Lewis, London
Leiba H, Ramot B, Many A 1965 Heredity and coagulation studies in ten families with factor XI (plasma thromboplastin antecedent) deficiency. British Journal of Haematology 11: 654–665
Lorand L, Losowsky M S, Miloszewski K J M 1980 Human factor XIII: fibrin stabilising factor. Progress in hemostasis and thrombosis 5: 245–290
Ludlam C A, Peake I R, Allen N, Davies B L, Furlong R A, Bloom A L 1980 Factor VIII and fibrinolytic response to deamino-8-d-arginine vasopressin in normal subjects and dissociate response in some patients with haemophilia and von Willebrand's disease. British Journal of Haematology 45: 499–511
Lutcher C L 1976 Reid trait: a new expression of high molecular weight kininogen deficiency. Clinical Research. 24: 440 (abstract)
Macfarlane R G 1938 A boy with no fibrinogen. Lancet i: 309–312
Macfarlane R G 1978 Blood coagulation and haemostasis. In: Biggs R (ed) The treatment of haemophilia A and B and von Willebrand's disease. Blackwell Scientific, Oxford p 26
Mannucci P M, Ruggeri Z M 1976 Haemophilia care in Italy. Thrombosis and Haemostasis 35: 531–536
Mannucci P M, Lombardi R, Pareti F I, Solinas S, Mazzucconi M G, Mariani G 1983 A variant of von Willebrand's disease characterised by recessive inheritance and missing triplet structure of von Willebrand factor multimers. Blood 62: 1000–1005
Mannucci P M, Bloom A L, Larrieu M J, Nilsson I M, West R R 1984 Atherosclerosis and von Willebrand factor. 1. Prevalence of severe von Willebrand's disease in Western Europe and Israel. British Journal of Haematology 57: 163–169
Manotti C, Quintavalla R, Pini M, Jeran M, Paolicelli M, Dettori A G 1989 Thromboembolic manifestations and congenital factor V deficiency: a family study. Haemostasis 19: 331–334
Marder V J, Shulman N R 1964 Clinical aspects of congenital factor VII deficiency. American Journal of Medicine 37: 182–194
Mazzucconi M G, Mandelli F, Mariani G, Briet E, Veltkamp J J 1977 A CRM- positive variant of factor VII deficiency and the detection of heterozygotes with the assay of factor-like antigen. British Journal of Haematology 36: 127–135
Menache D 1964 Constitutional and familial abnormal fibrinogen. Thrombosis et Diathesis Haemorrhagica 13: 173–185
Merskey C 1951 The occurrence of haemophilia in the human female. Quarterly Journal of Medicine 20: 299–312
Mielke C H Jr, Britten A F H 1970 Use of aspirin or acetaminophen in hemophilia. New England Journal of Medicine 282: 1270
Nachman R, Levine R, Jaffe E A 1977 Synthesis of factor VIII antigen by cultured guinea pig megakaryocytes. Journal of Clinical Investigation 60: 914–921
Nilsson I M 1976 Management of haemophilia in Sweden. Thrombosis and Haemostasis 35: 510–521
Nilsson I M, Blomback M, Jorpes E J, Blomback B, Johansson S A 1957 von Willebrand's disease and its correction with human fraction I-O. Acta Medica Scandinavica 159: 179–188
Nilsson I M, Bergman S, Reitalu J, Waldenstrom J 1959 Haemophilia in a 'girl' with male sex chromatin pattern. Lancet 2: 264–266
Nilsson I M, Holmberg L, Aberg M, Vilhardt H 1980 The release of plasminogen and factor VIII after injection of DDAVP in healthy volunteers and in patients with von Willebrand's disease. Scandinavian Journal of Haematology 24: 351–359
Nossel H L 1964 The contact phase of blood coagulation. Blackwell Scientific, Oxford
Nossel H L, Niemetz J, Mibashan R S, Schulze W G 1966 The measurement of factor XI (plasma thromboplastin antecedent). Diagnosis and therapy of the congenital deficiency state. British Journal of Haematology 12: 133–144
Oeri J, Matter M, Isenschmid H, Hauser F, Koller F 1954 Angeborener Mangel an Faktor V (parhaemophilie) verbunden mit echter haemophilie A bei zwei brudern. Bibliotheca Paediatrica 58: 575–588
Orstavik K H, Osterud B, Prydz H, Berg K 1975 Electroimmunoassay of factor IX in hemophilia B. Thrombosis Research 7: 373–382
Owen C A, Henriksen R A, McDuffie F C, Mann K G 1978 Prothrombin Quick: a newly identified dysprothrombinemia. Mayo Clinic Proceedings 53: 29–33
Owren P A 1947 The coagulation of blood. Investigations on a new clotting factor. Acta Medica Scandinavica Suppl 194
Peake I R, Bloom A L, Giddings J C 1974 Inherited variants of factor VIII related protein in von Willebrand's disease. New England Journal of Medicine 291: 113–117
Pettersson H, Ahlberg A, Nilsson I M 1980 A radiological classification of haemophilic arthropathy. Clinical Orthopaedics and Related Research 149: 153–159
Pinniger J L, Prunty F T G 1946 Some observations on the blood clotting mechanism. The role of fibrinogen and platelets with reference to a case of congenital afibrinogenaemia. British Journal of Experimental Pathology 27: 200–210
Potter J M 1965 Head injury and haemophilia. Acta Neurochirurgica 13: 380–387
Prentice A I D 1951 A case of congenital afibrinogenaemia. Lancet 1: 211–213
Prentice C R M, Lindsay R M, Barr R D, Forbes C D, Kennedy A C, McNicol G P, Douglas A S 1971 Renal complications in haemophilia and Christmas disease. Quarterly Journal of Medicine 40: 47–61
Rabe F, Salomon E 1920 Ueber Faserstoffmangel im Blute bei einem Falle von Hamophilie. Deutches Archiv fur Klinische Medizen 132: 240–244
Rapaport S I, Proctor R R, Patch M J, Yettra M 1961 The mode of inheritance of PTA deficiency: evidence for the existence of major PTA deficiency and minor PTA deficiency. Blood 18: 149–165
Ratnoff O D 1960 Bleeding syndrome. A clinical manual. C C Thomas, Springfield Illinois, p 72
Ratnoff O D, Colopy J H 1955 A familial hemorrhagic trait associated with a deficiency of clot promoting fraction of plasma. Journal of Clinical Investigation 34: 601–613
Ratnoff O D, Margolius A Jr 1957 On the epidemiology of hemophilia and Christmas disease. New England Journal of Medicine 256: 845–846

Ratnoff O D, Busse R J, Sheon R P 1968 The demise of John Hageman. New England Journal of Medicine 279: 760–761
Reitsma P H, Bertina R M, Ploos van Amstel J K, Riemens A, Briet E 1988 The putative factor IX promoter gene in hemophilia B Leyden. Blood 72: 1074–1076
Reitsma P H, Mandalaki T, Kasper C K, Bertina R M, Briet E 1989 Two novel point mutations correlate with an altered developmental expression of blood coagulation factor IX (hemophilia B Leyden phenotype). Blood 73: 743–746
Rimon A, Schiffman S, Feinstein D I, Rapaport S I 1976 Factor XI activity and factor XI antigen in homozygous and heterozygous factor XI deficiency. Blood 48: 165–174
Rizza C R, Spooner R J D 1983 Treatment of haemophilia and related disorders in Britain and Northern Ireland during 1976–1980: report on behalf of the directors of haemophilia centres in the United Kingdom. British Medical Journal 286: 929–933
Robbins K C 1944 A study on the conversion of fibrinogen to fibrin. American Journal of Physiology 142: 581–588
Roberts H R, Grizzle J E, McLester W D, Penick G D 1968. Genetic varients of hemophilia B: detection by means of specific inhibitor. Journal of Clinical Investigation 47: 360–365
Roberts G M, Evans K T, Bloom A L, Al-Gailani F 1983 Renal papillary necrosis in haemophilia and Christmas disease. Clinical Radiology 34: 201–206
Rosenthal R L, Dreskin O H, Rosethal M 1953 A new hemophilia-like disease caused by deficiency of a third plasma thromboplastin factor. Proceedings of the Society for Experimental Biology and Medicine 82: 171–174
Ruggeri Z M, Mannucci P M, Lombardi R, Federici A B, Zimmerman T S 1982a Multimeric composition of factor VIII/von Willebrand factor following administration of DDAVP: implications for pathophysiology and therapy of von Willebrand's disease subtypes. Blood 59: 1272–1278
Ruggeri Z M, Nilsson I M, Lombardi R, Holmberg L, Zimmerman T S 1982b Aberrant multimeric structure of von Willebrand's factor in a new variant of von Willebrand's disease (Type IIc). Journal of Clinical Investigation 70: 1124–1127
Rush B, Ellis H 1965 Treatment of patients with factor V deficiency. Thrombosis et Diathesis Haemorrhagica 14: 74–82
Saito H, Ratnoff O D, Waldmann R, Abraham J P 1975 Fitzgerald trait. Deficiency of a hitherto unrecognised agent, Fitzgerald factor, participating in surface-mediated reactions of clotting, fibrinolysis, generation of kinins and the property of diluted plasma enhancing vascular permeability (PF/Dil). Journal of Clinical Investigation 55: 1082–1089
Saito H, Goodenough L T, Soria J, Soria C, Aznar J, Espana F 1981 Heterogeneity of human pre-Kallikrein deficiency (Fletcher trait). Evidence that five of 18 cases are positive for cross-reacting material. New England Journal of Medicine 305: 910–914
Salzman E W 1963 Measurement of platelet adhesiveness. A simple in vitro technique demonstrating an abnormality in von Willebrand's disease. Journal of Laboratory and Clinical Medicine 62: 724–735
Schwartz M L, Pizzo S V, Hill R I, McKee P A 1973 Human factor XIII from plasma and platelets. Molecular weights, subunit structures, proteolytic activation and cross-linking of fibrinogen and fibrin. Journal of Biological Chemistry 248: 1395–1407
Seeler R A 1972 Parahemophilia. Factor V deficiency. Medical Clinics of North America 56: 119–125
Seligsohn U 1978 High gene frequency of factor XI (PTA) deficiency in Ashkenazi Jews. Blood 51: 1223–1228
Seligsohn U, Zivelin A, Zwang E 19821 Combined factor V and factor VIII deficiency among non-Ashkenazi Jews. New England Journal of Medicine 307: 1191–1197
Shapiro S S, Martinez J, Holburn R R 1969 Congenital dysprothrombinemia: an inherited structural disorder of human prothrombin. Journal of Clinical Investigation 48: 2251–2259
Shoa'i I, Lavergne J M, Ardaillou N, Obert B, Ala F, Meyer D 1977 Heterogeneity of von Willebrand's disease: study of 40 Iranian cases. British Journal of Haematology 37: 67–83
Small M, Rose P E, McMillan N, Belch J J F, Rolfe E B, Forbes C D, Stuart J 1982 Haemophilia and the kidney: assessment after 11 year follow up. British Medical Journal 285: 1609–1611
Smit Sibinga C Th, Gokemeyer J D M, Ten Kate L P, Bos van Zwol F 1972 Combined deficiency of factor V and factor VIII: Report of a family and genetic analysis. British Journal of Haematology 23: 467–481
Soff G A, Leoin J, Bell W R 1981 Familial multiple coagulation factor deficiencies II. Combined factor VIII, IX and XI deficiency and combined factor IX and XI deficiency: two previously uncharacterized familial multiple factor deficiency syndromes. Seminars in Thrombosis and Hemostasis 7: 149–169
Stuart J, Davies S H, Cumming R A, Girdwood R H, Darg A 1966 Haemorrhagic episodes in haemophilia: a 5-year prospective study. British Medical Journal 2: 1642–1662
Swanton M C 1957 The pathology of hemarthrosis in hemophilia. In: Brinkhous K M (ed) Hemophilia and hemophilioid disease. University of North Carolina Press, Chapel Hill, p 219–224
Swanton M C, Wysocki G P 1957 Pathology of joints in canine hemophilia A. In: Brinkhous K M, Hemker H C (eds) Handbook of hemophilia. Excerpta Medica, Amsterdam, p 313–332
Takahashi H 1980 Studies on the pathophysiology and treatment of von Willebrand's disease. IV. Mechanism of increased ristocetin-induced platelet aggregation in von Willebrand's disease. Thrombosis Research 19: 857–867
Takase T, Rotblat F, Goodall A H, Kernoff P B A, Middleton S, Chand S, Denson K W E, Austen D E G, Tuddenham E G D 1987 Production of factor VIII deficient plasma by immunodepletion using three monoclonal antibodies. British Journal of Haematology 66: 497–502
Telfer T P, Denson K W, Wright D R 1956 A 'new' coagulation defect. British Journal of Haematology 2: 308–316
Thompson A R 1977 Factor IX antigen by radioimmunoassay. Abnormal factor IX protein in patients on warfarin therapy and with hemophilia B. Journal of Clinical Investigation 59: 900–910
Treves F 1886 A case of haemophilia; Pedigree through five generations. Lancet II: 533–534
Triplett D A, Brandt J T, Batard M A Mc M, Dixon J L S, Fair D S 1985 Hereditary factor VII deficiency: heterogeneity defined by combined functional and immunochemical analysis. Blood 66: 1284–1287
UK Haemophilia Centre Directors Statistics (unpublished) 1990
US Department of Health Education and Welfare Publication no (NIH) 77–1274 1980 Study to evaluate supply demand relationships for AHF and PTC through 1980 p 77–1274
Valderrama J A F, Matthews J M 1965 The haemophilic pseudo-tumour or haemophilic subperiosteal haematoma. Journal of Bone and Joint Surgery 47B: 256–265
van Trotsenburg L 1975 Neurological complications of haemophilia. In: Brinkhous K M, Hemker H C (eds) Handbook of haemophilia. Excerpta Medica, Amsterdam, p 389–404
Veltkamp J J, Meiloff J, Remmelts H G, van der Vlerk D, Loeliger E A 1970 Another genetic variant of haemophilia B: haemophilia B Leyden. Scandinavian Journal of Haematology 7: 82–90
von Willebrand E A 1926 Hereditare pseudo hemofili. Finska Lakaresallskapets Handlingar 67: 7–12
Waldmann R, Abraham J P 1974 Fitzgerald factor: A heretofore unrecognised coagulation factor. Blood 44: 934 (abstract)
Wall R L, McConnell J L, Moore D, MacPherson C R, Marson A 1967 Christmas disease colour blindness and blood group Xg[a]. American Journal of Medicine 43: 214–226
Weiss A S, Gallin J I, Kaplan A 1974 Fletcher factor deficiency. A diminished rate of Hageman factor activation caused by absence of pre-kallikrein with abnormalities of coagulation, fibrinolysis, chemotactic activity and kinin generation. Journal of Clinical Investigation 53: 622–633
Weiss H J, Meyer D, Rabinowitz, Pietu G, Girma J-P, Vicic W J, Rogers J 1982 Pseudo-von Willebrand's Disease. An intrinsic platelet defect with aggregation by unmodified human factor VIII/von Willebrand factor and enhanced adsorption of its high molecular weight multimers. New England Journal of Medicine 306: 326–333
Wilkinson J F, Nour-Eldin F, Israels M C G, Barrett K E 1961 Haemophilia syndromes. A survey of 267 patients. Lancet 2: 947–950
Wright F W, Matthews J M, Brock L G 1971 Complications of haemophilic disorders affecting the renal tract. Radiology 98: 471–476

Wuepper K D 1973 Pre-kallikrein deficiency in man. Journal of Experimental Medicine 138: 1345–1355
Yang H C 1978a Immunological studies of factor IX (Christmas factor) II. Counter immuno electrophoresis method for factor IX antigen. Thrombosis Research 13: 97–109
Yang H C 1978b Immunological studies of factor IX (Christmas factor). II. Immunoradiometric assay of factor IX antigen. British Journal of Haematology 39: 215–224
Zimmerman T S, Abildgaard C F, Meyer D 1979 The factor VIII abnormality in severe von Willebrand's disease. New England Journal of Medicine 301: 1307–1310
Zimmerman T S, Ratnoff O D, Powell A E 1971 Immunological differentiation of classic hemophilia (factor VIII deficiency) and von Willebrand's disease with observations on combined deficiencies of antihemophilic factor and pro accelerin and on acquired circulating anticoagulant against antihemophilic factor. Journal of Clinical Investigation 50: 244–254

35. von Willebrand disease

J. E. Sadler

In 1926, von Willebrand published a description of an inherited bleeding disorder that now bears his name. The proband came to his attention as a five-year-old girl with severe spontaneous bleeding. She belonged to a large family living on the Åland Islands in the Gulf of Bothnia between Finland and Sweden. Three of her sisters died by the age of four years of severe bleeding; her parents, two brothers, and many relatives of both sexes had mild bleeding histories. The disease was clearly different from classical haemophilia, and also from Glanzmann's thrombasthenia. By the time that this first report was published, another sister had died at the age of five years of massive haematemesis (von Willebrand 1931). The proband died with her fourth menstrual period at the age of thirteen (von Willebrand & Jürgens 1933).

These early descriptions illustrated clearly the salient clinical features of von Willebrand disease (vWD). Mild vWD was inherited as an autosomal dominant trait, whereas severe, life-threatening vWD was inherited as an autosomal recessive trait. Both patterns of inheritance were observed in the same affected Åland family. Bleeding from skin and mucous membranes, and after trauma, was very common. In contrast to classical haemophilia, bleeding into joints and soft tissues was uncommon.

The bleeding tendency of vWD was consistent with a platelet abnormality, or a defect in the vasculature, but the pathophysiology of the disorder was not understood for many decades following its discovery. In 1953, a prolonged bleeding time was found to be associated with autosomally inherited deficiency of blood coagulation factor VIII, which suggested that a blood plasma defect caused vWD (Alexander & Goldstein 1953, Larrieu & Soulier 1953, Quick & Hussey 1953). This interpretation was confirmed by demonstrating that the haemostatic defect of vWD was corrected by transfusion with plasma fractions from normal individuals (Nilsson et al 1957a,b) or from patients with haemophilia A (Nilsson et al 1959).

The genetic relationship between haemophilia A and vWD remained controversial until both factor VIII and von Willebrand factor (vWF) were resolved chromatographically, purified to homogeneity, and shown to be structurally distinct. By the mid 1980s, the structure of both proteins had been determined by protein chemistry and recombinant DNA methods. We now know that vWF consists of a series of multimers that range in size from dimers of ≈500 KDa to species of ≥20 000 KDa, and that vWF and factor VIII circulate in blood plasma as a noncovalently associated complex. Approximately 99% of the mass of the factor VIII-vWF complex consists of vWF (Ch. 15). This association is required for the normal survival of blood coagulation factor VIII in the circulation. In haemophilia A, a defect in the factor VIII gene causes a decreased level of factor VIII activity, and vWF levels remain normal. In vWD, a defect in the vWF gene causes a decrease in the level of vWF activity and usually this is accompanied by a decrease in the level of vWF protein. Because the survival of factor VIII requires association with vWF, deficiency of vWD protein causes a secondary deficiency of factor VIII. This mechanism appears to explain the observed variations of vWF and factor VIII levels in both vWD and haemophilia A.

The clinical heterogeneity of vWD was appreciated from the earliest reports. The first evidence for biochemical heterogeneity of vWD was provided by Holmberg & Nilsson (1972) who distinguished quantitative and qualitative abnormalities of vWF. Since then, many qualitative variants of vWD have been identified. The characterization of vWD mutations has provided insight into the structure–function relationships of vWF, and specific molecular defects appear to correlate with distinct pathogenetic mechanisms.

MOLECULAR BIOLOGY

The vWF gene spans approximately 180 kb of DNA and contains 52 exons (Fig. 35.1) (Mancuso et al 1989). The vWF gene is located on chromosome 12p12-pter, and is the most telomeric marker known on the short arm of chromosome 12 (Ginsburg et al 1985, Verweij et al 1985).

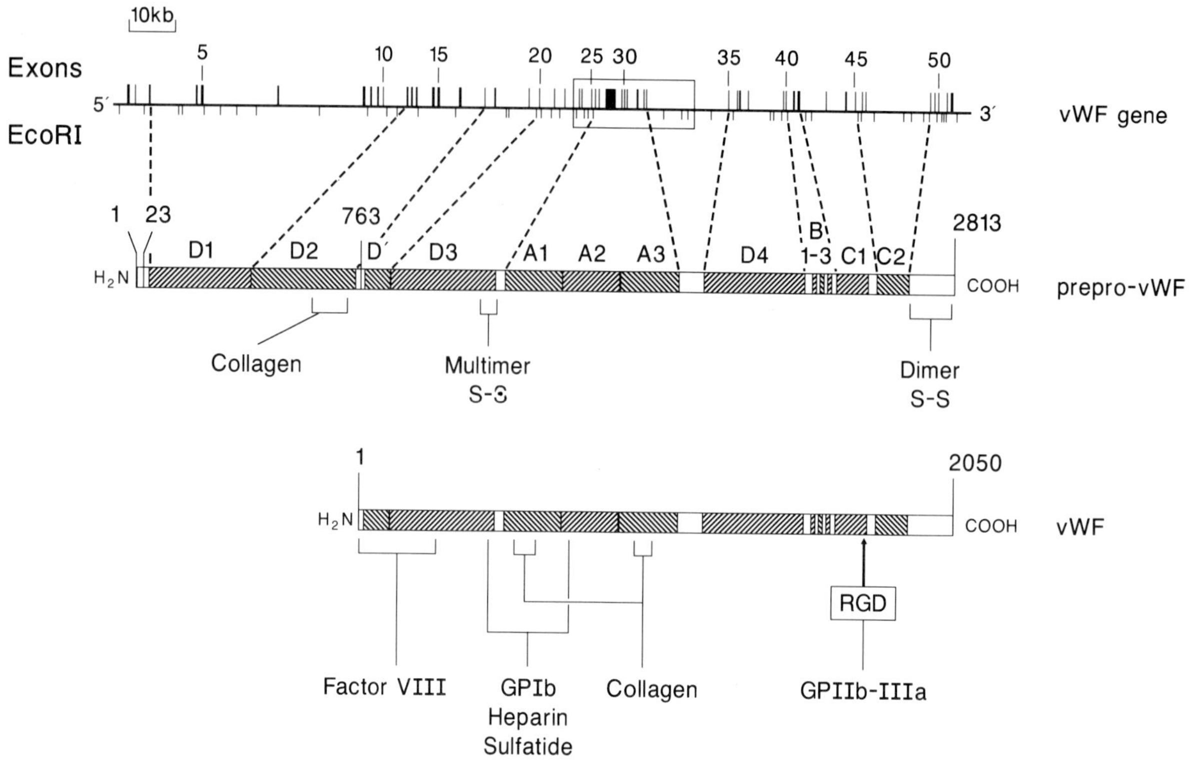

Fig. 35.1 Structure of the vWF gene and the encoded vWF protein. *vWF gene*: The structure of the vWF gene is shown with the position of exons and of EcoRI sites indicated. The box outline shows the region that is duplicated in the vWF pseudogene. *Prepro-vWF*: The structure of the *prepro-vWF* protein is shown below the structure of the vWF gene. The relationship between the exons and the repeated domains of the prepro-vWF amino acid sequence is indicated by dashed lines. The prepro-vWF consists of 2813 amino acid residues, of which residues 1–22 constitute a prepeptide or signal peptide, residues 23–762 constitute a propeptide that is cleaved from the majority of the subunits, and residues 763–2813 constitute the mature subunit. The propeptide is also known as von Willebrand antigen II. A collagen-binding site has been identified within the propepetide. Intersubunit disulphide bonds are formed between the C-terminal ends of pro-vWF to form dimers. Additional intersubunit disulphide bonds are formed near the N-terminal ends to form multimers. *vWF*: The mature vWF subunit consists of 2050 amino acids. Binding sites within the subunit have been localized as indicated for several macromolecules (Ch. 16). The glycoprotein IIb–IIIa complex of activated platelets binds vWF through a segment that includes the tripeptide sequence Arg-Gly-Asp (RGD).

The vWF gene lies within an interval of the genetic map for which recombination frequency is higher in males than in females. This contrasts with most other parts of the human linkage map, for which recombination is higher in females. The basis for this unusual genetic behaviour is not known (O'Connell et al 1987).

A partial pseudogene for vWF is located on chromosome 22 (Shelton-Inloes et al 1987). The pseudogene spans approximately 30 kb DNA and corresponds to exons 23–24 of the vWD gene. The presence of splice site and nonsense mutations indicates that this pseudogene cannot give rise to a functional transcript. The vWF gene and pseudogene have diverged approximately 3.1% in nucleotide sequence. This suggests a relatively recent origin for the vWF pseudogene within the last 10–15 million years, at about the time of divergence of Old World monkeys from the ancestors of the great apes and humans (Mancuso et al 1991c).

The vWF precursor is composed of four types of repeated domain, each present in two to five copies. Together these repeated domains constitute more than 90% of the subunit sequence (Ch. 16). The gene structure of vWF shows that intron-exon boundaries tend to occur in similar positions in homologous domains; this correspondence is consistent with the evolution of the current distribution of repeated domains by repeated gene segment duplications.

The evolution of vWF also appears to have involved exon shuffling, and vWF can be considered a mosaic protein. Homologues of the vWF A domains are found in at least 14 otherwise unrelated proteins that belong to at least six distinct protein superfamilies (reviewed in Colombatti & Bonaldo 1991). These families include vWF itself, several members of the integrin family of cell adhesion molecules, cartilage matrix protein, the non-fibrillar collagen types VI and XII (Yamagata et al 1991), the complement protease zymogens factor B and component C2, and undulin (Just et al 1991). In vWF, the A domains mediate binding to other macromolecules such as platelet glycoprotein Ib, fibrillar collagens, heparin, and sulphatides. Many of the proteins that contain vWF A domains also bind to other proteins, and it is tempting to speculate that this binding activity is dependent on the vWF A domains in these proteins.

The vWF gene and the encoded protein are highly polymorphic. More that 32 polymorphic marker systems have been described for the vWF gene, among which approximately one half alter the encoded amino acid sequence (Sadler & Ginsburg 1993). These amino acid sequence polymorphisms are not known to affect the function of vWF, but subtle differences in function potentially could be associated with sequence variations that are considered normal at the present time. In principle, such variation in the function of apparently normal vWF alleles could affect the severity of vWF.

Genetic polymorphisms provide powerful tools for the tracking of mutant vWF alleles within families, and for the prenatal diagnosis of affected infants. Genetic counselling for vWD is relatively straightforward. For severe vWD, genetic counselling is as for any autosomal recessive disorder. For the milder autosomal dominant forms of vWD, genetic counselling is possible and should be offered to affected families. Because of the relatively mild phenotype of most forms of dominant vWD, however, prospective parents generally do not elect to alter their reproductive plans.

CLINICAL FEATURES

Prevalence

Although vWD appear to be the most common human inherited bleeding disorder, precise data concerning prevalence are difficult to obtain. This lack of precision reflects the extreme variability in clinical presentation of milder forms of vWD. Inherited abnormalities of vWF function can be detected by laboratory testing in approximately 8000 persons per million population (Rodeghiero et al 1987), but most of these persons are asymptomatic and cannot be said to have a disease.

Clinically significant vWD appears to affect approximately 125 per million population (Holmberg & Nilsson 1985). Almost all of these individuals are affected by relatively mild, autosomal dominant variants of vWD. Severe, autosomal recessive vWD affects 0.5–5 persons per million. The prevalence in the United States and most of Europe appears to be approximately 1.4–1.6 per million (Weiss et al 1982a, Mannucci et al 1984a). Slightly higher values were reported for Scandinavia and for selected populations in the Middle East (Berliner et al 1986).

Symptoms

Bleeding symptoms in vWD often begin soon after birth and are lifelong. The pattern of bleeding tends to be similar to that seen in disorders of platelet function. The most common symptoms are nose bleeding, bleeding after tooth extraction, bleeding from minor skin wounds, gingival bleeding, and postoperative bleeding. Gastrointestinal bleeding is not common, but when it occurs it is usually serious. Most women with vWD suffer from menometrorrhagia (Buchanan & Leavell 1956, Larrieu et al 1968, Silwer 1973). Haemorrhage during labour and delivery is less frequent that might be expected due to the increase in vWF levels that accompanies pregnancy, but may be especially troublesome for variants of vWD (type II) with a dysfunctional vWF protein (Mannucci et al 1983, 1986, Kinoshita et al 1984, Mazurier et al 1986). Spontaneous bleeding into joints or soft tissues is distinctly uncommon, but does occur in severe vWD. There is a tendency for symptoms to decrease with advancing age.

Laboratory evaluation

The bleeding symptoms associated with vWD are not at all specific, therefore the diagnosis depends upon proper laboratory evaluation. Quantitative assays of plasma vWF concentration are commonly referenced to a standard normal plasma, which is defined to contain 1 unit/ml of vWF. One unit corresponds to approximately 5–10 μg of vWF.

Bleeding time. The template bleeding time provides a measure of platelet plug formation, which depends upon vWF. Several bleeding time methods are in common use, and the test results are notoriously variable and difficult to standardize (Triplett 1991). An abnormal bleeding time is not, however, specific for a defect in vWF, but may be caused by defects in platelets, connective tissue, or by faulty technique. The bleeding time is prolonged at some time in almost all patients with clinically significant vWD, but often is intermittently normal in milder vWD variants (Abildgaard et al 1980).

Ristocetin cofactor activity. A convenient laboratory test for vWF function was described in 1971 by Howard & Firkin, who discovered that the agglutination of platelets by the antibiotic ristocetin was dependent upon the presence of vWF. With increasing concentration, ristocetin dimerizes and binds both to platelets and to vWF (Coller 1978, Scott et al 1991). These interactions promote the binding of vWF to platelet glycoprotein Ib (Ch. 16); because platelets and vWF are polyvalent, this leads to platelet agglutination. Ristocetin cofactor activity (RiCoF) is assayed by mixing samples of patient platelet-poor plasma, washed formalin-fixed platelets and a high concentration of ristocetin. The maximal rate of platelet agglutination is determined by aggregometry and compared to the rates obtained with dilutions of a standard plasma (MacFarlane et al 1975). The distribution of vWF: RiCoF values in normal subjects is broad, from approximately 0.5–2.0 units/ml (Rodeghiero et al 1987), and this can cause difficulty in the identification of mild vWF.

Ristocetin-induced platelet agglutination. A second

ristocetin-based assay is employed to discriminate between certain gain-of-function and loss-of-function variants of vWD. To measure ristocetin-induced platelet aggregation (RIPA), ristocetin is added to patient platelet-rich plasma, and the rate and extent of platelet agglutination are determined as a function of ristocetin concentration. Detection is based on aggregometry, following an increase in light transmission (Weiss 1975).

Factor VIII. The maintenance of a normal plasma factor VIII concentration requires the interaction of factor VIII with vWF. Consequently, factor VIII levels indirectly reflect vWF levels or function. A discrepancy between the factor VIII level and the ristocetin cofactor level can provide evidence for a qualitative abnormality of vWF.

vWF antigen. Plasma vWF antigen level (vWF:Ag) can be assayed conveniently by electroimmunoassay (Laurell 1966, Zimmerman et al 1975), immunoradiometric assay (Hoyer 1972, Ruggeri et al 1976), or a variety of immunoenzymatic methods. The sensitivity depends on the precise method, but can be made to be less than 0.0002 units/ml. The range of normal values is similar to that for RiCoF.

vWF multimers. The multimer distribution of plasma or platelet vWF is determined by gel electrophoresis methods (Hoyer & Shainoff 1980, Ruggeri & Zimmerman 1980, 1981) (Fig. 35.2). Decreased vWF concentration with a normal multimer distribution is consistent with a quantitative deficiency of vWF. Structural abnormalities, such as a loss of high molecular weight multimers, are consistent with qualitative defects of vWF. The distinction between type I vWD and most forms of type II vWD is made conveniently on so-called low resolution agarose gels. These contain 1.0–1.4% agarose, and clearly distinguish the presence or absence of high molecular weight vWF multimers. The subclassification of many vWD type II variants requires the use of high resolution gel systems, which usually employ higher concentrations of agarose (2–3%) to resolve the structure of the smallest multimers and minor associated intervening or 'satellite' bands (Mannucci et al 1986).

Other assays. Crossed immunoelectrophoresis can demonstrate alterations in vWF multimer patterns (Zimmerman et al 1982), although this method is less sensitive than multimer gel electrophoresis. A protein found in the venom of *Bothrops jararaca*, termed 'botrocetin', induces platelet agglutination by promoting the binding of

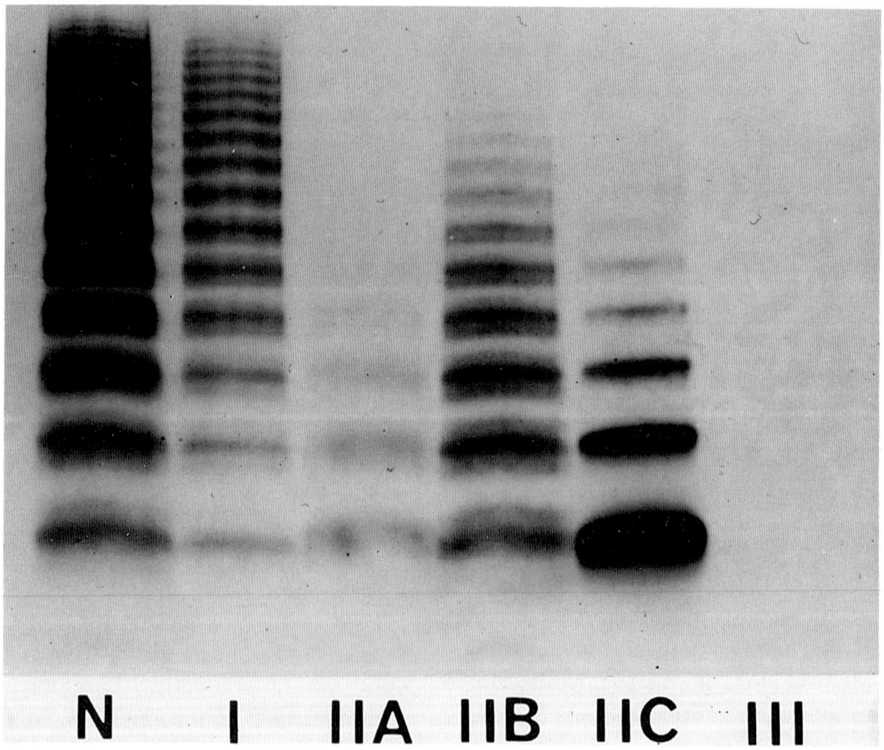

Fig. 35.2 Patterns of vWF multimers in several types of vWD Samples of plasma from a normal individual (N) and from patients with vWD types I, IIA, IIB, IIC, and III were electrophoresed on a 1.3% agarose/SDS gel, blotted by capillary action onto a polyvinylidene difluoride membrane, and the vWF multimers were visualized by an enzymatic method employing rabbit antihuman vWF antibodies (Raines et al 1990). Quantitative abnormalities of vWF are characterized by partial (type I) or complete (type III) deficiency of all vWF multimers. Qualitative abnormalities of vWF (type II) often are characterized by deficiencies of larger vWF multimers; some variants exhibit abnormal intensity or spacing of intervening bands (type IIC).

vWF to platelet glycoprotein Ib (Read et al 1978) and this property has been used to assay 'botrocetin cofactor activity' in a manner analogous to RiCoF (Brinkhous & Read 1980). Assays have been described for vWF binding to collagens (Brown & Bosak 1986, Aihara et al 1988), heparin (de Romeuf et al 1991), and factor VIII (Nishino et al 1989, Mazurier et al 1990a). Defective interaction between vWF and factor VIII can cause symptomatic factor VIII deficiency, as discussed below.

Diagnostic approach

The diagnosis of vWD should be considered in any patient with bleeding mainly from the skin and mucous membranes, especially if the family history suggests an autosomal pattern of inheritance. A complete evaluation of vWF structure and function would require at least a platelet count, bleeding time, assays of plasma and platelet vWF:Ag, plasma RiCoF and factor VIII, RIPA, and plasma and platelet vWF multimer analysis. In a more cost effective approach, the initial laboratory evaluation of a new patient suspected to have vWD could include a platelet count, bleeding time, and assays of plasma vWF:Ag, RiCoF, and factor VIII. Still less testing may be appropriate for a patient from a family with a well characterized form of vWD.

Thrombocytopenia does not exclude the diagnosis of vWD, particularly of variants with enhanced affinity of vWF for platelets, but a platelet count $\leq 100 \times 10^9$/l may prolong the bleeding time independently of vWF and thus complicate the interpretation of an abnormal bleeding time. Plasma vWF and factor VIII levels are substantially lower in persons of blood type O, and separate normal ranges should be established for type O versus all other ABO blood types. Patients with low normal values should have their ABO blood type determined so that they can be evaluated against the proper control population (Graham et al 1986, Gill et al 1987, Rodeghiero et al 1987). Levels of vWF and factor VIII also increase slightly with age.

Severe type III vWD rarely poses a diagnostic problem, but the recognition of mild forms of vWD (type I and some type II) can be difficult because the bleeding time and values for other assays may occasionally lie within the normal range (Abildgaard et al 1980). The effects of physiological stress may contribute to this variability. Plasma levels of vWF and factor VIII are increased by a variety of stresses such as inflammation, adrenergic agonists, pregnancy, and exercise (Bloom 1979). Consequently, repeated testing may be required to elicit abnormal values that support the diagnosis of vWD. In such cases, examination of family members can be useful to identify symptomatic or asymptomatic relatives with abnormalities of vWF, and thereby to demonstrate the autosomal inheritance of a vWF defect.

If the RiCoF is not clearly low, or the patient is thrombocytopenic, RIPA should be determined. This assay is not a good screening test for vWD because it is not particularly sensitive to decreases in vWF concentration (Weiss 1975). RIPA is used mainly to identify the paradoxically increased response to low doses of ristocetin that characterizes vWD type IIB (Ruggeri et al 1980) and type I New York (Weiss & Sussman 1986), and also platelet-type or pseudo vWD (Miller & Castella 1982, Weiss et al 1982b). Patients with these disorders are important to recognize because the treatment of bleeding with 1-deamino-8-D-arginine vasopressin (DDAVP) is generally ineffective and may cause or exacerbate thrombocytopenia.

A qualitative loss-of-function defect in vWF is suggested by a disproportionately low value for RiCoF compared to the values for vWF:Ag and factor VIII. Such type II vWD variants are further categorized on the basis of multimer gel analysis. Most forms of type II vWD are associated with the absence of high molecular weight multimers from plasma vWF (Fig. 35.2). Comparison of the plasma and platelet multimer patterns is useful to distinguish certain variants, and high-resolution gels can demonstrate still more phenotypic heterogeneity.

CLASSIFICATION AND MOLECULAR DEFECTS

Three major categories of vWD are distinguished (Table 35.1). Type I refers to partial quantitative deficiency of vWF, and is inherited in an autosomal dominant fashion. Type II refers to qualitative abnormalities, most of which are associated with defects in vWF multimer structure. Type III refers to virtually complete absence of plasma vWF, and is inherited in an autosomal recessive fashion. Each of these categories is genetically heterogeneous.

Mutations have been characterized in the vWF gene of many patients with various types of vWD. These mutations are catalogued in a database that is updated regularly (Ginsburg & Sadler 1993).

Table 35.1 Classification of the major types of vWD

Type	Pathophysiology	Molecular defects
I	Partial deficiency, normal vWF protein (dominant inheritance)	Unknown
II	Abnormal vWF protein	Missense mutations, small in-frame deletions or insertions
IIA	Defective multimer biosynthesis Increased multimer degradation	Figure 35.3; see text Figure 35.3; see text
IIB	Increased binding to platelet GPIb	Figure 35.3
II 'Normandy'	Decreased binding to factor VIII	Figure 35.4
III	Total vWF deficiency (recessive inheritance)	Deletions, nonsense mutations

Laboratory findings characteristic of these vWD type are described in the text.

Type I vWD

Type I vWD is the most common form of vWD and accounts for approximately 70% of symptomatic cases (Hoyer et al 1983, Holmberg & Nilsson 1985). It is inherited in an autosomal dominant fashion, but penetrance or expressivity are variable. In one study of two large pedigrees, 11 of 26 persons who appeared to transmit the disease were themselves phenotypically normal (Miller et al 1979). Type I vWD is characterized by similar decreases in all assays of vWF protein concentration or function. Multimer gel electrophoresis shows a normal distribution of multimers, but with decreased intensity. This pattern is consistent with a simple quantitative deficiency of vWF, and probably is caused by a decreased rate of synthesis of a normal vWF protein.

Type I vWD has been divided further into several subtypes on the basis of the comparisons between plasma and platelet vWF multimer subbands or satellite bands (Ciavarella et al 1985, López-Fernández et al 1991), the presence of unusually large VWF multimers (Mannucci et al 1988), or persistence of large amount of the uncleaved vWF propeptide in plasma vWF (Montgomery et al 1986). Certain of these distinctions may have clinical utility; in particular, normal platelet vWF structure, concentrations, and function appears to be associated with a favourable therapeutic response to DDAVP (Mannucci et al 1985). In some of these type I subtypes the vWF clearly has abnormal function, and these variants should be classified as qualitative or type II disorders.

Candidate molecular defects have been described in two patients with apparent type I vWD. The vWF:Ag levels were decreased, but in each case the RiCoF was disproportionately and markedly decreased. One patient was found to have a deletion of 11 amino acids within the Cys^{509}–Cys^{695} disulphide loop of vWF domain A1 (Mancuso et al 1991a), and the other had a missense mutation Phe^{606} to Ile in the same loop (Mancuso et al 1991b). Thus, despite the normal appearance of the multimer structure, the vWF was altered structurally and had abnormal function. To date, no type I mutations have been reported that cause quantitative, symptomatic deficiency of vWF.

Type II vWD

Type II vWD refers to bleeding diathesis that is caused by a qualitative abnormality of vWF. These variants are often characterized by a disproportionately low value for RiCoF compared to the values for vWF:Ag or factor VIII. In most cases, qualitative defects in vWF are associated with the loss of high molecular weight multimers. This association provides a convenient means to distinguish type I vWD from most variants of type II vWD, i.e. by multimer gel electrophoresis. The correlation between abnormal multimer pattern and abnormal vWF protein is not perfect, however, and as the molecular pathogenesis of vWD becomes better understood, some variants that are now considered to be type I vWD will require reclassification as type II vWD.

Mutations have been characterized in several subtypes of type II vWD (Ginsburg & Sadler 1993). These include missense mutations, small insertions and deletions, and one rather large in-frame deletion that appears to result in the synthesis of a short, defective vWF subunit (Bernardi et al 1990). Many of the missense mutations have been identified in more than one unrelated family, and virtually all of these apparently recurrent mutations are C→T transitions within CG dinucleotides. The cytidine in CG dinucleotides is frequently methylated in human DNA, and the recurrence of vWD mutations in such dinucleotides is consistent with other evidence that the methylcytidine groups in CG dinucleotides are 'hotspots' for mutation by demethylation to thymidine (Barker et al 1984).

Type IIA

This variant accounts for approximately three-fourths of all type II vWD. It is characterized by autosomal dominant inheritance, decreased or normal vWF:Ag levels, and markedly decreased ristocetin cofactor activity. The vWF multimer pattern in plasma shows an absence of high molecular weight multimers, often with an increase in the intensity of the smallest multimer and fastest migrating satellite band (Ruggeri & Zimmerman 1980).

The vWD type IIA phenotype appears to be caused by at least two distinct pathophysiological mechanisms that may correlate with the multimer pattern observed for platelet vWF (Table 35.1). In some patients the platelet vWF lacks large multimers, and the biosynthesis and processing of vWF appears to be abnormal so that large multimers cannot be properly assembled or secreted. Other patients exhibit an essentially normal platelet vWF pattern, and the pathophysiological mechanism appears to be increased sensitivity of plasma vWF to proteolytic degradation. Large multimers are rapidly degraded to lower molecular weight species in the circulation. The protease responsible for this degradation is not known, but a major site of subunit cleavage was shown to be the Tyr^{842}–Met^{843} bond within vWF domain A2 (Dent et al 1990). The vWF in protected sites, such as platelet α granules or endothelial cells, has a normal multimer pattern (Ruggeri & Zimmerman 1980, Weiss et al 1983, Gralnick et al 1985a, Batlle et al 1986a).

With a few exceptions, mutations that cause vWD type IIA cluster within a segment of vWF that corresponds to domain A2 (Fig. 35.3). This proximity to the principle site of subunit cleavage may be related to the enhanced proteolysis that is characteristic of some type IIA mutations. Studies of recombinant mutant vWF indicate that the mutations Gly^{742} to Glu and Arg^{834} to Trp do not impair multimer assembly, and presumably cause type IIA

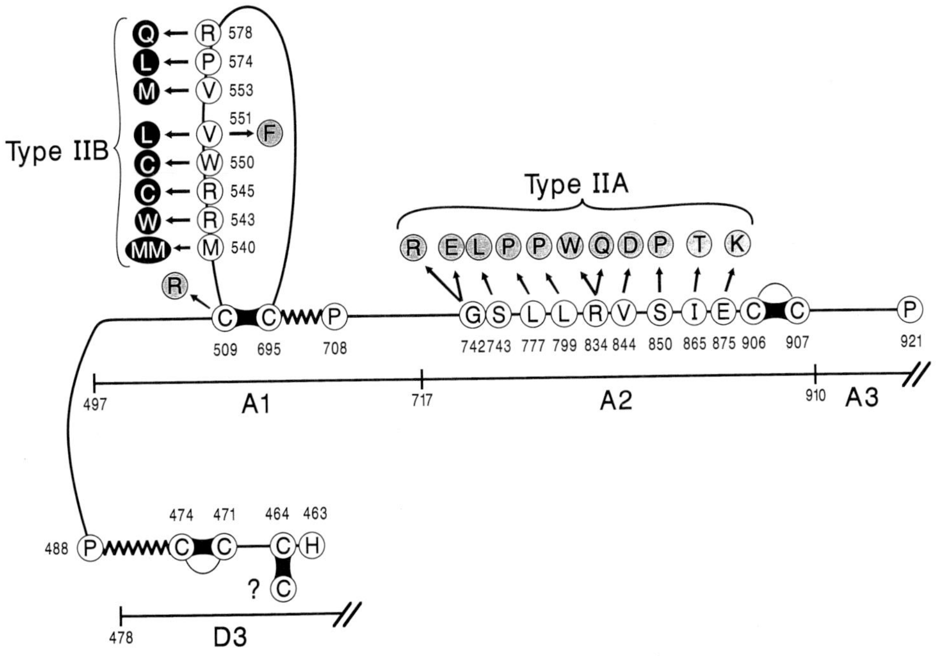

Fig. 35.3 Mutation within vWF exon 28 that cause vWD types IIA and IIB. Exon 28 encodes amino acid residues 463–921 of the mature vWF subunit. The positions of repeated domains D3, A1, A2, and A3 are indicated. Mutations reported to cause vWD type IIA (open circles) and type IIB (black circles) are indicated. Two proposed type IIA mutations occur in the region of the type IIB mutations. References to individual mutations are compiled in Ginsburg & Sadler (1993).

vWD by increasing susceptibility to proteolysis in vivo (Table 35.1) (Lyons et al 1992). In contrast, the mutations Gly^{742} to Arg, Ser^{743} to Leu, Val^{844} to Asp, and Ser^{850} to Pro result in the synthesis and secretion of small vWF multimers (Chang et al 1989, Lyons et al 1992). Interestingly, mutations that cause impaired multimer synthesis occur in the same region, and even in the same codon, as do mutations that cause enhanced sensitivity to proteolytic degradation (Lyons et al 1992). As yet, there is no explanation for why mutations cause vWD type IIA by one mechanism or the other.

The clustering of most vWD type IIA mutations in a small segment of the subunit sequence, and the relationship of specific mutations to distinct pathophysiological mechanisms, make screening for mutations an attractive idea. With recombinant DNA methods, it is feasible to identify mutations in most patients with vWD type IIA at relatively low cost. Knowledge of the mutation may have value for predicting the therapeutic response to DDAVP, although this remains to be demonstrated.

Type IIB

Type IIB vWD is a relatively uncommon variant, accounting for less than 20% of all type II vWD. The multimer pattern in plasma shows a loss of high molecular weight multimers, but the multimer pattern in platelets is normal (Ruggeri & Zimmerman 1980, Ruggeri et al 1980). The plasma vWF multimer pattern in vWF type IIB is often said to contain multimers of intermediate size that are absent in type IIA. However, the distribution of multimers does not reliably distinguish types IIA and IIB, Some patients with type IIB vWD have multimer patterns that are indistinguishable from type IIA on low-resolution gel systems, and the multimer distribution can vary for a single patient examined at different times.

This variant is characterized by normal to moderately decreased levels of vWF:Ag, normal to moderately decreased levels of RiCoF, but increased sensitivity to ristocetin in the RIPA assay. This apparent gain-of-function phenotype is paradoxically associated with bleeding. This appears to be explained by spontaneous binding of the mutant plasma vWF to platelet glycoprotein Ib, with subsequent clearance of the large multimers and platelets from the circulation. The remaining small multimers are not haemostatically effective.

Type IIB vWD is associated with variable thrombocytopenia that may be persistent or intermittent, and often is exacerbated by stress such as inflammation, surgery, or pregnancy (Holmberg et al 1983, Gralnick et al 1985b, Saba et al 1985, Rick et al 1987, Hultin & Sussman 1990). Families with this variant have been described in whom throbocytopenia is age dependent (Mazurier et al 1988), and this may by explained by the tendency of vWF levels to increase with age.

Mutations in vWD type IIB are clustered within the disulphide loop of domain A1, within the region of vWF that contains the binding site for platelet glycoprotein Ib

(Fig. 35.3). The mechanism by which these mutations enhance the binding of vWF to GPIb is not known. A small number of mutations appear to account for more than 80% of all cases of vWD type IIB. Thus, accurate molecular diagnosis of this variant is possible.

Type II 'Normandy'

This variant is characterized by normal levels of vWF:Ag, normal ristocetin cofactor activity, and a normal multimer pattern in both plasma and platelets, associated with a mildly to moderately decreased factor VIII level. The clinical characteristics resemble haemophilia A but the disorder is inherited as an autosomal recessive trait, and the plasma vWF from affected patients does not bind to factor VIII (Nishino et al 1989, Mazurier et al 1990a). This form of type type II vWD was tentatively named 'Normandy' after the birth province of one proband (Mazurier et al 1990a); this name is employed herein for convenience, in the absence of a generally accepted designation for this variant. Several mutations have been identified in the factor VIII binding site of vWF that abolish or markedly decrease the affinity of vWF for factor VIII and cause vWD Normandy (Fig. 35.4). Because normal factor VIII survival in the circulation requires binding to vWF, these defects result in a secondary deficiency of factor VIII.

The prevalence of vWD Normandy is not known, but at least 14 affected families have been reported since 1989. This diagnosis should be considered in any patient with factor VIII deficiency in whom the deficiency is not demonstrated to be X chromosome-linked. In contrast to patients with mild haemophilia, vWD Normandy does not respond to DDAVP with an increase of the plasma factor VIII level (López-Fernández et al 1992), and replacement therapy with highly purified factor VIII preparations is associated with decreased recovery and survival of factor VIII in vivo (Mazurier et al 1990b, López-Fernández et al 1992).

Several patients have been described in whom a vWD Normandy-like defect is associated with decreased vWF levels characteristic of vWD type I (Nishino et al 1989, Cacheris et al 1991, Kroner et al 1991, Peerlinck et al 1992). These patients appear to be compound heterozygous for a vWD Normandy allele and a vWD type I allele. The variable presentation of factor VIII binding defects in vWD illustrates the potential importance of compound heterozygosity in determining the clinical presentation of vWD variants.

Other type II variants

A bewildering variety of other qualitative abnormalities of

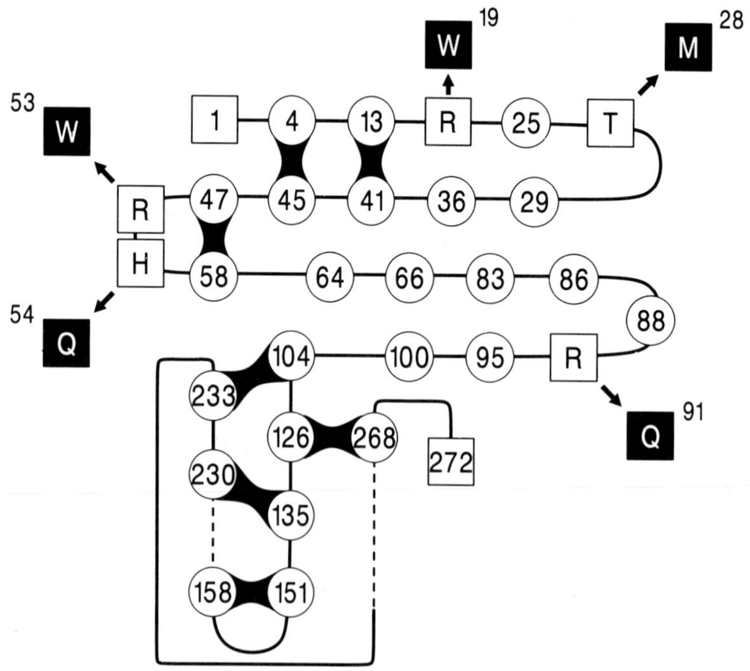

Fig. 35.4 Mutations of vWF that decrease binding to factor VIII. The numbered circles represent cysteine residues. The known disulphide pairings are indicated; the remaining cysteine residues form disulphide bonds within this fragment but the pairings have not been determined. The Arg(19)→Trp and His(54)→Gln mutations were found in the same allele of an affected patient; whether one or both are required to impair binding of factor VIII is not known. References to individual mutations are compiled in Ginsburg & Sadler (1993).

vWF have been described (reviewed in Ruggeri 1991). These include the variants originally designated as types IB (Hoyer et al 1983), IC (Ciavarella et al 1985), ID (López-Fernández et al 1991), I New York (Weiss & Sussman 1986), IIC (Ruggeri et al 1982b, Mannucci et al 1983, Batlle et al 1986b, c, Mazurier et al 1986), IID (Kinoshita et al 1984, Hill et al 1985), IIE (Zimmerman et al 1986), IIF (Mannucci et al 1986), IIG (Gralnick et al 1987), IIH (Federici et al 1989), and II-I (Castaman et al 1992), as well as type B (Howard et al 1982) and several unnamed variants.

The majority of these variants are characterized by abnormal vWF multimer patterns, usually with loss of high molecular weight multimers. These have been recognized chiefly on the basis of patterns observed on high resolution multimer gels. Defects have included variations in the number and spacing of minor bands that intervene between the major multimer bands. In most cases the inheritance is autosomal dominant. The underlying molecular defects and pathophysiology generally are not known; the exception is vWD type B, which is caused by a missense mutation in domain A1 Gly^{561} to Ser (Rabinowitz et al 1992) This variant is characterized by an interesting dissociation between two assays that reflect binding to platelet GPIb: RiCoF is absent, while botrocetin cofactor activity is normal (Howard et al 1982).

Almost all of these variants are represented by one or a few affected families, and recognition of similar patients requires not only exceptional technical facility with the electrophoretic analysis of vWF, but also access to reference plasma or platelet samples from the index patients. Since vWD is autosomally inherited, and most affected patients are compound heterozygous, some of the variation in multimer pattern may be due to interactions among different mutant alleles, or between one mutant allele and different normal alleles. As the molecular basis of vWD is understood in greater detail, classifications based principally on vWF multimer patterns may be replaced by a classification based upon specific molecular defects and pathophysiological mechanisms.

Type III vWD

Type III vWD is characterized by autosomal recessive inheritance, and by extremely low or undetectable levels of vWF in both plasma and platelets. As in vWD Normandy, the consequent failure to stabilize circulating factor VIII commonly results in moderate factor VIII deficiency. Occasional patients have severe factor VIII deficiency (Larrieu et al 1968, Italian Working Group 1977, Zimmerman et al 1979). Because of the combined defect of vWF and factor VIII, patients with vWD type III may have bleeding in patterns that are typical both of platelet dysfunction and of haemophilia A.

Type III vWD is quite uncommon, affecting 0.5 to 3 persons per million population (Mannucci et al 1984a). The expected prevalence of heterozygosity is, therefore, at least 1400 to 3500 per million. Since clinically significant vWD affects only about 125 per million, most heterozygous carriers of vWD type III must be asymptomatic. In fact, most parents and first degree relatives of patients with severe vWD are not symptomatic, although a large fraction do have abnormalities that can be detected by laboratory testing (Bloom & Peake 1979, Miller et al 1979, Mannucci et al 1989). One of the remaining mysteries in vWD is that mild quantitative deficiency of vWF is usually asymptomatic in the heterozygous relatives of patients with type III vWD, while apparently similar deficiencies are symptomatic in pedigrees affected by type I vWD.

Gene deletions and nonsense mutations have been characterized in several patients with type III vWD. Total gene deletions were found in three ostensibly unrelated families from Italy (Shelton-Inloes et al 1987, Ngo et al 1988). A small 2.3 kb deletion that contained exon 42 was found in a homozygous patient from Wales (Peake et al 1990). Larger partial gene deletions were found in members of two other unrelated families (Mannucci & Cattaneo 1991). Nonsense mutations were found in three patients, apparently caused by C→T transitions within the methylated CG dinucleotides of certain arginine codons (Bahnak et al 1991, Eikenboom et al 1991, Zhang et al 1992).

Gene deletions appear to predispose to the formation of inhibitory antibodies against transfused vWF. Inhibitor formation is a rare complication of therapy in vWD; only approximately 15 affected unrelated families have been reported (Mannucci & Mari 1984, Mannucci & Cattaneo 1991). Each of the six families with known gene deletions contains affected patients with such alloantibody inhibitors. In contrast, gene deletions have not been found in any patients who do not have alloantibody inhibitors.

DIFFERENTIAL DIAGNOSIS

The symptoms of vWD may include bleeding that is characteristic of platelet dysfunction or of factor VIII deficiency, and may range in severity from extremely mild to life-threatening. These symptoms are not specific, and occur in many conditions that otherwise do not resemble vWD. These include primary platelet disorders and the ingestion of antiplatelet drugs. Appropriate laboratory testing can distinguish most of these conditions, but a few provide special diagnostic challenges.

Haemophilia A

Mild haemophilia A can be confused with vWD, particularly if the vWF level is low for some reason, such as blood type O. The ingestion of antiplatelet drugs such as aspirin by patients with haemophilia A may produce a clinical picture that is very similar to vWD.

The potential for confusion between vWD Normandy and haemophilia A was discussed above (p. 850). Males with vWD Normandy have been misdiagnosed as having haemophilia A; their affected female relatives have been incorrectly identified as carriers of haemophilia A with symptomatic factor VIII deficiency attributed incorrectly to extreme lyonization (Mazurier et al 1990b, López-Fernández et al 1992). Correct diagnosis has significant implications for genetic counselling and also for therapy.

Platelet-type or pseudo-vWD

Platelet-type (Takahashi 1980, Miller & Castella 1982) or pseudo-vWD (Weiss et al 1982b) is an autosomal dominant disorder with clinical features that are very similar to vWD type IIB, but the defect is in platelet glycoprotein Ib rather than in vWF. The vWF concentration may be normal or decreased, but ristocetin-induced platelet agglutination (RIPA) occurs at relatively low concentrations of ristocetin. Plasma vWF is usually deficient in high molecular weight multimers. This condition can be distinguished from vWD type IIB by mixing experiments. Normal platelets suspended in patient plasma show normal sensitivity to ristocetin. In contrast, patient platelets suspended in normal plasma continue to exhibit increased sensitivity to ristocetin, whether measured as RIPA or as ristocetin-induced binding of vWF to platelets (Scott & Montgomery 1991). This condition is rare, but correct diagnosis is important so that appropriate therapy can be considered. The optimal treatment for bleeding is not obvious. Given alone, DDAVP or vWF preparations are often ineffective and may cause significant thrombocytopenia (Miller et al 1984, Takahashi et al 1984). Platelet transfusions may be necessary to compensate for the intrinsic platelet defect, and could be administered in combination with measures to increase plasma vWF.

Two candidate missense mutations in the GPIbα subunit gene have been characterized in this disorder: Gly^{233} to Val (Miller et al 1991) and Met^{239} to Val (Russell & Roth 1991).

Acquired von Willebrand syndrome

As discussed in Chapter 41 the acquired von Willebrand syndrome refers to vWF deficiency that is not inherited but is secondary to another cause (Mannucci & Mari 1984). In many cases the decrease in vWF function is presumably immunologically mediated, however antibodies to vWF can be demonstrated only in a small minority of patients. The condition is associated with recognized autoimmune disorders such as rheumatoid arthritis or systemic lupus erythematosus, with multiple myeloma and other lymphoproliferative disorders (Mannucci et al 1984b), and also with polycythaemia vera, essential thrombocythaemia, and other myeloproliferative disorders (Budde et al 1984, 1986, Fabris et al 1986). Several patients with hypothyroidism were reported with laboratory features of vWD, and some had bleeding symptoms (Dalton et al 1987, MacCallum et al 1987, Smith & Auger 1987, Takahashi et al 1987, Thornton et al 1987). In the acquired von Willebrand syndrome, the vWF concentration in plasma is low and the multimer distribution is often deficient in high molecular weight multimers, but platelet vWF multimers are normal. Without documentation of previously normal vWF function, the acquired von Willebrand syndrome may be very difficult to distinguish from inherited vWD. Successful treatment of the underlying disease may lead to correction of the vWF defect.

Other disorders

Type IIB vWD may cause progressive thrombocytopenia during pregnancy that can be confused with autoimmune thrombocytopenia. Such patients have received unnecessary treatment with corticosteroids (Giles et al 1987, Rick et al 1987) or intravenous immunoglobulins (Ieko et al 1990, Valster et al 1990). Two men, who were ultimately shown to have type IIB vWD, underwent splenectomy for presumed autoimmune thrombocytopenia that was unresponsive to prednisone (Saba et al 1985, Sakariassen et al 1985). Type IIB vWD has also presented as congenital thrombocytopenia (Donnér et al 1987).

TREATMENT

Aspects of therapy that reflect the unique characteristics of individual vWD subtypes are emphasized below. Therapeutic recommendations for specific clinical situations are discussed in detail in Chapter 38.

1-Deamino-8-D-arginine vasopressin (DDAVP)

The vasopressin analogue, 1-deamino-8-D-arginine vasopressin (DDAVP), promotes the release of vWF from endothelial cells, and can thereby increase the plasma level of vWF and factor VIII several fold. The response to DDAVP is rapid but transient; in most cases vWF and factor VIII levels are maximally increased within 1 hour after administration and decay to baseline over several hours to days (Mannucci et al 1977, Rodeghiero et al 1991).

An effective response to DDAVP requires that the patient can synthesize some vWF that functions normally, both in supporting platelet adhesion and in stabilizing factor VIII. Consequently, DDAVP is not effective in vWD type III, in which essentially no vWF is synthesized. Similarly, for patients with vWD Normandy, in which the mutant vWF does not bind factor VIII, DDAVP increases vWF levels but not factor VIII levels (López-Fernández et al 1992).

DDAVP is usually effective in type I vWD and ineffective in type II vWD; however, for each type of vWD the exceptions are sufficiently frequent that an elective diagnostic test dose should be considered. For example, a test dose of 0.3 μg/kg DDAVP, in a small volume of isotonic saline, is administered intravenously over 30 min. The factor VIII level is measured at 0, 30, 60, 120, and 240 min, and the bleeding time is measured at 0, 30, and 120 min. An increase in factor VIII to ⩾50% and correction of the bleeding time constitute a favourable response. The pattern of response to a trial infusion predicts future responsiveness and can be used as a guide to clinical management (Rodeghiero et al 1989, 1991).

For patients with type IIB vWD, the administration of DDAVP often causes or exacerbates thrombocytopenia, and usually does not normalize the bleeding time (Ruggeri et al 1982a, Holmberg et al 1983, Rodeghiero et al 1989); similar effects have been reported in platelet-type or pseudo-vWD (Takahashi et al 1984). Because of concerns that intravascular platelet agglutination may cause thrombosis, DDAVP is not recommended for use in type IIB vWD (or in platelet-type or pseudo-vWD). However, a few patients with type IIB vWD have had beneficial haemostatic responses to DDAVP, without significant thrombocytopenia (Kyrle et al 1988, Fowler et al 1989). The basis of this apparent phenotypic heterogeneity is not known.

The recommended therapeutic dosage of DDAVP is 0.3 μg/kg administered either intravenously over 30 min or by subcutaneous injection. Larger doses apparently are not more effective. Intravenous and subcutaneous DDAVP have similar pharmacokinetics and appear to be equally efficacious (Mannucci et al 1987). Intranasal administration of concentrated DDAVP by spray, at approximately ten times the recommended intravenous dose (300 μg), also appears to be effective (Lethagen et al 1990). Preparations sufficiently concentrated for subcutaneous or intranasal administration are not available in all countries, however. Doses can be repeated every 24–36 hours, or as often as every 8 hours in selected cases. Administration more frequently than every 48 hours is often associated with progressively decreasing responses, although some patients do not exhibit significant tachyphylaxis.

In responsive patients, DDAVP is the treatment of choice for spontaneous bleeding and for bleeding after minor trauma. DDAVP can also provide effective coverage for dental procedures and minor surgery. Experience in major surgery is limited, but in selected patients haemostasis has been obtained with DDAVP alone. DDAVP may be given safely with standard doses of antifibrinolytic agents, such as ε-aminocaproic acid or tranexamic acid, and this combination is useful for dental procedures or other oral surgery. For surgery outside the mouth, there is no consensus concerning the usefulness of antifibrinolytic agents combined with DDAVP. In general, DDAVP should be used primarily when a several-fold increase in vWF and factor VIII, for a period of at most a few days, is expected to be adequate for haemostasis.

Adverse side-effects of DDAVP are rare. Patients commonly experience a ≈20% increase in heart rate, a ≈10–15% decrease in mean blood pressure, and facial flushing (Bichet et al 1988). Transient headache, nausea and abdominal cramps occur infrequently. A very low incidence of acute thrombosis has been reported, approximately ten episodes among an estimated 433 000 treated persons (Mannucci & Lusher 1989). Thus, DDAVP probably should be used cautiously in patients with atherosclerosis or other risk factors for thrombosis. In such patients the risk of thrombosis might be increased by the simultaneous use of antifibrinolytic agents, although there is no direct evidence for this effect. The antidiuretic effect of DDAVP can predispose to hyponatraemia. This complication is uncommon in adults but is a significant risk for children. Accordingly, fluid and electrolyte balance should be monitored closely for at least 24 hours in children receiving DDAVP (Smith et al 1989, Weinstein et al 1989).

Blood products containing vWF

Cryoprecipitate traditionally has been the blood product of choice for the treatment of severe bleeding in vWD, despite the potential for transmission of various viral diseases. Now that effective virucidally-treated concentrates are available, the use of untreated plasma derivatives such as cryoprecipitate must be discontinued. Several intermediate purity factor VIII preparations have been demonstrated to be effective in the treatment of vWD (Fukui et al 1988, Berntorp & Nilsson 1989, Cumming et al 1990, Pasi et al 1990, Mannucci et al 1992, Rodeghiero et al 1992).

As factor VIII products for the treatment of haemophilia A become ever more purified, the vWF content decreases to the point that these concentrates are not suitable for treatment of vWD. This applies particularly to the so-called 'monoclonal' plasma-derived factor VIII preparations, and to recombinant factor VIII. These preparations lack sufficient vWF to support normal platelet adhesion, and may not contain enough vWF to bind and stabilize the coadministered factor VIII. When given to patients with type III vWD (Tuddenham et al 1982), or vWD Normandy (Mazurier et al 1990a, 1990b, López-Fernández et al 1992), highly purified factor VIII exhibits reduced initial recovery and rapid clearance from the circulation. To overcome these limitations, purified products specifically formulated for the treatment of vWD will be required. One such very high purity vWF concentrate which contains little factor VIII (vWF:VHP, Biotransfusion/CRTS Lille), was shown to be effective in several types of vWD (Lawrie et al 1991, Rothschild et al 1991).

REFERENCES

Abildgaard C F, Suzuki Z, Harrison J, Jefcoat K, Zimmerman T S 1980 Serial studies in von Willebrand's disease: Variability versus 'variants'. Blood 56: 712–716

Aihara M, Kimura A, Chiba Y, Yoshida Y 1988 Plasma collagen cofactor correlates with von Willebrand factor antigen and ristocetin cofactor but not with bleeding time. Thrombosis and Haemostasis 59: 485–490

Alexander B, Goldstein B 1953 Dual hemostatic defect in pseudohemophilia. Journal of Clinical Investigation 32:551

Bahnak B R, Lavergne J-M, Rothschild C, Meyer D 1991 A stop codon in a patient with severe type III von Willebrand disease. Blood 78: 1148–1149

Barker D, Schafer M, White R 1984 Restriction sites containing CpG show a higher frequency of polymorphism in human DNA. Cell 36: 131–138

Batlle J, López-Fernández M F, Campos M, Justica B, Berges C, Navarro J L, Diaz Cremades J M, Kasper C K, Dent J A, Ruggeri Z M, Zimmerman T S 1986a The heterogeneity of type IIA von Willebrand's disease: Studies with protease inhibitors. Blood 68: 1207–1212

Batlle J, López-Fernández M F, Lasierra J, Fernándex-Villamor A, López-Berges C, López-Borrasca A, Ruggeri Z M, Zimmerman T S 1986b von Willebrand disease type IIC with different abnormalities of von Willebrand factor in the same sibship. American Journal of Haematology 21: 177–188

Batlle J, López-Fernández M F, Fernández-Villamor A, López-Berges C, Zimmerman T S 1986c Multimeric pattern discrepancy between platelet and plasma von Willebrand factor in type IIC von Willebrand disease. American Journal of Hematology 22: 87–88

Berliner S A, Seligsohn U, Zivelin A, Zwang E, Sofferman G 1986 A relatively high frequency of severe (type III) von Willebrand's disease in Israel. British Journal of Haematology 62: 535–543

Bernardi F, Marchetti G, Guerra S, Sasonato A, Gemmati D, Patracchini P, Ballerihi G, Conconi F 1990 A de novo and heterozygous gene deletion causing a variant of von Willebrand disease. Blood 75: 677–683

Berntorp E, Nilsson I–M 1989 Use of a high-purity factor VIII concentrate (Hemate P) in von Willebrand's disease. Vox Sanguinis 56: 212–217

Bichet D G, Razi M, Lonergan M, Arthus M–F, Papukna V, Kortas C, Barjon J–N 1988 Hemodynamic and coagulation responses to 1-desamino[8-D-arginine] vasopression in patients with congenital nephrogenic diabetes insipidus. New England Journal of Medicine 318: 881–887

Bloom A L 1979 The biosynthesis of factor VIII. Clinics in Haematology 8: 53–77

Bloom A L, Peake I R 1979 Apparent 'dominant' and 'recessive' inheritance of von Willebrand's disease within the same kindreds. Possible biochemical mechanisms. Thrombosis Research 15: 505–512

Brinkhous K M, Read M S 1980 Use of venom coagglutinin and lyophilized platelets in testing for platelet-aggregating von Willebrand factor. Blood 55: 517–520

Brown J E, Bosak J O 1986 An ELISA test for the binding of von Willebrand antigen to collagen. Thrombosis Research 43: 303–311

Buchanan J C, Leavell B S 1956 Pseudohemophilia: Report of 13 new cases and statistical review of previously reported cases. Annals of Internal Medicine 44: 241–256

Budde U, Schaefer G, Mueller N, Egli H, Dent J, Ruggeri Z, Zimmerman T 1984 Acquired Von Willebrand's disease in the myeloproliferative syndrome. Blood 64: 981–985

Budde U, Dent J A, Berkowitz S D, Ruggeri Z M, Zimmerman T S 1986 Subunit composition of plasma von Willebrand factor in patients with the myeloproliferative syndrome. Blood 68: 1213–1217

Cacheris P M, Nichols W C, Ginsburg D 1991 Molecular characterization of a unique von Willebrand disease variant. A novel mutation affecting von Willebrand factor/factor VIII interaction. Journal of Biological Chemistry 266: 13499–13502

Castaman G, Rodeghiero F, Lattuada A, Mannucci P M 1992 A new variant of von Willebrand disease (type II I) with a normal degree of proteolytic cleavage of von Willebrand factor. Thrombosis Research 65: 343–351

Chang H-Y, Chen Y-P, Chediak J R, Levene R B, Lynch D C 1989 Molecular analysis of von Willebrand factor produced by endothelial cell strains from patients with type IIA von Willebrand disease. Blood 74 (suppl 1): 131a

Ciavarella G, Ciavarella N, Antoncecchi S, De Mattia D, Ranieri P, Dent J, Zimmerman T S, Ruggeri Z M 1985 High-resolution analysis of von Willebrand factor multimeric composition defines a new variant of type I von Willebrand disease with aberrant structure but presence of all size multimers (type IC). Blood 66: 1423–1429

Coller B S 1978 The effects of ristocetin and von Willebrand factor on platelet electrophoretic mobility. Journal of Clinical Investigation 61: 1168–1175

Colombatti A, Bonaldo P 1991 The superfamily of proteins with von Willebrand factor type A-like domains: One theme common to components of extracellular matrix, hemostasis, cellular adhesion, and defense mechanisms. Blood 77: 2305–2315

Cumming A M, Fildes S, Cumming I R, Wensley R T, Redding O M, Burn A M 1990 Clinical and laboratory evaluation of National Health Service factor VIII concentrate (8Y) for the treatment of von Willebrand's disease. British Journal of Haematology 75: 234–239

Dalton R G Dewar M S, Savidge G F, Kernoff P B A, Matthews K B, Greaves M, Preston F E 1987 Hypothyroidism as a cause of acquired von Willebrand's disease. Lancet 1: 1007–1009

de Romeuf C, Jorieux S, Mazurier C 1991 Measurement of vWF binding to heparin in patients with different subtypes of von Willebrand disease (vWD). Thrombosis and Haemostasis 65: 970

Dent J A, Berkowitz S D, Ware J, Kasper C K, Ruggeri Z M 1990 Identification of a cleavage site directing the immunochemical detection of molecular abnormalities in type IIA von Willebrand factor. Proceedings of the National Academy of Sciences, USA 87: 6306–6310

Donnér M, Holmberg L, Nilsson I M 1987 Type IIB von Willebrand's disease with probable autosomal recessive inheritance and presenting as thrombocytopenia in infancy. British Journal of Haematology 66: 349–354

Eikenboom J C J, Briët E, Reitsma P H, Ploos van Amstel H K 1991 Severe type III von Willebrand's disease in the Dutch population is often associated with the absence of von Willebrand factor messenger RNA. Thrombosis and Haemostasis 65: 1127

Fabris F, Casonato A, Del Ben M G, De Marco L, Girolami A 1986 Abnormalities of von Willebrand factor in myeloproliferative disease: a relationship with bleeding diathesis. British Journal of Haematology 63: 75–83

Federici A B, Mannucci P M, Lombardi R, Lattuada A, Colibretti M L, Dent J A, Zimmerman T S 1989 Type II H von Willebrand disease: new structural abnormality of plasma and platelet von Willebrand factor in a patient with prolonged bleeding time and borderline levels of ristocetin cofactor activity. American Journal of Hematology 32: 287–293

Fowler W E, Berkowitz L R, Roberts H R 1989 DDAVP for type IIB von Willebrand disease. Blood 74: 1859–1860

Fukui H, Nishino M, Terad S, Nishikubo T, Yoshioka A, Kinoshita S, Niinomi K, Yoshioka K 1988 Hemostatic effect of a heat-treated factor VIII concentrate (Haemate P) in von Willebrand's disease. Blut 56: 171–178

Giles A R, Hoogendoorn H, Benford K 1987 Type IIb von Willebrand's disease presenting as thrombocytopenia during pregnancy. British Journal of Haematology 67: 349–353

Gill J C, Endres-Brooks J, Bauer P J, Marks W J Jr, Montgomery R R 1987 The effect of ABO blood group on the diagnosis of von Willebrand disease. Blood 69: 1691–1695

Ginsburg D, Sadler J E 1993 von Willebrand disease: A database of point mutations, insertions, and deletions. Thrombosis and Haemostasis 69: 177–184

Ginsburg D, Handin R I, Bonthron D T, Donlon T A, Bruns G A P, Latt S A, Orkin S H 1985 Human von Willebrand factor (vWF): Isolation of complementary DNA (cDNA) clones and chromosome localization. Science 228: 1401–1406

Goudemand J, Mazurier C, Marey A, Caron C, Coupez B, Mizon P,

Goudemand M 1992 Clinical and biological evaluation in von Willebrand's disease of a von Willebrand factor concentrate with low factor VIII activity. British Journal of Haematology 80: 214–221
Graham J B, Rizza C R, Chediak J, Mannucci P M, Briét E, Ljung R, Kasper C K, Essien E M, Green P P 1986 Carrier detection in hemophilia A: A cooperative international study. I. The carrier phenotype. Blood 67: 1554–1559
Gralnick H R, Williams S B, MeKeown L P, Maisonneuve P, Jenneau C, Sultan Y, Rick M E 1985a In vitro correction of the abnormal multimeric structure of vWF in type IIA vWD. Proceedings of the National Academy of Sciences, USA 82: 5968–5972
Gralnick H R, Williams S B, McKeow L P, Rick M E, Maisonneuve P, Jenneau C, Sultan Y 1985b von Willebrand's disease with spontaneous platelet aggregation induced by an abnormal plasma von Willebrand factor. Journal of Clinical Investigation 76: 1522–1529
Gralnick H R, Williams S B, McKeown L P, Maisonneuve P, Jenneau C, Sultan Y 1987 A variant of type II von Willebrand disease with an abnormal triplet structure and discordant effects of protease inhibitors on plasma and platelet von Willebrand factor structure. American Journal of Hematology 24: 259–266
Hill F G H, Enayat M S, George A J 1985 Investigation of a kindred with a new autosomal dominantly inherited variant type von Willebrand's disease (possible type IID). Journal of Clinical Pathology 38: 665-670
Holmberg L, Nilsson I M 1972 Genetic variants of von Willebrand's disease. British Medical Journal 3: 317–320
Holmberg L, Nilsson I M 1985 von Willebrand disease. Clinics in Haematology 14: 461–488
Holmberg L, Nilsson I M, Borge L, Bunnarsson M, Sjorin E 1983 Platelet aggregation induced by 1-desamino-8-D-arginine vasopressin (DDAVP) in type IIB von Willebrand's disease. New England Journal of Medicine 309: 816–821
Howard M A, Firkin B G 1971 Ristocetin: A new tool in the investigation of platelet aggregation. Thrombosis et Diathesis Haemorrhagica 26: 362–369
Howard M A, Salem H H, Thomas K B, Hau L, Pekin J, Coghlan M, Firkin B G 1982 Variant von Willebrand's disease type B — Revisited. Blood 60: 1420–1428
Hoyer L W 1972 Immunologic studies of antihemophilic factor (AHF, factor VIII). IV. Radioimmunoassay of AHF antigen. Journal of Laboratory and Clinical Medicine 80: 822–833
Hoyer L W, Shainoff J R 1980 Factor VIII-related protein circulates in normal plasma as high molecular weight multimers. Blood 55: 1056–1059
Hoyer L W, Rizza C R, Tuddenham E G, Carta C A, Armitage H, Rotblat F 1983 Von Willebrand factor multimer patterns in von Willebrand's disease. British Journal of Haematology 55: 493–507
Hultin M B, Sussman II 1990 Postoperative thrombocytopenia in type IIB von Willebrand disease. American Journal of Hematology 33: 64–68
Ieko M, Sakurama S, Sagawa A, Yoshikawa M, Satoh M, Yasukouchi T, Nakagawa S 1990 Effect of a factor VIII concentrate on type IIb von Willebrand's disease-associated thrombocytopenia presenting during pregnancy in identical twin mothers. American Journal of Hematology 35: 26–31
Italian Working Group 1977 Spectrum of von Willebrand's disease: A study of 100 cases. British Journal of Haematology 35: 101–112
Just M, Herbst H, Hummel M, Dürkop H, Tripier D, Stein H, Schuppan D 1991 Undulin is a novel member of the fibronectin-tenascin family of extracellular matrix glycoproteins. Journal of Biological Chemistry 266: 17326–17332
Kinoshita S, Harrison J, Lazerson J, Abildgaard C F 1984 A new variant of dominant type II von Willebrand's disease with aberrant multimeric pattern of factor VIII-related antigen (type IID). Blood 63: 1369–1371
Kroner P A, Friedman D K, Fahs S A, Scott J P, Montgomery R R 1991 Abnormal binding of factor VIII is linked with the substitution of glutamine for arginine 91 in von Willebrand factor in a variant form of von Willebrand disease. Journal of Biological Chemistry 266: 19146–19149
Kyrle P A, Niessner H, Dent J, Panzer S, Brenner B, Zimmerman T S, Lechner K 1988 IIB von Willebrand's disease: Pathogenetic and therapeutic studies. British Journal of Haematology 69: 55–59
Larrieu M J, Soulier J P 1953 Déficit en facteur antihémophilique A chez une fille associé à un trouble du saignement. Nouvelle Revue Francaise d'Hématologie 8: 361–370
Larrieu M J, Caen J P, Meyer D O, Vainer H, Sultan Y, Bernard J 1968 Congenital bleeding disorders with long bleeding time and normal platelet count. II. Von Willebrand's disease (report of thirty-seven patients). American Journal of Medicine 45: 354–372
Lawrie A S, Goubran H A, Harrison P, Holland L J, Weston-Smith, S G, Savidge G F 1991 Comparison of factor VIII concentrates and vWF:THP for the treatment of von Willebrand's disease. Thrombosis and Haemostasis 65: 1128
Laurell C-B 1966 Quantitative estimation of proteins by electrophoresis in agarose gel containing antibodies. Analytical Biochemistry 15: 45–52
Lethagen S, Harris A S, Milsson I M 1990 Intranasal desmopressin (DDAVP) by spray in mild hemophilia A and von Willebrand's disease type I. Blut 60: 187–191
López-Fernández M F, González-Boullosa R, Blanco-López M J, Batlle J 1991 Abnormal proteolytic degradation of von Willebrand factor after desmopressin infusion in a new subtype of von Willebrand disease (ID). American Journal of Hematology 36: 163–170
López-Fernández M F, Blanco-López M J, Castiñeira M P, Batlle J 1992 Further evidence for recessive inheritance of von Willebrand disease with abnormal binding of von Willebrand factor to factor VIII. American Journal of Hematology 40: 20–27
Lyons S E, Bruck M E, Bowie E J W, Ginsburg D 1992 Impaired intracellular transport produced by a subset of type IIA von Willebrand disease mutations. Journal of Biological Chemistry 267: 4424–4430
MacCallum P K, Rodgers M, Taberner D A 1987 Hypothyroidism and von Willebrand's disease (letter). Lancet 1: 1314
Macfarlane D E, Stibbe J, Kirby E P, Zucker M B, Grant R A, McPherson J 1975 A method for assaying von Willebrand factor (Ristocetin cofactor) Thrombosis et Diathesis Haemorrhagica 34: 306–308
Mancuso D J, Tuley E A, Westfield L A, Worrall N K, Shelton-Inloes B B, Sorace J M, Alevy Y G, Sadler J E 1989 Structure of the gene for human von Willebrand factor. Journal of Biological Chemistry 264: 19514–19527
Mancuso D J, Adam P A, Kroner P A, Montgomery R R 1991a The molecular basis of a type I von Willebrand disease variant. Circulation 84 (suppl II): 418
Mancuso D J, Montgomery R R, Adam P 1991b The identification of a candidate mutation in the von Willebrand factor gene of patients with a variant form of type I von Willebrand disease. Blood 78 (suppl 1): 67a
Mancuso D J, Tuley E A, Westfield L A, Lester-Mancuso T L, Le Beau M M, Sorace J M, Sadler J E 1991c Human von Willebrand factor gene and pseudogene: Structural analysis and differentiation by polymerase chain reaction. Biochemistry 30: 253–269
Mannucci P M, Cattaneo M 1991 Alloantibodies in congenital von Willebrand's disease. Research in Clinical and Laboratory 21: 119–125
Mannucci P M, Lusher J M 1989 Desmopressin and thrombosis. Lancet 2: 675–676
Mannucci P M, Mari D 1984 Antibodies to factor VIII-von Willebrand factor in congenital and acquired von Willebrand's disease. In: Hoyer L W (ed) Factor VIII inhibitors. A R Liss New York, p 109–122
Mannucci P M, Ruggeri Z M, Pareti F I, Capitano A 1977 DDAVP, a new pharmacological approach to the management of haemophilia and von Willebrand's disease. Lancet 1: 869–872
Mannucci P M, Lombardi R, Pareti F I, Solinas S, Mazzucconi M G, Mariani G 1983 A variant of von Willebrand's disease characterized by recessive inheritance and missing triplet structure of von Willebrand factor multimers. Blood 62: 1000–1005
Mannucci P M, Bloom A L, Larrieu M J, Nilsson I M, West R R 1984a Atherosclerosis and von Willebrand factor. I. Prevalence of severe von Willebrand's disease in western Europe and Israel. British Journal of Haematology 57: 163–169
Mannucci P M, Lombardi R, Bader R, Horellou M H, Finazzi G, Besana C, Conard J, Samama M 1984b Studies of the pathophysiology of acquired von Willebrand's disease in seven

patients with lymphoproliferative disorders or benign monoclonal gammopathies. Blood 64: 614–621

Mannucci P M, Lombardi R, Bader R, Vianello L, Federici A B, Solinas S, Mazzucconi M G, Mariani G 1985 Heterogeneity of type I von Willebrand disease: Evidence for a subgroup with an abnormal von Willebrand factor. Blood 66: 796–802

Mannucci P M, Lombardi R, Federici A B, Dent J A, Zimmerman T S, Ruggeri Z M 1986 A new variant of type II von Willebrand disease with aberrant multimeric structure of plasma but not platelet von Willebrand factor (type IIF). Blood 68: 269–274

Mannucci P M, Vicente V, Alberca I, Sacchi E, Longo G, Harris A S, Lindquist A 1987 Intravenous and subcutaneous administration of desmopressin (DDAVP) to hemophiliacs: pharmacokinetics and factor VIII responses. Thrombosis and Haemostasis 58: 1037–1039

Mannucci P M, Lombardi R, Castaman G, Dent J A, Lattuada A, Rodeghiero F, Zimmerman T S 1988 von Willebrand disease 'Vicenza' with larger-than-normal (supranormal) von Willebrand factor multimers. Blood 71: 65–70

Mannucci P M, Lattuada A, Castaman G, Lombardi R, Colibretti M L, Ciavarella N, Rodeghiero F 1989 Heterogeneous phenotypes of platelet and plasma von Willebrand factor in obligatory heterozygotes for severe von Willebrand disease. Blood 74: 2433–2436

Mannucci P M, Tenconi P M, Castaman G, Rodeghiero F 1992 Comparison of four virus-inactivated plasma concentrates for treatment of severe von Willebrand disease: a cross-over randomized trial. Blood 79: 3130–3137

Mazurier C, Mannucci P M, Parquet-Gernez A, Goudemand M, Meyer D 1986 Investigation of a case of subtype IIC von Willebrand disease: Characterization of the variability of this subtype. American Journal of Haematology 22: 301–311

Mazurier C, Gernez-Parquet A, Goudemand J, Taillefer M F, Goudemand M 1988 Investigation of a large kindred with type IIB von Willebrand's disease, dominant inheritance, and age-dependent thrombocytopenia. British Journal of Haematology 69: 499–505

Mazurier C, Dieval J, Jorieux S, Delobel J, Goudemand M 1990a A new von Willebrand factor (vWF) defect in a patient with factor VIII (FVIII) deficiency but with normal levels and multimeric patterns of both plasma and platelet vWF. Characterization of abnormal vWF/FVIII interaction. Blood 75: 20–26

Mazurier C, Gaucher C, Jorieux S, Parquet-Gernez A, Goudemand M 1990b Evidence for a von Willebrand factor defect in factor VIII binding in three members of a family previously misdiagnosed mild haemophilia A and haemophilia A carriers: Consequences for therapy and genetic counselling. British Journal of Haematology 76: 372–379

Miller J L, Castella A 1982 Platelet-type von Willebrand's disease: Characterization of a new bleeding disorder. Blood 60: 790–794

Miller C H, Graham J B, Goldin L R, Elston R C 1979 Genetics of classic von Willebrand's disease. I. Phenotypic variation within families. Blood 54: 117–136

Miller J L, Boselli B D, Kupinski J M 1984 In vivo interaction of von Willebrand factor with platelets following cryoprecipitate transfusion in platelet-type von Willebrand's disease. Blood 63: 226–230

Miller J L, Cunningham D, Lyle V A, Finch C N 1991 Mutation in the gene encoding the α chain of paltelet glycoprotein Ib in platelet-type von Willebrand disease. Proceedings of the National Academy of Sciences, USA 88: 4761–4765

Montgomery R R, Dent J, Schmidt W, Kryle P, Hiessner H, Ruggeri Z M, Zimmerman T S 1986 Hereditary persistence of circulating pro von Willebrand factor (pro-vWF). Circulation 74(II): 406

Ngo K Y, Glotz T, Koziol J A, Lynch D, Gitscher J, Ranieri P, Ciavarella N, Ruggeri Z M, Zimmerman T S 1988 Homozygous and heterozygous deletions of the von Willebrand factor gene in patients and carriers of severe von Willebrand disease. Proceedings of the National Academy of Sciences, USA 85: 2753–2757

Nilsson I M, Blombäck M, Jorpes E, Blombäck B, Johansson S-A 1957a v. Willebrand's disease and its correction with human plasma fraction 1-0. Acta Medica Scandinavica 159: 179–188

Nilsson I M, Blombäck M, von Franken I 1957b On an inherited autosomal hemorrhagic diathesis with antihemophilic globulin (AHG) deficiency and prolonged bleeding time. Acta Medica Scandinavica 159: 35–57

Nilsson I M, Blombäck M, Blombäck B 1959 von Willebrand's disease in Sweden. Its pathogenesis and treatment. Acta Medica Scandinavica 164: 263–278

Nishino M, Girma J-P, Rothschild C, Fressinaud E, Meyer D 1989 New variant of von Willebrand disease with defective binding to factor VIII. Blood 74: 1591–1599

O'Connell P, Lathrop G M, Law M, Leppert M, Nakamura Y, Hoff M, Kumlin E, Thomas W, Elsner T, Ballard L, Goodman P, Azen E, Sadler J E, Lai G Y, Lalouel J-M, White R 1987 A primary genetic linkage map for human chromosome 12. Genomics 1: 93–102

Pasi K J, Williams M D, Enayat M S, Hill F G H 1990 Clinical and laboratory evaluation of the treatment of von Willebrand's disease patients with heat-treated factor VIII concentrate (BPL 8Y). British Journal of Haematology 75: 228–233

Peake I R, Liddell M B, Moodie P, Standen G, Mancuso D J, Tuley E A, Westfield L A, Sorace J M, Sadler J E, Verweij C L, Bloom A L 1990 Severe type III von Willebrand's disease caused by deletion of exon 42 of the von Willebrand factor gene: Family studies that identify carriers of the condition and a compound heterozygous individual. Blood 75: 654–661

Peerlinck K, Eikenboom J C J, Ploos van Amstel H K, Sangtawesin W, Arnout J, Reitsma P H, Vermylen J, Briët E 1992 A patient with von Willebrand's disease characterized by a compound heterozygosity for a substitution of Arg^{854} by Gln in the putative factor-VIII-binding domain of von Willebrand factor (vWF) on one allele and very low levels of mRNA from the second vWF allele. British Journal of Haematology 80: 358–363

Quick A J, Hussey V V 1953 Hemophilic condition in the female. Journal of Laboratory and Clinical Medicine 42: 929–930

Rabinowitz I, Tuley E A, Mancuso D J, Randi A M, Firkin B G, Howard, M A, Sadler J E 1992 von Willebrand disease type B: a missense mutation selectively abolishes ristocetin-induced von Willebrand factor binding to platelet glycoprotein Ib. Proceedings of the National Academy of Sciences, USA 89: 9846–9849

Raines G, Aumann G, Sykes S, Street A 1990 Multimeric analysis of von Willebrand factor by molecular sieving electrophoresis in sodium dodecyl sulphate agarose gel. Thrombosis Research 60: 201–212

Read M S, Shermer R W, Brinkhous K M 1978 Venom coagglutinin: An activator of platelet aggregation dependent on von Willebrand factor. Proceedings of the National Academy of Sciences, USA 75: 4514–4518

Rick M E, Williams S B, Sacher R A, McKeown L P 1987 Thrombocytopenia associated with pregnancy in a patient with type IIB von Willebrand's disease. Blood 69: 786–789

Rodeghiero F, Castaman G, Dini E 1987 Epidemiological investigation of the prevalence of von Willebrand's disease. Blood 69: 454–459

Rodeghiero F, Castaman G, Di Bona E, Ruggeri M 1989 Consistency of responses to DDAVP infusions in patients with von Willebrand's disease and hemophilia A. Blood 74: 1997–2000

Rodeghiero F, Castaman G, Mannucci P M 1991 Clinical indications for desmopressin (DDAVP) in congenital and acquired von Willebrand disease. Blood Reviews 5: 155–161

Rodeghiero F, Castaman G, Meyer D, Mannucci P M 1992 Replacement therapy with virus-inactivated plasma concentrates in von Willebrand disease. Vox Sanguinis 62: 193–199

Rothschild C, Fressinaud E, Wolf M, Dreyfus M, Laurian Y, Peynaud-Debayle E, Gazengel C, Meyer D, Larrieu M J 1991 Unexpected results following treatment of patients with von Willebrand disease with a new highly purified von Willebrand factor concentrate. Thrombosis and Haemostasis 65: 1126

Ruggeri Z M 1991 Structure and function of von Willebrand factor: Relationship to von Willebrand's disease. Mayo Clinic Proceedings 66: 847–861

Ruggeri Z M , Zimmerman T S 1980 Variant von Willebrand's disease. Characterization of two subtypes by analysis of multimeric composition of factor VIII/von Willebrand factor in plasma and platelets. Journal of Clinical Investigation 65: 1318–1325

Ruggeri Z M, Zimmerman T S 1981 The complex multimeric composition of factor VIII/von Willebrand factor. Blood 57: 1140–1143

Ruggeri Z M, Mannucci P M, Jeffcoate S L, Ingram G I C 1976 Immunoradiometric assay of factor VIII related antigen, with

observations in 32 patients with von Willebrand's disease. British Journal of Haematology 33: 221–232
Ruggeri Z M, Pareti F I, Mannucci P M, Ciavarella N, Zimmerman T S 1980 Heightened interaction between platelets and factor VIII/ von Willebrand factor in a new subtype of von Willebrand's disease. New England Journal of Medicine 302: 1047–1051
Ruggeri Z M, Mannucci P M, Lombardi R, Federici A B, Zimmerman T S 1982a Multimeric composition of factor VIII/von Willebrand factor following administration of DDAVP: Implications for pathophysiology and therapy of von Willebrand's disease subtypes. Blood 59: 1272–1278
Ruggeri Z M, Nilsson I M, Lombardi R, Holmberg L, Zimmerman T S 1982b Aberrant multimeric structure of von Willebrand factor in a new variant of von Willebrand's disease (type IIC). Journal of Clinical Investigation 70: 1124–1127
Russell S D, Roth G J 1991 A mutation in the platelet glycoprotein (GP) Ib alpha gene associated with pseudo-von Willebrand disease. Blood 78 (suppl 1): 281a
Saba H I, Saba S R, Dent J, Ruggeri Z M, Zimmerman T S 1985 Type IIB Tampa: A variant of von Willebrand disease with chronic thrombocytopenia, circulating platelet aggregates, and spontaneous platelet aggregation. Blood 66: 282–286
Sadler J E, Ginsburg D 1993 A database of polymorphisms in the von Willebrand factor gene and pseudogene. Thrombosis and Haemostasis 69: 185–191
Sakariassen K S, Nieuwenhuis H K, Sixma J J 1985 Differentiation of patients with subtype IIb-like von Willebrand's disease by means of perfusion experiments with reconstituted blood. British Journal of Haematology 59: 459–470
Scott J P, Montgomery R R 1991 The rapid differentiation of type IIB von Willebrand's disease from platelet-type (pseudo-) von Willebrand's disease by the 'neutral' monoclonal antibody binding assay. American Journal of Clinical Pathology 96: 723–728
Scott J P, Montgomery R R, Retzinger G S 1991 Dimeric ristocetin flocculates proteins, binds to platelets, and mediates von Willebrand factor-dependent agglutination of platelets. Journal of Biological Chemistry 266: 8149–8155
Shelton-Inloes B B, Chehab F F, Mannucci P M, Federici A B, Sadler J E 1987 Gene deletion correlate with the development of alloantibodies in von Willebrand disease. Journal Clinical Investigation 79: 1459–1465
Silwer J 1973 von Willebrand's disease in Sweden. Acta Paediatrica Scandinavica (suppl) 238: 5–159
Smith S R, Auger M J 1987 Hypothyroidism and von Willebrand's disease (letter) Lancet 1: 1314
Smith T J, Gill J C, Ambruso D R, Hathaway W E 1989 Hyponatremia and seizures in young children given DDAVP. American Journal of Hematology 31: 199–202
Takahashi H 1980 Studies on the pathophysiology and treatment of von Willebrand's disease. IV. Mechanism of increased ristocetin-induced platelet aggregation in von Willebrand's disease. Thrombosis Research 19: 857–867
Takahashi H, Nagayama R, Hattori A, Shibata A 1984 Platelet aggregation induced by DDAVP in platelet-type von Willebrand's disease. New England Journal of Medicine 310: 722–723
Takahashi H, Yamada M, Shibata A 1987 Acquired von Willebrand's disease in hypothyroidism (letter) Thrombosis and Haemostasis 58: 1095
Thornton J G, Parapia L A, Minford A M B 1987 Hypothyroidism and von Willebrand's disease (letter) Lancet 1: 1314–1315
Triplett D A 1991 Laboratory diagnosis of von Willebrand's disease. Mayo Clinic Proceedings 66: 832–840
Tuddenham E G D, Lane R S, Rotblat F, Johnson A J, Snape T J, Middleton S, Kernoff P B A 1982 Response to infusion of polyelectrolyte fractionated human factor VIII concentrate in human haemophilia A and von Willebrand's disease. British Journal of Haematology 52: 259–267
Valster F A A, Feijen H L M, Hutten J W M 1990 Severe thrombocytopenia in a pregnant patient with platelet-associated IgM and known von Willebrand's disease; a case report. European Journal of Obstetrics Gynecology and Reproducture Biology 36: 197–201
Verweij C L, de Vries C J M, Distel B, van Zonneveld A-J, van Kessel A G, van Mourik J A, Pannekoek H 1985 Construction of cDNA coding for human von Willebrand factor using antibody probes for colony-screening and mapping of the chromosomal gene. Nucleic Acids Research 13: 4699–4717
von Willebrand E A 1926 Hereditär pseudohemofili. Finska Läkarsällskapets Handlingar 68: 87–112
von Willebrand E A 1931 Über hereditar pseudohämophilie. Acta Medica Scandinavica 76: 521–550
von Willebrand E A, Jürgens R 1933 Über ein neues vererbbares Blutungsübel: Die konstitutionelle Thrombopathie. Deutsches Archiv fur Klinische Medizin 175: 453–483
Weinstein R E, Bona R D, Altman A J et al 1989 Severe hyponatremia after repeated intravenous administration of desmopressin. American Journal of Hematology 32: 258–261
Weiss H J 1975 Abnormalities of factor VIII and platelet aggregation — use of ristocetin in diagnosing the von Willebrand syndrome. Blood 45: 403–412
Weiss H J, Sussman II 1986 A new von Willebrand variant (Type I, New York): Increased ristocetin-induced platelet aggregation and plasma von Willebrand factor containing the full range of multimers. Blood 68: 149–156
Weiss H J, Ball A P, Mannucci P M 1982a Incidence of severe von Willebrand's disease. New England Journal of Medicine 307: 127
Weiss H J, Meyer D, Rabinowitz R, Piétu G, Girma J-P, Vicic W J, Rogers J 1982b Pseudo-von Willebrand's disease. An intrinsic platelet defect with aggregation by unmodified human factor VIII/von Willebrand factor and enhanced adsorption of its high-molecular-weight multimers. New England Journal of Medicine 306: 326–333
Weiss H J, Piétu G, Rabinowitz R, Girma J P, Roger J, Meyer D 1983 Heterogeneous abnormalities in the multimeric structure, antigenic properties, and plasma-platelet content of factor VIII/von Willebrand factor in subtypes of classic (type I) and variant (type IIA) von Willebrand's disease. Journal of Laboratory and Clinical Medicine 101: 411–425
Yamasata M, Yamada K M, Yamada S S, Shinomura T, Tanaka H, Nishida Y, Obara M, Kimata K 1991 The complete primary structure of type XII collagen shows a chimeric molecule with reiterated fibronectin type III motifs, von Willebrand factor A motifs, a domain homologous to a noncollagenous region of type IX collagen, and short collagenous domains with an Arg-Gly-Asp site. Journal of Cell Biology 115: 209–221
Zhang Z P, Falk G, Blombäck M, Egberg N, Anvret M 1992 Identification of a new nonsense mutation in the von Willebrand factor gene in patients with von Willebrand disease type III. Human Molecular Genetics 1: 61–62
Zimmerman T S, Hoyer L W, Edgington T S 1975 Determination of the von Willebrand's disease antigen (factor VIII-related antigen) in plasma by quantitative immunoelectrophoresis. Journal of Laboratory and Clinical Medicine 86: 152–159
Zimmerman T S, Abildgaard C F, Meyer D 1979 The factor VIII abnormality in severe von Willebrand's disease. New England Journal Medicine 301: 1307–1310
Zimmerman T S, Roberts J R, Ruggeri Z M 1982 Factor VIII-related antigen: Characterization by electrophoretic techniques. In: Bloom A L (ed) Methods in hematology 5, the hemophilias, Churchill Livingstone, Edinburgh, p 81–91
Zimmerman T S, Dent J A, Ruggeri Z M, Nannini L H 1986 Subunit composition of plasma von Willebrand factor. Cleavage is present in normal individuals, increased in IIA and IIB von Willebrand disease, but minimal in variants with aberrant structure of individual oligomers (types IIC, IID, and IIE). Journal of Clinical Investigation 77: 947–951

36. Molecular genetics of haemophilia A and B

E. G. D. Tuddenham   F. Giannelli

The two X-linked sublethal bleeding disorders – haemophilia A and B – have become a proving ground for techniques in molecular genetics able to localize mutations in large regions of the genome. Loss of disease alleles from the population means that new mutations are constantly maintaining the prevalence of these disorders and creating extreme heterogeneity at the DNA level.

Haemophilia A affects approximately 1 in 5000 males. It is caused by deleterious mutations in the factor VIII gene leading to deficiency of factor VIII, a co-factor for the activation of factor X by factor IXa. Characterization of these mutations was hampered by the large size of the human factor VIII gene and its complex structure (Fig. 36.1); the 9 kb mRNA is encoded by a gene comprising 26 exons spanning 186 kb of chromosomal DNA (Gitschier et al 1984, Tode et al 1984) located at Xq 2.8. However, the advent of rapid gene scanning and DNA sequencing techniques has greatly increased the number of characterized mutations, although it is clear that many remain to be identified.

Haemophilia B affects approximately 1 in 30 000 males and is due to mutations of the factor IX gene located at Xq 2.71. The gene (Fig. 36.2) spans 34 kb and contains 8 exons (Anson et al 1984, Yoshitake et al 1985). Much information on the regulation of this gene and on the structure and function of factor IX has been gained from the study of haemophilia B patients. In fact this disease is gaining a special place in molecular genetics because it is the first disease to offer a reasonably unbiased view of mutagenesis in man. Moreover, this disease offers a convenient model for developing and testing new strategies for the provision of genetic counselling in diseases of high mutational heterogeneity.

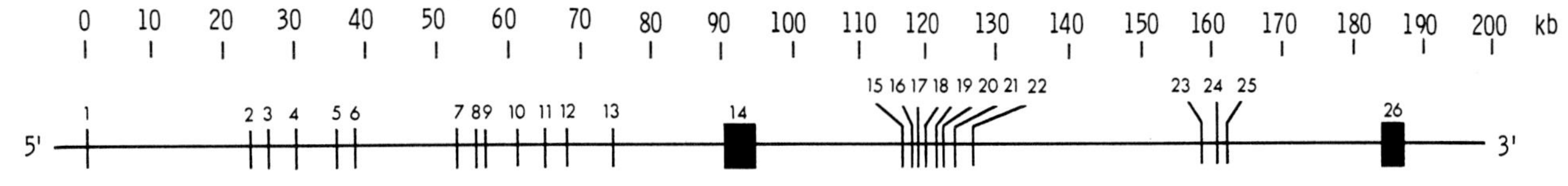

Fig. 36.1 Structure of the factor VIII gene. Filled in bars represent the 26 exons.

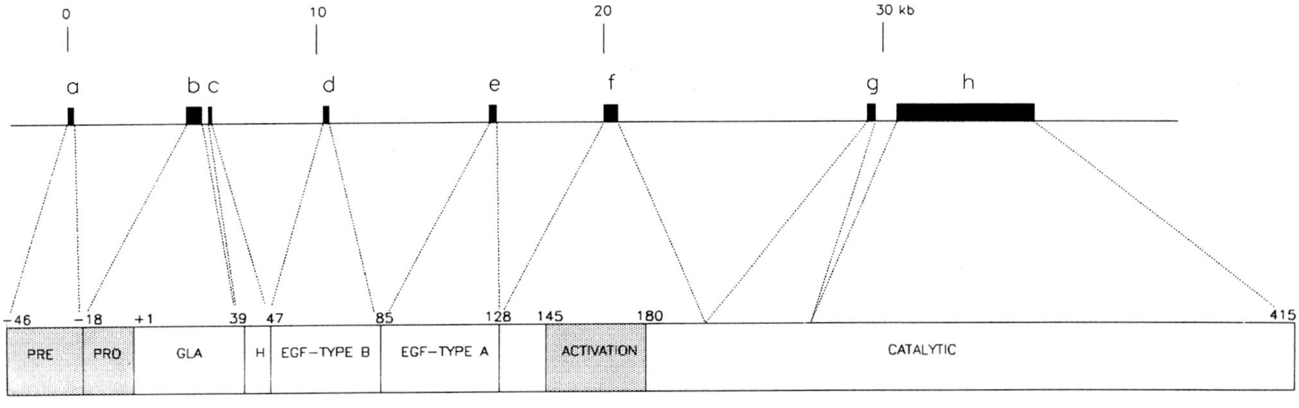

Fig. 36.2 The factor IX gene and protein. Exons are indicated by black boxes, dotted lines indicate segments of protein encoded by each exon. Shaded areas: segments of protein that are excised during maturation and activation.

METHODS OF DETECTING MUTATIONS

The desire to optimize genetic counselling and/or to take advantage of the wealth of different natural mutants led to the development of a variety of rapid procedures for the detection of factor VIII and factor IX gene mutations. Such methods include some entirely based on sequencing, and others based on more rapid screening procedures. The sequencing procedures either directly examine the products of polymerase chain reactions (PCR) (Green et al 1989) or entail PCR amplification followed by transcription of the amplified product and then transcript sequencing (Stoflet et al 1988). Among the screening procedures, two – amplification mismatch detection (AMD) (Montandon et al 1989) and denaturing gradient gel electrophoresis (DGGE) – are highly efficient.

Amplification mismatch detection is based on chemical modification of mismatched DNA heteroduplexes (Cotton et al 1988) and consists of the following steps:

1. Amplification of DNA from a control and a test factor IX gene
2. End-labelling of the two strands of control or test DNA
3. Melting and annealing of unlabelled and labelled DNA mixed at a 10:1 ratio
4. Treatment of the hybrid DNA with hydroxylamine (one half) and with osmium tetroxide (the other half) so as to modify, respectively, mismatched cytosines and thymines
5. Piperidine cleavage of the reacted DNA at the site of modified bases
6. Denaturating and sizing of reacted DNA by polyacrylamide denaturing gel electrophoresis.

Cleavage of the labelled DNA reveals the presence of a mismatch and the size of the cleavage product indicates its position. The precise nature of the sequence change can then be determined by direct sequencing of the amplified mismatch region (Green et al 1989).

DGGE is based on the concept that the migration of a DNA duplex is retarded when this enters a region of a gel with sufficient denaturant to melt its less stable domain (Fischer & Lerman 1983). Sequence changes that are not located in the highest or last melting domain can then be detected by their effect on the stability of the DNA duplex. Maximum efficiency with DGGE can be obtained by using a PCR primer containing a long segment of GC residues (G-C clamp) to create an artificial very high melting domain and also by forming heteroduplexes between normal and mutant DNA to exploit the lower melting point of mismatched sequences (Scheffield et al 1989, Abrams et al 1990). This method is limited to an optimum fragment length of 400–700 bp, it requires detailed analysis of the melting profile of each region to be studied, and does not indicate the site of the mutation within each amplified segment.

An easy but relatively inefficient mutation screening procedure relies on changes in secondary structure and the effect they may have on the migration of DNA single strands in neutral gradients (single strand conformational polymorphism, or in short SSCP). This method (Orita et al 1989) is expected to detect only a proportion of mutations and its efficiency rapidly decreases as the size of the region analysed increases above 150–200 bp. In the only large prospective, comparative study so far, SSCP detected only 35% of the haemophilia B mutations identified by sequencing, and a similar procedure employing RNA transcripts of amplified DNA segments (rSSCP) detected 75% (Sarkar et al 1992). This is well below the efficiency of AMD and DGGE, however, technical improvements in the SSCP protocol may enhance its sensitivity to a level comparable with AMD (Tuddenham 1992). AMD is not only extremely efficient (Green et al 1991b, Giannelli et al 1992b), but is also of great value in detecting mutations in very complex genes such as those for factor VIII and dystrophin where the ability to analyse long cDNA segments and obtain precise information on the position of mismatches results in dramatic increases in the speed of mutation detection (Naylor et al 1991, Roberts et al 1992).

MUTATIONS OF THE FACTOR VIII GENE

The origin of mutations causing haemophilia A

An estimate of the proportion of cases of haemophilia A that have arisen de novo is very important for risk assessment purposes. In families with a sporadic haemophiliac where de novo mutation can be proven by RFLP analysis the risk to subsequent offspring of the possible carrier mother can be said, in the absence of maternal mosaicism, to approximate to that in the population at large.

For the disease to be maintained in the population the loss of disease alleles from the population due to natural selection must not exceed the gain due to new mutations. Haldane (1935) showed that for any X-linked lethal disorder, assuming the mutation rate in males and females to be equal, the proportion of mutations which have occurred de novo will be one third. A lower proportion will however be found if the X-linked gene is not invariably lethal to males carrying it, if the mutation rate is higher in males than in females, or if the fitness of carrier females is somehow increased. While no evidence has been put forward for the greater fitness of female carriers of haemophilia A, the fitness of affected males is clearly greater than zero (Miller et al 1987). The latter fitness is currently very difficult to estimate since it will depend critically upon the net influence of such factors as improved treatment counterbalanced by the effects of HIV infection. However, an estimate of the fitness of affected males together with knowledge of the observed/expected frequency of genuinely sporadic mutations should in theory permit an indirect measurement of the relative mutation rate between the sexes. Based upon the observed rarity of such sporadic cases, Haldane (1947) concluded that the mutation rate in males could be as much as 10-fold higher than in females. This could be explained by the higher number of cell divisions undergone by a male compared to a female germ cell (i.e. ~15 times greater at the age of 28 (Vogel & Motulsky, 1986).

More recently, a considerable number of studies have been carried out to determine the proportion of cases of haemophilia A which are sporadic. Although a deficiency of sporadic cases has sometimes been found, a question mark has remained over the possibility of ascertainment bias and the reliability of carrier detection methods. Vogel (1977) reviewing these studies, concluded that a higher mutation rate in male germ cells was nevertheless likely, an assessment supported by data of Ananthakrishnan & D'Souza (1979). The largest study to date, of 949 families with haemophilia A (Barrai et al 1985) provided an estimate of 0.164 for the frequency of sporadic cases but no evidence for a significantly higher mutation rate in male germ cells (1.7 × that in female germ cells). Another study of 246 families showed that fewer than 12% of cases could have been due to new mutation (Miller et al 1987).

Clearly there are many problems associated with this type of study, not the least being able to distinguish between a true de novo mutation and one which has been transmitted matrilineally over several previous generations. In an attempt to overcome this problem, Winter et al (1983) conducted phenotypic carrier detection tests on 21 mothers of 'sporadic' haemophilia A patients (isolated affected males). A combination of linear discriminant analysis and prior probabilities calculated from pedigree data suggested that 16 (76%) were carriers. A conservative estimate of the fitness of affected males (0.7; the authors suggested that the true fitness might be as low as 0.3, a figure borne out by recent reproductive pattern data (Miller et al 1987)) was used to derive a maximum likelihood estimate of the male/female mutation ratio of 9.6 (95% confidence limits, 2.2–41.5). A lower value for the fitness of affected males would increase the size of this ratio still further. Whilst a much larger sample size could considerably reduce these wide confidence limits, the figure of 9.6 does agree with Haldane's (1947) prediction and with similar calculations carried out with data from Lesch–Nyhan disease families (Francke et al 1981). If this ratio is correct, then 97.4% of all mothers of haemophiliacs would be expected to be carriers.

In the past, it has been difficult to establish with certainty the precise origin of the haemophilia A mutation. Coagulation assays were the only tool available to assess carrier status. These assays are ~90–95% reliable due to the wide range of clotting activity values exhibited by both normal and especially carrier females. This inter-individual variation is due to the vagaries of X-inactivation (Graham et al 1975), possible allelic variation (Filippi et al 1984) or differences in age, exercise or blood group (Graham et al 1986). RFLP analysis, using both intragenic and extragenic probes can now be used in concert with coagulation assays to determine the origin of a novel haemophilia A mutation in a majority of cases. So, for example, when the chromosome bearing the haemophilia A allele is shown to have apparently originated in the haemostatically-normal maternal grandfather, a de novo mutation either in the proband or in his mother is indicated. Coagulation data from the mother can then distinguish between these alternatives allowing risk assessment for subsequent pregnancies.

This approach has proved successful in demonstrating cases of de novo mutation either in the maternal grandfather's gamete (Delpech et al 1986, Grover et al 1987, Pecorara et al 1987, Howard et al 1988) or in one of the mother's gametes (Grover et al 1987). The direct demonstration of a de novo mutation in haemophilia A has also been achieved by the detection of a CG→TG mutation in exon 24 of the factor VIII gene creating a premature stop in the proband's DNA, but absent from his mother's DNA (Gitschier et al 1985). A case of a GA→GG missense mutation in exon 7 of the factor VIII gene of the proband was detected by *Taq* I and this mutation was not present in DNA from the proband's mother (Youssoufian et al 1988b). A combination of oligonucleotide discrimination hybridization and DNA sequencing enabled Gitschier et al (1988) to demonstrate the presence of a CGC→TGC mutation at Arg^{1689} in a patient with haemophilia A and the absence of this mutation in his mother's DNA. Either the probands were new mutations or their mothers are germline mosaics for these lesions.

Such studies are also relevant to the question of a possible sex difference in the mutation rate of the factor VIII gene. Bernardi et al (1987a) studied 17 families of sporadic haemophilia A patients. In eight of these, RFLP analysis excluded the carrier status of the maternal grandmothers, while coagulation assays indicated that the mothers of the probands were themselves carriers. Six of these mutations were subsequently shown to be derived from a normal maternal grandfather and two from a maternal grandmother. Similarly, a study of 22 families of sporadic haemophilia A patients (Bröcker-Vriends et al 1987) identified seven in which the origin of the mutant chromosome was the maternal grandfather and three in which the origin was the maternal grandmother. Higuchi et al (1989) determined the origin of de novo mutation in five cases; three in the mother and two in the grandfather. Ljung et al (1989) reported eight mutations originating in the maternal grandfather and four in the maternal grandmother. These data are in keeping with the idea of a higher mutation rate in the male but suffer from imperfect carrier diagnoses and from biases that compromise a direct estimate of the ratio of the sex-specific mutation rates. Bröcker-Vriends et al (1991) used a computational method developed by Rosendaal et al (1990) which estimates the sex ratio of the mutation frequencies from pedigree data without assuming genetic equilibrium or knowledge of the relative fitness of haemophilia patients and carriers. They then reported a ratio for the sex-specific mutation rate of 5.2 (95% confidence limits, 1.8–15.1) which would yield a probability of carriership for the mothers of sporadic haemophiliacs of 86%. Further family studies tracking specific mutations in unselected populations of patients will be needed to arrive at direct estimates of the overall sex-specific mutation rates for haemophilia A.

Gross mutations

Large deletions

Over 60 different total or partial deletions of the factor VIII gene have been reported (Table 36.1). These vary considerably in size. All but three are associated with the severe phenotype. Two of the three exceptions involve exon 22 and result in moderately severe haemophilia (Youssoufian et al 1987a, Wehnert et al 1989). An in-frame deletion of exon 22 would remove 52 amino acids from the protein and presumably result in a protein with a shortened C1 domain. The specific activity of the resulting factor VIII molecule has not been reported. The re-

Table 36.1 Large deletions in the factor VIII gene of patients with haemophilia A

Patient/family	Exon(s) deleted	Size of deletion (kb)	FVIII: C U. dl^{-1}(%)	FVIII: Ag U.dl^{-1}(%)	Severity	Inhibitors	References
?	1–26	>210	?	?	Severe	No	Casarino et al 1986a
H1	1–26	>210	?	?	Severe	Yes	Casula et al 1990
H328	1–6	>55	<1	?	Severe	Yes	Millar et al 1990
484	1–5	>35	<1	?	Severe	No	Higuchi et al 1989
JH13	1	>2	<1	<1	Severe	No	Youssoufian et al 1988d
H309	1	>1	<1	?	Severe	No	Millar et al 1990
JH145	1	?	?	?	Severe	?	Higuchi et al 1991b
1067	Intron 1[b]	7	?	?	Severe	No	Levinson et al 1990
JH21	2–3	9–12	<1	<1	Severe	No	Youssoufian et al 1988d, Cutting et al 1988 Woods-Samuels et al 1991
JH22	3–13	60	<1	<1	Severe	Yes	Youssoufian et al 1988d, Cutting et al 1988
H151	3–5	11.7	<1	?	Severe	No	Millar et al 1990
656	3	1.7–2.0	<1	?	Severe	No	Higuchi et al 1988, 1989
JH23	4–25	133–145	<1	<1	Severe	No	Youssoufian et al 1988d, Cutting et al 1988
H571	5–13	57	<1	?	Severe	Yes	Millar et al 1990
?	5, 6	?	?	?	Severe	?	Gitschier et al 1989
2253	5, 6	2.5–10	?	?	Severe	Yes	Levinson et al 1990
H275	5	2	?	?	Severe	No	Bröcker-Vriends et al 1990
?	5 or 6	2	?	?	Severe	?	Bröcker-Vriends et al 1988
1059	6	10	?	?	Severe	No	Levinson et al 1990
JH6	6	7	<1	<1	Severe	No	Youssoufian et al 1987a
2213	6	3–6	?	?	Severe	No	Levinson et al 1990
H2	7–22	110	?	?	Severe	Yes	Casula et al 1990
JH24	7–14	40–56	<1	<1	Severe	No	Youssoufian et al 1988d
505	7–9	15–20	<1	?	Severe	Yes	Higuchi et al 1989
JH1	11–22	60	?	?	Severe	Yes	Antonarakis et al 1985, Cutting et al 1988, Woods-Samuels et al 1991
H20	14–22	>36	?	?	Severe	Yes	Nafa et al 1990
?	14–22	?	?	?	Severe	Yes	Lillicrap 1992[c]
H229	14–21	50	<1	?	Severe	Yes	Millar et al 1990
194/513	14	12–16	<1	?	Severe	Yes	Higuchi et al 1989
?	14	6	<1	<0.1	Severe	Yes	Mikami et al 1988b
580	14	2.3–3.0	<1	?	Severe	No	Higuchi et al 1989
JH7	14	2.5	<1	<1	Severe	No	Youssoufian et al 1987a, Woods-Samuels et al 1991
JH37	14	2.5	?	?	Severe	?	Woods-Samuels et al 1991
JH141	15–21	?	?	?	Severe	?	Higuchi et al 1991b
?	15–18	13	?	?	Severe	Yes	Camerino et al 1986, Bardoni et al 1988
JH29	15	?	?	?	Severe	?	Antonarakis et al 1992[c]
1.	17–19	?	?	?	Severe	No	Wehnert et al 1989
5	18, 19[a]?	?	?	?	Severe	?	Grover et al 1987
H58	19–21	4.7	<1	?	Severe	Yes	Millar et al 1990
JH10	22	5.5	2–5	?	Moderate	No	Youssoufian et al 1987a

Table 36.1 *Cont'd*

Patient/family	Exon(s) deleted	Size of deletion (kb)	FVIII: C U. dl^{-1}(%)	FVIII: Ag U.dl^{-1}(%)	Severity	Inhibitors	References
2.	Intron 22a	?	?	?	Severe	No	Wehnert et al 1989
3.	Intron 22a	?	?	?	Moderate	No	Wehnert et al 1989
?	23–26	?	?	?	Severe	Yes	Din et al 1986
HA664	23–26	?	?	?	Severe	Yes	Lavergne et al 1992[c]
JH9	23–25	>16	<1	<1	Severe	No	Youssoufian et al 1987a
H96	23–25	39	<1	?	Severe	Yes	Gitschier et al 1985
HA711	23–24	?	?	?	Moderate	No	Lavergne et al 1992[c]
JH8	24–25	>3.4	<1	<1	Severe	No	Youssoufian et al 1987a
H51	26	22	<1	?	Severe	No	Gitschier et al 1985
277	26	>18	<1	?	Severe	No	Higuchi et al 1989
JH26	26	14	<1	<1	Severe	No	Youssoufian et al 1988d
?	26	8.7	?	?	Severe	?	Bernardi et al 1987
H73	26	>2	?	?	Severe	No	Nafa et al 1990
?	26	>2	?	?	Severe	No	Youssoufian et al 1987b
H8	26	>2	?	?	Severe	?	Bernardi et al 1989
JH12	26	?	?	?	Severe	?	Antonarakis et al 1992[c]
HA364	26	?	?	?	Severe	No	Lavergne et al 1992[c]
HA544	26	?	?	?	Severe	No	Lavergne et al 1992[c]
HA599	26	?	?	?	Severe	No	Lavergne et al 1992[c]

[a]Precise extent unknown but includes at least region indicated.
[b]Not proven to be cause of disease phenotype although segregates with disease allele.
[c]Unpublished data.

maining patient, also with a moderately severe phenotype, possesses a deletion of exons 23 and 24 (Lavergne 1992) Again, the reading frame is unaltered.

34 gross deletions of the factor VIII gene have been found in a total of 1386 haemophilia A patients (2.5%) screened by Southern blotting according to a recent study of pooled data from a number of different groups (Millar et al 1990). In practice, the actual frequency of deletion will be rather higher than this since many deletions will only be detected by high resolution techniques such as DNA sequencing (see p. 869). Very small deletions will go undetected by Southern blotting unless they encompass one or more recognition sites for the restriction enzyme(s) used.

Reported gross gene deletions appear to be fairly heterogeneous both in terms of their size and position. No evidence for deletion hotspots is yet apparent from the distribution of deletion breakpoints. Deletion of the factor VIII gene is however associated with an approximately five-fold higher risk of developing inhibitors compared with other severe haemophiliacs without gene deletions (Millar et al 1990).

Large insertions

Examples of the insertional inactivation of the factor VIII gene are listed in Table 36.2. Two cases involving the insertion of non-factor VIII DNA sequences have been reported (Kazazian et al 1988). The inserted material was in both cases derived from a highly repetitive LINE element and gave rise to severe haemophilia A. Both insertions had occurred at different locations in exon 14 and both had probably occurred de novo. The frequency of

Table 36.2 Large insertions in the factor VIII gene of patients with haemophilia A

Patient	Exon	Nature of insertion	Severity	Reference
JH27	14	3.8 Kb LINE element	Severe	Kazazian et al 1988
JH28†	14	2.1 Kb LINE element	Severe	Kazazian et al 1988

LINE element insertion in the factor VIII gene is not very high, since no further examples of this type of lesion were found in a screen of over 800 haemophilia A patient DNA samples (Millar et al 1990, Pattinson et al 1990a).

Duplications

A partial factor VIII gene duplication has been reported by Gitschier (1988). The propositus possessed a deletion of 39 kb encompassing exons 23–25. However, his mother and sister possessed a different mutation: a 23 kb duplication of intron 22 inserted between exons 23 and 24. It was proposed that the duplicated allele was unstable and represented an intermediate stage in the deletion of this gene. Murru et al (1990) described an in-frame duplication of exon 13 giving rise to mild haemophilia A.

Point mutations and other small changes

Single nucleotide substitutions causing missense and nonsense mutations

Over 80 different point mutations have been reported in the factor VIII gene by a combination of Southern blotting, oligonucleotide discriminant hybridization, denaturing gradient gel electrophoresis, chemical cleavage and DNA sequencing. Table 36.3 lists the DNA and protein

Table 36.3 Single base substitutions found in the factor VIII gene of patients with haemophilia A

Exon/ intron	Codon[b]	Nucleotide change	Codon change	Number of unrelated cases	FVIII:C $U.dl^{-1}$(%)	FVIII:Ag $U.dl^{-1}$(%)	Clinical severity	Presence of inhibitors	Comments	References
Exon 1	−5	CGA→TGA	Arg→Term	1	<1	<1	Severe	No	Signal peptide	Pattinson et al 1990a
Exon 1	11	GAA→GTA	Glu→Val	1	?	?	Mild	No		Gitschier 1992
Intron 2	–	CGA→TGA	–	1	<1	?	Severe	No	Probably a neutral change ~300 bp 3′ to exon 2	Gitschier et al 1985
Exon 3	89	AAG→ACG	Lys→Thr	1	?	?	Mild	?		Higuchi et al 1991b
Exon 3	91	ATG→GTG	Met→Val	1	?	?	Mild	?		Higuchi et al 1991b
Exon 4	162	GTG→ATG	Val→Met	2	8/5	?	Moderate/Mild	No		Gitschier 1992
Exon 4	166	AAA→ACA	Lys→Thr	1	19	?	Mild	?		Higuchi et al 1991a
Exon 4	170	TCA→TTA	Ser→Leu	1	3.5	8.7	Moderate	No		Chan et al 1989
Intron 4	–	CGA→CAA	–	1	5–10	41	Mild	No	Proposed to activate cryptic splice site ~1 kb 3′ to exon 4	Youssoufian et al 1988c
Exon 5	205	G/gt..ag/GG→T/	Gly→Trp	1	3.2	?	Moderate	?		Higuchi et al 1991a
Intron 5		ag/→gg/	–	1	<1	?	Severe	No	+1 IVS5 acceptor splice site	Naylor et al 1991
Intron 6	–	ag/→ac/	–	1	?	?	Severe	?	+2 IVS6 acceptor splice site	Antonarakis et al 1992[a]
Exon 7	255	TGG→TGA	Trp→Term	1	?	?	Severe	?		Antonarakis et al 1992[a]
Exon 7	266	GTG→GGG	Val→Gly	1	?	?	Mild	?		Higuchi et al 1991b
Exon 7	272	GAA→GGA	Glu→Gly	1	2	3.5	Moderate	No		Youssoufian et al 1988b
Exon 7	282	CGC→CAC	Arg→His	3	?	?	Severe	?		Higuchi et al 1991b
Exon 7	293	TTC→TCC	Phe→Ser	1	?	?	Mild	?		Higuchi et al 1991b
Exon 7	295	ACT→GCT	Thr→Ala	1	14–16	?	Moderate	?		Higuchi et al 1991a
Exon 8	326	GTA→CTA	Val→Leu	1	?	?	Severe	No		Kogan & Gitschier 1990
Exon 8	326	GTA→CTA	Val→Leu	1	?	?	Moderate	?		Higuchi et al 1990
Exon 8	336	CGA→TGA	Arg→Term	7	0	<1	Severe	No	Activated protein C cleavage site	Gitschier et al 1988, Pattinson et al 1990a
Exon 8	372	CGC→TGC	Arg→Cys	3	3	70–80	Moderate	No	Thrombin activation site	Shima et al 1989, Pattinson et al 1990a,b, Lavergne et al 1992[a]
Exon 8	372	CGC→CAC	Arg→His	2	5	325	Mild	No	Thrombin activation site	Arai et al 1989, Pattinson et al 1990a
Exon 9	412	TTG→TTT	Leu→Phe	1	10.5	?	Mild	?		Higuchi et al 1991a
Exon 9	425	AAA→AGA	Lys→Arg	1	?	?	Severe	?		Higuchi et al 1991b
Exon 9	427	CGA→TGA	Arg→Term	1	<1	<1	Severe	No		Pattinson et al 1990a
Exon 10	473	TAT→CAT	Tyr→His	1	?	?	Mild	?		Higuchi et al 1991b
Exon 10	473	TAT→TGT	Tyr→Cys	1	2.7/3.5	?	Moderate	?		Higuchi et al 1991a
Exon 10	479	GGA→AGA	Gly→Arg	1	2	?	Moderate	No		Naylor et al 1993
Exon 11	504	CTG→CTT	Leu→Leu	3	?	?	Mild	?	Potential new acceptor site	Antonarakis et al 1992[a]
Exon 11	527	CGG→TGG	Arg→Trp	3	14.5–18 17–18	?	Mild	?		Higuchi et al 1991a
Exon 11	527	CGG→TGG	Arg→Trp	1	?	?	?	?		Antonarakis et al 1992[a]
Exon 11	531	CGC→TGC	Arg→Cys	3	6.7/4.2	?	Moderate	?		Higuchi et al 1991a, Antonarakis et al, 1992[a]
Exon 11	531	CGC→GGC	Arg→Gly	1	9.2	?	Moderate	?		Higuchi et al 1991a
Exon 11	535	AGT→GGT	Ser→Gly	2	?	?	?	?		Antonarakis et al 1992[a]
Exon 11	542	GAT→GGT	Asp→Gly	1	?	?	Severe	?		Higuchi et al 1991b
Exon 11	565	CAG/gt→AAG/gt	Gln→Lys	1	?	?	Moderate	?		Higuchi et al 1991a
Exon 12	566	ATA→ACA	Ile→Thr	1	<1	154	Severe	?	New N-glycosylation site N564	Hoyer et al 1991
Exon 12	577	TCT→CCT	Ser→Pro	1	?	?	?	?		Antonarakis et al 1992[a]
Exon 12	583	CGA→TGA	Arg→Term	1	<1	<1	Severe	No		Pattinson et al 1990a
Exon 12	584	AGC→ATC	Ser→Ile	1	?	?	?	?	Loss N-glycosylation site N582	Antonarakis et al 1992[a]
Exon 12	593	CGC→TGC	Arg→Cys	5	?	?	Mild	?		Higuchi et al 1991b, Antonarakis et al 1992[a]
Exon 12	612	AAC→AGC	Asn→Ser	1	?	?	?	?		Antonarakis et al 1992[a]

Table 36.3 *Cont'd*

Exon/ intron	Codon[b]	Nucleotide change	Codon change	Number of unrelated cases	FVIII:C U.dl^{-1}(%)	FVIII:Ag U.dl^{-1}(%)	Clinical severity	Presence of inhibitors	Comments	References
Intron 12	–	/gtgagt→gtgaat	–	1	?	?	Mild	?	+5 IVS 12 donor splice site	Antonarakis et al 1992[a]
Exon 13	644	GCA→GTA	Ala→Val	1	14	25	Mild/Moderate	?		Higuchi et al 1991a
Exon 14	704	[C]GCC→ACC	Ala→Thr	2	?	?	Mild	?		Higuchi et al 1991b
Exon 14	795	CGA→TGA	Arg→Term	1	<1	<1	Severe	No		Pattinson et al 1990a
Exon 14	1038	GAG→AAG	Glu→Lys	1	2.4	?	Mild/Moderate	?		Higuchi et al 1991a
Exon 14	1680	TAT→TTT	Tyr→Phe	2	10	20	Mild	No	Tyrosine sulphation/vWF interaction	Higuchi et al 1990, 1991b
Exon 14	1680	TAT→TGT	Tyr→Cys	1	?	?	Severe	No		Traystman et al 1990
Exon 14	1686	CAG→TAG	Gln→Term	1	<1	?	Severe	?		Higuchi et al 1990
Exon 14	1689	CGC→TGC	Arg→Cys	7	2–5	87–220	Moderate	No	Thrombin activation site	Arai et al 1990, Higuchi et al 1990, Pattinson et al 1990a, Schwaab et al 1991,
Exon 14	1689	CGC→TGC	Arg→Cys	1	0	96	Severe	No	Thrombin activation site	Gitschier et al 1988
Exon 14	1689	CGC→CAC	Arg→His	1	7	165	Mild	No	Thrombin activation site	Schwaab et al 1991
Exon 14	1696	CGA→TGA	Arg→Term	1	<1	?	Severe	Yes		Pattinson et al 1990a
Exon 14	1709	TAT→TGT	Tyr→Cys	1	18	?	Moderate	No		Traystman et al 1990
Exon 15	1772	ATG→ACG	Met→Thr	1	<1	72	Severe	?	New *N*-glycosylation site N1770	Hoyer et al 1991
Exon 16	1781	CGT→CAT	Arg→His	1	?	?	Mild/Moderate	?		Higuchi et al 1991a
Exon 16	1784	TCC→TAC	Ser→Tyr	1	?	?	Severe	?		Higuchi et al 1991b
Exon 16	1825	CCC→TCC	Pro→Ser	1	15	?	Moderate	?		Higuchi et al 1991a
Exon 16	1826	ACT→CCT	Thr→Pro	1	?	?	Mild	?		Antonarakis et al 1992[a]
Exon 16	1843	CTG/gt→CTA/gt	Leu→Leu	1	9–18	?	Moderate	?	–1 IVS16 donor splice site	Higuchi et al 1991a
Exon 17	1848	CAC→CGC	His→Arg	1	1–5	?	Mild/Moderate	?		Higuchi et al 1991a
Exon 18	1922	AAT→GAT	Asn→Asp	1	<1	?	Severe	Yes		Traystman et al 1990
Exon 18	1922	AAT→GAT	Asn→Asp	1	?	?	Moderate	?		Higuchi et al 1991b
Exon 18	1922	AAT→AGT	Asn→Ser	1	?	?	Moderate	?		Higuchi et al 1991b
Exon 18	1941	CGA→TGA	Arg→Term	8	<1	?	Severe	No 2 Yes 5 ? 1		Youssoufian et al 1986, Lavergne et al 1992[a], Schwaab et al 1992[a], Casula et al 1990, Antonarakis et al 1985a, 1992[a], Mathews et al 1987b, Higuchi et al 1989,
Exon 18	1941	CGA→CAA	Arg→Gln	4	5	20	Moderate/Mild	No		Levinson et al 1990, Antonarakis et al 1992[a], Naylor et al 1993, Inaba et al 1992[a]
Exon 19	1997	CGG→TGG	Arg→Trp	2	3.4/2.6	?	Mild/Moderate	?		Higuchi et al 1991a
Exon 22	2101	TTT→TTG	Phe→Leu	1	11	?	Mild/Moderate	?		Higuchi et al 1991a
Exon 22	2116	CGA→TGA	Arg→Term	5	<1	?	Severe	No		Youssoufian et al 1986, Naylor et al 1993 Lavergne et al 1992[a], Millar et al 1991
Exon 22	2116	CGA→CCA	Arg→Pro	1	<1	?	Severe	?		Levinson et al 1987
Exon 22	2119	TCC→TAC	Ser→Tyr	1	5–8	?	Mild/Moderate	?		Higuchi et al 1991a
Exon 23	2147	CGA→TGA	Arg→Term	7	<1	<0.1	Severe	No 2 Yes 3 ? 1		Levinson et al 1987 Millar et al 1991 Matthews et al 1987b, Mikami et al 1988a, Youssoufian et al 1988a, Levinson et al 1990 Higuchi et al 1991b

Table 36.3 *Cont'd*

Exon/ intron	Codon[b]	Nucleotide change	Codon change	Number of unrelated cases	FVIII:C $U.dl^{-1}$(%)	FVIII:Ag $U.dl^{-1}$(%)	Clinical severity	Presence of inhibitors	Comments	References
Exon 23	2150	CGT→CAT	Arg→His	5	5–7	?	Mild/Moderate	?		Higuchi et al 1991a,b, Antonarakis et al 1992[a]
Exon 23	2159	CGC→TGC	Arg→Cys	1	7.4–12	2	Mild/Moderate	No		Gitschier 1992[a] Higuchi et al 1991a, Naylor et al 1993
Exon 23	2163	CGC→CAC	Arg→His	2	?	?	Moderate	?		Antonarakis et al 1992[a]
Exon 23	2166	GTT→GCT	Leu→Ser	1	<1	?	Severe	No		Levinson et al 1990
Exon 24	2209	CGA→CTA	Arg→Leu	1	3	2.5	Moderate	No		Millar et al 1991
Exon 24	2209	CGA→TGA	Arg→Term	10	0	?	Severe	Yes 3 No 4 ? 3		Gitschier et al 1985 Schwaab et al 1992[a] Youssoufian et al 1988a, Antonarakis et al 1992[a], Lavergne et al 1992[a]
Exon 24	2209	CGA→CAA	Arg→Gln	7	<1	?	Severe	No		Bernardi et al 1988, 1989 Youssoufian et al 1988a, Casula et al 1990, Schwaab et al 1990, Traystman et al 1990, Higuchi et al 1991b
Exon 24	2209	CGA→CAA	Arg→Gln	4	2–5	?	Moderate	No		Levinson et al 1990, Antonarakis et al 1992[a], Inaba et al 1992[a]
Exon 24	2209	CGA→CAA	Arg→Gln	1	7	130	Mild	Yes		Schwaab et al 1992[a]
Exon 25	2229	TGG→TGT	Trp→Cys	1	3	?	Mild/Moderate	Yes		Naylor et al 1991
Intron 25	–	CAA→CGA	–	1	<1	?	Severe	No	Probably a neutral change ~1.9 kb 5′ to exon 26	Gitschier et al 1985
Exon 26	2300	CCG→CTG	Pro→Leu	1	7.5	?	Mild	?		Higuchi et al 1991b
Exon 26	2304	CGC→TGC	Arg→Cys	1	?	?	Mild	?		Higuchi et al 1991b
Exon 26	2307	CGA→TGA	Arg→Term	6	0	?	Severe	No		Gitschier et al 1985, 1986, Levinson et al 1990, Higuchi et al 1991b, Millar et al 1991, Antonarakis et al 1992[a], Schwaab et al 1992[a]
Exon 26	2307	CGA→CTA	Arg→Leu	1	2	4	Mild	No		Inaba et al 1989
Exon 26	2307	CGA→CTA	Arg→Leu	2	<1	?	Severe	No		Schwaab et al 1992[a]
Exon 26	2307	CGA→CAA	Arg→Gln	1	10	6	Mild	No		Gitschier et al 1986
Exon 26	2307	CGA→CAA	Arg→Gln	1	2	?	Moderate	No		Casula et al 1990

[a] Unpublished data.
[b] Codons numbered after scheme of Vehar et al 1984, i.e. starts at mature N-terminus and 19 signal peptide residues numbered negatively.

locations and phenotypic data connected with these mutations. Only where phenotype varies for mutations at a given location are cases listed separately. Otherwise a number indicates those cases thought to be independent, although doubt may remain as between recurrent mutation or identity by descent for some of these. Of the different point mutations so far characterized, 27 result in severe haemophilia A, 29 result in moderately severe haemophilia A and 18 result in mild haemophilia A. All nonsense mutations resulted in severe haemophilia A and indeed the majority of known point mutations causing severe haemophilia A are of this type. All examples of point mutations causing moderate and mild haemophilia are of the missense type.

Only in the cases reported from three groups (Higuchi et al 1991a,b, Naylor et al 1991, 1993, Gitschier 1992) has the entire factor VIII gene coding region been screened for other lesions. Absence of any other lesion in the entire coding region is good evidence that a given base change is causative. In the majority of cases evidence for causality comes from one or more of the following sources:

1. The occurrence of the mutation in a region of known importance for function
2. The previous independent occurrence of the mutation in haemophilia A
3. The novel appearance and subsequent co-segregation of the gene lesion and disease phenotype through a family pedigree
4. The failure to observe such a mutation in a large sample of normal controls (a weak criterion in the absence of other evidence)
5. In vitro expression studies.

The clinical phenotype exhibited by haemophilia A patients with the same point mutation is not always the same. For example, Pattinson et al (1990a) noted that one patient with a C→T mutation at codon 1689 was severely affected whilst two others were only moderately affected. Schwaab et al (1992) have observed a similar situation with a G→A transition at codon 2209 causing either severe (FVIII:C is less than 1%) or moderate (FVIII:C = 7%) haemophilia. These workers also also observed a G→T mutation (Arg→Leu) in codon 2307 causing severe haemophilia (FVIII:C = <1%) which contrasts with the mild (FVIII:C = 2%) phenotype exhibited by a patient described by Inaba et al (1989) with the same mutation. Inspection of Table 36.3 reveals several other examples of variable phenotype between unrelated patients with the same mutation. Thus individuals with mutations in codons 162, 372 (Arg→His), 2159 and 2307 (Arg→Gln) exhibit either a moderate or a mild phenotype while a Val→Leu substitution at residue 326 is associated with either a severe or a moderately severe phenotype. The reasons for these differences are unknown but may be due to the epistatic effects of other loci on the expression of factor VIII. Alternatively, some of these patients may have a second hitherto undetected mutation/polymorphic variant in their factor VIII genes. Differences between assays employed in different laboratories may also play a role but are less likely to account for cases of variable phenotype detected in the same laboratory. Life style of an individual patient could affect clinical assessment of bleeding severity. Whatever the explanation, only missense mutations are involved, nonsense mutations always resulting in clinically severe haemophilia.

Another aspect of phenotype heterogeneity can be seen in the presence or absence of inhibitors to therapeutically administered factor VIII. Inhibitors have so far been found in 12 of the patients with characterized point mutations. Ten of these patients possess a nonsense mutation and exhibit a severe phenotype. The remaining two missense mutations found in patients with inhibitors are intriguing and may indicate that such mutations alter an epitope required for the state of immune tolerance. One of these patients has an Arg→Gln substitution at residue 2209 associated with a mild phenotype; the other a Trp→Cys substitution at residue 2229 resulting in a mild/moderate phenotype, but his inhibitors have now proved to be transient. There also appears to be some association between specific mutations and the presence of inhibitors. Nonsense mutations at codons 1941 and 2147 together account for eight of the 12 inhibitor patients with point mutations so far reported. The reasons for such apparent biases are not clear. However, one interesting observation has been made recently in one of four patients, all inhibitor-free, with a nonsense mutation at codon 2116. Naylor et al (1993) have observed that a patient with this mutation has two mRNAs for factor VIII. One mRNA is normally spliced and therefore codes for a protein truncated at residue 2116. The other mRNA is misspliced and lacks exon 22. This defect, apparently a secondary effect of the nonsense mutation, results in factor VIII missing only the amino acids encoded by exon 22. Since patients with deletions involving only exon 22 have moderate rather than severe haemophilia (Youssoufian et al 1987a, Wehnert et al 1989) it is possible that the latter factor VIII is relatively stable and may reduce the patient's predisposition to the inhibitor complication. Nevertheless it is clear that possession of a particular mutation by itself is insufficient to specify inhibitor status, since both inhibitor positive and negative cases occur with certain mutations (e.g. in codons 1960 and 2228 among others).

The majority of point mutations so far detected are located in exons 8, 11, 14, 18, 23, 24 and 26. This is due to the fact that exons 14 and 26 between them comprise 55% of the length of the factor VIII mRNA and to the presence of CGA (Arg) codons within readily screened *Taq* I restriction sites in exons 18, 23, 24 and 26. If we look instead at the distribution of mutations detected in systematic screening studies, the short exons 7, 11, 12 and 16 appear to harbour a disproportionate number of mutations (Higuchi et al 1991a,b).

About 5% of patients with haemophilia A have an excess of factor VIII antigen over functional activity due to the presence of a factor VIII molecule with reduced specific activity. These cases are termed **C**ross **R**eacting **M**aterial **P**ositive (CRM$^+$). They have often been specifically selected for study in the hope of gaining information on the functionally critical regions of the factor VIII protein. For example, mutations producing a CRM$^+$ phenotype have been identified in the two arginine residues (372 and 1689) adjacent to the scissile bonds cleaved upon activation. The defect in function of these molecules has been clearly demonstrated to be associated with resistance to cleavage by thrombin of the heavy and light chains respectively (Arai et al 1989, 1990, O'Brien & Tuddenham 1989, O'Brien et al 1990). This result was anticipated by site-directed mutagenesis in vitro (Pittman & Kaufman 1988) but other CRM$^+$ variants identify functionally important regions of factor VIII not previously defined in this way. Thus Arg^{2209} appears critical for function since its substitution by Gln produced a CRM+ phenotype (FVIII:C = 7%, FVIII:Ag = 130%). As noted above this genotype is associated with a variable phenotype. An interesting example of a mutation almost certainly affecting stability of the protein in the circulation is that converting Tyr1680 to Phe. This residue is normally sulphated and is critical for the interaction of factor VIII with von Willebrand factor (Leyte et al 1991); loss of this interaction would lead to rapid clearance from the circulation. The lower activity (FVIII:C = 10%) than antigen (FVIII:Ag = 20%) in the case reported suggests an additional effect on function. The few other missense mutations where information is available produce a CRM reduced or CRM– phenotype with low amounts of residual activity and protein. This is most probably due to effects on stability due to interference with protein folding, often because the substituted residues are in the hydrophobic core of a domain, but could be due to interference with any stage of the expression pathway, which in the case of factor VIII involves complex post-translational modifications (Kaufman et al 1988). Precise localization of structurally and of functionally important regions of factor VIII should be possible from data accumulated by screening a fraction of the haemophilia A population of the planet (about 200 000 cases).

Of the different point mutations listed in Table 36.3, 38% are C→T or G→A transitions in a CpG dinucleotide. This doublet is already known to be hypermutable as a consequence of methylation-mediated deamination of 5-methyl cytosine; indeed about one third of all point mutations causing human genetic disease are CG→TG or CG→CA transitions consistent with this postulate (Cooper & Youssoufian 1988, Cooper & Krawczak 1990). The high proportion of CpG mutations among those listed in Table 36.3 is however at least in part due to the deliberate screening of these sites with restriction enzymes (Gitschier et al 1985) or by oligonucleotide discriminant hybridization (Gitschier et al 1988, Pattinson et al 1990a). A relatively unbiased estimate may be obtained from the data of Higuchi et al (1991a,b) where 32% of these mutations occurred in CG dinucleotides. Recurrent mutation at CpG dinucleotides appears to have occurred in at least 16 sites (codons 282, 336, 372(2), 527, 1689, 1941, 2116, 2147, 2150, 2159, 2209(2), 2228 and 2307(2)). This assertion is made on the basis either of RFLP haplotyping data or of extreme geographical separation (e.g. Pattinson et al 1990a). Multiple mutations have been reported at four further CpG sites at codons 531, 593, 704 and 1997. Identity by descent may however be suspected in the case of the five Arg^{593}→Cys mutations in (apparently unrelated) patients, all of whom originate from Tennessee and all of whom possess an identical RFLP haplotype (Antonarakis et al 1992). For the other CpG mutations at codons 531, 704 and 1997, it is at present difficult to distinguish recurrent mutation from identity by descent.

Mutations affecting mRNA splicing

A number of point mutations that putatively interfere with mRNA splicing have been detected in the factor VIII genes of haemophiliacs (Table 36.3). Since the factor VIII gene is transcribed in fairly inaccessible tissues, formal confirmation of a splicing defect is not available in most cases. However, 'ectopic' transcription has been successfully employed to demonstrate aberrant splicing in lymphocyte factor VIII mRNA (Naylor et al 1991). The putative splicing defects reported to date may be divided into three categories:

1. Mutations of the invariant GT and AG dinucleotides at the donor and acceptor splice junctions respectively
2. Mutations within the extended consensus sequences of the donor and acceptor splice junctions
3. Mutations which create a novel donor or acceptor splice site.

In the first category, the invariant AG dinucleotide in the IVS5 and IVS6 acceptor sites were mutated to GG and AC respectively; both resulted in a severe phenotype. In the second category, four mutations in donor splice site consensus sequences have been reported. In two cases, the altered nucleotide is the last base (–1) of an exon (Gly^{205} and Leu^{1843}) and in a third case is located at position –3 (Gln^{565}). These lesions result in either a mild or a moderate phenotype. Only in the case of the Gly^{205} mutation is the encoded amino acid changed; it is not yet possible to dissect the relative contribution of amino acid substitution and altered splicing to the clinical phenotype in this patient.

Table 36.4 Small deletions in the factor VIII gene of patients with haemophilia A

Patient/ family	FVIII:C ($U.dl^{-1}$)	FVIII:Ag ($U.dl^{-1}$)	Codons	Size in bp (nucleotides deleted)	Severity	Inhibitors	Comments	References
JH72	?	?	104–111	23	Severe	?	Includes IVS3 donor splice site	Higuchi et al 1991b
H23	?	?	340–341	4(AATG)	Severe	No	Frameshift in exon 8	Kogan & Gitschier 1988, 1990
JH31	?	?	341	2(GA)	Severe	?	Frameshift in exon 8	Antonarakis et al 1992[a]
MH	?	?	1212	1(C)	Severe	No	Frameshift in exon 14	Naylor et al 1993
JH142	?	?	1439	1(A)	Severe	?	A8→A7, frameshift in exon 14	Antonarakis et al 1992[a]
JH80	?	?	1535–6	2(GA)	Severe	?	Frameshift in exon 14	Higuchi et al 1991b
JH69	?	?	2136	2(AA)	Severe	?	A4→A2, frameshift in exon 23	Antonarakis et al 1992[a]
JH90	?	?	2204–5	3(CTC)	Moderate	?	Deletes 2205 Pro	Antonarakis et al 1992[a]

[a] Unpublished data.

Only two potential examples of the activation of cryptic splice sites have been reported, one in intron 4 (novel donor site) and the other at codon 504 (no amino acid substitution) in exon 11 (novel acceptor site). Both are reportedly associated with mild haemophilia suggesting that use of the novel splice site is <95%. Proof that these mutations do indeed give rise to aberrant splicing could be obtained either from ectopic transcript analysis or by the demonstration of de novo mutation.

Short deletions

The frequency of short gene deletions detectable by novel screening methods and by DNA sequencing may be rather higher than that found for gross gene deletions. A total of seven such deletions have so far been reported ranging in size between 1 and 23 bp (Table 36.4). The relative frequency of this type of lesion may be roughly estimated from the systematic screening studies undertaken by The Johns Hopkins Group (Higuchi et al 1991a,b, Antonarakis et al 1992): of all patients without a gross gene rearrangement, in whom a mutation was found, 7% possessed a short gene deletion of a few base-pairs. All were severely affected, no doubt due to frameshift causing premature termination of translation.

Two of the seven known short deletions occurred at the same location at amino acid residues Asn^{340}/Glu^{341} (Higuchi et al 1990, Kogan & Gitschier 1990). Significantly these deletions (2 bp and 4 bp respectively) occurred within a TGAAGA sequence which matches the postulated deletion hotspot consensus sequence (TGA/GA/G G/TA/C) of Krawczak & Cooper (1991).

Small insertions

Four examples of the insertion of a single base (three of them A residues) have also been noted causing frameshift and consequent premature termination of translation (Table 36.5). The introduction of an A into an existing string of A residues is consistent with slipped mispairing at the replication fork (Cooper & Krawczak 1991).

Mutations in the 5′-flanking region

Only one example of this type of mutation has been found to date. A mutation detected by SSCP has been located within the 1 kb 5′-flanking region of the factor VIII gene in a patient with another established mutation (R2209→Q) but clinically severe disease unlike all other reported examples of this missense mutation (Michaelides & Schwaab 1992). This type of lesion is probably infrequent since Higuchi et al (1990) and Kogan & Gitschier (1992) failed to find any base changes in 529 bp of the factor VIII 5′-flanking regions of 127 and 100 haemophilia A patients which they respectively screened.

Undetected mutations

In a survey of 30 cases of severe haemophilia A screened by denaturing gradient gel electrophoresis of PCR-amplified genomic DNA comprising 99% of the coding region and 94% of the normal intron–exon boundaries, Higuchi et al (1991b) could find causative mutations in only 16 patients. By contrast, they found a mutation, plausibly causing the phenotype, in 16 of 17 patients with mild or moderate haemophilia A.

A faster approach for the analysis of factor VIII mutations was developed in one of our laboratories (Naylor et al 1991). This technique, essentially based on the screening of the factor VIII mRNA found in peripheral lympho-

Table 36.5 Small insertions in the factor VIII gene of patients with haemophilia A

Patient	Exon	Nature of Insertion	Severity	Reference
JH100	11	1 bp (G at codon 513)	Severe	Antonarakis et al 1992[a]
JH77	14	1 bp (TCA→TCAA at codon 1395)	Severe	Higuchi et al 1991b
JH81	14	1 bp (A in stretch of 8A residues at codon 1439)	Severe	Higuchi et al 1991b
JH129	17	1 bp (A in stretch of 4A residues in codon 1888)	Severe	Higuchi et al 1991b

[a] Unpublished data.

cytes, has revealed an abnormality in every one of the 30 patients so far analysed (Naylor et al 1992). These patients include six mildly or moderately affected individuals, and 24 severely affected. Fourteen of the severely affected patients analysed by Naylor et al (1993) have mutations that could have been detected by genomic DNA analysis, i.e. exon deletions, small deletions or insertions and base substitutions in the coding sequence. One further patient had a splicing defect resulting in exon skipping that might or might not be detected by genomic DNA screening depending on whether the appropriate splice signals were analysed, and finally ten patients have abnormalities that definitely could not be detected by genomic analysis and probably largely account for the proportion of haemophilia A mutations undetected by Higuchi et al (1991b). These abnormalities affected the factor VIII transcript and prevent the normal splicing of exon 22 to 23 in the mRNA but do not affect the normal splice signals. They must be due to changes in intron 22. This 32 kb region therefore makes an unexpected contribution to the spectrum of mutations causing severe haemophilia A.

MUTATIONS OF THE FACTOR IX GENE

The haemophilia B mutation rate

The population genetics of haemophilia B is similar to that of haemophilia A and the disease has been maintained in the population by the equilibrium between loss and gain of detrimental genes proposed by Haldane (1935). As for haemophilia A, therefore, the question of whether male and female mutation rates are similar or not is of considerable biological interest and in some parts of the world of practical importance. In the UK, the development and application of rapid methods for carrier diagnoses based on the direct detection of the gene defect is eliminating the need to estimate the probability of carrier status and hence to consider the ratio of the sex-specific mutation rates for providing genetic counselling to the mother and other ascendant relatives of isolated patients.

Indirect methods for estimating the ratio of the sex-specific mutation rates such as those that have been used in haemophilia A have not been successfully applied to haemophilia B, due to the lower incidence of this disease relative to haemophilia A (Barrai et al 1985). However, the development of rapid methods of mutation analysis suited to the analysis of large populations of patients has allowed a direct approach to obtain estimates of mutation rates that are independent of any assumption about the Haldane equilibrium, genetic fitness and carrier status of any individual. The first estimates by this method were made on the Swedish population (Montandon et al 1992) and indicated an overall rate of 4.1×10^6 mutations per gene per gamete per generation in keeping with a previous indirect estimate (Ferrari & Rizza 1986) and also suggested a higher mutation rate in males than in females.

Gross mutations

Haemophilia B mutations are usually single base substitutions or small deletions or insertions (<20 bp) and rarely gross changes. Thus large deletions or duplications of the factor IX gene (Table 36.6) probably account for no more than 1–3% of all cases, but they represent a much larger proportion of the mutations found in patients with clinically relevant antibodies against factor IX (inhibitor patients) (Giannelli et al 1983, Green et al 1991a). The largest deletions comprise the whole gene and adjacent DNA including the mcf2 gene that belongs to the broad and heterogeneous group of transforming genes (Anson et al 1988). Such large deletions however are not associated with symptoms other than those of haemophilia B. Smaller deletions affect different regions of the gene and their functional consequences are difficult to predict in detail. Of course deletions result in loss of the domains coded by the missing exons, but in addition they may alter the reading frame, affect the splicing of adjacent exons or lead to unstable mRNA or protein. Only one deletion patient has been reported to have significant factor IX antigen in his circulation (Vidaud et al 1986). This patient had a deletion of exon d. Deletion junctions have been examined only in three patients: in the first no homologous sequences were found and the deletion is a clear example of non-homologous recombination (Green et al 1988). In the second case a complex rearrangement resulted in a deletion interrupted by the retention of a gene segment in inverted orientation (Peake et al 1989), and in the third case a recombination appeared to have occurred within a short homologous (14 bp) sequence (Chen & Scott 1990). Two insertions have also been reported (Chen et al 1988, Vidaud et al 1989).

Point mutations and other small changes

The 574 patients found so far to carry this type of mutation comprise 38 deletions, nine insertions and three additions plus deletions of a few bases (less than 20) (Giannelli et al 1992a). There are also a number of repeats of the same mutation. Such repeats in some cases may be shown, or have been shown, to represent independent changes at sites particularly prone to mutation (see for example Green et al 1992b) or, by contrast, they may represent replications of the same ancestral mutation. In fact few mutations appear to have enjoyed conditions that allowed them to achieve relatively high frequencies in specific populations. Thus founder effects have been claimed for $Thr^{296} \rightarrow Met$ and $Ile^{397} \rightarrow Thr$ in North America (Thompson et al 1990, Ketterling et al 1991).

The results obtained so far clearly demonstrate that haemophilia B mutations may exert their detrimental effects by several different mechanisms, that is: by impairing transcription, RNA processing or mRNA translation or, indeed by altering individual residues of the factor IX protein.

Table 36.6 Factor IX gene deletions

Mutation name (or reference, if no name)	Defect	Haematologic group	Reference
1 Malmö 34	complete	no inhibitor	Green et al 1991b
2 Manchester 1	complete	inhibitor	Giannelli et al 1983, Anson et al 1988
3 Manchester 2	complete	inhibitor	Giannelli et al 1983, Anson et al 1988
4 Jersey 1	complete	inhibitor	Matthews et al 1987a
5 Pisa 1	complete	inhibitor	Bernardi et al 1985
6 Boston 1	complete	inhibitor	Matthews et al 1987a
7 Malmö 2	complete	inhibitor	Green et al 1991b
8 Mikami et al 1987:1	complete	inhibitor	
9 Mikami et al 1987:2	complete	inhibitor	
10 Tanimoto et al 1988:1	complete	inhibitor	
11 Tanimoto et al 1988:2	complete	inhibitor	
12 Tanimoto et al 1988:3	complete	inhibitor	
13 Taylor et al 1988	complete	+/– inhibitor[b]	
14 Wadelius et al 1988	complete	no inhibitor	
15 Ludwig et al 1989	complete	no inhibitor	
16 B7: Thompson 1990	complete	no inhibitor	
17 Ludwig et al 1989	exon a	?	
18 Bari 1	exons a to h	inhibitor	Hassan et al 1985
19 Ludwig et al 1989	exons a,b,c	inhibitor	
20 Malmö 45	at least exon b–h	♀ heterozygous	Green et al 1991b
21 B19: Thompson 1990	exons b–h	no inhibitor	
22 Strasbourg 1	exon d	no inhibitor CRM^{+}	Vidaud et al 1986
23 Ludwig et al 1989	exons d,e	no inhibitor	
24 Seattle 1[a]	exons e,f	no inhibitor $CRM^{+/-}$	Bray & Thomson 1986
25 Chicago 1	exons e,g,h	inhibitor	Matthews et al 1987a
26 London 1	exons f,g,h	inhibitor	Giannelli et al 1983, Green et al 1988
27 Ludwig et al 1989	exon g	no inhibitor	
28 Casarino et al 1986b	at least exon d	inhibitor	
29 McGraw et al 1985	at least exon h	inhibitor	

[a] This patient has material in the urine reacting with antibodies against factor IX.
[b] One relative with transient antibody response and one with no inhibitor.
NB: A large intron deletion removing the donor splice site of exon d has been reported by Solera et al 1992.
CRM, cross reacting material.

Mutations affecting transcription, RNA processing and translation (Table 36.7)

Transcription is affected by promoter mutations (Table 36.7: 1–11). These have been found in a number of patients, singled out initially because they begin life with severe or moderate factor IX deficiency and then improve in an age-related manner, especially after puberty, becoming asymptomatic (Reitsma et al 1988, 1989, Crossley et al 1989, 1990). Such a course of the disease has been tentatively explained by suggesting that the mutations impair the factor IX promoter so that it becomes capable of sufficient activity only under androgen stimulation.

Recent experimental data have indicated that promoter mutations impair the binding of different transcription factors including C/EBP- or C/EBP-like proteins and that a weak androgen response element is present in the promoter region (Crossley & Brownlee 1990, 1992, Hirosawa et al 1990).

RNA processing is impaired by splicing mutations. These so far have been found at all splice sites except those at the 3′ end of intron 5 and at the 5′ end of intron 7 (Table 36.7: 12, 15–19, 21, 31–34, 37–40, 43–46, 51–52, 55–57, 64, 66–69, 72). Frequently such mutations affect the highly conserved GT and AG consensuses of the donor and acceptor sites at the start and end of introns (Table 36.7: 18, 19, 31, 38–40, 43, 45, 46, 56, 66–69, 72) but more unusual and interesting mutations also occur; for example a 10 bp deletion in the polypyrimidine tract preceding the acceptor site in intron 2 (Table 36.7: 34). Since polypyrimidine tracts are important to the assembly and function of the spliceosome (Helfman & Ricci 1989, Reed 1989) this mutation is consistent with the severe reduction in factor IX protein observed in the patient. Other mutations affect the wider splice-site consensuses and in this case they may (Table 36.7: 15, 37, 55) or may not alter the coding sequence. In some patients single base substitutions generating new potential splice sites have been observed (Table 36.7: 21, 51, 52, 64).

Mutations causing defective translation comprise single base substitutions generating translation stop signals and deletions or insertions of a few bases causing frameshifts. Interestingly the patients with such mutations show at best traces of factor IX protein even when the stop codon occurs very close to the end of the protein (codon 411; Table 36.7: 99) (Attree et al 1989) and only one frameshift, at codon 402 (Table 36.7: 95) and resulting in a substantial lengthening of the factor IX protein, is associated with significant factor IX antigen in the patient's circulation (Rao et al 1990). This suggests either that the truncated factor IX is markedly unstable or that the mRNA

Table 36.7 Haemophilia B; mutations affecting the transcription and translation of the factor IX gene[a]

Mutation name	Nucleotide change	Nucleotide position	Amino acid change	FIX:C (%)	FIX:Ag (%)	In	Reference	Comment
1 Brandeburg	G→C	–26		<1	<1		Giannelli et al 1992a	
2 Leyden 1	T→A	–20		1 var			Reitsma et al 1988	
3 Marseille	T→C	–20		9 var			Giannelli et al 1992a	
4 High Wycombe	G→A	–6		13 var			Crossley et al 1990	
5 Toulouse	G→C	–6		1–30	1–30		Gispert et al 1989	
6 Toronto 20	A→T	–5		3			Giannelli et al 1992a	
7 Leyden USA 2	T→A	6		2–37			Freedenberg & Black 1991	
8 Leyden, NZ	T→C	8		1–32			Royle et al 1991	
9 Leyden 3	1 bp del	13		1 var			Reitsma et al 1989	
10 Norwich	A→G	13		1 var			Crossley et al 1989	C/EBP binding site
11 Aachem	A→C	13		<1			Giannelli et al 1992a	
12 UK 36	10 bp del	111–120	f/s Cys-19	<1	<1		Giannelli et al 1992a	Donor splice site deleted
13 Meaux	1 bp del	112	f/s Cys-19	<1			Giannelli et al 1992a	
14 Recklinghausen	2 bp Ins	114	f/s Thr-18	<1	<1		Giannelli et al 1992a	
15 HB64	G→A	117	Val-17→lle	<1	2		Bottema et al 1991a	exon a donor splice (–1)
16 Malmö 33	G→A	122		3	2		Green et al 1991b	exon a donor splice (+5)
17 HB 135	T→G	6320					Bottema et al 1991b	exon b acceptor site (–6)
18 UK 70	G→A	6325		<1			Giannelli et al 1992a	exon b acceptor site (–1)
19 Spain	G→T	6325		<1			Giannelli et al 1992a	exon b acceptor site (–1)
20 Autun	1 bp del	6379	f/s Asn2	<1			Giannelli et al 1992a	
21 HB47	A→G	6390		7			Koeberl et al 1990 a	exon b new donor splice site (–99)
22 UK 12	1 bp del	6392	f/s Leu6	<1		y	Green et al 1989	
23 Malmö 8	2 bp del	6398–9	f/s Glu8	<1	<0.1		Green et al 1991b	
24 Madrid 3	10 bp del	6401–10	f/s Phe9	<1	<1	y	Giannelli et al 1992a	
25 Bonn 2	5 bp del	6402–6	f/s Phe9	<1	<1	y	Ludwig et al 1992a	
26 Oxford b3	C→T	6406	Gln11→stop	<0.5	0.2		Winship & Dragon 1991	
27 Mülheim/Ruhr	2 bp del	6416–17	f/s Leu14	4	4		Giannelli et al 1992a	?somatic mosaic
28 Malmö 4	C→T	6460	Arg29→stop	<1	<0.1	y	Green et al 1989	
29 Malmö 9	1 bp del	6466	f/s Val31	<1	<0.1		Green et al 1991b	
30 UK 180	2 bp Ins	6472	f/s Glu33				Giannelli et al 1992a	
31 Ursem	4 bp del	6492–5 or 6491–4		<1	<1		Poort et al 1990	exon b donor splice site (+1 to +4 or +2 to +5)
32 Paris 1	G→A	6494					Giannelli et al 1992a	exon b donor splice site (+5)
33 HB74/77	T→C	6495		1	1		Bottema et al 1990	exon b donor splice site (+6)
34 Malmö 10	10 bp del	6666–75		<1	0.2		Green et al 1991b	exon c acceptor splice site (–12 to –3)
35 HB7, Japan	2 bp del	6680–1	f/s Thr39	<1	<1	y	Matsushita et al 1990	
36 Malmö 52	C→T	6693	Gln44→Stop	<1			Giannelli et al 1992a	
37 UK 25	G→A	6702	Asp47→Asn	<1	<1		Giannelli et al 1992a	exon c donor splice site (–1)
38 Pirmasens	T→C	6704		<1	<1		Giannelli et al 1992a	exon c donor splice site (+2)
39 Oxford 2	T→G	6704		<0.5			Winship 1986	exon c donor splice site (+2)
40 Toronto 16	G→A	10391		3			Koeberl et al 1990a	exon d acceptor splice site (–1)
41 UK 86	3 bp del Ins A	10397–9	f/s Asp49	15			Giannelli et al 1992a	♀ heterozygous for f/s
42 HB97	G→T	10406	Glu52→Stop	<1	20		Bottema et al 1991a	
43 UK 132	4 bp del	10507–10					Giannelli et al 1992a	exon d donor splice site (+2 to +5)
44 HB6	4 bp del	17660–3		20			Koeberl et al 1989	exon e acceptor splice site (–9 to –6)
45 Toronto 14	A→G	17667		3	3		Koeberl et al 1990a	exon e acceptor splice site (–2)
46 Malmö 11	G→C	17668		<1	<1		Green et al 1991b	exon e acceptor splice site (–1)
47 Seattle 2	1 bp del	17669	f/s Asp85	<1	<0.2		Schach et al 1987	
48 Edmonton 1	C→A	17700	Cys95→Stop	<1			Giannelli et al 1992a	
49 NZ 4	1 bp Ins	17718	f/s Asn101	<1			Giannelli et al 1992a	
50 UK 50	2 bp Ins	17727	f/s Asn105	<1	<1		Giannelli et al 1992a	
51 Malmö 35	G→A	17736	Val107→silent	21	14		Green et al 1991b	exon e new acceptor splice site (–62)
52 UK 28	C→A	17761	Arg116→silent	5	5		Giannelli et al 1992a	exon e new acceptor splice site (–37)
53 Malmö 7	C→T	17761	Arg116→stop	<1	<0.1		Montandon et al 1990	double mutant (see His257 Table 36.8)

Table 36.7 *Cont'd*

Mutation name	Nucleotide change	Nucleotide position	Amino acid change	FIX:C (%)	FIX:Ag (%)	In	Reference	Comment
54 Wurzburg	Ins C	17763–4	f/s Leu117	<1			Ludwig et al 1992a	
55 HB68	G→A	17797	Val128→Met	1			Bottema et al 1991a	exon e donor splice site (−1)
56 Nortingen	G→T	17798		<1			Ludwig et al 1992a	exon e donor splice site (+1)
57 Toronto 13	A→G	17810		10			Koeberl et al 1990a	exon e donor splice site (+3)
58 Malmö 44	1 bp del	20398	f/s Thr140				Green et al 1991b	
59 HB23	13 bp del	20466–78	f/s Ala161	<1			Koeberl et al 1989	
60 HB17	C→T	20497	Gln173→stop	<1			Koeberl et al 1989	
61 HB78	1 bp del	20501	f/s Ser174				Bottema et al 1990	
62 Malmö 13	1 bp del	20510	f/s Asp177	<1	0.5		Green et al 1991b	
63 HB5 Japan	C→T	20551	Gln 191→stop	<1	<1	y	Matsushita et al 1990	
64 Seattle J	A→G	20553	Gln191→silent	3	2		Thompson et al 1992	exon f new donor splice (−13)
65 Malmö 5	G→A	20561	Trp194→stop	<1	<0.1	y	Green et al 1989	
66 Rotenburg	G→A	20566		<1	<1		Giannelli et al 1992a	exon f donor splice site (+1)
67 Oxford 1	G→T	20566		<0.5	0.3		Rees et al 1985	exon f donor splice site (+1)
68 UK 171	G→A	30038		<1			Giannelli et al 1992a	exon g acceptor splice site (−1)
69 HB102	G→C	30038		<1	<1		Bottema et al 1991a	exon g acceptor splice site (−1)
70 Bottrop 2	G→T	30090	Glu213→Stop	<1	<1		Giannelli et al 1992a	
71 unnamed	G→A	30097	Trp215→stop	<1	<1		Chen et al 1991	
72 HB6 Japan	G→A	30821		<1	<1	y	Matsushita et al 1990	exon h acceptor splice site (−1)
73 UK 140	1 bp del	30857	f/s Gln246	<1			Giannelli et al 1992a	
74 Malmö 3	C→T	30863	Arg248→stop	<1	<0.1	y	Green et al 1989	
75 Leiria	C→T	30875	Arg252→stop	<1	<1		Siguret et al 1988	
76 UK 48	1 bp del	30942	f/s Glu274				Giannelli et al 1992 a	♀heterozygous for f/s
77 Malmö 1	8 bp del	30950–7	f/s Glu277	<1	<0.1	y	Green et al 1989	
78 HB100	G→T	31001	Glu294→Stop	<1	<1		Bottema et al 1991a	
79 Seattle 0	T→A	31039	Tyr306→Stop	<1	<1		Thompson et al 1992	
80 unnamed	G→A	31051	Trp310→stop	<1	<1		Wang et al 1990a	
81 UK 11	2 bp del	31059–60	f/s Val313	<1	<2		Green et al 1989	
82 Riegelsberg	7 bp del	31084–90	f/s Leu321	<1	<1		Ludwig et al 1992a	
83 HB82	C→T	31091	Gln324→Stop	4	4		Bottema et al 1991a	
84 HB122	C→G	31096	Tyr325→Stop	4			Bottema et al 1991a	
85 HB29	C→T	31118	Arg333→stop	<1	<1		Koeberl et al 1990b	
86 UK 20	C→T	31133	Arg338→stop	2	<1		Green et al 1990	
87 UK170	2 bp Ins	31141, 2 or 3	f/s Lys341 or 340				Giannelli et al 1992a	
88 Samli	3 bp del 5 bp del 1 bp Ins	31149–51 31158–62 31158	f/s Thr343	<1	<1		Giannelli et al 1992a	
89 unnamed	2 bp Ins	31157, 8 or 9	f/s Asn346	<1	<1		Giannelli et al 1992a	
90 Offenbach	1 bp del	31166 or 7	f/s Phe 349	<1			Ludwig et al 1992a	
91 UK 144	G→T	31208	Gly363→Stop	<1			Giannelli et al 1992a	
92 Hong Kong 4	1 bp del	31261	f/s Thr380	<1	<10		Chan et al 1991	
93 Malmö 49	G→A	31276	Trp385→Stop	<1			Giannelli et al 1992a	
94 UK 29	14 bp del	31307–20	f/s Gly396	<1			Giannelli et al 1992a	
95 Lincoln Park	2 bp del, 10 bp Ins	31327–8	f/s Ser402	3	9		Rao et al 1990	
96 UK 53	G→A	31342	Trp407→stop	<1	<1		Giannelli et al 1992a	
97 Oxford 41	1 bp del	31344 or 45	f/s lle408	<1	0.2		Winship and Dragon 1991	
98 HB62	4 bp Ins	31346	f/s lle408				Bottema et al 1989	
99 Bordeaux	A→T	31352	Lys411→stop	<1	<1		Attree et al 1989	

[a] Repeats of any mutation are not shown, but they are listed in Giannelli et al 1992a. Nucleotide position and amino acid change, both numbered as in Yoshitake et al 1985. FIX:C, Factor IX coagulant; FIX:Ag, Factor IX antigen. Both levels are expressed in international units/dl and units/dl respectively. In, refers to the presence (y) of inhibitory antibodies; Del, deletion; Ins, insertion.

with a premature stop codon is very labile. Puzzling, in this context, is the report of a patient with a translation stop at codon 52 and significant factor IX antigen in circulation (Bottema et al 1991a) (Table 36.7: 42).

Missense mutations and single amino acid deletions

Alterations of individual residues of the factor IX protein include single amino acid deletions and amino acid substitutions (Table 36.8: 9). Five single amino acid deletions have been reported so far (Giannelli et al 1992a and Table 36.8: 25, 79, 80, 131, 142) together with 182 amino acid substitutions. Among the latter, five appear to be neutral (Table 36.9) because they accompany a second mutation thought or proven to be the cause of the disease and three are due to base substitutions that alter splice consensuses (Table 36.8: 3, 29, 64). In the latter it is difficult to tell whether the detrimental effects are a consequence of the amino acid substitution, the splice defect or both. The remaining 174 amino acid substitutions affect 124 different residues out of the 415 of the mature protein and the 46 or 41 or 39 of the signal peptide.

Table 36.8 Haemophilia B mutations causing single amino acid changes in factor IX[a]

	Mutation name	Nucleotide change	Nucleotide position	Amino acid change	FIX:C	FIX:Ag	Reference	Comment
1	UK 22	T→A	79	Ile-30→Asn	2	<1	Giannelli et al 1992a	
2	HB130	T→C	111	Cys-19→Arg	20		Bottema et al 1991b	
3	HB64	G→A	117	Val-17→Ile	<1	2	Bottema et al 1991a	exon a donor splice site (−1)
4	Malmö 6	C→T	6364	Arg-4→Trp	<1	26–34	Green et al 1989	
5	Oxford 3	G→A	6365	Arg-4→Gln	<0.5	69[b]	Bentley et al 1986	
6	Kingston 1	G→T	6365	Arg-4→Leu	<1	27	Koeberl et al 1990a	
7	Seattle E	G→T	6372	Lys-2→Asn	<1	37	Thompson et al 1992	
8	Cambridge	G→C or T	6375	Arg-1→Ser	<1	80	Diuguid et al 1986	
9	London, Ont 1	A→G	6379	Asn2→Asp	6		Koeberl et al 1990a	
10	Oxford b2	A→C	6395	Glu7→Ala	5	5	Winship & Dragon 1991	
11	HB151	A→G	6398	Glu8→Gly	2	45	Bottema et al 1991b	
12	UK 84	T→A	6400	Phe9→Ile	14	118	Giannelli et al 1992a	
13	Hong Kong 1	G→C	6410	Gly12→Ala	3		Chan et al 1991	
14	Unnamed	G→A	6424	Glu17→Lys	<1		Giannelli et al 1992a	
15	Zutphen	T→C	6427	Cys18→Arg	<1	100	Ludwig et al 1992a	
16	HB116	G→A	6428	Cys18→Tyr	<1		Bottema et al 1991a	
17	Nagoya 4	G→A	6436	Glu21→Lys	<1	52	Hamaguchi et al 1991	
18	JieLong	T→C	6442	Cys23→Arg	<1	35	Lin & Shen 1991	
19	UK 115	G→A	6443	Cys23→Tyr	<1	19	Giannelli et al 1992a	
20	Rheidt	T→C	6449	Phe25→Ser	2	32	Ludwig et al 1992a	
21	Seattle 3	G→A	6454	Glu27→Lys	<1	30	Chen et al 1989	
22	Chongqing	A→T	6455	Glu27→Val	<1	3	Wang et al 1990b	
23	HB2	G→A	6461	Arg29→Gln	30	70	Koeberl et al 1989	
24	HB9	A→C	6474	Glu33→Asp	4		Koeberl et al 1989	
25	UK 10	3 bp del	6484→6	Arg37 del	<1	12	Green et al 1989	
26	unnamed	C→G	6488	Thr38→Arg	<1		Giannelli et al 1992a	
27	UK89	C→T	6488	Thr38→Ile	7		Giannelli et al 1992a	
28	Hoogeveen	A→G	6690	Lys43→Glu	14	96	Giannelli et al 1992a	
29	UK 25	G→A	6702	Asp47→Asn	<1	<1	Giannelli et al 1992a	exon c donor splice site (−1)
30	Alabama	A→G	10392	Asp47→Gly	10	100	Davis et al 1987	
31	HB75	T→A	10393	Asp47→Glu	14	80	Bottema et al 1990	
32	Tainan	G→A	10394	Gly48→Arg	28	101	Lin & Shen 1991	
33	Malmö 27	G→T	10395	Gly48→Val	19	108	Green et al 1991b	
34	New London	A→C	10401	Gln50→Pro	<1	114	Lozier et al 1990	
35	Malmö 21	C→T	10415	Pro55→Ser	12	52	Green et al 1991b	
36	UK 7	C→G	10415	Pro55→Ala	10–12	49	Green et al 1989	
37	Malmö 22	C→T	10416	Pro55→Leu	20,32		Green et al 1991b	
38	Basel	T→C	10418	Cys56→Arg	<1		Alkan et al 1991	
39	Kleve	G→C	10419	Cys56→Ser	<1	<1	Ludwig et al 1991	
40	Toronto 2	G→A	10419	Cys56→Tyr	1	2	Koeberl et al 1990a	
41	UK 160	G→A	10427	Gly59→Ser	18		Giannelli et al 1992a	
42	HB141	G→T	10428	Gly59→Val	2		Bottema et al 1991b	
43	Durham	G→A	10430	Gly60→Ser	14	26[b]	Denton et al 1988	
44	HB154	G→C	10430	Gly60→Arg	<1	6	Bottema et al 1991b	
45	Toronto 6	G→A	10431	Gly60→Asp	1	2	Koeberl et al 1990a	
46	Oxford d1	G→A	10442	Asp64→Asn	3	117	Winship & Dragon 1991	
47	UK 6	A→G	10443	Asp64→Gly	8	87	Green et al 1989	
48	Trier	A→G	10458	Tyr69→Cys	<1		Giannelli et al 1992a	
49	UK 67	G→T	10479	Gly76→Val	6	12	Giannelli et al 1992a	♀ haemophiliac
50	UK 19	T→G	10482	Phe77→Tyr			Giannelli et al 1992a	
51	Konigswinter	G→C	17678	Cys88→Ser	<1		Giannelli et al 1992a	
52	Fukuoka	A→C	17689	Asn92→His	2	66	Nishimura et al 1991	

Table 36.8 *Cont'd*

Mutation name	Nucleotide change	Nucleotide position	Amino acid change	FIX:C	FIX:Ag	Reference	Comment
53 Chelles	T→A	17691	Asn92→Lys	<1		Giannelli et al 1992a	
54 HB106	A→T	17697	Arg94→Ser	1	84	Bottema et al 1991b	
55 HB134/157	G→A	17699	Cys95→Tyr	3[b]	6	Bottema et al 1991b	
56 Malmö 51	C→G	17700	Cys95→Trp	<1		Giannelli et al 1992a	
57 Hamilton 1	T→C	17710	Cys99→Arg	<1		Koeberl et al 1990a	
58 Unnamed	T→C	17738	Val107→Ala	20	120	Chen et al 1991	
59 HB111	T→C	17743	Ser110→Pro	<1	<1	Bottema et al 1991a	
60 Oxford e1	G→C	17756	Gly114→Ala	5	4	Winship & Dragon 1991	
61 UK 123	A→G	17759	Tyr115→Cys	2	1	Giannelli et al 1992a	
62 UK 9	A→T	17773	Asn120→Tyr	<1	0.4	Green et al 1989	
63 HB88	G→A	17786	Cys124→Tyr	2		Bottema et al 1991a	
64 HB68	G→A	17797	Val128→Met	1		Bottema et al 1991a	exon e donor splice site (–1)
65 Dakar	T→C	20374	Cys132→Arg	<1	<1	Giannelli et al 1992a	
66 Malmö 12	G→T	20375	Cys132→Phe	<1	<0.1	Green et al 1991b	
67 HB115	G→A	20375	Cys132→Tyr	<1		Bottema et al 1991a	
68 Cardiff 1	C→T	20413	Arg145→Cys	<1	48[b]	Liddell et al 1989	
69 Chapel Hill	G→A	20414	Arg145→His	8	110[b]	Noyes et al 1983	
70 Toronto 21	G→T	20414	Arg145→Leu	7	60	Giannelli et al 1992a	
71 Brest	C→G	20518	Arg180→Gly[c]	<1	85	Giannelli et al 1992a	
72 Deventer	C→T	20518	Arg180→Trp[c]	<1	130	Bertina et al 1990	
73 Hilo	G→A	20519	Arg180→Gln[c]	<1	120	Huang et al 1989	
74 Creston	G→C	20519	Arg180→Pro	<2		Giannelli et al 1992a	
75 Milano	G→T	20521	Val181→Phe[c]	<1	130	Bertina et al 1990	
76 Cardiff 2	G→C	20524	Val182→Leu[c]	15	132	Taylor et al 1990	
77 Kashihara	G→T	20524	Val182→Phe[c]	1	120	Sakai et al 1989	
78 Tokyo	T→C	20525	Val182→Ala[c]	23	100	Giannelli et al 1992a	
79 UK 54	3 bp del	20527–9	Gly183 del	<1	97	Giannelli et al 1992a	
80 Bottrop	3 bp del	20531–3	Gly184 del	<1	92	Giannelli et al 1992a	
81 Unnamed	C→A	20551	Gln191→Lys	<1	<1	Chen et al 1991	
82 Seattle K	T→C	20560	Trp194→Arg	4	4	Thompson et al 1992	
83 Unnamed	A→G	20564	Gln195→Arg	<1	<1	Giannelli et al 1992a	
84 UK 192	T→G	30046	Leu198→Trp	2		Giannelli et al 1992a	
85 Toronto 19	G→C	30070	Cys206→Ser	<1	<1	Taylor et al 1990	
86 HB142	G→A	30070	Cys206→Tyr	<1		Bottema et al 1991b	
87 UK 43	G→A	30072	Gly207→Arg	<1		Giannelli et al 1992a	
88 UK 37	G→A	30076	Gly208→Asp	1		Giannelli et al 1992a	
89 Wultschkau	G→T	30084	Val211→Phe	7		Giannelli et al 1992a	
90 HB72	T→C	30096	Trp215→Arg	4	<1	Bottema et al 1990	
91 Malmö 39	T→C	30100	lle216→Thr	4	4	Green et al 1991b	
92 HB65	T→G	30101	lle216→Met	15	4	Bottema et al 1991a	
93 Toronto 5	C→T	30112	Ala220→Val	<1	3	Koeberl et al 1990a	
94 UK 93	T→A	30117	Cys222→Ser	2		Giannelli et al 1992a	
95 HB24	T→G	30119	Cys222→Trp	1		Koeberl et al 1989	
96 HB1	G→A	30150	Ala233→Thr	12	13[b]	Koeberl et al 1989	
97 Spijkenisse	G→A	30854	Glu245→Lys	2	74	Giannelli et al 1992a	
98 Monschau	A→T	30855	Glu245→Val	3	39	Ludwig et al 1992b	
99 Seattle 4	G→A	30864	Arg248→Gln	3	4	Chen et al 1989	
100 UK 16	G→T	30876	Arg252→Leu	13		Giannelli et al 1992a	
101 HB131	A→G	30897	Tyr259→Cys	<1	<1	Bottema et al 1991b	
102 HB8	A→G	30900	Asn260→Ser	24		Koeberl et al 1989	
103 UK 88	A→G	30924	His268→Arg	7		Giannelli et al 1992a	
104 Malmö 50	A→T	30927	Asp269→Val	<1		Giannelli et al 1992a	
105 UK 15	A→T	30929	lle270→Phe	2	2	Giannelli et al 1992a	
106 Beuren	T→C	30930	lle270→Thr	<1	<1	Giannelli et al 1992a	
107 Toronto 1	C→T	30933	Ala271→Val	1	4	Koeberl et al 1990a	
108 HB143	T→G	30936	Leu272→Arg	<1	2	Bottema et al 1991b	
109 San Antonio	T→C	30945	Leu275→Pro	<1	14	Giannelli et al 1992a	
110 Zoeterwoude	T→A	30956	Leu279→lle	13	13	Giannelli et al 1992a	
111 Unnamed	C→T	30981	Pro287→Leu	<1	<1	Chen et al 1991	
112 HB109	T→G	30985	lle288→Met	<1	<1	Bottema et al 1991a	
113 Oxford h2	G→C	30992	Ala291→Pro	2	3	Winship & Dragon 1991	
114 UK 13	G→A	30992	Ala291→Thr	4–16	13[b]	Montandon et al 1989	
115 HB19	C→T	31008	Thr296→Met	5[b]	9[b]	Koeberl et al 1989	
116 Malmö 18	G→A	31035	Gly305→Asp	<1	<1	Green et al 1991b	
117 Malmö 26	T→G	31041	Val307→Gly	3	4	Green et al 1991b	
118 HB27	T→C	31041	Val307→Ala	18	46	Koeberl et al 1990a	
119 UK 122	G→A	31044	Ser308→Asn	5		Giannelli et al 1992a	
120 Emsdetten	T→G	31045	Ser308→Arg	<1		Giannelli et al 1992a	

Table 36.8 *Cont'd*

	Mutation name	Nucleotide change	Nucleotide position	Amino acid change	FIX:C	FIX:Ag	Reference	Comment
121	Oxford h3	G→A	31046	Gly309→Ser	<1	65	Winship & Dragon 1991	
122	Unnamed	G→T	31047	Gly309→Val	<1	58	Giannelli et al 1992a	
123	Toronto 21	T→C	31049	Trp310→Arg	<1	86	Giannelli et al 1992a	
124	HB139	G→A	31052	Gly311→Arg	2	100	Bottema et al 1991b	
125	Amagasaki	G→A	31053	Gly311→Glu[c]	<1	100	Miyata et al 1991	
126	UK 137	T→G	31059	Val313→Gly	<1	100	Giannelli et al 1992a	
127	Goldbach	G→C	31070	Gly317→Arg	<1		Giannelli et al 1992a	
128	Toronto 7	C→A	31080	Ala320→Asp	<1	90	Koeberl et al 1990a	
129	Oxford h5	G→T	31103	Val328→Phe	4	4	Winship 1990	
130	UK 90	T→C	31110	Leu330→Pro	7		Giannelli et al 1992a	
131	Ratingen 2	3 bp del	31110–2	Val331→del	<1	<1	Giannelli et al 1992a	
132	Oxford h1	T→C	31113	Val331→Ala	7	96	Winship & Dragon 1991	
133	Brünov	G→T	31115	Asp332→Tyr	4		Giannelli et al 1992a	
134	HB153/83	C→G	31118	Arg333→Gly	1 (13)	63 (70)	Bottema et al 1990	
135	HB110	G→T	31119	Arg333→Leu	1	150	Bottema et al 1991a	
136	UK 2	G→A	31119	Arg333→Gln	<1	135[b]	Tsang et al 1988	
137	Hong Kong 6	C→A	31122	Ala334→Asp	9	100	Chan et al 1991	
138	UK 8	T→C	31127	Cys336→Arg	2	2	Green et al 1989	
139	Malmö 24	G→A	31128	Cys336→Tyr	<1	<1	Green et al 1991b	
140	Calgary 3	C→A	31130	Leu337→lle	4	120	Fraser et al 1992	
141	Gladbeck	A→T	31151	lle344→Phe	4	87	Giannelli et al 1992a	
142	UK 135	3 bp del	31157–9 or 31160–2	Asn346→del or Asn347→del			Giannelli et al 1992a	
143	HB108	A→T	31161	Asn347→lle	<1	2	Bottema et al 1991a	
144	Unnamed	A→G	31163	Met348→Val	3	103	Chen et al 1991	
145	HB124	G→A	31165	Met348→lle	<1	40	Bottema et al 1991a	
146	Kingston 4	G→C	31170	Cys350→Ser	35	45	Taylor et al 1991	Somatic mosaic
147	UK 17	G→A	31170	Cys350→Tyr	<1	<1	Giannelli et al 1992a	
148	Unnamed	C→T	31200	Ser360→Leu	2	130	Chen et al 1991	
149	Los Angeles	G→A	31208	Gly363→Arg	<1	110	Giannelli et al 1992a	
150	Eagle Rock	G→T	31209	Gly363→Val	1–5	100	Bajaj et al 1990	
151	UK 35	G→A	31209	Gly363→Glu	2	53	Giannelli et al 1992a	
152	Seattle S	G→C	31209	Gly363→Ala	3	100	Thompson et al 1992	
153	HB80	G→C	31211	Asp364→His	2	95	Bottema et al 1990	
154	UK 30	G→A	31211	Asp364→Asn[c]	2		Giannelli et al 1992a	
155	Unnamed	A→T	31212	Asp364→Val	<1	130	Chen et al 1991	
156	Varel	TA→CG	31213–4	Ser365→Gly	<1	89	Ludwig et al 1992b	Inhibitor?
157	Schmallenberg	G→T	31215	Ser365→lle	<1		Ludwig et al 1992b	
158	Toronto 4	T→A	31216	Ser365→Arg	1	90	Koeberl et al 1990a	
159	HB87	G→A	31218	Gly366→Glu	<1	32	Bottema et al 1991a	
160	Unnamed	G→A	31220	Gly367→Arg	<1	14	Chen et al 1991	
161	Bergamo	C→A	31223	Pro368→Thr[c]	<1	156	Bertina et al 1990	
162	UK 190	C→T	31224	Pro368→Leu	3		Giannelli et al 1992a	
163	HB73	A→G	31227	His369→Arg	<1	<1	Bottema et al 1990	
164	Malmö 16	C→A	31248	Thr376→Asn	15	13	Green et al 1991b	
165	Unnamed	T→C	31253	Phe378→Leu	<1	<1	Chen et al 1991	
166	Brantford	A→C	31258	Leu379→Phe	5		Giannelli et al 1992a	
167	Barcelos	A→C	31259	Thr380→Pro	<1		Giannelli et al 1992a	
168	Hong Kong 5	C→G	31260	Thr380→Ser	7	<10	Chan et al 1991	
169	UK 76	C→T	31260	Thr380→lle	<1	1	Giannelli et al 1992a	
170	HB86	A→G	31281	Glu387→Gly	2	95	Bottema et al 1991a	
171	UK 42	G→A	31287	Cys389→Tyr	4	7	Giannelli et al 1992a	
172	Unnamed	C→A	31290	Ala390→Glu	2	30	Wang et al 1990a	
173	Niigata	C→T	31290	Ala390→Val[c]	2	140	Sugimoto et al 1988	
174	Angers	G→A	31307	Gly396→Arg[c]	<1	90	Attree et al 1989	
175	Long Beach	T→C	31311	lle397→Thr[c]	3	62	Ware et al 1988	
176	HB43	C→T	31326	Ser402→Phe	8		Koeberl et al 1990a	
177	Unnamed	T→C	31331	Tyr404→His	4		Giannelli et al 1992a	
178	Seattle T	G→T	31334	Val405→Phe	23	26	Thompson et al 1992	
179	HB92	T→C	31340	Trp407→Arg	<1	2	Bottema et al 1991a	
180	HB66	C→A	31356	Thr412→Lys			Bottema et al 1991a	

[a] Repeats of any mutation are not shown, but are listed in Giannelli et al 1992a.
Nucleotide and amino acid position both numbered as in Yoshitake et al 1985. Factor IX coagulant (FIX:C) and antigen (FIX:Ag) levels are expressed in international units/dl and units/dl respectively.
[b] FIX:Ag levels representing an average over several individuals with the same mutation rather than the value of the first reported case (see Giannelli et al 1992a for individual values).
[c] Substitutions found in patients with the Bm phenotype.

Table 36.9 Factor IX: neutral or probably neutral amino acid substitutions

Mutation name	Nucleotide change	Nucleotide position	Amino acid change	Reference
1 Riegelsberg	G→A	37	Arg-44→His	Ludwig et al 1992a
2 Calgary 4	A→T	48	lle-40→Phe	Giannelli et al 1992a
3 Brest	T→C	20512	Phe178→Leu	Giannelli et al 1992a
4 Malmö 7	C→T	30890	His257→Tyr	Montandon et al 1990
5 Ursem	G→A	31103	Val328→lle	Poort et al 1990

Association with different clinical phenotypes

Single amino acid substitutions or deletions may cause:

1. Similar decreases in factor IX activity and concentration in blood (Class III)
2. Greater decrease in activity than concentration (Class II)
3. Only a reduction in activity (Class I).

The first mutations presumably affect the stability, secretion and, possibly, synthesis of the protein; the second affect the function of factor IX but to some extent also impair its stability, secretion and possibly synthesis; the third purely affect factor IX function. Interestingly the first group comprises all the substitutions of cysteine participating in disulphide bridges except Cys^{18} and Cys^{23} (Table 36.8: 15, 16, 18, 19) that form a disulphide bridge in the Gla region where information on prothrombin (Soriano-Garcia et al 1992) suggests that Ca^{2+} co-ordination may play a major role in folding and maintenance of tridimensional structure. Of particular interest also is the substitution lle^{-30} → Asn (Table 36.8: 1), because inactivation of the prepeptide should result in defective secretion of factor IX. A charged residue at the amino end and a hydrophobic core are the only conserved features of prepeptides. The lle^{-30} → Asn substitution produces a significant interruption of the hydrophobic core of the factor IX prepeptide because Asn with the flanking Thr^{-31} and Cys^{-29} creates a block of hydrophilic residues. Such a mutation is the only change found in the essential regions of the factor IX gene of a severely affected patient (2% FIX:C; <1% FIXAg), and offers the clearest confirmation so far of the functional importance of the hydrophobic core of the prepeptide (Green et al 1992a).

In the second group of mutations the deletion of Arg^{37} illustrates how information on the three-dimensional structure of a factor IX homologue (prothrombin) may help in understanding the functional consequences of factor IX mutation (Green et al 1989). The crystal structure of prothrombin indicates the Arg37 should be part of an amphipathic α helix. A wheel plot diagram shows that the deletion of Arg^{37} destroys the amphipathic nature of the α helix (Fig. 36.3). This is consistent with marked effects on the stability of factor IX and also with some functional impairment as suggested by the patient's haematologic data (Table 36.8: 25). Mutations that only impair factor IX function should involve residues of marked functional significance, and in fact these include substitutions at activation cleavage sites and at residues essential to catalytic function such as Asp^{269} and Ser^{365}. Some of these mutations however affect residues with less well known functional importance. Interesting among these is Arg^{333}. Tsang et al (1988) noted that this residue is part of a strong electrostatic feature conserved among some serine proteases of blood coagulation and recent work on factor VII suggests that this region in the factor IX homologue may be

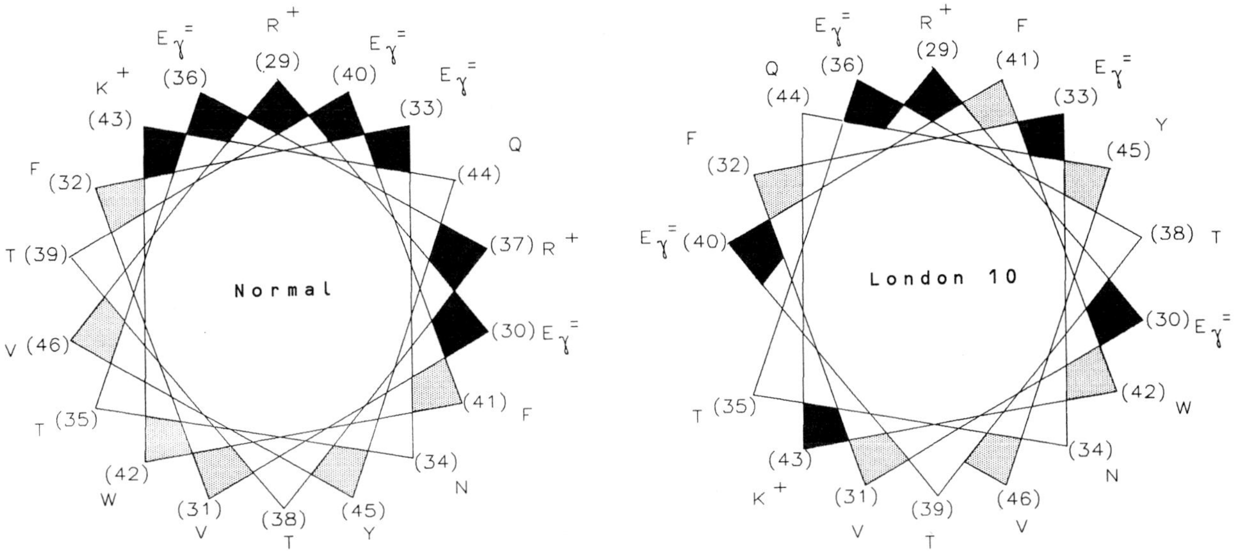

Fig. 36.3 Wheel plot of amino acid residues forming an α helix in the gla region of factor IX in normal (left) and patient with deletion of Arg37. Black, grey and white represent respectively charged, hydrophobic and neutral residues.

important for its interaction with tissue factor (O'Brien et al 1991). It is thus conceivable that, by analogy, Arg^{333} may be important to the interaction of factors VIII and IX. A number of mutations in this class show a moderately prolonged bovine prothrombin time. This phenotypic feature, usually referred to as Bm is not systematically tested, but it is interesting that cases reported so far have involved residues 180, 181, 182, 311, 364, 368, 390, 396 and 397 (Giannelli et al 1992a). It has been suggested that the distribution of mutations causing a Bm phenotype may reflect rather specific structural defects (Bertina et al 1990).

Distribution of mutations among different protein domains

Single amino acid changes have been observed at similar density in all domains of factor IX except in the signal and activation peptide domains which show fewer changes. This suggests that all domains of factor IX except the last two are similarly and fairly highly constrained.

So far only two detrimental amino acid substitutions have been found in the prepeptide: the $Ile^{-30} \rightarrow$ Asn mentioned above and $Cys^{-19} \rightarrow$ Arg (Bottema et al 1991b). The latter affects the cleavage site between the pre- and propeptide (Cys^{-19}/Thr^{-18}).

Five missense mutation have been reported in the propeptide besides one that may affect mRNA splicing. The former are in a region of the propeptide important for its cleavage from the mature protein (Table 36.8: 4–8). Conservation among homologues and site-directed mutagenesis indicate that the amino end of the propeptide contains residues important for the gamma carboxylation of glutamates in the Gla region (e.g. Phe^{-16}, Ala^{-10} and Leu^{-6}) (Jorgensen et al 1987, Handford et al 1991b) but mutations of such residues have not yet been detected in haemophilia B patients.

Nineteen substitutions and the Arg^{37} deletion mentioned above have been detected in the Gla region (Table 36.8: 9–28). Seven of these affect Gla residues and four Cys^{18} plus Cys^{23}. Interestingly, all the mutations at Gla residues result in significant reduction of FIXAg, thus indirectly confirming the importance of the Ca^{2+} binding sites formed by these residues and Ca^{2+} in the achievement and maintenance of normal FIX structure.

The first EGF domain shows 21 amino acid substitutions besides one ($Asp^{47} \rightarrow$ Asn) that could be accompanied by RNA missplicing (Table 36.8: 29–50). Five such mutations affect the N-terminal consensus: Asp^{47}GlyAsp GlnCys^{51} (Przyziecki et al 1987; Rees et al 1988), and two affect Asp^{64} which contributes to the high affinity Ca^{2+} binding site at the amino end of this domain (Handford et al 1991a). Furthermore, the 11 substitutions at Pro^{55}, Cys^{56}, Gly^{59} and Gly^{60} underline the importance of these residues in the tridimensional structure of this domain (Baron et al 1992).

Only 13 substitutions have been found in the second EGF domain in addition to one that may be accompanied by RNA missplicing (Table 36.8: 51–64). Five of these substitutions affect cysteines involved in the three disulphide bridges characteristic of the EGF domains.

The activation peptide region has shown 17 substitutions and two single amino acid deletions (Table 36.8: 65–83). Such substitutions are concentrated at: the cysteine that contributes to the disulphide bridge holding together the light and heavy chains of factor IXa (Cys^{132}), the cleavage sites of the activation peptide (Arg^{145}, Arg^{180}, Val^{181}) and the amino end of the heavy chain of factor IXa (Val^{181}–Gly^{184}). Since Val^{181} is thought to interact with Asp^{364} in the active centre of the serine protease domain (Titani & Fujikawa 1982) it is reasonable to assume that residues at the amino end of the heavy chain are important to the structure and activity of such a site.

The segment of the catalytic region encoded by exon g has shown 13 substitutions (Table 36.8: 84–96) and 11 of these affect two cysteines forming a disulphide bridge (Cys^{206}, Cys^{222}) and the amino acids intervening between them. The remainder of the catalytic region, which is coded by exon h, has shown 82 amino acid substitutions and two single amino acid deletions (Table 36.8: 97–180). A cluster of six substitutions (His^{268}–Leu^{272}) is found in the residues surrounding Asp^{269}, one of the cardinal residues of the active site. 11 substitutions are found in the peptide delimited by Gly^{305} and Val^{313}. 17 substitutions and two single amino acid deletions are clustered in the peptide Val^{328} – Cys^{350}, and indicate that the region immediately preceding and comprising the peptide loop, delimited by the cysteines Cys^{336} and Cys^{350} which form a disulphide bridge, is of structural and functional importance. 15 substitutions occur in the region Gly^{363} – His^{369} which include the cardinal Ser^{365}, thus confirming the importance of this region in the catalytic site of factor IX. 17 substitutions have been detected in the remainder of the catalytic region (Val^{370} – Thr^{415}).

Conservation of mutated residues

Alignment of the amino acid sequence of factor IX, VII, X and protein C according to the method of Higgins & Sharp (1988) shows that 107 of the factor IX residues are absolutely conserved, 73 show only one or two conservative substitutions and 45 only one non-conservative substitution, while the remaining 229 residues are less conserved. Haemophilia B mutations affect unequally the above four groups of residues since of the 174 substitutions claimed to be the cause of the disease, 90 affect the first, 38 the second, 15 the third and 29 the fourth, so that the frequency of substitutions per residue in the four groups is: 0.84, 0.52. 0.33 and 0.13 respectively. Furthermore of the 44 substitutions affecting residues poorly conserved among the factor IX homologues, 41 are at amino acids conserved in the factor IX of the mammalian species examined so far.

Different substitutions at the same residue (Table 36.10)

39 factor IX residues have shown more than one substitution. This clearly demonstrates the importance of the individual wild type residues and offers the opportunity to compare the phenotypic consequence of different substitutions of the same amino acid. For mutations at some sites the severity of the disease correlates with the degree of chemical discrepancy between the wild type residue and each of its substituents (Table 36.10: Group A), while at other sites, any substituent produces similar detrimental effects as if the loss of the wild type residue rather than the nature of the mutant ones dominated the pheno-

Table 36.10 Haemophilia B: comparison of phenotypes in patients with different substitutions of the same amino acid

Mutation	Severity	Haematological class
Group A		
Gla27→Lys	Severe	II
Gla27→Val	Severe	III
Gly59→Ser	Mild	?
Gly59→Val	Severe	?
Gly60→Ser	Mild	II
Gly60→Asp	Severe	III
Gly60→Arg	Severe	III
Arg145→Cys	Severe	II
Arg145→His	Moderate	I
Arg145→Leu	Moderate	I/II
Val182→Leu	Mild	I
Val182→Phe	Severe	I
Val182→Ala	Mild	I
Ile216→Thr	Moderate	III
Ile216→Met	Mild	III
Glu245→Lys	Severe	I
Glu245→Val	Severe	II
Ala291→Pro	Severe	III
Ala291→Thr	Moderate	III
Val307→Ala	Mild	II
Val307→Gly	Severe	III
Ser308→Asn	Moderate	?
Ser308→Arg	Severe	?
Val328→Phe	Severe/moderate	III
Val328→Ile	Normal	Normal
Val331→del	Severe	III
Val331→Ala	Moderate	I
Thr380→Ser	Moderate	III
Thr380→Ile	Severe	III
Thr380→Pro	Severe	?
Ala390→Val	Severe	I
Ala390→Glu	Severe	II
Group B		
Arg-4→Trp	Severe	II
Arg-4→Leu	Severe	II
Arg-4→Gln	Severe	I/II
Cys18→Arg	Severe	I
Cys18→Tyr	Severe	?
Cys23→Arg	Severe	II
Cys23→Tyr	Severe	II
Gly48→Arg	Mild	I
Gly48→Val	Mild	I
Pro55→Ala	Mild	II
Pro55→Ser	Mild	II
Pro55→Leu	Mild	?
Cys56→Arg	Severe	III
Cys56→Ser	Severe	III
Cys56→Tyr	Severe	III
Asp64→Asn	Severe/moderate	I
Asp64→Gly	Moderate	I
Cys132→Arg	Severe	III
Cys132→Phe	Severe	III
Cys132→Tyr	Severe	?
Arg180→Trp	Severe	I
Arg180→Gly	Severe	I
Arg180→Gln	Severe	I
Arg180→Pro	Severe	?
Cys206→Ser	Severe	III
Cys206→Tyr	Severe	?
Cys222→Trp	Severe	?
Cys222→Ser	Severe	?
Ile270→Phe	Severe	III
Ile270→Thr	Severe	III
Gly309→Ser	Severe	I/II
Gly309→Val	Severe	I/II
Cys336→Arg	Severe	III
Cys336→Tyr	Severe	III
Gly363→Val	Severe	I
Gly363→Glu	Severe	I/II
Gly363→Arg	Severe	I
Gly363→Ala	Severe	I
Asp364→His	Severe	I
Asp364→Asn	Severe	?
Asp364→Val	Severe	I
Ser365→Gly	Severe	I
Ser365→Ile	Severe	?
Ser365→Arg	Severe	I
Group C		
Thr38→Arg	Severe	?
Thr38→Ile	Moderate	?
Asp47→Asn	Severe	III (may affect splicing)
Asp47→Gly	Mild	I
Asp47→Glu	Severe (1)	I
	Mild (1)	I
Asn92→HIs	Severe	III
Asn92→Lys	Severe	?
Cys95→Tyr	Severe	III
Cys95→Trp	Severe	?
Gly311→Arg	Severe	I
Gly311→Glu	Severe	I
Arg333→Gly	Mild (1)	I
	Severe (1)	I
Arg333→Gln	Severe	I
Arg333→Leu	Severe	I
Met348→Ile	Severe	I
Met348→Val	Severe	II
Cys350→Ser	?	? (somatic mosaic)
Cys350→Tyr	Severe	III
Pro368→Thr	Severe	I
Pro368→Leu	Severe/moderate	?

Disease is defined as severe (<3% FIX:C), moderate (3–10% FIX:C) and mild (11–30% FIX:C). Haematological class is defined in text: the seriousness of the effects of mutations increases in the order mild → severe and haematological class I → III. Group A have effects that correlate with the difference in the substituents; group B have the same phenotype regardless of the substituent amino acid; in group C there are either insufficient data or other factors are expected to affect the phenotype as specified in brackets.
Data from Giannelli et al 1992a.

typic effect (Table 36.10: Group B). 14 residues fall in the first category and 17 in the second, while at the nine remaining either the observed substituents are chemically similar or the patients' haematologic data are incomplete (Table 36.10: Group C). Appropriately the group of residues in the second category include Arg^{-4} and Arg^{180} which are part of essential cleavage sites, Cys^{18}, Cys^{23}, Cys^{56}, Cys^{132}, Cys^{206}, Cys^{222} and Cys^{336} that are involved in disulphide bridges, Asp^{64} of the Ca^{2+} binding site of the first EGF domain, and Asp^{364} and Ser^{365} that are key residues of the active centre. Interesting also is the apparent specific requirement for Gly^{48} and Pro^{55} of the first EGF domain and Ile^{270} and Gly^{309} in the catalytic domain.

Neutral mutations and the functional intepretation of sequence changes

In the sample of 574 patients studied so far, 14 trivial sequence changes were observed: three of these caused amino acid substitutions in the circulating factor IX and two in a region of the prepeptide that may exist if translation starts at Met^{-46} rather than Met^{-39}, while the remainder were silent changes (Giannelli et al 1992a). The above figures probably represent an underestimate of the true frequency of trivial sequence changes within the essential regions of the factor IX gene (promoter, exons and RNA processing signals) because probably not all essential regions of the gene were examined in all patients listed so far and some under-reporting of trivial changes may be expected. Probably, therefore, not less than 3% of the factor IX gene has trivial changes in the 'essential' regions. Some of these neutral mutations may be mistaken for detrimental changes in patients where the true cause of the disease is not detected. This is unlikely if all the essential regions of the factor IX gene are examined by a fully effective procedure, since at Guy's Hospital, UK, only one of the 170 patients analysed has not shown a mutation in the essential regions of the gene. However, it is imprudent and scientifically unsatisfactory to examine only some of the essential sequences or to use a detection procedure that does not closely approach 100% efficiency.

The detrimental nature of many mutations is immediately obvious: for example stop codons, frameshifts and several amino acid substitutions at residues that are known to be essential to the structure and function of factor IX. Information on the last point is growing steadily and in a few years a full spectrum of the amino acid substitutions capable of producing haemophilia B will be available. Meanwhile some positive information will also be obtained on substitutions that are phenotypically neutral, for example $His^{257} \rightarrow Tyr$ (Montandon et al 1990). The mutations most difficult to interpret, in the absence of mRNA analysis, are those that alter the weak consensus sequences at splice sites or create new potential splice signals. The detrimental nature of these mutations, or any other change of uncertain functional importance, may be suggested by the absence of other abnormalities in the essential region of the factor IX gene, evidence that the mutation is of recent origin, or independent occurrence of the same mutation two or more times. The last may be demonstrated for example by the presence of the mutation in factor IX genes with different combinations (haplotypes) of RFLP markers (Green et al 1992b).

Recurrence of the same mutation

A number of mutations have been observed to occur independently in several families. These are usually CpG to TpG transitions due presumably to the deamination of methylated cytosines to thymidine. A detailed analysis of these mutations has suggested a rate of 1.05×10^{-7} $^{me}C \rightarrow T$ transitions per base per gamete per generation (Green et al 1990).

Repeated mutations provide some information on the degree of concordance between the phenotypic characteristics of patients with the same mutation. Data collected so far from laboratories in many parts of the world show, in spite of their heterogeneous origin, a good deal of uniformity and suggest that most mutations are associated with a specific phenotype. This in turn indicates that information on the factor IX mutation is of prognostic value in haemophilia B.

Type of mutation and risk of the inhibitor complication

Inhibitor patients show a restricted spectrum of mutations. Our analysis of an unbiased sample of the Swedish population indicates that, while the overall risk of the inhibitor complication is 3%, patients with gross deletions or mutations causing gross functional loss of coding information (i.e. stop codons and frameshifts) have a 20% risk while, by contrast, patients with other mutations have a risk close to zero (Green et al 1991b; unpublished observations).

A STRATEGY TO OVERCOME THE GENETIC COUNSELLING DIFFICULTIES RESULTING FROM HIGH MUTATIONAL HETEROGENEITY IN HAEMOPHILIA B

The mutational heterogeneity of haemophilia B prevents the use of mutation-specific probes for direct DNA-based carrier and prenatal diagnosis. Indirect diagnoses based on the familial segregation, within haemophilia B families, of factor IX-specific polymorphic DNA markers have several flaws. They fail in approximately 40% of families due to lack of either informative markers, family history or key live family members; are expensive because each one requires the analysis of a complete family group and often paternity testing; their accuracy is limited by the universality of the markers and hence the low chance of detecting sample identification errors and also by the possibility of recombination between the marker and the site of mutation; finally they do not provide information on the root cause of the disease and cannot contribute to progress in the understanding and treatment of the disease. For these reasons diagnoses based on the direct detection of the gene defect were advocated (Giannelli 1987).

In fact haemophilia B is a convenient model for the development of new strategies for the provision of genetic counselling in diseases of high mutational heterogeneity (e.g. haemophilia A, Duchenne muscular dystrophy and many others) because:

1. The frequency of the disease is high enough to make it clinically relevant but not so high as to slow progress excessively
2. The gene is of reasonable size and complexity
3. Factor IX consists of a number of domains, shared by large families of proteins
4. Three close homologues of the factor IX gene, factor VII, X and protein C, also exist (O'Hara et al 1987).

Features 3 and 4 allow identification of important residues that have been conserved in evolution, thus helping the functional interpretation of the haemophilia B mutations. They also allow inferences on the structure of factor IX based on the three-dimensional information available on homologous proteins. Conversely the existence of homologues increases the value of any information obtained on factor IX as this is relevant to other genes (e.g. factor VII, X and protein C) that are not equally endowed with easily detectable natural mutants.

The procedure used in one of our laboratories (Giannelli) to characterize haemophilia B mutations allows the analysis of all essential regions of the factor IX gene (promoter, exons and RNA processing signals) in 4–5 person working days. It is therefore possible to make carrier and prenatal diagnoses by the direct detection of the gene defect virtually in every case (Green et al 1991b). This abolishes the need for cumbersome family studies and paternity testing, increases the expected diagnostic success from 60% to virtually 100%, and reveals the root cause of the disease. Furthermore, once the haemophilia B mutation of an individual has been identified, carrier and prenatal diagnoses for the genetic counselling of his blood-relatives can be done for generation after generation by examining only the region that is affected in the index individual. This reduces by at least ten-fold the cost of such diagnoses and cuts the waiting time for a result down to 2 days.

In order to maximize such benefits, it was proposed to characterize the mutation of an index patient from each haemophilia B family in the UK and to construct a national haemophilia B register containing mutational, haematologic and pedigree information (see Giannelli et al 1992b for more details). In formulating such a proposal it was reasoned that the preliminary systematic characterization of mutations in index patients would very rapidly advance our understanding of the molecular biology of the disease, and also ensure a sound theoretical basis for the provision of diagnostic services. Furthermore the analysis of a large number of patients verifies the efficiency and reliability of the technical procedures; it yields data that help assess the functional consequences of any observed sequence change and reveals correlations between mutations and phenotypes that offer prognostic information valuable to genetic counselling. Diagnoses based on direct detection of gene defects are not dependent on the functional interpretation of the observed changes but such interpretations are needed when examining collateral or ascendant relatives of isolated ('sporadic') patients. It was also believed that the construction of a national database is the best way to inform even the most remote clinical centre of the new opportunities for diagnosis and genetic counselling, and to offer such centres access to state-of-the-art technology. Finally we were aware that the individuality of the mutations of different families ensures the automatic self-verification of the mutations in the register because whenever the abnormality identified in the index patient is found in one of his relatives the data in the register are confirmed.

Application of the above strategy to a pilot sample (the patients registered with the Malmö haemophilia centre) (Green et al 1991b) and then to the UK population, has so far led to the characterization of 170 haemophilia B mutations and to the provision of carrier and prenatal diagnoses to several families that could not have been helped by the indirect RFLP-based method (Green et al 1991b, 1992 Giannelli et al 1992b).

SUMMARY

Rapid methods for the detection of factor VIII and factor IX mutations have confirmed the expected high degree of mutational heterogeneity. The mutations identified affect the expression of factors VIII or IX or impair the maturation and translation of the mRNA or cause amino acid substitutions important to the structure and function of the corresponding proteins. A number of features important to the expression and function of factor VIII and factor IX have thus been delineated and fairly soon the spectrum of amino acid substitutions causing haemophilia B will be fully defined. Fairly precise genotype/phenotype correlations are emerging that provide useful prognostic information for the genetic counselling of haemophilia A and B patients. The establishment of national registers of mutational and pedigree data will allow accurate, rapid and economical carrier and prenatal diagnoses in every family with haemophilia B and will optimize genetic counselling. Once the model strategy prepared for haemophilia B is fully validated it may be possible to extend it to haemophilia A and other diseases of high mutational heterogeneity. The high proportion of undetected mutations in severe haemophilia A may however limit the mutation-specific approach to diagnosis. Meanwhile an impressive catalogue of mutations will continue to accumulate for the two sex-linked haemophilias with great benefit to genetic counselling services and to our understanding of underlying mechanisms of mutation, the structure and function of two clinically important proteins, and the phenotypic expression of diverse genotypes.

REFERENCES

Abrams, E S, Murdaugh S E, Lerman L S 1990 Comprehensive detection of single base changes in human genomic DNA using denaturing gradient gel electrophoresis and a GC clamp. Genomics 7: 463–475

Alkan M, Rodriguez Ponte M, Malik N J et al 1991 Factor IX Basel: a Swiss family with severe haemophilia B having a point mutation in EGF type B domain. Nucleic Acids Research 19: 409

Ananthakrishnan R, D'Souza S 1979 Some aspects of the occurrence of new mutations in haemophilia. Human Heredity 29: 90–94

Anson D S, Choo K H, Rees D J G et al 1984 The gene structure of human anti-haemophilic factor IX. European Molecular Biology Organization Journal 3: 1053–1060

Anson D S, Blake D J, Winship P R, Birnbaum D, Brownlee G G 1988 Nullisomic deletion of the mcf2 transforming gene in two haemophilia B patients. European Molecular Biology Organization Journal 7: 2795–2799

Antonarakis S E et al 1992 Unpublished data

Antonarakis S E, Waber P G, Kittur S D et al 1985 Hemophilia A: Detection of molecular defects and of carriers by DNA analysis. New England Journal of Medicine 313: 842–848

Arai M, Inaba H, Higuchi M et al 1989 Direct characterization of factor VIII in plasma: Detection of a mutation altering a thrombin cleavage site (arginine 372 histidine). Proceedings of the National Academy of Science, USA 86: 4277–4281

Arai M, Higuchi M, Antonarakis S E et al 1990 Characterization of a thrombin cleavage site mutation (Arg1689 to Cys) in the factor VIII gene of two unrelated patients with cross-reacting material-positive hemophilia A. Blood 75: 384–389

Attree O, Vidaud D, Vidaud M et al 1989 Mutations in the catalytic domain of human coagulation factor IX: rapid characterization by direct genomic sequencing of DNA fragments displaying an altered melting behaviour. Genomics 4: 266–272

Bajaj S P, Spitzer S G, Welsh W J et al 1990 Experimental and theoretical evidence supporting the role of Gly 363 in blood coagulation factor IXa (Gly 193 in Chymotrypsin) for proper activation of the proenzyme. Journal of Biological Chemistry 265: 2956–2961

Bardoni B, Sampietro M, Romano M et al 1988 Characterization of a partial deletion of the factor VIII gene in a haemophiliac with inhibitor. Human Genetics 79: 86–88

Baron M, Norman D G, Harvey T S et al 1992 The 3-dimensional structure of the first EGF-like module of human factor IX – comparison with EGF and TGF-α. Protein Science 1: 81–90

Barrai I, Cann H M, Cavalli-Sforza L L, Barbujan G, De Nicola P 1985 Segregation analysis of hemophilia A and B. American Journal of Human Genetics 37: 680–699

Bentley A K, Rees D J G, Rizza C, Brownlee G G 1986 Defective propeptide processing of blood clotting factor IX caused by mutation of arginine to glutamine at position –4. Cell 45: 343–348

Bernardi F, Del Senno L, Barbieri R et al 1985 Gene deletion in an Italian haemophilia B subject. Journal of Medical Genetics 22: 305–307

Bernardi F, Marchetti G, Bertagnolo V et al 1987 RFLP analysis in families with sporadic hemophilia A; estimate of the mutation ratio in male and female gametes. Human Genetics 76: 253–256

Bernardi F, Legnani C, Volinia et al 1988 A Hind III RFLP and a gene lesion in the coagulation factor VIII gene. Human Genetics 78: 359–362

Bernardi F, Volinia S, Patracchini et al 1989 A recurrent missense mutation (Arg→Gln) and a partial deletion in factor VIII gene causing severe haemophilia A. British Journal of Haematology 71: 271–276

Bertina R M, van der Linden I K, Manucci P M et al 1990 Mutations in hemophilia B_m occur at the Arg180–Val activation site or in the catalytic domain of factor IX. Journal of Biological Chemistry 265: 10876–10883

Bottema C D K, Ketterling R P, Cho H I, Sommer S S 1989 Hemophilia B in a male with a four-base insertion that arose in the germline of his mother. Nucleic Acids Research 17: 10139

Bottema C D K, Ketterling R P, Yoon H S, Sommer S S 1990 The pattern of factor IX germ-line mutations in Asians is similar to that of Caucasians. American Journal of Human Genetics 47: 835–841

Bottema C D K, Ketterling R P, Li S et al 1991a Missense mutations and evolutionary conservation of amino acids: evidence that many of the amino acids in factor IX function as 'spacer' elements. American Journal of Human Genetics 49: 820–838

Bottema C D K, Bottema M J, Ketterling R P et al 1991b Why does the human factor IX gene have a G + C content of 40%? American Journal of Human Genetics 49: 839–850

Bray G L, Thompson A R 1986 Partial factor IX protein in a pedigree with hemophilia B due to a partial gene deletion. Journal of Clinical Investigation 77: 1194–1200

Bröcker-Vriends A H J T, Briët E, Dreesen J C F M et al 1987 The origin of the mutation in families with an isolated case of haemophilia A. Thrombosis and Haemostasis 58: 337

Bröcker-Vriends A H J T, Dreesen J C F M, Bakker B, Briët E 1988 Somatic mosaicism for a deletion in the clotting factor VIII gene Circulation (Suppl. 2) 78: 254

Bröcker-Vriends A H J T, Briët E, Dreesen J C F M 1990 Somatic origin of inherited haemophilia A. Human Genetics 85: 288–292

Bröcker-Vriends A H J T, Rosendaal F R, van Hauwelingen J C et al 1991 Sex ratio of the mutation frequencies in haemophilia A. Coagulation assays and RFLP analysis. Journal of Medical Genetics 28: 672–680

Camerino G, Bardoni B, Sampietro M et al 1986 Molecular basis of haemophilias. Ric. Clin. Lab. 16: 227

Casarino L, Pecorara M, Mori P G et al 1986a Molecular basis for hemophilia A in Italians. Ric. Clin. Lab. 16, 227

Casarino L, Sangiorgi S, Pecorara M et al 1986b Carrier detection of haemophilia B with factor IX DNA specific probe. Preliminary results. In: Ciavarella N L, Ruggeri Z M, Zimmerman T S (eds) Factor VIII/von Willebrand factors — biological and clinical advances. Wichtig Editore, Milan, p 201–205

Casula L, Murru S, Pecorara M et al 1990 Recurrent mutations and three novel rearrangements in the factor VIII gene of hemophilia A patients of Italian descent. Blood 75: 662–670

Chan V, Chan T K, Tong T M F, Todd D 1989 A novel missense mutation in exon 4 of the factor VIII: C gene resulting in moderately severe hemophilia A. Blood 74: 2688–2691

Chan V, Yip B, Tong T M F et al 1991 Molecular defects in haemophilia B: detection by direct restriction enzyme analysis. British Journal of Haematology 79: 63–69

Chen S-H, Scott C R 1990 Recombination between two 14 base pair homologous sequences is the mechanism for the gene deletion in factor IX Seattle 1. American Journal of Human Genetics 47: 1020–1022

Chen S-H, Scott C R, Edson J R, Kurachi K 1988 An insertion within the Factor IX gene: haemophilia B El Salvador. American Journal of Human Genetics 42: 581–584

Chen S H, Thompson A R, Zhang M, Scott C R 1989 Three point mutations in the factor IX genes of five haemophilia B patients. Journal of Clinical Investigation 84: 113–118
Chen S H, Zhang M, Lovrien E W, Scott C R, Thompson A R 1991 CG dinucleotide transitions in the factor IX gene account for about half of the point mutations in hemophilia B patients: a Seattle series. Human Genetics 87: 177–182
Cooper D N, Krawczak M 1990 The mutational spectrum of single base-pair substitutions causing human genetic disease: Patterns and predictions. Human Genetics 85: 55–74
Cooper D N, Krawczak M 1991 Mechanisms of insertional mutagenesis in human genes causing genetic disease. Human Genetics 87: 409–415
Cooper D N, Youssoufian 1988 The CpG dinucleotide and human genetic disease. Human Genetics 78: 151–155
Cotton R G H, Rodrigues N R, Campbell R D 1988 Reactivity of cytosine and thymine in single-base-pair mismatches with hydroxylamine and osmium tetroxide and its application to the study of mutations. Proceedings of the National Academy of Sciences, USA 85: 4397–4401
Crossley P M, Winship P R, Black A, Rizza C R, Brownlee G G 1989 An unusual case of haemophilia B. Lancet i: 960
Crossley M, Brownlee G G 1990 Disruption of a C/EBP binding site in the factor IX promoter is associated with Haemophilia B. Nature 345: 444–446
Crossley M, Winship P R, Austen D E G, Rizza C R, Brownlee G G 1990 A less severe form of haemophilia B Leyden. Nucleic Acids Research 18: 4633
Crossley M, Ludwig M, Stowell K M et al 1992 Recovery from haemophilia B Leyden. Androgen-responsive element in the factor IX promoter. Science 257: 377–379
Cutting G R, Antonarakis S E, Youssoufian H, Kazazian H H 1988 Accuracy and limitations of pulsed field gel electrophoresis in sizing partial deletions of the factor VIII gene. Molecular Biology and Medicine 5: 173–184
Davis L M, McGraw R A, Ware J L, Roberts H R, Stafford D W 1987 Factor IX Alabama: a point mutation in a clotting protein results in hemophilia B. Blood 69: 140–143
Delpech M, Deburgrave N, Baudis M et al 1986 De novo mutation in hemophilia A established by DNA haplotype analysis and precluding prenatal diagnosis. Human Genetics 74: 316–317
Denton P H, Fowlkes D M, Lord S T, Reisner H M 1988 Hemophilia B Durham: a mutation in the first EGF-like domain of factor IX characterized by PCR technology. Blood 72: 1407–1411
Din N, Schwartz M, Kruse T et al 1986 Factor VIII gene specific probes used to study heritage and molecular defects in hemophilia A. Ric. Clin. Lab. 16: 182
Diuguid D L, Rabiet M J, Furie B C, Liebman H A, Furie B 1986 Molecular basis of haemophilia B: a defective enzyme due to an unprocessed propeptide is caused by a point mutation in the factor IX precursor. Proceedings of the National Academy of Sciences, USA 83: 5803–5807
Ferrari N, Rizza C R 1986 Estimation of genetic risks of carriership for possible carriers of Christmas disease (haemophilia B). Brazilian Journal of Genetics 9: 87–99
Filippi G, Mannucci P M, Coppola R, Farris A, Rinaldi A, Siniscalco M 1984 Studies on hemophilia A in Sardinia bearing on the problems of multiple allelism, carrier detection and differential mutation rate in the two sexes. American Journal of Human Genetics 36: 44–71
Fischer S G, Lerman L S 1983 DNA fragments differing by single basepair substitutions are separated in denaturing gradient gels: correspondence with melting theory. Proceedings of the National Academy of Sciences, USA 80: 1579–1583
Francke U, Winter R M, Lin D et al 1981 Use of carrier detection tests to estimate male to female ratio of mutation rates in Lesch–Nyhan disease. In: Hook E B, Porter I H (eds) Population and biological aspects of human mutation. Academic Press, London, p 117–130
Fraser B M, Poon M C, Hoar D I 1992 Identification of factor IX mutations in haemophilia B: application of polymerase chain reaction and single strand conformation analysis. Human Genetics 88: 426–430
Freedenberg D L, Black B 1991 Altered developmental control of the factor IX gene: a new T to A mutation at position +6 of the FIX gene resulting in haemophilia B Leyden. Thrombosis and Haemostasis 65: 964
Giannelli F 1987 The identification of haemophilia B mutations. In: Peeters H (ed) Protides of the biological fluids, Pergamon Press, Oxford, vol 35: 29–32
Giannelli F, Choo K H, Rees D J G, Boyd Y, Rizza C R 1983 Gene deletions in patients with haemophilia B and anti factor IX antibodies. Nature 303: 181–182
Giannelli F, Green P M, High K A et al 1992a Haemophilia B: database of point mutations and short additions and deletions – third edition. Nucleic Acids Research 20 (suppl): 2027–2063
Giannelli F, Saad S, Montandon A J, Bentley D R, Green P M 1992b A new strategy for the genetic counselling of diseases of marked mutational heterogeneity: haemophilia B as a model. Journal of Medical Genetics 29: 602–607
Gispert S, Vidaud M, Vidaud D et al 1989 A promoter defect correlates with an abnormal coagulation factor IX gene expression in a French family (Haemophilia B Leyden). American Journal of Human Genetics 45: A189
Gitschier J 1988 Maternal duplication associated with gene deletion in sporadic hemophilia. American Journal of Human Genetics 43: 274–279
Gitschier J 1992 unpublished data
Gitschier J, Wood W I, Goralka T M et al 1984 Characterization of the human factor VIII gene. Nature 312: 326–330
Gitschier J, Wood W I, Tuddenham E G D et al 1985 Detection and sequence of mutations in the factor VIII gene of haemophiliacs. Nature 315: 427–430
Gitschier J, Wood W I, Shuman M A, Lawn R M 1986 Identification of a missense mutation in the factor VIII gene of a mild hemophiliac. Science 232: 1415–1416
Gitschier J, Kogan S, Levinson B, Tuddenham E G D 1988 Mutations of factor VIII cleavage sites in hemophilia A. Blood 72: 1022–1028
Gitschier J, Levinson B, Lehesjoki A -E, de la Chapelle A 1989 Mosaicism and sporadic haemophilia A: Implications for carrier determination. Lancet i: 273–274
Graham J B, Barrow E S, Roberts H R et al 1975 Dominant inheritance of hemophilia A in three generations of women. Blood 46: 175–188
Graham J B, Rizza C R, Chediak J et al 1986 Carrier detection in hemophilia A: A cooperative international study I. The carrier phenotype. Blood 67: 1554–1559
Green P M et al 1992 Unpublished data
Green P M, Bentley D R, Mibashan R S, Giannelli F 1988 Partial deletion by illegitimate recombination of the factor IX gene in a family with two inhibitor patients. Molecular Biology and Medicine 5: 95–106
Green P M, Bentley D R, Mibashan R S, Nilsson I M, Giannelli F 1989 Molecular pathology of haemophilia B. European Molecular Biology Organization Journal 8: 1067–1072
Green P M, Montandon A J, Bentley D R et al 1990 The incidence and distribution of CpG → TpG transitions in the coagulation factor IX gene. A fresh look at CpG mutational hotspots. Nucleic Acids Research 18: 3227–3231
Green P M, Montandon A J, Bentley D R, Giannelli F 1991a Genetics and molecular biology of haemophilia A and B. Blood Coagulation and Fibrinolysis 2: 539–565
Green P M, Montandon A J, Ljung R et al 1991b Haemophilia B mutations in a complete Swedish population sample. A test of new strategy for the genetic counselling of diseases with high mutational heterogeneity. British Journal of Haematology 78: 390–397
Green P M, Mitchell V E, McGraw A, Goldman E, Giannelli F 1992a Haemophilia B caused by a missense mutation in the prepeptide sequence of factor IX. Human Mutation (in press)
Green P M, Montandon A J, Ljung R, Nilsson I-M, Giannelli F 1992b Haplotype analysis of identical factor IX mutants using PCR. Thrombosis and Haemostasis 67: 66–69
Grover H, Phillips M A, Lillicrap D P et al 1987 Carrier detection of haemophilia A using DNA markers in families with an isolated affected male. Clinical Genetics 32: 10–19
Haldane J B S 1935 The rate of spontaneous mutation of a human gene. Journal of Genetics 31: 317–326

Haldane J B S 1947 The mutation of the gene for haemophilia and its segregation ratios in males and females. Annals of Eugenics 13: 262–271

Hamaguchi M, Matsushita T, Tanimoto M et al 1991 Three distinct point mutations in the factor IX gene of three Japanese CRM$^+$ hemophilia B patients (factor IX BM Nagoya 2, factor IX Nagoya 3 and 4). Thrombosis and Haemostasis 65: 514–520

Handford P A, Mayhew M, Baron M et al 1991a Key residues involved in calcium-binding motifs in EGF-like domains. Nature 351: 164–167

Handford P A, Winship P R, Brownlee G G 1991b Protein engineering of the propeptide of human factor IX. Protein Engineering 4: 319–323

Hassan H J, Leonardi A, Guerriero R et al 1985 Haemophilia B with inhibitor: molecular analysis of subtotal deletion of the factor IX gene. Blood 66: 728–730

Helfman D M, Ricci W M 1989 Branch point selection in alternative splicing of tropomyosin pre mRNA. Nucleic Acids Research 17: 5633–5650

Higgins D G, Sharp P M 1988 CLUSTAL: a package for performing multiple sequence alignment on a microcomputer. Gene 73: 237–244

Higuchi M, Kochhan L, Olek K 1988 A somatic mosaic for haemophilia A detected at the DNA level. Molecular Biology and Medicine 5: 23–27

Higuchi M, Kochhan L, Schwaab R et al 1989 Molecular defects in hemophilia A: Identification and characterization of mutations in the factor VIII gene and family analysis. Blood 74: 1045–1051

Higuchi M, Wong C, Kochhan L et al 1990 Characterization of mutations in the factor VIII gene by direct sequencing of amplified genomic DNA. Genomics 6: 65–71

Higuchi M, Antonarakis S E, Kasch et al 1991a Towards complete characterization of mild-to-moderate hemophilia A: Detection of the molecular defect in 25 of 29 patients by denaturing gradient gel electrophoresis. Proceedings of the National Academy of Sciences, USA 88: 8307–8311

Higuchi M, Kazazian H H, Kasch L et al 1991b Molecular characterization of severe haemophilia A: Detection of the molecular defect in 25 or 29 patients by denaturing gradient gel electrophoresis. Proceedings of the National Academy of Sciences, USA 88: 7405–7409

Hirosawa S, Fahner J B, Salier J P et al 1990 Structural and functional basis of the developmental regulation of human coagulation factor IX gene: Factor IX Leyden. Proceedings of the National Academy of Sciences, USA 87: 4221–4225

Howard P L, Hoag J B, Bovill E G, Heintz N H 1988 Spontaneous mutation in the male gamete as a cause of hemophilia A: Clarification of a case using DNA probes. American Journal of Hematology 28: 167–169

Hoyer L W, Ashraf M A, Higuchi M, Kaspen, Kazazian H H, Antonarakis S E 1991 Haemophilia A due to mutations that create new N-glycosylation sites. Thrombosis and Haemostasis 65: 727 (abstract)

Huang M -N, Kasper C K, Roberts H R, Stafford D W, High K A 1989 Molecular defect in factor IX Hilo, A hemophilia B variant: Arg to Gln at the carboxy terminal cleavage site of the activation peptide. Blood 73: 718–721

Inaba H et al 1992 Unpublished data

Inaba H, Fujimaki M, Kazazian H H, Antonarakis S E 1989 Mild hemophilia A resulting from Arg-to-Leu substitution in exon 26 of the factor VIII gene. Human Genetics 81: 335–338

Jorgensen M J, Cantor A B, Furie B C et al 1987 Recognition site directing vitamin K-dependent gamma-carboxylation resides on the propeptide of factor IX. Cell 48: 185–191

Kaufman R J, Wasley L C, Dorner A J 1988 Synthesis, processing and secretion of recombinant human factor VIII expressed in mammalian cells. Journal of Biological Chemistry 263: 6352–6362

Kazazian H H, Wong C, Youssoufian et al 1988 Haemophilia A resulting from de novo insertion of L1 sequences represents a novel mechanism for mutation in man. Nature 332: 164–166

Ketterling R P, Bottema C D K, Philips J A, Sommer S S 1991 Evidence that descendants of three founders constitute about 25% of hemophilia B in the United States. Genomics 10: 1093–1096

Koeberl D D, Bottema C D K, Buerstedde J M, Sommer S S 1989 Functionally important regions of the factor IX gene have a low rate of polymorphism and a high rate of mutation in the dinucleotide CpG. American Journal of Human Genetics 45: 448–457

Koeberl D D, Bottema C D K, Ketterling R P et al 1990a Mutations causing haemophilia B: direct estimate of the underlying rate of spontaneous germ-line transitions, transversions and deletions in a human gene. American Journal of Human Genetics 47: 202–217

Koeberl D D, Bottema C D K, Sarkar G et al 1990b Recurrent nonsense mutations at arginine residues cause severe hemophilia B in unrelated hemophiliacs. Human Genetics 84: 387–390

Kogan S, Gitschier J 1990 Mutations and a polymorphism in the factor VIII gene discovered by denaturing gradient gel electrophoresis. Proceedings of the National Academy of Sciences, USA 87: 2092–2096

Kogan S, Gitschier J 1992 Unpublished data

Krawczak M, Cooper D N 1991 Gene deletions causing human genetic disease: Mechanisms of mutagenesis and the role of the local DNA sequence environment. Human Genetics 86: 425–441

Lavergne 1992 Unpublished data

Levinson B, Janco R, Phillips J, Gitschier J 1987 A novel missense mutation in the factor VIII gene identified by analysis of amplified haemophilia DNA sequences. Nucleic Acids Research 15: 9797–9805

Levinson B, Lehesjoki A-E, de la Chapelle A, Gitschier J 1990 Molecular analysis of hemophilia A mutations in the Finnish population. American Journal of Human Genetics 46: 53–62

Leyte A, van-Schijndel H B, Niehrs C 1991 Sulfation of Tyr 1680 of human blood coagulation factor VIII is essential for the interaction of factor VIII with von Willebrand factor. Journal of Biological Chemistry 266: 740–746

Liddell M B, Peake I R, Taylor S A M 1989 Factor IX Cardiff: a variant factor IX protein that shows abnormal activation is caused by an arginine to cysteine substitution at position 145. British Journal of Haematology 72: 556–560

Lillicrap D P 1992 Unpublished data

Lin S W, Shen M C 1991 Characterization of genetic defects of hemophilia B of Chinese origin. Thrombosis and Haemostasis 66: 459–463

Ljung R, Kling S, Sjörin E, Nilsson I M 1989 The majority of isolated cases of hemophilia A are caused by a recent mutation. Thrombosis and Haemostasis 62: 202

Lozier J N, Monroe D M, Stanfield-Oakley S et al 1990 Factor IX New London: substitution of proline for glutamine at position 50 causes severe hemophilia B. Blood 75: 1097–1104

Ludwig M, Schwaab R, Eigel A et al 1989 Identification of a single nucleotide C to T transition and five different deletions in patients with severe hemophilia B. American Journal of Human Genetics 45: 115–122

Ludwig M, Brackman H H, Olek K 1991 Prenatal diagnosis of haemophilia B by the use of polymerase chain reaction and direct sequencing. Klinische Wochenschrift 69: 196–200

Ludwig M, Grimm T, Brackmann H H, Olek K 1992a Parental origin of factor IX gene mutations, and their distribution in the gene. American Journal of Human Genetics 50: 164–173

Ludwig M, Sabharwal A K, Brackmann H H et al 1992b Hemophilia B caused by five different nondeletion mutations in the protease domain of factor IX. Blood 79: 1225–1232

McGraw R A, Davis L M, Lundblad R L, Stafford D W, Roberts H R 1985 Structure and function of factor IX: defects in haemophilia B. Clinical Haematology 14: 359–383

Matsushita T, Tanimoto M, Yamamoto K et al 1990 DNA sequence analysis of three inhibitor-positive hemophilia B patients without gross gene deletion: identification of four novel mutations in factor IX gene. Journal of Laboratory and Clinical Medicine 116: 492–497

Matthews R J, Anson D S, Peake I R, Bloom A L 1987a Heterogeneity of the factor IX locus in nine haemophilia B inhibitor patients. Journal of Clinical Investigation 79: 746–753

Matthews R J, Peake I R, Bloom A L 1987b Point mutation of factor VIII coding sequences in haemophilia A. Thrombosis and Haemostasis 58: 336

Michaelides K, Schwaab R 1992 Unpublished data

Mikami S, Nishino M, Nishimura T, Fukui H 1987 RFLPs of factor IX gene in Japanese haemophilia B families and gene deletion in two

high-responder-inhibitor patients. Japanese Journal of Human Genetics 32: 21–31
Mikami S, Nishimura T, Naka H et al 1988a Nonsense mutation in factor VIII gene of a severe haemophiliac patient with anti-factor VIII antibody. Japanese Journal of Human Genetics 33: 409–415
Mikami S, Nishimura T, Naka H, Kuze K, Fukui H 1988b A deletion involving intron 13 and exon 14 of factor VIII gene in a haemophiliac with anti-factor VIII antibody. Japanese Journal of Human Genetics 33: 401–407
Miller C H, Hilgartner M W, Aledort L M 1987 Reproductive choices in hemophilic men and carriers. American Journal of Medical Genetics 26: 591–598
Millar D S, Steinbrecher R A, Wieland K et al 1990 The molecular genetic analysis of haemophilia A; characterization of six partial deletions in the factor VIII gene. Human Genetics 86: 219–227
Millar D S, Zoll B, Martinowitz U, Kakkar V V, Cooper D N 1991 The molecular genetics of haemophilia A; screening for point mutations in the factor VIII gene using the restriction enzyme Taq I. Human Genetics 87: 607–612
Miyata T, Sakai T, Sugimoto M et al 1991 Factor IX Amagasaki: a new mutation in the catalytic domain resulting in the loss of both coagulant and esterase activities. Biochemistry 30: 11286–11291
Montandon A J, Green P M, Giannelli F, Bentley D R 1989 Direct detection of point mutations by mismatch analysis: application to haemophilia B. Nucleic Acids Research 17: 3347–3358
Montandon A J, Green P M, Bentley D R et al 1990 Two factor IX mutations in the family of an isolated haemophilia B patient. Direct carrier diagnosis by amplification mismatch detection (AMD). Human Genetics 85: 200–204
Montandon A J, Green P M, Bentley D R et al 1992 Direct estimate of the haemophilia B (factor IX deficiency) mutation rate and of the ratio of the sex-specific mutation rates in Sweden. Human Genetics 89: 319–322
Murru S, Casula L, Pecorara M, Mori P, Cao A, Pirastu M 1990 Illegitimate recombination produced a duplication within the FVIII gene in a patient with mild hemophilia. Genomics 7: 115–118
Nafa K, Meriane F, Reghis A et al 1990 Investigation of factor VIII: C gene restriction fragment length polymorphisms and search for deletions in hemophilic subjects in Algeria. Human Genetics 84: 401–405
Naylor J A, Green P M, Montandon A J, Rizza C R, Giannelli F 1991 Detection of three novel mutations in two haemophilia A patients by rapid screening of whole essential region of factor VIII gene. Lancet 337: 635–639
Naylor J A, Green P M, Rizza C R, Giannelli F 1992 Factor VIII gene explains all cases of haemophilia A. Lancet 340: 1066–1067
Naylor J A, Green P M, Rizza C R, Giannelli F 1993 Analysis of factor VIII in RNA reveals defects in every one of 28 haemophilia A patients. Human Molecular Genetics 2: 11–17
Nishimura H, Takeya H, Suehiro K et al 1991 Characterisation of factor IX Fukuoka with substitution of Asn 92 by His into second epidermal growth factor-like domain. Thrombosis and Haemostasis 65: 712
Noyes C M, Griffith M J, Roberts H R, Lundblad R L 1983 Identification of the molecular defect in factor IX Chapel Hill: Substitution of histidine for arginine at position 145. Proceedings of the National Academy of Sciences, USA 80: 4200–4202
O'Brien D P, Tuddenham E G D 1989 Purification and characterization of factor VIII 1689 Cys: A non-functional cofactor occurring in a patient with severe haemophilia A. Blood 73: 2117–2122
O'Brien D P, Pattinson J K, Tuddenham E G D 1990 Purification and characterization of factor VIII 372-Cys: A hypofunctional cofactor from a patient with moderately severe haemophilia A. Blood 75: 1664–1672
O'Brien D P, Gale K M, Anderson J S 1991 Purification and characterisation of factor VII 304-Gln: a variant molecule with reduced activity isolated from a clinically unaffected male. Blood 78: 132–40
O'Hara P J, Grant F J, Haldman B et al 1987 Nucleotide sequence of the gene coding for human factor VII, a vitamin K-dependent protein participating in blood coagulation. Proceedings of the National Academy of Sciences, USA 84: 5158–5162
Orita M, Suzuki Y, Sekiya T, Hayashi K 1989 Rapid and sensitive detection of point mutations and DNA polymorphisms using the polymerase chain reaction. Genomics 5: 874–879
Pattinson J, Millar D S, McVey J et al 1990a The molecular genetic analysis of haemophilia A; a directed-search strategy for the detection of point mutations in the human factor VIII gene. Blood 76: 2242–2248
Pattinson J K, McVey J H, Boon M, Ajani A, Tuddenham E G D 1990b CRM$^+$ haemophilia A due to a missense mutation (372 Cys) at the internal heavy chain thrombin cleavage site. British Journal of Haematology 75: 73–77
Peake I R, Matthews R J, Bloom A L 1989 Haemophilia B Chicago: severe haemophilia B caused by two deletions and an inversion within the factor IX gene. British Journal of Haematology 71 (suppl): 1
Pecorara M, Casarino L, Mori P G et al 1987 Hemophilia A: Carrier detection and prenatal diagnosis by DNA analysis. Blood 70: 531–535
Pittman D D, Kaufman R J 1988 Proteolytic requirements for thrombin activation of anti-haemophilic factor (factor VIII). Proceedings of the National Academy of Sciences, USA 85: 2429–2433
Poort S R, Briët E, Bertina R M, Reitsma P H 1990 Two mutations of the factor IX gene including a donor splice consensus deletion and a point mutation in a Dutch patient with severe hemophilia B. Thrombosis and Haemostasis 64: 379–384
Przysiecki C T, Staggers J E, Ramjit H G et al 1987 Occurrence of β-hydroxylated asparagine residues in non-vitamin K dependent proteins containing epidermal growth factor-like domains. Proceedings of the National Academy of Sciences, USA 84: 7856–7860
Rao K J, Lyman G, Hamsabhushanam K, Scott J P, Jagadeeswaran P 1990 Human factor IX (Lincoln Park): a molecular characterization. Molecular and Cellular Probes 4: 335–340
Reed R 1989 The organisation of 3′ splice site sequences in mammalian introns. Genes and Development 3: 2113–2123
Rees D J G, Rizza, C R, Brownlee G G 1985 Haemophilia B caused by a point mutation in a donor splice junction of the human factor IX gene. Nature 316: 643–645
Rees D J G, Jones I M, Handford P A et al 1988 The role of beta-hydroxy-aspartate and adjacent carboxylate residues in the first EGF domain of human factor IX. European Molecular Biology Organization Journal 7: 2053–2061
Reitsma P H, Bertina R M, Ploos van Amstel J K, Riemans A, Briët E 1988 The putative factor IX gene promotor in hemophilia B Leyden. Blood 72: 1074–1076
Reitsma P H, Mandalaki T, Kasper C K, Bertina R M, Briët E 1989 Two novel point mutations correlate with an altered developmental expression of blood coagulation factor IX (hemophilia B Leyden phenotype). Blood 73: 743–746
Roberts R G, Bobrow M, Bentley D R 1992 Point mutations in the dystrophin gene. Proceedings of the National Academy of Sciences, USA 89: 2331–2335
Rosendaal F R, Bröcker-Vriends A H J T, van Houwellingen J C et al 1990 Sex ratio of the mutation frequencies in haemophilia B: Estimation and meta-analysis. Human Genetics 86: 139–146
Royle G, van de Water N S, Berry E, Ockelford P A, Browett P J 1991 Haemophilia B Leyden arising de novo by point mutation in the putative factor IX promoter region. British Journal of Haematology 77: 191–194
Sakai T, Yoshioka A, Yanamoto K, et al 1989 Blood clotting factor IX Kashihara: amino acid substitution of valine-182 by phenylalanine. Journal of Biochemistry 105: 756–759
Sarkar G, Yoon H-S, Sommer S S 1992 Screening for mutations by RNA single-strand conformation polymorphism (rSSCP): comparison with DNA-SSCP. Nucleic Acids Research 20: 871–878
Schach B G, Yoshitake S, Davie E W 1987 Haemophilia (Factor IX Seattle 2) due to a single nucleotide deletion in the gene for factor IX. Journal of Clinical Investigation 80: 1023–1028
Scheffield V C, Cox D R, Lerman L S, Myers R M 1989 Attachment of a 40 base pair G + C rich sequence (GC clamp) to genomic DNA fragments by the polymerase chain reaction results in improved detection of single base changes. Proceedings of the National Acedemy of Sciences, USA 86: 232–236

Schwaab R et al 1992 Unpublished data
Schwaab R, Ludwig M, Oldenburg J et al 1990 Identical point mutations in the factor VIII gene that have different clinical manifestations of hemophilia A. American Journal of Human Genetics 47: 743–744
Schwaab R, Ludwig M, Kochhan L et al 1991 Detection and characterization of two missense mutations at a cleavage site in the factor VIII light chain. Thrombosis Research 61: 225–234
Shima M, Ware J, Yoshioka A, Fukui H, Fulcher C A 1989 An arginine to cysteine amino acid substitution at a critical thrombin cleavage site in a dysfunctional factor VIII molecule. Blood 74: 1612–1617
Siguret V, Amselem S, Vidaud M et al 1988 Identification of a CpG mutation in the coagulation factor IX gene by analysis of amplified DNA sequences. British Journal of Haematology 70: 411–416
Solera J, Magallon M, Martin-Villar J, Coloma A 1992 Factor $IX_{Madrid\ 2}$: A deletion/insertion in factor IX gene which abolishes the sequence of the donor junction at the exon IV-intron d splice site. American Journal of Human Genetics 50: 434–437
Soriano-Garcia M, Padmanabhan K, de Vos A M, Tulinsky A 1992 The Ca2+ ion and membrane binding structure of the gla domain of Ca-prothrombin fragment 1. Biochemistry 31: 2554–2566
Stoflet E S, Koeberl D D, Sarkar S S, Sommer S S 1988 Genomic amplification with transcript sequencing. Science 239: 491–494
Sugimoto M, Miyata T, Kawabata S et al 1988 Blood clotting factor IX Niigata: substitution of alanine 390 by valine in the catalytic domain. Journal of Biochemistry 104: 878–880
Tanimoto M, Kojima T, Kamiya T et al 1988 DNA analysis of seven patients with hemophilia B who have anti-factor IX antibodies: relationship to clinical manifestations and evidence that the abnormal gene was inherited. Journal of Laboratory and Clinical Medicine 112: 307–313
Taylor S A M, Lillicrap D P, Blanchette V et al 1988 A complete deletion of the factor IX gene and new Taq I variant in a haemophilia B kindred. Human Genetics 79: 273–276
Taylor S A M, Liddell M B, Peake I R, Bloom A L, Lillicrap D P 1990 A mutation adjacent to the beta cleavage site of factor IX (valine 182 to leucine) results in mild haemophilia. British Journal of Haematology 75: 217–221
Taylor S A M, Deugau K V, Lillicrap D P 1991 Somatic mosaicism and female-to-female transmission in a kindred with hemophilia B (factor IX deficiency). Proceedings of the National Academy of Sciences, USA 88: 39–42
Thompson A R 1990 Molecular biology of the haemophilias. Progress in Haemostasis and Thrombosis 10: 175–214
Thompson A R, Bajaj S P, Chen S H, McGillivray R T A 1990 'Founder' effect in different families with haemophilia B mutations. Lancet i: 418
Thompson A R, Schoof J M, Weinmann A F, Chen S H 1992 Factor IX mutations: rapid, direct screening methods for 20 new families with hemophilia B. Thrombosis Research 65: 289–295
Titani K, Fujikawa K 1982 The structural aspects of vitamin K-dependant blood coagulation factors. Acta Haematologica Japonica 45: 807–816
Toole J J, Knoff J L, Wozney J M et al 1984 Molecular cloning of a cDNA encoding human antihaemophilic factor. Nature 312: 342–347
Traystman M D, Higuchi M, Kasper C K, Antonarakis S E, Kazazian H H 1990 Use of denaturing gradient gel electrophoresis to detect point mutations in the factor VIII gene. Genomics 6: 293–301
Tsang T C, Bentley D R, Mibashan R S, Giannelli F 1988 A factor IX mutation, verified by direct genomic sequencing, causes haemophilia B by a novel mechanism. European Molecular Biology Organization Journal 7: 3009–3015
Tuddenham E G D 1992 Unpublished data
Vehar G A, Keyt B, Eaton D et al 1984 Structure of human factor VIII. Nature 312: 337–342
Vidaud M, Chabret C, Gazengel C et al 1986 A de novo intragenic deletion of the potential EGF domain of the factor IX gene in a family with severe hemophilia B. Blood 68: 961–963
Vidaud M, Vidaud D, Siguret V, Lavergne J M, Goossens M 1989 Mutational insertion on an Alu sequence causes haemophilia B. American Journal of Human Genetics 45: A226
Vogel F 1977 A probable sex difference in some mutation rates. American Journal of Human Genetics 29: 312–319
Vogel F, Motulsky A 1986 Human genetics: problems and approaches, 2nd edn. Springer Verlag, Berlin, p 435
Wadelius C, Blombäck M, Pettersson U 1988 Molecular studies of haemophilia B in Sweden: identification of patients with total deletion of the factor IX gene and without inhibitory antibodies. Human Genetics 81: 13–17
Wang N S, Chen S H, Thompson A R 1990a Point mutations in four hemophilia B patients from China. Thrombosis and Haemostasis 64: 302–306
Wang N S, Zhang N S, Thompson A R, Chen S H 1990b Factor IX Chongqing: a new mutation in the calcium-binding domain of factor IX resulting in severe hemophilia B. Thrombosis and Haemostasis 63: 24–26
Ware J, Davis L, Frazier D, Bajaj S P, Stafford D W 1988 Genetic defect responsible for the dysfunctional protein fator IX Long Beach. Blood 72: 820–822
Wehnert M, Herrmann F H, Wulff K 1989 Partial deletions of factor VIII gene as molecular diagnostic markers in haemophilia A. Disease Markers 7: 113–117
Winship P R 1986 Carrier detection and patient studies in haemophilia B D Phil thesis, Oxford University
Winship P R 1990 Haemophilia B caused by mutation of a potential thrombin cleavage site in factor IX. Nucleic Acids Research 18: 1310
Winship P R, Dragon A C 1991 Identification of haemophilia B patients with mutations in the two calcium binding domains of factor IX: importance of a beta-OH Asp-64 → Asn change. British Journal of Haematology 77: 102–109
Winter R M, Tuddenham E G D, Goldman E, Matthews K B 1983 A maximum likelihood estimate of the sex ratio of mutation rates in haemophilia A. Human Genetics 64: 156–159
Woods-Samuels P, Wong C, Mathias S L et al 1989 Characterization of a non deleterious L1 insertion in an intron of the human factor VIII. Genomics 4: 290–296
Woods-Samuels P, Kazazian H H, Antonarakis S E 1991 Non-homologous recombination in the human genome: Deletions in the human factor VIII gene. Genomics 10: 94–101
Yoshitake S, Schach B G, Foster D C, Davie E W, Kurachi K 1985 Nucleotide sequence of the gene for human factor IX (antihemophilic factor B). Biochemistry 24: 3736–3750
Youssoufian H, Kazazian H H, Phillips D G et al 1986 Recurrent mutations in haemophilia A give evidence for CpG mutation hotspots. Nature 324: 380–382
Youssoufian H, Antonarakis S E, Aronis S et al 1987a Characterization of five partial deletions of the factor VIII gene. Proceedings of the National Academy of Sciences, USA 84: 3772–3776
Youssoufian H, Patel A, Phillips D, Kazazian H H, Antonarakis S E 1987b Recurrent mutations and an unusual deletion in haemophilia A. Thrombosis and Haemostasis 58: 336
Youssoufian H, Antonarakis S E, Bell W, Griffin A M, Kazazian H H 1988a Nonsense and missense mutations in hemophilia A: Estimate of the relative mutation rate at CG dinucleotides. American Journal of Human Genetics 42: 718–725
Youssoufian H, Wong C, Aronis S, Platokoukis H, Kazazian H H, Antonarakis S E 1988b Moderately severe hemophilia A resulting from Glu→Gly substitution in exon 7 of the factor VIII gene. American Journal of Human Genetics 42: 867–871
Youssoufian H, Kazazian H H, Patel et al 1988c Mild hemophilia A associated with a cryptic donor splice site mutation in intron 4 of the factor VIII gene. Genomics 2: 32–36
Youssoufian H, Kasper C K, Phillips D G, Kazazian H H, Antonarakis S E 1988d Restriction endonuclease mapping of six novel deletions of the factor VIII gene in hemophilia A. Human Genetics 80: 143–148

37. Linkage analysis in the diagnosis of haemostatic disorders

I. Peake

The accurate detection of carriers and the reliable performance of prenatal diagnosis (when appropriate) can make a significant contribution to the overall impact of any inherited disease, particularly if the disease is inherited in a recessive mode. This may also be true in dominantly inherited conditions where variable phenotypic expression of the condition is observed. Of the major inherited haemostatic bleeding disorders, haemophilia A and B (factor VIII and factor IX deficiency) fall into the first category, and von Willebrand's disease (vWd, von Willebrand factor deficiency) falls into the second.

In practice there are two methodologies which can be used to track a defective gene through a family and so identify carriers of the condition and be used in prenatal diagnosis. The first of these is by identification within an affected individual of the precise gene defect within the risk factor gene (point mutation, deletion, insertion), followed by the analysis of all family members at risk for the particular defect. The second procedure is to utilize DNA polymorphisms to identify and track defective genes (linkage analysis). This type of analysis is the main topic of this chapter.

The first of these procedures (direct defect detection) is dependent upon the finding of the defect and requires the use of technically-demanding DNA analysis procedures. Since the advent of the polymerase chain reaction (PCR, Saiki et al 1988) and associated DNA analysis techniques, it is now possible to analyse all coding and essential non-coding regions in smaller genes (e.g. factor IX) and to detect defects in the majority of patients. A database has been established for factor IX gene defects in patients with haemophilia B and to date 206 unique mutations have been reported (Giannelli et al 1991). Attempts to assemble similar data for haemophilia A (Tuddenham et al 1991) and von Willebrand's disease are also in hand and these studies, like haemophilia B, are covered elsewhere in the volume (Chs 35, 36).

Until recently the identification of the precise gene defect causing a bleeding disorder was difficult and, even with the introduction of PCR, sophisticated DNA analysis procedures are required. The observation that there are many different mutations within a particular gene that can cause the disease (i.e. there are in general no hot spots for mutation) also means that the analysis will be different in most families.

The methodology which has been of most use to date in family studies of the inherited bleeding disorders has been linkage analysis using the identification and tracking of DNA polymorphisms. These changes in DNA sequence are not related to the defect itself and occur throughout the general population. However they are present within or close to the defective gene and can therefore be used, if informative (p. 889), to track that gene through a kindred both to detect carriers and to perform prenatal diagnosis.

POLYMORPHISMS

DNA polymorphisms are variations in DNA sequence which have no discernible effect on the expression of any gene or genes within the genome. By definition they occur at a frequency of greater than 1% in the normal population. Such changes are usually within extragenic sequence or within introns. They can also be within exons when the change, usually a nucleotide transition or transversion at the third position of a codon, does not change the amino acid code. Occasionally the change can result in a conservative amino acid change which has no effect on the function of the protein expressed (e.g. the alanine/threonine dimorphism at amino acid 148 within the activation peptide of factor IX).

The majority of polymorphisms are single nucleotide changes and where this change removes or creates a cutting site for a restriction endonuclease then it is termed a **R**estriction **F**ragment **L**ength **P**olymorphism or RFLP. Since such polymorphisms will alter the digestion pattern of DNA they are readily detectable. Single nucleotide changes that do not affect restriction endonuclease digestion fragments can also be detected using specific oligonucleotide probes (allele-specific oligonucleotides ASO; p. 888).

A second type of DNA polymorphism, which is being observed and utilized increasingly, depends on variable physical length of a region of DNA. This is due to the presence of a varying number of tandem repeats of DNA sequence (Variable Number Tandem Repeats or VNTR). The length of one repeat can be from a single base to 50 or more bases, and these repeat regions of DNA are most widely utilized as the basis of the mini satellite regions detected in DNA fingerprinting techniques (Jefferies et al 1985). VNTR sequences at specific loci within the genome can be readily analysed by PCR amplification of the sequence of interest and are proving to be very useful polymorphic markers, particularly since they are usually multiallelic and therefore potentially very informative.

METHODS OF POLYMORPHISM ANALYSIS

The Southern blot procedure was the method of RFLP detection prior to the introduction of PCR amplification, and is still the only method of detection for anonymous RFLPs where the exact locus and therefore the DNA sequence is unknown. Indeed PCR is not possible without knowledge of at least some DNA sequence flanking the polymorphism so that the necessary primers can be designed. Southern blotting involves the isolation of DNA, its digestion with the appropriate restriction endonuclease (to reveal the polymorphic site), gel electrophoresis of the digested DNA, blotting of the separated fragments onto a suitable membrane and finally probing of the fragments on the membrane with a tagged (usually with ^{32}P) single-stranded DNA or RNA probe. The probe is specific for the region of the RFLP and the fragments detected show the presence or absence of the polymorphic site.

PCR amplification of the region of DNA containing the RFLP followed by restriction endonuclease digestion and analysis of the products by agarose or polyacrylamide gel electrophoresis has rapidly replaced Southern blotting where the DNA sequence surrounding the RFLP is known. PCR-based analysis is quick and does not involve the use of probes, radioactivity, blotting, etc. Where a Southern blot analysis can take a week or more, PCR-based studies can be completed in a day. PCR also enables polymorphic nucleotide substitutions which do not affect restriction enzyme sites to be detected by probing the amplified material with allele-specific oligonucleotides probes or by the use of the **A**mplification **R**efractory **M**utation **S**ystem (ARMS) where one of the PCR primers is designed to bind at the site of the polymorphism and to be allele specific (Newton et al 1989). As a result amplification will only occur for one of the alleles. A primer designed to bind to the other allele sequence is also used to give a negative control.

Of increasing significance is the use of PCR to detect gene-specific VNTRs. In this case the actual amplified product will vary in length depending on the number of repeats preset in the amplified fragment. Generally, where the size difference is four bases or more the alleles can be visualized by electrophoresis on polyacryamide or agarose gels followed by staining with ethidium bromide and visualization under UV light. For dinucleotide repeats the alleles are identified using DNA sequencing gels and are radiolabelled by the end labelling of one of the primers prior to PCR amplification. The amplified fragments are then detected by autoradiography.

Quality control aspects of polymorphism analysis are of considerable importance. A major problem for RFLP analysis can be partial digestion of the DNA by the restriction endonuclease which can lead to, for example, an apparent heterozygous pattern (+/–) in a homozygous individual (+/+). The problem is usually readily detected in Southern blot procedures where several 'unusual' fragments are seen. However with PCR-amplified material where a single fragment is seen which, after digestion with enzyme, is either completely, partially or not cut at all, then the detection of a partial digestion is difficult. Several procedures have been introduced to help identify this problem including the occurrence within the amplified fragment of a second non-polymorphic invariant site for the same restriction endonuclease (e.g. PCR amplification of the intragenic *Hind*III factor VIII gene RFLP; Graham et al 1990). Cleavage at this site can be used as a monitor of the enzyme digestion. Where such a site is not available then the inclusion within the PCR reaction of a second set of primers to amplify an unrelated area of the genome which contains an invariant site for the restriction endonuclease has also been reported (e.g. a control for the *Bcl*I factor VIII intragenic RFLP by co-amplification of a region of the beta globin gene cluster; Sampietro et al 1990). Cleavage of the second fragment is then used as an internal control of complete enzyme digestion. Finally the simple addition of a DNA fragment obtained either by cloning or by prior PCR amplification can also provide an internal control for digestion.

THE USEFULNESS OF POLYMORPHISMS

Linked probes

Polymorphisms within the gene of interest can be assumed to be genetically very close to the defect within that gene. As a result the chance of a crossover occurring between the defect locus and polymorphism at meiosis is very small. However where the polymorphism is at a different locus which is linked to the gene then a potential crossover (recombination) rate must be considered. For example two informative polymorphisms have been extensively used in the study of haemophilia A. They are at loci DXS15 (probe DX13; Harper et al 1984) and

DXS52 (probe ST14; Oberle et al 1985) and have been shown to have a potential crossover rate of about 5%. Thus any carrier status assessment made on the basis of one of these polymorphisms alone will carry a probability of 95%. A prenatal diagnosis similarly based would carry an error rate of 5%.

Allelic frequency

Any individual will only be potentially informative for a given polymorphism if they are heterozygous for that polymorphism. That is, the alleles for each of their gene pair are different. In the case of X chromosome-inherited conditions this applies to female carriers. The frequency of heterozygosity depends upon the allele frequency within the overall population and, with RFLP analysis, where only two alleles occur (+ or – the cutting enzyme site) then the maximum frequency of heterozygosity (or heterozygosity rate) can be only 50%, and this will only occur when both alleles occur at equal frequency within the population. This is not generally the case and therefore heterozygosity rates for given RFLPs tend to be lower than 50%. Where the polymorphism is a VNTR and the number of alleles is more than two then the heterozygosity rate can be greater than 50%. For example one of the intron 40 von Willebrand factor gene VNTRs described below (Peake et al 1990) has eight alleles and shows a heterozygosity rate of greater than 75%. Clearly the number of alleles observed determines the overall usefulness of a polymorphism as does the relative frequency of the alleles.

Linkage disequilibrium

Where an individual or family are non-informative for a particular RFLP then it is logical to use a second with the highest possible frequency. Although it is possible to calculate the probability of the second polymorphism being informative, several studies have shown that this often an overestimate, and in some cases the second RFLP is no more useful than the first. This is particularly true for polymorphisms that are physically close, for example within the same gene, and is a result of linkage disequilibrium, or the non-random assocation of alleles. This effect is a result of both the closeness of the polymorphisms and the time when the original DNA alteration occurred. Both these effects limit the number of crossovers which can have occurred through time between the two polymorphic loci and which lead to randomization of allele association. Examples of linkage disequilibrium are given below (p. 891).

Ethnic variation

While some polymorphisms are present at about the same frequency in many different ethnic groups, this is not always the case. Indeed, of the RFLPs within the factor IX gene found to be useful for family studies in haemophilia B in European and North American white populations, few are of use in far eastern groups, including Japanese and Chinese. The incidence of the three diseases discussed below (haemophilia A, B and vWd) seems to be similar in all racial groups that have been studied.

Sporadic cases and new mutations

Some 30% of cases of haemophilia A and B have no family history of the disease. In such cases polymophorphism-based gene tracking and analysis is of limited use, even when combined with phenotypic analysis (carriers of these diseases will on average have 50% of the normal plasma level of the particular factor). Diagnosis of non-carrier status is possible by allelic exclusion and is also often useful in families where all the required family members are not available. In sporadic cases, direct defect detection is probably the only satisfactory approach, given that there is now evidence that new mutations can have arisen either in the patient or the germinal tissue of his mother, grandfather or grandmother. Germline mosaicism has also been reported in the haemophilias and vWd and this is a situation where family studies based on polymorphisms or gene defect detection are inappropriate.

HAEMOPHILIA A

A series of nine useful DNA polymorphisms have been described within the factor VIII gene, of which seven are RFLPs, one is a dinucleotide repeat VNTR (CA repeats; eight alleles) and one is a sequence polymorphism which may be detected by allele-specific oligonucleotides (ASO). Details of the polymorphisms, together with alleles, allelic frequencies and heterozygosity rates, and relevant references are given in Table 37.1. Figures are given for white European/North American populations unless otherwise stated. The second *Msp*I RFLP listed (Inaba et al 1990) is the only polymorphism which is useful in Japanese (and Asian Indian) populations and is not found in white populations. As shown in Table 37.2, where ethnic variations in the frequencies of these factor VIII polymorphisms are shown, frequencies in non-white populations appear to be lower than those in white groups and this is particularly true for factor IX gene polymorphisms. This probably only reflects the fact that the initial detection of these polymorphisms was performed in white populations and the reverse situation would have occurred if initial studies had been performed in non-white groups when, presumably, different polymorphisms would have been detected.

Extragenic (or linked polymorphic loci) which can be

Table 37.1 Factor VIII gene DNA polymorphisms

Type	Restriction endonuclease	Probe Southern blot	Alleles (kb) –	Alleles (kb) +	Allelic frequency[1] (%) –	Allelic frequency[1] (%) +	Heterozygosity[1] (%)	Locus	Reference
RFLP	*BclI*	p114.12	1.1	0.8	29	71	42	Int 18	Gitschier et al 1985
RFLP	*XbaI*	p482.6	6.2	4.8 (1.4)	41	59	48	Int 22	Wion et al 1988
RFLP	*BglI*	Probe C	20	5	10	90	18	3′ exon 26	Antonarakis et al 1985
RFLP	*HindIII*	F8e16/19	2.7	2.6	70	30	42	Int 19	Ahrens et al 1987
RFLP	*MspI*	p625.3	7.5	4.3 + 3.2	68	32	43.5	3′ flank	Youssoufian et al 1987
RFLP	*MspI*	Probe B	4.0	3.8	–	–	45[2]	Int 22	Inaba et al 1990
RFLP	*TaqI*	p701.1	9.5	4.0	72	28	40	5′ Flank	Kenwick et al 1991
VNTR	($CA_{(n)}$ repeat: PCR detection: 8 alleles)				–	–	91[3]	Int 13	Lalloz et al 1991
Sequence polymorphism		(ASO detection after PCR)			–	–	–	Int 7	Kogan & Gitschier 1988

[1] White European/North American population unless otherwise stated; [2] Japanese population only; [3] observed frequency.

Table 37.2 Factor VIII gene polymorphisms; ethnic variations

Ethnic group	Heterozygosity % *BclI*	*XbaI*	*BglI*	*HindIII*	*MspI*	*BglII*[1]	*TaqI/MspI*[2]
White, European and North American	42[a]	49[a]	24[a]	42[a]	0[d]	50[a]	70a
American Black	29,32[b,c]	u	38[b]	34[c]	0[d]	u	u
Asian Indian	42,44[b,c]	u	11[b]	41[c]	13[d]	u	u
Chinese	29,38[c,e]	49[e]	0[e]	36[c]	u	u	u
Japanese	42[g]	48[g]	16[g]	u	45[d]	27[g]	u
Malay	33[c]	u	u	35[c]	u	u	u
Polynesian	49[f]	50[f]	2[f]	u	u	u	daf[f]
Maori	44[c]	49[f]	11[f]	u	u	u	daf[f]
Thai	34[h]	48[h]	0[h]	u	u	36[h]	u

u = unknown; daf = different allele frequency; [1] DX13 – DXS15 locus; [2] ST14 – DXS52 locus; [a] Combined data, published and unpublished; collected for ISTH SSC Factor IX/VIII Subcommittee; [b] Antonarakis et al 1985; [c] Graham et al 1990; [d] Inaba et al 1990; [e] Chan et al 1988; [f] Van der Water et al 1991; [g] Suehiro et al 1988; [h] Chuansumrit et al Personal communication.

used in factor VIII gene tracking studies are detailed in Table 37.7, together with those for factor IX. Of these loci, detailed analysis of crossover rates have been performed for the polymorphisms detected by the probes DX13 (DXS15) and ST14 (DXS52). In an analysis by the author of 286 meioses (from published and non-published data), 11 crossovers (3.85%) between the ST14 locus and the factor VIII gene locus were observed, and for DX13, eight crossovers were seen in 182 meioses (4.39%). It would seem reasonable to assign a crossover rate of about 5% to polymorphisms detected at these loci when performing family studies in haemophilia A and therefore to counsel an appropriate level of probability.

Those factor VIII polymorphisms which can be detected by PCR-based DNA amplification techniques are shown in Table 37.3, with details of the primers used in the reference quoted. Detection of the *XbaI* RFLP by this technique is complicated by the presence of homologous

Table 37.3 Factor VIII gene: PCR-based polymorphism analysis

Polymorphisms	Site	Primers	Fragment (bp)	Digest fragments (bp)	Reference
BclI	Int 18	5′-TAAAAGCTTTAAATGGTCTAGGC – 3′ 5′-TTCGAATTCTGAAATTATCTTGTTC – 3′	142	99 + 43	Kogan et al 1987
XbaI	Int 22	5′-CACGAGCTCTCCATCTGAACATG – 3′ 5′-GGGCTGCAGGGGGGGGGACAACAG – 3′	96	68 + 28	Kogan et al 1987
HindIII	Int 19	5′-GGCGAGCATCTACATGCTGGGATGAGC – 3′ 5′-GTCCAGAAGCCATTCCCAGGGGAGTCT – 3′	717	469[1] + 167 + 81	Graham et al 1990
VNTR	Int 13	5′-TGCATCACTGTACATATGTATCTT – 3′ 5′-CCAAATTACATATGAATAAGCC – 3′	8 alleles		Lalloz et al 1991
VNTR	DXS52	5′-GGCATGTCATCACTTCTCTCATGTT – 3′ 5′-CACCACTGCCCTCACGTCACTT – 3′	14 alleles		Richards et al 1991
Sequence polymorphism	Int 7	–	–		Kogan and Gitschier 1988

[1] Invariant fragment.

regions to intron 22 present elsewhere on the X chromosome (Paterson et al 1989), and indeed other *XbaI* polymorphisms within these homologous regions have now been shown to be of potential use in haemophilia A family studies, although crossover rates are as yet unknown (Chan et al 1989).

The VNTR at DXS52, previously detected by Southern blotting as a multiallelic locus using restriction endonucleases *Taq*I and *Msp*I, has now been shown to consist, at least in part, of an almost perfectly reproduced repeat of 60 bp (Richards et al 1991). Ten major and four minor alleles have been described. The intragenic VNTR recently described by Lalloz et al (1991) is potentially the most useful polymorphism so far reported for haemophilia A family studies.

As discussed, the limiting factor regarding overall heterozygosity rates for a series of polymorphisms is the level of linkage disequilibrium. Although calculations can be made to quantitate this effect, within a group of available polymorphisms close to or within a particular gene, it is probably important only to note those which are in complete, or almost complete, linkage disequilibrium, and those in complete equilibrium. Thus, with the factor VIII gene polymorphisms there is strong linkage disequilibrium between the *Bcl*I RFLP and those detected by *Hind*III, *Msp*I and *Bgl*I. The level of disequilibrium between *Bcl*I and *Xba*I is less but is still appreciable. Linkage disequilibrium between the intron 13 VNTR and the intragenic RFLPs has yet to be estimated, but given the multiallelic nature of the VNTR, it is by no means certain that any association of alleles will necessarily be detrimental to the overall combined informativeness.

The overall informativeness of the intragenic factor VIII RFLPs (*Bcl*I {or *Hind*III}, *Xba*I, and *Msp*I {3′ flanking region}) in white European/North American populations is reported to be about 75%. With the inclusion of the intron 13 VNTR this figure will be in excess of 90% and, if the extragenic/linked polymorphisms are used, it is unlikely that any family would not be informative for at least one polymorphism.

HAEMOPHILIA B

A list of the nine useful RFLPs detected within the factor IX gene locus is given in Table 37.4. Those detected by the restriction endonucleases *Taq*I, *Xmn*I, *Dde*I, *Msp*I, and *BamH*I (two RFLPs although there is some evidence that they may be the same) were initially analysed by Southern blotting techniques. All are the result of single nucleotide changes except for the *Dde*I RFLP which results from a 50 bp inset/deletion within intron 1 and therefore this polymorphism can also be detected by digestion with other restriction endonucleases, e.g. *Hinf*I. The *Hha*I RFLP, described by Winship et al (1989) is only detected in PCR-amplified DNA. Conventional Southern blotting cannot be used because methylation of the cytosine residue at the CpG dinucleotide within this *Hha*I recognition site in genomic DNA protects it from cleavage by the enzyme. The *Mnl*I RFLP in exon six results from an amino acid dimorphism at position 148 within the activation peptide (alanine or threonine). This polymorphism can be detected using epitope-specific monoclonal antibodies (Thompson et al 1988), by ASO procedures (Winship & Brownlee 1986) and more recently by PCR amplification and *Mnl*I digestion (Graham et al 1989). The MseI RFLP, recently described by Winship & Peake (1991), results from a nucleotide change (C to T) at position –698 in the 5′ flanking region of the factor IX gene.

The factor IX gene polymorphisms show considerably more ethnic variation in heterozygosity rates when compared to the factor VIII gene polymorphisms as shown in Table 37.5. Indeed, the only polymorphisms which occur at significant frequencies in the non-white or American black communities are those detected by *Hha*I, *Mse*I and the linked RFLP at DXS99 detected by *Sst*I (see also Table 37.7). A second potentially useful linked RFLP at DXS102 has also been reported, detected by *Taq*I digestion (Table 37.7), but to date the crossover rate between this RFLP, that at DXS99 and the factor IX gene locus has not been estimated.

Table 37.4 Factor IX gene DNA polymorphisms

Type	Restriction endonuclease	Probe Southern blot	Alleles (kb) –	Alleles (kb) +	Allelic frequency[1] –	Allelic frequency[1] +	Heterozygosity[1]	Locus	Reference
RFLP	*Taq*I	VIII	1.8	1.3	65	35	45	Int 4	Giannelli et al 1984
RFLP	*Xmn*I	VIII	11.5	6.5	71	29	41	Int 3	Winship et al 1984
RFLP	*Dde*I	XIII	1.75 (50 bp insert)	1.7	24	76	36	Int 1	Winship et al 1984
RFLP	*Msp*I	cDNA	5.8	3.4 + 2.4	22	78	34	Int 4	Camerino et al 1985
RFLP	*Hha*I	(PCR)	–	–	61	39	48	3′ flank	Winship et al 1989
RFLP	*BamH*I	Genomic	25	23	94	6	11	5′ flank	Hay et al 1986
RFLP	*BamH*I	VIII	15	13	52	48	50[2]	Int 3	Driscoll et al 1988
RFLP	*Mnl*I	(ASO)	–	–	33	67	45	Amino Acid 148 Ala/Thr	Winship & Brownlee 1986
RFLP	*Mse*I	(PCR)	–	–	67	33	45	5′ flank	Winship & Peake 1991

[1] White European/North American population unless otherwise stated; [2] American Black population.

Since the complete DNA sequence of the factor IX gene has been reported, PCR-based RFLP analysis can be readily established for all the intragenic polymorphisms. Examples of these are given in Table 37.6. Bowen et al (1991) have combined three of these polymorphisms (for *Taq*I, *Xmn*I and *Dde*I) into a multiplex PCR reaction allowing for the rapid assessment of these three polymorphisms in one amplification reaction.

Linkage disequilibrium between several of the factor IX gene RFLPs has been assessed by Winship et al (1984).

Table 37.5 Factor IX gene polymorphisms: ethnic variations

	Polymorphisms (heterozygosity %)									
Ethnic group	*Taq*I	*Xmn*I	*Dde*I	*Msp*I	*BamH*I	*BamH*I	*Mnl*I	*Hha*I	*Mse*I	*Sst*I[1]
White European and North American	43[a]	37[a]	36[a]	36[a]	0–13[b,i,d]	0[b]	43[a]	50[d]	44[k]	49[j]
American Blacks	18–27[b,c,d]	8–21[b,c,d]	45[b]	48–50[b,g]	33–50[b,d,g]	23[b]	21[2,b,d]	49[d]	u	u
Asian Indian	0–16[c,d,e]	0–11[c,d,e]	u	0[g]	0[g]	u	0–8[c,d]	30[d]	u	u
Chinese	2–6[c,d]	8[c,d]	u	u	0[d]	u	6[d]	30[d]	u	u
Japanese	0[h]	0[h]	0[h]	u	u	u	u	u	u	50[j]
Malay	2[c,d]	0[c,d]	u	u	0[d]	u	6[d]	11[d]	u	u
Polynesian	1[f]	0[f]	u	u	u	u	u	u	u	u
Maori	7[f]	6[f]	u	u	u	u	u	u	u	u
Thai	4[l]	4[l]	13[l]	u	u	u	u	u	32[l]	u

u, unknown; [1]DXS99 locus; [2]8% in South African Blacks; [a] Combined data published and unpublished, collected for ISTH SSC factor IX/VIII subcommittee; [b] Driscoll et al 1988; [c] Lubahn et al 1987; [d] Graham et al 1991; [e] Scott et al 1987; [f] Van der Water et al 1991; [g] Cullen et al 1986; [h] Kojima et al 1987; [i] Hay et al 1986; [j] Tanimota et al 1989; [k] Winship and Peake 1991; [l] Chuansumrit et al Personal communication.

Table 37.6 Factor IX gene: PCR-based polymorphism analysis

RFLP	Site	Primers	Fragment (bp)	Digest fragments (bp)	Reference
*Taq*I	Int 4	5′-CTGGAGTATGACTGGCCAATTATCC – 3′ 5′-GGTACACAAGGATTCTAAGGTTG – 3′	163	124 + 39	Bowen et al 1991
*Xmn*I	Int 3	5′-AATCAGAGACTGCTGATTGACTT – 3′ 5′-GAAACAGCCAGATAAAGCCTCCA – 3′	222	154 + 88	Bowen et al 1991
*Dde*I	Int 1	5′-GGGACCACTGTGGTATAATGTGG – 3′ 5′-CTGGAGGATAGATGTCTCTATCTG – 3′	369 or 319		Bowen et al 1991
*Hha*I	3′ flank	5′-ACAGGCACCTGCCATCACTT – 3′ 5′-AGATTTCAAGCTACCAACAT – 3′	230	150 + 80	Winship et al 1989
*BamH*I	5′ flank	not reported	356	216 + 140	Zhang et al 1989
*Mnl*I	Ex 6	5′-GATTTGAAAACTGTCCATGAAAATAAC – 3′ 5′-AAGTACCTGCCAAGGGAATTGACCTGG – 3′	405	126[1] + 120 + 159 (or 279)	Graham et al 1989
*Mse*I	5′ flank	5′-GATAGAGAAACTGGAAGTAGACCC – 3′ 5′-CAATGTATGAGTGGTCCAGTTAGT – 3′	523	57 + 26 (or 83) (184, 73, 54, 50, 42, 37)[1]	Winship & Peake 1991

[1] Invariant band.

Table 37.7 Extragenic/Linked polymorphisms: factor VIII and IX genes

Type	Restriction endonuclease	Probe Southern blot	Alleles (kb) –	Alleles (kb) +	Allelic Frequency[1] –	Allelic Frequency[1] +	Heterozygosity[1] (%)	Locus and linkage	Reference
RFLP	*Bgl*II	DX13	5.8	2.8	50	50	50	DXS15 FVIII	Harper et al ;1984
RFLP	*Msp*I	767	11.8	6.0 + 5.8	86	14	24	DXS115 FVIII	Jedlicka et al 1990
RFLP	*Ace*I	767	9	4	10	90	18	DXS115 FVIII	Jedlicka et al 1990
RFLP	PstI	767	1.8	1.75	77	23	35	DXS115 FVIII	Paterson et al 1989
RFLP	*BstX*1	767	6.4	4.25	86	14	24	DXS115 FVIII	Arveiler et al 1988
VNTR	*Taq*I/*Msp*I	ST14 (or PCR)	(60 bp repeats: 14 alleles)				>70	DXS52 FVIII	Oberle et al 1985 Richards et al 1991
RFLP	*Sst*I	PX58dIIIa	8.8	5.9	57	43	49	DXS99 FIX	Mulligan et al 1987
RFLP	*Taq*I	CX38.1	11.8	1.65(3.9)	85	15	26	DXS102 FIX	Arveiler et al 1988

[1] White European/North American population unless otherwise stated.

Thus for the RFLPs detected by *Taq*I, *Xmn*I and *Dde*I, a theoretical overall heterozygosity rate of 75% calculated from allelic frequency data is replaced by an observed rate of 66%. Taking linkage disequilibrium into account, in white populations the seven RFLPs detected by *Taq*I, *Xmn*I, *Dde*I, *Msp*I, *Hha*I, *Mnl*I and *Mse*I should result in 94% of families being informative. However, using only three polymorphisms (*Mse*I, *Taq*I and *Hha*I) as the initial screen, 84% will already be informative (Winship & Peake 1991). This is because there is complete linkage equilibrium between *Hha*I and both *Taq*I and *Mse*I, and only a low level of disequilibrium between *Mse*I and *Taq*I. This in turn probably results from the fact that these 3 polymorphisms are situated in the 5′ flanking region, the centre of the gene, and in the 3′ flanking region respectively, i.e. with a maximum distance between them.

VON WILLEBRAND'S DISEASE (VWD)

Unlike the haemophilias, vWd is an autosomally inherited disease, generally in a dominant fashion. Recessive disease is seen however and those individuals homozygous or compound heterozygous for this condition are severely affected. The overall size and complexity of the von Willebrand factor (vWf) gene (178 kb with 52 exons) make the identification of gene defects a difficult procedure although some success has been reported (Ch. 35). In practice, in the majority of cases gene tracking using DNA polymorphisms is the only option to confirm inheritance of a defective gene.

A series of polymorphisms have been found within the vWf gene of which 19 are itemized in Table 37.8. All are RFLPs apart from two VNTRs found close together within intron 40. These VNTRs are comprised of the same repeat sequence (ATCT) and are within a BKm type repetitive region of the gene (Mancuso et al 1989). They are by far the most informative single polymorphisms within the gene and are not in linkage disequilibrium. As indicated above, they are readily detectable by PCR amplification of the region of intron 40, and the various alleles can be distinguished by electrophoresis on 6 or 8% polyacrylamide gels and visualization following ethidium bromide staining, under UV light. The first of these VNTRs has been used both in prenatal diagnosis of severe vWd (Peake et al 1990) and in family studies (Standen et al 1990).

Ethnic variations in polymorphism heterozygosity rates within the vWf gene have only been reported, to date, for the *Rsa*I RFLP (Kunkel et al 1990). This RFLP results in an amino acid dimorphism at codon 789 (alanine or threonine) and frequencies range from 46% (Anglo-Americans) to 11% (Chinese).

SUMMARY

This chapter has reviewed the use of DNA polymorphisms and identified those which have been and are being used in family studies in the three most important inherited bleeding disorders, haemophilia A and B and von Willebrand's disease. Throughout the 1980s their use in the haemophilias in particular has provided for the first time precise carrier detection and prenatal diagnosis (based on CVS analysis). The introduction of PCR-based analysis has also considerably simplified the analyses and

Table 37.8 Von Willebrand factor gene: DNA polymorphisms

Type	Restriction endonuclease	Probe Southern blot	Alleles (kb) −	+	Allelic frequency[2] (%) −	+	Heterozygosity	Locus	Reference
RFLP	*Bgl*II	pvWF1100	9	7.4	69	31	43	Intragenic	Verweij et al 1985
RFLP	*BamHI*	pDL34	7.8	7.2	18	82	29	Intragenic	Nishino & Lynch 1986
RFLP	*Xba*I	pvWF1210[1]	6.9	5.2	87	13	23	Intragenic	Quadt et al 1986
RFLP	*Taq*I	vWFcDNA[1]	3.3	2.6	51	49	50	Intragenic	Bernardi et al 1987
RFLP	*Taq*I	"	4.5	2.3	95	5	9	Intragenic	Bernardi et al 1987
RFLP	*Rsa*I	pvWE6[1]	1.0	0.6	22	78	34	Intragenic	Iannuzzi et al 1987
RFLP	*Sac*I	pvWE6[1]	14.2	10.5 + 3.7	62	38	47	Intragenic	Konkle et al 1987
RFLP	*Xba*I	pvWF1100	36	10.5	8	92	15	Intragenic	Lavergne et al 1987
RFLP	*Taq*I	pvWF1PC8	2.3	1.0	24	76	36	Intragenic	Lavergne et al 1988
RFLP	*EcoRI*	pDL34[1]	7.1	5.3	93	7	13	Intragenic	Lindstedt et al 1989
RFLP	*Taq*I	cDNA[1]	2.2	1.0	22	78	34	Intragenic	Marchetti et al 1989
RFLP	*Taq*I	cDNA[1]	1.8	0.7	14	86	24	Intragenic	Marchetti et al 1989
RFLP	*EcoRI*	cDNA[1]	7.0	5.3	86	14	24	Intragenic	Ewerhardt et al 1989
VNTR	(8 alleles: ATCT repeat: PCR detection)						>75	Intron 40	Peake et al 1990
VNTR	(6 alleles: ATCT repeat: PCR detection)						–	Intron 40	Ploos van Amstel & Reitsma 1990
RFLP	*Stu*I	pvWH22[1]	5.6	4.8	30	70	42	Intragenic	Inbal and Handin 1990
RFLP	*Stu*I	pvWH22[1]	3.8	3.3	60	40	48	Intragenic	Inbal and Handin 1990
RFLP	*Rsa*I	(PCR)			35	65	46	Codon 789 (Thr/Ala)	Kunkel et al 1990
RFLP	*Kpn*I	cDNA[1]	9.0	4.0	44	56	49	Intragenic	Driscoll et al 1990

[1] Derived from this clone -see reference; [2] White European/North American population.

reduced the time required to produce a result. Although polymorphism-based gene tracking is not possible in all cases due to lack of essential family members, questions of paternity, lack of an informative polymorphism and the high incidence of 'new' mutations, it is still an important technique.

The rapid technical advances in recent years in DNA sequence analysis now allows for the detection of the precise DNA defect in many of the smaller genes and this is now possible for the factor IX gene (haemophilia B). Further rapid advances in this area are to be expected and in many countries these procedures will become standard practice. However the application of polymorphism analysis, with its universal applicability in all cases irrespective of the structural gene defect itself, will no doubt continue to be an important procedure in genetic studies in these bleeding disorders which are equally prevalent throughout all countries of the world.

REFERENCES

Ahrens P, Kruse T A, Schwartz M, Rasmussen P B, Din N 1987 A new HindIII restriction fragment length polymorphism in the haemophilia A locus. Human Genetics 76: 127–128

Antonarakis S E, Waber P G, Kittur S D et al 1985 Hemophilia A: Detection of molecular defects and of carriers by DNA analysis. New England Journal of Medicine 313: 842–848

Arveiler B, Oberle I, Vincent A, Hofker M H, Pearson P L, Mandel J L 1988 Genetic mapping of the Xq27-q28 region: New RFLP markers useful for diagnosis applications in fragile-X and haemophilia B families. American Journal of Human Genetics 42: 380–389

Bernardi F, Marchetti G, Bertagnolo V, Faggioli L, Del Senno L 1987 Two TaqI RFLPs in the human von Willebrand Factor gene. Nucleic Acids Research 15: 1347

Bowen D J, Thomas P, Webb C E, Bignell P, Peake I R, Bloom A L 1991 Facile and rapid analysis of the DNA polymorphisms within the human factor IX gene using the polymerase chain reaction. British Journal of Haematology 17: 559-560

Camerino G, Oberle I, Drayna O, Manel J L 1985 A new MspI restriction fragment length polymorphism within the haemophilia B locus. Human Genetics 71: 79–81

Chan V, Chan T K, Lui V W S, Wong A C K 1988 Restriction fragment length polymorphisms associated with factor VIII:C gene in Chinese. Human Genetics 79: 128–131

Chan V, Tong T M F, Chan T P T et al 1989 Multiple XbaI polymorphisms for carrier detection and prenatal diagnosis of haemophilia A. British Journal of Haematology 73: 497–500

Chuansumrit et al 1992 Personal communication

Cullen C R, Hubberman P, Kaslow D C, Migeon B R 1986 Comparison of factor IX methylation on human active and inactive X-chromosomes: implications for X inactivation and transcription of tissue-specific genes. European Molecular Biology Organisation Journal 5: 2223–2229

Driscoll M C, Dispenzieri A, Tobias E, Miller C H, Aledort L M 1988 A second BamHI DNA polymorphism and haplotype association in the factor IX gene. Blood 72: 61–65

Driscoll M C, Chui C, Hilgartner M W 1990 A KpnI DNA polymorphism in the human von Willebrand factor (vWF) gene. Nucleic Acids Research 18: 4962

Ewerhardt B, Ludwig M, Schwaab R, Schneppenheim R, Olek K 1989 An EcoRI polymorphism in the human von Willebrand factor (vWF) gene. Nucleic Acids Research 17: 5416

Giannelli F, Anson D S, Choo K H et al 1984 Characterisation and use of an intragenic polymorphic marker for detection of carriers of haemophilia B (factor IX deficiency). Lancet i: 239-241

Giannelli F, Green P M, High K A et al 1991 Haemophilia B database of point mutations and short additions and deletions — second edition. Nucleic Acids Research 19: 2193–2220

Gitschier J, Drayna D, Tuddenham E G D, White R L, Lawn R 1985 A BclI polymorphism in the factor VIII gene enables genetic mapping diagnosis of haemophilia A. Nature 314: 730–734

Graham J B, Kunkel G R, Tennyson G S, Lord S T, Foulkes D N 1989 The Malmo polymorphism of factor IX: Establishing the genotypes by rapid analysis of DNA. Blood 73: 2104–2107

Graham J B, Kunkel G R, Fowlkes D N, Lord S T 1990 The utility of a HindIII polymorphism of factor VIII examined by rapid DNA analysis. British Journal of Haematology 76: 75–79

Graham J B, Kunkel G R, Egilmez N K, Wallmark A, Fowlkes D M, Lord S T 1991 The varying frequences of five DNA polymorphisms of X-linked coagulant factor IX in eight groups. American Journal of Human Genetics (in press)

Harper K, Pembrey M E, Winter R M, Hartley D, Tuddenham E G D 1984 A clinically useful DNA probe closely linked to haemophilia A. Lancet ii: 6–8

Hay C W, Robertson K A, Young S-L, Thompson A R, Growe G H, MacGillivray R T A 1986 Use of a BamHI polymorphism in the factor IX gene for the determination of hemophilia B carrier status. Blood 67: 1508–1511

Iannuzzi M C, Konkle B A, Ginsburg D, Collins F S 1987 RsaI RFLP in the human von Willebrand factor gene. Nucleic Acids Research 15: 5909

Inaba H, Fujimaki M, Kazazian H H, Antonarakis S E 1990 MspI polymorphism site in intron 22 of the factor VIII gene in the Japanese population. Human Genetics 84: 214–215

Inbal A, Handin R I 1990 StuI polymorphisms in the vWF gene. Nucleic Acids Research 18: 4959

Jedlicka P, Greer S, Millar D S et al 1990 Improved carrier detection of haemophilia A using novel RFLPs at the DXS115 (767) locus. Human Genetics 85: 315–318

Jefferies A J, Wilson V, Thein S L 1985 Hypervariable minisatellite regions in human DNA. Nature 314: 67–69

Kenwick S, Bridge P, Lillicrap D, Lehesjoki A E, Bainton J, Gitschier J 1991 A TaqI polymorphism adjacent to the factor VIII gene (F8C). Nucleic Acids Research 19: 2513

Kogan S C, Doherty N, Gitschier J 1987 An improved method for prenatal diagnosis of genetic diseases by analysis of amplified DNA sequences: Application to hemophilia A. New England Journal of Medicine 317: 985–990

Kogan S C, Gitschier J 1988 Detection of hemophilia A mutations near the acidic region of factor VIII by DNA amplification and denaturing gel electrophoresis. Blood 72: 300a

Kojima T, Tanimoto M, Kamiya T et al 1987 Possible absence of common polymorphisms in coagulation factor IX gene in Japanese subjects. Blood 69: 349–352

Konkle B A, Kim S, Iannuzzi M C, Alani R, Collins F S, Ginsburg D 1987 SacI RFLP in the human von Willebrand factor gene. Nucleic Acids Research 15: 6766

Kunkel G R, Graham J B, Fowlkes D M, Lord S T 1990 RsaI polymorphism in von Willebrand factor (vWF) at codon 789. Nucleic Acids Research 18: 4961

Lalloz M R A, McVey H H, Pattinson J K, Tuddenham E G D 1991 Haemophilia A diagnosis by analysis of a hypervariable dinucleotide repeat within the human factor VIII gene. Lancet ii: 207–211

Lavergne J M, Bahnak B R, Verveij C L, Pannekoek H, Meyer D 1987 A second XbaI polymorphic site within the human von Willebrand factor (vWF) gene. Nucleic Acids Research 15: 9099

Lavergne J M, Bahnak B R, Assouline Z et al 1988 A TaqI polymorphism in the 5′ region of the von Willebrand factor (vWF) gene. Nucleic Acids Research 16: 2742

Linstedt M, Anvret M 1989 An EcoRI polymorphism of the human von Willebrand factor cDNA (vWF). Nucleic Acids Research 17: 2882

Lubahn D B, Lord S T, Bosco J et al 1987 Population genetics of coagulation factor IX: Frequencies of two DNA polymorphisms in five ethnic groups. American Journal of Human Genetics 40: 527–536

Mancuso D J, Tuley E A, Westfield L A et al 1989 Structure of the gene for human von Willebrand factor. Journal of Biological Chemistry 264: 19514–19527

Marchetti G, Sacchi E, Patracchini P, Randi A M, Sampietro M, Bernardi F 1989 Two additional TaqI RFLPs in von Willebrand factor gene (vWF) and pseudogene. Nucleic Acids Research 17: 3229

Mulligan L, Holden J J A, White B N 1987 A DNA marker closely linked to the factor IX (haemophilia B) gene. Human Genetics 75: 381–383

Newton C R, Graham A, Heptinstall L E et al 1989 Analysis of any point mutation in DNA. The amplification refractory mutation system. Nucleic Acids Research 17: 2503–2516

Nishino K, Lynch D C 1986 A polymorphism of the human von Willebrand factor (vWF) gene with BamHI. Nucleic Acids Research 14: 4697

Oberle I, Camerino G, Heilig R 1985 Genetic screening for hemophilia A (classic hemophilia) with a polymorphic probe. New England Journal of Medicine 312: 682–686

Paterson M N, Gitschier J, Bloomfield J et al 1989 An intronic region within the human factor VIII gene is duplicated within Xq29 and is homologous to the polymorphic locus DXS115 (767). American Journal of Human Genetics 44: 679–685

Peake I R, Bowen D, Bignell P et al 1990 Family studies and prenatal diagnosis in severe von Willebrand's disease by polymerase chain reaction amplification of a variable number tandem repeat region of the von Willebrand factor gene. Blood 76: 555–561

Ploos van Amstel H K, Reitsma P H 1990 Tetranucleotide repeat polymorphisms in the vWF gene. Nucleic Acids Research 18: 4957

Quadt R, Verweij C L, de Vries C J M, Briet E, Pannekoek H 1986 A polymorphic XbaI within the human von Willebrand factor (vWF) gene identified by a vWF cDNA clone. Nucleic Acids Research 14: 7139

Richards B, Heilig R, Oberle I, Storjohann L, Horn G T 1991 Rapid PCR analysis of the ST14 (DXS52) VNTR. Nucleic Acids Research 91: 1944

Saiki R K, Gelfand D H, Stoffel S et al 1988 Primer-directed enzymatic amplification of DNA with a thermostable DNA polymerase. Science 239: 487–491

Sampietro M, Yang Y Y, Sacchi E, Mannucci P M 1990 Restriction of polymerase chain reaction products for carrier detection and prenatal diagnosis of haemophilia A: description of an internal control. Thrombosis and Haemostasis 63: 527–528

Scott C R, Chen S H, Schoof J, Kurachi K 1987 Hemophilia B: population differences in RFLP frequencies useful for carrier detection. American Journal of Human Genetics 41: A262 (suppl)

Standen G R, Bignell P, Bowen D J, Peake I R, Bloom A L 1990 Family studies in von Willebrands disease by analysis of restriction fragment length polymorphisms and an intragenic variable number tandem repeat (VNTR) sequence. British Journal of Haematology 76: 242–249

Suehiro K, Tanimoto M, Hamaguchi M et al 1988 Carrier detection in Japanese hemophilia A by use of three intragenic and two extragenic Factor VIII probes: A study of 24 kindreds. Journal of Laboratory Clinical Medicine 112: 314–318

Tanimoto A, Kojima T, Ogata K et at 1989 Extragenic factor IX gene RFLP is useful for detecting carriers of Japanese haemophilia B. Acta Haematology 52: 92–95

Thompson A R, Chen S H, Smith K J 1988 Diagnostic role of an immunoassay detected polymorphism of factor IX for potential carriers of hemophilia B. Blood 72: 1633–1638

Tuddenham E G D, Cooper D N, Gitschier J et al 1991 Haemophilia A database of nucleotide substitutions, deletions, insertions and rearrangements of the factor VIII gene. Nucleic Acids Research 19: 4821–4833

Van Der Water N S, Ridgway D, Ockelford P A 1991 Restriction fragment length polymorphisms associated with the factor VIII and factor IX genes in Polynesians. Journal of Medical Genetics 28: 171–176

Verweij C L, Hofker M, Quadt R, Briet E, Pannekoek H 1985 RFLP for a human von Willebrand factor (vWF) cDNA clone, pvWF1100. Nucleic Acids Research 13: 8289

Winship P R, Brownlee G G 1986 Diagnosis of haemophilia B carriers using intragenic oligonucleotide probes. Lancet ii: 218–219

Winship P R, Peake I R 1991 A clinically useful RFLP in the 5′ flanking region of the factor IX gene. Proceedings British Society for Haemostasis and Thrombosis, September, London.

Winship P R, Anson D S, Rizza C R, Brownlee G G 1984 Carrier detection in haemophilia B using two further intragenic restriction fragment length polymorphisms. Nucleic Acids Research 12: 8861–8872

Winship P R, Rees D J G, Alkan M 1989 Detecting polymorphisms at CpG dinucleotides using the polymerase chain reaction procedure: Application to the diagnosis of haemophilia B carriers. Lancet i: 631–634

Wion K L, Tuddenham E G D, Law R M 1986 A new polymorphism in the factor VIII gene for prenatal diagnosis of hemophilia A. Nucleic Acids Research 14: 4535–4542

Youssofian H, Phillips D E, Kazazian H H, Antonarakis S E 1987 MspI polymorphism in the 3′ flanking region of the human factor VIII gene. Nucleic Acids Research 15: 6312

Zhang M, Chen S-H, Scott C R, Thompson A R 1989 The factor IX BamHI polymorphism: CpG transversion at the nucleotide sequence -561. Human Genetics 82: 283–284

38. The management of patients with inherited blood coagulation disorders

A. L. Bloom

It has often been emphasized that successful management of patients with inherited disorders of blood coagulation is heavily dependent on obtaining normal or reasonably normal circulating levels of the biological activity of the appropriate coagulation factor, thereby correcting defective haemostasis. However it must be realized that coagulation factor replacement is not the be all and end all of patient management. As more refined and purified coagulation factor replacement becomes available, true prophylactic therapy will be more easily achieved but this or somatic gene therapy is still some way off and many problems remain to be solved or managed. Locomotor or other lesions can progress even with effective factor replacement and inhibitor development and resistance to treatment, dental and general surgery, problems of viral infections, their sequelae and prevention, as well as genetic investigation and specialized counselling and a host of general problems face the haemophilia practitioner. Haemophilia management is not just a matter of factor replacement but must encompass and co-ordinate all these aspects. Comprehensive haemophilia diagnostic, treatment and management centres remain as necessary as ever and will do so for the foreseeable future.

It is the object of this chapter to review these aspects of haemophilia management commencing with the principles of factor replacement and the nature of factor concentrates and progressing to the management of individual types of bleeding and to the more general aspects of haemophilia care.

PRINCIPLES OF COAGULATION FACTOR REPLACEMENT

Coagulation factor deficiencies reflect different types of gene defects. Where the genetic lesion is severe, such as deletion or frame shift, mRNA is not produced and severe cross-reacting material negative (CRM^-) deficiency results. Less severe genetic lesions from, for instance, point mutations which are not critically located result in secretion of CRM^+ protein with reduced biological activity. The phenotypic expression also depends on the inheritance pattern. Men with haemophilia A and B are hemizygous and the gene defect if inherited will be fully expressed. This must be distinguished from the severity of the coagulation defect since this can be mild or severe. In the autosomal disorders, severity depends not only upon the nature of the genetic lesion but also on hetero- or homozygosity. A severe gene defect can be dominantly or recessively inherited and this will influence the clinical expression. The net results are greater or lesser deficiencies of clotting factor activity but there is no evidence in most cases of haemophilia A and B that the CRM^+ protein, if present, modifies the haemostatic action of transfused normal factor. The aim of replacement therapy is thus to raise the level of the patient's clotting factor activity (hereinafter called the 'factor level') to one that will bring about haemostatis and to maintain it until healing is substantially complete. If the initiation of effective treatment is delayed, wound healing may be interrupted, the wound may disrupt and more treatment than usual will be required.

The basic principles of replacement therapy are similar for deficiencies of any of the coagulation factors but the main experience is with haemophilia A, B and von Willebrand's disease (vWD). The amount of treatment depends upon the plasma concentration of the coagulation factor needed for haemostatis, the recovery in blood and the half life of the transfused material, in other words the conventional pharmacokinetics, but this is complicated in the case of vWD since transfused von Willebrand factor (vWF) interacts with endogenous vWF and also stabilizes factor VIII. The relevant properties of the other coagulation factors in concentrates when transfused are shown in Table 38.1 and these should be considered in planning replacement therapy.

COAGULATION FACTOR REPLACEMENT

Haemophilia A and B

As commented on above, haemophilia occurs in all degrees of severity. The patient with no detectable factor

Table 38.1 Properties of blood clotting factors in vivo

Factor	Plasma concentration required for normal haemostasis (u or iu/dl ≡ %)	Half life after transfusion	Recovery in blood (% amount infused)
I	100 mg/dl	4–6 days	50
II	40	3 days	40–50
V	15	12 h	80
VII	10	4–6 h	70–80
VIII	> 30	≈ 12 h	80–100
IX	> 30	≈ 18 h	≈ 40
X	≈ 15	24 h	50
XI	30	2 days	90–100
XII	–	–	–
XII	1–5	7 days	?

Modified from Rizza & Jones 1987.

Table 38.2 Severity of haemophilia related to factor VIII or IX levels

Severity	Factor Level (%)	Type of presentation
Severe	0–1	Apparently spontaneous bleeds. Severe bleeding
Moderate	2–5	Few bleeds. Haemarthroses mainly traumatic
Mild	5–30	Post-traumatic, post-surgical, post-dental extraction bleeding. Few episodes

Table 38.3 Approximate levels of factor VIII or IX required for haemostasis in different lesions

Lesion	Plasma concentration of factor (iu/dl) VIII	IX	Initial dose (iu/kg body weight) VIII	IX
Minor spontaneous haemarthrosis:				
home treatment	30	20	15	20
hospital treatment	40	30	20	30
Severe haemarthrosis:				
Minor surgery	60	55	30	45
Major surgery	100	80	45	70

VIII (or IX) is usually severely affected and bleeds into muscles and joints on minimal trauma and sometimes apparently spontaneously (Table 38.2). A small amount of factor VIII (or IX) gives considerable protection so that patients with 2–5% of factor VIII usually suffer only post-traumatic bleeding and less severe bleeding into muscles and joints etc. and are often said to be moderately affected. Patients with over 5% of factor VIII usually bleed only after significant trauma or surgery and are said to be mildly affected. It must be realised that this classification of bleeding does not always hold good. Some patients with very low factor VIII levels rarely bleed whilst others even with over 5% factor VIII may bleed repeatedly into a 'target joint' damaged originally by a traumatic haemarthrosis and appear to be 'severely' affected. As a generalization however, bleeding symptoms are less obvious with higher factor levels so that abnormal bleeding does not usually occur at factor VIII levels over 35–40%. Rather lower levels of factor IX seem to be adequate to control haemostasis but this is a generalization that does not always hold good. The general correlation between factor levels and symptoms in haemophilia A and B is shown in Table 38.2. Experience over many years of transfusing factor VIII to patients who are bleeding or undergoing dental extraction or surgery have confirmed that if factor VIII levels are maintained over 30–40% until healing is complete then normal haemostasis is usually maintained. However other considerations are also important. Movement of the affected part such as a haemarthrosis, coughing or walking after abdominal surgery may promote bleeding. Physiotherapy or manipulation may require rather higher levels whilst immobilization of mild lesions may allow control of bleeding with relatively modest factor levels. The increased availability of concentrates has allowed safer and more liberal replacement therapy. Approximate target levels which can be aimed for in various situations and the doses of concentrate needed are shown in Table 38.3. Recovery of factor VIII after infusion, approaches or equals 100%. Recovery of factor IX in haemophilia B is very much lower, about 30–50%. The exact reason for this is not known but it may be due to a combination of binding to endothelial receptors (Stern et al 1983) and extravascular loss.

In calculating the dose of factor needed, various formulae have been used (see Rizza & Jones 1987) but it must be realised that these give only approximate estimations. It is always better to err on the side of higher doses than risk re-bleeding. Older factor IX concentrates also contained factors X and II with or without significant factor VII. Prothrombin, in particular has a long half life and dangerously high levels can result from over-enthusiastic treatment. Highly purified preparations of factor IX are now becoming available and these should be safer.

As a rule of thumb an approximate estimate of plasma volume can be determined empirically by determining the weight in kilograms and multiplying this by 41. A dose of factor VIII concentrate equivalent to the plasma volume in units will generally give a plasma concentration of about 100 u/dl (100%) since one international unit is approximately equivalent to the activity of 1 ml of fresh human plasma. Subsequent doses can be modified according to requirements.

With regard to factor IX the calculation is rather more speculative, partly because the international factor IX standard unit has varied over the years and is no longer equivalent to that in 1 ml of plasma but is equivalent to that contained in about 1.2 ml plasma. Furthermore in vivo recovery is reduced compared to that of factor VIII to 30–50%. Thus for a 70 kg man the expected plasma volume would be 70 × 41 ml = 3000 ml (approximately) and a dose of factor VIII of 3000 u would be expected to produce a rise of plasma factor VIII to approximately 100% or in the case of factor IX to about 50%. The response to the initial dose of factor VIII or IX tends to be lower than subsequent doses (in a course) because of equilibration with extravascular factor or because of utilization in the case of factor VIII or due, hypothetically, to binding to the vascular endothelium in the case of factor IX. Doses subsequent to the first one can be adjusted to the required intensity of treatment. Theoretically since the fall of factor activity after infusion is exponential the most effective and economic way of delivering treatment would be by continuous infusion to maintain the lowest haemostatic level required. However certain technical problems may render this form of therapy difficult especially the promotion of venous thrombosis in the vein draining the catheter. As a practical compromise the author tends to administer factor VIII therapy as needed in divided doses often morning and evening in order to prevent the risk of bleeding overnight. Factor IX levels can be more easily maintained on a once a day infusion regime because of the longer half life of factor IX.

Therapeutic Materials

Although the use of fresh frozen plasma was a notable advance in therapy, it was soon realised that in order to avoid circulatory overload a concentrated form of factor VIII or IX would be needed. Crude concentrates produced by Cohn fractionation, alcohol and ether precipitation, became available yet supplies were limited and potency low. Early preparations of animal factor VIII were pioneered in Oxford by Macfarlane's group. Reactions, thrombocytopenia due to von Willebrand factor (vWF) analogue and immunological resistance, limited the value of the original animal concentrate but it allowed operative treatment to be relatively safely performed. Judith Pool's development of cryoprecipitate (Pool & Shannon 1965) marked a turning point in haemophilia management. It not only allowed efficient on-demand therapy but formed the starting point for the development of high potency freeze-dried concentrates for home treatment and comprehensive care. Of course the economic and practical need for large plasma pools to prepare these and more sophisticated concentrates has led to virus complications, but with efficient partition and sterilization processes we are at last emerging from this decade of concentrate-transmitted HIV and hepatitis and setting new targets. At the same time the spread of these infections in the general population and potentially in blood donors has led to the abandonment of untreated frozen plasma and cryoprecipitate as a treatment modality except in situations where the viral safety of these products can be guaranteed with reference to the lesions treated. In the United Kingdom and most parts of North America and Western Europe, plasma and cryoprecipitates have been abandoned for the treatment of haemophilia and readers wishing details of these materials are referred to earlier editions of this book. It must be realised that donors tested for HIV antibody and found to be negative theoretically can still be infected since there is a 'window' between infection and seroconversion during which time viral transmission can occur. Similar considerations may be relevant in the case of non A non B hepatitis (hepatitis C). The older concentrates of factor VIII were well reviewed by Roberts & Macik (1987) and the general features of blood infectivity were described. An up-to-date classification of factor VIII concentrates is given in Table 38.4 which is adapted from Bloom (1991) but this is a developing subject which will

Table 38.4 Factor VIII concentrates

Type	Names	Production	Sterilization method	Specific activity (u/mg)
Crude	–	Cryoprecipitate Cryo-ethanol precipitation	none or SD	0.1–0.9
Intermediate	8Y (BPL)		Dry heat (80°C–72 h)	
	Profilate SD (Alpha)	Various, PEG – amino acid	SD	
	Hemate P (Behring)	ppt, chromatography, etc.	Wet pasteurization	
	Beriate P (Behring) (reduced vWF)		Wet pasteurization	up to 10
	Kryobulin (Immuno)		Vapour heat	
'High' purity	FVIII: CP high purity (Behring)	Precipitation and ion-exchange glucose/saccharose stabilization	Wet pasteurization	25
	Octa VI (Octapharma)	Chromatography	SD	
	FVIII VHP (Biotransfusion)	Chromatography	SD	up to 250
	Monoclate P(Armour)	Immunoaffinity on monoclonal	Pasteurization	15 (diluted from
	Hemofil M (Baxter)	antibodies	SD	3000 with albumin)
	8SM (BPL)		SD	
	Recombinate (Baxter)	Recombinant technology	Aseptic technology	15 (diluted from
	Kogenate (Cutter)	Recombinant technology	SD	3000 with albumin)

SD, solvent/detergent.

no doubt change very rapidly. Crude concentrates such as freeze-dried cryoprecipitates or cryo-alcohol precipitated factor VIII really represent other plasma proteins especially fibrinogen and fibronectin more or less contaminated with factor VIII. Specific activities range from 0.1 to 1 u/mg. This type of concentrate is no longer produced by commercial suppliers but is still produced by some voluntary or national organisations. Single donor cryoprecipitate is not amenable to sterilization and is no longer used in the United Kingdom. Intermediate purity concentrates have specific activities of 1–10 u/mg and are produced by various chromatographic and precipitation techniques. High purity concentrates are of two types. Those produced by more conventional chromatographic techniques have specific activities of up to 250 u/mg but still contain many plasma proteins albeit in very low concentration compared to intermediate concentrates. The second type of high purity concentrate is produced by immunoaffinity purification on immobilized monoclonal antibodies either to factor VIII or to von Willebrand factor with subsequent elution or dissociation and further chromatographic purification. Theoretically these 'monoclonally purified' concentrates have specific activity of 3000 u/mg, i.e. approaching the theoretical maximum but in practice for pharmaceutical reasons and stability they are diluted in human albumin so that the final specific activity is about 15 u/mg. The high purity concentrates have less contaminating proteins than the previously described preparations but it should be noted that albumin may contain low concentrations of several other human proteins and murine proteins from the monoclonal antibodies may be present in minute amounts. Similar principles apply to recombinant factor VIII. It should also be noted that the monoclonally purified and recombinant concentrates contain virtually no vWF but significant and therapeutically useful amounts are present in crude and in some intermediate factor VIII concentrates and at least one high purity concentrate of vWF has been prepared. These will be discussed below (p. 903).

Virucidal Processes

The realisation that blood and blood products transmitted infectious diseases has led to the development of virucidal processes to sterilize factor concentrates. These were originally developed for hepatitis viruses but were found to be effective against the human immunodeficiency viruses (HIV) (Levy et al 1984).

Although albumin has been successfully sterilized by a form of pasteurization in aqueous solution and has been in clinical use for over 40 years with a good safety record, extension of this technique to coagulation factor concentrates proved to be more difficult because of their heat-lability. Moreover addition of various stabilizers tends also to stabilize viruses.

A pasteurized factor VIII concentrate was developed by 1981 (Heimberger et al 1981), but supplies were restricted to the German domestic market. In any case the yield of factor VIII at that time was unacceptably low. Also, in retrospect, adequate clinical evidence of sterilization of hepatitis viruses and in due course HIV was not available although subsequent evidence suggests that the process was effective (Schimpf et al 1987, 1989, Mannucci et al 1990b). Also available in Germany at that time was a preparation of factor IX concentrate sterilized by β-propiolactone and ultraviolet light (Heinrich et al 1982). Recent evidence has thrown doubt on the effectiveness and consistency of this process (Kleim et al 1990) and it has appeared occasionally to transmit HIV. Apart from these preparations, other first generation concentrates included those dry-heated at 60–80°C for periods of time varying between 24 and 72 hours. Second generation concentrates were heated in water vapour under pressure or in organic solvent to dissolve lipid viral envelopes. An extension of the latter principle, but not involving heat, is the use of organic solvent such as tri(n-butyl)phosphate (TNBP) and a detergent such as sodium cholate or 'Tween' 80 (Prince et al 1986). These cold methods have the advantage of high yield of factors VIII or IX. In the United Kingdom, dry heat at high temperatures (80°C) for 72 hours has been remarkably successful with no apparent failure and high yield for intermediate grade concentrates sterilized in this way. An advantage of this method is that the individual vials are endsterilized thus reducing the risk from in-process contamination or cross-contamination but the solvent-detergent method has also been remarkably successful.

The effectiveness of these processes has been the subject of many reports. Until very recently one problem in assessing non A non B (NANB) hepatitis has been the lack of markers of infection which necessitated the detection of raised transaminases in previously unexposed patients as an indication of infection. Hanley & Lippman-Hand (1983) described the 'rule of three' to give a statistical assessment of the risk if all tests remain negative and Mannucci & Columbo (1989), applying this to haemophilia, re-emphasized the strict requirements of clinical trials for these products but it is to be hoped that with the development of serological tests for hepatitis C these requirements may be somewhat relaxed (Mannucci et al 1990b). Table 38.5 summarizes the broad significance of virucidal processes and the status of various types of concentrates. Immunoaffinity processes alone are not sufficient to remove viruses entirely and effective sterilization processes are needed especially as volume scale up occurs to meet increasing requirements. Care must be taken also in extrapolating information obtained with one product to similar sterilization processes which may be used during the course of production of another. Subtle differences may be present which could modify the virucidal effects.

Table 38.5 Viral inactivation processes and the status of factor concentrates

Viral inactivation method	Clinical safety HCV	HBV	HIV
Dry heat 60–68°C, 24–72 h	Ineffective	Partially effective	Effective
Heptane suspension 60°C, 20 h	Partially effective	Effective	Effective
Vapour-treated	Effective	Some transmission	Effective
Wet pasteurized	Effective	Occasional transmission reported	Effective
Dry heat 80°C, 72 h	Effective	*	Effective
Solvent-detergent	Effective	*	Effective
Monoclonal + dry heat	Partially effective	*	Effective
Monoclonal pasteurized	Effective	*	Effective
Monoclonal SD	Effective	*	Effective

* probably effective but patients vaccinated.

Important advances are occurring in the testing for exposure of donors and patients to hepatitis viruses and in the treatment of acute and chronic hepatitis in patients with haemophilia. These important aspects of haemophilia therapy are considered in more detail in Chapter 34.

With regard to HIV, most virucidal processes used at present seem to be effective but dry heat at only 60°C for 30 hours has been associated with several seroconversions, a handful of cases have been associated with other heat-treated products (MMWR 1988) and as stated above sterilization with β-propiolactone and UV light has also failed on at least one occasion. It remains to be seen if more recent techniques such as PCR for integrated DNA and transcribed viral RNA will be of value in excluding more HIV-infected donors (Loche & Mach 1988, Gibbons et al 1990, Dannatt et al 1992). The relative risk of donor infection in various populations must also be considered. It has been estimated that by 1991, 50% of lots of factor VIII concentrate in the USA could be considered to be infected with HIV (before sterilization) whereas only 1% of lots in the UK could be similarly considered (Bloom 1991) Clinical assessment of seroconversion must take this into account and it is unlikely that any method of sterilization will be 100% foolproof for each vial all of the time. It is important therefore to counsel patients accordingly without frightening them and to include serological tests for HIV and hepatitis in routine follow-up protocols.

Parvovirus. There is evidence that this virus may contaminate blood products. Parvovirus B19 is a very heat-resistant organism at temperatures up to 120°C and is apparently not sensitive to solvent-detergent. There is clinical evidence that a factor IX concentrate dry-heated at 80°C for 72 hours transmitted the virus (Lyon et al 1989). The clinical sequelae of B19 infection include erythema infectiosum, aplastic crisis and aplastic anaemia, arthropathy and fetal infection and hydrops fetalis. The virus is not only transmitted parenterally but more typically via the respiratory tract as well as by nosocomial contact.

Factor VIII concentrate and immune modulation

The problems of immunity and HIV in haemophilia will be discussed in Chapter 40 but it is important to consider here some of the immunological features of various concentrates since they impact on haemophilia therapy. It has been suggested that crude, and even newer, intermediate purity factor VIII concentrates down-regulate immune function in haemophilia irrespective and independently of HIV infection (Madhok et al 1986). This has been presumed to be due to the effect of impurities other than factor VIII. The immunological changes which have been observed are summarized in Table 38.6 and the in vitro effects seem to be independent of the method of heat sterilization used (Thorpe et al 1989). The clinical significance of these observations is open to debate. Clinical immune impairment was not a feature of haemophilia during the heyday of therapy with crude concentrates such as cryoprecipitate before the HIV era. On the other hand in the Edinburgh cohort exposed to one lot of factor VIII concentrate infected with HIV, seroconversion was related to pre-existing T4 cell counts and to the amount of concentrate received (Ludlam et al 1985). In a group of children exposed to open tuberculosis in a childrens' ward, those on immunosuppressive therapy or with haemophilia (HIV antibody-negative) contracted the disease (Beddal et al 1985). One explanation that could account for the differential transmission of disease to HIV-negative haemophiliacs in both these series was that they were immunosuppressed by intermediate purity factor VIII concentrates.

Table 38.6 Factor VIII concentrates and immune modulation

In vitro effects on peripheral blood mononuclear cells (PBMC)
Down regulation of Fc receptors
Inhibition of IL2 production
MLR and PHA transformation impaired
Modified T cell activation and receptor expression
In vivo effects in HIV-negative haemophiliacs
Reduction of T4 cells
Reduced production of IFN-gamma by PBMC
Reduced cutaneous hypersensitivity
Clinical evidence
High purity factor VIII stabilizes immune parameters in HIV Ab-positive haemophiliacs?
Low purity factor VIII associated with increased susceptibility to infections in HIV-negative haemophiliacs?

Although these findings suggest that some component of intermediate purity factor VIII concentrate may impair clinical immunity this impairment was not detected in a series of HIV-negative haemophiliacs treated with an intermediate purity concentrate (Evans et al 1991).

The importance of these observations in clinical practice is controversial. Brettler et al (1989) suggested that a high purity monoclonal product stabilized T4 cell counts and skin hypersensitivity tests in HIV-infected patients and similar results have been reported in full (de Biasi et al 1991, Goldsmith et al 1991) or in abstract form (Fukatake et al 1991). Thus although a relationship between high purity concentrates and immunoprotection seems likely, proof is still lacking and will depend on the results of ongoing clinical trials. Nevertheless, haemophiliacs are deficient only in factor VIII (or IX) and the long-term aim must be towards specific replacement or genetic cure.

Factor VIII concentrates and inhibitors

Before discussing recommendations for therapy one more consideration must enter the equation. Recently, concern has been raised regarding the incidence of inhibitors appearing in patients treated with monoclonal purified (Kessler & Sachse 1990, Lusher et al 1990) and recombinant factor VIII products (Schwartz et al 1990). Many of these inhibitors were very mild, did not require cessation of therapy and occurred most frequently in previously unexposed patients, especially children. Further experience is needed to assess this risk but experience does not suggest that this is going to be a problem more severe than that observed with previous intermediate or crude products.

Factor IX concentrates

The general features of treatment of haemophilia B with factor IX concentrates have been touched on above. For the main part the specific treatment of haemophilia B to date has consisted of administration of various types of prothrombin complex concentrates (PCC) which are produced by chromatographic methods. They contain not only factor IX but also other vitamin K-dependent clotting factors. Some, such as PPSB (prothrombin, proconvertin, Stuart factor, antihaemophilic factor B) contained four factors (II, VII, X, IX) whilst others such as BPL 9D do not contain significant factor VII, but a useful factor VII concentrate is a by-product.

One of the problems of these concentrates is that they may result in high levels of circulating prothrombin and contain activated factors such as factor Xa which may render them thrombogenic (Kasper 1975) especially during surgery. This is especially so for orthopaedic surgery of the lower limbs. In order to avoid these complications, factor IX concentrates devoid of other coagulation factors have been prepared either by conventional chromatographic or monoclonal antibody immunoaffinity techniques (Ménaché et al 1984, Burnouf et al 1989, Kim et al 1990) and sterilized by methods similar to those used for factor VIII. These concentrates have specific activity up to 200 u/mg and are much less thrombogenic than the older three or four factor concentrates in in vitro tests and animal models as well as in an in vivo study (Mannucci et al 1990a). There can be little doubt that these concentrates will rapidly replace PCCs for the treatment of haemophilia B.

Other coagulation factor concentrates

Concentrates of factor VII and factor X have been prepared and will be useful for the treatment of rare cases of haemophilia due to deficiency of these factors. Factor VIIa has been prepared chromatographically and by recombinant techniques and its use in the management of patients with inhibitors will be described below (p. 910). Factor XI concentrate is prepared by the Bio Products Laboratory (BPL). This has not yet undergone published clinical trials but is available for compassionate use on a named patient basis. A concentrate of factor XIII has been available for several years and is sterilized by a wet pasteurization process. It is of human placental origin and has been used very successfully for inherited deficiency of this factor (Lorand et al 1980). Concentrates of protein C (Immuno) antithrombin III (BPL) and plasminogen (BPL) are also available but a discussion of these is beyond the scope of this chapter.

Recombinant clotting factors

The current status of haemophilia therapy could shortly be changed by the application of recombinant genetic techniques. Biogenetic expression of factor VIII has been achieved in mammalian, usually hamster, cells (Toole et al 1984, Wood et al 1984). Although coexpression of vWF promoted production, similar promotion has been achieved by other means. However purification using immunoaffinity and conventional chromatography is just as demanding as for plasma factor VIII. Toxicity and animal trials in normal animals and haemophilic dogs have been undertaken. Decay curves and half life ($t_{1/2}$) in haemophilic dogs closely resembled those of plasma-derived (pd) human factor VIII (Giles et al 1988b).

White et al (1989) described two subjects who were successfully treated with rFVIII concentrate and formal clinical trials of rFVIII produced separately by Baxter Health Care and Cutter Biologicals, Miles Inc. are well advanced and results of the latter trial have been published (Schwartz et al 1990, Harrison et al 1991). Clinical and laboratory responses were excellent, and adverse reactions, mild in nature, occurred in only 1% of episodes treated. New inhibitors were uncommon, developing in only one of 85 previously-treated patients. Rather more worrying was the development of inhibitor in five out of 20 previously untreated children and in one child previously treated only with fresh frozen plasma. The inhibitors were usually of low titre and continued treatment was usually possible. The occurrence of inhibitors after use of highly purified factor VIII, whether monoclonally purified or recombinant, is worrying but must be viewed in perspective. The incidence of inhibitors in haemophilia after treatment is generally accepted as being up to about 20% but they have not previously been sought prospectively in such demanding trials. Further experience suggests that they are not observed more frequently than with older concentrates.

Recombinant factor IX poses more difficult problems especially post-translational γ-carboxylation. In addition the normal plasma concentration of factor IX in absolute terms is much higher than that of factor VIII, 5000 ng/ml versus 100–200 ng/ml. Moreover patients with haemophilia B are far less numerous than those with haemophilia A. It remains to be seen if it will be economically viable to produce increased material for fewer patients.

Therapeutic concentrates for von Willebrand's disease

Most patients with von Willebrand's disease (vWD) are heterozygous and much less severely affected than those with severe hemizygous haemophilia A but those with homozygous or compound heterozygous disease can be severely affected.

Until the early 1980s treatment was relatively straight forward. Factor VIII levels seemed to be most important for control of surgical bleeding and although mucous membrane bleeding, epistasis and menorrhagia could be troublesome, most of the crude concentrates and cryoprecipitate then available contained enough high molecular weight vWF to control this type of bleeding and stabilize endogenous factor VIII — the so-called secondary rise. The advent of deamino-D-arginine vasopressin (DDAVP) also promised to be a useful adjunct to treatment. Since then several developments have complicated the issue.

The advent of HIV infection was a considerable stimulus to fractionation technology in order to produce factor VIII products with high specific activity and which could be adequately sterilized. Although donor screening has done much to render single donor cryoprecipitate relatively safe from HIV and hepatitis B, the value of HCV antibody screening remains to be fully assessed. Although sterilization processes are available for freeze-dried cryoprecipitate, in many Western countries the use of single donor frozen cryoprecipitate has been abandoned. At the same time many of the high purity factor VIII concentrates, such as those produced using monoclonal antibodies or sophisticated chromatography, lack vWF. Although it is possible to overemphasize the importance of heterozygous vWD as a therapeutic challenge there is no doubt that a concentrate of vWF would be of considerable assistance in some circumstances and for surgery as well as for the severe type III disease. A commercial, intermediate-purity factor VIII concentrate heat-treated in aqueous solution (Hemate P, Behring) contains a reasonable amount of HMW vWF and is effective (Schmipf et al 1987, Fukui et al 1988, Berntop & Nilsson 1989, Rose et al 1990). Factor VIII 8Y (BPL, UK) is also claimed to be effective (Cumming et al 1990, Pasi et al 1990) but the evidence for this is not convincing. Biotransfusion, the fractionation arm of the French blood transfusion service, has produced a concentrate of vWF and similar concentrates are under study elsewhere (Table 38.7).

Table 38.7 Concentrates for vWD

Concentrate	Comments
Single donor cryoprecipitate	Risk of infections. No longer used in many countries
Intermediate purity factor VIII concentrates	
BPL 8Y (UK)	Most are ineffective
Hemate P (Behringwerke) (Humate P in USA)	Some effect Effective
High purity factor VIII concentrates	Ineffective. Contain little vWF
Concentrates of vWF	
vWF/FVIII VHP (Biotransfusion, France)	50–100 u/mg FVIII and vWF
vWF (Biotransfusion, France)	
von Willebrand factor (Behringwerke)	100 u/mg vWF (little FVIII)

Pharmacological agents for the management of haemophilia

These materials are fully described in Chapter 45 but are put here more into the context of haemophilia and vWD.

Tranexamic acid. This is replacement for the original antifibrinolytic agent ε-aminocaproic acid (EACA). The latter required large doses which sometimes caused gastrointestinal side-effects. Tranexamic acid is administered intravenously or orally. It inhibits the fibrinolytic enzyme plasmin and interferes with its binding to fibrin. Its main use is in combination with factor VIII in oral and dental bleeding (p. 907) since the buccal mucosa has high fibrinolytic potential. It will also be of value in this situation with the new single factor IX high purity concentrates. There is little evidence that tranexamic acid is of significant value in haemophilic bleeding elsewhere and it is contraindicated in upper urinary tract bleeding where consolidated clots may cause colic and obstruction.

D-amino D-arginine vasopressin (DDAVP). This substance was found serendipitously to raise factor VIII levels in normal individuals and in those with mild haemophilia and von Willebrand's disease (Mannucci et al

1977). The primary action may be on release of vWF with stabilization of factor VIII. DDAVP is not active in severe haemophilia and vWD and may act by releasing existing stores. In patients with mild haemophilia administration of DDAVP has an unpredictable, but reasonably constant, effect in individual patients (Rodeghiero et al 1989). In some patients it is virtually ineffective but generally in usual therapeutic doses of 3–4 μg/kg it leads to a 2–3 times rise of factor VIII levels and sometimes rather higher rise in vWD. Except in some patients with severe vWD it also stimulates a rise of plasminogen activator presumably from endothelial cells (Ludlam et al 1980) It is therefore logical but not essential to add tranexamic acid to the regimen.

The demonstration of different types of vWD has clouded the issue regarding the indications for DDAVP. In type I with production of reduced but normal vWF it is likely to be most effective. In type II vWD, other than type IIB where there is production of abnormally polymerized vWF, DDAVP could be expected to be less effective because it may merely raise levels of abnormal vWF. However, DDAVP may partially correct haemostasis via other mechanisms and it may be effective even in type II or type III vWD (Cattaneo et al 1985). In type IIB and pseudo-vWD (platelet-type) its value is more controversial since in these diseases it may cause platelet agglutination and thrombocytopenia. However, the clinical significance of this apparent fall of platelet count is not clear and it is not an absolute contraindication to a trial of DDAVP in an appropriate clinical setting.

Originally DDAVP was promoted as a factor-sparing therapy mainly on economic grounds, but the occurrence of virus infections transmitted by blood products has given it a new lease of life. Nevertheless it has several drawbacks and limitations and it should be remembered that the doses needed to raise factor VIII levels are very much higher than those used for diabetes insipidus (Table 38.8). The induced factor VIII level may have a very short half life and assay control is essential for treatment of significant lesions. The response to DDAVP has been said to wane after a few days — a process known as tachyphylaxis — but recent evidence suggests that this occurs mainly after the first dose and that DDAVP effects on factor VIII are thereafter maintained (Mannucci 1992). Even so the factor VIII levels usually fall below 30 u/dl so that its role in surgery is strictly limited. There are few reports of its safety and efficacy in infants and young children but hyponatraemia and seizures may occur (Smith et al 1989, Weinstein et al 1989). On the positive side, an aerosol preparation at much higher dosage is absorbed via the mucosa and can be useful for the domicilliary treatment of menorrhagia in women with vWD.

Table 38.8 Limitations of DDAVP in haemophilia and vWD

Only of value in mildly-affected patients
Unpredictable effect except by trial
Effect may be temporary (tachyphylaxis) and reduced after the first dose
Flushing, headaches
Osmolality changes after prolonged course
Hyponatraemia and seizures especially in children
Thrombocytopenia in type IIB and pseudo vWD
Myocardial ischaemia (not advised over 40 years of age or with relevant history)

General therapeutic recommendations

Having considered the materials available and their characteristics, it is appropriate to formulate some general principles regarding replacement therapy before going on to describe the management of individual lesions. One must bear in mind that the detailed recommendations are constantly evolving as new materials appear and that they apply mainly to the situation in developed countries. Unfortunately in many countries the health services cannot afford sophisticated therapeutic products. In that case more simple therapeutic measures must be adopted but with the spread of HIV and the prevalence of hepatitis it is inadvisable that non-virucidally-treated blood products are used except in case of life-threatening emergency.

All patients who may possibly require blood products including those with mild haemophilia or vWD should be tested for hepatitis B antibody, immunized as necessary, and the immunization status periodically reviewed. Patients who have mild haemophilia or vWD and who require treatment could with advantage be tested in advance for their response to DDAVP and this drug used if appropriate in order to avoid blood products. With regard to other patients it is the author's practice to offer treatment with high purity concentrates to HIV-positive patients who do or do not have symptoms of HIV infection especially if they have deteriorating markers of infection such as falling T4 cell count or rising levels of β_2-microglobulin.

In HIV-negative individuals, the evidence for adverse and clinically significant immune impairment due to intermediate purity concentrates is much less clear cut. These concentrates are much cheaper than those of high purity and the incidence of inhibitors, especially in children, with the latter is still being assessed. At the present time there seems to be little reason definitely to advise high purity materials for this group but the natural tendency will be towards specific replacement.

For patients with haemophilia B, treatment where possible should be with high purity factor IX concentrate. Where these are not available three or four factor PCC concentrates which have been adequately virucidally treated can be safely used for ordinary non-surgical lesions. Non-urgent especially orthopaedic surgery of the lower limb should be postponed pending attempts to obtain high purity single factor concentrate of factor IX.

THE MANAGEMENT OF SPECIFIC TYPES OF BLEEDING

The general principles of management of specific lesions have changed little since the previous edition of this volume but will be summarized here for completeness.

Acute haemarthroses

Bleeding into joints is the most common feature of severe haemophilia A or B. Prompt and effective treatment is important to ensure resorption of the blood and return of normal joint function. Many haemophiliacs have prodromal symptoms such as generalized sweating, tingling around or within the joint and other symptoms before there are physical signs. An experienced haemophiliac knows when he is bleeding and medical and nursing staff should accept this and not stand on their dignity. Indeed this is the basis of on-demand home therapy. There are four main aims of therapy:

1. To stop bleeding as soon as possible
2. To relieve pain
3. To maintain and restore joint function
4. To prevent the onset of chronic arthropathy.

If adequate replacement therapy is given early enough, all these aims can be achieved even with only one or two treatments. If treatment is delayed, especially if the lesion is due to injury, then immobilization, analgesic drugs and physiotherapy may be required. Aspiration is rarely needed. A single dose of 10–15 u of factor VIII/kg body weight will control most early haemarthroses where there is no significant injury. Most concentrates are supplied in bottles of about 250, 500 and 1000 units and it is convenient to go to the number of bottles of the same batch (lot) nearest to and above the calculated unit requirement. It is almost always better to err on the side of liberal dosage within economic constraints rather than to give too little.

For more severe haemarthroses especially when treatment has been delayed, or in the case of injury, rather larger doses of factor VIII may be needed on successive days. Usually a splint is unnecessary and often not tolerated by the patient. However recurrence of bleeding sometimes occurs at night and a simple foam plastic backslab splint can be of help. At first the limb should be held in the position of rest with no attempt to straighten it until this is painless and comfortable. A further night splint can then be constructed and the patient can save these for future use at home. As the joint recovers, gentle physiotherapy can be constituted such as quadriceps exercises leading to straight leg raising and exercises in the hydrotherapy pool. Physiotherapy is conveniently and more safely given after a dose of factor VIII. This can be in the region of 20 u/kg body weight daily at first, gradually reducing as the joint recovers and muscle power returns. At the same time walking can be gradually allowed and it may be helpful if small doses of factor VIII are continued at home if training in home therapy has been given.

Aspiration of the joint is sometimes recommended. This should only be attempted for tense, very painful joints and should be covered by factor VIII therapy before and for a few days after. It has been suggested that the first dose of factor VIII should be administered as the blood is aspirated in order to limit coagulation within the joint before aspiration. In the author's experience aspiration is rarely if ever needed.

Chronic haemophilic arthropathy

If all joint bleeds are treated promptly as soon as they develop and with adequate replacement then theoretically they should resolve and normal joint function and anatomy should be maintained. This is the aim of modern therapy, home treatment and prophylaxis (p. 909). Unfortunately this counsel of perfection is not always attained. Bleeding may occur at inopportune moments so that treatment is delayed; or the bleeding is due to trauma and resolution is slow. If the blood is not rapidly resorbed chronic inflammation may develop and the presence of fragile intra-articular granulation tissue leads to repeated bleeding and the development of a 'target' joint. This may be a feature even in less severe haemophilia and give a mistaken impression of general severity of the haemophilia. The natural history of a developing chronic haemarthropathy varies. Some joints gradually develop chronic arthropathic changes with muscular wasting and quite severe pain. Others go through a phase of marked synovial thickening with the formation of a 'boggy' joint, usually a knee, and a silent effusion. Pain is then not a feature even when recurrent bleeding occurs. Aspiration often yields thick viscous blood stained synovial fluid but does little to halt the progression of the lesion. Gradually intra-articular adhesions develop, the joint shrinks and, at the end stage, very painful chronic arthropathy results.

Treatment of a boggy almost painless arthropathy is very difficult. Prophylactic factor VIII therapy will often lead to some regression but the lesion then recurs especially if the patient neglects it due to lack of pain. Medical or surgical synovectomy may sometimes be successful. Medical synovectomy involves the intra-articular injection of a sclerosing agent but great care should be taken in HIV-positive individuals in whom there is a raised incidence of septic arthritis.

The final stage of chronic arthropathy becomes mainly an orthopaedic problem. At one time anti-inflammatory drugs were held to be contraindicated in haemophilia and this still applies to aspirin which permanently acetylates platelet cyclo-oxygenase for the platelet life span. The effect of other non-steroidal antiinflammatory drugs (NSAIDS) on the platelets are short acting and more gentle. NSAIDS such as ibuprofen and naproxyn given at the lower end of the usual therapeutic doseages and preferably in enteric-coated form can give considerable relief from pain and early morning stiffness but it is wise to warn patients of the risks of bleeding. The orthopaedic management of chronic haemophilia arthropathy includes physiotherapy, non-surgical methods and appliances and reconstructive surgery.

Physiotherapy. The main aim of physiotherapy is to prevent chronic arthropathy occurring after acute bleeds and to maintain joint and muscle function. It is essential that the physiotherapist is experienced in dealing with haemophilic patients, knows the principles of antihaemophilic therapy and prophylaxis and has a working knowledge of HIV infection. Indeed one of the in-patient functions of the haemophilia centre physiotherapist is to help in the management of chest infections and in obtaining sputum for microbiological diagnosis. In patients with chronic arthropathy there is a limit to what can be achieved by physiotherapy but the physiotherapist can help considerably in maintaining and improving muscle power and joint function by means of graded exercises, appliances such as the Flowtron and graded splints, hydrotherapy and supervising correction of flexion deformities. Moreover, all these functions require the physiotherapist to have expert knowledge of haemophilia and its therapy without which physiotherapy can be counter-productive.

Non surgical orthopaedic management. Before the availability of effective and safe concentrates, the use of braces, callipers and other orthopaedic devices were of considerable importance. A full description of these is beyond the scope of this volume and readers are referred to specialized texts such as the monograph of Duthie et al (1970) and more recently Smith (1989) but development of light plastic splints and braces have made these much more acceptable to patients. Other non-surgical corrective procedures include wedging plasters, serial plasters and various forms of casts which can be used to straighten joints and improve function. The reversed dynamic sling (Stein & Dickinson 1975) is one which can easily be set up and is quite useful for gently straightening knees with flexion deformities.

Orthopaedic surgery. The main indication for arthrodesis is pain which is often worse at night. Various muscle sliding and tendon-lengthening operations are useful for improving both muscle and joint function. Joint replacement operations are often extremely successful in alleviating pain, improving movements and reducing the number of haemarthroses. Hip replacements are now quite a common operation in haemophiliacs and are usually very effective. With improvements in materials and techniques it can be recommended even for comparatively young haemophiliacs who are appropriately disabled. Knee replacement operations are technically satisfactory but are not as successful in the long-term as those of the hip. They tend to be more successful in older, less active, individuals than in young active persons and the latter especially should be warned that re-operation may be needed.

Muscle haematoma

Muscle haematoma is the second most common type of lesion in haemophilia. Bleeding may occur into almost any group of muscles but those following trauma to the calves, thigh, gluteal region and arms are most common. Bleeding may also occur in the ilio-psoas muscle and in the sublingual and retropharyngeal region. Bleeding into muscles, e.g. of the calf, if not treated may lead to nerve involvement and arterial compression. Whereas bleeding into a joint rarely gives rise to chronic extra-articular problems other than quadriceps wasting, bleeding into a muscle can lead to widespread damage and contractures. Muscle bleeding often responds only slowly to factor replacement and treatment may need to be more intense than for haemarthroses.

Retroperitoneal haematoma. This is a common and important lesion. The patient develops abdominal pain perhaps with fever, pallor and occasionally backache. Typically he lies with his leg flexed on the affected side and it is important to exclude compensaory lordosis when asking him to straighten the leg. Often there is neurological involvement with loss of sensaion, especially over the patella on the affected side. If treatment is delayed quadriceps wasting may occur and the knee becomes destabilized with resultant frequent haemarthroses. Rarely the haematoma extends upwards into the thorax or downwards from the perinephric region to the pelvis. Vomiting may occur and pain in the right inguinal fossa may mimic acute appendicitis. Differentiation of this lesion is vital and if doubt exists an abdominal ultrasound or CT scan will resolve the issue.

Sublingual and retropharyngeal haematomas. This group of lesions are quite common and potentially very dangerous. Bleeding occurs from dental trauma, under the tongue and extends downwards into the neck or from the tonsillar region extending retropharyngeally. These are real medical emergencies and high level therapy should be given as soon as possible. If neglected, bleeding may extend leading to respiratory obstruction.

Haematuria

Bleeding from the renal tract is quite common in severe haemophilia and does not require repeated renal tract investigation unless it occurs in mildly-affected patients or in the presence of other indications. The most effective treatment is with factor concentrate 20–30 u/kg 12 hourly for 2 or 3 days. Rarely urinary infection or clot colic occur. Treatment with fibrinolytic inhibitors has been associated with colic and ureteric obstruction and these drugs are not indicated except perhaps if the bleeding is known to be below the ureter when they can counteract urinary fibrinolysis. Drinking and diuresis should be encouraged. In the author's experience steroid hormones, although sometimes recommended, are of no additional value. If haematuria persists or recurs frequently, formal investigation of the urinary tract should be undertaken.

Cerebral haemorrhage

Before the onset of AIDS, cerebral haemorrhage was the commonest cause of death in haemophilia and is still an important cause. Patients should be advised to avoid contact sports, cricket and dangerous occupations and to report if there is the slightest risk of intracranial bleeding. Diagnosis can be assisted by CAT scan and other investigations can be undertaken with appropriate concentrate cover. Treatment is by high doses of factor VIII coupled with usual investigation and treatment as in a non-haemophiliac.

Surgery in haemophilia

Surgery in haemophilia can be safely carried out, but it is advisable that this is supervised by an experienced team. In the first place the diagnosis should be confirmed, factor VIII level assessed and inhibitor excluded. The haemophilia team should liaise with the surgical team, the nature of the operation determined and the treatment plan decided, preferably with broadly described written details of factor VIII cover, certain precautions and copies made available to all concerned. The plan however, should allow a flexible approach to allow for unexpected eventualities. The factor VIII dose is calculated to produce a preoperative level of 100 u/dl (100%). During operation, consumption of factor VIII may be increased and supplementary doses according to assays may be needed. Thereafter factor VIII is given two to three times a day to keep levels above 40–50%. Doses should be arranged so that the morning dose is given early to allow optimum cover for nursing, physiotherapy and minor surgical procedures and the evening dose is given late enough to last all night. Short cuts and delay especially at weekends must be avoided. Although the first few days are most important, bleeding sometimes occurs at 7–10 days after operation. This is particularly undesirable as the skin wound may have healed over and a deep haematoma can result. Physiotherapy, minor procedures, toilet and bed baths should be covered by factor concentrate and not done first thing in the morning when levels are at their lowest ebb. Factor VIII therapy should be continued until healing is complete. Generally the patient is best kept in bed with gentle physiotherapy but if all seems well after the first few days he can be allowed up for a short while after a dose of factor VIII. Antibiotics should be given if there is a risk of infection.

One of the most severe operations in haemophilia is removal of a haemophilic cyst. This is a potentially fatal complication of a muscle or sub-periosteal haematoma leading to a locally-invasive blood cyst which may point, discharge and become infected. Regression is usually unlikely even with continued factor replacement and radiotherapy. Often the cyst wall is very thick and unless removed completely becomes the nidus of a recurrent cyst. These operations are best undertaken at a major centre.

Dental extraction

At one time dental extraction was extremely hazardous but with the development of factor concentrates and antifibrinolytic drugs it has become routine. Construction of dental splints are no longer routinely required. Factor concentrates can be given for the whole period of healing as with any surgery but the use of antifibrinolytic drugs enables the amount of concentrate needed to be reduced considerably since fibrinolytic activity in the buccal mucosa is marked. Effective regimes were described by Walsh et al (1971) and Forbes et al (1972). Factor VIII is given to raise the factor VIII level to 50 u/dl and tranexamic acid 15 mg/kg given intravenously for the first dose and subsequently three times a day by mouth. The factor VIII ensures an effective haemostatic plug and tranexamic acid stops it dissolving. An oral antibiotic is given, e.g. penicillin 250 mg three times a day and treatments continued for 7–10 days. No further factor VIII is given after the first dose, unless bleeding occurs when a supplementary dose is administered and the patient is usually managed as an outpatient or with only one or two days in hospital. Of course a soft diet and reduced activity is recommended so that the clot is not disturbed. In haemophilia B the full use of this regime could be criticised if PCCs are used because concomitant use of tranexamic acid could aggravate thromboembolic complications. The arrival of purified factor IX concentrate will be reassuring in this regard.

Analgesia in haemophilia

Pain is very common in haemophilia both in acute and chronic arthropathies and in other lesions. The safest and most effective analgesic is to achieve haemostatic factor levels; this rapidly reduces oedema and inflammation due to extravasated blood. If pain is severe, analgesic drugs may be needed. Aspirin must be avoided since it poisons platelets and other non-steroidal antiflammatory drugs (NSAIDS) should also be avoided in the presence of acute bleeding. Paracetamol may suffice for mild pain but its frequent and repeated use should be avoided especially if there is any evidence of chronic hepatitis. Dihydrocodeine (DF 118) in a dose of 30–60 mg orally is useful for moderate pain but may cause dizziness and constipation. It can be repeated every 4–6 hours. This type of alkaloid therapy should be used with caution in patients with a history of drug dependence but it would be wrong to permit patients to undergo severe pain for fear of drug dependence. It is sometimes necessary to prescribe a limited dosage of pethidine or dextromoramide but care should be taken to ensure that apparent symptoms match the nature of the lesion and strictly to limit the duration of therapy particularly when there is a history of drug abuse or dependence.

Treatment in haemophilia B (Christmas disease)

The inheritance pattern, clinical presentation and the varying degrees of severity of haemophilia B are the same as those for haemophilia A except that the haemostatic defect is of factor IX and not factor VIII and the incidence is only about 20% that of haemophilia A. The principles of treatment, also, are the same as for haemopholia A but the half life of factor IX is a little longer than that of factor VIII, about 18–24 hours compared to 10–14 hours. Treatment may, therefore, be given a little less frequently. The three or four factor PCCs which have hitherto been used have a slight incidence of thromboembolic complications particularly after surgery on the lower limbs. These concentrates are being replaced by high purity virucidally treated single factor concentrates of factor IX which have much less thrombogenic potential. It is common practice to administer prophylactic factor IX therapy in severe haemophilia B. Because of the long half life of the therapeutic materials, relatively widely-spaced injections seem to suffice, e.g. 20 u/kg once or twice a week.

Treatment of carriers of haemophilia A or B

In accordance with Lyons hypothesis of inactivation of the X chromosome, the level of factor VIII or IX may be more or less reduced in some women who are heterozygous for the gene defect. Such women may have a mild bleeding tendency, and can have excessive bleeding after surgery. They should be assessed for their response to DDAVP and have treatment with this or factor VIII concentrate as would a mildly-affected haemophiliac. Factor VIII levels rise during pregnancy and may reach safe levels but they fall rapidly in the postpartum period and treatment may be needed for episiotomy or other lesion. Factor IX levels do not rise during pregnancy and treatment, preferably with high purity single factor concentrate, may be needed in the intra- and postpartem period.

Treatment in von Willebrand's disease

von Willebrand's disease is probably the commonest, inherited disorder. Many of those patients diagnosed however are very mild and do not require treatment being identified during epidemiological studies (Rodeghiero et al 1989a). On the other hand homozygous recessive, or compound heterozygous inheritance leads to the extremely severe type III phenotype. The availability of DDAVP and the development of specific concentrates of vWF have been discussed (pp 899, 903) All that remains to be done here, is to put this information into the context of tactical aspects of therapy.

When bleeding is primarily due to defective primary (i.e. capillary) haemostasis such as epistaxis, menorrhagia and gastrointestinal bleeding, DDAVP should be considered first. For out-patient treatment, e.g. domiciliary management of severe menorrhagia, a nasal atomiser spray seems to be effective and can produce adequate absorption of DDAVP. If DDAVP is contraindicated, or ineffective after a therapeutic trial, then a concentrate providing at least some HMW vWF multimers should be used. Local considerations concerning the safety of single donor cryoprecipitate should be borne in mind especially the prevalence of HIV and hepatitis virus carriers in the population. In the United Kingdom, single donor cryoprecipitate is no longer recommended. When surgical intervention is planned, the response to a test dose of DDAVP, if not already determined, should be obtained. For relatively minor surgery, such as herniorrhaphy etc., if a good response is obtained with DDAVP then this can be used throughout the postoperative period until healing is complete, but close assay control at least of factor VIII levels is essential. For secondary haemostasis after surgery it seems that factor VIII levels are the most important determinants. When surgical intervention is planned in patients not expected to respond sufficiently to DDAVP it is probably wise to correct both primary and secondary haemostasis with an appropriate concentrate such as Haemate P (p. 899), at least during the first few days. Subsequently adequate levels of factor VIII for secondary haemostasis are most important and concentrates which are relatively depleted of HMW vWF will suffice. These may contain sufficient vWF to stabilize the patient's endogenous factor VIII and, except in type III vWD, treatment may be needed less frequently than in haemophilia, e.g. once a day. High potency factor VIII concentrates containing no vWF should be avoided. Hopefully fractionators will maintain a supply of concentrates containing adequate HMW vWF as well as factor VIII for the treatment of vWD. Of course it goes without saying that these concentrates should be treated during manufacture to render them safe from pathogenic viruses.

A few patients with severe, probably homozygous, type III vWD develop antibodies after treatment (Stratton et al 1975, Mannucci et al 1976). Some of these patients have partial gene deletions (Peake et al 1990). The antibodies usually, but not always, are precipitating and act primarily against vWF. Factor VIII levels may respond more favourably to high potency concentrate rather than to crude preparations which contain vWF (Bloom et al 1979) and which will react with the antibody.

Home treatment

Home treatment is now an established method of treatment for most patients with severe haemophilia A, B or vWD. The term refers to treatment administered by parents, guardians or the patient himself outside the hospital or primary care setting. After the child is diagnosed the parents bring him to hospital for treatment and gradually learn the nature of bleeding episodes and when they need to be treated. As the child grows older venous access improves and the parents are taught the technique of venepuncture, safe disposal of equipment, when to seek medical help, etc., so that by the time venous access is suitable and they are confident, then they can undertake administration of treatment first under supervision in hospital and then at home. The age at which this is feasible varies with venous access and capability and intelligence of the parents but by the time the child is 5-years-old many can be established on home treatment. Later perhaps at the age of 10–12 years the child can be gradually instructed to administer the material himself. Patients presenting for the first time as adults can usually be established on home therapy and taught to administer their factor.

The main advantage of home therapy include:

- Early administration of treatment which aborts bleeding episodes and limits tissue and joint damage
- Allows the patient to go to school or work
- Reduces the need to go to hospital
- Allows freedom to travel
- Facilitates prophylactic treatment if this is indicated
- Psychological effect giving parents and patient some control over activities and treatment.

When home therapy is established the main indications for treatment are:

- Bleeding into a joint or muscles
- Head injury or cerebral symptoms (notify haemophilia centre or attend)
- All open wounds which may require suturing (notify haemophilia centre or attend)
- Any injury that may lead to bleeding.

The parents or patient should seek medical advice in the event of recurrent bleeding at one site or if a single bleed does not promptly respond. Regular follow-up at the Haemophilia Centre is important to assess the patient and to complete documentation. It is the author's practice to issue a home-treatment form to document doses, lot (batch) number and type of material, lesion, response and date. Further treatment is only issued against receipt of a satisfactorily completed form.

Contraindications to home therapy are uncommon and include:

- Presence of an inhibitor, however recombinant factor VIIa is being assessed for home treatment
- Lack of suitable domestic facilities such as a refrigerator
- Lack of intellectual capacity in patient or parents in order to maintain asepsis etc
- If bleeding episodes are too infrequent to keep in practice.

Prophylactic therapy

Prophylactic therapy means the administration of concentrate on a more or less regular basis even in the absence of bleeding. There are two types. Intermittent prophylaxis may be given to prevent bleeding during stressful situations such as examinations or to prevent recurrence after treatment of a bleeding episode. The logical extension and possible aim of prophylaxis is to administer it more permanently to try to normalize the patient's haemostatic mechanism continuously. Various schedules have been adopted for this purpose but with the development of high-purity plasma-derived or recombinant materials this aim may become a reality. The difference between haemophilia and say, diabetes, in this respect is that without prophylaxis on a daily basis the diabetic will die whereas the severe haemophiliac will just develop frequent bleeds which can be treated on an 'on demand' basis. Nevertheless as purified products develop there will no doubt be a move to long-term prophylaxis for severe haemophilia which may well be limited mainly by economic considerations or by complications such as the development of an inhibitor.

Prophylactic therapy is undergoing re-evaluation with the advent of virus-safe high purity concentrates. If the level of factor VIII or IX can be maintained in the 2–5 u/dl range, especially in children, then much joint disability may be prevented. Because of its longer half life this is easier with factor IX in haemophilia B and it is convenient to administer about 20 u/kg once or twice a week. Prophylactic factor VIII therapy requires rather more frequent doses. Venous access is a problem and the use of a central line with subcutaneous access such as a 'portacath' or construction of an arterio-venous fistula may be a partial answer particularly during early childhood which is a period of life during which it is very important to prevent the onset of chronic arthropathy.

THE MANAGEMENT OF PATIENTS WITH INHIBITORS

Factor VIII or IX inhibitors are antibodies that develop

in patients in whom transfused factor is recognised as 'foreign', either because the patient has a severe gene defect with lack of mRNA for the appropriate factor or because a mutated factor is present which differs sufficiently from the transfused factor. Factor VIII inhibitors inactivate factor VIII in a time-dependent fashion showing simple or complex reaction kinetics (Biggs et al 1972a,b. Allain & Frommel 1974, Gawryl & Hoyer 1982). Most factor VIII inhibitors exhibit simple kinetics and can be measured by an inactivation method and expressed in units (such as Bethesda units) per ml (Kasper 1975). Factor IX inhibitors are instantaneously reacting, cannot validly be measured by the Bethesda method and are often expressed simply as a dilution titre.

The presence of an inhibitor is, after AIDS and hepatitis, the most serious complication of haemophilia treatment and renders the patient more or less resistent to specific factor replacement. Inhibitors are most common in severe haemophilia A (up to 20% of patients) but are rare in haemophilia B (about 1%). They occasionally occur, usually at low strength, in mild or moderate haemophilia A when they may exhibit complex reaction kinetics. Similar inhibitors of factor VIII sometimes develop in non-haemophiliacs, following pregnancy, in association with rheumatoid arthritis and other diseases, or in elderly people for no apparent reason. They are autoantibodies which lead to acquired (non-inherited) haemophilia (see Chapter 34).

The management of patients with inhibitors has been the subject of several comprehensive reviews (Bloom 1987, Kasper 1989, 1991) and involves two broad approaches:

1. Attempts to reduce the inhibitor permanently by immunosuppression and immunotolerance.
2. Treatment of acute bleeds in the presence of the inhibitor.

The discussion that follows refers mainly to factor VIII inhibitors but the principles apply also to those of factor IX.

Reducing factor VIII inhibitors permanently

The following methods have been used:

1. Immunosuppression with drugs
2. Immunodepletion plus immunosuppression
3. Immunosuppression plus factor plus intravenous IgG.

Immunotolerance has been achieved using very high doses of factor VIII concentrate, use of low dose factor plus steroids as well as low dose factor alone. Immunomodulation using anti-idiotypes is a possibility yet to be achieved although this may be a mechanism of action of intravenous IgG via the presence of anti-idiotypes in the treatment of acute bleeding especially in patients with autoimmune-acquired inhibitors.

Immunosuppression and immunotolerance regimes

The Malmo regimen. Theoretically, immunosuppressive drugs would be most effective if given during the primary immunizing phase combined with the dose of factor, but this phase is rarely detectable (Dormandy & Sultan 1975). At best they can only delay an anamnestic response (Nilsson & Hedner 1976) or possibly convert a high immunological responder to a low one (Hedner & Tengborn 1985). Nevertheless, derived from this experience together with the use of extracorporeal immunodepletion for acute bleeding and the serendipitous use of intravenous IgG both to replace IgG and to suppress the inhibitor activity, Nilsson and colleagues (Nilsson et al 1983, 1988, Nilsson & Sundqvist 1984) developed a successful regime to suppress factor VIII and IX antibodies. The method which Nilsson and her colleagues eventually developed is as follows. At first immunodepletion was performed on an extracorporeal circuit incorporating protein A or antigen adsorbed to a solid phase. Following this, for adults, cyclophosphamide was given intravenously at first in 500 mg doses daily for 2 days, and then 50 mg orally three times a day for 8 days. At the same time intravenous immunoglobulin 0.4 g/kg per day was given for 5 days together with factor VIII (or IX) in moderate doses, e.g. 3000 u daily for 14 days. An inhibitor assay was then performed. Factor VIII or IX was reduced on alternate days for 2 weeks and further reduced depending on inhibitor assays and factor recovery. It appeared that an immune complex of antibody and factor appears that is not inhibitory in coagulation (Nilsson et al 1990). Adolescents and parents should be warned of the possible delay of puberty due to cyclophosphamide.

The Bonn regimen. In an alternative immunotolerating regime Brackmann and colleagues (1984) described their regimen of using very high doses of factor VIII over a period of about a year or so. The treatment was divided into four phases. In *phase 1* 100 u/kg factor VIII were administered twice daily together with an activated prothrombin complex concentrate FEIBA (Immuno) in doses of 50 u/kg twice daily until the inhibitor was reduced to 0.5 u/ml. The FEIBA was given to prevent bleeding during the induction phase but its use is not essential (Brackmann, 1992). In *phase 2,* factor VIII 100 u/kg was administered alone until the inhibitor disappeared. In *phase 3,* the factor VIII therapy was slowly reduced until the half life of factor VIII was normal for 8 weeks and in *phase 4* the patient went on to an 'on-demand regimen'. There seems to be little doubt that this regimen is successful but the main drawback is the extremely high cost. As a result, various teams have turned to less demanding and less expensive forms of immunotoleration. Rizza & Matthews (1982) reported on the serendipitous observation that in patients treated with various doses of factor VIII over 1–5 years in a certain proportion the in-

Table 38.9 Methods for controlling acute bleeding in patients with factor VIII inhibitors

Local measures
Pharmacological methods, e.g. DDAVP
Factor VIII concentrates, human and porcine
Plasmapheresis
Extracorporeal immunodepletion
Intravenous IgG
Methods of bypassing factor VIII and its inhibitors:
Non-activated PCCs
Activated PCCs
rFVIIa
Experimental methods

hibitors disappeared or were reduced in titre. Wensley et al (1986) reported success in 50% of inhibitor patients with doses as low as 250 u of factor VIII on alternate days and similar findings have been reported by Ewing et al (1988) and, with the addition of a 3-week course of low dose steroids, by Aznar et al (1984). These methods are of course not always effective but may be worth a try.

The management of acute bleeds in inhibitor patients

This subject has been reviewed by Bloom (1987, 1991) and by Kasper (1989, 1991). In general the methods are as outlined in Table 38.9. Local measures such as immobilization of joints and muscles and topical applications such as thrombin or Russell's viper venom for external bleeding points are only of limited value. Fibrinolytic inhibitors such as tranexamic acid 15 mg/kg three times a day by mouth are helpful for intraoral bleeding but not for other lesions such as haemarthroses. Theoretically DDAVP should not be effective. Most inhibitor patients are severely affected and any rise of factor VIII would be neutralized. However, DDAVP may have other effects on haemostasis, e.g. on platelets, and it is worth a try in an unresponsive patient.

However, there is no doubt that when it can be achieved, circulating active factor VIII is most effective. This can sometimes be achieved with low titre inhibitor patients who are low immunological responders and sometimes factor VIII is effective instantaneously before it is neutralized.

Antibodies can have species specificity and thus may not neutralize porcine factor VIII. The original preparation of porcine factor VIII caused severe reactions and thrombocytopenia probably due to the analogue of vWF, moreover resistance developed after about a week probably due to the development of antibodies to that analogue. More recently high purity porcine factor VIII has been prepared and is relatively free from side-effects. If the inhibitor does not react with porcine factor VIII, this will be an extremely effective therapeutic concentrate for factor VIII inhibitor patients (Kernoff et al 1984).

It may be possible to reduce the level of factor VIII antibodies temporarily by plasmapheresis, replacing with plasma protein fraction to avoid viral exposure or an amnestic response before factor VIII replacement therapy is given. A similar effect can be obtained with extracorporeal immunoabsorption (Nilsson et al 1981). In this technique blood is circulated through an extracorporeal circuit in which protein A adsorbed to a solid medium absorbs factor VIII (or IX) inhibitors from the patient's plasma and allows replacement with factor VIII or factor IX. A disadvantage of this technique is that it requires special equipment and is rather elaborate for repeated minor bleeds. It has the advantages that the patient's own plasma is returned, that immunoglobulin can be replaced and it can form part of an immunosuppressive regime.

Methods of bypassing factor VIII and its inhibitors include the use of activated PCC and its possible components, factor Xa-phospholipid, tissue factor and factor VIIa. The role of PCC in inhibitor patients has been described. In clinical trials non-activated PCC was effective in about 50% of episodes (Lusher et al 1980). Activated PCC such as FEIBA (Immuno) was effective in about 65% of episodes but not to the extent seen with factor VIII in ordinary haemophilia and, as expected, a placebo effect with albumin was noted (Sjamsoedin et al 1981). It appears that heat treatment does not impair clinical efficacy (Hilgartner et al 1991).

The possible active principles of APCC could include activated factor IX, X or factor VII or possibly phospholipid which could act in concert with Xa or by protecting factor VIII. Thus phospholipid protected factor VIII from interaction with anti-factor VIII (Barrowcliffe et al 1981, Yoshioka et al 1983). Giles et al (1988a) showed that phospholipid and Xa may be determinants of thrombogenicity of factor IX-PCC concentrates and carefully formulated mixtures of Xa and phospholipid are under experimental trial as factor VIII by-passing agents. The therapeutic threshold for intravascular coagulation, however, seems to be low.

A third approach to the factor VIII inhibitor by-passing problem involves the tissue factor pathway. This may represent a pathway alternative to the intrinsic system to induce haemostasis at the site of injury without (theoretically) involving factor VIII. Although recombinant tissue factor is under experimental study, there is considerable experimental and clinical evidence concerning the efficacy of activated factor VII. Factor VII acts with tissue factor in the extrinsic coagulation system and it has been hoped that this would induce haemostasis locally without systemic effect. Hedner & Kisiel (1983) first used plasma derived (pd) factor VIIa for successful management of two inhibitor patients and therapeutic concentrates of pd FVIIa have been prepared (Chabbat et al 1989, Hedner et al 1989). However, the treatment has been placed on a more realistic basis by the development by Thim and colleagues (Thim et al 1988) of Novo Industrii (Copenhagen, now Novo-Nordisk) of recombinant human factor VIIa (rFVIIa) in transfected baby hamster kidney cells. It is almost fully carboxylated and with similar glycosylation to human pd FVIIA.

Successful use of rFVIIa has been reported in massive doses for synovectomy and in more modest doses for a sublingual haematoma (Hedner et al 1988, Macik et al 1989). A multicentre international trial of rVIIa is in progress. Our initial experience has been encouraging. The half life of rVIIa is only about 2–3 hours (Harrison & Bloom 1991) so that repeated infusions are needed but our initial experience using doses of 35 to 70 μg/kg every 3–4 hours has been encouraging (Bloom 1991). Treatment was successful if plasma levels of factor VII exceeded 6 u/ml when measured by a one-stage method using rabbit brain tissue extract and were maintained over 3.5 u/ml for 24 hours. It should be pointed out that rVIIa may be dangerous in the presence of tissue destruction due to induction of disseminated intravascular coagulation (Stein et al 1990) and that it is not always effective in surgical patients (Gringeri et al 1991). However, although we observed an occasional minor fall of antithrombin III level we have never seen signs of DIC and we have successfully used rVIIa to cover surgery. Interestingly not only does shortening of the prothrombin time occur but also marked shortening of the activated partial thromboplastin time (aPTT; KCCT). Possibly supraphysiological concentrations of VIIa activate factor X (Telgt et al 1989, Rao & Rappaport 1990). It is of interest to note that rVIIa does not contain human blood derivatives and could represent an acceptable form of treatment for haemophilia A or B in Jehovah's Witnesses.

TREATMENT OF LESS COMMON INHERITED COAGULATON FACTOR DEFICIENCIES

Fibrinogen deficiency

It is generally believed that the haemostatic level of fibrinogen is 100 mg/dl but for major surgery it is probably wise to aim for a rather higher level. The half life of plasma fibrinogen is about 4–5 days so that, provided an acceptable therapeutic material is available, this can be given infrequently by infusion every 3–4 days. Until the recent problems with HIV and realisation of the importance of hepatitis viruses, plasma cryoprecipitate and freeze dried concentrates were an acceptable source of fibrinogen. It is no longer acceptable in the United Kingdom to administer fresh frozen plasma or cryoprecipitate to correct inherited coagulation factor deficiencies even if tested for the presence of antibodies to HIV or various forms of hepatitis, since these products are not usually subjected to virucidal processes. However, a preparation of heat-treated fibrinogen is available commercially from Immuno.

Factor XIII

Inherited deficiency of factor XIII is very uncommon but may be associated with abnormal bleeding after injury, delayed wound healing and dehiscence and a high incidence of miscarriage (Kitchen & Newcomb 1979). Prolonged bleeding from the umbilical cord at birth and intracranial bleeding may occur. Factor XIII has a very long half life of up to 10 days so that prophylactic therapy every 3–6 weeks has been recommended (Losowksy & Miloszweski 1976). A pasteurized preparation of placental factor XIII is obtainable from Hoechst and seems to be acceptably safe.

Factor XI deficiency

Factor XI deficiency was originally termed plasma thromboplastin antecedent deficiency or haemophilia C. The haemorrhagic tendency is usually mild and is not necessarily related to the level of factor XI. Excessive bruising and menorrhagia may occur in women. Until fairly recently the only effective treatment was by fresh frozen plasma but fortunately a heat-treated concentrate produced by Bio Products Laboratory (BPL, UK) is now available. This is apparently effective and virologically safe and is available on a named-patient compassionate basis. The biological half life of factor XI is long, about 60 hours, which makes it easy to maintain effective levels with the concentrate.

No concentrates of other contact factors such as prekallikrein and factor XII are available but deficiencies of these factors are rarely associated with abnormal bleeding.

Factor V deficiency

Although factor V has been purified for biochemical studies (Chiu et al 1983) no therapeutic concentrate is available. It seems that the minimum levels needed for haemostasis are variable, between 15–20% (Melliger & Duckert 1971, Breederveld et al 1974). Recovery of factor V in the circulation after plasma transfusion is reported to be only about 50% of theoretical so that replacement needs to be given frequently. Since no virologically safe concentrate is available the best that can be done is to use fresh or fresh frozen plasma that has been carefully selected from known donors and tested virologically. The in vivo half life reported by Rizza & Jones (1987) was 11.4 hours and they recommended 15 ml/kg of fresh (frozen) plasma every 12 hours.

Factor VII deficiency

This deficiency is uncommon but can be associated with abnormal bleeding. On the other hand surgical procedures have been reported to be well tolerated even without treatment but it would be unwise to rely on this. The half life of factor VII is very short, about 3 hours, so that, although recovery in the circulation is almost complete, frequent infusions are needed.

There are several sources of virally-inactivated factor VII concentrates (BPL, Elstree; Biotransfusion, France) so that recourse to fresh frozen plasma is not needed and usually not practical because of overloading of the circulation. In addition pd and rFVIIa are available (p. 912) and some (but not all) PCCs contain factor VII. Adequate levels of factor VII may be obtained by infusing about 10 u/kg since levels needed for maintaining haemostasis may be as low as 15% but this should be regarded as the minimum.

Factor X deficiency

This is a rare disorder but can lead to excessive bleeding apparently spontaneously and after accident or surgery. Fortunately factor X is present in several virally secure PCCs. It has a half life about 24 hours, recovery is about 50% and, for major surgery, levels should be maintained over 30%.

Prothrombin deficiency

This is one of the most uncommon of the inherited coagulation factor deficiencies. Most of the patients described have had levels over 10% but levels over 40% are needed for normal haemostasis. Replacement therapy is relatively easy. Recovery in the circulation is about 50% but the half life of transfused prothrombin is long; about 2 to 3 days. Prothrombin is present in most virucidally-treated prothrombin complex concentrates which can therefore be used for treatment. Care should be taken not to over-treat in case of inducing thromboembolic complications.

THE ORGANISAION OF HEAEMOPHILIA CARE

It is salutary to consider that in spite of the vast amount of knowledge concerning factor VIII and factor IX, haemophilia and related disorders which is described in this volume the majority of the world's haemophiliacs do not have access to any specific diagnosis or therapy. Nevertheless it is important to describe the optimum conditions for haemophilia care in the broadest sense as a target towards which emerging treatment systems can aim. The concept and development of comprehensive haemophilia care have been well described by Boone (1976) Hilgartner & Pochedly (1989) and Jones (1990).

Haemophilia care is not just a matter of administering therapeutic concentrates but involves the close interaction of a number of experts. The family of the haemophiliac is closely involved and needs expert and informed counselling not only on therapeutic options but on the impact of HIV and hepatitis viruses and on their infectivity and sexual transmission. The latter is linked to the question of genetic options and it is essential that counsellors are aware of these interacting problems. On the more physical side, centres dealing with a large number of haemophilia referrals should have the sevices of a dedicated physiotherapist who becomes experienced in the rehabilitation of the locomotor lesions of haemophilia. When orthopaedic correction is needed, it is essential that the surgeon is aware of the problems of haemophilia control such as inhibitors and the use of factor concentrates. Similar considerations apply to general and dental surgery.

Haemophiliacs have always been disadvantaged in education and employment and have needed the services of specialized social workers. As these problems have been ameliorated by the development of concentrates and home therapy the many aspects of AIDS and hepatitis have emerged. The duties of the social worker have thus expanded not only to include the problems of work and school and financial assistance but now also to the harrowing problems of AIDS in the context not only of the patient but also of his whole family. In the author's centre the need for social work has expanded from one dedicated social worker to three during the last 6 years. This work is so demanding and distressing that the social workers themselves need professional counselling and regular psychiatric sessions for patients have been added to the comprehensive care system.

The core team of a large haemophilia treatment centre is outlined in Figure 38.1 together with the input needed from other advisers. In the United Kingdom, each region is served by a large comprehensive centre originally described as a Reference Centre. Within the region are several other haemophilia centres each capable of undertaking regular therapy on a 24 hour basis, conducting a home treatment programme, diagnosing and registering new patients and detecting and quantitating inhibitors. Whilst most day to day local haemophilia care is supervised from these centres, special problems such as genetic diagnosis, major surgery, etc. are referred to the reference centre which collates regional data that are collected nationally. Smaller associated treatment units, for example dealing with less than 10 severely-affected patients each year, undertake day to day treatment but refer more difficult problems to larger centres as considered to be appropriate. Of course in addition to offering initial examination, counselling and treatment haemophilia centres offer regular medical, physiotherapeutic and social follow-up as well as testing and assessment for the progression of HIV-related and liver disease. The whole country is thus covered by an integrated system of management for haemophilic patients and their families. It is not the practice in the United Kingdom for factor concentrates to be available from private pharmacies (druggists) but they are only available from haemophilia centres in hospitals. Family doctors do not therefore offer initial therapy for acute lesions but they are kept fully informed and may be involved with helping in home therapy and vaccination programmes as well as in the general care of patients.

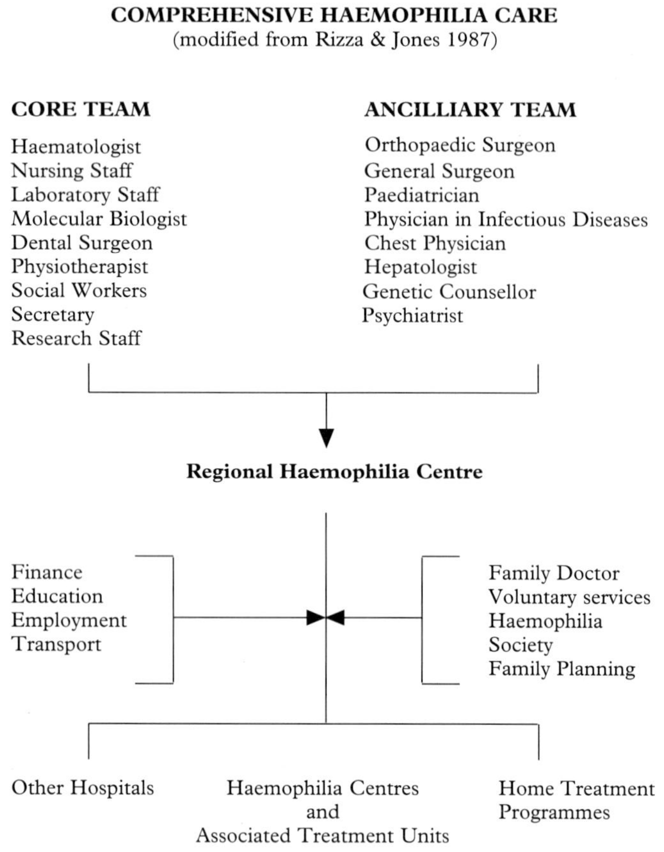

Fig. 38.1 Comprehensive haemophilia care. (Modified from Rizza & Jones 1987.)

In addition to day to day management it is important formally to discuss patients' problems. In the author's centre, a system of regular and frequent multidisciplinary case conferences has been established. The aim is to review all patients on the register at least once a year including severely-affected and mild patients. Some patients are reviewed more frequently as needed. These conferences are attended by the core team and other carers even if they are not directly involved. The conferences are primarily held to serve the functional needs of the patients but they also have an important educational component.

Haemophilia care as described above is expensive. Financial arrangements vary in different countries and too often no financial provision at all is possible. The capital outlay for the centre and its staff is considerable but this is dwarfed by the revenue consequences of haemophilia therapy. Intermediate purity concentrates are expensive but are only half the cost of high purity concentrates, prescription of which is becoming increasingly necessary. In addition, the high cost of antiviral agents such as zidovudine for HIV, antibiotics and anti-fungal agents means that haemophilia is one of the most expensive conditions to treat. Furthermore, haemophilia centres are frequently situated in haematology departments which are responsible also for high cost leukaemia therapy although there is little in common between the two groups of diseases. Hopefully as the economies of emergent countries improve the use of these expensive materials will rise and their cost will accordingly fall until comprehensive haemophilia care worldwide becomes a reality.

REFERENCES

Allain J P, Frommel D 1974 Antibodies to factor VIII: specificity and kinetics of iso- and hetero antibodies in haemophilia A. Blood 44: 313-322

Aznar J A, Jorquera J I, Peiro A 1984 The importance of corticoids added to continued treatment with factor VIII concentrates in the suppression of inhibitors in haemophilia A. Thrombosis and Haemostasis 51: 217–221

Barrowcliffe T W, Kemball-Cook G, Gray E 1981 Factor VIII inhibitor bypassing activity: suggested mechanism of action. Thrombosis Research 21: 181–186

Beddal A C, Hill F G H, George R H, Williams M D, Al-Rubei K 1985 Unusually high incidence of tuberculosis among boys with haemophilia during an outbreak of the disease in hospital. Journal of Clinical Pathology 38: 1163–1165

Bell B A, Kerczynski E M, Bergman G 1990 Inhibitors to monoclonal antibody purified factor VIII Lancet 336: 638

Berntorp E, Nilsson I M 1989 Use of a high-purity factor VIII concentrate (Hemate P) in von Willebrand's disease. Vox Sanguinis 56: 212–217

Biggs R, Austen D E G, Denson K W E, Rizza C R, Borret R 1972a. The mode of action of antibodies which destroy factor VIII-I antibodies which have second order concentration graphs. British Journal of Haematology 23: 125–135

Biggs R, Austen D E G, Denson K W E, Borret R, Rizza C R 1972b The mode of action of antibodies which destroy factor VIII-II antibodies which give complex concentration graphs. British Journal of Haematology 23: 137–155

Bloom A L 1987 The treatment of factor VIII inhibitors. Verstraete M, Vermylen J, Lijnen R, Arnout J (eds) Thrombosis and haemostasis, Leuven University Press, Leuven, p 441–471

Bloom A L 1989 The treatment of factor VIII inhibitors. In Verstraete M, Vermylen J, Lijnen H R, Arnout J (eds) Thrombosis and haemostasis. International Society of Haemostasis and Thrombosis. Leuven University Press, Leuven, p 447–471

Bloom A L 1991 Progress in the clinical management of haemophilia. Thrombosis and Haemostasis 61: 166–171

Bloom A L, Peake I R, Furlong R A, Davis B L 1979 High potency factor VIII concentrate: more effective than cryoprecipitate in a patient with von Willebrand's disease and inhibitor. Thrombosis Research 16: 847–852

Boone D C (ed) 1976 Comprehensive management of hemophilia. F A Davies, Philadelphia

Brackmann H H 1984 Successful treatments of haemophilia A inhibitor patients with induced immunotolerance. In: Proceedings fourth international symposium on hemophilia treatment, Tokyo, p 187–196

Breederveld K, van Royen E A, ten Cate J W 1974 Severe factor V deficiency with a prolonged bleeding time. Thrombosis et Diathesis Haemorrhagica 32: 538–548

Brackmann H H 1992 Personal communication

Brettler D B, Forsberg A D, Levine P H et al 1989 Factor VIII: C concentrate purified from plasma using monoclonal antibodies: Human studies. Blood 73: 1859–1863

Burnouf T, Michalski E, Goudemand M, Huart J J 1989 Properties of a highly purified human plasma factor IX: C therapeutic concentrate prepared by conventional chromatography. Vox Sanguinis 57: 225–232

Cattaneo M, Moia M, Della Valle P, Castellana P, Mannucci P M 1989 DDAVP shortens the prolonged bleeding times of patients with severe von Willebrand disease treated with cryoprecipitate. Evidence for a mechanism independent of released von Willebrand factor, Blood 74: 1972–1976

Chabbat J, Hampikian-Lenin S, Toully Y et al 1988 A human factor VIIa concentrate and its effects in the hemophilia A dog. Thrombosis Research 54: 603–612

Chiu H C, Whitaker E, Colman R W 1983 Heterogenity of human factor V deficiency: Evidence for the existence of antigen-positive variants. Journal of Clinical Investigation 72: 493

Cumming A M, Fildes S, Cumming I R et al 1990 Clinical and laboratory evaluation of National Health Service factor VIII concentrate (8Y) for the treatment of von Willebrand's disease. British Journal of Haematology 75: 234–239

Dannatt A H G, Goodwin S J, Dasani H, Bowen D J, Peake I R, Bloom A L 1992 The relationship of HIV-1 viral sequences detected by the polymerase chain reaction in haemophilic patients to clinical and other markers of infection. Clinical and Laboratory Haematology 14 in press

de Biasi R, Rocino E M, Mastrullo L, Quirion A A 1991 The impact of a very high purity factor VIII concentrate on the immune system of human immunodeficiency virus-infected haemophiliacs: A randomised, prospective two-year comparison with an intermediate purity concentrate. Blood 78: 1919–1922

Dormandy K M, Sultan Y 1975 The suppression of factor VIII antibodies in haemophilia. Pathologie et Biologie 23 (suppl): 17–23

Duthie R B, Matthews J M, Rizza C R, Steel W M 1972 The management of musculo-skeletal problems in the haemophilias, Blackwell Scientific, Oxford

Evans J A, Pasi K, Williams M D, Hill F G H 1991 Consistently normal CD4+, CD8+ levels in haemophilic boys only treated with a virally safe factor VIII concentrate (BPL8Y). British Journal of Haematology 79: 457–461

Ewing N P, Sanders N L, Dietrich S L, Kasper C K 1988 Induction of immune tolerance to factor VIII in hemophiliacs with inhibitors. Journal of the American Medical Association 259: 65–68

Forbes C D, Barr R D, Reid G, Thomson C, Prentice C R M, McNicol G P, Douglas A S 1972 Tranexamic acid in control of haemorrhage after dental extraction in haemophilia and Christmas disease. British Medical Journal 2: 311–313

Fukatake K, Fujimaki M, Hanabusa S, Inagaki M, Mimaya J, Shirahat A 1991 Multicentre study on the influence of long-term continuous use of ultra-purified factor VIII preparation on the immunological status of HIV-infected and non-infected haemophilia A patients. Thrombosis and Haemostasis 65: 996

Fukui H, Nishino M, Terada S et al 1988 Hemostatic effect of a heat-treated factor VIII concentrate (Hemate P) in von Willebrand's disease. Blut 56: 171–178

Gawryl M S, Hoyer L W 1982 Inactivation of factor VIII coagulant activity by two different types of human antibodies. Blood 60: 1103

Gibbons J, Cory J M, Hewlett I K et al 1990 Silent infections with human immunodeficiency virus type 1 are highly unlikely in multitransfused seronegative haemophiliacs. Blood 76: 1924–1926

Giles A R, Mann K G, Nesheim M E 1988a A combination of factor Xa and phosphatidylcholine-phosphatidylserine resides bypasses factor VIII in vivo. British Journal of Haematology 69: 491–497

Giles A R, Tinlin S, Hoogedoorn H et al 1988b In vivo characterisation of recombinant factor VIII in a canine model of haemophilia A (factor VIII deficiency). Blood 72: 335–339

Goldsmith J M, Deutsche J, Tang M, Green D 1991 CD4 cells in HIV-1 infected hemophiliacs: Effect of factor VIII concentrates. Thrombosis and Haemostasis 66 (4): 415–419

Gringeri A, Santagostino E, Mannucci P M 1991 Failure of recombinant activated factor VII during surgery in a haemophiliac with high-titer factor VIII antibody. Haemostasis 21: 1–4

Hanley J D, Lippman-Hand A 1983 If nothing goes wrong, is everything all right? Journal of American Medical Association 249: 1743–1745

Harrison J F M, Bloom A L 1991 Pharmacokinetics and coagulation changes after administration of recombinant human activated factor VII (rVIIa NOVO). Proceedings of the British Society for Haematology. British Journal of Haematology 77 (suppl 1): 26

Harrison J F M, Bloom A L, Abildgaard C G for the rFactor VIII Clinical Trial Group 1991 The pharmacokinetics of recombinant factor VIII. Seminars in Hematology 28 (suppl 1): 29–35

Hedner U, Kisiel W 1983 Use of human factor VIIa in the treatment of two hemophilia A patients with high-titer inhibitors. Journal of Clinical Investigation 71: 1836–1841

Hedner U, Tengborn L 1985 Management of haemophilia A with antibodies — the effect of combined treatment with factor VIII, hydrocortisone and cyclophosphamide. Thrombosis and Haemostasis 54: 776–779

Hedner U, Bjoern S, Bernvil S S et al 1989 Clinical experience with human plasma-derived factor VIIa in patients with hemophilia A and high titre inhibitors. Haemostasis 19: 335–343

Hedner U, Glazer S, Pnegel K et al 1988 Successful use of recombinant factor VIIa in patient with severe haemophilia A during synovectomy. Lancet ii: 1193

Heimburger N, Schwinn H, Cratz P, Luben G, Kumpe G, Herchenhahn B 1981 A factor VIII concentrate highly purified and heat treated in solution. Arzneim Forsch 41: 619–622

Heinrich D, Kotische R, Berthold H 1982 Clinical evaluation of the hepatitis safety of a β-propioalactone/ultraviolet treated factor IX concentrate (PPSP). Thrombosis Research 28: 75–83

Hilgartner M W, Pochedly C 1989 Hemophilia in the child and adult, 3rd edn. Raven Press, New York

Hilgartner M, Aledort L, Andes A, Gill J 1990 Efficacy and safety of vapor-heated anti-inhibitor coagulant complex in hemophilia patients. FEIBA Study Group. Transfusion 30: 626–630

Jones P 1990 Living with haemophilia, 3rd edn. Castle House Publications, Kent, UK

Kasper C K 1975 Clinical use of factor IX concentrates: Report on thromboembolic complications. Thrombosis et Diathesis Haemorrhagica 33: 640–644

Kasper C K 1989 Treatment of factor VIII inhibitors. Progress in Haemostasis and Thrombosis 9: 57–86

Kasper C K 1991 Complications of Hemophilia A treatment: factor VIII inhibitors. In: Progress in vascular biology, haemostasis and thrombosis. Annals of the New York Academy of Sciences 614: 97–105

Kasper C K, Aledort L M, Counts R B et al 1975 A more uniform measurement of factor VIII inhibitors. Thrombosis et Diathesis Haemorrhagica 34: 875–876

Kernoff P B A, Thomas N D, Lilley P A, Matthew K B, Gadman E, Tuddenham E G D 1984 Clinical experience with polyelectrolyte fractionated porcine factor VIII concentrate in the treatment of haemophiliacs with antibodies to factor VIII. Blood 63: 31–41

Kessler C M, Sachse F 1990 Factor VIII: C inhibitor associated with monoclonal-antibody purified factor VIII concentrate Lancet 335: 1403

Kim H C, McMilan C W, White G C et al 1990 Clinical experience of a new monoclonal antibody purified factor IX: Half-life recovery and safety in patients with hemophilia B. Seminars in Hematology 27 (suppl 2): 30–35

Kitchen C S, Newcomb T F 1979 Factor XIII. Medicine 58: 413–429

Kleim J P, Bailly E, Schneweis K T et al 1990 Acute HIV-1 infection in patients with haemophilia B treated with β-propiolactone – UV – inactivated clotting factor. Thrombosis and Haemostasis 64: 336–337

Levy J A, Mitra G, Mozen M M 1984 Recovery and inactivation of infectious retroviruses added to factor VIII concentrate. Lancet ii: 722–723

Loche M, Mach B 1988 Identification of HIV-infected seronegative individuals by a direct diagnostic test based on hybridisation to amplified viral DNA. Lancet ii: 418–421

Lorand L, Losowsky M S, Miloszewski K J M 1980 Human factor XIII. Fibrin stabilising factor. Progress in Haemostasis and Thrombosis 5: 245–290

Losowsky M S, Miloszewski K J A 1976 Management of patients with congenital deficiency of fibrin stabilising factor (Factor XIII). 16th International Congress of Haematology, Kyoto 1966. Excerpta Medical International Congress series

Ludlam C A, Peake I R, Allen N, Davies B C, Furlong R A, Bloom A L 1980 Factor VIII and fibrinolytic response to deamino-8-D arginine vasopressin in normal subjects and dissociate response in some patients with haemophilia and von Willebrand's disease. British Journal of Haematology 45: 499–511

Ludlam C A, Tucker J, Steel C M et al 1985 Human T-lymphotropic virus type III (HTLVIII) infection in seronegative haemophiliacs after transfusion of factor VIII. Lancet ii: 233–236

Lusher J M, Shapiro S S, Palascak J E, Rao A V, Levine P H, Blatt P M 1980 Efficacy of prothrombin-complex concentrates in hemophiliacs with antibodies for factor VIII. A multicentre trial. New England Journal of Medicine 303: 421–425

Lusher J M, Salzman P M and the Monoclate Study Group 1990 Viral safety and inhibitor development associated with factor VIIIC concentrates. Seminars in Hematology 27 (suppl 2): 1–7

Lyon D J, Chapman C S, Martin C et al 1989 Symptomatic parvovirus B19 infection and heat-treated factor IX concentrate. Lancet i: 105

Macik B G, Hohneker J, Roberts H R, Griffin A M 1989 Use of recombinant activated factor VII for treatment of a retropharyngeal haemorrhage in a haemophilic patient with a high titer inhibitor. American Journal of Haematology 32: 232–234

Madhok R, Gracie A, Lowe G D O et al 1986 Impaired cell mediated immunity in haemophilia in the absence of infection with human immunodeficiency virus. British Medical Journal 293: 978–980

Mannucci P M 1992 Personal communication

Mannucci P M, Meyer D, Ruggeri Z M, Koutts J, Ciaverella N, Lavergne J-M 1976 Precipitating antibodies in von Willebrand's disease. Nature 262: 141–142

Mannucci P M, Ruggeri Z M, Pareti F I, Capitanio A 1977 1-deamino-8-D-arginine vasopression: a new pharmacological approach to the management of haemophilia and von Willebrand's disease in haemophilia. Lancet 2: 1171–1172

Mannucci P M, Colombo B 1989 Revision of the protocol recommended for studies of safety from hepatitis of clotting factor concentrates. Thrombosis and Haemostasis 61: 552–534

Mannucci P M, Bauer K A, Gringeri A et al 1990a Thrombin generation is not increased in the blood of hemophilia B patients after the infusion of a purified factor IX concentrate. Blood 76: 2540–2545

Mannucci P M, Zanetti A R, Colombo M et al 1990b Antibody to hepatitis C virus after a vapour-heated factor VIII concentrate. Thrombosis and Haemostasis 64: 232–234

Mannucci P M, Schimpf K, Brettler B et al 1990c Low risk for hepatitis C in haemophiliacs given a high-purity, pasteurised factor VIII concentrate. Annals of Internal Medicine 13(1): 27–32

Melliger E J, Duckert F 1971 Major surgery in a subject with factor V deficiency. Thrombosis et Diathesis Haemorrhagica 25: 438–446

Ménaché D, Behre H E, Orthner C L et al 1984 Coagulation factor IX concentrate: Method of preparation and assessment of potential in vivo thrombogenicity in animal models. Blood 64: 1220–1227

MMWR 1988 Safety of therapeutic products used for haemophilia patients. Morbidity and Mortality Weekly Reports 37: 441–450

Nilsson I M, Hedner U 1976 Immunosuppressive treatment in haemophiliacs with inhibitors to factor VIII and factor IX. Scandinavian Journal of Haematology 16: 369–382

Nilsson I M, Sundqvist S-B 1984 Suppression of secondary antibody response by intravenous immunoglobulin and development of tolerance in a patient with haemophilia B and antibodies. Scandinavian Journal of Haematology 33: 203–206

Nilsson I M, Jonsson S, Sundqvist S-B, Ahlberg A, Bergentz S-E 1981 A procedure for removing high titer antibodies by extra corporeal protein A-Sepharose adsorption in hemophilia: Substitution therapy and surgery in a patient with hemophilia B and antibodies. Blood 58: 38–44

Nilsson I M, Sundqvist S-B, Ljung R, Holmberg L, Freiburghaus C, Bjorling G 1983 Suppression of secondary antibody response by intravenous immunoglobulin and development of tolerance in a patient with haemophilia B and antibodies. Scandinavian Journal of Haematology 30: 459–464

Nilsson I M, Berntorp E, Zetterwall O 1988 Induction of immune tolerance in patients with haemophilia and antibodies to factor VIII by combined treatment with intravenous IgG, cyclosphosphamide and factor VIII. New England Journal of Medicine 328: 947–950

Nilsson I M, Berntorp E, Zetterwall O, Dählbäck B 1990 Non coagulation inhibitory factor VIII antibodies after induction of tolerance to factor VIII in haemophilia A patients. Blood 75: 378–383

Pasi K J, Williams M D, Enayat M S 1990 Clinical and laboratory evaluation of the treatment of von Willebrand's disease patients with heat-treated factor VIII concentrate (BPL8Y) British Journal of Haematology 75: 228–233

Peake I R, Furlong B L, Bloom A L 1984 Carrier detection by direct gene analysis in a family with haemophilia B (Factor IX deficiency) Lancet 1: 242-243

Peake I R, Liddell M B, Moodie PM et al 1990 Severe type III von Willebrand's disease caused by deletion of exon 42 of the von Willebrand factor gene: family studies that identify carriers of the condition and a compound heterozygous individual. Blood 75: 654–661

Pool J G, Shannon A E 1965 Production of high-potency antihemophilic globulin in a closed bag system. New England Journal of Medicine 273: 1443–1447

Prince A M, Horowitz B, Brotman B 1986 Sterilization of hepatitis and HTL VIII viruses by exposure to tri (N-butyl) phosphate and sodium cholate. Lancet i: 706–710

Rao L V M, Rapaport S I 1990 Factor VIIa — catalysed activation of factor X independent of tissue factor: Its possible significance for control of hemophilic bleeding by infused factor VIIa. Blood 75: 1069–1073

Rizza C R, Jones P 1987 Management of patients with inherited blood coagulation defects. In: Bloom A L, Thomas D H (eds) Coagulation defect management. Haemostasis and thrombosis. Churchill Livingstone, Edinburgh, p 465–493

Rizza C R, Matthews J M 1982 Effect of frequent factor VIII replacement on the level of factor VIII antibodies in haemophiliacs. British Journal of Haematology 52: 13–24

Roberts H R, Macik B G 1987 Factor VIII and IX concentrates: clinical efficacy as related to purity. In: Verstraete M, Vermylen J, Lijnen H R, Arnout J (eds) Thrombosis and haemostasis. Leuven University Press, Leuven, p 563–581

Rodeghiero F, Castaman G, Dini E 1987 Epidemiological investigation of the prevalence of von Willebrand's disease Blood 69: 454–459

Rodeghiero F, Castaman G, Di Bona E, Ruggeri M 1989 Consistency of responses to repeated DDAVP infusions in patients with von Willebrand's disease and hemophilia A. Blood 74: 1997–2000

Rose E, Forster A, Aledort L M 1990 Correction of prolonged bleeding time in von Willebrand's disease with Humate P. Transfusion 30: 381

Schimpf K, Mannucci P M, Kreutz W et al 1987 Absence of hepatitis after treatment with a pasteurised factor VIII concentrate in patients with haemophilia and no previous transfusions. New England Journal of Medicine 316: 918–922

Schimpf K, Brackmann H H, Kreutz W et al 1989 Absence of anti-human immunodeficiency virus types 1 and 2 seroconversion after the treatment of haemophilia A or von Willebrand's disease with pasteurised factor VIII concentrate. New England Journal of Medicine 321: 1148–1152

Schwartz R S, Abildgard C F, Aledort L M et al 1990 Human recombinant DNA-derived antihemophilic factor (factor VIII) in the treatment of haemophilia A. New England Journal of Medicine 323: 1800–1805

Sjamsoedin L J M, Heijnen L, Mauser-Bunschoten E P, van Geijlswisk J L, van Houwelingen H, van Asteb P, Sixma J J 1981 The effect of activated prothrombin complex concentrate (FEIBA) on joint and muscle bleeding in patients with hemophilia A and antibodies to factor VIII. A randomised double blind clinical trial. New England Journal of Medicine 305: 171–721

Smith M A 1989 Orthopaedic management in hemophilia. In: Seghatchian M J, Savidge G F (eds) Factor VIII — von Willebrand factor, CRC Press, Boca Raton p 183–221

Smith T J, Gill J C, Ambruso D R, Hathaway W E 1989 Hyponatremia and seizures in young children given DDAVP. American Journal of Medicine 31: 199–202

Stein H, Dickson R A 1975 Reversed dynamic slings for knee flexion contractures in the haemophiliac. Journal of Bone and Joint Surgery 57A: 282

Stein S F, Duncan A, Cutler D, Glaser S 1990 Disseminated intravascular coagulation (DIC) in a hemophiliac treated with recombinant factor VIIa. Blood 176 (suppl 1): 438a

Stern D M, Drillings M, Nossel H L, Hurlet-Jensen A, LaCamma K, Owren J 1983 Binding of factors IX and IXa to cultured vascular endothelial cells. Proceedings of the National Academy of Sciences, USA 80: 4119–4123

Stratton R D, Wagner R H, Webster W P, Brinkhous K M 1975 Antibody nature of circulating inhibitor of plasma von Willebrand's factor. Proceedings of the National Academy of Sciences, USA 72: 4167–4171

Telgt D S C, Macik B G, McCord D M et al 1989 Mechanism by which recombinant factor VIIa shortens the aPTT: Activation of factor X in the absence of tissue factor. Thrombosis Research 56: 603–609

Thim L, Bjoern S, Christensen M et al 1988 Amino acid sequence and post-translational modifications of human factor VIIa from plasma and transfected baby hamster kidney cells. Biochemistry 27: 7785–7793

Thorpe R, Dilger P, Dawson N J, Barrowcliffe T W 1989 Inhibition of interleukin-2 secretion by factor VIII concentrates: A possible cause of immunosuppression in haemophiliacs. British Journal of Haematology 71: 387–391

Toole J J, Knopf J L, Wozey J M et al 1984 Molecular cloning of a cDNA encoding human antihaemophilic factor. Nature 312: 342–347

van Leeuen E F, Mauser-Bunschoten E P, van Dijken P J, Kok A J, Sjamsoedin-Visser E J M, Sixma J J 1986 Disappearance of factor VIII: C antibodies in patients with haemophilia A upon frequent administration of factor VIII in intermediate or low dose. British Journal of Haematology 64: 291–297

Walsh P N, Rizza C R, Matthews J M et al 1971 Epsilon-amino caproic acid therapy for dental extraction in haemophilia and Christmas disease: a double blind controlled trial. British Journal of Haematology 20: 463–475

Weinstein R E, Bona R D, Altman A J, Quinn J J, Weisman S J, Bartolomeo A, Rickles F R R 1989. Severe hyponatremia after repeated intravenous administration of desmopressin. American Journal of Hematology 32: 258–261

Wensley R T, Burns A M, Reading O M 1986 Induced tolerance to factor VIII in haemophilia A with inhibitor using low dose of human factor VIII. Ricerca in Clinica e Laboratoria 16: 104

White G CII, McMilan C W, Kingdom H S, Shoemaker C B 1989 Use of recombinant antihemophilic factor in the treatment of two patients with classic hemophilia. New England Journal of Medicine 320: 166–170

Wood W I, Capon D J, Simonsen C C et al 1984 Expression of active human factor VIII from recombinant DNA clones. Nature 312: 330–336

Yoshioka A, Peake I R, Furlong B L, Furlong R A, Giddings J C, Bloom A L 1983 The interaction between factor VIII clotting antigen (VIIIC Ag) and phospholipid. British Journal of Haematology 55: 27–36

39. Hepatitis in blood product recipients

M. Makris F. E. Preston

Although the first description of epidemic jaundice can be traced to the writings of Hippocrates from the 4th century BC, blood product-transmitted hepatitis was not reported for another 2000 years. In 1883, 191 of 1339 workers in a factory in Bremen, Germany developed jaundice following vaccination against smallpox. The inoculum used was cowpox virus in the form of glycerinized human serum from previously vaccinated individuals and Lurman elegantly showed that the hepatitis was related to one batch of presumably infected inoculum (Lurman 1885). Large outbreaks of hepatitis occurred in the late 1930s and early 1940s in recipients of yellow fever vaccine, which contained pooled human plasma to stabilize the vaccine (Zuckerman 1983). By far the largest outbreak occurred during the second world war when 28 585 American soldiers developed hepatitis following yellow fever vaccination (Journal of the American Medical Association 1942).

During the first part of this century, jaundice was reported in patients treated with arsenicals, diabetics treated with insulin and rheumatoid arthritis patients treated with gold. Although at first this was thought to be due to direct toxicity of the injected compound, MacCullam suggested that jaundice could be transmitted by means of unsterile syringes (MacCullam 1943). In the same year Beeson reported for the first time the development of jaundice in seven patients following blood transfusion (Beeson 1943). Post-transfusion hepatitis (PTH) is today the commonest serious complication of blood transfusion.

THE HEPATITIS VIRUSES

PTH can be caused by a number of different blood-borne viruses (Table 39.1). In terms of number and morbidity hepatitis A (HAV), Epstein Barr virus (EBV) and Cytomegalovirus (CMV) are responsible for only a very small proportion of PTH. Other hepatotropic viruses which could theoretically be transmitted by blood include hepatitis E, herpes simplex, coxsackie B, echovirus and yellow fever virus. None of them causes chronic hepatitis and since, with the exception of CMV and EBV, they have relatively short periods of viraemia, the proportion of the donor pool likely to be infected at any time is thus very small. Of much greater importance in terms of PTH are the hepatitis B, D and C viruses.

Table 39.1 Viruses transmitted by blood and blood products

Virus	Acute hepatitis	Chronic hepatitis
Hepatitis A	+	–
Hepatitis B	+	+
Hepatitis C	+	+
Hepatitis D	+	+
Hepatitis E*	+	–
Cytomegalovirus	+	–
Epstein Barr virus	+	–

* Theoretical, no reports of transmission by blood.

Hepatitis B

Hepatitis B, a double-stranded DNA virus, was the first virus to be identified as a cause of PTH. It can be transmitted by blood and blood products, through the use of contaminated needles, and through sexual contact. Hepatitis B causes acute (sometimes fulminant) as well as chronic hepatitis. 5–10% of patients with acute hepatitis B become chronic carriers and remain infectious. The risk of chronic carriage of hepatitis B is increased in the immunocompromised, in males and in the young. It has been estimated that there are 300 million chronic HBsAg carriers world-wide (Maynard et al 1988). 25% of these develop chronic active hepatitis with ultimate progression to cirrhosis and hepatocellular carcinoma (Alter et al 1991).

Since the introduction of sensitive assays for the hepatitis B surface antigen (HBsAg) and screening of all blood donations, the incidence of post-transfusion hepatitis due to this virus has been reduced enormously. Some cases still occur due to very low levels of circulating HBsAg which fall below the sensitivity of the assays (Alter et al 1991). A few of these cases are due to mutations in the precore region of the HBV genome, the so-called precore mutants which have high levels of circulating HBV viraemia with low HBsAg expression (Kojima et al 1991). Despite the absence of detectable HBsAg, anti-HBc often at high titre is found in most of these potentially infectious cases (Hoofnagle et al 1978, Kojima et al 1991).

Hepatitis D

Hepatitis D is a defective DNA virus that requires the surface antigen of the hepatitis B virus to replicate and infect the host. Originally described in Italy (Rizzetto et al 1979), its occurrence has been demonstrated world-wide (Rizzetto 1982). Hepatitis D virus infection is endemic in Italy, the Middle East and some areas of South America such as the Amazon basin, but relatively rare in Western Europe and North America (Lau et al 1991). It is parentally transmitted, and is associated with a more severe hepatitis than that seen in patients infected with hepatitis B alone.

Hepatitis C

Following the widespread introduction of immunological markers for the detection of hepatitis B and hepatitis A it became clear that another major agent was responsible for the majority of PTH. The agent responsible was called non-A, non-B hepatitis (NANBH) and, even before its formal identification, its physicochemical properties were characterized by cross-challenge experiments on chimpanzees (Bradley 1985).

The virus responsible, hepatitis C (HCV), has recently been identified and sequenced by a group at the Chiron Corporation in California (Choo et al 1989). At approximately the same time and using similar techniques, Arima and colleagues (Arima et al 1989) independently reported the cloning of a related, but not identical, HCV isolate from Japan. The Chiron group cloned cDNA from a chronically-infected chimpanzee into the bacteriophage lambda-gt11 and used the serum of patients with chronic non-A, non-B hepatitis (NANBH) to screen the polypeptides produced by the cDNA clones. The first specific clone C100, (now known to represent most of the NS4 region of the HCV genome) (Fig. 39.1) was fused to the human superoxide dysmutase gene (SOD) and expressed in yeast. Fusion to human SOD facilitates the expression of heterologous proteins in yeast (Choo et al 1990). Thus large amounts of the fusion polypeptide C100-3 were produced. The C100-3 was used as the antigen in the first generation of anti-HCV assays (Kuo et al 1989).

The hepatitis C virus is a single positively-stranded RNA virus of around 10 000 nucleotides and is 32 ± 3 nm in size (Muchmore et al 1991). It shares aminoacid and nucleotide homology with the flaviviruses such as yellow fever virus and with pestiviruses such as hog cholera virus (Houghton et al 1991). The functional domains of the HCV genome are shown in Figure 39.1. A number of groups have isolated and sequenced different strains of HCV and these have now been subdivided into three groups on the basis of nucleotide homology. Most strains found in Western populations belong to group 1 (Houghton et al 1991). Marked variability of the HCV genome occurs between amino acid positions 384–414 and this region has now been designated the E2 hypervariable region (E2HV). In infected subjects, rapid HCV mutation may occur within the E2HV region and this may explain how the virus escapes host immunological surveillance resulting in the development of chronic infection (Ogata et al 1991).

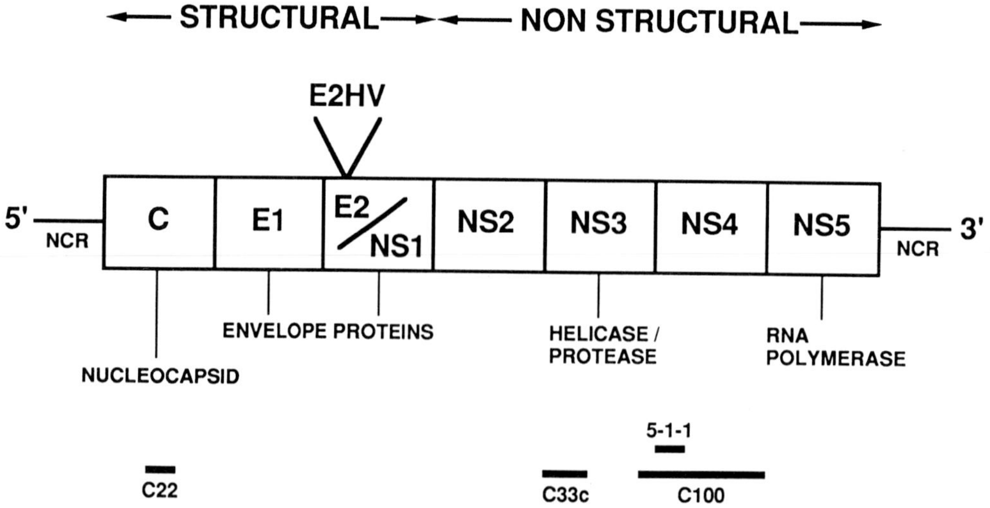

Fig. 39.1 The hepatitis C genome showing the structural (C, E1 and E2/NS1) and non-structural components (NS2-5). The hypervariable region (E2HV) is located within the E2/NS1 region. Non-coding regions (NCR) are found at both ends of the genome. The lower part of the figure shows the proteins commonly used for HCV testing and their relationship to the genome.

Testing for hepatitis C

The first HCV antibody assay, which was never commercially marketed, utilized the C100-3 antigen in a radioimmunoassay system (Kuo et al 1989, Makris et al 1990). Shortly afterwards an ELISA system using the same antigen was marketed by Ortho Diagnostics (Raritan, USA). Using these first generation assays it has been demonstrated that HCV antibodies are found in most cases of chronic and some cases of acute NANBH. Antibodies to C100-3 develop at around 3–4 months (Fig. 39.2) but may be delayed up to a year or more especially in immunocompromised patients. False positive results are not uncommon. These may reflect antibodies to the superoxide dismutase part of the C100-3 fusion protein (Ikeda et al 1990) or may be due to rheumatoid factor (Theilmann et al 1990). False positive results also occur with autoimmune chronic active hepatitis (McFarlane et al 1990) and paraproteinaemia (Boudart et al 1990). Although the use of a urea wash with the first ELISA step may reduce the number of false positives (Goeser et al 1990), it does not completely abolish them.

More recently a number of manufacturers have introduced second generation ELISA assays, employing antigens from both the structural and non-structural parts of the HCV genome. These have a higher specificity and sensitivity than first generation assays and are now in routine use in the screening of all blood donations in Europe, North America, Australia and Japan. The introduction of a second generation recombinant immunoblot assay (RIBA-2) has enhanced the diagnostic accuracy of currently available tests. In this system, four different recombinant HCV antigens (C22, C33c, 5-1-1 and C-100) are used thus increasing the specificity of the assay (van der Poel et al 1991).

There is little doubt that over the next few years, new assays will be developed and marketed which will be much more specific and sensitive than those available today. A disadvantage of all the current antibody assays is that they are not informative as to whether they reflect immunity from infection or whether they are indicative of continuing infection. The development of serological assays for HCV antigen detection is at present difficult since viral expression in the circulation is low. The detection of viral RNA by the polymerase chain reaction (PCR) overcomes this problem (Weiner et al 1990) and the use of nested primers for PCR amplification increases the specificity and sensitivity of this technique (Garson et al 1990a). It is now recognised that there is considerable sequence variation in the HCV genome and selection of primers for the two stages of the PCR is therefore critical (Garson et al 1990b, Cristiano et al 1991). The use of primers from the highly conserved 5′ non-coding region of the virus where there is >99% homology between all viral strains so far reported (Han et al 1991) offers the most reliable approach to the detection of HCV RNA. Pozzato and colleagues have recently shown a relationship between HCV genome structure and clinical outcome (Pozzato et al 1991).

In acute NANBH, HCV viraemia can been demonstrated within 2 weeks of infection (Fig. 39.3) which is several months before the appearance of antibody to C100-3 (Garson et al 1990c, Farci et al 1991). Patients with chronic infection remain viraemic while those with self-limiting acute hepatitis become HCV RNA negative.

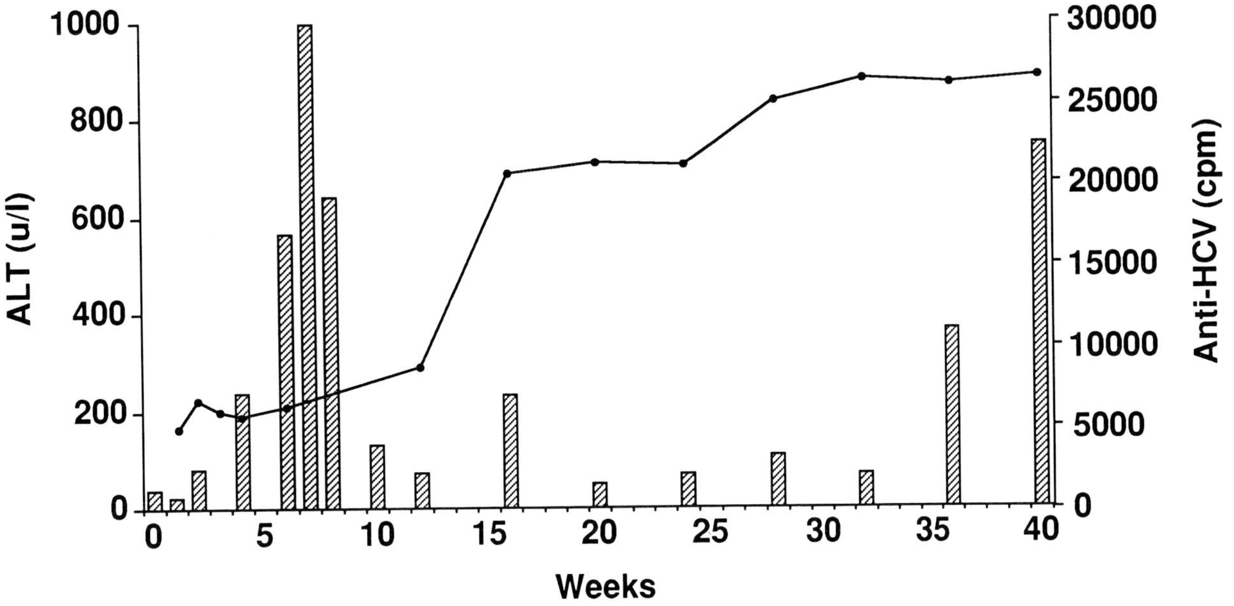

Fig. 39.2 The development of acute hepatitis C in a haemophiliac treated for the first time with factor VIII at time 0. HCV seroconversion occurred between 3–4 months. HCV antibody was detected with the Chiron first generation radioimmunoassay. ALT levels are indicated by the shaded bars and HCV antibody by the line.

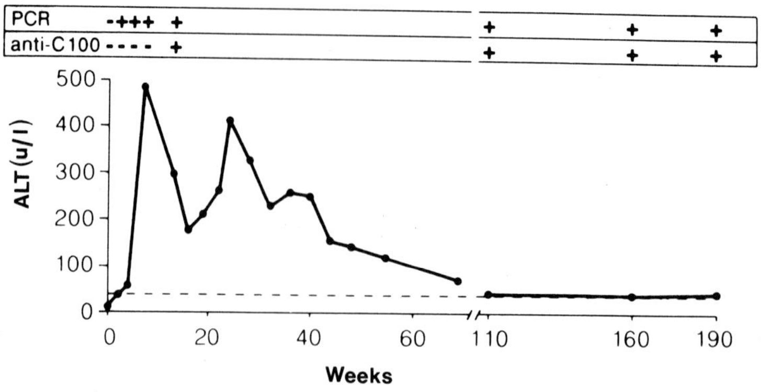

Fig. 39.3 Haemophilic patient receiving his first exposure to factor VIII. HCV RNA was detected at 2 weeks and seroconversion for C100 antibody occurred at 13 weeks. This patient continues to be viraemic despite normal ALT. (Reproduced with permission from Garson et al 1990C.)

However ongoing HCV infection may still be present even in previously infected subjects with normal liver enzymes (Garson et al 1990c). In high prevalence populations, such as haemophiliacs, more than 90% of HCV antibody-positive patients are viraemic, whereas in blood donors only one in six is viraemic (Garson et al 1990a, Tedder et al 1991, Watson 1991). Garson and colleagues have shown that PCR-positive donors are much more likely to be associated with PTH in the recipient than PCR-negative, anti-C100-3-positive donors (Garson et al 1990a).

Table 39.2 Factors shown to influence the incidence of post-transfusion hepatitis

Anti-HCV incidence in the donor population
Exclusion of high-risk donors
Number of exposures to blood or blood products
Number of donors used in pooled products
Type of donors (volunteer or paid)
Intensity of follow-up of recipients
Hepatitis B vaccination of recipients
ALT and Anti-HBc testing of donor units
Anti-HCV testing of donor units
Method of viral inactivation of pooled products

HEPATITIS IN RECIPIENTS OF BLOOD TRANSFUSION

With the more widespread practice of transfusion medicine since the Second World War, post-transfusion hepatitis has been increasingly identified. Prior to 1970 the incidence of post-transfusion hepatitis in the USA, where paid donors were used, was as high as 33% (Alter et al 1975). This incidence was markedly reduced, down to 10%, following the introduction of testing for HBsAg and the shift from paid to volunteer donors (Aach et al 1978). A further reduction was seen following the exclusion of donors considered to be at high risk for HIV (Mattsson et al 1988). Retrospective analysis of cases of PTH showed that donors likely to transmit the agent were more likely to have anti-HBc antibodies and have elevated liver enzymes. In the absence of a test for NANBH, tests for these two surrogate markers, anti-HBc and ALT, were introduced in the USA in 1986 and 1987 respectively. These measures however did not gain widespread acceptance in countries with a lower incidence of PTH such as the UK. Table 39.2 lists some of the factors which affect the rate of post-transfusion hepatitis. Figure 39.4 shows the value of the introduction of different measures in reducing PTH in the USA.

Following the identification of the hepatitis C virus, it became clear that the majority of cases of post-transfusion NANBH were due to this virus. Many countries quickly introduced tests for HCV antibody in an attempt to reduce the incidence of PTH further. The problem with the first generation assay was the high number of false positives leading to wastage of collected donor units and false negatives leading sometimes to hepatitis C in the recipient despite screening of all units. With the introduction of second generation and confirmatory assays it is hoped that this problem will be overcome.

PTH is a serious disease associated with significant morbidity and mortality (Alter 1989). In contrast to the serious nature of chronic HCV, the acute event is often trivial and frequently goes unnoticed. Only a small minority of infected patients develop jaundice and an even smaller number feel unwell. Until the recent introduction of HCV testing, the only way of demonstrating acute infection was with frequent ALT estimation in the recipient. This, however, was rarely done outside the setting of formal studies and thus the incidence of PTH was underestimated. The clinical importance of NANBH lies in its tendency to produce chronic liver disease which occurs in 50% of infected subjects. This is characterized by fluctuating or by persistently raised liver enzymes. In PTH patients who have undergone liver biopsy chronic active hepatitis was present in 36% and cirrhosis in 20% (Alter 1989). Figure 39.5 illustrates the possible histological outcomes following acute NANBH. In contrast to the cirrhosis of alcohol-associated liver disease, PTH cirrhosis

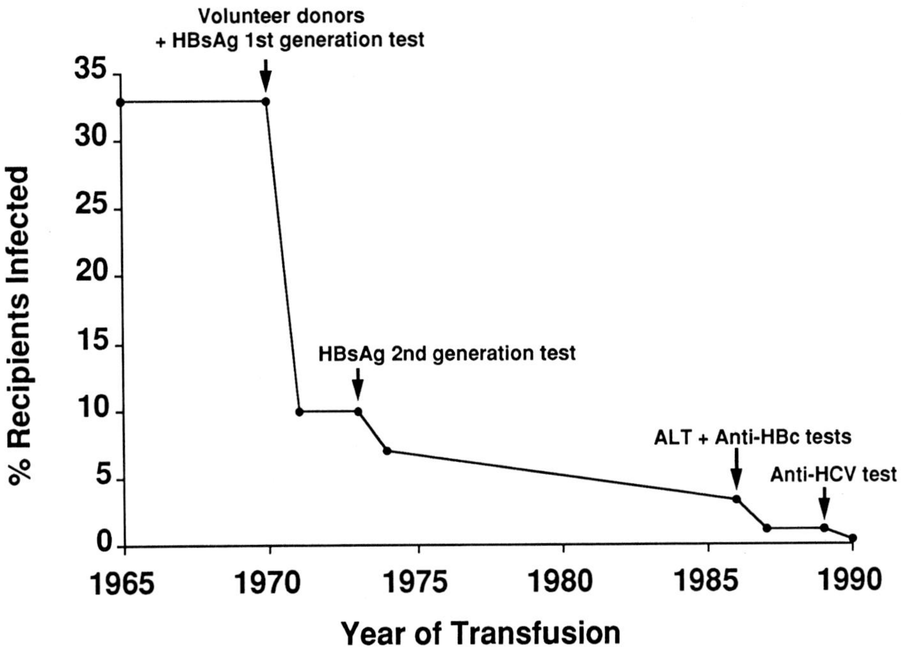

Fig. 39.4 The incidence of PTH in the USA in relation to the introduction of different measures. (Data from Alter et al 1985, and Donahue et al 1992.)

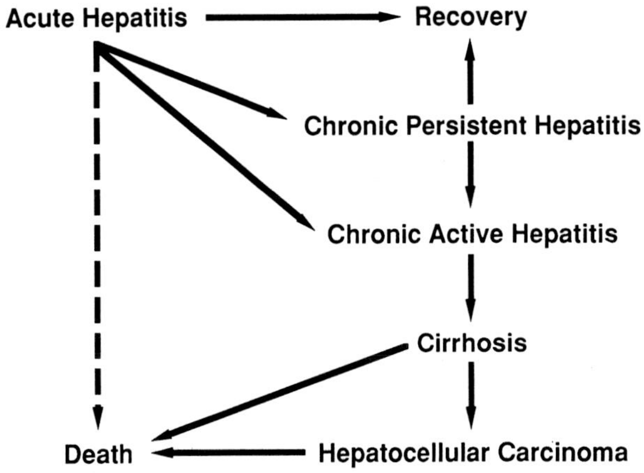

Fig. 39.5 Possible outcomes of acute NANBH. The development of fulminant hepatitis following acute NANBH is rare.

pursues a more indolent course and symptoms are a late manifestation of the disorder.

HEPATITIS IN RECIPIENTS OF IMMUGLOBULIN

Concentrated immunoglobulin preparations are available in intramuscular (IMIG) and intravenous (IVIG) forms. They are widely used for specific passive immunization, replacement in hypo-gammaglobulinaemic subjects and for the management of a wide variety of conditions where autoimmune aetiology has been demonstrated or postulated. Apart from a few early reports of hepatitis B and particularly since the introduction of donor screening for this virus, the IMIG preparation has proved to be remarkably safe. Recently, the intravenous form has gained widespread acceptance and although it is generally believed to be as safe as the intramuscular preparation, transmissions of NANBH have been attributed to its use (Williams et al 1989), and to date two major and three minor outbreaks of NANBH after IVIG have been reported (Anonymous 1991). There is no clear explanation why IVIG and not IMIG has transmitted NANBH. In one instance of products prepared from the same donor pool, the intravenous preparation transmitted non-A, non-B hepatitis whilst the intramuscular form did not (Lane 1983). These events have led to the production of a newer generation of IVIG products which involve additional virucidal steps. It remains to be seen whether this produces the expected elimination of hepatitis. Although the overall safety record of intramuscular immunoglobulin is good, constant surveillance is nevertheless still necessary. This is highlighted by the recent report from East Germany where several hundred women were infected with HCV by a single batch of intramuscular anti-D, an immunoglobulin preparation used to prevent rhesus sensitization (Durkop et al 1990).

HEPATITIS IN HAEMOPHILIACS

With the introduction of pooled concentrates in the early 1970s it was recognised that a small but significant number of patients developed jaundice (Kasper & Kipnis 1972). In the decade that followed, many workers have indirectly attempted to quantify the problem of hepatitis in haemophilia by measuring circulating levels of alanine aminotransferase (ALT). The incidence of reported ALT abnormalities varied between 45–81% of all patients treated with clotting factor concentrate (Mannucci et al 1975, Hasiba et al 1977, Preston et al 1978, Cederbaum et al 1982). The wide difference in the reported figures reflects methodological differences. The ALT levels in chronic NANBH liver disease are known to fluctuate and may be only intermittently raised. It is therefore not surprising that the quoted incidence of chronic liver disease is lower when single point determinations have been carried out (Mannucci et al 1975) than when repeated liver enzyme determinations have been undertaken (Hasiba et al 1977, Preston et al 1978, Cederbaum et al 1982). In the largest study to date involving 1332 US haemophiliacs, where conclusions were based on the results of the three most recent liver enzyme determinations, 23.6% had persistently raised ALT, 47.5% intermittently raised ALT and 28.9% had normal ALT (Cederbaum et al 1982).

The incidence of chronic hepatitis appears to relate to the number of donors to which recipients have been exposed. Hasiba found that 95% of HBsAg-negative haemophiliacs exposed to more than three lots of unheated concentrate had abnormal LFTs compared to 75% in those who had received less concentrate and only 8% in those who had received only cryoprecipitate (Hasiba et al 1977). Although the use of volunteer donors reduced the incidence of PTH in blood transfusion recipients, this was not the case with clotting factor concentrates. This was clearly shown by two studies from England in which the reported incidence of acute hepatitis following a first exposure to concentrate was almost 100%, with concentrates from both commercial and volunteer donors being equally implicated (Fletcher et al 1983, Kernoff et al 1985).

In the late 1970s a number of groups performed liver biopsies in haemophiliacs with biochemical evidence of chronic liver disease. The majority of biopsies showed chronic persistent hepatitis (CPH), which was considered to be benign and non-progressive. A substantial proportion however had serious chronic liver disease such as chronic active hepatitis and cirrhosis (Lesesne et al 1977, Preston et al 1978, Spero et al 1978). Some of the observed differences may be attributable to the criteria for patient selection, since some groups biopsied only patients with persistent enzyme abnormalities (Lesesne et al 1977, Preston et al 1978) while others studied those with either intermittent abnormalities (Mannucci et al 1978, Stevens et al 1983) or with a combination of the two (Schimpf 1986).

The natural history of chronic liver disease in haemophilia has been the subject of much debate and in the 1980s there were a number of conflicting reports on its clinical significance and its rate of progression. Mannucci rebiopsied the patients of their earlier study and found no evidence of progression (Mannucci 1982), while Stevens and colleagues found only mild disease in patients having a first biopsy (Stevens et al 1983). White et al reported on biopsies from a group selected specifically because they had intermittent enzyme abnormalities and found almost exclusively chronic persistent hepatitis (White et al 1982). They concluded that since intermittent ALT abnormalities were the most common pattern seen in their haemophilic population, and since CPH is a non-progressive form of liver disease, most haemophiliacs were unlikely to have or develop serious liver disease. In contrast to these, two later studies from the UK and Germany suggest that chronic liver disease in haemophilia was progressive and potentially serious. The Sheffield (UK) group who rebiopsied patients with persistent ALT abnormalities showed that rapid progression to severe liver disease had occurred in the majority of the patients studied. They also demonstrated progression of chronic persistent hepatitis, a form of liver disease usually considered to be benign, to chronic active hepatitis and even cirrhosis (Hay et al 1985). The German group who biopsied haemophiliacs who were not selected on the basis of ALT abnormalities found 32% of their patients had chronic active hepatitis and 9% cirrhosis (Schimpf 1986, 1990). By far the largest series of liver biopsies in haemophilia is that reported by Aledort and his coworkers in 1985 (Aledort et al 1985). They collected data on 155 patients from haemophilia centres throughout the world. Although many of the biopsies are included in the previously published studies, and most biopsies were considered to show mild changes, 22% showed either severe chronic active hepatitis or cirrhosis. In this study the frequency of severe liver disease in patients receiving large, pooled concentrates was no greater than in patients treated principally with cryoprecipitate or plasma implying that the concentration of the initial infective viral load was not important in the course of the disease.

There is an understandable reluctance to carry out biopsies on haemophiliacs because of the risk of bleeding (Aledort et al 1985). Alternative non-invasive approaches to study liver disease have been reported. Using CT scanning Miller and colleagues in 1988 found splenomegaly in 28 of 47 patients with abnormal liver function tests and collateral oesophageal veins in seven of 28 haemophiliacs (Miller et al 1988). Dynamic tests of liver function such as galactose elimination and bromsulphthalein clearance have been considered but early promising results have not yet been confirmed in haemophilia (Stevens et al 1983). Serum procollagen III peptide has been suggested as a marker of hepatic fibrosis, and although levels in haemophiliacs are significantly higher than in controls, it is not possible to differentiate between cirrhosis and less severe liver disease (Evely et al 1987). A step wise increase in serum IgG levels commensurate with liver disease progression has been reported in UK haemophiliacs. However in HIV antibody-positive patients this relationship is complicated by concomitant HIV-related hypergammaglobulinaemia (Hay et al 1987). Despite the range of non-invasive tests available, the liver biopsy remains the only reliable method of assessing the severity of liver disease in haemophilia.

Chronic liver disease in haemophilia is common and can progress to cirrhosis and, possibly, hepatocellular carcinoma. What is its aetiology? Although 44–90% of haemophiliacs who received non-heat-treated concentrates have serological evidence of previous hepatitis B infection, very few are chronic carriers (Holsteen et al 1977, Sterling et al 1983, Lee & Kernoff 1990). In the UK it is estimated that only 2–5% of haemophiliacs are HBsAg positive. As chronic liver disease is not seen in patients who lose the HBsAg, hepatitis B plays only a minor role in haemophilic liver disease in this country. Most HBsAg-positive patients are also infected with the hepatitis C virus and it is difficult to evaluate the individual contribution of these two hepatotropic viruses to chronic liver disease. As already discussed, hepatitis D only occurs in HBsAg-positive patients. Rizetto reported the incidence of anti-delta (hepatitis D) antibodies in Italian HBsAg-positive haemophiliacs to be 49% in adults in 25% in children (Rizzetto et al 1982). Overall chronic liver disease due to hepatitis D is rare in the UK.

It was clear long before the identification of hepatitis C that the majority of haemophilic hepatitis was due to non-A, non-B hepatitis. Many investigators reported the incidence of anti-HCV in their haemophilic cohorts. With the first generation tests, 59–85% of patients were found to be positive (Ludlam et al 1989, Makris et al 1990). The difference in the figures reflects the selection of patients to be tested and the type of test employed.

If the incidence of non-A, non-B hepatitis after first exposure to concentrate is 100%, why is this not the case with antibodies to hepatitis C? The most likely explanations are that the first generation HCV assay was relatively insensitive and that some HCV haemophiliacs do not have antibody despite high levels of circulating HCV viraemia (Simmonds et al 1990). Newer second generation assays employing structural HCV antigens indicate that the incidence of anti-HCV in haemophiliacs treated with non-virally-inactivated concentrates is >95% (Watson 1992). Using PCR and a nested primer technique, Garson et al have demonstrated viral sequences in the serum of >90% of haemophiliacs with abnormal liver function tests (Garson et al 1990b). Although no large study of HCV viraemia in haemophiliacs with normal liver function tests has been reported, there is evidence that it can occur (Garson et al 1990c).

MORBIDITY AND MORTALITY DUE TO LIVER DISEASE

If chronic liver disease due to hepatitis C is common, how does it affect morbidity and mortality in haemophilia? Although no report to date directly addresses morbidity, the data from mortality studies, and from reports of liver transplantation in haemophiliacs clearly show that a proportion of these patients are suffering serious morbidity.

Aronson analysed data from death certificates on 949 patients with haemophilia A dying during 1968–79 in the United States (Aronson 1988). Eight deaths directly due to hepatitis were recorded. Cirrhosis however, was the primary or associated cause of death in 8% of all cases in the study. Eyster and colleagues, also in the USA, followed up 79 patients identified in the late 1970s as having persistent lymphocytopenia or thrombocytopenia (Eyster et al 1985). 5 years later ten patients (12.6%) died, in five of these the cause of death was cirrhosis. Similarly in Germany, cirrhosis was the cause of death of 17% of haemophiliacs dying in the period 1978–87 (Lanbeck 1987).

Much lower figures have been reported from the United Kingdom. Rizza and Spooner reporting on all haemophilic deaths during 1976–80 found hepatitis to be responsible for 2% of all deaths (Rizza & Spooner 1983) whilst in Sweden Larsson found liver disease to have been responsible for 4% of deaths in the period 1957–68 and 9.1% during 1969–80 (Larsson & Wiechel 1983). It is not clear whether these differences do in fact represent real differences in morbidity and mortality. At least in the UK the lack of objective confirmation through autopsy data almost certainly underestimates the problem.

PREVENTION OF POST-TRANSFUSION HEPATITIS

Donor selection

Since many blood-borne viruses share common risk factors they frequently coexist in infected individuals. The HIV epidemic of the 1980s led blood transfusion services to exclude donors at high risk of HIV such as homosexuals, intravenous drug abusers and visitors to sub-Saharan Africa. The reduction in HIV transmission was accompanied by a simultaneous reduction in the incidence of post-transfusion hepatitis as many of the hepatitis C-positive donors were from these same high risk groups (Mattsson et al 1988). Another important factor in the reduction of PTH has been the use of volunteer rather than paid donors. In a study from the United States in 1975, Goldfield et al reported the incidence of post-transfusion hepatitis to be 28.7% of recipients of paid donors compared to 7.7% of recipients of volunteer donor blood (Goldfield et al 1975). In this study all donor units were screened for HBsAg. In contrast to this, there did not appear to be a difference in the transmission of HCV by non-viral inactivated concentrates derived from paid and volunteer donors (Makris et al 1990). This is almost certainly a reflection of the very large size of the donor pool for these products.

Screening of donor units

There is little doubt that the introduction of HBsAg screening greatly reduced the incidence of PTH in the early 1970s (Alter et al 1972, 1975). Screening for ALT and anti-HBc was introduced in 1986 and 1987 as surrogate markers for NANBH. The introduction of anti-HBc may have contributed further to the reduction in the incidence of hepatitis B in cases of viraemic donors who do not express HBsAg (Hoofnagle et al 1978). The effectiveness of surrogate marker screening was demonstrated by a collaborative study from the United States where the introduction of these tests reduced the incidence of PTH in cardiac surgery patients from 3.4% to 1.2% (Nelson et al 1991). The incidence of PTH was further reduced to 0.4% following the introduction of anti-HCV testing (Nelson et al 1991). It is not yet possible to say whether the new second generation anti-HCV tests will render surrogate marker screening unnecessary. Although in retrospective studies, anti-HCV assays performed remarkably well in identifying potentially infective units, it remains to be seen whether they perform equally well in prospective studies. The early experience suggests that even first generation prospective anti-HCV screening is effective. In a study from Japan, the incidence of PTH was reduced from 4.9% to 1.9% following screening for anti-HBc and anti-HCV (C-100). Interestingly, in this study anti-HBc positive units were only excluded if the antibody was of high titre, the authors having previously identified this as a risk factor for HBV viraemia (Japanese Red Cross Non-A Non-B Hepatitis research group 1991).

Product sterilization

The recent introduction of viral inactivation procedures in the manufacture of clotting factor concentrates has greatly reduced their viral infectivity. The number of viral elimination techniques used today is almost as large as the number of manufacturers of blood products. Although the early methods of dry heat treatment at 60–68°C for 32–72 h were largely ineffective in preventing NANBH transmission (Colombo et al 1985, Preston et al 1985) other methods have proved far superior. Whilst most manufacturers have introduced a step of wet heating, solvent detergent treatment or monoclonal antibody purification, the Bio Products Laboratory (Elstree, UK) continues to use super dry heat (80°C for 72 h) with excellent results (Study Group 1988). Despite the markedly improved safety record of the newer clotting factor concentrates there is no place for complacency as cases of hepatitis can still occur with processes previously reported to be 100% effective (Berntorp et al 1990).

Proof of safety can only be assessed through carefully conducted clinical trials. It should be appreciated that the lack of observed events in a particular study, however well controlled is not in itself a guarantee of absolute safety (Mannucci & Colombo 1989). The power of any safety trial depends on the number of patients treated. The 'rule of three' is a simple calculation which estimates the risk of an event occurring in trials with no positive events (Hanley & Lippman-Hand 1983). For example if no cases of hepatitis were observed in a trial involving 30 patients the risk of an event occurring is three in 30, i.e. less than 10%. Despite improvements in the methods of viral elimination we will perhaps have to wait for the widespread introduction of recombinant concentrates before the hepatitis worry can be ignored.

Hepatitis B vaccination

Despite screening for HBsAg of all donor units and the introduction of viral inactivation procedures for clotting factor concentrates, rare cases of hepatitis B transmitted by heat-treated factor VIII have continued to occur (Brackman & Egli 1988, Mannucci et al 1988). In an effort to reduce the risk further, previously unexposed patients likely to be exposed to blood products should be vaccinated with the plasma-derived or recombinant hepatitis B vaccine. The effectiveness of hepatitis B vaccination has been demonstrated by carefully controlled studies in exposed populations such as homosexual men (Szmuness et al 1980) and haemodialysis patients (Stevens et al 1984). Factors likely to lead to suboptimal response to the hepatitis B vaccine are given in Table 39.3.

TREATMENT OF POST-TRANSFUSION HEPATITIS

Many attempts have been made to treat PTH, with the aim of halting and perhaps reversing disease progression. Of the first agents to be tried, corticosteroids (Stocks et al 1987) and acyclovir (Pappas et al 1985) have been shown to be ineffective.

The success of recombinant interferon-alpha in some patients with hepatitis B, prompted Hoofnagle and colleagues to examine its effect in chronic NANBH (Hoofnagle et al 1986). In an uncontrolled study, the transaminases of eight of ten patients with chronic NANBH were normalized by subcutaneous interferon alpha-2b at a dose of 3 million units three times weekly. A flurry of controlled

Table 39.3 Factors likely to cause suboptimal responsiveness to hepatitis B vaccine

Age
Obesity
Alcoholism
Chronic illness (e.g. chronic renal failure)
HIV infection
Immunosuppression
Route of administration

Reproduced with permission from Harrison et al 1991.

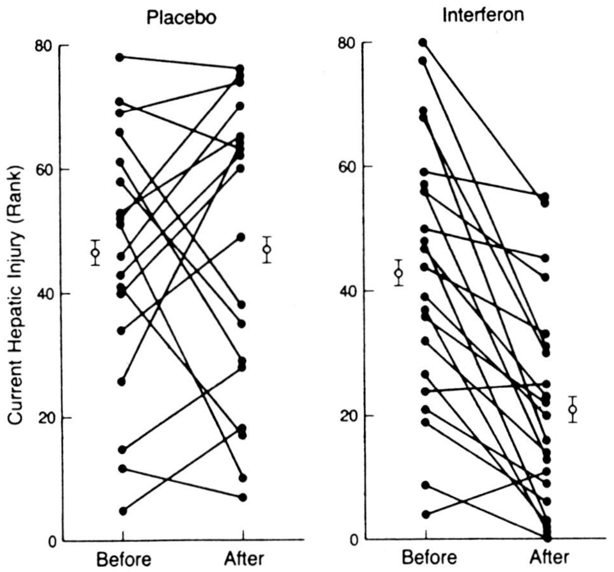

Fig. 39.6 Changes in ranking of hepatic injury on histologic examination in patients with chronic hepatitis C before and after receiving interferon or placebo. The open circles indicate the mean ± SE values at each time in each group (reproduced with permission from Davis et al 1989.)

and uncontrolled trials followed, confirming the value of low dose alpha interferon for post-transfusion chronic hepatitis. The largest controlled multicentre trial to date (Davis et al 1989) showed a 38% complete response rate in patients treated for 6 months with 3 million units thrice weekly, compared with a 16% response rate in those treated with 1 million units and 4% in the untreated controls. However, following discontinuation of the drug, 50% of the 3 million unit and 44% of the 1 million unit-treated patients relapsed. Figure 39.6 illustrates the improvement in liver histology seen following interferon in this trial. Despite many completed studies, the optimum treatment regimen has yet to be established. It appears that at present interferon alpha-2b at 3 million units thrice weekly is likely to induce complete remission in 50% of patients treated, with half of these responders relapsing on discontinuing treatment (Tine et al 1991).

Most reports on the use of interferon have been in patients acquiring hepatitis C through blood transfusion. Three reports, one in hypogammaglobulinaemic patients (Thomson et al 1987) and two in haemophilia (Lee et al 1989, Makris et al 1991b) have confirmed the value of alpha interferon in chronic HCV acquired through other blood products. Figure 39.7 shows the biochemical response to interferon in a haemophilic patient.

Patients who develop cirrhosis with portal hypertension are managed in the same way as patients with liver failure of other aetiology. For patients with documented cirrhosis, endoscopy is useful in identifying patients with oesophageal varices, and abdominal ultrasound with alpha fetoprotein estimation are of value in the detection of early hepatocellular carcinoma.

Liver transplantation is a therapeutic option in patients in whom medical management of liver failure has failed. The success rate of liver transplantation in non-haemophiliacs is in excess of 70% one-year survival (Busuttil et al 1987) but, although widely practised for patients with blood transfusion-acquired NANBH, relatively few haemophiliacs have had liver transplants. The first successful liver transplant in a haemophiliac was reported by Lewis

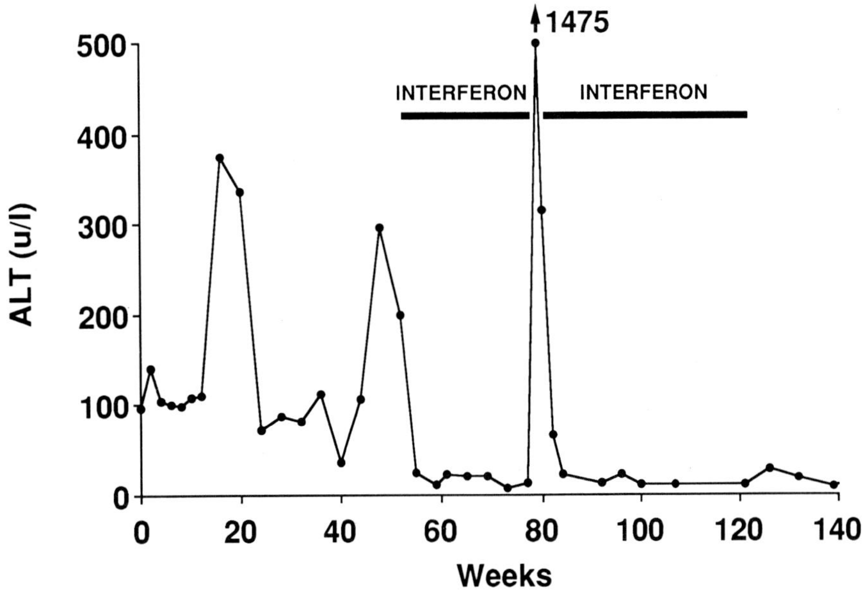

Fig. 39.7 ALT levels in a haemophilic patient with chronic active hepatitis normalizing during a 6-month course of interferon. Rapid relapse on stopping responded promptly to further interferon. Normal ALT is maintained following cessation of further treatment.

and colleagues in 1985 (Lewis et al 1985) and since then there are reports of 12 other such transplants in patients with both haemophilia A and haemophilia B as well as in a patient with type III von Willebrand's disease (Mannucci et al 1991). An added bonus in haemophilia is that not only does the transplant correct the liver failure it also reverses the phenotypic expression of haemophilia since the new liver produces enough factor VIII/IX to keep the level in the normal range. Coexistent HIV infection generally precludes liver transplantation. A potential problem is that many patients are viraemic for hepatitis C at the time of transplantation and post-transplant they may reinfect the new liver with HCV (Makris et al 1991a).

For patients receiving their first exposure of blood products in the 1990s the risk of hepatitis has never been smaller. With the increased understanding of the biology of hepatitis C and B the risk will hopefully be reduced to almost zero. For patients unfortunate to have been already infected with chronic hepatitis C the use of interferon offers encouraging prospects.

REFERENCES

Aach R D, Lander J J, Sherman L A et al 1978 Transfusion transmitted viruses: interim analysis of hepatitis among transfused and non transfused patients. In: Vyas G N, Cohen S N, Schmid R (eds) Viral hepatitis. Franklin Institute Press, Philadelphia, 383–396

Aledort L M, Levine P H, Hilgartner M et al 1985 A study of liver biopsies and liver disease among hemophiliacs. Blood 66: 367–372

Alter H J 1985 Post transfusion hepatitis: Clinical features, risk and donor testing. Progress in Clinical and Biological Research 182: 47–61

Alter H J 1989 Chronic consequences of non-A, non-B hepatitis. In: Seeff L B, Lewis J H (eds) Current perspectives in hepatology Plenum Publishing, New York, p 83–97

Alter H J, Holland P V, Purcell R H et al 1972 Posttransfusion hepatitis after exclusion of commercial and hepatitis B antigen-positive donors. Annals of Internal Medicine 77: 691–699

Alter H J, Purcell R H, Holland P V, Feinstone S M, Morrow A G, Moritsugu Y 1975 Clinical and serological analysis of transfusion associated hepatitis. Lancet 2: 838–841

Alter H J, Evatt B L, Margolis H S et al 1991 Public health service inter-agency guide-lines for screening donors of blood, plasma, organs, tissues, and semen for evidence of hepatitis B and hepatitis C. Morbidity and Mortality Weekly Report 40: 1–17

Anonymous 1991 Immunoglobulin therapy. Lancet 338: 157–158

Arima T, Nagashima H, Murakami S et al 1989 Cloning of a cDNA associated with acute and chronic hepatitis C infection generated from patients serum RNA. Gastroenterology (Japan): 540–544

Aronson D L 1988 Cause of death in hemophilia A patients in the United States from 1968–1979. American Journal of Hematology 27: 7–12

Beeson P B 1943 Jaundice occurring one to four months after transfusion of blood or plasma. Journal of the American Medical Association 121: 1332

Berntorp E, Nilsson I M, Ljung R, Widel A 1990 Hepatitis C virus transmission by monoclonal antibody purified factor VIII concentrate. Lancet 335: 1531–1532

Boudart D, Lucas J C, Muller J Y et al 1990 False positive hepatitis C antibody tests in paraproteinaemia. Lancet 336: 63

Brackman H H, Egli H 1988 Acute hepatitis B infection after treatment with heat-inactivated factor VIII concentrate. Lancet 2: 967

Bradley D W 1985 Research perspectives in posttransfusion non-A, non-B hepatitis. Progress in Clinical and Biological Research 182: 81–97

Busuttil R W, Colonna J O, Hiatt J R et al 1987 The first 100 liver transplants at UCLA. Annals of Surgery 206: 387–402

Cederbaum A I, Blatt P M, Levine P H 1982 Abnormal serum transaminase levels in patients with hemophilia A. Archives of Internal Medicine 142: 481–484

Choo Q L, Kuo G, Weiner A J, Overby L R, Bradley D W, Houghton M 1989 Isolation of cDNA clone derived from a blood borne non-A, non-B viral hepatitis genome. Science 244: 359–362

Choo Q L, Weiner A J, Overby L R, Kuo G, Houghton M, Bradley D W 1990 Hepatitis C virus: The major causative agent of viral non-A, non-B hepatitis. British Medical Bulletin 46: 423–441

Colombo M, Mannucci P M, Carnelli V, Savidge G F, Gazengel C, Schimpf K 1985 Transmission of non-A, non-B hepatitis by heat treated factor VIII concentrate. Lancet 2: 1–4

Cristiano K, Di Bisceglie A M, Hoofnagle J H, Feinstone S M 1991 Hepatitis C viral RNA in serum of patients with chronic non-A, non-B viral hepatitis: Detection by the polymerase chain reaction using multiple primer sets. Hepatology 14: 51–55

Davis G L, Balart L A, Schiff E R et al 1989 Treatment of chronic hepatitis C with recombinant interferon alpha. A multicentre randomized controlled trial. New England Journal of Medicine 321: 1501–1506

Donahue J G, Munoz A, Ness P M et al 1992 The declining risk of post-transfusion hepatitis C virus infection. New England Journal of Medicine 327: 369–373

Durkop et al 1990 Zeitschrift Klinische Medizinische 45: 1833–1835

Evely R S, Hay C R M, Preston F E, Triger D R, Greaves M, Underwood J C E 1987 Type III pro-collagen peptide in liver disease in haemophilia. Thrombosis and Haemostasis 58: 338

Eyster M E, Whitehurst D A, Catalano P M et al 1985 Long term follow-up of hemophiliacs with lymphocytopenia or thrombocytopenia. Blood 66: 1317–1320

Farci P, Alter H J, Wong D et al 1991 A long-term study of hepatitis C virus replication in non-A, non-B hepatitis. New England Journal of Medicine 325: 98–104

Finlayson J S, Tankersley D L 1990 Anti-HCV screening and plasma fractionation: the case against. Lancet 335: 1274–1275

Fletcher M L, Trowell J M, Craske J, Pavier K, Rizza C R 1983 Non-A, non-B hepatitis after transfusion of factor VIII in infrequently treated patients. British Medical Journal 287: 1754–1757

Garson J A, Tedder R S, Briggs M et al 1990a Detection of hepatitis C viral sequences in blood donations by 'nested' polymerase chain reaction and prediction of infectivity. Lancet 335: 1419–1422

Garson J A, Ring C, Tuke P, Tedder R S 1990b Enhanced detection by PCR of hepatitis C virus RNA. Lancet 336: 878–879

Garson J A, Tuke P W, Makris M et al 1990c Demonstration of viraemia patterns in haemophiliacs treated with hepatitis C virus contaminated factor VIII concentrates. Lancet 336: 1022–1025

Goeser T, Blazek M, Gmelin K, Kommerell B, Theilmann L 1990 Washing with 8mol/l urea to correct false-positive anti-HCV results. Lancet 336: 878

Goldfield M, Black H C, Bill J, Srihongse S, Pizzuit W 1975 The consequence of administering blood pretested for HBsAg by third generation techniques: a progress report. American Journal of Medical Science 270: 335–342

Han J K, Shymala V, Richman K M et al 1991 Characterization of the terminal regions of hepatitis-C viral RNA: identification of conserved sequences in the 5′-untranslated region and poly (A) tails at the 3′ end. Proceedings of the National Academy of Sciences, USA 88: 1711–1715

Hanley J A, Lippman-Hand A 1983 If nothing goes wrong, is everything all right? Journal of the American Medical Association 249: 1743–1745

Harrison P M, Lau J Y N, Williams R 1991 Hepatology. Postgraduate Medical Journal 67: 719–741

Hasiba U W, Spero J A, Lewis J H 1977 Chronic liver dysfunction in multitransfused haemophiliacs. Transfusion 17: 490–494

Hay C R M, Preston F E, Triger D R, Underwood J C E 1985 Progressive liver disease in haemophilia: An understated problem? Lancet i: 1495–1498
Hay C R M, Preston F E, Triger D R, Greaves M, Underwood J C E, Westlake L 1987 Predictive markers of chronic liver disease in hemophilia. Blood 69: 1595–1599
Holsteen V, Skinjoj P, Cohn 1977 Hepatitis type B in haemophiliacs: relation to source of clotting factor concentrates. Scandinavian Journal of Haematology 18: 214–218
Hoofnagle J H, Seef L B, Buskell Bales Z, et al 1978 Type B hepatitis after transfusion with blood containing antibody to hepatitis B core antigen. New England Journal of Medicine 298: 1379–1383
Hoofnagle J H, Mullen K D, Jones D B et al 1986 Treatment of chronic non-A, non-B hepatitis with recombinant human alpha interferon: A preliminary report. New England Journal of Medicine 315: 1575
Houghton M, Weiner A, Han J, Kuo G Choo Q L 1991 Molecular biology of the hepatitis C viruses: Implications for diagnosis, development and control of viral disease. Hepatology 14: 381–388
Ikeda Y, Toda G, Hashimoto N, Kurokawa K 1990 Antibody to superoxide dismutase, autoimmune hepatitis and antibody tests for hepatitis C virus. Lancet 335: 1345–1346
Japanese Red Cross Non-A, Non-B Hepatitis Research Group 1991 Effect of screening for hepatitis C virus antibody and hepatitis B virus core antibody on incidence of post-transfusion hepatitis. Lancet 338: 1040–1041
Journal of the American Medical Association 1942 Jaundice following yellow fever vaccination. Journal of the American Medical Association 119: 110
Kasper C K, Kipnis S A 1972 Hepatitis and clotting factor concentrates. Journal of the American Medical Association 211: 510
Kernoff PBA, Lee C A, Karayiannis P, Thomas H C 1985 High risk of non-A, non-B hepatitis after a first exposure to volunteer or commercial clotting factor concentrates: effect of prophylactic immune serum globulin. British Journal of Haematology 60: 469–479
Kojima M, Shimizu M, Tsuchimochi T et al 1991 Posttransfusion fulminant hepatitis B associated with Precore-defective HBV mutants. Vox Sanguis 60: 34–39
Kuo G, Choo Q L, Alter H J et al 1989 An assay for circulating antibodies to a major etiologic virus of human non-A, non-B hepatitis. Science 244: 362–364
Landbeck G 1987 HIV-1 Infektion. AIDS-Manifestation und Todesursachen der Bundesrepublik Deutschland. Die ellipse p 156–158
Lane R S 1983 Non-A, non-B hepatitis from intravenous immunoglobulin. Lancet 2: 974–975
Larsson S A, Wiechel B, 1983 Deaths in Swedish hemophiliacs, 1957–1980. Acta Medica Scandinavica 214: 199–206
Lau J Y N, Alexander G J M, Alberti A 1991 Viral Hepatitis. Gut Supplement S47–S62
Lee C A, Kernoff P B A 1990 Viral hepatitis and haemophilia. British Medical Bulletin 46: 408–422
Lee C A, Kernoff P B A, Karayiannis P, Thomas H C 1989 Interferon therapy for chronic non-A, non-B and delta liver disease in haemophilia. British Journal of Haematology 72: 235–238
Lesesne H R, Morgan J E, Blatt P M et al 1977 Liver biopsy in Hemophilia A. Annals of Internal Medicine 86: 703–707
Lewis J H, Bontempo F A, Spero J A, Ragni M V, Starlz T E 1985 Liver transplantation in a hemophiliac. New England Journal of Medicine 312: 1189–1190
Ludlam C A, Chapman D, Cohen B, Litton P A 1989 Antibodies to hepatitis C virus in haemophilia. Lancet 2: 560–561
Lurman 1985 Eine icterusepidemie. Berlin Klinische Wochenschrift 22: 20
MacCallum F O 1943 Jaundice in syphilitics. British Journal of Venereal Diseases 19: 63
McFarlane I G, Smith H M, Johnson P J, Bray G, Vergani D, Williams R 1990 Significance of possible anti-HCV antibodies in autoimmune chronic active hepatitis. Lancet i: 754–757
Makris M, Preston F E, Triger D R, et al 1990 Hepatitis C antibody and chronic liver disease in haemophilia. Lancet 335: 1117–1119
Makris M, Preston F E, Triger D R, Neuberger J, Franklin I, Garson J A 1991a Liver transplantation in haemophilia. Thrombosis and Haemostasis 65: 1157
Makris M, Preston F E, Triger D R, Underwood J C E, Westlake L, Adelman M I 1991b A randomized controlled trial of recombinant interferon alpha in chronic hepatitis C in hemophiliacs. Blood 78: 1672–1677
Mannucci P M, Capitanio A, Del Ninno E, Colombo M, Pareti F, Ruggeri Z M 1975 Asymptomatic liver disease in haemophilia. Journal of Clinical Pathology 28: 620–624
Mannucci P M, Ronchi G, Rota L et al 1978 A clinicopathological study of liver disease in haemophiliacs. Journal of Clinical Pathology 31: 779–783
Mannucci P M, Colombo M, Rizzetto M, et al 1982 Nonprogressive course of non-A, non-B chronic hepatitis in multitransfused haemophiliacs. Blood 60: 655–658
Mannucci P M, Zanetti A R, Colombo M and the Study Group of the Fondazione dell' Emofilia 1988 Prospective study of hepatitis after factor VIII concentrate exposed to hot vapour. British Journal of Haematology 68: 427–430
Mannucci P M, Colombo M 1989 Revision of the protocol recommended for studies of safety from hepatitis of clotting factor concentrates. Thrombosis and Haemostasis 61: 532–534
Mannucci P M, Federici A, Cattaneo M, Fassati R, Galmarini D 1991 Liver transplantation in severe von Willebrand disease. Lancet 337: 1105
Mattsson L, Aberg B, Weiland O, Sellman M, Davilen J 1988 Non-A, non-B hepatitis after open heart-surgery in Stockholm: declining incidence after introduction of restrictions for blood donations due to human immunodeficiency virus. Scandinavian Journal of Infectious Diseases 20: 371–376
Maynard J E, Kane M A, Alter M J, Hadler S C 1988 Control of hepatitis B by immunization: global prospective. In: Zuckerman A J (ed) Viral hepatitis and liver disease. A R Liss, New York, p 967
McFarlane I G, Smith H N, Johnson P J et al 1990 False-positivity for antibodies to hepatitis C virus in chronic active hepatitis. Lancet 335: 754–757
Miller E J, Lee C A, Karayiannis O, Hamilton-Dutoit S J, Dick R, Thomas H C, Kernoff P B A 1988 Non-invasive investigation of liver disease in haemophilia patients. Journal of Clinical Pathology 41: 1039–1043
Muchmore E, Manabe S, Alter H et al 1991 Hepatitis C virus particle size as determined by Bemberg Microporous Membrane removal of infectivity, confirmed by chimpanzee inoculation tests. Third International Symposium on HCV, abstract book p 64
Ogata N, Alter H J, Miller R H, Purcell R H 1991 Nucleotide sequence and mutation rate of the H strain of hepatitis C virus. Proceedings of the National Academy of Sciences, USA 88: 3392–3396
Pappas S C, Hoofnagle J H, Young N et al 1985 Treatment of chronic non-A, non-B hepatitis with Acyclovir: pilot study. Journal of Medical Virology 15: 1
Pozzato G, Moretti M, Franzin F et al 1991 Severity of liver disease with different hepatitis C viral clones. Lancet 338: 509
Preston F E, Triger D R, Underwood J C E et al 1978 Percutaneous liver biopsy in chronic liver disease in haemophiliacs. Lancet 2: 592–594
Preston F E, Hay C R M, Dewar M S et al 1985 Non-A, non-B hepatitis and heat-treated factor VIII concentrates. Lancet 2: 213
Rizza C R, Spooner R J D 1983 Treatment of haemophilia and related disorders in Britain and Northern Ireland during 1976–1980: report on behalf of the directors of haemophilia centres in the United Kingdom. British Medical Journal 286: 929–933
Rizzetto M, Shih JW-K, Gocke D J, Purcell R H, Verme G, Gerin J L 1979 Incidence and significance of antibodies to delta antigen in hepatitis B virus infection. Lancet 2: 986–990
Rizzetto M, Morello C, Mannucci P M et al 1982 Delta infection and liver disease in haemophilic carriers of hepatitis B surface antigen. Journal of Infectious Diseases 145: 18–22
Schimpf K 1986 Liver disease in haemophilia. Lancet 1: 323
Schimpf K 1990 Liver disease in haemophilia. Transfusion Science 11: 15S–22S
Simmonds P, Zhang L Q, Watson H G et al 1990 Hepatitis C

quantification and sequencing in blood products, haemophiliacs, and drug users. Lancet 336: 1469–1472

Spero J A, Lewis J H, Van Thiel D H et al 1978 Asymptomatic structural liver disease in haemophilia. New England Journal of Medicine 298: 1373–1378

Stevens C E, Alter H J, Taylor P E, Zang E A, Harley E J, Szmuness W 1984 Hepatitis B vaccine in patients receiving haemodialysis: Immunogenicity and efficacy. New England Journal of Medicine 311: 496–501

Stevens R F, Cuthbert A C, Perera P R et al 1983 Liver disease in haemophiliacs: An overstated problem? British Journal of Haematology 55: 649–655

Stirling M L, Murray J A, Mackay P, Black S H, Peuterer J F, Ludlam C A 1983 Incidence of infection with hepatitis B virus in 56 patients with haemophilia A 1971–1977. Journal of Clinical Pathology 36: 577–580

Stocks P, Lopez W C, Balart L A 1987 Effects of short term corticosteroid therapy in patients with chronic non-A, non-B hepatitis. Gastroenterology 92: 1783

Study Group of the UK Haemophilia Centre Directors on Surveillance of Virus Transmission by Concentrates 1988 Effect of dry-heating of coagulation factor concentrates at 80°C for 72 hours on transmission of non-A, non-B hepatitis Lancet 2: 814–816

Szmuness W, Stevens C E, Harley E J et al 1980 Hepatitis B vaccine: Demonstration of efficacy in a controlled trial on a high risk population in the United States. New England Journal of Medicine 303: 833–841

Tedder R S, Briggs M, Ring C, Tuke P W, Jones P, Savidge G F, Rodgers B, Garson J A 1991 Hepatitis C antibody profile and viraemia prevalence in adults with severe haemophilia. British Journal of Haematology 79: 512–515

Theilmann L, Blazek M, Goeser T et al 1990 False positive anti-HCV tests in rheumatoid arthritis. Lancet 335: 1346

Thomson B J , Doran M, Lever A M L, Webster ADB 1987 Alpha-interferon therapy for non-A, non-B hepatitis transmitted by gammaglobulin replacement therapy. Lancet 1: 539–541

Tine F, Magrin S, Craxi A, Pagliaro L 1991 Interferon for non-A, non-B chronic hepatitis; A meta-analysis of randomised clinical trials. Journal of Hepatology 13: 192–199

van der Poel C L, Cuypers H T M, Reesink H W et al 1991 Confirmation of hepatitis C virus infection by new four-antigen recombinant immunoblot assay. Lancet 337: 317–319

Watson H G, Ludlam C A, Rebus S, Zhang L Q, Pentherer J F, Simmonds P 1992 Use of several second generation serological assays to determine the true prevalence of hepatitis C virus infection in haemophiliacs treated with non-virus inactivated factor VIII and IX concentrates. British Journal of Haematology 80: 514–518

Weiner A J, Kuo G, Bradley D W et al 1990 Detection of hepatitis C viral sequences in non-A, non-B hepatitis. Lancet 335: 1–5

White G C, Zeitler K D, Lesesne H R et al 1982 Chronic hepatitis in patients with haemophilia A: Histologic studies in patients with intermittently abnormal liver function tests. Blood 60: 1259–1262

Williams P E, Yap P L, Gillon J et al 1989 Transmission of non-A, non-B hepatitis by pH4-treated intravenous immunoglobulin. Vox Sanguis 57: 15–18

Zuckerman A J 1983 The history of viral hepatitis from antiquity to the present. In: Deinhardt F, Deinhardt J (eds) Viral hepatitis: laboratory and clinical science p 3–32

40. Immunity and HIV infection in haemophilia

C. A. Ludlam

Prior to 1982 the immune system of individuals with haemophilia was considered to be essentially normal. Following the first reporting of cases of AIDS associated with haemophilia (Centre for Disease Control (CDC) 1982a) a number of studies were undertaken which demonstrated that severe immune modulation was widespread in recipients of coagulation factor concentrates. Initially it was unclear whether the observed abnormalities were due to subclinical infection with the putative AIDS virus, secondary to repeated transfusion of non-factor VIII protein in the therapeutic concentrates, or other transfused viruses (Table 40.1). It had also been considered that in haemophilia, as well as a deficiency of coagulant activity, there might be a previously unrecognised congenital aberration of the immune system.

Before the AIDS era, however, observations suggestive of immunological activation were recognised in haemophiliacs secondary to a variety of possible stimuli. Splenomegaly had been observed in some individuals, and although this was most probably secondary to hepatic pathology, in some it was considered to represent an immunological response to repeated concentrate infusions (Levine et al 1977). A not unexpected immunological response is the development of anti-factor VIII antibodies in approximately 10–30% of severe haemophiliacs consequent on factor VIII concentrate infusions. That more patients do not develop such inhibitors raises the possibility that an immunosuppressive component of the concentrate might inhibit specific antibody production particularly as the use of highly purified factor VIII concentrate may be associated with a higher incidence of such antibodies (Bell et al 1990), or that the factor VIII molecule may be partially denatured during purification to reveal neo-antigens. A recent report, however, indicates that the true rate of anti-factor VIIIC appearance may approach 50% of severe haemophiliacs treated with intermediate purity factor VIII concentrate. This indicates that the apparent high rate found recently with high purity concentrate may be no greater than formerly with those of lower purity (Ehrenforth et al 1992).

Table 40.1 Viruses transmitted by coagulation factor concentrates

Hepatitis A virus
Hepatitis B virus
Hepatitis C virus
Hepatitis D virus
Human immunodeficiency virus
Parvovirus

Since the early 1980s it has clearly emerged that HIV is responsible for most of the clinically significant immune deficiency arising in haemophiliacs. What is still unresolved is the extent to which immune changes in HIV-negative haemophiliacs are due to non-factor VIII/IX protein components of the coagulation factor concentrates, and which may be secondary to other blood transmissible viruses, e.g. hepatitis B virus (HBV) and HCV, either directly or secondary to chronic hepatitis.

In this chapter the reports relating to immune changes in HIV-negative haemophiliacs will be considered (Watson & Ludlam, 1992). This will include immune modulation observed in patients as well as the effect of factor VIII/IX concentrates on lymphocyte, monocyte and polymorph function in vitro. Thereafter the effects of HIV in haemophiliacs will be described with particular reference to differences compared to other risk groups (de Biasi et al 1991a).

IMMUNE CHANGES IN HIV-NEGATIVE HAEMOPHILIACS

The initial reports in the early 1980s of reduced levels of circulating CD4 cells and cell-mediated immunity in haemophiliacs, prompted by the reporting of the first cases of AIDS, were almost certainly referring mainly to HIV-positive patients (Jones et al 1983, Lederman et al 1983, Menitove et al 1983, Weintrub et al 1983, Lee et al 1985, Moffat et al 1985). It was not until the identification of HIV and the development of reliable specific antibody tests in 1984 that it became possible to ascertain which patients were infected. Although many haemo-

Table 40.2 Immune abnormalities in HIV-negative haemophiliacs

T cell subsets	Decreased CD4 count Decreased CD4/CD8 ratio
Lymphocyte functional abnormalities	Decreased response to mitogens Decreased natural killer cell response to interferon Decreased cell-mediated immunity Hypergammaglobulinaemia Increased secretion of B cell growth and differentiation factors
T cell activation	Increased β2-microglobulin Increased soluble interleukin-2 receptors Cell surface markers of T cell activation
Monocyte dysfunction	Decreased monocyte phagocytic function Defective antigen handlling

philiacs who were exposed to HIV became infected, some remained anti-HIV negative. There has for a long time been some doubt as to whether such individuals are truly not infected or whether they may be infected but have failed to produce specific anti-HIV antibodies. As time has passed the evidence in favour of their being free of HIV has accumulated, e.g. none has developed clinical stigmata of HIV infection, CD4 counts have remained stable, and neither viraemia nor viral genome by PCR has been detected. It seems reasonable to conclude, therefore, that anti-HIV-negative haemophiliacs are probably free of HIV infection (Gibbons et al 1990, Peutherer et al 1990). Table 40.2 lists the principal immune changes that have been reported in HIV-negative haemopholiacs.

Lymphocyte abnormalities

The initial reports in 1983–85 of decreased circulating CD4 counts in haemophiliacs did not differentiate between those invividuals who were HIV infected and those who were not because the studies were undertaken prior to the development of anti-HIV testing, but it is likely that the majority of patients investigated were infected. It subsequently became clear, however, that CD4 counts, and CD4/CD8 ratio, were also reduced in HIV-negative haemophiliacs and that these were more pronounced in recipients of factor VIII than factor IX concentrates (Carr et al 1984, Teitel et al 1989, Cuthbert et al 1992). The circulating concentration of CD8 cells was normal, or in some, slightly increased (Sullivan et al 1986, Freedman et al 1987). Although recipients of infrequent infusions of cryoprecipitate may have CD4 counts close to normal it has not been possible to demonstrate a relationship between annual factor VIII use and the degree of depression of CD4 counts in HIV-negative haemophiliacs (Carr et al 1984). The concentrate component which may cause the reduction in CD4 cells is unknown although β2-microglobulin has been considered a candidate because of its relatively high concentration in factor VIII preparations, compared to factor IX concentrates (Lee et al 1984). Recent studies in HIV- and HCV-negative children treated exclusively with virally inactivated intermediate purity factor VIII concentrate have failed to observe any lymphoctye changes during a relatively short follow-up period (Evans et al 1991).

The function of circulating lymphocytes in HIV-negative haemophiliacs is also impaired, as revealed by their impaired response to non specific T cell mitogens, PHA and conconavalin A ex vivo (Sullivan et al 1986). This is not due to excessive T suppressor activity as removal of CD8 cells does not restore to normal the proliferative response. Studies on CD4 cells have revealed that during PHA stimulation there is less IL-2 secretion and reduced IL-2 receptor expression (Thorpe et al 1989, Hay et al 1990). Addition of IL-2 to the cell cultures did not restore transformation to normal indicating that the reduced IL-2 receptor expression was not secondary to lack of IL-2 production. When added to lymphocytes in vitro, factor VIII concentrates can reduce or enhance proliferative response and IL-2 receptor expression (p. 933).

The proliferative response to the more physiological stimulation of *Escherischia coli*-loaded monocytes, is also reduced indicating either impaired antigen presentation or failure of its recognition (Mannhalter et al 1986). In support of these possibilities several studies have reported defective monocyte function in HIV-negative haemophiliacs (p. 933).

Although the CD4 counts and function ex vivo are depressed, there is evidence of overall immune activation as reflected by increased plasma concentrations of β2-microglobulin, immunoglobulins and T cells bearing activation markers (DR and CD3/38) (Cuthbert et al 1992). This immune activation may reflect, at least in part, HCV infection.

Cell-mediated immunity can be assessed in vivo by measuring the cutaneous response to intradermal injection of antigens. These can be to de novo antigens, e.g. DNCB, which measures the overall immune responsiveness from recognition of foreign antigen to development of a specific T cell response, i.e. both afferent and efferent loops. Recall activity, or efferent loop, can be measured by intradermal exposure to previously encountered antigens, e.g. candida, tetanus toxoid etc. The Merieux Multitest device allows the quantitation of response to the intradermal injection of seven recall antigens. Such studies have demonstrated that the response is depressed in HIV-negative haemophiliacs (Brettler et al 1986, Madhok et al 1986, Cuthbert et al 1992). This reduction is inversely proportional to annual factor VIII (but not factor IX) use. This is of particular interest because it is one of the few quantifiable assessments of immune dysfunction in haemophiliacs that is related to factor VIII usage, indicating that the immunomodulation seen in this group may be directly due to concentrate use rather than HCV infection or liver disease.

B cells

Raised serum immunoglobulin levels were first noted in haemophiliacs in the mid 1970s. There is evidence that elevated IgG levels, in particular, may reflect chronic hepatitis and that rising concentrations may indicate its progression (Hay et al 1987, Brieva et al 1985). It appears that the B cells are chronically activated as they spontaneously secrete immunoglobulin as well as B cell growth and differentiation factors in vitro (Brieva et al 1985, Biagiotti et al 1986, Ragni et al 1987, Cuthbert et al 1992). As the cells are already activated, only limited further stimulation can be achieved with pokeweed mitogen (Matheson et al 1987). The relationship between hepatitis (Madhok et al 1991), HCV and the B cell system remains to be elucidated but it is possible that the active HCV replication stimulates B cells.

Natural killer cells

Natural killer cells, which recognise foreign viral or tumour antigens on cell membranes, are present in normal numbers but have reduced function in haemophiliacs (Matheson et al 1986b). Their activity is reduced and their response to β and α interferon depressed.

Monocytes

Ex vivo studies of monocytes from haemophiliacs have demonstrated reduced chemotaxis and adhesion, although the ability to phagocytose candida is reported to be both augmented and diminished (Eibl et al 1987, Mannhalter et al 1988, Pasi & Hill 1990). There is also evidence of impaired antigen handling and/or presentation.

The ability to phagocytose Rh(D) erythrocytes sensitized with anti-D is impaired after infusion of intermediate and high purity factor VIII concentrate (Pasi & Hill 1990). The mechanism remains unknown although incubation of factor VIII concentrate with monocytes leads to down regulation of IgG Fc receptors. This is more marked when intermediate or high purity ion exchange purified factor VIII is used rather than monoclonal antibody purified concentrate (Pasi & Hill 1990). The reduction in Fc receptors may be secondary to circulating immune complexes which can be found in many haemophiliacs (Mannhalter et al 1988).

Lymphocyte reactions in vitro to factor VIII concentrates

As leukocytes from haemophiliacs have demonstrated a range of abnormalities ex vivo investigators have attempted to ascertain which ones might be due to components of the therapeutic concentrates acting directly upon circulating cells. In these studies peripheral blood mononuclear cells (PBMC) have been stimulated in the presence of factor VIII/IX concentrate. PHA or tetanus toxoid or anti-CD3 stimulation of PBMC is inhibited in a dose-dependent fashion by factor VIII concentrate and cryoprecipitate (Lederman et al 1986, Matheson et al 1986a). Inhibitation, in general, is greater with intermediate purity concentrates compared to those prepared with monoclonal antibodies. Attempts to identify the inhibitory component(s) have been unsuccessful although it appears not to be fibrinogen or fibronectin.

The one way mixed lymphocyte reaction (MLR), in which the stimulant is allogeneic HLA antigens, is perhaps a situation that might pertain in vivo, particularly as patients may be transfused with components of the class I and II antigens, including β_2-microglobulin, as contaminants in factor concentrates. Monoclonally purified factor VIII products have no effect on the MLR but some intermediate purity products augment the response (Batchelor et al 1992). Furthermore, it has been reported that even small amounts of concentrate may stimulate lymphocytes directly without the addition of irradiated lymphocytes or other mitogen (Matheson et al 1986a). These studies are potentially of importance clinically because, if factor VIII concentrate stimulates circulating lymphocytes, this could result in enhanced HIV replication in infected patients leading to further accelerated immune damage.

Some factor VIII concentrates inhibit IL-2 production after mitogen stimulation (Thorpe et al 1989); subsequently it has been observed that mitogen stimulation in the presence of factor VIII results in reduced exposure of both early and late activation markers, e.g. IL-2 receptor expression (IL-2R, CD25), transferrin receptor (CD71) and DR positivity. IL-2R expression is promoted by the presence of IL-2 from activated helper lymphocytes. The addition, however, of IL-2 to the cultures failed to enhance IL-2R expression, thus demonstrating that some factor VIII concentrates inhibit IL-2R expression by a mechanism other than decreasing IL-2 secretion (Hay et al 1990). The inhibitory effect was apparent with concentrates prepared by a variety of processes and did not appear to be related to total protein content, method of preparation or viral inactivation process.

Monocyte function

As monocyte function ex vivo is apparently defective in haemophiliacs, studies have examined the effect of concentrates on their function when added to cells in vitro. The results demonstrated that Fc receptor expression was depressed as was their ability to kill bacteria (Eibl et al 1987, Mannhalter et al 1988, Pasi & Hill 1990). Oxygen radical release after mixing the cells with opsonized zymogen or aggregated IgG was also impaired. The ability of monocytes from haemophiliacs, ex vivo to phagocytose Rh(D) cells sensitized with anti-D was also reduced particularly with intermediate purity concentrates. The component(s) of the concentrates responsible for inhibiting monocyte function is unknown but one candidate might be aggregated IgG or immune complexes (Mannhalter et al 1990). Recently, inhibitors of Fc receptor expression by a monoclonal antibody purified concentrate has been demonstrated, possibly due to an VIII/anti-VIII complex (Mannhalter et al 1990).

Clinical significance of immune modulation

The potential clinical importance of immune changes due to factor VIII/IX concentrate infusion should be considered separately in HIV-negative and positive haemophilics; the latter are considered in a later section of this chapter (p. 935).

In HIV-negative haemophiliacs, the best evidence for clinically significant immune suppression secondary to factor VIII concentrate use was an outbreak of tuberculosis in a ward of the Birmingham Children's Hospital in 1981 (Beddall et al 1985). Following the identification of an index case of open pulmonary tuberculosis, other children, both in- and out-patients, were screened for evidence of acquiring infection. Of these exposed, 39% developed evidence of infection, a rate similar to other children in the ward who were severely immunosuppressed as a result of intensive chemotherapy for leukaemia or solid tumours. The haemophiliac children developed evidence of self-limiting primary infection whereas some of those with treated malignancy succumbed to milliary tuberculosis. Of further interest was the observation that the children who had previously used more factor VIII concentrate had a greater chance of becoming infected after exposure.

Review of causes of haemophiliac deaths, particularly in the pre-AIDS era, provides some evidence of increased incidence of malignancies and also deaths from infection (Rizza & Spooner 1983, Aronson 1988). In both the UK and USA, reviews of haemophiliac deaths prior to HIV indicates that approximately 5% were due to infection whereas in the non-haemophilic individuals it was 0.9%. These figures may not be entirely reliable because they are based on causes as given on death certificates.

The death rate from malignancy, again as given on death certificates, has been reviewed in several studies. In the USA the incidence of fatal malignancies was approximately a quarter of that expected, whereas in a Dutch study the rate was two and a half times that for the general population. This latter study is a result that might be anticipated if cell-mediated immunity, and particularly natural killer cell function, was impaired as a result of repeated concentrate infusions as suggested by several studies.

A study of postoperative wound infections in haemophiliacs found that the rate was similar to that in other patients receiving comparable surgery (Buehrer et al 1990). Thus although there is some evidence of impaired polymorph function in haemophiliacs when the cells are tested ex vivo, this did not appear to predispose to post-operative bacterial infections.

The haemophiliacs response to HBV and particularly HCV infection has been difficult to study because, since 1985, patients have been treated almost exclusively with HCV-negative concentrates and are thus not being repeatedly re-exposed to one or more strains of this virus. This reduced exposure may have modified hepatitis progression as evidenced by the observation that since 1985, IgG levels in a small group of HIV-negative patients have fallen (Cuthbert et al 1992). Furthermore it is of interest to note that in patients reported with hepatocellular carcinoma, or cirrhosis requiring liver transplantation, there would appear to be an excess of patients with mild haemophilia (Bontempo et al 1987). This is consistent with intermediate purity concentrates having a suppressive effect on either HBV or HCV replication, or that repeated concentrate infusion reduces the development of cirrhosis. It is therefore potentially of concern that if, by whatever mechanism, the progression of liver disease is retarded by immunosuppressive effect of factor concentrates then the switch to higher purity products might be accompanied by more rapid progression to end stage cirrhosis.

ACQUIRED IMMUNODEFICIENCY SYNDROME

The first cases of AIDS were reported in 1981 in homosexual men (CDC 1981a, b) but, when further cases were discovered in intravenous drug abusers and haemophiliacs in the following year it was clear that the responsible agent might be transmissible by blood or blood products (CDC 1982b). The epidemiology appeared identical to that of hepatitis B virus and some claimed that the pathogen was even a mutant form of this virus (Ravenholt 1983).

Studies in those with AIDS quickly characterized an abnormality in cell-mediated immunity which was consistent with the opportunist infections being observed. The principal defect appeared to be a deficiency of circulating CD4 lymphocytes and an accompanying marked impairment of cell-mediated immunity as evidenced by a reduced cutaneous response to de novo and recall antigens. Further studies in asymptomatic individuals from the three risk groups revealed that many had significant abnormalities of their immune systems. In the case of haemophiliacs, it was unclear whether many were infected asymptomatically with a putative AIDS virus, or whether the immune changes could have been secondary to the non-factor VIII proteins in the therapeutic concentrates, or other viruses, e.g. HCV. During 1982–83 two further cases of AIDS in haemophiliacs were reported in the USA and seven from elsewhere and, as none of those affected belonged to other known risk groups, it became increasingly apparent that a putative virus was being transmitted by factor concentrates. With only a handful of cases reported out of a total haemophiliac population of several tens of thousands in North America and Europe it was difficult to know the true extent of the putative virus infection.

The first identification of the virus now known as HIV-1, also previously known as human lymphotropic virus III (HTLV-III), lymphadenopathy-associated virus (LAV), and AIDS-related virus (ARV), was made from a patient with haemophilia B and homosexual men in 1983 (Vilmer et al 1984). Initial attempts to measure specific antibody to the virus, assessed reaction to HTLV-I (Essex et al 1983) the virus causing T cell ALL/lymphoma in Japan and the West Indies. It was not until specific antibody tests were devised in 1984, when initial reports indicated that up to 94% of severe haemophiliacs were anti-HIV positive (Kitchen et al 1984), that the extent of HIV infection in haemophiliacs became apparent. As the majority of individuals were clinically well it was not clear whether the presence of specific antibody indicated only previous exposure or whether such individuals continued to harbour live but dormant virus. It soon became clear that anti-HIV-positive individuals possessed virus as it could be cultured from their PBMCs. Although it became apparent that many haemophiliacs were infected by early 1985, less than 1% had developed AIDS by that time, and it was unclear what proportion would eventually succumb to clinical disease. Subsequent events are well known and have indicated that many HIV infected haemophiliacs will eventually develop AIDS.

In the early 1980s it became accepted that many haemophiliacs had been infected with one or more virus(es) resulting in the development of hepatitis and studies published in 1983 indicated that virtually every recipient of factor VIII/IX concentrate developed HCV (Fletcher et al 1983, Kernoff et al 1985). These clinical observations have now been confirmed by finding evidence of HCV infection by serological tests or PCR in virtually all patients (Watson et al 1992). Meanwhile manufacturers of therapeutic concentrates had been attempting mainly by heat treatment, to destroy viable viruses in concentrates without inactivating the factor VIII or altering its antigenic structure which might lead to the development of neoantigens. In late 1984 it became apparent that HIV was heat sensitive and this knowledge was immediately used to reduce infectivity by dry heat-treating factor VIII concentrates (Levy et al 1984, CDC, 1984). This, along with the other measures that were being taken to exclude high risk donors, which eventually included anti-HIV donor screening, led to blood pooled products being rendered virtually sterile for HIV. Occasional HIV transmission occurred subsequently from heat treated concentrates and these regrettable incidents have allowed the definition of the stringent conditions necessary for inactivation of HIV (CDC 1988, Brettler & Levine 1989). A recent report indicates that hepatitis A, a non-lipid coated virus, may be transmitted by solvent-detergent treated concentrate (Mannucci 1992).

Human immunodeficiency virus

Transmission of HIV occurs horizontally by blood and sexual transmission, and vertically from mother to fetus. Although haemophiliacs were infected initially by blood products, secondary sexual spread to partners and then to off-spring has been observed (Goedert et al 1987).

In the majority of individuals, infection occurs without symptoms although a minority develop a seroconversion illness which may range from mild malaise with a sore throat, pyrexia and rash to a severe life-threatening glandular fever-like condition (Tucker et al 1985). Most individuals become viraemic within a few weeks of exposure and this can be identified by detection of p24 antigenaemia, HIV RNA by PCR, or culture of the virus in vitro (Cuthbert et al 1989, Simmonds 1990). At a variable time thereafter specific antibody responses to components of the virus become detectable, e.g. anti-core (anti-p24) or anti-envelope (anti-Gp120) (Simmonds et al 1988, Eyster et al 1989). In some individuals specific IgM is initially detected, followed later by IgG antibody. Thereafter the degree of apparent viraemia may decline such that p24 antigen is no longer detectable for a period of time; later in the illness the patient may again become p24 antigenaemic. It may be that viraemia persists throughout the infection but that the virus forms a circulating complex with specific antibody rendering it undetectable by antigen assays in vitro. It may, however, still be detectable, either by dissociating virus from antibody by culture or by RNA PCR. As well as the HIV being present free in plasma it, along with the DNA provirus integrated into the host genome, is present in circulating mononuclear cells. By PCR amplification of the viral RNA and proviral DNA it is possible to follow, within one individual, the appearance of viral subtypes over a period of time. After initial infection marked genomic change can be observed, particularly in the genes coding for parts of the envelope protein, e.g. V3 loop, which are more likely to mutate than those coding for the core proteins (Balfe et al 1991). Furthermore within one individual only certain subtypes proliferate indicating that there is selective pressure probably by the immune system preventing replication of certain mutants (Simmonds et al 1990a, Leigh Brown 1992). From studies on a group of haemophiliacs infected from a single batch of HIV-contaminated factor VIII concentrate, only limited divergence of HIV has been observed over a 7-year period and the virus subtypes discernible within each individual are all clearly recognizable as having originated from a common source (Balfe et al 1991). It is of interest to note that HIV RNA in plasma may differ from integrated DNA of provirus in the circulating mononuclear cells. Individual subtypes are detectable as circulating free plasma viral RNA and at some time subsequently appear in PBMC as proviral DNA. One inference from this observation is that at some place in the immune system, other than circulating lymphocytes, HIV is proliferating and being shed into the plasma and it is only later that it becomes integrated within blood lymphocytes. Whereas subtypes in plasma may be relatively transient they are observable as provirus over much longer periods of time extending to many years.

In addition to qualitative changes in the viral genome being detectable, the quantity of circulating virus differs markedly between individuals (Schechter et al 1991, Simmonds et al 1990b). Quantitation is possible by PCR amplification of dilutions to the limit of detection. In general, as HIV disease progresses, the number of circulating infected lymphocytes increases. Early in HIV infection, during the initial period of viraemia, it is possible to culture virus from blood, thereafter during the long asymptomatic phase it is harder to obtain positive cultures. As the patient's immune system collapses and HIV-associated symptoms appear, the virus is again more readily isolated (Cuthbert et al 1989). From these observations it is clear that there is a close inter-relation between the virus and its attempts at genomic drift which is specifically constrained, at least for a period of time, by the immune system.

There is both a specific humoral and cellular immune response to HIV (Valentine & Jacobson 1990). The relationship of these to viral antigenic epitopes is complex not only because of the relatively high mutation rate of the envelope but also because it infects the immune system ultimately causing its collapse.

Specific IgM, G and A responses are discernable against epitopes of many of the viral components. Evidence is emerging that the nature of the humoral response may predict the subsequent rate of clinical deterioration (Simmonds et al 1991). Specific immunity against envelope may only react with some subtypes allowing others to proliferate unhindered. Such diversity is not evident in *gag* components and hence monoclonal antibodies developed against core components can be used in reliable screening tests for the detection of viraemia.

Much interest has centred around the identification of epitopes which induce the development of specific neutralizing antibody. This is of major importance because such antibodies may help contain infection. Research has therefore been directed at the identification of epitopes to which neutralizing antibodies develop, because if conserved ones can be identified their presentation to an HIV naive host may have value as a vaccine (Autran & Letvin 1992, Moore & Nara 1992).

As well as a humoral response, a cellular reaction to the virus is detectable. Cytotoxic lymphocytes can be identified which have, like the immunoglobulin response, specificity for viral epitopes. Such reactions are MHC restricted (Walker & Plata, 1990, Autran et al 1991, Biberfield & Emini 1992). This cytotoxic immunity is responsible for the lysis of infected host cells expressing both the specific epitope along with Class I antigens.

As became evident early in HIV research, the virus has a propensity to infect CD4 positive T lymphocytes (T helper cells) because the virus binds to the CD4 molecule before becoming internalized (Habeshaw et al 1990). However, within the peripheral blood, only a tiny proportion of lymphocytes are infected although the number increases as disease progresses (Simmonds et al 1990b). The absolute number however of CD4 lymphocytes may temporarily fall at seroconversion but thereafter there is a steady linear decline punctuated by marked flutuations for inapparent reasons (Eyster et al 1987, Goedert et al 1989, Lee et al 1989, Cuthbert et al 1990). It is therefore imprudent to attach too much significance to single CD4 counts, rather it is important to perform serial measurements over a period of several months to discern a trend. As will be discussed below, the level of CD4 cell count is one of the best predictions of prognosis (p. 943).

In the healthy individual approximately 10–30% of circulating T lymphocytes are CD8 positive. Many of these cells have suppressor and cytotoxic activity. Following infection with viruses other than HIV, e.g. EBV, these cells proliferate to contain the immune response. In early HIV infection there is also acute proliferation of $CD8^+$ cells which appear on a blood film as 'glandular fever', or activated T cells, during the seroconversion illness. Thereafter, usually over a period of years, the absolute number of CD8 cells increase in the peripheral blood before declining as the patient becomes clinically ill. Furthermore as the patients become progressively less well, the number and also percentage of such cells expressing activation marker increases (Simmonds et al 1991). CD4 positive cells during activation, increase CD4 expression on the cell surface thus augmenting the potential for HIV infection. It is for this reason that some have advocated the use of immunosuppressive therapy to reduce immune activation. Further evidence for immune activation and proliferation following HIV infection is the observed increase in the plasma concentration of β_2-microglobulin, part of the MHC class I antigen, and neopterin, a purine metabolic product of activated macrophages (Cuthbert et al 1990).

As well as a B cell response to HIV as demonstrated by the appearance of specific immunoglobulin to viral components, there is progressive pan B cell activation as evidenced by polyclonal hypergammaglobulinaemia. The total levels of IgG, M and A do not increase in parallel and each is clearly under separate control (Simmonds et al 1991). The usual response is to observe a gradual rise in total IgG which accelerates as disease progresses, whereas IgA levels tend to rise sharply when patients become symptomatic. The mechanisms responsible for this polyclonal antibody response are at present unclear although it is in part due to loss of B cell suppression by T cell-dervied cytokines. There is evidence that HIV can also infect B cells and this may also promote their nonspecific activation.

Clinical presentation of HIV infection

HIV infection may cause clinical conditions which are directly due to the virus, e.g. glandular fever-like illness at seroconversion, whereas other clinical stigmata are secondary to immunological decline, e.g. opportunistic infections like *Pneumocystis carinii* pneumonia. The clinical consequences of HIV infection in haemophiliacs are very similar to its effects in non-haemophiliacs. There are, however, some important differences and these will be discussed below.

Following HIV infection the majority of individuals remain asymptomatic for a prolonged period. Only a small minority develop the glandular fever-like illness (Tucker et al 1985), which may be indistinguishable, both clinically and on blood film appearances, from that due to EBV, CMV or toxoplasmosis. Those who experience this seroconversion illness have a less good prognosis and progress to AIDS more quickly.

The period of asymptomatic infection can extend from a few weeks to many years, and during this period the individual may feel well. Serial studies, during this time do, however, demonstrate progressive deterioration of immune competence. This is perhaps best reflected by the declining peripheral blood CD4 count and development of cutaneous anergy.

Some patients develop persistent generalized lymphadenopathy (PGL) in which there is symmetrical painless discrete lymphadenopathy mainly in the neck and axilla; this is not associated with a poor prognosis. Whereas in many the size of the nodes remains fairly constant, in others they may change in size quite dramatically over short periods of time and when this occurs it indicates a poor prognosis. In some, particularly where the lymphadenopathy is very asymmetrical, it may be necessary to perform a lymph node biopsy to exclude lymphoma. In PGL the histology is that of intense reactive hyperplasia with prominent follicle development. When marked immune deterioration has occurred, the lymphadenopathy and splenomegaly disappear concomitantly with the appearance of AIDS.

As immunological decline progresses patients become more susceptible to bacterial infections particularly of the respiratory and urinary tracts as well as septicaemia. The appearance of oral candida indicates that the immune system is severely compromised.

Thrombocytopenia is observed in 5–10% of asymptomatic HIV-infected individuals. It may arise from a variety of causes (Table 40.3) and, when of immune origin, is not associated with a poor prognosis. The mechanism is thought to be due to autoimmune thrombocytopenia as well as the presence of immune complexes which become attached to platelet Fc receptors leading to their premature removal by the monocyte-macrophage system (Karpatkin 1990, Ragni et al 1990). Thrombocytopenia may also arise because HIV infects megakaryocytes.

Table 40.3 Causes of thrombocytopenia in HIV

1. Auto-immune thrombocytopenia
2. Circulating immune complexes
3. Infection of megakaryocytes by HIV
4. Infiltration of bone marrow by
   1. opportunistic infection
   2. lymphoma
5. Anti-microbial therapy
   1. Anti-viral, e.g. zidovudine
   2. Antibiotic, e.g. cotrimoxazole
   3. Antifungal

As HIV infection progresses, a stage is reached when the individual is sufficiently immunocompromised that opportunistic infections or malignancies occur, e.g. *Pneumocytis carinii* pneumonia or non-Hodgkin's lymphoma. This may be accompanied by marked weight loss, associated with malabsorption and/or diarrhoea, and night sweats. With the use of zidovudine, pentamidine or other prophylaxis against PCP, and fluconazole, patients feel relatively well and survive for much longer periods, with very few circulating CD4 cells, without developing clinical AIDS. As a result of improved prophylaxis and treatment of opportunistic infections, many patients survive longer, and now appear to be dying later with HIV but before an AIDS-defining condition occurs. Many succumb to the HIV wasting syndrome in which the patient's weight rapidly declines often associated with persistent watery diarrhoea without an infective organism being identified.

AIDS was originally defined on broad clinical criteria set out by the Centre for Disease Control, Atlanta, in 1981 to include individuals with an infection characteristic of immune deficiency but without an otherwise known cause for immune depression. The definition also included B cell immunoblastic lymphomas and Kaposi's sarcoma. In 1987, following the accumulation of much more experience of the clinical consequences of HIV, the definition of AIDS was revised to include a long definitive list of many opportunistic infections and tumours (CDC 1987). In addition the HIV status of the individual was taken into account.

The CDC classification of HIV-associated disease (CDC 1986) identifies four stages which do not necessarily follow sequentially the decline in CD4 counts (Table 40.4). Furthermore, there is not a clear relationship between different subsections of stage IV and the categorization of an individual having AIDS. Several other

Table 40.4 CDC classification system for HIV-associated disease

Group I	Acute symptomatic infection
Group II	Asymptomatic infection
Group III	Persistent generalized lymphadenopathy (PGL)
Group IV	Other disease
Subgroup A	Constitutional disease (fever or diarrhoea for 1 month or 10% weight loss)
Subgroup B	Neurologic disease (dementia, myelopathy or neuropathy)
Subgroup C	Secondary infectious diseases
Category C-1	Specified secondary infectious diseases listed in the CDC surveillance definition for AIDS, e.g. PCP, cryptosporadiosis, toxoplasmosis etc.
Category C-2	Other specified secondary infectious disease, e.g. oral hairy leukoplakia, multidermatome zoster, tuberculosis
Subgroup D	Secondary cancers, e.g. Kaposi's sarcoma, non-Hodgkin's lymphoma
Subgroup E	Other conditions, e.g. thrombocytopenia

schemes have been developed which take into account clinical symptomatology along with measurement of immune status. These include the Walter Reed staging (Redfield et al 1986) and WHO classification. Other more simplified schemes have been proposed which may have clinical utility (Royce et al 1991).

Kaposi's sarcoma and non-Hodgkin's lymphomas are found with greatly increased incidence in HIV-infected individuals and are AIDS-defining illnesses. The aetiology of Kaposi's sarcoma remains obscure although it may be due to a second virus co-transmitted with HIV. Of importance is the observation that this sarcoma is hardly ever observed in haemophiliacs and intravenous drug abusers, but it is usually only found in those who acquired HIV sexually. Recent evidence indicates that the pathogen may be spread by faeces. Of further interest is the observation that the incidence of Kaposi's sarcoma appears to be declining. It is diagnosed at a higher CD4 count that many other AIDS-defining illnesses and in a third of homosexual men is the feature that leads to diagnosis of AIDS.

LYMPHOMAS

In HIV-positive individuals, non-Hodgkin's lymphoma (NHL) is 60 times commoner than in those without infection. The principal features are summarized in Table 40.5. So far as is known, the spectrum of NHL disease in haemophiliacs is similar to that observed in other risk groups except that its incidence is higher (Beral et al 1990, Rabkin et al 1992). Approximately half the lymphomas seen are of high grade B cell immunoblastic type which develop when the mean CD4 is less than 50×10^6/l. The mechanism by which the lymphoma develops is unclear although it arises from a polyclonally expanded B cell system which may become multiclonal before finally developing into a monoclonal tumour. The incidence of NHL rises progressively with age. Prognosis is better in those with a CD4 count greater than 100×10^6/l at diagnosis and in those who are asymptomatic of HIV infection. Primary lymphoma of the brain occurs in a quarter of the lymphoma patients and is 1000 times commoner than in HIV-negative individuals; the incidence does not vary with age. A diagnosis of Burkitt's lymphoma is made in the remaining quarter of lymphoma patients, it tends to occur in teenage patients and to be diagnosed when the CD4 count is in the region of 2–400 $\times 10^6$/l. The incidence of NHL is much increased in other immunosuppressed patients, e.g. following renal transplantations, and the finding of primary brain lymphomas or other NHLs in severely immunocompromised subjects is therefore not unexpected. At present there is no good explanation as to why individuals get Burkitt's lymphoma particularly when this occurs at a relatively high CD4 count. HIV-positive individuals with Hodgkin's disease have a poor prognosis and there is some evidence to suggest that the virus may predispose to the development of the lymphoma (Gold et al 1991). The importance of EBV or prior zidovudine therapy in the aetiology of NHL in HIV-positive individuals remains to be determined (Pluda et al 1990).

Table 40.5 Features of HIV-associated lymphomas

Histology	Large B cell immunoblastic non-Hodgkin's lymphoma (older adults) Burkitt's lymphoma (young adults) Hodgkin's disease
Site	Extranodal often disseminated at diagnosis Presence of 'B' symptoms common Intracranial
Prognosis	Immunoblastic: may respond to chemotherapy Burkitt's lymphoma: relatively good prognosis Intracranial lymphoma: poor

Epidemiology of HIV in haemophiliacs

When reliable specific antibody tests for HIV became available in 1984 it rapidly became apparent that the prevalence of infection in haemophiliacs largely reflected the infection rate in the countries in which the source plasma for concentrate manufacture was collected and the amount of concentrate used by individual patients. The prevalence of HIV seropositivity was found to be 60–90% in severe haemophiliacs with much lower rates in those with moderate and mild disease (United Kingdom Haemophilia Directors 1988a) (Table 40.6). Haemophiliacs in those countries which depended heavily on the purchase of factor VIII from United States blood donors had higher rates of infection. Elsewhere, in addition to a country's dependence on US commercial product, the time of entry of HIV into the local population determined the extent of infection in haemophiliacs treated with locally manufactured products. Because of the long asymptomatic latency with HIV infection and absence initially of reliable anti-

Table 40.6 Prevalence in UK of HIV in haemophilia A, B and von Willebrand's disease

Inherited disorder		No.	%
Haemophilia A:	Severe	782	59
	Moderate	136	20
	Mild	34	11
	Total	952	41
Haemophilia B:	Severe	21	11
	Moderate	4	3
	Mild	1	3
	Total	26	6
von Willebrand's disease:		12	4

body tests, some countries originally considered to have uncontaminated blood supply were subsequently found to have widespread infection. For example in Australia, a country which prohibits the importation of commercial factor VIII, it was initially considered that the blood supply was not infected (Rickard et al 1983, Wearne et al 1984). Subsequently it transpired that HIV was relatively widespread and many haemophiliacs had become infected (Garsia et al 1987). In Europe, with the exception of France, the prevalence of HIV in the general population lagged behind that of North America. Those countries, therefore, which relied principally on locally collected plasma for the manufacture of factor VIII had low rates of infection in haemophiliacs in 1984. As can be seen from Table 40.7 it is principally those countries in Northern and Eastern Europe which have a low HIV infection risk in haemophiliacs and in some it is virtually absent.

By retrospectively testing frozen stored serum samples, the first HIV seroconversions in haemophiliacs were found in samples collected in 1978 (Goedert et al 1989, Lee et al 1989). The prevalence increased during the succeeding 8 years but with a particular rise in 1981–83 in individuals treated with coagulation concentrates derived from US donors (Eyster et al 1985). (Fig. 40.1). Patients treated only with products derived from local donors tended to seroconvert later at a time when HIV, often

Table 40.7 Anti-HIV prevalence in haemophiliacs by country

Country	% Positive
Europe	
Belgium	6
Bulgaria	9
Czechoslovakia	17
Denmark	30
Germany	20
Finland	1
France	45
Greece	34
Italy	28
Netherlands	19
Norway	7
Poland	1
Portugal	28
Spain	48
Sweden	24
Switzerland	20
United Kingdom	39
Yugoslavia	38
Other Countries	
Argentina	35
Australia	23
Brazil	55
Canada	47
Costa Rica	40
Japan	40
Malaysia	4
New Zealand	13
United States	47
Venezuela	20

Source: World Haemophilia AIDS Centre and elsewhere.

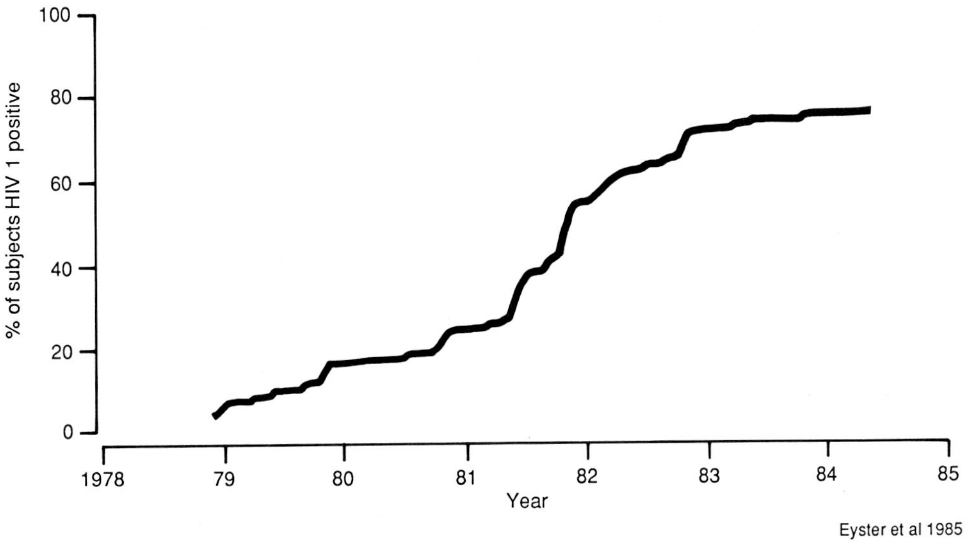

Fig. 40.1 Estimate of percentage of patients seroconverting to HIV since 1978 (Eyster et al 1985).

asymptomatically, entered the donor population. The use of various virucidal treatments for the concentrates became widespread in 1984, although the efficiency of heat treatment was only demonstrated in the closing months of that year (Levy et al 1984). During early 1985 most Western countries changed to the use of such concentrates, effecting a dramatic fall in the incidence of new infections. Seroconversion to HIV was still observed for many months after switching to virucidally treated concentrates because of the relatively long latency observed in some individuals between exposure to HIV and development of a specific antibody response. However it became apparent from the study of seroconversions occurring after the change to virucidally treated concentrates that not all inactivation procedures were equally effective in preventing HIV infection (Brettler & Levine 1989). The efficacy of the virucidal processes were examined by 'spiking' experiments in which live virus, e.g. either model resistant viruses or HIV, were added to concentrates in vitro prior to treatment. The virucidal effect was dependent upon such factors as the temperature and duration of the procedure, the degree of moisture in the 'dry' heated concentrates and the presence of stabilizers to protect factors VIII/IX from inactivation. The ultimate test of viral safety has been the careful follow-up of HIV-negative patients with serial anti-HIV tests (Mannucci & Colombo 1989). Careful evaluation of patients who seroconverted after the change to virucidally treated concentrates has allowed characterization of treatment procedures which are unsafe (Mannucci & Colombo 1988, Thomas, 1988, Horowitz, 1990). It is now generally agreed that protection against HIV infection is afforded best by dry heat treatment at 80°C for 72 hours (United Kingdom Haemophilia Directors 1988b), heat treatment in solution for 10 hours at 60°C (Schimpf et al 1989), heated vapour (Mannucci et al 1988), heptane and heat (Kernoff et al 1987), or the use of solvent/detergent regimes (Horowitz et al 1988) (Table 40.8).

Since 1988, there has only been one major HIV transmission episode which was due to a factor IX concentrate treated with B propiolactone and UV light (Kleim et al 1990) the product has now been withdrawn from the market.

Pari pasu with the introduction of viral inactivation procedures in the mid 1980s was the discouragement of donors at high risk of HIV infection from giving blood and the screening of individual donations for anti-HIV. The potential HIV viral load now in plasma, therefore, is much lower and hence it is more difficult to assess the efficacy of virucidal treatments. Traditional pasteurization of albumin solutions at 60°C for 10 hours has rendered this product free from virus transmission and it is noteworthy that one factor VIII concentrate so heated from 1980 has not been associated with any documented case of HIV transmission during a period when the plasma source was likely to have been significantly contaminated (Schimpf et al 1989). As the chance of HIV transmission by factor VIII and IX concentrates is now very small, attention has focused on the prevention of transmission of other viruses particularly hepatitis C and parvo virus (Williams et al 1990). This important topic is further considered below.

The use of large plasma pool coagulation factor concentrates has led to the rapid dissemination of HIV amongst haemophiliacs because it is possible that a single infected donation may render a pool of 25 000 donors infectious and the resultant individual vials of product may be used to treat many hundreds of patients. The extent to which use of cryoprecipitate has resulted in less HIV infection is difficult to determine because this form of therapy has been reserved, in some countries, mainly for mild and moderate haemophiliacs who only need treatment occasionally. In the early 1980s such treatment was used primarily to prevent hepatitis transmission. Furthermore it is difficult to judge the safety of cryoprecipitate because those countries using significant amounts of it, or very small plasma pools, were those in which the donor population became infected relatively late (Gringeri & Mannucci 1988, de Biasi et al 1991a). That the exclusive use of cryoprecipitate was not inherently safe was demonstrated by the finding that 40% of severe haemophiliacs treated only with this product in Seattle became infected; this reflecting the prevalence of HIV in the donor population and the frequent requirement for treatment.

The infectivity of blood products depends upon the viral load administered with each transfusion episode. Whereas all recipients of HIV-infected red cells or platelets probably become infected, not all vials of potentially infectious concentrate have resulted in HIV transmission (Ludlam et al 1985). The extent to which HIV, or other viruses co-purify with factor VIII or IX in their manufacture, is one variable which determines the potential for its transmission. The prevalence of HIV infection in haemophilia B is much lower than in haemophila A (Table 40.6) in most countries. This is likely to be due to less viral contamination in factor IX concentrates; this may be related to such products in general being of higher purity. Countries which used less pure PPSB concentrates, prepared by PEG precipitation (Gringeri & Mannucci 1988), e.g. Italy, have higher HIV prevalence in haemophilia B

Table 40.8 Techniques for sterilizing coagulation factor concentrates

Treatment	Temperature (°C)	Duration (h)
Dry heat	80	72
Wet pasteurization	60	10
Heptane	60	60
Vapour	60/80	10/1
Solvent/detergent (TNBT/cholate, Tween 80)		
β propiolactone + UV light* — now withdrawn		

* Only used for factor IX concentrate.

patients than those that used fractionation procedures based on alcohol precipitation to produce a purer product. Whether it was the repeated use over many years of a lower purity product leading to a greater immune modulating effect that increased the susceptibility of the recipient to infection, or that such products contained more virus, or that the alcohol had some virucidal effect remains unknown. It has been argued that monoclonally purified products are less liable to result in virus transmission because of the highly specific nature of the purification process, however such concentrates have resulted in virus transmission even despite inclusion of a viral inactivation step (Berntorp et al 1990).

To date all human immunodeficiency virus infection in haemophilia has been with HIV-1. No infection by HIV-2 from factor VIII/IX concentrate has been reported. Although there has been overwhelming epidemiological evidence for infectious HIV being present in coagulation factor concentrates prior to 1985 it is only recently that direct proof has been obtained by detection of PCR amplified fragments of HIV-1 from freeze-dried concentrates which were available in the early 1980s (Zhang et al 1991). Furthermore sequence analysis has demonstrated that the HIV-1 was likely to have been of North American origin.

HIV disease in haemophiliacs

There is much evidence that HIV disease in haemophiliacs is very similar to that observed in individuals who acquire the virus by intravenous drug abuse or sexually. There have been many studies to identify possible cofactors that might influence progression of HIV disease. Although many of these were originally identified in haemophiliacs they are also probably associated with HIV progression in non-haemophiliacs.

Table 40.9 Clinical manifestations of HIV in haemophiliacs which differ from non-haemophiliac infected individuals

Faster rate of HIV clinical progression in older inidividuals *
Pyogenic arthritis
Increased incidence of lymphoma
Lack of Kaposi's sarcoma
Use of high purity concentrates may be associated with slower progression of HIV disease

* This may also apply to individuals infected by non-coagulation factor concentrates.

There are several consequences of HIV in haemophiliacs (Table 40.9), however, that are different from the infection in other individuals. Disease in haemophiliacs is similar to that observed in others who also became infected intravenously. Intravenous drug abusers, for example, like haemophiliacs rarely develop Kaposi's sarcoma. This multifocal tumour is usually observed only in those who become infected sexually. The aetiological agent for Kaposi's sarcoma is unknown, it is possibly a passenger virus co-transmitted with HIV which is not infectious by the intravenous route. An alternative explanation is that the endothelial proliferation characteristic of Kaposi's sarcoma is a response to intense immune stimulation by factors with angiogenic activity, but this does not explain its absence in haemophiliacs.

There is evidence to suggest that lymphomas may be more common in HIV-positive haemophiliacs than in other infected individuals (Beral et al 1990). Whether this represents a true increase, or whether it merely represents more accurate diagnosis and reporting because haemophiliacs, as a group, are more consistently followed by

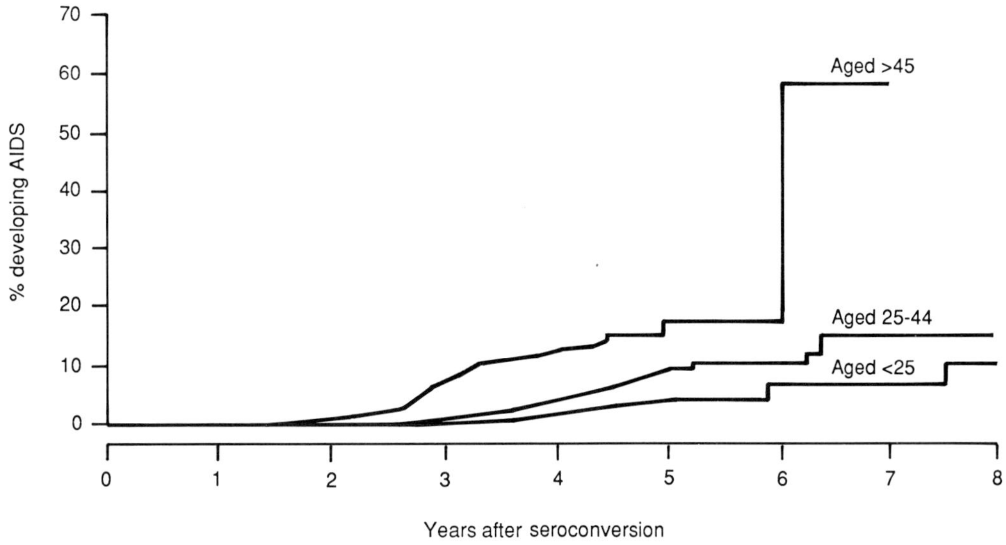

Fig. 40.2 Estimated percentage of patients developing AIDS in the UK by time, since estimated date of seroconversion (Dary et al 1989a).

haematologists who may be more likely to diagnose, treat and report a lymphoma, is currently unknown. An alternative explanation is that another agent, possibly viral is also transmitted by coagulation factor concentrates and is involved in the pathogenesis of lymphoma. As discussed above non-HIV-related immune modulation in haemophiliacs might predispose to lymphomas.

Pyogenic arthritis, particularly due to *Staphylococcus aureus* is a well recognised complication of HIV infection only observed in haemophiliacs (Goldsmith et al 1984, Scott et al 1985, Ragni & Hanley 1989). The diagnosis should be suspected in any painful joint, in which the symptoms seem atypical of a bleed particularly if it does not settle promptly with factor VIII/IX therapy. Without appropriate antibiotic therapy the symptoms progress and the patient will become pyrexial and systematically unwell. Patients are often bacteraemic and the organism can be cultured and identified from blood cultures as well as by direct aspiration of the joint. As infection of prosthetic joints has also been observed, it is probably prudent to avoid the implantation of new arthroplasties in HIV-positive haemophiliacs unless these are essential for mobility or reasonable social functioning.

Originally the prognosis of HIV-positive haemophiliacs appeared better than other infected subjects but this was probably due to many being relatively young. Several studies have demonstrated that older age is associated with a worse prognosis (Fig. 40.2) (Goedert et al 1989, Dary et al 1990a). It has not, however, been possible to demonstrate the same age effect for other risk groups, probably because of the narrower age range of infected adults. Young individuals are able to tolerate HIV viraemia and their CD4 cells also decline at a slower rate (Goedert et al 1989).

Study of individuals in whom the date of seroconversion is accurately known has demonstrated that the time from HIV infection to the development of PCP is the same for all risk groups, when the data are corrected for age. The diagnosis of AIDS in homosexuals is often at an earlier stage than in haemophiliacs as in many the AIDS-defining illness is Kaposi's sarcoma which generally occurs at a higher CD4 count than an opportunistic infection (Biggar 1990).

One of the potential cofactors relating to HIV disease progression in haemophiliacs is the purity of factor VIII or IX concentrate used in treatment (Table 40.10). Many of the studies on the effect of concentrates in vitro indicate that some of both lower and high purity, can inhibit lymphocyte and monocyte function (p. 933). It has been argued that treatment of HIV-positive haemophiliacs with such products may hasten immune decline. Following HIV infection the rate of decline is independent of the severity of haemophilia, and the amount of annual treatment, and is similar for haemophilia A and B (Goedert et al 1989). Most patients with haemophilia B have been treated with factor IX concentrates of higher specific activity than factor VIII products, and therefore the similar rates of decline in haemophilia A and B is evidence against a deleterious effect of immunomodulating components of concentrates on HIV progression. Trials comparing the effect of high and low purity concentrates on the rate of CD4 cell decline have given conflicting results. This is in part due to the small number of patients included in several of the studies. Recent reports, however, indicate that CD4 decline may be less rapid in patients treated with high purity concentrates although others indicate that purity does not influence the rate (de Biasi et al 1991b, Goldsmith et al 1991, Mannucci et al 1992). With the greater availability of high purity concentrates there is an increasing trend towards their use in HIV-positive haemophiliacs. It is unlikely, therefore, that large prospective studies to assess the potential value of high purity products in HIV-positive patients will ever be undertaken.

Table 40.10 Evidence for and against coagulation factor concentrates influencing HIV progression

Evidence suggestive of an effect of concentrate

1. CD4 cells decline slower in patients receiving high purity factor VIII concentrates

Evidence suggestive that factor VIII concentrate purity does ***not*** *influence HIV progression*

1. The rate of clinical progression
   a. Similar for haemophilia A and B
   b. Independent of severity of haemophilia
   c. Time to develop PCP same for haemophiliacs as non-haemophiliacs (after correction for age)
2. CD4 cell decline is not slower in patients on high purity concentrates

The effect on disease progression of immune abnormalities (as described above) predating HIV infection is largely unknown. Recent evidence suggests that haemophiliacs with higher total serum IgM levels prior to HIV infection (Simmonds et al 1991) progressed to CDC IV disease quicker after infection. Whether the raised IgM levels were a response to previous concentrate infusions, the presence of other viral infections, e.g. HCV, or were genetically determined, at present remains unknown.

There is evidence from studies that some viruses may transactivate HIV expression in cell culture systems. For example, if CMV and HIV co-infect lymphocytes in vitro enhanced HIV replication is observed. There is some evidence that HIV-positive individuals co-infected with CMV may progress more rapidly to AIDS (Webster et al 1989) although this has been disputed.

Monitoring of HIV infected haemophilacs

It is essential that the HIV status of all haemophiliacs is reliably known. The diagnosis can be made by detecting anti-HIV antibody against p24 and confirming the diagnosis by Western or immuno-blot containing envelope antigens specific for HIV-1 and HIV-2.

The single most useful immunological investigation is serial CD4 counts. Although when cohorts of HIV-positive haemophiliacs are studied the mean rate of CD4 decline appears linear, individual patients may exhibit marked temporary fluctuations for inapparent reasons (Eyster et al 1989, Goedert et al 1989, Phillips et al 1989, Teitel et al 1989). Reliance therefore should not be placed on single determinations, instead the trend of sequential counts should be considered.

After a period of HIV infection when there has been a gradual decline in CD4 number the count may rapidly plummet (Eyster et al 1987) and, in the days prior to anti-retroviral therapy and anti-microbial prophylaxis, this was followed relatively quickly by the development of AIDS.

One of the principal clinical reasons for assessing serial CD4 counts is to determine when treatment with antiviral and antimicrobial drugs should be started. Once the CD4 has fallen below $200 \times 10^6/l$ the risk of developing AIDS rises and as a result this level has been used by many clinicians as a threshold for starting treatment with zidovudine, anti-PCP and antifungal and anti-toxoplasmal prophylaxis. With such therapy many patients are surviving longer, many for several years with almost undetectable levels of CD4 cells (Lee et al 1991).

The next most useful parameter to measure is the serum β2-microglobulin concentration. The plasma concentration rises progressively and is higher in individuals who are at greater risk of developing symptoms. There is less agreement about the value of serial neopterin levels although some studies indicate that this parameter has useful prognostic value, others have found that the levels within a single individual vary too widely for it to be informative (Fuchs et al 1988, Valentine & Jacobson 1990).

Serial immunoglobulin concentrations have revealed a steady increase in IgG, however IgA levels only increase as the patients become symptomatic and are thus of limited predictive value. IgM levels gradually increase but do not predict imminent clinical deterioration.

Cell-mediated immunity to recall antigens, e.g. PPD, tetanus toxoid or candida, is normal shortly after HIV infection but as disease progresses cutaneous anergy becomes apparent (Brettler et al 1986). The use of repeated skin testing as a prognostic indicator in HIV-positive patients has not been evaluated.

Prognostic markers in HIV-positive haemophiliacs

Studies of haemophiliacs cohorts have resulted in identification of patient characteristics which may influence both susceptibility to infection and the subsequent prognosis (Table 40.11). Such studies have been easier to perform in haemophiliacs because they are mostly registered at treatment centres where they are reviewed regularly. Although several of the prognostic factors have only been identified as of being of value in haemophiliacs it is likely that they will be applicable to other infected individuals.

Table 40.11 Prognostic indications in HIV infected haemophiliacs

Factor affecting the chance of infection after HIV exposure
1. Dose of infective inoculum
2. HLA haplotype
Factors associated with poor prognosis after HIV infection
1. Older age
2. Possession of A1B8DR3 haplotype or DR3 alone
3. Increased total serum IgM level prior to infection
4. Occurrence of 'glandular fever' illness at seroconversion
5. Presence of IgM anti-HIV at seroconversion

Several factors have been identified that appear to predispose to HIV infection after exposure to the virus. There is clearly a dose effect in that individuals receiving a greater amount of infectious concentrate are more likely to seroconvert (Ludlam et al 1985). Certainly not all individuals treated with HIV-contaminated factor concentrates have become infected.

There is evidence that particular HLA antigens may be associated with a greater propensity to seroconversion after exposure to HIV. In one Italian study, possession of the haplotype A2 (Fabio et al 1990) was associated with a higher incidence of seroconversion in haemophiliacs. In a separate study there was an indication that A1 B8 DR3 might predispose to infection although, possibly because of small numbers in the study, the level of risk did not quite reach statistical significance (Steel et al 1988).

Following the establishment of HIV infection, several prognostic actors have been identified. Age is the factor that influences the course of infection more than any other known variable (Fig. 40.2). Several studies have indicated that older individuals have a poorer prognosis (Brookmeyer & Goedert 1989, Eyster et al 1989, Goedert et al 1989, Darby et al 1990b, Schinaia et al 1991). Over a 7-year period those under 25 years have a 6% chance of developing AIDS whereas individuals over 45 years have a 30% risk. This effect of age is probably due to the gradual immune decline that occurs with age in healthy individuals. Those with HIV are either less able to mount such an effective specific immune response or the immune system is less able to regenerate from HIV-induced damage.

Evidence has accumulated that certain host haplotypes may be associated with a less good prognosis. HLA AI B8 DR3 or DR3 alone has been reported in several studies to be associated with a more rapid decline in CD4 numbers and the earlier appearance of clinical symptoms (Steel et al 1988, Fabio et al 1990, Kaslow et al 1990, Donald et al 1992,). It is particularly noteworthy that this haplotype is also associated with autoimmune diseases, e.g. SLE, conditions which may result from a 'hyperactive' immune system.

The host response at, or shortly after HIV infection,

may identify individuals who will progress to earlier symptomatic disease. As discussed above those individuals who have raised total serum IgM levels prior to HIV exposure have a worse prognosis (Simmonds et al 1991). However, so far as assessing the prognosis for an individual patient is concerned, the IgM level prior to infection is not likely to be known. Shortly after infection, specific anti-HIV antibodies become detectable. In some individuals the initial specific antibody response is by IgG, however as with many other infections, the first detectable antibody may be IgM type. Individuals who develop this specific IgM response prior to IgG antibodies have a worse prognosis (Simmonds et al 1991). The reason for this is currently unknown.

Individuals who develop the glandular fever-like illness progress to AIDS sooner than those whose initial infection occurs asymptomatically. Marked IgG- and IgA-specific anti-HIV responses are noted to be associated with poor prognosis in other groups.

Management of HIV-positive haemophiliacs

The prognosis for HIV-positive individuals has steadily improved during the past 5 years due to the application of knowledge gained from clinical trials of anti-viral therapy. The increase in life expectancy has probably been more influenced, however, by an increased understanding of prevention, diagnosis and treatment of opportunistic infections. New more sensitive diagnostic tests, e.g. monoclonal antibody or PCR techniques for detection of *Pneumocystis carinii*, along with novel approaches to therapy, e.g. nebulized pentamidine, and the availability of new anti-microbial drugs, e.g. fluconazole, have radically improved the outlook.

Management of HIV-positive haemophiliacs requires a range of skills only available in an integrated and coordinated multidisciplinary team. Patients continue to require effective treatment for their haemophilia and in most instances this is similar to HIV-negative individuals. There are, however, additional complications related to both the propensity to bleeds and infections arising in arthritic or prosthetic joints. The frequency of haemophilic bleeds may increase particularly when patients start to lose weight and muscle bulk. Factor VIII consumption may also rise because additional infusions will be needed to cover invasive diagnostic procedures which may be necessary to identify infective organisms. HIV-associated ITP, further compromises the haemostatic system and will predispose particularly to gastrointestinal and intracranial haemorrhage.

Regular clinical review is essential and it is important to have readily available base line data. Although the serological response to infection is impaired in HIV, it is useful to know what organisms the patients has been exposed to previously, particularly those that may become active as immunity declines e.g. toxoplasmosis. Objective assessment of the respiratory system is helpful as minor radiographic changes, or deterioration of function, may be of great significance, particularly in the diagnosis of PCP. Regular investigations which should be performed are listed in Table 40.12. The frequency with which these are carried out varies between centres but in those who are asymptomatic every 3 months is probably adequate.

Table 40.12 Laboratory monitoring of HIV-infected haemophiliacs

1. Full blood count
2. Absolute CD4 cell count
3. β_2-microglobulin
4. Neopterin
5. Total serum IgG and IgA
6. p24 antigen

The overall aim must be to allow the individual to function as normally as possible in their social environment. Some will manage this with little help but others will require extensive psychological and social help. The importance of avoiding sexual transmission must be stressed and sympathetic counselling may be necessary (Goldman et al 1992). Some couples will wish to consider artificial insemination or adoption in order to have children. Support and counselling must be available to the partners and other family members.

In the early days of the AIDS pandemic, patients only received anti-HIV or anti-microbial therapy when they became symptomatically ill from HIV or developed an acute bacterial infection. However current practice is to give specific anti-HIV therapy before patients become symptomatic and anti-microbial prophylaxis against organisms which are likely to cause symptomatic infection. There are no rigid guidelines to indicate when the various therapies should be started. One approach is to start zidovudine therapy when patients are asymptomatic (Fischl et al 1987, Fischl et al 1990, Volberding et al 1990) with a CD4 count below $200 \times 10^9/1$, on two consecutive occasions, or if, constitutional symptoms due to HIV, e.g. night sweats or weight loss, begin even when the CD4 count is above this level. A dose of 100 mg five times daily appears to be efficacious (Nordic Medical Research Councils' HIV Therapy Group 1992) and is much less likely than a larger dose started later to cause bone marrow depression. When on such therapy it is important to monitor monthly the full blood count and creatine phosphokinase (CPK) (to detect myositis).

In approximately one third of HIV-infected individuals, PCP is the first AIDS-defining illness. As the risk of developing PCP rises significantly when the CD4 count falls below $200 \times 10^6/1$ prophylactic therapy should be started at this time. Studies have demonstrated that nebulized pentamidine 300 mg monthly (immediately preceded by salbutamol 5 mg), or cotrimoxazole 480 mg three times weekly are both effective prophylaxes (Leoung et al 1990,

Ruskin & LaRiviere 1991). The cotrimoxazole may have the additional benefit of offering some degree of prophylaxis against toxoplasmosis.

Oral hygiene should be encouraged and nystatin (or amphotericin lozenges) daily should be started as soon as candida is detected. If candida persists, fluconazole 50 mg can be started. Initially a once weekly dose may be adequate but if the thrush persists the frequency can be increased to daily therapy. Such treatment will substantially delay oesophageal or systemic infection but may result in the development of resistant strains.

The above regimen of zidovudine, pentamidine and nystatin has enabled HIV-positive patients to remain feeling relatively well for prolonged periods even when CD4 counts have fallen to almost undetectable level. Other specific anti-retroviral drugs are under evaluation and it is likely that either combinations or sequential courses of treatment with several therapies may offer better suppression of HIV than zidovudine alone. It is likely that other anti-microbial drugs will be used prophylactically in future. The recommendations given above have been devised for patients in Europe and North America. In other continents different organisms result in opportunistic infection with an AIDS-defining illness. In sub-Saharan Africa, for example, tuberculosis and cryptococcal infection is prevalent and prophylaxis against these organisms is therefore indicated.

Treatment of opportunistic infections

Treatment of opportunistic infections, as far as reasonably practical, must be based on accurate identification of the infective organism. This requires close cooperation between clinician and diagnostic laboratory to ensure that the correct samples are delivered promptly. A detailed description of treatment regimes for opportunistic infections is beyond the scope of this chapter. The chance of specific therapy being effective is much higher if it is started early. Furthermore, even when patients are symptomatically better from an opportunistic infection there is a high likelihood of recurrence unless prophylactic long-term specific anti-microbial therapy is started immediately after the acute infection has settled, e.g. following cerebral toxoplasmosis patients should be treated with long-term maintenance therapy.

Treatment of lymphomas

High grade B cell lymphomas are often widely disseminated at diagnosis when the patient is likely to have symptoms. In such patients, with stage IV disease 20–30% will have marrow involvement. A variety of anti-lymphoma therapies have been tried ranging from single drug to standard anti-lymphoma chemotherapeutic cocktails (Levine 1990). Most regimens are based on the CHOP (cyclophosphamide, adriamycin, vincristine and prednisolone) combination to which bleomycin or methotrexate has been added. By the time immunoblastic lymphoma develops, 30–50% of patients will have had a previous AIDS-defining illness and the prognosis, even without the lymphoma, is therefore limited. In some reported series, with treatment up to 50% have entered remission and survival of these individuals may be up to 2 years. Those who fail to enter remission have a poor prognosis.

Those with primary intracranial lymphoma treated with radiotherapy have an approximately 50% chance of obtaining remission but this is usually short lived.

Patients with Burkitt's lymphoma potentially have a better prognosis because they occur in young individuals with a relatively high CD4 count. Treatment should be as for B-ALL with intracranial prophylaxis. Although initial reports of therapy were disappointing more aggressive chemotherapy has led to lasting remissions and relative success following syngeneic transplantation has been reported (Turner et al 1992).

REFERENCES

Aronson D L 1988 Cause of death in hemophilia A patients in the United States from 1968 to 1979. American Journal of Hematology 27: 7–12

Autran B, Plata F, Debre P 1991 MHC-restricted cytotoxicity against HIV. Journal of Acquired Immune Deficient Syndromes 4: 361–367

Autran B, Letvin N L 1992 HIV epitopes recognized by cytotoxic T-lymphocytes. In: Adler M W, Gold J W M, Levy J A, Groupman J E, AIDS 1991. Current Science, London

Balfe P, Simmonds P, Ludlam C A, Bishop J O, Leigh Brown A J 1991 Concurrent evolution of human immunodeficiency virus type 1 in patients infected from the same source: Rate of sequence change and low frequency of inactivating mutations. Journal of Virology 64: 6221–6233

Batchelor A, Steel C M, Ludlam C A 1992 Enhancement of human T-cell responses to allogenic stimulation by factor VIII concentrates. British Journal of Haematology (in Press)

Beddall A C, Hill F G, George R H, Williams M D, al-Rubei K 1985 Unusually high incidence of tuberculosis among boys with haemophilia during an outbreak of the disease in hospital. Journal of Clinical Pathology 38: 1163–1165

Bell B A, Kurczynski E M, Bergman G 1990 Inhibitors to monoclonal antibody purified factor VIII letter. Lancet 336: 638

Beral V, Peterman T A, Berkelman R L, Jaffe H W 1990 Kaposi's sarcoma among persons with AIDS: a sexually transmitted infection? Lancet 335: 123–128

Berntorp E, Nilsson I M, Ljung R, Widell A 1990 Hepatitis C virus transmission by monoclonal antibody purified factor VIII concentrate letter. Lancet 335: 1531–1532

Biagiotti R, Giudizi M G, Almerigogna F et al 1986 Abnormalities of in vitro immunoglobulin production in apparently healthy haemophiliacs: relationship with alterations of T cell subsets and with HTLV-III seropositivity. Clinical and Experimental Immunology 63: 354–358

Biberfield G, Emini E A 1992 Progress with HIV vaccines. In: Adler M W, Gold J W M, Levy J A, Groopman J E (eds) AIDS 1991. Current Science, London

Biggar R J 1990 AIDS incubation in 1891 HIV seroconvertors from different exposure groups. Aids 4: 1059–1066
Bontempo F A, Lewis J H, Gorenc T J et al 1987 Liver transplantation in hemophilia A. Blood 69: 1721–1724
Brettler D B, Forsberg A D, Brewster F, Sullivan J L, Levine P H 1986 Delayed cutaneous hypersensitivity reactions in hemophiliac subjects treated with factor concentrate. American Journal of Medicine 81: 607–611
Brettler D B, Levine P H 1989 Factor concentrates for treatment of hemophilia: which one to choose? Blood 73: 2067–2073.
Brieva J A, Sequi J, Zabay J M et al 1985 Abnormal B cell function in haemophiliacs and their relationship with factor concentrates administration. Clinical and Experimental Immunology 59: 491–498
Brookmeyer R, Goedert J J 1989 Censoring in an epidemic with an application to hemophilia-associated AIDS. Biometrics 45: 325–335
Buehrer J L, Weber D J, Meyer A A et al 1990 Wound infection rates after invasive procedures in HIV-1 seropositive versus HIV-1 seronegative hemophiliacs. Annals of Surgery 211: 492–498
Carr R, Veitch S E, Edmond E et al 1984 Abnormalities of circulating lymphocyte subsets in haemophiliacs in an AIDS-free population. Lancet 1: 1431–1434
Center for Disease Control 1981a Pneumocystis Pneumonia–Los Angeles. Morbidity and Mortality Weekly Report 30: 250–252
Center for Disease Control 1981b Kaposi's sarcoma and pneumocystis pneumonia among homosexual men–New York City and California. Morbidity and Mortality Weekly Report 30: 305–308
Center for Disease Control 1982a Pneumocystis carinii pneumonia among persons with hemophilia A. Morbidity and Mortality Weekly Report 31: 365–367
Center for Disease Control 1982b Update on acquired immune deficiency syndrome (AIDS) among patients with hemophilia A. Morbidity and Mortality Weekly Report 31: 644–652
Center for Disease Control 1984 Update: acquired immunodeficiency syndrome (AIDS) in persons with hemophilia. Morbidity and Mortality Weekly Report 33: 589–591
Center for Disease Control 1986 Classification System for Human T-lymphotropic Virus Type III/Lymphadenopathy-Associated Virus Infections. Morbidity and Mortality Weekly Report 35: 334–339
Center for Disease Control 1987 Revision of the CDC Surveillance Case Definition for Acquired Immunodeficiency Syndrome. Morbidity and Mortality Weekly Report 36: 3S–15S
Center for Disease Control 1988 Safety of therapeutic products used for hemophilia patients. Morbidity and Mortality Weekly Report 37: 441–451
Cuthbert R J, Ludlam C A, Rebus et al 1989 Human immunodeficiency virus detection: correlation with clinical progression in the Edinburgh haemophiliac cohort. British Journal of Haematology 72: 387–390
Cuthbert R J, Ludlam C A, Tucker et al 1990 Five year prospective study of HIV infection in the Edinburgh haemophiliac cohort. British Medical Journal 301: 956–961
Cuthbert R J, Ludlam C A, Steel C M et al 1992 Immunological studies in HIV seronegative haemophiliacs: relationships to blood product therapy. British Journal of Haematology 80: 364–369
Darby S C, Doll R, Thakrar B et al 1990a Time from infection with HIV to onset of AIDS in patients with haemophilia in the UK. Statistics and Medicine 9: 681–689
Darby S C, Doll R, Thakrar B, et al 1990b Time from infection with HIV to onset of AIDS in patients with haemophilia in the UK. Statistics and Medicine 9: 681–689
de Biasi R, Rocino A, Miraglia E, Mastrullo L, Carola A 1991a AIDS and hemophilia. Antibiotics and Chemotherapy. 43: 156–172
de Biasi R, Rocino A, Miraglia E, Mastrullo L, Quirino A A 1991b The impact of a very high purity factor VIII concentrate on the immune system of human immunodeficiency virus-infected hemophiliacs: A randomized prospective, two-year comparison with an intermediate purity concentrate. Blood 78: 1919–1922
Donald J A, Rudman K, Cooper D W et al 1992 Progression of HIV-related disease is associated with HLA DQ and DR alleles defined by restriction fragment length polymorphisms. Submitted for publication
Ehrenforth S, Kreuz W, Scharrer I et al 1992 Incidence of development of factor VIII and factor IX inhibitors in haemophiliacs. Lancet 339: 594–598
Eibl M M, Ahmad R, Wolf H M et al 1987 A component of factor VIII preparations which can be separated from factor VIII activity, down modulates human monocyte functions. Blood 69: 1153–1160
Essex M, McLane M F, Lee T H et al 1983 Antibodies to cell membrane antigens associated with human T-cell leukemia virus in patients with AIDS. Science 220: 859–862
Evans J A, Pasi K J, Williams M D, Hill F G 1991 Consistently normal CD4+, CD8+ levels in haemophilic boys only treated with a virally safe factor VIII concentrate (BPL 8Y). British Journal of Haematology 79: 457–461
Eyster M E, Goedert J J, Sarngadharan M G et al 1985 Development and early natural history of HTLV-III antibodies in persons with hemophilia. Journal of the American Medical Association 253: 2219–2223
Eyster M E, Gail M H, Ballard J O et al 1987 Natural history of human immunodeficiency virus infections in hemophiliacs: effects of T-cell subsets, platelet counts, and age. Annals of Internal Medicine 107: 1–6
Eyster M E, Ballard J O, Gail M H, Drummond J E, Goedert J J 1989 Predictive markers for the acquired immunodeficiency syndrome (AIDS) in hemophiliacs: persistence of p24 antigen and low T4 cell count. Annals of Internal Medicine 110: 963–969
Fabio G, Smeraldi R S, Gringeri A et al 1990 Susceptibility to HIV infection and AIDS in Italian haemophiliacs is HLA associated. British Journal of Haematology 75: 531–536
Fischl M A, Richman D D, Grieco M H et al 1987 The efficacy of azidothymidine (AZT) in the treatment of patients with AIDS and AIDS-related complex. A double-blind, placebo-controlled trial. New England Journal of Medicine 317: 185–191
Fischl M A, Richman D D, Hansen N et al 1990 The safety and efficacy of zidovudine (AZT) in the treatment of subjects with mildly symptomatic human immunodeficiency virus type 1 (HIV) infection. A double-blind, placebo-controlled trial. The AIDS Clinical Trials Group Annals of Internal Medicine 112: 727–737
Fletcher M L, Trowell J M, Craske J et al 1983 Non-A non-B hepatitis after transfusion of factor VIII in infrequently treated patients. British Medical Journal 287: 1754–1757
Freedman J, Mazaheri R, Read S et al 1987 Humoral and cellular immune abnormalities in adult hemophiliacs followed over a 2-year period. Diagnostic Clinical Immunology 5: 30–40
Fuchs D, Hausen A, Reibnegger G et al 1988 Neopterin as a marker for activated cell-mediated immunity: Application in HIV infection. Immunology Today 9: 150–155
Garsia R J, Gatenby P A, Basten A et al 1987 Australian hemophiliac recipients of voluntary donor blood products longitudinally evaluated for AIDS. A clinical and laboratory study, 1983–1986. Australian and New Zealand Journal of Medicine 17: 371–378
Gibbons J, Cory J M, Hewlett I K et al 1990 Silent infections with human immunodeficiency virus type 1 are highly unlikely in multitransfused seronegative hemophiliacs. Blood 76: 1924–1926
Goedert J J, Eyster M E, Biggar R J, Blattner W A 1987 Heterosexual transmission of human immunodeficiency virus: association with severe depletion of T-helper lymphocytes in men with hemophilia. AIDS Research into Human Retroviruses 3: 355–361
Goedert J J, Kessler C M, Aledort L M et al 1989 A prospective study of human immunodeficiency virus type 1 infection and the development of AIDS in subjects with hemophilia. New England Journal of Medicine 321: 1141–1148
Gold J E, Altarac D, Ree H J et al 1991 HIV-associated Hodgkin disease: a clinical study of 18 cases and review of the literature. American Journal of Haematology 36: 93–99
Goldman E, Miller R, Lee C A 1992 Counselling HIV positive haemophiliac men who wish to have children. British Medical Journal 304: 829–830
Goldsmith J C, Silberstein P T, Fromm R E Jr, Walker D Y 1984 Hemophilic arthropathy complicated by polyarticular septic arthritis. Acta Haematologica (Basel) 71: 121–123
Goldsmith J M, Deutsche J, Tang M, Green D 1991 CD4 cells in HIV-1 infected hemophiliacs: Effect of factor VIII concentrates. Thrombosis and Haemostasis 66: 415–419
Gringeri A, Mannucci P M 1988 National survey of human

immunodeficiency virus infection in Italian hemophiliacs: 1983–1987. The Medical-Scientific Committee of the Fondazione dell'Emofilia. Ricerca in Clinica e in Laboratorio 18: 275–280
Habeshaw J A, Dalgleish A G, Bountiff L et al 1990 AIDS pathogenesis: HIV envelope and its interaction with cell proteins. Immunology Today 11: 418–425
Hay C R, Preston F E, Triger D R et al 1987 Predictive markers of chronic liver disease in hemophilia. Blood 69: 1595–1599
Hay C R, McEvoy P, Duggan-Keen M 1990 Inhibition of lymphocyte IL2-receptor expression by factor VIII concentrate: a possible cause of immunosuppression in haemophiliacs. British Journal of Haemotology 75: 278–281
Horowitz B 1990 Blood protein derivative viral safety: observations and analysis. Yale Journal of Biology and Medicine 63: 361–369
Horowitz M S, Rooks C, Horowitz B, Hilgartner M W 1988 Virus safety of solvent/detergent-treated antihaemophilic factor concentrate. Lancet 2: 186–189
Jones P, Proctor S, Dickinson A, George S 1983 Altered immunology in haemophilia letter. Lancet 1: 120–121
Karpatkin S 1990 HIV-I-related thrombocytopenia. In: Costello C (ed) Baillière's clinical haematology, haematology in HIV disease. vol 3(1): 115–138
Kaslow R A, Duquesnoy R, VanRaden M et al 1990 A1, Cw7, B8, DR3 HLA antigen combination associated with rapid decline of T-helper lymphocytes in HIV-1 infection. A report from the Multicenter AIDS Cohort Study Lancet 335: 927–930
Kernoff P B, Lee C A, Karayiannis P, Thomas H C 1985 High risk of non-A non-B hepatitis after a first exposure to volunteer or commercial clotting factor concentrates: effects of prophylactic immune serum globulin. British Journal of Haematology 60: 469–479
Kernoff P B, Miller E J, Savidge G F 1987 Reduced risk of non-A, non-B hepatitis after a first exposure to 'wet heated' factor VIII concentrate. British Journal of Haematology 67: 207–211
Kitchen L W, Barin F, Sullivan J L et al 1984 Aetiology of AIDS — antibodies to human T-cell leukaemia virus (type III) in haemophiliacs. Nature 312: 367–369
Kleim J P, Bailly E, Schneweis K E 1990 Acute HIV-1 infection in patients with haemophilia B treated with B-propiolactone-UV-inactivated clotting factor. Thrombosis and Haemostasis 64: 336–337
Lederman M M, Ratnoff O D, Scillian J J et al 1983 Impaired cell-mediated immunity in patients with classic hemophilia. New England Journal of Medicine 308: 79–83
Lederman M M, Saunders C, Toossi Z et al 1986 Antihemophilic factor factor VIII preparations inhibit lymphocyte proliferation and production of interleukin-2. Journal of Laboratory and Clinical Medicine 107: 471–478
Lee C A, Kernoff P B, Bofill M 1984 HTLV and haemophilia letter. Lancet 1: 1028
Lee C A, Bofill M, Janossy G, Thomas H C et al 1985 Relationships between blood product exposure and immunological abnormalities in English haemophiliacs. British Journal of Haematology 60: 161–172
Lee C A, Phillips A, Elford J et al The natural history of human immunodeficiency virus infection in a haemophilic cohort. British Journal of Haematology. 73: 228–234
Lee C A, Phillips A N, Elford J et al 1991 Progression of HIV disease in a haemophilic cohort followed for 11 years and the effect of treatment. British Medical Journal 303: 1093–1096
Leigh Brown A J 1992 Sequence variability in human immunodeficiency viruses: pattern and process in viral evolution. Groopman J E (eds) In: Adler M W, Gold J W M, Levy J A, AIDS 1991. Current Science, London
Leoung G S, Feigal D W Jr, Montgomery A B et al 1990 Aerosolized pentamidine for prophylaxis against Pneumocystis carinii pneumonia. The San Francisco community prophylaxis trial New England Journal of Medicine 323: 769–775
Levine A M 1990 Lymphoma in acquired immunodeficiency syndrome. Seminars in Oncology 17: 104–112
Levine P H, McVerry B A, Attock B, Dormandy K M 1977 Health of the intensively treated hemophiliac, with special reference to abnormal liver chemistries and splenomegaly. Blood 50: 1–9
Levy J A, Mitra G, Mozen M M 1984 Recovery and inactivation of infectious retroviruses from factor VIII concentration. Lancet 2: 722–723
Ludlam C A, Tucker J, Steel C M et al 1985 Human T-lymphotropic virus type III (HTLV-III) infection in seronegative haemophiliacs after transfusion of factor VIII. Lancet 2: 233–236
Madhok R, Gracie A, Lowe G D et al 1986 Impaired cell mediated immunity in haemophilia in the absence of infection with human immunodeficiency virus. British Medical Journal 293: 978–980
Madhok R, Gracie J A, Forbes C D Lowe G D 1991 B cell dysfunction in haemophilia in the absence or presence of HIV-1 infection. Thrombosis and Haemostasis 65(1): 7–10
Mannhalter J W, Ahmad R, Leibl H et al 1988 Comparable modulation of human monocyte functions by commercial factor VIII concentrates of varying purity. Blood 71: 1662–1668
Mannhalter J W, Ahmad R, Eibl M M, Leibl H 1990 Modulation of human monocyte functions by factor VIII-anti-factor VIII complexes present in an affinity-purified factor VIII product letter. Blood 75: 810–811
Mannhalter J W, Zlabinger G J, Ahmad R et al 1986 A functional defect in the early phase of the immune response observed in patients with hemophilia A. Clinical Immunology and Immunopathology 38: 390–397
Mannucci P M 1992 Outbreak of hepatitis A among Italian patients with haemophilia (Letter). Lancet 339: 819
Mannucci P M, Colombo M 1988 Virucidal treatment of clotting factor concentrates. Lancet 2: 782–785
Mannucci P M, Colombo M 1989 Revision of the protocol recommended for studies of safety from hepatitis of clotting factor concentrates. International Society for Thrombosis and Hemostasis. Thrombosis and Haemostasis 61: 532–534
Mannucci P M, Zanetti A R, Colombo M 1988 Prospective study of hepatitis after factor VIII concentrate exposed to hot vapour. British Journal of Haematology 68: 427–430
Mannucci P M, Gringeri A, de Biasi R et al 1992 Immune status of asymptomatic HIV-infected hemophiliacs: Randomized, prospective, two-year comparison of treatment with a high-purity or an intermediate-purity factor VIII concentrate. Thrombosis and Haemostasis 67: 310–313
Matheson D S, Green B J, Poon M C et al 1986a T lymphocytes from hemophiliacs proliferate after exposure to factor VIII product. Vox Sanguinis 51: 92–95
Matheson D S, Green B J, Poon M C et al 1986b Natural killer cell activity from hemophiliacs exhibits differential responses to various forms of interferon. Blood 67: 164–167
Matheson D S, Green B J, Fritzler M J et al 1987 Humoral immune response in patients with haemophilia. Clinical Immunology and Immunopathology 4: 41–50
Menitove J E, Aster R H, Casper J T et al 1983 T-lymphocyte subpopulations in patients with classic hemophilia treated with cryoprecipitate and lyophilized concentrates. New England Journal of Medicine 308: 83–86
Moffat E H, Bloom A L, Jones et al 1985 A study of cell mediated and humoral immunity in haemophila and related disorders. British Journal of Haematology 61: 157–167
Moore J P, Nara P L 1992 The role of the V3 loop of gp120 in HIV infection. In: Adler M W, Gold J W M, Levy J A, Groopman J E (eds) AIDS 1991. Current Science, London
Nordic Medical Research Councils' HIV Therapy Group 1992 Double blind dose-response study of zidovudine in AIDS and advanced HIV infection. British Medical Journal 304: 13–17
Pasi K J, Hill F G 1990 In vitro and in vivo inhibition of monocyte phagocytic function by factor VIII concentrates: correlation with concentrate purity. British Journal Haematology 76: 88–93
Peutherer J F, Rebus S, Barr P et al 1990 Confirmation of non-infection in persistently HIV-seronegative recipients of contaminated factor VIII (letter). Lancet 336: 1008
Phillips A, Lee C A, Elford J et al 1989 Prediction of progression to AIDS by analysis of CD4 lymphocyte counts in a haemophilic cohort. Aids 3: 737–741
Pluda J M, Yarchoan R, Jaffe E S et al 1990 Development of non-Hodgkin lymphoma in a cohort of patients with severe human immunodeficiency virus (HIV) infection on long-term antiretroviral therapy. Annals of Internal Medicine 113: 276–282
Rabkin C S, Hilgartner M W, Hedberg K W et al 1992 Incidence of lymphomas and other cancers in HIV-infected and HIV-uninfected

patients with hemophilia. Journal of the American Medical Association 267 :1090–1094

Ragni M V, Hanley E N 1989 Septic arthritis in hemophilic patients and infection with human immunodeficiency virus (HIV) letter. Annals of Internal Medicine 110: 168–169

Ragni M V, Ruben F L, Winkelstein et al 1987 Antibody responses to immunization of patients with hemophilia with and without evidence of human immunodeficiency virus (human T-lymphotropic virus type III) infection. Journal of Laboratory Medicine 109: 545–549

Ragni M V, Bontempo F A, Myers D J, Kiss J E, Oral A 1990 Hemorrhagic sequelae of immune thrombocytopenic purpura in human immunodeficiency virus-infected hemophiliacs. Blood 75: 1267–1272

Ravenholt R T 1983 Role of hepatitis B virus in acquired immunodeficiency syndrome. Lancet ii: 885–886

Redfield R R, Wright D C, Tramont E C 1986 The Walter Reed staging classification for HTLV-III/LAV infection. New England Journal of Medicine 314: 131–132

Rickard K A, Joshua D E, Campbell J et al 1983 Absence of AIDS in haemophiliacs in Australia treated from an entirely voluntary blood donor system letter. Lancet 2: 50–51

Rizza C R, Spooner R J 1983 Treatment of haemophilia and related disorders in Britain and Northern Ireland during 1976–80: report on behalf of the directors of haemophilia centres in the United Kingdom. British Medical Journal 286: 929–933

Royce R A, Luckmann R S, Fusaro R E, Winkelstein W Jr 1991 The natural history of HIV-1 infection: staging classifications of disease. Aids 5: 355–364

Ruskin J, LaRiviere M 1991 Low-dose co-trimoxazole for prevention of Pneumocystis carinii pneumonia in human immunodeficiency virus disease. Lancet 337: 468–471

Schechter M T, Neumann P W, Weaver M S et al 1991 Low HIV-1 proviral DNA burden detected by negative polymerase chain reaction in seropositive individuals correlates with slower disease progression. Aids 5: 373–379

Schimpf K, Brackmann H H, Kreuz W et al 1989 Absence of anti-human immunodeficiency virus types 1 and 2 seroconversion after the treatment of hemophilia A or von Willebrand's disease with pasteurized factor VIII concentrate. New England Journal of Medicine 321: 1148–1152

Schinaia N, Ghirardini A, Chiarotti F, Gringeri A, Mannucci P M & Italian Group 1991 Progression to AIDS among Italian HIV-seropositive haemophiliacs. Aids 5: 385–391

Scott J P, Maurer H S, Dias L 1985 Septic arthritis in two teenaged hemophiliacs. Journal of Pediatrics 107: 748–751

Simmonds P 1990 Variation in HIV virus load of individuals at different stages in infection: Possible relationship with risk of transmission. Aids 4: S77–S83

Simmonds P, Lainson F A, Cuthbert R et al 1988 HIV antigen and antibody detection: variable responses to infection in the Edinburgh haemophiliac cohort. British Medical Journal 296: 593–598

Simmonds P, Balfe P, Ludlam C A et al 1990a Analysis of sequence diversity in hypervariable regions of the external glycoprotein of human immunodeficiency virus type 1. Journal of Virology 64: 5840–5850

Simmonds P, Balfe P, Peutherer J F et al 1990b Human immunodeficiency virus-infected individuals contain provirus in small numbers of peripheral mononuclear cells and at low copy numbers. Journal of Virology 64: 864–872

Simmonds P, Beatson D, Cuthbert R J G et al 1991 Determinants of HIV disease progression: six year longitudinal study in the Edinburgh haemophilia/HIV cohort. Lancet 338: 1159–1163

Steel C M, Ludlam C A, Beatson D et al 1988 HLA haplotype A1 B8 DR3 as a risk factor for HIV-related disease. Lancet 1: 1185–1188

Sullivan J L, Brewster F E, Brettler D B et al 1986 Hemophiliac immunodeficiency: influence of exposure to factor VIII concentrate, LAV/HTLV-III, and herpesviruses. (Published erratum appears in Journal of Pediatrics 1986 109(6): 1075.) Journal of Pediatrics. 108: 504–510

Teitel J M, Freedman J J, Garvey M B, Kardish M 1989 Two-year evaluation of clinical and laboratory variables of immune function in 117 hemophiliacs seropositive or seronegative for HIV-1. American Journal of Hematology 32: 262–272

Thomas D P 1988 Reducing the risk of virus transmission by blood products. British Journal of Haematology. 70: 393–395

Thorpe R, Dilger P, Dawson N J, Barrowcliffe T W 1989 Inhibition of interleukin-2 secretion by factor VIII concentrates: a possible cause of immunosuppression in haemophiliacs. British Journal of Haematology 71: 387–391

Tucker J, Ludlam C A, Craig A et al 1985 HTLV-III infection associated with glandular-fever-like illness in a haemophiliac (letter). Lancet 1: 585

Turner M L, Watson H G, Russell L et al 1992 An HIV positive haemophiliac with acute lymphoblastic leukaemia successfully treated with intensive chemotherapy and syngeneic bone marrow transplantation. Bone Marrow Transplantation 9: 183–191

United Kingdom Haemophilia Directors 1988a Prevalence of antibody to HIV in haemophiliacs in the United Kingdom: a second survey. AIDS Group of the United Kingdom Haemophila Centre Directors with the co-operation of the United Kingdom Haemophilia Centre Directors. Clinical and Laboratory Haematology 10: 187–191

United Kingdom Haemophilia Directors 1988b Effect of dry-heating of coagulation factor concentrates at 80 degrees C for 72 hours on transmission of non-A, non-B hepatitis. Study Group of the UK Haemophilia Centre Directors on Surveillance of Virus Transmission by Concentrates. Lancet 2: 814–816

Valentine F T, Jacobson M A 1990 Immunological and virological surrogate markers in the evaluation of therapies for HIV infection. Aids 4 (suppl 1): 5201–5207

Vilmer E, Barre-Sinoussi F, Rouzioux C et al 1984 Isolation of new lymphotropic retrovirus from two siblings with haemophilia B, one with AIDS, Lancet 1: 753–757

Volberding P A, Lagakos S W, Koch M A et al 1990 Zidovudine in asymptomatic human immunodeficiency virus infection. A controlled trial in persons with fewer than 500 CD4-positive cells per cubic millimeter. The AIDS Clinical Trials Group of the National Institute of Allergy and Infectious Disease New England Journal of Medicine 322: 941–949

Walker B D, Plata F 1990 Cytotoxic T lymphocytes against HIV. Aids 4: 177–184

Watson H G, Ludlam C A 1992 Immunological abnormalities in haemophiliacs. Blood Reviews 6: 26–23

Watson H G, Ludlam C A, Rebus S et al 1992 Use of several second generation serological assays to determine the true prevalence of hepatitis C virus infection in haemophiliacs treated with non-virus inactivated factor VIII and IX concentrates. British Journal of Haematology 80: 514–518

Wearne A, Joshua D E, Rickard K A, Kronenberg H 1984 Abnormal T-cell subpopulations in hemophilic patients receiving factor VIII concentrates from voluntary donors. Australian and New Zealand Journal of Medicine. 14: 149–153

Webster A, Lee C A, Cook D G et al 1989 Cytomegalovirus infection and progression towards AIDS in haemophiliacs with human immunodeficiency virus infection. Lancet 2: 63–66

Weintrub P S, Koerper M A, Addiego J E Jr et al 1983 Immunologic abnormalities in patients with hemophilia A. Journal of Pediatrics. 103: 692–695

Williams M D, Cohen B J, Beddall A C et al 1990 Transmission of human parvovirus B19 by coagulation factor concentrates. Vox Sanguinis 58: 177–181

Zhang L Q, Simmonds P, Ludlam C A, Leigh Brown A J 1991 Detection, quantification and sequencing of HIV-1 from the plasma of seropositive individuals and from factor VIII concentrates. AIDS 5: 675–681

41. Acquired disorders of coagulation

P. M. Mannucci   P. L. F. Giangrande

Acquired disorders of haemostasis may present in a number of ways, ranging from sudden life-threatening bleeding after surgery or childbirth at one end of the spectrum to minor purpura or an increased bruising tendency at the other. It is important to establish from a personal history whether there have been spontaneous haemorrhagic problems, e.g. epistaxis, haemarthrosis, gastrointestinal bleeding, in the past or bleeding after surgery, e.g. tonsillectomy, appendicectomy, or dental extractions. The family history should also be elicited. Symptoms of congenital disorders of haemostasis usually appear early in life. However, it should be borne in mind that mild forms of congenital disorders such as haemophilia may only become evident after surgery or major trauma. Equally, postoperative bleeding is a common cause of referral for subsequent investigation to exclude a disorder of haemostasis: it must not be forgotten that failure to tie off blood vessels is frequently the underlying cause!

In this chapter, abnormalities of haemostasis in relation to hepatic and renal disease, malignancy, vitamin K deficiency, cardiopulmonary bypass, massive blood transfusion and drug therapy are discussed, as well as acquired inhibitors of coagulation. Disseminated intravascular coagulation is discussed separately in Chapter 42.

DISORDERS OF HAEMOSTASIS IN RENAL DISEASE

Patients with renal diseases often have many alterations of haemostasis. As a result of these alterations patients with chronic renal failure tend to have a bleeding tendency. Those with nephrotic syndrome, by contrast, may develop thrombotic complications such as renal vein thrombosis and deep venous thrombosis in the limbs. Thrombosis of the vascular access site is a frequent problem for patients requiring haemodialysis. For a review on disorders of haemostasis in renal disease, see Deykin (1983) and Remuzzi (1988).

Uraemic bleeding

Symptoms

The most frequent haemorrhagic manifestations observed in uraemic patients, whether on chronic haemodialysis or not, are usually from mucosal surfaces (gastrointestinal bleeding, epistaxis, menorrhagia). Soft tissue bleeding (large ecchymoses, haematomas) is rarer. Even though the bleeding tendency in these patients is usually not severe, life-threatening episodes are sometimes encountered. These include retroperitoneal haemorrhage, bleeding into the pericardial and pleural spaces and intracranial haemorrhage (particularly subdural haematomas). Patients do not usually bleed after surgical procedures, but renal biopsies are sometimes complicated by the formation of an intrarenal haematoma.

Pathogenesis

Prolongation of the skin bleeding time, associated with a normal or only slightly reduced platelet count and normal coagulation tests are the usual findings in uraemia, indicating a defect in platelet plug formation at the transected ends of blood vessels (Steiner et al 1979). Several possible mechanisms have been proposed. Severe thrombocytopenia is rare. Some studies indicate that platelet aggregation in response to various aggregating agents is impaired (Castaldi et al 1966, Evans et al 1972), although others have found no significant defect in aggregation (Jorgensen & Ingeberg 1979). The intraplatelet content of serotonin and nucleotides, stored within the dense granules, may be reduced (Eknoyan & Brown 1981), but this finding is neither consistent nor marked. Another biochemical defect in platelets is an elevation in cyclic AMP content (Vlachoyannis & Schoeppe 1982), which reduces the availablity of intraplatelet calcium and thereby inhibits platelet function. Platelet arachidonate metabolism is also abnormal, with defective synthesis of prostaglandin endoperoxides and thromboxane, perhaps due to inhibition of cyclo-oxygenase function (Remuzzi et al 1983). Synthesis of prostacyclin (PGI_2), a potent vasodilator and inhibitor of platelet aggregation, is increased in uraemic vessels (Remuzzi et al 1977). Recent experimental data indicate that excessive production of the vasodilator nitric oxide by the endothelium might contribute to the prolongation of the bleeding time in uraemia (Remuzzi et al 1990). Erythrocytes are also clearly implicated in the pathogenesis of the haemostatic defect. There is an inverse relationship between the haematocrit and the bleeding time in uraemic subjects (Livio et al 1982). This is probably because erythrocytes promote transport of centrally flowing platelets in the blood vessels towards the vessel wall, hence increasing platelet adhesion to the subendothelium. It thus appears that the pathogenesis of abnormal bleeding in uraemia is multifactorial, and it is difficult to determine which factor, if any, is more important than the others.

Management of uraemic bleeding

The choice of therapeutic agents in uraemia for management or prevention of bleeding is usually based on the capacity to shorten or normalize the bleeding time. The rationale behind this approach is that the degree of prolongation of the bleeding time correlates quite closely with the bleeding tendency (Steiner et al 1979). Haemodialysis or transfusion of platelet concentrates may produce transient shortening of the bleeding time, but these measures are not uniformly effective in all patients (Stewart & Castaldi 1967). Cryoprecipitate is a plasma fraction which contains large amounts of factor VIII (FVIII) and von Willebrand factor (vWF), as well as fibrinogen, fibronectin and smaller amounts of virtually all plasma proteins. The infusion of 8–10 bags of cryoprecipitate in uraemic patients is usually followed by shortening or even normalization of the bleeding time. The effect is delayed (being maximal 4–6 hours after infusion) and transient (lasting 24–36 hours) (Janson et al 1980). The administration of cryoprecipitate is not entirely without hazard, as there is the possibility of transmission of blood-borne viruses. 1-deamino-8-D-arginine vasopressin (DDAVP, desmopressin) is a synthetic derivative of antidiuretic hormone and produces a short-lasting release of autologous factor VIII and vWF from storage sites into the circulation. DDAVP at a dose of 0.3–0.4 μg/kg usually restores the bleeding time to normal in uraemic subjects one hour after intravenous infusion (Mannucci et al 1983). The bleeding time returns to the original baseline value after 8 hours. DDAVP is thus of limited use when long-term control of bleeding is required (gastrointestinal bleeding, menorrhagia) as the effect only lasts 4–8 hours. Conjugated oestrogens provide an attractive alternative in these conditions, improving the bleeding time within 6 hours of an intravenous dose. Furthermore, the effect of repeated intravenous doses divided over 5 consecutive days usually lasts as long as 14 days (Livio et al 1986). Transfusion of washed red cell concentrates in uraemic subjects in order to correct anaemia and maintain the haematocrit above 0.30 shortens the bleeding time and results in a corresponding improvement in bleeding symptoms (Livio et al 1982). Diminished production of erythropoietin is the most important factor in the development of anaemia in uraemia. The increase in erythrocyte count induced by administration of human recombinant erythropoietin is also parallelled by shortening of the bleeding time (Moia et al 1987). Shortening of the bleeding time with corresponding improvement of the bleeding tendency is evident when the haematocrit is only partially corrected to values above 0.30: there is little further improvement even when higher haematocrits are attained (Moia et al 1987).

In conclusion, there are several therapeutic options for the management of abnormal bleeding in uraemic subjects. DDAVP is indicated prior to biopsies and for the treatment of acute bleeding, as its onset of action is rapid. The duration of its effect is limited to some 4–8 hours. DDAVP is preferable to infusions of cryoprecipitate because of the possible risk of transmission of infection with a plasma product. Conjugated oestrogens are preferable for the treatment of subacute or recurrent bleeding, as their effect persists for up to 15 days. Erythropoietin may be used for long-term correction of a bleeding tendency, as its onset of action is delayed but sustained for long periods.

Thrombotic complications of the nephrotic syndrome

Thrombotic complications are not infrequent in the nephrotic syndrome, particularly renal vein thrombosis but also deep venous thrombosis in the lower limbs and cerebral vein thrombosis. It is thought that thrombosis occurs because of an imbalance in the haemostatic system. The haemostatic abnormalities most commonly found in patients with the nephrotic syndrome are hyperaggregability of platelets (Bang et al 1973), high levels of clotting zymogens (particularly vitamin K-dependent factors II, VII, IX and X) and cofactors (VIII) (Vaziri et al 1980), low levels of the main naturally-occurring anticoagulant, antithrombin III (Kauffmann et al 1978), and hypofibrinolysis. Platelet 'hyperactivity' (as expressed by enhanced platelet aggregation in response to arachidonic acid and other agents, shortened platelet survival and increased production of thromboxane B_2) is usually attributed to hyperlipidaemia and the urinary loss of proteins such as albumin which control normal platelet function (Silver et al 1973, Remuzzi et al 1979, Stuart et al 1980, Schieppati et al 1984). In addition, plasma levels of von Willebrand factor and fibrinogen may be very high (Takeda & Chen 1967, Coppola et al 1981). Enhanced synthesis of these proteins, through acute phase reactions or other mechanisms, in conjunction with low levels of antithrombin III secondary to urinary loss clearly favour a tendency to the formation of thrombin (Kauffmann et al 1978), even though levels of other anticoagulant proteins such as protein C are usually normal or even high in these patients (Mannucci et al 1986a). Hypofibrinolysis is mainly related to an increase in the plasma level of the two main inhibitors of fibrinolysis, α_2-antiplasmin and plasminogen activator inhibitor type 1, although the effect on fibrinolysis of these abnormalities tends to be counteracted by low plasminogen levels, owing to urinary loss of the protein (Du et al 1985).

Overall, these complex abnormalities tend to tilt the haemostatic balance in favour of thrombus formation. However, it is possible that these abnormalities may be the result of thrombotic events, rather than the cause. Only prospective studies can establish their causal role, and determine whether haemostatic measurements have any useful role in predicting thrombosis in patients with the nephrotic syndrome.

Thrombosis of vascular access for haemodialysis

Despite technical advances in the form of vascular access and the use of materials of low thrombogenicity, thrombosis of the shunt has been a major complication ever since the introduction of arteriovenous shunts for maintenance haemodialysis.

The early (1 year) failure rate of the shunts due to thrombosis is around 8–10%, with an overall failure rate at 4–5 years of 20–30% (del Greco et al 1989). Thrombotic occlusion of shunts may be due to a number of factors, of which hypercoagulability (e.g. in the nephrotic syndrome) and inadequate heparinization during haemodialysis are probably the least important. Narrowing of the arterial lumen is an important structural factor of particular importance in patients with diabetes mellitus, hyperlipidaemia and the elderly (del Greco et al 1989). Haemodynamic factors which impair arterial flow or venous return (hypotension, congestive cardiac failure) are equally important (del Greco et al 1989). Shunt occlusion can be avoided by preventing the development of such conditions and through the use of antiplatelet agents. Sulphinpyrazone (800 mg/day) is effective (Kaegi et al 1974), but results with aspirin (160 mg/day) are also excellent (Harter et al 1979). Some have also attempted to lyse the thrombi with fibrinolytic agents such as streptokinase or urokinase. Although such attempts are often successful, thrombosis tends to recur so that the cost and the side-effects do not appear to be justified.

DISORDERS OF HAEMOSTASIS IN LIVER DISEASE

The liver is the principal site of synthesis and clearance of coagulation factors, components of the fibrinolytic system and naturally-occurring anticoagulants such as antithrombin III and proteins C and S. Both acute and chronic liver diseases are thus frequently associated with haemostatic abnormalities. The main abnormalities present, usually in combination, are multiple defects of clotting zymogens and anticoagulant proteins, thrombocytopenia, platelet function defects and hyperfibrinolysis. As a general rule, the severity of the haemostatic abnormalities is directly proportional to the extent of hepatocellular damage.

Liver disease is associated with haemorrhagic problems. The most frequent are oesophageal and gastrointestinal haemorrhage, as well as bleeding from biopsy sites and during and after surgery. Bleeding into soft tissues is only rarely encountered. Although the abnormalities in the haemostatic system may contribute in some instances to the bleeding tendency in patients with liver disease, anatomical and haemodynamic alterations are of greater importance. The presence of portal hypertension is particularly important. In fact, even though some abnormalities may predispose to bleeding (such as low levels of clotting factors and hyperfibrinolysis), they tend to be counterbalanced by low levels of naturally-occurring anticoagulant proteins, such as antithrombin III and protein C. The net result of these changes is likely to be a haemostatic balance set at a lower level.

Multiple coagulation defects

Although the majority of patients with uncomplicated infectious or toxic acute hepatitis do not have marked abnormalities of haemostatic parameters, fulminant hepatitis is often associated with dramatic abnormalities associated with haemorrhagic symptoms, which often dominate the clinical picture. The most common laboratory findings are a marked reduction in the plasma levels of all coagulation factors except factor VIII, thrombocytopenia and increased levels of fibrinogen/fibrin degradation products (FDP) and of cross-linked fibrin derivatives (XDP). It has been suggested that this constellation of laboratory abnormalities is the result of disseminated intravascular coagulation induced by the release of necrotic hepatic tissue into the circulation, impaired removal of activated coagulation factors by the damaged liver and decreased levels of naturally-occurring anticoagulant proteins (Rake et al 1970). This hypothesis has not been universally accepted (Straub 1977), and the evidence implicating disseminated intravascular coagulation is indirect, since intravascular microthrombi are only infrequently found at autopsy.

Patients with chronic liver disease usually have multiple coagulation defects, the severity of which are roughly correlated with the reduced capacity of the liver to synthesize proteins (Biland et al 1978). The use of simple coagulation tests, such as the prothrombin time, to evaluate the extent of hepatic damage exploits this correlation. It has been suggested, however, that coagulation defects are due, at least in part, to disseminated intravascular coagulation (Verstraete et al 1974). When there is portal hypertension endotoxins absorbed from the gastrointestinal tract into the portal system bypass the liver and enter the systemic circulation unaltered, where they may be responsible for initiating platelet aggregation and triggering thrombin formation (Wilkinson 1977). The occurrence of disseminated intravascular coagulation in chronic liver disease is suggested by the finding of a shortened half life of radio-labelled fibrinogen, prothrombin, and plasminogen and by the reported ability of heparin to correct these alterations (Tytgat et al 1971, Coleman et al 1975). However, as in fulminant hepatitis, the precise role of disseminated intravascular coagulation in chronic liver disease has not been firmly established.

Quantitative and qualitative platelet defects

In acute viral or toxic hepatitis, thrombocytopenia is unusual or only of modest severity ($100–150 \times 10^9$/l) and not clinically significant. Thrombocytopenia is more severe ($50–100 \times 10^9$/l) in patients with chronic liver disease. A number of factors contribute to the development of thrombocytopenia. Hypersplenism is probably the most important, causing increased platelet pooling and sequestration in the spleen (Toghill et al 1977, Karpatkin & Freedman 1978). Other factors may also contribute, since there is no relationship between the platelet count and the size of the spleen. In some patients thrombocytopenia may be caused by alcoholism or folic acid deficiency.

Qualitative defects of platelet function have been reported in patients with chronic liver disease (Ballard & Marcus 1976, Thomas et al 1967). It is unlikely, however, that platelet dysfunction is of clinical importance in liver disease, except when the skin bleeding time is prolonged out of all proportion to the degree of thrombocytopenia (Blake et al 1990).

Hyperfibrinolysis

Although it is well established that hyperfibrinolysis is present in patients with liver disease (O'Connell et al 1964, Merskey et al 1966, Fletcher et al 1969), the contribution of increased fibrinolysis to the overall haemostatic defect in liver disease is uncertain. Patients with liver disease have a decreased plasma level of naturally occurring α_2-antiplasmin (Aoki & Yamanaka 1978, Collen & Wiman 1978) (due, presumably, to defective synthesis) and delayed removal of circulating plasminogen activators (Das & Cash 1969). Portacaval shunt surgery (Grossi et al 1962) and liver transplantation are considered to be the only clinical situations associated with truly pathological fibrinolysis.

Haemostasis and cholestasis

The hepatic synthesis of biologically active (γ-carboxylated) forms of factors II, VII, IX and X requires vitamin K. Coagulation defects due to impaired absorption of vitamin K are not frequently encountered in patients with obstructive jaundice due to pancreatic tumours or gallstones, probably because many of these patients undergo prompt investigation and are treated early with parenteral vitamin K. On the other hand, high levels of fibrinogen, impaired fibrinolysis and increased plasma levels of factors V and VIII are often found in these conditions, presumably due to a non-specific rise in 'acute-phase' glycoproteins in response to inflammation (Dioguardi et al 1973, Cederblad et al 1976). Despite such laboratory evidence of hypercoagulability the prevalence of deep venous thrombosis after biliary surgery is no greater than after surgical operations of comparable severity (personal observations, PMM).

Haemostatic problems during liver transplantation

An acute disorder of haemostasis is well documented during liver transplantation (Bohmig 1977). It is characterized by multiple coagulation defects and by signs of hyperfibrinolysis, reflected by high plasma levels of tissue plasminogen activator. The most critical periods are the anhepatic phase and the phase of revascularization of the graft. It is likely that the acute coagulopathy is due to loss of the ability to clear activators of fibrinolysis, which are released into the circulation during surgical trauma. The ability to clear such activators is an important property of the intact liver. Normal haemostasis is rapidly restored if the graft subsequently functions well. However, the abnormalities persist or worsen if the graft does not function well. Liver transplantation may be complicated by portal vessel thrombosis in children (Harper et al 1988). It has been suggested that thrombosis is due to procoagulant imbalance in the postoperative period, when relatively high plasma levels of coagulation zymogens (particularly factors II and X) are found in association with low levels of the naturally-occurring anticoagulant protein C (Harper et al 1988). Therapeutic trials currently in progress will establish whether plasma-derived concentrates of protein C can prevent this complication.

Management of haemostatic failure in liver disease

Besides vitamin K, which is indicated only when the defect is associated with deficiency or unavailability of the vitamin, therapeutic measures which have been proposed are transfusion of fresh frozen plasma or prothrombin-complex concentrates, or the administration of synthetic inhibitors of fibrinolysis, desmopressin (DDAVP) or heparin.

Fresh frozen plasma contains all of the coagulation factors and inhibitors present in blood and, therefore, is theoretically the most suitable agent for the correction of the multiple abnormalities associated with liver disease. In practice, however, replacement may prove difficult because the large volume of plasma required to correct the defects (1–1.5 litres) is frequently not tolerated by patients with severe liver disease (Mannucci et al 1976).

Prothrombin-complex concentrates are commercially available and contain high concentrations of factors II, IX and X. The content of factor VII is very variable and depends upon the particular product: some brands contain a negligible amount. The administration of prothrombin-complex concentrates does not usually completely correct abnormal coagulation tests since other coagulation factors that are also lacking in liver disease (e.g. factors V and XI) are not present in significant quantities in these concentrates (Mannucci et al 1976). Concentrates made from large plasma pools may transmit hepatitis, which may have particularly serious consequences in patients with pre-existing liver disease. There is also a risk of thrombotic complications, including deep venous thrombosis, pulmonary embolism and disseminated intravascular coagulation. Thrombosis is probably related to the presence in the concentrates of activated coagulation factors which are not adequately neutralized because of poor hepatic clearance. Concentrates are therefore best avoided in liver disease.

Platelet concentrates are ineffective in patients with liver disease, even in the presence of severe thrombocytopenia, because the infused platelets are rapidly removed from the circulation by the liver and spleen. When there is prolongation of the bleeding time, indicative of associated platelet dysfunction, desmopressin (DDAVP) at a dose of 0.3 μg/kg can be used to shorten the bleeding time before invasive procedures such as biopsy or laparoscopy (Mannucci et al 1986b).

The administration of synthetic inhibitors of fibrinolysis, such as ε-amino caproic acid and tranexamic acid, may be considered because of the possible role of hyperfibrinolysis in the pathogenesis of the bleeding tendency associated with liver disease. These drugs may be useful in the management of upper gastrointestinal bleeding because they inhibit local hyperfibrinolysis (Nilsson et al 1975b), and to reduce blood loss before and after surgery to create a portacaval shunt (Grossi et al 1964). The role of such drugs in the general management of bleeding associated with liver disease must be evaluated by controlled therapeutic trials before their use can be recommended.

In conclusion, there is little indication for the use of haemostatic agents in the management of the most frequent haemorrhagic complications encountered in patients with liver disease (i.e. oesophageal and gastrointestinal bleeding), since haemodynamic and anatomical factors are of greater importance than haemostatic defects in their pathogenesis. The judicious use of plasma is advised when the coagulation defects themselves are felt to play an important role (e.g. surgical bleeding). DDAVP can be used to shorten the bleeding time before invasive surgical procedures.

VITAMIN K DEFICIENCY

Vitamin K: biochemistry and physiology

In 1929 Henrik Dam of Copenhagen observed that chicks fed on an ether-extracted diet developed a haemorrhagic disorder. Subsequent work by him, rewarded with the Nobel prize for medicine in 1943, led to the isolation of a substance he termed vitamin K (Koagulationsvitamin). Vitamin K is necessary for post-translational modification of coagulation factors II (prothrombin), VII, IX and X, as well as proteins C and S. In the presence of the vitamin, certain glutamic acid residues at the N-terminal end of the nascent polypeptides are converted to gamma-carboxyglutamic acid. This confers the ability to bind calcium (and other metals) upon the protein, a property essential for physiological function of the molecules. Vitamin K is required as a co-factor for the carboxylase enzyme involved, which is an integral membrane protein (for review, see Furie & Furie 1990). In the absence of vitamin K, protein precursors devoid of function called PIVKA (Proteins Induced by Vitamin K Absence) may be detected by immunoelectrophoresis. There are two main forms of vitamin K : vitamin K_1 (phylloquinone) is found in plants and cereals, particularly in green leafy vegetables, and vitamin K_2 (the menaquinones) is actually a family of related substances produced by bacteria, including those colonizing the human intestine. Vitamin K (like vitamins A, D and E) is fat-soluble and is absorbed effectively only in the presence of bile salts. The recommended daily intake of vitamin K in adults is 70–140 μg. Little vitamin K is stored in the body and in experimental conditions, symptoms of deficiency may become evident within a few weeks.

Consequences of vitamin K deficiency

Deficiency of vitamin K is associated with prolongation of both the prothrombin time and the partial thromboplastin time. The thrombin time and plasma fibrinogen concentration are normal, which helps in the exclusion of disseminated intravascular coagulation, and the platelet count is normal. Typical haemorrhagic manifestations are easy bruising, and bleeding from sites of injury or from the gums or gastrointestinal tract.

Dietary deficiency and malabsorption

Dietary deficiency of vitamin K may result in haemorrhagic problems (Colvin & Lloyd 1977). Elderly patients, often with psychiatric disturbances, are particularly vulnerable and there may well be deficiencies of other important vitamins, such as folic acid, ascorbic acid (vitamin C) and iron. Debilitated patients undergoing surgery are also particularly vulnerable, as dietary deficiency may be compounded by the administration of broad-spectrum antibiotics which kill off gut bacteria that synthesize the vitamin (Pineo et al 1973, Hooper et al 1980).

Vitamin K will not be effectively absorbed from the gastrointestinal tract when there is obstruction of the bile duct. The administration of the anion exchange resin cholestyramine for symptomatic relief of pruritus associated with subtotal biliary tree obstruction further impairs vitamin K absorption, and may precipitate haemorrhage (Gross & Brotman 1970). Malabsorption of vitamin K may also occur in coeliac disease (gluten-sensitive enteropathy). It is essential to check the prothrombin time (as well as the platelet count) before diagnostic jejunal biopsy when this condition is suspected. Cystic fibrosis, biliary atresia, abetalipoproteinaemia and α_1-antitrypsin deficiency are other congenital disorders which may be associated with malabsorption of vitamin K (Payne & Hasegawa 1984). Acute gastroenteritis in infancy may also be associated with transient malabsorption of vitamin K and prolongation of the prothrombin time (Matoth 1950, Merskey & Hansen 1957). Vitamin K deficiency as a consequence of partial biliary tree obstruction may contribute to the development of impaired haemostasis in chronic hepatic disorders such as cirrhosis. An injection of vitamin K may shorten an abnormally long prothrombin time in such cases. Venom from the snake *Echis carinatus* may be used to predict the response to vitamin K in such cases (Solano et al 1990). The venom contains proteases capable of activating both normal and decarboxylated forms of prothrombin (factor II). Comparison of the conventional prothrombin time and the Echis clotting time can be used to predict responsiveness to vitamin K, as the Echis time is normal in the presence of decarboxyprothrombin associated with vitamin K deficiency.

Haemorrhagic disease of the newborn (see also Ch. 44)

Haemorrhagic disease of the newborn usually presents 2–4 days after delivery with gastrointestinal bleeding, purpura or bleeding from the umbilical stump. True gastrointestinal bleeding must be distinguished from swallowed maternal blood, ingested during parturition: blood eluted from the stool will be denatured with alkali in the case of swallowed maternal (adult) blood, but not in the case of true gastrointestinal haemorrhage, as fetal haemoglobin is resistant to denaturation (Apt's test) (Apt & Downey 1955). Various factors contribute to the deficiency of vitamin K in this condition. Hepatic immaturity is an important factor, and premature babies are particularly at risk. Maternal consumption of anticonvulsants (especially phenytoin) or antituberculous medication induces fetal hepatic metabolism of vitamin K, and is another risk factor. The gastrointestinal tract of neonates is not colonized with bacteria, and there is no significant endogenous production of vitamin K. Breast-fed babies are thus particularly vulnerable in comparison to bottle-fed babies, as milk powders are artificially fortified with vitamin K. It is recommended that all newborn infants should receive a single intramuscular injection of 1 mg vitamin K_1 after birth in order to prevent haemorrhagic disease of the newborn (American Academy of Pediatrics 1961, Canadian Paediatric Society 1988). Oral vitamin K supplementation in the neonatal period may prevent early haemorrhagic manifestations, but appears not to be as effective in preventing later haemorrhagic complications, including serious intraventricular haemorrhage (McNinch & Tripp 1991, Handel & Tripp 1991).

Oral anticoagulants (see also Ch. 65)

Warfarin and its congeners are competitive inhibitors of vitamin K (review: Hirsh 1991b). Patients taking oral anticoagulants should be monitored regularly in order to ensure that the INR (International Normalized Ratio) is within the therapeutic range of 2.0–4.5. More specific ranges have been recommended depending upon the clinical indication (Haemostasis and Thrombosis Task Force, BCSH 1990). In one series, the incidence of haemorrhagic problems was 4.3% per treatment year (Forfar 1979). However, the risk of bleeding is influenced by the intensity of anticoagulant therapy (Hull et al 1982, Turpie et al 1988, Saour et al 1990). Typical problems include epistaxis, ecchymoses, haematuria and subconjunctival haemorrhage. More serious problems which are occasionally encountered include gastrointestinal haemorrhage, intracranial haemorrhage and retroperitoneal bleeding. Bleeding may be provoked by the introduction of additional drugs which potentiate the action of coumarin anticoagulants, change in alcohol consumption, or diet. The possibility of underlying disease, such as peptic ulceration or gastrointestinal neoplasia, should be considered when there is unexpected bleeding and the INR is within the conventional therapeutic range.

Haemorrhagic problems due to surreptitious consumption of warfarin have been reported, particularly in medically trained personnel (O'Reilly et al 1962, Bowie et al 1965, O'Reilly & Aggeler 1976).

Measures which have been recommended to reverse anticoagulant therapy are shown in Table 41.1 (Haemostasis and Thrombosis Task Force, BCSH 1990).

The use of a prothrombin-complex concentrate rather than fresh frozen plasma was recommended in order to minimize the risk of transmission of HIV and hepatitis C. However, it should be borne in mind that concentrate is

Table 41.1 Recommendations on reversal of oral anticoagulant therapy

A. *Life-threatening haemorrhage:* Immediately give 5 mg vitamin K_1 by slow intravenous infusion and a concentrate of factor II, IX, X, with factor VII concentrate (if available). The dose of concentrate should be calculated based on 50 iu factor IX/kg body weight. If no concentrate is available fresh frozen plasma should be infused (about one litre for an adult) but this may not be as effective
B. *Less severe haemorrhage such as haematuria and epistaxis:* Withhold warfarin for 1 or more days and consider giving vitamin K_1 0.5–2.0 mg intravenously
C. *INR of greater than 4.5 without haemorrhage:* Withdraw warfarin for one or two days and then review
D. *Unexpected bleeding at therapeutic levels:* Investigate possibility of underlying cause such as unsuspected renal or alimentary tract disease

much more expensive. Furthermore, screening of plasma for anti-hepatitis C antibody has been introduced in many countries since these recommendations were drawn up.

Prior to introduction into clinical use, warfarin was originally widely employed as a rodenticide. Owing to the emergence of warfarin resistance, new and extremely potent long-acting anticoagulants have been developed and are now readily available in several over-the-counter rodenticide products. The 'superwarfarin' brodifacoum has a half life of some 30 days. Both accidental and deliberate consumption of the drug have been reported (Weitzel et al 1990, Routh et al 1991). Serious haemorrhage may subsequently ensue, and extremely large doses of vitamin K may be required to reverse the effects of the drug. Such therapy will also need to be continued for a long time in order to prevent haemorrhage.

DISORDERS OF HAEMOSTASIS IN PATIENTS WITH SOLID TUMOURS

Complex disturbances of haemostasis are frequently found in patients with solid tumours. The prevalence varies according to the type and extent of the tumour, but some abnormality is present in about 50% of all patients, rising to over 90% among those with metastatic disease (Slichter & Harker 1974). Such alterations include both quantitative and/or qualitative platelet changes and defects in the plasma components of haemostasis (coagulation factors, naturally-occurring anticoagulant proteins, and components of the fibrinolytic system). Whilst there are often no related clinical symptoms, up to 15–20% of patients experience clinically evident haemorrhage and/or thrombosis (for reviews, see Donati et al 1981, Rickles & Edwards 1983, Goldsmith 1984, Markus 1984, Dano et al 1985).

Platelet defects

Alterations in the production and survival of platelets are observed in association with a wide range of solid tumours. Such changes are usually found alongside other haematological abnormalities. There are three types of platelet defect observed in patients with tumours: thrombocytopenia, thrombocytosis and abnormal platelet function. Of these, thrombocytopenia is the most frequent abnormality and this may result in severe haemorrhage from mucosal surfaces, particularly when the platelet count is below 20×10^9/l. Thrombocytopenia may be the result of either reduced platelet production in the bone marrow (amegakaryocytic) or increased platelet sequestration and/or destruction (megakaryocytic) in the periphery. Amegakaryocytic thrombocytopenia is usually the consequence of neoplastic infiltration of the bone marrow, or bone marrow suppression following chemotherapy or radiotherapy. Platelet destruction in megakaryocytic thrombocytopenia may be mediated by anti-platelet antibodies, often associated with lymphomas and only rarely in association with solid tumours, or by consumption, through a mechanism similar to that operating in disseminated intravascular coagulation.

A high platelet count is commonly found in association with several types of tumour. The platelet count usually ranges from $400–600 \times 10^9$/l with normal platelet function (Levin & Conley 1964). The picture in this condition of reactive, or secondary, thrombocytosis thus differs from that seen in myeloproliferative disorders where the platelet count often exceeds 700×10^9/l and there are often functional abnormalities. However, a prolonged bleeding time may be found in patients with tumours, even when the platelet counts and coagulation factor levels are normal, indicating abnormal platelet function. This usually indicates underlying acquired storage pool deficiency, as reflected by low platelet content of dense granule components such as serotonin and ADP (Boneu et al 1984, Mannucci et al 1989).

Changes in coagulation

Solid tumours often produce changes in plasma factors involved in haemostasis. The most frequent of these changes are dysfibrinogenaemia, the production of circulating anticoagulants and activation of the coagulation cascade that can, in some cases, trigger full-blown disseminated intravascular coagulation.

Acquired dysfibrinogenaemia may be present in association with hepatocellular carcinoma, as well as other chronic liver disorders (Martinez et al 1978). A modified fibrinogen molecule with excessive sialic acid content is produced. The thrombin time and reptilase time are prolonged, reflecting abnormal fibrin polymerization. There is also a discrepancy between functional and immunological assays for fibrinogen, which yield higher results with immunoassays than with functional assays.

Circulating anticoagulants may appear in association

with various types of tumour, although they are most frequently associated with lymphoid tumours. Circulating anticoagulants may be directed against specific coagulation proteins (e.g. factor VIII inhibitors). Alternatively, they may have a more generalized effect upon phospholipids, similar to the so-called lupus anticoagulant (for more details, see section below relating to acquired inhibitors of coagulation, p. 957).

Disseminated intravascular coagulation is frequently encountered, as tumour cells produce substances that activate coagulation and liberate them into the blood stream. Coagulation factors, plasminogen, platelets and anticoagulant proteins may accordingly be consumed in association with malignant disease, and products of fibrinogen and fibrin degradation are formed as a consequence of secondary fibrinolysis. This consumptive coagulopathy translates into a prolonged prothrombin time, activated partial thromboplastin time and thrombin time. Thrombocytopenia is also frequent. Erythrocytes may be fragmented, reflecting fibrin deposition in the microcirculation. A distinction between acute and chronic forms of disseminated intravascular coagulation may be made (Al-Mondhiry 1975, Sack et al 1977, Slichter & Harker 1979). The acute form occurs in patients with tumours with rapid cell replication and necrosis. This condition may be considered as one aspect of the so-called 'tumour lysis syndrome', in which tumour lysis is a result of specific cytotoxic therapy. In addition, disseminated intravascular coagulation may be the result of other complications associated with neoplasia and related therapy, such as infection, severe hypotension and haemolytic transfusion reactions. When acute disseminated intravascular coagulation is very severe there will be rapid consumption of the principal coagulation factors, with haemorrhage. Chronic disseminated intravascular coagulation is seen in patients with slowly growing tumours, where there is little lysis. The process of activation of coagulation typical of this variety of disseminated intravascular coagulation may last for weeks or months. Sometimes the only sign of activation cascade is the presence of high plasma levels of fibrinopeptide A, a fragment cleaved by thrombin from the α-chain of fibrinogen (Peuscher et al 1980). A high fibrinopeptide A level is often the only coagulation abnormality in patients with a solid tumour, particularly in the early stages. There may be a paradoxical but compensatory increase in the levels of some coagulation factors, particularly fibrinogen and factor V, owing to increased synthesis (Mannucci et al 1985).

Changes in fibrinolysis

There tends to be a modest enhancement of fibrinolysis in patients with solid tumours. This is revealed by the presence of high plasma levels of cross-linked fibrin degradation products and of the fibrinogen fragment Bβ 15–42, which reflect the action of plasmin on both stabilized fibrin and recently formed fibrin (Mannucci et al 1990). Other findings are high plasma levels of plasminogen activator inhibitor type 1, tissue plasminogen activator and, particularly in the cases of breast and gastric carcinomas, urokinase-type plasminogen activator (de Jong et al 1987, Kirchheimer et al 1987). On the whole, these changes in the fibrinolytic system hardly affect the overall haemostatic balance, and they are likely to play only a minor role in the development of the haemorrhagic and thrombotic complications associated with neoplasia. The role of fibrinolysis is more important in the metastatic spread of solid tumours. High fibrinolytic activity of the primary tumour facilitates local invasion and the release of neoplastic cells into the circulation (Dano et al 1985). Since fibrinolysis can be inhibited by synthetic agents, it is quite possible that such drugs may acquire therapeutic relevance.

Hypercoagulability and thrombosis

Deep venous thrombosis is an established complication of neoplastic disease. The overall frequency of thrombosis that is either clinically evident or detected postmortem has been variably reported as being between 2% and 58% (Lieberman et al 1961, Ambrus et al 1975). Symptoms of venous thromboembolism may even be the initial clinical presenting manifestation of neoplasia. In addition, there is a very high prevalence of asymptomatic deep venous thrombosis in patients with cancer undergoing surgery: this may be as high as 60% when sensitive diagnostic methods are used. Compression of the large vessels by tumour mass, prolonged bed rest, and therapeutic administration of oestrogens are other important predisposing factors. Venous thrombosis is most frequent in the deep venous system of the lower limbs. Occasionally, there may be thrombosis in other vessels such as the inferior or superior vena cava, portal venous system, upper hepatic veins or cerebral veins. Venous thrombosis in an apparently healthy patient who does not seem to have any risk factors for thrombosis should always trigger suspicion of occult neoplasia. Some patients present with one or more features of Trousseau's syndrome, characterized by migratory thromboembolism in the superficial and/or deep venous system and arterial thrombosis, sometimes associated with disseminated intravascular coagulation (Sack et al 1977).

Thrombotic microangiopathy is a complication which may develop in patients with cancer. The main vessels involved are the small vessels of the kidney and brain. The symptoms are very similar to those seen in thrombotic thrombocytopenic purpura and haemolytic uraemic syndrome (see Ch. 33). Haemolytic anaemia associated with the presence of fragmented erythrocytes in the peripheral blood film is a constant feature, together with a variable degree of thrombocytopenia. Renal insufficiency and neurological signs and symptoms may be prominent clinical features. The plasma fibrinogen level is often normal, since fibrinogen turnover is increased. Infusion of fresh frozen plasma is probably the most effective therapy.

ACQUIRED INHIBITORS OF COAGULATION

Acquired inhibitors of coagulation, also known as 'circulating anticoagulants', are pathological moieties that inactivate single clotting factors or interfere with the interactions of multiple clotting factors during fibrin formation. The majority of these are autoantibodies. Unlike alloantibodies which develop in patients with congenital disorders of coagulation, they usually arise de novo, although frequently in association with autoimmune disease. They may develop in individuals with no underlying immunological disorder, particularly among young women and older individuals of both sexes. Such antibodies can be associated with a serious bleeding tendency, or in some instances a thrombotic tendency. However, an inhibitor may be picked up quite by chance during routine screening, perhaps before surgery, since many patients with inhibitors have absolutely no symptoms.

Lupus anticoagulant

The lupus anticoagulant is a pathological moiety which interferes with phospholipid-dependent tests of coagulation. It was first described in two patients with systemic lupus erythematosus, who had a prolonged prothrombin time and evidence of anticoagulant activity (Conley & Hartman 1952). It was subsequently shown that the coagulation test most often showing abnormal prolongation is not the prothrombin time but the activated partial thromboplastin time (APTT) (Mannucci et al 1979), although other phospholipid-dependent tests may show abnormal prolongation. The same abnormality could be found in patients with no evidence of systemic lupus erythematosus, and even in apparently healthy individuals. Interest in the lupus anticoagulant has grown considerably recently, since an association with an increased risk of recurrent thromboembolic events (both venous and arterial) and spontaneous abortions has become evident. Recent reviews on the subject are those of Lechner (1987) and Creagh & Greaves (1991).

The incidence of the lupus anticoagulant in the general population is unknown, although it is without doubt one of the most frequent causes of a prolonged APTT in clinical laboratories. The prevalence among patients with systemic lupus erythematosus has been reported as between 20% and 60%, probably depending upon the varied sensitivity of the diagnostic methods (Shapiro & Thiagarajan 1982). A very high prevalence of the lupus anticoagulant (30% or more) is found in patients receiving long-term treatment with chlorpromazine and related psychotropic drugs (Canoso & Hutton 1977). The lupus anticoagulant is also found with a relatively high frequency among patients with rheumatoid arthritis and other connective tissue diseases and in patients with malignant disease, particularly lymphomas and other lymphoproliferative disorders.

The production of the lupus anticoagulant may be viewed as an autoimmune disorder, in which pathological immunoglobulins (IgG, IgM or both) are generated. Phospholipids are the most likely target of the antibodies (Yin & Gaston 1965, Thiagarajan et al 1980). The specificity of the lupus anticoagulant for phospholipids is demonstrated by the fact that the inhibitor slows prothrombin activation by factor V and factor X_a only in the presence of phospholipid vesicles (Dahlback et al 1983). It is likely, however, that the mechanisms whereby the lupus anticoagulant inhibits coagulation are varied. The mechanism by which thrombosis is facilitated is not well established. Interactions with phospholipids in the endothelial cells of the vessel wall and its interference with important antithrombotic mechanisms such as the protein C/thrombomodulin system, the antithrombin III-heparin system and the availability of prostacyclin (Carreras & Vermylen 1982) have been proposed as possible mechanisms (reviewed by Lechner 1987).

The uncertainties about the prevalence of the lupus anticoagulant in patients with systemic lupus erythematosus or other populations of interest are probably due to differing diagnostic approaches amongst laboratories. Test systems that are used to diagnose the presence of the anticoagulant can be divided into screening procedures, meant to identify the existence of a coagulation abnormality and its probable nature, and confirmation procedures, which identify the dependence of the antibody upon phospholipid. The Scientific and Standardization Committee of the International Society for Thrombosis and Haemostasis has recently proposed a set of diagnostic criteria (Exner et al 1991). Testing should be carried out on fresh plasma which has either been filtered or strongly centrifuged, as inadequate removal of platelets in the test plasma adversely affects results (Exner et al 1991, Haemostasis and Thrombosis Task Force, BCSH 1991). The screening criterion is the prolongation of one of several phospholipid-dependent clotting tests, i.e. APTT, kaolin clotting time, dilute Russell's viper venom time or tissue thromboplastin inhibition test. With either test the clotting time of a mixture of patient and normal plasma should be more than two standard deviations longer than that of normal plasma mixed with plasma from patients with no anticoagulants. The confirmatory criterion is a relative correction of the clotting time defect after the addition of lysed, washed platelets or phospholipid liposomes to either of the aforementioned tests. Other secondary diagnostic criteria for the lupus anticoagulant are its lack of specificity for single coagulation factors, loss of anticoagulant activity on dilution of plasma and lack of time-dependency on anticoagulant activity. Several immunological methods employing antibodies to cardiolipin or other phospholipids have been used recently to identify patients with lupus anticoagulant (Harris 1990). The results obtained with these immunoassays do not always coincide with those obtained using coagulation assays. Since the association between clinical events and the lupus anticoagulant was originally established using coagulation assays, immunological tests should not be used as the screening test of choice until their association with disease is fully established.

The presence of a lupus anticoagulant is usually not associated with haemorrhage, unless there is concomitant thrombocytopenia or hypoprothrombinaemia. Hypoprothrombinaemia is quite rare (Shapiro & Thiagarajan 1982). The low plasma level of prothrombin is usually the result of complex formation between the antibodies and prothrombin, which is subsequently cleared from the circulation (Bajaj et al 1983). Autoimmune thrombocytopenia is more frequent, which probably reflects the underlying tendency in these patients to produce autoantibodies (Shapiro & Thiagarajan 1982). It is the association between thrombosis and the lupus anticoagulant which underlies the clinical interest in this phenomenon. The evidence for such an association is quite strong, even though there are very few prospective studies. In one study of 219 subjects with the lupus anticoagulant, but without evidence of systemic lupus erythematosus, 25% had experienced thrombotic episodes (Gastineau et al 1985). Screening for the lupus anticoagulant is therefore warranted in patients with unexplained thrombosis, particularly among young subjects. Related thrombotic events have mainly involved the deep veins of the limbs, from which pulmonary emboli may arise, but occlusion of cerebral arteries and veins have also been reported (Slater 1981). Other clinical problems linked to the lupus anticoagulant are pulmonary hypertension and recurrent abortion (Nilsson et al 1975a Firkin et al 1980). This latter complication is probably the result of thrombosis in placental or intervillous vessels (Nilsson et al 1975a).

Thrombosis in patients with the lupus anticoagulant should be treated in exactly the same way as in other patients without the inhibitor. Attempts to eradicate the lupus anticoagulant with steroids or other potent immunosuppressive agents are usually unsuccessful. Limited experience would suggest a trial of prednisone (at doses of 4–50 mg/day) and low-dose aspirin (75 mg/day) to prevent recurrent abortions (Lubbe et al 1983) . The role of this preventative therapy, however, is still not firmly established.

Factor VIII inhibitors

Although factor VIII inhibitors are found more commonly in multitransfused haemophiliacs, they may also develop de novo in patients who previously had normal levels of factor VIII and result in 'acquired haemophilia'. They are usually autoantibodies (IgG, or more rarely IgM) which bind to limited epitopes within the heavy or light chains of the factor VIII molecule, destroying coagulant activity (Scandella et al 1989). The resulting acquired deficiency of FVIII is usually accompanied by haemorrhagic problems which can be very severe.

The development of a factor VIII inhibitor is a rare phenomenon, being diagnosed in 0.2 to 1 per million of the population per year (Duran Suarez 1982, Lottenberg et al 1987). 215 cases were found in a large worldwide survey of haemophilia centres in 1981 (Green & Lechner 1981), although many cases were undoubtedly not reported centrally.

The pathogenesis of the inhibitors is not understood. It is believed that they arise as a consequence of derangement of the immune system with the emergence of lymphocyte clones that produce antibodies against the patients' own factor VIII. Immunological disorders most frequently associated with the development of an acquired factor VIII inhibitor are rheumatoid arthritis, systemic lupus erythematosus, inflammatory bowel disease, lymphoproliferative disorders (especially lymphomas) and multiple sclerosis. An association with certain drugs, and penicillin in particular, has been described. They may appear in the postpartum period, usually in previously healthy women although a minority may have evidence of underlying autoimmune disease. They may also arise in otherwise normal individuals, especially in old age.

The presence of an inhibitor is usually heralded by the appearance of haemorrhagic manifestations in elderly individuals with no prior history. The spectrum of symptoms is similar but not identical to that observed in congenital factor VIII deficiency. Haemarthrosis, for example, is very rare in patients with acquired inhibitors, whereas it is the hallmark of congenital haemophilia. Symptoms more frequently encountered are the development of haematomas, ecchymoses, and postoperative bleeding. Life-threatening intracranial haemorrhage and retroperitoneal bleeding are rarer manifestations. The natural history of the inhibitor is extremely variable. In some cases the antibody may disappear within a few months, especially when it first appears in the postpartum period, whereas in others it may persist for years (particularly in association with autoimmune diseases).

The typical findings suggestive of an inhibitory antibody against factor VIII are a prolonged APTT with normal prothrombin time, and very low factor VIII levels. Mixtures of patient plasma must be incubated with normal plasma and residual factor VIII activity measured after a period of incubation in order to confirm that the inhibitor specifically inactivates factor VIII. The finding of a lower factor VIII level than expected when normal plasma is incubated with the test plasma is evidence of a specific inhibitor, and the method can be modified to yield semiquantitative results. Although the kinetics of the reaction between normal factor VIII and acquired inhibitors are different from those seen in the case of congenital haemophiliacs with inhibitory antibodies (Green 1968), the assays are still of clinical use in determining the potency of acquired inhibitors. The tendency of the patients to develop an anamnestic rise in the antibody titre after replacement therapy is variable. Some patients behave like true haemophiliacs with alloantibodies to infused factor VIII, and respond with marked rises in titre, whereas in others there is little or no anamnestic response.

Therapy has two main goals: eradication of the inhibitor and management of ongoing bleeding episodes. Attempts to eradicate the inhibitor with immunosuppressive drugs (steroids, azathioprine or cyclophosphamide) appear to be more successful than in congenital haemophiliacs with inhibitors (Green & Lechner 1981). Prednisone is the drug of choice, at a dose of 1–2 mg/kg. Inhibitors tend to disappear within 2–3 weeks in certain categories of patients, particularly in women who develop a low titre inhibitor in the postpartum period. The inhibitor often persists and proves resistant to steroid therapy in patients with associated autoimmune disease. Cyclophosphamide (50–150 mg daily) and azathioprine (100–200 mg daily) may be tried in such patients. The results are usually disappointing, particularly when the antibody is of high titre (Green et al 1980, Green & Lechner 1981).

Bleeding episodes should be treated promptly since they are associated with considerable morbidity and mortality. It may be possible to achieve measurable levels of factor VIII in plasma with large doses of human factor VIII concentrate (50–100 U/kg or more). A satisfactory response may be achieved more often with porcine factor VIII concentrates, since the inhibitors cross-react poorly or not at all with porcine factor VIII (Gatti & Mannucci 1984). Prothrombin-complex concentrates (Kurczynski & Penner 1974) or activated factor VIIa (Hedner & Kisiel 1983), which is now produced through recombinant DNA technology, may be tried when measurable factor VIII levels cannot be achieved in plasma after infusion of human or porcine factor VIII. These materials bypass the function of factor VIII in the intrinsic coagulation pathway. Results are usually less satisfactory than those obtained with factor VIII concentrates. Plasma exchange or immunoadsorption of the inhibitory immunoglobulins to immobilized ligands such as protein A have been employed with some success (Gjorstrup & Watt 1990).

Inhibitors to von Willebrand factor

A syndrome that resembles congenital von Willebrand's disease sometimes occurs in patients without a family history or previous symptoms of abnormal bleeding. The main laboratory hallmarks of this form of acquired von Willebrand's disease are low plasma levels of von Willebrand factor (vWF), a prolonged bleeding time and a low factor VIII level secondary to deficiency of vWF which normally protects factor VIII from proteolysis in the circulation. This syndrome occurs most often in association with autoimmune or lymphoproliferative disorders, with or without associated monoclonal gammopathy. Angiodysplasia has been reported in association with some cases of acquired von Willebrand's disease but it is not established whether these vascular malformations are causally related or the result of the condition (Rosborough & Swaim 1978, Wautier et al 1976). The most typical clinical features are mild or moderately severe mucosal bleeding and bleeding after surgery, as seen in patients with congenital von Willebrand's disease (for review, see Mannucci & Mari 1984).

Three general mechanisms have been proposed concerning the pathogenesis of acquired von Willebrand's syndrome. Firstly, there may be selective adsorption of von Willebrand factor (and factor VIII) by abnormal lymphocyte clones or malignant cells. Alternatively, monoclonal immunoglobulins may bind the two proteins and induce rapid clearance from the circulation through formation of non-specific complexes. Finally, autoantibodies which interact specifically with von Willebrand factor may develop in these patients. Eradication of underlying disease will result in cure, but the syndrome may reappear if the underlying disorder recurs. The bleeding tendency in this acquired disorder is usually not difficult to control. In our experience, desmopressin (DDAVP) is a useful alternative to cryoprecipitate or other plasma-derived products, although its effect is only transient as factor VIII and von Willebrand factor are rapidly cleared from the circulation (Mannucci et al 1984).

These forms of acquired von Willebrand's disease with an immunological basis must be distinguished from that associated with hypothyroidism (Dalton et al 1987, Smith & Auger 1987). In this acquired disorder it is believed that reduced synthesis of von Willebrand factor by endothelial cells reflects general slowing of metabolism in hypothyroidism, and indeed treatment with thyroxine will restore normal haemostasis.

Inhibitors of other clotting factors

A reduction in the plasma level of coagulation factors other than factor VIII and von Willebrand factor may be caused by one of four general mechanisms:

1. Abnormal proteins, usually monoclonal immunoglobulins, bind coagulation factors and inhibit their activity.
2. Abnormal proteins may bind to factors without inhibiting their action in vitro, but there is rapid clearance of the complex from the circulation.

3. Abnormal proteins deposited in the extravascular space may bind coagulation factors.

4. Circulating heparin-like substances may arise which inhibit coagulation.

Usually only one coagulation factor is affected, although sometimes several may be affected.

The process of fibrin formation and stabilization is a frequent target of inhibitors. Inhibitors may retard cleavage of fibrinopeptides or aggregation of monomers or inhibit the cross-linking of the α and β chains of fibrin by factor XIII. The inhibitor may be an immunoglobulin (Cohen et al 1970, Coleman et al 1972, Marciniak & Greenwood 1979) or a heparin-like substance (Khoory et al 1980, Palmer et al 1984, Kaufman et al 1989). Often, there are no haemorrhagic problems related to the presence of such an inhibitor. Both the prothrombin time and the APTT may be prolonged, but the laboratory hallmark of these inhibitors is prolongation of the thrombin and reptilase times, with lack of correction by the addition of normal plasma. If the inhibitor is an antibody, the thrombin and reptilase times of normal plasma will be prolonged by the addition of patient plasma heated to 56°C or a semipurified immunoglobulin fraction derived from patient plasma.

Inhibitors of other factors are encountered very rarely (reviewed by Shapiro 1979). Inhibitors to factors V and XI are probably those most frequently reported. There is often a related bleeding tendency, albeit less severe than that seen in association with inhibitors directed against factor VIII. Whilst inhibitors against factor VIII and factor IX will result in isolated prolongation of the APTT, both the APTT and prothrombin time will be prolonged in the presence of an inhibitor directed against factor V. The stimulus for the appearance of such inhibitors is unclear. The most frequent conditions temporally related to the emergence of the inhibitor are drug therapy (particularly streptomycin and penicillin), major surgery and autoimmune disorders. Factor IX inhibitors are much more rarely encountered than factor VIII inhibitors. There is no report so far of acquired factor X deficiency related to the development of an inhibitor. However, low factor X levels are sometimes found in patients with systemic amyloidosis. Amyloid fibrils in the spleen, liver and other tissues may bind circulating factor X (Furie et al 1981). Similarly, factor IX deficiency has been reported in association with Gaucher's disease (Boklan & Sawitsky 1976): it is believed that factor IX is bound by glucocerebroside deposits.

The treatment of bleeding episodes in patients with inhibitors is somewhat empirical because these cases are so rare that no single centre can accumulate sufficient experience. It is always worth trying to replace the deficient factor with plasma or concentrates, as measurable circulating levels may be obtained when the inhibitor is not very potent or if complexes dissociate to make the coagulation factor available locally for haemostasis. When such therapy is ineffective, prothrombin-complex concentrates or recombinant activated VII may be tried. If an underlying disease can be identified and treated the inhibitor may be eradicated. An infusion of protamine sulphate may be used to neutralize a heparin-like inhibitor (Palmer et al 1984, Kaufman et al 1989). Immunosuppressive therapy may be tried when it is not feasible to treat an underlying disease but the development of the inhibitor is felt to have an immunological basis.

CARDIOPULMONARY BYPASS

Cardiopulmonary bypass for open heart surgery is now commonly performed in hospitals throughout the world, mainly for coronary artery bypass surgery. A large proportion of banked blood and derived products in hospitals may be dedicated to cardiac surgery. Although overall mortality from such major surgery has now fallen to between 1–4%, excessive bleeding is not infrequently a problem. Several factors contribute to this problem (for review see Woodman & Harker 1990).

Thrombocytopenia

Thrombocytopenia is often present during cardiopulmonary bypass (Bloom 1961). The platelet count may drop by as much as one third (Porter & Silver 1968), although the count usually remains above $100\,000 \times 10^9/l$ during the operation (Milam et al 1981). There is also impairment of platelet function, associated with prolongation of the bleeding time. Platelet dysfunction is related to contact with the synthetic surface of the oxygenator, and probably the induced hypothermia. Aggregation in response to the agonists ADP, collagen and ristocetin is impaired (Mohr et al 1986). The contents of α-granules are released into the circulation, although the number of dense bodies (and hence platelet nucleotide content) is not affected (Harker et al 1980). Many patients with coronary artery disease may be taking aspirin. Patients taking aspirin before cardiopulmonary bypass surgery are at risk of excessive blood loss during the procedure (Michelson et al 1978, Torosian et al 1978). It is therefore recommended that aspirin be discontinued at least 5 days before cardiopulmonary bypass.

Despite abnormalities in platelet number and function, there is no evidence that *routine* perioperative transfusion of platelet concentrates is necessary (Office of Medical Applications of Research, National Institutes of Health 1987, UK Health Departments 1989).

Coagulation factor levels

Cardiopulmonary bypass is associated with a drop in the plasma levels of most coagulation factors, which is primarily attributable to haemodilution (Milam et al 1981). The fall in the level of factor VIII is not as much as for the other factors, although the level of all factors remains well within the range considered satisfactory for haemostasis. As with platelet concentrates, it is not necessary routinely to transfuse fresh frozen plasma during cardiopulmonary bypass. Inappropriate use of fresh frozen plasma in cardiothoracic surgery is common, and has logistic and economic implications (Thomson et al 1991). There may also be a modest fall in the level of von Willebrand factor, although again the level remains adequate for haemostasis (Weinstein et al 1988). Selective deficiency of high molecular weight von Willebrand factor multimers and associated prolongation of the bleeding time with a haemorrhagic tendency have been described in both adults and children with valvular heart disease or congenital cardiac defects (Gill et al 1986, Weinstein et al 1988). Surgical correction of the cardiac defect results in normalization of the multimeric pattern.

Heparin-related problems

Heparin is routinely administered in order to prevent extracorporeal clotting in the oxygenator. The activated clotting time may be monitored during surgery. An activated clotting time of between 400 and 600 seconds maintains adequate anticoagulation. Protamine sulphate is administered at the end of surgery in order to neutralize remaining heparin: typically, 1 mg of protamine is injected for every 100 units of heparin infused. Allergic reactions to protamine have been reported. Susceptible individuals include those who have received the drug before, perhaps in the setting of previous cardiac surgery. Furthermore, in gross excess, protamine itself acts as an anticoagulant. Following initial adequate heparin neutralization, the reappearance of active heparin in the bloodstream may occur 2–6 hours later. This rebound effect is caused by the delayed return of sequestered extravascular heparin which occurs when peripheral perfusion improves, and possibly through the release of some free heparin from bound heparin-protamine complexes. Thrombocytopenia may complicate heparin therapy in about 5% of patients receiving the drug (King & Kelton 1984). The onset of thrombocytopenia is variable, but is typically between 6–12 days after exposure to the drug. Thrombocytopenia may develop more rapidly in those who have received heparin before. The development of thrombocytopenia is associated with the development of an antiheparin IgG antibody, which binds to the platelet surface and induces platelet activation with degranulation (Kelton et al 1988, Chong et al 1989a). The possibility of heparin-induced thrombocytopenia should always be considered in the differential diagnosis when thrombocytopenia develops after cardiopulmonary bypass. Platelet concentrates should only be transfused if there are bleeding complications. Acute arterial thrombosis has been reported after transfusion of platelets for treatment of heparin-induced thrombocytopenia (Babcock et al 1976, Cimo et al 1979).

Reduction of blood loss: aprotinin, DDAVP and fibrin glues

Bovine aprotinin is a polypeptide of 58 amino acid residues which inhibits serine proteases such as kallikrein and plasmin. The administration of aprotinin significantly reduces intraoperative and postoperative blood loss associated with cardiopulmonary bypass (Royston et al 1987, Royston 1990). The requirement for blood transfusion is reduced, and the actual operating time is also shortened. The dramatic reduction in blood loss may be particularly useful where blood conservation is important, e.g. Jehovah's witnesses, patients with rare blood groups and/or unusual anti-erythrocyte antibodies, and patients infected with HIV. Aprotinin has a plasma half life of around 2 hours. After an initial loading dose, aprotinin is administered by continuous infusion during cardiopulmonary bypass. Allergic reactions have been reported, as the protein is of bovine origin. Although aprotinin inhibits fibrinolysis, there is no evidence of an associated increased incidence of coronary graft occlusion or thromboembolism.

Randomized trials of desmopressin (DDAVP) have not shown a similarly significant reduction in the requirement for blood transfusion during cardiopulmonary bypass (Rocha et al 1988, Hackman et al 1989). It is interesting to note that the use of DDAVP during cardiopulmonary bypass has not been associated with an increased incidence of thrombotic events (Mannucci & Lusher 1989).

Fibrin glues have been used in cardiothoracic surgery in order to secure good local haemostasis. The basic ingredients of such kits include bovine fibrinogen, which is painted on locally, and topical thrombin (review: Gibble & Ness 1990). There is no evidence that absorption may provoke disseminated intravascular coagulation. Antibodies to thrombin and factor V may develop after the use of such a fibrin glue during cardiac surgery, although only rarely do there appear to be related haemorrhagic problems (Flaherty et al 1989, Zehnder & Leung 1990).

MASSIVE BLOOD TRANSFUSION

Changes in blood upon storage

Blood collected in citrate phosphate dextrose with added adenine (CPDA1) has a shelf life of 35 days at 4°C. However, levels of all the coagulation factors decline during storage. Factors V and VIII are particularly labile. Levels of factor VIII decline in a biphasic manner with a rapid initial 50% reduction in content after only 24 hours (Pepper et al 1978, Nilsson et al 1983). After 1–2 weeks at 4°C, the factor VIII content falls to around one third of the original content and the factor V content falls to about 60% of the original content. Levels of fibrinogen and factors II, VII, IX, X, XII, and XIII also decline with storage, but to a lesser extent. Even after 35 days the levels of these factors remain above the low end of the normal range (Nilsson et al 1983). It is thought that proteolytic enzymes released from platelets and erythrocytes are responsible, at least in part, for the degradation of coagulation factors in stored blood since the fall in coagulation factor levels in plasma stored at 4°C is much less (Nilsson et al 1983).

Platelets in donated blood also rapidly lose their viability, reflected by poor recovery and shortened life span in the recipient after transfusion, when stored at 4°C (Murphy & Gardner 1969).

Clinical problems associated with massive blood transfusion

As a result of changes during storage, haemorrhagic problems may develop when a patient's blood is replaced by large quantities of stored blood within a short period of time (Lim et al 1973, Counts et al 1979). Dilution of coagulation factors will be exacerbated if plasma-reduced blood or red cells suspended in optimal additive solution are used. Microvascular bleeding is a typical manifestation of the impaired haemostasis. Examples include bleeding from mucous membranes, oozing from catheter sites which persists after application of pressure, continuous oozing from surgical wounds and generalized petechiae.

Impaired haemostasis is, of course, only one of several important problems encountered in patients receiving a massive blood transfusion. These include hypocalcaemia due to citrate overload, hyperkalaemia and hypothermia (Collins 1976, Blood Transfusion Task Force, BCSH 1988). Such patients are often very ill with serious underlying medical problems (Sawyer & Harrison 1990), and the situation may be complicated by the development of disseminated intravascular coagulation.

Management of haemostatic problems

When there is no underlying medical complication, replacement of up to one blood volume (8–10 units of blood in an adult) is not likely to be associated with significant haemostatic problems. Laboratory tests of coagulation may help to identify patients who need additional blood components to improve haemostasis when larger volumes of blood are transfused. A platelet count of less than 50×10^9/l, prothrombin time ratio of 1.8 or more and a plasma fibrinogen level of 0.5 g/l or less are strongly associated with microvascular bleeding (Blood Transfusion Task Force, BCSH 1988). Platelet support may be required once the patient has received 15 or more units of blood. Fresh frozen plasma is a source of coagulation factors, including fibrinogen.

Haemostatic changes associated with plasma exchange

Plasma exchange is increasingly used to treat a number of medical conditions. Up to 4 or more litres of plasma may be removed during a single session. Plasma levels of coagulation factors remain well within the normal range after a single large exchange, even when albumin and saline alone are used as replacement fluids, and levels return to their original values within 24 hours (Volkin et al 1980). Repeated exchanges of plasma may, however, significantly reduce levels of circulating immunoglobulins, fibrinogen (Volkin et al 1980) and other coagulation factors (Flaum et al 1979) if no fresh plasma is administered. Levels of antithrombin III may also fall significantly after repeated plasma exchange. This may be of importance in subjects who already have borderline plasma levels, and could provoke thrombosis (Sultan et al 1979).

Healthy subjects may volunteer to donate plasma by plasmapheresis for the manufacture of such products as factor VIII concentrates or anti-D immunoglobulin. No significant changes in plasma levels of coagulation factors would be anticipated, as only some 500 ml of plasma are removed at each session. Furthermore, the number of donations allowed in one year is regulated: in the United Kingdom, healthy donors may donate not more than 600 ml on one occasion, and no more than 15 litres in one year.

DRUG THERAPY

Oral anticoagulants

Oral anticoagulants are discussed in the earlier section in this chapter on vitamin K (p. 954), and more comprehensively in Chapter 65.

Antiplatelet drugs

Antiplatelet drugs are discussed in chapter 67.

Heparin

Heparin is widely used for the prophylaxis and initial treatment of thromboembolism (review: Hirsh 1991a and Ch. 64). As with oral anticoagulants, therapy carries some risk of haemorrhage, and the risk can be minimized by careful monitoring of therapy. Haemorrhagic problems associated with excessive heparin therapy include purpura, haematuria and gastrointestinal bleeding. Rarely, there may be retroperitoneal or intracerebral haemorrhage.

Prophylactic use of heparin to prevent thromboembolism after surgery at doses of 5000 iu twice daily is associated with an increased incidence of wound haematomas, but there is no increased risk of significant perioperative haemorrhage (Kakkar et al 1975, Collins et al 1988). It is sensible to avoid epidural anaesthesia during labour in women who have been taking prophylactic heparin during pregnancy.

In most patients, haemorrhage may be controlled merely by interrupting the administration of heparin since the half life is of the order of 60 minutes. Protamine sulphate may be infused when urgent neutralization of heparin is required: 1 mg of protamine is infused for each 100 iu of remaining heparin. Rapid injection of protamine may provoke hypotension, flushing and dyspnoea, and so the drug must be infused slowly over 10–20 minutes.

Accidental administration of heparin may also result in unexpected bleeding (Glueck et al 1965, Pachman 1965). This might happen when, for example, concentrated heparin rather than heavily diluted heparin is used to flush an intravenous cannula. Once the diagnosis is suspected, it can be confirmed by the finding of a prolonged thrombin time but normal Reptilase time. Reptilase (Pentapharm Ltd, Basel) is a thrombin-like venom from the snake *Bothrops atrox*, which is not inhibited by the presence of heparin. Surreptitious self-administration of heparin in order to produce haemorrhagic problems has also been recorded (Martin et al 1970).

Equally, it is very important to consider whether abnormal coagulation test results on a laboratory sample might be due to contamination with heparin. This is a very common problem in hospital laboratories, where samples for laboratory testing may be drawn from heparinized indwelling venous catheters. Recognition of the problem will save considerable time and expense.

Thrombocytopenia may complicate heparin therapy in about 5% of patients receiving the drug (King & Kelton 1984). The onset of thrombocytopenia is variable, but is typically between 6–12 days after exposure to the drug. Thrombocytopenia may develop more rapidly in those who have received heparin before. The development of thrombocytopenia is associated with the development of an antiheparin IgG antibody, which binds to the platelet surface and induces platelet activation with degranulation (Kelton et al 1988, Chong et al 1989a). If it is not possible to rely on warfarin for adequate anticoagulation, alternatives include low-molecular weight heparin (Vitoux et al 1986) and the snake venom ancrod (Demers et al 1991). However, thrombocytopenia may persist with low molecular weight heparins, as there is some degree of crossover in reactivity of the antibody responsible. Heparinoids have been employed successfully in a limited number of cases, as there is minimal cross-reactivity with the antibody (Chong et al 1989b). It is hoped that the polypeptide anticoagulant hirudin will also be useful in this situation in future. Platelet concentrates should only be transfused if there are bleeding complications. Acute arterial thrombosis has been reported after transfusion of platelets for treatment of heparin-induced thrombocytopenia (Babcock et al 1976, Cimo et al 1979).

Thrombolytic agents

Thrombolytic agents (see also Ch. 66) have an established role in the treatment of many disorders, including acute myocardial infarction, massive pulmonary embolism and extensive deep vein thrombosis. Haemorrhage is the principal adverse side-effect of this therapy (review: Sane et al 1989). The risk of haemorrhage is comparable with all thrombolytic agents currently employed. The majority (around 70%) of significant haemorrhages in earlier trials actually occurred at sites of vessel puncture, although this will become less of a problem as the drugs are now administered by intravenous bolus and without any need for invasive monitoring such as cardiac catheterization. However, it is intracranial haemorrhage which is most feared. This complication arises in around 0.2–0.6% of cases. It is clear that concomitant infusion of heparin is associated with an increased risk of bleeding. It is also evident that the risk of haemorrhage is greater when thrombolytic agents are utilized to treat pulmonary embolism or venous thrombosis as opposed to myocardial infarction. This is related to the duration of therapy, as a single bolus is administered for myocardial infarction, whilst thrombolytic agents may be infused for up to 72 hours in other clinical settings. In order to minimize the risk of serious bleeding it is vital to identify potential contraindications prior to therapy with thrombolytic agents (Table 41.2).

A number of factors contribute to the development of haemorrhage in association with the use of thrombolytic agents. None of the agents currently used has restricted specificity for fibrin, and degradation of fibrinogen is an important factor. However, other contributory factors may include disaggregation of platelets through proteolysis of cohesive fibrinogen bridges between platelets (Loscalzo & Vaughan 1987), degradation of platelet surface glycoproteins (Adelman et al 1986, Stricker et al 1986), and degradation of plasma von Willebrand factor (Federici et al 1992).

Appropriate laboratory screening before thrombolytic therapy will help reduce the incidence of bleeding, al-

Table 41.2 Contraindications to thrombolytic therapy

It is important to identify patients at risk from bleeding prior to therapy with thrombolytic agents

Contraindications:
Recent surgery (within last 10 days)
Recent invasive procedures (within last 10 days)
Gastrointestinal bleeding within last 6 months
Thrombocytopenia, or any other known haemorrhagic diathesis
Significant renal or hepatic impairment
Uncontrolled hypertension
Pregnancy
Recent parturition (within last 10 days)
Serious trauma
Visceral carcinoma
Ulcerative colitis

though this is often not feasible if early treatment is to be initiated after myocardial infarction. Invasive procedures, such as cardiac catheterization, are best avoided. In most patients, coagulation tests are not routinely warranted after treatment.

Local external bleeding may be controlled with pressure alone. If a thrombolytic agent is being given by infusion, this should be interrupted. Significant bleeding may require transfusion of fresh frozen plasma and platelets. The aim should be to achieve a plasma fibrinogen level of at least 1 g/l. If bleeding persists despite such measures, an antifibrinolytic agent should be given. If heparin has been administered after thrombolysis, the infusion should be stopped and protamine sulphate may be required. It is important to maintain an adequate blood volume in these patients, who may have a severely compromised haemodynamic state.

Other drug therapy

Dextrans. It is well established that infusions of dextrans may prolong the bleeding time. The effect is related to molecular weight of the dextran, with larger forms (now no longer used in clinical practice) having a proportionally greater effect on the bleeding time. The maximal effect is delayed, and peaks 3–6 hours after the infusion (Langdell et al 1958, Åberg et al 1979). Spontaneous bruising and bleeding may occasionally develop with large doses. Impaired platelet adhesion is seen after dextran infusion, but no such change is evident when dextran is added directly to blood in vitro (Weiss 1967). These findings are suggestive of an indirect effect of dextran upon platelets. The infusion of dextran causes a significant decrease in von Willebrand factor antigen and in ristocetin-induced platelet aggregation (Åberg et al 1979). However, there should be no significant clinical problems as long as the maximum recommended dosage of dextran is not exceeded.

Penicillins. The administration of penicillins at high dosage via intravenous infusion may be associated with haemorrhagic problems due to platelet dysfunction (McClure et al 1970, Brown et al 1974). The bleeding time may be prolonged, and impaired platelet aggregation in response to ADP has been documented (Brown et al 1976). Platelet dysfunction has been recorded in association with penicillin G as well as a number of derivatives, including ampicillin, carbenicillin, ticarcillin, piperacillin and mezlocillin (Fass et al 1988). There are often other contributing factors, such as thrombocytopenia or renal failure. It should also be remembered that broad-spectrum antibiotics may precipitate haemorrhagic problems related to vitamin K deficiency in vulnerable individuals.

Asparaginase. The enzyme asparaginase is often used in conjunction with other cytotoxic agents to induce remission in acute lymphoblastic leukaemia. The enzyme inhibits the synthesis of a number of proteins, including vitamin K-dependent coagulation factors and proteins C and S (Bezeaud et al 1986). Both haemorrhagic and thrombotic complications have been documented in association with the use of this cytotoxic agent as a consequence of these changes in the haemostatic balance.

REFERENCES

Åberg M, Hedner U, Bergentz S-E 1979 Effect of dextran on factor VIII (antihemophilic factor) and platelet function. Annals of Surgery 189: 243–247

Adelman B, Michelson A D, Greenberg J, Handin R I 1986 Proteolysis of platelet glycoprotein Ib by plasmin is facilitated by plasmin lysine-binding regions. Blood 68: 1280–1284

Al-Mondhiry H 1975 Disseminated intravascular coagulation: experience in a major cancer centre. Thrombosis et Diathesis Haemorrhagica 34: 181–193

Ambrus J L, Ambrus C M, Mink I B, Pickren J W 1975 Causes of death in cancer patients. Journal of Medicine 6: 61–64

Aoki N, Yamanaka T 1978 The α_2-plasmin inhibitor levels in liver diseases. Clinica Chimica Acta 84: 99–105

Apt L, Downey W S 1955 'Melena' neonatorum: the swallowed blood syndrome. A simple test for the differentiation of adult and fetal hemoglobin in bloody stools. Journal of Pediatrics 47: 6–12

Babcock R B, Dumper C W, Scharfman W B 1976 Heparin-induced immune thrombocytopenia. New England Journal of Medicine 295: 237–241

Bajaj S P, Rapaport S I, Fierer D S, Herbst K D, Schwartz D B 1983 A mechanism for the hypoprothrombinemia of the acquired hypoprothrombinemia-lupus anticoagulant syndrome. Blood 61: 684–692

Ballard H S, Marcus A J 1976 Platelet aggregation in portal cirrhosis. Archives of Internal Medicine 136: 316–319

Bang N U, Trygstad C W, Schroeder J, Heidenreich R D, Csiscko B M 1973 Enhanced platelet function in glomerular renal disease. Journal of Laboratory and Clinical Medicine 81: 651–660

Bezeaud A, Drouet L, Leverger G, Griffin J H, Guillin M C 1986 Effect of L-asparaginase therapy for acute lymphoblastic leukemia on plasma vitamin K-dependent coagulation factors and inhibitors. Journal of Pediatrics 108: 698–701

Biland L, Duckert F, Prisender S, Nyman D 1978 Quantitative estimation of coagulation factors in liver disease. The diagnostic and prognostic value of factor XIII, factor V and plasminogen. Thrombosis and Haemostasis 39: 646–649

Blake J C, Sprengers D, Grech P, McCormick P A, McIntyre N, Burroughs A K 1990 Bleeding time in patients with hepatic cirrhosis. British Medical Journal 301: 12–15

Blood Transfusion Task Force, British Committee for Standardization in Haematology 1988 Guidelines for transfusion for massive blood loss. Clinical and Laboratory Haematology 10: 265–273

Bloom A L 1961 Changes in the blood after using an extracorporeal circulation. British Medical Journal 2: 16–20

Bohmig H 1977 The coagulation disorder of orthotopic hepatic transplantation. Seminars in Thrombosis and Hemostasis 4: 57–69

Boklan B F, Sawitsky A 1976 Factor IX deficiency in Gaucher's disease: an in vitro phenomenon. Archives of Internal Medicine 136: 489–492

Boneu B, Bugat R, Boneu A, Eche N, Sie P, Combes P F 1984 Exhausted platelets in patients with malignant solid tumours without evidence of active consumption coagulopathy. European Journal of Cancer and Clinical Oncology 20: 899–905

Bowie E J W, Todd M, Thompson J H, Owen C A, Wright I S 1965 Anticoagulant malingerers (the 'dicoumarol-eaters'). American Journal of Medicine 39: 855–864

Brown C H, Natelson E A, Bradshaw M W, Williams T W, Alfrey C P 1974 The hemostatic defect produced by carbenicillin. New England Journal of Medicine 291: 265–270
Brown C H, Bradshaw M W, Natelson E A, Alfrey C P, Williams T W 1976 Defective platelet function following the administration of penicillin compounds. Blood 47: 949–956
Canadian Paediatric Society 1988 The use of vitamin K in the neonatal period. Canadian Medical Association Journal 139: 127–130
Canoso R T, Hutton R A 1977 A chlorpromazine-induced inhibitor of blood coagulation. American Journal of Hematology 2: 183–191
Carreras L O, Vermylen J G 1982 'Lupus' anticoagulant and thrombosis. Possible role of inhibition of prostacyclin formation. Thrombosis and Haemostasis 48: 38–40
Castaldi P A, Rozenberg M C, Stewart J H 1966 The bleeding disorder of uraemia. Lancet 2: 66–69
Cederblad G, Korsan-Bengsten K, Olsson R 1976 Observation of increased levels of blood coagulation factors and other plasma proteins in cholestatic liver disease. Scandinavian Journal of Gastroenterology 11: 391–396
Chong B H, Castaldi P A, Berndt M C 1989a Heparin-induced thrombocytopenia: effects of rabbit IgG, and Fab and Fc fragments on antibody-heparin-platelet interaction. Thrombosis Research 55: 291–295
Chong B H, Ismail F, Cade J, Gallus A S, Gordon S, Chesterman C N 1989b Heparin-induced thrombocytopenia: studies with a new molecular weight heparinoid, Org 10172. Blood 73: 1592–1596
Cimo P L, Moake J L, Weinger R S, Ben-Menachem Y, Khalil K G 1979 Heparin-induced thrombocytopenia: association with a platelet aggregating factor and arterial thromboses. American Journal of Hematology 6: 125–133
Cohen I, Amir J, Ben-Shaul Y, Pick A, de Vries A 1970 Plasma cell myeloma associated with an unusual myeloma protein causing impairment of fibrin aggregation and platelet function in a patient with multiple malignancy. American Journal of Medicine 48: 766–776
Coleman M, Vigliano E N, Weksler M E, Nachman R L 1972 Inhibition of fibrin monomer polymerization by lambda myeloma globulins. Blood 39: 210–223
Coleman M, Finlayson N, Bettigole R E, Sadula D, Cohn M, Pasmantier M 1975 Fibrinogen survival in cirrhosis: improvement by 'low dose' heparin. Annals of Internal Medicine 83: 79–81
Collen D, Wiman B 1978 Physiological inhibitors of fibrinolysis. In: Gaffney P J, Balkuv-Ulutin S (eds) Fibrinolysis: fundamental and clinical concepts. Academic Press, London, p 12–26
Collins J A 1976 Massive blood transfusion. Clinics in Hematology 5: 201–222
Collins R, Scrimgeour A, Yusuf S, Peto R 1988 Reduction in fatal pulmonary embolism and venous thrombosis by perioperative administration of subcutaneous heparin: overview of results of randomized trials in general, orthopedic, and urologic surgery. New England Journal of Medicine 318: 1162–1173
Colvin B T, Lloyd M J 1977 Severe coagulation defect due to a dietary deficiency of vitamin K. Journal of Clinical Pathology 30: 1147–1148
Conley C L, Hartman R C 1952 A hemorrhagic disorder caused by circulating anticoagulant in patients with disseminated lupus erythematosus. Journal of Clinical Investigation 31: 621–622
Coppola R, Guerra L, Ruggeri Z M, Tarantino A, Mannucci P M, Ponticelli C 1981 Factor VIII/von Willebrand factor in glomerular nephropathies. Clinical Nephrology 16: 217–22
Counts R B, Haisch C, Simon T L, Maxwell N G, Heimbach D M, Carrico C J 1979 Hemostasis in massively transfused trauma patients. Annals of Surgery 190: 91–99
Creagh M D, Greaves M 1991 Lupus anticoagulant. Blood Reviews 5: 162–167
Dahlbäck B, Nilsson I M, Frohm B 1983 Inhibition of platelet prothrombinase activity by a lupus anticoagulant. Blood 62: 218–225
Dalton R G, Dewar M S, Savidge G F et al 1987 Hypothyroidism as a cause of acquired von Willebrand's disease. Lancet 1: 1007–1009
Dano K, Andreasen P A, Grondahl-Hansen J, Kinstensen P, Nielsen L S, Shriver L 1985 Plasminogen activators, tissue degradation and cancer. Advances in Cancer Research 44: 139–255
Das P C, Cash J D 1969 Fibrinolysis at rest and after exercise in hepatic cirrhosis. British Journal of Haematology 17: 431–443
de Jong E, Knot E A R, Piket D et al 1987 Increased plasminogen activator inhibition levels in malignancy. Thrombosis and Haemostasis 57: 140–143
del Greco F, Soper W S, Krumlovsky F A, Levin M L, Boske R 1989 Thrombosis of vascular access for haemodialysis. In: Remuzzi G, Rossi E C (eds) Haemostasis and the kidney. Butterworth, London, p 303–308
Demers C, Ginsburg J S, Brill-Edwards P et al 1991 Rapid anticoagulation using ancrod for heparin-induced thrombocytopenia. Blood 78: 2194–2197
Deykin D 1983 Uremic bleeding. Kidney International 24: 698–705
Dioguardi N, Mari D, Del Ninno E, Mannucci PM 1973 Fibrinolysis in cholestatic jaundice (letter). British Medical Journal 2: 778–779
Donati M B, Poggi A, Semeraro N 1981 Coagulation and malignancy. In: Poller L (ed) Recent advances in blood coagulation. Churchill Livingstone, vol 3: 227–254
Du X H, Glass-Greenwalt P, Kani K S 1985 Nephrotic syndrome with renal vein thrombosis: pathogenetic importance of α_2 plasmin inhibitor (α_2 antiplasmin). Clinical Nephrology 24: 186–191
Duran-Suarez J R 1982 Incidence of circulating anticoagulants in a normal population. Acta Haematologica 67: 217–219
Eknoyan G, Brown C H 1981 Biochemical abnormalities of platelets in renal failure. American Journal of Nephrology 1: 17–23
Evans E P, Branch R A, Bloom A L 1972: A clinical and experimental study of platelet function in chronic renal failure. Journal of Clinical Pathology 25: 745–753
Exner T, Triplett D A, Taberner D, Machin S J 1991 Guidelines for testing and revised criteria for lupus anticoagulant. Thrombosis and Haemostasis 65: 320–322
Fass R J, Copelan E A, Brandt J T, Moeschberger M L, Ashton J J 1987 Platelet-mediated bleeding caused by broad-spectrum penicillins. Journal of Infectious Diseases 155: 1242–1248
Federici A B, Berkowitz S D, Zimmerman T S, Mannucci P M 1992 Proteolysis of von Willebrand factor after thrombolytic therapy in patients with acute myocardial infarction. Blood 79: 38–44
Firkin B G, Howard M A, Radford N 1980 Possible relationship between lupus inhibitor and recurrent abortion in young women (letter). Lancet 2: 366
Flaherty M J, Henderson R, Wener M H 1989 Iatrogenic immunization with bovine thrombin: a mechanism for prolonged thrombin times after surgery. Annals of Internal Medicine 111: 631–634
Flaum M A, Cuneo R A, Appelbaum F R, Deisseroth A B, Engel W K, Gralnick H R 1979 The hemostatic imbalance of plasma-exchange transfusion. Blood 54: 694–702
Fletcher A P, Biedman O, Moore D, Alkajaersig N, Sherry S 1969 Abnormal plasminogen-plasmin system activity (fibrinolysis) in patients with hepatic cirrhosis. Journal of Clinical Investigation 43: 681–689
Forfar J C 1979 A 7-year analysis of haemorrhage in patients on long term anticoagulant treatment. British Heart Journal 42: 128–132
Furie B, Furie B C 1990 Molecular basis of vitamin K-dependent gamma carboxylation. Blood 75: 1753–1762
Furie B, Voo L, McAdam K P W J, Furie B C 1981 Mechanism of factor X deficiency in systemic amyloidosis. New England Journal of Medicine 304: 827–830
Gastineau D A, Kazmier F L, Nichols W L, Bowie E J W 1985 Lupus anticoagulant: an analysis of the clinical and laboratory features of 219 cases. American Journal of Hematology 19: 265–275
Gatti L, Mannucci P M 1984 Use of porcine factor VIII in the management of seventeen patients with factor VIII antibodies. Thrombosis and Haemostasis 51: 379–384
Gibble J W, Ness P M 1990 Fibrin glue: the perfect operative sealant? Transfusion 30: 741–747
Gill J C, Wilson A D, Endres-Brooks J, Montgomery R J 1986 Loss of the largest von Willebrand factor multimers from the plasma of patients with congenital cardiac defects. Blood 67: 758–761
Gjorstrup P, Watt R M 1990 Therapeutic protein A immunoadsorption. A review. Transfusion Sciences 11: 281–302
Glueck H I, Light I J, Flessa H, Sutherland J M 1965 Inadvertent sodium heparin administration to a newborn infant. Journal of the American Medical Association 191: 1031–1032

Goldsmith G H 1984 Hemostatic disorders associated with neoplasia. In: Disorders of hemostasis. Grune and Stratton, p 351–366
Green D 1968 Spontaneous inhibitors of factor VIII. British Journal of Haematology 15: 57–75
Green D, Lechner K 1981 A survey of 215 non-hemophilic patients with inhibitors to factor VIII. Thrombosis and Haemostasis 45: 200–203
Green D, Schuette PT, Wallace WH 1980 Factor VIII antibodies in rheumatoid arthritis: effect of cyclophosphamide. Archives of Internal Medicine 140: 1232–1235
Gross L, Brotman M 1970 Hypoprothrombinemia and hemorrhage associated with cholestyramine therapy. Annals of Internal Medicine 72: 95–96
Grossi C E, Rousselot L M, Panke W F 1962 Coagulation defects in patients with cirrhosis of the liver undergoing portasystemic shunts. American Journal of Surgery 104: 512–526
Grossi C E, Rousselot L M, Panke E W F 1964 Control of fibrinolysis during portacaval shunts. Study of patients with cirrhosis of the liver. Journal of the American Medical Association 187: 1005–1008
Hackmann T, Gascoyne R D, Naiman S C et al 1989 A trial of desmopressin (1-desamino-8-d-arginine vasopressin) to reduce blood loss in uncomplicated cardiac surgery. New England Journal of Medicine 321: 1437–1443
Haemostasis and Thrombosis Task Force, British Committee for Standardization in Haematology 1990 Guidelines on oral anticoagulation, 2nd ed. Journal of Clinical Pathology 43: 177–183
Haemostasis and Thrombosis Task Force, British Committee for Standardization in Haematology 1991 Guidelines on testing for the lupus anticoagulant. Journal of Clinical Pathology 44: 885–889
Handel J, Tripp J H 1991 Vitamin K prophylaxis against haemorrhagic disease of the newborn in the United Kingdom. British Medical Journal 303: 1109
Harker L, Malpass T W, Branson H E, Hessel E A, Slichter S A 1980 Mechanism of abnormal bleeding in patients undergoing cardiopulmonary bypass: acquired transient platelet dysfunction associated with selective A granule release. Blood 56: 824–834
Harper P L, Edgar P F, Luddington R J et al 1988 Protein C deficiency and portal thrombosis in liver transplantation in children. Lancet 2: 924–927
Harris E N 1990 Antiphospholipid antibodies. British Journal of Haematology 74: 1–9
Harter H R, Burch J W, Majerus P W et al 1979 Prevention of thrombosis in patients on hemodialysis by low-dose aspirin. New England Journal of Medicine 301: 577–579
Hedner U, Kisiel W 1983 Use of human factor VIIa in the treatment of two hemophilia A patients with high-titer inhibitors. Journal of Clinical Investigation 71: 1836–1841
Hirsh J 1991a Heparin. New England Journal of Medicine 324: 1565–1573
Hirsh J 1991b Oral anticoagulant drugs. New England Journal of Medicine 324: 1865–1875
Hooper A C, Haney B B, Stone H H 1980 Gastrointestinal bleeding due to vitamin K deficiency in patients on parenteral cefamandole (letter). Lancet 1: 39–40
Hull R, Hirsh J, Jay R et al 1982 Different intensities of oral anticoagulant therapy in the treatment of proximal-vein thrombosis. New England Journal of Medicine 307: 1676–1681
Janson P A, Jubelirer S J, Weinstein M J, Deykin D 1980 Treatment of the bleeding tendency in uremia with cryoprecipitate. New England Journal of Medicine 303: 1318–1322
Jorgensen K A, Ingerberg S 1979 Platelets and platelet function in patients with chronic uremia on maintenance hemodialysis. Nephron 23: 233–236
Kaegi A, Pineo GF, Shimizu A, Trivedi H, Hirsh J 1974 Arteriovenous shunt thrombosis. Prevention by sulfinpyrazone. New England Journal of Medicine 290: 304–306
Kakkar V V, Corrigan T P, Fossard D P et al 1975 Prevention of fatal postoperative pulmonary embolism by low doses of heparin. Lancet 2: 45–51
Karpatkin S, Freedman M L 1978 Hypersplenic thrombocytopenia differentiated from increased peripheral destruction by platelet volume. Annals of Internal Medicine 89: 200–203
Kauffmann R H, Veltkamp J J, van Tilburg N H, van Es L A 1978 Acquired antithrombin III deficiency and thrombosis in the nephrotic syndrome. American Journal of Medicine 65: 607–613
Kaufman P A, Gockerman J P, Greenberg C S 1989 Production of a novel anticoagulant by neoplastic plasma cells: report of a case and review of the literature. American Journal of Medicine 86: 612–616
Kelton J G, Sheridan D, Santos A et al 1988 Heparin-induced thrombocytopenia: laboratory studies. Blood 72: 925–930
Khoory M S, Nesheim M E, Bowie E J W, Mann K G 1980 Circulating heparan sulphate proteoglycan anticoagulant from a patient with a plasma cell disorder. Journal of Clinical Investigation 65: 666–674
King D J, Kelton J G 1984 Heparin-associated thrombocytopenia. Annals of Internal Medicine 100: 535–540
Kirchheimer J C, Huber K, Wagner O, Binder B R 1987 Pattern of fibrinolytic parameters in patients with gastrointestinal carcinomas. British Journal of Haematology 66: 85–89
Kurczynski E M, Penner J A 1974 Activated prothrombin concentrate for patients with factor VIII inhibitors. New England Journal of Medicine 291: 164–167
Langdell R D, Adelson E, Furth F W, Crosby W H 1958 Dextran and prolonged bleeding time: results of a sixty-gram, one liter infusion given to one hundred sixty three normal human subjects. Journal of the American Medical Association 166: 346–351
Lechner K 1987 Lupus anticoagulant and thrombosis. In: Verstraete M, Vermylen J, Lijnen H R, Arnout J (eds) Thrombosis and haemostasis. ISTH and Leuven University Press, Leuven p 525–547
Levin J, Conley C L 1964 Thrombocytosis associated with malignant disease. Archives of Internal Medicine 114: 497–500
Lieberman J S, Borrero J, Urdaneta E, Wright I S 1961 Thrombophlebitis and cancer. Journal of the American Medical Association 177: 542–545
Lim R C, Olcott C, Robinson A J, Blaisdell F W 1973 Platelet response and coagulation changes following massive blood replacement. Journal of Trauma 13: 577–582
Livio M, Gotti E, Marchesi D, Mecca G, Remuzzi G, de Gaetano G 1982 Uraemic bleeding: role of anaemia and beneficial effect of red cell transfusions. Lancet 2: 1013–1015
Livio M, Mannucci P M, Viganò G L et al 1986 Conjugated estrogens for the management of bleeding associated with renal failure. New England Journal of Medicine 315: 731–735
Loscalzo J, Vaughan D E 1987 Tissue plasminogen activator promotes platelet disaggregation in plasma. Journal of Clinical Investigation 79: 1749–1755
Lottenberg R, Kentro T B, Kitchens C S 1987 Acquired hemophilia. Archives of Internal Medicine 147: 1077–1081
Lubbe W F, Butler W S, Palmer S J, Liggins G C 1983 Fetal survival after prednisone suppression of maternal lupus anticoagulant. Lancet 1: 1361–1363
McClure P D, Casserly J G, Monsier C, Crozier D 1970 Carbenicillin-induced bleeding disorder (letter). Lancet 2: 1307–1308
McNinch A W, Tripp J H 1991 Haemorrhagic disease of the newborn in the British Isles: two year prospective study. British Medical Journal 303: 1105–1109
Mannucci P M, Lusher J M 1989 Desmopressin and thrombosis (letter). Lancet 2: 675–676
Mannucci P M, Mari D 1984 Antibodies to factor VIII-von Willebrand factor in congenital and acquired von Willebrand's disease. Progress in Clinical and Biological Research 150: 109–122
Mannucci P M, Franchi F, Dioguardi N 1976 Correction of abnormal coagulation in chronic liver disease by combined use of fresh-frozen plasma and prothrombin complex concentrates. Lancet 2: 542–545
Mannucci P M, Canciani M T, Mari D, Meucci P 1979 The varied sensitivity of partial thromboplastin and prothrombin time reagents in the demonstration of the lupus-like anticoagulant. Scandinavian Journal of Haematology 22: 423–432
Mannucci P M, Remuzzi G, Pusineri F et al 1983 Deamino-8-d-arginine vasopressin shortens the bleeding time in uremia. New England Journal of Medicine 308: 8–12
Mannucci P M, Lombardi R, Bader R et al 1984 Studies on the pathophysiology of acquired von Willebrand's disease in seven patients with lymphoproliferative disorders or benign monoclonal gammopathies. Blood 64: 614–621
Mannucci P M, Vaglini M, Maniezzo M, Magni E, Mari D, Cascinelli

N 1985 Hemostatic alterations are unrelated to the stage of tumor in untreated malignant melanoma and breast carcinoma. European Journal of Cancer and Clinical Oncology 21: 681–685
Mannucci P M, Valsecchi C, Bottasso B, D'Angelo A, Casati S, Ponticelli C 1986a High plasma levels of protein C activity and antigen in the nephrotic syndrome. Thrombosis and Haemostasis 55: 31–33
Mannucci P M, Vicente V, Vianello L et al 1986b Controlled trial of desmopressin in liver cirrhosis and other conditions associated with a prolonged bleeding time. Blood 67: 1148–1153
Mannucci P M, Cattaneo M, Canciani M T, Maniezzo M, Vaglini M, Cascinelli N 1989 Early presence of activated ('exhausted') platelets in malignant tumors (breast adenocarcinoma and malignant melanoma). European Journal of Cancer and Clinical Oncology 25: 1413–1417
Mannucci PM, Cugno M, Bottasso B et al 1990 Changes in fibrinolysis in patients with localized tumors. European Journal of Cancer and Clinical Oncology 26: 83–87
Marciniak E, Greenwood M F 1979 Acquired coagulation inhibitor delaying fibrinopeptide release. Blood 53: 81–92
Markus G 1984 The role of hemostasis and fibrinolysis in the metastatic spread of cancer. Seminars in Thrombosis and Hemostasis 10: 61–70
Martin C M, Engstrom P F, Barrett O 1970 Surreptitious self-administration of heparin. Journal of the American Medical Association 212: 475–476
Martinez J, Palascak J E, Kwasniak D 1978 Abnormal sialic acid content of the dysfibrinogenemia associated with liver disease. Journal of Clinical Investigation 61: 535–538
Matoth Y 1950 Plasma prothrombin in infantile diarrhoea. American Journal of Diseases in Childhood 80: 944–954
Merskey C, Hansen J D L 1957 Blood coagulation defects in kwashiorkor and infantile gastroenteritis. British Journal of Haematology 3: 39–49
Merskey C, Kleiner G J, Johnson A J 1966 Quantitative estimation of split products of fibrinogen in human serum, relation in diagnosis and treatment. Blood 28: 1–18
Michelson E L, Morganroth J, Torosian M, MacVaugh H 1978 Relation of preoperative use of aspirin to increased mediastinal blood loss after coronary artery bypass graft surgery. Journal of Thoracic and Cardiovascular Surgery 76: 694–697
Milam J D, Austin S F, Martin R F, Keats A S, Cooley D A 1981 Alteration of coagulation and selected clinical chemistry parameters in patients undergoing open heart surgery without transfusions. American Journal of Clinical Pathology 76: 155–162
Mohr R, Golan M, Martinowitz U, Rosner E, Goor D A, Ramot B 1986 Effect of cardiac operation on platelets. Journal of Thoracic and Cardiovascular Surgery 92: 434–441
Moia M, Mannucci P M, Vizzotto L, Casati S, Cattaneo M, Ponticelli C 1987 Improvement in the haemostatic defect of uraemia after treatment with recombinant human erythropoietin. Lancet 2: 1227–1229
Murphy S, Gardner F H 1969 Platelet preservation: effect of storage temperature on maintenance of platelet viability – deleterious effect of refrigerated storage. New England Journal of Medicine 280: 1094–1098
Nilsson I M, Åstedt B, Hedner U, Berezin D 1975a Intrauterine death and circulating anticoagulant ("antithromboplastin"). Acta Medica Scandinavica 197: 153–159
Nilsson I M, Bergentz S E, Hedner U, Kullensberg K 1975b Gastric fibrinolysis. Thrombosis et Diathesis Haemorrhagica 34: 409–418
Nilsson L, Hedner U, Nilsson I M, Robertson B 1983 Shelf-life of bank blood and stored plasma with special reference to coagulation factors. Transfusion 23: 377–381
O'Connell R A, Grossi C E, Rousselot L M 1964 Role of inhibitors of fibrinolysis in hepatic cirrhosis. Lancet 1: 990–993
Office of Medical Applications of Research, National Institutes of Health 1987 Platelet transfusion therapy. Journal of the American Medical Association 257: 1777–1780
O'Reilly R A, Aggeler P M, Gibbs J O 1962 Hemorrhagic state due to surreptitious ingestion of bishydroxycoumarin: a detailed case study. New England Journal of Medicine 267: 19–24
O'Reilly R A, Aggeler P M 1976 Covert anticoagulant ingestion: study of 25 patients and review of the world literature. Medicine 55: 389–399
Pachman D J 1965 Accidental heparin poisoning in an infant. American Journal of Diseases in Children 110: 210–212
Palmer R N, Rick P D, Zeller J A, Gralnick H R 1984 Circulating heparan sulfate anticoagulant in a patient with a fatal bleeding disorder. New England Journal of Medicine 310: 1696–1699
Payne N R, Hasegawa D K 1984 Vitamin K deficiency in newborns: a case report in α_1-antitrypsin deficiency and a review of factors predisposing to haemorrhage. Pediatrics 73: 712–716
Pepper M D, Learoyd P A, Rajah S M 1978 Plasma factor VIII, variables affecting stability under standard blood bank conditions and correlation with recovery in concentrates. Transfusion 18: 756–760
Peuscher F W, Cleton F J, Armstrong L, Stoepman-van Dalen E A, von Mourik J A, van Aken W G 1980 Significance of plasma fibrinopeptide A (fpA) in patients with malignancy. Journal of Laboratory and Clinical Medicine 96: 5–14
Pineo G F, Gallus A S, Hirsh J 1973 Unexpected vitamin K deficiency in hospitalized patients. Canadian Medical Association Journal 109: 880–883
Porte R J, Bontempo F A, Knot E A R, Lewis J H, Kang Y G, Starzl T E 1989 Systemic effects of tissue plasminogen activator-associated fibrinolysis and its relation to thrombin generation in orthotopic liver transplantation. Transplantation 47: 978–984
Porter J M, Silver D 1968 Alterations in fibrinolysis and coagulation associated with cardiopulmonary bypass. Journal of Thoracic and Cardiovascular Surgery 56: 869–878
Rake M O, Flute P T, Pannell G, Williams R 1970 Intravascular coagulation in acute hepatic necrosis. Lancet 1: 533–537
Remuzzi G 1988 Bleeding in renal failure. Lancet 1: 1205–1208
Remuzzi G, Cavenaghi A E, Mecca G, Donati M B, de Gaetano G 1977 Prostacyclin-like activity and bleeding in renal failure. Lancet 2: 1195–1197
Remuzzi G, Mecca G, Marchesi D, Livio M, de Gaetano G, Silver M J 1979 Platelet hyperaggregability and the nephrotic syndrome. Thrombosis Research 16: 345–354
Remuzzi G, Benigni A, Dodesini P et al 1983 Reduced platelet thromboxane formation in uremia. Evidence for a functional cyclooxygenase defect. Journal of Clinical Investigation 71: 762–768
Remuzzi G, Perico N, Zoja C, Corna D, Macconi D, Viganò G 1990 Role of endothelium-derived nitric oxide in the bleeding tendency of uremia. Journal of Clinical Investigation 86: 1768–1771
Rickles F R, Edwards R L 1983 Activation of blood coagulation in cancer: Trousseau's syndrome revisited. Blood 62: 14–31
Rocha E, Llorens R, Paramo J A, Arcas R, Cuesta B, Trenor A M 1988 Does desmopressin acetate reduce blood loss after surgery in patients on cardiopulmonary bypass? Circulation 77: 1319–1323
Rosborough T K, Swaim W R 1978 Acquired von Willebrand's disease, platelet release defect and angiodysplasia. American Journal of Medicine 65: 96–100
Routh C R, Triplett D A, Murphy M J, Felice L J, Sadowski J A, Bovill E G T 1991 Superwarfarin ingestion and detection. American Journal of Hematology 36: 50–54
Royston D 1990 The serine anti-protease aprotinin: a novel approach to reducing post-operative bleeding. Blood Coagulation and Fibrinolysis 1: 55–69
Royston D, Bidstrup B P, Taylor K M, Sapsford 1987 Effect of aprotinin on need for blood transfusion after repeat open heart surgery. Lancet 2: 1289–1291
Sack G H, Levin J, Bell W R 1977 Trousseau's syndrome and other manifestations of chronic disseminated coagulopathy in patients with neoplasms: clinical, pathophysiologic and therapeutic features. Medicine 56: 1–37
Sane D C, Califf R M, Topol E J, Stump D C, Mark D B, Greenberg C S 1989 Bleeding during thrombolytic therapy for acute myocardial infarction. Annals of Internal Medicine 111: 1010–1022
Saour J N, Sieck J O, Mamo L A R, Gallus A S 1990 Trial of different intensities of anticoagulation in patients with prosthetic heart valves. New England Journal of Medicine 322: 428–432
Sawyer P R, Harrison C R 1990 Massive transfusion in adults. Diagnoses, survival and blood bank support. Vox Sanguinis 58: 199–203

Scandella D, Mattingly M, de Graaf S, Fulcher C 1989 Localization of epitopes for human factor VIII inhibitor antibodies by immunoblotting and antibody neutralization. Blood 74: 1618–1626

Schieppati A, Dodesini P, Benigni A et al 1984 The metabolism of arachidonic acid by platelets in nephrotic syndrome. Kidney International 5: 671–676

Shapiro S S 1979 Antibodies to blood coagulation factors. Clinics in Haematology 8: 207–214

Shapiro S S, Thiagarajan P 1982 Anticoagulants. Progress in Haemostasis and Thrombosis 6: 263–285

Silver M J, Smith J B, Ingerman C M, Kocsis J J 1973 Arachidonic acid-induced human platelet aggregation and prostaglandin formation. Prostaglandins 4: 863–875

Slater D 1981 'Lupus' and prostacyclin formation (letter). Lancet 1: 393

Slichter S J, Harker L A 1974 Hemostasis in malignancy. Annals of the New York Academy of Sciences 230: 252–261

Smith S R, Auger M J 1987 Hypothyroidism and von Willebrand's disease (letter). Lancet 1: 1314

Solano C, Cobcroft R G, Scott D C 1990 Prediction of vitamin K response using the Echis time and Echis-prothrombin time ratio. Thrombosis and Haemostasis 64: 353–357

Steiner R W, Coggins C, Carvalho A C A 1979 Bleeding time in uremia: a useful test to assess clinical bleeding. American Journal of Hematology 7: 107–117

Stewart J W, Castaldi P A 1967 Uraemic bleeding: a reversible platelet defect corrected by dialysis. Quarterly Journal of Medicine 36: 409–423

Straub P W 1977 Diffuse intravascular coagulation in liver disease. Seminars in Thrombosis and Hemostasis 4: 29–39

Stricker R B, Wong D, Shiu D T, Reyes P T, Shuman M A 1986 Activation of plasminogen by tissue plasminogen activator on normal and thrombasthenic platelets: effects on surface proteins and platelet aggregation. Blood 68: 275–280

Stuart M J, Spitzer R E, Nelson D A, Sills R H 1980 Nephrotic syndrome: increased platelet prostaglandin endoperoxide formation, hyperaggregability, and reduced platelet life span. Reversal following remission. Pediatric Research 14: 1078–1081

Sultan Y, Bussel A, Maisonneuve P, Poupeney M, Sitty X, Gajdos P 1979 Potential danger of thrombosis after plasma exchange in the treatment of patients with immune disease. Transfusion 19: 588–593

Takeda Y, Chen A Y 1967 Fibrinogen metabolism and distribution in patients with the nephrotic syndrome. Journal of Laboratory and Clinical Medicine 70: 678–685

Thiagarajan P, Shapiro S S, de Marco L 1980 Monoclonal immunoglobulin M coagulation inhibitor with phospholipid specificity. Journal of Clinical Investigation 66: 397–405

Thomas D P, Ream V J, Stuart R K 1967 Platelet aggregation in patients with Laennec's cirrhosis of the liver. New England Journal of Medicine 276: 1344–1348

Thomson A, Contreras M, Knowles S 1991 Blood component treatment: a retrospective audit in five major London hospitals. Journal of Clinical Pathology 44: 734–737

Toghill P J, Green S, Ferguson R 1977 Platelet dynamics in chronic liver disease with special reference to the role of the spleen. Journal of Clinical Pathology 30: 367–371

Torosian M, Michelson E L, Morganroth J, MacVaugh H 1978 Aspirin- and coumadin-related bleeding after coronary artery bypass graft surgery. Annals of Internal Medicine 89: 325–328

Turpie A G G, Gunstensen J, Hirsh J, Nelson H, Gent M 1988 Randomised comparison of two intensities of oral anticoagulant therapy after tissue heart valve replacement. Lancet 1: 1242–1245

Tytgat G N, Collen D, Verstraete M 1971 Metabolism of fibrinogen in cirrhosis of the liver. Journal of Clinical Investigation 50: 1690–1701

United Kingdom Health Departments 1989 Handbook of Transfusion Medicine, HMSO, p 12

Vaziri N D, Branson H E, Ness R 1980 Changes of coagulation factors IX, VIII, VII, X and V in the nephrotic syndrome. American Journal of Medical Science 280: 167–171

Verstraete M, Vermylen J, Collén D 1974 Intravascular coagulation in liver disease. Annual Review of Medicine 25: 447–455

Vitoux J F, Mathieu J F, Roncato M, Fiessinger J N, Aiach M 1986 Heparin-associated thrombocytopenia: treatment with low molecular weight heparin. Thrombosis and Haemostasis 55: 37–39

Vlachoyannis J, Schoeppe W 1982 Adenylate cyclase activity and cAMP content of human platelets in uremia. European Journal of Clinical Investigation 12: 379–381

Volkin R L, Starz T W, Winkelstein A et al 1982 Changes in coagulation factors, complement, immunoglobulins, and immune complex concentrations with plasma exchange. Transfusion 22: 54–58

Wautier J L, Caen J R, Rymer R 1976 Angiodysplasia in acquired von Willebrand's disease (letter). Lancet 2: 973

Weinstein M, Ware J A, Troll J, Salzman E 1988 Changes in von Willebrand factor during cardiac surgery: effect of desmopressin. Blood 71: 1648–1655

Weiss H J 1967 The effect of clinical dextran on platelet aggregation, adhesion, and ADP release in man: in vivo and in vitro studies. Journal of Laboratory and Clinical Medicine 69: 37–46

Weitzel J N, Sadowski J A, Furie B C et al 1990 Surreptitious ingestion of a long-acting vitamin K antagonist/rodenticide, brodifacoum: clinical and metabolic studies of three cases. Blood 76: 2555–2559

Wilkinson S P 1977 Endotoxins and liver disease. Scandinavian Journal of Gastroenterology 12: 385–387

Woodman R C, Harker L A 1990 Bleeding complications associated with cardiopulmonary bypass. Blood 76: 1680–1697

Yin E T, Gaston L W 1965 Purification and kinetic studies on a circulating anticoagulant in a suspected case of lupus erythematosus. Thrombosis et Diathesis Haemorrhagica 14: 88–115

Zehnder J L, Leung L L K 1990 Development of antibodies to thrombin and factor V with recurrent bleeding in a patient exposed to topical bovine thrombin. Blood 76: 2011–2016

42. Disseminated intravascular coagulation

A. R. Giles

There cannot be many topics in haemostasis and thrombosis that have generated such a diversity of opinion and controversy as the topic of this chapter. Since the original experimental description during the latter part of the 19th century (Nauyn 1873, Foa & Pellacani 1884), of diffuse intravascular coagulation following the infusion of homogenized tissue or erythrocyte stroma, there has been an increasing number of reports in the medical and scientific literature documenting the relevance of these original observations to clinical medicine and exploring the elusive issues involved in its pathogenesis. Many excellent review articles have been written on the subject. A selection is included in a separate bibliography at the end of this chapter. The list is not exhaustive but does provide historical perspective and has served as a substantial source of information to supplement the author's clinical and experimental experience. Some of the texts obviously reflect a bias influenced by information on the syndrome itself and the understanding of the basic mechanisms of haemostasis, available at the time of writing. This discussion is no exception to this. Central to the difficulties in understanding the condition is the failure to recognize that this is not a pathology in isolation. With possibly the only exception being the direct activation of coagulation by the injection of venom, DIC is a secondary response to a preexisting primary pathology, i.e. it is 'an intermediary mechanism of disease' (McKay 1965). Although the primary conditions may be grouped into general categories, the diversity between and within these groups, both with regard to their individual pathology, the magnitude of the coagulant response and the consequences that may occur, is broad. Therefore, it is not surprising that it has been extremely difficult to unravel the interacting pathologies in order to develop either faithful experimental models or conduct well-controlled and appropriate clinical trials. In the discussion that follows, an attempt will be made to reflect what is believed to be a consensus on the approach to this condition, particularly with regard to diagnosis and management. In the discussion of its pathogenesis, some emphasis will be placed on experimental model systems that take account of recent improvements in our understanding of basic haemostatic mechanisms. Given the difficulties involved in detailed characterization in the clinical situation, which is unpredictable and frequently life-threatening, the use of such models probably presents the only rational way to identify key issues that can be subsequently validated or refuted in humans.

Equally as controversial as the disease itself is the nomenclature used. Much has been written favouring one descriptive title over another. The author's own bias favours the title chosen: Disseminated intravascular coagulation (DIC). The hallmark of normal haemostasis is the exquisite regulation of a focused event, i.e. the formation of a haemostatic plug, at the site of injury to a blood vessel. The antithesis of this is what occurs in DIC. The events are not confined to achieving haemostasis, i.e. they are widely disseminated, albeit that this may be confined to a local pathology, such as a haemangioma, or totally systemic, as in Gram-negative shock. Similarly, the haemostatic plug is predominantly extravascular and thus intravascular implies a perturbation of the normal haemostatic mechanism. Finally, as will be expanded upon later, the process is initiated by a procoagulant event. Alternative terms that are used interchangeably are 'consumptive coagulopathy', 'consumptive thrombohaemorrhagic disorder' and 'defibrination syndrome'. Although not descriptively incorrect they do not provide the same level of insight into the mechanisms involved and may be misleading. For example, defibrination may not occur and consumption, although occurring, may not be apparent. Finally, in discussing the nomenclature of the condition, it is worth differentiating between an inappropriate and an unwanted side-effect of an appropriate haemostatic response. Not infrequently, DIC is described as inappropriate when in fact in most cases it represents an appropriate response to a haemostatic challenge threatening the viability of the individual. As will be further discussed, the best example of this is the activation of the fibrinolytic system that occurs in such patients. Although the response is initially directed at clearing the vasculature of unwanted deposits of fibrin, due to the lack of specificity of plasmin and the consequent proteolytic degradation of essential co-factors of coagulation such as factors V and VIII, it may eventually compromise haemostasis. Nonetheless, appreciation of the fact that this is an unwanted side-effect rather than an inappropriate response directs attention to the importance of regulating the procoagulant rather than the fibrinolytic event in all but very rare instances.

PATHOGENESIS

It would appear that one shared characteristic of all the primary conditions, both experimental and clinical, that are known to be associated with DIC, is the provision of conditions which either directly provide or favour the development of a procoagulant stimulus. Although the pathways by which this develops may vary both between and within conditions, the generation of thrombin, the terminal enzyme of the coagulation cascade, is the final expression. As our knowledge of the biochemistry and molecular biology of haemostasis increases, so does our appreciation of the ubiquity of thrombin's actions in the process overall. Table 42.1 summarizes these activities.

In the context of this discussion, its classic procoagulant activities, i.e. the conversion of the sol protein, fibrinogen, to the gel fibrin and the activation of fibrin- stabilizing factor (factor XIII), which converts the gel fibrin from a relatively weak hydrogen bond linked polymer to the more stable covalent state, are obviously relevant (Greenberg et al 1987). In addition, as the principal activator of the essential co-factors VIII and V, it has a profound effect on the potency of the *tenase* and *prothrombinase* complexes in generating factor Xa and thrombin, respectively (Mann 1984). Thrombin's ability to 'activate' platelets inducing platelet aggregation and release has been apparent for some years (Deykin 1974). More recently, the ability of thrombin activated as opposed to resting platelets to provide specific binding sites for individual coagulation factors as well as a coagulant active phospholipid surface on which enzymatic complexes are assembled, has been demonstrated (Tracy et al 1979, Nesheim et al 1988, Mann et al 1990). The amplification of the initial procoagulant stimulus that these events support illustrate the propensity that thrombin has to promote dramatically its own generation following the initial triggering of the coagulation cascade (Nesheim & Mann 1979). Conversely, we are now aware of potent mechanisms which either down-regulate its generation or antagonize its activity. An apparent paradox is that they themselves rely on thrombin generation to promote their activities. In the presence of an endothelial cell co-factor, thrombomodulin, thrombin activates the vitamin K-dependent zymogen protein C to the serum protease, activated protein C (APC), which demonstrates specific substrate specificity for the activated forms of factors V and VIII (factor Va/VIIIa) (Walker et al 1990). As a consequence of this activity, thrombin generation is drastically curtailed. The fibrinolytic system, via its terminal enzyme plasmin, has a relative specificity for fibrin and thus clears, by proteolysis, the major product of thrombin generation, fibrin (Wiman & Collen 1978). It has been suggested by some that in normal haemostasis a balance exists between the coagulation and fibrinolytic systems (Astrup 1956). Experimental evidence suggests that the availability of tissue plasminogen activator (tPA), required for conversion of the inactive zymogen plasminogen to the active serine protease plasmin, is also regulated by thrombin promoting either directly or indirectly its release from endothelial cell stores (Levin et al 1986). In experimental studies in non-human primates, profound increases in tPA release and fibrinolysis occur following the generation of thrombin in vivo (Giles et al 1990). Appreciation of the many thrombin-mediated activities which may either be co-operative or antagonistic to each other is fundamental to the appreciation of the principals involved in the understanding of the pathogenesis and the management of this condition. Although many issues relating to the inter-regulation of these events remain unresolved, experimental studies and extrapolation of the findings to clinical cases suggest that appreciation of the role of more recently characterized haemostatic mechanisms such as protein C and the tissue factor pathway inhibitor (TFPI) (Rapaport 1991) may soon improve our comprehension of the condition and in turn our ability to manage it. In the remainder of this discussion, the activation and inhibitory pathways of coagulation and fibrinolysis will be discussed in the context of this condition.

Table 42.1 Effect of thrombin

Procoagulant
- Converts fibrinogen to fibrin
- Activates factor XIII
- Activates factors V and VIII
- 'Activates' platelets

Anticoagulant
- Activates protein C
- Stimulates fibrinolysis

Initiation of coagulation

Extrinsic (tissue factor) pathway-dependent stimulus

In the very earliest experimental studies, a condition strongly resembling DIC was induced by the infusion of organ extracts (Foa & Pellacani 1884) and is probably analogous to the most dramatic forms of acute DIC seen clinically in association with obstetric accidents and major brain trauma. It is reasonable to assume that this relates to tissue factor being directly released into the circulation. During the last 5 years, enormous progress has been made in the characterization of the biochemistry and molecular biology of the extrinsic pathway of coagulation in general and tissue factor in particular. Excellent reviews have become available recently (Nemerson 1988, Rapaport 1989, 1991). It is now apparent that, although tissue factor-rich materials may obtain gross access to the circulation as previously described, its availability may be more subtly regulated. Leukocytes express tissue factor-like activity following exposure to endotoxin (Muhlfelder et al 1978) and their ability to express the apoprotein has recently been confirmed (Edgington 1991). Monocytes from individuals with neoplastic conditions possess tissue factor-like activity (Rickles & Edwards 1983) as do promyelocytic leukaemic cell lines (Gralnick & Abrell 1973). Endothelial cells do not normally synthesize tissue factor but this may become up-regulated (Edgington 1991). Of interest is that this is associated with down-regulation of the expression of thrombomodulin, the essential co-factor required for the activation of protein C by thrombin (Moore et al 1987). This information suggests that the tissue factor-dependent extrinsic pathway of coagulation may well provide the procoagulant stimulus in the development of DIC in conditions such as obstetric accidents or trauma, particularly head injuries, where tissue factor rich material gains direct access to the circulation. Alternatively, tissue factor expression is up-regulated either due to stimulation of cells competent in tissue factor synthesis or by the availability of neoplastic cells where the generation of such activity is unregulated.

Intrinsic pathway-dependent stimulus

The role of contact activation as an initiating mechanism in normal haemostasis remains elusive (Kaplan 1978). Congenital deficiencies of factor XII, prekallikrein (Fletcher factor), and high molecular weight kininogen (Fitzgerald factor) are not associated with a haemostatic deficit, suggesting that either they have no role in the normal haemostatic response to vascular injury or that their role is normally bypassed by alternative mechanisms (Ratnoff 1987). It has been suggested that this may be achieved via the tissue factor-dependent extrinsic pathway consequent to the observation that tissue factor/factor VIIa is an effective activator of factor IX and that this may represent the principal haemostatic event in response to injury (Repke et al 1990). More recently, a further role for thrombin has been suggested by the finding that, in the presence of an anionic surface, it can activate factor XI which then proceeds through the classically characterized intrinsic pathway of coagulation to thrombin generation (Gailani & Broze 1991). This may explain why patients with factor XI deficiency do have a bleeding tendency, although this is relatively mild in comparison to the deficiencies of factors IX and VIII. In both cases, however, the integrity of the contact system is not a pre-requisite for haemostatic function. Nonetheless, this does not exclude a pathogenetic role in the development of DIC. Activation of factor XII occurs following exposure to natural materials, from which it is normally excluded by the endothelial cell barrier, or to artificial surfaces such as those used in vascular prostheses or extra-corporeal systems in cardiopulmonary bypass procedures. Injury to the endothelium, induced for example by endotoxin exposure or burns, would promote contact with collagen and other connective tissue components which have been demonstrated to promote the activation of factor XII (Niewiarowski et al 1966, Wilner et al 1968). The presence of a factor XII activator in endothelial cells has been suggested and this may also become available following endothelial cell lysis (Wiggins et al 1980). The activation of factor XII has a number of consequences that are reviewed in detail elsewhere in this book but it should be emphasized that, as well as providing the initial trigger to thrombin generation, it promotes the generation of bradykinin and thus contributes to the vasodilatation and hypotension commonly found in association with the coagulant or fibrin generating characteristics of this syndrome (Mason et al 1970, Newball et al 1978). Finally, activation of factor XII has been shown to directly promote plasminogen activation in vitro (Heimark et al 1980) but the importance of this mechanism in vivo remains controversial (Wiman & Collen 1978). In support of these theoretical considerations of the role of the contact system in DIC is the observation of decreased levels of factors XII, prekallikrein and kallikrein inhibitors and an increase in levels of bradykinin and kallikrein-inhibitor complexes in patients with hypotensive septicaemia (Mason et al 1970, O'Donnell et al 1976, Colman et al 1978).

Direct (non-physiological) activation of coagulation

Factor X and prothrombin may in certain circumstances be activated directly or non-physiologically, i.e. by agents that are not components of the classically described intrinsic, extrinsic or common coagulation pathways. Pineo and co-workers have demonstrated direct activation of factor X by purified mucin and proposed this mechanism as an explanation for the association of thromboembolic disease with mucin-producing tumours (Pineo et al 1973). Similarly, Gordon and co-workers have demonstrated the presence of a protease in tumour cells which apparently directly activates factor X (Gordon & Cross 1981). A number of venoms have been characterized as showing specificity for different components of the coagulation cascade. *Echis carinatus* venom directly activates prothrombin to thrombin (Franza et al 1975). The venom of *Vipera russelli* (Russell viper) directly activates factor X to factor Xa (Kisiel et al 1976). It is therefore reasonable to assume that the DIC-like syndrome that ensues following the bite of such snakes is directly related to this procoagulant activity that the venoms contain. A more subtle promotion of procoagulant activity may be exercised by proteolytic enzymes of broad specificity such as elastase and plasmin. Plasmin has been demonstrated to activate and inactivate factor V in vitro (Lee & Mann 1989). It also inactivates factor VIII and preliminary data suggest activation occurs prior to this event (Rick & Krizek 1986, Taylor et al 1982). Similarly, both neutrophil and pancreatic elastase activate and subsequently inactivate factor V (Oates & Salem 1987, Lyon & Giles 1991). By extrapolation, it is also possible that it exercises similar activities over factor VIII. In activating these two co-factors, an increased enzymatic efficiency of both the *tenase* and *prothrombinase* complexes may be expected and amplification of factor Xa and thrombin generation would result (Marciniak 1973). As the levels of elastase may be significantly elevated in association with septicaemias (Abbink et al 1991), this mechanism may be influential in amplifying the response to marginal or threshold coagulant stimuli and result in the association of DIC with these conditions. It is possible that the observation relating elastase levels to fibrin degradation in patients undergoing therapy for promyelocytic leukaemia could be explained on this basis (Sterrenberg et al 1985). Similarly, this activity of plasmin could be a further example of an unwanted side-effect of an appropriate fibrinolytic response directed at clearing the circulation of fibrin but inadvertently indirectly promoting its further generation.

Increased availability of coagulant active phospholipid

The essential role of negatively charged phospholipids in providing a surface for the assembly of enzymatically active complexes is well established (Mann 1984). Under normal physiological circumstances, this facility is provided by the platelet which is exquisitely regulated by mechanisms, defined and undefined, which normally ensure that its contribution is focused at the site of vascular injury. Similar phospholipids may become available, however, from cells that do not normally function as a source. For example, erythrocytes are richly endowed with negatively charged phospholipids on their inner leaflet but these would not normally be externalized in contrast to the platelet which undergoes 'flip-flop' of its membrane to expose negatively charged phospholipids following activation (Rosing et al 1988). Nonetheless, haemolysis, as would occur during an incompatible blood transfusion reaction, would make such lipids available and could explain the intravascular coagulation that occurs in such situations (Krevans et al 1957). It would seem, however, that additional mechanisms must also be involved as chemical unlike immune haemolysis is not associated with activation of coagulation (Mannucci et al 1969). In light of the previous discussion of the role of the contact system, it is possible that immune complex formation and complement activation and their known interactions with the contact activation system may provide a threshold procoagulant stimulus that is subsequently amplified by the availability of increased quantities of coagulant active phospholipid (Giles et al 1982b). Experimentally, this has been shown to be potently thrombogenic in combination with factor Xa and to induce a syndrome in experimental animals which is strikingly similar to the clinical condition of DIC (Giles et al 1984b, 1990).

In summary, there are a number of candidate mechanisms for initiating the procoagulant stimulus that leads to thrombin generation and fibrinogen to fibrin conversion. In individual cases of clinical DIC, the mechanism may be singular and clearly determined, e.g. envenomation following a snake bite. In other situations, the mechanism may be less clear cut and involve one or more of the mechanisms described. By clinical association, e.g. in severe head injury, a tissue factor-dependent pathway may appear more likely and, as will be discussed below, study of the inhibitory mechanisms involved may reinforce that hypothetical view.

Inhibition of coagulation

Inhibitors of coagulation can be categorized conveniently as inhibitors of thrombin generation or inhibitors of thrombin action.

Inhibitors of thrombin generation

The protein C/protein S system, due to its regulation of the co-factors V and VIII (Esmon 1989), would be seen in the traditional concept of coagulation as regulating the generation of thrombin via the intrinsic/common pathways. In light of the more recent reappraisal of the role of tissue factor/factor VIIa, as a potential primary activator of factor IX (Østerud & Rapaport 1980), this may no longer be appropriate. Consequently, the protein C/S system would clearly play a pivotal role in regulating thrombin generation resulting either from increased tissue factor availability or contact activation. Excellent reviews of the system have been published (Esmon 1989) and it is discussed in detail elsewhere in this book (Ch. 30). Evidence for its involvement in both clinical and experimental models of DIC come from observation of reduced levels of the zymogen (Heeb et al 1989, Madden et al 1989) and appearance of the activated product in complex with its inhibitors, protein C inhibitor (PCI), α1-antitrypsin and α_2-macroglobulin (Hoogendoorn et al 1990, 1991). Experimental models of its participation have been particularly useful in demonstrating a good correlation between the magnitude of the procoagulant stimulus, the degree of protein C activation and its subsequent partitioning between its inhibitors. PCI appears to be its primary inhibitor but as the procoagulant stimulus is increased or prolonged, the degree of protein C activation exceeds the availability of PCI to inhibit it and α_1-antitrypsin and

α_2-macroglobulin become more prominent as overflow inhibitors (Hoogendoorn et al 1990). Their appearance in patients with DIC appears to be associated with a poor prognosis (Scully et al 1992). This observation linked with the established association between a pre-thrombotic state and congenital deficiency states of this system (Broekmans et al 1983) would suggest that an acquired deficiency related to consumption may be a critical factor in the pathogenesis of this syndrome and thus has potential implications for its management (see p. 980).

The tissue factor pathway inhibitor (TFPI), previously termed the intrinsic pathway inhibitor (EPI) by Rapaport and co-workers and the lipoprotein associated coagulation inhibitor (LACI) by Broze and co-workers, has been a subject of major interest in recent years following its detailed characterization by them and others. The topic has recently been reviewed (Rapaport 1991) and is discussed in detail elsewhere in this book (Ch. 15). It is an unusual inhibitor in that, although possessing inhibitory activity of the tissue factor/factor VIIa complex itself, this is significantly amplified when it forms a complex with activated factor X (Sanders et al 1985). Thus, it is another example of an inhibitor whose activity is promoted by the availability of the product of the pathway upon which it acts. Experimental evidence has been presented by Rapaport and co-workers that strongly suggests a role for TFPI as a physiological anticoagulant, presumably by limiting tissue factor/factor VIIa activity to the immediate environment of the forming normal haemostatic plug (Sandset et al 1991). It has been suggested that the failure of the extrinsic pathway to bypass the need for factor VIII in haemophilia A may reflect the restraint exercised on this pathway by TFPI (Repke et al 1990). Support for this comes from clinical and experimental studies suggesting that such a bypass may be achieved by the infusion of pharmacological levels of tissue factor (apoprotein) (O'Brien et al 1988) and factor VIIa (Hedner & Kisiel 1983). As TFPI would be expected to be cleared during such a process, either as TFPI/factor Xa complexes or as a quaternary TFPI/factor Xa/factor VIIa/TF complex, it may be predicted that TFPI levels would be reduced in patients with DIC. It is of interest that in most cases this has not proven to be the case (Warr et al 1989). In one patient with massive brain injury investigated by Rapaport and co-workers, the plasma TFPI functional activity was reduced to 20% of normal and this was associated with the classic clinical and laboratory features of DIC including a major reduction in protein C functional activity (Rapaport 1991). Although this was interpreted by them as suggesting that in most patients DIC occurs as a result of the continuing formation of factor VIIa/tissue factor complexes rather than the depletion of TFPI, it may also suggest that TFPI exercises a significant regulatory role in DIC only in those situations where the tissue factor pathway is involved and it may be less relevant where alternative pathways predominate. In contrast, participation of protein C would be independent of this variable. These considerations have major implications for the study, diagnosis and management of this syndrome.

Inhibitors of thrombin activity

Antithrombin III and heparin co-factor II inhibit thrombin and this activity is significantly enhanced in the presence of heparin (Damus et al 1973, Tollefson & Blank 1981). In the case of antithrombin III, factors IXa, Xa and XIa are also inhibited (Griffith 1983). The resistance of the normal endothelialized vessel wall to thrombus formation has been attributed to the presence of heparin-like substances associated with the endothelium (Marcum et al 1986). Congenital deficiency of antithrombin III is associated with evidence of a pre-thrombotic state and a malignant thrombotic tendency in some individuals (Marciniak et al 1974). Reductions in levels of both antithrombin III and heparin co-factor II in DIC have been presumed to result from consumption following the clearance of thrombin inhibitor complexes (Bauer & Rosenberg 1984). These observations have formed the basis for the use of antithrombin III concentrates in this condition.

Consideration of the role of thrombomodulin is usually confined to its participation in the process of protein C activation. As its name suggests, however, in vitro characterization has demonstrated a 'switching' by thrombomodulin of thrombin's procoagulant effects on fibrin generation and platelet activation to an anticoagulant effect mediated by protein C activation. Exposure of endothelial cells in culture to endotoxin results in down-regulation of thrombomodulin and up-regulation of tissue factor synthesis (Edgington 1991). Although of theoretical interest, the relevance of these observations in human pathophysiology has yet to be established.

Reduced activity of the reticuloendothelial system (RES)

A role for the reticuloendothelial cell system in general and the liver in particular has been proposed in the clearance of activated clotting factors from the circulation (Wessler & Yin 1968). In experimental systems, RES blockade induced by agents such as thoratrast have been demonstrated to sensitize experimental animals to both systemic and localized intravascular coagulation (McKay 1973). As there is evidence that relative RES blockade may exist in a number of the clinical situations associated with the development of DIC, it has been suggested that these experimental observations are of clinical relevance (Rabiner & Friedman 1968, Lahnborg et al 1976). In particular, individuals with liver disease appear to be at particular risk and have a reduced tolerance in regulating procoagulant challenges. Although this may also reflect decreased levels of the physiological inhibitors, protein C and antithrombin III, it is reasonable to suppose that reduced reticuloendothelial cell capacity is an additional major pathogenetic factor in the development of DIC in such individuals.

Fibrinolysis

With the exception of the use of heparin in the management of DIC, which will be discussed later (p. 981), there is probably no issue more contentious than whether or not the role of the fibrinolytic system is as a primary or secondary participant in this syndrome. The issue is certainly not academic as the conclusion reached and the management decisions made consequent to this have significant implications for the overall outcome. The inappropriate or untimely use of anti-fibrinolytic therapy may have disastrous consequences and yet unrestrained plasmin activity may promote a calamitous haemorrhagic diathesis. Demonstration of the products of the activity of the fibrinolytic system, i.e. fibrin/fibrinogen split products are the sine qua non of the syndrome and the diagnostic efficiency for DIC has improved substantially with the development of specific tests (Merskey et al 1966). In recent years, such tests have been improved through the development of immunological reagents that recognize epitopes on fragments that result from plasmin cleavage of cross-linked fibrin rather than fibrinogen and thus differentiate between fibrinolysis and fibrinogenolysis (Nieuwenhuizen 1986). It would appear that the consensus of recent reviews is that, in the majority of cases and irrespective of the source of the procoagulant stimulus, the fibrinolytic system is activated in response to the procoagulant stimulus leading successively to thrombin generation and fibrin deposition in the intravascular space. It would seem to be the exception rather than the rule that haemorrhagic manifestations of this syndrome occur as a result of primary fibrinolysis although well-documented cases of this have been reported in the literature (Davidson et al 1969). Whilst this assessment does not detract from the role that the non-specific proteolytic activity of plasmin plays in the pathogenesis of the haemorrhagic manifestations, it does dictate that the management approach should be weighted in favour of regulating the procoagulant activity rather than the fibrinolytic response. Moreover, if the clinical situation dictates that the latter approach should be adopted, this should never be instituted without concurrent therapy directed at inhibiting either thrombin generation or activity.

In summary, available clinical and experimental data suggest that the primary event that occurs in DIC is the development of a procoagulant stimulus and the generation of thrombin consequent to that. The outcome of this will be predicated by both the intensity of the stimulus and the level of competence of the physiological anticoagulant systems. These activities will be further modulated by the response of the fibrinolytic system. Although initially directed at the maintenance of the patency of the vascular tree, under circumstances of continued procoagulant activity, it may be associated with unwanted proteolytic activity leading to depletion of haemostatic factors and convert the net response from a thrombotic to a haemorrhagic diathesis. These events are illustrated in simplified form in Figure 42.1. This figure summarizes the major events discussed in this section but is by no means all inclusive. For example, the role of plasmin and elastase in promoting and then demoting procoagulant activity via the proteolysis of factors V and VIII has not been included. The figure should be taken as a minimal rationalization of a complex sequence of diverse and interacting events.

CLINICAL PRESENTATION

Disseminated intravascular coagulation is an intermediary mechanism of disease (McKay 1965). The relevance of emphasizing this point relates both to difficulties in making generalizations with regard to its clinical and laboratory features when these are frequently clouded by the signs and symptoms of the primary disorder but also to seek and recognize the diagnosis in patients with conditions classically predisposed to its development. Table 42.2 is extracted from a large and probably representative retrospective survey of patients presenting with clinical and laboratory evidence of DIC grouped into their primary disease categories (Spero et al 1980). The strong association with malignancy and infection is noted and accounts for 50% of the cases diagnosed. As for the reasons given, the clinical presentation may vary in relationship to the primary condition; this will be first discussed in general and then in the context of individual primary disease settings.

General considerations

In evaluating a patient with clinical and laboratory evidence of DIC, a judgement must be made as to whether the condition is:

1. acute or chronic
2. systemic or localized
3. the fibrinolytic activity is a primary or secondary manifestation of the condition.

The relevance of defining the condition as acute versus chronic relates to the urgency of management decision making and is usually a priority in the patient presenting with laboratory rather than clinical evidence of the condition. Although a significant number of patients with subclinical acute DIC will show spontaneous reversal, it is individuals in this group who may show the most gratifying response to rapid confirmation of the diagnosis and urgent institution of therapeutic intervention.

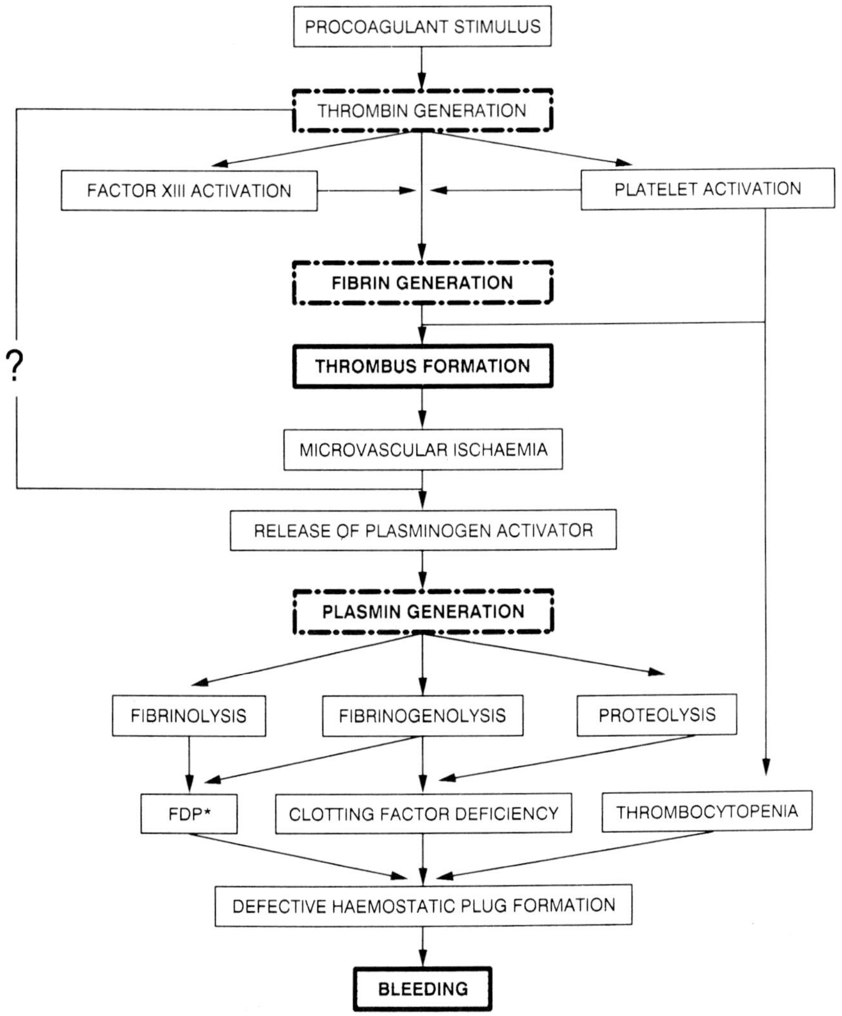

Fig. 42.1 Interaction of the coagulation and fibrinolytic systems in DIC. *Fibrin(ogen) degradation products (FDP).

Table 42.2 Primary disease categories of patients presenting with DIC

Disease entity	Total (%)	Survival
Infection	26	24
Malignancy	24	31
Miscellaneous (including obstetric)	23	42
Surgery	19	32
Liver disease	8	39

Taken from Spero et al 1980.

The hallmark of this condition is the disseminated nature of the perturbed haemostatic response as opposed to the focused events of normal haemostasis. Nonetheless, this process may not be systemic but localized anatomically, e.g. to an organ such as the kidney. In such individuals, although laboratory testing may provide systemic evidence of the condition, the pathological effects may be confined locally and the therapeutic approach may be optimally directed to this. Examples are aortic aneurysm and cavernous haemangiomas. Although the condition may be localized, the systemic effects may be profound and some individuals may develop major evidence of consumption of platelets and coagulation factors and develop life-threatening haemorrhage (Fine et al 1967). The importance of recognizing the relevance of the localized nature of this condition is underscored by the evidence that such patients may respond dramatically to surgical removal or medical ablation of the local pathology.

Activation of the fibrinolytic system occurs to a greater or lesser extent in all cases whether DIC is acute or chronic, systemic or localized. As previously discussed, the appearance of split products is the hallmark of the condition. The primary issue in the clinical manifestation rests with a decision as to whether this response represents primary (spontaneous) fibrin/fibrinogenolysis or is secondary to the development of thrombin generation and microvascular thrombus formation. As will be discussed later, laboratory testing is not helpful as in each case the consequences of unrestrained plasmin-induced proteolysis of various coagulation factors is the same. The clinical context may be useful, however, in that certain conditions such as prostatic surgery, are classically associated with primary fibrinolysis. Overall, the most common sequence of events appear to be those described in Figure 42.1.

Specific conditions associated with disseminated intravascular coagulation

Infection

A wide spectrum of infectious agents, from viruses to protozoa, are associated with the risk of developing DIC (Dennis et al 1967, McKay & Margaretten 1967, Preston et al 1973). As described in Table 42.2, in most practitioners' experience, it represents the single largest at-risk group (Spero et al 1980). In some cases, it presents as the most florid manifestation of the condition and is responsible for the high mortality of these conditions. For example in fatal cases of meningococcal sepsis, postmortem evidence of diffuse intravascular thrombosis may be determined and haemorrhagic necrosis of the adrenal glands, the Waterhouse–Friderichsen syndrome, is one of the most feared outcomes of this condition, resulting in acute circulatory collapse (Ferguson & Chapman 1948). Gram-negative bacteria are more frequently associated with this complication than Gram-positive although cases of purpura fulminans have been documented in streptococcal infections (Hall 1965) and less frequently with staphylococcus (Murray et al 1977). A number of viruses and rickettsial infections are associated with haemorrhagic, DIC-like presentations of which Rocky Mountain Spotted Fever is a well-established example (Schaffner et al 1965).

The mortality associated with DIC complicating infection remains high (Table 42.2) and its management remains controversial. As previously discussed, the diversity of the primary conditions has probably defeated attempts to perform adequately controlled clinical trials in order to address specific issues such as the benefit of heparin anticoagulation, etc. It is sobering that although one of the fundamental principals of treating DIC is to address and control the primary condition, despite the enormous advances with regard to the availability of potent and specific antibiotics, the mortality remains high and does not appear to have shown substantial improvement over the years.

Obstetric accidents

Of all the areas of speciality medicine, there is probably no group more familiar with the rare but constant risk of this complication in a previously healthy individual. The presentation may vary from the acute fulminating and devastating haemorrhage associated with amniotic fluid embolism to the more chronic presentation associated with the dead fetus syndrome. Excellent reviews are available on the changes that take place in coagulation and fibrinolysis during pregnancy and immediately after parturition (Bonnar 1973). It has been suggested that, at term, the mother in fact demonstrates a pre-thrombotic state and thus is at greater risk of thromboembolic disease in general (Bonnar 1976). In the author's opinion, although this situation may reinforce the event when it occurs, it would seem logical to assume that the event itself is the development of a procoagulant stimulus and, in the obstetric situation, this probably represents thromboplastic material gaining direct access to the maternal circulation. Of all the primary conditions associated with DIC, this group appears to provide the most gratifying confirmation of the benefit of moving quickly to remove the provocative stimulus. Removal of the products of conception by simple procedures such as curettage or, less frequently, by more radical procedures such as hysterectomy are frequently associated with spontaneous remission of the condition and even substantial replacement therapy may not be required. Even in the devastating haemorrhagic cases associated with abruptio placentae or amniotic fluid embolism, bleeding may be self-limiting. Unfortunately, however, the acute and severe hypovolaemia that ensues may have produced irreversible major organ damage by the time that this occurs.

In the dead fetus syndrome and not infrequently following therapeutic termination of pregnancy, evidence of chronic DIC may exist but, again, an abrupt beneficial response follows the removal of the products of conception either by surgical procedure or spontaneous delivery. Septic abortion is more complicated as it combines the additional feature of infection which is associated with DIC in its own right. Given the previous comments on the response of patients with infection alone, it is interesting that this is generally considered to be a condition that is relatively refractory to the classical management approach used in other obstetric complications.

Trauma

Major trauma is frequently associated with the development of DIC. This is particularly frequent in major head injuries and appears to represent an example of a tissue factor-mediated procoagulant stimulus. Autopsy findings on such individuals suggest that the sequence of events described in Figure 42.1 generally occur. In patients succumbing early, thrombosis may predominate, whereas later deaths are associated with haemorrhagic manifestations, presumably secondary to reactive fibrinolysis.

DIC is also associated with severe burns and heat stroke which seems to reflect diffuse endothelial cell damage. (Weber & Blakeley 1969, Ekoe et al 1985). For reasons discussed previously, it would be interesting to monitor the fate of the tissue factor pathway inhibitor in such patients but this information is not presently available.

Leukaemia

DIC may complicate certain forms of leukaemia as a presenting feature or following the initiation of chemotherapy. Acute promyelocytic leukaemia is frequently associated with a DIC-like syndrome. This is usually expressed haemorrhagically but both venous and arterial thrombosis may occur in a minority of patients (Gralnick et al 1972). Interestingly, the prothrombin time may be prolonged in the face of a normal activated partial thromboplastin time and we have personally reviewed three patients where this appeared to reflect a relatively discrete deficiency of factor VII. These data suggest an extrinsic pathway-mediated procoagulant stimulus which would be in line with the observation of a tissue factor-like activity in promyeloblasts (Gralnick & Abrell 1973).

Although commonly observed in this type of leukaemia, DIC has been described in acute myelogenous leukaemia (Baker et al 1964), acute lymphoblastic leukaemia (Guarini et al 1980), acute myelomonocytic leukaemia (Mangal et al 1984), chronic myeloid leukaemia (Gingrich & Burns 1979), angioimmunoblastic lymphadenopathy (Minerbrook et al 1983) and malignant histiocytosis (Salz-Steiner et al 1984). In some cases, DIC occurs after the initiation of chemotherapy and in those patients at highest risk, i.e. with acute promyelocytic leukaemia, concomitant therapy with heparin has been proposed to decrease haemorrhagic complications (Gralnick et al 1972). It should be emphasized that the thrombocytopenia associated with primary marrow dysplasia, further exacerbated by chemotherapy, etc. presents an additional challenge to haemostasis.

Neoplasia

Patients with malignant neoplastic disease, particularly when disseminated, may show evidence of a low grade or chronic DIC (Sack et al 1977). In many cases, this is subclinical and only detectable by laboratory tests such as a peripheral blood smear showing microangiopathic features and evidence of enhanced fibrinolysis resulting in increased levels of fibrin split products. The condition may exacerbate, however, into an acute fulminating disorder either spontaneously or following an intervention such as surgery. The manifestations may be either primarily thrombotic or haemorrhagic although usually the former appears to predominate. The classic description of Trousseau of thrombosis migrans in association with neoplasms of the pancreas is presumed to be an example of this (Trousseau 1865). As this condition exemplifies, evidence of chronic DIC may be the first indication of an underlying neoplastic disorder. Of particular importance with regard to the previous discussion of primary fibrinolysis is consideration of the diagnosis of prostatic carcinoma which reflects the presence of high concentrations of plasminogen activators in this organ. The use of low dose subcutaneous heparin has been advocated for the management of the chronic DIC observed in this association. Generally speaking, although this approach does have some merit in modulating the intensity of the DIC, the decision must be taken in the context of the general palliative approach adopted to patients with what is usually terminal disease. Nonetheless, symptomatic improvement in the development of thrombotic complications may be particularly valuable in this context.

Surgery

DIC may complicate certain surgical procedures more frequently than others, e.g. as an associated complication of Gram-negative sepsis complicating surgical conditions of the biliary system. Reference has already been made to the risk in trauma patients and the local consequences related to aortic aneurysms. Of particular importance is the high frequency of this complication in patients undergoing cardiopulmonary bypass (Harker 1986). In the survey reported by Spero and co-workers, summarized in Table 42.2, 52% of the surgical patients were in this category (Spero et al 1980). In 12 patients recently studied by us whilst undergoing cardiopulmonary bypass for valve replacement and coronary artery bypass procedures, we observed significant laboratory evidence of thrombin generation and protein C activation/inactivation in all 12 cases despite heparinization (Scully et al 1991). Postoperatively, most patients had a reversible depression of factor V but in no case was there overt clinical evidence of a haemorrhagic diathesis. Nonetheless, it is well-established that occasional patients do develop clinically overt DIC and our data would suggest that in all cases a significant procoagulant stimulus is generated during such procedures.

Liver disease

The association of DIC with liver disease appears to be controversial. In severe hepatic deficiency there is essentially a balanced state of coagulation due to the liver's synthetic responsibility for producing both procoagulant and anticoagulant proteins. Autopsy studies of patients, without additional complications to their liver disease leading to death, do not apparently demonstrate evidence of active DIC (Oka & Tanaka 1977). Nonetheless, in our own experience, some of the most fulminating examples of DIC have been observed in patients with severe liver disease where one may presume that a procoagulant stimulus has 'tipped' the haemostatic balance in favour of coagulation. Examples of this are patients receiving prothrombinase complex concentrates (Cederbaum et al 1976) and those undergoing procedures to reduce an ascitic load, such as the Leveen shunt, where ascitic fluid is returned to the vascular circuit via a venous shunt (Leveen

1985). Our experience and that of others suggest that DIC is an invariable consequence of such interventions and presumably relates to the patient's deficiency in the physiological anticoagulant proteins C/S and antithrombin III (Ragni et al 1983, Hoffman & Hultin 1986).

Complications of therapy

A number of therapeutic interventions, biological and non-biological, may be associated with the development of DIC. As previously discussed, some of the earliest observations on this condition related to the consequences of incompatible blood transfusions (Krevans et al 1957). The procoagulant activity appears to relate to the erythrocyte stroma as the infusion of haemoglobin alone is not associated with this condition (Rabiner & Friedman 1968, Rabiner et al 1970). Of interest, is the lack of association of chemical haemolysis as observed in patients with glucose-6-phosphate dehydrogenase deficiency (Mannucci et al 1969), in contrast to that observed following incompatible blood transfusion or the haemolysis associated with other immune-mediated conditions such as paroxysmal nocturnal haemoglobinuria (Crosby & Stefanini 1952). Although differences in RES-mediated clearance in these conditions have been suggested as an explanation for this, an alternative explanation could be that, whereas both situations require increased availability of coagulant active phospholipid from the inner leaflet of the erythrocyte membrane, only in the immune-mediated event is the coagulation cascade activated via the contact system.

DIC has been a recognized complication of the use of prothrombin complex concentrates since their original development (Triantaphyllopoulos, 1972). Patients with liver disease appear to be particularly at risk and their use is now generally contraindicated in such patients (Cederbaum & Roberts 1973, Kasper 1975). Whilst this side effect has been attributed to the known contamination with activated products of the component zymogens, using experimental approaches we have demonstrated that it is the presence of coagulant active phospholipid derived from platelet and erythrocyte lysis during plasma collection that appears to be the primary determinant of this activity (Giles et al 1982a, 1984a). Although non-thrombogenic in its own right, a powerful synergism develops when co-infused with activated factor X which is an invariable contaminant of all available PCC preparations (Giles et al 1981). The development of purified IX preparations promises greater security for the management of isolated factor IX deficiency (haemophilia B) (Mannucci et al 1990) but a multiple factor concentrate with comparable safety for use in patients with liver disease is not available.

Finally, the association of DIC in patients following initiation of chemotherapy has been discussed previously (p. 977).

Neonate

Neonates appear to be at particular risk of developing this condition and, in any given primary condition, the mortality is significantly higher (Spero et al 1980, Dairaku et al 1982). The basic mechanism and associated conditions have features in common with the adult variety of the condition. The increased risk presumably reflects immaturity of the physiological anticoagulants which is exacerbated in prematurity together with the difficulties in providing active intensive care as compared to their adult counterparts.

Snake bites

As previously discussed (p. 971), a number of venoms activate coagulation at specific points in the cascade. Although specifying the precise nature of the venom involved is of major relevance with regard to the use of specific anti-venoms, the overall procoagulant response is for the most part common to all and thus the management with regard to diagnosis and therapy follows the principles outlined in the following sections.

LABORATORY EVALUATION

In approaching the laboratory evaluation of DIC, it is important to discriminate between an approach directed at:

1. Establishing a data base that confirms or improves our understanding of the pathogenetic factors involved in DIC.
2. Establishing the diagnosis of DIC in an individual patient with particular reference to the source of the procoagulant stimulus in a given primary condition.
3. Monitoring the progress/severity of the condition with particular reference to the response to therapeutic intervention.

As previously discussed, despite intensive investigation in both experimental and clinical DIC, much remains to be learned about this condition. Experimental models have provided important information particularly when new basic information on the biochemistry and molecular biology of haemostasis have been incorporated into their design and analysis. Scrutiny of clinical cases of DIC on the basis of such information has confirmed its relevance and it is reasonable to assume that as a consequence clinical management will improve in due course. The technological armoury available to the clinical investigator has expanded enormously since the early 1980s, particularly with regard to immunologically based testing which now enables detailed characterization of any particular component or pathway considered to be involved. For example, specific fibrin/fibrinogen split product assays can delineate between plasmin cleavage of cross-linked fibrin as opposed to fibrinogen (Nieuwenhuizen 1986). Activation of protein C and its partition between its inhibitors may be characterized qualitatively by Western blotting and quantitatively by ELISA (Scully et al 1992). Unfortunately, many of these approaches require a level of stringency with regard to sample collection and performance that is not usually attainable for a number of reasons in the clinical setting. For example, the traditional anticoagulants used may not control thrombin generation and action ex vivo. Consequently the results obtained may not reflect in vivo changes and activity. In view of this, detailed investigations of this type will probably be limited to specialized centres where the appropriate resources and facilities are available, or in those clinical situations where the presentation or course of the condition permits a more controlled approach to laboratory evaluation. Nonetheless, it is important to emphasize the need for the diligent collection of epidemiological, clinical and laboratory data if our understanding and our subsequent management approach of this condition is to be improved.

In making the diagnosis of DIC, as in many other clinical situations, recognizing the clinical context in which DIC may occur is essential. Recognition of the frequency of association of this complication with certain primary conditions will suggest both the need for appropriate screening tests and the frequency of follow-up. In other situations, the presenting feature requiring investigation will be those of DIC. For example, in the case of unexpected haemorrhage in a surgical patient, it will be required to establish DIC as the mechanism involved. The preferred approach in our laboratory is to rely on the classical screening tests, i.e. the activated partial thromboplastin time (APTT), the prothrombin time (PT), the thrombin clotting time (TCT), platelet count and peripheral blood smear examination, and reserve more or less specific tests for patients demonstrating abnormalities in these. Fibrin split product (FSP) determinations are not included in our routine screening battery as, in our experience, this is not cost effective. The initial screening thrombin clotting time used (final concentration of thrombin 0.3 units/ml) is sensitive to elevations of FSP as well as qualitative and quantitative deficiencies in fibrinogen. Repeat testing of samples giving abnormal results using an increased thrombin concentration of 1.6 u/ml (final) will usually correct the TCT when this is prolonged due to the presence of FSP whereas the abnormality will remain in the presence of fibrinogen deficiency. In comparison to FSP determination, this test is cheap and relatively easy to perform and permits the further evaluation of patients showing abnormalities by both general and specific assay of split products, e.g. D-dimer. The one stage PTT is a sensitive indicator of clotting factor deficiency and this can be confirmed simply by repeating the test with a 50/50 mix of patient and control plasma, upon which the test time should correct back into the normal range. Generally speaking, the PT using the traditional rabbit brain thromboplastins is less frequently affected except where fibrinogen, the substrate of the test system, is drastically reduced. The exceptions to this rule are in cases previously discussed where the extrinsic pathway may be the exclusive provider of the procoagulant stimulus. Thrombocytopenia is a primary feature of the vast majority of patients with DIC and in approximately 50% the count will be less than 50×10^9/litre (Colman et al 1972, Spero et al 1980). Given the accuracy and facility of modern particle counters, this test is one of the most useful screening tests available except in those patients with conditions such as leukaemia where other factors may be involved. Classically, the microangiopathic blood picture and the associated anaemia have been considered hallmarks of the condition (Bull & Brain 1968). It should be realized, however, that this is a relatively non-specific finding that is frequently seen in the primary conditions associated with the risk of developing DIC, e.g. metastatic malignancy, vascular prostheses, etc., without DIC actually being present.

Patients demonstrating abnormalities in the screening tests, particularly if associated with the primary conditions previously discussed, qualify for further investigation. These may include repetition of the screening tests with greater frequency and/or the use of more specific assay procedures. With regard to repeating the screening assays, it should be emphasized that normal findings do not exclude a significant consumptive process. For example, in pregnancy, a normal PTT and TCT does not exclude significant consumption of clotting factors such as factor VIII and fibrinogen due to the substantial elevation of these factors during the final stages of normal pregnancy (Bonnar 1973). For example, a factor VIII or fibrinogen level within the normal range for a non-pregnant female is not a normal finding at the time of parturition. It is therefore essential to recognize this phenomenon in such patients and institute repetitive and frequent testing if the diagnosis of DIC is to be excluded.

In resorting to specific tests, the need is to establish the diagnosis, determine the severity and pace of progress of the condition and exclude primary fibrinogenolysis as the underlying condition.

In order to establish the diagnosis, the levels of fibrinogen and FSP should be determined. For the reasons previously discussed, the use of the thrombin clotting time as described may provide a more rapid and reasonable approximation should the rate of the process put time at a premium. As currently performed in most laboratories, determination of fibrinogen as thrombin clottable protein may be unreliable, giving a spuriously low result due to interference with fibrin polymerization in the presence of high levels of FSP. Although of importance from a mechanistic point of view, this does not present major difficulties in making management decisions as the two events, i.e. reduced level of fibrinogen and increased levels of FSP, are normally highly correlated. Demonstration of reduced levels of factors VIII and V are not necessary from a diagnostic point of view but may be useful in assessing the efficiency of replacement therapy. Time restraints again may preclude this and the use of the screening tests may prove adequate. In fact, the experience of Spero and coworkers suggests that factor VIII levels may even be misleading in contrast to the widely held view that levels are invariably reduced in this condition (Spero et al 1980). The explanation for these findings is not clear but may represent the selection criteria used in their survey. Measurement of other coagulation parameters such as tPA, plasminogen, tPA inhibitors (PAI-1), α_2-antiplasmin, protein C, protein C inhibitor complexes, antithrombin III and antithrombin III in factor Xa/thrombin complexes are all feasible but usually unnecessary in the common clinical setting. At the present time, management decisions are not usually influenced by these specific findings. It is possible however that, as our understanding of the pathogenesis of the disorder improves, the correctness of the management approach adopted may well be influenced by such findings. For example, although it is critically important to discriminate between primary and secondary generated plasmin activity, the clinical correlates, i.e. the primary disease state, are probably a more reliable indicator than any of the above tests. As the technology improves, however, evidence of fibrinolytic activation in the absence of evidence of thrombin generation may be possible but, given the evidence of plasmin's ability to activate coagulation via activation cleavage of factors V and VIII, this may prove to be extremely difficult.

The approach to the use of laboratory testing for monitoring treatment will be governed in large part by the pace of the condition. In the acute fulminating form, the test systems used must be robust, simple and rapid in performance in order for the physician to make appropriate decisions with regard to replacement and anticoagulant therapy. In the author's experience, this precludes most of the more specific assays and thus reliance is placed on the screening tests such as the PT, PTT and TCT and full blood counts in particular. Such testing should be performed frequently during the acute phase of the condition and then at spaced intervals dictated by the overall clinical response of the patient. It is our practice to keep frozen plasma aliquots from all specimens obtained to permit the retrospective performance of specific assays to assist in the subsequent management of the patient and provide data for retrospective analysis of the pathogenesis of the individual case.

MANAGEMENT

Acute disseminated intravascular coagulation

As DIC usually complicates other pathologies, it is important to recognize the need to institute appropriate therapeutic measures directed at the primary disease as well as attending to basic life support considerations such as fluid and electrolyte balance, adequate oxygenation, etc. Fundamental to the management of the complicating DIC is the implementation of aggressive therapy directed at forestalling or eradicating the primary pathology as the source of the procoagulant stimulus. For example, institution of appropriate antibiotic therapy in specific infections may bring about a spontaneous reversal of the DIC process without additional therapy directed at DIC itself. Removal of the products of conception in obstetric accidents may be the only therapeutic manoeuvre required. Confirmation of this reversal will be gained by clinical assessment and laboratory monitoring using the screening tests previously described. In those patients where the primary pathology is not so amenable to correction or where DIC continues despite an apparently appropriate intervention, therapeutic measures directed at the DIC itself will be required. The overall approach is to restrain and eventually eliminate thrombin generation and replace blood components whose deficiency might either promote the haemorrhagic tendency or diminish the physiological anticoagulant response in endogenously regulating thrombin generation.

Clearly, removal of the procoagulant stimulus markedly influences the degree of thrombin generation. Consequently, this should be the primary objective of therapy wherever this is feasible. At times, this may only be achieved by making procedures such as surgical intervention possible by aggressive blood component replacement therapy to reverse hypotension, anaemia, etc. The use of heparin to limit thrombin's procoagulant effects remains controversial. There are many reports of apparent success attending its use (Colman et al 1974). In particular, purpura fulminans, a fulminating and lethal form of DIC has been shown to be dramatically responsive to heparin by a number of investigators after the initial observation by Little in 1959. Subsequent experience of its use in other forms of acute DIC have been supported by some and rejected by others (Corrigan et al 1973, Colman et al 1979, Corrigan 1977). One of the principal difficulties lies with the absence of adequate means of monitoring dosage. In normal circumstances, patients on heparin therapy are monitored by laboratory tests such as the PTT and TCT and clinically for evidence of bleeding, suggesting overdosage (Hirsh 1991). In patients with DIC, neither approach is feasible as the tests are already abnormal and the justification for heparin usage is commonly related to existing excessive haemorrhage. Arbitrary protocols of an initial bolus of 10 000 units intravenously followed by 1000 units per hour are advocated (Colman et al 1972) but evidence of increased heparin resistance in some patients makes the institution of a fixed protocol approach unreliable (Hanada et al 1985) and may explain the marked disagreement in opinion with regard to modifying outcome. There is a clear need to develop laboratory tests for measuring thrombin generation directly that are rapid, easy to perform and monitor the efficacy of heparin in this condition. It may well be feasible to develop such systems for the measurement of prothrombin activation products such as fragment 1 + 2 (Bauer & Rosenberg 1987). At the present time a reasonable compromise is to consider the use of heparin in those patients where it is clear that the source of the procoagulant stimulus cannot be readily contained or where the rate of DIC is so fulminant that replacement therapy cannot keep pace with the loss through haemorrhage. As an alternative to therapy directed at inhibiting thrombin activity, there is currently major interest in the use of replacement therapy with concentrates of protein C. This approach is based on the evidence that protein C is activated and consumed during DIC (Griffin et al 1982). Given its essential physiological role in regulating thrombin generation, on theoretical grounds alone it would be reasonable to assume that restoration of depleted levels of this physiological anticoagulant may be beneficial. In studies in an animal model of Gram-negative shock, Taylor and co-workers have provided persuasive evidence that this is indeed the case (Taylor et al 1987). Infusion of baboons with thrombin to provide endogenous activation of protein C or the infusion of pre-activated protein C offered significant protection from the gram-negative shock induced by the infusion of lethal doses of *Escherischia coli*. Furthermore, inhibition of protein C activation by the pre-infusion of a monoclonal antibody, that prevents protein C activation and promotes thrombin generation (Taylor et al 1992), increased the toxicity of sub-lethal doses of *Esch.coli*. Of particular interest was the finding that the protective effects of activated protein C were apparently not limited to the prevention of the coagulant component of the syndrome, suggesting that protein C plays an additional role to that of limiting thrombin generation (Esmon et al 1991). Alternatively, the effects of thrombin may have pathological significance beyond its role in generating fibrin. These studies strongly suggest the beneficial role for protein C replacement therapy in patients with DIC. To date, clinical experience with such an approach is extremely limited but appears promising (Okajima et al 1990). In the same context the association of antithrombin III deficiency that occurs in such patients has also suggested the need to consider replacement therapy with a concentrate of antithrombin III. Such concentrates are available but to date their efficacy in the management of patients with DIC has not been clearly established (Schipper & ten Cate 1982, Buller & ten Cate 1983, Blauhut et al 1985).

Replacement of factors V and VIII and fibrinogen using fresh frozen plasma or cryoprecipitate is clearly essential in the acutely bleeding patient with evidence of major consumption of these factors. Nonetheless, such therapy is not without controversy. This relates to the concern that the result of replacing such factors is to 'stoke the fire' inferring that the hypocoagulable state induced by DIC protects the individual from further thrombin generation. There is now a consensus that not only is this view theoretically questionable but the exchange for a life-threatening haemorrhagic diathesis is unacceptable. Currently, opinion rests between either replacement after initiating anticoagulant therapy (except in those situations where the source of the procoagulant stimulus has clearly been removed), or replacement therapy as a primary approach. In the latter, anticoagulation is instituted only in those patients where replacement alone may be predictably inadequate or proves to be so as the condition progresses. Examples would be women with DIC associated with choriocarcinoma where with modern chemotherapy the prospects for eradicating the tumour and the associated procoagulant activity are excellent but cannot be achieved with immediacy. Other examples may occur in association with any of the known primary disease conditions where the severity and rate of consumption is so great that it becomes physically impossible to keep pace with replacement. Patients with amniotic fluid embolism are classic examples of this situation. Of the two approaches, the author currently favours the latter, i.e. reserving heparinization for selected patients. This approach relates specificly to concerns related to the control of therapy in an acutely bleeding and compromised patient and not to the basic principle of controlling thrombin activity which should be emphasized as the ultimate goal of therapy in this condition. Despite the reservations relating to therapeutic control, in those conditions where the thrombotic tendency appears to predominate, such as purpura fulminans, the use of heparin may be life-saving (Little 1959). This observation together with the association of this condition with homozygous deficiency of protein C underlines the physiological importance of the protein C system and suggests that the use of protein C concentrates may assume a significant role in the management of these conditions in the future. Moreover, although optimal replacement would not be achieved with the use of fresh frozen plasma alone, some degree of replacement would be achieved which could explain why, in the author's experience, supplementation of replacement therapy by heparin is not always necessary despite theoretical predictions to the contrary. One other difficulty of replacement therapy deserves a mention. Materials that contain fibrinogen, factor VIII and V such as fresh frozen plasma and cryoprecipitate are difficult to sterilize and may therefore contain viruses such as HIV, HBV and HCV. Although sterilized concentrates of fibrinogen and factor VIII are available, if they are not the decision to expose patients to viral infections must be made on clinical grounds in the light of prevailing local blood donor safety.

It has also been suggested that reduction in the levels of

fibronectin compromise RES activity which theoretically would reduce the clearance of activated clotting factors and other products of coagulation and fibrinolysis (Mosesson & Amrani 1980). Reduced levels of fibronectin have been reported in patients with DIC and low concentrations appear to correlate with a poor prognosis (Cembrowski & Mosherb 1984, O'Connell et al 1984). Replacement with fibronectin-rich products such as cryoprecipitate has been advocated (Saba et al 1978). As with many other treatment modalities in this condition, well-controlled clinical studies directed at confirming the validity of this approach do not appear to be available.

The approach recommended is summarized in Figure 42.2. The overall goal of therapy is to remove the source of the procoagulant stimulus. In some situations, this will be the sole approach required. In the majority, however, a balanced approach is required to restrain either thrombin generation or activity and restore the level of consumed haemostatic factors that promote the haemorrhagic tendency. The use of heparin remains controversial primarily due to difficulties in the clinical and laboratory monitoring of its effects. In the future, it is possible that test systems will become available that will remedy these difficulties and dramatically change the efficacy of this approach. Even more promising is the potential for controlling the coagulant response by the use of therapeutic concentrates of physiological inhibitors such as protein C and tissue factor pathway inhibitor. Furthermore, as our knowledge of the basic mechanisms of haemostasis improve, a less empirical approach to the problem may result. It is sobering to realize that the overall mortality of this condition is still of the order of 70% despite the major improvements that have occurred in the intensive care setting, infection control, etc. Unfortunately, the comments that the letters 'DIC' could be taken as standing for 'Death Is Coming' (Spero et al 1980) is not an unreasonable reminder of the progress that remains to be made in our understanding and management of this not uncommon condition.

Chronic disseminated intravascular coagulation

Patients with laboratory evidence of DIC alone, rarely require therapeutic intervention. The basic approach is to institute clinical and laboratory monitoring in order to intercept acute exacerbations of the condition. As this occurs not infrequently in the presence of terminal and/or metastatic malignancy, clearly judgement must be exercised with regard to the intensity of surveillance in the context of the overall approach to palliation. Where the condition becomes symptomatic, and thrombotic and/or haemorrhagic manifestations require treatment, anticoagulation with heparin has been used with good effect.

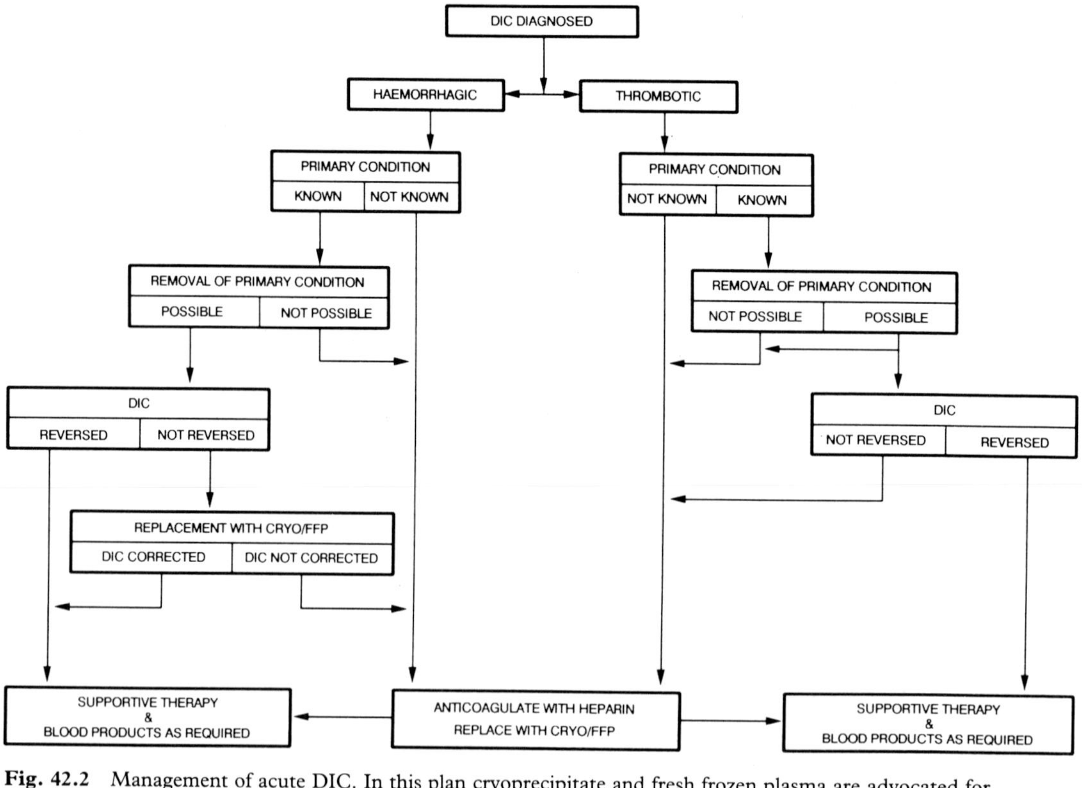

Fig. 42.2 Management of acute DIC. In this plan cryoprecipitate and fresh frozen plasma are advocated for replacement purposes. These may be contaminated with viruses and their use should balance the clinical requirement against the risk from local donors. CRYO, cryoprecipitate; FFP, fresh frozen plasma.

It is generally recommended that the subcutaneous route be used and the lowest possible dose of heparin, required to contain the condition, employed. The use of oral anticoagulants, although more convenient, appears to be less effective (Mosesson et al 1968). Antifibrinolytic therapy, although advocated by some, is, in the author's opinion, contraindicated in this situation as it is highly likely that it would convert a relatively sub-clinical condition into an acute thrombotic disease.

Primary fibrinolysis

As previously discussed (p. 974) anti-fibrinolytic therapy is now rarely, if ever, used in DIC. The concern with its use relates to documented evidence of major thrombotic risk following the use of such agents (Naeye 1962, Gralnick & Greipp 1971). Moreover, there is increasing evidence that the fibrinolytic response, although associated with some undesirable side-effects, is an essential physiological response to the thrombotic state. Consequently, regulation of this will in turn regulate fibrinolysis and its associated side-effects. As previously discussed, in some instances there would appear to be evidence of primary fibrinogenolysis. The key issue then becomes the validity of diagnosis which will rest largely on the assessment of the clinical history given that laboratory testing at the present time cannot discriminate between the primary and secondary states. Recent evidence suggests the prophylactic use of trasylol in surgical patients reduces the incidence and severity of postoperative bleeding (Woodman & Harker 1990). This agent has broad specificity antiproteolytic activity including inhibition of the enzymes of the fibrinolytic system (Dubber et al 1968). These data are consequently of major interest but further investigation is required before any recommendation can be made with regard to its use in patients with established DIC.

REVIEW ARTICLES

Bick R L 1978 Disseminated intravascular coagulation and related syndromes: etiology, pathophysiology, diagnosis and management. American Journal of Hematology 5: 265

Bowie E J W, Owen C A 1983 The clinical pathology of intravascular coagulation. Bibliotheca Haematologica 49: 217

Colman R W, Robboy S J, Minna J D 1972 Disseminated intravascular coagulation (DIC): an approach. American Journal of Medicine 52: 679

Colman R W, Robboy S J, Minna J D 1979 Disseminated intravascular coagulation: a reappraisal. Annual Reviews in Medicine 30: 359

Deykin D 1970 The clinical challenge of disseminated intravascular coagulation. New England Journal of Medicine 283: 636

Feinstein D I 1982 Diagnosis and management of disseminated intravascular coagulation: the role of heparin therapy. Blood 60: 284

Hamilton P J, Stalker A L, Douglas A S 1978 Disseminated intravascular coagulation: A review. Journal of Clinical Pathology 31: 609

Hardaway R M 1966 Syndromes of disseminated intravascular coagulation with special reference to shock and hemorrhage, C C Thomas, Springfield

McKay D G 1965 Disseminated intravascular coagulation. Harper-Hoeber, New York p 493

Merskey C, Johnson A J, Kleiner G J et al 1967 The defibrination syndrome: Clinical features and laboratory diagnosis. British Journal of Haematology 13: 528

Merskey C 1973 Defibrination syndrome or . . . ? Blood 41: 599

Sharp A A 1977 Diagnosis and management of disseminated intravascular coagulation. British Medical Bulletin 33: 265

Verstraete M, Vermylen C, Vermylen J et al 1965 Excessive consumption of blood coagulation components as cause of hemorrhagic diathesis. American Journal of Medicine 35: 899

REFERENCES

Abbink J J, Kamp A M, Swaak A J G et al 1991 Production of monoclonal antibodies against inactivated alpha-1-antitrypsin. Journal of Immunological Methods 143: 197

Astrup T 1956 The biological significance of fibrinolysis. Lancet 2: 565

Baker W G, Bang N U, Nachman R L et al 1964 Hypofibrinogenemic hemorrhage in acute myelogenous leukemia treated with heparin: With autopsy findings of widespread intravascular clotting. Annals of Internal Medicine 61: 116

Bauer K A, Rosenberg R D 1984 Thrombin generation in acute promyelocytic leukemia. Blood 64: 791

Bauer K A, Rosenberg R D 1987 The pathophysiology of the prethrombotic state in humans: Insights gained from studies using markers of hemostatic system activation. Blood 70: 343

Blauhut B, Kramar H, Vinazzer H et al 1985 Substitution of antithrombin III in shock and DIC: A randomized study. Thrombosis Research 39: 81

Bonnar J 1973 Blood Coagulation and Fibrinolysis in Obstetrics. Clinical Haematology 2: 213

Bonnar J 1976 Coagulation Disorders. Journal of Clinical Pathology 29 (suppl 10): 35

Broekmans A W, Veltkamp J J, Bertina R M 1983 Congenital protein C deficiency and venous thromboembolism. New England Journal of Medicine 309: 340

Bull B S, Brain M C 1968 Experimental models of microangiopathic haemolytic anaemia. Proceedings of the Royal Society of Medicine 61: 1134

Buller H R, ten Cate J W 1983 Antithrombin III infusion in patients undergoing peritoneovenous shunt operation: failure in the prevention of disseminated intravascular coagulation. Thrombosis and Haemostasis 49: 128

Cederbaum A I, Roberts H R 1973 Complications of the use of prothrombin complex concentrates in liver diseases. Clinical Research 21: 92

Cederbaum A I, Blatt P M, Roberts H R 1976 Intravascular coagulation with use of human prothrombin complex concentrates. Annals of Internal Medicine 84: 683

Cembrowski G S, Mosherb D F 1984 Plasma fibronectin concentration in patients with acquired consumptive coagulopathies. Thrombosis Research 36: 437

Colman R W, Robboy S J, Minna J D 1972 Disseminated intravascular coagulation (DIC): An approach. American Journal of Medicine 52: 679

Colman R W, Robboy S J, Minna J D 1974 Therapy of clinically significant disseminated intravascular coagulation. In: Ingelfinger F J et al (eds) Controversy in internal medicine II. Saunders, Philadelphia, p 633

Colman R W, Edelman R, Scott G F et al 1978 Plasma kallikrein

activation and inhibition during typhoid fever. Journal of Clinical Investigation 61: 287
Colman R W, Robboy S J, Minna J D 1979 Disseminated intravascular coagulation: A reappraisal. Annual Review of Medicine 30: 359
Corrigan J J 1977 Heparin therapy in bacterial septicemia. Journal of Pediatrics 91: 695
Corrigan J J, Jordan C M, Bennett B B 1973 Disseminated intravascular coagulation in septic shock: Report of three cases not treated with heparin. American Journal of Diseases in Childhood 126: 629
Crosby W H, Stefanini M 1952 Pathogenesis of the plasma transfusion reaction with special reference to the blood coagulation system. Journal of Laboratory and Clinical Medicine 40: 374
Dairaku M, Sueishi K, Tanaka K 1982 Disseminated intravascular coagulation in newborn infants: Prevalence in autopsies and significance as a cause of death. Pathology, Research and Practice 174: 106
Damus P S, Hicks M, Rosenberg R D 1973 Anticoagulant action of heparin. Nature 246: 355
Davidson J F, McNicol G P, Frank G L et al 1969 Plasminogen-activator-producing tumour. British Medical Journal 1: 88
Dennis L H, Eichelberger J W, Inman M M et al 1967 Depletion of coagulation factors in drug-resistant Plasmodium falciparum malaria. Blood 29: 713
Deykin D 1974 Emerging concepts of platelet function. New England Journal of Medicine 290: 144
Dubber A H C, McNicol G P, Uttley D et al 1968 In vitro and in vivo studies with trasylol, an anticoagulant and a fibrinolytic inhibitor. British Journal of Haematology 14: 31
Edgington T S 1991 The structural biology of expression and function of tissue factor. Thrombosis and Haemostasis 66: 67
Ekoe J M, Cunningham M, Jaques O et al 1985 Disseminated intravascular coagulation and acute myocardial necrosis caused by lightning. Intensive Care Medicine 11: 160
Esmon C T 1989 The roles of protein C and thrombomodulin in the regulation of blood coagulation. Journal of Biological Chemistry 264: 4743
Esmon C T, Taylor F B, Snow T R 1991 Inflammation and coagulation: Linked processes potentially regulated through a common pathway mediated by protein C. Thrombosis and Haemostasis 66: 160
Ferguson J H, Chapman O D 1948 Fulminating meningococcic infections and the so-called Waterhouse–Friderichsen syndrome. American Journal of Pathology 24: 763
Fine N L, Applebaum J, Elguezabal A et al 1967 Multiple coagulation defects in association with dissecting aneurysm. Archives in Internal Medicine 119: 522
Foa P, Pellacani P 1884 Sul fermento fibrinogeno: Sulle azioni tossiche, escercitate da alcuni organi freschi. Archivio per le Scienze Mediche (Torino) 7: 113
Franza B R, Aronson D L, Finlayson J B 1975 Activation of human prothrombin by procoagulant factor from the venom of Echis carinatus. Journal of Biological Chemistry 250: 7057
Gailani D, Broze G J 1991 Factor XI activation in a revised model of blood coagulation. Science 253: 909
Giles A R, Hoogendoorn H, Blajchman M A 1981 The thrombogenicity of prothrombin complex concentrates: III. The relationship of in vivo thrombogenicity to the nature of the starting plasma. Thrombosis Research 21: 255
Giles A R, Nesheim M E, Hoogendoorn H et al 1982a The coagulant-active phospholipid content is a major determinant of in vivo thrombogenicity of prothrombin complex (factor IX) concentrates in rabbits. Blood 59: 401
Giles A R, Nesheim M E, Hoogendoorn H et al 1982b Stroma-free human platelet lysates potentiate the in vitro thrombogenicity of factor Xa by the provision of coagulant-active phospholipid. British Journal of Haematology 51: 457
Giles A R, Hoogendoorn H, Tinlin S 1984a The thrombogenicity of prothrombin complex concentrates: IV. The source of coagulant-active phospholipid. Thrombosis Research 34: 567
Giles A R, Nesheim M E, Mann K G 1984b Studies of factors V and VIII: C in an animal model of disseminated intravascular coagulation. Journal of Clinical Investigation 74: 2219
Giles A R, Nesheim M E, Herring S W et al 1990 The fibrinolytic potential of the normal primate following the generation of thrombin in vivo. Thrombosis and Haemostasis 63: 476
Gingrich R D, Burns C P 1979 Disseminated coagulopathy in chronic myelomonocytic leukemia. Cancer 44: 2249
Gordon S G, Cross B A 1981 A factor X-activating cysteine protease from malignant tissue. Journal of Clinical Investigation 67: 1665
Gralnick H R, Abrell E 1973 Studies of the procoagulant and fibrinolytic activity of promyelocytes in acute promyelocytic leukaemia. British Journal of Haematology 24: 89
Gralnick H R, Greipp P 1971 Thrombosis with epsilon aminocaproic acid therapy. American Journal of Clinical Pathology 56: 151
Gralnick H R, Bagley J, Abrell E 1972 Heparin treatment for the hemorrhagic diathesis of acute promyelocytic leukemia. American Journal of Medicine 52: 167
Greenberg C S, Achyuthan K E, Fenton J W 1987 Factor XIIIa formation promoted by complexing of alpha-thrombin, fibrin and plasma factor XIII. Blood 69: 867
Griffin J H, Mosher D F, Zimmerman T S et al 1982 Protein C, an antithrombotic protein, is reduced in hospitalized patients with intravascular coagulation. Blood 60: 261
Griffith M J 1983 Heparin-catalyzed inhibitor/protease reactions: Kinetic evidence for a common mechanism of action of heparin. Proceedings of the National Academy of Sciences, USA 80: 5460
Guarini A, Baccarani M, Corbelli G et al 1980 Defibrination in adult acute lymphoblastic leukaemia: Report of four cases. Nouvelle Revue de Françoise d'Hematologie 22: 115
Hall W H 1965 Purpura fulminans with group B β-hemolytic streptococcal endocarditis. Archives in Internal Medicine 116: 594
Hanada T, Abe T, Takita H 1985 Antithrombin III concentrates for treatment of disseminated intravascular coagulation in children. American Journal of Pediatric Hematology and Oncology 7: 3
Harker L A 1986 Bleeding after cardiopulmonary bypass. New England Journal of Medicine 314: 1446
Hedner U, Kisiel W K 1983 Use of human factor VIIa in the treatment of two hemophilia A patients with high-titre inhibitors. Journal of Clinical Investigation 71: 1836
Heeb M J, Mosher D, Griffin J H 1989 Activation and complexation of protein C and cleavage and decrease of protein S in plasma of patients with intravascular coagulation. Blood 73: 455
Heimark R L, Kurachi K, Fujikawa K et al 1980 Surface activation of blood coagulation, fibrinolysis and kinin formation. Nature 286: 456
Hirsh J 1991 Heparin. New England Journal of Medicine 324: 1565
Hoffman C, Hultin M B 1986 Factor IX concentrate therapy and thrombosis: relation to changes in antithrombin III. Thrombosis Research 43: 143
Hoogendoorn H, Nesheim M E, Giles A R 1990 A qualitative and quantitative analysis of the activation and inactivation of protein C in vivo in a primate model. Blood 75: 2164
Hoogendoorn H, Toh C H, Nesheim M E et al 1991 Alpha-2 macroglobulin binds and inhibits activated protein C. Blood 78: 2283
Kaplan A P 1978 Initiation of the intrinsic coagulation and fibrinolytic pathways of man: The role of surfaces, Hageman factor, prekallikrein, high molecular weight kininogen and factor XI. In: Spaet T H (ed) Progress in hemostasis and thrombosis. Grune & Stratton, New York p 127–175
Kasper C K 1975 Thromboembolic complications. Thrombosis et Diathesis Haemorrhagica 33: 640
Kisiel W K, Hermodson M A, Davie E W 1976 Factor X activating enzyme from Russell's viper venom: Isolation and characterization. Biochemistry 15: 4901
Krevans J R, Jackson D P, Conley C L et al 1957 The nature of the hemorrhagic disorders accompanied by hemolytic transfusions in man. Blood 12: 834
Lahnborg G, Berghem L, Lagergren H et al 1976 Influence of thrombin-induced disseminated intravascular coagulation on RES functions in rabbits. Thrombosis Research 9: 653
Lee C D, Mann K G 1989 Activation/inactivation of human factor V by plasmin. Blood 73: 185
Leveen H H 1985 The LeVeen Shunt. Annual Reviews in Medicine 36: 453
Levin E G, Stern D M, Nawroth P P et al 1986 Specificity of the thrombin-induced release of tissue plasminogen activator from

cultured human endothelial cells. Thrombosis and Haemostasis 56: 115
Little J R 1959 Purpura fulminans treated successfully with anticoagulation: Report of a case. Journal of the American Medical Association 169: 36
Lyon M E, Giles A R 1991 The characterisation of the anticoagulant effect of activated protein C resulting from the generation of thrombin in vivo (unpublished work)
McKay D G 1965 Disseminated intravascular coagulation. Harper-Hoeber New York p 493
McKay D G 1973 Vessel wall and thrombogenesis – endotoxin. Thrombosis et Diathesis Haemorrhagica 29: 11
McKay D G, Margaretten W 1967 Disseminated intravascular coagulation in virus disease. Archives of Internal Medicine 120: 129
Madden R M, Ward M, Marlar R A 1989 Protein C activity levels in endotoxin-induced disseminated intravascular coagulation in a dog model. Thrombosis Research 55: 297
Mangal A K, Grossman L, Vickars L 1984 Disseminated intravascular coagulation in acute monoblastic leukemia: Response to heparin therapy. Canadian Medical Association Journal 130: 731
Mann K G 1984 Membrane-bound enzyme complexes in blood coagulation. In: Spaet T H (ed) Progress in hemostasis and thrombosis. Grune & Stratton, Orlando, p 1–23
Mann K G, Nesheim M E, Church W R et al 1990 Surface-dependent reactions of the vitamin K-dependent enzyme complexes. Blood 76: 1
Mannucci P M, Lubina G F, Caocci L et al 1969 Effect on blood coagulation of massive intravascular haemolysis. Blood 33: 207
Mannucci P M, Bauer K A, Gringeri A et al 1990 Thrombin generation is not increased in the blood of hemophilia B patients after the infusion of a purified factor IX concentrate. Blood 76: 2540
Marciniak E 1973 Factor-Xa inactivation by antithrombin III: Evidence for biological stabilization of factor Xa by factor V-phospholipid complex. British Journal of Haematology 24: 391
Marciniak E, Farley C H, De Simone P A 1974 Familial thrombosis due to antithrombin III deficiency. Blood 43: 219
Marcum J A, Atha D H, Fritze L M S et al 1986 Cloned bovine aortic endothelial cells synthesize anticoagulantly active heparan sulfate proteoglycan. Journal of Biological Chemistry 268: 7507
Mason J W, Kleeberg U, Dolan P et al 1970 Plasma kallikrein and Hageman factor in Gram-negative sepsis. Annals of Internal Medicine 73: 545
Merskey C, Kleiner G J, Johnson A J 1966 Quantitative estimation of split products of fibrinogen in human serum: Relation to diagnosis and treatment. Blood 28: 1
Minerbrook M, Budman D R, Schulman P et al 1983 De novo disseminated intravascular coagulation in angioimmunoblastic lymphadenopathy (AILD). Cancer 51: 1927
Moore K L, Andreoli S P, Esmon N L et al 1987 Endotoxin enhances tissue factor and suppresses thrombomodulin expression of human vascular endothelium in vitro. Journal of Clinical Investigation 79: 124
Mosesson M W, Amrani D L 1980 The structure and biologic activities of plasma fibronectin. Blood 56: 145
Mosesson M W, Colman R W, Sherry S 1968 Chronic intravascular coagulation syndrome: Report of a case with special studies of an associated plasma cryoprecipitate ('cryofibrinogen'). New England Journal of Medicine 278: 815
Muhlfelder T W, Khan I, Niemetz J 1978 Factors influencing the release of procoagulant-tissue factor activity from leukocytes. Journal of Laboratory and Clinical Medicine 92: 65
Murray H W, Tuazon C V, Sheagren J N 1977 Staphylococcal septicemia and disseminated intravascular coagulation. Archives of Internal Medicine 137: 844
Naeye R L 1962 Thrombotic state after a hemorrhagic diathesis, a possible complication of therapy with epsilon-aminocaproic acid. Blood 19: 694
Nauyn B 1873 Unterschungen Ober Blutgerinnung I.M. Lebenden Tiere und Ihre Folgen. Archiv for Experimentalle Pathologie und Pharmakologie 1: 1
Nemerson Y 1988 Tissue Factor and Hemostasis. Blood 71: 1
Nesheim M E, Mann K G 1979 Thrombin-catalyzed activation of single chain bovine factor V. Journal of Biological Chemistry 254: 1326
Nesheim M E, Pittman D D, Wang G H et al 1988 The binding of 35S-labeled recombinant factor VIII to activated and unactivated human platelets. Journal of Biological Chemistry 263: 16467
Newball H H, Revak S D, Cochrane C G 1978 Activation of human Hageman factor by a leukocytic protease. In: Fuju S, Muriya H, Suzuki T (eds) Kinins-II systemic proteases and cellular function. Plenum Press, New York, vol 120B: 139
Nieuwenhuizen W 1986 The use of monoclonal antibodies in demonstrating different fibrinogen derivatives. In: Berghaus-Muller G, Scheefers-Borchel U, Selmayr E, Henschen A (eds) Fibrinogen and its derivatives. Elsevier Science, Amsterdam, p 245–256
Niewiarowski S, Stuart R K, Thomas D P 1966 Activation of intravascular coagulation by collagen. Proceedings of the Society for Experimental Biology and Medicine 123: 196
Oates A M, Salem H H 1987 The regulation of human factor V by a neutrophil protease. Blood 70: 832
O'Brien D P, Giles A R, Tate K M et al 1988 Factor VIII-bypassing activity of bovine tissue factor using the canine hemophilic model. Journal of Clinical Investigation 82: 206
O'Connell M T, Becker D M, Steele B W et al 1984 Plasma fibronectin in medical ICU patients. Critical Care medicine 12: 479
O'Donnell T F Jr, Clowes G H A, Talamo R C et al 1976 Kinin activation in the blood of patients with sepsis. Surgical Gynecology and Obstetrics 143: 538
Oka K, Tanaka K 1977 Intravascular coagulation in autopsy cases with liver diseases. Thrombosis and Haemostasis 4: 29
Okajima K, Imamura H, Koga S et al 1990 Treatment of patients with disseminated intravascular coagulation by protein C. American Journal of Hematology 33: 277
Østerud B, Rapaport S I 1980 Activation of 125-I-factor IX and 125-I-factor X: Effect of tissue factor and factor VII, factor Xa and thrombin. Scandinavian Journal of Haematology 24: 213
Pineo G F, Regoeczi E, Hatton M W C et al 1973 The activation of coagulation by extracts of mucus: a possible pathway of intravascular coagulation accompanying adenocarcinomas. Journal of Laboratory and Clinical Medicine 82: 255
Preston E F, Malia R G, Sworn M J et al 1973 Intravascular coagulation and E. coli septicaemia. Journal of Clinical Pathology 26: 120
Rabiner S F, Friedman L H 1968 The role of intravascular haemolysis and the reticulo-endothelial system in the production of a hypercoagulable state. British Journal of Haematology 14: 105
Rabiner S F, O'Brien K, Peskin G W et al 1970 Further studies with stroma-free hemoglobin solution. Annals of Surgery 171: 615
Ragni M V, Lewis J H, Spero J A 1983 Ascites-induced LeVeen shunt coagulopathy. Annals of Surgery 198: 91
Rapaport S I 1989 Inhibition of factor VIIa/tissue factor-induced blood coagulation: with particular emphasis upon a factor Xa-dependent inhibitory mechanism. Blood 73: 359
Rapaport S I 1991 The extrinsic pathway inhibitor: a regulator of tissue factor dependent blood coagulation. Thrombosis and Haemostasis 66: 6
Ratnoff O D 1987 John Hageman (1916–1968). Journal of Laboratory and Clinical Medicine 109: 519
Repke D, Gemmell C H, Guha A et al 1990 Hemophilia as a defect of the tissue factor pathway of blood coagulation: Effect of factors VIII and IX on factor X activation in a continuous-flow reactor. Proceedings of the National Academy of Sciences, USA 87: 7623
Rick M E, Krizek D M 1986 Platelets modulate the proteolysis of factor VIII:C protein by plasmin. Blood 67: 1649
Rickles F R, Edwards R L 1983 Activation of blood coagulation in cancer: Trousseau's syndrome revisited. Blood 62: 14
Rosing J, Speijer H, Zwaal R F A 1988 Prothrombin activation on phospholipid membranes with positive electrostatic potential. Biochemistry 27: 8
Saba T M, Blumenstock F A, Scovill W A et al 1978 Cryoprecipitate reversal of opsonic alpha-2-surface binding glycoprotein deficiency in septic surgical and trauma patients. Science 201: 622
Sack G H, Levin J, Bell W R 1977 Trousseau's syndrome and other manifestations of chronic disseminated coagulopathy in patients with neoplasms: Clinical, pathologic and therapeutic features. Medicine (Baltimore) 56: 1

Salz-Steiner D, Eldor A, Vangrover D et al 1984 Disseminated intravascular coagulation in two patients with histiocytic medullary reticulosis. American Journal of Clinical Pathology 82: 119

Sanders N L, Bajaj S P, Zivelin A et al 1985 Inhibition of Tissue factor/factor VIIa activity in plasma requires factor X and an additional plasma component. Blood 66: 204

Sandset P M, Warn-Cramer B J, Rao L V M et al 1991 Depletion of extrinsic pathway inhibitor (EPI) sensitizes rabbits to disseminated intravascular coagulation induced with tissue factor: Evidence supporting a physiological role for EPI as a natural anticoagulant. Proceedings of the National Academy of Sciences, USA 88: 708

Schaffner W, McLeod A C, Koenig M G 1965 Thrombocytopenic Rocky Mountain spotted fever. Archives in Internal Medicine 116: 857

Schipper H G, ten Cate J W 1982 Antithrombin III transfusion in patients with hepatic cirrhosis. British Journal of Haematology 52: 25

Scully M F, Hoogendoorn H, Solymoss S et al 1991 Decrease in factor V activity associated with protein C activation and complex formation during cardio-pulmonary bypass surgery. Thrombosis and Haemostasis 65(6): 1028 (abstract)

Scully M F, Toh C H, Hoogendoorn H et al 1992 Activation of protein C and its distribution between its inhibitors, protein C Inhibitor, alpha-1 antitrypsin and alpha-2 macroglobulin, in patients with disseminated intravascular coagulation. (in press)

Spero J A, Lewis J H, Hasiba U 1980 Disseminated intravascular coagulation: findings in 346 patients. Thrombosis and Haemostasis 43: 28

Sterrenberg L, Haak H L, Brommer E J et al 1985 Evidence of fibrinogen breakdown by leukocyte enzymes in a patient with acute promyelocytic leukemia. Haemostasis 15: 126

Taylor F B, Chang A, Esmon C T et al 1987 Protein C prevents the coagulopathic and lethal effects of Escherichia coli infusion in the baboon. Journal of Clinical Investigation 79: 918

Taylor F B, Hoogendoorn H, Chang A C K et al 1992 Anticoagulant and fibrinolytic activities are promoted not retarded in vivo following thrombin generation in the presence of a monoclonal antibody that inhibits activation of protein C. Blood (in press)

Tollefsen D M, Blank M K 1981 Detection of a new heparin-dependent inhibitor of thrombin in human plasma. Journal of Clinical Investigation 68: 589

Tracy P B, Peterson J M, Nesheim M E et al 1979 Interaction of coagulation factor V and factor Va with platelets. Journal of Biological Chemistry 254: 10354

Triantaphyllopoulos D C 1972 Intravascular coagulation following injection of prothrombin complex. American Journal of Clinical Pathology 57: 603

Trousseau A 1865 Phlegmasia alba dolens. Clinique Medicale de l'Hotel-Dieu de Paris London, The New Sydenham Society 3: 94

Walker F J, Scandella D, Fay P J 1990 Identification of the binding site for activated protein C on the light chain of factors V and VIII. Journal of Biological Chemistry 265: 1484

Warr T A, Rao L V M, Rapaport S I 1989 Human plasma extrinsic pathway inhibitor activity: II. Plasma levels in disseminated intravascular coagulation and hepatocellular disease. Blood 74: 994

Weber M B, Blakeley J A 1969 The hemorrhagic diathesis of heat stroke: a consumption coagulopathy successfully treated with heparin. Lancet 1: 1190

Wessler S, Yin E T 1968 Experimental hypercoagulable state induced by factor X: comparison of the nonactivated and activated forms. Journal of Laboratory and Clinical Medicine 72: 256

Wiggins R C, Loskutoff D J, Cochrane C G et al 1980 Activation of rabbit Hageman factor by homogenates of cultured rabbit endothelial cells. Journal of Clinical Investigation 65: 197

Wilner G D, Nossel H L, Leroy E D 1968 Activation of Hageman factor by collagen. Journal of Clinical Investigation 47: 2608

Wiman B, Collen D 1978 Molecular mechanism of physiological fibrinolysis. Nature 272: 549

Woodman R C, Harker L A 1990 Bleeding complications associated with cardiopulmonary bypass. Blood 76: 1680

43. Haemostasis and thrombosis in pregnancy

I. A. Greer

PHYSIOLOGICAL CHANGES IN THE COAGULATION SYSTEM IN PREGNANCY

Normal pregnancy is associated with major changes in the coagulation and fibrinolytic systems. These have traditionally been thought to represent an adaptive and preparatory mechanism for the haemostatic challenge of delivery. The physiological changes in each of the components of the haemostatic system in normal pregnancy will be examined in turn.

Platelets

Platelet count does not change significantly during pregnancy (Hellgren & Blomback 1981, Beller & Ebert 1982, Stirling et al 1984), although there may be a slight fall towards the end of the 3rd trimester (Fay et al 1983) in keeping with reports of a trend towards a reduction in platelet lifespan (Wallenburg & van Kessel 1978, Rakoczi et al 1979). The increase in mean platelet volume and volume distribution width (Fay et al 1983, Sill et al 1985, Singer et al 1986, Tygart et al 1986) also suggests that a compensated state of progressive platelet destruction occurs during the 3rd trimester. This may be supported by the enhanced platelet reactivity reported by some studies in normal pregnancy (Morrison et al 1985, Burgess-Wilson et al 1986), although others have reported that platelet reactivity is unchanged (Whigham et al 1978, Greer et al 1988). However, as studies of platelet reactivity ex vivo are unlikely to be an ideal representation of platelet function in vivo, these discrepancies may largely reflect different methodologies. O'Brien et al (1986) have shown that circulating platelet aggregates are increased in normal pregnancy, in keeping with enhanced reactivity in vivo, while ex vivo platelet reactivity was simultaneously reduced, probably reflecting a degree of platelet exhaustion secondary to enhanced activation in vivo. In vivo activation in late pregnancy is also supported by increased plasma levels of β-thromboglobulin (reflecting in vivo platelet activation and degranulation) in the 2nd and 3rd trimester compared to the 1st trimester and non-pregnant levels (Douglas et al 1982). Thus, normal pregnancy is associated with a degree of enhanced platelet destruction which is compensated for by increased production. Following the haemostatic challenge of delivery, platelet count increases (Hellgren & Blombäck 1981) in reaction to, and in compensation for, platelet consumption.

Coagulation system changes

Factor XIII, high molecular weight kininogen and prekallikrein increase in pregnancy although reports on the last have not been entirely consistent with some authors reporting no change in prekallikrein levels (Hellgren & Blombäck 1981, Sayama et al 1981, Adam et al 1985). Factor XI levels fall gradually through pregnancy reaching their nadir at term (Hellgren & Blombäck 1981). Factor IX remains static or increases slightly (Beller & Ebert 1982). Both factor VIII coagulant activity and von Willebrand factor antigen increase progressively as pregnancy advances (Hellgren & Blombäck 1981, Stirling et al 1984). These increases in the two components of the factor VIII complex appear to occur in parallel in the first half of pregnancy, but then diverge due to a greater increase in von Willebrand factor antigen. This increases the ratio of von Willebrand factor antigen:factor VIII coagulant activity (Hellgren & Blombäck 1981, Inglis et al 1982, Stirling et al 1984) from one (the non-pregnant and early pregnancy value) to around two. Factor VII also increase in pregnancy (Stirling et al 1984, Beller & Ebert 1982).

Factor X increases while factors II and V do not change in pregnancy (Hellgren & Blombäck 1981, Stirling et al 1984). Fibrinogen increases substantially and progressively with gestation and a significant change is evident from the 1st trimester with an almost two-fold increase over non-pregnant levels by term (Hellgren & Blombäck 1981, Stirling et al 1984). Factor XIII shows an initial increase but then falls to normal non-pregnant values in late pregnancy (Persson et al 1980).

The endogenous inhibitor of coagulation, antithrombin III, was initially thought to decrease in pregnancy; however, more recent studies show that levels do not appear to change in pregnancy (Hellgren & Blombäck 1981, Weiner & Brandt 1982, Stirling et al 1984). Although antithrombin III may increase following delivery (Hellgren & Blombäck 1981), this has not been a consistent finding (Weenink et al 1982). Protein C levels remain constant or increase slightly (Mannucci et al 1984, Gonzalez et al 1985, Malm et al 1988). Protein S normally exists in plasma in two forms; the functionally active, free protein S and protein S complexed with C4b-binding protein which is functionally inactive. Normally an equilibrium exists in plasma between these two forms. In normal pregnancy there is a reduction in protein S activity and this appears to be due to a reduction in total protein S as measured antigenically rather than a change in C4b-binding protein (Comp et al 1986).

Fibrinolysis

Overall fibrinolytic activity is impaired during pregnancy, but returns rapidly to normal following delivery (Bonnar et al 1969, 1970, Stirling et al 1984). This is due to placentally derived plasminogen activator inhibitor type 2 (PAI-2) which is present in substantial quantities during pregnancy (Lecander & Astedt 1986, Nilsson et al 1986, Booth et al 1988). The endothelial-derived inhibitor of plasminogen activator (PAI-1) increases in pregnancy by around three-fold. Increased levels of t-PA and u-PA have also been reported, although this study was out of keeping with most previous studies as it found no change in overall fibrinolytic activity (Kruithof et al 1987). Plasminogen increases during pregnancy (Bonnar et al 1969, Hellgren & Blombäck 1981, Beller & Ebert 1982) as does antiplasmin. Despite the reduction in fibrinolytic activity, fibrinolysis cannot be completely shut down as FDPs remain present in the plasma with several studies showing that FDPs increase as pregnancy progresses (Woodfield et al 1968, Bonnar et al 1969, Thorburn et al 1982, Stirling et al 1984).

The activity of the fibrinolytic system in response to stimulation of fibrinolysis by venous occlusion has been assessed in pregnancy. Total t-PA release is significantly reduced in pregnancy with free t-PA remaining below the limit of detection of the assay following occlusion (Ballegeer et al 1987). This is in contrast to the non-pregnant situation where both total and free t-PA increase significantly following venous occlusion. These data suggest that t-PA release is impaired in pregnancy and that free t-PA is rapidly inhibited, in keeping with the high levels of plasminogen activator inhibitors noted in pregnancy (p. 988). Despite this impairment in the response to venous occlusion, D-dimer fragment of cross-linked fibrin was substantially increased in the 1st, 2nd, and 3rd trimesters as compared to non-pregnant women (Ballageer et al 1987). This indicates that fibrinolysis is still occurring and clearly is not impaired to the extent suggested by the reduced levels of t-PA and increased PAI-1 and PAI-2.

Impaired fibrinolysis can be found in some patients with a history of deep venous thrombosis (Isacson & Nilsson 1972) and the physiological impairment of fibrinolysis seen in pregnancy may contribute to the increased thrombotic risk associated with pregnancy. Overall, the data discussed in relation to changes in the coagulation and fibrinolytic systems in pregnancy suggest that activation of both systems is occurring with deposition of fibrin and subsequent fibrinolysis with increased levels of FDPs. These changes are compatible with a compensated state of low grade disseminated intravascular coagulation. This is supported by other studies where increased fibrinopeptide A, FDPs and platelet-release products have been found in normal pregnancies indicating coagulation, fibrinolysis and in vivo platelet activation respectively (Gerbasi et al 1990), in keeping with compensated low grade disseminated intravascular coagulation. It is interesting that this study found that fibronectin levels were not increased indicating that despite the low grade disseminated intravascular coagulation, there was no evidence of endothelial damage in contrast to disorders such as pre-eclampsia where low grade disseminated intravascular coagulation is associated with endothelial injury.

The physiological reasons underlying these changes in pregnancy are unclear, but they may be important for the maintenance of the placento-uterine interface or the haemostatic challenge of delivery.

Changes in coagulation and fibrinolysis following delivery

The majority of the pregnancy-related changes in the haemostatic systems revert to normal following separation of the placenta. There is evidence of contact system activation and platelet consumption immediately following delivery, then an increase in fibrinogen, factor VIII:C and platelet count a few days later (Bonnar et al 1970, Hellgren & Blombäck 1981). The fibrinolytic system rapidly returns to normal in keeping with the loss of the placental source of PAI-2 (Wiman et al 1984). The normal non-pregnant state is regained by around 4 weeks after delivery.

CHANGES ASSOCIATED WITH PRE-ECLAMPSIA

Widespread deposition of fibrin associated with vascular damage such as acute atherosis in the placental bed or glomerular endotheliosis, has long been known to be a pathological feature of pre-eclampsia, suggesting that the coagulation system is activated (Davies & Prentice 1992, Greer 1992). This is unlikely to be a primary phenomenon, and probably represents a secondary phenomenon consequent upon vascular damage. Nonetheless it will still contribute to this damage, promoting a positive feedback loop. There is a degree of physiological coagulation system activation in normal pregnancy, and pre-eclampsia may represent an exaggerated form of this process. Routine coagulation tests are essentially normal, unless pre-eclampsia is complicated by full blown disseminated intravascular coagulation (Davies & Prentice 1992). The normal prothrombin time and activated partial thromboplastin time and slightly prolonged thrombin time do not imply that significant coagulation activation is not occurring, as these tests are relatively insensitive. Elevated levels of fibrinopeptide A (Douglas et al 1982), a sensitive indicator of coagulation activation resulting from cleavage of fibrinogen by the action of thrombin, suggest that fibrinogen breakdown occurs in severe disease. Fibrinogen itself also increases in hypertensive compared to normal pregnancy (Howie et al 1971), although this may simply be an acute phase reactant increasing in response to the disease in general. There is an increase in factor VIIIc activity (Howie et al 1971, 1976) but the increase in von Willebrand factor antigen (previously termed factor VIII-related antigen) is greater (Redman et al 1977b). This increased ratio of von Willebrand factor antigen to factor VIIc was initially thought to reflect consumption of factor VIIIc after activation; however, we now know that these two substances are distinct entities which join together in the circulation to form a macromolecular complex. Factor VIII is produced by the liver while von Willebrand factor is synthesized by the vascular endothelium in response to damage. This increase in von Willebrand factor may therefore reflect endothelial damage.

There are no major changes in most of the individual coagulation factors. A prospective study showed that there was slight increase in factor XII and a slight reduction in factors X and XI in women who went on to develop pre-eclampsia (Condie 1976). Antithrombin III is reduced, in keeping with the low grade disseminated intravascular coagulation which occurs (Howie et al 1971, Weiner & Brandt 1987), and correlates with disease severity (Weiner & Brandt 1982). Protein C is also reduced in severe disease (Aznar et al 1986). These data suggest that in general, only minimal coagulation activation occurs, although this may progress to complete disseminated intravascular coagulation in some severe cases.

Activation of the coagulation cascade is usually associated with activation of the fibrinolytic system, and this is true for pre-eclampsia (Davies & Prentice 1991). Concentrations of fibrinogen-fibrin degradation products (Howie et al 1971 and soluble fibrinogen-fibrin complexes (Edgar et al 1977) are increased. The activity of plasminogen activators initially appeared to be normal or slightly reduced in pre-eclampsia compared to normal pregnancy (Bonnar et al 1971, Howie et al 1971), but more precise assays of plasminogen activators and their inhibitors have recently shown unchanged plasma plasminogen activator, but increased levels of tissue plasminogen activator in plasma (Estellés et al 1987). This may be due to stimulation of, or damage to, the endothelium. This increase in tissue plasminogen activator is accompanied by an increase in plasminogen activator inhibitors 1 and 2 (Estellés et al 1987), a feature which had previously been noted as a reduction in urokinase activity (Howie et al 1971). Plasminogen activator inhibitor 2 is produced only from the placenta and is not found in plasma from non-pregnant subjects. The increase in this placental plasminogen activator inhibitor may again reflect placental vascular damage and would predispose to local thrombosis by local inhibition of fibrinolysis in the abnormal vessels of the placental bed. All studies have not been consistent however; de Boer et al (1988) found an increase in total plasminogen activator inhibitor in pre-eclampsia with a reduction in the placentally-derived inhibitor component compared to normal. They also showed that low levels of placental plasminogen activator inhibitor are associated with poor fetal outcome and might, therefore, simply be a measure of placental function.

The increase in fibrinopeptide Bβ 1–42 provides additional evidence of fibrinolytic activation. This peptide is generated by plasmin degradation of fibrin I, a soluble intermediate between fibrinogen and the spontaneously polymerizing fibrin II (Borok et al 1984). This study also measured levels of the peptides cleaved from fibrinogen by the action of thrombin, and suggested that fibrinolysis is more pronounced than fibrin formation in patients with severe disease. Plasminogen (Spencer et al 1983) and the inhibitor of plasmin, α_2-antiplasmin (Oian et al 1985), have also been found to be reduced, in keeping with fibrinolytic activation. This increase in fibrinolysis may be a response to intravascular coagulation which may be prevented from reaching its full potential due to the concomitant increase in intravascular inhibitors of plasminogen activation.

Platelets play a crucial role in the pathophysiology of pre-eclampsia by promoting vascular damage and obstruction, leading to tissue ischaemia and further damage (Greer 1992). Thromboxane A_2, the major product of arachidonic acid metabolism in platelets, is a potent vasoconstrictor and platelet aggregating agent. As it has a short half life, it is normally measured as its stable hydration product, thromboxane B_2. The effects of thromboxane A_2 are normally counterbalanced by prostacyclin, a potent vasodilator and antiplatelet prostanoid which is the major product of arachidonic acid metabolism in vascular endothelium and which plays an important role in protecting the endothelium and limiting damage by inhibiting platelet aggregation and promoting vasodilation. These two substances function as local hormones and are thought to be important in the control of the platelet–endothelium interaction. They oppose each other through the regulation of platelet adenylate cyclase, which controls cAMP production and thereby platelet free calcium concentration; this links receptor occupancy with cellular response. Pro-aggregatory substances such as thromboxane A_2 inhibit adenylate cyclase, allowing free intracellular calcium to rise, while prostacyclin stimulates adenylate cyclase thus increasing cAMP, reducing free intracellular calcium and inhibiting platelet activation.

There is considerable evidence implicating platelets in the pathophysiology of pre-eclampsia. The circulating platelet count is reduced (Redman et al 1978), reflecting a reduced platelet lifespan (Rakoczi et al 1979), and an inverse relationship between platelet count and fibrinogen degradation products has been noted, suggesting that the reduction in platelet count is due to increased platelet consumption associated with low grade DIC (Howie et al 1971). The platelet specific protein, β-thromboglobulin, a marker of platelet activation in vivo, has also been found to be increased in pregnancy-induced hypertension (Redman et al 177a, Douglas et al 1982, Socol et al 1985). This correlates with proteinuria and serum creatinine (Socol et al 1985), linking platelet activation with renal microvascular damage.

The platelet content of 5-hydroxytryptamine is reduced in pre-eclampsia indicating platelet aggregation and stimulation of the platelet release reaction in vivo. Low platelet 5-hydroxytryptamine levels have also been associated with loss of platelet responsiveness to various aggregating agents in vitro. The explanation suggested for these findings is that platelets are activated in the micro-circulation of the placenta, kidney and liver, release their products such as β-thrombogobulin and 5-hydroxytryptamine, and then re-enter the system in an 'exhausted' state, unable to respond normally to aggregating agents and containing lower levels of 5-hydroxytryptamine (Howie 1977). In support of this hypothesis, placentae from patients with pre-eclampsia have been shown to contain high levels of 5-hydroxytryptamine, possibly of platelet origin. Other studies using platelet aggregation in platelet-rich plasma have also noted 'platelet exhaustion' (Ahmed et al 1991). This platelet exhaustion phenomenon has also been noted in molar pregnancy complicated by severe hypertension, where anti-platelet therapy corrected the hypofunctional platelet response (Greer et al 1987).

Platelets have also been shown to be less sensitive to the anti-aggregatory effects of prostacyclin in pre-eclampsia, and this may contribute to the platelet consumption seen in this disease, especially as deficiency of prostacyclin production may coexist, as discussed below. Increased platelet thromboxane A_2 production ex vivo has been shown to occur in pre-eclampsia complicated by intra-uterine growth retardation (Wallenburg & Rotmans 1982). More recently, a whole blood platelet aggregation technique has been used to study platelet reactivity (Greer et al 1988). This technique, which leaves platelets in their natural milieu, surrounded by red cells and white cells which may themselves influence the aggregation response, may be a more physiological method than the traditional turbidometric techniques which use platelet-rich plasma. This study showed that platelet reactivity is enhanced in pregnancy-induced hypertension compared to normal pregnant and non-pregnant women. However, Louden et al (1991) found reduced platelet reactivity in whole blood in women with pre-eclampsia compared to normal controls, although there was no difference in thrombaxane B_2 production ex-vivo. The report of Louden et al (1991) would be in keeping with platelet exhaustion as discussed above, and the differences in results between studies may reflect differences in patient severity as platelet reactivity may vary according to the stage of the disease process with increased reactivity perhaps occurring in the early stages of the disease and platelet exhaustion in advanced disease. The role of platelets in the pathophysiology of the disease is also emphasized by the recent success of antiplatelet therapy in the treatment of high risk pregnancies (Beufils et al 1985, Wallenburg et al 1986).

The changes in the coagulation system and in platelet function support the concept that disseminated intravascular coagulation occurs in patients with pregnancy-induced hypertension. A 'coagulation index' of serum fibrin-fibrinogen degradation products, platelets count and plasma factor VIII has been shown to correlate with a 'clinical index' of disease severity (Howie et al 1976), highlighting the association of the two conditions.

Prostacyclin and the endothelium in pre-eclampsia

Platelet activity is normally limited by the vascular endothelium. The endothelium is not simply an inert container for circulating blood; it plays a role in the control not only of haemostasis and thrombosis, but also of vascular tone (Greer 1992). It produces prostacyclin, which can inhibit the activation of platelets and neutrophils, and substances such as tissue plasminogen activator which prevent or limit vascular damage. Conversely, the endothelium can render itself thrombogenic by secreting von Willebrand factor, platelet activating factor and plasminogen activator inhibitor, which promote local coagulation and repair at the site of injury. The endothelium contributes to the regulation of vascular tone by release of prostacyclin and the recently characterized endothelium-derived relaxing factor. In the normal situation, the endothelium, platelets, and neutrophils will interact homeostatically. Although it has long been appreciated that denudation of the endothelium will result in thrombosis, endothelial dysfunction may have similar effects and could transform the endothelium from a non-thrombogenic to a thrombogenic surface. There is now considerable evidence linking endothelial dysfunction to pre-eclampsia (Greer 1992).

Prostacyclin is a potent, vasodilator, inhibitor of platelet aggregation and a stimulator of renin secretion. The pathological features of pregnancy-induced hypertension are the opposite to these; vasoconstriction, platelet consumption and low renin secretion. In addition women with pre-eclampsia are very sensitive to exogenous angiotensin II infusions when compared to normal pregnant women (Gant et al 1973); the insensitivity to angiotensin II seen in normal pregnancy can be abolished by treatment with a cyclo-oxygenase inhibitor such as indomethacin (Everett et al 1978), and enhanced by infusion of prostacyclin (Broughton-Pipkin et al 1984) or prostaglandin E_2 (Broughton-Pipkin et al 1982). These experiments suggest that in normal pregnancy angiotensin II may be balanced by the action of vasodepressor prostaglandins such as prostacyclin. A deficiency of prostacyclin might therefore result in the angiotensin II sensitivity seen in pre-eclampsia.

Maternal vascular prostacyclin production is reduced in pre-eclampsia (Bussolino et al 1980), and plasma and urinary prostacyclin metabolites are significantly lower, particularly in those with severe disease (Goodman et al 1982, Greer et al 1985, Moodley et al 1984). On the other side of the equation, platelet thromboxane A_2 production may be increased in pre-eclampsia complicated by intrauterine growth retardation (Wallenburg & Rotmans 1982) although Loudon et al (1991) found no difference in thromboxane production between normal and hypertensive pregnancies. Placentae taken from pregnancies complicated by pre-eclampsia have been shown to produce more thromboxane A_2 and less prostacyclin than those from normal pregnancies (Walsh 1985). The resulting imbalance between prostacyclin and thromboxane is likely to contribute to the enhanced platelet reactivity and vascular damage seen in pre-eclampsia.

On the fetal side, production of prostacyclin from placenta and cord vessels is reduced in pre-eclampsia (Remuzzi et al 1979, Downing et al 1980, Walsh 1985). Intact umbilical arteries taken from pregnancies complicated by pre-eclampsia have been shown to be unresponsive to a stimulus of prostacyclin production when compared with normal umbilical arteries (McLaren et al 1986, 1987) suggesting that the ability of the vascular endothelium to produce prostacyclin in response to a physiological stimulus is absent or substantially diminished in pre-eclampsia. Since the umbilical artery lacks any innervation it may depend on humoral control of blood flow by prostanoids (Tuvemo 1980) to maintain the low pressure–high flow feto-placental circulation. Failure of the vessel to produce prostacyclin in response to physiological stimulation may result in increased umbilical artery resistance due to vasocontriction, especially in the face of increased thromboxane production by the placenta. The deficiency of prostacyclin and resulting prostanoid imbalance may also allow vascular damage to occur unchecked. The mechanism underlying prostacyclin deficiency is unclear, but it may be due to reduced activity of enzyme systems required for its production. These enzymes could be inactivated by free radicals or proteolytic enzymes, making the prostacyclin deficiency a feature of endothelial damage and dysfunction. Other such markers, such as elevated levels of fibronectin, endothelin (Greer et al 1991c, Nova et al 1991), increased concentrations of von Willebrand factor and plasminogen activator inhibitors, can be found in pre-eclampsia.

Neutrophil activation in pre-eclampsia

Neutrophils are involved in the pathophysiology of vascular damage in non-pregnant individuals. Activated neutrophils release a variety of substances capable of mediating vascular damage, including the contents of neutrophil granules such as elastase and other proteases. These can destroy the integrity of the endothelial cells, vascular basement membrane and subendothelial matrix (Harlan 1987). Toxic oxygen species are also released, and can produce membrane lipid peroxidation, lysis of endothelial cells, and increased vascular permeability and reactivity (Harlan 1987). Leukotrienes are also synthesized and released following neutrophil activation and they too will increase vascular permeability, induce vasoconstriction, and promote further neutrophil activation and adherence (Bray 1983).

Neutrophil elastase, a marker of neutrophil activation in vivo, is elevated in pre-eclampsia, indicating the presence of neutrophil activation (Greer et al 1989a), but this is confined to the maternal circulation (Greer et al 1991b). As elevated neutrophil elastase is found in both mild/moderate and severe disease, it may be an early part of the disease process (Greer et al 1989a). The elevated levels of neutrophil elastase seen in pre-eclampsia correlate with the increase in plasma von Willebrand factor and are associated with an increase in the endothelial-derived vasoconstrictor, endothelin (Greer et al 1991c). Neutrophil activation may therefore contribute directly to the vascular lesions seen in pre-eclampsia, such as those noted in the placental bed. Elastase-positive neutrophils can be found in significantly increased numbers in the decidua of the placental bed in women with pre-eclampsia compared to normal pregnancies and this correlates with plasma urate, an established marker of disease severity (Butterworth et al 1991). In addition to directly bringing about endothelial damage, neutrophils will interact with platelet, coagulation and complement systems. The activation of neutrophils in pre-eclampsia is likely to be a secondary phenomenon, possibly triggered by the immunological mechanisms which have been implicated in the aetiology of this disorder, or simply secondary to vascular damage per se; nonetheless it may be an important contributor to the pathogenesis of this disease.

It is of interest that neutrophil granule enzymes (Miller

et al 1985), reactive oxygen species (Ager & Gordon 1984), and leukotrienes (Pologe et al 1984) have been shown to stimulate prostacyclin release from endothelial cells. This seems paradoxical since pregnancy-induced hypertension is associated with a deficiency of prostacyclin production which is thought to contribute to the platelet consumption and vasoconstriction seen in the condition. It is known that low concentrations of reactive oxygen species can stimulate cyclo-oxygenase, which is essential for prostacyclin production, but higher concentrations will inhibit both this enzyme and prostacyclin synthase (Warso & Lands 1983). Furthermore high concentrations of reactive oxygen species can reorientate the arachidonic acid pathway in the cell away from the production of the cytoprotective and vasodilator agent prostacyclin towards thromboxane A_2 (Warso & Lands 1983). Thus neutrophil activation may account for the necrotizing arteriopathy of pre-eclampsia which has been hitherto poorly explained, and may also explain several other features of the disease, such as prostacyclin deficiency and enhanced thromboxane production. Such neutrophil activation is not specific to pre-eclampsia as increased neutrophil elastase has been found in diabetic pregnancy (Greer et al 1989b) and in mothers with pregnancies complicated by intrauterine growth retardation (Johnston et al 1991). It has also been noted that serum from women with pre-eclampsia has a greater cytotoxic effect on cultured endothelial cells than serum from normal pregnancies (Rodgers et al 1988). Although the nature of this factor is unclear the authors suggest that, as this effect diminishes following delivery, it may be released from the placenta, but it may equally well be related to neutrophil activation. There is also evidence of a serum factor in pre-eclampsia which can increase vascular reactivity to angiotensin II in vitro (Tulenko et al 1987).

From the foregoing discussion, it is clear that endothelial damage and dysfunction is a common feature of all of the pathological features of pre-eclampsia whether in the uteroplacental bed or in the renal microcirculation. The biochemical evidence of endothelial damage includes elevated von Willebrand factor and fibronectin levels, which are released when endothelial cell injury occurs, and reduced prostacyclin production. Functionally, the vessels have an exaggerated response to angiotensin II and there is increased capillary permeability. Endothelial damage and dysfunction stimulates activation of platelets and the coagulation system, promoting further vascular damage. Neutrophils can also be activated by dysfunctional endothelium. Activation of platelets and the coagulation system can cause endothelial damage directly, and also indirectly by activation of neutrophils. If neutrophils are activated they will produce endothelial damage directly, and also indirectly, by platelet activation. Thus, endothelial damage, the platelets and coagulation system, and neutrophils all interact; once one of these systems is triggered a positive feedback loop will promote vascular damage. The trigger which initiates this vicious circle is unclear. It appears to originate in the placenta or utero-placental bed and is probably linked to the failure of trophoblast invasion which is characteristic of the disease. This process leads to tissue ischaemia which in turn activates the vicious circle described above to produce widespread endothelial damage and dysfunction. It is also obscure which facet of the vicious circle, endothelial damage, neutrophil activation or platelet activation is triggered first.

Antiplatelet therapy in the treatment and prevention of pre-eclampsia

Prostacyclin Infusion

Perhaps the most obvious intervention is to replace the deficient prostacyclin by an exogenous infusion and so compensate for the dysfunctional endothelium. This has been used in pre-eclampsia (Belch et al 1985; Greer & Belch 1986), where it has been shown to lower blood pressure, reduce platelet consumption and increase urinary output in oliguric patients in the short term. However, relatively large amounts of prostacyclin are required and dose-related side-effects, including flushing, headache, nausea, and vomiting, are severe enough to limit the dose which could be given. Furthermore tachyphylaxis rapidly develops, with loss of blood pressure control even at the maximum tolerated dose. In the situation the use of antihypertensive agents such as labetalol may temporarily restore blood pressure control. Prostacyclin also has a short half-life, and continuous intravenous infusions are required. Other therapeutic possibilities must, therefore, be explored.

Aspirin

Aspirin is the most practicable and effective agent presently available for clinical use as antiplatelet therapy. It has been used successfully in the prevention of pre-eclampsia and intrauterine growth retardation. The biggest problem with regard to its use is perhaps that of identifying patients who will require such therapy; this is especially true in pre-eclampsia, where those with the most severe disease are often primigravidae.

Aspirin acts by irreversibly inhibiting cyclo-oxygenase, which is required for prostaglandin and thromboxane production, and reducing thromboxane generation and platelet activation. However, the beneficial effects of aspirin may be offset by its inhibition of vascular prostacyclin production, as cyclo-oxygenase is required for the production of both substances (Greer et al 1986). This is clearly undesirable in pre-eclampsia. However, low-dose aspirin may selectively block thromboxane production. Aspirin is extensively metabolized by the liver, and low doses given orally are thought to produce pharmacologically active drug concentrations in the portal circulation and not in the systemic circulation. Since platelet cyclo-oxygenase is irreversibly inhibited by aspirin, effective inhibition of platelet function would result as the platelet passes through the portal circulation, while systemic vascular prostacyclin production might remain unaffected due to lower concentrations in the systemic circulation. In addition the nucleated vascular endothelial cells, unlike anucleate platelets, can synthesize new protein and are therefore able to replace any inactivated enzyme in a matter of hours (Heavey et al 1985), thus maintaining prostacyclin production. The efficacy of low dose aspirin in reducing thromboxane A_2 production has largely been demonstrated in non-pregnant patients; doses as low as 20 mg/day reduce thromboxane A_2 production by up to 95% (Sinzinger et al 1989). However, it appears unlikely that any dose of aspirin can produce maximal inhibition of platelet thromboxane A_2 production without affecting prostacyclin production to some extent, although there appears to be a high degree of relative sparing of prostacyclin production with low-dose aspirin (Fitzgerald et al 1983, 1987).

Perhaps the biggest concern regarding the use of aspirin in pregnancy is that of aspirin reaching the fetus and impairing haemostasis or closing the ductus arteriosus, especially near to the time of delivery. Stuart et al (1982) have documented haemostatic problems in neonates whose mothers received large doses (5–10 g) of aspirin up to 5 days before delivery. Ritter et al (1987) found that 37.5 mg of aspirin administered daily for 2 weeks prior to the expected date of delivery significantly lowered maternal thromboxane A_2 but had no significant effect on thromboxane A_2 in neonatal blood or on prostacyclin production by the umbilical artery ex vivo. This differential effect is likely to reflect the extensive first pass metabolism of aspirin in the liver, although significant levels of active aspirin can be detected in maternal plasma 1 hour after doses as low as 37.5 and 75 mg (Greer et al 1991a). Chronic maternal intake of 60 mg of aspirin daily was also shown to have no significant effect on neonatal platelet function (Louden et al 1989). Sibai et al (1989) have also shown that chronic maternal therapy with aspirin (20–80 mg/day) has no effect on neonatal platelet function or on the ductus arteriosus. Thus, it would appear that low-dose aspirin has a selective effect on maternal platelet function, sparing fetal platelet function and prostacyclin production. It is also reassuring that there is no obvious effect on the ductus arteriosus.

There have now been several studies examining the clinical efficacy of low-dose aspirin in the prevention of pre-eclampsia. The first was that of Beaufils et al (1985), who randomized 102 women at high risk of pre-eclampsia to receive either no therapy or aspirin 15 mg in combination with dipyridamole 300 mg daily. The patients were selected on the basis of their past medical and obstetric histories, such as essential hypertension or a series of complicated pregnancies, and 99 of the women were parous. Spontaneous abortions and loss of patients to follow-up left 93 patients for inclusion in the analysis. There was a significant reduction of pre-eclampsia and improved perinatal outcome in the treated group; six of 45 patient in the control group compared to none of the 48 patients in the treatment group developed pre-eclampsia. The incidence of growth retardation and fetal/neonatal loss was also significantly reduced and there was a significant prolongation of pregnancy. There were no side-effects except headache associated with dipyridamole therapy, and no haemorrhagic complications were encountered. This study, however, used relatively small numbers of patients and the groups were unbalanced with regard to several variables of prognostic significance, which could bring the results into question. In addition it tested two drugs, aspirin and dipyridamole, in combination, although there is no evidence to suggest that dipyridamole will enhance the clinical effect of aspirin alone. Finally 150 mg/day of aspirin was used; this is substantially more than is required to produce effective inhibition of platelet thromboxane A_2 production.

Wallenburg et al (1986) reported their findings on low-dose (60 mg/day) aspirin therapy in women at risk of pre-eclampsia. Patients were selected for inclusion in the double-blind, placebo-controlled trial by screening 207 women with angiotensin II infusions. The 46 who were sensitive to angiotensin II at 28 weeks gestation were recruited to the study; 44 were included in the analysis. While there was a significant reduction in the development of hypertensive complications (two of 21 in the treatment group versus 12 of 23 in the placebo group) there was no significant effect on length of gestation at delivery or number of growth-retarded infants, although there was a tendency to a lower incidence of these conditions in the treatment group.

Schiff et al (1989) selected patients on the basis of the 'roll over test' (Gant et al 1974), although the predictive value of this test is disputed (Phelen et al 1977). After blood pressure has been measured in the left lateral position, the patient rolls on to her back, and after a few minutes the blood pressure measurement is repeated. An increase in diastolic blood pressure of more than 15 mmHg after 'rolling over' is considered positive. After screening 791 women, 65 with positive tests were randomized to receive aspirin 100 mg/day or placebo in a prospective double-blind manner. The patients were of mixed parity. There was a significant reduction in hypertensive complications, an increase in gestation at delivery, and an increase in adjusted birthweight centile compared to the placebo group. There were no maternal side-effects and no maternal or neonatal haemorrhagic effects.

Benigni et al (1989) studied the effects of 60 mg aspirin

or placebo in 33 women judged to be at risk of pre-eclampsia on the basis of their past obstetric history or past medical history such as chronic hypertension. Treatment was started from the 12th week single-blind. The infants of the treatment group had a significantly greater birthweight and longer gestation than those of the placebo group but no other differences were noted. Aspirin also significantly and substantially reduced urinary thromboxane B_2 levels, but there was no effect on prostacyclin production, measured as its metabolites in urine, indicating that a selective effect on platelets was occurring, with sparing of the endothelium. Again, no haemorrhagic complications were found in the newborn infants, although there was a significant reduction in serum thromboxane B_2 in the neonates in the treatment group but this was not as great as the reduction which occurred in the mothers. However, this suggests that even with a dose as low as 60 mg aspirin/day the fetus is still exposed to some active aspirin.

The potential efficacy of antiplatelet therapy with low-dose aspirin is not limited to pre-eclampsia. Pregnancies at risk of intrauterine growth retardation also appear to benefit from such therapy (Wallenburg & Rotmans 1987, Trudinger et al 1988, Uzan et al 1991), as do pregnancies at risk of intrauterine growth retardation and fetal loss because of maternal systemic lupus erythematosus (Elder et al 1988). This is not surprising; all of these disorders are associated with vascular damage in the placental bed.

Finally, as identification of patients, especially primigravidae, is a major problem, the reports raising the possibility that platelet angiotensin II receptors may identify high-risk women (Baker et al 1989, 1991) are an interesting development as such a simple test could be widely employed, and a positive results used as an indication for low dose aspirin therapy. Until effective objective techniques for identification of patients at risk are available, the obstetrician must weigh up the available evidence for aspirin's benefits (and potential hazards) against the patient's risk of significant clinical problems and treat the patient as is felt appropriate.

THROMBOTIC PROBLEMS IN PREGNANCY

Incidence

While it is clear that pregnancy substantially increases the risk of thromboembolism (Royal College of General Practitioners 1967), there are wide variations in the reported incidence of thromboembolic complications during pregnancy. This reflects diagnostic difficulties and the inclusion of various clinical entities within the disease classification. However, reliable data exist on fatal thromboembolic complications in pregnancy due to the thorough and detailed reports of the Confidential Enquiries into Maternal Deaths in England and Wales which more recently have also included Scotland and Northern Ireland (Department of Health 1989, 1991). Since 1952 when these data were first collected the incidence of fatal pulmonary thromboembolism (PTE) has fallen dramatically (Fig. 43.1), but PTE remains the most common cause of maternal death in the United Kingdom today (Department of Health et al 1991). Fatal PTE is more common following caesarean section. Although the rate has fallen by almost 90% between the 1955–57 report and the 1978–81 report, the relative risk of fatal PTE following caesarean section has increased compared to vaginal delivery where the reduction has been greater (Fig. 44.1). The majority of these deaths occur in the first 2 weeks after delivery, but almost 40% occur between 15 and 42 days following delivery (Table 43.1). Thus, most of these fatalities will occur after the initial discharge from hospital and practitioners caring for women in the puerperium must be aware of, and alert to, the possibility of postpartum PTE. The ratio of fatal PTE occuring postpartum to those occurring antepartum has also decreased so that they now have similar frequencies. It is also of concern

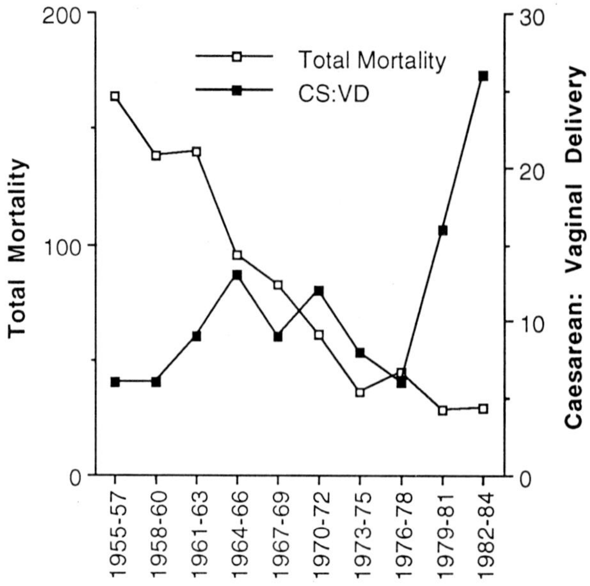

Fig. 43.1 Total maternal mortality from PTE in pregnancy and the ratio of postpartum deaths following caesarean section (CS) versus vaginal delivery (VD).

Table 43.1 Time between delivery and fatal pulmonary embolism following vaginal delivery and caesarean section (data for England and Wales 1970–87)

Time after delivery (days)	Vaginal delivery	Caesarean section
Up to 7	27 (39.7%)	19 (36.5%)
8 to 14	14 (20.6%)	12 (23.1%)
15 to 42	27 (39.7%)	21 (40.4%)

Source: Report on confidential enquiries into maternal deaths in the United Kingdom 1985–87, London, HMSO.

that many of these antepartum deaths occur in the 1st and 2nd trimesters. The most recent Confidential Enquiries Report contained six deaths in the 1st trimester and four in the 2nd trimester with all but two of the 17 deaths occurring by 32 weeks' gestation. Furthermore, eight of these antepartum deaths were associated with early pregnancy problems such as hyperemesis.

In contrast to the reliable figures for fatal PTE, the reported incidence of deep venous thrombosis (DVT) and non-fatal PTE varies considerably. The most reliable diagnostic techniques of venography and radio-iodine labelled fibrinogen are unsuitable for screening an obstetric population. In the past, the use of clinical diagnostic criteria has estimated the incidence of DVT in pregnancy between 0.05% and 1.8% (Hiilesmaa 1960, Aaro & Juergens 1971, Coon et al 1973), increasing to between 0.08–1.2% following a vaginal delivery (Daniel et al 1967, Husni et al 1967, Aaro & Juergens 1971, Flessa et al 1974), and to 2.2–3.0% (Hiilesmaa 1960, Husni et al 1967) following caesarean section. The clinical diagnosis of DVT is notoriously inaccurate (Genton & Turpie 1980) and there has only been one sizeable study using ^{125}I-labelled fibrinogen (Friend & Kakkar 1970), which reported an incidence of 2.6% following vaginal delivery suggesting that underdiagnosis was occurring using clinical criteria alone. A more recent Swedish study which confirmed the clinical diagnosis by objective means — plethysmography, thermography, and venography — found an incidence of 0.07% during pregnancy in their population (Bergqvist et al 1983). The same group, using plethysmography, screened 169 women following caesarean section and found an incidence of DVT of 1.8% (Bergqvist et al 1979). The diagnosis of DVT is of course crucial as PTE will occur in 16% of patients with untreated DVT resulting in a 13% mortality (Villa Santa 1965). Anticoagulation will substantially reduce the risk of PTE and subsequent mortality, the latter being reduced to 0.7% (Villa Santa 1965).

The incidence of PTE in pregnancy has been estimated at 0.3–1.2% (Villa Santa 1965, Friend & Kakkar 1970), although more recently the risk of postpartum PTE has been placed at 0.04–0.05% (Weiner 1985). A retrospective review of 35 000 pregnancies at Queen Charlotte's Hospital, London, found an overall incidence of DVT and PTE of 0.09% (Letsky & de Swiet 1984).

Long term morbidity from DVT associated with pregnancy

DVT during pregnancy increases the risk of a future thrombosis both within and outwith pregnancy, with a 15% risk of recurrence during pregnancy and the puerperium and a 33% risk of DVT not associated with pregnancy over a median follow-up time of over 10 years (Bergqvist et al 1991). These data are similar to those obtained from a retrospective review of the literature (Bergqvist et al 1991) and other retrospective studies (Tengborn et al 1989). However, prospective studies (de Swiet et al 1987) suggest that this may be an overestimate with regard to recurrence in pregnancy as discussed later in this chapter.

In addition to the risk of recurrent DVT, there is the risk of developing deep venous insufficiency secondary to the damage and destruction of the valves in the deep veins during the thrombotic process. Deep venous insufficiency is manifest clinically as pain, leg swelling, varicose veins, pigmentation and ulceration. It can be diagnosed objectively with techniques such as venous pressure measurement, plethysmography and Doppler ultrasound. The frequency of objectively diagnosed deep venous insufficiency has been studied in women with a history of proven DVT in pregnancy after a median follow-up period of 7 years (Lindhagen et al 1986). The frequency of deep venous insufficiency in the previously thrombosed leg was 65% compared to 22% in the healthy leg, the latter acting as a control. There was no correlation between size of thrombosis and development of venous insufficiency. Venous insufficiency occurred despite all patients being treated with anticoagulation during the acute episode. Futhermore, this frequency of 65% is significantly greater (Bergqvist et al 1991) than that found after postoperative DVT diagnosed by radio-labelled fibrinogen uptake testing (32%) or after clinically suspected acute DVT confirmed by venography (49%) (Lindhagen et al 1984, 1985). In view of the young age of the pregnant group relative to the other groups studied, DVT in pregnancy with subsequent deep venous insufficiency is likely to pose a significant health problem for these women. This is supported by a questionnaire study following up a group of women who had developed DVT in pregnancy or the puerperium (Bergqvist et al 1991). This study, with a median follow-up time of around 10 years, examined the frequency of subjective complaints associated with deep venous insufficiency. Only 24% were asymptomatic, while 55% complained of leg swelling, 34% of varicose veins, 27% of skin discoloration, 15% required regular use of a compression bandage and 4% had leg ulceration. Thus DVT in pregnancy is not simply associated with risk of PTE and mortality, but also with a risk of deep venous insufficiency and further DVT.

The pathogenesis of thrombosis

In 1846 Virchow put forward his original concepts on the pathogenesis of thrombosis (Virchow 1846). He proposed that three main factors were involved; venous stasis, vascular damage and hypercoagulability of the blood. Virchow's triad remains true today although we now have a better understanding of the pathophysiological changes which underlie these features in the pregnant situation and these are reflected in the risk factors for thrombosis in pregnancy.

Physiological adaptation of the coagulation system in pregnancy. In normal pregnancy the balance between the coagulation and fibrinolytic systems changes in favour of coagulation as discussed above. The overall effect from these changes in an increased thrombotic potential which is most marked around term and the immediate postpartum period.

Mode of delivery. As can be seen from Figure 43.1 the risk of fatal PTE following caesarean section is around 26 times greater than after vaginal delivery and risk appears greater after an emergency procedure. This may be due to reduced mobility, and trauma to pelvic veins at the time of operation. It is likely that there is an increased risk following forceps deliveries since one study has shown that 25% of cases of thromboembolism occurred in complicated pregnancies which included difficult forceps deliveries and prolonged labour (Aaro & Juergens 1974).

Age and parity. The Confidential Enquiries into Maternal Deaths for England and Wales show that age and parity are important, with risk increasing more sharply with age, especially in those over 35-years-old, than with increasing parity. The risk of fatal PTE in a 40-year-old para 4 being 263.6 per million maternities compared to 11.3 per million maternities in a 20–24 year old para 4 (Department of Health 1989).

Obesity. Obesity is undoubtedly an important risk factor for DVT/PTE as obese patients have impaired fibrinolytic activity and increased likelihood of venous stasis and poor mobility.

Immobilization. Restricted activity, often associated with hospitalization and bed rest for complications of pregnancy such as hypertension, is also an important risk factor especially when the patient may have an increased likelihood of other risk factors such as operative delivery.

Suppression of lactation by oestrogens. The relationship between suppression of lactation with oestrogen (stilboestrol) and thromboembolism was first highlighted by Daniel et al (1967). There is no place in modern obstetrics for such therapy.

Venous flow in pregnancy. The venous tone appears to be reduced in pregnancy resulting in diminished flow prior to physical obstruction by the gravid uterus, although physical obstruction of the inferior vena cava also occurs later in pregnancy due to uterine size and is exacerbated by engagement of the fetal head (Wright et al 1950, Flessa et al 1974).

Surgical procedures in pregnancy. If a surgical procedure is carried out during pregnancy or the puerperium, such as postpartum sterilization, then there is an increased risk of thrombotic problems.

Previous thrombotic episode. If the patient has a history of a previous thrombotic problem then the risk of a further problem is increased. This risk has been estimated from restrospective studies at 12–15% (Badaracco & Vessey 1974, Bergqvist et al 1991). In a prospective randomized study of anticoagulant therapy in pregnancy in such patients, only one patient in the control group of 20 developed a DVT (Howell et al 1983). More recently de Swiet's group have reported 59 pregnancies in women with a history of thrombosis who received no anticoagulant therapy antenatally (although intrapartum and postpartum prophylaxis was given). None of these women had any thromboembolic complication (de Swiet et al 1987). These figures suggest that the risk is much lower than previously thought.

Other risk factors. Other risk factors include a hypertensive problem in pregnancy, excessive blood loss (Department of Health 1989), sickle cell anemia (Thomas et al 1982, van Dinh et al 1982), dehydration and to have a blood group other than O (Jick et al 1969, Bergqvist et al 1983). Hereditary thrombotic problems such as ATIII or protein C deficiency, and acquired thrombotic problems such as lupus anticoagulant also place the patient at increased risk and these are discussed below.

Diagnosis of DVT

The diagnosis of DVT is crucial as the presence of a DVT places the woman at substantial risk of PTE, while anticoagulant therapy without a firm diagnosis may subject the woman to unnecessary and potentially dangerous therapy. The clinical diagnosis of DVT, however, is notoriously unreliable. The most common symptoms and signs are pain, tenderness, swelling, oedema, Homan's sign, a change in leg colour and temperature, and a palpable thrombosed vein. It is of interest that over 80% of DVT in pregnancy are left sided (Lindhagen et al 1986). However, clinical examination has both a low sensitivity and a low specificity for DVT diagnosis. Less than 50% of cases of DVT including those involving major proximal veins are recognisable clinically, while venography substantiates the diagnosis in only about 40% of patients with clinical findings compatible with DVT (Genton & Turpie 1980, Ramsey 1983). It is also noteworthy that the majority of women dying from PTE had no clinical evidence of DVT, yet thrombus was found in leg and pelvic veins at postmortem (Department of Health et al 1991). Objective assessment of the diagnosis is therefore required. Despite this, a survey among general physicians in Scotland in 1982 showed that 47% were diagnosing (and presumably treating) DVT on clinical diagnosis alone (Prentice et al 1982) and one might presume that obstetricians may be no different. Ramsay (1983) has estimated that, by using clinical diagnostic criteria alone, two patients out of every three would receive anticoagulants unnecessarily. The causes of pseudothrombo-phlebitis include ruptured Baker's cyst, muscular injury and cellulitis, although the presence of such diagnoses does not exclude DVT as a Baker's cyst and DVT not uncommonly coexist (Belch et al 1981). In view of the low sensitivity and specificity of clinical diagnosis outlined above, it is crucial that an objective assessment of DVT is performed. Perhaps the biggest contribution the clinician can make is to be aware of the presence of risk factor and alert to the possibility of the diagnosis. He should not depend on clinical examination to exclude thrombosis. There has been a reluctance to use venography in pregnancy and while this should be avoided in the first half of pregnancy if possible, it can be used in the second half of pregnancy with shielding being used to protect the uterus so that the direct radiation dose to the fetus is small and less than with X-ray pelvimetry (Laros & Alger 1979). Furthermore, the use of ultrasound in the diagnosis of DVT (Greer et al 1990) in pregnancy will largely avoid the need for venography, so allowing clinicians to proceed to objective diagnosis without regard to the potential risks of X-ray exposure. This should encourage the use of objective assessment in patients thought to be at risk.

Venography

Venography remains the 'gold standard' of the objective tests for DVT. It is an invasive technique but has the greatest degree of sensitivity and specificity of all the objective tests, and is the technique against which other techniques are compared. In the hands of a skilled radiologist it will probably detect up to 95% of peripheral thrombi (Browse 1978).

The diagnosis of thrombosis is made by the identification of a constant filling defect in more than one film. If the vein is completely occluded, contrast media will be seen above and below the occluded segments, with an abrupt termination of the column of contrast medium. The diagnosis may also be supported by the visualization of contrast medium in collateral vessels. It is often difficult to obtain good opacification, and visualization of all the veins in the muscle of the calf and also the tributaries of the profunda femoris and internal iliac veins. This along with technical failures will account for the small false negative rate associated with venography (Browse 1978). False positive results can occur due to inadequate mixing of blood and contrast, and streaming of the contrast medium. As with all invasive techniques, there are risks associated with venography. These include pain at the time of injection of contrast, hypersensitivity to the medium, or, rarely, extravasation of the medium resulting in damage to the skin of the foot. Thrombosis can occur secondary to venography due to the irritant effects of the hyperosmolar media on the venous endothelium. However this should be uncommon, and can be lessened by elevating the legs and flushing the legs with isotonic saline. It has been suggested that a single dose of heparin after the examination may reduce the incidence of thrombosis following venography, however studies have not confirmed this (Cranley 1975, Bettman & Paulin 1977). Lowering the osmolality of contract media will reduce the irritant effects and subsequent DVT formation (Bettman & Paulin, 1977) although it will not be abolished. The use of a non-ionic low osmolality medium (metrizamide) has been shown not to provoke thrombosis compared to an ionic hyperosmolar medium (Albrechtsson & Olsson 1979).

There has been a reluctance to employ venography in pregnancy because of the radiation hazard to the fetus. However, the risks of unwarranted anticoagulation must also be considered. In addition the uterus can be shielded so that the direct radiation dose to the fetus is small and less than with X-ray pelvimetry (Laros & Alger 1979).

Impedence plethysmography

Impedence plethysmography (IPG) is a non-invasive technique. It indirectly measures changes in the volume of a limb by the change in electrical resistance across it. Following inflation of a thigh cuff the venous outflow of the limb is occluded. In the absence of any obstruction to venous flow, release of the cuff will result in a rapid outflow of blood and an associated change in electrical resistance as measured between two electrodes placed round the limb. In the presence of venous thrombosis the rate of emptying will be reduced. In the non-pregnant this technique is both sensitive and specific in the detection of proximal occlusive venous thrombi (Hull et al 1976). Despite the physiological changes in venous flow in pregnancy due to reduced venous tone, and obstruction to flow by the gravid uterus, this technique can still be successfully employed in pregnancy provided the physiological changes are taken into account (Clarke-Pearson & Jolovsek, 1981). In view of the risk of a false positive result from external compression, however, it would seem prudent to confirm the diagnosis by venography. The main disadvantage of this technique is its very poor sensitivity in detecting calf vein thrombosis (Hull et al 1876) and non-occlusive thrombi.

Doppler ultrasound

Doppler ultrasound will detect changes in venous blood flow in the limb. Flow can be assessed in the femoral and popliteal veins during respiration and following compression of the calf. Flow will be absent in the presence of occlusive thrombi. While this technique is sensitive to proximal thrombosis, like IPG it is poorly sensitive to distal thrombus and non-occlusive thrombus (Hirsh et al 1981). It also has the disadvantage of relying on a subjective interpretation of flow.

Real time ultrasound diagnosis of DVT

Recently real time ultrasound scanning has been successfully employed in the diagnosis of DVT. It has the advantage of being non-invasive, quick, and utilizing standard scanning equipment which is available in most obstetric units. With this technique the veins and thrombi can be directly visualized (Sulliven et al 1984, Aitken & Godden 1987). The normal femoral and popliteal veins appear free of soft tissue echoes and are easily compressed during an ultrasound examination. When a thrombus is present a relatively echogenic soft tissue mass is seen within the vein which will prevent the vein collapsing on compression. The normal response of an increase in diameter of the vein in association with the Valsalva manoeuvre is also diminished or absent with venous occlusion by thrombus (Effeney et al 1984). Acute and chronic thrombi may also be distinguished on scanning as the latter are usually highly echogenic (Coelho et al 1982). A recent study comparing venography with real time ultrasound has shown that the latter technique has a sensitivity of 94% and a specificity of 100% (Aitken & Godden 1987), with similar results being obtained by other workers (Sulliven et al 1984, Cronan et al 1987). The disadvantages of this technique are that the calf veins, except the most proximal segments, cannot be visualized and neither can the iliac veins (Cronan et al 1987). The popliteal-femoral segment within the adductor hiatus may also be difficult to visualize (Aitken & Godden 1987). Although there are no comparative studies in the literature on the use of this technique in pregnancy, it is now being successfully employed for DVT diagnosis in pregnancy (Greer et al 1990, Polak & Wilkinson 1991). It can also be combined with pulsed Doppler ultrasound, but this is unlikely to contribute to the diagnosis in the majority of cases. A further advantage of this technique is its ability to diagnose other problems such as a Baker's cyst which might mimic DVT. In view of its non-invasiveness, safety and high degree of sensitivity and specificity it seems likely that this technique will become the first choice for DVT diagnosis in pregnancy in the future.

^{125}I-fibrinogen scanning

This technique is now only of historical interest and depends on the incorporation of radiolabelled fibrinogen into a developing thrombus. Subsequent scintillation scanning will pick up a 'hot spot' if thrombosis is present. It is accurate in picking up thrombus in the lower thigh and calf but false positive results can be obtained due to inflammation and oedema (Browse 1978). It is inaccurate above the mid-thigh region as the background count is high making diagnosis difficult. This technique of course cannot be used during pregnancy or lactation as ^{125}I will cross the placenta and the breast and will accumulate in the fetal or neonatal thyroid. In the non-lactating mother it could be used postpartum as employed by Friend & Kakkar (1970). The mother's thyroid can be protected by the concomitant administration of potassium iodide to prevent uptake of radioactive iodine. There is a theoretical possibility of viral transmission.

Other imaging techniques

Thermography has been employed in DVT diagnosis. While it may have some value as a screening tool more accurate techniques are required to confirm the diagnosis. Isotope venography using radiolabelled albumin or platelets has been used in the non-pregnant however these techniques have not been fully evaluated and in view of the radiation hazards are unlikely to find any place in the diagnosis of DVT in pregnancy.

Diagnosis of PTE

The signs and symptoms of PTE depend on the number and size of the emboli and arise from mis-matching of ventilation and perfusion, reduced cardiac output due to arterial obstruction, and infarction or collapse of lung segments. Clinical features are non-specific and include dyspnoea, pleurisy haemoptysis, chest pain, abdominal pain, hypertension, fever, collapse and sudden death. The differential diagnosis will include chest infection, pneumothorax, aspiration, amniotic fluid embolism and myocardial infarction. Like DVT, the bedside diagnosis of PTE is unreliable. The classic triad of dyspnoea, pleuritic pain and haemoptysis is present in only a fifth of patients with major PTE (Wenger et al 1972) and pulmonary embolus is diagnosed in less than one third of episodes (Windebank 1987). In view of these non-specific symptoms the clinician must remain vigilant to the possibility of PTE. Traditionally, initial investigations, include ECG, chest X-ray and blood gases. However, these tests are of no diagnostic value for PTE (Robin 1977). They may initially be normal and the ECG may show changes resulting from the effects of pregnancy itself on the heart in the absence of PTE. The main use of these tests is in helping to exclude other pathology. Chest X-rays, ECG and arterial blood gases not in keeping with the diagnosis of PTE were the principal reasons for treatment not being given in many of the cases in the Confidential Enquiries (Department of Health et al 1991) yet symptoms or signs such as dyspnoea, chest pain, hyperventilation and cyanosis were present. A ventilation-perfusion isotope lung scan should be obtained if PTE is suspected. The radiation dose to the fetus is low. Perfusion is assessed by intravenous administration of technetium-99 microspheres. This is best performed supine to increase apical perfusion and imaged erect for good visualization of the bases. Ventilation is assessed with radioactive xenon or krypton.

A ventilation perfusion mismatch is suggestive of PTE. A normal result effectively excludes the possibility of PTE. An abnormal result showing normal ventilation and a perfusion defect which is segmental or larger in size is diagnostic of PTE (Windebank 1987). With smaller defects the diagnosis is far from certain (Hull et al 1986b, McBride et al 1986) as other conditions can cause sub-segmental mis-match. In addition matched defects do not always indicate a chest problem other than PTE, as one third of patients with matched defects have been shown to have PTE (Windebank 1987).

Pulmonary angiography is the 'gold standard' for PTE diagnosis. It is highly invasive, involving injection of contrast media into the pulmonary artery but gives accurate imaging of the pulmonary circulation. In patients in whom the ventilation-perfusion scan shows sub-segmental mismatching, angiography should be considered. If this is unavailable or the patient is too ill for the procedure then venography should be performed as this may help reach a decision regarding treatment (Genton & Turpie 1980) although it must be remembered that one third of patients with PTE have no evidence of DVT (Hull et al 1986b).

Techniques other than imaging may also have a role in the diagnosis of DVT and PTE. Plasma markers which reflect activation of the coagulation or fibrinolytic systems have been used in the past (Ludlam et al 1975, Genton & Turpie 1980) but were found to lack specificity. This may be especially true if conditions such as pre-eclampsia coexist. However, more recently the measurement of D-Dimer in plasma has been found to aid the diagnosis of suspected DVT and PTE (Bounameaux et al 1989, 1991). In a study of 171 patients with suspected PTE (Bounameaux et al 1991), the authors found that a plasma concentration of D-Dimer of 500 μg/l or above provided a sensitivity of 98% and a specificity of 39%. The sensitivity was also found to remain high (93%) 7 days after the initial presentation. Thus, D-dimer which can be readily measured in plasma using monoclonal antibodies, may provide a useful test to exclude the presence of DVT or PTE or aid the diagnosis where other investigations such as the ventilation/perfusion lung scan is equivocal. Although this technique has not been assessed in a pregnant population it is still likely to provide assistance with the diagnosis in this situation, at least in the absence of other complications, such as severe pre-eclampsia or major haemorrhage with disseminated intravascular coagulation. This technique is worthy of further evaluation in the clinical situation.

Treatment of thrombotic problems: anticoagulants

The treatment of DVT and PTE is anticoagulation. This will not remove the clot already present but prevents further deposition of fresh clot which is likely to embolize. The two anticoagulants which are relevant to clinical practice in the UK are heparin and warfarin. Both these agents have special considerations regarding their hazards and safety during pregnancy which must be taken into account prior to their use.

Heparin

Neither unfractionated standard heparin nor low-molecular weight (LMW) heparins (see Ch. 10) cross the placenta (Flessa 1965, Forestier et al 1984, 1987, Andrew et al 1985, Omri et al 1989) or the breast. Heparin is thus particularly suited in this respect for use in pregnancy. Although it might increase the risk of haemorrhage in the mother and utero-placental bed, as it does not cross the placenta there is no risk of fetal haemorrhage per se or of any teratogenic effect. There are, however, other risks associated with the use of heparin in pregnancy. Perhaps the most worrying of these is heparin-induced osteoporosis. This was first described in 1965 in non-pregnant patients on long term subcutaneous (SC) heparin for ischaemic heart disease (Griffith et al 1965). There have been several reports of heparin-induced osteoporosis in patients on long-term heparin therapy during pregnancy with resultant problems such as vertebral collapse (Squires & Pinch 1979, Wise & Hall, 1980). This was initially thought to be an idiosyncratic phenomenon. However, de Swiet et al (1983) have shown objectively that the effects are dose related and that significant bone demineralization occurs in women taking subcutaneous heparin 20 000 iu daily in pregnancy and 16 000 iu daily after delivery for greater than 22 weeks compared to women on short-term therapy (less than 7 weeks). In addition, an intermediate effect may be seen in patients on therapy for 10–22 weeks (de Swiet et al 1983). However, there was no correlation between loss of bone mass and symptoms which might be attributable to this (de Swiet et al 1983). In a small randomized study of prophylactic heparin therapy during pregnancy compared to no prophylaxis during pregnancy, one of the 20 patients on therapy developed severe debilitating osteopenia (Howell et al 1983).

The mechanism behind heparin-induced osteopenia is unclear but appears to be related to a deficiency of 1,25 dihydroxy vitamin D (Aarskog et al 1980) which returns to normal several weeks after stopping heparin. Heparin may be able to increase serum calcium with subsequent inhibition of parathyroid hormone (PTH) secretion. Since PTH is the major stimulus to conversion of 25-hydroxy vitamin D to 1,25-dihydroxy vitamin D in the kidney this may be the mechanism responsible for this deficiency especially since 25-hydroxy vitamin D and 24, 25-dihydroxy vitamin D levels are normal (Aarskog et al 1980). This raises the possibility that heparin-induced osteopenia may be preventable with vitamin D supplements although this hypothesis remains to be explored. It is not known if LMW heparins will confer any benefit in this regard.

However, they seem unlikely to do so as in animal studies, chronic dosing with unfractionated and LMW heparin given in comparable doses both resulted in osteoporosis of a similar degree (Matzch et al 1987). Whether or not the osteopenia induced by heparin is reversible is yet to be established, however, osteopenic effects could still be demonstrated up to 2 years after cessation of treatment in de Swiet's study (de Swiet et al 1983), suggesting that short-term reversal is unlikely.

Heparin can also cause thrombocytopenia, allergic reactions and alopecia, but these appear to be uncommon. The incidence of heparin-induced thrombocytopenia has been estimated at between 0–30% (King & Kelton 1984). However, most recent studies have reported an incidence of between 1 and 5%. There appear to be two types of thrombocytopenia associated with heparin. The first is a relatively mild form of early onset which is due to a minor degree of platelet aggregation induced by heparin itself (Salzman et al 1980, Chong et al 1982). This does not occur in all patients and therefore suggests that other factors may be involved which, when combined with the presence of heparin, may provoke aggregation and benign thrombocytopenia. The second is a severe thrombocytopenia which occurs later during heparin therapy. It may be due to heparin acting as a hapten inducing an antibody against the platelet-heparin complex (King & Kelton 1984) and a heparin-dependent IgG antibody has been identified in these patients (Chong et al 1982). The thrombocytopenia occurs 6–12 days after starting heparin. It is important not because of haemostatic problem, but because it is associated with thrombotic problems related to platelet stimulation and thromboxane production triggered by the antibody. Should this complication develop, heparin should be stopped and platelet count will usually return to normal within several days. An alternative anticoagulant may be required especially if a thrombotic problem has developed. As these thrombotic problems are related to platelet activation, anti-platelet therapy may be of benefit (King & Kelton 1984). There has been one report of such a thrombotic problem occurring with heparin therapy in pregnancy, where replacing the heparin with a different brand of the same agent resulted in reversal of the problem and clinical improvement (Meytes et al 1986). There have also been two recent reports of LMW heparins being used successfully in pregnancies complicated by heparin allergy and thrombocytopenia (Henny et al 1986, Harenberg et al 1987).

It has been reported that heparin is associated with an adverse fetal outcome in up to one third of pregnancies associated with its use (Hall et al 1980). This is surprising as heparin does not cross the placenta and bleeding complications are not common enough to explain it. However, this finding was based on a literature survey which did not control for the presence of other conditions which could be associated with fetal loss independently of heparin therapy. For example, many of the patients in this study were given heparin for treatment of hypertension in pregnancy. A recent literature review of 186 studies which reported 1325 pregnancies associated with anticoagulant therapy and which took into account factors such as maternal co-morbid conditions, found that heparin therapy was not associated with any adverse fetal or infant outcome (Ginsberg et al 1989, Ginsberg 1992).

Warfarin

In view of its high degree of protein binding, warfarin does not significantly cross the breast (Orme et al 1977) and is therefore safe to use during lactation. However, it is a small molecule and crosses the placenta. Warfarin is a known teratogen. It produces a specific warfarin embryopathy which may occur following exposure to the drug in the 1st trimester, with the period between 6 and 9 weeks gestation (Hall et al 1980) being the most vulnerable time. It is difficult to estimate the incidence of warfarin embryopathy as most studies have been retrospective, however, an extensive recent literature review has placed the incidence at 4.6% (45 of 970 pregnancies associated with oral anticoagulant therapy) (Ginsberg et al 1989, Ginsberg 1991). The only prospective study of coumarin anticoagulation in pregnancy was performed in patients with valvular heart disease (Iturbe-Alessio et al 1986). This study showed an incidence of fetal abnormality of almost 30% in infants exposed to a coumarin between 6 and 12 weeks gestation. Furthermore, when heparin was substituted for warfarin between the 6th and 12th weeks, none of the infants were found to have warfarin embryopathy. Thus, warfarin embryopathy appears to be a significant but potentially preventable problem for mothers requiring anticoagulation in pregnancy.

The warfarin embryopathy takes the form of abnormal bone and cartilage formation: chondrodysplasia punctata. This is characterized by nasal and midface hypoplasia, frontal bossing, short stature and stippled chondral calcification. Other abnormalities have also been documented in association with warfarin therapy, including microcephaly, central nervous system abnormalities, optic atrophy, cardiac defect and the asplenia syndrome (Cox et al 1977, Hall et al 1980, Stevenson et al 1980, Ginsberg 1992). It should be noted, however, that central nervous system abnormalities may occur with warfarin exposure at any stage of pregnancy (Hall et al 1980, Ginsberg 1992). The mechanism behind central nervous system abnormalities is thought to be related to small intracerebral bleeds and subsequent scarring in utero. As the fetal liver enzyme systems are immature, the levels of vitamin K-dependent coagulation factors are low. Consequently, warfarin therapy maintained in the therapeutic range in the mother is likely to be associated with excessive anticoagulation and subsequent bleeding in the fetus. The incidence of CNS abnormalities has been estimated at around 3% from retrospective studies (Hall et al 1980, Ginsberg 1991) based on literature reviews. A recent study has not shown any intellectual or developmental difference between a group of 22 infants whose mothers took warfarin during the 2nd and 3rd trimesters compared to matched controls (Chong et al 1984). This is also supported by a study of Chen et al (1982) which found no developmental problems in infants exposed to warfarin in the 2nd and 3rd trimester except in one infant with congenital hydrocephalus. These latter two studies suggest that the incidence of CNS abnormalities may be much lower than previously thought. The outcome of affected infants is variable due to varying severity of the warfarin embryopathy syndrome. However, around 50% of survivors with the embryopathy appear to do well while those with haemorrhages or CNS abnormalities do poorly (Hall et al 1980).

The use of warfarin also places both mother and fetus at increased risk of haemorrhagic complications in later pregnancy, during delivery and in the early postpartum period (de Swiet et al 1977). Early reports found a high incidence of fetal intracerebral haemorrhage in late pregnancy (Villa Santa 1965). There is a substantial risk of major haemorrhagic complications for both mother and fetus during delivery, especially if this is carried out by operative means, even with optimal anticoagulant control. As warfarin has such a long duration of action it will take several hours for any reversal of anticoagulation to occur following parenteral vitamin K administration, and fresh frozen plasma will be required to correct the haemostatic defect in an emergency situation.

Warfarin has also been associated with an increase in spontaneous abortion rates when administered in the 1st trimester, ranging from 28–44% (Lutz et al 1978, Chen et al 1982, Salazar et al 1984). There is some evidence to suggest that if heparin is substituted for coumarin derivatives, the spontaneous abortion rate may be lessened. Larrea et al (1983) found an abortion rate of 34.6% in women who received a coumarin in the 1st trimester compared with 9.5% of women treated with heparin over the same period. However, the study of Iturbe-Alessio et al (1986) found no significant difference in spontaneous abortion rates for women who received a coumarin throughout the 1st trimester compared to those who were changed to heparin before 6 weeks gestation. Clearly, more information is required to confirm this possibility.

The management for established thrombosis

The aim of anticoagulant therapy is to prevent further thromboembolic complications and extension of any existing thrombus. The effectiveness of such therapy is evidenced by the study of Villa Santa (1965) which showed a substantial reduction in mortality from 13% to 0.7% with the use of anticoagulant therapy for thromboembolism.

The acute therapy for DVT/PTE is heparin. Many regimes exist for its use and most are satisfactory provided that monitoring of heparin activity and adjustment of the dose is carried out to establish and maintain therapeutic levels. Most regimens employ intravenous administration of a bolus of 5000–10 000 iu followed by a continuous infusion of 1000–1600 iu per hour for 5–10 days. The continuous infusion can be made up in saline and given by syringe pump. Continuous intravenous administration is preferable to intermittent intravenous injections as comparative studies have shown the former to be safer in terms of major haemorrhagic complications (Salzman et al 1975, Glazier & Crowel 1976). However, subcutaneous therapy may be a satisfactory alternative as it is a more practicable treatment regime for patients and staff by avoiding the continuous intravenous infusion. The risk of haemorrhagic complications with subcutaneous therapy does not appear to be any greater than with continuous intravenous infusion (Bentley et al 1980, Andersson et al 1982, Hull et al 1986a) and the efficacy appears to be equally good in terms of recurrent thromboembolism (Bentley et al 1980, Andersson et al 1982).

A variety of tests is available for monitoring heparin therapy. These include the activated partial thromboplastin time (APTT), the heparin level measured by the protamine sulphate neutralization test (PSNT), the thrombin clotting time and factor Xa inhibitory activity (anti-Xa). Perhaps the most commonly used of these is the APTT. This should be maintained in the range 1.5–2.0 times the normal result. This therapeutic range for the APTT has been obtained from animal models (Zucker & Cathay 1969) and from retrospective studies examining the development of recurrent thromboembolic episodes while on continuous heparin and relating this to the APTT (Basu et al 1972). Both these animal and clinical studies related an APTT of less than 1.5 times the normal level to thromboembolic recurrence while on therapy. On the other hand, the risk of haemorrhagic complications does not correlate well with APTT (Pitney et al 1970, Hirsh 1986) and haemorrhagic complications appear to be related more to other factors such as heparin level, an underlying haemorrhagic tendency, or recent surgery. The anti-platelet effects of unfractionated heparin may also contribute to the haemorrhagic effects of high heparin levels. In some patients with venous thrombosis, very high doses of heparin are required: in excess of 50 000 iu/day, to prolong the APTT by 1.5–2.0 times the normal mean. Such patients are often termed heparin resistant. However, this may be a laboratory phenomenon especially in late pregnancy. This may result from dissociation of the APTT from the heparin levels as determined from the PSNT. The latter may be well inside the therapeutic range while the former is subtherapeutic. This phenomenon may be related to high concentration of procoagulant factors particularly factor VIII (Hirsh 1986) as found in late pregnancy. It has been shown that the anticoagulant effect of heparin is markedly decreased in late pregnancy with approximately 1.5 times as much heparin being required in pregnancy to double the APTT compared to the non-pregnant situation (Whitfield et al 1983). In addition, Bonnar has found that a 5000 iu subcutaneous dose of heparin at 14 weeks gestation is equivalent to a 10 000 iu dose at 35 weeks, in terms of plasma heparin concentration (Bonnar 1976) and this may be related to the increased plasma volume of pregnancy. True heparin resistance may also occur but in this situation the APTT and the PSNT will both be subtherapeutic despite high doses of heparin. This is usually seen in the early stages of treatment of patients with large venous thrombosis or PTE, due to increased heparin clearance (Hirsh 1986) related to the size of the thrombus.

In view of these difficulties some workers suggest that the PSNT is more useful (Letsky & de Swiet 1984) as a monitoring test in pregnancy. This test calculates the heparin concentration from the amount of protamine sulphate required to neutralize the effect of heparin on the thrombin clotting time (therapeutic range 0.6–1.0 iu/ml). These workers have found this technique a much more reliable and satisfactory method in pregnancy than the APTT (de Swiet 1985), and, if available, seems preferable to the APTT in pregnancy. This is supported by animal work which has shown that the anti-thrombotic effects of heparin correlate better with the heparin level than with the APTT when FVIII and fibrinogen are elevated (Chiu et al 1977).

Following the acute phase of therapy, chronic anticoagulation is required. The options lie between subcutaneous heparin and warfarin. In view of the problems of warfarin in pregnancy the former is clearly preferable. This is given as 10 000 iu heparin twice daily subcutaneously and can be administered in a small volume if a concentrated heparin solution (50 000 iu/ml) is employed. Recently in the UK a pre-loaded subcutaneous preparation has been introduced containing 10 000 iu in 0.2 ml which is especially useful in pregnancy, and avoids the hazards of measuring small volumes. Since such low-dose heparin does not affect the conventional coagulation tests, therapy is monitored by the anti-Xa activity method of Denson & Bonnar (1973), and levels should be maintained at less than 0.4 u/ml. This is very rarely exceeded with a dose of 20 000 iu a day in pregnancy. It is unnecessary to employ any more than this in pregnancy (de Swiet 1985) and there appears to be no risk of bleeding in labour if anti-Xa levels are less than 0.4 u/ml (Howell et al 1983, Hathaway & Bonnar 1987). Blood loss during Caesarean section performed following subcutaneous low-dose heparin has been shown to be no different from that following placebo (Hill et al 1988). It has been suggested that the combination of heparin and an anti-platelet agent such as aspirin or a nonsteroidal anti-inflammatory drug may be associated with increased risk of bleeding. However, there is no evidence of any haemostatic drug interaction between these agents (Spowart et al 1988), although particular care should obviously be taken if these agents are prescribed together.

As heparin is cleared by the kidney, care should be taken in patients with renal impairment or pre-eclampsia as high heparin levels and haemorrhagic complications may occur. In the puerperium, the heparin dosage can be reduced to 7500 iu twice daily subcutaneously as recommended by de Swiet (1985) or 5000 iu three times daily. In view of the risk of haemorrhage if warfarin is employed in the early puerperium, heparin should be continued for at least 7–10 days. After this time warfarin may safely be used. The duration of anticoagulant therapy is quite arbitrary. In the case of an antenatal thrombosis, treatment should be continued throughout pregnancy and for at least 6 weeks following delivery as it takes some time for the 'physiological coagulopathy' of pregnancy to disappear. 6 weeks therapy seems satisfactory for a simple post partum DVT but a longer period of 3 months or more may be required in the case of a PTE or a very extensive DVT.

If warfarin is employed, it should be started approximately 3 days prior to stopping heparin, due to the time required for its maximal effect to occur. Various regimens exist for warfarin loading. A satisfactory one is 20 mg on the 1st day of warfarin therapy, 10 mg on the 2nd day, then stop the heparin and maintain anticoagulation with a maintenance dose of warfarin which should be titrated against the prothrombin time which is the most satisfactory test for warfarin's anticoagulant effect. The heparin should not be stopped until the prothrombin time is in the therapeutic range (2.0–4.0 times the normal control plasma). To allow international comparison, the prothrombin time may be expressed as the International Normalized Ratio (INR) to take into account the differing sensitivies of the varying thromboplastins used in this test throughout the world (Hirsh 1986).

Thrombolytic therapy

Thrombolytic therapy with streptokinase has been employed in pregnancy complicated by major PTE (Pfeiffer 1970, Hall et al 1972, Ludwig 1973, McTaggart & Ingram 1977) with some success as regards thrombolysis. However, major haemorrhagic problems may be encountered, especially from the placental site or any surgical wounds if it is employed around the time of delivery or the early puerperium. It should, therefore, only be employed after due consideration of these major risks, in the most life-threatening situation. Recently, recombinant tissue plasminogen activator tPA has become available and has been successfully employed in the thrombolysis of arterial and venous thrombosis. This is superior to streptokinase and urokinase both in terms of its specific activity and lack of systemic fibrinolytic activation (Collen 1985). It has not been assessed in pregnancy but may be a possible therapeutic option in the future.

Surgical management

Should heparin therapy fail to prevent recurrent thromboembolism despite adequate anticoagulation, surgical interruption of the vena cava may be required. Open ligation or plication can for the most part be avoided by the use of filters which can be inserted into the inferior vena cava and lodged below the renal veins. These can be inserted via the femoral vein and the procedure carries less risk than open ligation (Donaldson et al 1980, Jones et al 1986), although it may be associated with femoral venous thrombosis and chronic venous stasis. It has been employed in the pregnant situation (Hux et al 1986).

Surgical embolectomy under cardiopulmonary bypass may be required in patients with severe life-threatening PTE associated with sustained hypotension and hypoxia. Prompt surgical referral and pulmonary angiography are required, and it is best to involve the vascular or cardiothoracic surgeons as early a possibly in the management of patients who potentially may require surgical intervention.

Prophylaxis

Until recently, long-term administration of anticoagulants was employed in the antenatal period as the established prophylactic therapy for women with a past history of thromboembolism occurring within or outwith pregnancy. This was because the incidence of recurrence of this potentially lethal complication was thought to be around 12–15% (Badaracco & Vessey 1974, Bergqvist et al 1991) and the risks of long-term anticoagulants in pregnancy were not appreciated. Nonetheless 52% of UK obstetricians would still use prophylaxis antenatally in women with a previous DVT outwith pregnancy, rising, to 81% if the previous DVT had occurred during pregnancy (Greer & de Swiet 1993). This view of routine prophylaxis has, justifiably, been challenged in the last few years, principally by de Swiet's group at Queen Charlotte's Hospital, London. They have published two studies where anticoagulant therapy was not used in the antenatal period. The first was a randomized study of 40 women with a history of previous thromboembolic problems. They were randomized to receive heparin 10 000 iu subcutaneously twice per day antenatally or no anticoagulant therapy antenatally. Both groups were given heparin postpartum. One DVT occurred in the control group and none in the treatment group, while one patient in the treatment group developed severe debilitating osteopenia (Howel et al 1983). The second study involved 26 patients with a past history of thromboembolism (Lao et al 1985). None received anticoagulants antenatally but dextran was used intrapartum and heparin or heparin followed by warfarin was used postpartum for 6 weeks to cover the increased risk associated in the puerperium. Only one patient had a possible thromboembolic event antenatally and none had any problems postnatally. There were no significant problem from the therapy. These figures have recently been updated (de Swiet et al 1987) and no thromboembolic problems have occurred either antenatally or postnatally in 59 patients with this regimen. These studies clearly suggest that the risk of antenatal thromboembolism in these women is much lower than previously thought. When this is balanced against the hazards of anticoagulation, prophylactic therapy is questionable and perhaps is best reserved for those with recurrent severe problems, congenital or acquired thrombophilia or those with postphlebitic insufficiency. Additionally, pregnancy is not contraindicated in women with such a history. Some authorities, however, still advise prophylactic anticoagulant therapy if the previous problem occurred in pregnancy, starting 4–6 weeks before the gestational age when the previous thromboembolic problem occurred (Rutherford & Phelen 1986, Hathaway & Bonnar 1987). If subcutaneous heparin prophylaxis is employed, then it should be used in similar manner as chronic therapy following a thromboembolic problem as discussed above (p. 999). As thromboembolism is a potentially fatal condition and prophylaxis is not without hazard, it seems prudent to discuss the various risks of these problems pre-pregnancy, or at least in early pregnancy, with the patient, no matter which prophylactic philosophy is taken, especially since neither approach has been fully evaluated in a large controlled clinical study. All authorities do agree, however, on postnatal prophylactic therapy in patients with a past history of thromboembolism.

Increasingly, short-term prophylactic heparin is being used postpartum in patients with significant risk factors such as operative delivery, obesity, age over 35-years-old, and restricted activity prior to deliver. Such prophylaxis must be encouraged if we wish to impact upon the morbidity and mortality associated with DVT and PTE in the puerperium.

The role of low molecular weight heparins in thromboprophylaxis in pregnancy has yet to be established. However, their efficacy in the non-pregnant situation, potentially lower risk of haemorrhagic complications and better bioavailability suggest that they will be of value. There are anecdotal reports of the use of these compounds in pregnancy (Priollet et al 1986), and in our own practice we have found that the low molecular weight heparin, enoxaparine (Rhone-Poulenc-Rorer, UK), has better bioavailability than unfractionated heparin as determined by anti-Xa levels (unpublished data). While low molecular weight heparin may only require to be given once a day in the non-pregnant situation, we have noted that twice daily administration may be required in pregnancy to provide satisfactory anti-Xa levels over a 24 hour period (unpublished observation). Thus, if low molecular weight heparin is employed in pregnancy for thromboprophylaxis, we would recommend, at least until more experience is gained, that anti-Xa levels are monitored and dosage adjusted to achieve a satisfactory anti-Xa level. In the puerperium once daily administration may provide adequate thromboprophylaxis, but again anti-Xa levels should be monitored to determine if this sufficient.

Dextran may also be considered for intrapartum or intraoperative prophylaxis. Its precise mode of action is unknown but may be due to haemodilution and improved flow as well as its effects on the haemostatic system which include anti-platelet effects, a fall in factor VIII and possibly enhanced plasminogen activators (Bergqvist 1983). Its disadvantage is the small risk of anaphalactoid reaction, but this can be markedly reduced by pre-treatment with the low molecular weight hapten, dextran (Bergqvist 1983). Although widely used in Europe, surprisingly this is not available in the UK. There is also evidence to suggest that heparin and dextran may be associated with haemorrhagic problems if used together (Bergqvist 1983). Physical methods of prophylaxis such as intermittent calf compression are also useful intraoperatively.

Anticoagulants and spinal and epidural anaesthesia

There is no doubt that full anticoagulation with heparin or warfarin, or recent thromblysis with streptokinase or tissue-plasmonigen activator are clear contraindications to the use of spinal or epidural anaesthesia. However, the situation with low dose heparin is much more controversial and the traditional conservative philosophy (Crawford 1978) is increasingly being challenged with the increase in epidural and spinal anaesthesia in general and in particular in labour and caesarean section (Wildsmith & McClure 1991). However, many anaesthetists and obstetricians still feel that low dose heparin is a contraindication to epidural or spinal anaesthesia. A recent Danish Study (Wille-Jorgensen et al 1991) of anaesthetists found that 38% of them felt this combination was contraindicated, and a survey of consultant obstetricians in the UK found that 48% of them shared that view (Greer & de Swiet 1993). There are few data to support or refute this practice. The major concern of employing spinal or epidural anaesthesia in the presence of low-dose heparin, is the risk of spinal haematoma, which may be associated with substantial and often permanent neurological damage. Spinal haematoma is a very rare condition and there are no data providing a reliable estimate of the incidence of this problem. In addition it can occur spontaneously in patients who have had neither spinal instrumentation nor anticoagulant therapy including a report of such an occurrence in the puerperium (Crawford 1975). Thus spinal instrumentation and haematoma development may not be causally related, although a review of the literature has shown that the majority of reports of spinal haematoma occurring after spinal or epidural nerve blockade were in patients with coagulation disorders (Sage 1990). However, against this extremely low risk of spinal haematoma we must balance the risk of thrombosis which is likely to be substantially greater. Each case, therefore, has to be judged on its own merits. Guidelines for anaesthetists have recently been suggested (Wildsmith & McClure 1991). These include delaying the siting of a block until 4–6 hours after the last administration of low-dose heparin, as some patients have significant systemic concentrations of heparin within 2 hours of administration, or delaying administration until the block has been sited. In addition, as regional blockade reduces the risk of DVT (Thorburn et al 1980), heparin prophylaxis could be delayed until the operation is completed.

ANTICOAGULANT PROPHYLAXIS IN PATIENTS WITH ARTIFICIAL HEART VALVES IN PREGNANCY

Patients with prosthetic valves require prophylactic anticoagulants to avoid the risk of systemic embolism and valve thrombosis (Cheeseboro et al 1986). It is established that inadequate anticoagulation is associated with a substantial increase in risk, which is also related to the position and number of valves involved, the type of replacements, the presence of an enlarged atrium and perhaps, most importantly, atrial fibrillation (Cheseboro et al 1986).

It is clearly essential that patients with artificial valves receive anticoagulants throughout pregnancy to avoid the increased risk from the physiological coagulopathy of pregnancy. In the non-pregnant state these women are managed on warfarin. However, as discussed above, this poses problems for mother and fetus in terms of early pregnancy loss, fetal abnormality and haemorrhage. In one study, an attempt was made to avoid anticoagulants in pregnancy. Of nine women who were managed without anticoagulants through 11 pregnancies, one died from cerebral embolism and another had a thrombosed valve (Chen et al 1982), compared to one non-fatal embolus postnatally in 30 mothers given anticoagulants, thus emphasizing the need for prophylactic therapy. This has led to the exploration of alternative anticoagulant regimes.

It is known that anti-platelet agents such as dipyridamole will enhance the anti-thrombotic effects of warfarin in these patients (Cheeseboro et al 1986). However, there is reliable evidence from a randomized controlled trial that anti-platelet agents alone are not effective in this situation (Mok et al 1985) despite sporadic reports of their successful use in pregnancy (Chen et al 1982). In the pregnant situation, Salazar et al 1984 studied 68 pregnancies in which anti-platelet therapy replaced coumarin therapy in the 1st trimester and compared this to 128 pregnancies where coumarins were continued until 38 weeks. The former group was complicated by three maternal deaths from valve thrombosis and a 25% incidence of cerebral emboli, compared to only a 2.3% incidence of emboli in the latter group. The former group was, however, associated with a much smaller fetal loss rate and avoided warfarin embryopathy. Clearly, anti-platelet therapy alone must not be used in this situation.

The other alternative is heparin. When given in the 1st trimester and in the weeks immediately prior to delivery in a fixed dose of 5000 iu twice in the day, warfarin embryopathy was avoided (Iturbe-Alessio et al 1986) but unfortunately it was associated with a high incidence of valve thrombosis and thromboembolism (Wang et al 1983, Iturbe-Alessio et al 1986). However, there have been more recent reports employing higher doses of heparin with adjustments to maintain the APTT, or PSNT in the therapeutic range. Using such a regimen, both warfarin embryopathy and thromboembolic problems have been avoided (Lee et al 1986). In all these studies, warfarin was reintroduced following the 1st trimester and replaced again with heparin in the weeks immediately prior to delivery. In the latter study, there was still a high spontaneous abortion rate which may be related to warfarin therapy in very early pregnancy. The possibility of switching to heparin prior to conception should therefore be considered.

The safest regimen for the mother at least, until more information is available on therapeutic long-term heparinization, is warfarin therapy continuously in pregnancy until 37 weeks gestation. This means accepting the risk of fetal loss and abnormality. After 36 weeks, the risk of fetal and maternal bleeding with approaching delivery is too high with warfarin and therapeutic doses of heparin should be substituted. This can be given by continuous intravenous infusion or subcutaneous injections and should be monitored appropriately. The dose should be reduced for delivery which can be carried out safely on prophylactic doses of heparin, provided heparin levels are less than 0.4 iu/ml (de Swiet 1985). Following delivery by whatever route, therapeutic doses of heparin should be reinstituted with a switch to warfarin after 7–10 days when the risk of postpartum haemorrhage associated with warfarin is reduced.

The alternative to this approach is to use therapeutic heparinization in the 1st trimester and possibly from before conception as suggested by Lee et al (1986), or possibly continuing this throughout pregnancy and avoiding warfarin altogether as recommended by Hathaway & Bonnar (1987). In these situations, heparin will probably need to be given three times daily to maintain the APTT in the therapeutic range. The latter of these regimens also carries all the maternal risks of long-term heparin therapy.

Whatever regime is employed, it is clearly essential to discuss the risks and options with the couple prior to or at least very early in pregnancy. This will allow them information to decide whether to embark on, or continue with a pregnancy and will allow them to see the importance of adequate anticoagulation and monitoring. It is clearly important that the couple should be involved in the decision-making process regarding which anticoagulant regime to use.

Bioprosthetic heart valves do not carry the same risks as mechanical ones (Salazar et al 1984, Cheeseboro et al 1986). However, anticoagulation may still be required for association risk factors such as atrial fibrillation. Unfortunately, the poor durability of these valves means that they are not commonly used in young women.

CONGENITAL THROMBOTIC PROBLEMS

The main congenital thrombotic problems are deficiencies of the endogenous coagulation inhibitor, ATIII, protein C and protein S although abnormalities of fibrinolysis, hereditary dysfibrinogenaemias, and homocystinuria may also be responsible for recurrent thromboembolism (Winter & Douglas 1991). These conditions should be considered and preferably evaluated pre-pregnancy in women with recurrent thrombosis. In view of the pregnancy-associated changes in the coagulation system, it is not surprising that pregnancy may unmask such underlying problems in young women.

ATIII deficiency

Deficiency of ATIII was first described in 1965 (Egeberg 1965). It may be a quantitative defect with a marked reduction in both immunoreactive and functional levels of ATIII, or a qualitative defect with normal immunoreactive ATIII and deficient functional ATIII (Sas et al 1974). It is usually inherited as an autosomal dominant disorder with the gene locus being located on the long arm of chromosome one (Winter et al 1982a). With the advent of DNA probes, early prenatal diagnosis of the disorder has become possible. The incidence is around 1:5000 (Odegard & Abildgaard 1978). Anti-thrombin III deficiency usually presents with DVT or mesenteric thrombosis.

Pregnancy is a major precipitant for thromboembolism in women with this deficiency (Winter & Douglas 1991). The risk of such problems developing during pregnancy and the puerperium is substantial in the absence of anticoagulant therapy. Winter et al (1982b) reporting 16 pregnancies in 7 patients found an incidence of 81% in pregnancy and 12% in the puerperium, while a Scandanavian report (Hellgren et al 1982) of 47 pregnancies in 29 patients found an incidence of 51% and 17% for pregnancy and the puerperium respectively. This pattern contrasts with that reported from France where 63 pregnancies in 25 patients were included (Conard et al

1990). This report found a lower incidence of thrombosis overall with the majority of thrombosis occurring in the puerperium (18% incidence of thrombosis in pregnancy, 33% incidence in the puerperium). In any case, the risk of thrombosis is substantial and long-term prophylactic anticoagulant therapy is clearly justified. However, management should start with pre-pregnancy counselling and carrier detection in affected families, discussing the risks of thrombosis, hazards of anticoagulants and the hereditary nature of the disease. The mainstay of prophylactic therapy is subcutaneous heparin, and prophylactic treatment appears to reduce the incidence of thrombosis (Douglas et al 1990).

If the patient is already on warfarin, this is switched to heparin before pregnancy if possible. The management in pregnancy has been previously discussed (Hellgren et al 1982, Samson et al 1984, Douglas et al 1990, Winter & Douglas 1991). Briefly, the patient should receive 10 000 iu heparin subcutaneously initially. This dose should be adjusted to maintain the APTT (the PSNT is unsuitable in this disorder) 5–10 seconds above the normal value on a sample taken immediately prior to heparin administration. Monitoring of APTT and platelet count should be carried out at least fortnightly. When delivery is imminent, the heparin is reduced to 5000 iu twice daily and ATIII concentrate infused on alternate days to maintain the ATIII level greater than 80% of normal. Following delivery, ATIII infusions and heparin are continued for 7 days, then warfarin can be employed as the risk of postpartum haemorrhage will have diminished by that time. Low molecular weight heparins have been successfully employed for prophylaxis in ATIII-deficient women (Henny et al 1986, Manson et al 1991) and may be superior to unfractionated heparin (Manson et al 1991). However, further and more extensive evaluation of these compounds is required in this situation. Warfarin should continue for 6–8 weeks or indefinitely if there is a past history of thromboembolism. Oestrogen-containing contraceptives should be avoided as they are associated with thrombosis. However, the progesterone-only pill appears suitable. An umbilical cord blood sample should be checked for ATIII level to determine whether the infant is affected, although this may not be conclusive. Thrombotic problems are much less common in neonates than in adults with this disorder. Established thrombosis is treated by therapeutic doses of heparin and ATIII concentrate for 7–10 days, then prophylactic heparin as above. If a thrombosis develops while on heparin, warfarin should be employed.

Protein C and protein S deficiency

Again both these disorders appear to be autosomal dominant and may be quantitative or qualitative deficiencies, the former being more common. Protein C deficiency was first described by Griffin et al (1981). It is found in 8% of young people with thrombosis (Broekmans et al 1983), although the incidence has been reported at 1:16 000 (Broekmans et al 1983) in Holland. Proteins S deficiency only came to light in 1984 (Comp et al 1984) and there is therefore little knowledge about this problem. Both disorders present with thrombosis, although this appears to be much less common than with ATIII deficiency, although superficial thrombophlebitis is more common. A particular association is coumarin-induced skin necrosis. This starts several days following the commencement of coumarins. It is thought to be due to a rapid fall in protein C and factor VII due to their short half lives. This results in thrombosis of the microcirculation of the skin and infarction which becomes haemorrhagic with further inhibition of the coagulation system. Conard et al (1990) have reported on 93 pregnancies in 36 patients with protein C deficiency and 44 pregnancies in 17 patients with protein S deficiency. In the absence of anticoagulant therapy the incidence of thrombosis during pregnancy was 7% and 0%, and during the puerperium 19% and 17% for protein C and protein S deficiency respectively. As protein S levels fall during pregnancy it is perhaps surprising that thrombotic problems are so infrequent during pregnancy in women with protein S deficiency, however, there are occasional reports of thrombosis occurring in these women during pregnancy (Schwartz et al 1984). There is little information on prophylactic therapy. There have been successful reports of therapy with subcutaneous heparin (Gonzalez et al 1985, Carter & Bellem 1988) with warfarin being employed in the puerperium. Although there have been successful reports of prophylactic therapy with warfarin in patients with protein S deficiency (Broekmans et al 1985, Michiels et al 1987), prophylactic heparin therapy is likely to be satisfactory as for ATIII deficiency. The data discussed above on the incidence of thrombosis in pregnancy and the puerperium in protein C and protein S deficient women suggest that prophylaxis is essential in the purpeurium, but during pregnancy, especially in protein S deficiency, prophylaxis may not be required and each case must be individually assessed until more experience is obtained (Conard et al 1990).

LUPUS ANTICOAGULANT AND PREGNANCY

Lupus anticoagulant is an autoantibody, usually of the IgG class but sometimes of the IgM class, which is directed against negatively charged phospholipids in cell membranes, such as platelets. It can therefore interfere with activation of prothrombin by the prothrombin activator complex of factor Xa, factor V, platelet phospholipid and Ca^{2+}. Thus the phospholipid-dependent coagulation tests such as the APTT and prothrombin time (PT) are prolonged and suggest that an endogenous inhibitor of coagulation is present. The name lupus anticoagulant derives from the original description of the phenomenon in patients with SLE (Conley & Hartman, 1952). However, it is found in only 5–10% of patients with SLE, although around 40–50% of patients with lupus anticoagulant will have underlying SLE. It is also found in association with other auto-immune conditions. The name is something of a misnomer as it is rarely associated with bleeding except when accompanied by thrombocytopenia or hypoprothrombinaemia. It is more commonly, and paradoxically, associated with arterial and venous thrombosis which are often recurrent (Bowie et al 1963, Mueh et al 1980). The mechanism behind the thrombotic tendency is unclear. Lupus anticoagulant has been shown to inhibit endothelial PGI_2 production (Carreras et al 1981), although more recent studies have not confirmed this (Walker et al 1988). It has been suggested that the thrombotic effect may be due to inhibition of endothelial cell mediated protein C activation (Cariou et al 1986). This hypothesis is somewhat unsatisfactory as protein C deficiency is usually associated with venous thrombosis. The mechanism does however, appear to be, at least in part, platelet mediated as platelet count falls with thrombotic episodes. It appears likely that several mechanisms exist whereby lupus anticoagulant can induce thrombosis (Walker et al 1988). Lupus anticoagulant may be associated with the presence of other autoantibodies such as anti-cardiolipin antibody and anti-nuclear antibody (Harris et al 1985) and is also associated with false-positive syphilis serology. There is a strong association between anticardiolipin antibody and lupus anticoagulant with the former being present in between 80–100% of women with lupus anticoagulant. However, these antibodies can be dissociated with steroid therapy, when prolonged coagulation tests return to normal while anticardiolipin antibody may be unaltered (Derksen et al 1986). High titers of this antibody may predict thrombotic problems (Lockshin et al 1985, Harris et al 1986). Anticardiolipin antibody is not the only phospholipid antibody to be found, a variety exists such as antiphosphatidylinositol or antiphosphatidylserine antibodies. Antiphosphatidylinositol antibodies appear to be associated with thrombosis even in the absence of anticardiolipin antibody and lupus anticoagulant (Falcon et al 1990).

In obstetrics, lupus anticoagulant is associated not only with thrombotic problems per se but also with recurrent fetal loss and intrauterine death (Nilsson et al 1975). Scott et al (1987) recently reported the results of 242 untreated pregnancies in 65 women with lupus anticoagulant. The incidence of spontaneous abortion or intrauterine death was 91%. These losses may occur late in pregnancy and become progressively earlier in future pregnancies. Affected women may also have a history of recurrent DVT, renal, axillary and occular vein thrombosis, arterial thrombosis and even the Budd–Chiari syndrome (Hughes 1988). The mechanism underlying the fetal losses appears to be placental infarction. Pathologically, infarction of the spiral arteries of the basal plate of the placenta, with fibrinoid necrosis, acute atherosis and intraluminal thrombosis are seen (de Wolf et al 1982). These findings are non-specific, however, and are similar to those seen with pre-eclampsia and growth retardation. Fetal loss has also been associated with presence of anti-cardiolipin antibodies, and high titres of this antibody appear to predict thrombotic complications, fetal distress and fetal loss (Lockshin et al 1985, Harris et al 1986). In patients with such a history who are negative for lupus anticoagulant and anti-cardiolipin antibodies, it may be useful to screen for antiphosphatidylinositol antibodies as these have been associated with thrombotic problems and fetal loss in the absence of lupus anticoagulant and anticardiolipin antibodies (Falcon et al 1990). The presence of lupus anticoagulant is also associated with pre-eclampsia, growth retardation and chorea gravidarum (Lubbe & Walker 1983, Lubbe et al 1984, Branch et al 1985). The diagnosis of lupus anticoagulant is made by finding a prolonged phospholipid-dependent coagulation test with failure of this to correct after the addition of normal plasma. The kaolin cephalin clotting time (KCCT) and dilute prothrombin time are the most commonly used tests. The latter is more sensitive, with increasing prolongations of the test being found with increasing dilution (Boxer et al 1976). The APTT has a variable sensitivity (Mannucci et al 1979) and is therefore best avoided. Mixing curves for a test such as the KCCT should also be performed to exclude a coagulation factor deficiency (Exner et al 1978). More recently the dilute Russell Viper venom time has been employed and this has been shown to be sensitive, reproducible and easy to perform (Thiagarajan et al 1986). The presence of other auto-antibodies in particular anticardiolipin antibody should also be sought.

The treatment of lupus anticoagulant in pregnancy is based on the report of Lubbe et al (1983) who described the first successful therapeutic regime in this condition. They reported six women with a history of 14 pregnancy losses between them, who subsequently had five out of six successful pregnancies on a combination of prednisone 40–60 mg a day and aspirin 75 mg a day. The aim of this regime is to suppress autoantibody production with steroids and inhibit platelet function with aspirin. A coagulation test such as the KCCT should be monitored and when this returns to normal, steroids may be reduced to a maintenance dose. Branch et al (1985) reported eight patients with a past history of 31 pregnancies between them with 30 of these ending in spontaneous abortion or fetal death. These patients were subsequently treated with prednisone and aspirin with resultant shortening of their APTTs and reduction of the pregnancy loss to 37.5%, although pre-eclampsia and growth retardation were common in these women with successful pregnancies.

Women with lupus anticoagulant must be carefully assessed and monitored throughout pregnancy to assess disease activity, to look for complications such as pre-eclampsia and to monitor fetal growth and wellbeing. Recently Trudinger et al (1988) have reported the use of Doppler measurement of umbilical artery flow velocity waveforms to monitor the fetus in pregnancies complicated by lupus anticoagulant. In view of the placental vasculopathy associated with this condition this may be a potentially useful investigation. In Trudinger's study (Trudinger et al 1988) delivery was guided by the detection of deteriorating umbilical artery flow velocity waveforms and although all patients were delivered early, all six pregnancies were successful despite no therapy being given for lupus anticoagulant. Although the outcome appears to be improved with steroids and aspirin there are no controlled data on the efficacy of this regimen. A recent study has questioned the value of steroid therapy. Lockshin et al (1989) observed patients with anti-phospholipid antibodies and a history of previous fetal loss. These women received either no therapy, prednisone alone, aspirin alone or predinisone and aspirin. Nine of the 11 pregnancies treated with steroids ended in fetal loss, although three were in the 1st trimester around the time steroids were started, while five of the ten pregnancies where steroids were not employed ended in fetal loss, with only one of these occurring in the 1st trimester. This difference was statistically significant, but with small numbers and a non-randomized design it is difficult to make any firm recommendations on the basis of such observational studies. Feinstein (1985) has urged for a randomized, prospective controlled trial of this therapy to be conducted with both groups receiving intensive fetal monitoring to assess accurately the usefulness of therapy compared to intensive monitoring alone. Additionally it may be important to assess the use of aspirin alone as this appears to be associated with a much improved outcome in patients with SLE and anticardiolipin antibody or lupus anticoagulant (Elder et al 1988).

CEREBRAL THROMBOSIS

Cerebral arterial and venous thrombosis are uncommon conditions in pregnancy. A survey of women aged 15–45 years between 1956 and 1967 in Glasgow showed that 35% of the 65 women in this age group with ischaemic stroke were pregnant or in the puerperium (Cross et al 1968) giving a rate of around 1:20 000 live birth. A more recent study form Rochester has put the incidence lower than this with only one cerebral infarction in over 26 000 live births (Wiebers & Whisnant 1985). Srinivasan (1983), in India, has reported 135 patients out of around 65 000 deliveries with cerebrovascular accidents in pregnancy, of which six were arterial thrombosis, while 120 were cerebral venous thrombosis (CVT). Of the arterial thrombotic lesions, middle cerebral artery occlusion is the commonest lesion in pregnancy while internal carotid occlusion appears more common in the puerperium. The pathological basis of these lesions is uncertain but in some cases may have been related to an underlying thrombotic problem which may not have been apparent when these studies, most of which were conducted over 20 years ago, were performed. Once the occlusion occurs, management is identical to that in the non-pregnant, with supportive measures being taken and possibly steroid therapy being used to reduce cerebral oedema.

CVT appears to be a rare complication of pregnancy in the western world. Cross et al (1968) did not encounter a single case in their 10-year survey during which 23 pregnant women were found with arterial occlusion. The presenting features are often non-specific and include headache, a focal neurological deficit — often a hemiplagia or dysphasia — seizures, papilloedema, fever and coma. The development of a DVT may herald the subsequent development of a CVT (Srinivasan 1983). Risk factors other than pregnancy include diabetes, dehydration, sickle cell anaemia, haemolytic anaemia and cardiac failure (Halpern et al 1984). The diagnosis may be hampered by CVT simulating other neurological problems such as viral encephalitis, benign intercranial hypertension, arterial stroke and tumours. The diagnosis usually requires bilateral carotid angiography. Isotope brain scan and computerized tomography may be helpful although the signs are non-specific and these investigations may be normal even in the presence of CVT. Treatment consists of anticonvulsant therapy and the use of steroids and mannitol to reduce the intracranial pressure. Anticoagulation with heparin appears to prevent extension, and reduces the risk of PTE which is a common mode of death in patients with CVT (Bousser et al 1984). There is however a risk of bleeding as intracranial haemorrhage and subarachnoid haemorrhage can be found in patients dying from CVT (Barnett & Hyland 1953). Thus the use of anticoagulants is controversial. Halpern et al (1984) have suggested that anticoagulation should be considered in patients with no objective evidence of cerebral haemorrhage, which will usually require computerized tomography. Bousser et al (1984) suggest that heparin be employed in patients who deteriorate despite symptomatic measures, and 23 of the 38 patients in the series they reported received heparin and all survived. In view of the rarity of CVT the mortality is difficult to gauge, however survivors appear to do reasonably well and often have only minimal neurological sequelae (Srinivasan 1983).

PELVIC THROMBOPHLEBITIS

This condition can occur following vaginal or Caesarean delivery or after abortion. The incidence of this condition is around 0.05% (Josey & Stagger 1974, Dunnihoo et al

1991), but figures as high as 0.9% have been reported following caesarean section (Mulkamy 1980). It usually starts in the ovarian veins and may extend into the vena cava, renal veins or iliac veins with around 13% of patients developing PTE (Dunnihoo et al 1991). It usually presents with persistent fever and leukocytosis following delivery which may be unresponsive to antibiotics, and pelvic or flank pain. Nausea and vomiting and an ileus may also be seen. It is often associated with endometritis. Most episodes are right sided, possibly due to the right ovarian vein crossing over the ureter at the pelvic brim making it more susceptible to compression with dextrorotation of the uterus. Patients may also have urologic symptoms due to ureteric compression. Symptoms usually start within the first 5 days after delivery, commonly on day 1 or day 2. On examination, the abdomen will be tender over the site of thrombosis and a mass may be palpable. The differential diagnosis will include appendicitis.

Objective diagnosis may be made with computerized tomography (Khurana et al 1988) and duplex ultrasound (Baran & Frisch 1987) may have a role. The characteristic findings on computerized tomography which have been described are: a sausage-shaped mass in the paracolic gutter which disappears at the level of the renal veins, a grossly dilated ovarian vein, associated thrombus in the vena cava, iliac and femoral veins, which may be enhanced with contrast material, and an inflammatory mass around the affected veins (Khurana et al 1988). Treatment depends on the clinician being alert to the possibility of the diagnosis, in particular in patients with persistent and apparently unexplained pyrexia following delivery. Anticoagulation and antibiotics should be employed. This condition has recently been extensively and well reviewed (Dunihoo et al 1991).

CONCLUSION

Thromboembolism contributes substantially to maternal mortality and morbidity. The clinician must be aware of the risk factors for thromboembolism as these are often present in patients who go on to develop DVT or PTE. The risk can be reduced by thromboprophylaxis with agents such as low dose heparin, and the wider use of such prophylaxis in high and moderate risk situations associated with pregnancy should be encouraged. Furthermore, the clinician must be alert to the possible diagnosis of DVT or PTE in pregnancy or the puerperium. In view of the poor reliability of clinical diagnosis, objective investigations such as ultrasound examination should be employed to confirm or refute the presence of thrombosis and guide further management. Such an increased awareness and greater use of prophylaxis may allow us to reduce the mortality from PTE in pregnancy and the puerperium.

REFERENCES

Aaro L A, Juergens J L 1971 Thrombophlebitis associated with pregnancy American Journal of Obstetrics and Gynecology 109: 1128–1133

Aaro L A, Juergens J L 1974 Thrombophlebitis and pulmonary embolism as a complication of pregnancy. Medical Clinics of North American 58: 829–834

Aarskog A, Aksnes L, Lehmann V 1980 Low 1,25-dihydroxyvitamin D in heparin-induced osteopaenia. The Lancet ii: 650–651

Adam A, Albert A, Boulanger J et al 1985 Influence of oral contraceptives and pregnancy on constituents of the kallikrein-kininogen system in plasma. Clinical Chemistry 31: 1533–1536

Ager A, Gordon J L 1984 Differential effects of hydrogen peroxide on indices of endothelial cell function. Journal of Experimental Medicine 159: 592–603

Ahmed Y, Sullivan M H F, Elder M G 1991 Detection of platelet desensitization in pregnancy-induced hypertension is dependent on the agonist used. Thrombosis and Haemostasis 65(5): 474–477

Aitken A G F, Godden D J 1987 Real time diagnosis of deep venous thrombosis: a comparison with venography. Clinical Radiology 38: 309–313

Albrechtsson U, Olsson C G 1979 Thrombosis after phlebography: a comparison of two contrast media. Cardiovascular Radiology 2: 9–18

Andersson G, Fagrell B, Holmgren K, Johnsson H, Ljungberg B, Nilsson, E, Wilhelmsson S, Zetterquist S 1982 Subcutaneous administration of heparin. A randomized comparison with intravenous administration of heparin to patients with deep-vein thrombosis. Thrombosis Research 27: 631–639

Andrew M, Boneu B, Cade J et al 1985 Placental transport of low molecular weight heparin in the pregnant sheep. British Journal of Haematology 59: 103–108

Aznar J, Gilabert J, Estellés A, España F 1986 Fibrinolytic activity and protein C in pre-eclampsia. Thrombosis and Haemostasis 55: 314–317

Badaracco M A, Vessey M 1974 Recurrence of venous thromboembolism disease and use of oral contraceptives. British Medical Journal 1: 215–17

Baker P N, Broughton Pipkin F, Symonds E M 1989 Platelet angiotensin II binding sites in hypertension in pregnancy. Lancet ii: 1151 (letter)

Baker P N, Broughton-Pipkin F, Symonds E M 1991 Platelet angiotensin II binding sites in normotensive and hypertensive women. British Journal of Obstetrics and Gynaecology 98: 436–440

Ballegeer V, Mombaerts P, Declerk P J et al 1987 Fibrinolytic response to venous occlusion and fibrin fragment D-Dimer levels in normal and complicated pregnancy. Thrombosis and Haemostasis 58: 1030–1032

Baran G W, Frisch K M 1987 Duplex Doppler evaluation of puerperal ovarian vein thrombosis. American Journal of Radiology 149: 321–325

Barnett H J M, Hyland H H 1953 Non-infective intracranial venous thrombosis. Brain 76: 36–49

Basu D, Gallus A, Hirsh J, Cade J F 1972 A prospective study of the value of monitoring heparin treatment with the activated thromboplastin time. New England Journal of Medicine 287: 324–327

Beaufils M, Uzan S, Donsimoni R, Colau J C 1985 Prevention of pre-eclampsia by early anti-platelet therapy. Lancet i: 840–842

Belch J J F, McMillan N C, Fogelman I, Capell H, Forbes C.D 1981 Combined phlebography and arthrography in patients with painful swollen calf. British Medical Journal 282: 949

Belch J J F, Thorburn J, Greer I A, Sarfo S, Prentice C R M 1985 Intravenous prostacyclin in the management of pregnancies complicated by severe hypertension. Clinical and Experimental Hypertension B4: 75–86

Beller F K, Ebert C 1982 The coagulation and fibrinolytic enzyme systems in normal pregnancy and the puerperium. European Journal of Obstetrics and Gynecology and Reproductive Biology 13: 177–197

Benigni A et al 1989 Effect of low dose aspirin on fetal and maternal generation of thromboxane by platelets in women at risk for pregnancy induced hypertension. New England Journal of Medicine 321: 357–362

Bentley P G, Kakkar V V, Scully M F et al 1980 An objective study of alternative methods of heparin administration. Thrombosis Research 18: 177–187

Bergqvist D 1983 Post-operative thromboembolism. Springer Verlag, New York, p 106–107.

Bergqvist A, Bergqvist D, Hallbrook T 1979 Acute deep venous thrombosis after caesarean section. Acta Obstetricia et Gynecologica Scandinavica 58: 473–476

Bergqvist A, Bergqvist D, Hallbrook T 1983 Deep vein thrombosis during pregnancy. Acta Obstetricia et Gynecologica Scandinavica 62: 443–448

Bergqvist D, Bergqvist A, Lindhagen A, Matzsch T 1991 Long term outcome of patients with venous thromboembolism during pregnancy. In: Greer I A, Turpie A G G, Forbes C D (eds) Haemostasis and thrombosis in obstetrics and gynaecology. Chapman and Hall, London, p 349–360

Bettman M A, Paulin S 1977 Less phlebography: The incidence, nature and modification of undesirable side effects. Radiology 122: 101–104

Bonnar J 1976 Long-term self-administered heparin therapy for prevention of thromboembolic complications in pregnancy. In: Kakkar V V, Thomas D P (eds) Heparin: chemistry and clinical usage. Academic Press, London, p 247–260

Bonnar J, McNicol, G P, Douglas A S et al 1969 Fibrinolytic enzyme system and pregnancy British Medical Journal 3: 387–389

Bonnar J, McNicol G P, Douglas A S et al 1970 Coagulation and fibrinolytic mechanisms during and after normal childbirth British Medical Journal 2: 200–203

Bonnar J, McNicol G P, Douglas A S 1971 Coagulation and fibrinolytic systems in pre-eclampsia. British Medical Journal 2: 12–16

Booth N, Reith A, Bennett B et al 1988 A plasminogen activator inhibitor (PAI-2) circulates in two molecular forms during pregnancy. Thrombosis and Haemostasis 59: 77–79

Borok Z, Weitz J, Owen M, Auerbach M, Nossel H L 1984 Fibrinogen proteolysis and platelet-granule release in pre-eclampsia/eclampsia. Blood 63: 525–531

Bounameaux H, Schneider P-A, Rober G, de Moerloose P, Krahenbuhl B 1989 Measurement of D-Dimer for diagnosis of deep venous thrombosis. American Journal of Clinical Pathology 91: 82–85

Bounameaux H, Cirafici P, de Moerloose P, Schneider P A, Slosman D, Reber G, Unger P F 1991 Measurement of D-dimer in plasma as diagnostic aid in suspected pulmonary embolism. Lancet 337: 196–200

Bousser M G, Chiras J, Bories J, Castaigne P 1985 Cerebral venous thrombosis — a review of 38 cases. Stroke 16: 199–213

Bowie E J W, Thompson J H, Pascuzzi C A, Owen C A 1963 Thrombosis in systemic lupus erythematosis despite circulating anticoagulants. Journal of Laboratory Clinical Medicine 62: 416–430

Boxer M, Ellman L, Carvalho A 1976 The lupus anticoagulant. Arthritis and Rheumatism 19: 1244–1248

Branch D W, Scott J R, Kochenour N K, Hershgold E 1985 Obstetric complications associated with the lupus anticoagulant. New England Journal of Medicine 313: 1322–1326

Bray M A 1983 The pharmacology and pathophysiology of leukotriene B4. British Medical Bulletin 39: 249–254

Broekmans A W, Veltkampm J J, Bertina R M 1983 Congenital protein C deficiency and venous thromboembolism. New England Journal of Medicine 309: 340–344

Broekmans A W, Bertina R M, Reinalda-Poot J, Engesser L, Muller H P, Leeuw J A, Michiels J J, Brammer E J P, Brier E 1985 Hereditary protein S deficiency and venous thrombo-embolism. Thrombosis and Haemostasis 53: 273–277

Broughton-Pipkin F, Hunter J C, Turner S R, O'Brien P M S 1982 Prostaglandin E2 attenuates the pressor response to angiotensin II in pregnant, but non-pregnant humans. American Journal of Obstetrics and Gynecology 142: 168

Broughton-Pipkin F, Morrison R, O'Brien P M S 1984 Effects of prostacyclin on the pressor response to angiotensin II in human pregnancy. European Journal of Clinical Investigation 14: 3

Browse N 1978 Diagnosis of deep venous thrombosis. British Medical Bulletin 34: 163–167

Burgess-Wilson M E, Morrison R, Heptinstall S 1986 Spontaneous platelet aggregation in heparinised blood during pregnancy. Thrombosis Research 37: 385–393

Bussolino F, Benedetto C, Massobrio M, Comussi G 1980 Maternal vascular prostacyclin activity in pre-eclampsia. Lancet ii: 702 (letter)

Butterworth B, Greer I A, Liston W D et al 1991 Immunocytochemical localization of neutrophil elastase in term placenta decidua and myometrium in pregnancy-induced hypertension. British Journal of Obstetrics and Gynaecology 98: 929–933

Cariou R, Tobelem G, Soria C et al 1986 Inhibition of protein C activation by endothelial cells in the presence of lupus anticoagulants. New England Journal of Medicine 314: 1193–1194

Carreras L O, Vermylen J, Spitz B, van Asche A 1981 Lupus anticoagulant and inhibition of prostacyclin formation in patients with recurrent abortion, intra-uterine growth retardation and intra-uterine death. British Journal of Obstetrics and Gynaecology 88: 890–894

Carter C J, Bellem P J 1988 Management of protein C deficiency in pregnancy. Fibrinolysis Supplement I: 161, Longman Group

Chen W C C, Chan C S Lee P K, Wang R Y C, Wong V C W 1982 Pregnancy in patients with prosthetic heart valves: an experience with 45 pregnancies. Quarterly Journal of Medicine LI: 358–365

Cheeseboro J H, Adams P C, Fuster V 1986 Antithrombotic therapy in patients with valvular heart disease and prosthetic heart valves. Journal of the American College of Cardiology 8: 41–56

Chiu H M, Hirsh J, Yung W L, Regoeczi E, Gent M 1977 Relationship between the anticoagulant and antithrombotic effects of heparin in experimental venous thrombosis. Blood 49: 171–184

Chong B H, Pitney W R, Castaldi P A 1982 Heparin-induced thrombocytopenia: Association of thrombotic complications with heparin dependent IgG antibody that induces thromboxane synthesis and platelet aggregation. Lancet ii: 1246–1249

Chong M K B, Harvey D, de Swiet M 1984 Follow up of children whose mothers were treated with warfarin during pregnancy. British Journal of Obstetrics and Gynaecology 91: 1070–1073

Clarke-Parson D L, Jolovesek F R 1981 Alterations of occlusive cuff impedence plethysmography results in obstetric patients. Surgery 89: 594–598

Coelho J C, Sigel B, Ryva J C, Machi J, Renigers S A 1982 B-Mode sonography of blood clots. Journal of Clinical Ultrasound 10: 323–327

Collen D 1985 Fibrinolysis: mechanism and clinical aspects. In: Bowie E J W, Sharp A A (eds) Haemostasis and thrombosis. Butterworths London, p 237–258

Comp P C, Nixon R R, Cooper M R, Esmon C T 1984 Familial protein S deficiency is associated with recurrent thrombosis. Journal of Clinical Investigation 74: 2082–2088

Comp P C, Thurneau G R, Welsh J, Esmon C T 1986 Functional and immunologic protein S levels are decreased during pregnancy. Blood 68: 881–885

Conard J, Horellou M H, van Dreden P, Lecompte T, Samama M 1990 Thrombosis and pregnancy in congenital deficiencies in ATIII, protein C or protein S: Study of 78 women. Thrombosis and Haemostasis 63: 319–320

Condie R G 1976 A serial study of coagulation factors XII, XXI and X in normal pregnancy and in pregnancy complicated by pre-eclampsia. British Journal of Obstetric and Gynaecology 83: 636–639

Conley C L, Hartman R C 1952 A haemorrhagic disorder caused by circulating anticoagulant in patients with disseminated lupus erythematosis. Journal of Clinical Investigation 31: 651–652

Coon W, Willis P, Keller J 1973 Venous thromboembolism and other venous disease in the Tecumesh community health study. Circulation 48: 839–846

Cox D R, Martin L, Hall B D 1977 Asplenia syndrome after fetal exposure to warfarin. Lancet ii: 1134–1134

Cranley J J 1975 Venous thrombosis secondary to phlebography. In:

Vascular surgery Harper and Row, Hagerstown, Maryland vol 2: 70–71
Crawford J S 1975 Pathology in the extradural space. British Journal of Anaesthesia 47: 412–415
Crawford J S 1978 Principles and practice of obstetric anaesthesia, 4th Edn. Blackwell, Oxford, p 182–183
Cronan K K, Dorfman G S, Scola F M, Schepps B, Alexander J 1987 Deep venous thrombosis: US assessment using vein compression. Radiology 162: 191–194
Cross J N, Castro P O, Jennett W B 1968 Cerebral strokes associated with pregnancy and the puerperium. British Medical Journal 3: 214–218
Daniel D G, Campbell H, Turnbull A C 1967 Puerperal thromboembolism and suppression of lactation. Lancet ii: 287–289
Davies J A, Prentice C R M 1992 Coagulation changes in pregnancy-induced hypertension and growth retardation. In: Greer I A, Turpie A G G, Forbes (eds) Haemostasis and thrombosis in obstetrics and gynaecology. Chapman & Hall, London, p 143–162
de Boer K, Lecander I, ten Cate J W, Borm J J J, Treffers P E 1988 Placental type plasminogen activator inhibitor in pre-eclampsia. American Journal of Obstetrics and Gynecology 158: 518–522
de Swiet M 1985 Thromboembolism. Clinics in Haematology 14: 643–661
de Swiet M, Letsky E, Mellow H 1977 Drug treatment and prophylaxis of thromboembolism in pregnancy. In: Lewis P J (ed) Therapeutic problems in pregnancy. MTP, Lancaster, p 81–89
de Swiet M, Dorrington Ward P, Fidler J, Horsman A, Katz D, Letsky E, Peacock M, Wise P H 1983 Prolonged heparin therapy in pregnancy causes bone demineralisation (heparin-induced osteopenia). British Journal of Obstetrics and Gynaecology 90: 1129–1134
de Swiet M, Floyd E, Letsky E 1987 Low risk of recurrent thromboembolism in pregnancy. British Journal of Hospital Medicine 38: 264
de Wolf F, Carreras L O, Moerman P, Vermylen J, van Assche A, Renaer M 1982 Decidual vasculopathy and extensive placental infarction in a patient with repeated thromboembolic accidents, recurrent fetal loss, and a lupus anticoagulant. American Journal of Obstetrics and Gynecology 142: 829–834
Denson K W E, Bonnar J 1973 The measurement of heparin: a method based on the potentiation of anti-factor Xa. Thrombosis Diathesis Haemorhagica 30: 471–479
Department of Health 1989 Confidential enquiries into maternal deaths in England and Wales 1982–84. HMSO, London
Department of Health, Welsh Office, Scottish Home and Health Department and Department of Health and Social Services, Northern Ireland 1991 Confidential enquiries into maternal deaths in the United Kingdom 1985–87. HMSO, London
Derksen R H W M, Bieswa D, Bouma B N et al 1986 Discordant effects of prednisone on anticardiolipin antibodies and the lupus anticoagulant. Arthritis and Rheumatism 29: 1295–1296
Donaldson M C, Wirthlin L S, Donaldson G A 1980 Thirty year experience with surgical interruption of the inferior vena cava for prevention of pulmonary embolism. Annals of Surgery 191: 367–372
Douglas J T, Shah M, Lowe G D O et al 1982 Plasma fibrinopeptide A and betathromboglobulin in pre-eclampsia and pregnancy hypertension. Thrombosis and Haemostasis 47: 54–55
Douglas A S, Walker I D, Bennett N B 1990 A Scottish Hebridean antithrombin III deficient family — twelve years on. Scottish Medical Journal 35: 108–113
Downing I, Shepherd G L, Lewis P J 1980 Reduced prostacyclin production in pre-eclampsia. Lancet ii: 1374 (letter)
Dunnihoo D R, Gallapsy J W, Wise R B, Otterson W N 1991 Postpartum ovarian vein thrombophlebitis : A review. Obstetrical and Gynecological Survey 46: 415–427
Edgar W, McKillop C, Howie P W, Prentice C R M 1977 Composition of soluble fibrin complexes in pre-eclampsia. Thrombosis Research 10: 567–574
Effeney D J, Friedman M B, Gooding G A W 1984 Ileofemoral venous thrombosis: real time ultrasound diagnosis, normal criteria clinical application. Radiology 150: 787–792
Egeberg O 1965 Inherited anti-thrombin deficiency causing thrombophilia. Thrombosis et Diathesis Haemorrhagica 13: 516–530
Elder M G, de Swiet M, Robertson A, Elder M A, Floyd E, Hawkins D F 1988 Low dose aspirin in pregnancy. Lancet i: 410 (letter)
Estellés A, Gilabert J, Esapana F, Aznar J, Gomez-Lechon M J 1987 Fibrinolysis in pre-eclampsia. Fibrinolysis 1: 209–214
Everett R B, Worley R J, MacDonald P C, Gant N F 1978 Oral administration of theophyline to modify pressor responsiveness to angiotensin II in women with pregnancy-induced hypertension. American Journal of Obstetrics and Gynecology 132: 359–362
Exner T, Richard R A, Kronenberg H 1978 A sensitive test demonstrating lupus anticoagulant and its behavioural patterns. British Journal Haematology 40: 143–151
Falcon C R, Hoffer A M, Carreras L O 1990 Antiphosphatidylinositol antibodies as markers of the antiphospholipid antibody syndrome. Thrombosis and Haemostasis 63: 321–322
Fay R A, Hughes A O, Farron N T 1983 Platelets in pregnancy: Hyperdestruction in pregnancy. Obstetrics and Gynecology 61: 238–240
Feinstein D I 1985 Lupus anticoagulant thrombosis and fetal loss New England Journal of Medicine 313: 348–1350
Fitzgerald G A, Oates J A, Hawiger J, Mass R L et al 1983 Endogenous biosynthesis of prostacyclin and thromboxane and platelet function during chronic administration of aspirin in man. Journal of Clinical Investigation 71: 676–688
Fitzgerald D J, Mayo G, Catella F, Entman S S, Fitzgerald G A 1987 Increased thromboxane biosynthesis in normal pregnancy is mainly derived from platelets. American Journal of Obstetrics and Gynecology 157(2): 325–330
Flessa H C, Kapstrom A B, Glueck H I, Will J J 1965 Placental transport of heparin. American Journal of Obstetrics and Gynecology 93: 570–573
Flessa H C, Glueck H I, Dritschilo A 1974 Thromboembolic disorders in pregnancy. Clinical Obstetrics and Gynaecology 17: 195–235
Forestier F, Daffos F, Capella-Pavlovsky M 1984 Low molecular weight heparin (PK 10169) does not cross the placenta during the second trimester of pregnancy: Study by direct fetal blood sampling under ultrasound. Thrombosis Research 34: 557–560
Forestier F, Daffos F, Rainaux M, Toulemonde F 1987 Low molecular weight heparin (CY216) does not cross the placenta during the third trimester of pregnancy. Thrombosis and Haemostasis 57: 234
Friend J R, Kakkar V V 1970 The diagnosis of deep venous thrombosis in the puerperium. Journal of Obstetrics and Gynaecology of the British Commonwealth 77: 820–823
Gant N F, Daley G L, Chand S, Whalley P J, Macdonald P C 1973 A study of angiotensin II pressor response throughout primigravid pregnancy. Journal of Clinical Investigation 52: 2682–2689
Gant N F, Chand S, Worley R J, Whalley P J, Crosby U D, Macdonald P C 1974 A clinical test useful for predicting the development of acute hypertension in pregnancy. American Journal of Obstetrics and Gynecology 120: 1–7
Genton E, Turpie A G G 1980 Venous thromboembolism associated with gynaecologic surgery. Clinical Obstetrics and Gynaecology 23: 209–241
Gerbasi F R, Bottoms S S, Farag A et al 1990 Increased intravascular coagulation associated with pregnancy. Obstetrics and Gynecology 75: 385–389
Ginsberg J S 1992 Fetal abnormalities and anticoagulants. In: Greer I A, Turpie A G G, Foibes C D (eds) Haemostasis and thrombosis in obstetrics and gynaecology. Chapman and Hall, London, p 361–369
Ginbergs J S, Hirsh J, Turner D C et al 1989 Risks to the fetus of anticoagulant therapy during pregnancy. Thrombosis and Haemostasis 61: 197–203
Glazier R L, Crowel E B 1976 Randomised prospective trial of continuous versus intermittent heparin therapy. Journal of the American Medical Association 236: 1365–1367
Gonzalez R, Alberca I, Sala N, Vicente V 1985 Protein C deficiency–response to danazol and DDAVP. Thrombosis and haemostasis 53: 320–322
Goodman R P, Killam A P, Brash A R, Branch R A 1982 Prostacyclin production during pregnancy: comparison of production during normal pregnancy and pregnancy complicated by hypertension. American Journal of Obstetrics and Gynecology 142: 817–822
Greer I A 1985 The effect of anti-hypertensive agents on platelets,

prostacyclin and thromboxane and observation on prostacyclin and thromboxane in normal and hypertensive pregnancy. MD Thesis, University of Glasgow

Greer I A 1992 Pathological processes in pregnancy-induced hypertension and intrauterine growth retardation: 'an excess of heated blood' In: Greer I A, Turpie A G G, Forbes C D (eds) Haemostasis and thrombosis in obstetrics and gynaecology. Chapman & Hall, London, p 163–202

Greer I A, Belch J J F 1986 Prostacyclin in pregnancy induced hypertension, Raynaud's phenomenon and haemolytic uraemic syndrome. In: William E B (ed) Current clinical concepts, prostacyclin past, present and future. MCS, Kent, p 37–45

Greer I A, de Swiet M 1993 Thrombosis prophylaxis in obstetrics and gynaecology. British Journal of Obstetrics and Gynaecology 100: 37–40

Greer I A, Walker J J, Cameron A D, McLaren M, Calder A A, Forbes C D 1985 A prospective longitudinal study of immunoreactive prostacyclin and thromboxane metabolites in normal and hypertensive pregnancies. Clinical and Experimental Hypertension B4: 167–182

Greer I A, Walker J J, Forbes C D, Calder A A 1986 The low dose aspirin controversy solved at last? British Medical Journal 391: 1277–1278

Greer I A, Walker J J, Forbes C D, Calder A A 1987 Platelet function in pregnancy-induced hypertension following treatment with labetalol and low dose aspirin. Thrombosis Research 46: 667–612

Greer I A, Calder A A, Walker J J, Lunan C B, Tulloch I 1988 Increased platelet reactivity in pregnancy-induced hypertension and uncomplicated diabetic pregnancy: an indication for anteplatelet therapy? British Journal of Obstetrics and Gynaeocology 95: 1204–1208

Greer I A, Haddad N G, Dawes J, Johnstone F D, Calder A A 1989a Neutrophil activation in pregnancy induced hypertension British Journal of Obstetrics and Gynaecology 96: 978–982

Greer I A, Haddad N G, Dawes J, Johston, T A, Johnstone F D, Steel J 1989b Increased neutrophil activation in diabetic pregnancy and non-pregnant diabetic women. Obstetrics and Gynecology 74: 878–81

Greer I A, Barry J, Macklon N, Allan P 1990 Diagnosis of deep venous thrombosis in pregnancy; a new role for diagnostic ultrasound. British Journal of Obstetrics and Gynaecology 97: 53–57

Greer I A, Gibson J, Brennand J, Calder A A 1991a Does low dose aspirin provide a totally selective effect in pregnancy? British Journal of Haematology 77 (suppl 1): 5

Greer I A, Dawes J, Johnston T A, Calder A A 1991b Neutrophil activation is confined to the maternal circulation in pregnancy induced hypertension. Obstetrics and Gynecology 78: 28–32

Greer I A, Leask R, Hodson B A et al 1991c Endothelin, elastase and endothelial dysfunction in pre-eclampsia. Lancet i: 558

Griffin J H, Evatt B, Zimmerman T S, Kleiss A J, Wildeman C 1981 Deficiency of protein C in congenital thrombotic disease. Journal of Clinical Investigation 68: 1370–1375

Griffith G C, Nichols G, Asher J D, Flanagan B 1965 Heparin osteoporosis. Journal of the American Medical Association 193: 85–88

Hall R J, Young C, Sutton G C, Campbell S 1972 Treatment of acute massive pulmonary embolism by streptokinase during labour and delivery. British Medical Journal 4: 647–649

Hall J G, Pauli R M, Wilson K M 1980 Maternal and fetal sequelae of anticoagulation during pregnancy. American Journal of Medicine 68: 122–140

Halpern J P, Morris J G L, Driscoll G L 1984 Anticoagulants and cerebral venous thrombosis. Australian and New Zealand Journal of Medicine 14: 643–648

Harlan J D 1987 Neutrophil-mediated vascular injury. Acta Medica Scandinavica (supp) 715: 123–129

Harenberg J, Leber G, Zimmerman R, Schmidt W 1987 Thromboembolеprophylaxe mit nieder molekularem Heparin in der Schwangenschaft. Geburtshilfe und Frauenheilkunde 47: 15–18

Harris E N, Gharavi A E, Loizou S et al 1985 Cross reactivity of antiphospholipid antibodies. Journal of Clinical Laboratory Immunology 16: 1–6

Harris E N, Chan J K H, Asherson R A, Aber V R, Gharavi A E 1986 Thrombosis recurrent fetal loss, and thrombocytopenia. Archives of International Medicine 146: 2153–2156

Hathaway W E, Bonnar J 1987 Haemostatic disorders of the pregnant woman and newborn infant. Elsevier, New York

Heavey D J, Barrow S E, Hickling N E, Ritter J M 1985 Aspirin causes short-lived inhibition of bradykinin-stimulated prostacyclin production in man. Nature 318: 186–188

Hellgren M, Blombäck M 1981 Studies on blood coagulation and fibrinolysis in pregnancy, during delivery and in the puerperium I Normal condition. Gynaecological and Obstetrical Investigation 12: 141–154

Hellgren M, Tengborn L, Abildgaard V 1982 Pregnancy in women with congenital ATIII deficiency. Experience of treatment with heparin antithrombin. Gynaecological and Obstetrical Investigation 14: 127–141

Henny C P, ten Cate H, ten Cate J W, Prummel M F, Peters M, Buller H R 1986 Thrombosis prophylaxis in an ATIII-deficient pregnant woman: application of low molecular weight heparinoid. Thrombosis and Haemostasis 55: 301

Hiilesmaa V 1960 Occurrence and anticoagulant treatment of thromboembolism in gravidas, parturients and gynecological patients. A study of 678 cases treated in the Women's Clinic of the University of Helsinki. Acta Obstetricia et Gynaecologica Scandinavica Suppl 2: 1953–1957

Hill N C W, Hill J G, Sargent J M, Taylor C G, Bush P V 1988 Effect of low dose heparin on blood loss at caesarean section. British Medical Journal 296: 1505–1506

Hirsh J 1986 Mechanism of action and monitoring of anticoagulants. Seminars in Thrombosis and Haemositasis 12: 1–11

Hirsh J, Genton E, Hull R 1981 Venous thromboembolism. Grune & Stratton, New York

Howell R, Fidler J, Letsky E, de Swiet M 1983 The risks of antenatal subcutaneous heparin prophylaxis; a controlled trial. British Journal of Obstetrics and Gynaecology 90: 1124–1128

Howie P W 1977 The haemostatic mechanisms of pre-eclampsia. Clinics in Obstetrics and Gynaecology 4: 595–609

Howie P W, Prentice C R M, McNicol G P 1871 Coagulation, fibrinolysis and platelet function in pre-eclampsia, essential hypertension and placental insufficiency. Journal of Obstetrics and Gynaecology of the British Commonwealth 78: 992–1003

Howie P W, Begg C B, Purdie D W, Prentice C R M 1976 Use of coagulation test to predict the clinical progress of pre-eclampsia. Lancet ii: 323–325

Hughes G R V 1988 Vascular disease, thrombosis and recurrent abortion British Medical Journal 297: 700–701

Hull R, van Aken W G, Hirsh J, Gallus A S, Hoicka G, Turpie A G G, Walker I, Gent M 1976 Impedence plethysmography using the occlusive cuff technique in the diagnosis of venous thrombosis. Circulation 53: 696–700

Hull R D, Raskob G E, Hirsh J et al 1986a Continuous intravenous heparin compared with intermittent subcutaneous heparin in the initial treatment of proximal-vein thrombosis. New England Journal of Medicine 315: 1109–114

Hull R D, Roskob G E, Hirsh J 1986b The diagnosis of clinically suspected pulmonary embolism. Chest 89: (supp) 417–425

Husni E, Pena L, Lenhert E 1967 Thrombophlebitis in pregnancy. American Journal of Obstetrics and Gynecology 97: 901–905

Hux C H, Wapner R J, Clayen B, Ratton P, Jarrell B, Grenfield L 1986 Use of the Greenfield filter for thromboembolic disease in pregnancy. American Journal of Obstetrics and Gynecology 155: 734–737

Inglis T C M, Stuart J, George A J, Davies A J 1982 Haemostatic and rheological changes in normal pregnancy and pre-eclampsia. British Journal of Haematology 50: 461–465

Isacson S, Nilsson I M 1972 Defective fibrinolysis in blood and vein walls in recurrent idiopathic venous thrombosis. Acta Chirurgica Scandinavia 138: 313–319

Iturbe-Alessio I, del Carmen Fonseca M, Mutchinik O, Santos M A, Zajarias A, Salazar E 1986 Risks of anticoagulant therapy in pregnant women with artificial heart valves. New England Journal of Medicine 315: 1390–1393

Jick H, Slone D, Westerholm B et al 1969 Venous thromboembolic disease and ABO blood type. A co-operative study. Lancet i: 539–542

Johnston T A, Greer I A, Dawes J, Calder A A 1991 Neutrophil activation in small for gestational age pregnancies. British Journal of Obstetrics and Gynaecology 98: 104–105
Jones T K, Barnes R W, Greenfield L J 1986 Greenfield vena caval filter: Rationale and current indications. Annals of Thoracic Surgery 42(suppl 1): 48–55
Josey W E, Staggers S R 1974 Heparin therapy in septic pelvic thrombophlebitis. A study of 46 cases. American Journal of Obstetrics and Gynecology 196: 309–313
Khurana B K, Rao J, Friedman S A et al 1988 Computed tomographic features of puerperal ovarian vein thrombosis. American Journal of Obstetrics and Gynecology 159: 905–909
King D J, Kelton J G 1984 Heparin associated thrombocytopenia. Annals of Internal Medicine 100: 535–540
Kruithof E K O, Chien T T, Gudinchet A et al 1987 Fibrinolysis in pregnancy; a study of plasminogen activation inhibitors. Blood 69: 460–466
Lao T T, de Swiet M, Letsky E, Walters B N J 1985 Prophylaxis of thromboembolism in pregnancy: an alternative. British Journal of Obstetrics and Gynaecology 92: 202–206
Laros R K, Alger L S 1979 Thromboembolism in pregnancy. Clinics in Obstetrics and Gynaecology 22: 871–873
Larrea J L, Nunez L, Reque J A, Gil Aguado M, Matarros R, Minguez J A 1983 Pregnancy and mechanical valve prostheses: A high risk situation for the mother and the fetus. Annals of Thoracic Surgery 36: 459–463
Lecander I, Astedt B 1986 Isolation of a new specific plasminogen activator inhibitor from pregnancy plasma. British Journal of Haematology 62: 221–228
Lee P R, Wang R Y C, Chow J S F, Cheung K L, Wong Y C W, Chan T R 1986 Combined use of warfarin and adjusted sodium heparin during pregnancy in patients with an artificial heart valve. Journal of the American College of Cardiology 8: 221–224
Letsky E, de Swiet M 1984 Thromboembolism in pregnancy and its management. British Journal of Haematology 57: 543–552
Lindhagen A, Bergqvist D, Hallbook T 1984 Deep venous insufficiency after postoperative thrombosis diagnosed with ^{125}I-labelled fibrinogen uptake test. British Journal of Surgery 71: 511–515
Lindhagen A, Bergqvist D, Hallbook T, Elsing H O 1985 Venous function five to eight years after clinically suspected deep venous thrombosis. Acta Medica Scandinavica 217: 389–395
Lindhagen A, Bergqvist A, Bergqvist D, Hallbook T 1986 Late venous function in the leg after deep venous thrombosis occurring in relation to pregnancy. British Journal of Obstetrics and Gynaecology 93: 348–352
Lockshin M D, Druzin M L, Goei S et al 1985 Antibody to cardiolipin as a predictor of fetal distress or death in pregnant patients with systemic lupus erythematosus. New England Journal of Medicine 313: 152–156
Lockshin M D, Druzin M L, Qamar T 1989 Prednisone does not prevent recurrent fetal death in women with antiphospholipid antibody. American Journal of Obstetrics and Gynecology 160: 439–443
Louden K A, Heptinstall S, Broughton-Pipkin F, Mitchell J R A, Symonds E M 1989 The effect of low dose aspirin on platelet reactivity on pregnancy, PIH and neonates. Clinical and Experimental Hypertension B8: 398
Louden K A, Broughton-Pipkin F, Heptinstall S, Fox S C, Mitchell J R A, Symonds E M 1991 Platelet reactivity and serum thromboxane B_2 production in whole blood in gestational hypertension and pre-eclampsia. British Journal of Obstetrics and Gynaecology 98: 1239–1244
Lubbe W F, Walker E B 1983 Chorea gravidarum associated with circulating lupus anticoagulant: successful treatment of pregnancy with prednisone and aspirin therapy. British Journal of Obstetrics and Gynaecology 90: 487–490
Lubbe W F, Butler W S, Palmer S J, Liggins G C 1984 Lupus anticoagulant in pregnancy. British Journal of Obstetrics and Gynaecology 91: 357–363
Lubbe W F, Butler W S, Palmer S J, Liggins G C 1983 Fetal survival after prednisone suppression of maternal lupus-anticoagulant. Lancet i: 1361–1363
Ludlam C A, Moore S, Bolton A E, Cash J D 1975 New rapid method for diagnosis of deep venous thrombosis. Lancet ii: 259–260
Ludwig H 1973 Results of streptokinase therapy in deep vein thrombosis during pregnancy. Postgraduate Medical Journal (suppl 5) 49: 65–67
Lutz D J, Noller K L, Spittell J A, Danielson G K, Fish C R 1978 Pregnancy and its complications following cardiac value prostheses. American Journal of Obstetrics and Gynecology 131: 460–468
McBride K, La Morte W W, Menzoian J O 1986 Can ventilation-perfusion scans accurately diagnose pulmonary embolism? Archives of Surgery 121: 754–757
McLaren M, Greer I A, Walker J J, Forbes C D 1987 Reduced prostacyclin production by umbilical arteries from pregnancy complicated by severe pregnancy induced hypertension. Clinical and Experimental Hypertension B6: 365–374
McLaren M, Greer I A, Walker J J et al 1986 Umbilical artery perfusion: a method to measure prostacyclin production in vitro. Progress in Lipid Research 25: 311–315
McTaggart D R, Ingram T G 1977 Massive pulmonary embolism during pregnancy treated with streptokinase. Medical Journal of Australia 1: 18–20
Malm J, Laurell M, Dahlbäck B 1988 Changes in the plasma levels of Vitamin K-dependent proteins C and S and of C4b-binding protein during pregnancy and oral contraception. British Journal of Haematology 68: 437–443
Mannucci P M, Canciani M T, Mari D et al 1979 The varied sensitivity of partial thromboplastin and prothrombin reagents in the demonstration of the lupus-like anticoagulant. Scandinavian Journal of Haematology 22: 423–432
Mannucci P M, Vigano S, Bottasso B et al 1984 Protein C antigen during pregnancy, delivery and the puerperium. Thrombosis and Haemostasis 52: 217 (letter)
Manson L M, Bisland M P, Greer I A, Ludlam C A 1991 Unfractionated and low molecular weight heparin prophylaxis in congenital antithrombin III deficiency. British Journal of Haematology 77 (suppl 1): 65
Matzsch T, Bergqvist D, Hedner U, Nilsson B, Ostergaard P 1987 Induction of osteoporosis in rats by standard heparin and low molecular weight heparin. Thrombosis and Haemostasis 58: 36
Meytes D, Ayalou H, Virag I, Weisbort Y, Zakut H 1986 Heparin induced thrombocytopenia and recurrent thrombosis in pregnancy. A case report. Journal of Reproductive Medicine 31: 993–996
Michiels J J, Stibbe J, Bertina R, Broekman A 1987 Effectiveness of long term oral anticoagulant therapy in preventing venous thrombosis in hereditary protein S deficiency. British Medical Journal 295: 641–643
Miller D K, Sandowski S, Soderman, D D, Kuel F A Jr 1985 Endothelial cell prostacyclin production induced by activated neutrophils. Journal of Biological Chemistry 260: 1006–1014
Mok C K, Boey J, Wang R et al 1985 Warfarin versus dipyriamole-aspirin + pentoxifylline-aspirin for the prevention of prosthetic heart valve thromboembolism — a prospective randomized clinical trial. Circulation 72: 1059–1063
Moodley J, Norman R J, Reddi K 1984 Central venous concentrations of immunoractive prostaglandin E, F and 6-keto-prostaglandin F_1 in eclampsia. British Medical Journal 288: 1487–1489
Morrison R, Crawford J, MacPherson M et al 1985 Platelet behaviour in normal pregnancy, pregnancy complicated by essential hypertension and pregnancy induced hypertension. Thrombosis and Haemostasis 54: 607–611
Mueh J R, Herbst K D, Rapaport S I 1980 Thrombosis in patients with the lupus anticoagulant. Annals of Internal Medicine 92: 156–159
Mulkamy H 1980 Heparin therapy in post caesarean septic pelvic thrombophlebitis. International Journal of Gynecology and Obstetrics 17: 564–566
Nilsson I M, Astedt B, Hedner U, Berezin D 1975 Intrauterine death and circulating anticoagulant. Acta Medica Scandinavica 197: 153–159
Nilsson I M, Felding P, Lecander I et al 1986 Different types of plasminogen activator inhibitors in plasma and platelets in pregnant women. British Journal of Haematology 62: 215–220
Nova A, Sibai B M, Barton J R, Mercer B M, Mitchell M D 1991

Maternal plasma level of endothelin is increased in pre-eclampsia. American Journal of Obstetrics and Gynecology 165: 3: 724–727
O'Brien W F, Saba H I, Knuppel R A et al 1986 Alterations in platelet concentration and aggregation in normal pregnancy and pre-eclampsia. American Journal of Obstetrics and Gynecology 155: 486–490
Odegard O R, Abildgaard U 1978 Anti-thrombin III; critical review of assay methods. Haemostasis 7: 127–134
Oian P, Omsjo I, Maltau J M, Østerud B 1985 Increased sensitivity to thromboplastin synthesis in blood monocytes from pre-eclamptic patients. British Journal of Obstetrics and Gynaecology 92: 511–517
Omri A, Delaloye J F, Anderson H, Bachman F 1989 Low molecular weight heparin Novo (LHN-1) does not cross the placenta during the second trimester of pregnancy. Thrombosis and Haemostasis 61: 55–56
Orme M, L'E Lewis P J, de Swiet M J, Sibeon R, Baty J D, Breckenbridge A M 1977 May mothers given warfarin breast-feed their infants? British Medical Journal 1: 1564–1565
Persson B L, Stenberg P, Holmberg L et al 1980 Transamidating enzymes in maternal plasma and placenta in human pregnancies complicated by intrauterine growth retardation. Journal of Development Physiology 2: 37–46
Pfeiffer G W 1970 The use of thrombolytic therapy in obstetrics and gynaecology. Australian Annals of Medicine (suppl): 28–31
Phelen J P, Everidge G J, Wilder T L, Newman C 1977 Is the supine pressor test an adequate means of predicting acute hypertension in pregnancy? American Journal of Obstetrics and Gynecology 128: 173–176
Pitney W R, Pettit J E, Armstrong L 1970 Control of heparin therapy. British Medical Journal 4: 139–141
Polak J F, Wilkinson D L 1991 Ultrasonographic diagnosis of symptomatic deep venous thrombosis in pregnancy. American Journal of Obstetrics and Gynecology 165: 625–629
Pologe L G, Cramer E V, Pawlowski N A et al 1984 Stimulation of human endothelial cell prostacyclin synthesis by select leukotrienes. Journal of Experimental Medicine 160: 1043–1053
Prentice A G, Lowe G D O, Forbes C D 1982 Diagnosis and treatment of venous thromboembolism by consultants in Scotland. British Medical Journal 285: 630–632
Priollet P, Roncato M, Aiach M, Housset E, Poissonnier M H, Chavinie J 1986 Low molecular weight heparin in venous thrombosis during pregnancy. British Journal of Haematology 63: 605–606
Rakoczi I, Talian F, Bagdany S et al 1979 Platelet life-span in normal pregnancy and pre-eclampsia as determined by a non-radioisotope technique. Thrombosis Results 15: 553–556
Ramsey L E 1983 Impact of venography on the diagnosis and management of deep venous thrombosis. British Medical Journal 286: 698–699
Redman C W G, Allington M J, Bolton F G, Stirrat G M 1977a Plasma β-thromboglobulin in pre-eclampsia. Lancet i: 248
Redman C W G, Denson K W E, Beikin L J, Bolton F G, Stirrat G M 1977b Factor VIII Consumption in pre-eclampsia. Lancet ii: 1249–1252
Redman C W G, Bonnar J, Beilin L J 1978 Early platelet consumption in pre-eclampsia. British Medical Journal 1: 467–469
Remuzzi G et al 1979 Prostacyclin and human foetal circulation Prostaglandins 18: 341–348
Ritter J M, Farquar C, Rodin A, Thom M H 1987 Low dose aspirin treatment in late pregnancy differentially inhibits cyclo-oxygenase in maternal platelets. Prostaglandins 34: 717–722
Robin E D 1977 Overdiagnosis and over-treatment of pulmonary embolism: The emperor may have no clothes. Annals of Internal Medicine 87: 775–781
Rodgers G M, Taylor R N, Roberts J M 1988 Pre-eclampsia is associated with a serum factor cytoxic to human endothelial cells. American Journal of Obstetrics and Gynecology 159: 908–914
Royal College of General Practitioners 1967 Oral contraception and thromboembolic disease. Journal of Royal College of General Practitioners 13: 267–279
Rutherford S E, Phelan J P 1986 Thromboembolic disease in pregnancy. Clinics in Perinatology 13: 719–739
Sage D J 1990 Epidurals, spinals and bleeding disorders in pregnancy. Anaesthesia and Intensive Care 18: 319–326
Salazar E, Zajarias A, Gutierrez N, Iturbe I 1984 The problem of cardiac valve prostheses anticoagulants and pregnancy. Circulation 70 (suppl 1): 169–177
Salzman E W, Deykin D, Shapiro R M, Rosenberg R 1975 Management of heparin therapy. New England Journal of Medicine 292: 1046–1050
Salzman E W, Rosenberg R D, Smith M H, Linden J N, Favreau L 1980 Effect of heparin and heparin fractions on platelet aggregation. Journal of Clinical Investigation 65: 54–73
Samson D, Stirling Y, Woolf L, Howarth D, Seghatchian M. J, de Chazal R 1984 Management of planned pregnancy in a patient with congenital anti-thrombin III deficiency. British Journal of Haematology 56: 243–249
Sas G, Blasko G, Banhegyi D, Jako J, Palos L A 1974 Abnormal antithrombin III as a cause of familial thrombophilia. Thrombosis et Diathesis Haemorrhagica 32: 105–115
Sayama S, Kashiwagi H, Ogawa T et al 1981 Circulating levels of prekallikrein and kallikrein in pregnancy and labor. Biological Research in Pregnancy 2: 90–94
Schiff E, Peleg E, Goldenberg M, Rosenthal T et al 1989 The use of aspirin to prevent pregnancy-induced hypertension and lower the ratio of thromboxane A_2 to prostaglandin in relatively high risk pregnancies. New England Journal of Medicine 322: 204–205
Schwartz H P, Fischer M, Hopmeier P, Batard M A, Griffin J D 1984 Plasma protein S deficiency in familial thrombotic disease. Blood 64: 1297–1300
Scott J R, Rote N S, Branch D W 1987 Immunologic aspects of recurrent abortion and fetal death. Obstetrics and Gynecology 60: 645–656
Sibai B M, Mirro R, Chesney C M, Leffler C 1989 Low dose aspirin in pregnancy, Obstetrics and Gynecology 74: 551–557
Sill P R, Lind T, Walker et al 1985 Platelet values during normal pregnancy. British Journal of Obstetrics and Gynaecology 92: 480–483
Singer C R J, Walker J J, Cameron A et al 1986 Platelet studies in normal pregnancy and pregnancy induced hypertension Clinical Laboratory Haematology 8: 27–32
Sinzinger H, Virgolini I, Peskar B A 1989 Response of thromboxane B_2 malondialdehyde and platelet sensitivity to 3 weeks low dose aspirin in health volunteers. Thrombosis Research 53: 261–269
Socol M L, Weiner C P, Louis G, Rehnberg K, Rossi E C 1985 Platelet activation in pre-eclampsia. American Journal of Obstetrics and Gynecology 151: 494–497
Spencer J A D, Smith M J, Cederholm-Williams S A, Wilkinson A R 1983 Influence of pre-eclampsia on concentrations of haemostatic factors in mothers and infants. Archives of Disease of Children. 58: 739–741
Spowart K, Greer I A, McLaren M, Lloyd J, Bullingham R, Forbes C D 1988 Haemostatic effects of ketorolac with and without heparin. Thrombosis and Haemostasis 60: 382–386
Squires J W, Pinch L W 1979 Heparin induced spinal fractures. Journal of the American Medical Association 241: 2417–2418
Srinivasan K 1983 Cerebral venous and arterial thrombosis in pregnancy and puerperium. Angiology Journal and Vascular Disease. 34: 731–746
Stevenson R E, Burton M, Ferlauto G J, Taylor H A 1989 Hazards of oral anticoagulants during pregnancy. Journal of the American Medical Association 243: 1549–1551
Stirling Y, Woolf L, North W R S, Seghatchian M J, Meade T W 1984 Haemostasis in normal pregnancy. Thrombosis and Haemostasis 52: 176–182
Stuart M J, Gross S J, Elrad H, Groeber J E 1982 Effects of acetylsalicylic acid ingestion on maternal and neonatal haemostasis. New England Journal of Medicine 307: 909–912
Sulliven E D, Peter D J, Cranley J J 1984 Real time B-mode venous ultrasound. Journal of Vascular Surgery i: 465–471
Tengborn L, Bergqvist D, Matzsch T, Bergqvist A, Hednar V 1989 Recurrent thromboembolism in pregnancy and puerperium. Is there a need for thromboprophylaxis? American Journal of Obstetrics and Gynecology 160: 90–95
Thiagarajan P, Pengo V, Shapiro S 1986 The use of the dilute Russel Viper venom time for the diagnosis of lupus anticoagulant. Blood 68: 869–874

Thomas A N, Pattison C, Serjeant G R 1982 Causes of death in sickle-cell disease in Jamaica. British Medical Journal 285: 633–635
Thorburn J, Louden J, Vallance R 1980 Spinal and general anaesthesia in total hip replacement: frequency of deep venous thrombosis. British Journal of Anaesthesia 52: 1117–1121
Thorburn J, Drummond M M, Whigham K A et al 1982 Blood viscosity and haemostatic factors in late pregnancy, pre-eclampsia and fetal growth retardation. British Journal of Obstetrics and Gynaecology 89: 117–122
Trudinger B J, Stewart G J, Cook C M, Connelly A, Exner T 1988 Monitoring lupus anticoagulant positive pregnancies with umbilical flow velocity waveforms. Obstetrics and Gynecology 72: 215–218
Tulenko T, Schneider J, Floro C, Sicilla M 1987 The in vitro effect on arterial wall function of serum from patients with pregnancy induced hypertension. American Journal of Obstetrics and Gynecoloy 156: 817–823
Tuvemo T 1980 Role of prostaglandins, prostacyclin and thromboxanes in the control of the umbilical-placental circulation. Seminars in Perinatology 4: 91–95
Tygart S G, McRoyan D K, Spinnato J A et al 1986 Longitudinal study of platelet indices during normal pregnancy. American Journal of Obstetrics and Gynecology 154: 883–887
Uzan S, Beaufils M, Breart G, Bazin B, Capitant C, Paris J 1991 Prevention of fetal growth retardation with low-dose aspirin: findings of the EPREDA trial. Lancet 337: 1427–1431
van Dinh T, Boor P J, Gazra J R 1982 Massive pulmonary embolism following delivery of a patient with sickle cell trait. American Journal of Obstetrics and Gynecology 143: 722–724
Villa Santa U 1965 Thromboembolic disease in pregnancy. American Journal of Obstetrics and Gynecology 93: 142
Virchow R 1846 Die verstopfung den lungen arterie und ihre folgen. Beitrage zur esperimantallen Pathologie und Physiologie, part 2 p 1–90
Walker T S, Triplett D A, Javed N, Musgrave K 1988 Evaluation of lupus anticoagulants. Thrombosis Research 51: 267–281
Wallenburg H C S, Rotmans N 1982 Enhanced reactivity of the platelet thrombaxane pathway in normotensive and hypertensive pregnancies with insufficient fetal growth. American Journal of Obstetrics and Gynecology 144: 523–528
Wallenburg H C S, Rotmans N 1987 Prevention of recurrent idiopathic fetal growth retardation by low-dose aspirin and dipyridamole. American Journal of Obstetrics and Gynecology 157: 1230–1235
Wallenburg H C S, van Kessel P H 1978 Platelet lifespan in normal pregnancy as determined by a nonradioisotopic technique. British Journal of Obstetrics and Gynaecology 85: 33–36
Wallenburg H C S Dekker G A, Mokovitz J W, Rotmans P 1986 Low dose aspirin prevents pregnancy induced hypertension and pre-eclampsia in angiotensin-sensitive primigravidae. Lancet i: 1–3
Walsh S W 1985 Pre-eclampsia: an imbalance in placental prostacyclin and thromboxane production. American Journal of Obstetrics and Gynecology 152: 335–340
Wang R Y C, Lee P K, Chow J S F, Chen W W C 1983 Efficacy of low dose, subcutaneously administered heparin in treatment of pregnant women with artificial heart valves. Medical Journal of Australia 2: 126–128
Warso M A, Lands W E M 1983 Lipid peroxidation in relation to prostacyclin and thromboxane physiology and pathophysiology. British Medical Bulletin 39: 277–280
Weenink G H, Treffers P E, Kahle L H et al 1982 Antithrombin III in normal pregnancy. Thrombosis Results 26: 282–287
Weiner C P 1985 Diagnosis and management of thromboembolic disease during pregnancy. Clinical Obstetrics and Gynaecology 28: 107–117
Weiner C P, Brandt J 1980 Plasma antithrombin III activity in normal pregnancy. Obstetrics and Gynaecology 56: 601–603
Weiner C P, Brandt J 1982 Plasma antithrombin III activity: an aid in the diagnosis of pre-eclampsia/eclampsia. American Journal of Obstetrics and Gynecology 142: 275–281
Wenger N K, Stein P D, Willis P W 1972 Massive acute pulmonary embolism. The deceivingly non-specific manifestations. Journal of the American Medical Association 220: 843–844
Whigham K A E, Howie P W, Drummond A H et al 1978 Abnormal platelet function in pre-eclampsia. British Journal of Obstetrics and Gynaecology 85: 28–32
Whitfield L R, Lele A S, Levy G 1983 Effect of pregnancy on the relationship between concentration and anticoagulant actin of heparin. Clinical Pharmacology Therapeutics 34: 23–28
Wiebers D O, Whisnant J P 1985 The incidence of stroke among pregnant women in Rochester, Minn, 1955–1979. Journal of the American Medical Association 254: 3055–3057
Wildsmith J A W, McClure J M 1991 Anticoagulant drugs and central nervous system blockade. Anaesthesia 46: 613–614
Wille-Jorgensen P, Jorgensen L N, Rasmussen L S 1991 Lumbar regional anaesthesia and prophylactic anticoagulation therapy. Is the combination safe? Anaesthesia 46: 624–628
Wiman B, Csemiczky G, Marsk L, Robbe H 1984 The fast inhibitor of tissue plasminogen activator in plasma during pregnancy. Thrombosis and Haemostasis 52: 124–126
Windebank W J 1987 Diagnosis pulmonary thromboembolism. British Medical Journal 292: 1369–1370
Winter J H, Douglas A S 1991 Congenital thrombotic problems in obstetrics and gynaecology. In: Greer I A, Turpie A C G, Forbes C D (eds) Haemostasis and thrombosis in obstetrics and gynaecology. Chapman and Hall, London, p 431–458
Winter J H, Bennett B, Watt J L, Brown T, San Roman C, Schnizel A, King J, Cook P J L 1982a Confirmation of linkage between anti-thrombin III and Duffy blood group and assignment of ATIII to lq22/1q25. Annals of Human Genetics 46: 29–34
Winter J H, Fenech A, Ridley W, Bennett B, Cumming A M, Mackie M, Douglas A S 1982b Familial antithrombin III deficiency. Quarterly Journal of Medicine 51: 373–395
Wise P H, Hall A J 1980 Heparin-induced osteopenia in pregnancy. British Medical Journal 281: 110–111
Woodfield D G, Cole S K, Allan A G E et al 1968 Serum fibrin degradation products throughout normal pregnancy. British Medical Journal 4: 665–668
Wright H P, Osborn S B, Edmonds O G 1950 Changes in the rate of flow of venous blood in the leg during pregnancy measured with radioactive sodium. Surgery Gynecology and Obstetrics 90: 481–485
Zuker S, Cathey M H 1969 Control of heparin therapy. Journal of Laboratory and Clinical Medicine 73: 320–326

44. Neonatal haemostasis

Sara Israels   Maureen Andrew

The discovery of individual components of haemostasis over the past century has been accompanied by the realization that there are profound differences in the haemostatic system of newborns compared to adults. Because neither haemorrhagic nor thromboembolic complications occur in healthy infants, one can argue that the haemostatic system of infancy is physiologic, even though it is profoundly different from the adult system. In some cases the haemostatic system of infancy appears to offer advantages over the adult system. For example, thrombotic complications from inherited heterozygote forms of antithrombin III, protein C, and protein S rarely present in infancy. Rather these patients present with thrombotic complications in early adulthood. In contrast the haemostatic system of infancy has little reserve capacity for other disorders. For example, the borderline vitamin K status at birth places otherwise healthy infants at risk for haemorrhagic disease of the newborn if vitamin K intake is low during the first days of life.

Congenital and acquired disorders of haemostasis frequently present in newborns with either haemorrhagic or thrombotic complications. The correct diagnosis of these haemostatic problems can be difficult for several reasons. The circulating plasma concentrations of some coagulation proteins are physiologically low and overlap with values considered pathologic in adults. In addition, plasma concentrations of coagulation proteins are rapidly changing. The latter necessitates multiple reference ranges which reflect the postnatal and gestational age of infants (Andrew et al 1987a, 1988d, 1989a). The infant's small size limits the sample available for assaying and requires microtechniques for an indepth evaluation (Johnston et al 1980). Recent systematic evaluation of the haemostatic system of infancy has produced reliable reference ranges which allow the clinician to confirm the presence of specific haemostatic problems. However the efficacy and safety of a variety of commonly used therapeutic interventions have not been rigorously evaluated in newborns. In most instances case reports and case series are used to justify clinical practice. An important step in the management of infants with haemostatic problems will be the use of randomized controlled trials to test the merits of specific therapeutic modalities. In this chapter, conclusions from well-designed studies are given greater weight than conclusions from studies with weaker designs (Sackett 1986).

Procoagulant proteins

All components of haemostasis are synthesized by fetuses and do not cross the placenta from mothers. Plasma concentrations of coagulation proteins increase with gestational age with an initial appearance at approximately 10 weeks of age (Cade et al 1969, Kisker et al 1981, Andrew et al 1988b, Holmberg et al 1974, Jensen et al 1973, Barnard et al 1979, Mibashan et al 1979, Forestier et al 1985, 1986ab, 1988, Nossel et al 1966, Toulon et al 1986). When selecting valid reference ranges it is important that the population studied is completely healthy. For this reason reference ranges from extremely premature infants (less than 30 weeks gestation) are not available. Samples obtained at fetoscopy provide the closest assessment of normal for these infants (Table 44.1). The neonatal subcommittee to the International Congress on Thrombosis and Haemostasis recently published guidelines for the determination of normal ranges in newborns (Hathaway & Corrigan 1991). In brief, subjects must be described for gestational age, health, postnatal age, and use of vitamin K. The site from which the sample was drawn must be specified and details of sample handling must be given. The methods used for analysis should be described and data analysis provided (Hathaway & Corrigan 1991). Reference ranges for premature infants of 30–36 weeks gestational age and for fullterm infants are available (Andrew et al 1987a, 1988d, 1990) (Tables 44.2–5). Additional normal data for cord values and day one values are also available (Hathaway 1987, Hathaway & Corrigan 1991, Corrigan 1991). The reference ranges provided in Tables 44.2–5 were generated from consecutive cohorts of healthy infants that had to meet rigorous inclusion criteria. The value of each protein was based on a minimum

Table 44.1 Reference values for components of the coagulation system in healthy fetuses (19–27 weeks GA) and premature infants at birth (28–31 weeks GA)

Test	Gestational age (weeks) 19–27	28–31
PT (s)	–	15.4 (14.6–16.9)[d]
APTT (s)	–	108 (80–168)[d]
Fibrinogen (gl)	1.00 (± 0.43)[e]	2.56 (1.60–5.50)[d]
II (U/ml)	0.12 (± 0.02)[b]	0.31 (0.19–0.54)[d]
V (U/ml)	0.41 (± 0.10)[a]	0.65 (0.43–0.80)[d]
VII (U/ml)	0.28 (± 0.04)[b]	0.37 (0.24–0.76)[d]
VIII (U/ml)	0.39 (± 0.14)[a]	0.79 (0.37–1.26)[d]
vWF (U/ml)	0.64 (± 0.13)[a]	1.41 (0.83–2.23)[d]
IX (U/ml)	0.10 (± 0.01)[b]	0.18 (0.17–0.20)[d]
X (U/ml)	0.21 (± 0.03)[b]	0.36 (0.25–0.64)[d]
XI (U/ml)	–	0.23 (0.11–0.33)[d]
XII (U/ml)	0.22 (±0.03)	0.25 (0.05–0.35)[d]
PK (U/ml)	–	0.26 (0.15–0.32)[d]
HMWK (U/ml)	–	0.32 (0.19–0.52)[d]
ATIII (U/ml)	0.24 (± 0.03)[c]	0.28 (0.20–0.38)[d]
HCII (U/ml)	0.27 (± 0.05)[c]	–
Protein C (U/ml)	0.11 (± 0.03)[b]	–

PT, prothrombin time; APTT, activated partial thromboplastin time; VIII, factor VIII procoagulant; vWF, von Willebrand factor; PK, prekallikrein; HK, high molecular weight kininogen. All factors except fibrinogen are expressed as units per millilitre (U/ml) where pooled plasma contains 1.0 U/ml. All values are extrapolated from designated reference: [a] Forestier et al 1986b; [b] Forestier et al 1985; [c] Toulon et al 1986; [d] Barnard & Hathaway 1979; [e] Holmberg et al 1974, and expressed as a mean followed by the lower and upper boundary. Reproduced with permission.

of 40 infant samples. The large sample size was necessary to address the problem of population variability. Cord blood was not used because it may not completely reflect the haemostatic system of infants during the first day of life. The entire study population was studied longitudinally over the first 6 months of life. The data for some coagulation proteins required correction for skewing. The ranges of normal in the Tables (44.2–5) reflect 95% of the population.

The screening tests used most frequently to evaluate infants for a haemostatic abnormality are the prothrombin time (PT), activated partial thromboplastin time (APTT), thrombin clotting time (TCT), and fibrinogen concentration (Tables 44.2, 3). The published values for the PT, and APTT are highly variable probably reflecting the source of the sample (cord versus infant), the reagent used, the method of clot detection and ethnic population (Koepke 1986). The PT values in the tables were measured with an insensitive reagent. For clarity the International Normalized Ratio is provided in addition to the PT values in seconds. The PT and APTT are prolonged in newborns during the first weeks of life. Although mean values become similar to adults by 1 month of age the range of normal remains wider for infants than for adults. The TCT was performed as a 2 unit thrombin time with calcium in the buffering system therefore it was not sensitive to the presence of 'fetal' fibrinogen, but was sensitive to heparin and a low fibrinogen concentration (Ockelford et al 1982). If a 2 unit TCT is performed without calcium it is prolonged in newborns (Witt et al 1969, Gralnick et al 1978, Hamulyak et al 1983). The prolonged APTT in newborns reflects low plasma concentrations for the four contact factors (high molecular weight kininogen ((HMWK), prekallikrein (PK), factor XII, and factor XI) and the four vitamin K-coagulant factors (factors II, VII, IX, X) (Aballi & de Lamerens 1962, Bleyer et al 1971, Strothers et al 1975, Gross & Stuart 1977, Buchanan,

Table 44.2 Reference values for coagulation tests in the healthy fullterm infant during the first 6 months of life

Tests	Day 1	Day 5	Day 30	Day 90	Day 180	Adult
PT (sec)	13.0 (10.1–15.9)*	12.4 (10.0–15.3)*	11.8 (10.0–14.3)*	11.9 (10.0–14.2)*	12.3 (10.7–13.9)*	12.4 (10.8–13.9)
INR	1.00 (0.53–1.62)	0.89 (0.53–1.48)	0.79 (0.53–1.26)	0.81 (0.53–1.26)	0.88 (0.61–1.17)	0.89 (0.64–1.17)
APTT (sec)	42.9 (31.3–54.5)	42.6 (25.4–59.8)	40.4 (32.0–55.2)	37.1 (29.0–50.1)*	35.5 (28.1–42.9)*	33.5 (26.6–40.3)
TCT (sec)	23.5 (19.0–28.3)*	23.1 (18.0–29.2)	24.3 (19.4–29.2)*	25.1 (20.5–29.7)*	25.5 (19.8–31.2)*	25.0 (19.7–30.3)
Fibrinogen (gl)	2.83 (1.67–3.99)*	3.12 (1.62–4.62)*	2.70 (1.62–3.78)*	2.43 (1.50–3.79)*	2.51 (1.50–3.87)*	2.78 (1.56–4.00)
II (U/ml)	0.48 (0.26–0.70)	0.63 (0.33–0.93)	0.68 (0.34–1.02)	0.75 (0.45–1.05)	0.88 (0.60–1.16)	1.08 (0.70–1.46)
V (U/ml)	0.72 (0.34–1.08)	0.95 (0.45–1.45)	0.98 (0.62–1.34)	0.90 (0.48–1.32)	0.91 (0.55–1.27)	1.06 (0.62–1.50)
VII (U/ml)	0.66 (0.28–1.04)	0.89 (0.35–1.43)	0.90 (0.42–1.38)	0.91 (0.39–1.43)	0.87 (0.47–1.27)	1.05 (0.67–1.43)
VIII (U/ml)	1.00 (0.50–1.78)*	0.88 (0.50–1.54)*	0.91 (0.50–1.57)*	0.79 (0.50–1.25)*	0.73 (0.50–1.09)	0.99 (0.50–1.49)
vWF (U/ml)	1.53 (0.50–2.87)	1.40 (0.50–2.54)	1.28 (0.50–2.46)	1.18 (0.50–2.06)	1.07 (0.50–1.97)	0.92 (0.50–1.58)
IX (U/ml)	0.53 (0.15–0.91)	0.53 (0.15–0.91)	0.51 (0.21–0.81)	0.67 (0.21–1.13)	0.86 (0.36–1.36)	1.09 (0.55–1.63)
X (U/ml)	0.40 (0.21–0.68)	0.49 (0.19–0.79)	0.59 (0.31–0.87)	0.71 (0.35–1.07)	0.78 (0.38–1.18)	1.06 (0.70–1.52)
XI (U/ml)	0.38 (0.10–0.66)	0.55 (0.23–0.87)	0.53 (0.27–0.79)	0.69 (0.41–0.97)	0.86 (0.49–1.34)	0.97 (0.67–1.27)
XII (U/ml)	0.53 (0.13–0.93)	0.47 (0.11–0.83)	0.49 (0.17–0.81)	0.67 (0.25–1.09)	0.77 (0.39–1.15)	1.08 (0.52–1.64)
PK (U/ml)	0.37 (0.18–0.69)	0.48 (0.20–0.76)	0.57 (0.23–0.91)	0.73 (0.41–1.05)	0.86 (0.56–1.16)	1.12 (0.62–1.62)
HK (U/ml)	0.54 (0.06–1.02)	0.74 (0.16–1.32)	0.77 (0.33–1.21)	0.82 (0.30–1.46)*	0.82 (0.36–1.28)*	0.92 (0.50–1.36)
XIII_a (U/ml)	0.79 (0.27–1.31)	0.94 (0.44–1.44)*	0.93 (0.39–1.47)*	1.04 (0.36–1.72)*	1.04 (0.46–1.62)*	1.05 (0.55–1.55)
XIII_b (U/ml)	0.76 (0.30–1.22)	1.06 (0.32–1.80)	1.11 (0.39–1.73)*	1.16 (0.48–1.84)*	1.10 (0.50–1.70)*	0.97 (0.57–1.37)

PT, prothrombin time; APTT, activated partial thromboplastin time; TCT thrombin clotting time; VIII, factor VIII procoagulant; vWF, von Willebrand factor; PK, prekallikrein; HK, high molecular weight kininogen; INR, international normalized ratio. All factors except fibrinogen are expressed as units per millilitre (U/ml) where pooled plasma contains 1.0 U/ml. All values are expressed as mean followed by the lower and upper boundary encompassing 95% of the population. Between 40 to 77 samples were assayed for each value for the newborn. Some measurements were skewed due to a disproportionate number of high values. The lower limit which excludes the lower 2.5% of the population has been given. Reproduced with permission (Andrew et al 1990a). *Values that are indistinguishable from those of the adult.

Table 44.3 Reference values for coagulation tests in the healthy premature infant (30–36) weeks gestation) during the first 6 months of life

	Day 1	Day 5	Day 30	Day 90	Day 180	Adult
PT (sec)	13.0 (10.6–16.2)*	12.5 (10.0–15.3)*	11.8 (10.0–13.6)*	12.3 (10.0–14.6)*	12.5 (10.0–15.0)*	12.4 (10.8–13.9)
INR	1.0 (0.61–1.7)	0.91 (0.53–1.48)	0.79 (0.53–1.11)	0.88 (0.53–1.32)	0.91 (0.53–1.48)	0.89 (0.64–1.17)
APTT (sec)	53.6 (27.5–79.4)+	50.5 (26.9–74.1)	44.7 (26.9–62.5)	39.5 (28.3–50.7)*	37.5 (27.1–53.3)*	33.5 (26.6–40.3)
TCT (sec)	24.8(19.2–30.4)*	24.1 (18.8–29.4)*	24.4 (18.8–29.9)*	25.1 (19.4–30.8)*	25.2 (18.9–31.5)*	25.0 (19.7–30.3)
Fibrinogen (gl)	2.43 (1.50–3.73)*+	2.80 (1.60–4.18)*+	2.54 (1.50–4.14)*	2.46 (1.50–3.52)*	2.28 (1.50–3.60)	2.78 (1.56–4.00)
II (U/ml)	0.45 (0.20–0.77)	0.57 (0.29–0.85)+	0.57 (0.36–0.95)+	0.68 (0.30–1.06)	0.87 (0.51–1.23)	1.08 (0.70–1.46)
V (U/ml)	0.88 (0.41–1.44)*+	1.00 (0.46–1.54)*	1.02 (0.48–1.56)*	0.99 (0.59–1.39)*	1.02 (0.58–1.46)*	1.06 (0.62–1.50)
VII (U/ml)	0.67 (0.21–1.13)	0.84 (0.30–1.38)	0.83 (0.21–1.45)	0.87 (0.31–1.43)	0.99 (0.47–1.51)*	1.05 (0.67–1.43)
VIII (U/ml)	1.11 (0.50–2.13)	1.15 (0.53–2.05)*+	1.11 (0.50–1.99)*+	1.06 (0.58–1.88)*+	0.99 (0.50–1.87)*+	0.99 (0.50–1.49)
vWF (U/ml)	1.36 (0.78–2.10)	1.33 (0.72–2.19)	1.36 (0.66–2.16)	1.12 (0.75–1.84)*	0.98 (0.54–1.58)*	0.92 (0.50–1.58)
IX (U/ml)	0.35 (0.19–0.65)+	0.42 (0.14–0.74)+	0.44 (0.13–0.80)	0.59 (0.25–0.93)	0.81 (0.50–1.20)	1.09 (0.55–1.63)
X (U/ml)	0.41 (0.11–0.71)	0.51 (0.19–0.83)	0.56 (0.20–0.92)	0.67 (0.35–0.99)	0.77 (0.35–1.19)	1.06 (0.70–1.52)
XI (U/ml)	0.30 (0.08–0.52)+	0.41 (0.13–0.69)+	0.43 (0.15–0.71)+	0.59 (0.25–0.93)+	0.78 (0.46–1.10)	0.97 (0.67–1.27)
XII (U/ml)	0.38 (0.10–0.66)+	0.39 (0.09–0.69)+	0.43 (0.11–0.75)	0.61 (0.15–1.07)	0.82 (0.22–1.42)	1.08 (0.52–1.64)
PK (U/ml)	0.33 (0.09–0.57)	0.45 (0.25–0.75)	0.59 (0.31–0.87)	0.79 (0.37–1.21)	0.78 (0.40–1.16)	1.12 (0.62–1.62)
HK (U/ml)	0.49 (0.09–0.89)	0.62 (0.24–1.00)+	0.64 (0.16–1.12)+	0.78 (0.32–1.24)	0.83 (0.41–1.25)*	0.92 (0.50–1.36)
XIII_a (U/ml)	0.70 (0.32–1.08)	1.01 (0.57–1.45)*	0.99 (0.51–1.47)*	1.13 (0.71–1.55)*	1.13 (0.65–1.61)*	1.05 (0.55–1.55)
XIII_b (U/ml)	0.81 (0.35–1.27)	1.10 (0.68–1.58)*	1.07 (0.57–1.57)*	1.21 (0.75–1.67)	1.15 (0.67–1.63)	0.97 (0.57–1.37)

PT, prothrombin time; APTT, activated partial thromboplastin time; TCT, thrombin clotting time; VIII, factor VIII procoagulant; vWF, von Willebrand factor; PK, prekallikrein; HK, high molecular weight kininogen; INR, international normalized ratio. All factors except fibrinogen are expressed as units per millilitre (U/ml) where pooled plasma contains 1.0 U/ml. All values are given as a mean followed by the lower and upper boundary encompassing 95% of the population. Between 40 to 96 samples were assayed for each value for the newborn. Some measurements were skewed due to a disproportionate number of high values. The lower limit which excludes the lower 2.5% of the population has been given. *Values that are indistinguishable from the adult. +Values different from those of the fullterm infants. Reproduced with permission (Andrew et al 1990a).

1978, 1986, Hathaway & Bonner 1978, Zipursky & Jaber 1978, Gobel et al 1979, Andrew et al 1982, 1987a, 1988d, 1990, McDonald & Hathaway 1983, Montgomery et al 1985, Gibson 1989, Bahakim et al 1990). Of these, low plasma concentrations of the four contact factors have the most profound effect on the APTT (Andrew et al 1982).

The values for the four vitamin K-dependent procoagulants in Table 44.2 and 44.3 are derived from infants who received intramuscular vitamin K at birth. During the first 6 months of life the plasma concentrations for the contact and vitamin K-dependent procoagulant factors gradually increase towards adult values. However, at 6 months of age only the plasma concentration of HMWK is statistically indistinguishable from adult values. The haemostatic system during childhood has recently been studied in detail (Andrew et al 1991e). Many of the coagulation proteins do not achieve adult levels until much later in childhood.

Plasma concentrations of factor VIII and von Willebrand factor are higher in newborns than adults (Aballi et al 1962, Bleyer et al 1971, Strothers et al 1975, Gross & Stuart 1977, Buchanan 1978, 1986, Hathaway & Bonner 1978, Gobel et al 1979, McDonald & Hathaway 1983, Montgomery et al 1985, Andrew et al 1987, 1988, 1990, Gibson 1989, Katz et al 1989, Weinstein et al 1989, Bahakim et al 1990). The values in Tables 44.2 and 44.3 have been adjusted to provide an accurate lower limit of normal because of skewing to high values. Factor VIII deficiency or haemophilia A is of particular importance because it is one of the most important and common inherited deficiencies. The normal data used to generate Tables 44.2 and 44.3 had less than 1% of infants with values for factor VIII less than 0.40 units/ml, and all values were above 0.30 units/ml. In addition to the increased plasma concentrations of vWF, the multimeric structure of vWF is altered in newborns with increased amounts of unusually large vWF multimers (Katz et al 1989, Weinstein et al 1989). These forms of vWF disappear in the first weeks of life (Katz et al 1989).

Plasma concentrations of factor V, factor XIII, and fibrinogen in newborns are similar to adults (Aballi et al 1962, Bleyer et al 1971, Strothers et al 1975, Gross & Stuart 1977, Buchanan 1978, 1986, Hathaway & Bonner 1978, Zipursky & Jaber 1978, Gobel et al 1979, McDonald et al 1983, Montgomery et al 1985, Hathaway & Bonner 1987, Gibson 1989, Bahakim et al 1990, Corrigan 1991, Hathaway & Corrigan 1991). However plasma concentrations of fibrinogen increase during the first week of life reaching levels 4.62 g/l. In addition there is convincing evidence for a fetal fibrinogen. Fetal fibrinogen is similar to adult fibrinogen in amino acid structure but has an increased content of sialic acid which is responsible for prolonging the thrombin clotting time in newborns (Witt et al 1969, Galanakis & Mosesson 1976, Hamulyak et al 1983).

Procoagulant inhibitors

Plasma concentrations of antithrombin III (ATIII), the most important inhibitor of coagulation in adults, is low in fullterm infants (0.63 units/ml) and even lower in premature infants (0.38 units/ml) (Aballi et al 1962, Bleyer et al 1971, Strothers et al 1975, Gross & Stuart 1977,

Table 44.4 Reference values for the inhibitors of coagulation in the healthy fullterm and premature infant during the first 6 months of life

	Day 1	Day 5	Day 30	Day 90	Day 180	Adult
Fullterm infants						
ATIII (U/ml)	0.63 (0.39–0.87)	0.67 (0.41–0.93)	0.78 (0.48–1.08)	0.97 (0.73–1.21)*	1.04 (0.84–1.24)*	1.05 (0.79–1.31)
α_2M (U/ml)	1.39 (0.95–1.83)	1.48 (0.98–1.98)	1.50 (1.06–1.94)	1.76 (1.26–2.26)	1.91 (1.49–2.33)	0.86 (0.52–1.20)
CT-INH (U/ml)	0.72 (0.36–1.08)	0.90 (0.60–1.20)*	0.89 (0.47–1.31)	1.15 (0.71–1.59)	1.41 (0.89–1.93)	1.01 (0.71–1.31)
α_1AT (U/ml)	0.93 (0.49–1.37)*	0.89 (0.49–1.29)*	0.62 (0.36–0.88)	0.72 (0.42–1.02)	0.77 (0.47–1.07)	0.93 (0.55–1.31)
HCII (U/ml)	0.43 (0.10–0.93)	0.48 (0.00–0.96)	0.47 (0.10–0.87)	0.72 (0.10–1.46)	1.20 (0.50–1.90)	0.96 (0.66–1.26)
Protein C (U/ml)	0.35 (0.17–0.53)	0.42 (0.20–0.64)	0.43 (0.21–0.65)	0.54 (0.28–0.80)	0.59 (0.37–0.81)	0.96 (0.64–1.28)
Protein S (U/ml)	0.36 (0.12–0.60)	0.50 (0.22–0.78)	0.63 (0.33–0.93)	0.86 (0.54–1.18)*	0.87 (0.55–1.19)*	0.92 (0.60–1.24)
Premature infants (30–36 weeks gestation)						
ATIII (U/ml)	0.38 (0.14–0.62)+	0.56 (0.30–0.82)	0.59 (0.37–0.81)+	0.83 (0.45–1.21)+	0.90 (0.52–1.28)+	1.05 (0.79–1.31)
α_2 (U/ml)	1.10 (0.56–1.82)+	1.25 (0.71–1.77)	1.38 (0.72–2.04)	1.80 (1.20–2.66)	2.09 (1.10–3.21)	0.86 (0.52–1.20)
CT-INH (U/ml)	0.65 (0.31–0.99)	0.83 (0.45–1.21)	0.74 (0.40–1.24)+	1.14 (0.60–1.68)*	1.40 (0.96–2.04)	1.01 (0.71–1.31)
α_1AT (U/ml)	0.90 (0.36–1.44)*	0.94 (0.42–1.46)*	0.76 (0.38–1.12)+	0.81 (0.49–1.13)*+	0.82 (0.48–1.16)*	0.93 (0.55–1.31)
HCII (U/ml)	0.32 (0.10–0.60)+	0.34 (0.10–0.69)	0.43 (0.15–0.71)	0.61 (0.20–1.11)	0.89 (0.45–1.40)*+	0.96 (0.66–1.26)
Protein C (U/ml)	0.28 (0.12–0.44)+	0.31 (0.11–0.51)	0.37 (0.15–0.59)+	0.45 (0.23–0.67)+	0.57 (0.31–0.83)	0.96 (0.64–1.28)
Protein S (U/ml)	0.26 (0.14–0.38)+	0.37 (0.13–0.61)	0.56 (0.22–0.90)	0.76 (0.40–1.12)+	0.82 (0.44–1.20)	0.92 (0.60–1.24)

ATIII, antithrombin III; α_2M, α_2-macroglobulin; C_1-INH, C_1-esterase inhibitor α_1-AT, α_1-antitrypsin; HCII, heparin cofactor II. All values are expressed in units per millilitre (U/ml) where pooled plasma contains 1.0 U/ml and are given as a mean followed by the lower and upper boundary encompassing 95% of the population. Between 40–75 samples were assayed for each value for the newborn. Some measurements were skewed due to a disproportionate number of high values. The lower limit which excludes the lower 2.5% of the population has been given. *Values that are indistinguishable from those of the adult, +Values different from those of the fullterm infant. Reproduced with permission (Andrew et al 1990a).

Buchanan 1978, 1986, Hathaway & Bonner 1978, Gobel et al 1979, McDonald et al 1983, Peters et al 1984, Montgomery et al 1985, Hathaway & Bonner 1987, Gibson 1989, Manco-Johnson 1989, Bahakim et al 1990, Corrigan 1991, Hathaway & Corrigan 1991) (Table 44.4). Similarly, plasma concentrations of protein C, protein S, and heparin cofactor II are also low with levels less than 50% of adult values (Aballi et al 1962, Bleyer et al 1971, Strothers et al 1975, Gross & Stuart 1977, Buchanan 1978, 1986, Hathaway & Bonner 1978, Gobel et al 1979, McDonald et al 1983, Montgomery et al 1985, Karpatkin et al 1986, Andersson et al 1988, Gibson 1989, Takamiya et al 1989, Bahakim et al 1990). Indeed, levels of these inhibitors are all in the range where spontaneous thrombotic complications occur in heterozygous adults. Levels of antithrombin III in fullterm infants reach adult values by 3 months of life although the range of normal remains wider than for adults. Plasma concentrations of protein C remain low well into early childhood and do not achieve adult values until the early teen years (Karpatkin et al 1986, Andrew et al 1991). Recently the composition of adult and fetal protein C were compared (Greffe et al 1989). Protein C in cord plasma was identical to adult plasma, except that there was a two-fold increase in single chain protein C compared to adults. The authors suggested that the processing of fetal protein C may be developmentally influenced.

In contrast, newborn plasma concentrations of inhibitors of lesser importance in the adult haemostatic system are either similar to adult values or increased above adult values (Aballi et al 1962, Bleyer et al 1971, Strothers et al 1975, Gross & Stuart 1977, Buchanan 1978, 1986, Hathaway & Bonner 1978, Gobel et al 1979, McDonald et al 1983, Montgomery et al 1985, Andrew et al 1987, 1988, 1990, Hathaway & Bonner et al 1987, Gibson 1989, Bahakim et al 1990, Corrigan 1991, Hathaway & Corrigan 1991). These include CT esterase inhibitor, α_2-macroglobulin (α_2M) and α_1-antitrypsin inhibitor. By 6 months of age the plasma concentrations of α_2-macroglobulin are at least two-fold higher than adult values and remain elevated throughout childhood (Ganrot et al 1967, Andrew et al 1991).

Thrombin regulation

An important assessment of overall function of the coagulation system is the ability to generate the enzyme thrombin. Thrombin is a key enzyme in haemostasis with many important coagulant and some anticoagulant functions. Thrombin generation is delayed and decreased in newborn plasma compared to adult plasma and prothrombin is completely consumed (Schmidt et al 1989) (Fig. 44.1). This impaired thrombin generation varies with gestational age. When prothrombin levels are increased to adult values, in vitro or in vivo, the amount of thrombin generated similarly increases and the rate of thrombin generation is dependent on the concentration of other procoagulant proteins (Andrew et al 1990).

Thrombin is inhibited in the fluid phase by three inhibitors, ATIII, α_2M, and heparin cofactor II (HCII). When thrombin is added to defibrinated plasma, the rate of thrombin inhibition is slower than for adult plasma and significantly more thrombin is inhibited by α_2M than ATIII in newborn plasma (Schmidt et al 1989, Shah et al 1991). There is evidence that increased binding to α_2M also occurs in vivo (Levine et al 1987). In addition to the

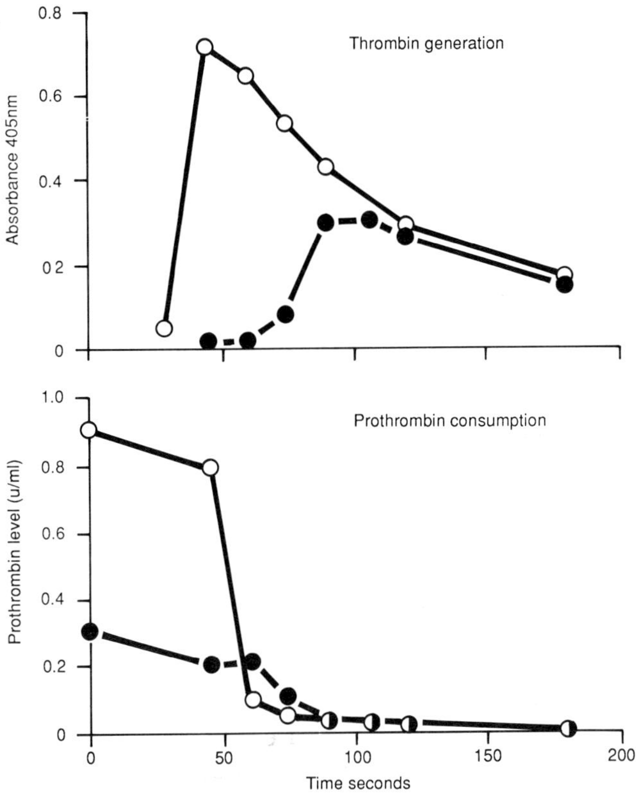

Fig. 44.1 Thrombin generation and prothrombin consumption following activation in the APTT system in plasma from adults (o) and from fullterm infants (●) at birth. The amount of thrombin generated was determined by its ability to cleave a chromogenic substrate, resulting in a change in the absorbance reading at 405 nm. Prothrombin was measured by ELISA.

enhanced thrombin inhibition by α_2M, there is also more thrombin inhibited by HCII. The latter is due to a circulating glycosaminoglycan that catalyzes thrombin inhibition by the natural inhibitor HCII (Andrew et al 1991d). This fetal anticoagulant has properties similar to dermatan sulphate, not heparin sulphate (Muller & van Doorm 1977, Andrew et al 1991d, Matzch et al 1991), and is also present in plasma from pregnant women (Andrew et al 1991d). In addition to fluid phase differences in thrombin inhibition, endothelial cell surface glycosaminoglycans potentiate thrombin inhibition more readily in adult plasma than newborn plasma (Xu et al 1991). Overall this information suggests that newborns have a reduced ability to inhibit thrombin once it is formed, despite a partial compensation by high levels of α_2M and a circulating glycosaminoglycan with anticoagulant activity.

Fibrinolysis

Screening tests of fibrinolysis show evidence of accelerated activity in cord blood compared to adults (Markarian et al 1967, Ekelund et al 1970, Reverdiau-Moalie et al 1991). Whole blood clotting times and euglobulin lysis times are short in cord blood and newborns following delivery. Plasma concentrations of components of the fibrinolytic system are very different from adults (Table 44.5) (Aballi et al 1962, Bleyer et al 1971, Strothers et al 1975, Gross & Stuart 1977, Buchanan, 1978, 1986, Hathaway & Bonner 1978, Gobel et al 1979, McDonald et al 1983, Montgomery et al 1985, Andrew et al 1987, 1988, 1990, Kolindewala et al 1987, Corrigan 1988, Corrigan et al 1989, Gibson 1989, Runnebaum et al 1989, Bahakim et al 1990). Plasminogen, the zymogen for the critical enzyme, plasmin, is only half adult concentrations (Aballi et al 1962, Ambrus et al 1979, Andrew et al 1987, 1988, 1990, Kolindewala et al 1987, Corrigan 1988, Corrigan et al 1989, Runnebaum et al 1989). Recent studies provide evidence for a fetal form of plasminogen in cord blood (Edelberg et al 1990). Like adults, newborns have two glycoforms of plasminogen, however both fetal forms had

Table 44.5 Reference values for the components of the fibrinolytic system in the healthy fullterm and premature infant during the first 6 months of life

	Day 1	Day 5	Day 30	Day 90	Day 180	Adult
Fullterm infant						
Plasminogen (U/ml)	1.95 (1.25–2.65)	2.17 (1.41–2.93)	1.98 (1.26–2.70)	2.48 (1.74–3.22)	3.01 (2.21–3.81)	3.36 (2.48–4.24)
TPA (ng/ml)	9.6 (5.0–18.9)	5.6 (4.0–10.0)*	4.1 (1.0–6.0)*	2.1 (1.0–5.0)*	2.8 (1.0–6.0)*	4.9 (1.4–8.4)
α_2AP (U/ml)	0.85 (0.55–1.15)	1.00 (0.70–1.30)*	1.00 (0.76–1.24)*	1.08 (0.76–1.40)*	1.11 (0.83–1.39)*	1.02 (0.68–1.36)
PAI_1 (U/ml)	6.4 (2.0–15.1)	2.3 (0.0–8.1)*	3.4 (0.0–8.8)*	7.2 (1.0–15.3)	8.1 (6.0–13.0)	3.6 (0.0– 11.0)
Premature infant (30–36 weeks gestation)						
Plasminogen (U/ml)	1.70 (1.12–2.48)+	1.91 (1.21–2.61)+	1.81 (1.09–2.53)	2.38 (1.58–3.18)	2.75 (1.91–3.59)+	3.36 (2.48–4.24)
TPA (ng/ml)	8.48 (3.00–16.70)	3.97 (2.00–6.93)*	4.13 (2.00–7.79)*	3.31 (2.00–5.07)*	3.48 (2.00–5.85)*	4.96 (1.46–8.46)
α_2AP (U/ml)	0.78 (0.40–1.16)	0.81 (0.49–1.13)+	0.89 (0.55–1.23)+	1.06 (0.64–1.48)*	1.15 (0.77–1.53)	1.02 (0.68–1.36)
PAI_1 (U/ml)	5.4 (0.0–12.2)*+	2.5 (0.0–7.1)*	4.3 (0.0–10.9)*	4.8 (1.0–11.8)*+	4.9 (1.0–10.2)*+	3.6 (0.0–11.0)

TPA, tissue plasminogen activator; α_2AP, α_2-antiplasmin; PAI_1, plasminogen activator inhibitor. α_2AP, values are expressed as units per millilitre (U/ml) where pooled plasma contains 1.0 U/ml. Plasminogen units are those recommended by the Committee on Thrombolytic Agents. Values for PAI_1 are given as units per ml where one unit of PAI_1 activity is defined as the amount of PAI_1 that inhibits one international unit of human single chain TPA. All values are given as a mean followed by the lower and upper boundary encompassing 95% of the population. *Values that are indistinguishable from those of the adult. +Values that are different from those of the fullterm infant. Reproduced with permission (Andrew et al 1990a).

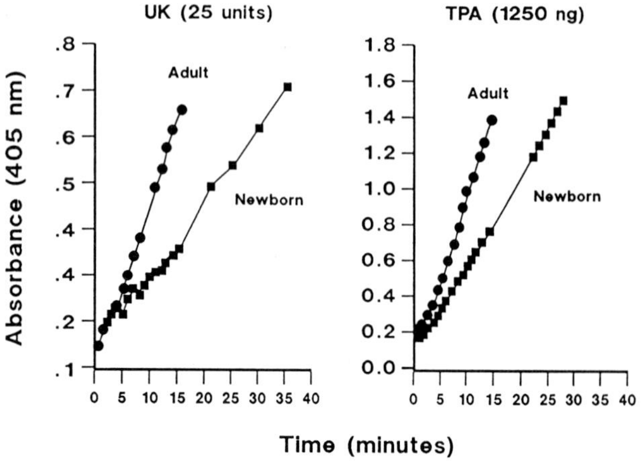

Fig. 44.2 Plasmin generation, chromogenic method. Urokinase (UK) or tissue-type plasminogen activator (tPA) were added to undiluted acid-treated plasma containing S-2251. The change in absorbance over time is shown. (Reproduced with permission, Corrigan et al 1989).

increased amounts of mannose and sialic acid. The same authors reported decreased functional activity of fetal plasminogen and decreased binding to cellular receptors. Other investigators concluded that fetal and newborn plasminogen were identical in function (Summaria 1989). Further studies will be needed to confirm that a fetal form of plasminogen exists. Plasma concentrations of tissue plasminogen activator (tPA), an important activator of plasminogen, and plasminogen activator inhibitor (PAI), an inhibitor of tPA, are increased in plasma from infants (Table 44.5). (Andrew et al 1990). The latter likely reflects release from endothelial cells following the birth process, as cord values for tPA and PAI are not increased (Corrigan et al 1989, Reverdiau-Moalie et al 1991). Plasma concentrations of the major inhibitor of plasmin, α_2-antiplasmin (α_2AP), is approximately 80% of adult values (Kolindewala et al 1987, Corrigan 1988, Corrigan et al 1989, Runnebaum et al 1989, Andrew et al 1990). The ability of the newborn's fibrinolytic system to generate plasmin in vitro is decreased compared to adults probably predominantly due to low plasma concentrations of plasminogen (Corrigan et al 1989, Andrew et al 1991) (Fig. 44.2). The reduced ability to generate plasmin impairs the overall ability of the newborn's fibrinolytic system to lyse fibrin clots (Andrew et al 1991). Increasing plasma concentrations of plasminogen, either with purified plasminogen or with plasma supplementation enhances the fibrinolytic capacity of the newborn system to adult values (Andrew et al 1991) (Fig. 44.3).

Mechanisms of regulation of coagulation proteins

Potential mechanisms responsible for differences in plasma concentrations of coagulation components are: decreased synthesis, increased clearance, consumption, and presence of proteins with decreased activity. Hassan and coworkers measured RNA and protein level for factors

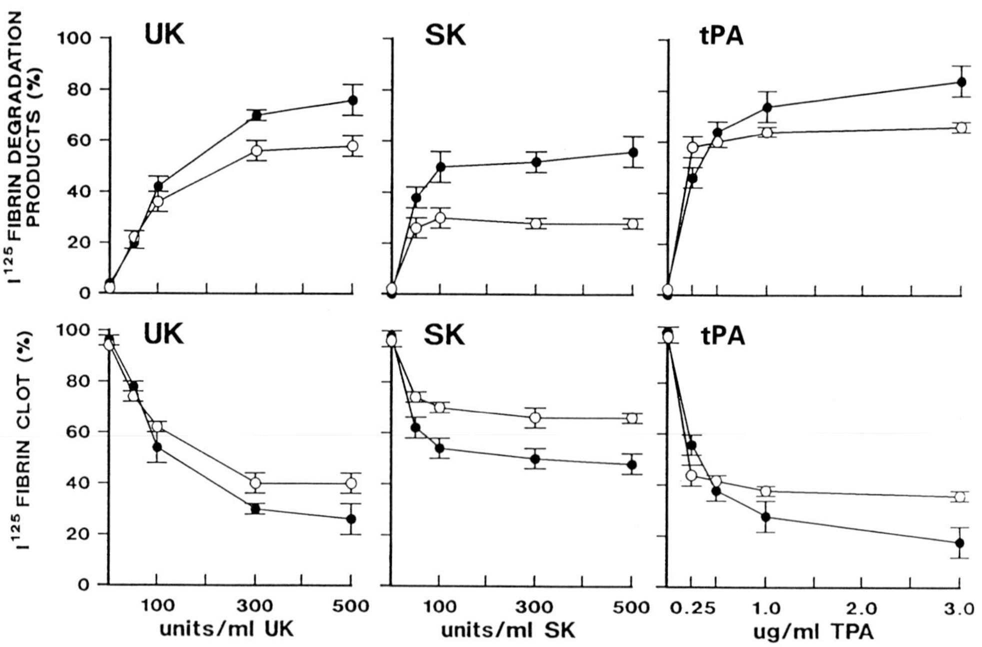

Fig. 44.3 The ^{125}I-labelled fibrin degradation products (%) released into the bathing labelled plasma (upper panel) and ^{125}I-labelled fibrin clot lysis (%) in the cord system (washed cord ^{125}I-labelled fibrin clots placed in cord plasma (C/C, ○–○) compared to the similar adult system (A/A, ●–●) in the presence of increasing amounts of urokinase (UK), streptokinase (SK) and tissue plasminogen activator (tPA). The cord system was resistant to the effects of all three thrombolytic agents compared to the adult system (●–●) mean ± 1 SEM, $p < 0.01$).

VII, VIII, IX, X, fibrinogen, antithrombin III, and protein C in hepatocytes from 5 to 10-week-old human embryos and fetuses (Hassan et al 1990). They reported similar size of embryonic-fetal transcripts and adult mRNAs and an identical nucleotide sequence of factor IX and factor X mRNA. They concluded that the expression of RNA was variable, with adult values for some coagulation proteins and decreased expression for others (Fig. 44.4). Other investigators reported similar concentrations of prothrombin mRNA in newborn and adult rabbit livers (Karpatkin et al 1991). Only one study has reported lower mRNA concentrations for prothrombin in a sheep model (Kisker et al 1988).

At least some coagulation proteins are cleared more rapidly in newborns than adults (Karitzky et al 1971, Feusner et al 1983, Schmidt et al 1984, Andrew et al 1988a). The half life of fibrinogen is significantly shorter in newborn animals and in infants with respiratory distress syndrome than for corresponding adults (Karitzky et al

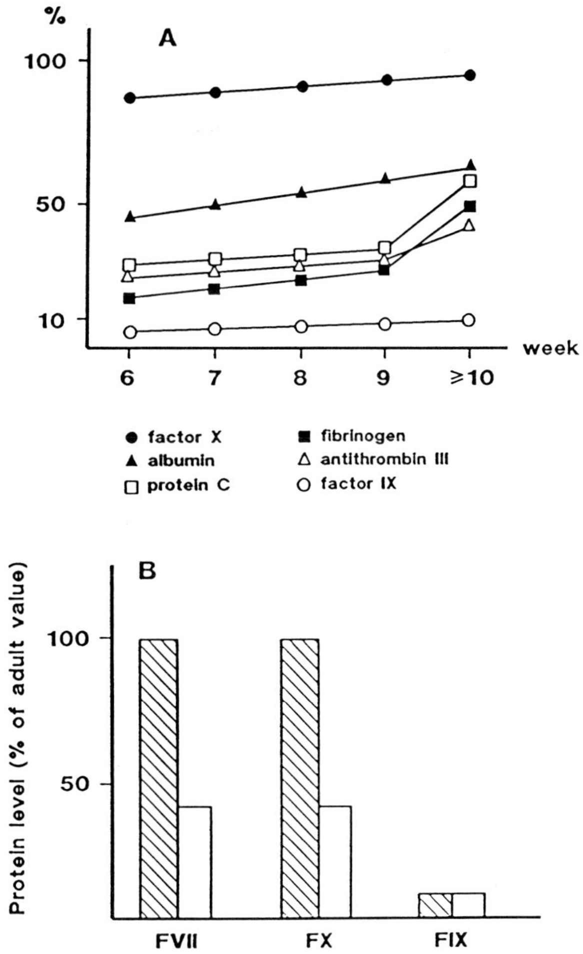

Fig. 44.4 Expression of blood coagulation factors during onotogeneic development A RNA level in the 5–10 week post-conception period, and B protein level at 7–8 weeks in liver (□ bar) and plasma (⊣). Values are percentage of adult level. (Reproduced with permission, Bleyer et al 1971.)

1971, Feusner et al 1983, Andrew et al 1988a). The half life of ATIII is shorter in infants requiring an exchange transfusion for hyperbilirubinaemia than for healthy adults (Schmidt et al 1984). Reasons for faster clearance of these proteins in newborns are incompletely understood but may be due in part to an increased basal metabolic rate in newborns (Pencharz et al 1977).

Activation of coagulation occurs at birth, as evidenced by elevated levels of fibrinopeptide A, and thrombin-antithrombin III complexes in cord blood (Suarez et al 1984, 1988, Yuen et al 1989). However activation does not provide an explanation for low concentrations of coagulation proteins in newborns (Kisker et al 1981, Andrew et al 1988). Similarly there is no evidence that fetal proteins are significantly affecting functional measurements of coagulation proteins and thereby contributing to low plasma concentrations of the proteins involved.

Newborns compensate for the immaturity of their haemostatic system in unexpected ways. For example, plasma concentrations of protein S are markedly reduced in newborns compared to adults (Moalic et al 1988, Schwarz et al 1988). However protein S circulates completely in the free, active form in newborns (Moalic et al 1988, Schwarz et al 1988), due to an absence of C4b-binding protein. vWF circulates with increased plasma concentrations of the active high molecular weight multimeric forms (Katz et al 1989, Weinstein et al 1989). The latter may provide part of the explanation for short bleeding times in newborns (Andrew et al 1987, 1989).

CONGENITAL DEFICIENCIES OF COAGULATION PROTEINS

Coagulant proteins

Inherited deficiencies of coagulant proteins can present clinically in either severe or mild forms. Frequently these patients present with their first bleeding complication as infants or in early childhood. Prenatal diagnosis is possible for most coagulant protein deficiencies but is largely confined to severe haemophilia A (factor VIII) and haemophilia B (factor IX) (Firshein et al 1979, Forestier et al 1986a, Daffos et al 1988). Prenatal diagnosis of deficiencies of factors V, VII, XIII and vWF have also been described. Recombinant technology is the method of choice if it can be used, whereas fetal blood sampling offers an alternative method in some patients. These topics are discussed in detail in other chapters.

Severe deficiencies of coagulation factors usually present in otherwise healthy fullterm infants with spontaneous bleeding or excessive bleeding from minor trauma. Although acquired problems are more frequent than congenital deficiencies, the latter must be seriously considered because of their early presentation in infancy (Girolami et al 1985). These infants may present with oozing from the umbilicus, bleeding into the scalp resulting in large cephalohaematomas, persistent bleeding following heel puncture, bleeding following circumcision, or bleeding into the skin. Unfortunately, the first clinical manifestation may be an intracranial haemorrhage (Silverstein 1960, Struwe 1970, Mariani et al 1983, Girolami et al 1985, Abbondanzo et al 1988, Yoffe & Buchanan 1988). The risk of intracranial haemorrhage in infants with severe haemophilia A or B is 2–8% (Silverstein 1960, Baehner & Strauss 1966, Yoffe & Buchanan 1988). In one review of 75 cases of factor VII deficiency, 12 patients bled intracranially, and these occurred in early infancy (Ragni et al 1986). Intracranial haemorrhage can occur in the absence of an inherited coagulation deficiency. However, any otherwise-well, fullterm infant with an intracranial haemorrhage should be evaluated for an inherited bleeding disorder (Hayden et al 1985). Occasionally, congenital coagulation deficiencies occur in combination with other disorders. Examples are factor VII deficiency in infants with Dubin–Johnson syndrome and Gilbert syndrome (Seligsohn et al 1970, Levanon et al 1972).

von Willebrand's disease (vWD) is the most common inherited bleeding disorder in adults. However, vWD rarely presents in newborns, with bleeding unlikely because plasma concentrations of vWF are increased in the early postnatal period. In addition, high molecular weight multimeric forms of vWF are disproportionately increased in newborns (Andrew et al 1987, 1988, 1990a, Katz et al 1989, Weinstein et al 1989). Thus most forms of vWD cannot be diagnosed in newborns by assays reflecting vWF activity or protein concentration. There are rare forms of vWD, usually homozygous, associated with marked decreases of both vWF and factor VIII, that can present with bleeding in newborns, and can be identified by specific assays of factor VIII and vWF (Donner et al 1987).

The most common congenital coagulation defects to present clinically in newborns are the haemophilias (Silverstein 1960, Baehner & Strauss 1966, Girolami et al 1985, Yoffe et al 1988). Severe (less than 0.01 units/ml), and moderate (0.01–0.05 units/ml) forms of both haemophilia A (factor VIII deficiency), and haemophilia B (factor IX deficiency) can be diagnosed at the time of birth because physiological levels do not overlap with pathological values. Mild forms of haemophilia A can also be diagnosed at birth, however mild forms of haemophilia B may overlap with the lower physiological limit of normal for infants (0.15 units/ml). Usually patients with severe forms of haemophilia present during the first months of life when their level of physical activity increases. Factor XI deficiency, sometimes called haemophilia C, in contrast to haemophilia A and B, is inherited autosomally (Rapaport et al 1961). Distinguishing inherited factor XI deficiency from physiological deficiencies can be difficult because the lower limit of normal is 0.05 units/ml. Patients with severe forms of factor XI deficiency could potentially have plasma concentrations of factor XI in the physiological range. Because infants with factor XI deficiency are rarely tested at birth, it is unknown if physiological and congenital deficits in combination result in levels less than 0.05 units/ml for all affected infants. Infants at risk should be retested later in the postnatal period for confirmation of the diagnosis. Elective surgical procedures such as circumcision should be delayed until the diagnosis is made.

Other autosomally inherited coagulation deficiencies that may cause bleeding in newborns include factors II, V, VII, and X (Mariani & Mazzucconi 1983, Mammen, 1983a,b,c, Triplett et al 1985, Ragni et al 1986). Homozygous forms of these factor deficiencies are very rare and number only a few hundred in the literature. Homozygous forms for factors V and VII are characterized by plasma concentrations less than 0.10 and 0.03 units/ml respectively. These levels are easily distinguished from physiological values (Mariani & Mazzucconi 1983, Girolami et al 1985, Ragni et al 1986). In contrast, homozygous deficiencies of factors II and X result in plasma levels less than 0.20 and 0.10 units/ml respectively, which overlap with physiological levels (Mammen 1983a,c, Girolami et al 1985). Heterozygote forms for factors II, V, VII, and X deficiency may be more difficult to diagnose in newborns because plasma concentrations overlap with physiological levels (Girolami et al 1985, Mariani & Mazzucconi 1983, Ragni et al 1986, Mammen 1983a,b,c, Triplett et al 1985). Rarely an inherited combined deficiency of factors II, VII, IX, and X occurs, presumably caused by defective γ-carboxylation (Johnson et al 1980, Goldsmith et al 1982). Deficiencies of factor XII, HMWK, and PK do not cause bleeding complications in infants or adults.

The goals of treatment for infants with inherited deficiencies of factors II, VII, V, and X are similar to adults. Usually factor replacement is achieved with either stored plasma (except for factor V), or fresh frozen plasma but rarely with factor concentrates. The recovery of coagulation factors has not been studied in a rigorous fashion in newborns and it is likely that it will be less than for adults. This is due, in part, to a faster clearance of proteins (Pencharz et al 1977). Administering 10 ml/kg of a plasma product should raise the factor level by approximately 0.10 units/ml. The latter should be directly measured in infants, particularly if there is no clinical response. Target replacement levels depend upon the underlying disorder and/or haemostatic challenge.

Defects in fibrinogen are comprised of hypo- and afibrinogenaemias, and dysfibrinogenaemias (Mammen 1983d, Girolami et al 1985). Usually only homozygous patients are symptomatic whereas heterozygous patients are asymptomatic. Plasma concentrations of fibrinogen are similar in newborns, to adults, therefore the afibrinogenaemias can be easily diagnosed. However many of the functional assays used to demonstrate the presence of a dysfibrinogenaemia are also affected by the physiological 'fetal' fibrinogen in infancy (Galanakis et al 1976, Witt et al 1969, Hamulyak et al 1983). Cryoprecipitate is the plasma product of choice to treat these patients because of its high fibrinogen concentration.

Persistent umbilical bleeding is a frequent presentation of homozygous factor XIII deficiency (Lorand et al 1980, Girolami et al 1985, Abbondanzo et al 1988). Plasma concentrations of factor XIII are less than 0.01 units/ml in homozygous patients and are readily differentiated from physiological values. It is important to remember that factor XIII deficiency does not prolong the common screening tests and must be measured specifically. Identification of infants with factor XIII deficiency is important because these infants should be treated prophylactically to prevent spontaneous intracranial haemorrhage. This may occur in up to a third of patients who are not treated. The half life of factor XIII is long and only very low levels of factor XIII are required for haemostasis. These features facilitate prophylactic treatment of these patients with either cryoprecipitate, fresh frozen plasma, or factor XIII concentrate.

Procoagulant inhibitors

Heterozygous deficiencies of the inhibitors, antithrombin III, protein C, protein S, and heparin cofactor II may predispose to thrombotic complications in adults but rarely in childhood except in the presence of another pathological event (Bjarke et al 1974, Shapiro et al 1981, Mannino & Travers 1983, de Stefano et al 1987, Israels et al 1987b). In contrast, the homozygous form of protein C deficiency presents in newborns with extensive life-threatening thrombotic complications (Griffin et al 1981, Marciniak et al 1985, Marlar et al 1989). The diagnoses of homozygous protein C deficiency is made in the presence of the appropriate clinical picture, a protein C plasma concentration below normal for age and heterozygous state in the parents. In the absence of clinical symptoms, a low plasma concentration of protein C is not diagnostic of congenital protein C deficiency because physiological plasma concentrations of protein C are as low as 0.12 units/ml. A combination of this physiological deficiency and an acquired pathological deficiency, as may occur in sick premature infants, may further decrease plasma concentrations of protein C to unmeasurable values (Manco-Johnson et al 1991). The clinical significance of this remains to be clarified. For congenital homozygous protein C deficiency, replacement therapy with plasma products is the initial management. Treatment options for long-term therapy include oral anticoagulant therapy, replacement therapy with protein C concentrates (Riess et al 1985, Vukovich et al 1988, Dreyfus et al 1991), and liver transplantation (Griffin et al 1981, Casella et al 1988, Marlar et al 1989). Homozygous forms of the other inhibitors have not been reported.

ACQUIRED COAGULOPATHIES

Although any infant presenting with bleeding should be considered to have either an acquired or congenital haemostatic deficit (Aballi et al 1962, Strothers et al 1975, Gross & Stuart 1977, Buchanan 1978, 1986, Hathaway & Bonner 1978, Gobel et al 1979, McDonald et al 1983, Montgomery et al 1985, Gibson 1989, Bahakim et al 1990), acquired problems are far more frequent. The most common acquired defects to present in sick infants are disseminated intravascular coagulation (DIC), liver failure, and vitamin K deficiency. The laboratory evaluation of these infants should initially include a PT, APTT, TCT, fibrinogen level, and platelet count. Depending on the results of these tests and the clinical presentation additional tests may be indicated.

Disseminated intravascular coagulation

Disseminated intravascular coagulation (DIC), was the name originally given to the observation of pathological, diffuse fibrin deposition in the microvasculature in patients who suffered haemorrhagic and thrombotic complications prior to death (Boyd 1966, 1967, 1969). As an understanding of haemostasis evolved, the relationship between the clinicopathological findings in DIC and decreased plasma concentrations of coagulation proteins was recognized (Rodriguez-Erdmann 1965, Phillips 1967, Abildgaard 1969, Hathaway et al 1969, Dube et al 1986). DIC is a secondary process initiated by a variety of underlying diseases (Rodriguez-Erdmann 1965, Phillips 1967, Abildgaard 1969, Hathaway et al 1969, Dube et al 1986). These differ in newborns from those in children and adults, and frequently involve the fetal placental unit (Markarian et al 1967a,b, Edson et al 1968, Chessells & Wigglesworth 1971a,b, 1972, Anderson et al 1974, Corrigan 1979, Watkins et al 1980, Dudley & Dalton 1986, Conover et al 1990). For example, adverse events related to the birth process may result in asphyxia and shock, two of the most common predisposing events for DIC in newborns. Other neonatal disorders that may initiate DIC include extreme prematurity associated with respiratory distress syndrome (RDS), viral or bacterial infections, hypothermia, and meconium or amniotic fluid aspiration syndromes.

The clinical presentation of DIC in infancy is highly variable reflecting the intensity and duration of activation of the haemostatic system, the degree of impaired blood flow and hepatic function (Corrigan 1979). Early descriptions of DIC in infancy were of overt haemorrhagic or thrombotic complications frequently followed by death. However, the clinical spectrum of DIC is changing with the majority of infants surviving, reflecting the ever improving perinatal case of sick infants. For an increasing number of infants, DIC is a laboratory diagnosis with few manifestations of the problem and no apparent clinical significance.

In the 1960s and 1970s, the diagnosis of DIC was characterized by prolonged screening tests; low plasma concentrations of fibrinogen, factors V and VIII, elevated levels of fibrinogen/fibrin degradation products, thrombocytopenia and red cell fragmentation (Rodriguez-Erdmann 1965, Phillips 1967, Abildgaard 1969, Hathaway et al 1969, Corrigan 1979). This pattern of coagulation abnormalities was usually seen in infants who were clinically symptomatic from the haemostatic defects. More recently, assays of inhibitors of coagulation (Tollefsen & Pestka 1985, Chuansumrit et al 1989), and sensitive laboratory tests for thrombin and plasmin generation have been developed and used for newborns. The latter tests include the measurement of thrombin-antithrombin III complexes, cross-linked fibrin (D-dimer), fibrinopeptide A, and plasmin-α_2-antiplasmin complexes. These sensitive tools have facilitated the diagnosis of milder, and sometimes clinically asymptomatic cases of DIC. Further, many of these tests are abnormal in cord blood from healthy infants probably reflecting activation of coagulation during the normal birth process (Suarez et al 1984, 1985, 1988, Yuen et al 1989). Clearly positive results for these sensitive tests do not always indicate the presence of DIC nor the need to therapeutically intervene. In practice, no single laboratory test can be used to confirm or exclude DIC.

Successful management of DIC requires successful treatment of the underlying disease. The treatment of secondary haemostatic problems is frequently controversial and reflects the lack of relevant and current controlled trials in this area of transfusion medicine. One approach is to intervene with coagulation factor replacement therapy for infants with overt evidence of haemorrhagic or thrombotic complications in addition to laboratory confirmation of DIC. In contrast, there is no evidence that infants with no apparent clinical manifestations of DIC and only mild laboratory abnormalities, benefit from coagulation factor replacement therapy. For infants between these two extremes, coagulation factor replacement therapy is dictated by the severity of the haemostatic and laboratory measured impairment. In making the decision to intervene with plasma products, it is important to remember that newborns do not have the same reserve capacity as adults because of the immaturity of their coagulation system. Thus, they may deteriorate rapidly, developing overt haemostatic problems if the underlying disorder is poorly controlled.

Replacement of coagulation factors may be accomplished in newborns by simple transfusions of plasma products, or by exchange transfusions. Several controlled studies have documented an improvement in laboratory tests following coagulation factor replacement (Gross & Melhorn 1971, De Lemos et al 1973, Hambleton & Appleyard 1973, Waltt et al 1973, Snydor et al 1977, Woods et al 1979, Turner et al 1981, Gross et al 1982, Yamada et al 1983, Beverley et al 1985a,b). Fresh frozen plasma is the most commonly used plasma product because it contains adult levels of factors V and VIII in addition to all other coagulation proteins. Cryoprecipitate is a very useful product because of the high concentration of fibrinogen and factor VIII. Occasionally, in very severe cases, exchange transfusions can be helpful in restoring haemostasis, at least on a temporary basis. Exchange transfusions are not without risk, and are only transiently helpful if the underlying problem does not resolve. Prothrombin complex concentrates have been used in the past in newborns, however they are not generally recommended because of potential thrombotic and infectious side-effects (Waltt et al 1973). Platelet concentrates are helpful in maintaining platelet counts at least above 50×10^9/l.

Anticoagulant therapy has been used in some infants with DIC. There is no convincing clinical data supporting the general use of heparin for infants with DIC (Corrigan & Jordan 1970, Markarian et al 1971, Corrigan 1977, Gobel et al 1980, Yamada et al 1983, von Kries et al 1985). Plasma concentrations of inhibitors ATIII and HCII that are already physiologically low are further decreased in DIC (Andrew et al 1983a, Tollefsen & Pesta 1985, Chuansumrit et al 1989). ATIII concentrates have been tested recently in small trials in infants with DIC without demonstrating any benefit (Hanada et al 1985, von Kries et al 1985). Although these trials were too small to come to any reliable conclusions, ATIII concentrates must at this time be considered investigational for infants with DIC.

Vitamin K deficiency

Townsend described the clinical features of Haemorrhagic Disease of the Newborn (HDN) in 1894 (Townsend 1894). The features consisted of haemorrhage from multiple sites on days 1 to 5 of life, in otherwise healthy infants, in the absence of trauma, asphyxia, or infection. During the first decades of this century a causal link between HDN and abnormal blood clotting was made (Kugelmass 1932, Sanford et al 1932, Clifford 1941, Aballi et al 1962). Early attempts at treatment were made with intravenous, intramuscular and subcutaneous injection of blood or serum into infants. One of the first controlled trials was conducted in 1938 to determine if intramuscular blood was helpful (Sanford & Leslie 1938). Not surprisingly this modality was not helpful. In 1929, Dam reported the link between vitamin K deficiency and spontaneous haemorrhaging in chicks fed a vitamin K-deficient diet (Dam 1929). Vitamin K deficiency was rapidly implicated in HDN (Brinkhous et al 1937, Dam et al 1939, Bruchsaler 1941, Aballi et al 1962) and treatment of affected infants with vitamin K followed (Nygaard 1939, Quick & Grossman 1939a,b, Waddell & Guerry 1939, Aballi et al 1962).

During the 1930s when the association between vitamin K deficiency and HDN was recognized, an important screening test of coagulation, the PT, was developed by Quick and subsequently used in assessing newborns (Quick & Grossman 1939a,b). The PT was prolonged in newborns compared to adults, further prolonged in newborns with HDN and corrected when vitamin K was administered. Physiologically, plasma concentrations of prothrombin decreased in newborns on days 2 to 4 of life, with corresponding increases for the PT. The results returned to normal by days 5 to 7 of life (Nygaard, 1939, Quick & Grossman 1939a,b, Waddell & Guerry 1939, Dam et al 1942, Aballi et al 1957, 1962) (Fig. 44.5). Decreases in plasma prothrombin concentrations during the first days of life could be prevented by giving prophylactic vitamin K to either mothers or infants (Nygaard 1939, Fitzgerald & Webster 1940, Bruchsaler 1941, Hellman & Shettles 1942, Aballi et al 1962). These data together suggested that newborns were deficient in vitamin K during the first days of life and that prophylactic vitamin K was helpful in preventing HDN (Sanford et al 1932, Nygaard 1939, Waddell & Guerry 1939, Fitzgerald & Webster 1940, Gellis & Lyon 1941, Mull et al 1941, Hellman & Shettles 1942, Motohara et al 1984, 1989). Unfortunately, few controlled trials were performed, rather vitamin K prophylaxis was introduced in some populations and not in others. Thus the debate over the benefits and risks of prophylactic vitamin K began. This controversy underscores the need for carefully controlled, epidemiologically-sound clinical trials when a potentially helpful form of therapy is being evaluated.

The policy of administering vitamin K prophylactically became less clear for a number of reasons. First, there was

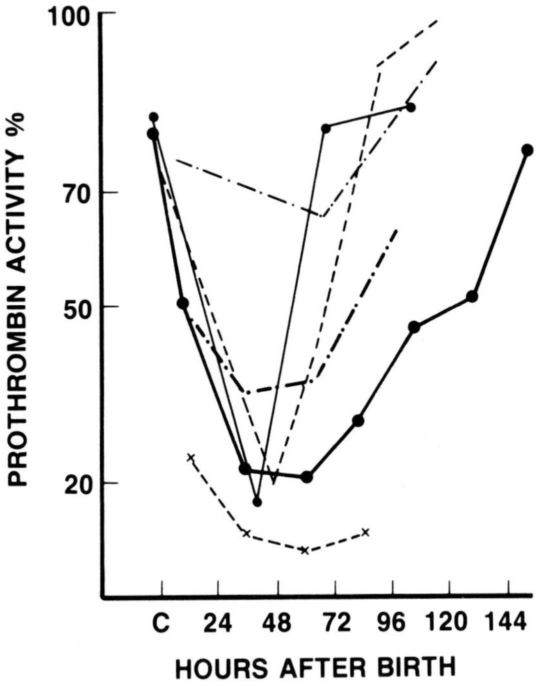

Fig. 44.5 The pattern of prothrombin levels in otherwise healthy fullterm infants who did not receive prophylactic vitamin K at birth. ●–●, Sanford et al 1942; ●—● Grossman et al; x---x, Dam et al 1942; -·-·-, Aballi et al 1957; ---, Quick & Grossman 1939a, Waddell & Guerry 1939; -·-·- Nygaard 1939. (Reproduced with permission, Andrew et al 1991d.)

recognition that newborns bled from disorders that were not due to vitamin K deficiency (Kugelmass 1932, Clifford 1941, Potter 1945, Aballi et al 1959, 1962). Second, other coagulation proteins that were not vitamin K-dependent, were discovered and found to be low in newborns. Third, some infants received a water-soluble form of vitamin K in high amounts (50–70 mg) which caused a haemolytic anaemia with kernicterus (Lucey & Dolan 1959, Committee on Nutrition 1961, Aballi et al 1962). These adverse outcomes in conjunction with a view that not all healthy fullterm infants needed vitamin K prophylaxis, led to the suspension of vitamin K prophylaxis in some countries (Parks & Sweet 1942, Potter 1945, Waddell & Whitehead 1945, Malia et al 1980). Over the past several decades numerous studies have been published supporting or refuting the need for vitamin K prophylaxis. These trials are reviewed in a subsequent section (p. 1029).

Diagnosis of vitamin K deficiency in newborns

At birth the plasma concentrations of the four vitamin K procoagulants (factors II, VII, IX, X) are physiologically half adult values in otherwise healthy infants (Aballi et al 1962, Andrew et al 1987, 1990, Andrew & Schmidt 1988). When infants become vitamin K deficient, plasma concentrations of vitamin K-dependent procoagulants rapidly decrease to values below critical haemostatic levels. The result can be serious haemorrhagic complications in otherwise healthy infants (Lehmann 1944, Kries et al 1988). The clinical presentation of vitamin K deficiency can be classified into three patterns based on the timing of the complications (MacElfresh 1961, Aballi et al 1962, Hathaway 1986, 1987, Shapiro et al 1986, Fetus and Newborn Committee, Canadian Pediatric Society 1988). The original description of HDN was severe clinical bleeding in breast-fed, otherwise healthy fullterm infants on days 2–5 of life (Aballi et al 1962, Lane & Hathaway 1985, Rose 1985, Shapiro et al 1986, Hall & Pairaudeau 1987, Hathaway 1987, Hanawa et al 1988, Kries et al 1988). Newborns are relatively vitamin K deficient compared to adults because of low placental transfer of vitamin K (Hamulyak et al 1987, Hiraike et al 1988a,b, Mandelbrot et al 1988), low stores of vitamin K in the liver, low intake of vitamin K in the first days of life due to small feeds, low concentration of vitamin K in breast milk (less than 20 μg/l), and a sterile gut (Gellis & Lyon 1941, Lawson 1941, Aballi et al 1962, Haroon et al 1982, Shearer et al 1982, Shirahata et al 1982, Widdershoven et al 1986, Allison et al 1987, Olson 1987, von Kries et al 1987a,c, Greer et al 1988, Shinzawa et al 1989). Commercially available formulas and cow's milk have higher concentrations of vitamin K than breast milk, approximately 830 mg/l, and 15 mg/l respectively (Haroon et al 1982, von Kries et al 1987a). Therefore vitamin K deficiency does not occur as frequently in formula-fed infants. The classic form of HDN is rarely seen in countries in which vitamin K is given prophylactically to all infants. The frequency of HDN when vitamin K prophylaxis is not given varies in different parts of the world depending upon the use of formula supplementation, the nutritional status of mothers, and frequency of breast milk feeding. Some estimates place the frequency of vitamin K deficiency as high as 1/200 infants (Aballi et al 1962, Sutherland & Glueck 1967).

Infants born to mothers who have been taking drugs that interfere with vitamin K metabolism may present with bleeding events in the first 24 hours of life. Frequently these complications are serious and include intracranial haemorrhage. The drugs implicated are warfarin, anticonvulsants, rifampin and isoniazid (Mountain et al 1970, Srinivasan et al 1982, Laosombat 1988). A third pattern of vitamin K deficiency presents later in the postnatal period, beyond the first weeks of life (Muntean et al 1979, Forbes 1983, Martin-Bouyer et al 1983, Chaou et al 1984, Payne & Hasagawa 1984, Editorial 1985, Motohara et al 1986, 1987, Goldschmidt et al 1988, Matsuda et al 1989). Unfortunately many of these infants also present with intracranial haemorrhage. Usually these infants have underlying diseases that compromise the supply of vitamin K. Some examples are: chronic diarrhoea, cystic fibrosis, α_1-antitrypsin deficiency, hepatitis, and celiac disease.

There are several laboratory tests that can help confirm the occurrence of vitamin K deficiency when it is clinically suspected. These include: specific factor assays, measurements of decarboxylated forms of the vitamin K-dependent factors, and measurements of the plasma concentration of vitamin K. The correct diagnosis of pathological vitamin K deficiency is dependent on comparing the results of these tests in affected infants to values from age-matched, healthy, controls. Vitamin K-dependent proteins induced in the absence of vitamin K (PIVKA), are decarboxylated and can be quantitated by direct measurement (Bloch et al 1984, Fujimura et al 1984, Kotohara & Endo 1985, Motohara et al 1985, 1987, Widdershoven et al 1986, 1988). The presence of PIVKA can also be inferred when a discrepancy occurs between coagulant activity and immunological concentration of vitamin K-dependent proteins (Fujimura et al 1982). A rapid, and therefore clinically useful test for documenting vitamin K deficiency is the Echis assay (Corrigan & Kryc 1980). Because the snake venom from *Echis carinatum* cleaves both decarboxylated and carboxylated forms of prothrombin, it measures total prothrombin concentration (Corrigan & Kryc 1980). Discrepancies between the traditional calcium-dependent prothrombin assay and the Echis prothrombin assay provides confirmation of vitamin K deficiency.

Prevention and treatment

Low fetal stores of vitamin K and occurrence of HDN form the rationale for administering vitamin K prophylactically to newborns. The controversy over the benefits and risks of prophylactic vitamin K reflects, in part, the apparently conflicting results from several different studies. Studies supporting or refuting the benefits or prophylactic vitamin K can be grouped by their design. There are no randomized controlled trials using clinical outcomes that refute the benefits of prophylactic vitamin K, administered to infants. In contrast, there are two randomized controlled trials that report a significant decrease in clinical bleeding for infants receiving vitamin K prophylaxis (Vietti et al 1960, Sutherland & Glueck 1967). In the study by Sutherland & Glueck, 3338 healthy infants were randomized to receive placebo or vitamin K intramuscularly (Sutherland & Glueck 1967). The clinical outcomes were both minor and major bleeding as assessed by health care personnel who were unaware of which therapy the infants had received. Bleeding events occurred in infants receiving placebo at a rate of 7.5% compared to a rate of 5.5% for infants receiving vitamin K. Serious bleeding, such as intracranial bleeding, occurred in 0.7% of infants receiving placebo but was not observed in vitamin K-treated infants. Further, infants with clinical bleeding had prolonged PTs that corrected when vitamin K was administered. A second study by Vietti and coworkers randomized male infants who were to be circumcised to receive prophylactic vitamin K or no treatment (Vietti et al 1960). Only six of 240 infants who received vitamin K bled following circumcision compared to 32 of 470 infants who did not receive vitamin K. Vietti conducted a further study that was smaller and not blinded with the same results (Vietti et al 1961). Although the study by Sutherland & Glueck (1967) did not use objective tests of intracranial haemmorhage (because they were not available at that time), and the study by Vietti randomized infants by day rather than individually, these two studies still provide strong evidence of benefit from vitamin K prophylaxis.

The use of vitamin K prophylaxis is further supported by many case control studies that used surrogate laboratory outcomes as evidence of vitamin K deficiency (Astrowe & Palmeston 1941, Lehmann 1944, Aballi et al 1962, Wefring 1962, Keenan et al 1971, O'Connor & Addiego 1986, Widdershoven et al 1986, Motohara et al 1987, von Kries et al 1987, Ogata et al 1988). In these studies infants given vitamin K prophylaxis were compared to concurrent untreated control infants. These studies showed that laboratory evidence of vitamin K deficiency occurred less frequently in infants who received vitamin K prophylaxis compared to infants who did not receive vitamin K prophylaxis. Further support for vitamin K prophylaxis comes from studies that evaluated and reported biochemical evidence of vitamin K deficiency at birth in large groups of infants (Shearer et al 1982, Bloch et al 1984, Hall & Pairandeau 1987, Motohara et al 1987, Greer et al 1988, Hiraike et al 1988a,b). In some countries vitamin

K prophylaxis was instituted and then withdrawn with the subsequent reoccurrence of HDN (Waddell & Guerry 1939, Lawson 1941, Lehmann 1941, MacElfresh 1961, Aballi et al 1962, Hanawa et al 1988). In other studies, a clinical or biochemical beneficial effect was observed following administration of vitamin K to the mother (Fitzgerald et al 1940, Mull et al 1941, Hellman & Shettles 1942, Fresh et al 1959, Lucey & Dolan 1959, Aballi et al 1962). Weak but supportive data come from higher frequencies of HDN in countries not administering vitamin K prophylaxis when compared to countries that do (MacElfresh 1961, Aballi et al 1962). Finally case reports continue to be published describing the occurrence of HDN in infants who, for a variety of reasons, did not receive vitamin K at birth (Lane & Hathaway 1983, Chaou et al 1984, Behrmann et al 1985, Binder 1986).

The evidence against the need for vitamin K prophylaxis is weak and in some cases has been misinterpreted (Sanford et al 1942, Gobel et al 1977, Mori et al 1977, Corrigan & Kryc 1980, Malia et al 1980). As mentioned there are no randomized controlled trials using clinical outcomes that have failed to demonstrate a beneficial effect. The case control studies have small sample sizes, sequential rather than concurrent controls (Potter 1945) and the frequency of breast-feeding may not have been considered. Some investigators could not demonstrate biochemical evidence of vitamin K deficiency in cord blood (Sanford et al 1942, Gobel et al 1977, Mori et al 1977, Corrigan & Kryc 1980, Malia et al 1980). However this may reflect insensitivity of the assays used and does not provide evidence that HDN does not occur in subsequent days. In some studies, mothers rather than infants received vitamin K prophylaxis (Parks & Sweet 1942). One would anticipate variability in placental transport affecting delivery of vitamin K to fetuses in these studies. Some studies did show biochemical evidence of benefit from vitamin K prophylaxis but not clinical benefit. Small sample sizes likely provide at least part of the explanation for these discrepancies (Sanford et al 1942). Concerns over potential adverse effects of vitamin K prophylaxis have been raised (Freeman et al 1987, Israels et al 1987a), however their clinical importance is still speculative (Cornelissen et al 1991). In summary, a reasonably strong recommendation for vitamin K prophylaxis in newborns can be made based on available information.

Prophylactic vitamin K administration

Vitamin K exists in three forms: vitamin K_1 (phytonadione), which is present in green leafy vegetables, vitamin K_2 (menaquinone), which is synthesized by intestinal bacterial flora, and vitamin K_3 (menadione), a synthetic, water-soluble form. Vitamin K_3 is not used in newborns because it can cause a haemolytic anaemia, with resulting jaundice, if used in high doses (Lucey & Dolan 1959, Committee on Nutrition 1961, Aballi et al 1962). Most countries that have a policy on vitamin K prophylaxis, recommend a single dose of 0.5–1.0 mg intramuscularly or an oral dose of 2–4 at birth (Aballi et al 1962, Dunn 1982, McNinch et al 1983, Hathaway 1986, 1987, Shapiro et al 1986, Tripp & McNinch 1987, Fetus and Newborn Committee, Canadian Pediatric Society 1988, Brown et al 1989, Motohara et al 1989). Newborns' daily requirements for vitamin K are approximately 1–5 μg/kg body weight (Sells et al 1941, Hardwicke 1944, Sann et al 1985a,b). Although oral vitamin K prophylaxis is effective, less expensive and less traumatic than intramuscular vitamin K, it is not clear whether the oral route is as efficacious as the intramuscular route. Although there are several studies that report similar biochemical outcomes for oral and intramuscular vitamin K prophylaxis, the general applicability of these findings is not completely clear (McNinch et al 1985, Sann et al 1985,a,b, O'Connor & Addiago 1986, von Kries et al 1987, Jorgensen et al 1991). The absorption of oral vitamin K varies widely among infants (Shinzawa et al 1989) and, outside of controlled studies, one can anticipate that some infants will not swallow all of a dose. HDN has occurred in some infants who received oral vitamin K prophylaxis. These problems suggest that oral vitamin may not be as efficacious as intramuscular vitamin K, however, the magnitude of the problem is unclear and requires further study.

Prophylactic vitamin K should also be given to pregnant women who are at high risk of delivering vitamin K-deficient infants. For example, women taking oral anticonvulsant therapy require additional vitamin K prophylaxis. One approach is to give these women oral vitamin K in their third trimester of pregnancy. In addition, certain high risk groups of infants (i.e. infants with α_1-antitrypsin deficiency, chronic diarrhoea, cystic fibrosis, coeliac disease) require additional vitamin K prophylaxis.

Treatment of vitamin K deficiency

Infants with haemorrhagic complications that are suspected to be due to vitamin K deficiency should be treated immediately with vitamin K either subcutaneously or intravenously but not intramuscularly. The last may result in haematoma formation at the site of injection. The subcutaneous route is often preferred in adults because the rapid intravenous administration of vitamin K may cause an anaphylactoid reaction. Although this has not been described in newborns, it seems prudent to give intravenous vitamin K slowly to these patients as well. Infants with serious but non-life-threatening bleeding, secondary to vitamin K deficiency, should additionally be treated with plasma. It takes approximately 2 hours for systemically administered vitamin K to increase the plasma concentrations of vitamin K dependent proteins. If an infant has an intracranial haemorrhage or other form of life-threatening bleed, treatment with prothrombin complex concentrates should be considered. These concentrates will immediately increase the plasma concentrations of the vitamin K dependent factors to safe values. These products are not routinely recommended for treatment of bleeding secondary to vitamin K deficiency because there is a high risk of hepatitis and the potential to develop DIC. Infants that are given prothrombin complex concentrates should also receive hepatitis B immunoglobulin and hepatitis B vaccination.

Liver disease

Impaired haemostasis secondary to liver failure is complex and multifactorial. Decreased production of proteins involved in haemostasis occurs because the liver is the main site of synthesis with a few exceptions (vWF, tPA, PAI). Both procoagulant and fibrinolytic systems may be activated in liver failure generating by-products such as fibrin/fibrinogen degradation products, and enzyme-inhibitor complexes. The latter increase in concentration because of poor hepatic clearance. The turnover of haemostatic proteins may be accelerated, in part due to loss of these proteins into ascitic fluid (Roberts & Cederbaum 1972, Joist 1982, Kelly & Summerfield 1987). Abnormal platelet function and presence of abnormally glyscoslyated proteins are also characteristic of liver failure. Common causes of liver failure in newborns include viral hepatitis, hypoxia, fetal hydrops, and damage from long-term total parenteral nutrition (Johnson et al 1976, Odievre et al 1976, Hoskova & Mrskos 1977, Hey & Jones 1979, Laffi et al 1986). The goal of haemostatic management for these infants is to sustain them until the liver recovers normal function or, rarely, a liver transplantation is performed. Because these patients are usually long-term management problems and frequently have prolonged periods in which they do not bleed despite abnormal coagulation tests, replacement therapy is usually reserved for intermittent episodes of bleeding. Replacement of coagulation proteins with plasma products and platelets with platelet concentrates are the mainstay of therapy. In more severe cases, exchange transfusions may be temporarily helpful.

Intracranial haemorrhage

Intracranial haemorrhage (ICH) may occur in either fullterm or premature infants, although the incidence is considerably higher in small premature infants weighing less than 1500 grams. Germinal layer and intraventricular haemorrhage (IVH) are the most frequent sites of ICH in premature infants. The use of computed tomography and bedside ultrasound through the anterior fontanelle revolutionized the diagnosis of ICH, which had, prior to the late 1970s, been diagnosed clinically or at autopsy (White 1979, Bejar et al 1980, Mack et al 1981, Dolfin et al 1983, Pape et al 1983, Perlman et al 1983b, Graziani et al 1985, Sinha et al 1985, Trounce et al 1986).

Although relatively rare, ICH can occur spontaneously in fullterm infants. These infants should be carefully evaluated for congenital or acquired haemostatic defects, however they are rarely present (Cartwright et al 1979, Chaplin et al 1979, Palma et al 1979, Serfontein et al 1980, Guckos-Thoeni et al 1982, Scher et al 1982, Jackson & Blumhagen 1983, Mackay et al 1984, Girolami et al 1985, Gunn et al 1985). Case reports indicate that perinatal asphyxia and birth trauma may result in ICH in fullterm infants. In the only prospective study published, smaller birth weights, younger gestational ages and racial group were identified as risk factors (Hayden et al 1985). ICH are most frequently subependymal in location and require supportive care only. On occasion some infants require surgical intervention and have long-term neurological morbidity.

IVH occurs primarily in premature infants (Burnstein et al 1977, Shinnar et al 1982, Tarby & Volpe 1982, Volpe 1981, 1983, Goddard-Finegold 1984, Ment et al 1987). Initially IVH was a pathologic diagnosis, however, the availability of computerized tomography (White 1979, Volpe 1981) and ultrasound allow accurate diagnosis of IVH in infants (Bejar et al 1980, Mack et al 1981, Dolfin et al 1983, Pape et al 1983, Perlman et al 1983, Graziani et al 1985, Sinha et al 1985, Trounce et al 1986). These tools have been effectively utilized to determine the natural history of IVH and to assess the outcome of specific therapeutic interventions.

The incidence of IVH is decreasing, probably reflecting improved neonatal care. Approximately 40% of infants with a birth weight less than 1500 g develop an IVH. The IVH occurs early, usually within the first 72 hours of age (Tsiantos et al 1974, Hambleton & Wigglesworth 1976, Papile et al 1978, Dolfin et al 1983, Szymonowicz & Yu 1984, Ment et al 1987). The bleeding occurs from the fragile microvasculature of the subependymal germinal matrix, and may, in approximately 10–20% of infants, extend into the lateral ventricles or into the brain parenchyma (Tsiantos et al 1974, Papile et al 1978, Ahmann et al 1980, Shinnar et al 1982, Levene & de Vries 1984). The etiology of IVH in premature infants is incompletely understood and likely multifactorial. It is associated with prenatal asphyxia, assisted ventilation, respiratory distress syndrome, hypercarbia, acidosis, hypoxia, pneumothorax, and prematurity (Simmons & Adcock 1974, Tsiantos et al 1974, Dykes et al 1980, Kosmetatos et al 1980, Clark et al 1981, Cooke 1981, Lipscomb et al 1981, Goddard-Finegold 1984, Szymonowicz & Yu 1984, Perlman et al 1985, Ment et al 1987). Decreased perfusion of brain tissue due to abnormal regulation of cerebral blood flow is probably the mechanism of primary importance to subsequent long-term morbidity (Goddard et al 1980, Lou 1980, Perlman et al 1981, 1983, Greisen et al 1984, Ment et al 1984, Tweed et al 1986, Sonesson et al 1987). In addition, increased fragility of the germinal matrix capillaries, oxidative damage to endothelium, and impairment of haemostasis are other potential contributing mechanisms (Gilles et al 1971, Beverley et al 1984a, 1985, McDonald et al 1984).

There are numerous clinical trials testing a variety of therapeutic interventions directed at decreasing the frequency and severity of IVH. These trials tested a variety of agents that enhance haemostasis, drugs that affect cell membranes and drugs that affect blood flow. Only therapeutic interventions that affect haemostasis are discussed here. The association of pathological alterations of haemostasis with IVH has formed the rationale for intervention studies with plasma, drugs that enhance haemostasis in a variety of ways and platelet concentrates (Gray et al 1968, Waltt et al 1973, Turner et al 1981, Gross et al 1982, Beverley et al 1984a, 1985, Andrew et al 1987b, 1991b,c, Lupton et al 1988). Early intervention studies with plasma products used, by necessity, clinical or pathological documentation of IVH as outcome measures and are not considered further. The studies conducted after objective measurements of ICH were available are summarized in Table 44.6.

In a randomized controlled trial performed in 1985, treated infants received 10 ml per kg of FFP on admission to the nursery and at 24 hours of age (Beverley et al 1985). The control group was treated with usual management only. Five of 36 treated infants developed ICH compared to 15 of 37 control infants, a significant difference. Another group administered factor XIII concentrates to premature infants and reported a significant reduction in ICH (Shirahata et al 1990). However the analysis was performed on a small subset of infants entered into the study. Another strategy used to enhance haemostasis in premature infants was to administer vitamin K antenatally to mothers to ensure that infants were not vitamin K deficient (Pomerance et al 1987, Morales et al 1988, Kazzi et al 1989). Three clinical studies have been reported in the literature, two reported a benefit and one did not. Infants whose mothers received vitamin K were born with increased plasma concentrations of vitamin K-dependent factors in the positive studies.

Some investigators have suggested that IVH may be due to enhanced local fibrinolytic activity (Gilles et al 1971). To test this hypothesis, infants were treated with an inhibitor of fibrinolysis, tranexamic acid (Hensey et al 1984). However no benefit could be shown. The association of IVH and thrombocytopenia formed the rationale for an intervention study with platelet transfusions (Andrew et al 1991b,c). Thrombocytopenic infants were randomized to receive platelet concentrates in the first 72 hours of life to maintain a platelet count in the normal range, that is greater than 150 000. The control group was treated

Table 44.6 Prevention studies in intracerebral haemorrhage (ICH)

Study	Number	Weight (kg)	Dose mg/kg	Dose Route	Duration Frequency (hourly)	Duration Period (days)	Effect on ICH
I. Indomethacin							
Ment et al 1985	48	0.600–1.250	0.5–0.6	IV	12	5	Decreased
Rennie et al 1986	50	≤1.750	0.2	IV	24	3	No change
Hanigan et al 1988	33	0.550–0.999	0.4	IV	12	4	No change
	78	1.000–1.500	0.4	IV	24	3	Decreased
Ment et al 1988a	36	0.600–1.250	0.1	IV	24	3	Decreased
Bandstra et al 1988	199	≤1.300	0.2	IV	12	1	Decreased
Bada et al 1989	141	≤1.500	0.2	IV	6 (Single dose)		Decreased
			0.1	IV	18 h & 30 h		
II. Ethamsylate							
Morgan et al 1981	70	<1.500	12.5	IM	6	4	Decreased
Benson et al 1986	330	<1.500	12.5	IM/IV	6	4	Decreased
III. Vitamin K							
Pomerance et al 1987	53	<1.500	10	IM	4	1	Decreased
Morales et al 1988	100	<1.500	10	IM	Every 5 days		Decreased
Kazzi et al 1989	98	0.370–2.550	10	IM	4 days	12	No change
IV. Other treatments							
Hensey et al 1984 (tranexamic acid)	100	<1.250	25	IV	6	5	No change
Beverley et al 1985 (fresh frozen plasma)	73	<1.500	10 ml	IV	24	2	Decreased
Shirahata et al 1990 (factor XIII)	21	not clear	70–100 μ	IV		1	Decreased
Andrew et al 1991b (plateles)		0.500–1.500	10 ml/kg	IV		1–3	No change

IV, intravenous IM, intramuscular.

in the usual fashion. This study did not show a significant effect on the extent of IVH and the study was constructed to detect a 25% effect or greater.

Ethamsylate is a drug used for decades in some countries to reduce capillary bleeding during selected surgical interventions (ear, nose and throat surgery). Ethamsylate enhances platelet adhesiveness and capillary resistance by inhibiting individual enzymes in the prostaglandin pathways. Two randomized controlled trials and one controlled trial reported a reduction in IVH with ethamsylate (Morgan et al 1981, Cooke & Morgan 1984, Benson et al 1986).

Cerebral blood flow is regulated in part by prostaglandins such as prostacylin (PGI_2), and thromboxane A_2 (TXA_2). PGI_2 is a potent vasodilator that also inhibits platelet aggregation, and TXA_2 is a potent vasoconstrictor that promotes platelet aggregation. In the Beagle puppy model, indomethacin, a drug which blocks the enzyme cyclooxygenase, significantly decreased the incidence of IVH. Indomethacin reduced plasma concentrations of 6-keto-$PGF_1\alpha$ and TXB_2, the stable metabolites of PGI_2 and TXA_2 (Ment et al 1983). Four randomized controlled trials have been conducted with indomethacin, three of which described a beneficial effect (Ment et al 1985, 1988, Hanigan et al 1988) and one which did not detect a change (Rennie et al 1986).

There are several confounding variables that may have contributed to differing results in the trials discussed. Of particular importance is the apparently declining incidence of IVH during the 1980s probably reflecting improved perinatal management of newborns. Ongoing clinical studies are necessary to test potentially beneficial therapeutic agents. At this time no firm recommendations can be made for any of the intervention modalities discussed because of a lack of consistent results (Ment et al 1988).

Respiratory distress syndrome

Respiratory distress syndrome (RDS) is an acute lung disorder characterized by diffuse atelectasis, high permeability oedema, hyaline membrane formation and right to left shunting of pulmonary blood flow (Strang 1966). RDS is primarily due to increased pulmonary surface tension due to surfactant deficiency (Avery & Mead 1959). A prominent pathologic feature of RDS is fibrin deposition intra-alveolarly and intravascularly (Gajl-Paczalska 1964). This characteristic has prompted studies of haemostasis in infants with RDS (Liebermann 1961, Ambrus et al 1966, Stark et al 1968, El-Bardeesy & Johnson 1971, Markarian et al 1971, Mahasandana & Hathaway 1973, Watkins et al 1980, Andrew et al 1983b, 1985, Peters et al 1984, Arnold et al 1985, van den Berg et al 1989). RDS is often characterized by prolonged screening tests, low levels of coagulation factors and inhibitors of coagulation (Markarian et al 1971, Mahasandana & Hathaway 1973, Peters et al 1984, Andrew et al 1985, van den Berg et al 1989). A recent prospective cohort study has carefully documented a strong association between the severity of RDS and the generation of thrombin as reflected by plasma concentrations of thrombin-antithrombin III complexes (Schmidt et al 1991). In addition to these descriptive studies, there are four intervention studies testing the effects of antithrombotic or thrombolytic therapy in RDS (Ambrus et al 1966, Markarian et al 1971, 1977, Gobel et al 1980). In two studies, the potential benefits of heparin therapy were tested but did not improve outcome. The lack of benefit with heparin may be because heparin's antithrombotic effectiveness is mediated by endogenous antithrombin III, which is decreased in infants with RDS. Another study tested the potential benefits from increasing the plasma concentration of antithrombin III by using antithrombin III concentrates (Muntean & Rosseger 1989). In this trial, 45 infants were randomized to receive ATIII concentrates and heparin, and 53 infants were randomized to receive standard care. There was no beneficial effect from the intervention for frequency and duration of ventilation, nor for frequency of IVH. Two trials conducted in 1966 and 1977 reported a significant benefit from the infusion of plasminogen (Ambrus et al 1966, 1977). The study conducted in 1977 was a double-blind, randomized study of 500 premature infants who were treated with either plasminogen or placebo intravenously within 60 minutes of birth (Ambrus et al 1977). The authors reported a highly significant decrease in severe respiratory distress and death caused by hyaline membrane disease. These results were impressive at the time they were published, however, the relevance of these forms of therapy to infants managed in modern neonatal units is unknown. Future clinical trials are needed to assess the potential benefits of anticoagulant and antithrombotic agents in RDS.

Extracorporeal membrane oxygenation

Extracorporeal membrane oxygenation (ECMO) consists of a semi-permeable membrane that permits the transfer of oxygen to infants with life-threatening respiratory insufficiency. ECMO is used in the treatment of meconium aspiration syndrome, severe RDS, congenital diaphragmatic hernia, persistent pulmonary hypertension and other disorders characterized by severe respiratory failure. Several hundred infants have been treated with ECMO with an overall survival rate of approximately 60% (White et al 1971, Heiden et al 1975, Andrews et al 1983, 1984, Bartlett et al 1985, 1986, Short & Pearson 1986, Trento et al 1986). The long-term follow-up studies are encouraging with a majority of infants developmentally normal (Krummel et al 1984, Townes et al 1985). Unfortunately ECMO was introduced without rigorous critical evaluation resulting in considerable controversy over its use. Only two controlled trials assessing its efficacy have been published (Bartlett et al 1985, O'Rourke et al 1989, Chalmers 1990). One used a 'play the winner' study design which showed a statistical benefit from ECMO over conventional therapy (Bartlett et al 1985). However only one infant was treated conventionally and 11 with ECMO. The second trial was a conventional randomized controlled trial. However the study was halted after nine infants treated with ECMO survived compared to six of ten in the conventional medical group.

Unfortunately, intracranial haemorrhage (ICH) occurs in some infants treated with ECMO and is a leading cause of death (Bartlett et al 1985, Short & Pearson 1986). The etiology of ICH is multifactorial. The use of heparin, the presence of thrombocytopenia, and vascular alterations all contribute to ICH. There is no single predictor of ICH, although infants with thrombocytopenia and low birth-weight infants appear to be at higher risk. For this reason the platelet count is usually maintained over $100 \times 10^9/l$ and small premature infants are not eligible for ECMO.

Heparin is used in ECMO to prevent clot formation in the membrane system and microthrombi in the infants. Heparin is used in full systemic doses with a bolus of 100 to 150 units/kg followed by a continuous infusion of heparin at 20–70 units/kg/hour. Heparinization is monitored at the bedside by an activated clotting time (ACT) at two to three times baseline values (240–280 seconds) (Hattersley 1966). These guidelines are extrapolated from adults without determining whether this degree of anticoagulation is necessary. The role of potentially safer anticoagulant drugs such as the low molecular weight heparins, dermatan sulphate, or hirudin and its anologues remains to be determined. Minor haemostatic morbidity can often be treated locally.

Miscellaneous acquired disorders

There are other disorders such as hyperviscosity, and small for gestational age that are also linked to impaired haemostasis (Perlman & Dvilansky 1975, Rivers 1975, Katz et al 1982, Sibai et al 1984, Fuse 1986).

ACQUIRED PROTHROMBOTIC STATES

Catheter-related complications

Secondary thromboembolic complications occur in infants with serious underlying problems (Barnard et al 1979, Schmidt & Zipursky 1984, Schmidt & Andrew 1988). The risk factors for these events include abnormalities in vessel walls, poor perfusion and acquired coagulation abnormalities. Recent studies show that thrombin generation is relatively preserved in sick newborns but the ability to inhibit thrombin is impaired (Shah et al 1991). Other studies report that there is evidence of ongoing thrombin generation in premature infants with RDS (Schmidt et al 1991) and an acquired protein C deficiency (Manco-Johnson et al 1991) that may contribute to these secondary thrombotic complications. In these same infants, blood flow may be impaired due to increased blood viscosity secondary to the high haematocrit, dehydration and poor deformability of physiologically large red cells (Aarts et al 1983).

Indwelling arterial catheters, frequently umbilical in location, are necessary for the management of sick premature infants. Unfortunately, these catheters are the leading causes of large vessel thrombi in newborns, regardless of the type of catheter used or its location (Barnard et al 1979, Turrito & Weiss 1980, O'Neill et al 1981, Schmidt & Zipursky 1984, Jackson et al 1987, Schmidt & Andrew 1988). The most frequent vessel involved is the aorta, however thrombotic complications have been described in all vessels accessed. Catheters promote thrombus formation by providing a foreign surface, damaging the vessel wall (Chidi et al 1983), and delivering substances that may cause local damage to the vessel (Cohen et al 1977, Clawson & Boros 1978, Tooley & Myerberg 1978, Wesstrom et al 1979).

Based on a retrospective study of the period between 1971 and 1980 and involving approximately 4000 infants with an umbilical artery catheter in place symptomatic obstruction occurred in 1% of infants (O'Neill et al 1981). Asymptomatic catheter thromboses occur more frequently based on postmortem examination (3–59%), and prospective angiographic studies (10–90%) (Neal et al 1972, Goetzman et al 1975, Olinsky et al 1975, Mokrohisky et al 1978).

Catheter-related thrombotic complications can cause immediate and/or long-term problems. Symptomatic, acute thrombi cause severe organ or limb impairment, or death (Wigger et al 1970, Marsh et al 1975). The long-term morbidity may manifest as hypertension, abnormal renal function, and/or discrepancies in leg measurements. Follow-up studies of asymptomatic catheter-related thrombotic complications are needed to delineate fully the magnitude of the problem. The presence or absence of significant long-term morbidity from catheter-related thrombi will dictate the approach to initial management.

Placement of arterial catheters is one of the very few instances where heparin prophylaxis is used in childhood. Both the need to maintain catheter patency and to prevent symptomatic thrombi provide the rationale for heparin prophylaxis. A survey of American nurseries reported that 75% of nurseries used heparin prophylaxis (Gilhooly et al 1987). Four controlled trials all report that heparin prophylaxis prolonged catheter patency (Rajani et al 1979, David et al 1981, Alpan et al 1984, Bosque & Weaver 1986). However none of these trials adequately assessed catheter-related thrombosis or the risk of bleeding, particularly ICH. A retrospective case control study reported a four-fold increase in the risk of ICH when heparin was used for catheter prophylaxis (Lesko et al 1986). Although the design of this study was weak, future studies must address the issue of increased bleeding secondary to heparin prophylaxis in newborns.

Indwelling venous catheters, frequently in the umbilical vein, also cause large vessel thrombotic complications (Symansky & Fox 1972). Autopsy studies report an incidence of catheter-related thrombi in 20–65% of cases. Correct placement of venous catheters is critical to prevent portal vein thrombosis and hepatic necrosis. Hyperosmolar solutions may cause hepatic necrosis if injected directly into the portal or hepatic system (Scott, 1965; Enger et al 1976). There are no comprehensive long-term studies of infants who had umbilical venous catheters. However there are case reports of long-term sequelae which include portal hypertension (Tizard 1962, Oski et al 1963, Obladen et al 1975), splenomegaly (Tizard 1962, Vos et al 1974) gastric and oesophageal varices (Vos et al 1974), and hypertension (Evans et al 1981).

Spontaneous thrombosis

Although very rare, spontaneous thrombosis of arterial vessels does occur in some very sick infants. The clinical presentation depends on the site and degree of occlusion. In the most severe cases, gangrene and loss of the affected limb or ischaemic organ damage may occur (Barnard & Hathaway 1979, Schmidt & Zipursky 1984, Schmidt & Andrew 1988). Systemic hypertension secondary to renal artery thrombosis is an example of a long-term complication. Spontaneous thrombosis in the venous system may also occur in sick infants. The most frequent site affected is the renal vein (Kaufmann 1958, Lowry et al 1970, Arneil et al 1973, Editorial 1974, Duncan et al 1977, Rasoulpour & McLean 1980, Rosenberg et al 1980, Gonzalez et al 1982, Jobin et al 1982). Indeed the majority of renal vein thrombi in childhood occur in children less than one year of age (Arneil et al 1973, Kaufmann 1958, Gonzalez et al 1982). Both the physiologically decreased renal flow and small diameter of the renal vessels contribute to the high risk of renal thrombosis in this age group (Editorial 1974). Classically, infants with renal vein thrombosis present with haematuria, an enlarged kidney, and thrombocytopenia. Oedema and cyanosis of the legs may occur when the inferior vena cava is also involved. Supportive care, including dialysis if necessary, is the cornerstone of management. Anticoagulant and thrombolytic therapy are used by some investigators. However the benefit from the latter remains to be demonstrated (Arneil et al 1973, Duncan et al 1977, Rasoulpour & McLean 1980, Gonzalez et al 1982, Jobin et al 1982). Some infants with bilateral renal vein thrombosis have benefited from thromboectomy (Lowry et al 1970, Duncan et al 1977, Gonzalez et al 1982). Other sites that may be thrombosed include the vena cava (Arneil et al 1973, Gonzalez et al 1982), adrenal vein (de Sa & Nicholls 1972), portal vein, and hepatic vein (Thompson & Sherlock 1964). The last are most frequently secondary to omphalitis.

Pulmonary embolism from a distant venous site is a diagnosis rarely made in newborns. The clinical symptoms are easily confused with RDS and until recently only a perfusion scan could be performed in newborns. Recently ventilation scans using a submicronic radiolabelled aerosol have been developed and used in newborns (O'Brodovich & Coates 1984, Arnold et al 1985). The ability to perform both a perfusion and ventilation scan should increase the number of pulmonary emboli diagnosed antemortem.

Diagnosis of prothrombotic disorders

Validation of diagnostic techniques in newborns with thrombotic complications is more difficult than in children or adults because of the rarity of the problems and the multiple sites that may be affected. Recent guidelines published by the neonatal subcommittee to the International Congress of Thrombosis and Haemostasis recommend that contrast angiography be considered the gold standard reference test in the absence of studies that validate non-invasive approaches (Schmidt & Andrew 1991). Non-invasive tests such as doppler/ultrasound offer important advantages for the diagnosis of large vessel thrombosis in newborns. However, clinical trials to determine their sensitivity and specificity compared to contrast angiography have not been published to date. The importance of validating these non-invasive approaches was illustrated by a review of 20 newborns with aortic thrombosis in which ultrasound failed to identify thrombi in four patients, three of whom had complete obstruction (Vailas et al 1986). The observer agreement and reproducibility have not been determined for these highly subjective operator-dependent tests (Seibert et al 1987).

The diagnosis of renal vein thrombosis poses a special problem because there is no commonly agreed reference test to which newer diagnostic tests can be compared (Rasoulpour & McLean 1980, Rosenberg et al 1980, Schmidt & Andrew 1988). Selective renal venography is technically difficult and potentially hazardous in small infants. The techniques commonly used to diagnose renal vein thrombosis are contrast venography, renal scintigraphy, excretory urography, ultrasonography with or without doppler, computed tomography and magnetic resonance imaging.

Prophylaxis/treatment of thrombotic disorders

Prophylactic therapy for thrombotic complications in newborns includes supportive care and in some cases heparin. Arterial catheter-related thrombi are the only example where heparin prophylaxis is commonly used. As discussed previously, a majority of American nurseries use heparin prophylaxis based on four controlled trials that all demonstrated benefit from this approach but did not adequately determine safety (Rajani et al 1979, David et al 1981, Alpan et al 1984, Bosque & Weaver 1986, Lesko et al 1986, Gilhooly et al 1987). Further studies are needed to clarify the risks and benefits of heparin prophylaxis for catheters.

Therapeutic options for newborns with large vessel thrombotic complications include supportive care alone, anticoagulant therapy, thrombolytic therapy and surgical thrombectomy (Schmidt & Andrew 1991). The low incidence and complex presentation of thrombotic complications in newborns has, to date, prevented clinical trials with strong designs from being conducted. This lack of controlled trials has prevented a consensus for the management of thromboembolic complications in newborns. In most nurseries, catheters are not routinely screened for associated thrombi, so by exclusion most infants with clinically silent thrombi receive supportive care alone (Barnard & Hathaway 1979, Schmidt & Zipursky 1984, Schmidt & Andrew 1988).

The decision to treat a clinically apparent thrombotic complication with active intervention therapy can be difficult. Recent guidelines published by the neonatal subcommittee to the International Congress on Thrombosis and Haemostasis suggest that anticoagulant and/or thrombolytic therapy may be helpful when significant limb or organ impairment is present (Schmidt & Andrew 1991). The doses and duration of therapy are summarized in Table 44.7. These guidelines are completely extrapolated from protocols validated in adults and used in case reports in newborns. The validation of these protocols has been hindered in newborns by the rarity of symptomatic thrombotic complications and the pressing need to treat when a catastrophic thrombotic complication occurs.

Table 44.7 Treatment of neonatal thrombosis

General
Maintain platelet count above 50 × 10^9/l
Maintain fibrinogen concentration above 1 g/l
Supportive care
Suitable for clinically 'silent' thrombosis
Anticoagulants
Heparin is the drug of choice
Loading dose of 50 unit/kg by bolus followed by 20 units/kg/hr
No valid therapeutic range established
Closely monitor clinical response and by serial non-invasive techniques
Use laboratory monitoring to avoid excessive heparinization
No evidence that further treatment with oral anticoagulants are needed for most infants
Thrombolytic therapy
Consider in life or limb- or organ-threatening circumstances urokinase as 4400 units/kg over 20 min followed by 4400 units/kg/hr for no more than 48 h
Monitor fibrinogen and/or fibrinogen/fibrin degradation products to confirm a laboratory response
Follow thrombolytic therapy with heparin

From Schmidt & Andrews 1991.

In vitro studies and newborn animal models have provided valuable preclinical sources of information which clarify the responses to be anticipated from anticoagulant and thrombolytic drugs in newborns. For example, in newborn plasma, test such as the APTT, PT, and thrombin generation assays display an apparent 'sensitivity' to heparin compared to adults (Barnard & Hathaway 1979, Schmidt et al 1989b, Vieira et al 1989). In contrast, newborn plasma is relatively 'resistant' to the effects of heparin in assays where exogenous factor Xa or thrombin are added to plasma (Schmidt et al 1988, 1989). The apparent 'sensitivity' and 'resistance' of newborn plasma to heparin reflects the ratio of antithrombin III to enzyme in the assay system. Which of these in vitro anticoagulant tests most closely reflects the in vivo antithrombotic effect of heparin is unknown and can only be established in clinical trials. If therapeutic ranges for heparin therapy are simply extrapolated from adult literature to newborns, the APTT will systematically overestimate the amount of heparin present and heparin assays will systematically underestimate the amount of heparin present (Schmidt et al 1988, 1989). In the absence of clinical trials, assessing the response to heparin therapy consists of monitoring the clinical course in combination with non-invasive monitoring such as duplex ultrasound. Measurement of the APTT and/or heparin level may be helpful to ensure that the amount of heparin present is not excessive (McDonald & Hathaway 1982, Levine & Hirsch 1986, Andrew et al 1988). When heparin levels are used, it is important to determine whether a thrombin-based or Xa-based assay is being used by the laboratory because the therapeutic ranges for the two assays differ (van den Besselaar et al 1990). In the absence of clinical trials, animal models provide the only in vivo assessment of heparin's effect in an immature haemostatic system. The coagulation system of newborn piglets is similar to human infants (Massicotte-Nolan et al 1986). Both the pharmacokinetics and activity of heparin as an antithrombotic agent have been tested in this model (Andrew et al 1988c, 1989b, Schmidt et al 1988a). Heparin is cleared more quickly in newborn pigs compared to adults due, primarily, to an increased volume of distribution (Andrew et al 1988c). In addition, heparin was less effective in preventing a jugular vein thrombus in newborns compared to adults (Schmidt et al 1988a). The heparin resistance in newborn pigs could be overcome by either increasing the plasma concentration of ATIII, or by increasing the amounts of heparin given.

New anticoagulants have been developed and are being tested in adults with large vessel thrombi. These drugs all inhibit thrombin, however some, heparin, low molecular weight heparins (LMWH), and dermatan sulphate (DS), potentiate the antithrombin effect of endogenous inhibitors, whereas others directly inhibit thrombin (hirudin, and its derivatives). Some of these anticoagulants may offer therapeutic advantages over standard heparin (Thomas 1984). These anticoagulants may have a role in adult patients when the use of standard heparin is problematic. These patients require antithrombotic protection but are particularly vulnerable to bleeding complications. Sick newborns can be considered vulnerable because of the immaturity of their coagulation system, frequency of thrombocytopenia, and risk of IVH.

Only LMWHs have been assessed in newborn systems. LMWHs are prepared from standard heparin and are equally efficacious as antithrombotic agents compared to standard heparin (Thomas 1984). Low molecular weight heparins are particularly helpful in adults when patients require antithrombotic protection but are also particularly at risk for bleeding complications. LMWHs are currently being evaluated in animal models and in vitro. LMWHs are cleared more quickly from newborn piglets than from adult pig (Andrew et al 1989b). However, just as in adults, the clearance of LMWHs is significantly slower than for standard heparin in newborn piglets. In vitro, the recovery of anti-factor Xa activity is also limited by the ATIII concentration in newborn plasma for LMWHs (Vieira et al 1989).

Although relatively rare, newborns may develop thrombotic complications that impair organ function or threaten limb viability. Unfortunately, there are only case reports of treatment with thrombolytic therapy in newborns. In vitro studies show that the rate of plasmin generation in newborn plasma in response to thrombolytic therapy is slower than for adults (Corrigan et al 1989). Furthermore, thrombolysis of fibrin clots in vitro is impaired in newborns compared to adults in response to streptokinase, urokinase, and tissue plasminogen activator (tPA) (Andrew et al 1991). The decreased fibrinolytic response was improved when the plasma concentration of plasminogen was increased to adult values. Of the three agents, tPA was the most effective in vitro. Whether these in vitro findings are also true in vivo remains to be shown. The clinical reports of the newborn's response to thrombolytic therapy have been variable (Corrigan 1988), and a variety of protocols have been used. Guidelines for the use of thrombolytic agents in newborns have recently been published by the neonatal subcommittee of the International Congress of Thrombosis and Haemostasis (Table 44.7) (Schmidt & Andrew 1991). If an infant does not respond to a particular thrombolytic agent, increasing the plasma concentration of plasminogen may be helpful. Surgical removal of a clot in a major vessel in infants may be curative, however, it is technically difficult and poses a considerable life-threatening risk to these infants who often are premature with many other problems (Braly 1965, Fee et al 1977, Flanigan et al 1982). Therefore thrombolytic therapy for these infants is usually preferred.

PHYSIOLOGY OF NEONATAL PLATELETS

Platelet number and size

Platelet counts in fullterm newborns are not different from adult values. Although the average count in premature infants is slightly lower it is still within the normal range of 150–450 $\times$ 10^9/l (Beverly et al 1984b). Values obtained for fetuses between 18 and 30 weeks of gestation also fall within this range with a mean of 250 $\times$ 10^9/l and do not change during this period (Forestier et al 1986b). The mean platelet volume is similar in both fullterm and premature infants compared to adults, averaging 7–9 fl (Kipper & Sieger 1982, Arad et al 1986).

Platelet function

Most studies of platelet function in newborns were performed on cord platelets not platelets from newborns following delivery. Because cord platelets and platelets from newborns may have differences in function they are designated separately in this review. There are some well characterized differences in cord platelet function compared to adult platelets as studied by standard in vitro methods. Although studies agree that functional differences occur, the details are contentious. This probably reflects differences in methodology, the use of cord blood versus venous blood from infants, and the timing and methods of collection (Ahlsten et al 1983, Gader et al 1988, Saving et al 1991). Under normal circumstances platelets circulate as disc-shaped structures that are not adherent to vessel walls or to other cells. Following vascular injury platelets adhere to damaged endothelium and change shape by extending pseudopods. Adhesion initiates the secretion of platelet granule contents that include ADP and adhesive proteins such as von Willebrand factor (vWF) and fibrinogen. These substances promote both adhesion and formation of aggregates. Platelets also participate in coagulation by providing a lipoprotein surface on which the soluble coagulation factor complexes can form, with the ultimate generation of thrombin and formation of fibrin. Thrombin itself is a potent stimulus of platelet aggregation. Platelet fibrin clots seal the sites of injury and following injury retract to reopen vessels.

Bleeding time

Bleeding times provide an important screen for the interaction between platelets and blood vessel walls. Devices available to perform bleeding times in adults and older children are not satisfactory for newborns. Devices modified for neonates make reproducible small incisions, making this test widely applicable to this age group. Studies with these devices report shorter bleeding times for infants compared to normal ranges for adults. This enhanced platelet/vessel wall interaction likely reflects higher plasma concentrations of vWF (Andrew et al 1987a, 1988, Katz et al 1989, Weinstein et al 1989) enhanced vWF function (Katz et al 1989, Weinstein et al 1989) and/or high haemocrits in newborns (Gerrard et al 1989).

Platelet adhesion

When endothelial cells lining vessel walls are injured, platelets adhere to subendothelium. This process involves a specific receptor on platelet surfaces, glycoprotein Ib (GPIb) and an adhesive protein, vWF. vWF is secreted by endothelial cells and platelets, and is present in both subendothelium and plasma. GPIb is present on membranes of fetal platelets in normal adult amounts (Gruel et al 1986). vWF is present in neonatal plasma in increased concentration (Andrew et al 1987a, 1988). Ristocetin-induced platelet agglutination, which reflects functional vWF as well as plasma concentrations of vWF, is enhanced in cord platelets (Ts'ao et al 1976). Neonatal plasma will promote platelet agglutination at lower concentrations of ristocetin (Fig. 44.6) which can be explained by a relative increase in the most functional high molecular weight multimers of vWF in fetal and neonatal plasma (Katz et al 1989, Weinstein et al 1989). In vitro measurements of platelet adhesion have not shown consistent abnormalities (Hrodek 1966).

Platelet aggregation

Platelet–platelet interaction, mediated by fibrinogen, requires activation of platelets to expose binding sites for fibrinogen on GPIIb/IIIa. These glycoproteins are present on fetal platelet membranes (Gruel et al 1986). Results of in vitro aggregation studies of cord platelets with a variety of agonists including ADP, epinephrine, collagen, thrombin and arachidonic acid have all demonstrated differences from adult platelets (Fig. 44.7). The aggregation response to epinephrine is markedly impaired due to decreased numbers of alpha-adrenergic receptors on cord platelets (Corby & O'Barr 1981, Stuart et al 1984). It is unclear whether this is due to delayed maturation of these receptors or to their occupation by the elevated levels of catecholamines that occur during birth.

Responses to other agonists in vitro have been variable. As normal aggregation responses are dependent on secretion of platelet granule contents, cord platelets have been examined for the presence of secretory granules and defects in release mechanisms. Electron microscopy studies have demonstrated normal numbers of granules (Ts'ao et al 1976, Saving et al 1991) but serotonin and ADP, which are stored in dense granules, are present at concentrations that are less than 50% adult levels (Flachaire et al 1990). Cord platelets can, however, bind and concentrate exogenous ADP and serotonin in their granules normally (Whaun 1973, 1980). Release of granule contents is decreased in cord platelets particularly in response to collagen (Whaun 1973, Israels et al 1990). Studies of activation pathways leading to release have not identified specific abnormalities. Inositol phosphate production and protein phosphorylation are normal (Israels et al 1990), as well as

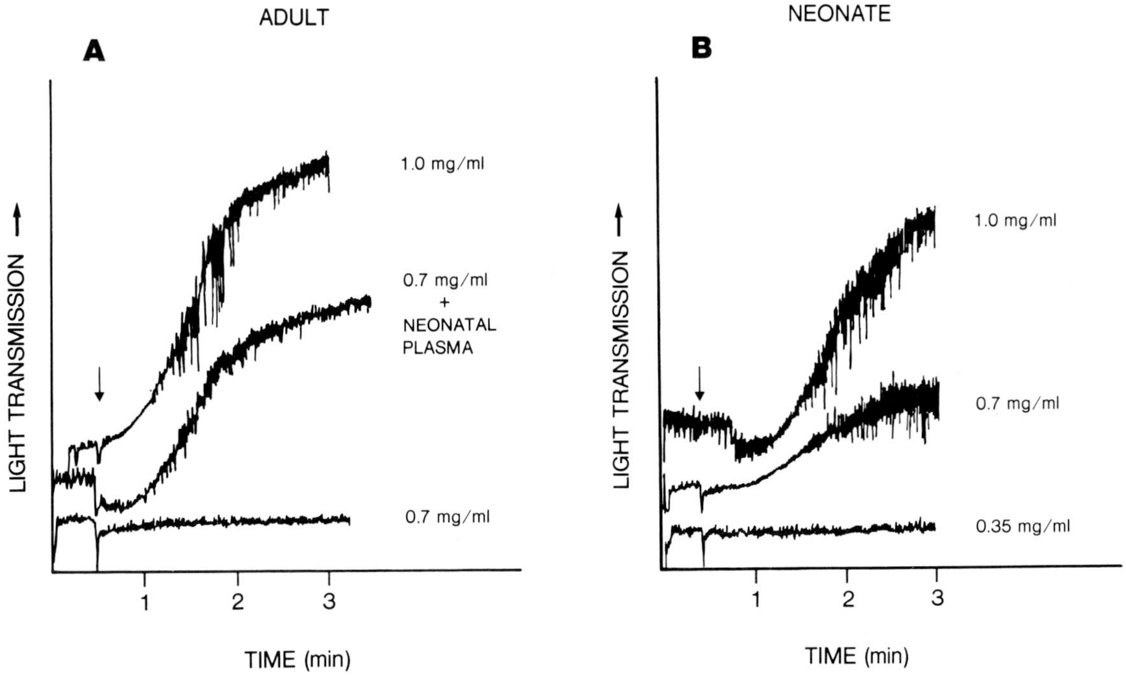

Fig. 44.6 Ristocetin-induced platelet aggregation. Newborn plasma cause increased platelet agglutination.

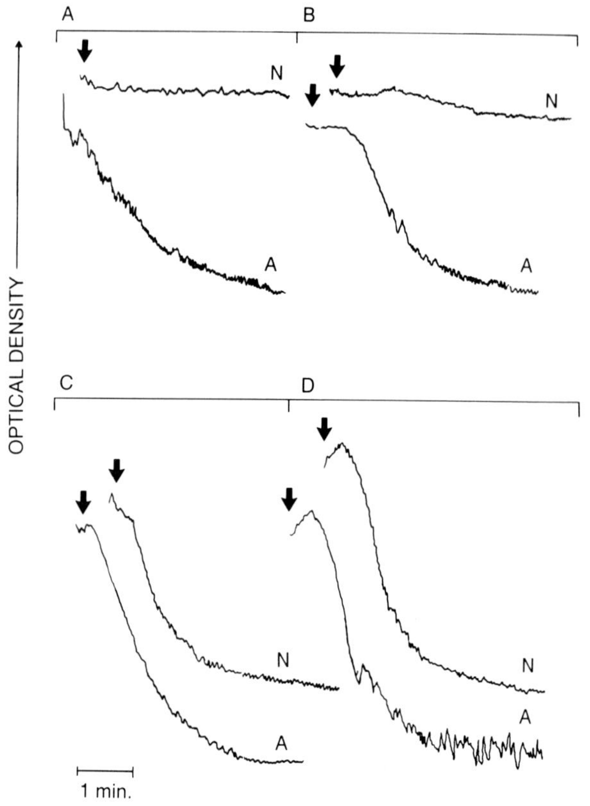

Fig. 44.7 Platelet aggregation studies with cord platelets (N) and adult platelets (A) in response to A, adrenaline; B, collagen; C, arachidonic acid and D, thrombin.

production of arachidonic acid and its metabolites (Stuart et al 1984). In fact, cord platelets release more arachidonic acid than adult platelets in response to stimulation by thrombin. This may be due to platelet membranes made more reactive by low levels of vitamin E (Stuart & Oski 1979, Stuart & Dusse 1985). Agonist receptors, with the exception of the alpha-adrenergic receptor, do not appear to be decreased in number. Despite a poor response to collagen stimulation, cord platelets have normal amounts of the collagen receptor GPIa/IIa present on platelet membranes (Israels et al 1990). Coupling of agonist receptors to phospholipases may be the site of the transient activation defect (Corby & Barr 1981b).

Although earlier studies suggested abnormalities in clot contraction (Mull & Hathaway 1970), recent quantitative studies have shown no difference between adult and cord platelets (Israels et al 1987b). The latter suggest normal functioning of both fibrinogen receptors and contractile cytoskeleton.

Platelet activation during delivery

Evidence that delivery induces platelet activation is supported by increased cord plasma levels of thromboxane B_2, β-thromboglobulin and platelet factor 4 (Suarez et al 1988). Consistent with these observations, Saving et al (1991) noted decreased numbers of granules in platelets from cord blood. However, Suarez et al (1988) did not observe differences in platelet ultrastructure. Thus transient platelet dysfunction at birth for some infants, may be due to refractoriness post-activation. Mechanisms of activation are likely multi-factorial and include thermal changes, hypoxia, acidosis, adrenergic stimulation and thrombogenic effects of amniotic fluid (Stuart et al 1987).

ABNORMALITIES OF NEONATAL PLATELET FUNCTION

Congenital abnormalities

Inherited disorders of platelet function are discussed elsewhere. Two rare but severe hereditary disorders, Bernard–Soulier syndrome and Glanzmann's thrombasthenia, can cause bleeding from birth. Bernard–Soulier syndrome is characterized by thrombocytopenia, large platelets and deficient ristocetin-induced platelet agglutination. The platelets are deficient in several membrane glycoproteins including Ib, IX and V. The bleeding abnormality results from defective vWF binding by platelets in the absence of GPIb. Glanzmann's thrombasthenia is characterized by severe clinical bleeding, absent platelet aggregation in response to ADP and other physiological agonists, and poor clot contraction. Thrombasthenic platelets are deficient in the GPIIa/IIIb complex which forms the receptor for adhesive proteins such as fibrinogen, vWF and fibronectin on activated platelets. Diagnosis of these disorders is not often made in the newborn period unless a family history suggests investigation.

Acquired abnormalities

Acquired abnormalities of platelet function from drug effects or pathological states are more common causes of platelet dysfunction. Despite transient abnormalities identified in tests of cord platelet function, healthy newborns rarely bleed. Addition of secondary factors such as drugs taken by either mother or infant, maternal diabetes, nutritional deficits, hyperbilirubinaemia and phototherapy, amniotic fluid aspiration and renal failure may contribute to clinical bleeding.

Prenatal drug administration can lead to impaired platelet function in newborns, however, the clinical significance of this is uncertain (Whaun et al 1980). For example, salicylates cross the placenta and affect platelet function and thromboxane production in the fetus (Corby & Shulman 1971, Levy & Garrettson 1974, Ylikorkala et al 1986). Maternal aspirin ingestion has been linked to clinical bleeding in neonates in some case reports (Haslam et al 1974, Stuart et al 1982) but low dose aspirin has been used to treat pregnancy-induced hypertension without adverse effects to newborns (Benigni et al 1989, McFarland et al 1990). Infants do not appear to be at greater risk than adults from the effects of aspirin (Ts'ao 1977, Stuart & Dusse 1985). Indomethacin which is used in premature infants to promote closure of patent ductus arteriosus, also interferes with platelet thromboxane production and platelet aggregation and prolongs the bleeding time (Setzer et al 1982, Corrazza et al 1984). As discussed earlier, there is controversy about the role of indomethacin in intraventricular haemorrhage (Ment et al 1988a). Maternal smoking and ethanol ingestion can also affect thromboxane production in neonatal platelets and prostacyclin production in umbilical arteries (Ahlsten et al 1985, 1986, Ylikorkala et al 1987).

The reactivity and prostaglandin production of platelets of diabetics is increased in response to aggregating agents (Colwell et al 1983). Increased prostaglandin production is associated with increased thromboxane production in infants of diabetic mothers and may lead to platelet hyperfunction (Stuart et al 1979, Kaapa et al 1986). In addition, decreased prostacyclin synthesis (Stuart et al 1981) may contribute to the occurrence of thrombosis in these infants (Cowett & Schwartz 1982).

Nutritional alterations in mothers and infants may also affect platelet function. For example, changes in maternal intake of saturated and unsaturated fat can alter thromboxane synthesis in mothers and breast-fed infants (Kaapa et al 1986) Infants with essential fatty acid deficiency can develop decreased thromboxane production and platelet dysfunction (Friedman et al 1977). The lipid composition of platelets can be transiently altered during infusion of lipid emulsions used for parenteral nutrition. A decrease in cholesterol content and an increase in triglyceride and phospholipid content were found during and shortly after infusions of lipid (Aviram & Deckelbaum 1989). The significance of these changes in terms of platelet function is questionable as Herson et al (1989) found no effect on bleeding times or collagen-induced platelet aggregation.

Plasma levels of vitamin E are lower in normal newborns than adults. Vitamin E acts as an anti-oxidant decreasing lipid peroxidation and damage to cell membranes. As a result it stabilizes platelet membranes and decreases lipid release from platelet membranes on stimulation (Cox et al 1980). In neonates, the presence of low levels of vitamin E may explain the increased arachidonic acid release seen on activation of neonatal platelets (Khurshid et al 1975, Stuart et al 1979, Stuart & Allen 1982).

Amniotic fluid enhances platelet thromboxane production (Stuart et al 1987). This proaggregatory effect may contribute to platelet thrombi seen in the pulmonary microcirculation at autopsy in instances where pulmonary hypertension has complicated perinatal aspiration (Levin et al 1983). Platelet recruitment to the pulmonary vasculature by thromboxane A_2 may contribute to both thrombocytopenia and the persistent pulmonary hypertension associated with this syndrome.

Finally platelet dysfunction has been reported both in association with hyperbilirubinaemia (Suvansri et al 1969, Kaapa 1985) and its treatment with phototherapy (Maurer et al 1976, Karim et al 1981).

THROMBOCYTOPENIA

Incidence and impact of thrombocytopenia

Thrombocytopenia, defined as a platelet count less than $150 \times 10^9/l$, is a common problem in sick neonates. For many infants this thrombocytopenia is relatively mild and will not require therapy but may provide evidence of an underlying disease process. Evaluation of infants with thrombocytopenia should include a family history, determining whether the infant is sick or well, the severity and site of bleeding, size and morphology of platelets, and response to therapy. Because artifactually low automated platelet counts may occur, low platelet counts should always be confirmed by examination of blood smears. Pseudothrombocytopenia caused by agglutination of platelets in blood samples collected in EDTA can be ruled out by collecting blood in citrate anticoagulant (Pegels et al 1982).

In a prospective cohort study by Castle et al (1986), 22% of sick neonates in an intensive care nursery developed thrombocytopenia. More than 50% of these had counts less than $100 \times 10^9/l$ and 20% had platelet counts less than $50 \times 10^9/l$. In this population the course of the thrombocytopenia showed a nadir on the 4th day of life and recovery by day 10 for the majority of infants. Platelet counts less than $100 \times 10^9/l$ were associated with an increased incidence of clinical bleeding and increased incidence and severity of intraventricular haemorrhage when compared to age and illness-matched controls without thrombocytopenia (Andrew et al 1987b).

Pathogenesis

Thrombocytopenia can be caused by increased platelet destruction, decreased production, splenic pooling or combinations of these mechanisms. Elucidation of the mechanism is important as it has implications both for therapy and prognosis. Disease states related to these mechanisms are listed in Table 44.8.

Platelet destruction

Increased destruction is the most common mechanism of thrombocytopenia (Castle et al 1986, 1987). Evidence of destruction includes shortened platelet survival of radiolabelled platelets (Castle et al 1987, 1988) and increasing platelet volumes over the first week of life. The major causes of destruction can be divided into immune and

Table 44.8 Causes of neonatal thrombocytopenia

I. Increased destruction
  A. Immune-mediated
    1. Passive
      a. Maternal ITP
      b. Maternal SLE
      c. Maternal drugs
      d. Maternal preeclampsia
    2. Active
      a. Neonatal alloimmune thrombocytopenia
  B. Non-immune, associated DIC
    1. Asphyxia
    2. Sepsis
    3. Perinatal aspiration
    4. Necrotizing enterocolitis
    5. Respiratory distress syndrome
    6. Giant haemangiomas (Kasabach–Merritt syndrome)
    7. Thrombosis
  C. Other
    1. Hyperbilirubinaemia
    2. Phototherapy
    3. Polycythaemia
    4. Haemolytic disease of the newborn
    5. Exchange transfusion
    6. Parenteral nutrition (lipid emulsions)
    7. Amino acidurias
  D. Ineffective thrombopoiesis
    1. Wiskott–Aldrich syndrome
    2. Isolated X-linked thrombocytopenias
    3. Familial thrombocytopenias with autosomal inheritance

II. Decreased production
  A. Bone marrow infiltrative disorders
    1. Congenital leukaemia
    2. Neuroblastoma
    3. Histiocytosis
    4. Osteopetrosis
  B. Megakaryocytic hypoplasia
    1. Thrombocytopenia with absent radii
    2. Amegakaryocytic thrombocytopenia
    3. Thrombocytopenia associated with trisomy 13 and 18
    4. Thrombocytopenia with microcephaly
    5. Drug - induced aplasia
    6. Congenital infection

III. Hypersplenism
  A. Congenital infection
  B. Osteopetrosis
  C. Other causes

non-immune events. Immune-mediate thrombocytopenias are the result of increased platelet clearance caused by antiplatelet antibody. Tests for platelet-associated-immunoglobulin (PAIgG) are highly sensitive for immune thrombocytopenias but have low specificity (Kelton et al 1982). Increased PAIgG can be detected not only in alloimmune and autommune thrombocytopenia but also in thrombocytopenia associated with sepsis (Tate et al 1981) and maternal preeclampsia (Rote & Lau 1985, Pritchard et al 1987). The basis for the elevated PAIgG remains obscure in many cases.

Immune thrombocytopenias

Neonatal alloimmune thrombocytopenia (NATP)

NATP is the result of maternal antibodies directed against paternally-derived antigens present on fetal platelets causing immune destruction of platelets in utero; analogous to haemolytic disease of the newborn. Mothers themselves have normal platelets counts and have no bleeding history. The most common cause is fetomaternal Pl^{A1} (Zw^a) incompatibility which can result in maternal production of IgG antibodies reactive with Pl^{A1} antigens inherited from the father and present on fetal platelets. This particular antigen is present on platelets of 98% of the Caucasian population, and accounts for approximately 75% of cases of NATP (Pearson et al 1964, von dem Borne et al 1981, Mueller-Eckhardt et al 1989). Other implicated antigens are listed in Table 44.9. Platelet antigen incompatibility between mother and fetus does not invariably result in alloimmunization. It appears that sensitization is associated with immune response genes of the major histocompatibility complex. For example, the HLA-B8, -DR3 phenotype in Pl^{A1}-negative women has been associated with an increased incidence of alloantibody formation (Reznikoff-Etievant et al 1983, Mueller-Echkhardt et al 1985). Alloimmunization occurs in approximately 1/1000 pregnancies but not all will result in NATP (Blanchette et al 1990).

Table 44.9 Platelet antigens involved in neonatal alloimmune thrombocytopenia (NATP)

Antigen	Localization (glycoprotein)	Alleles	Antigen incidence (%)	Involvement NATP (Reference)
74Pl^A (Zw)	GP IIIa	Pla^{A1} (Zwa)	98	most common,
		Pl^{A2} (Zwb)	27	Mueller-Eckhardt et al 1986, 1987
Br	GP Ia/IIa	Br^a	20	Kaplan et al 1991, Bussel et al 1991a,b
		Br^b		
Bak (Lek)	GP IIb	Bak^a	90	von dem Borne & von Riesz 1980
		Bak^b		
Pl^E	GP Ib/IX	Pl^{E1}	99	Pearson et al 1964
		Pl^{E2}	5	
Yuk (Pen)	GP IIIa	Yuk^a	1.0	Shibata et al 1986a,b
		Yuk^b	99.9	
Ko		Ko^a	14	Bizzaro & Dianese 1988
		Ko^b	99	

The incidence of NATP is 1/2000–1/5000 births (Blanchette et al 1986, 1990). 50% of cases occur with the first pregnancy and the rate of recurrence in subsequent pregnancies is 75–90%. Most infants are otherwise healthy but petechiae and thrombocytopenia are present at birth or develop within a few hours. The thrombocytopenia is often profound and bleeding may occur from any site. Of most concern is the occurrence of intracranial haemorrhage in as many as 10–20% (Bussel et al 1991a,b) often associated with neurological complications and death. Long-term sequelae also include hydrocephalus and porencephalic cysts. Trauma at the time of delivery is probably an important contributor but antenatal haemorrhage is well recognized (Zalneraitis et al 1979, Friedman & Aster 1985, Burrows & Kelton 1988, Reznikoff-Etievant 1988). Thrombocytopenia usually develops in utero as maternal antibodies can cross the placenta as early as 14 weeks gestation and platelet antigens are fully expressed by 18 weeks gestation (Gruel et al 1986). Thrombocytopenic fetuses have been identified at 20 weeks gestation (Bussel et al 1988, Kaplan et al 1988). Bleeding may be aggravated by platelet dysfunction caused by the binding of antibody to the Pl^{A1} antigen which is located on glycoprotein IIIa, a component of the platelet fibrinogen receptor.

The diagnosis is confirmed when neonatal or fetal thrombocytopenia occurs associated with maternal alloantibody reacting to the infant's platelets. Typing of maternal and paternal platelets is important as testing of the infant's platelets is often impossible because of the severe thrombocytopenia. Antibodies can be detected in maternal serum (McFarland et al 1989) in the majority of cases using sensitive techniques including immunofluorescence and immunoprecipitation (von dem Borne et al 1981, Kiefel et al 1987). However in about 20% of cases alloantibodies cannot be detected in maternal sera even when fetal PAIgG is elevated (Kaplan et al 1988).

Management of unexpected, profound thrombocytopenia depends on the correct diagnosis and should include prompt laboratory investigation of the causes. However, treatment is usually begun based on a clinical diagnosis and not delayed while awaiting laboratory confirmation (Blanchette et al 1986). Optimal treatment is the transfusion of compatible, antigen-negative platelets. These are most easily provided by transfusion of maternal platelets, washed (to remove antibodies) and irradiated (to prevent graft-versus-host disease). In urgent situations random donor platelets can be given while awaiting the matched platelets. The response to the random transfusion may help to confirm the diagnosis. Intravenous immunoglobulin has been shown to be of benefit alone or in addition to compatible platelets (Sidiropoulous & Straume 1984, Mueller-Eckhardt et al 1989, Pietz et al 1991). Steroids and exchange transfusion are of little value.

Management of subsequent pregnancies in a mother with a previously affected child starts with antenatal monitoring for fetal thrombocytopenia in an attempt to prevent intracranial haemorrhage in utero. Fetal blood sampling by cordocentesis has made it possible to obtain a platelet count as early as 20 weeks and to transfuse compatible platelets to treat the thrombocytopenia from 26 weeks onwards. This may require one or repeated transfusions depending on gestational age and platelet count (Kaplan et al 1988, Nicolini et al 1988). Delivery can be by elective caesarean section or in selected cases, vaginally, following in utero transfusion. A less invasive alternative involves administration of high dose intravenous immunoglobulin to mothers when fetal thrombocytopenia is diagnosed and monitoring fetal platelet counts to determine response. Although initial single case reports showed no effect from this therapy (Waters et al 1987, Bussel et al 1988, Kaplan et al 1988, Mir et al 1988), other groups were successful in raising neonatal platelet counts using immunoglobulin with or without the addition of dexamethasone (Bussel et al 1991a,b, Levine & Berkowitz 1991). The approach to antenatal management is still being refined.

Autoimmune thrombocytopenia (ITP)

Placental transfer of antiplatelet antibodies can result in thrombocytopenia in newborns of mothers with autoimmune thrombocytopenia, either isolated or as part of other autoimmune diseases such as systemic lupus erythematosis (de Swiet 1985). The antibodies are directed at antigens common to maternal and neonatal platelets. Maternal ITP must be distinguished from the frequent occurrence of mild gestational thrombocytopenia in healthy pregnant women which appears to have no adverse affect on mother or infant and does not require intervention (Burrows & Kelton 1988, Aster 1990, Bussel et al 1991a).

The risk of severe thrombocytopenia leading to in utero or perinatal haemorrhage is less than for alloimmune thrombocytopenia. A retrospective study of consecutive women with ITP (Burrows & Andrews 1990, Burrows & Kelton 1990) found 4.9% of infants had a cord blood platelet count less than 50×10^9/l and 14.7% had a count of less than 150×10^9/l. Neonatal platelet counts tend to reach their nadir several days following birth so that intracranial haemorrhage rarely occurs prenatally or with delivery. The actual risk of intracranial haemorrhage is unclear from the older literature because of inclusion of mothers with disorders other than simple ITP. Prenatal management remains controversial because of the problem of predicting which fetuses are most at risk and therefore in need of intervention (Blanchette et al 1989b). Maternal platelet counts do not correlate with fetal platelet counts. Women with normal platelet counts post-splenectomy may still deliver thrombocytopenic infants. Direct determination of fetal platelet counts in fetal blood obtained by cordocentesis or fetal scalp sampling (Scott et al 1980) can provide the information required. Neither of these techniques is without drawbacks as there are risks to the fetus with cordocentesis which may equal the risk of bleeding in utero (Moise et al 1988) and fetal scalp sampling can be technically difficult and sometimes inaccurate (Christiaens & Helmerhorst 1987, Burrows & Andrew 1990, Burrows & Kelton, 1990). A method of identifying which women require this invasive testing and which women can be allowed to give birth without intervention is still lacking. A study by Samuels et al (1990) suggested that absence of a maternal history of ITP before gestation and negative results of circulating antibody testing identifies a group with minimal risk of significant neonatal thrombocytopenia.

The efficacy of prenatal therapy to elevate the fetal platelet count is uncertain. Karpatkin et al (1981) reported that prednisone given to mothers antenatally improved platelet counts of infants at birth. The effectiveness of steroids to raise neonatal platelet counts was not confirmed by Christiaens et al (1990) in a randomized study of low dose betamethasone administered to mothers in the last few weeks of pregnancy, and steroids cannot presently be recommended for this purpose.

Clinically these infants are usually healthy at birth with mild manifestations of thrombocytopenia. Other causes of thrombocytopenia should be excluded on the basis of maternal history and clinical examination. Serological studies can confirm the basis of the thrombocytopenia (Kelton et al 1980, Pao et al 1991). Therapeutic intervention for infants with platelet counts less than $50 \times 10^9/l$ have included platelet transfusions, exchange transfusions and corticosteroids (Karpatkin et al 1981). Recently, high-dose intravenous immunoglobulin has been used after delivery and has been safe and effective. Response rates to immunoglobulin with or without steroids has been approximately 75% (Chirico et al 1983, Ballin et al 1988, Blanchette et al 1989b, Linder et al 1990) and is similar to the response in acute ITP in older children. It is unclear what added benefit steroids have in the response to immunoglobulin. Infants must be followed carefully for recurrence of thrombocytopenia as some may require retreatment before permanent resolution of thrombocytopenia occurs.

Non-immune destruction

Thrombocytopenia caused by the dilutional effect of exchange transfusion (Podolsak 1973, Austin & Darlow 1988) depends on the amount of blood transfused. Recovery usually occurs by a week post-transfusion. Platelet consumption, with or without disseminated intravascular coagulation (DIC), is a frequent cause of thrombocytopenia and associated with a variety of disease states in neonates. Some of the more common causes are described.

Asphyxia at birth is associated with thrombocytopenia and DIC. This is supported by animal studies that demonstrate decreased platelet survival in the presence of hypoxia (Castle et al 1988). Chronic hypoxia may contribute to thrombocytopenia seen in infants with intrauterine growth retardation. Hypertensive disorders of pregnancy are associated with an increased risk of thrombocytopenia particularly in premature infants with growth retardation (Burrows & Andrew 1990).

Infections, either congenital (rubella, HSV, CMV, toxoplasmosis, syphilis, ECHO virus, HIV) or acquired can cause thrombocytopenia. The mechanism is multifactorial. In bacterial sepsis these mechanisms include DIC, platelet activation initiated by bacterial damage of endothelium, and an immune-mediated mechanism (Tate et al 1981). Rapid increases in platelet volumes in the presence of bacteraemia support a primarily consumptive thrombocytopenia (Patrick & Lazarchick 1990). Infants with congenital infection and severe thrombocytopenia may also have decreased thrombopoiesis (Weinblatt et al 1987) and increased splenic pooling related to hypersplenism. 45–80% of infants with congenital rubella may have thrombocytopenia which usually resolves by 2 months of age (Cooper et al 1965).

Thrombocytopenia in sick premature infants may be associated with multiple risk factors (Mehta et al 1980) including respiratory distress syndrome, mechanical ventilation (Ballin et al 1987), necrotizing enterocolitis (Tudehope & Yu 1977) and phototherapy (Maurer et al 1976). Perinatal aspiration syndrome and persistent pulmonary hypertension have been associated with thrombocytopenia. Platelet activation (Horgan et al 1985, Stuart et al 1987) and deposition of platelet-fibrin thrombi in the pulmonary vasculature may be responsible for this syndrome.

Giant haemangiomas can be associated with a localized consumptive coagulopathy (Kasabach–Merritt syndrome) characterized by thrombocytopenia, hypofibrinogenaemia, elevated fibrin degradation products and microangiopathic haemolysis. These vascular tumours are present at birth but may enlarge rapidly during the first few months of life (Fig. 44.8). They can occur anywhere on the body surface or in the viscera, especially bowel and liver, and may be multiple. Thrombocytopenia can be profound and some infants have severe bleeding manifestations while others are asymptomatic. The natural history of these lesions is one of slow regression over years. For children who are symptomatic because of their coagulopathy, therapeutic options include surgery (Shim 1968), steroids (Fost & Easterly 1968, Brown et al 1972), embolization (Johnson et al 1984) or alpha-interferon (Orchard et al 1989, White et al 1991). Irradiation should be avoided if possible because of long-term sequelae. Supportive therapies for the coagulopathy have included blood product replacement with platelets, cryoprecipitate and plasma and anti-coagulation therapy with heparin, antiplatelet agents (Hagerman et al

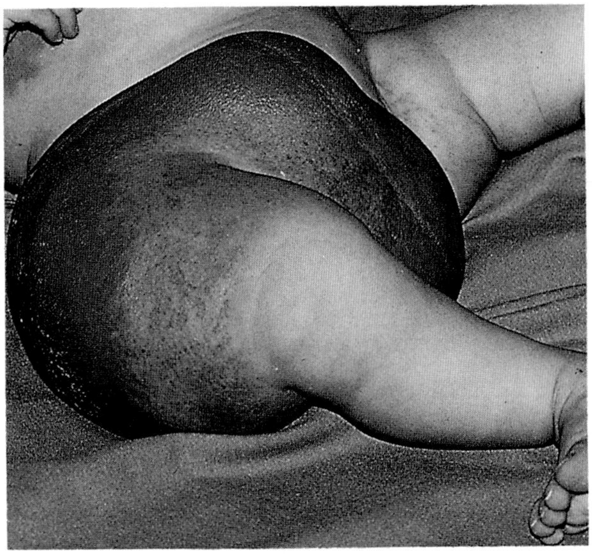

Fig. 44.8 An infant with a giant haemangioma; Kasabach–Merritt syndrome.

1975) and antifibrinolytic agents (Shim 1968, Hanna & Bernstein 1989).

Acute thrombosis, particularly renal vein thrombosis, can be associated with thrombocytopenia as can polycythaemia with haematocrits greater than 0.70. Such infants often have other abnormalities that may contribute to thrombocytopenia. There are rare case reports of a congenital syndrome with features of thrombotic thrombocytopenic purpura (TTP) including thrombocytopenia, microangiopathic haemolytic anaemia and neurological abnormalities (Monnens & Retera 1967, Upshaw 1978).

Familial causes of thrombocytopenia are often associated with ineffective thrombopoiesis. The best defined of these rare syndromes is Wiskott–Aldrich syndrome, an X-linked disorder characterized by severe thrombocytopenia, eczema and immunodeficiency. It is often apparent by the first month of life if the thrombocytopenia is severe. Major risks are related to intracranial haemorrhage and infections. In the newborn period it may be confused with immune thrombocytopenia as platelet survival is decreased (Baldini 1972) but can be differentiated by a markedly decreased platelet volume (Baldini 1972, Murphy et al 1972), bleeding disproportionate to the platelet count and evidence of abnormalities in cell-mediated immunity (Ochs et al 1980). Bone marrow evaluation usually shows normal numbers of megakaryocytes with atypical morphology. Platelet function is also abnormal with evidence of impaired energy generation (Verhoeven et al 1989). Therapy includes supportive care in the form of platelet transfusions and immunoglobulin supplementation. Splenectomy is often successful in alleviating the thrombocytopenia but carries a serious risk of life-threatening infection (Lum et al 1980). Treatment with allogenic bone marrow transplantation is curative (Parkman et al 1978, Kapoor et al 1981). Variants of Wiskott–Aldrich without the immunodeficiency have also been described (Stormorken et al 1991). Other familial thrombocytopenias may rarely present with clinical bleeding in the newborn period.

Decreased production of platelets

Thrombocytopenia due to decreased production is relatively uncommon in the neonatal period (Pearson & McIntosh 1978, Gill 1983). This includes infants with infiltrative disorders of bone marrow such as congenital leukaemia, transient myeloproliferative syndrome in infants with Down syndrome, neuroblastoma and histiocytosis (Letterer–Siwe).

Congenital megakaryocytic hypoplasia may be isolated or associated with congenital anomalies, the best described syndrome being thrombocytopenia with absent radii (TAR) (Hall et al 1969 Hedberg & Lipton 1988). The defect appears to be the absence or arrested development of the committed megakaryocyte progenitor cell (Homans et al 1988; Freedman & Estrov 1990). Infants can be at risk of severe bleeding including intracranial haemorrhage and supportive care in the form of platelet transfusions is often necessary. For infants with TAR syndrome, responses to splenectomy and steroids have not been consistent (Hedberg & Lipton 1988) and a single case report showed no response of the thrombocytopenia to intravenous immunoglobulin (Sopo et al 1991). The platelet count often improves over the course of the first year of life.

Decreased production may also be the result of bone marrow suppressive effects of infection particularly congenital viral infection or drugs.

Hypersplenism

Thrombocytopenia associated with hypersplenism alone is rarely severe. However it may complicate a number of disorders that also cause decreased production or consumption of platelets including congenital leukaemia, histiocytosis, congenital infection or osteopetrosis. Recovery of ^{111}Indium oxine-labelled-platelets is a sensitive indicator of hypersplenism and is low in many thrombocytopenic infants (Castle et al 1985).

THROMBOCYTOSIS

Elevated platelet counts occur frequently in premature infants at 4–6 weeks postnatal age (Chan et al 1989). Reactive thrombocytosis may also occur in association with other disorders, most commonly infection. There are no clinical manifestations of this thrombocytosis, no increased risk of thrombosis and no intervention is indicated.

REFERENCES

Aarts P A M M, Bolhuis P A, Sakariassen K S, Heethaar R M, Sixma J J 1983 Red blood cell size is important for adherence of blood platelets to artery subendothelium Blood 62: 214–217

Aballi A J, de Lamerens S 1962 Coagulation changes in the neonatal period and in early infancy. Pediatric Clinics of North America 9: 785–817

Aballi A J, Banus V L, de Lamerens S, Rozengvaig S 1957 Coagulation studies in the newborn period. I. Alterations of thromboplastin generation and effects of vitamin K on fullterm and premature infants. American Journal of Diseases of Children 94: 589–600

Aballi A J, Lopez Banus V et al 1959 The coagulation defect of fullterm infants. Pediatria Internazionale 9: 315–319

Abbondanzo S L, Gootenberg J E, Lofts R S, McPherson R A 1988 Intracranial hemorrhage in congenital deficiency of factor XIII. American Journal of Pediatric Hematology and Oncology 10: 65–68

Abildgaard C F 1969 Recognition and treatment of intravascular coagulation. Journal of Pediatrics 74: 163–176

Ahlsten G, Ewald G, Tuvemo T 1983 Cord blood platelet aggregation: Quality control by a two-sample technique. Upsala Journal of Medical Sciences 88: 9–15

Ahlsten G, Ewald U, Kindahl H, Tuvemo T 1985 Aggregation of and thromboxane B2 synthesis in platelets from newborn infants of smoking and non-smoking mothers. Prostaglandins Leukatriemes Medicine 19: 167–176

Ahlsten G, Ewald U, Tuvemo T 1986 Maternal smoking reduces prostacyclin formation in human umbilical arteris. A study on strictly selected pregnancies. Acta Obstetrica Gynecologica Scandinavica 65: 645–649

Ahmann Pa, Lazzara A, Dykes F D, Brann A W, Schwartz J F 1980 Intraventricular hemorrhage in the high-risk preterm infant: Incidence and outcome. Annals of Neurology 7: 118

Allison P M, Mummah-Schendel L L, Kindberg C G, Harms C S, Bang N U, Suttie J W 1987 Effects of a vitamin K-deficient diet and antibiotics in normal human volunteers. Journal of Laboratory and Clinical Medicine 110: 180–188

Alpan G, Eyal F, Springer C, Glick B, Goder K, Armon J 1984 Heparinization of alimentation solutions administered through peripheral veins in premature infants. A controlled study. Pediatrics 74: 375–378

Ambrus C, Jung O, Ambrus J, Mirand E, Choi T, Bartfay-Szabo A 1979 The fibrinolysin system and its relationship to disease in the newborn. American Journal of Pediatric Hematology/Oncology 1(3): 251–260

Ambrus C M, Weinstraub D H, Ambrus J L 1966 Studies on hyaline membrane disease. III Therapeutic trial of urokinase-activated human plasmin. Pediatrics 38: 231–243

Ambrus C M, Choi T S, Cunnanan E et al 1977 Prevention of hyaline membrane disease with plasminogen. A cooperative study. Journal of the American Medical Association 237(17): 1837–1841

Anderson J M, Brown J K, Cockburn F 1974 On the role of disseminated intravascular coagulation on the pathology of birth asphyxia. Developmental Medicine and Childhood Neurology 16: 581–591

Andersson T R, Bangstad H, Larsen M L 1988 Heparin cofactor II and antithrombin and protein C in plasma from term and preterm infants. Acta Paediatrica Scandinavica 77: 485–488

Andrew M, Karpatkin M 1982 A simple screening test for evaluating prolonged partial thromboplastin times in newborn infants. Journal of Pediatrics 101: 610–612

Andrew M, Schmidt B 1988 The use of heparin in newborn infants. Seminars in Thrombosis and Haemostasis 14: 28–32

Andrew M, Massicotte-Nolan P M, Karpatkin M 1983a Plasma protease inhibitors in premature infants: Influence of gestational age, postnatal age and health status. Proceedings of the Society for Experimental Biology and Medicine 173: 495–500

Andrew M, Massicotte-Nolan P, Mitchell L, Cassidy K 1985 Dsyfunctional antithrombin III in sick premature infants. Pediatric Research 19: 237–239

Andrew M, Paes B, Milner R et al 1987a The development of the human coagulation system in the fullterm infant. Blood 70: 165–172

Andrew M, Castle V, Saigal S, Carter C, Kelton J G 1987b. Clinical impact of neonatal thrombocytopenia. Journal of Pediatrics 110: 457–464

Andrew M, Mitchell L, Berry L, Schmidt B, Hatton M W C 1988a Fibrinogen has a rapid turnover in the healthy newborn lamb. Pediatric Research 23: 249–252

Andrew M, O'Brodovich H, Mitchell L 1988b The fetal lamb coagulation system during normal birth. American Journal of Hematology 28: 116–118

Andrew M, Ofosu F A, Schmidt B, Brooker L, Hirsh J, Buchanan M R 1988c Heparin clearance and ex vivo recovery in newborn piglets and adult pigs. Thrombosis Research 52: 517–527

Andrew M, Paes B, Milner R, et al 1988d Development of the human coagulation system in the healthy premature infant. Blood 72: 1651–1657

Andrew M, Castle V, Mitchell L, Paes B 1989a A modified bleeding time in the infant. American Journal of Hematology 30: 190–191

Andrew M, Ofosu F, Brooker L, Buchanan M 1989b The comparison of the pharmacokinetics of a low molecular heparin in the newborn and adult pig. Thrombosis Research 56: 529–539

Andrew M, Paes B, Johnston M 1990a Development of the hemostatic system in the neonate and young infant. American Journal of Pediatric Hematology/Oncology 12: 95–104

Andrew M, Schmidt B, Mitchell L, Paes B, Ofosu F 1990b Thrombin generation in newborn plasma is critically dependent on the concentration of prothrombin. Thrombosis and Haemostasis 63: 27–30

Andrew M, Brooker L, Leaker M, Paes B, Weitz J 1991a Fibrin clot lysis by thrombolytic agents is impaired in newborns due to a low plasminogen concentration. Thrombosis and Haemostasis 66: 325–330

Andrew M, Caco C, Vegh P et al 1991b Benefits of platelet transfusions in premature infants: A randomized controlled trial. Thrombosis and Haemostasis 65(6): 721 (abstract)

Andrew M, Caco C, Vegh P et al 1991c A multicentre randomized controlled trial of platelet infusions in premature infants. Pediatric Research 29 (4) part 2: 272A (abstract)

Andrew M, Mitchell L, Paes B et al 1991d An anticoagulant dermatan sulphate proteoglycan circulates in the pregnant woman and her fetus. Journal of Clinical Investigation 89: 321–326

Andrew M, Vegh P, Johnston M, Bowker J, Ofosu F, Mitchell L 1991 Maturation of the hemostatic system during childhood. Unpublished observations

Andrews A F, Klein M D, Toomasian J M, Roloff D W, Bartlett R H 1983 Venovenous extracorporeal membrane oxygenation in neonates with respiratory failure. Journal of Pediatric Surgery 18: 339

Andrews A F, Roloff D M, Bartlett R H 1984 Use of extracorporeal membrane oxygenation in persistent pulmonary hypertension of the newborn. Clinics in Perinatology 11: 729–735

Arad I D, Alpan G, Sznajderman S D, Eldor A 1986 The mean platelet volume (MVP) in the neonatal period. American Journal of Perinatology 3: 1–3

Arneil G C, MacDonald A M, Morphy A V, Sweet E M 1973 Renal venous thrombosis. Clinics in Nephrology 1: 119–131

Arnold J, O'Brodovich H, Whyte R, Coates G 1985 Pulmonary thromboemboli after neonatal asphyxia. Journal of Pediatrics 106: 806–809

Aster R H 1990 'Gestational' thrombocytopenia, a plea for conservative management. New England Journal of Medicine 323: 264–266

Astrowe P S, Palmerton E S 1941 Clinical studies with vitamin K in newborn infants. Journal of Pediatrics. 18: 507–515

Austin N, Darlow B A 1988 Transfusion-associated fall in platelet count in very low birthweight infants. Australian Paediatric Journal 24: 354–356

Avery M E, Mead J 1959 Surface properties in relation to atelectasis and hyaline membrane disease. American Journal of Diseases of Children 97: 517–523

Aviram M, Deckelbaum R J 1989 Intralipid infusion into humans reduces in vitro platelet aggregation and alters platelet lipid composition. Metabolism 38: 343–347

Bada H S, Green R S, Pourcyrous M et al 1989 Indomethacin reduces

the risks of severe intraventricular hemorrhage. Journal of Pediatrics 115: 631–637
Baehner R L, Strauss H S 1966 Hemophilia in the first year of life. New England Journal of Medicine 275: 524–528
Bahakim H, Garder A, Galil A, Babbar FA-A, Gaafar T H, Edrees Y B 1990 Coagulation parameters in maternal and cord blood at delivery. Annals of Saudi Medicine 10: 149–155
Baldini M G 1972 Nature of the platelet defect in the Wiskott–Aldrich syndrome. Annals of the New York Academy of Science 201: 437–444
Ballin A, Koren G, Kohelet D et al 1987 Reduction of platelet counts induced by mechanical ventilation in newborn infants. Journal of Pediatrics. 111: 445–449
Ballin A, Andrew M, Ling E, Perlman M, Blanchette V 1988 High-dose intravenous gammaglobulin therapy for neonatal autoimmune thrombocytopenia. Journal of Pediatrics 112: 789–792
Bandstra E S, Montalvo B M, Goldberg R N et al 1988 Prophylactic indomethacin for prevention of intraventricular hemorrhage in premature infants. Pediatrics 82(4): 533–542
Barnard D R, Hathaway W E 1979 Neonatal thrombosis. American Journal of Pediatric Hematology/Oncology 1: 235–244
Barnard D R, Simmons M A, Hathaway W E 1979 Coagulation studies in extremely premature infants. Pediatric Research 13: 1330–1335
Bartlett R H, Roloff D W, Cornell R G, Andrews A F, Dillon P W Zwischenberger J B 1985 Extracorporeal circulatory support in neonatal respiratory failure: A prospective randomized study. Pediatrics 76: 749
Bartlett R H, Gazzaniga A B, Corwin A G, Roloff D, Rucker R, Toomasian J M 1986 Extracorporeal membrane oxygenation (ECMO) in neonatal respiratory failure: 100 cases. Annals of Surgery 204: 236
Behrmann B A, Chan W K, Finer N N 1985 Resurgence of hemorrhagic disease of the newborn, a report of three cases. Canadian Medical Association Journal 133: 884–885
Bejar R, Curbelo V, Coen R W, Leopold G, James H, Gluck L 1980 Diagnosis and follow-up of intraventricular and intracerebral hemorrhages by ultrasound studies of infant's brain through the fontanelles and sutures. Pediatrics 66: 661
Benigni A, Gregorini G, Frusca T et al 1989 Effect of low-dose aspirin on fetal and maternal generation of thromboxane by platelets in women at risk for pregnancy-induced hypertension. New England Journal of Medicine 321: 357–362
Benson J W T, Drayton M R, Hayward C et al 1986 Multicentre trial of ethamsylate for prevention of periventricular haemorrhage in very low birthweight infants. Lancet ii: 1297–1300
Beverley D W, Chance G W, Inwood M J, Schaus M, O'Keefe B 1984a Intraventricular haemorrhage and haemostasic defects. Archives of Disease in Childhood 59: 444–448
Beverley D W, Inwood M J, Chance G W, Schaus M, O'Keefe B 1984b 'Normal' haemostasis parameters: A study in a well-defined unborn population of preterm infants. Early Human Development 9: 249–257
Beverley D W, Pitts-Tucker T J, Congdon J, Arthur R J, Tate I G 1985 Prevention of intraventricular haemorrhage by fresh frozen plasma. Archives of Diseases in Childhood 60: 710–713
Binder L 1986 Hemorrhagic disease of the newborn: An unusual etiology of neonatal bleeding. Annals of Emergency Medicine 15: 935–938
Bizzaro N, Dianese G 1988 Neonatal alloimmune amegakaryocytosis. Case report. Vox Sanguinis 54: 112
Bjarke B, Herin P, Blomback M 1974 Neonatal aortic thrombosis. A possible clinical manifestation of congenital antithrombin III deficiency. Acta Paediatrica Scandinavica 63: 297–301
Blanchette V S, Peters M A, Pegg-Feige K 1986 Alloimmune thrombocytopenia. Review from a neonatal intensive care unit. Current Studies in Hematology and Blood Transfusions 52: 87–96
Blanchette V, Andrew M, Perlman M, Ling E, Ballin A 1989a Neonatal autoimmune thrombocytopenia: role of high-dose intravenous immunoglobulin G therapy. Blut 59: 139–144
Blanchette V S, Sacher R A, Ballem P J, Bussell J B, Imbash P 1989b Commentary on the management of autoimmune thrombocytopenia during pregnancy and in the neonatal period. Blut 59: 121–123
Blanchette V S, Chen L C, Salomon de Friedberg Z, Hogan V A, Trudel E, Decary F 1990 Alloimmunization to the P1A1 platelet antigen: results of a prospective study. British Journal of Hematology 74: 209–218
Bleyer W A, Hakami N, Shepard T H 1971 The development of hemostasis in thc human fetus and newborn infant. Journal of Pediatrics 79: 838–853
Bloch C A, Rothberg A D, Bradlow B A 1984 Mother-infant prothrombin precursor status at birth. Journal of Pediatric Gastroenterology and Nutrition 3: 101–103
Bosque E, Weaver L 1986 Continuous versus intermittent heparin infusion of umbilical artery catheters in the newborn infant. Journal of Pediatrics 108: 141–143
Boyd J F 1966 Disseminated fibrin thromboembolism in stillbirths; a histological picture similar to one form of maternal hypofibrinogenemia. Journal of Obstetrics and Gynaecology in the British Commonwealth 73: 629–639
Boyd J F 1967 Disseminated fibrin thromboembolism among neonates dying within 48 hours of birth. Archives of Diseases in Childhood 42: 401–409
Boyd J F 1969 Disseminated fibrin thromboembolism among neonates dying more than 48 hours after birth. Journal of Clinical Pathology 22: 663–671
Braly B D 1965 Neonatal arterial thrombosis and embolism. Surgery 58: 869–873
Brinkhous K M, Smith H P, Warner E D 1937 Plasma prothrombin level in normal infancy and in hemorrhagic disease of the newborn. American Journal of Medical Science 193: 475 (abstract)
Brown S G, McHugh G M, Shapleski J, Wotherspoon P A, Taylor B J, Gillett W R 1989 Should intramuscular vitamin K prophylaxis for haemorrhage disease of the newborn be continued? A decision analysis. New Zealand Medical Journal 102: 3–5
Brown S H, Neerhout R C, Fonkalsrud E W 1972 Prednisone therapy in the management of large hemangiomas in infants and children. Surgery 71: 168–173
Bruchsaler F S 1941 Vitamin K and the prenatal and postnatal prevention of hemorrhagic disease in newborn infants. Journal of Pediatrics 18: 317
Buchanan G R 1978 Neonatal coagulation: normal physiology and pathophysiology. Clinical Haematology 1: 85–109
Buchanan G R 1986 Coagulation disorders in the neonate. Pediatric Clinics of North America 33: 203–220
Burnstein J, Papile L et al 1977 Subependymal germinal matrix and intraventricular hemorrhage in premature infants: Diagnosis by CT. American Journal of Roetgenology 128: 971–976
Burrows R F, Andrew M 1990 Neonatal thrombocytopenia in the hypertensive disorders of pregnancy. Obstetrics and Gynecology 76: 234–238
Burrows R F, Caco C C, Kelton J G 1988a Neonatal alloimmune thrombocytopenia: Spontaneous in utero intracranial hemorrhage. American Journal of Hematology 28: 98–102
Burrows R F, Kelton J G 1988b. Incidentally detected thrombocytopenia in healthy mothers and their infants. New England Journal of Medicine 319: 142–145
Burrows R F, Kelton J G 1990 Low fetal risks in pregnancies associated with idiopathic thrombocytopenic purpura do not justify obstetrical interventions. American Journal of Obstetrics and Gynecology 163: 1147–1150
Bussel J P, Berkowitz R L, McFarland J G, Lynch L, Chitkara U 1988 Antenatal treatment of neonatal alloimmune thrombocytopenia. New England Journal of Medicine 319: 1374–1378
Bussel J, Kaplan C, McFarland J, Working Party on Neonatal Immune Thrombocytopenia of the Neonatal Hemostasis Subcommittee of the Scientific and Standardization Committee of the ISTH 1991a Recommendations for the evaluation and treatment of neonatal autoimmune and alloimmune thrombocytopenia. Thrombosis and Haemostasis 65(5): 631–634
Bussel J B, Tanli S, Peterson H C 1991b Favorable neurological outcome in 7 cases of perinatal intracranial hemorrhage due to immune thrombocytopenia. American Journal of Pediatric Hematology/Oncology 13(2): 156–159
Cade J F, Hirsh J, Martin M 1969 Placental barrier to coagulation factors: Its relevance to the coagulation defect at birth and to haemorrhage in the newborn. British Medical Journal 2: 281–283

Cartwright G W, Culbertson K, Schreiner R L, Garg B P 1979 Changes in clinical presentation of term infants with intracranial hemorrhage. Developmental Medicine and Childhood Neurology 21: 730

Casella J F, Bontempo F A, Markel H, Lewis J H, Zitell B J, Starzl T E 1988 Successful treatment of homozygous protein C deficiency by hepatic transplantation. Lancet 1: 435–437

Castle V, Coates G, Mitchell L, O'Brodovich H, Andrew M 1985 Platelet survivals in the newborn: effect of hypoxia. Blood 66: 301 (abstract)

Castle V, Andrew M, Kelton J G, Carter C, Giron D, Johnston M 1986 Frequency and mechanism of neonatal thrombocytopenia. Journal of Pediatrics 108: 749–755

Castle V, Coates G, Kelton J, Andrew M 1987 ^{111}Indium oxime platelet survivals in the thrombocytopenic infant. Blood 70: 652–656

Castle V, Coates G, Mitchell L, O'Brodovich H, Andrew M 1988 The effect of hypoxia on platelet survival and site of sequestration in the newborn rabbit. Thrombosis and Haemostasis 59: 45–48

Chalmers T C 1990 A belated randomized control trial. Pediatrics 85: 366–369

Chan K W, Kaikov Y, Wadsworth L D 1989 Thrombocytosis in childhood: A survey of 94 patients. Pediatrics 84: 1064–1067

Chaou W-T, Chou M-L, Eitzman D V 1984 Intracranial hemorrhage and vitamin K deficiency in early infancy. Journal of Pediatrics 105: 880–884

Chaplin E R Jr, Goldstein G W, Norman D 1979 Neonatal seizures, intracerebral hematoma, and subarachnoid hemorrhage in fullterm infants. Pediatrics 63: 812

Chessells J M, Wigglesworth J S 1971a Coagulation studies in severe birth asphyxia. Archives of Diseases in Childhood 46: 253–256

Chessells J M, Wigglesworth J S 1971b Haemostatic failure in babies with rhesus isoimmunization. Archives of Diseases in Childhood 46: 38–45

Chessells J M, Wigglesworth J S 1972 Coagulation studies in preterm infants with respiratory distress and intracranial hemorrhage. Archives of Diseases in Childhood 47: 564–570

Chidi C C, King D R, Bales E T Jr 1983 An ultrastructural study of the intimal injury by an indwelling umbilical catheter. Journal of Pediatric Surgery 18: 109–115

Chirico G, Duse M, Ugazio A, Rondini G 1983 High-dose intravenous gamma-globulin therapy for passive immune thrombocytopenia in the neonate. Journal of Pediatrics 103: 654–655

Christiaens G C M L, Helmerhorst F M 1987 Validity of intrapartum diagnosis of fetal thrombocytopenia. American Journal of Obstetrics and Gynecology 157(4) part 1: 864–865

Christiaens G C, Nieuwenhuis H K, von dem Borne A E 1990 Idiopathic thrombocytopenic purpura in pregnancy: a randomized trial on the effect of antenatal low dose corticosteroids on neonatal platelet count. British Journal of Obstetrics and Gynaecology 97: 893–898

Chuansumrit A, Manco-Johnson M J, Hathaway W E 1989 Heparin cofactor II in adults and infants with thrombosis and DIC. American Journal of Haematology 31: 109

Clark C E, Clyman R I, Roth R S, Sniderman S H, Lane B, Ballard R A 1981 Risk factor analysis of intraventricular haemorrhage in low-birth-weight infants. Journal of Pediatrics 99: 625

Clawson C C, Boros S J 1978 Surface morphology of polyvinyl chloride and silicone elastomer umbilical artery catheters by scanning electron microscopy. Pediatrics 62: 702–705

Clifford S H 1941 Hemorrhagic disease of the newborn. A critical consideration. Journal of Pediatrics 18: 333–336

Cohen I T, Dahms B, Hays D M 1977 Peripheral total parenteral nutrition employing a lipid emulsion (Intralipid): Complications encountered in pediatric patients. Journal of Pediatric Surgery 12: 837–845

Colwell J A, Wincour P D, Halushka P A 1983 Do platelets have anything to do with diabetic microvascular disease? Diabetes 32 (suppl 2): 14–19

Committee on Nutrition Academy of Pediatrics 1961 Vitamin K compounds and water-soluble analogues: Use in therapy and prophylaxis in pediatrics. Pediatrics 28: 501–507

Conover P T, Abramowsky C, Beyer-Patterson P 1990 Immunohistochemical diagnosis of disseminated intravascular coagulation in newborns. Pediatric Pathology 10: 707–716

Cooke R W I 1981 Factors associated with periventricular haemorrhage in very low birthweight infants. Archives of Diseases in Children 56: 425

Cooke R W I, Morgan M E I 1984 Prophylactic ethamsylate for periventricular haemorrhage. Archives of Diseases in Childhood 59: 82–83

Cooper L Z, Green R H, Krugman S, Giles J P, Mirick G S 1965 Neonatal thrombocytopenic purpura and other manifestations of rubella contracted in utero. American Journal of Diseases in Childhood 110: 416–427

Corby D G, O'Barr T P 1981a Decreased alpha-adrenergic receptors in newborn platelets. Cause of abnormal response to epinephrine. Developmental Pharmacology and Therapeutics 2: 215–225

Corby D G, O'Barr T P 1981b Neonatal platelet function: A membrane-related phenomenon? Haemostasis 10: 177–185

Corby D G, Schulman I 1971 The effects of antenatal drug administration on aggregation of platelets of newborn infants. Journal of Pediatrics 79: 307–313

Cornelissen M, Smeets D, Merkx G, De Abreu R, Kollee L, Monnens L 1991 Analysis of chromosome aberrations and sister chromatid exchanges in peripheral blood lymphocytes of newborns after vitamin K prophylaxis at birth. Pediatric Research 30(6): 550–553

Corrazza M S, Davis R F, Merritt A, Bejar R, Cvetnic W 1984 Prolonged bleeding time in preterm infants receiving indomethacin for patent ductus arteriosus. Journal of Pediatrics 105: 292–296

Corrigan J 1988 Neonatal thrombosis and the thrombolytic system. Pathophysiology and therapy. American Journal of Pediatric Hematology and Oncology 10: 83–91

Corrigan J J 1977 Heparin therapy in bacterial septicemia. Journal of Pediatrics 91: 695–700

Corrigan J J 1979 Activation of coagulation and disseminated intravascular coagulation in the newborn. American Journal of Pediatric Hematology and Oncology 1: 245–249

Corrigan J J 1991 Normal hemostasis in fetus and newborn. Coagulation. In: Polin R A, Fox W W (eds) Neonatal and fetal medicine. Physiology and pathophysiology. Grune and Stratton, New York

Corrigan J J, Earnst D 1980 Factor II antigen in liver disease and warfarin induced vitamin K deficiency: Correlation with coagulation activity using echis venom. American Journal of Haematology 8: 249–255

Corrigan J J, Jordan C M 1970 Heparin therapy in septicemia with disseminated intravascular coagulation: Effect on mortality and on correction of hemostatic defects. New England Journal of Medicine. 283: 778

Corrigan J, Kryc J J 1980 Factor II (prothrombin) levels in cord blood. Correlation of coagulant activity with immunoreactive protein. Journal of Pediatrics 97: 979–983

Corrigan J, Sluth J J, Jeter M, Lox C D 1989 Newborn's fibrinolytic mechanism: Components and plasmin generation. American Journal of Hematology 32: 273–278

Cowett R M, Schwartz R 1982 The infant of the diabetic mother. Pediatric Clinics of North America 29: 1213–1231

Cox A C, Rao G H R, Gerrard J M, White J G 1980 The influence of vitamin E quinone on platelet structure, function and biochemistry. Blood 55: 907–914

Daffos F, Forestier F, Kaplan C, Cox W 1988 Prenatal diagnosis and management of bleeding disorders with fetal blood sampling. American Journal of Obstetrics and Gynecology 158: 939–946

Dam C P H 1929 Cholesterinstoffwechsel in Huhnereierin und Huhnchen. Biochemischeschrift Zeitschrift 215: 475–492

Dam H, Tage-Hansen E, Plum P 1939 K-avitaminose hos spaede born som aarag til hemorrhagisk diathese. Ugeskrift for Laeger 101: 896–904

Dam H, Glavind J, Larsen E H, Plum P 1942 Investigations into the cause of the physiological hypoprothrombinemia in new-born children. IV. The vitamin K content of woman's milk and cow's milk Acta Medica Scandinavica 112: 210–216

David R J, Merten D F, Anderson J C, Gross S 1981 Prevention of umbilical artery catheter clots with heparinized infusates. Developmental Pharmacology and Therapeutics 12: 117–126

de Lemos R A, McLaughlin G W, Koch H F, Diserens H W 1973 Abnormal partial thromboplastin time and survival in respiratory distress syndrome. Effect of exchange transfusion. Pediatric Research 7: 396 (abstract)
de Sa D J, Nicholls S 1972 Haemorrhagic necrosis of the adrenal gland in perinatal infants: A clinico-pathological study. Journal of Pathology 106: 133–149
de Stefano V, Leone G, Carolis M P et al 1987 Antithrombin III in fullterm and preterm newborn infants: Three cases of neonatal diagnosis of AT III congenital defect. Thrombosis and Haemostasis 57: 329–331
de Swiet M 1985 Maternal autoimmune disease and the fetus. Archives of Diseases in Childhood 60: 794–797
Dolfin T, Skidmore M B, Fong K W, Hoskins E M, Shennan A T 1983 Incidence, severity and timing of subependymal and intraventricular hemorrhages in preterm infants born in a perinatal unit as detected by serial real-time ultrasound. Pediatrics 71: 541–546
Donner M, Holmberg L, Nilsson I M 1987 Type IIB von Willebrand's disease with probable autosomal recessive inheritance and presenting as thrombocytopenia in infancy British Journal of Haematology 66: 349–354
Dreyfus M, Magny J F, Bridey F et al 1991 Treatment of homozygous protein C deficiency and neonatal purpura fulminans with a purified protein C concentrate. New England Journal of Medicine 325 (22): 1565–1568
Dube B, Bhargava V, Dube R K, Das B K, Abrol P, Kolindewala J K 1986 Disseminated intravascular coagulation in neonatal period. Indian Pediatrics 23: 925–931
Dudley D K, Dalton M E 1986 Single fetal death in twin gestation. Seminars in Perinatology 10: 65–72
Duncan R E, Evans A T, Martin L W 1977 Natural history and treatment of renal vein thrombosis in children. Journal of Pediatric Surgery 12: 639–645
Dunn P M 1982 Vitamin K for all newborn babies (letter). Lancet 2: 770
Dykes F D, Lazzara A, Ahmann P, Blumenstein B, Schwartz J, Brann A W 1980 Intraventricular haemorrhage: A prospective evaluation of etiopathegenesis. Pediatrics 66: 42–49
Edelberg J M, Enghild J J, Pizzo S V, Gonzalez-Gronow M 1990 Neonatal plasminogen displays altered cell surface binding and activation kinetics. Correlation with increased glycosylation of the protein. Journal of Clinical Investigation 86: 107–112
Editorial 1974 Renal vascular damage after birth. British Medical Journal 3: 296–297
Editorial 1985 Late onset of hemorrhagic disease of the newborn. Nutrition Reviews 43: 303–305
Edson J R, Blaese R M, White J G et al 1968 Defibrination syndrome in an infant born after abruptio placentae. Journal of Pediatrics 72: 342–346
Ekelund H Hedner U, Nilsson I 1970 Fibrinolysis in newborns. Acta Paediatrica Scandinavia 59: 33–43
El-Bardeesy M W, Johnson A M 1971 Serum proteinase inhibitors in infants with hyaline membrane disease. Journal of Pediatrics 81: 579–587
Enger E, Jacobsson B, Sorensen S E 1976 Tissue toxicity of intravenous solutions: A phlebographic and experimental study. Acta Pediatrica Scandinavica 65: 248–252
Evans D J, Silverman M, Bowley N B 1981 Congenital hypertension due to unilateral renal vein thrombosis. Archives of Diseases in Childhood 56: 306–308
Fee H J, McAvoy R A, Dainko E A 1977 Neonatal arterial occlusion. Journal of Pediatric Surgery 12: 711–713
Fetus and Newborn Committee, Canadian Pediatric Society 1988 The use of vitamin K in the perinatal period. Canadian Medical Association Journal 139: 127–130
Feusner J H, Slichter S J, Harker L A 1983 Acquired haemostatic defects in the ill newborn. British Journal of Haematology 53: 73–84
Firshein S I, Hoyer L W, Lazarchick J et al 1979 Prenatal diagnosis of classic hemophilia. New England Journal of Medicine 300: 937–941
Fitzgerald J E, Webster A 1940 Effect of vitamin K administered to patients in labor. American Journal of Obstetrics and Gynecology 40: 413–422
Flachaire E, Beney C, Berthier A, Salandre J, Quincy C, Renaud B 1990 Determination of reference values for serotonin concentration in platelets of healthy newborns, children, adults, and elderly subjects by HPLC with electrochemical detection. Clinical Chemistry 36: 2117–2120
Flanigan D P, Stolar C J H, Pringle K C, Schuler J J, Fisher E, Vidyasager D 1982 Aortic thrombosis after umbilical artery catheterization: successful surgical management. Archives of Surgery 117: 371–374
Forbes D 1983 Delayed presentation of haemorrhagic disease of the newborn. Medical Journal of Australia 2: 136–138
Forestier F, Daffos F, Rainaut M, Sole Y, Amiral J 1985 Vitamin K Dependent proteins in fetal hemostasis at mid trimester pregnancy. Thrombosis and Haemostasis 53: 401–403
Forestier F, Daffos E, Sole Y, Rainaut M 1986a Prenatal diagnosis of hemophilia by fetal blood sampling under ultrasound guidance. Haemostasis 16: 346 (abstract)
Forestier F, Daffos F, Galacteros F, Bardakjian J, Rainaut M, Berezard Y 1986b Hematological values of 163 normal fetuses between 18 and 30 weeks of gestation. Pediatric Research 20: 342–346
Forestier F, Cox W L, Daffos F, Rainaut M 1988 The assessment of fetal blood samples. American Journal of Obstetrics and Gynecology 158: 1184 (abstract)
Fost N C, Esterly N B 1968 Successful treatment of juvenile hemangiomas with prednisone. Journal of Pediatrics 72: 351–357
Freedman M H, Estrov Z 1990 Congenital amegakaryocytic thrombocytopenia: An intrinsic hematopoietic stem cell defect. American Journal of Pediatric Hematology/Oncology 12:225–230
Freeman B A, Tanswell A K, Cunningham M K 1987 Vitamin K_1 stimulates endothelial free radical production. American Review of Respiratory Disease 135: A98 (abstract)
Fresh J W, Adams H, Morgan F M 1959 Vitamin K — blood clotting studies during pregnancy and prothrombin and proconvertin levels in the newborn. Obstetrics and Gynecology 13: 37–40
Friedman J M, Aster R H 1985 Neonatal alloimmune thrombocytopenic purpura and congenital porencephaly in two siblings associated with 'new' maternal antiplatelet antibody. Blood 65: 1412–1415
Friedman Z, Lamberth E L Jr, Stahlman M T 1977 Platelet dysfunction in the neonate with essential fatty acid deficiency. Journal of Pediatrics 90: 439–443
Fujimura Y, Mimura Y, Kinoshita S, Yoshioka A, Kitawaki T, Yoshioka K 1982 Studies on vitamin K-dependent factor deficiency during early childhood with special reference to prothrombin activity and antigen level. Haemostasis 11: 90–95
Fujimura Y, Okubo Y, Sakai T et al 1984 Studies on precursor proteins PIVKA-II, -IX, and -X in the plasma of patients with 'hemorrhagic disease of the newborn'. Haemostasis 14: 211–217
Fuse Y 1986 Small for gestational age (SGA) neonates: a study of blood coagulation and fibrinolysis. Asia Oceania Journal of Obstetrics and Gynaecology 12: 291–299
Gader A M A, Bahakim H, Jabber F A, Lambourne A L, Gaafar T H 1988 Dose-response aggregometry in maternal/neonatal platelets. Thrombosis and Haemostasis 60: 314–318
Gajl-Paczalska K 1964 Plasma protein composition of hyaline membrane in the newborn as studies by immunofluorescence. Archives of Disease in Childhood 39: 226–231
Galanakis D K, Mosesson M W 1976 Evaluation of the role of in vivo proteolysis (fibrinogenolysis) in prolonging the thrombin time of human umbilical cord fibrinogen. Blood 48: 109–118
Ganrot P O, Schersten B 1967 Serum α_2-macroglobulin concentration and its variation with age and sex. Clinica Chimica Acta 15: 113–120
Gellis S S, Lyon R A 1941 The influence of the diet of the newborn infant on the prothrombin index. Journal of Pediatrics 19: 495–502
Gerrard J M, Docherty J C, Israels S J 1989 A reassessment of the bleeding time: Association of age, hematocrit, platelet function, von Willebrand factor, and bleeding time thromboxane B2 with the length of the bleeding time. Clinical and Investigative Medicine 12: 165–171
Gibson B 1989 Neonatal haemostasis. Archives of Diseases in Childhood 64: 503–506
Gilhooly J T, Lindenberg J A, Reynold J W 1987 Survey of umbilical catheter practices. Clinical Research 34: 142a

Gill F M 1983 Thrombocytopenia in the newborn. Seminars in Perinatology 7: 201–212

Gilles F H, Price R A, Kevy S V, Berenberg W 1971 Fibrinolytic activity in the ganglionic eminence of the premature human brain. Biology of the Neonate 18: 426–431

Girolami A, De Marco L, Dal Bo Zanon R, Patrassi R, Cappellato M G 1985 Rarer quantitative and qualitative abnormalities of coagulation. Clinics in Haematology 14: 385–411

Gobel U, Sonnenschein-Kosenow S, Petrich C, von Voss H 1977 Vitamin-K deficiency in the newborn (letter). Lancet 2: 187

Gobel U, Voss H C, Petrich C, Jurgens H, Oliver A 1979 Etiopathology and classification of acquired coagulation disorders in the newborn infant. Klinische Wochenschrift 57: 81–86

Gobel U, von Voss H et al 1980 Efficiency of heparin in the treatment of newborn infants with respiratory distress syndrome and disseminated intravascular coagulation. European Journal of Pediatrics 133: 47

Goddard J, Lewis R M, Armstrong D L, Zeda R S 1980 Moderate, rapidly induced hypertension as a cause of intraventricular hemorrhage in the newborn beagle model. Journal of Pediatrics 96: 1057

Goddard-Finegold J 1984 Periventricular, intraventricular hemorrhages in the premature newborn. Update on pathologic features, pathogenesis and possible means of prevention. Archives of Neurology 41: 766–771

Goetzman B W, Stadalnik R C, Bogren H G, Blankenship W J, Ikeda R M, Thayer J 1975 Thrombotic complications of umbilical artery catheters: a clinical and radiographic study. Pediatrics 56: 374–379

Goldsmith G H Jr, Pence R F, Ratnoff O D, Adelstein D J, Furie B 1982 Studies on a family with combined functional deficiencies of vitamin K-dependent coagulaton factors. Journal of Clinical Investigation 69: 1253–1260

Goldschmidt B, Bors S, Szabo A 1988 Vitamin K-dependent clotting factors during longterm parenteral nutrition in fullterm and preterm infants. Journal of Pediatrics 112: 108–111

Gonzalez R, Schwartz S, Sheldon C A, Fraley E E 1982 Bilateral renal vein thrombosis in infancy and childhood. Urology Clinics of North America 9: 279–283

Gralnick H R, Gilverber H, Abrams E 1978 Dysfibrinogenemia associated with hepatoma. Increased carbohydrate content of the fibrinogen molecule. New England Journal of Medicine 299: 221–226

Gray O P, Ackerman A, Fraser A J 1968 Intracranial hemorrhage and clotting defects in low birth weight infants. Lancet 1: 545–551

Graziani L J, Pasto M, Stanley C et al 1985 Cranial ultrasound and clinical studies in preterm infants. Journal of Pediatrics 106: 269–276

Greer F R, Mummah-Schendel L L, Marshall S, Suttie J W 1988 Vitamin K_1 (phylloquinone) and Vitamin K_2 (menaquinone) status in newborns during the first week of life. Pediatrics 81: 137–140

Greffe B S, Marlar R A, Manco-Johnson M 1989 Neonatal protein C: Molecular Composition and distribution in normal term infants. Thrombosis Research 56: 91

Greisen G, Johansen K, Ellison P H, Fredriksen P S, Mali J, Friis-Hansen B 1984 Cerebral blood flow in the newborn infant: Comparison of Doppler ultrasound and ^{133}Xenon clearance. Journal of Pediatrics 104: 411–418

Griffin J H, Evatt B, Zimmerman T S, Kleiss A J, Wideman C 1981 Deficiency of protein C in congenital thrombotic disease. Journal of Clinical Investigation 68: 1370–1373

Gross S, Melhorn D K 1971 Exchange transfusion with citrated whole blood for disseminated intravascular coagulation. Journal of Pediatrics 78: 415–419

Gross S J, Stuart M J 1977 Hemostasis in the premature infant. Clinics in Perinatology 4: 259–304

Gross S, Filston H C, Anderson J C 1982 Controlled study of treatment for disseminate intravascular coagulation in the neonate. Journal of Pediatrics 100: 445–448

Gruel Y, Boizard B, Daffos F, Forestier F, Caen J, Wautier J L 1986 Determinations of platelet antigens and glycoproteins in the human fetus. Blood 68: 488–492

Guckos-Thoeni U, Boltshauser E, Willi U V 1982 Intraventricular hemorrhage in fullterm neonates. Developmental Medicine and Childhood Neurology 24: 704–707

Gunn T R, Mok P M, Becroft D M O 1985 Subdural hemorrhage in utero. Pediatrics 76: 605–610

Hagerman L J, Czapek E E, Donnellan W L, Schwartz A D 1975 Determination of platelet antigens and glycoproteins in the human fetus. Journal of Pediatrics 87: 766–768

Hall M A, Pairaudeau P 1987 The routine use of vitamin K in the newborn. Midwifery 3: 170–177

Hall J G, Levin J, Kuhn J P, Ottenheimer E J, van Berkum K A P, McKusick K A 1969 Thrombocytopenia with absent radius. Medicine 48: 411–439

Hambleton G, Appleyard W J 1973 Controlled trial of fresh frozen plasma in asphyxiated low birthweight infants. Archives of Diseases in Childhood 48: 31–35

Hambleton G, Wigglesworth J S 1976 Origin of intraventricular hemorrhage in the preterm infant. Archives of Diseases in Childhood 51: 651–659

Hamulyak K, de Boer-van den Berg M A G 1987 The placental transport of [^{3}H] vitamin K_1 in rats. British Journal of Haematology 65: 335–338

Hamulyak K, Nieuwenhuizen W, Deville P P, Hemker H C 1983 Re-evaluation of some properties of fibrinogen purified from cord blood of normal newborns. Thrombosis Research 32: 301–320

Hanada T, Abe T, Takita H 1985 Antithrombin III concentrates for treatment of disseminated intravascular coagulation in children. American Journal of Pediatric Hematology/Oncology 7: 3–8

Hanawa Y, Maki M, Murata B et al 1988 The second nation-wide survey in Japan of vitamin K deficiency in infants. European Journal of Pediatrics 147: 472–477

Hanigan W C, Kennedy G, Roemisch F, Anderson R, Cusack T, Powers W 1988 Administration of indomethacin for the prevention of periventricular-intraventricular hemorrhage in high-risk neonates. Journal of Pediatrics 112: 941–947

Hanna B D, Bernstein M 1989 Tranexamic acid in the treatment of Kasabach–Merritt syndrome in infants. American Journal of Pediatric Hematology/Oncology 11: 191–195

Hardwicke S H 1944 Studies on the minimal effective dose of a water-soluble vitamin K substitute in the prevention of hypoprothrombinemia in the newborn infant. Journal of Pediatrics 24: 259–269

Haroon Y, Shearer M J, Rahim S, Gunn W G, McEnery G, Barkhan P 1982 The content of phylloquinone (vitamin K_1) in human milk, cow's milk and infant formula foods determined by high-performance liquid chromatography Journal of Nutrition 112: 1105–1117

Haslam R R, Ekert H, Gillam G L 1974 Hemorrhage in a neonate possibly due to maternal ingestion of salicylate. Journal of Pediatrics 84: 556–557

Hassan H, Leonardi C, Chelucci C, et al 1990 Blood coagulation factors in human embryonic-fetal development: Preferential expression of the FVII/Tissue factor pathway. Blood 76(6): 1158–1164

Hathaway W E 1986 ICTH Subcommittee on Neonatal Hemostasis. Thrombosis and Haemostasis 55: 145

Hathaway W E 1987 New insights on vitamin K. Hematology/Oncology Clinics of North America 1: 367–379

Hathaway W E, Bonnar J 1978 Bleeding disorders in the newborn infant. In: Oliver T K (ed) Perinatal coagulation, monographs in neonatology. Grune and Stratton, New York, p 115–169

Hathaway W E, Bonnar J 1987 Hemostatic disorders of the pregnant woman and newborn infant. Elsevier Science, New York

Hathaway W, Corrigan J 1991 Report of scientific and standardization subcommittee on neonatal hemostasis. Thrombosis and Haemostasis 65 (3): 323–325

Hathaway W E, Mull M M, Pechet G S 1969 Disseminated intravascular coagulation in the newborn. Pediatrics 43: 233–238

Hattersley P 1966 Activated coagulation time of whole blood. Journal of the American Medical Association 196 (5): 150–154

Hayden C K, Shattuck K E, Richardson C J, Ahrendt D K, House R, Swischu K 1985 Subependymal germinal matrix hemorrhage in fullterm neonates. Pediatrics 75: 714–718

Hedberg V A, Lipton J M 1988 Thrombocytopenia with absent radii. A review of 100 cases. American Journal of Pediatric Hematology and Oncology 10: 51–64

Heiden D, Mielke C H, Rodvien R, Hill J D 1975 Platelets, hemostasis and thromboembolism during treatment of accute respiratory insufficiency with extracorporeal membrane oxygenation. Journal of Thoracic and Cardiovascular Surgery 70: 644–655

Hellman L M, Shettles L B 1942 The prophylactic use of vitamin K in obstetrics. Southern Medical Journal 35: 289–293

Hensey O J, Morgan M E I, Cooke R W I 1984 Tranexamic acid in the prevention of periventricular hemorrhage. Archives of Diseases in Childhood 59: 519–721

Herson V C, Block C, Eisenfeld L, Maderazo E G, Krause P J 1989 Effects of intravenous fat infusion on neonatal neutrophil and platelet function. Journal of Parenteral and Enteral Nutrition 13: 620–622

Hey E, Jones P 1979 Coagulation failure in babies with rhesus isoimmunization. British Journal of Haematology 42: 441–454

Hiraike H, Kimura M, Itokawa Y 1988a Determination of K vitamins (phylloquinone and menaquinones) in umbilical cord plasma by a platinum-reduction column. Journal of Chromotography 430: 143–148

Hiraike H, Kimura M, Itokawa Y 1988b Distribution of K vitamins (phylloquinone and menaquinones) in human placenta and maternal and umbilical cord plasma. American Journal of Obstetrics and Gynecology 158: 564–569

Holmberg L, Henriksson P, Ekelund H, Astedt B 1974 Coagulation in the human fetus, comparison with term newborn infants. Journal of Pediatrics 85: 860–864

Homans A C, Cohen J L, Mazur E M 1988 Defective megakaryocytopoiesis in the syndrome of thrombocytopenia with absent radii. British Journal of Haematology 70: 205–210

Horgan M J, Carrasco N J M, Risemberg H 1985 The relationship of thrombocytopenia to the onset of persistent pulmonary hypertension of the newborn in the meconium aspiration syndrom. New York State Journal of Medicine 85: 245–247

Hoskova A, Mrskos A 1977 Haemorrhagic diathesis as a possible early sign of hereditary fructose intolerance. European Journal of Pediatrics 127: 63–65

Hrodek O 1966 Blood platelets in the newborn: their function in haemostasis and haemocoagulation. Acta Universitatis Carolinae Monograph 22

Israels S J, Seshia S S 1987 Childhood stroke associated with protein C or S deficiency. Journal of Pediatrics 111: 562–564

Israels L G, Friesen E, Jansen A H, Israels E D 1987a Vitamin K1 increases sister chromatid exchange in vitro in human leukocytes and in vivo in fetal sheep cells: A possible role for 'vitamin K deficiency' in the fetus. Pediatric Research 22: 405–408

Israels S J, Gowen B, Gerrard J M 1987b Contractile activity of neonatal platelets. Pediatric Research 21: 293–295

Israels S J, Daniels M, McMillan E M 1990 Deficient collagen-induced activation in the newborn platelet. Pediatric Research 27: 337–343

Jackson J C, Blumhagen J D 1983 Congenital hydrocephalus due to prenatal hemorrhage. Pediatrics 72: 344–346

Jackson J C, Truog W E, Watchko J F, Mack L A, Cyr D R, van Belle G 1987 Efficacy of thromboresistant umbilical artery catheters in reducing aortic thrombosis and related complications. Journal of Pediatrics 110: 102–105

Jensen A H, Josso S, Zamet P, Monset-Couchard M, Minkowski A 1973 Evolution of blood clotting factors in premature infants during the first ten days of life: A study of 96 cases with comparison between clinical status and blood clotting factor levels. Pediatric Research 7: 638–644

Jobin J, O'Regan S, Demay G, Mongeau J G, Robitaille P 1982 Neonatal renal vein thrombosis–long term follow-up after conservative management. Clinical Nephrology 17: 36–40

Johnston M, Zipursky A 1980 Microtechnology for the study of the blood coagulation system in newborn infants. Canadian Journal of Medical Technology 42: 159–164

Johnson C A, Sobrinho T C M, Aziz E M, Rogers S B 1976 Refractory coagulopathy in an infant with loss of clotting proteins into ascitic fluid Acta Pediatrica Scandinavica 65: 773–775

Johnson C A, Chung K S, McGrath K M, Bean P E, Roberts H R 1980 Characterization of a variant prothrombin in a patient congenitally deficient in factors II, VII, IX and X. British Journal of Haematology 44: 461–469

Johnson D H, Vinson A M, Wirth F H 1984 Management of hepatic hemangioendotheliomas of infancy by transarterial embolization: A report of two cases. Pediatrics 73: 546–549

Joist J J 1982 Hemostatic abnormalities in liver disease. In: Colman R W, Hirsh J et al (eds) Hemostasis and thrombosis. J B Lippincott, Philadelphia, p 861–872

Jorgensen F S, Fedding P, Vinther S, Andersen G E 1991 Vitamin K in neonates. Peroral versus intramuscular administration. Acta Paediatrica Scandinavica 80 (3): 304–307

Kaapa P 1985 Immunoreactive thromboxane B_2 and 6-keto-prostaglandin $F_1\alpha$ in neonatal hyperbilirubinemia. Prostaglandins Leukotrienes Medicine 17: 97–105

Kaapa P, Knip M, Viinikka L, Ylikorkala O 1986a Increased platelet thromboxane B_2 production in newborn infants of diabetic mothers. Prostaglandins Leukotrienes Medicine 21: 299–304

Kaapa P, Uhari M, Nikkari J, Viinikka L, Ylikorkala O 1986b Dietary fatty acid and platelet thromboxane production in puerperal women and their offspring. American Journal of Obstetrics and Gynecology 155: 146–149

Kaplan C, Daffos F, Forestier F et al 1988 Management of alloimmune thrombocytopenia: Antenatal diagnosis and in utero transfusion of maternal platelets. Blood 72: 340–343

Kaplan C, Morel-Kopp M C, Kroll H 1991 HPA-5b (Bra) neonatal alloimmuno thrombocytopenia: clinical and immunological analysis of 39 cases. British Journal of Haematology 78: 425–429

Kapoor N, Kirkpatrick D, Blaese R M 1981 Reconstitution of normal megakaryocytopoiesis and immunologic functions in Wiskott–Aldrich syndrome by marrow transplantation following myeloablation and immunosuppression with busulfan and cyclophosphamide. Blood 57: 692–696

Karim M A G, Clelland I A, Chapman I V, Walker C H M 1981 B-thromboglobulin levels in plasma of jaundiced neonates exposed to phototherapy. Journal of Perinatal Medicine 3: 141–144

Karitzky D, Kleine N, Pringsheim W, Kunzer W 1971 Fibrinogen turnover in the premature infant with and without idiopathic respiratory distress syndrome. Acta Paediatrica Scandinavica 60: 465–470

Karpatkin M, Porges R F, Karpatkin S 1981 Platelet counts in infants of women with autoimmune thrombocytopenia: Effects of steroid administration to the mother. New England Journal of Medicine 305: 936–939

Karpatkin M, Manucci P M, Bhogal M, Vigano S, Nardi M 1986 Low protein C in the neonatal period. British Journal of Haematology 62: 137–142

Karpatkin M, Blei F, Hurlet A, Greco A, Tang Z 1991 Prothrombin expression in the adult and fetal rabbit liver. Pediatric Research 30: 266–269

Katz J, Rodriguez E, Mandani G, Branson H E 1982 Normal coagulation findings, thrombocytopenia, and peripheral hemoconcentration in neonatal polycythemia. Journal of Pediatrics 101: 99–102

Katz J A, Moake J L, McPherson P D, Weinstein M J, Moise K J 1989 Relationship between human development and disappearance of unusually large von Willebrand factor multimers from plasma. Blood 73: 1851–1858

Kaufmann H J 1958 Renal vein thrombosis. American Journal of Diseases of Children 95: 377–384

Kazzi N J, Ilagen M B, Liang K C 1989 Maternal administration of vitamin K does not improve the coagulation profile of preterm infants. Pediatrics 84: 1045–1050

Keenan W J, Jewett T, Glueck H I 1971 Role of feeding and vitamin K in hypoprothrombinemia of the newborn. American Journal of Diseases of Children 121: 271–277

Kelly D A, Summerfield J A 1987 Hemostasis in liver disease. Seminars in Liver Disease 7: 182–191

Kelton J G, Blanchette V S, Wilson W E et al 1980 Neonatal thrombocytopenia due to passive immunization. Prenatal diagnosis and distinction between maternal platelet alloantibodies and autoantibodies. New England Journal of Medicine 302: 1401–1403

Kelton J G, Powers P J, Carter C J 1982 A prospective study of the usefulness of the measurement of platelet associated IgG for the diagnosis of idiopathic thrombocytopenia purpura. Blood Vol 60: 1050–1053

Khurshid M, Lee T J, Pealre I R, Bloom A L 1975 Vitamin E

deficiency and platelet function defect in a jaundiced infant. British Medical Journal 4: 19–21
Kiefel V, Santoso S, Weisheit M, Mueller-Eckhardt C 1987 Monoclonal antibody-specific immobilization of platelet antigens (MAIPA): a new tool for the identification of platelet-reactive antibodies. Blood 70: 1722–1726
Kipper S, Sieger L 1982 Whole blood platelet volumes in newborn infants. Journal of Pediatrics 101: 763–766
Kisker C T, Robillard J E et al 1981 Development of blood coagulation-a fetal lamb model. Pediatric Research 15: 1045–1050
Kisker C T, Perlman S, Bohlken D, Wicklund D 1988 Measurement of prothrombin mRNA during gestation and early neonatal development. Journal of Laboratory and Clinical Medicine 112: 407–412
Koepke J A 1986 Partial thromboplastin time test — proposed performance guidelines. ICSH panel on the APTT. Thrombosis and Haemostasis 55: 143–144
Kolindewala J K, Das B K, Dube B, Bhargava B 1987 Blood fibrinolytic activity in neonates: Effect of period of gestation, birth weight, anoxia and sepsis. Indian Pediatrics 24: 1029–1033
Kosmetatos N, Dinter C, Williams M L, Lourie H, Berne A S 1980 Intracranial haemorrhage in the premature: Its predictive features and outcome. American Journal of Diseases of Children 13: 855–859
Kotohara K, Endo F 1985 Effect of vitamin K administration of acarboxy prothrombin (PIVKA-II) levels in newborns. Lancet 2: 242–244
Kries R V, Shearer M J, Gobel U 1988 Vitamin K in infancy. European Journal of Pediatrics 147: 106–112
Krummel T M, Greenfield L J, Kirkpatrick B V et al 1984 The early evaluation of survivors after extracorporeal membrane oxygenation for neonatal pulmonary failure. Journal of Pediatric Surgery 19: 585–590
Kugelmass I N 1932 The management of hemorrhagic problems in infancy and childhood. Journal of the American Medical Association 99: 895–897
Laffi G, La Villa G, Pinzani M 1986 Altered renal and platelet arachidonic acid metabolism in cirrhosis. Gastroenterology 90: 274–282
Lane P A, Hathaway W E 1985 Medical Progress: Vitamin K in infancy. Journal of Pediatrics 106: 351–359
Lane P A, Hathaway W E, Githens J H, Krugman R D, Rosenberg P A 1983 Fatal intracranial hemorrhage in a normal infant secondary to vitamin K deficiency. Pediatrics 72: 562–564
Laosombat V 1988 Hemorrhagic disease of the newborn after maternal anticonvulsant therapy: A case report and literature review. Journal of the Medical Association of Thailand 71: 643–648
Lawson R B 1941 Treatment of hypoprothrombinemia (hemorrhagic disease) of the newborn infant. Journal of Pediatrics 18: 224–234
Lehmann J 1944 Vitamin K as a prophylactic in 13 000 infants. Lancet i: 493–494
Lesko S M, Mitchell A A, Eopstein M F, Louik C, Gracoia G P, Shapiro S 1986 Heparin use a risk factor for intraventricular hemorrhage in low birth weight infants. New England Journal of Medicine 314: 1156–1160
Levanon M, Rimon S, Shani M, Ramot B, Goldberg E 1972 Active and inactive factor VII in Dubin–Johnson syndrome with factor VII deficiency, hereditary factor VII deficiency and on coumadin administration. British Journal of Haematology 23: 669–677
Levene M I, de Vries L 1984 Extension of neonatal intraventricular hemorrhage. Archives of Diseases in Childhood 59: 631–636
Levine D L, Weinberg A G, Perin R M 1983 Pulmonary microthrombi syndrome in newborn infants with unresponsive persistent pulmonary hypertension. Journal of Pediatrics 102: 299–303
Levine A B, Berkowitz R L 1991 Neonatal alloimmune thrombocytopenia. Seminars in Perinatology 15 (suppl 2): 35–40
Levine M N, Hirsh J 1986 Hemorrhagic complications of anticoagulant therapy. Seminars in Thrombosis and Haemostasis 12: 39–57
Levine J J, Udall J N, Evernden B A, Epstein M F, Bloch K J 1987 Elevated levels of α_2-macroglobulin-protease complexes in infants. Biology of the Neonate 51: 149
Levy G, Garrettson L K 1974 Kinetics of salicylate elimination by newborn infants of mothers who ingested aspirin before delivery Pediatrics 53: 201–209
Liebermann J 1961 The nature of the fibrinolytic enzyme defect in hyaline membrane disease. New England Journal of Medicine 265: 363–369
Linder N, Shapiro S C, Moser A M, Roitman J, Engelhard D 1990 Treatment of neonatal immune thrombocytopenia with high dose intravenous gamma-globulin. Developmental Pharmacology and Therapeutics 14: 205–208
Ling X, Delorme M, Berry L, Brooker L, Mitchell L, Andrew M 1991 Thrombin generation in newborn and adult plasma in the presence of an endothelial surface. Thrombosis and Haemostasis 65(6): 1230 (abstract)
Lipscomb A P, Thorburn R J, Reynolds E O R 1981 Pneumothorax and cerebral haemorrhage in preterm infants. Lancet 1: 414
Lorand L, Losowsky M S, Miloszewski K J M 1980 Human factor XIII: Fibrin stabilizing factor. Progress in Haemostasis and Thrombosis 5: 245–290
Lou H C 1980 Perinatal hypoxic-ischaemic brain damage and intraventricular haemorrhage: A pathogenic model. Archives of Neurology 37: 585
Lowry M F, Mann J R, Abrams L D, Chance G W 1970 Thrombectomy for renal venous thrombosis in infant of diabetic mother. British Medical Journal 3: 687
Lucey J F, Dolan R G 1959 Hyperbilirubinemia of newborn infants associated with the parenteral administration of a vitamin K analogue to the mothers. Pediatrics 23: 553–560
Lum L G, Tubergen D G, Corash L, Blaese R M 1980 Splenectomy in the management of the thrombocytopenia of the Wiskott–Aldrich syndrome. New England Journal of Medicine 302: 892–896
Lupton B A, Hill A, Whitfield M F, Carter C J, Wadsworth L D, Roland E H 1988 Reduced platelet count as a risk factor for intraventricular haemorrhage. American Journal of Diseases of Children 142: 1222–1224
McDonald M M, Hathaway W E 1982 Anticoagulant therapy by continuous heparinization in newborn and older infants. Journal of Pediatrics 101: 451–457
McDonald M M, Hathaway W E 1983 Neonatal haemorrhage and thrombosis. Seminars in Perinatology 7: 213–225
McDonald M M, Johnson M L, Rumack C M et al 1984 Role of coagulopathy in newborn intracranial haemorrhage. Pediatrics 74: 26–31
MacElfresh M E 1961 Coagulation during the neonatal period. American Journal of Medical Science 242: 77
McFarland J G, Frenzke M, Aster R H 1989 Testing of maternal sera in pregnancies at risk for neonatal alloimmune thrombocytopenia. Transfusion 29: 128–133
Mack L A, Wright K et al 1981 Intracranial hemorrhage in premature infants: Accuracy of sonographic evaluation. American Journal of Roentgenology 137: 245–250
Mackay R J, Crespigny L, Laurence J, Morton R, Neil D 1984 Intraventricular haemorrhage in term neonates: Diagnosis by ultrasound. Australian Paediatric Journal 18: 205–209
McNinch A W, Orme R L, Tripp J W 1983 Haemorrhagic diseases of the newborn returns. Lancet 1: 1089–1093
McNinch A W, Upton C, Samuels M et al 1985 Plasma concentrations after oral or intramuscular vitamin K_1 in neonates. Archives of Disease in Childhood 60: 814–818
McParland P, Pearce J M, Chamberlain G V 1990 Doppler ultrasound and aspirin in recognition and prevention of pregnancy-induced hypertension. Lancet: 1552–1555
Mahasandana C, Hathaway W E 1973 Circulating anticoagulants in the newborn: Relation to hypercoagulability and the idiopathic respiratory distress syndrome. Pediatric Research 7: 670–673
Malia R G, Preston F E et al 1980 Evidence against vitamin K deficiency in normal neonates. Thrombosis and Haemostasis 44: 159–160
Mammen E F 1983a Factor II abnormalities. Seminars in Thrombosis and Haemostasis 9: 13–16
Mammen E F 1983b Factor V deficiency. Seminars in Thrombosis and Haemostasis 9: 17–18
Mammen E F 1983c Factor X abnormalities. Seminars in Thrombosis and Haemostasis 9: 31–33
Mammen E F 1983d Fibrinogen abnormalities. Seminars in Thrombosis and Haemostasis 9: 1–9

Manco-Johnson M 1989 Neonatal antithrombin III deficiency. American Journal of Medicine 87 (suppl 3B): 49S–52S
Manco-Johnson M, Abshire T C, Jacobson L J, Marlar R A 1991 Severe neonatal protein C deficiency: Prevalence and thrombotic risk. Journal of Pediatrics 119: 793–798
Mandelbrot L, Guillaumont M, Forestier F et al 1988 Placental transfer of vitamin K_1 and its implications in fetal haemostasis. Thrombosis Haemostasis 60: 39–43
Mannino F L, Travner D A 1983 Stroke in neonates. Journal of Pediatrics 102: 605–610
Marciniak E, Wilson H D, Marlar R A 1985 Neonatal purpura fulminans: A genetic disorder related to the absence of protein C in blood. Blood 65: 15–20
Mariani G, Mazzucconi M G 1983 Factor VII congenital deficiency. Haemostasis 13: 169–177
Markarian M, Lindley A, Jackson J J, Bannon A 1967a Coagulation factors in pregnant women and premature infants with and without the respiratory distress syndrome. Thrombosis Diathesis Haemorrhagica 17: 585–594
Markarian M, Githens J, Jackson J et al 1967b Fibrinolytic activity in premature infants. Relationship of the enzyme system to the respiratory distress syndrome. American Journal of the Diseased Child 113: 312–321
Markarian M, Githens J H, Fernandez F et al 1971a Hypercoagulability in premature infants with special reference to the respiratory distress syndrome and haemorrhage. 1. Coagulation studies. Biology of the Neonate 17: 84–97
Markarian M, Luchenco L O, Rosenblut E 1971b Hypercoagulability in premature infants with special reference to the respiratory distress syndrome and hemorrhage. II. The effect of heparin. Biology of the Neonate 17: 98
Marlar R A, Montgomery R R, Broekmans A W, and the working party 1989 Diagnosis and treatment of homozygous protein C deficiency. Journal of Pediatrics 114: 528–534
Marsh J L, King W, Barrett C, Fonkalsrud E W 1975 Serious complications after umbilical artery catheterization for neonatal monitoring. Archives of Surgery 110: 1203
Martin-Bouyer G, Linh P D, Tuan L C 1983 Epidemic of haemorrhagic disease in Vietmanese infants caused by warfarin-contaminated talcs. Lancet 1: 230–233
Massicotte-Nolan P, Mitchell L et al 1986 Animal models of neonatal coagulation. Pediatric Research 20: 961
Matsuda I, Nishiyama S, Motohara K, Endo F, Ogata T, Futagoishi Y 1989 Late neonatal vitamin K deficiency associated with subclinical liver dysfunction in human milk fed infants. Journal of Pediatrics 114: 602–605
Matzch T, Bergqvist D, Bergqvist A et al 1991 No transplacental passage of standard heparin or an enzymatically depolymerized low molecular weight heparin. Blood Coagulation and Fibrinolysis 2: 273–278
Maurer H M, Haggins J C, Still W J S 1976 Platelet injury during phototherapy. American Journal of Hematology 1: 89–96
Mehta P, Vasa R, Newman L, Karpatkin M 1980 Thrombocytopenia in the high risk infant. Journal of Pediatrics 97: 791–794
Ment L R, Stewart W, Scott D, Duncan C 1983 Beagle puppy model of intraventricular hemorrhage: Randomized indomethacin prevention trial. Neurology 33: 179–184
Ment L R, Duncan C C, Ehrenkranz R A et al 1984 Intraventricular hemorrhage in the preterm neonate: Timing and cerebral blood flow changes. Journal of Pediatrics 104: 419–425
Ment L R, Duncan C C, Ehrenkranz R A 1985 Randomized indomethacin trial for prevention of intraventricular hemorrhage in very low birth weight infants. Journal of Pediatrics 107: 937–943
Ment L R, Duncan C C, Ehrenkranz R A 1987 Intraventricular hemorrhage of the preterm neonate. Seminars in Perinatology 11: 132–141
Ment L R, Duncan C C, Ehrenkranz R A 1988a Randomized low dose indomethacin trial for prevention of intraventricular hemorrhage in very low birth weight neonates. Journal of Pediatrics 112: 948–955
Ment L R, Ehrenkranz R A et al 1988b Intraventricular hemorrhage of the preterm neonate: prevention studies. Seminars in Perinatology 12: 359–372
Mibashan R S, Rodeck C H, Thumpson J K, Edwards R J, Singer J D, White J M 1979 Plasma assay of fetal factors VIIIc and IX for prenatal diagnosis of haemophilia. Lancet 1: 1309–1311
Mir N, Samson D, House M J, Kavan I Z 1988 Failure of antenatal high-dose immunoglobulin to improve fetal platelet count in neonatal alloimmune thrombocytopenia. Vox Sanguinis 55: 188–189
Moalic P, Gruel Y, Body G, Foloppe P, Dalahousse B, Leroy J 1988 Levels and plasma distribution of free and C4b-BP-bound Protein S in human fetuses and fullterm newborns. Thrombosis Research 49: 471–480
Moise K J, Carpenter R J, Cotton D B, Wasserstrom N, Kirshon B, Cano L 1988 Percutaneous umbilical cord blood sampling in the evaluation of fetal platelet counts in pregnant patients with autoimmune thrombocytopenia purpura. Obstetrics and Gynecology 72: 346–350
Mokrohisky S T, Levin R, Blumhagen J B, Wesenberg R L, Simmons S A 1978 Low positioning of umbilical artery catheters increases associated complications in newborn infants. New England Journal of Medicine 299: 561–564
Monnens L A H, Retera F J M 1967 Thrombotic thrombocytopenia purpura in a neonatal infant. Journal of Pediatrics 71: 118–123
Montgomery R R, Marlar R A, Gill J C 1985 Newborn haemostasis. Clinical Haematology 14: 443–460
Morales W J, Angel J L, O'Brien W F, Knuppel R A, Marsalisi F 1988 The use of antenatal vitamin K in the prevention of early neonatal intraventricular hemorrhage. American Journal of Obstetrics and Gynecology 159(3): 774–779
Morgan M E I, Ben J W T, Cooke R W I 1981 Ethamsylate reduces the incidence of periventricular haemorrhage in very low birth weight babies. Lancet 2: 830–831
Mori P G, Bisogni S, Odini S et al 1977 Vitamin K deficiency in the newborn (letter). Lancet 2: 188
Motohara K, Kuroki Y, Kan H, Endo F, Matsuda I 1985 Detection of vitamin K deficiency by use of an enzyme-linked immunosorbent assay for circulating abnormal prothrombin. Pediatric Research 19: 354–357
Motohara K, Matsukura M, Matsuda I, Irbe K, Tsuchiya F 1984 Severe vitamin K deficiency in breast-fed infants. Journal of Pediatrics 105: 943–945
Motohara K, Endo F, Matsuda I 1986 Vitamin K deficiency in breast-fed infants at one month of age. Journal of Pediatric Gastroenterological Nutrition 5: 931–933
Motohara K, Endo F, Matsuda I 1987 Screening for late neonatal vitamin K deficiency by acarboxyprothrombin in dried blood spots. Archives of Disease in Childhood 62: 370–375
Motohara K, Matsukane I, Endo F, Kiyota Y, Matsuda I 1989 Relationship of milk intake and vitamin K supplementation to vitamin K status in newborns. Pediatrics 84: 90–93
Mountain K R, Hirsh J, Gallus A S 1970 Neonatal coagulation defect due to anticonvulsant drug treatment in pregnancy. Lancet 1: 265–268
Mueller-Eckhardt C, Mueller-Eckhardt G, Willen-Ohff H 1985 Immunogenicity and immune-response to the human platelet antigen Zwa is strongly associated with HLA-B8 and DR3. Tissue Antigens 26: 71–76
Mueller-Eckhardt C, Becker T, Weishert M, Witz C, Santosa S 1986 Neonatal alloimmune thrombocytopenia due to fetomaternal Zw^b incompatibility. Vox Sanguinis 50: 94–96
Mueller-Eckhardt C, Kiefel V, Grubert A et al 1989 348 cases of suspected neonatal alloimmune thrombocytopenia. Lancet 1: 363–366
Mull M M, Hathaway W E 1970 Altered platelet function in newborns. Pediatric Research 4: 229–237
Mull J W, Bill A H et al 1941 Effect on the newborn of vitamin K administered to mothers in labor. Journal of Laboratory and Clinical Medicine 26: 1305–1309
Muller A D, van Doorm J M 1977 Heparin like inhibitor of blood coagulation in normal newborn. Nature 267: 616–617
Muntean W, Rosseger H 1989 Antithrombin III concentrate in preterm infants with IRDS: An open, controlled, randomized clinical trial. Thrombosis and Haemostasis 62: 288 (abstract)
Muntean W, Petck W, Rosanelli K, Mutz I D 1979 Immunologic studies of prothrombin in newborns. Pediatric Research 13: 1262–1265

Murphy S, Oski F A, Naiman J L, Lusch C J, Goldberg S, Gardner F H 1972 Platelet size and kinetics in hereditary and acquired thrombocytopenia. New England Journal of Medicine 286: 499–504
Neal W A, Reynolds J W, Jarvis C W, Williams H J 1972 Umbilical artery catheterization: demonstration of arterial thrombosis by aortography. Pediatrics 50: 6–13
Nicolini U, Rodeck C H, Kochenour N K, Greco P, Fisk N M, Letsky E 1988 In utero platelet transfusion for alloimmune thrombocytopenia (letter). Lancet 2: 506
Nossel H L, Lanzkowsky P, Levy S, Mibashan R S, Hansen J D L 1966 A study of coagulation factor levels in women during labour and in their newborn infants. Thrombosis Diathesis Haemorrhagica 16: 185–197
Nygaard K K 1939 Prophylactic and curative effect of vitamin K in hemorrhagic disease of the newborn (hypothrombinemia hemorrhagica neonatorum). A preliminary report. Acta Obstetrica Gynecologica Scandinavica 19: 361–370
Obladen M, Ernst D, Fiest D 1975 Portal hypertension in children following neonatal umbilical disorders. Journal of Perinatal Medicine 3: 101–104
O'Brodovich H, Coates J 1984 Quantitative ventilation perfusion lung scans in infants and children: Utility of a submicronic radiolabelled aerosol to assess ventilation. Journal of Pediatrics 105: 377–383
Ochs H D, Slichter S J, Harker L A, Von Behrens W E, Clark R A, Wedgewood R J 1980 The Wiskott–Aldrich syndrome: Studies of lymphocytes, granulocytes and platelets. Blood 55: 243–252
O'Connor M E, Addiego J E 1986 Use of oral vitamin K_1 to prevent hemorrhagic disease of the newborn infant. Journal of Pediatrics 108: 616–619
Ockelford P A, Carter C J 1982 Disseminated intravascular coagulation: The application and utility of diagnostic tests. Seminars in Thrombosis and Haemostasis 8: 198–216
Odievre M, Hadchouel P, Dupuy J M, Alagille D 1976 Coagulation intravasculaire et insuffisance hepatique grave du nourrison. Archives Francaises Pediatriques 33: 31–36
Ogata T, Motohara K, Endo F et al 1988 Vitamin K effect in low birth weight infants. Pediatrics 81: 423–427
Olinsky A, Aitken F G, Isdale J M 1975 Thrombus formation after umbilical arterial catherization: an angiographic study. South African Medical Journal 49: 1467–1470
Olson J A. 1987 Recommended dietary intakes (RDI) of vitamin K in humans. American Journal of Clinical Nutrition 45: 687–692
O'Neill J A, Neblett W W III, Born M L 1981 Management of major thromboembolic complications of umbilical artery catheters. Journal of Pediatric Surgery 16: 972–978
Orchard P J, Smith C M III, Woods W G, Day D L, Dehner L P, Shapiro R 1989 Treatment of haemangioendotheliomas with alpha interferon. Lancet: 565–567
O'Rourke P P, Crone R K, Vacanti J P 1989 Extracorporeal membrane oxygenation (ECMO) and conventional medical therapy in neonates with persistent pulmonary hypertension of the newborn: A prospective randomized study. Pediatrics 84: 957–963
Oski F A, Allen D M, Diamond L K 1963 Portal hypertension–A complication of umbilical vein catherization. Pediatrics 31: 297–302
Palma P A, Miner M E et al 1979 Intraventricular hemorrhage in the neonate at term. American Journal of Diseases of Children 133: 941–944
Pao M, Karlowicz M G, Kickler T S, Zinkhan W H 1991 Importance of platelet serologic testing for defining the cause of neonatal thrombocytopenia. American Journal of Pediatric Hematology/ Oncology 13: 71–76
Pape K E, Bennett-Britton S, Szywonowicz W, Martin D J, Fitz C R, Becker L 1983 Diagnostic accuracy of neonatal brain imaging: A postmortem correlation of computed tomography and ultrasound scans. Journal of Pediatrics 102: 275–280
Papile L-A, Burstein J et al 1978 Incidence and evolution of subependymal and intraventricular hemorrhage: A study of infants with birth weights less than 1500 gm. Journal of Pediatrics 92: 529–534
Parkman R, Rappaport J, Geha R 1978 Complete correction of the Wiskott–Aldrich syndrome by allogeneic bone-marrow transplantation. New England Journal of Medicine 298: 921–927
Parks J, Sweet L K 1942 Does the antenatal use of vitamin K prevent hemorrhage in the newborn infant? American Journal of Obstetrics and Gynaecology 44: 432–442
Patrick C H, Lazarchick J 1990 The effect of bacteremia on automated platelet measurements in neonates. American Journal of Clinical Pathology 93: 391–394
Payne N R, Hasegawa D K 1984 Vitamin K deficiency in newborns: A case report in α-1-antitrypsin deficiency and a review of factors predisposing to hemorrhage. Pediatrics 73: 712–716
Pearson H A, McIntosh S 1978 Neonatal thrombocytopenia. Clinical Haematology 7: 111–122
Pearson H A, Shulman N R, Marder V J, Cone T E 1964 Isoimmune neonatal thrombocytopenic purpura. Clinical and therapeutic considerations. Blood 23: 154–177
Pegels J G, Bruynes E C E, Engelfriet C P, von dem Borne A E G Kr 1982 Pseudothrombocytopenia: An immunologic study on platelet antibodies dependent on ethylene diamine tetra-acetate. Blood 59: 157–161
Pencharz P B, Steffee W P, Cochran W, Scrimshaw N S, Rand W M, Young V R 1977 Protein metabolism in human neonates: Nitrogen-balance studies, estimated obligatory losses of nitrogen and whole-body turnover of nitrogen. Clinical Science and Molecular Medicine 52: 485–498
Perlman J M, Dvilansky A 1975 Blood coagulation status of small-for-dates and postmature infants. Archives of Diseases in Childhood 50: 424
Perlman J M, Hill A, Volpe J J 1981 The effect of patent ductus arteriosus on flow velocity in the anterior cerebral arteries: Ductal steal in the premature newborn infant. Journal of Pediatrics 99: 767–771
Perlman J M, McMenamin J B, Volpe J J 1983a Fluctuating cerebral blood-flow velocity in respiratory distress syndrome. New England Journal of Medicine 309: 204
Perlman J M, Nelson J S, McAlister W H, Volpe J J 1983b Intracerebellar haemorrhage in a permature newborn: Diagnosis by real-time ultrasound and correlation with autopsy findings. Pediatrics 71: 159–162
Perlman J M, Goodman S, Kreuser K L, Volpe J J 1985 Reduction in intraventricular hemorrhage by elimination of fluctuating cerebral blood-flow velocity in preterm infants with respiratory distress syndrome New England Journal of Medicine 312: 1353–1357
Peters M, Jansen E, ten Cate J W, Kahle L H, Ockelford P, Breederveld C 1984a Neonatal antithrombin III. British Journal of Haematology 58: 579–587
Peters M, ten Cate J W, Breederveld C, De Leeuw R, Emeis J, Koppe J 1984b Low antithrombin III levels in neonates with idiopathic respiratory distress syndrome: Poor prognosis. Pediatric Research 18: 273–276
Phillips L L 1967 Alterations in blood clotting system in disseminated intravascular coagulation. American Journal of Cardiology 20: 174
Pietz J, Kiefel V, Sontheimer D, Kobialka B, Linderkamp O, Mueller-Eckhardt C 1991 High-dose intravenous gammaglobulin for neonatal alloimmune thrombocytopenia in twins. Acta Paediatrica Scandinavica 80: 129–132
Podolsak B 1973 Thrombopoeisis in newborn infants after exchange blood transfusion. Zeitschrift fur Kinderheilkdam 114: 13–26
Pomerance J J, Teal J G, Gogdok J F, Brown S, Stewart M E 1987 Maternally administered antenatal vitamin K_1: Effect on neonatal prothrombin activity, partial thromboplastin time, and intraventricular hemorrhage. Obstetrics and Gynecology 70: 235–241
Potter E L 1945 The effect on infant mortality of vitamin K administered during labor. American Journal of Obstetrics and Gynecology 50: 235–247
Pritchard J A, Cunningham F G, Pritchard S A, Mason R A 1987 How often does maternal preeclampsia-eclampsia incite thrombocytopenia in the fetus? Obstetrics and Gynecology 69: 292–295
Quick A J, Grossman A M 1939 Concentration of prothrombin in blood of babies (3 to 7 days old). Proceedings of the Society for Experimental Biology and Medicine 40: 647–648
Ragni M V, Lewis J J, Spero J A, Hasiba U 1986 Factor VII deficiency. American Journal of Hematology 10: 79–88
Rajani K, Goetzman B W, Wennberg R P, Turner E, Abildgaard C 1979 Effect of heparinization of fluids infused through an umbilical artery catheter on catheter patency and frequency of complications. Pediatrics 63: 552–556

Rapaport S I, Proctor R R, Patch J J, Yettra M 1961 The mode of inheritance of PTA deficiency: Evidence for the existence of major PTA deficiency and minor PTA deficiency. Blood 18: 149–165
Rasoulpour M, McLean R H 1980 Renal venous thrombosis in neonates. Initial and follow-up abnormalities. American Journal of Diseases of Children 134: 276–279
Rennie J M, Doyle J, Cooke R W I 1986 Early administration of indomethacin to preterm infants. Archives of Diseases in Childhood 61: 233–238
Reverdiau-Moalie P, Gruel Y, Delahousse B et al 1991 Comparative study of the fibrinolytic system in human fetuses and in pregnant women. Thrombosis Research 61: 489–499
Reznikoff-Etievant M F 1988 Management of alloimmune neonatal and antenatal thrombocytopenia. Vox Sanguinis 55: 193–201
Reznikoff-Etievant M F, Muller J Y, Julien F, Patereau C 1983 An immune response gene linked to HLA in man. Tissue Antigens 22: 312–313
Riess H, Binsack T, Hiller E 1985 Protein C antigen in prothrombin complex concentrates: content, recovery, and half life. Blut 50: 303–306
Rivers R P A 1975 Coagulation changes associated with a high haematocrit in the newborn infant. Acta Pediatrica Scandinavica 64: 449
Roberts H R, Cederbaum A I 1972 The liver and blood coagulation: Physiology and pathology. Gastroenterology 63: 297–320
Rodriguez-Erdmann F 1965 Bleeding due to increased intravascular blood coagulation. Hemorrhagic syndrome caused by consumption of blood clotting factors (Consumption coagulopathies). New England Journal of Medicine 273: 1370–1378
Rose S J 1985 Neonatal hemorrhage and vitamin K. Acta Haematologica 74: 121
Rosenberg E R, Trought W S, Kirks D R, Sumner T E, Grossman H 1980 Ultrasonic diagnosis of renal vein thrombosis in neonates. American Journal of Roentgenology 134: 35
Rote N S, Lau R J 1985 Immunologic thrombocytopenic purpura. Clinical Obstetrics and Gynecology 28: 84–100
Runnebaum I B, Maurer S M, Daly L, Bonnar J 1989 Inhibitors and activators of fibrinolysis during and after childbirth in maternal and cord blood. Journal of Perinatal Medicine 17: 113–119
Sackett D L 1986 Rules of evidence and clinical recommendations on the use of agents. Archives of Internal Medicine 146: 464–465
Samuels P, Bussel J B, Braitman L E 1990 Estimation of the risk of thrombocytopenia in the offspring of pregnant women with presumed immune thrombocytopenic purpura. New England Journal of Medicine 323: 229–235
Sanford H N, Leslie E I 1938 Blood coagulation factors in hemorrhagic disease of the newborn and the value of intramuscular injections of father's and mother's blood. Journal of Pediatrics 12: 16–20
Sanford H N, Gasteyer T H, Wyatt L 1932 The substances involved in the coagulation of the blood of the newborn. American Journal of Diseases of Children 43: 566–568
Sanford H N, Shmigelsky I, Chapin J M 1942 Is administration of vitamin K to the newborn of clinical value? Journal of the American Medical Association 118: 697–702
Sann L, Leclercq M, Guillaumont M, Trouyez R, Bethenod M, Bourgeay-Causse M 1985a Serum vitamin K1 concentrations after oral administration of vitamin K_1 in low birth weight infants. Journal of Pediatrics 107: 608–611
Sann L, Leclercq M et al 1985b Pharmacokinetics of vitamin K_1 in low-birth-weight neonates. Developmental Pharmacology and Therapeutics 8: 269–275
Saving K, Aldag J, Jennings D, Caughey B, Regan M, Powers W 1991 Electron microscopic characterization of neonatal platelet ultrastructure: Effects of sampling techniques. Thrombosis Research 61: 65–80
Scher M S, Wright F S, Lockman L A, Thompson T R 1982 Intraventricular hemorrhage in the fullterm neonate. Archives of Neurology 39: 769–772
Schmidt B, Andrew M 1988 Neonatal thrombotic disease: Prevention, diagnosis and therapy. Journal of Pediatrics 113: 407–410
Schmidt B, Andrew M 1992 Report of scientific and standardization subcommittee on neonatal hemostasis diagnosis and treatment of neonatal thrombosis. Thrombosis and Haemostasis 67: 381–382
Schmidt B, Zipursky A 1984. Thrombotic disease in newborn infants. Clinics in Perinatology 11: 461–488
Schmidt B, Wais U, Pringsheim W, Kunzer W 1984 Plasma elimination of antithrombin III is accelerated in term newborn infants. European Journal of Pediatrics 141: 225–227
Schmidt B, Buchanan M R, Ofosu F, Brooker L, Hirsh J, Andrew M 1988a Antithrombotic properties of heparin in a neonatal piglet model of thrombin induced thrombosis. Thrombosis Haemostasis 60: 289–292
Schmidt B, Mitchell L, Ofosu F, Andrew M 1988b Standard assays underestimate the concentration of heparin in neonatal plasma. Journal of Laboratory and Clinical Medine 112: 641–643
Schmidt B, Mitchell L, Ofosu F, Andrew M 1989a Alpha-2-macroglobulin is an important progressive inhibitor of thrombin in neonatal and infant plasma. Thrombosis Haemostasis 62: 1074–1077
Schmidt B, Ofosu F A, Mitchell L, Brooker L A, Andrew M 1989b Anticoagulant effects of heparin in neonatal plasma. Pediatric Research 25: 405–408
Schmidt B K, Vegh P, Weitz J, Johnston M, Caco C, Roberts R 1991 Thrombin/antithrombin III complex formation in the neonatal respiratory distress syndrome. Unpublished observations
Schwarz H P, Muntean W, Watzke H, Richter B, Griffin J H 1988 Low total protein S antigen but high protein S activity due to decreased C_4b-binding protein in neonates. Blood 71: 562–565
Scott J M 1965 Iatrogenic lesions in babies following umbilical vein catheterization. Archives of Disease in Childhood 40: 426–429
Scott J R, Cruikshank D P, Kochenouri N K, Pitkin R M, Warenski 1980 Fetal platelet counts in the obstetric management of immunologic purpura. American Journal of Obstetrics and Gynecology 136: 495–499
Seibert J J, Taylor B J, Williamson S L, Williams B T, Szabo J S, Corbitt S L 1987 Sonographic detection of neonatal umbilical-artery thrombosis. American Journal of Roentgenology 148: 965–968
Seligsohn U, Shani M et al 1970 Gilbert syndrome and factor VIII deficiency. Lancet 1: 1398
Sells R L, Walker S A, Owen C A 1941 Rouncen K requirement of the newborn infant. Proceedings of the Society for Experimental Biology and Medicine 47: 441–445
Serfontein G L, Rom S, Stein S 1980 Posterior fossa subdural hemorrhage in the newborn. Pediatrics 65: 40
Setzer E S, Webb I B, Wassenaar J W, Reeder J D, Mehta P S, Eitzman D V 1982 Platelet dysfunction and coagulopathy in intraventricular hemorrhage in the premature infant. Journal of Pediatrics 100: 599–605
Shah J K, Mitchell L G, Paes B, Ofosu F A, Schmidt B, Andrew M 1991 Thrombin inhibition is impaired in plasma of sick neonates. Pediatric Research 31: 391–395
Shapiro M E, Riodvien R, Bauer K A, Salzman E W 1981 Acute aortic thrombosis in antithrombin III deficiency. Journal of the American Medical Association 245: 1759–1761
Shapiro A D, Jacobson L J, Aramon M E et al 1986 Vitamin K deficiency in the newborn infant: Prevalence and perinatal risk factors. Journal of Pediatrics 109: 675–680
Shearer M J, Barkhan P, Rahim S, Stimmler L 1982 Plasma vitamin K_1 in mothers and their newborn babies. Lancet 2: 460–463
Shibata Y, Matsuda I, Miyaji T, Ichikawa Y 1986a Yuk^a, a new platelet antigen involved in two cases of neonatal alloimmune thrombocytopenia. Vox Sanguinis 50: 117–180
Shibata Y, Miyaji T, Ichikawa Y, Matsuda I 1986b A new platelet antigen system, Yuk^a/Yuk^b. Vox Sanguinis 51: 334–336
Shim K T 1968 Hemangiomas of infancy complicated by thrombocytopenia. American Journal of Surgery 116: 896–906
Shinnar S, Molteni A, Gammon K, D'Souza B J, Altman J, Freeman J M 1982 Intraventricular hemorrhage in the premature infant: A changing outlook. New England Journal of Medicine 306: 1464–1468
Shinzawa T, Mura T, Tsunei M, Shiraki Z 1989 Vitamin K absorption capacity and its association with vitamin K deficiency. American Journal of Diseases of Children 143: 686–689
Shirahata A, Nojiri T, Takaragi S, Horiuchi T, Yamada K 1982 Normotest screenings and prophylactic oral administration for idiopathic vitamin K deficiency in infancy. Acta Haematologica (Japan) 45: 867–875
Shirahata A, Nakamura T, Shimono M, Kaneko M, Tanaka S, 1990 Blood coagulation findings and the efficacy of factor XIII concentrate

in premature infants with intracranial hemorrhages. Thrombosis Research 57: 755–763
Short B L, Pearson G D 1986 Neonatal extracorporeal membrane oxygenation: A review. Journal of Internal Care Medicine 1: 48–50
Sibai B M, Spinnato J A, Watson D L, Hill G A, Anderson G D 1984 Pregnancy outcome in 303 cases with severe preeclampsia. Obstetrics and Gynecology 64: 319–325
Sidiropoulous C, Straume B 1984 Treatment of neonatal isoimmune thrombocytopenia with intravenous immunoglobulin (IgG iv). Blut 48: 383–386
Silverstein A 1960 Intracranial bleeding in hemophilia. Archives of Neurology 3: 141–157
Simmons M A, Adcock E W 1974 Hypernatremia and intracranial hemorrhage in neonates. New England Journal of Medicine 291: 6–10
Sinha S K, Davies J M, Sims D G, Chiswick M L 1985 Relation between periventricular haemorrhage and ischaemic brain lesions diagnosed by ultrasound in very preterm infants. Lancet 2: 1154
Syndor M S, Weaver R L, Johnson C A 1977 Effects of fresh frozen plasma infusions on coagulation screening tests in sick neonates. Pediatric Research 11: 542 (abstract)
Sonesson S-V, Winberg P, Lundell B P W 1987 Early postnatal changes in intracranial arterial blood flow velocities in term infants. Pediatric Research 22: 461–464
Sopo S M, Pesaresi M A, Celestini E, Stabile A M, Stabile A 1991 Intravenous immunoglobulins in thrombocytopenia with absent radii. Acta Haematology 85: 105–106
Srinivasan G, Seeler R A, Tiruvury A, Pildes R S 1982 Maternal anticonvulsant therapy and hemorrhagic disease of the newborn. Obstetrics and Gynecology 59: 250–252
Stark C R, Abramson D, Erkan V 1968 Intravascular coagulation and hyaline membrane disease of the newborn. Lancet 1: 1180–1181
Stormorken H, Helleum B, Egeland T, Abrahamsen T G, Hovig T 1991 X-linked thrombocytopenia and thrombocytopathia: Attenuated Wiskott-Aldrich syndrome. Thrombosis and Haemostasis 65: 300–305
Stothers J, Boulton F, Wild R et al 1975 Neonatal coagulation (letter). Lancet 1: 408–409
Strang L B 1966 The pulmonary circulation in the respiratory distress syndrome. Pediatric Clinics of North America 13: 693–730
Struwe F E 1970 Intracranial hemorrhage and occlusive hydrocephalus in hereditary bleeding disorders. Developmental Medicine and Childhood Neurology 12: 165–169
Stuart M J, Allen J B 1982 Arachidonic acid metabolism in the neonatal platelet. Pediatrics 69: 714–718
Stuart M J, Dusse J 1985 In vitro comparison of the efficacy of cyclooxygenase inhibitors on the adult versus neonatal platelet. Biology of the Neonate 47: 265–269
Stuart M J, Oski F A 1979 vitamin E and platelet function. American Journal of Pediatric Hematology/Oncology 1: 77–81
Stuart M J, Elrad H, Graeber J E, Hakanson D O, Sunderi S G, Barvirchak M N 1979 Increased synthesis of prostaglandin endoperoxides and platelet hyperfunction in infants of mothers with diabetes mellitus. Journal of Laboratory and Clinical Medicine 94: 12–26
Stuart M J, Sunderji S J et al 1981 Decreased prostacyclin production in the infants of the diabetic mothers. Journal of Laboratory and Clinical Medicine 98: 412–416
Stuart M J, Gross S J, Elrad H, Graeber J E 1982 Effects of acetylsalicylic acid ingestion on maternal and neonatal hemostasis. New England Journal of Medicine 307: 909–912
Stuart M J, Dusse J, Clark A D, Walenga R W 1984 Differences in thromboxane production between neonatal and adult platelets in response to arachidonic acid and epinephrine. Pediatric Research 18: 823–826
Stuart M J, Wu J, Sunderji S, Cranley C 1987 Effect of amniotic fluid on platelet thromboxane production. Journal of Pediatrics 110: 289–292
Suarez C R, Menendez C E, Walenga J M, Fareed J 1984 Neonatal and maternal hemostasis. Value of molecular markers in the assessment of hemostatic status. Seminars in Thrombosis and Haemostasis 10: 280–284
Suarez C R, Walenga J, Mangogna L C, Fareed J 1985 Neonatal and maternal fibrinolysis: Activation at time of birth. American Journal of Haematology 19: 365–372
Suarez C R, Gonzalez J, Menendez C, Fareed J, Fresco R, Walenga J 1988 Neonatal and maternal platelets: Activation at time of birth. American Journal of Hematology 29: 18–21
Summaria L 1989 Comparison of human normal, full-term, fetal and adult plasminogen by physical and chemical analyses. Haemostasis 19: 266–273
Sutherland J M, Glueck H I 1967 Hemorrhagic disease of the newborn; breast feeding as a necessary factor in the pathogenesis. American Journal of Diseases of Children 113: 524–533
Suvansri U, Cheung W H, Sawitzky A 1969 The effect of bilirubin on the human platelet. Journal of Pediatrics 74: 240–246
Symansky M R, Fox H A 1972 Umbilical vessel catheterization: indications, management, and evaluation of the technique. Journal of Pediatrics 80: 820–826
Szymonowicz W, Yu V Y H 1984 Timing and evolution of periventricular haemorrhage in infants weighing 1250 g or less at birth. Archives of Diseases in Childhood 59: 7–12
Szymonowicz W, Yu V Y H, Wilson F E 1984 Antecedents of periventricular hemorrhage in infants weighing 1250 g or less at birth: Archives of Diseases in Childhood 59: 13–17
Takamiya O, Kinoshita S, Niinomi K, Yshioka K 1989 Protein C in the neonatal period. Haemostasis 1: 45–58
Tarby T J, Volpe J J 1982 Intraventricular hemorrhage in the premature infant. Pediatric Clinics of North America 29: 1077–1104
Tate D Y, Carlton G T, Johnson D et al 1981 Immune thrombocytopenia in severe neonatal infections. Journal of Pediatrics 98: 449–453
Thomas D P 1984 Heparin, low molecular weight heparin and heparin analogues. British Journal of Haematology 58: 385–390
Thompson E, Sherlock S 1964 The aetiology of portal vein thrombosis with particular reference to the role of infection and exchange transfusion. Quarterly Journal of Medicine 33: 465–480
Tizard J P 1962 Portal hypertension following exchange transfusion through the umbilical vein. Proceedings of the Society for Experimental Biology and Medicine 55: 772
Tollefsen D M, Pestka C A 1985 Heparin cofactor II activity in patients with disseminated intravascular coagulation and hepatic failure. Blood 66: 769–774
Tooley W H, Myerberg D C 1978 Should we put catheters in the umbilical artery? Pediatrics 66: 853
Toulon P, Rainaut M, Aiach M, Roncato M, Daffos F, Forestier F 1986 Antithrombin III (ATIII) and heparin cofactor III (HCII) in normal human fetuses (21st–27th week) (letter). Thrombosis Haemostasis 56: 237 (abstract)
Townes B H, Lott I T, Hicks D A, Hegley T 1985 Long term follow-up of infants and children treated with extracorporeal membrane oxygenation (ECMO): A preliminary report. Journal of Pediatric Surgery 20: 410–414
Townsend C W 1894 The haemorrhagic disease of the newborn. Archives of Pediatrics 11: 559–561
Trento A, Griffith B P, Hardesty R L 1986 Extracorporeal membrane oxygenation experience at the University of Pittsburg. Annals of Thoracic Surgery 42: 56–59
Triplett D A, Brandt J T, Batard M A, McG et al 1985 Hereditary factor VII deficiency heterogeneity defined by combined functional and immunochemical analysis. Blood 66: 1284–1287
Tripp J H, McNinch A W 1987 Haemorrhagic disease and vitamin K (E). Archives of Diseases in Childhood 62: 436–437
Trounce J Q, Fagan D, Levene M I 1986 Intraventricular haemorrhage and periventricular leucomalacia: ultrasound and autopsy correlation. Archives of Diseases in Childhood 61: 1203–1207
Ts'ao C H 1977 Comparable inhibition of P R P of neonates and adults by aspirin. Haemostasis 6: 118–126
Ts'ao C H, Green D, Schultz K 1976 Function and ultrastructure of platelets of neonates; enhanced ristocetin aggregation of neonatal platelets. British Journal of Haematology 32: 225–233
Tsiantos A, Victorin L, Relier J P 1974 Intracranial hemorrhage in the prematurely born infant: Timing of clots and evaluation of clinical signs and symptoms. Journal of Pediatrics 85: 854
Tudehope D I, Yu V Y H 1977 The haematology of neonatal necrotizing enterocolitis. Australian Paediatric Journal 13: 193–199
Turner T, Prouse C V, Prescott R J, Cash J D 1981 A clinical trial on the early detection and correction of haemostatic defects in selected high-risk neonates. British Journal of Haematology 47: 65–75

Turrito V T, Weiss H J 1980 Red blood cells: Their dual role in thrombus formation. Science 207: 541–543
Tweed A, Cote J, Lou H, Gregory G, Wade J 1986 Impairment of cerebral blood flow autoregulation in the newborn lamb by hypoxia. Pediatric Research 20: 516–519
Upshaw J D 1978 Congenital deficiency of a factor in normal plasma that reverses microangiopathic haemolysis and thrombocytopenia. New England Journal of Medicine 298: 1350–1352
Vailas G N, Brouillette R T, Scott J P, Shkolnik A, Conway J, Wiringa K 1986 Neonatal aortic thrombosis: recent experience. Journal of Pediatrics 109: 101–108
van den Berg W, Breederveld C, ten Cate J W, Peters M, Borm J J J 1989 Low antithrombin III: accurate predictor of idiopathic respiratory distress syndrome in premature neonates. European Journal of Pediatrics 148: 455–458
van den Besselaar A, Meeuwisse-Braun J, Bertina R M, 1990 Monitoring heparin therapy: Relationship between the activated partial thromboplastin time and heparin assays based on ex-vivo heparin samples. Thrombosis and Haemostasis 63(1): 16–23
Verhoeven J M, van Oostrum I E A, van Haarlem H, Akkerman J W N 1989 Impaired energy metabolism in platelets from patients with Wiskott–Aldrich syndrome. Thrombosis and Haemostasis 61: 10–14
Vieira A, Ofosu A, Andrew M 1989 Heparin sensitivity and resistance in the newborn: an explanation. Pediatric Research 25: 274
Vietti T J, Murphy T P, James J A, Pritchard J A 1960 Observation on the prophylactic use of vitamin K in the newborn. Journal of Pediatrics 56: 343–346
Vietti T J, Stephens J C, Bennett K R 1961 Vitamin K_1 prophylaxis in the newborn. Journal of the American Medical Association 176: 791–793
Volpe J J 1981 Neonatal intraventricular hemorrhage. New England Journal of Medicine 304: 886–891
Volpe J J 1983 Intraventricular hemorrhage: Incidence, neuropathology, and pathogenesis. Neonatology Letter 1: 1
von dem Borne A E G K, von Riesz E 1980 Bak[a], a new platelet-specific antigen involved in neonatal alloimmune thrombocytopenia. Vox Sanguinis 39: 113–120
von dem Borne A E G K, van Leeuwen E F, von Reisz L E, van Boxtel C J, Engelfriet C P 1981 Neonatal alloimmune thrombocytopenia: Detection and characterization of the responsible antibodies by the platelet immunofluorescent test. Blood 57: 649–656
von Kries R, Stannigel H, Gobel U 1985 Anticoagulant therapy by continuous heparin-antithrombin III infusion in newborns with disseminated intravascular coagulation. European Journal of Pediatrics 114: 191–194
von Kries R, Becker A, Gobel U 1987a Vitamin K in the newborn: Influence of nutritional factors on acarboxy-prothrombin detectability and factor II and VII clotting activity. European Journal of Paediatrics 146: 123–127
von Kries R, Kreppel S, Becker A, Gobel U, Tangermann R 1987b Acarboxyprothrombin activity after oral prophylactic vitamin K. Archives of Diseases in Childhood 62: 938–940
von Kries R, Shearer M J, McCarthy P T, Haug M, Hanzer G, Gobel U 1987c Vitamin K_1 content of maternal milk: Influence of the stage of lactation, lipid composition, and vitamin K_1 supplements given to the mother. Pediatric Research 22: 513–517
Vos L J M, Potocky V, Broker F W L, de Vries J A, Postma L, Edens E 1974 Splenic vein thrombosis with oesophageal varices. A late complication of umbilical vein catheterization. Annals of Surgery 180: 152–156
Vukovich T, Auberger K, Weil J, Engelmann H, Knobl P, Hadorn H B 1988 Replacement therapy for a homozygous protein C deficiency-state using a concentrate of human protein C and S. British Journal of Haematology 70: 435–440
Waddell W W, Guerry D 1939 The role of vitamin K in the etiology, prevention, and treatment of hemorrhage in the newborn infant. Part II. Journal of Pediatrics 15: 802–811
Waddell W W Jr, Whitehead B W 1945 Neonatal mortality rates in infants receiving prophylactic doses of vitamin K. Southern Medical Journal 38: 349–351
Waltt H, Kurz R, Mitterstieler G, Fodisch J H, Hohenauer L, Rossler H 1973 Intracranial haemorrhage in low birth weight infants and prophylactic administration of coagulation factor concentrates. Lancet 1: 1284–1288
Waters A H, Ireland R, Mibashan R S 1987 Fetal platelet transfusions in the management of alloimmune thrombocytopenia. Thrombosis and Haemostasis 58: 323a
Watkins M N, Swan S, Caprini J A, Gardner T H, Zuckerman L, Vagher J P 1980 Coagulation changes in the newborn with respiratory failure. Thrombosis Research 17: 153–175
Wefring K W 1962 Hemorrhage in the newborn and vitamin K prophylaxis. Journal of Pediatrics 61: 686–692
Weinblatt M E, Scimeca P G, James-Herry A G, Pahwa S 1987 Thrombocytopenia in an infant with AIDS. American Journal of Diseases in Childhood 141: 15–22
Weinstein M J, Blanchard R, Moake J L, Vosburgh E, Moise K 1989 Fetal and neonatal von Willebrand factor (vWF) is unusually large and similar to the vWF in patients with thrombotic thrombocytopenia purpura. British Journal of Haematology 72: 68–72
Wesstrom G, Finnstrom O, Stenport G 1979 Umbilical artery catheterization in newborns. I. Thrombosis in relation to catheter type and position. Acta Pediatrica Scandinavica 68: 575–581
Whaun J 1973 The platelet of the newborn infant: 5-hydroxytryptamine uptake and release. Thrombosis Diathesis Haemorrhagica 30: 327–333
Whaun J H 1980 The platelet of the newborn infant: Adenine nucleotide metabolism and release. Thrombosis and Haemostasis 43: 99–103
Whaun J M, Smith Gr, Sochor V A 1980 Effect of prenatal drug administration on maternal and neonatal platelet aggregation and PF4 release. Haemostasis 9: 226–237
White L W 1979 CT brain scanning in neonates: indications and practices. Applied Radiology 58: 16–25
White J J, Andrews H J, Risenberg H, Mazur D, Waller J A 1971 Prolonged respiratory support in newborn infants with a membrane oxygenator. Surgery 70: 288–296
White C W, Wolf S J, Korones D N, Sondheimer H M, Tosi M F, Yu A 1991 Treatment of childhood angiomatous diseases with recombinant interferon alfa-2a. Journal of Pediatrics 118: 59–66
Widdershoven J, Kollee L, van Munster P, Bosman A M, Monnens L 1986a Biochemical vitamin K deficiency in early infancy: diagnostic limitation of conventional coagulation tests. Helvetica Paediatrica Acta 41: 195–201
Widdershoven J, Motohara K, Endo F, Matsuda I, Monnens L 1986b Influence of the type of feeding on the presence of PIVKA-II in infants. Helvetica Paediatrica Acta 41: 25–29
Widdershoven J, Lambert W, Motohara K, et al 1988 Plasma concentrations of vitamin K_1 and PIVKA-II in bottle-fed and breast-fed infants with and without vitamin K prophylaxis at birth. European Journal of Pediatrics 148: 139–142
Wigger H J, Bransilver B R, Blanc W A 1970 Thromboses due to catheterization in infants and children. Journal of Pediatrics 76: 11
Witt I, Muller H, Kunter L J 1969 Evidence for the existence of fetal fibrinogen. Thrombosis Diathesis Haemorrhagica 22: 101–109
Woods W G, Luban N L C, Hilgartner M W, Miller D R 1979 Disseminated intravascular coagulation in the newborn. American Journal of Diseases of Children 133: 44–46
Yamada K, Shirahata A, Inagaki M, Miyaji Y, Mori N, Horiuchi I 1983 Therapy for DIC in newborn infants. Biblica Haematalogica 49: 329–341
Ylikorkala O, Makila U M, Kaapa P, Viinikka L 1986 Maternal ingestion of acetyl-salicylic acid inhibits fetal and neonatal thromboxane in humans. American Journal of Obstetrics and Gynecology 155: 345–349
Ylikorkala O, Halmesmaki E, Viinikka L 1987 Effect of ethanol on thromboxane and prostacyclin synthesis by fetal platelets and umbilical artery. Life Sciences 41: 371–376
Yoffe G, Buchanan G R 1988 Intracranial haemorrhage in newborn and young infants with hemophilia. Journal of Pediatrics 113: 333–336
Yuen P M P, Yin J A, Lao T T H 1989 Fibrinopeptide A levels in maternal and newborn plasma. European Journal of Obstetrics and Gynecology 30: 239–244
Zalneraitis E L, Young R S K, Krishnamoorthy K S 1979 Intracranial haemorrhage in utero as a complication of isoimmune thrombocytopenia. Journal of Pediatrics 95: 611–614
Zipursky A, Jaber H M 1978 The hematology of bacterial infection in newborn infants. Clinics in Hematology 7: 175–193

45. Haemostatic drugs

M. Verstraete

In patients with a congenital deficiency of a coagulation factor, bleeding can be prevented or treated by intravenous transfusion of a concentrate of the missing factor(s). In addition, acquired defects of blood coagulation factors can usually be corrected by administration of the missing factor(s) or of platelets, and in some instances by administering vitamin K. Prolonged bleeding in patients with preoperatively normal haemostasis frequently occurs during operation. This complication can be due to errors in surgical technique, certain anesthetic procedures, errors in drug administration (e.g. heparin, some antibiotics in patients with renal insufficiency), administration of mismatched blood, or massive transfusion of blood or plasma expanders.

Bleeding may also occur without apparent surgical, haematological, vascular or other cause. A direct approach to the prevention or reduction of bleeding during surgery consists of electrocoagulation, suture ligation, reduction of systemic blood pressure (carrying the risk of cerebral and myocardial infarction in elderly men), towel application and the use of gauze packs, and sometimes, cooling of the irrigation fluid in certain operations or blockade of the sympathic nervous system. When these measures fail, when bleeding is located at sites which are inaccessible, or when no technical or other cause for faulty haemostasis can be found, a drug which reduces bleeding is indicated. Although many of the presently available haemostatic drugs are reported to reduce blood loss during and after surgery, recent and stringent clinical trials have often been unable to support this clinical claim (Verstraete 1977). Critical re-evaluation of these drugs is therefore a timely exercise.

EFFECTIVENESS AND SIDE-EFFECTS OF SPECIFIC HAEMOSTATIC DRUGS

Desmopressin

Desmopressin (1-deamino-8-D-arginine vasopressin, DDAVP) is a synthetic analogue of the naturally occurring antidiuretic hormone vasopressin[1].

The pharmacokinetics of desmopressin have been well studied in terms of the drug itself and its effects on factor VIII/von Willebrand factor, plasminogen activator and the bleeding time. Bioavailability of desmopressin given by the subcutaneous route compares reasonably well with desmopressin administered via the intravenous route. The bioavailability of the drug given by concentrated intranasal spray is approximately 10%. The dosage of desmopressin for haemostatic purposes is approximately 15 times that used for antidiuretic effects. Maximum response in factor VIII/von Willebrand factor and plasminogen activator release is obtained with a dosage of 0.3 μg/kg intravenously, while the response to 300 μg given by concentrated intranasal spray is as effective as 0.2 μg/kg intravenously. While there is considerable inter-individual variation in maximal factor VIII/von Willebrand factor response, it appears to be reasonably consistent in individual subjects (Richardson & Robinson 1985, Lusher 1990).

Desmopressin is regarded as the treatment of choice for persons with mild haemophilia A (factor VIII deficiency) and classical (type 1) von Willebrand's disease (Mannucci et al 1977, 1987, de la Fuente et al 1985, Mannucci 1986, Lethagen et al 1990, Muhm et al 1990, Rose & Aledort 1991). This drug has also been used to enhance haemostasis in a wide variety of clinical situations including bleeding associated with certain platelet function defects, uraemia, and hepatic cirrhosis (clinical conditions in which there are haemostatic abnormalities, but not of factor VIII/von Willebrand factor) (Mannucci et al 1983, 1986, Kobrinsky et al 1987, Mannucci 1986, Kentro et al 1987, Lens et al 1988, Nieuwenhuis & Sixma 1988). Additionally, desmopressin reportedly has been of benefit in reducing blood loss (thus reducing the need for blood transfusions) in haemostatically normal individuals undergoing certain orthopaedic, cardiovascular and neurosurgical procedures that are usually associated

[1] Minrin, Minirin.

substantial blood loss (Salzman et al 1986, Czer et al 1987, Kobrinsky et al 1987, Rocha et al 1988, Salzman 1990). While the precise mechanism by which desmopressin enhances haemostasis in conditions other than mild haemophilia A and type I von Willebrand's disease is not known with certainty (Barnhart et al 1983, Mannucci 1986, Cattaneo et al 1989), it has been postulated that desmopressin causes release of high molecular weight multimers of von Willebrand factor from endothelial cells, thereby enhancing platelet spreading and adhesion at injury sites of the vessel wall (Czer & Capon 1990).

Adverse effects of desmopressin, facial flushing, headache, a slight fall in blood pressure, and a rise in the pulse rate, occur with rapid infusions and are generally mild and infrequent. These effects can usually be reduced by slowing the rate of infusion. Transient gastrointestinal complaints have been noted in some patients. Water intoxication with resultant hyponatraemia has been reported only rarely. Severe hyponatraemia can cause seizures (Shepherd et al 1989, Czer & Capon 1991).

A possible prothrombotic effect has been a source of concern, especially in patients with coronary or cerebral atherosclerosis. There have been three isolated case reports of myocardial infarction after desmopressin infusion (Bond & Bevan 1988, O'Brien et al 1989, van Dantzig et al 1989). To evaluate the risk of thrombosis with desmopressin in patients undergoing cardiac surgery, data from all known published and unpublished clinical trials in cardiac surgery were pooled by Mannucci & Lusher (1989). Thrombotic events (myocardial infarction, stroke, venous thromboembolism) occurred in 15 (3.9%) of 382 desmopressin-treated patients compared with 11 (2.9%) of 381 untreated patients ($p = 0.43$). It was concluded that desmopressin does not significantly increase the incidence of thrombosis. Nevertheless, close monitoring of patients with coronary or cerebral atherosclerosis may be warranted (Mannucci & Lusher 1989). In cardiac surgery, concomitant use of antifibrinolytic agents is not recommended, since they blunt the fibrinolytic effect of desmopressin (Mannucci & Lusher 1989).

TISSUE EXTRACTS

It is well known that tissue extracts[2] have a thromboplastin-like action and shorten the in vitro coagulation times of blood and plasma as well as increase prothrombin consumption. The same effects can be observed in vivo during the first hour after intravenous administration of the substance but not after intramuscular or oral administration. However, all routes have been recommended by the manufacturers (Kommerell 1960, Haiböck 1972).

A micellar suspension of at least six phospholipids extracted from animal brains and mixed in fixed proportions is commercially available as a haemostatic agent[3]. This substance accelerates in vitro coagulation, but in certain concentrations only (Deutsch 1952, Deutsch & Fischer 1963). Shortening of the coagulation time of blood and plasma was also obtained after slow intravenous administration in man (Schimpf et al 1972).

OXALIC AND MALONIC ACID

An aqueous acid solution of oxalic and malonic acid[4] was at one time proposed as a haemostatic substance for systemic use. Its clinical efficacy was never demonstrated and this substance now seems to have been almost abandoned.

TETRAGALACTURONIC ACID ESTER

Colloidal polygalacturonic acid esters from apple pectin (tetragalacturonic acid ester)[5] have been recommended as a haemostatic agent for topical and oral use. This substance has no effect on coagulation in vitro but was claimed to shorten the coagulation time in vivo in rabbits and man. Subsequently it became evident that pectin-like substances have an in vivo inhibitory effect on fibrinolysis (Nilsson et al 1961). Controlled trials of blood loss with tetragalacturonic acid are not available.

BUTANOL

A mixture of butyl alcohol, citric acid and disaccharides is known as the haemostatic substance named after Dr E. Revici, who postulated that bleeding occurs at places of local alkalosis in injured or diseased tissue[6]. Whether the small amount of citric acid present in the preparation could induce the desired change is highly questionable. The few experiments performed in rats and rabbits did not result in a significant decrease of the bleeding time after either oral or intravenous administration of the substance (Kuschinsky et al 1968). There are no controlled clinical trials giving sound results, but a rich harvest of anecdotal reports.

SODIUM 4-AMINONAPHTHALENE-1-SULPHONATE

It is known that Congo Red can induce thrombophlebitis of the vein into which it is injected; naphtionine[7] is related to Congo Red and has been reported to reduce the blood coagulation and bleeding time slightly in normal and thrombocytopenic subjects (Poller 1955, Poller & More 1964). This effect was believed to be due to a decrease

[2] Clauden, Coagulen, Hémostatique Ercé Hémocoagulene, Manétol, Thrombocytine.
[3] Tachostyptan, 'Hämostypticum 733 Schoch'.
[4] Koagamin.
[5] Arrhémapectine, Coagucit, Sangostop, Strypturon.
[6] Haemostypticum 'Revici'.
[7] Emostane, 101 Estéve, Hémorragine, Naphtionine.

of the isoelectric point of fibrinogen, whereby its gel state is favoured. No sound clinical trials support the extravagant claims made for naphthionine in earlier days.

ETHAMSYLATE

This is a derivative of Congo Red (diethylammonium 2, 5-dihydroxybenzenesulphate)[8], a synthetic water-soluble drug which is absorbed and excreted unchanged (Deacock & Birley 1969). Ethamsylate has been shown to increase platelet adhesiveness to glass beads, to increase capillary resistance and to reduce the bleeding time in animals, normal subjects and patients with a moderately prolonged bleeding time. Surprisingly, the reduction in bleeding time in patients appears to be unrelated to the number of platelets (Louis & Paulus 1967). Ethamsylate appears to have an antihyaluronidase activity and to inhibit prostacyclin directly (Vinazzer 1980). Nevertheless, there is still uncertainty concerning the mode of action of the drug.

From a clinical point of view, two of four double-blind trials indicated that ethamsylate significantly reduces blood loss in primary or IUD-induced menorrhagia (Jaffé & Wickham 1973, Kasonde & Bonnar 1975, Harrison & Campbell 1976, Kovacs & Annus 1978). The clinical benefit in patients without bleeding disorders undergoing dental extraction, adenotonsillectomy or transuretheral prostatectomy, is well established in controlled trials. The recommended dose in adults is 500 mg three or four times a day; the paediatric dosage is half of this. For surgery or emergency use, 750 mg should be given intravenously or per cannula in an adult, followed if necessary by a further 250 mg during or at the end of operation.

There is limited evidence that ethamsylate might improve survival in low birth weight infants where intraventricular haemorrhage is the major cause of death and handicap among survivors (Harrison & Matthews 1984, Benson et al 1986, Cooke 1987).

AMINAPHTONE

This is a synthetic agent with the chemical formula 2-hydroxy-3 methyl-1,4-naphthohydroquinone-2-(*p*-aminobenzoate)[9] which is believed to be a vasoactive drug because it significantly shortens the bleeding time in normal and heparinized rabbits and mice (Pepeu 1975), and possibly also in patients with or without a bleeding defect. Not all the clinical reports are in agreement and no double-blind trial with objective end-points has been performed with this substance.

β-NAPHTHOQUINONE SEMICARBAZONE

Naftazone[10] is prepared by diazotization of sulphonic acid with β-naphthol and is similar to adrenochrome (Derouaux 1961). Naftazone significantly reduces the normal bleeding time (72%) and blood loss in rabbits and dogs (Dermaut & Gilson 1963). In many ways, this drug resembles adrenochrome but it may have, in addition, certain effects at a cellular level. The results of only one double-blind controlled trial with an objective end-point are available; this was performed in patients undergoing prostatectomy (Charles & Coolsaet 1972). Urinary blood loss and blood transfusion requirements were significantly lower in the group treated with naftazone. More double-blind randomized trials with objective end-points are desirable before this agent can be recommended.

ADRENOCHROME

Adrenochrome, an oxidation product of adrenaline, becomes stable when combined with monosemicarbazone (adrenochrome, monosemicarbazide)[11]. When complexed with sodium salicylate this substance is much more soluble (carbazochrome salicylate)[12] and is administered as a hypertonic solution which causes a brief painful stinging sensation when injected intramuscularly. Experiments in animals demonstrate a significant reduction of the normal bleeding time when adrenochrome monosemicarbazide is given (Roskam et al 1944). Because of rapid destruction and elimination in the gastrointestinal tract, the oral absorption is approximately one-third of the parenteral dose. There is evidence to show that some effects of adrenochrome are inhibited by the action of antihistamines.

The two forms of this drug were marketed at a time when the requirements of clinical pharmacology were not so stringent. A comparison of cases treated with and without the drug was, however, made and the minimal effect was to be confirmed by more refined testing. Six recent double-blind randomized trials in surgical situations failed to reveal a reduction in blood loss, and the efficacy of the substance, at least for this indication, is unproved.

HYDROXYTRYPTAMINE CREATININE

Platelets are the main carriers of 5-hydroxytryptamine (5-HT), which they possibly sequester when this amine escapes from the enterochromaffin system. Aggregating platelets release their 5-HT, and this was considered to be responsible in part for the vasoconstrictor activity of

[8] Aglumin, cyclonamine, Dicynene, Dicynone, Eselin, Mediaven, OM-Dicinoma.
[9] Baldena, Capillarema.
[10] Haemostop, Karbinone.
[11] Adona AC-17, Adrenoxyl, Emex.
[12] Adrenosem, Adrenosemsalicylate, Stadren.

platelets. For this reason 5-HT creatinine sulphate[13] was proposed as a haemostatic agent (Correll et al 1952, Djerassi et al 1958). That 5-HT is essential for haemostasis is now seriously in doubt, because patients who have 5-HT-depleted platelets during prolonged reserpine treatment have no haemostatic defect (Haverback et al 1957). The clinical value of this substance is unproven, as no meaningful clinical trials have been performed.

CONJUGATED OESTROGENS AND OESTRIOL SUCCINATE

A mixture of the sodium salts of sulphate esters of oestrogenic substances, principally oestrone and equilin of the type that are excreted by pregnant mares, are the main constituents of a haemostatic agent recommended for systemic use.[14] It has been shown to increase the number and polymerization of acid mucopolysaccharides, which may alter the local gel–sol equilibrium of the ground substance in favour of the gel phase (Wayne et al 1964).

The majority of controlled, mainly double-blind, clinical studies with Premarin, in which an attempt was made to quantify blood loss, demonstrated no significant effect of Premarin in the prophylaxis or treatment of bleeding, although in patients with chronic renal failure a reduction in bleeding time was noted (Liu et al 1984, Bronner et al 1986, Livio et al 1986; Shemin et al 1990). The most striking early case reports of its successful use were for epistaxis, but in the only single-blind trial of its use in severe epistaxis, Premarin was not superior to placebo.

Oestriol disodium succinate[15] is a natural weak oestrogen. The haemostatic effect of natural oestrogen is possibly related to an increase in the proportion of acid mucopolysaccharides, due to the hyaluronidase-inhibiting effect of the drug. Hyaluronidase causes the breakdown of mucopolysaccharides in the ground substance of the capillary wall. Such breakdown, accompanied by measurable and consistent increase in capillary fragility, apparently occurs in normal women premenstrually and during the first 2 or 3 days of the menstrual cycle. This is attributed to the currently low circulating levels of oestrogens. Further work has indeed revealed that oestriol improves reduced capillary resistance, decreases capillary fragility and tends to normalize increased capillary permeability (Poliwoda 1965, Staubesand et al 1966).

Most of the clinical trials with oestriol were performed 25 years ago according to standards not likely to be accepted at the present time. There are various studies with control groups, but apparently none with a double-blind approach and proper quantitation of blood loss. Although oestrogens do affect the vascular wall, their clinical usefulness as a haemostatic agent has not been convincingly demonstrated.

PURIFIED SNAKE VENOMS

For many years extracts of snake venoms have been prepared for their coagulatory properties and used as haemostatic agents.[16] The venoms of different species of snakes have been used and the subspecies used for the commercial preparations have varied somewhat over the years. Commercial fractions are free from neurotoxin and other toxic components.

Botropase *(Bothrops jararaca)*

Botropase converts fibrinogen to fibrin by removal of fibrinopeptide A only (des A-fibrin) and, in vivo, produces low grade diffuse intravascular coagulation associated with the formation of soluble fibrin monomer complexes (Blombäck et al 1957). Moreover, the drug has a thromboplastin-like activity but the generated thrombin is probably neutralized by the plasma antithrombin system (de Nicola et al 1969).

Botropase shortens the coagulation time and induces low grade intravascular coagulation, which may have harmful consequences (Gaffney & Brasher 1974). Its effectiveness as a haemostatic agent is supported only by a double-blind clinical trial in ENT surgery, the end-point of which was a subjective one (Nicoumar 1975). In another controlled and randomized trial in patients subjected to transvesical prostatic adenomectomy, measured blood loss revealed a significant reduction but only during the first postoperative day (Gamba et al 1979). The benefits and disadvantages not being known, Botropase cannot be recommended as a general haemostatic agent and it is advisable to conduct appropriate and stringent clinical trials.

Reptilase *(Bothrops atrox)*

Reptilase also contains a thrombin-like activity and a platelet-activating enzyme called 'thrombocytin', which has been isolated (Niewiarowski et al 1977). As Reptilase is not neutralized by antithrombin, it splits peptide A from fibrinogen at very low levels. Due to circulating soluble fibrin monomer-fibrinogen complexes, a hypercoagulable state is produced. Two out of three trials in normal patients undergoing surgery revealed a decrease in measured blood loss. The effect of Reptilase on patients with a bleeding disorder or menorrhagia/metrorrhagia

[13] Antemovis.
[14] Equigyne, Estradurin, Premarin.
[15] Presomen, Stryptanon.
[16] Botropase, Haemocoagulase, Ophidiase, Reptilase.

is open to conjecture until more valid clinical data are assembled.

APROTININ

This is a well-defined serine protease inhibitor, isolated from bovine lung and is identical to the basic pancreatic trypsin inhibitor[17] (Werle 1968). Its chemical structure is known precisely and its inhibitory effect on trypsin, plasmin, kallikrein and chymotrypsin has been extensively studied. Moreover, aprotinin has an anticoagulant effect, its action being specifically directed against the activation of factor XII and XI (Blombäck et al 1967, Prentice et al 1970). The overall half life in the blood in man is 37–50 minutes.

Clinical efficacy of aprotinin

In this indication it is mainly the antifibrinolytic effect that is being utilized. Aprotinin has been recommended for use in the acute acquired defects of the coagulation mechanism, arising secondary to a variety of clinical situations.

Gynaecology and obstetric application

In a prospective, randomized study conducted in patients with abruptio placentae complicated by fetal death, diffuse intravascular coagulation and uterine inertia, aprotinin was found to decrease the consumption of coagulation factors and to reduce the overall complication rate. There was enhanced contraction of uterine muscle in all but one patient of the aprotinin group (n = 18) whereas 13 of 18 control patients had no resumption of uterine activity and required Caesarean section (Sher 1980). The rapid relief of uterine inertia in such cases is due probably to neutralization of excess kinin production (Haberland & McConn 1979), but this remains to be proven. In patients with dead fetus syndrome (Pfeifer 1968) and with amniotic fluid embolism (Graeff et al 1978, Oeney et al 1982), aprotinin has been used with apparent success to stop haemorrhage secondary to intense activation of the coagulation and fibrinolytic system.

Women with an intrauterine device may have excessive blood loss. Intrauterine application of aprotinin or tranexamic acid was tried in 34 women with an IUD complaining of menorrhagia and the results were compared with those of a placebo group. Both inhibitors reduced the length of the menstrual period by about 50% (Tauber et al 1977). Whereas in this study intrauterine instillation of 1 ml concentrated aprotinin solution of 50 000 to 100 000 KIU/ml was used, it was confirmed later that the commercial preparations(20 000 KIU/ml) are also suitable (Tauber 1979).

Prostatic surgery application

Blood loss during and after surgery of the prostate was investigated by haemoglobin measurements in a comparative trial of different antifibrinolytic drugs (Kösters & Wand 1973). After administration of 200 000 KIU aprotinin in combination with either 5 g ε-aminocaproic acid or 1 g tranexamic acid, there was a significantly reduced blood loss compared to controls or to patients given either drug alone. It should be noted that patients with transvesical prostatectomy did not respond to antifibrinolytic treatment, whereas in transurethral resection, blood loss was reduced by 50% when the combined drug schemes were applied.

It is desirable to use the lowest effective dose of synthetic fibrinolytic inhibitors because these can produce stable fibrin deposits obstructing the urinary tract. This is not the case for aprotinin, which is not cleared by the kidney and therefore does not inhibit the lysis by urokinase of fibrin in the urogenital tract.

Use in neurosurgery and neurology

While a number of randomized controlled trials suggest that tranexamic acid may be effective in preventing or delaying rebleeding in patients with ruptured intracranial aneurysm, antifibrinolytic agents can also produce delayed cerebral ischaemic complications. A reduction has been noted in the frequency of recurrent haemorrhage following the combined treatment with a low dose of tranexamic acid (1 g) and 500 000 KIU aprotinin three times daily (Beck & Oeckler 1981). The different mode of action of aprotinin and its additional effects via the kallikrein-kinin system might avoid the delayed vasospastic effects of tranexamic acid in this clinical setting (Guidetti & Spallone 1981).

Use in cardiovascular surgery, extracorporeal circulation

Although excessive blood loss has considerably decreased with more refined cardiac bypass methodology and equipment, there is still a concern for reducing postoperative bleeding in cardiac surgery.

Earlier studies have shown that aprotinin could reduce blood loss by an average of 21% during open heart surgery with extracorporeal circulation (Tice et al 1964) at a dose (400 000 KIU in adults) that had little effect on the levels of coagulation factors (Mammen 1968, Ambrus et al 1971, Pilbrant et al 1981, Popov-Cenic et al 1982, Hack et al 1983). However, when aprotinin was administered at the end of bypass time, i.e. immediately

[17] Antagosan, Anticrein, Antilysin, KIR, Midran, Iniprol, Onquinon, Repulson, Traskolan, Trasylol, Trazinine, Zymofren.

before neutralization of heparin by protamine, no distinct effect on coagulation parameters could be found (Köstering et al 1973). This would indicate that any therapeutic intervention should begin when the cardiopulmonary bypass is started. Pilot studies to determine its effect in open heart surgery in children with congenital cardiac defects (Popov-Cenic et al 1982) and in adults subjected to aortic or mitral valve replacement (Hack et al 1983) have been published. At a dose of 5000 KIU/kg given prior to institution of cardiopulmonary bypass, myocardial protection from global ischaemia has been noted (Sunamori et al 1980). It is also worth noting that aprotinin has been used successfully to prevent leakage of fibrin-coated aortic allografts (Borst et al 1982, Haverich et al 1983).

In another study 2 million KIU of aprotinin was given over 30 minutes at the start of anaesthesia, followed by 500 000 KIU per hour during cardiopulmonary bypass. This high-dose treatment resulted in platelet preservation and prevented thromboxane and neutrophil elastase release; postoperative blood loss was also significantly decreased (by circa 50%) compared with an untreated control group (357 ml versus 674 ml) ($p < 0.01$) (van Oeveren et al 1987).

In a prospective controlled trial in 22 patients undergoing repeat open heart surgery through a previous median sternotomy (Royston et al 1987, Bidstrup et al 1988, 1989, Markland et al 1988, van Oeveren et al 1988, Clozel et al 1990, Bethune 1991, Locatelli et al 1991), an ultra high-dose of 5 million KIU aprotinin (700 mg) was given intravenously from the start of anaesthesia to the end of the procedure. The patients' mean drainage blood loss was reduced by an average of 81%, from 1509 ml in the controls to 286 ml in the patients receiving aprotinin ($p < 0.001$). The mean haemoglobin losses were 78 and 8.3 g, respectively, a reduction of 89% ($p < 0.001$). Blood transfusion requirements were eight-fold higher in the control group than in the aprotinin group (reduction of 91%), seven of whom received only the single unit of their own blood taken before cardiovascular bypass.

It is postulated that this beneficial effect of aprotinin is related to the preservation of two platelet receptors that are removed by plasmin; the von Willebrand glycoprotein Ib receptor required for platelet adhesion and the fibrinogen receptor IIb/IIIa on platelets required for aggregation (Adelman 1985, Peerschke & Wainer 1985, George et al 1986, van Oeveren et al 1988, John et al 1991, Lu et al 1991). Aprotinin seems also to inhibit activated protein C (Espãna et al 1989).

It is to be stressed that with the technical improvement on membrane oxygenators, the activation of haemostasis is becoming less of a problem and the need for and the regimens of aprotinin in cardiopulmonary bypass must be evaluated for each oxygenator (Vandenvelde et al 1991).

Use in liver transplantation

Liver transplantation is frequently complicated by severe coagulopathy and blood loss. Accelerated fibrinolysis has been identified as an important component of the haemostatic disorders that contribute to perioperative bleeding (Porte et al 1985). Aprotinin (2 000 000 KIU loading dose followed by an infusion of 500 000 KIU/h until the patient's return to the intensive care unit) has been reported to reduce blood loss by several (Neuhaus et al 1989, Mallett et al 1990) but not by all (Hunt et al 1990) surgical groups.

SYNTHETIC FIBRINOLYSIS INHIBITORS

ε-Aminocaproic acid (EACA) (6-aminohexanoic acid)[18] was the first synthetic representative of a new class of drugs, the antifibrinolytic agents. The potency of the antifibrinolytic effects of aminocarboxylic acids depends on the presence of free amino and carboxylic groups and on the distance between the COOH-groups and the carbon atoms to which the NH_2-group is attached (Markwardt 1978). The study of the antifibrinolytic activity of a series of cyclic compounds with terminal amino or carboxylic groups led to the identification of *p*-aminomethylbenzoic acid (PAMBA) (Lohmann et al 1963). The comparison of EACA and PAMBA showed that the latter is about 3 times more active. Tranexamic acid is the trans-stereo-isomer of 4-aminomethylcyclohexane carboxylic acid (AMCHA)[19]. The initial investigations were made using a preparation containing a mixture of isomers, but it was subsequently found that only the trans-stereo-isomer has antifibrinolytic activity.

The antifibrinolytic effect of the synthetic compounds EACA, PAMBA and tranexamic acid is mainly related to a reversible complex formation with a modified plasminogen associated with conformational changes of this proenzyme (Thorsen 1975). Human plasminogen contains structures called 'lysine-binding sites' which are of importance not only for plasminogen interaction with synthetic antifibrinolytic amino acids but also its interaction with α_2-antiplasmin and with fibrin (Thorsen 1975). Native human plasminogen contains one lysine-binding site with high affinity for tranexamic acid and four or five with low affinity. The binding of plasminogen and of the heavy chain of plasmin to fibrin monomer is also mediated through the lysine-binding sites of plasminogen to specific lysine residues of fibrin; this interaction is virtually completely blocked by synthetic antifibrinolytic amino acids. It is primarily the high affinity lysine-binding

[18] Acikaprin, Afibrin, Amicar, Capracid, Capramol, Caprocid, Caprolest, Caprolisin, EACA-Roche, Eacina, Ecapron, Apsikapron, Epsilon-Tachostyptan, Hemocaprol.

[19] Anvitoff, Espercil, Exacyl, Frenolyse, Hemostan, Pridemon, Tranex, Tranexamico-Labaz, Transamin, Transamine, Transamcha, Ugurol.

site of plasminogen which is involved in its binding to fibrin; saturation of this binding site with tranexamic acid displaces plasminogen from the fibrin surface (Hoylaerts et al 1981). This results in a retardation of fibrinolysis, because no matter how rapidly plasmin is formed, it cannot bind to fibrinogen or fibrin monomers, thereby precluding the proteolytic action by the serine-histidine enzyme site. Conversely, when the lysine-binding sites of plasmin are blocked by tranexamic acid, inactivation by α_2-antiplasmin is virtually impossible.

Due to subtle chemical differences tranexamic acid is, on a molar basis, 7–10 times more potent than EACA and twice as potent as PAMBA, but has the same low acute and chronic toxicity (Andersson et al 1965). As tranexamic acid also displays a considerably higher and more sustained antifibrinolytic activity in tissues than does EACA and has a longer half-life, tranexamic acid is more often used in therapeutics at the present time.

Clinical efficacy of tranexamic acid in individuals without a generalized bleeding disorder

After tonsillectomy and adenoidectomy

The most common complication of tonsillectomy is rebleeding, the frequency varying with the surgical technique used. In two double-blind trials comparing tranexamic acid (10 mg/kg intravenous) and placebo injected intravenously 30 minutes before surgery, a significant reduction in measured blood loss (28%) during the procedure was achieved with less recurrence of bleeding (27% compared with 67% in the control group) (Castelli & Vogt 1977, Verstraete et al 1977).

In prostatic surgery

The urine contains the plasminogen activator urokinase, which induces the breakdown of blood clots, thereby enhancing bleeding in the urinary tract. Moreover, prostatic tissue contains large amounts of plasminogen activator. These are two reasons for haemorrhages occurring from time to time in connection with prostatectomy.

The effects of tranexamic acid on the frequence of haemorrhage in the first days after prostatectomy or in the following 4 weeks have been demonstrated in several controlled trials (Hedlund 1969, Kaufman & Siefker 1969, Rö et al 1970, Gamba et al 1979, Miller et al 1980). The incidence of secondary bleeding was reduced from 50% in the control group to 24% in the treatment group. For this indication, the recommended dose, starting immediately after surgery, is 10–15 mg/kg weight given intravenously 2–3 times daily during the first 3 postoperative days, and thereafter 1–1.5 g orally three to four times daily until macroscopic haematuria is no longer present. If high bleeding is also present, there is a risk of clot retention in the kidney, in the ureter with subsequent urinary obstruction, or in the bladder. One may question whether the blood saving is of clinical relevance set against these potential complications.

The usefulness of antifibrinolytic drugs has also been tested in children after unilateral or bilateral reimplantation of ureters for vesicoureteric reflux (Rö et al 1970). Postoperative blood loss was significantly reduced but some children passed large blood clots. There are anecdotal reports on the use of tranexamic acid to reduce bleeding in haemorrhagic cystitis and after renal biopsy. Antifibrinolytic drugs are not recommended in patients with idiopathic haematuria originating from the upper urinary tract because of the risk of ureteric obstruction or transient bladder retention.

After cervical conization

This operation has become more common for non-invasive cancer of the cervix. Postoperative bleeding requiring extra measures occurs in about 14% of cases when using the open technique (Kinn 1970). Since the uterine cervix contains a high concentration of plasminogen activator, it is logical to treat these patients with fibrinolytic inhibitors. Two double-blind trials (one with open surgical technique without suturing and one with suturing) revealed a significant reduction in blood loss (average of 70%) in patients who received 1.5 g tranexamic acid daily for at least 12 days postoperatively (Rybo & Westerberg 1972, Landin & Werner 1975).

Treatment of primary or IUD-induced menorrhagia

In a random population 9–11% of the women have menstrual blood loss in excess of 80 ml per period. Four controlled clinical trials, three of which were randomized, double-blind, cross-over trials with tranexamic acid and one a controlled study, showed a dose-dependent reduction (35–51%) of menstrual blood loss in essential menorrhagia (Nilsson & Rybo 1967, 1971, Vermylen et al 1968, Callender et al 1970, Rö et al 1970). The dose recommended is 1–1.5 g of tranexamic acid orally three to four times daily for 3–4 days. The treatment is started when the bleeding has become profuse.

Tranexamic acid has been shown to reduce blood loss more effectively than the prostaglandin synthetase inhibitor flurbiprofen, in 15 women with idiopathic menorrhagia (ADIS Press 1990). Both treatments significantly reduced blood loss compared with control values, but tranexamic acid had a greater effect. Nonetheless, values below 80 ml were not attained with either therapy. Since the two drugs act through different mechanisms, it would be of interest to investigate the efficacy of a combined regimen.

A second situation frequently associated with excessive menstrual blood loss is the use of inert or, to a lesser degree, copper intrauterine devices. Weström & Bengtsson (1970) in a well-designed controlled trial with random allocation of women with inert or copper-loaded intrauterine devices, demonstrated that 6 g of tranexamic acid daily reduced very significantly uterine blood loss after insertion of an IUD; the reduction observed was from 82.7% to 11.5%.

In another double-blind trial tranexamic acid and a prostaglandin synthesis inhibitor were compared in women with an intrauterine contraceptive device (Ylkiorkala & Viinikka 1983). Mean menstrual blood loss before treatment was 135 ml and fell to 102 ml with the prostaglandin synthesis inhibitor and to 59 ml with tranexamic acid. More women on tranexamic acid complained of side-effects but in none was the drug withdrawn.

Bleeding during or after pregnancy

Bleeding during pregnancy is associated with three to four-fold increase in perinatal mortality. Bleeding from small vessels at the borders of the placenta may be due to defective sealing of the microcirculation. Tranexamic acid crosses the placental barrier and may secure local haemostasis and reduce premature labour.

Tranexamic acid has been used in a limited number of cases of threatened placental abruption with a low perinatal mortality (8%) and no maternal mortality (Astedt & Nilsson 1978, Svandberg et al 1980, Walzman & Bonnar 1982).

One is always reluctant to use drugs during pregnancy. Reproduction studies performed in mice, rats and rabbits at doses up to 75 times the human dose of tranexamic acid, have revealed no evidence of impaired fertility or harm to the fetus. Limited experience from treatment of pregnant women did not reveal harmful effects to the fetus.

Treatment of gastric and intestinal haemorrhage

In six randomized, double-blind studies, the effect of tranexamic acid was evaluated in patients with bleeding in the upper gastrointestinal tract (Cormack et al 1973, Biggs et al 1976, Engqvist et al 1979, Bergqvist et al 1980, Barer et al 1983, Stael von Holstein et al 1987). Bleeding was distal to the oesophagogastric junction and presumably most often due to diffuse gastritis and erosive gastroduodenitis. The effect of tranexamic acid was judged on the need for blood transfusion, continuous or recurrent bleeding, surgery and death. The results obtained indicate that tranexamic acid reduces transfusion requirements. Henry & O'Connell (1989) performed a meta-analysis of these six double-blind placebo-controlled trials involving a total of 126 patients and estimated a 20 to 30% reduction in the rate of rebleeding in association with tranexamic acid, as well as a 30 to 40% reduction in the need for surgery, and a 40% reduction in mortality.

In the light of the published studies it would appear appropriate to give antifibrinolytic drugs in addition to customary forms of treatment in patients with gastroduodenal bleeding. Treatment can be started with intravenous administration of 1 g tranexamic acid four to six times daily for 2–3 days, followed by 1.5 g orally three to four times daily. In view of the local fibrinolytic activity in the walls of the stomach, oral administration at the same dosage is the preferable route.

Local fibrinolytic activity also occurs in the colon, more particularly around small submucosa vessels as noted in biopsy material of patients with ulcerative colitis in an active phase. A group of such patients was treated with enemas containing 5 g tranexamic acid dissolved in 100 ml of warm water, twice daily for 6 months; in all patients with pathologically increased fibrinolytic activity in the mucosa, remission of the disorder was obtained (Kondo et al 1981, Miglioli et al 1989, McElligot et al 1991). In addition to uncontrolled trials, there are two double-blind trials, one with equivocal results (Mowatt et al 1973). The second one was conducted in patients with ulcerative colitis in a stable phase and revealed that oral tranexamic acid (1.5 g thrice daily) results in a significant reduction of rectal haemorrhages but is without effect on stool frequency or consistency (Hollanders et al 1983). Further studies are needed in this difficult field to determine the place of tranexamic acid in the treatment of upper and low intestinal tract bleeding.

In summary, although further investigation in larger trials is required, tranexamic acid appears useful in the treatment of gastrointestinal bleeding. It has been suggested that the benefit obtained is comparable to that observed with histamine H_2-antagonists (Langman 1987).

Treatment of recurrent epistaxis

Recurrent nose-bleeds are rather common, and external trauma or a vascular change on the anterioseptum is most frequently the cause. In other instances the aetiology is not quite clear and several factors, such as hypertension, common cold or upper respiratory infection and the intake of salicylic acid, have been reported to play a role. In a randomized double-blind trial, tranexamic acid reduced significantly the severity of idiopathic nose-bleeds and the rebleeding frequency when used at the usual dose of 1.5 g three times daily (Petruson 1974).

After ocular trauma

Ocular trauma, accidental or surgical, is often accompanied

by haemorrhage in the anterior chamber of the eye. The most serious complication of traumatic hyphaema is secondary bleeding, usually occurring in the 2nd to 7th post-traumatic day in 38% of the patients (Pandolfi 1978). Impaired vision or blindness may be the disastrous consequence. The purpose of antifibrinolytic therapy is to prevent rebleeding in the anterior chamber and the vitreous body.

The results of two controlled trials show that tranexamic acid treatment (1 g three times daily) significantly reduces the frequence of secondary haemorrhage (Jerndal & Frisén 1976, Varnek et al 1980). These findings support the favourable impression of five other trials with historical controls.

Prevention of postoperative corneal oedema

Two double-blind trials in postoperative corneal oedema after cataract operation (Bramsen et al 1978) and trabeculectomy (Bramsen 1977) revealed that tranexamic acid is effective in reducing corneal thickness and is associated with improved visual activity. In a third, randomized non-blind study, it was reported that tranexamic acid plus naproxen was no more effective than either drug alone in postoperative corneal oedema after cataract removal and implantation of anterior chamber lens (Norrelykke Nissen & Ehlers 1986).

Prevention of bleeding after thyroid surgery

Only one study investigating the effect of tranexamic acid on intraoperative and postoperative bleeding in patients undergoing thyroid surgery has been published (Auvinen et al 1987). This double-blind trial used a 0.5 g dose of tranexamic acid at the induction of anaesthesia, followed by 1.5 g infused over the 24 hours during and after thyroid surgery. Bleeding was not significantly reduced in the active treatment group compared with controls.

Prevention of bleeding after extracorporeal circulation

Haemorrhage is a major complication after surgery utilizing extracorporeal circulation. Collier et al (1988) investigated the efficacy of tranexamic acid (10 mg/kg intravenously over 20 minutes, followed by 1 mg/kg/hour for 10 hours) in decreasing postoperative bleeding after such surgery. Plasminogen availability was reduced by more than half in the 14 evaluable patients receiving tranexamic acid ($p < 0.001$ vs placebo), and fibrin split products were present much less frequently ($p < 0.00005$). Blood loss was nearly 50% greater in patients treated with placebo ($p < 0.05$). Thus, tranexamic acid, used prophylactically, significantly reduces blood loss after extracorporeal circulation, so that exposure to potentially infectious agents in transfused blood may be minimized.

Prevention of rebleeding of subarachnoid haemorrhage

Patients who have survived the initial rupture of an intracranial aneurysm run a 20% risk of rebleeding and of developing delayed ischaemic cerebral deficits. In contrast to the cerebral tissue, the meninges and the choroid plexus are rich in tissue plasminogen activator. The aim of treating these patients with antifibrinolytic agents is to prolong the duration of the blood clot formed within and about the wall of the aneurysm and thus to reduce the critical period of surgical delay.

In addition to an American co-operative study (Nibbelink 1975), 11 randomized controlled clinical trials using tranexamic acid in the management of ruptured cerebral aneurysm have been published. Five of them were in favour of the drug (Chandra 1978, Fodstad et al 1978, Maurice-Williams 1978, Vermeulen et al 1984, Chowdhary & Sayed 1986), while six question its benefit (van Rossum et al 1977, Kaste & Ramsey 1979, Gelmers 1980, Fodstad et al 1981, Irthum et al 1986, Muizelaar et al 1988). Interpretation of at least some of the trials is confounded by flaws inherent in their design and methodology, including failure to use concurrent rather than historical control groups, lack of objective confirmation of rebleeding, absence of double-blinding or randomization, small patient numbers, and failure to begin therapy as soon as possible. Nevertheless, the problem remains that the reduction in mortality and morbidity from rebleeding is offset by an increase in incidence of ischaemic complications. The challenge is to find ways of eliminating the ischaemic complications, while the preventive effect on rebleeding is preserved (van Gijn 1991).

In conclusion, antifibrinolytic treatment can be considered during the first 10 days, and initial benefit appears sometimes to be lost due to delayed cerebral ischaemic deficits. The most suitable candidates for antifibrinolytic therapy are those in whom surgery is contraindicated and the risk of vasospasm is minimal (Adams 1987, Weir 1987). Consequently, it may be seriously argued whether tranexamic acid should be used routinely in the pre-operative management of patients with recently ruptured intracranial aneurysms. In any case, the drug should not be given over 10 days after the primary aneurysm rupture and should be immediately withdrawn if symptoms of delayed cerebral ischaemia appear.

There is a suggestion that low-dose tranexamic acid (3 g daily) with aprotinin (400 000 KIU daily) would be a more rational combination for lowering the rebleeding incidence without late ischaemic complications and post-subarachnoid haemorrhage (Guidetti & Spallone 1981, Spallone et al 1987). Another possible solution is to combine antifibrinolytic therapy with drugs that reduce the risk of cerebral ischaemia. The calcium entry blocker nicardipine has been administered together with antifibrinolytic drugs (EACA) in a preliminary study with promising results (Beck et al 1988).

Clinical efficacy of tranexamic acid in patients with a generalized bleeding disorder

Prevention of spontaneous bleeding in haemophilia

Antifibrinolytic drugs have been used as prophylaxis against spontaneous bleeding episodes in haemophilia with a daily dose of 2 g of tranexamic acid. One well designed long-term (12 months) double-blind study failed to show benefit (Bennett et al 1973) while another trial using 3 g daily (Rainsford et al 1973) in a double-blind, crossover study found a reduction in spontaneous bleeding episodes, significant at the 5% level.

Further studies are needed to elucidate the effect of tranexamic acid as long-term prophylactic drug against spontaneous bleeding episodes in haemophilia.

After tooth extraction in patients with haemophilia

The oral mucosa and the salivary gland have been found to contain a high concentration of plasminogen activators. This may explain why haemorrhage after oral surgical procedures may be caused by local fibrinolytic activity. Bleeding may be particularly marked in patients with a haemorrhagic diathesis (Vinckier & Vermylen 1984).

Forbes et al (1972), in a prospective randomized double-blind study, found that tranexamic acid, 1 g three times daily for 5 days, given in conjunction with factor VIII or IX, significantly reduced blood loss and transfusion requirements after dental extraction in patients with haemophilia. Other controlled trials (Taverner 1973, Ramström & Blombäck 1975) and a world-wide experience have in the meantime confirmed the favourable conclusion of the initial reports. Before dental extraction tranexamic acid, 15–25 mg per kg body weight, is given intravenously together with a factor VIII or IX concentrate. Before suturing, the site is irrigated with 4.8% tranexamic acid, and repeated mouth washes with the same solution for 2 minutes are recommended (Sindet-Pedersen et al 1988, 1989a,b). After surgery 15–25 mg/kg tranexamic acid are administered orally three to four times daily for 8 days. Usually, there is no further substitution therapy with coagulation factor concentrates required after surgery. The use of tranexamic acid has reduced the need for factor VIII or IX concentrates after dental extractions by 80%, also avoiding potential hazards inherent to blood products.

The combination of 1-deamino-8-D-arginine vasopressin (DDAVP) and tranexamic acid for dental extractions in mild to moderate haemophilia has also been advocated (Prince 1987). Similarly, Baudo et al (1988) have suggested that combined use of tranexamic acid and tissucol, a preparation of plasma containing a high concentration of fibrinogen, factor XIII and other plasma proteins, may obviate the need for replacement blood products for the management of oral bleeding in haemophiliacs. Subsequent analysis of their data has indicated that tranexamic acid exerts a statistically significant haemostatic effect (Sindet-Pedersen et al 1989b).

Treatment of bleeding in acute promyelocytic leukaemia

Acute promyelocytic leukaemia is commonly associated with a severe bleeding diathesis, which is fatal in 15% of patients. In a double-blind study, 12 consecutive patients with acute promyelocytic leukaemia were randomized either to tranexamic acid or to placebo for 6 days. In patients treated with tranexamic acid there were fewer haemorrhagic episodes (three versus 42, $p = 0.0045$), fewer red cell transfusions (28 versus 56, $p = 0.016$) were needed, and fewer platelet concentrates (69 versus 267, $p = 0.045$) were required (Avvisati et al 1989).

Side-effects of tranexamic acid

Side-effects of tranexamic acid are rare and mainly limited to nausea or diarrhoea, and occasionally an orthostatic reaction. It is likely that the better tolerance of tranexamic acid compared with EACA is due to the lower daily dose required with the former (3–6 g) than with the latter (18–30 g). As the antifibrinolytic activity with the recommended doses of each drug is of the same magnitude, the predisposition to thrombosis should be similar. It is well known that extravascular blood clots formed when the inhibitor is in the circulation may be resistant to physiological fibrinolysis (e.g. thrombi in the renal pelvis or bladder in patients with haematuria). In addition, there is the theoretical risk of an increased incidence of thrombosis, and a few patients have developed intracranial thrombosis (Naeye 1962, Sonntag & Stein 1974, Rydin & Lundberg 1976, Hoffman & Koo 1979) during treatment with EACA or tranexamic acid, or evidence of thrombosis in other vascular areas (Fletcher et al 1962, Naeye 1962, Gibbon & Camishion 1964, Lewis & Doyle 1964, Sharp 1964, Davies & Howell 1977). Although it has been shown that tranexamic acid does not deplete plasminogen levels, it does have an inhibitory effect on the activation of plasminogen. Theoretically, therefore, the administration of this antifibrinolytic agent could facilitate the development of thrombosis.

This association may be fortuitous and the reality of this

potential hazard is not clear. Indeed, the adverse reaction follow-up data of the Swedish National Board of Health and Welfare, correlated with the actual consumption over a period of 19 years, provide no evidence that tranexamic acid increases the risk of thromboembolic complications in the treatment of heavy menstrual periods. From 1969 to 1987, treatment of menorrhagia with tranexamic acid comprised 238 000 women-years. During the same period of time, 11 thromboembolic complications were reported to the Board. In two of these cases tranexamic acid was not implicated. 11 complications in 238 000 women-years, or an annual incidence of 0.005%, is no higher than the spontaneous incidence of thrombosis in fertile women (KabiVitrum AB, Survey Report 88.96.477; Astedt & Bekassy 1990).

In a retrospective study of 256 patients treated with tranexamic acid during pregnancy for various types of bleeding, 66% had been delivered by Caesarian section. Only two of 256 patients had a thromboembolic complication while the incidence of thrombosis during pregnancy is 0.5–1.0 per thousand and at surgery 1.8–5% (Lindoff et al 1992).

An adapted dosage to patients with decreased renal function will decrease the incidence of gastrointestinal side-effects in this disorder. Thus, in patients with serum creatinine concentration of 120–250 μmol/l, 10 mg tranexamic acid/kg body weight may be administered intravenously twice daily. In those with levels between 250 and 500 μmol/l, the same dose may be given at 24-hour intervals, and in those with a creatinine concentration of over 500 μmol/l the same dose may be given at 48-hour intervals (Andersson et al 1978). Although undue accumulation of the drug will be avoided, this precaution will not in theory reduce the risk of intravascular thrombosis if this potential hazard is a real clinical possibility.

HAEMOSTATIC AGENTS FOR TOPICAL USE

A topical haemostatic procedure is important in the management of local and superficial minor bleeding.

PURIFIED THROMBIN

Purified thrombin[20] can be used as a topical haemostatic agent either in a diluted solution (100–1000 NIH units/ml) or as a lyophilized powder. After topical application, the surface blood comes into contact with thrombin and the area is immediately filled with a firm coagulum. Thrombin was shown to control capillary bleeding and promote adhesion of tissue surfaces, e.g. fixation of tissue-transplants or skin grafts. Bovine thrombin is usually used as, despite its origin, antigenicity is rare when it is employed topically. The usual content of a vial is 1000, 5000 or 10 000 NIH units (one unit is that amount of thrombin required to clot 1 ml of standard fibrinogen solution in 15 seconds at 28°C). A thrombin solution can be sprayed with a syringe and a fine needle or can be used in conjunction with absorbable gelatin sponges or other, e.g. gingival, packing. For many years a weak thrombin preparation prepared from rabbit blood has been used in America.[21] A thrombin solution can also be taken by mouth in cases of gastrointestinal bleeding, provided its destruction is prevented by dissolving it in a phosphate buffer.

A new suturing system using physiologic substances for microneural and microvascular anastomoses, for closure of dural defects in bone surgery and for haemostasis, is based on the application of a fibrin adhesive system[22]. To this end, plasma cryoprecipitate in high concentrations is used as a source of fibrinogen and factor XIII, and thrombin solution enriched with calcium ions and a fibrinolysis inhibitor (aprotinin) are sprayed simultaneously in the surgical area. The solution firmly adheres to the wound surface and is quickly transformed into a rubberlike mass, which gains in strength in the hours following application.

TOPICAL USE OF APROTININ

Aprotinin is an essential component of the fibrin-adhesive mixture that is also being used in neurosurgery (Kletter et al 1978, Gastpar et al 1979) and in surgery of liver and spleen. The logic is that high local concentrations of the plasmin inhibitor (about 1000 KIU/ml) are required to stabilize the artificial fibrin glue. In brain surgery, haemostasis may sometimes become a problem due to the high concentration of plasminogen activitors in meningiomas, medulloblastomas, and cerebellar sarcomas. Aprotinin solutions have been applied topically to stop oozing and to prevent postoperative rebleeding (Tschesche 1974).

The haemostatic effect of local application of aprotinin (about 1 000 KIU/ml) in surgery of the brain was further investigated in an animal experiment and superiority against hydrogen peroxide solution has been demonstrated (Leheta et al 1982).

SOME SNAKE VENOMS

Some snake venoms[23] have a thrombin-like action, as they can coagulate fibrinogen directly. The fibrin formed is, however, chemically different (only fibrinopeptide A

[20] Thrombase (ISH, Paris), Thrombin Topical (Parke-Davis), Thrombo-Tuffon (Ligner and Fisher), Topostasin (Hoffman-La Roche).
[21] Haemostatic rabbit globulin or Parfentjev.
[22] Tisseel and Tissucol (Immuno), Beriplast P (Hoecast), Biocol (CATS).
[23] Botropase (Ravizza), Reptilase (Pentapharm).

is split off) from thrombin-generated fibrin (fibrinopeptide A and B are split off), and the clot formed does not completely resemble a normal clot.

Purified extracts of viper venoms

Purified extracts of viper venoms such as Russell's viper venom[24] are prepared as a dry powder; when reconstituted with water in a dilute solution (1/10 000), this substance acts as a powerful thromboplastin and rapidly activates prothrombin. Its action is even faster in the presence of lipids and supersedes that of the previously used tissue thromboplastin suspensions, which were acetone extracts of rabbit brain or lung tissue. These materials had the advantage of being harmless, but were almost inactive as topical haemostatics. Venoms prepared from other snakes such as the Australian tiger snake and the fer-de-lance have also been used as local haemostatics.

ABSORBABLE MATERIALS

Absorbable sponges of skin gelatin[25] are sterile, water insoluble, foamy materials which are usually moistened with saline or soaked in a thrombin solution before use.

Gelatin sponges do not have the disadvantage of conventional cotton wool, namely the frequent occurrence of rebleeding when the dressing is removed. Most of the gelatin sponges are completely absorbed in 4–6 weeks and may therefore be left in place after closure of the wound. Gelatin is easily destroyed if an inflammatory reaction occurs.

Methyl cellulose[26]

This is the water-soluble, cotton-like methyl ether of cellulose. It is non-allergenic and capable of absorbing eight times its weight of fluid. It exerts its physical effect by mechanical pressure; with the absorption of fluid the material swells and compresses the bleeding capillaries. Once in position, the methyl cellulose pad attains the consistency of moist blotting paper; it can be removed easily and painlessly, leaving a dry wound.

Oxidized cellulose[27]

This is a specially treated form of surgical gauze or cotton which is made absorbable by oxidation with nitrogen dioxide. This spongy substance is said to promote coagulation by a reaction between haemoglobin and cellulose acid; it also provides a large surface area at the site of haemorrhage, and the threads in the cotton provide reinforcement for the fibrin mesh. The absorption of oxidized cellulose may take 7 days to 7 weeks or longer. This material should not be used for implantation or packing in fractures, because it interferes with bone regeneration and may cause cyst formation. Oxidized cellulose also inhibits epithelialization and is therefore not a good surface dressing. Oxidized regenerated cellulose[28] is prepared from α-cellulose and is also a polyanhydroglucuronic acid. This product does not dissolve in water, salt solutions or plasma. Due to its negatively charged surface, clotting proceeds rapidly and the swollen material provides a matrix for fibrin, forming a partially artificial coagulum. Because of its low pH, oxidized cellulose interferes with the activity of thrombin unless this enzyme is dissolved in a 0.5% sodium bicarbonate solution. It does not cause local irritation.

Calcium alginate[29]

Upon hydrolysis of an extract of seaweed, algenic acid – a polymer of d-mannuronic acid – is obtained; its formula bears a striking resemblance to that of cellulose. Although salts of metals other than calcium can be used to coagulate alginates, calcium alginate has been found to be most useful, as its degree of contraction in drying is the lowest and it has excellent film-forming properties. Calcium alginate is absorbable and has the advantage of being heat-sterilizable. This material is used in the prevention of adhesion formation in the course of tissue repair and in the arrest of capillary haemorrhage.

Microcrystalline collagen[30]

This is an off-white flour-like powder prepared from bovine skin corium or from equine collagen fibrils. Its haemostatic activity can be ascribed to an inherent tissue-cohesive property of collagen itself, and to adhesion of platelets. This material is being used in cardiovascular surgery to arrest bleeding around arterial anastomoses. Several collagen preparations are made from pig or cattle skin and purified by proteolytic agents. This material is easy to handle, non-immunogenic and completely absorbable. It has been shown to be an effective topical haemostatic agent in orthopaedic surgery, vascular surgery, in the treatment of burns and atonic skin ulcers, and in the topical treatment of liver rupture.

---

[24] Stypven (Wellcome).
[25] Gelfilm (Upjohn), Gelfoam (Upjohn), Gelita-Tampon (Braun Melsungen), Sorbacel (Hartmann), Spongostan (Ferrosan), Sterispon (Allen and Hanbury).
[26] Colagel (Lilly), Hydrolose (Upjohn), Methocal (Dow Chemica Co).
[27] Oxycel[R] (Parke-Davis), Tabotamp Surgicel and Surgicel Nu-krit (Johnson and Johnson).
[28] Hemo-Pak (Johnson and Johnson), Oxycel (Parke-Davis), Sorbacel (Wander), Sorgical (Ethicon).
[29] Calgitex (Medical Alginates), Coalgan (Wallace, Cameron), Hemalgan (Delforge), Stop Hemo (Brothier), Trophiderm (Thiwissen), Ultraplast (Wallace, Cameron).
[30] Avitene (Avicon), Collagen Fleece (Pentapharm), Colgen (Interphar), Cutycol (Pharmacia), Tachotop (Hormon-Chemie).

ADDENDUM

The increasing use of large caliber new devices such as atherectomy catheters, stents or circulatory support systems is also associated with a greater risk of local bleeding. To shorten the compression times required to achieve haemostasis, a biodegradable collagen plug has been developed that enhances the formation of fibrin at the puncture site. Immediately after the end of the invasive procedure, collagen is delivered using a cartridge through a special applicator sheath and a second plug of collagen fills the place between the first plug and the skin (Ernst et al 1993). The procedure appears to be effective and safe. Theoretically, the insertion of collagen into the arterial lumen remains the major risk associated with this procedure.

REFERENCES

Adams H P 1987 Antifibrinolytics in aneurysmal subarachnoid hemorrhage; do they have a role? No. Archives in Neurology 44: 115–115

Adelman B, Michelson A D, Loscalzo J 1985 Plasmin effect on platelet glycoprotein Ib-von Willebrand's factor interaction. Blood 65: 32–40

ADIS Press 1990 Tranexamic Acid in Review. ADIS Press, Auckland, p 20

Ambrus J L, Schinnert G, Lajos T Z et al 1971 Effect of antifibrinolytic agents and estrogens on blood loss and blood coagulation factors during open heart surgery. Journal of Medicine, Experimental and Clinical 2: 65–81

Andersson L, Erikson O, Hedlund P O, Kjellman H, Lindqvist B 1978 Special considerations with regard to the dosage of tranexamic acid in patients with chronic renal diseases. Urological Research 6: 83–88

Andersson L, Nilsson I M, Nilehn J E, Hedner U, Grandstrand B, Melander B 1965 Experimental and clinical studies on AMCA, the antifibrinolytically active isomer of p-aminoethyl cyclohexane carboxylic acid. Scandinavian Journal of Haematology 2: 230–247

Astedt B, Nilsson I M 1978 Recurrent abruptio placentae treated with the fibrinolytic inhibitor tranexamic acid. British Medical Journal 1: 726–727

Astedt B, Bekassy Z 1990 Treatment with the fibrinolytic inhibitor tranexamic acid — risk for thrombosis? Acta Obstetrica et Gynecologica Scandinavica 69: 353–354

Auvinen O, Baer GA, Nordback I, Saaristo J 1987 Antifibrinolytic therapy for prevention of haemorrhage during surgery of the thyroid gland. Klinische Wochenschrift 65: 253–255

Avvisati G, ten Cate J W, Büller H R, Mandelli F 1989 Tranexamic acid for control of haemorrhage in acute promyelocytic leukemia. Lancet 1: 122–124

Barer D, Ogilvie A, Henry D et al 1983 Cimetidine and tranexamic acid in the treatment of acute upper-gastrointestinal tract bleeding. New England Journal of Medicine 308: 1571–1575

Barnhart M, Chen S, Lusher J M 1983 DDAVP: does the drug have a direct effect on the vessel wall? Thrombosis Research 31: 239–253

Baudo F, DeCataldo F, Landonio G, Muti G 1988 Management of oral bleeding in haemophilic patients. Lancet 2: 1082

Beck O J, Oeckler R 1981 Frühdiagnose und Therapie der Aneurysmablutungen. Münchner Medizinische Wochenschrift 123: 561–564

Beck D W, Adams H P, Flamm E S et al 1988 Combination of aminocaproic acid and nicardipine in treatment of aneurysmal subarachnoid hemorrhage. Stroke 19: 63–67

Bennett A E, Ingram G I C, Inglish P J 1973 Antifibrinolytic treatment in haemophilia: a controlled trial of prophylaxis with tranexamic acid. British Journal of Haematology 24: 83–88

Benson J W T, Drayton M R, Hayward C, Murphy J F, Osborne J P, Rennie J M, Schulte J F, Speidel B D, Cooke R W I 1986 Multicentre trial of ethamsylate for prevention of periventricular haemorrhage in very low birthweight infants. Lancet ii: 1297–2300

Bergqvist D, Dahlgren S, Hessman Y 1980 Local inhibition of the fibrinolytic system in patients with massive upper gastrointestinal hemorrhage. Uppsala Journal of Medical Sciences 85: 173–178

Bethune D W 1991 Aprotinin and cardiac surgery (Letter). British Medical Journal 303: 991

Bidstrup B P, Royston D, Taylor K M, Sapsford R N 1988 Effect of aprotinin on need for blood transfusion in patients with septic endocarditis having open-heart surgery. Lancet i: 336–337

Bidstrup B P, Royston D, Sapsford R N, Taylor K M 1989 Reduction in blood loss and blood use after cardiopulmonary bypass with high dose aprotinin (Trasylol). Journal of Thoracic and Cardiovascular Surgery 97: 364–372

Biggs C, Hugh T B, Dodds A J 1976 Tranexamic acid and upper gastrointestinal haemorrhage: a double blind trial. Gut 17: 729–734

Blombäck B, Blombäck M, Nilsson I M 1957 Coagulation studies on Reptilase, an extract of the venom from Bothrops Jararaca. Thrombosis et Diathesis Haemorrhagica 1: 1–13

Blombäck B, Blombäck M, Olsson P 1967 Action of a proteolytic enzymatic inhibitor on blood coagulation in vitro. Thrombosis et Diathesis Haemorrhagica 18: 2–9

Bond L, Bevan D 1988 Myocardial infarction in a patient with hemophilia treated with DDAVP. New England Journal of Medicine 318: 121

Borst H G, Haverich A, Walterbusch G, Maatz W 1982 Fibrin adhesive: an important hemostatic adjunct in cardiovascular operations. Journal of Thoracic and Cardiovascular Surgery 84: 548–553

Bramsen T 1977 Traumatic hyphaema treated with the antifibrinolytic drug tranexamic acid. II. Acta Ophthalmologica 55: 616–620

Bramsen T, Corydon L, Ehlers N 1978 A double-bind study of the influence of tranexamic acid on the central corneal thickness after cataract extraction. Acta Ophthalmologica 56: 121–126

Bronner M H, Pate M B, Cunningham J T, Marsh W H 1986 Estrogen progesterone therapy for bleeding gastrointestinal teleangiectasias in chronic renal failure. Annals of Internal Medicine 105: 371–374

Callender S T, Warner G T, Cope E 1970 Treatment of menorrhagia with tranexamic acid: a double blind trial. British Medical Journal 4: 214–216

Castelli G, Vogt E 1977 Der Erfolg einer antifibrinolytischen Behandlung mit Tranexamsaure zur Reduktion der Blutverlustes während und nach Tonsillektomien. Schweizerische Medizinische Wochenschrift 107: 780–784

Cattaneo M, Moia M, Della Valle P, Castellana P, Mannucci P M 1989 DDAVP shortens the prolonged bleeding times of patients with severe von Willebrand disease treated with cryoprecipitate. Evidence for a mechanism of action independent of release of von Willebrand factor. Blood 74: 1972–1975

Chandra B 1978 Treatment of subarachnoid haemorrhage from ruptured intracranial aneurysm with tranexamic acid: a double-blind clinical trial. Annals of Neurology 3: 502–504

Charles O, Coolsaet B 1972 Prévention des hémorragies en chirurgie prostatique. Annals of Urologie 6: 209–212

Chowdhary U M, Sayed K 1986 Prevention of early recurrence of aneurysmal subarachnoid haemorrhage by tranexamic acid: a controlled clinical trial. Vascular Surgery 20: 8–13

Clozel J P, Banken L, Roux S 1990 Aprotinin: an antidote for recombinant tissue-type plasminogen activator (rt-PA) active in vivo. Journal of the American College of Cardiology 16: 507–510

Collier W, Hlavacek J, Horrow J C, Goldman S, Goel I P 1988 Prophylactic tranexamic acid decreases blood loss after extracorporeal circulation. Anesthesiology 69: A135

Cooke R W I 1987 Effect of ethamsylate on cerebral blood flow (letter). Lancet i: 923–924

Cormack F, Chakrabarti R R, Jouhar A J, Fearnley G R 1973 Tranexamic acid in upper gastrointestinal haemorrhage. Lancet 1: 1207–1208

Correll J T, Lyth L F, Long S, Vanderpoel J C 1952 Some physiological responses to 5–hydroxytryptamine. American Journal of Physiology 169: 537

Czer L S, Bateman T M, Gray R J, Raymond M, Steward M E et al 1987 Treatment of severe platelet dysfunction and hemorrhage after cardiopulmonary bypass: reduction in blood product usage with desmopressin. Journal of the American College of Cardiology 9: 1139–1147

Czer L S C, Capon S M 1990 Clinical experience in disorders of haemostasis. Drug Investigation 2 (suppl 5): 32–44

Davies D, Howell D A 1977 Tranexamic acid and arterial thrombosis. Lancet 1: 49

Deacock A A, Birley D M 1969 The anti-hemorrhagic activity of ethamsylate (Dicynone). British Journal of Anaesthesiology 41: 18–24

de la Fuente B, Kasper C K, Rickless F R, Hoyer L W 1985 Response of patients with mild and moderate hemophilia A and von Willebrand's disease to treatment with desmopressin. Annals of Internal Medicine 103: 6–14

de Nicola P, Guccione G, Manara G, Cipolli P L 1969 Manifestazioni emorragiche in pazienti con reperti normali dell emocoagulazione e dell'emostasis. Minerva Otorinolaringica 17: 183–188

Dermaut G, Gilson M 1963 Etude expérimentale des propriétés hémostatiques et de l'activité vasculaire de la monosemicarbazone de la beta-naphtoquinone. Archives Internationales de Pharmacodynamie et de Thérapie 146: 517–528

Derouaux G 1961 Etude expérimentale des propriétés hémostatiques de la monosemicarbazone de la beta-naphtoquinone. Comptes Rendus des Séances de la Société de Biologie et de ses Filiales 155: 950–962

Deutsch E 1952 Der Wirkugsmechanismus von 'Hämostyptikum Schoch'. Arzneimittel-Forschung 2: 470–477

Deutsch E, Fischer M 1963 Die Verwendung eines stabilen Phospholipidpräparates als Thrombocytenersatz bei Gerinnungsanalysen. Arzneimittel-Forschung 13: 439–445

Djerassi I, Klein E, Farber S, Palmer D 1958 Effects of 5-hydroxytryptamine on some aspects of the hemorrhagic state in radiation-induced thrombocytopenia. Proceedings of the Society of Experimental Biology and Medicine 57: 552

Engqvist A, Broström O, von Feilitzen F et al 1979 Tranexamic acid in massive haemorrhage from the upper gastrointestinal tract. A double-blind study. Scandinavian Journal of Gastroenterology 14: 839–884

Ernst S M P G, Tjonjoegin M, Schräder R, Kaltenbach M, Sigwart V, Sanborn T A, Plokker W T 1993 Immediate sealing of arterial puncture sites after cardiac catheterization and coronary angioplasty using a biodegradable collagen plug: results of an international registry. Journal of the American College of Cardiology 15: 851–855

España F, Estelles A, Griffin J H, Aznar J, Gilabert J 1989 Aprotinin (Trasylol) is a competitive inhibitor of activated protein C. Thrombosis Research 56: 751–756

Fletcher A P, Alkjaersig N, Sherry S 1962 Fibrinolytic mechanisms and the development of thrombolytic therapy. American Journal of Medicine 33: 738–752

Fodstad H, Liliequist B, Schannong M, Thulin CA 1978 Tranexamic acid in the preoperative management of ruptured intracranial aneurysms. Surgical Neurology 10: 9–15

Fodstad H, Forsell A, Liliequist B, Schannong M 1981 Antifibrinolysis with tranexamic acid in aneurysmal subarachnoid haemorrhage: a consecutive controlled trial. Neurosurgery 8: 158–165

Forbes C D, Barr R D, Reid G, et al 1972 Tranexamic acid in control of hemorrhage after dental extraction in haemophilia and Christmas disease. British Medical Journal 2: 311–313

Gaffney P, Brasher M 1974 Mode of action of ancrod as a defibrinating agent. Nature 251: 53–54

Gamba G, Fornasari P M, Grignani G, Dolci D, Colloi D 1979 Haemostasis during transvesical prostatic adenomectomy. A controlled trial on the effects of drugs with antifibrinolytic and thrombin-like activities. Blut 39: 89–98

Gastpar H, Kastenbauer E R, Behbehani A A 1979 Erfahrungen mit einem humanen Fibrinkleber bei operativen Eingriffen im Kopf-Hals-Bereich. Laryngologie, Rhinologie, Otologie (Stuttgart) 58: 389–399

Gelmers J H 1980 Prevention of recurrence of spontaneous subarachnoid haemorrhage by tranexamic acid. Acta Neurochirurgica 52: 45–50

George J N, Pickett E B, Saucerman S, McEver R P, Kunucki T J, Kieffer N, Newman P J 1986 Platelet surface glycoproteins. Studies on resting and activated platelets and platelet membrane microparticles in normal subjects, and observations in patients with adult respiratory distress syndrome and cardiac surgery. Journal of Clinical Investigation 78: 340–348

Gibbon J H, Camishion R C 1964 Problems in hemostasis with extracorporeal apparatus. Annals of the New York Academy of Sciences 115: 195–198

Graeff H, Halter R, von Hugo R 1978 Akute Blutgerinnungsstörungen in der Geburtshilfe. Die Medizinische Welt 29: 212–216

Guidetti B, Spallone A 1981 The role of antifibrinolytic therapy in the preoperative management of recently ruptured intracranial aneurysms. Surgical Neurology 15: 139–148

Haberland G, McConn R 1979 A rationale for the therapeutic action of aprotinin. Federation Proceedings 38: 2760–2767

Hack G, Kirchhoff P G, Popov-Cenic S, Kulzer R, Schlemminger B, Piepho A 1983 Aprotinin bei Operationen am offenen Herzen. Die Medizinische Welt 34: 726–731

Haiböck H F 1972 Clinical and experimental investigations of a physiological haemostatic agent. Zeitschrift für Therapie 6: 339–342

Harrison R, Campbell S 1976 A double-blind trial of ethamsylate (Dicynene) in the treatment of excessive menstrual bleeding in patients with and without intrauterine contraceptive device. Lancet 2: 283–285

Harrison R F, Matthews T 1984 Intrapartum ethamsylate (letter). Lancet 2: 296

Haverback B J, Dutcher T F, Shore P A, Tomich E G, Terry L L, Brodie B B 1957 Serotonin changes in platelets and brain induced by small daily doses of reserpine-lack of effect of depletion of platelet serotonin on hemostatic mechanisms. New England Journal of Medicine 256: 343–345

Haverich A, Walterbusch G, Borst H G 1983 Abdichtung poröser Gefässprothesen under Teil-Heparinisierung und extrakorporaler Zirkulation. Angio 5: 215–220

Hedlund P O 1969 Antifibrinolytic therapy with Cyclokapron in connection with prostatectomy: a double blind study. Scandinavian Journal of Urology and Nephrology 3: 177–182

Henry D A, O'Connell D L 1989 Effects of fibrinolytic inhibitors on mortality from upper gastrointestinal haemorrhage. British Medical Journal 296: 1142–1146

Hoffman E P, Koo A H 1979 Cerebral thrombosis associated with Amicar. Radiology 131: 687–689

Hollanders D, Thomson J M, Schofield P F 1983 Tranexamic acid therapy in ulcerative colitis. Postgraduate Medical Journal 58: 87–91

Hoylaerts M, Lijnen H R, Collen D 1981 Studies on the mechanism of antifibrinolytic action of tranexamic acid. Biochimica et Biophysica Acta 673: 75–85

Hunt B J, Cottam S, Segal H, et al 1990 Inhibition by aprotinin of tPA-mediated fibrinolysis during orthotopic liver transplantation. Lancet 335: 381

Irthum B, Chazal J, Commun C, Chabannes J, Janny P 1986 Essai prospectif de traitement des hémorragies meningées anévrysmales par intervention differée sous couvert d'un traitement antifibrinolytique. Neurochirurgie 32: 122–126

Jaffé G, Wickham A 1973 A double-blind pilot study of Dicynene in the control of menorrhagia. Journal of International Medical Research 1: 127–129

Jerndal T, Frisén M 1976 Tranexamic acid (AMCA) and late hyphaemia – A double blind study in cataract surgery. Acta Ophthalmologica 54: 417–429

John L C H, Rees G M, Kovacs I B 1991 Aprotinin and cardiac surgery (letter). British Medical Journal 303: 991–992

Kasonde J M, Bonnar J 1975 Effects of ethamsylate and aminocaproic acid on menstrual blood loss in women using intrauterine devices. British Medical Journal 4: 21–22

Kaste M, Ramsay M 1979 Tranexamic acid in subarachnoid hemorrhage. A double-blind study. Stroke 10: 519–522

Kaufmann J, Siefker K 1969 Medikamentöse Senkung postoperativer Blutungen nach Prostatektomien. Urologie 8: 57–59

Kentro T B, Lottenbery R, Kitchens C S 1987 Clinical efficacy of

desmopressin acetate for hemostatic control in patients with primary platelet disorders undergoing surgery. American Journal of Hematology 24: 215–219
Kinn A C 1970 Konisation vid cancer in situ. Läkartidn 67: 2529–2532
Kletter G, Matras H, Dinges H P 1978 Zur partiellen Klebung von Mikrogefässanastomosen im intrakraniellen Bereich. Wiener Klinische Wochenschrift 90: 415–419
Kobrinsky N L, Letts R M, Patel L R, Israels E D, Monson R C, et al 1987 1-desamino-8-D-arginine vasopressin (desmopressin) decreases operative blood loss in patients having Harrington Rod spinal fusion surgery. A randomized, double-blind controlled trial. Annals of Internal Medicine 107: 446–450
Kommerell B 1960 The coagulation activation effect of Clauden as established by the Thrombokinase formation test. Münchener Medizinische Wochenschrift 102: 1332–1334
Kondo M, Fukumoto K, Yoshikawa T et al 1981 Tissue fibrinolysis in the digestive mucosa. III. Treatment of ulcerative colitis by the direct administration of an antifibrinolytic agent as an enema. Nippon Shokakibyo Gakkai Zasshi 3: 653–657
Köstering H, Kirchhoff P G, Völker P, Warmann E, Koncz J 1973 Untersuchungen der Blutgerinnungsveränderungen während und nach Operationen mit Hilfe der Herz-Lungen-Maschine. Thoraxchirurgie 21: 534–543
Kösters S, Wand H 1973 Ueber die Beeinflussung des Blutverlustes nach Prostata-operationen durch prä-operative Applikation von Antifibrinolytika. Urologie A 12: 295–296
Kovacs L, Annus J 1978 L'efficacité de l'etamsylate dans la ménorragie provoquée par les dispositifs intra-utérins. Gynecologic and Obstetric Investigation 9: 161–165
Kuschinsky G, Lang M, Wollert U 1968 Untersuchungen über die Wirkungen von Butanol als Hämostypticum. Deutsche Medizinische Wochenschrift 93: 1443–1445
Landin L E, Werner E 1975 Late bleeding after conization. The effect of tranexamic acid (Cyclokapron). Opuscula Medica 20: 280–284
Langman M J S 1987 Drug treatment of haematemesis and melaena. Scandinavian Journal of Gastroenterology 22 (suppl 137): 67–70
Leheta F, Lenz C, Welchenmeier I et al 1982 Die Beeinflussung der Fibrinolyse am traumatisierten Rattenhirn durch lokale Applikation von Aprotinin. Wasserstoffperoxid und physiologischer NaCl-Losüng. Medizinische Welt 33: 1802–1804
Lens X M, Casals F J, Oliva J A, Pascual R, Carrio J, et al 1988 Transfornos de la coagulacion en la insuficiencia renal: modificaciones por de la desamino-8-d-arginina vasopressin. Medicina Clinica (Barcelona) 90: 603–606
Lethagen S, Harris A S, Nilsson I M 1990 Intranasal desmopressin (DDAVP) by spray in mild hemophilia A and von Willebrand's disease type I. Blut 60: 187–191
Lewis J H, Doyle A P 1964 Effects of epsilon-aminocaproic acid on coagulation and fibrinolytic mechanisms. Journal of the American Medical Association 188: 56–63
Lindoff C, Rybo G, Astedt B 1992 Treatment with tranexamic acid during pregnancy; no evidence of any increase in the risk of thromboembolic complications. (submitted for publication)
Liu Y R, Kosfield R E, Marcum S G 1984 Treatment of uraemic bleeding with conjugated oestrogen. Lancet 2: 887–890
Livio M, Mannucci P M, Vigano G et al 1986 Conjugated estrogens for the management of bleeding associated with renal failure. New England Journal of Medicine 315: 731–735
Locatelli A, Ceriana P, Maurelli M, Bertollo D, Bianchi T, Mazza M P, Chiaudani G, Pagnin A 1991 Aprotinin in cardiac surgery (letter). Lancet 338: 254
Lohmann K, Markwardt F, Landmann H 1963 Ueber neue Hemmstoffe der Fibrinolyse. Naturwissenschaften 50: 502
Louis J, Paulus J M 1967 Essai d'un nouvel hémostatique: la Dicynone. Revue Médical de Liège 22: 649–651
Lu H, Soria C, Commin J P, Soria J, Piwnica A, Schumann F, Regnier O, Legrand Y, Caen J P 1991 Hemostasis in patients undergoing extracorporeal circulation: the effect of aprotinin (Trasylol). Thrombosis and Haemostasis 66: 633–637
Lusher J M 1990 Pharmacology and pharmacokinetics of desmopressin in haemostatic disorders. Drug Investigation 2 (suppl 5): 25–31
McElligot E, Quigley C, Hanks G W 1991 Tranexamic acid and rectal bleeding (letter). Lancet 337: 431
Mallett S V, Cox D, Burroughs A K, Rolles K 1990 Aprotinin and reduction of blood loss and transfusion requirements in orthotopic liver transplantation. Lancet 336: 886–887
Mammen E F 1968 Natural proteinase inhibitors in extracorporeal circulation. Annals of the New York Academy of Sciences 146: 754–761
Mannucci P M 1986 Desmopressin (DDAVP) for treatment of disorders of hemostasis. Progress in Hemostasis and Thrombosis 8: 19–45
Mannucci P M, Lusher J M 1989 Desmopressin and thrombosis. Lancet ii: 675–676
Mannucci P M, Ruggeri Z M, Pareti F I, Capitanio A 1977 DDAVP: a new pharmaceutical approach to the management of haemophilia and von Willebrand's disease. Lancet ii: 1171–1172
Mannucci P M, Remuzzi G, Pusineri F, Lombardi R, Valsecchi C et al 1983 Deamino-8-D-arginine vasopressin shortens the bleeding time in uremia. New England Journal of Medicine 308: 8–12
Mannucci P M, Vicente V, Vianello L 1986 Controlled trial of desmopressin in liver cirrhosis and other conditions associated with a prolonged bleeding time. Blood 67: 1148–1153
Mannucci P M, Vicente V, Alberca I, Sacchi E, Longo G et al 1987 Intravenous and subcutaneous administration of desmopressin (DDAVP) to hemophiliacs: pharmacokinetics and factor VIII response. Thrombosis and Haemostasis 58: 1037–1039
Markland C G, Strurridge M F, Hulf J F, Woodall N M 1988 Effect of aprotinin in blood loss in repeat open heart surgery. Lancet i: 711
Markwardt F 1978 Synthetic inhibitors of fibrinolysis. In: Markwardt F (ed): Fibrinolytics and antifibrinolytics. Springer-Verlag, Berlin, p 511–577
Maurice-Williams R S 1978 Prolonged antifibrinolysis: an effective non-surgical treatment for ruptured intracranial aneurysms? British Medical Journal 1: 945–947
Miglioli M, Barbara L, Di Febo G, Gozzetti G, Lauri A, Paganelli G M, Poggioli G, Santucci R 1989 Topical administration of 5-aminosalicylic acid: a therapeutic proposal for the treatment of pouchitis (letter). The New England Journal of Medicine 320: 257
Miller R A, May M W, Hendry W F, Whitfield H W, Wickham J E A 1980 The prevention of secondary haemorrhage after prostatectomy: the value of antifibrinolytic therapy. British Journal of Urology 52: 26–28
Mowatt M A G, Douglas A S, Brunt P W, McIntosh J A R, King P C, Boddy K 1973 Epsilon aminocaproic acid therapy in ulcerative colitis. Digestive Diseases 18: 959–965
Muhm M, Grois N, Kier P, Stümfplen A, Kyrle P, Pabinger I, Bettelheim P, Hinterberger W, Lechner K 1990 1-Deamino-8-D-arginine vasopressin in the treatment of non-haemophilic patients with acquired factor VIII inhibitor. Haemostasis 20: 15–20
Muizelaar J P, Vermeulen M, van Crevel H, Hijdra A, van Gijn J et al 1988 Outcome of aneurysmal subarachnoid hemorrhage in patients 66 years of age and older. Clinical Neurology and Neurosurgery 90: 203–207
Naeye L 1962 Thrombotic state after hemorrhagic diathesis, a possible complication of therapy with epsilon-aminocaproic acid. Blood 19: 694–701
Neuhaus P, Bechstein W O, Lefèbre B, Blumhardt G, Slama K 1989 Effect of aprotinin on intraoperative bleeding and fibrinolysis in liver transplantation. Lancet ii: 924–925
Nibbelinck D W 1975 Cooperative aneurysm study: anti-hypertensive and antifibrinolytic therapy following subarachnoid haemorrhage from ruptured intracranial aneurysm. In: Whisnant J P, Sandok B A (eds) Cerebral vascular disease. Grune & Stratton, New York, p 155–173
Nicoumar G 1975 L'utilisation prophylactique et thérapeutique de la Bothropase en Chirurgie ORL. Médecine et Hygiène (Genève) 33: 772
Nieuwenhuis H K, Sixma J J 1988 1-desamino-8-d-arginine vasopressin (desmopressin) shortens the bleeding time in storage pool deficiency. Annals of Internal Medicine 105: 65–67
Niewiarowski S, Kirby E P, Stocker K 1977 Thrombocytin — a novel platelet activating enzyme from Bothrops atrox venom. Thrombosis Research 10: 863–869
Nilsson L, Rybo G 1967 Treatment of menorrhagia with an antifibrinolytic agent, tranexamic acid (AMCA): a double-blind

investigation. Acta Obstetrica et Gynecologica Scandinavica 46: 572–580
Nilsson L, Rybo G 1971 Treatment of menorrhagia. American Journal of Obstetrics and Gynecology 110: 713–720
Nilsson I M, Björkman S E, Studnitz W, Hallen A 1961 Antifibrinolytic activity of certain pectins. Thrombosis et Diathesis Haemorrhagica 6: 177–187
Norrelykke Nissen J, Ehiers N 1986 No additive effect of tranexamic acid and naproxen on corneal deswelling. Acta Ophthalmologica 64: 291–294
O'Brien J R, Green P J, Salmon G, Weir P, Colin-Jones D et al 1989 Desmopressin and myocardial infarction. Lancet i: 664–665
Oeney T, Schander K, Müller N, Fromm G, Lang N 1982 Fruchtwasserembolie mit Gerinnungsstörung — ein kasuistischer Beitrag. Geburtshilfe und Frauenheilkunde 42: 25–28
Pandolfi M 1978 Intraocular haemorrhages: a haemostatic therapeutic approach. Survey of Ophthalmology 22: 322–334
Peerschke E I B, Wainer J A 1985 Examination of irreversible platelet-fibrinogen interactions. Cellular Physiology 17: C466
Pepeu G 1975 Toxicological and pharmacological investigations on aminonaphtone (2-hydroxy-2-methyl-14-naphtohydroquinone-2-amino-benzoate). Quaderni della Coagulazione 1: 19–25
Petruson B 1974 A double-blind study to evaluate the effect in epistaxis with oral administration of the antifibrinolytic drug tranexamic acid (Cyclokapron). Acta Otolaryngologica (suppl) 317: 57–61
Pfeifer G W 1968 Proteinasenblockade bei abgestorbener Schwangerschaft, dead fetus syndrome. Deutsche Medizinische Wochenschrift 93: 479–485
Pilbrant A, Shannong M, Vessman J 1981 Pharmacokinetics and bioavailability of tranexamic acid. European Journal of Clinical Pharmacology 20: 65–72
Poliwoda H 1965 Die medikamentöse Therapie von Blutungen unter Berucksichtigung ihrer Aetiologie und Pathogenese. Landartz 41: 1468–1472
Poller L 1955 A study of Naphthionin, a new haemostatic drug. Journal of Clinical Pathology 8: 331–333
Poller L, More J R S 1964 A study of Naphthionin in the management of the bleeding defect in patients with thrombocytopenia. Journal of Clinical Pathology 17: 680–684
Popov-Cenic S, Urban A E, Noë G 1982 Studies on the cause of bleeding during and after surgery with a heart-lung machine in children with cyanotic and acyanotic congenital cardiac defects and their prophylactic treatment. In: McConn (ed) Role of chemical mediators in the pathophysiology of acute illness and injury. Raven Press, New York, p 229–242
Porte R J, Bontempo F A, Knott E A R et al 1985 Tissue type plasminogen activator associated fibrinolysis in orthotopic liver transplantation. Transplantation Proceedings 21: 3542
Prentice C R M, Mc Nicol G P, Douglas A S 1970 Studies on the anticoagulant action of aprotinin (Trasylol). Thrombosis et Diathesis Haemorrhagica 24: 265–272
Prince S 1987 An alternative to blood product therapy for dental extractions in the mild to moderate haemophiliac patient. British Dental Journal 162: 256
Rainsford S G, Jouar A J, Hall A 1973 Tranexamic acid in the control of spontaneous bleeding in severe haemophilia. Thrombosis et Diathesis Haemorrhagica 30: 272–279
Ramström G, Blombäck M 1975 Tooth extraction in hemophiliacs. International Journal of Oral Surgery 4: 1–17
Richardson D W, Robinson A G 1985 Desmopressin. Annals of Internal Medicine 103: 228–239
Rö J S, Knutrud O, Stormorken H 1970 Antifibrinolytic treatment with tranexamic acid (AMCHA) in pediatric urinary tract surgery. Journal of Pediatric Surgery 5: 315–320
Rocha E, Llorens R, Paramo S A, Arcas R, Cuesta B et al 1988 Does desmopressin acetate reduce blood loss after surgery in patients on cardiopulmonary bypass? Circulation 77: 1319–1323
Rose E H, Aledort L M 1991 Nasal spray desmopressin (DDAVP) for mild hemophilia A and von Willebrand disease. Annals of Internal Medicine 114: 563–568
Roskam J, Derouaux G, Meys I, Swalue L 1944 Action hémostatique de la monomine et de la mono-semicarbazone d'adrénochrome chez l'homme. Archives Internationales de Pharmacodynamie et de Thérapie 69: 875–877
Royston D, Taylor K M, Bidstrup B P, Sapsford R N 1987 Effect of aprotinin on need for blood transfusion after repeat open-heart surgery. Lancet 2: 1289–1291
Rybo G, Westerberg H 1972 The effect of tranexamic acid (AMCA) in postoperative bleeding after conization. Acta Obstetrica et Gynecologica Scandinavica (suppl) 51: 347–350
Rydin E, Lundberg P O 1976 Tranexamic acid and intracranial thrombosis. Lancet 2: 49
Salzman E W 1990 Desmopressin and surgical hemostasis. New England Journal of Medicine 322: 1085 (Letter)
Salzman E W, Weinstein M J, Weintraub R M, Ware J A, Thurer R L et al 1986 Treatment with desmopressin acetate to reduce blood loss after cardiac surgery. A double blind randomized trial. New England Journal of Medicine 314: 1402–1406
Schimpf K, Hanf-Hoppe H W, Immich H 1972 Intravenous infusion of a standardised coagulation active phospholipid complex in uremic coagulation deficiency. Thrombosis et Diathesis Haemorrhagica 27: 554–558
Sharp A A 1964 Pathological fibrinolysis. British Medical Bulletin 20: 240–246
Shemin D, Elnour M, Amarantes B, Abuelo J G, Chazan J A 1990 Oral estrogens decrease bleeding time and improve clinical bleeding in patients with renal failure. American Journal of Medicine 89: 436–440
Shepherd L L, Hutchinson R J, Worden E K, Koopman C F, Coran A 1989 Hyponatremia and seizures after intravenous administration of desmopressin acetate for surgical hemostasis. Journal of Pediatrics 114: 470–472
Sher G 1980 Trasylol in the management of abruptio placentae with consumption coagulopathy and uterine inertia. Journal of Reproductive Medicine 25: 113–118
Sindet-Petersen S, Ingerslev J, Ramström G, Blombäck M 1988 Management of oral bleeding in haemophilic patients. Lancet 2: 566
Sindet-Petersen S, Ingerslev J, Ramström G, Blombäck M 1989a Management of oral bleeding in haemophilic patients. Lancet 1: 325
Sindet-Petersen S, Ramström G, Bernvil S, Blombäck M 1989b Hemostatic effect of tranexamic acid mouthwash in anticoagulant-treated patients undergoing oral surgery. New England Journal of Medicine 320: 840–843
Sonntag V K H, Stein B M 1974 Arteriopathic complications during treatment of subarachnoid haemorrhage with epsilon-aminocaproic acid. Journal of Neurosurgery 40: 480–485
Spallone A, Pastore F S, Rizzo A, Guidetti B 1987 Low-dose tranexamic acid combined with aprotinin in the pre-operative management of ruptured intracranial aneurysms. Neurochirurgia 30: 172–176
Stael von Holstein C, Eriksson S B S, Källen R 1987 Tranexamic acid as an aid to reducing blood transfusion requirements in gastric and duodenal bleeding. British Medical Journal 294: 7–10
Staubesand J, Schmidt-Matthiesen H, Poliwoda H 1966 Elektronmitroskopische und histochemische Befund zum Problem des sog. Gefässfaktors bei hämorrhagische Diathesen. Klinische Wochenschrift 44: 547–550
Sunamori M, Amano J, Kameda T, Okamura T, Ozeki M, Suzuki A 1980 Additive protection of aprotinin, protease inhibitor to cold cardioplegia from ischemic myocardium. Japanese Circulation Journal 44: 771–775
Svandberg L, Astedt B, Nilsson I M 1980 Abruptio placentae. Treatment with the fibrinolytic inhibitor tranexamic acid. Acta Obstetrica et Gynacologica Scandinavica 59: 127–130
Tauber P F 1979 Uterine Blutungen bei intrauteriner Kontrazeption. Die Medizinsche Welt 30: 1547–1553
Tauber P F, Wolf A S, Herting W, Zaneveld L J D 1977 Hemorrhage induced by intrauterine devices: control by local proteinase inhibition. Fertility and Sterility 28: 1375–1377
Taverner R W H 1973 The use of tranexamic acid in the control of haemorrhage after extraction of teeth in haemophilia and Christmas disease. British Medical Journal 2: 314–315
Thorsen S 1975 Differences in the binding to fibrin of native

plasminogen and plasminogen modified by proteolytic degradation. Influence of ω-aminocarboxylic acids. Biochimica et Biophysica Acta 393: 55–65
Tice D A, Worth M H, Clauss R H, Reed G H 1964 The inhibition of Trasylol of fibrinolytic activity associated with cardiovascular operations. Surgery, Gynecology and Obstetrics 119: 71–74
Tschesche H 1974 Biochemie natürlicher Proteinase-Inhibitoren. Angew Chemie 86: 21–40
van Dantzig J M, Durec D R, Witen C J W 1989 Desmopressin and myocardial infarction. Lancet i: 664
Vandenvelde C, Fondu P, Dubois-Primo J 1991 Low-dose aprotinin for reduction of blood loss after cardiopulmonary bypass (letter). Lancet 337: 1157–1158
van Gijn J 1991 Managing subarachnoid haemorrhage. Proceedings of the Royal College of Physicians of Edinburgh 21: 16–32
van Oeveren W, Jansen N J G, Bidstrup B P, Royston D, Estaby S, Neuhof H, Wildevuur C R H 1987 Effects of aprotinin on hemostatic mechanisms during cardiopulmonary bypass. Annals of Thoracic Surgery 44: 640–645
van Oeveren W, Eijsman L, Roozendaal K J, Wildevuur C R H 1988 Platelet preservation by aprotinin during cardiopulmonary bypass. Lancet 1: 644
van Rossum J, Wintzen A R, Enotz L J, Schoen J H R, Jorge H 1977 Effects of tranexamic aid on rebleeding after subarachnoid hemorrhage. A double-blind controlled clinical trial. Annals of Neurology 2: 238–242
Varnek L, Dalsgaard C, Hansen A, Klie F 1980 The effect of tranexamic acid on secondary haemorrhage after traumatic hyphaemia. Acta Ophthalmologica 58: 787–793
Vermeulen M, Lindsay K W, Murray G D, Chesh F, Hijdra A et al 1984 Antifibrinolytic treatment in subarachnoid hemorrhage. New England Journal of Medicine 311: 432–437
Vermylen J, Verhaegen-Declercq M L, Verstraete M, Fierens F 1968 A double-blind study of the effect of tranexamic acid in essential menorrhagia. Thrombosis et Diathesis Haemorrhagica 20: 583–587
Verstraete M (ed) 1977 Haemostatic drugs. A critical appraisal. Martinus Nijhoff, The Hague, p 155
Verstraete M, Vermylen J (eds) 1984 Thrombosis. Pergamon Press, Oxford
Verstraete M, Tyberghein J, Degreef V, Daems L, Van Hoof A 1977 Double-blind trials with ethamsylate, batroxobin or tranexamic acid on blood loss after adenotonsillectomy. Acta Clinica Belgica 32: 136–141
Vinazzer H 1980 Clinical and experimental studies on the action of ethamsylate on haemostasis and on platelet functions. Thrombosis Research 19: 783–791
Vinckier F, Vermylen J 1984 Wound healing following dental extraction in rabbits: effects of tranexamic acid, warfarin anticoagulation and socket packing. Journal of Dental Research 63: 646–649
Walzman M, Bonnar J 1982 Effects of tranexamic acid on coagulation and fibrinolytic systems in pregnancy complicated by placental bleeding. Archives of Toxicology (suppl) 5: 214–220
Wayne L, Glueck H I, Brodine C, Coots M 1964 Effect of intravenous estrogen on an inhibitor of hyaluronidase and on clotting factors in blood. Proceedings of the Society for Experimental Biology and Medicine 116: 85
Weir B 1987 Antifibrinolytics in subarachnoid hemorrhage: do they have a role? Archives of Neurology 44: 116–118
Werle E 1968 Contribution to the biochemistry of Trasylol. In: Haberland G L, Matis P (eds) New aspects of Trasylol therapy. The clinical significance of the vascular and circulatory action of Trasylol. Report on an international symposium. Schattauer, Stuttgart, p 51–62
Weström I, Bengtsson L P 1970 Effect of tranexamic acid (AMCA) in menorrhagia with intrauterine contraceptive devices. A double-blind study. Journal of Reproductive Medicine 5: 154–161
Ylkiorkala O, Viinikka L 1983 Comparison between antifibrinolytic and antiprostaglandin treatment in the reduction of increased menstrual blood loss in women with intrauterine contraceptive devices. British Journal of Obstetrics and Gynaecology 90: 78–83

46. Vascular and non-thrombocytopenic purpuras

C. D. Forbes

Purpura is the Latin word (purpura: purple) which is used to describe the eruption of multiple purple spots following extravasation of blood from capillaries. The name is derived from a genus of marine gasteropod (*Purpura lapillus*) which yields a purple dye (Jones & Tocantins 1933).

Haemostasis is probably the most important homeostatic mechanism of the intact animal and may be defined as the prevention of bleeding from damaged or cut vessels. The process is complex and requires normal vessel function, the presence of normal subendothelial collagen, normal platelet count and function, and normal blood coagulation. This chapter sets out to describe changes in haemostasis which are abnormal, primarily because of components of vessel structure, function or support. It is appreciated that because of the complex interactions of the systems involved, some aspects of platelet function, coagulation or fibrinolysis may also be covered.

Basic haemostasis, vessel function and platelet interaction have been reviewed in Chapters 1, 9, 11. The response of a vessel to injury has been extensively studied and reviewed (Macfarlane 1972, Gimbrone 1986.)

It seems clear that large vessels with muscular walls have the potential to contract and arrest bleeding, but the capillary is essentially an endothelial tube with a supporting fibrillary membrane. The relationship of individual endothelial cells and their supporting structure has been intensively researched (Barnhart & Baechler 1978). The integrity of the endothelial layer requires the presence of an intercellular cement, which is possibly hyaluronic acid, and large defects require plugging with fibrin or adherent platelets (Baumgartner et al 1976). Flow into the microcirculation is controlled by a precapillary sphincter (Chien & Tsai 1948), which is extremely sensitive to anoxia, accumulation of metabolites, and local hormones such as 5-hydroxytryptamine, adrenaline, nor-adrenaline, acetyl choline, histamine, vasopressin, oxytocin and bradykinin. The individual capillaries have no independent mechanism of contraction, but in the transected capillary, the endothelial cells may adhere and occlude the vessel (Sanders 1970). Maintenance of haemostatic integrity requires an active metabolic process with normal temperature, oxygen and carbon dioxide levels.

Disorders of vascular haemostasis may therefore be due to loss of endothelium function, increased permeability of vessels, reduction of 'strength', and failure to contract on injury. It is however usual to classify vascular disorders as primary or secondary (Table 46.1).

Table 46.1 Causes of non-thrombocytopenic purpuras

Primary:
Purpura simplex (simple easy bruising)
Senile purpura (age spots)
Hereditary haemorrhagic telangiectasia (Osler–Weber–Rendu syndrome)
Giant cavernous haemangioma (Kasabach–Merritt syndrome)
Hereditary connective tissue disorders
Ehlers–Danlos syndrome
Pseudoxanthoma elasticum
Marfan syndrome
Osteogenesis imperfecta
Ataxia telangiectasia
Noonan's syndrome
Secondary:
Mechanical purpura/factitial bleeding/non-accidental injury in children
Vascular spiders
Systemic sclerosis
Henoch–Schonlein (allergic) purpura
Metabolic purpuras
Scurvy
Diabetes mellitus
Homocystinuria
Albinism
Cushing's syndrome and steroid therapy
Pernicious anaemia
Uraemia (see Ch. 41)
Liver disease (see Chs 41, 44)
Dysproteinaemias
Amyloidosis
Loin pain–haematuria syndrome
Purpura associated with infectious disease
Purpura fulminans
Embolic purpura
Drug-induced vasculitis
Auto-erythrocyte sensitization
DNA sensitivity

HISTORY AND CLINICAL EXAMINATION

An accurate history is often the keystone to success in the diagnosis of vascular disorders, and in particular a positive family history of easy bruising, epistaxis in childhood, bleeding after dental treatment, after surgery and excess menstruation. Careful examination of the skin is essential. Lesions diagnostic of the basic disease may be very obvious, e.g. giant cavernous haemangioma, hereditary haemorrhagic telangiectasia, or scurvy. The most common features of vascular haemostatic abnormalities are petechiae, purpura and bruising.

Tests of defective vascular function are the most difficult of all the haemostatic tests to perform and interpret. Numerous tests have been published and recently reviewed (Owen et al 1975, Ingram 1977, Bowie & Owen 1984). The only investigation of some value is the bleeding time and its modifications (Quick 1975, Sutor et al 1977). A recent critical review of the bleeding time test has cast doubts on its general application as a clinical test. It is clearly affected by factors such as the haematocrit, uraemia, by drugs such as aspirin, by hypertension and by a raised serum bilirubin (Rodgers & Levin 1990, Anon 1991).

PRIMARY DISORDERS OF VESSELS

Purpura simplex (simple easy bruising)

Purpuric lesions and ecchymosis often appear in the skin of normal individuals, in particular in young women, on the upper arms, thighs, breasts and buttocks. The bruises are usually under 2 cm in diameter and fade rapidly. There are no other symptoms of bleeding elsewhere and a history of trauma is usually denied. These 'devil's pinches' or 'dead man's pinches' are of no consequence, except from the cosmetic point of view and the patient should be reassured that there is no serious underlying pathology. The condition has also been called 'hereditary familial purpura simplex' (Davis 1941), but the name has little to commend it and, as the condition is benign in nature, it is best called by a colloquial name. On occasion there is a strong family history, particularly on the female side, of easy bruisability. In previous studies (Lackner & Karpatkin 1975) a subgroup has been identified with impairment of platelet aggregation to collagen and to adrenaline. There is little evidence that any drug is effective in preventing the formation of such bruises (Vermylen & Blockmans 1992) or removing them when formed. It is however worthwhile reassuring such patients and recommending that they avoid aspirin and related drugs.

Senile purpura

This is a common benign disease of the elderly in which the characteristic purpuric spots develop spontaneously on the extensor surfaces of the forearms and backs of the hands and occasionally on the face and neck (Plate 46.1). The number of patients with lesions increases with advancing years and tends to be more common in men than women (Wong 1988). The defect seems to be due to lack of collagen support of small vessels, associated with loss of subcutaneous fat and elastic fibres (Shuster et al 1975, Shiozawa et al 1979). The lesions tend to last for a prolonged period and remain deep reddish-purple in colour. They often leave a brown stain in the skin ('age spots'). It has been suggested that there may be lack of macrophage activity (Shuster & Scarborough 1961), and this may be the cause of the slow resolution of the lesions. Other authors (Feinstein et al 1973) dispute this. In this respect the condition is similar to the purpura seen in Cushing's syndrome and after corticosteroid administration (Plate 46.2). Haemostatic tests are normal. Care should be taken when carrying out the bleeding time on the forearm as large ecchymosis may be produced by leakage of blood into the tissues. There may also be delayed skin healing. There is no evidence that any drug treatment is of value and the patient should be reassured about the benign nature of the lesions. Such elderly patients also have fine thready veins and care should be taken with routine venepunctures that adequate pressure is maintained after removal of the needle in order to ensure haemostasis.

Hereditary haemorrhagic telangiectasis (Osler–Webber–Rendu disease)

This disease is the most common of the hereditary vascular disorders (Osler 1901). There is often a family history and the disorder is transmitted as an autosomal dominant trait, both sexes being equally affected. Bleeding is from the vascular lesions on skin or mucosal surfaces. The lesions consist of dilated arterioles and capillaries lined by a thin endothelial layer. The commonest site is the nasal mucosa, where, in early childhood, epistaxis is the presenting feature. In the adult, typical lesions may develop on the lips, oral mucosa, tongue, face, hands, oesophagus, stomach and rectum and rarely in the eye, respiratory, gynaecological and urinary tracts (Plate 46.3). In some patients, chronic, recurrent hypochromic anaemia from occult alimentary blood loss may be the presenting feature and in occasional subjects the typical lesions may only be visible in the gastric mucosa at endoscopy (Plate 46.4).

The lesions are very typical: 1–3 mm in size, flat, round, red or violet in colour and blanching on pressure. There is evidence that the number of lesions tends to increase with advancing age. There is an association with pulmonary arteriovenous fistulae (20% of patients) and these may be multiple (Hodgson et al 1959). In addition, there is a significant association with cirrhosis of the liver, hepatomas, and splenomegaly (Fitz-Hugh 1931) and splenic arterial aneurysm (Schuster 1937). The basic pathology is not understood but the histology of the vessels shows deficiency of supporting elastic fibres in the dilated vessel wall; however, elastic fibres seem normal elsewhere in the body.

In addition to the obvious vascular malformation there may be abnormalities in blood coagulation, fibrinolysis and platelet function (Muntean et al 1978). In up to 50% of patients there may be low grade but continuous evidence of disseminated intravascular coagulation (DIC) which on occasion may become acute, the so-called 'mini Kasabach–Meritt syndrome' (Bick & Fekete 1978, Bick 1981). Several cases of an association with factor VIII deficiency have also been reported (Esham et al 1974, Harborough & Kickler 1975) and with von Willebrand's disease (Ramsay et al 1976, Conlan et al 1978). Abnormalities in platelet aggregation and adhesion (Muckle 1964, Quick 1966) are recorded but bleeding times are normal (Singer & Wolfson 1944).

Treatment of bleeding from the telangiectasia is non-specific. Nasal bleeding usually responds to local measures such as packing, balloon compression and topical thrombin. Cauterization of the nasal mucosa may be of transient value but repeated use can lead to mucosal atrophy and perforation of the septum. Oestrogen therapy has been used in an attempt to convert the nasal mucosa to a stratified squamous epithelium which overgrows the abnormal vessel (Koch et al 1952, Blackburn 1963, Vase 1981). However, the success rate of this method is not high and the mucosa may become dry and crusty (Harrison 1964, Vase & Lorentzen 1983). It is of interest that remission of bleeding tends to occur during pregnancy and this may represent a state with high oestrogen levels affecting the mucosa and also producing an elevated factor VIII level. Grafting of the nasal mucosa has been attempted (Sander 1960, Laurian et al 1979).

Recurrent haemorrhage from the gastrointestinal tract presents a major problem of investigation. Only if a site of persistent severe bleeding can be localized by endoscopy is it worthwhile undertaking local ablation of the lesions with a laser or resection of the intestine. Radiotherapy has also been attempted in the stomach for local lesions, but this is of unproven value (Schwartz et al 1982). The problem is even more difficult in the lung and is compounded by the presence of arteriovenous fistulae and the multiplicity of the lesions. There is evidence that new telangectasiae form even after resection of one lesion has been carried out.

The most important therapeutic problem is treatment of chronic iron deficiency, and many of the most severely affected patients are chronically anaemic despite routine administration of iron.

Giant cavernous haemangiomata (Kasaback–Merritt syndrome)

The Kasaback–Merritt syndrome is one of chronic DIC associated with the presence of giant haemangiomata (Kasaback & Merritt 1940, Inceman & Tangun 1969) (see also p. 1042). Such giant cavernous haemangiomata are benign tumours of blood vessels and consist histologically of masses of dilated, thin-walled venules (Fig. 44.8 in Ch. 44). The skin is usually involved but the haemangiomata may penetrate and connect with underlying tissues and may rarely be found in internal organs. The syndrome may present at any age, including the newborn (Shim et al 1968, Thatcher 1968). When the skin is not affected and the haemangioma is in an internal organ (liver or spleen), the presenting clinical feature may be bleeding because of consumption of fibrinogen and platelets (Bland et al 1974, Linderkamp et al 1976). The cause of the DIC is not clear, but blood is static in the venous sinusoids and both platelet and contact factors may be activated by the abnormal endothelium. Episodes of acute DIC may supervene on the chronic state and these are amenable to treatment with heparin (Hagerman et al 1975). When DIC is controlled, surgery, radiotherapy, steroids and aminocaproic or tranexamic acid may be given in an attempt to reduce tumour size; there is some evidence that thrombosis is the mechanism of regression (Kasubuchi et al 1973, Evans et al 1975, Bartochesky et al 1978, Neidhart & Roach 1982). Embolization of the tumour has also been attempted.

An association between giant cavernous haemangiomas and Ehlers–Danlos syndrome has been reported (Husebye & Getz 1958).

HEREDITARY CONNECTIVE TISSUE DISORDERS

These disorders are extremely rare and are easily recognized except for occasional patients with type IV Ehlers–Danlos syndrome. They do not present a therapeutic problem.

Ehlers–Danlos syndrome

The Ehlers–Danlos syndrome (EDS) is an uncommon syndrome which includes a range of symptoms, signs and biochemical disorders of connective tissue (Ehlers 1901, Danlos 1908). The condition may be transmitted as an autosomal dominant, recessive or X-linked trait and is manifested by a hyperextensible skin, hypermobile joints, joint laxity, fragile tissues and a bleeding tendency, mainly subcutaneous haematoma. 11 distinct varieties of the disease are recognized on the basis of clinical, genetic and biochemical evidence. The ecchymotic type is type IV. Both sexes are affected and the incidence is about 1: 200 000.

The skin changes are perhaps the most typical and these features are common to all the varieties. The skin is soft, like chamois leather, hyperextensible, and may be stretched for several inches before returning to normal. There is a liability for the skin to be easily broken and it then heals in paper-thin connective tissue scars. These wide papyraceous scars are present over bony prominences and may often be brownish in colour because of deposition of haemosiderin from recurrent haematomas. Such patients have a characteristic facies with large irregular scars on forehead and chin, lop ears, a crooked nose and uneven teeth. Molluscoid pseudotumours are common over elbows and knees.

The degree of joint laxity is variable but in extreme cases joint hypermobility in all direction is possible. There may be chronic dislocation of patellae, clavicles, shoulders and hips. Such people may be employed as 'India rubber men' in sideshows. In addition, abnormalities have been described in the cardiovascular, gastrointestinal, neurological, ocular and respiratory systems. For reviews of these associations see Beighton (1970) and Pope (1991).

The bleeding diathesis may be extremely severe and present with easy bruising, purpura, bleeding from gums after dental extraction, gastrointestinal bleeding and haemoptysis. Rupture of major arteries is seen in type IV disease and presents dramatically. It has usually been considered that the cause of the defect is an abnormal capillary structure with deficiency of perivascular collagen and an increase in elastic fibres (Uden 1982, Pope 1991). It has been suggested that in some patients there may be a qualitative disorder of collagen with deficiency of hydroxylysine (type VI) (Pinnell et al 1972) and this may be related to a platelet glucosyl transferase abnormality (Greenberg et al 1972). However type IV (ecchymotic) is associated with diminished levels of type III collagen, which predominates in blood vessels and the gastrointestinal tract (Pope et al 1975). Microscopy shows reduction of collagen fibres and there may be fragmentation of elastic tissues due to recurrent damage. Electron microscopy reveals a reduction in collagen fibre diameter.

Platelet abnormalities have also been reported in some patients (Roberts & Kroncke 1971). In individual patients there may be a positive tourniquet test (Frick & Kratchuk 1956), prolonged bleeding time and abnormal platelet adhesion/aggregation tests, as well as abnormalities in platelet ultrastructure (Kashiwagi et al 1965, Estes 1972, Dodds 1974, Hardisty 1975) as well as defective capillary structure (Uden 1982). There is also a single report of an association with acquired von Willebrand's disease (Clough et al 1979). In addition there have been case reports of patients with factor XII (Hageman) deficiency (Fantl et al 1961) factor VIII (Bertin et al 1989) and factor IX (Christmas factor) deficiency (Lisker et al 1960).

It is important in such patients to avoid any elective surgery, because of the likelihood of multiple haemostatic defects, friable tissues and delayed wound-healing.

Pseudoxanthoma elasticum

This is an extremely rare defect of elastic fibres and the clinical manifestations may occur only in the 2nd or 3rd decade of life. It is often transmitted as an autosomal recessive trait. In severely affected individuals there is a characteristic facies with redundant folds of skin in neck, face, axilla and inguinal regions. The skin changes are very suggestive, with small tan-yellow papules usually on the neck and axilla, and there are associated telangiectasiae. In the fundus oculi there are typical angioid streaks. Spontaneous haemorrhage, resulting from the defective vessels, may occur in any part of the body, most commonly into skin, eyes, kidney, joints, uterus and gastrointestinal tract. The common causes of death are subarachnoid and gastrointestinal haemorrhage. There is in addition a tendency to thrombosis in major arteries, with gangrene of the feet (Goodman et al 1963, Altman et al 1974, Scully et al 1983).

The cause of the vessel abnormality is not understood but it seems to be associated with a defect in the elastic fibres (Ross et al 1978). No specific treatment is available except when a bleeding point can be identified and excised, e.g. in gastrointestinal bleeding. There is no prolongation of standard bleeding times and no delay in wound-healing.

Marfan syndrome

Marfan syndrome is an autosomally dominant inherited connective tissue disorder with a prevalence of 1 in 10 000 of the population. The clinical expression of the disease is extremely variable and this often makes diagnosis difficult. Such patients are usually diagnosed on clinical grounds because of the obvious skeletal abnormalities (arachnodactyly: long limbs) cardiovascular abnormalities (aortic wall defects) and ocular defects (dislocation of the lens) (Pyeritz & McKusick 1979). Patients should have two of the three symptoms classically involved, plus a family history.

The molecular defect is in a 350 kDa glycoprotein called fibrillin which is reduced or defective. This is an essential component of the elastic elements of the extracellular matrix (Hollister et al 1990).

The natural history of the disease is now well documented, with a mean age of death in the mid-thirties due to aortic root dilatation and dissection (Marsalese et al 1989). In addition such patients may present with easy bruising and may bleed excessively at operation. Minor defects in platelet function (Bick 1979) and an associated deficiency of factor VIII have been described (Erdohazi et al 1964).

Osteogenesis imperfecta

This defect is transmitted as an autosomal dominant trait and presents clinically with deformation and brittleness of bones due to patchy lack of bone matrix. Few of the patients have a haemorrhagic problem which presents with bruising, epistaxis, haemoptysis and intracranial bleeding. In a few patients prolongation of the bleeding time, a positive Hess test and abnormalities of platelet function have been described (Siegel et al 1957), but such abnormalities have not been found by other investigators (Ratnoff 1968).

The basic abnormality seems to be a defect in the amino acid composition of collagen fibres and there is no specific therapy.

Ataxia telangiectasia

This is an extremely rare congenital disorder transmitted as an autosomal recessive. There is no generalized bleeding defect but there may be multiple cutaneous and conjunctival telangiectasia. The other clinical features include progressive ataxia, dementia, frequent infections, immune deficiency and lymphoid tumours.

Noonan's syndrome

Noonan's syndrome is inherited as an autosomal dominant and has a population incidence of about 1 in 2000 (Noonan & Ehmke 1963, Allanson 1987). It is characterized by short stature, a dysmorphic facies and congenital heart disease, usually pulmonary stenosis or hypertrophic cardiomyopathy. Many patients have a history of excessive bruising and bleeding both spontaneously and after surgery. This may be partly due to thrombocytopenia (Char et al 1972) and to a prolonged bleeding time in some patients (Witt et al 1988). Some patients with normal platelet counts also bleed excessively. A range of abnormalities of the intrinsic coagulation pathway have now been described, however there was a poor correlation between the severity of the measured defect and the clinical history of bleeding. Abnormalities include decreased levels of factor VIIIc, factor XII and factor XI alone and in combination (Sahrland et al 1992). It is of interest that these abnormalities are also found in first degree relatives. The abnormalities are thought to be genetic in origin and do not reflect the severity of the associated heart disease.

Mechanical purpura

Mechanical factors play an important role in the production of vascular trauma; even in the person with totally normal haemostatic mechanism, extensive lesion may be produced. The amount of pressure required to produce lesions declines with age and in the healthy young person ranges from 300–400 mm of mercury down to 150 mm in the elderly (Gough 1962). Such pressure changes are best measured by means of a suction cup connected to a mercury manometer.

Purpura due to a sudden increase in venous pressure resulting from coughing, vomiting, asphyxia and epileptic fits is well recognised. This usually involves the face and neck, particularly the periorbital skin. A similar purpura may be seen in the legs of patients with tight garters and with varicose veins (acroangiodermatitis). Direct skin trauma may be self-inflicted (factitial purpura) as part of a psychiatric syndrome and is usually easily recognised due to its distribution (see below) (Plate 46.5).

Skin suction commonly causes petechiae in adolescents (love bites) and these lesions tend to be elliptical or round and show evidence of teeth marks. The common sites are the neck, shoulder, breasts, abdomen, thighs and buttocks (Lowe 1991). Similar lesions may also be produced by sticking a sucker on the forehead or sucking air from a glass placed over the face (purpura cyclops) (Conrad 1964, Lovejoy et al 1971, Turnstall–Pedloe & Lightman 1982).

Factitial bleeding

Self injury is perhaps the most difficult of the purpuras to diagnose. It may take four forms.

1. True self-flagellation in which the patients usually present with bruising of the skin in accessible areas particularly in the thighs, breasts and legs.
2. Induction of skin petechiae by sucking the skin. The lesions are usually found on the upper limbs and breast and the area of the lesion is usually circumscribed.
3. Internal bleeding. Purpura and skin haemorrhage due to ingestion of anticoagulant drugs. This is a relatively rare condition and seems to be a condition of psychiatrically disturbed medical and paramedical personnel (for a review see Ratnoff 1984).
4. Application to the skin of corrosive materials to produce skin necrosis and stimulate a vasculitic disorder. Such situations are extremely difficult to prove and as the patients often have a major underlying psychiatric disturbance, must be handled with skill and tact (Plate 46.6).

Non-accidental injury in children

The cardinal features of child abuse are (Franklin 1978, Ellerstein 1978, O'Hare & Eden 1984):

- A discrepancy between the physical findings and history
- The bruises are in different stages of evolution despite a reported single injury
- The bruising may have a definite pattern (of a hand or an instrument).

All such children require to have an intensive investigation of their haemostatic mechanism, as in up to 15% of suspected cases an abnormality which might account for the bruising may be found (O'Hare & Eden 1984), e.g.

haemophilia, von Willebrand's disease (vWD), quantitative and qualitative platelet defect, and acquired circulating anticoagulants. Paradoxically the child with a bleeding defect is at particular risk of abuse and this presents a major problem in management (Darbyshire & Eden 1982). Battered children are often generally neglected with evidence of malnutrition and infestations. They rapidly cheer up on admission to hospital and resent returning home. Care of the family unit demands medical, psychiatric, social and legal help.

Vascular spiders

These skin lesion are often found in normal people, especially in females on the upper-trunk, forearms and face. They are said to be more frequent on areas exposed to sunlight. Pregnancy and oestrogen therapy increase the number and size in normal people and the number is increased in patients with chronic liver disease. (Plate 46.7). Occasionally they may bleed excessively if traumatized especially in patients with liver disease and a prolonged prothrombin time. Reassurance is often necessary in the pregnant patient that the lesions will regress after parturition. Occasionally cosmetic attention is necessary to ablate the central spiral artery.

Systemic sclerosis

Telangiectasia are frequently found in patients with systemic sclerosis – especially on the face and lips and on the fingers. Unlike spider naevi the lesions consist of a leash of dilated venules without a single supplying artery. They blanch on pressure. They are not associated with haemostatic abnormalities and routine tests are usually normal.

Henoch–Schonlein syndrome (allergic or anaphylactoid purpura)

This group of purpuras includes a variety of conditions caused by different pathological processes, the final common pathway of which is an allergic vasculitis, i.e. a leukoclastic vasculitis caused by circulating IgA immune complexes (for review see Duquesnoy 1991). The trigger is often unknown but may include drugs, foods, insect bites or bacterial infections. The original description of joint involvement with purpura was written by Schonlein in 1837, a condition which he called 'peliosis rheumatica', and purpura with gastrointestinal symptoms was described by Henoch in 1874. In the acute case there may be dominant joint or alimentary symptomatology and this may be associated with development of skin changes that start as a diffuse erythematous, macular rash which then becomes purpuric (Cream et al 1970). The purpuric spots may be palpable. Evidence may also be found of involvement of the brain and renal tract and up to 30% of cases have glomerulonephritis (Chantler 1976, Plate 46.8). In addition there may be pleurisy, pericarditis and pneumonia. The syndrome is most common in children under 10 years with the greatest incidence at springtime.

Histology of the skin lesions reveals diffuse perivascular infiltration with neutrophils, lymphocytes and macrophages typical of an allergic aetiology (Wedgewood & Klauss 1955). In renal biopsy material, fibrin-related antigen and IgA immunoglobulins can be demonstrated by immunofluorescence (Meadow et al 1972). Due to similar histological appearances it is suggested that Henoch–Schonlein purpura is the systemic form of IgA nephropathy (Waldo 1988). The platelet count is usually normal and no changes are found in conventional tests of blood coagulation. There may be present in the plasma increased levels of inhibitors to the production of PGI_2 (prostacyclin) (Turi et al (1989)). The sedmentation rate is elevated and this is because there is a reactive rise in the level of fibrinogen. Because of the clinical association between anaphylactoid purpura and preceding upper respiratory infection, about a third of cases will have elevation of the anti-streptolysin-O titre resulting from previous β-haemolytic streptococcal infection (Ayoub & Hayer 1969). In addition, a variety of drugs such as penicillins and sulphonamides have been implicated as has HLA type BW35. Clinical and laboratory criteria for the diagnosis of Henoch–Schonlein purpura have been agreed by the American College of Rheumatology (Hunder 1989). Treatment consists of penicillin, corticosteroids and cytotoxic drugs for progressive glomerulonephritis. No adequate controlled trials are available for these different regimes (Austin & Balow 1983).

METABOLIC PURPURAS

Scurvy

This is probably the most common bleeding problem in the history of mankind but is now an uncommon disease in clinical practice in the Western World although it is still relatively common in deprived, malnourished communities in which it is seen in association with other vitamin deficiencies. In Britain; it is occasionally seen in the extremes of life, in the malnourished, in the alcoholic and in food faddists (Wallerstein & Wallerstein 1976). Deficiency of ascorbic acid results in decreased quantity and quality of collagen, as ascorbic acid is needed to activate the enzyme proline hydroxylase which hydroxylates proline and lysine residues in collagen and stabilizes its helical structure. In the affected baby, subperiosteal bleeding is the common presentation and in the adult there may be gingival bleeding, and in the skin, perifollicular haemorrhages and purpura (Plate 46.9). Severe deficiency is associated with internal bleeding, particularly into the gastrointestinal tract and brain. The diagnosis is made on clinical grounds, by assessment of dietary ascorbic acid intake and by measurement of leukocyte ascorbic acid levels. The proof is the clinical response to therapy (50 mg ascorbic acid per day) which causes the bleeding to stop. The platelets of scorbutic individuals are deficient in platelet factor 3 (Cetingil et al 1958); in scorbutic guinea pigs there is defective collagen formation (Barkhan & Howard 1959) and in the human, reduced platelet adhesiveness (Wilson et al 1967). However, platelet aggregation and platelet plug formation may be normal (Harrison & Honour 1967, Purcell & Constantine 1972, Johnson et al 1981).

Diabetes mellitus

Abnormalities of the capillary bed are seen in diabetes, particularly in the retina and renal vessels, but all vessels may be affected. True purpura is rarely seen and there is no haemostatic abnormality found in the Hess test or bleeding time and other tests of clotting function. By use of fluorescein angiography, increased permeability of retinal capillaries has been shown. Retinal haemorrhages are frequently found. The cause of these is unknown. This may be associated with a hyperviscosity syndrome (Lowe et al 1980).

Homocystinuria

Homocystinuria is a rare disease affecting about 1: 100 000 births (Clayton 1976). It is due to a defect of sulphur metabolism and is transmitted as an autosomal recessive trait. In the classical case the child may appear normal for the first 2 years of life and the clinical features develop only gradually (Carson 1975). These include ectopia lentis, and skeletal abnormalities such as osteoporosis of spine, abnormal gait and muscle weakness. There is a deficiency in activity of cystathionine synthetase in liver, brain and fibroblasts and this is manifested as elevated plasma levels of homocysteine, homocystine, methionine and increased urinary excretion of homocystine. Homocystine interferes with the formation of the intermolecular cross-links, which normally stabilize the collagen macromolecular network by binding to the aldehydic functional groups of the collagen molecule.

The clinical manifestations include an increased tendency to gastrointestinal bleeding and thrombosis both in the venous and arterial trees (Hill-Zobel et al 1982). Coagulation studies are sparse but have shown deficiencies of factors VII and X and elevated levels of β-thromboglobulin. These abnormalities improve after therapy with folate and pyridoxine (Palareti & Coccheri 1989).

Albinism

This is a heterogeneous group of diseases in which there is an inherited defect in melanin metabolism. The clinical features are easily recognised (Witkop et al 1978).

A mild haemorrhagic disorder associated with total albinism has been recorded. This may manifest as easy bruising, menorrhagia, and prolonged bleeding after trauma and surgery. There have been reports of a prolonged bleeding time and an abnormality of platelet function (Hardisty & Hutton 1967). The Hermansky–Pudlak syndrome is a rare autosomal inherited trait consisting of tyrosinase-positive albinism, storage pool-deficient platelets and accumulation of pigment in macrophages, e.g. in bone marrow (see Ch. 21).

Cushing's syndrome

Easy bruising and petechiae are well-recognised features of Cushing's syndrome and of the prolonged therapeutic use of adrenocortical hormones. The skin lesions produced are diffuse but have a predilection for the arms and legs. The basic lesion is probably due to atrophy of dermal connective tissue and also deficient phagocytosis of extravasated red cells (Scarborough & Shuster 1960). This resembles the lesions of senile purpura (Rosenberg et al 1978) (Plate 46.2).

Pernicious anaemia

Purpura is an extremely rare manifestation of pernicous anaemia.

Dysproteinaemias

The dysproteinaemias include macroglobulinaemia, hyperglobulinaemia, cryoglobulinaemia and multiple myeloma. Bleeding is a common feature of these disorders and paradoxically there is, in addition, a high incidence of vasculitis and thrombotic disorders (Winkelman 1980) (Plate 46.10).

Macroglobulinaemia may arise as a primary or secondary condition associated with chronic illness. Bleeding may be the presenting and dominant clinical feature of this group of disorders and there may be associated lymphadenopathy, hepatosplenomegaly and retinal haemorrhages. There is usually gross elevation of the ESR and there may be an associated hyperviscosity syndrome (Preston 1980). Reduction of blood flow with tissue anoxia may alter capillary permeability.

Cryoglobulinaemia is a condition in which abnormal globulins gel when plasma is cooled. It is usually secondary, being associated with multiple myeloma, reticuloses, and collagen disorders. The usual presentation is circulatory impairment after exposure to cold. Gangrene of fingers, toes, ears or nose may result from arterial thrombosis. There may also be a mild generalized bruising and excess bleeding after surgery. Purpuric lesions may be provoked by cold and a simple test is to apply an ice cube to the dorsum of the hand.

Hypergammaglobulinaemic purpura is a rare disease affecting young and middle-aged females, and usually presents as recurrent crops of purpura on the legs. These may eventually leave residual patches of brown pigmentation. The condition is associated with a diffuse increase in gammaglobulins in patients who have features of related collagen disorders, e.g. Sjogren's syndrome, keratoconjunctivitis sicca and lupus erythematosus (Lee & Miotti 1975). Histology of the lesions shows evidence of vasculitis.

A variety of haemostatic disorders have been reported in the dysproteinaemias which may be present in isolation or in combination. These include thrombocytopenia, qualitative platelet disorders, abnormalities of fibrinolysis, abnormalities of individual clotting factors, and circulating anticoagulants (Deutsch et al 1976). In addition there is gross elevation of whole blood, plasma and serum viscosity (Preston et al 1978).

The mechanism by which macromolecules interfere with haemostasis is not clear, but they may inhibit the platelet-collagen interaction by coating the opposing surfaces and by direct inhibition of platelet aggregation (Pachter et al 1959). In a large review of such patients, Perkins et al (1970) found the incidence of bleeding to be greater in patients with IgA myeloma than those with the IgG type; there were also statistically lower levels of factors II, V, VII, X, XI, XIII. Platelet function tests of adhesion and aggregation were also abnormal, particularly in those patients with hyperviscosity syndrome. There is also evidence from other studies of failure of fibrin polymerization (Lackener et al 1970) and excess calcium binding (Glueck) et al 1962).

A temporary correction of some of these haemostatic variable may be found after plasmapheresis, which also corrects the defects associated with the hyperviscosity (Fahey et al 1965, Somer 1975).

Amyloidosis

This may be a primary disease or present as a complication of chronic infection (tuberculosis, osteomyelitis, bronchiectasis and malaria), or be associated with collagen disorders (rheumatoid arthritis, systemic lupus erythematosus, scleroderma and dermatomyostitis) (Kyle & Bayrd 1975). It is also found in a number of other conditions such as Hodgkin's disease, renal carcinoma, regional enteritis, ulcerative colitis and multiple myeloma (for review see Rosenthal & Franklin 1977). Haemorrhage is one of the common features with purpura (especially involving the face, neck and upper trunk), ecchymosis and spontaneous internal bleeding. Lesions may be induced by stroking or applying pressure to the skin. This may be, in part, the result of immune complexes directed against the endothelium and perivascular tissues (Snapper 1971).

In generalized amyloidosis a variety of different coagulation factor deficiencies have been reported and these have often been associated with excess bleeding, particularly after biopsy procedures. These include deficiency of factors IX and X (Furie et al 1977, McPherson et al 1977) which may be due to the presence of specific factor inhibitors (Mulhare et al 1991), altered antithrombin activity (Galbraith et al 1974), and factors V, VII and fibrinogen (Amir et al 1971, Gastineau et al 1991). There have also been sporadic cases with evidence of activation of fibrinolysis due to excessive production or release of urokinase-type plasminogen activator (u-PA) (Sane et al 1989).

Loin pain and haematuria syndrome

The syndrome of unexplained symptoms of loin pain and haematuria in the absence of renal pathology was originally described by Little (1967). Intravenous pyelography is usually normal and there is no evidence of obstructive uropathy or infection. Occasionally there may be minor pathological changes on renal biopsy (Burden et al 1975, Leaker et al 1990) and evidence of some spasm of the intravenal vessels on angiography (Burden et al 1975, 1979, Bergroth et al 1987). The clinical course may be aggravated by taking oral contraceptives (Aber & Higgins 1982). There has been no evidence of a generalized bleeding tendency (Burden et al 1979, Aber & Higgins 1982) but there is evidence of platelet activation (shortened platelet lifespan and increased platelet reactivity and platelet factor 3) as well as minor changes in fibrinolysis (elevation of D-dimer) (Jones et al 1977, Leaker et al 1990). No changes were found in levels of blood coagulation or fibrinolytic inhibitors, or, blood rheology parameters. In addition there were no changes to indicate endothelial damage (Leaker et al 1990). Other authors have reported deficiency of prostacyclin stimulating factor (Siegler et al 1988) and factor XII deficiency (Smellie et al 1987).

The causation of this syndrome is still obscure but has been likened to migraine, i.e. localized arterial spasm associated with increased platelet responsiveness and circulating platelet aggregates. It is of interest that attempts have been made to treat the condition by renal autotransplantation and that this may be associated with recurrence (Hutchison et al 1987, Sheil et al 1987).

PURPURA ASSOCIATED WITH INFECTIOUS DISEASES AND INFECTION

A variety of infectious agents may present with purpura during the course of the illness. These may be bacterial, viral, rickettsial or protozoal. Bacteria often implicated are meningococci (Plate 46.11), streptococci, *Salmonella typhi*, and *Corynebacterium diphtheria;* viruses include smallpox, influenza and measles; Rickettsiae include Rocky Mountain spotted spotted fever, typhus and epidemic haemorrhagic fever; protozoa include malaria and filariasis (Levin 1984).

Purpura may be due to a direct endothelial injury by the infectious agent, by an autoimmune process or by a toxin (see Ch. 41). Markers of the severity of the process include tumour necrosis factor (TNF), interleukin-1 and gamma-interferon. There is a positive correlation between elevation of these factors and subsequent death (Girardin et al 1988).

Purpura fulminans

The clinical features of this syndrome, which often follows an infectious illness, are fever, hypotension and a severe purpuric rash over all skin areas. It is probably an extreme form of disseminated intravascular coagulation. The pathogenesis of the disease parallels that of the Schwartzman reaction seen in experimental animals. In the affected skin there is venous and capillary thrombosis with evidence of DIC in the blood. In the past there has been confusion with Henoch–Schonlein purpura, but Hjory et al (1964) have now accurately defined the syndrome and at least 100 cases have been reviewed by Spicer & Rau (1976). It is clear that children are mainly affected and adults only rarely, the sex incidence is equal and there is no familial incidence. There is a seasonal variation in incidence with a peak in winter and spring. There are positive associations with varicella, streptococcal infection, rubella, roseola, diphtheria and smallpox vaccination. The onset of symptoms of purpura and bleeding occurs after a latent period of up to 4 weeks (Chu & Blaisdell 1982). In a small number of cases there is a history of exposure to penicillins for the primary disease. Also some patients, often newborn babies, are genetically deficient in protein C and S. (Ozsoylu et al 1988, Tuddenham et al 1989, Madden et al 1990).

The clinical course starts abruptly with areas of skin necrosis on the limbs, buttocks, nose, ears, cheeks, or genitalia. The patients are usually critically ill. New crops of lesions may appear in the ensuing weeks. If the patients survive the acute onset, the prime problem becomes organ failure: respiratory distress syndrome, renal and hepatic failure. These may be complicated by massive gastrointestinal haemorrhage. The basic clinical picture is due to septicaemia, shock and DIC.

The laboratory findings include a microangiopathic haemolytic process and leukocytosis with thrombocytopenia. The Hess test may be positive and bleeding times are prolonged in 50% of patients. The screening tests for coagulation (APTT and PT) are prolonged and there is often depletion of fibrinogen and factors V and VIII, protein C and S.

The histology of the lesions shows diffuse and extensive haemorrhage into skin with subsequent necrosis. Similar features may be found in internal organs, particularly bowel, bladder, brain and serosa. There may also be evidence of vasculitis, with perivascular cuffing of small vessels with polymorphonuclear leukocytes and focal fibrinoid necrosis of the walls of small arteries (Robboy et al 1973). The mortality from the disease is about 40%.

Treatment during the acute phase is a combination of supportive measures, heparin for the DIC, followed by a prolonged course of warfarin (Hartman et al 1989). Control of DIC does not, however, seem to affect the progression of the haemorrhagic skin lesions or the incidence of gangrene. In the long-term, skin grafting may be necessary and amputation may be occasionaly required.

In most of these diseases, purpura appears during the septicaemic or viraemic stage and later there may be diffuse bleeding from all mucous membranes. The defect is partly vascular, with a positive Hess test and prolonged bleeding time, and there may be thrombocytopenia with associated reduction in levels of factor II and VII (McKay & Margaretten 1967). Recently an inherited defect in protein C has been described in children with purpura fulminans (Branson et al 1983, Tuddenham et al 1989, Madden et al 1990).

Embolic purpura

This is usually associated with infective endocarditis, but may be found after insertion of prosthetic valves, in atrial myxoma and in a variety of carcinomas. In infective endocarditis the clinical associations of splinter haemorrhages, Osler's nodes and haematuria are well known and are probably due to anoxia in the capillary bed with a subsequent vasculitic reaction associated with small microemboli in the arterioles (Rubenfield & Min 1977). A similar picture may be found in patients with true DIC in which fibrin microthrombi form in the skin vessels and vasculitis may be induced (Robboy et al 1973) (Plate 46.12). An example of this is the rare condition of embolism following multiple fractures of long bones or insertion of prosthetic joints. Cases have also been decribed after severe burns, infections, sickle cell crises, renal transplant and after cardiopulmonary bypass. Marrow fat droplets enter the circulation and embolize to the brain, lung and heart to produce diffuse cerebral symptoms and respiratory failure. Purpura is usually seen in the upper half of the body and should be looked for in the conjunctivae. Histology of the various tissues shows microthrombi. The picture is complex and is probably a combination of actual fat embolism, asphyxia, disseminated intravascular coagulation, vasculitis due to free fatty acids (Kind et al 1971a, b) and trauma. After surgery in orthopaedic patients there is usually a fall in PaO_2 and this is associated with a fall in platelet count and a rise in fibrin degradation products (Riseborough & Herndon 1978). The value of antithrombotic therapy is still under debate and general supportive measures are required.

DRUG-INDUCED VESSEL DISEASE

Occasionally a non-thrombocytopenic purpuric reaction may be seen in association with food or drug administration (Mullick et al 1979). Drugs may produce an adverse effect on vessels in three ways (Stefanini & Mednicoff 1954, Criep & Cohen 1957).

1. Development of a specific antivessel antibody
2. Development of immune complexes
3. Changes in vessel permeability.

It has been suggested that there may be a similarity of antigens between platelets and endothelial cells. The precise mechanism of endothelial and platelet damage is unknown in most cases and drugs of similar chemical structure may have separate actions, e.g. diethylbromoacetylcarbamide (Carbromal) and allylisopropylacetylcarbamide (Sedormid). Carbromal produces a capillary reaction without a fall in platelet count and Sedormid produces thrombocytopenia.

A wide variety of drugs associated with the production of vasculitis is now known (Table 46.2, Plate 46.13). Treatment of such a reaction is to withdraw the drug immediately and see if the patient improves. To prove that the drug was in fact the cause of the purpura requires re-exposure and this may be difficult to do on ethical grounds, even if a patch-test procedure is used. The patient is best warned to avoid the drug and similar compounds.

IDIOPATHIC PURPURA

Auto-erythrocyte sensitization

In the past 100 years there have been numerous individual case reports of patients bleeding as a direct result of emotional stress. There seemed to be no evidence of a generalized haemostatic defect, the lesions being preceded by local erythema and prodromal sensation of pain. In addition many of these patients had psychiatric syndromes and the suspicion was always of self-inflicted injury. In 1955 Gardner & Diamond described a similar syndrome in four women. The characteristic lesion was a painful, raised bruise which is usually preceded by symptoms of pain, localized swelling and redness. The lesions were usually on the thighs, uncommonly on the arms and rarely on the trunk. Various related symptoms such as headache, dizziness, weakness, double vision, gastrointestinal symptoms, dysuria and menorrhagia may be present. There is often a previous history of major surgery, severe trauma and emotional instability. The psychiatric syndromes include masochism, depression, psychosexual problems and passive aggression towards men (Ratnoff 1984).

Table 46.2 Drugs associated with non-thrombocytopenic purpura

Aspirin	Iodides
Allopurinol	Isoniazid
Arsenicals	Mercury
Atropine	Meprobamate
Barbiturates	Methyldopa
Belladonna	Oestrogens
Chloral hydrate	Penicillins
Chloramphenicol	Phenacetin
Chlorothiazide	Piperazine
Chlorpropamide	Procaine
Coumarins	Quinine
Digoxin	Quinidine
Frusemide	Reserpine
Gold salts	Sulphonamides
Indomethacin	Tolbutamide

The disease appears to be due to sensitization of the patient to the stroma of her own red cells, and a typical lesion may be reproduced by injection of 0.1 ml of homologous blood. The lesions seem to be cyclical in nature and appear at times of major stress. They are not factitious in origin, as they may appear while the patient is being continuously observed. A variety of drugs have been used including steroids, antihistamines and desensitization with red cells (Gardner & Diamond 1955, Ratnoff & Agle 1968). Over 200 patients have now been described with auto-erythrocyte sensitivity (Ratnoff 1980, 1991).

Psychotherapy is perhaps the treatment of choice and it is of interest that hypnosis can inhibit a positive skin test but does not seem to produce long-term remissions (Ratnoff & Agle 1968). These authors suggest that a better term would be 'psychogenic purpura'.

DNA sensitivity

Pupura due to hypersensitization to deoxyribonucleoprotein has also been described (Levin & Pinkus 1961, Ratnoff 1980). The clinical presentation is identical to autoerythrocyte sensitivity with painful ecchymoses on the limbs. Therapy with chloroquine, however, seems to be successful (Schwartz et al 1962).

In addition, a similar condition has been described with sensitivity to red cell stroma or lipid (Groch et al 1966), and a remarkably similar clinical condition has been described in two patients with marked acceleration of fibrinolysis (Rowell 1974). This may represent a variant of the above conditions.

Purpura following cardiopulmonary bypass

A syndrome of mild non-thrombocytopenic purpura with splenomegaly and atypical lymphocytosis has been reported following cardiopulmonary bypass (Behrendt et al 1968). This purpura is usually benign but one patient in this series developed glomerulonephritis similar to that seen in allergic vasculitis. A similar type of fatal vasculitis was reported following coronary artery bypass surgery (Bick et al 1973).

The acute haemostatic changes in this situation result from platelet and clotting factor consumption and stimulation of fibrinolysis (Ch. 58).

CONCLUSION

The diagnosis of a primary vascular cause of purpura may be difficult and eventually may be made by exclusion of other causes. A family history and clinical examination may provide additional pointers. The laboratory tests of vascular function are primitive and non-specific and biopsy of a lesion may be equally unhelpful. There is little evidence that any of the group of haemostatic drugs is of value in the arrest of bleeding (see Ch. 45).

REFERENCES

Aber G M, Higgins P M 1982 Natural history and management of the loin pain/haematuria syndrome. British Journal of Urology 54: 613–615

Allanson J E 1987 Noonan Syndrome. Journal of Medical Genetics 24: 9–13

Altman L K, Fialkow P J, Parker F, Sagebiel R W 1974 Pseudoxanthoma elasticum, an underdiagnosed, genetically heterogeneous disorder with protean manifestations. Archives of Internal Medicine 134: 1048–1054

Amir J, Kessler E, de Vrelis A 1971 Skin and mucosal haemorrhage of prolonged duration in systemic amyloidosis. Blood 37: 530–533

Anon 1991 The bleeding time. Lancet 337: 1447–1448

Austin H A, Balow J E 1983 Henoch–Schonlein nephritis; prognostic features and the challenge of therapy. American Journal of Kidney Diseases 2: 512–520

Ayoub E M, Hayer J 1969 Anaphylactoid purpura. Streptococcal antibody titres and: gb_1-globulin levels. Journal of Pediatrics 75: 193–201

Barkhan P, Howard A N 1959 Some blood coagulation studies in normal and scorbutic guinea pigs. British Journal of Nutrition 13: 389–400

Barnhart M I, Baechler C A 1978 Endothelial cell physiology, perturbations and responses. Seminars in Thrombosis and Haemostasis 2: 50–87

Bartochesky L F, Bull M, Feingold M 1978 Corticosteroid treatment of cutaneous hemangiomas: how effective? A report of 24 children. Clinical Pediatrics 17: 627–38

Baumgartner H R, Muggli R, Tschopp T B, Turitto V T 1976 Platelet adhesion, release and aggregation in flowing blood: Effects of surface properties and platelet function. Thrombosis and Haemostasis 35: 124–138

Behrendt D M, Epstein S E, Morrow A G 1968 Post-perfusion non-thrombocytopenic purpura: an uncommon sequel of open heart surgery. American Journal of Cardiology 22: 631–635

Beighton P 1970 The Ehler–Danlos syndrome, Heineman Medical Books, London, p 1–194

Bergroth V, Konttinen Y, Nordstrom D, Laasonen L 1987 Loin pain and haematuria syndrome: possible associations with intravenal arterial spasms. British Medical Journal 294: 1657

Bertin P, Treves R, Julia A, Gaillard S, Desproges-Gotterion R 1989 Ehlers–Danlos syndrome, clotting disorders and muscular dystrophy. Annals of Rheumatic Disorders 48: 953–6

Bick R L 1979 Vascular disorders associated with thrombohemorrhagic phenomena. Seminars in Thrombosis and Hemostasis 5: 167–183

Bick R L 1981 Hereditary hemorrhagic telangiectasia and disseminated intravascular coagulation: a new clinical syndrome. Annals of the New York Academy of Sciences 370: 851–4

Bick R L, Fekete L F 1978 Hereditary haemorrhagic telangiectasia and associated defects in hemostasis. Blood 52 (suppl 1): 179 (abstract)

Bick R L, Comer T P, Arbegast N R 1973 Fatal purpura fulminans following total cardio-pulmonary bypass Journal of Cardiovascular Surgery (Torino) 1: 569–574

Blackburn E K 1963 Long-term treatment of epistaxis with oestrogens. British Medical Journal 2: 159–160

Bland K I, Abney H T, MacGregor A M C 1974 Hemangiomatosis of the colon and ano-rectum: case report and a review of the literature. American Surgeon 40: 626–635

Bowie E J W, Owen C A 1984 The clinical and laboratory diagnosis of hemorrhagic disorders. In: Ratnoff O D, Forbes C D (eds), Disorders of hemostasis, Grune & Stratton, New York, p 43–73

Branson H E, Katz J, Marble R 1983 Inherited protein C deficiency and coumarin-responsive relapsing purpura fulminans in a newborn infant. Lancet 3: 1165–1168

Burden R P, Booth L J, Ockenden B G, Boyd W N, Higgins P M, Aber G M 1975 Intravenal vascular changes in adult patients with recurrent haematuria and loin pain — a clinical, histological and angiographic study. Quarterly Journal of Medicine 175: 433–447

Burden R P, Dathan J R, Etherington M D. Guyer P B, Maclver A G 1979 The loin pain/haematuria syndrome. Lancet i: 897–900

Carson N A J 1975 Homocystinuria in the treatment of inherited metabolic disease. In: Raine D N (ed) Medical & technical publishing. Lancaster, p 33–369

Cetingil A I, Ulutin O N, Karaca M 1958 A platelet defect in a case of scurvy. British Journal of Haematology 4350–4354

Chantler C 1976 Management and prognosis of renal disease in childhood: Glomerulonephritis. In: Hull D (ed) Recent advances in pediatrics. Churchill Livingstone, Edinburgh, p 275

Char F, Rodriguez-Fernandez H L, Scott C I, Borgaonkar D S, Bell B B, Rowe R D 1972 The Noonan Syndrome — a clinical study of forty-five cases. Birth Defects 8: 110–118

Chien T I, Tsai C 1948 The mechanisms of haemostasis in peripheral vessels. Journal of Physiology 107: 280–288

Chu D Z, Blaisdell F W 1982 Purpura fulminans. American Journal of Surgery 143: 356–362

Clayton B E 1976 Screening and management of infants with amino acid disorder. In: Hull D (ed) Recent advances in paediatrics. Churchill Livingstone, Edinburgh, p 161

Clough V, MacFarlane I A, O'Connor J, Wood J K 1979 Acquired von Willebrand's syndrome and Ehlers–Danlos syndrome presenting with gastrointestinal bleeding. Scandinavian Journal of Haematology 22: 305–310

Conlan C L, Weinger R S, Cimo P L, Moak J L, Olson J D 1978 Telangiectasis and von Willebrand's disease. Annals of Internal Medicine 89: 921–4

Conrad M E 1964 Purpura cyclops. Blood 24: 316 (letter)

Cream J J, Gumpel J M, Peachey R D G 1970 Schonlein–Henoch purpura in the adult. Quarterly Journal of Medicine 39: 461–484

Criep L H, Cohen S G 1957 Purpura as a manifestation of penicillin sensitivity. Annals of Internal Medicine 34: 1219–1223

Danlos M 1908 Un cas de cutis laxa avec tumeurs par contusion chronique des coudes et des genous (xanthome juvenile pseudodiabetique de MM Hallopeau et Mace de Lepinay). Bulletine de la Societe Francaise de Dermatologie et de Syphiligraphic 19: 70–72

Darbyshire P, Eden O B 1982 Severe bleeding disorders in children with normal coagulation screening tests. British Medical Journal 285: 134 (letter)

Davis E 1941 Hereditary familial purpura simplex. Lancet 1: 145–146

Deutsch E, Neuman E, Niessner H 1976 Pathogenese der haemorrhagischen. Diathesen bei monoclonalen. Haematologie und Bluttransfusion (Munchen) 18: 357–65

Dodds W J 1974 Hereditary and acquired haemorrhagic disorders in animals. Progress in Haemostasis and Thrombosis 2: 215–247

Duquesnoy B 1991 Henoch–Schonlein purpura. Baillière's Clinical Rheumatology 5: 253–261

Ehlers E 1901 Cutis laxa, Neigung zu Haemorrhagien in der Haut

Lockerung mechrerer Artikulationum (case report). Dermatologische Zeitschrift 8: 173–174
Ellerstein N A 1978 The cutaneous manifestations of child abuse and neglect. American Journal of Diseases of Childhood 133: 906–9
Erdohazi M, Cowie V, Lo S S 1964 A case of haemophilia with Marfanos Syndrome. British Medical Journal 1: 102–103
Esham R H, Skilling F C, Dodson W H, Hammack W J 1974 Hereditary hemorrhagic telangiectasia and factor VIII deficiency. Archives of Internal Medical 134: 327–329
Estes J W 1972 Platelet abnormalities in heritable disorders of connective tissue. Annals of the New York Academy of Sciences 201: 445–450
Evans J, Batchelor A D R, Stark G, Uttley W S 1975 Hemangioma with coagulopathy. Sustained response to prednisolone. Archives of Diseases of Childhood 50: 809–812
Fahey J L, Barth W F, Solomon A 1965 Serum hyperviscosity syndrome. Journal of the American Medical Association 192: 464–467
Fantl P, Morris K N, Sawers R J 1961 Repair of cardiac defect in patient with Ehlers–Danlons syndrome and deficiency of Hageman factor. British Medical Journal 1: 1202–1204
Feinstein R J, Hallprin K M, Penney N S 1973 Senile purpura. Archives of Dermatology 108: 229–232
Fitz-Hugh T 1931 Splenomegaly and hepatic enlargement in hereditary hemorrhagic telangiectasia. American Journal of Medical Sciences 181: 261–268
Franklin A W 1978 Child abuse. Churchill Livingstone, New York
Frick P G, Kratchuk J D 1956 Studies of haemostasis in the Ehlers–Danlos syndrome. Journal of Investigative Dermatology 26: 453–457
Furie B, Greene E, Furie B C 1977 Syndrome of acquired factor X deficiency and systemic amyloid. New England Journal of Medicine 297: 81–85
Galbraith P A, Sharma N, Parker W L, Kilgour J M 1974 Acquired factor X deficiency. Altered plasma antithrombin activity and association with amyloidosis. Journal of the American Medial Association 230: 1658–1660
Gardner F H, Diamond L K 1955 Auto-erythrocyte sensitization: a form of purpura producing painful bruising following auto-sensitization to red cells in certain women. Blood 10: 675–690
Gastinaeu D A, Gertz M A, Daniels T M, Kyle R A, Bowie E J 1991 Inhibitor of the thrombin time in systemic amyloidosis: a common coagulation abnormality. Blood 77: 2637–2640
Gimbrone M A 1986 Vascular endothelium: nature's blood container in vascular endothelium. In: M A Gimbrone (ed) Hemostasis and thrombosis. Churchill Livingstone, Edinburgh, p 1–13
Giradin E, Grau G E, Dayer J M, Roux-Lombard P, Lambert P H 1988 Tumour necrosis factor and interleukin-1 in the serum of children with severe infectious purpura. New England Journal of Medicine 319: 397–400
Glueck H I, Wayne L, Goldsmith R 1962 Abnormal calcium binding associated with hyperglobulinaemia, clotting defects, and osteoporosis: A study of this relationship. Journal of Laboratory and Clinical Medicine 59: 40–64
Goodman R M, Smith E W, Paton D 1963 Pseudoxanthoma elasticum: A clinical and histopathological study. Medicine 42: 292–334
Gough K R 1962 Capillary resistance to suction in hypertension. Blood 28: 19–33
Greenberg J H, Urban C, Nigra T P, Owen C A, Jamieson G A 1972 Glucosyltransferase studies in Ehlers–Danlos syndrome. In: International Society on Thrombosis and Haemostasis, 3rd Congress, Washington DC, p 198 (abstract)
Groch G S, Finch S C, Rogoway W, Fischer D S 1966 Studies in the pathogenesis of auto-erythrocyte sensitization syndrome. Blood 28: 19–33
Hagerman L J, Czapek E E, Donnellan W L 1975 Giant haemangioma with consumption coagulopathy. Journal of Pediatrics 87: 766–768
Hartman K R, Manco-Johnson M, Rawlings J S, Bower D J, Marlar R A 1989 Homozygous protein C deficiency: early treatment with warfarin. American Journal of Pediatric Oncology 11: 395–401
Harborough E, Kickler T 1975 Hereditary hemorrhagic telangiectasia and factor VIII deficiency. Archives of Internal Medicine 135: 490 (letter)
Hardisty R M 1975 Platelets: recent advances in basic research and clinical aspects. In: Ulutin O N (ed) International Congress Series No 357. Excerpta Medica, Amsterdam. p 201
Hardisty R H, Hutton R A 1967 Bleeding tendency associated with 'new' abnormality of platelet behaviour. Lancet 1: 983–985
Harrison D F N 1964 Familial haemorrhagic telangiectasia: 20 cases treated with systemic oestrogen. Quarterly Journal of Medicine 33 (NS 1): 25–38
Harrison M J G, Honour A J 1967 Haemostatic plug in experimental scurvy. Nature 216: 1119–1120
Hartman K R, Manco-Johnson M, Rawlings J S, Bower D J, Marlar R A 1989 Homozygous protein C deficiency: early treatment with warfarin. American Journal of Pediatric Oncology 11: 395–401.
Henoch H 1874 Ueber eine eigenthumliche Form von Purpura. Berliner Klinische Wochenscrift 11: 641–643
Hill-Zobel R H, Pyeritz R E, Scheffel U et al 1982 Kinetics and distribution of ^{111}Indium-labelled platelets in patients with homocystinuria. New England Journal of Medicine 307: 781–786
Hjort P F, Papaport S F, Jorgensen I 1964 Purpura fulminans — report of a case successfully treated with heparin and hydrocortisone. Review of 50 cases from the literature. Scandinavian Journal of Haematology 1: 169–192
Hodgson D H, Birchell H B, Good C A, Clagett O T 1959 Hereditary hemorrhagic telangiectasia and pulmonary arterio-venous fistula. Survey of a large family. New England Journal of Medicine 261: 625–636
Hollister D W, Godfrey M, Sakai L Y, Pyeritz R E 1990 Immunohistological abnormalities of the microfibrillar — fiber system in the Marfan syndrome. New England Journal of Medicine 323: 152–159
Hunder G G 1989 New diagnostic criteria for vasculitis. American College of Rheumatology, Cincinnatti publication
Husebye K O, Getz K 1958 Ehlers–Danlos syndrome — collection of clinical and histopathological findings. American Medical Association Archives of Dermatology (Chicago) 78: 732–739
Hutchison S M, Doig A, Jenkins A M 1987 Recurrence of loin pain/haematuria syndrome after renal autotransplantation. Lancet 1: 1501–1502
Inceman S, Tangun Y 1969 Chronic defibrination syndrome due to a giant hemangioma associated with micro-angiopathic hemolytic anaemia. American Journal of Medicine 46: 997–1002
Ingram G I C 1977 Investigation of a long standing bleeding tendency. British Medical Bulletin 33: 261–264
Johnson G J, Holloway D E, Hutton S W, Duane W C 1988 Platelet function in scurvy and experimental human vitamin C deficiency. Thrombosis Research 24: 85–93
Jones H W, Tocantins L M 1933 The history of purpura hemorrhagica. Annals of Medical History 5: 349–364
Jones K, Naish P F, Aber G M 1977 Oestrogen-associated disease of the renal microcirculation. Clinical Science and Molecular Medicine 52: 33–42
Kasabach H H, Merritt K K 1940 Capillary haemangioma with extensive purpura — report of a case. American Journal of Diseases of Children 59: 1063–1070
Kashiwagi H, Riddle J M, Abraham J P, Frame B 1965 Functional and ultrastructural abnormalities of platelets in Ehlers–Danlos syndrome. Annals of Medicine 63: 249–254
Kasubuchi Y, Sawada T, Nakamura T 1973 Successful treatment of neonatal retroperitoneal hemangioma with corticosteroid. Journal of Pediatric Surgery 8: 59–62
King E G, Wagener W W Jr, Ashbaugh D G, Latham L P, Halsey D R 1971a Alterations in pulmonary microanatomy after fat embolism. Chest 59: 524–530
King E G, Weily H S, Genton E, Ashbaugh E G 1971b Consumption coagulopathy in the canine oleic acid model of fat embolism. Surgery 69: 533–541
Koch H J, Escher G L, Lewis J S 1952 Hormonal management of hereditary hemorrhagic telangiectasia. Journal of the American Medical Association 149: 1376–1380
Kyle R A, Bayrd E 1975 Amyloidosis. Review of 236 cases. Medicine 54: 271–299
Lackner H, Karpatkin S 1975 On the 'easy bruising' syndrome with normal platelet count. Annals of Internal Medicine 83: 190–196

Lackner H, Hunt V, Zucker M B, Pearson J 1970 Abnormal fibrin ultrastructure, polymerisation and clot reaction in multiple myeloma. British Journal of Haematology 18: 625–636
Laurian N, Kalmanovitch M, Shimberg R 1979 Amniotic graft in the management of severe epistaxis due to hereditary haemorrhagic telangiectasia. Journal of Laryngology and Otology 93: 589–95
Leaker B R, Gordge M P, Patel A and Neild G H 1990 Haemostatic changes in the loin pain and haematuria syndrome: secondary to renal vasospasm? Quarterly Journal of Medicine 281: 969–979
Lee S L, Miotti A B 1975 Disorders of hemostatic function in patients with systemic lupus erythematosis. Seminars of Arthritis and Rheumatism 4: 241–52
Levin J 1984 Bleeding with infectious diseases. In: Ratnoff O D, Forbes C D (eds) Disorders of hemostasis, Grune & Stratton, New York, p 367–378
Levin M B, Pinkus H 1961 Autosensitivity to deoxyribonucleic acid (DNA). Report of a case with inflammatory skin lesions controlled by chloroquine. New England Journal of Medicine 264: 533–537
Linderkamp O, Hopner F, Klose H 1976 Solitary hepatic haemangioma in a newborn infant complicated by cardiac failure, consumption coagulopathy microangiopathic haemolytic anaemia and obstructive jaundice. Case report and review of the literature. European Journal of Paediatrics 124: 23–29
Lisker R, Nogueron A, Sanchez-Medal L 1960 Plasma thromboplastin component in the Ehlers–Danlos syndrome. Annals of Internal Medicine 53: 388–395
Little P J, Sloper J S, De Wardener H E 1967 A syndrome of loin pain and haematuria associated with disease of peripheral renal arteries. Quarterly Journal of Medicine 142: 253–259
Lovejoy F H, Maraise E K, Landrigan P J 1971 Two examples of purpura factitia. Clinical Pediatrics 10: 183–184
Lowe G D O 1984 Vascular disease and vasculitis. In: Ratnoff O D, Forbes C D (eds) Disorders of hemostasis, Grune & Stratton, New York, p 527–547
Lowe 1991 Vascular disease and vasculitis. In: Ratnoff O D, Forbes C D (eds) Disorders of hemostasis, Saunders, Philadelphia, p 532–549
Lowe G D O, Lowe J M, Drummond M M et al 1980 Blood viscosity in young male diabetics with and without retinopathy. Diabetologia 18: 1–5
Macfarlane R G 1972 Haemostasis. In: Biggs R (ed) Human blood coagulation, haemostasis and thrombosis, Blackwell, Oxford, p 543
McKay D G, Margaretten W 1967 Disseminated intravascular coagulation in virus diseases. Archives of Internal Medicine 120: 129–152
McPherson R A, Oustad J W, Ugaretz R J, Wolf P L 1977 Coagulopathy in amyloidosis. Combined deficiency of factor IX and X. American Journal of Hematology 3: 225–235
Madden R M, Gill J C, Marlar R A 1990 Protein C and protein S levels in two patients with acquired purpura fulminans. British Journal of Haematology 75: 112–117
Marsalese D L, Moodie D S, Vacante M et al 1989 Marfan syndrome: natural history and long-term follow-up of cardiovascular involvement. Journal of the American College of Cardiology 14: 422–428
Meadow S R, Glasgow E F, White R H R, Moncrieff M W, Cameron J S, Ogg C S 1972 Schonlein-Henoch nephritis. Quarterly Journal of Medicine 41: 241–258
Muckle T J 1964 Low in-vivo adhesive-platelet count in hereditary haemorrhagic telangiectasia. Lancet 2: 880–882
Mulhare P E, Tracy P B, Golden E A, Branden R F, Bouill E G 1991 A case of acquired factor X deficiency with in-vivo and in-vitro evidence of inhibitor activity directed against factor X. American Journal of Clinical Pathology 96: 196–200
Mullick F G, McAllister H A, Waggoner B H, Fenoglio J J 1979 Drug related vasculitis: Clinicopathologic corrections in thirty patients. Human Pathology 10: 313–325
Muntean W, Kaspar G, Stoffler G, Petek W 1978 Die Hamostase bei der Telangiectasia Hereditaria. Paediatric und Paedologie (Vienna) 13: 205–210
Neidhart J A, Roach R W 1982 Successul treatment of skeletal haemangioma and Kasabach-Meritt syndrome with aminocaproic acid. Is fibrinolysis defensive? American Journal of Medicine 73: 434–8
Noonan J A, Ehmke D A 1963 Associated with congenital heart disease. Journal of Paediatrics 63: 468–70
O'Hare, Eden O B 1984 Bleeding disorders and non-accidental injury. Archives of Diseases in Childhood 59: 860–864
Osler W 1901 On a family form of recurrent epistaxis associated with telangiectasia of the skin and mucous membranes. Bulletin of the Johns Hopkins Hospital 12: 333–337
Owen C A, Bowie E J W, Thompson J H 1975 Tests of hemostasis and blood coagulation in the diagnosis of bleeding disorders. Little, Brown, Boston, p 85
Ozsoylu S, Cengiz B, Karabent A 1988 Purpura fulminans in a case of protein C deficiency. European Journal of Pediatrics 147: 209–210
Pachter M R, Johnson S A, Neblett T R, Truant J P 1959 Bleeding, platelets and macroglobulinaemia. American Journal of Clinical Pathology 31: 467–482
Palareti G, Coccheri S 1989 Lowered antithrombin 111 activity and other clotting changes in homocystinuria: effects of pyridoxine-folate regimen. Haemostasis 19 (Suppl): 24–28
Perkins H A, MacKenzie M R, Fudenberg H H 1970 Haemostatic defects in dysproteinemias. Blood 35: 695–707
Pinnell S R, Krane S, Kenzora J E, Glincher M J 1972 A new heritable disorder of connective tissue with hydroxylysine-deficient collagen. New England Journal of Medicine 286: 1013–1020
Pope F M 1991 Ehlers–Danlos Syndrome. Baillière's Clinical Rheumatology 5: 321–349
Pope F M, Martin G R, Lichtenstein J R et al 1975 Patients with EDS lack type III collagen. Proceedings of the National Academy of Sciences, USA 72: 1314–1316
Preston F E 1980 Circulatory complications of leukaemia and paraproteinaemia. In: Lowe G D O, Barbenel J C, Forbes C D (eds), Clinical aspects of blood viscosity, cell deformability and rheology. Springer-Verlag, London
Preston E, Cooke K B, Foster M E, Winfield D A, Lee D 1978 Myelomatosis and the hyperviscosity syndrome. British Journal of Haematology 38: 517–530
Priest R E, Moinuddin J F, Priest J H 1973 Collagen of Marfan syndrome is abnormally soluble. Nature 245: 264–266
Purcell I M, Constantine J W 1972 Platelets and experimental scurvy. Nature 235: 289–391
Pyeritz R A, McKusick V A 1979 The Marfan Syndrome: Diagnosis and management. New England Journal of Medicine 300: 772–777
Quick A J 1966 Telangiectasia. In: Hemorrhagic diseases and thrombosis. Lea & Febiger, Philadelphia, p 96
Quick A J 1975 The bleeding time as a test of haemostatic function. American Journal of Clinical Pathology 64: 87–94
Ramsay D M, MacLeod D A D, Buist T A S, Heading R C 1976 Persistent gastrointestinal bleeding due to angiodysplasia of the gut in von Willebrand's disease. Lancet 2: 275–278
Ratnoff O D 1968 Treatment of haemorrhagic disease. Hoeber, New York, p 221
Ratnoff O D 1980 The psychogenic purpuras. A review of auto-erythrocyte sensitization, auto-sensitization to DNA, 'hysterical' and factitial bleeding and the religious stigmata. Seminars in Haematology 17: 192–213
Ratnoff O D 1984 Psychogenic Bleeding. In: Ratnoff O D, Forbes C D (eds) Disorders of haemostasis, Grune & Stratton, New York, p 549–554
Ratnoff O D 1991 Psychogenic bleeding. In: Ratnoff O D, Forbes C D (eds) Disorders of hemostasis, 2nd edn. Saunders, Philadelphia, p 532–549
Ratnoff O D, Agle D P 1968 Psychogenic purpura. A re-evaluation of the syndrome of auto-erythrocyte sensitization. Medicine 47: 475–500
Riseborough E J and Herndon J H 1976 Alterations in pulmonary function, coagulation and fat metabolism in patients with fractures of the lower limbs. Clinical Orthopedics 15: 248–267
Robboy S J, Mihm M C, Colman R W 1973 The skin in disseminated intravascular coagulation. Prospective analysis of 36 cases. British Journal of Dermatology 88: 221–229
Roberts H R, Kroncke F G 1971 The platelet tests of platelet activity.

In: Brinkhous K W, Shermer R W, Mastofi F K (eds) Application to clinical diagnosis, Williams & Wilkins, Baltimore, p 251
Rodgers R P C and Levin J A 1990 A critical review of the bleeding time. Seminars in Thrombosis and Hemostasis 16: 1–20
Rosenberg E M, Hahn T J, Ortho D N, Deftos L J, Tanaka K 1978 ACTH-secreting medullary carcinoma of the thyroid presenting as a severe idiopathic osteoporosis and senile purpura: report of a case and review of the literature. Journal of Clinical Endocrinology and Metabolism 47: 255–262
Rosenthal C J, Franklin E C 1977 Amyloidosis and amyloid proteins. In: Thompson R A (ed) Recent advances in clinical immunology. Churchill Livingstone, Edinburgh p 41
Ross P, Failkow P J, Altman L K 1978 Fine structure alterations of elastic fibres in pseudoxanthoma elasticum. Clinical Genetics 13: 221–223
Rowell N R 1974 A painful bleeding syndrome associated with increased fibrinolytic activity. British Journal of Dermatology 91: 591–596
Rubenfield S, Min K W 1977 Leukocytoclastic vasculitis in subacute bacterial endocarditis. Archives of Dermatology 113: 1033–1074
Sanders A G 1970 In vivo observations on haemostasis in the hamster. In: MacFarlane R G (ed) The haemostatic mechanism in man and other animals. Academic Press, London, p 109
Sane D C, Pizzo S V, Greenberg C S 1989 Elevated urokinase-type plasminogen activator level and bleeding in amyloidosis: case report and literature review. American Journal of Hematology 31: 53–57
Saunders W H 1960 Permanent control of nosebleeds in patients with hereditary haemorrhagic telangiectasia. Annals of Internal Medicine 53: 147–152
Scarborough H, Shuster S 1960 Corticosteroid purpura. Lancet 1: 93–94
Schonlein J L 1837 Pelliosis rheumatica (Peliosis Circumscripta) In: Allgemeine und speckelle Pathologie und Therapie, 3rd edn. Herisau, Switzerland, p 48–49
Schuster N H 1937 Familial haemorrhagic telangiectasia associated with multiple aneurysms of the splenic artery. Journal of Pathology and Bacteriology 44: 29–39
Schwartz J T, Patton G A, Graham D Y, Cain G D 1982 Gastric radiotherapy as a treatment of hereditary haemorrhagic telangiectasia. American Journal of Gastroenterology 77: 53–4
Schhwartz R S, Lewis F B, Dameshek W 1962 Hemorrhagic cutaneous anaphylaxis due to auto-sensitization in deoxyribonucleic acid. New England Journal of Medicine 267: 1105–1111
Scully R E, Mark E J, McNeely B U 1983 Case records of the Massachusetts General Hospital. Weekly clinicopathological exercises. New England Journal of Medicine 308: 579–85
Sharland M, Patton M A, Talbot S, Chitolie A, Bevan D H 1992 Coagulation-factor deficiencies and abnormal bleeding in Noonan's syndrome. Lancet 339: 19–21
Sheil A G, Ibels L S, Pollock C, Graham J C, Short J 1987 Treatment of loin pain/haematuria syndrome by renal autotransplantation. Lancet 17: 907–908
Shim W K 1968 Haemangiomas of infancy complicated by thrombocytopenia. American Journal of Surgery 116: 898–906
Shiozawa S, Tanaka T, Miyahara T, Murai A, Kameyamma M 1979 Age-related change in the reducible cross-link of human skin and aorta collagens. Gerontology 25: 247–254
Shuster S, Scarborough H 1961 Senile purpura. Quarterly Journal of Medicine 30: 33–40
Shuster S, Black M M, McVitie E 1975 Influence of age and sex on skin thickness, skin collagen and density. British Journal of Dermatology 96: 639–643
Siegel B M, Briedman I A, Schwartz S O 1957 Hemorrhagic disease in osteogenesis imperfecta; studies of platelet function defect. American Journal of Medicine 22: 315–321
Siegler R L, Brewer E D, Hammond E 1988 Platelet activation and prostacyclin supporting capacity in the loin pain haematuria syndrome. American Journal of Kidney Disease 12: 156–160
Singer K, Wolfson W Q 1944 Hereditary hemorrhagic telangiectasia. An analysis of capillary heredopathies. New England Journal of Medicine 230: 637–642
Smellie S W, Lambert M, Lavenne E, van Cangh P J 1987 Factor XII deficiency associated with loin pain/haematuria syndrome. Lancet 2: 1330
Snapper I 1971 Amyloidosis. In: Snapper I, Kah A (eds) Myelomatosis. University Park Press, Baltimore, p 238
Somer T 1975 Hyperviscosity syndrome in plasma cell dycrasias. Advances in Microcirculation 6: 1–55
Spicer T E, Rau J M 1976 Purpura fulminans. American Journal of Medicine 61: 566–571
Stefanini M, Mednicoff I B 1954 Demonstration of antivessel agents in serum of patients with anaphylactoid purpura and periarteritis nodosa. Journal of Clinical Investigation 33: 967 (abstract)
Sutor A H, Bowie E J, Owen C A 1977 Quantitative bleeding time (hemorrhagometry). A review. Mayo Clinic Proceedings 52: 238–240
Thatcher L G, Chatanoff D V, Stiehm E R 1968 Splenic haemangioma with thrombocytopenia and afibrinogenemia. Journal of Pediatrics 73: 343–354
Tuddenham E G, Takase T, Thomas A E et al 1989 Homozygous protein C deficiency with delayed onset of symptoms at 7 to 10 months. Thrombosis Research 53: 475–484
Tunstall-Pedoe H, Lightman S 1982 Sucker-daddy (Purpura cyclops). Lancet 1: 632 (letter)
Turi S, Nagy J, Haszon I, Havass Z, Nemeth M, Bereczki C 1989 Plasma factors influencing PGI_2-like activity in patients with IgA nephropathy and Henoch–Schonlein purpura. Pediatric Nephrology 3: 61–67
Uden A 1982 Collagen and bleeding diathesis in Ehlers–Danlos syndrome. Scandinavian Journal of Haematology 28: 425–30
Vase P 1981 Estrogen treatment of hereditary hemorrhagic telangiectasia: A double-blind controlled clinical trial. Acta Medica Scandinavica 209: 393–396
Vase P, Lorentzen M 1983 Histological findings following oestrogen treatment of hereditary haemorrhagic telangiectasia. A controlled double-blind investigation. Journal of Laryngology and Otology 97: 427–429
Vermylen J, Blockmans D 1992 In: Forbes C D, Cushieri A (eds) Drugs used in bleeding in surgical practice. Blackwell, Oxford, p 321–337
Verstraete M 1977 Haemostatic drugs: A critical appraisal, Nijhoff, The Hague
Waldo F B 1992 Is Henoch–Schonlein purpura the systemic form of IgA nephropathy? American Journal of Kidney Diseases 12: 373–377
Wallerstein R O, Wallerstein R O Jr 1976 Scurvy. Seminars in Haematology 13: 211–218
Wedgewood R J P, Klaus M H 1955 Anaphyllactoid purpura (Henoch-Schonlein). A long-term follow-up with special reference to renal involvement. Pediatrics 16: 196–205
Wilson P A, McNicol G P, Douglas A S 1967 Platelet abnormalities in human scurvy. Lancet 1: 975–978
Winkelman R K 1980 Classification of vasculitis. In: Wolff K, Winkelmann R K (eds) Vasculitis. Lloyd-Luke, London
Witkop C J, Quevedo W C, Fitzpatrick T B 1978 Albinism. In: Stanbury J B, Syngardero J B, Fredrickson D S (eds) The metabolic basis of inherited disease, 4th edn. McGraw-Hill, New York, p 328
Witt D R, McGillvray B C, Allanson J E et al 1988 Bleeding diathesis in Noonan syndrome: a common association. American Journal of Medical Genetics 31: 305–317
Wong Hy 1988 Hypothesis: senile purpura is a prognostic feature in elderly patients Age-Ageing 17: 422–424

47. White cells, free radicals and scavengers

Jill Belch

'Unlike erythrocytes and platelets, the leukocytes are merely passengers in the bloodstream.'
Oxford Textbook of Medicine, 1983

Intense study within the field of coagulation and thrombosis has elucidated many of the mechanisms of ischaemic vascular disease. Over the past 3 decades, the role of the platelet and red blood cell (RBC) has become increasingly recognised, as has the importance of plasma coagulation factors such as fibrinogen. Little attention, however, has been paid to the white blood cell (WBC). It is the object of this chapter to present current evidence for a new hypothesis on the mechanisms of tissue injury in ischaemia. In addition to the classical picture of atherosclerosis, vascular spasm, platelet and fibrin thrombus and embolus formation, there is increasing evidence that another key event may take place: obstruction of blood vessels in the microcirculation and tissue injury by the WBC, more particularly the polymorphonuclear cells (PMNs) (Table 47.1).

The role of the PMN in the inflammatory response to ischaemia is well-recognised. Neutrophil infiltration of tissues during the first 12–24 hours following infarction has been well-documented, where a migrating population of inflammatory cells at the margin of the damaged tissue progresses towards the centre as necrosis and repair progress in the same direction. However, recent evidence suggests a broader and earlier role for the neutrophil in the acute injury process and these cells may be mediators of cell damage during ischaemia.

Table 47.1 White blood cells

Phagocyte	Lymphocyte
Polymorphonuclear cell (PMN) or granulocyte 1. Neutrophils 2. Basophils 3. Eosinophil Neutrophils with a diameter of 10–20 μm, are probably most important in modifying microcirculatory flow	Small round cells (20–50% of leukocytes) Lymphocytes often present within advanced human atherosclerotic plaques. As yet there is little evidence to support a role in ischaemic vascular disease
Monocytes/macrophage Monocytes migrate to tissues where, as macrophages they remove unwanted particulate matter. Probable role in atherogenesis	

THE TOTAL LEUKOCYTE COUNT AS A RISK FACTOR FOR ARTERIAL DISEASE

The blood white cell count (WCC) is a consistent and powerful predictor of cardiovascular events in epidemiological studies. A number of large studies have found that an increased WCC within the 'normal range' following myocardial infarction (MI) is predictive of further coronary events. (Friedman et al 1974, Schlant et al 1982, Haines et al 1983).

Haines et al (1983) reviewed 272 patients with MI. They found that the 68 who died within 1 year had significantly higher WCCs. The peak creatine kinase (CK) was also significantly higher in those who died compared to the survivors and a significant correlation between CK and WCC was detected. In the PARIS I study (Persantin-Aspirin Reinfarction Study) 2026 patients with MI were studied (Lowe et al 1985). A positive correlation with WCC, sudden death and reinfarction was detected. It might be suggested that the increase in WCC in these studies merely reflected the severity of the first infarct: the larger the initial area of tissue damage, the brisker the acute phase response following MI, including an increase in WCC. However, Friedman et al (1974) measured WCCs in the 2 years preceding a first MI in 464 patients. These patients were compared with two control groups, one of which was matched for gender, race and age and the other additionally matched for the more conventional risk factors. The WCC was found to be a strong predictor of infarction with a predictive value similar to that of a serum cholesterol measurement or a single determinant of blood pressure (BP).

Cigarette smoking increases the WCC and in the study by Friedman et al (1974) the WCC did correlate positively with cigarette smoking. However, only two thirds of the excess risk of the high count patients was explicable on the basis of such cigarette smoking. In the Paris prospective study, Zalokar et al (1981) followed over 7000 male employees of a branch of the Paris city government for an average of 6.5 years after an initial examination. The leukocyte count at the initial examination was a highly significant predictor of MI (104 cases), however this effect was confined to subjects who inhaled cigarette smoke. Within the smoking group, however, the 17% of inhalers who had leukocyte counts above $9 \times 10^9/l$ had nearly four times the incidence of MI among the 48% of smokers with counts under $7 \times 10^9/l$. Thus, although smoking may partly explain the correlation of WCC with MI, it is unlikely to be the full explanation.

Prentice et al (1982) investigated survivors of the Japanese atomic bomb blasts. They were able to relate total WCC and differential counts to the risk of coronary artery disease (CAD). The total WCC correlated positively with CAD. This was independent of cholesterol, BP, smoking and gender. Examination of the differential counts showed the likely culprit to be the neutrophil. Additionally, eosinophil and monocyte counts were also predictive while lymphocyte counts were not. In the MRFIT study (Multiple Risk Factor Intervention Trial) (Grimm et al 1985) there was also a strong correlation between the WCC and CAD prevalence, risk of non-fatal MI and risk of sudden cardiac death. This was independent of other risk factors such as smoking. Moreover, if a WCC declined during the study so did the risk of CAD events. A fall of 1×10^9 WBC/l was associated with a 14% fall in risk of cardiac death, not explained by changes in other risk factors.

This suggestion, that a lower count lowers the risk, is supported by studies of neutropenic states. Laboratory work investigating animals treated with a neutrophil antiserum experienced myocardial infarctions that were on average 43% smaller than infarcts in animals treated with non-immune rabbit serum or saline (Romson et al 1983). Histopathological examination revealed that the infarcted myocardium from the control animals had a substantial neutrophilic infiltrate which was virtually absent in the tissue from animals treated with neutrophil antiserum. In a similar study, Engler et al (1986) reported fewer arrythmias in the neutrophil-depleted animals. These animal studies are complemented by a study of the Yemenite Jews (Shoenfeld & Pinkhas 1981). This group frequently have a benign constitutional neutropenia and they rarely experience ischaemic vascular events.

This correlation between WCC and vascular disease is likely to be meaningful. Two smaller studies provide further evidence for this. Maisel et al (1985) have shown that the initial WCC is an independent predictor of primary ventricular fibrillation. Of 20 variables examined, the initial PMN count was the best predictor for the arrhythmia, better than both systolic blood pressure or heart rate. Kuzuya et al (1988) extended this work by demonstrating that the WCC of patients immediately following MI was positively related to the severity of ventricular arrhythmias. Patients who had PMN counts of around $13 \times 10^9/l$ all had severe ventricular arrhythmias within 8 ± 2 hours of their MI. Patients whose counts were around $10 \times 10^9/l$ or lower did not. Kostis et al (1984) showed a positive association between PMN count and the presence and extent of coronary atherosclerosis as determined by coronary arteriography. In their study of 573 patients with stable ischaemic heart disease this was considered to be an independent contribution from the WCC after accounting for effects of age, sex, cholesterol and triglycerides. As with the other previously mentioned studies, smoking weakened the contribution of the WCC but did not fully explain it.

The risks associated with a high WCC are not limited to the heart. The total WCC also correlates with the risk of thrombotic stroke (Prentice et al 1982) and possibly with re-thrombosis following peripheral vascular grafting (Dormandy et al 1988). There is, therefore, convincing evidence to suggest that an elevation of the WCC in the peripheral blood is associated with an increased risk of vascular disease. To understand the possible mechanisms involved in such a process it is necessary to be aware of the normal morphology and behaviour patterns of WBC.

LEUKOCYTE TYPES

Five different types of leukocyte are found in the peripheral blood (Table 47.1), however, it is convenient to separate them into two groups: the phagocytes which are able to engulf particles such as micro-organisms, and the lymphocytes which are concerned with the immune response. The phagocytes can be further subdivided into the polymorphonuclear leukocytes (PMNs) which are cells that have lost the capacity to replicate and whose nuclei consist of two or more separate lobes, and the monocytes which are precursors of the much longer-lived tissue macrophage. The different appearances of the cytoplasmic granules after staining allow further subdivision of the PMNs into neutrophils, eosinophils and basophils. The term granulocyte can also be used to refer to these cells as a group or, more specifically, to the neutrophils which are by far the most numerous.

LEUKOCYTES IN DISEASE: MONOCYTES, MACROPHAGES AND ATHEROSCLEROSIS

The observation that most or all of the foam cells in atherosclerotic plaques are macrophages helps to explain aspects of atherogenesis previously not understood. Monocytes may increase transport of LDL into the intima as they migrate from the blood (Mitchinson & Ball 1987).

Macrophages can secrete factors that are chemo-attractants which increase medial smooth muscle cell migration into the intima. The secretion of a growth factor resembling platelet-derived growth factor (PDGF) by macrophages might then lead to proliferation of the smooth muscle cells. The secretion of neutral proteases contributes to the degradation of tissue matrix within the plaques and the production of oxygen radicals contributes further to tissue damage extending the lesion and increasing the permeability of the endothelium. The resultant oxidized lipids are cytotoxic and adversely effect the production of prostaglandins (PGs) and leukotrienes (LTs) (Belch 1990) and may lead to the production of ceroid, the hard insoluble cuff around lipid droplets which seems to render them difficult to disperse.

GRANULOCYTES AND VASCULAR DISEASE

There are several possible explanations as to why the WCC, particularly the granulocyte count, appears as a risk factor for arterial disease. One explanation is that the WCC may serve as a marker for one or more other disease processes that lead to vascular injury. For example, the marginal pool of PMNs can be rapidly mobilized into the circulating pool by such stimuli as adrenaline and exercise and it may be stimuli such as these that produce the vascular damage with the elevation in WCC occurring as a consequence. However, another more exciting possibility is that WCCs play a pathogenic role in thrombosis and evidence is accumulating to suggest that this is so, particularly for the neutrophil.

The adhesive, locomotory, secretory and invasive properties of neutrophils have been known for over 100 years. Their role is one of a clearance system which removes damaged or dying tissue and also bacterial pathogens and small foreign bodies. They can also, however, cause vascular damage in a number of ways: (1) by physical obstruction (2) by release of noxious chemicals and (3) by their interaction with other blood constituents.

1. Physical obstruction

Deformability

Granulocytes are large cells with a diameter of about 8 µm and they require considerable deformation to pass through capillaries which have typical diameters of about 5–6 µm (Fig. 47.1a). In the passive state the plasma membranes of individual cells have numerous small folds resulting in an excess of membrane surface area. It is this excess surface area that allows deformation/change of shape of the cell during capillary passage or during migration across the vascular wall. Thus the amount of deformation is limited by the amount of membrane available for unfolding. When leukocytes pass through post-capillary venules they

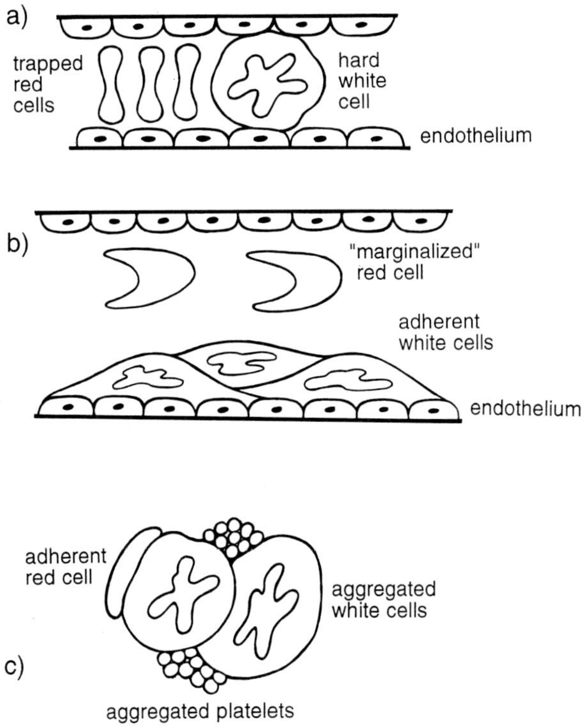

Fig. 47.1 Microcirculatory effects of neutrophils.

are able to emigrate across vascular endothelium by the projection of pseudopods. However, when they are trapped in capillaries, they are already elongated, their membranes fully unfolded and they fill the lumen of the capillary. Under these conditions the formation of pseudopods for migration is opposed by the membrane tension and the WBC remains trapped in the lumen rather than migrating to the tissue. If the PMN is already activated when it reaches the capillary, the prior projection of pseudopods has taken up all membrane slack and its rigidity increases still further. Trapped granulocytes are frequently located at the entry of capillaries or at local bulging of endothelial cell nuclei. Several details of the rheological properties of PMNs have been described in recent years (Schmid-Schönbein & Engler 1986). Most striking is the fact that they are about 2000 times less deformable than the erythrocyte. Thus, although red cell deformability contributes to microvascular flow by virtue of the cell's large number, the less numerous WBC can still have profound effects by virtue of its intense rigidity.

In support of this concept, poorly deformable WBCs have been found in patients with vascular disease. In a study investigating the filterability of granulocytes in patients with MI, increases in cell rigidity were found in patients aged less than 60 years predominantly in the granulocyte population (Nash et al 1989). A control group of chest-pain patients without evidence of MI showed no increase in cell rigidity. Whether cause of or consequent on the initial ischaemic event, the effect may be detrimental to the remaining myocardium. The importance of WBC deformability is further emphasized by a finding of impaired leukocyte filtration in acute cerebral infarction with no change in red blood cell deformability (Mercuri et al 1989). Patients with chronic cerebrovascular disease also have rigid WBCs (Vermes & Strik 1988) as do patients with lower limb peripheral vascular disease (Ciuffetti et al 1989). A further increase in granulocyte rigidity occurs at the time of onset of intermittent claudication symptoms. It is also probable that flow elsewhere in the body is also dependent on WBC deformability as shown by animal studies in other organs such as the kidney (Braide et al 1986).

Margination and Adhesion

Another property of PMNs which has important implications with respect to microcirculatory flow is adhesion to endothelium. White blood cells do not normally adhere to the walls of blood vessels and tend, because of their size, to be in the axial part of the bloodstream. In order to leave the vessel a PMN must first enter the marginal flow and form an adhesive contact which is strong enough to withstand the shearing stresses generated by the flowing blood. This localization can occur through several possible mechanisms such as a local change in blood flow, a local change in the endothelium, activation of circulating leukocytes or indeed a combination of these.

This wall shear stress is likely to be adversely affected where there is atheroma, partly because of turbulent flow and partly because of decreased lumen size. An increase in the local vascular permeability will produce oedema, thicken the blood and make flow more sluggish. This in turn increases the probability of an adhesive interaction. Whether the leukocyte remains trapped in the capillary is dependent on the strength of the adhesion as even a relatively stiff granulocyte will eventually pass through the capillary since its cytoplasm is visco-elastic. In the presence of adhesion a new situation arises since now the flowing blood must not only deform the cell, but overcome this adhesion. A single granulocyte may thus occlude capillaries completely and by adhering to the vascular endothelium of arterioles or venules significantly increase microvascular resistance (Fig. 47.1b) (Lackie 1982).

In the same way, adhesion to other granulocytes (aggregation) or other blood cell type can lead to the formation of cellular microemboli (Fig. 47.1c). It is of interest to note that thrombotic events appear to have a circadian rhythm, being more frequent in the early morning.There is a matching circadian variation in granulocyte aggregation (Bridges et al 1992a). Although other factors may contribute to this early morning thrombotic tendency, such an increase in WBC aggregation may be relevant. There is an increase in PMN aggregation in whole blood taken from patients with MI (Fisher et al 1989) and increased pseudopod formation and clumping has been described in isolated WBCs taken from patients with unstable angina (Mehta et al 1989). Cigarette smoking further increases PMN aggregation (Bridges et al 1993a) even in normal controls and may be a further mechanism whereby smoking exerts its prothrombotic effects.

All the above work suggests that activated and thus more rigid and adherent granulocytes are to be found in thrombotic vascular diseases. What is not yet clear are the mechanisms leading to such activation. It is possible, though unlikely, that patients are 'earmarked' for vascular disease by a genetically determined high level of WBC activity. This has yet to be investigated and such studies will have difficulty in separating the genetic and environmental factors, e.g. smoking parents tend to have children who smoke, passive smoking has effects on non-smoking offspring and diet tends to be similar within the family group, etc. Although such studies, if undertaken, will be of interest, it is likely that the WBC activation is a secondary event. Chronic cigarette smoking, a well-recognised risk factor for vascular disease is a likely candidate for WBC activation. However, in the epidemiological studies described above, the WCC effect appeared to be partly independent of smoking habit. The enhanced neutrophil function may, therefore, relate to other factors such as complement activation. Membrane interaction and complement-mediated neutrophil activation result in enhanced leukocyte adherence, diminution of microvascular flow and endothelial injury. Cholesterol and other atheroma lipids have been shown to be capable of activating complement (Hammerschmidt et al 1981). Other mechanisms may also be involved. Even a small concentration of platelet activating factor (PAF) activates PMNs (Worthen et al 1988) as do activated platelets themselves (see p. 1098). Thrombin is chemotactic for granulocytes (Bar-Shavit et al 1983) and is probably responsible for the movement of leukocytes into clots.

Alternatively, it may not be a question of excessive activation of PMNs but of compromised inhibition. Since transient ischaemia does not always lead to infarction it seems reasonable to suggest that there may be an inhibitory feedback on granulocytes that has physiological significance. Prostacyclin (PGI_2) decreases PMN adhesion and aggregation (Boxer et al 1980, Belch et al 1986). It is possible that in minor degrees of endothelial cell injury there is a transient decrease in PGI_2 production sufficient to allow leukocytes to adhere and tissue repair to occur. A later increase in PGI_2 from the repaired area permits normal endothelial function thereafter. In atheroma where PGI_2 formation appears to be absent, the neutrophil may be further activated and vascular damage enhanced (Gryglewski et al 1978). A further mechanism for white cell inhibition is through the adenosine pathway. The adenosine receptors also inhibit WBC activation and adenosine addition in vitro inhibits both platelet and white cell loss (Cronstein et al 1983). However, regardless of the precise stimulus, enhanced neutrophil rigidity and adhesion may provide a milieu for the progression of stable arterial disease to unstable critical ischaemia.

2. Release of noxious chemicals

Once the PMN has become fixed in the microvasculature it can deliver a variety of further insults to the vessel lining. In normal circumstances this capability of the WBC allows emigration of the cell from the circulation to the site of tissue damage and later phagocytosis and the destruction of noxious material found therein. If the cell is trapped in the circulation, however, vascular damage can result. Many of the chemicals released from neutrophils can have effects on thrombus formation and dissolution (Table 47.2). Of those listed, probably the most important are the neutral hydrolases, the biologically active lipids and the toxic oxygen metabolites.

Neutral hydrolases biologically active lipids and other WBC granule contents

One mechanism by which activated neutrophils can induce cell damage is through the release of potent proteolytic enzymes. Elastase is one of the serine proteases released from the granules of PMNs after activation of the cell. It has a wide range of substrates including collagen, elastin, fibrinogen and other matrix macromolecules and is implicated in the pathophysiology of several human diseases (Malech & Gallin 1987). Cathepsin G is also released from neutrophils and studies of both elastase and cathepsin G have shown many wide ranging effects on coagulation and thrombosis. Both these neutral proteases inactivate plasma clotting factors I, II, V, VII, VIII, XII and XIII as well as plasma inhibitors of coagulation and fibrinolysis such as anti-thrombin III (ATIII), C1 inactivator and α_2-antiplasmin (for review see Bykowska et al 1985). Recently it has been suggested that elastase in particular may mediate some of the vascular damage produced by PMNs in ischaemic states. Elastase can cause digestion of basement membrane and increase endothelial cell adhesiveness, permeability and tissue oedema (Mehta et al 1989). Both elastase and cathepsin G will damage platelets enhancing ADP aggregation particularly in the presence of fibrinogen (Bykowska et al 1985). Interestingly, inhibition of elastase by α_1-antitrypsin is attenuated by other WBC release products such as free radicals (Mehta et al 1988). Elevated plasma elastase levels occur in MI patients (Bell et al 1990). This increase is independent of the MI-induced elevation in WCC and appears to reflect true WBC activation. Mehta et al (1989) studied various categories of patients with CAD. They measured the peptide Bβ 30–43 suggesting that this fibrinogen fragment was produced in blood by the action of released neutrophil elastase on fibrin(ogen). Elevated levels were detected in patients with unstable angina and myocardial infarction compared to control subjects and those with stable angina.

Table 47.2 Chemicals released by neutrophils with effects on coagulation and thrombosis

Toxic oxygen metabolites
Superoxide
Hydroxyl radical
Hydrogen peroxide
Singlet oxygen
Neutral hydrolases
Elastase
Collagenase
Plasminogen activator
Acid hydrolases
Protease
Lipase
Phosphatase
Coagulation factors
Factor V
Factor VII
Factor IX
Factor X
Lipids
Prostaglandins and thromboxane
Leukotrienes
Platelet activating factor
Others
α_2-macroglobulin
Fibronectin
Histamine

Activation of neutrophils also results in the release of the 5-lipoxygenase metabolites of arachadonic acid, principally leukotriene B_4 (LTB_4). This very potent chemoattractant causes neutrophils to accumulate in the area of ischaemic injury and also initiates neutrophil aggregation and degranulation. LTB_4 can stimulate the release of lysosomal enzymes and superoxide anion from PMNs and promote endothelial permeability and plasma leakage (Belch 1988). Small amounts of LTD_4 C_4 and E_4 are also released from PMNs and these have been shown to increase vascular resistance and reduce blood flow in the microcirculation (Wargovich et al 1985). Additionally, both LTC_4 and LTD_4 promote adhesion of neutrophils to endothelial cells and their extravasation through the blood vessel wall. Other lipoxygenase products such as hydroxyeicosatetraenoic acid (HETE) are also formed during PMN activation allowing secondary augmentation of PMN activity. PMN LTB_4 production in patients with MI is increased and there is a correlation between this elevated LTB_4 production and increased severity of ventricular arrythmias following MI (Kuzuya et al 1988). LTB_4 production is also increased in unstable angina (Mehta et al 1989) and in patients with PAD manifest by Raynaud's phenomenon (Lau et al 1992).

Other white cell release products have also been implicated in vascular damage. For example, thromboplastin, one of the most potent triggers of blood coagulation known, can be released from WBCs particularly those of the monocyte population (Lyberg & Pruydz 1982). Interleukin I and tumour necrosis factor (TNF) from PMNs can also induce release of thromboplastin by endothelial cells and this may also have a potentially important role in thrombogenesis (Bevilacqua et al 1984, Nawroth & Stern 1986, Shapiro et al 1986). Histamine, another WBC release product, is thought also to contribute to vascular damage and atherosclerosis by increasing permeability of the vascular wall and allowing passage of large molecules such as cholesterol and growth factor. Patients with atherosclerotic PAD have an increased histamine content of their WBCs which is further augmented by the presence of diabetes mellitus (Gill et al 1988) suggesting a role for histamine in vascular damage. The mechanism whereby histamine is increased in these patients is not yet clear; whether it reflects increased synthesis, decreased catabolism or even increased uptake has yet to be determined.

OXYGEN FREE RADICALS

In the course of bacterial killing and phagocytosis, PMNs consume large quantities of oxygen which may be transformed into reactive oxygen species (ROS) of which some are free radicals (FRs). FRs are normally used in the protection of the organism against microbial invaders but such defence mechanisms can also be prothrombotic.

A normal chemical bond consists of paired electrons sharing a single molecular orbital. A free radical is simply a species which contains one or more unpaired electrons in its outermost shell. It can be positive, negative or neutrally charged. The odd electron is often represented in the formula as a dot. FRs may thus be considered to contain an open bond rendering them chemically very reactive. Since molecules achieve their stability by electron pairing, radicals are inheritently unstable capable of undergoing both oxidation and reduction. Thus, if two radicals meet they combine their unpaired electrons and join to form a covalent bond.

$$R^{\cdot} + R^{\cdot} \longrightarrow R - R$$

If a radical reacts with a non-radical by either taking or donating an electron, that other molecule itself becomes a radical:

$$R^{\cdot} + CH \longrightarrow RH + C^{\cdot}$$

This enables FRs to participate in chain reactions and contributes to their extreme toxicity. These reactions can be propagated by transition metal ions or terminated either by the random collision of two FRs to form a stable molecule or by one of the cellular defence mechanisms outlined below.

Molecular oxygen as a source of free radicals

Molecular oxygen, O_2, is itself a bi-radical as it has two unpaired electrons. The biological reduction of molecular oxygen in cells is accompanied by the production of both FRs and active non-radical oxygen species. The term reactive oxygen species (ROS) is used in preference to FRs since hydrogen peroxide (H_2O_2) and singlet oxygen are not radicals but have important functions within the area of thrombosis (Halliwell 1990). Molecular oxygen is a relatively slowly reacting molecule which can accept electrons one at a time to produce in turn the superoxide radical ($O_2^{\cdot -}$), hydrogen peroxide, the hydroxyl radical ($OH^{\cdot}$) and finally water (Fig. 47.2). Under normal physiological conditions approximately 95% of molecular oxygen is reduced tetravalently by the mitochondrial electron transport chain to water. The remaining 5% undergoes the reaction shown in Figure 47.2. The superoxide radical is not particularly active, it acts physiologically as a mild reducing agent and cannot penetrate the membranes of surrounding cells. In pathological conditions it is important as a source of H_2O_2 which can easily penetrate cell membranes and initiate damage in places distant to its site of formation. This conversion of $O_2^{\cdot -}$ to H_2O_2 is catalysed by superoxide dismutase enzymes (SOD) (Fridovich 1989). However, in the presence of trace amounts of free iron, $O_2^{\cdot -}$ and H_2O_2 are also rapidly converted to $OH^{\cdot}$ by the Haber–Weiss reaction and the Fenton reaction (Fig. 47.3). Fenton type oxidation can also be catalysed by other transition metal ions such as copper.

Formation of reactive oxygen species

The white blood cell is an important source of FRs. Neutrophil activation allows the formation of $O_2^{\cdot -}$ by NADH oxidase during the respiratory burst. The $O_2^{\cdot -}$ released, stimulates other PMNs and thus any response to tissue injury is enhanced and augmented. The $O_2^{\cdot -}$ generating

$$\underset{\text{molecular oxygen}}{O_2} \xrightarrow{e^-} \underset{\text{superoxide}}{O_2^{\cdot -}} \xrightarrow{2e^- + 2H^+} \underset{\text{hydrogen peroxide}}{H_2O_2} \xrightarrow{2e^- + 2H^+} \underset{\text{hydroxy radical}}{OH^{\cdot}} \xrightarrow{2e^- + 2H^+} \underset{\text{water}}{H_2O}$$

Fig. 47.2 Reduction of molecular oxygen to free radicals and water.

$$\underset{\text{superoxide}}{O_2^{\cdot -}} + Fe^{3+} \longrightarrow O_2 + Fe^{2+}$$

$$\underset{\text{hydrogen peroxide}}{H_2O_2} + Fe^{2+} \longrightarrow Fe^{3+} + OH^- + OH^{\cdot} \quad \text{Fenton Reaction}$$

Fig. 47.3 Free iron and hydroxyl radical production; the Fenton reaction.

oxidase of the phagocytic cell is a membrane-bound enzyme system. This oxidase is present in an inactive or resting state in all the phagocytic white cells and can be activated by a large number of agents to consume oxygen, the so-called repiratory burst. The source of electrons is NADPH formed by the hexose monophosphate pathway, the activity of which is greatly stimulated during the PMN respiratory burst.

$$NADPH + 2O_2 \longrightarrow NADP^- + H^+ + 2O_2^{\cdot -}$$

NADPH oxidase is only in the active state following stimulation of the cell surface. Recently the mechanisms whereby it is transformed from a resting to an active state have become clearer although not yet fully defined. After exposure to the stimulating agent a complex series of biochemical events takes place which include rises in intracellular free calcium, changes in membrane potential due to ion movements, phospholipid hydrolysis, altered cyclic nucleotide levels, protein phosphorylation and activation of GTP-binding proteins. These alterations result in activation of certain phagocytic functions dependent on the pathway evoked, such as chemotaxis, phagocytosis, degranulation, adhesion and respiratory burst. Various natural inhibitors of this activation reaction exist such as bilirubin, thiols, adenosine and zinc (Cross 1990). Additionally, certain drugs may mediate some of their anti-inflammatory effects at this level, for example, aspirin, diclofenac, ebselen, chloroquine and gold.

ROS production is not, however, limited to the neutrophil. FRs are produced in small amounts by four other normal cellular processes (Fig. 47.4). Purine metabolism is also a major pathway for the production of ROS. This pathway is potentiated by ischaemia during which ATP is degraded stepwise to its purine substrate and endothelial xanthine dehydrogenase is transformed to xanthine oxidase (McCord 1985) (Fig. 47.5). During reperfusion of an ischaemic area (re-oxygenation), xanthine oxidase catalyses $O_2^{\cdot -}$ production from the purine substrates xanthine and hypoxanthine. This forms the basis for the so-called reperfusion injury where return of blood to a previously ischaemic tissue, as occurs with spontaneous or drug-induced thrombolysis, produces a burst of toxic FRs (Belch et al 1988). Interestingly, their production is critically dependent on the pO_2 of the reperfusing solution. Reperfusion with hyperoxic solution increases FR-

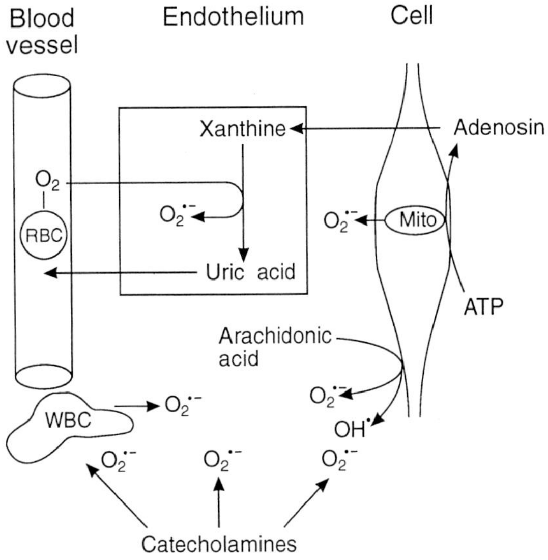

Fig. 47.4 Sources of reactive oxygen species.

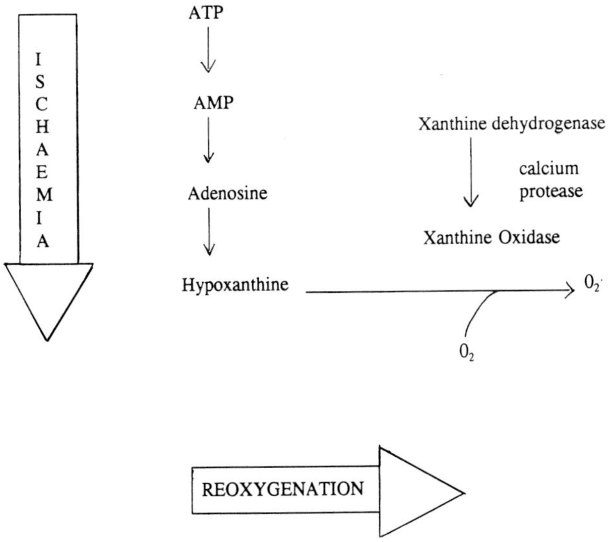

Fig. 47.5 Ischaemia – reperfusion production of superoxide anion.

mediated damage (Wolbarsht & Fridovitch 1989) whereas reperfusion with hypoxic solutions (pO_2 = 10 mmHg) prevents FR production (Garlick et al 1987). It has been suggested that this reperfusion system of radical production is important to human disease. However, its exact

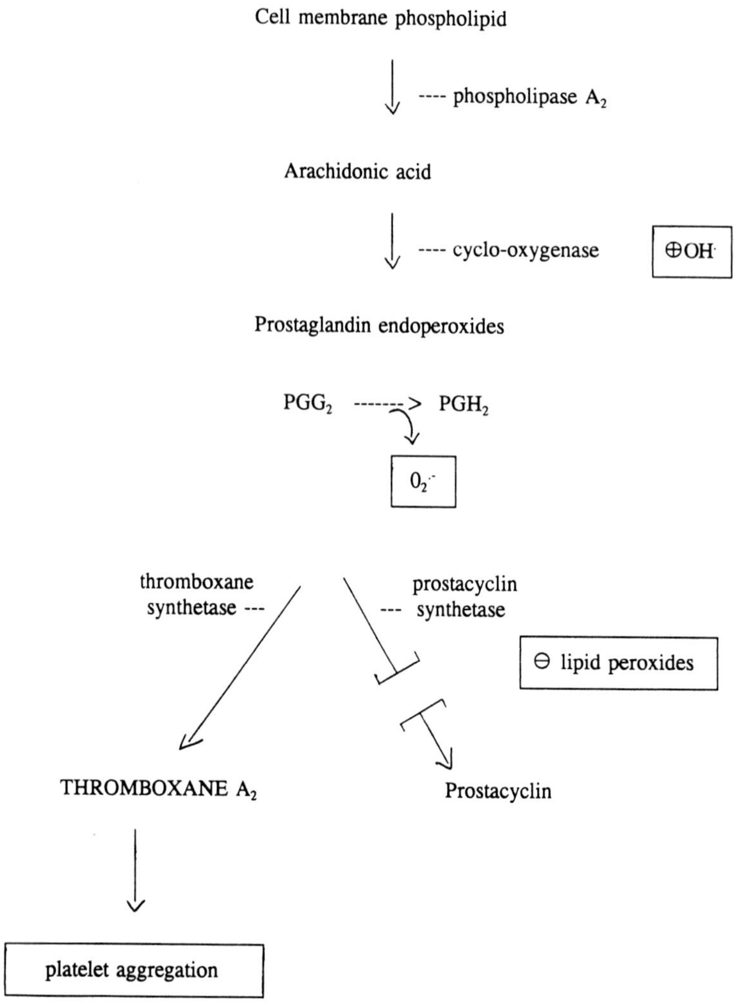

Fig. 47.6 The arachidonic acid cascade.

relevance is unknown as there are marked species variations in the tissue levels of xanthine oxidase and since the level of this enzyme in the human heart does not appear to be very high it may be of lesser importance in man (Muxfelat & Schaper 1987).

The synthesis of prostaglandins (PGs) through the arachidonic acid cascade also generates $O_2^{\cdot -}$ when PGG_2 converts to PGH_2 (Fig. 47.6). Although this process can occur in health, any type of tissue trauma, including ischaemia, which leads to AA release can amplify this pathway. Ischaemia further potentiates this reaction via enhanced accumulation of reduced nucleotides which then facilitate $O_2^{\cdot -}$ production during reperfusion.

Cell respiration within the mitochondria also yields $O_2^{\cdot -}$. This pathway operates during normal metabolism with the stepwise addition of four electrons to molecular oxygen reducing it to water. However 'leaks' in the system allow O_2 to accept single electrons forming $O_2^{\cdot -}$. This is also promoted by re-oxygenation following ischaemia. Auto-oxidation of catecholamines is another mechanism for ROS production. Such auto-oxidation leads to production of electrons which can reduce molecular oxygen to $O_2^{\cdot -}$. Isoprenaline can induce FR lipid damage in the rat heart and if endogenous catecholamines have a similar effect, this could contribute to their detrimental effects on the heart (Singal et al 1983). This pathway may be less relevant to ischaemic damage but probably contributes to the FR pathology seen in heart failure (Belch et al 1991a).

Prothrombotic effects of ROS

A consequence of uncontrolled ROS production is damage to biomolecules leading to altered function and disease. Free radicals can react with and damage proteins, nucleic acids, lipids and other classes of molecules such as the extracellular matrix glycosaminoglycans.

The sulphur-containing amino acids and the polyunsaturated fatty acids (PUFAs) are particularly vulnerable. FRs such as $OH^{\cdot}$ can fragment and cross-link proteins (Wolff & Dean 1986). The oxidation of protein in cell membranes, particularly sulphydryl groups, or the proteins of ion pumps and ion channels will have serious consequences for membrane function. Furthermore, FR-mediated damage of DNA will affect cell function by interfering with DNA's protein synthesis (McCord 1985).

Damage to cell membrane lipid, lipid peroxidation, will affect cell membrane function also (Halliwell & Gutteridge 1984). This occurs when the $OH^{\bullet -}$ is generated close to the cell membrane and attacks the FA sidechains of membrane phospholipids. It selects the FA sidechains with several double bonds such as those in AA. Accumulation of lipid peroxides in a membrane disrupts its function and can cause it to collapse. This is relevant in the area of thrombosis as damage to the red blood cell can encourage ADP release which in turn will aggregate platelets, and minor degrees of peroxidation of the red cell membrane increases its stiffness (Pfafferott et al 1982). A further consequence of increased lipid hydroperoxides is that they can decompose to yield a range of highly cytotoxic products such as the aldehydes (Esterbauer et al 1988). PUFAs undergoing peroxidation give rise to the formation of lipid breakdown products such as malondialdehyde (MDA) and diene-conjugates. These have become useful markers of oxidative lipid damage. Increased or uncontrolled ROS production therefore has the capacity for widespread cellular damage. This has implications in the field of thrombosis and coagulation when the damaged cells are those involved in the maintenance of blood flow (Fig. 47.7)

Reactive oxygen species and endothelium

FR damage to the endothelial cell can occur via the WBC trapped in the circulation as described earlier or via reperfusion injury, for example following thrombolysis (Fig. 47.8). This can lead to altered endothelial cell function and even cell death. Direct oxidative damage will increase the likelihood of thrombosis occurring over the damaged area. Additionally, production of endothelium-derived anti-thrombotic substances can be altered by ROS and their products. $O_2^{\bullet -}$ enhances the breakdown of endothelium-derived relaxant factor (EDRF) (Gryglewski et al 1987). This endogenous vasodilator regulates vascular tone and its rapid destruction may lead to an increase in tone which may be critical in situations of already compromised blood flow. EDRF mediates the action of endothelium-dependent vasodilators such as acetylcholine bradykinin and vasopressin (Kosaka et al 1989). EDRF is nitric oxide (NO) (Palmer et al 1987). NO is itself a free radical and promotes intracellular accumulation of cGMP. In this context NO synergizes with prostacyclin (PGI_2) which inhibits platelet aggregation by increasing intracellular levels of cAMP. In addition NO inhibits platelet adhesion in vitro (May et al 1990). The exact role of NO in the regulation of platelet behaviour in vivo remains unclear because oxyhaemoglobin in red blood cells (RBC) would be expected to bind and destroy free

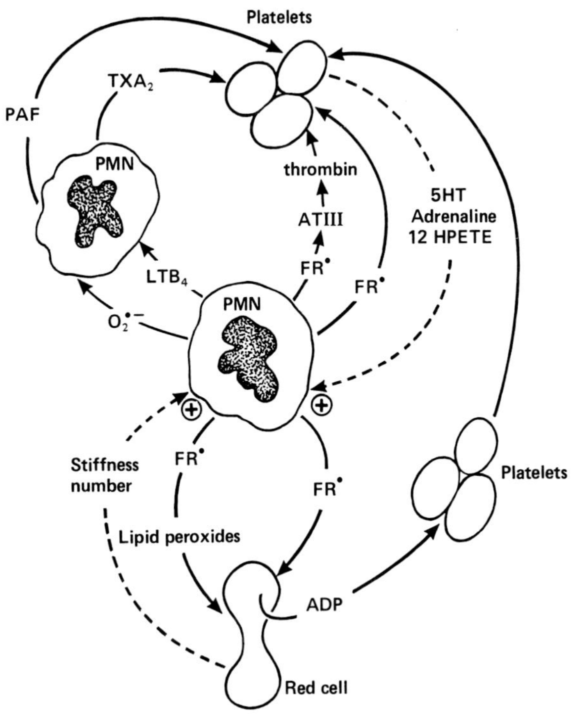

Fig. 47.7 Prothrombotic mechanisms of reactive oxygen species.

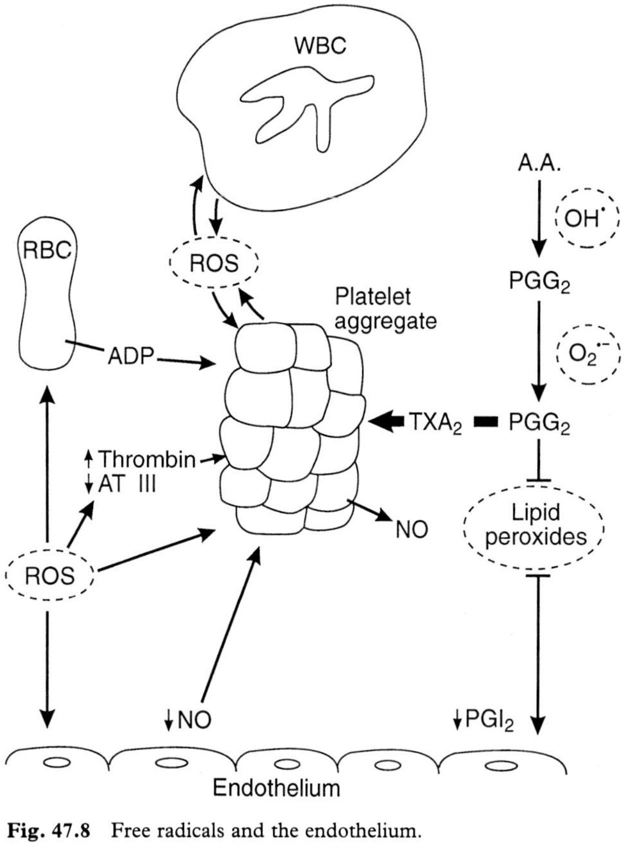

Fig. 47.8 Free radicals and the endothelium.

NO in the bloodstream. Recent work in the pulmonary circulation of rabbits, however, does suggest that NO has a role in vivo probably through altering platelet adhesion (Salvemini et al 1989). A negative feedback exists whereby the rate of breakdown of the NO is enhanced by $O_2^{\bullet -}$ (Kosaka et al 1989). The recent finding that platelets themselves produce NO and may thus have the capacity to control aggregation/adhesion within blood vessels will no doubt open new avenues. Neutrophils also synthesize NO, which inhibits both platelet aggregation and that of other neutrophils (Salvemini et al 1989). Thus it can be seen that any $O_2^{\bullet -}$-mediated breakdown of NO will be prothrombotic.

PGI_2 is another endothelial product affected by FR behaviour. PGI_2 is a most potent inhibitor of platelet aggregation produced by the endothelium. Thus, any damage to endothelial cell function will decrease PGI_2 production. In addition, the FR-produced lipid peroxides block PGI_2 formation (Moncada et al 1976) (Fig. 47.6). The hydroxyl radical also interacts in the AA cascade by augmenting the action of the cyclo-oxygenase enzyme. The combined effects of increasing cyclo-oxygenase activity and decreasing PGI_2 synthesis produces a net effect of selective enhancement of thromboxane A_2 (TXA_2) production (Tate et al 1984). This decreased PGI_2 production brought about by FRs is attenuated by the addition of anti-oxidants (Wang et al 1989), and low PGI_2 synthesis in vitamin E-deficient animals correlates with elevated lipid peroxide levels (Karpen et al 1981). As PGI_2 may itself protect against FR attack perpetuation of events can occur. Furthermore, PGI_2 inhibits PMN adhesion and prevents PMN aggregation so its decreased production leads to further WBC accumulation.

Vessel wall damage is further augmented by lipid peroxides increasing the cholesterol-donating ability of LDL and inhibiting the cholesterol accepting capacity of HDL, thus promoting cholesterol accumulation in blood vessel cells and subsequent atherosclerosis (Azizova et al 1989).

Reactive oxygen species, blood cells and plasma factors

In addition to the above neutrophil- and platelet-activating activities, FRs can directly affect blood cell behaviour. ROS attack on platelets will promote platelet aggregation and the peroxidative breakdown of RBC membrane lipids allows leaching of the potent platelet aggregant ADP and probably contributes to shear-induced platelet aggregation seen in whole blood (Jen & McIntire 1984, Saniabadi et al 1984). Lipid peroxidation of the membrane alters cell fluidity and a direct correlation between lipid peroxides and red cell deformability in peripheral arterial disease has been demonstrated (Pfafferott et al 1982).

There is evidence that other ROS in addition to NO are produced within the platelet itself (Dikskit et al 1989) and early work suggested that the platelets of patients with aspirin-induced asthma synthetized ROS to excess (Ameisen et al 1985). Later work, however, although confirming the ability of the platelet to produce ROS, could not confirm the increase in this disease (Schmutz-Schumann et al 1989). These ROS can activate both the platelet and the nearby PMN. Considerable evidence exists which indicates that platelets adherent to a damaged vascular surface contribute to the local recruitment and activation of PMNs and, although the sequence of events leading to such a phenomenon is not entirely understood, it is thought to include platelet-generated ROS (Belch 1992). As with any homeostatic process, mechanisms exist to limit the extent of the reaction. Platelets are in turn able to remove ROS primarily by consuming PMN-derived H_2O_2 via their glutathione cycle (Dallegri et al 1989). This supports a dual or regulatory role of platelets in their interaction with PMNs, initially interacting and activating the influx of PMNs at sites of vascular injury then down-regulating the PMN inflammatory and thrombotic effects by consuming H_2O_2. This capacity is consistent with the well-known commitment of platelets to vascular wall defence and repair.

Plasma coagulation factors are also affected by FRs. Thrombin generation is enhanced via the effects of lipid peroxides on lipoproteins and ATIII (Barrowcliffe et al 1985). Incubating phospholipid chylomicrons with lipid peroxide promotes its procoagulant activity. This suggests a direct interaction of lipid peroxides with the phospholipid in the outer coat of the lipoprotein possibly through an increase in negative charge. This in turn would promote the binding of coagulation factors. Inhibition of ATIII by lipid peroxides occurs principally at its heparin-binding site (Gray & Barrowcliffe 1984). A further procoagulant effect comes from the lipid peroxide-stimulated thromboplastin production from PMNs (Dean & Prydz 1983).

PROTECTIVE MECHANISMS

The abundance of ROS substrate, that is molecular oxygen, with such potent toxic effects of ROS as outlined above has required the concomitant development of a complex series of defence mechanisms to safeguard tissues against ROS attack. It is only when these fail, due either to excessive FR formation or impairment of the defence system, that damage occurs. The body has a number of sophisticated defence mechanisms at its disposal. These can be divided into two broad categories of primary and secondary mechanisms. In the primary group are superoxide dismutase (SODs), catalase, peroxidase enzyme and glutathione, and transition metal-binding proteins. The secondary mechanisms are those of cell anti-oxidants.

Primary defence mechanisms

The cytochrome oxidase system localized on the inner mitochondrial membrane reduces the major portion of oxygen produced by aerobic cells. However, SODs are essential for defence against oxygen toxicity. They are metalloenzymes that catalyse the dismutation of $O_2^{\bullet -}$.

$$O_2^{\bullet -} + O_2^{\bullet -} + 2H \xrightarrow[SOD]{} H_2O_2 + O_2$$

This reaction can proceed spontaneously but the enzyme increases this rate by more than 10 000 fold. $O_2^{\bullet -}$ is therefore no longer available as substrate for the Haber–Weiss reaction. There are three classes of SOD; containing manganese, iron, or both copper and zinc. Manganese SOD is located in the mitochondria and copper-zinc SOD in the cytosol. SOD activity in the plasma is low although a copper-zinc enzyme called extracellular SOD exists in human plasma (Marklund et al 1982). It has been proposed that extracellular SOD is normally attached to the surface of endothelial cells offering localized protection (Karlsson & Marklund 1987). This ability of extracullar SOD to bind to cell surfaces does suggest that it might act as an effective anti-oxidant in protecting from reperfusion injury. SOD is, however, primarily an intracellular defence. It is found within most cell types including the RBC. Low SOD activity in RBCs has been reported in patients with ischaemic vascular disease such as angina and atherosclerotic PAD (Belch et al 1989). Interestingly, aluminium decreases SOD activity and one of the mechanisms of aluminium-induced pre-senile dementia may be through increased FR activity (Shainkin-Kestenbaum et al 1989) and may also go some way in explaining the early onset of vascular disease seen in patients with uraemia.

The subsequently formed H_2O_2 is removed intracellularly by catalases and peroxidases to form H_2O. In the heart, glutathione peroxidase is the important enzyme as very little catalase is present. H_2O_2 is reduced by glutathione peroxidase in the presence of glutathione (Fig. 47.9). The oxidized glutathione produced by this reaction is then reduced by glutathione reductase in the presence of NADPH, the co-factor for the reaction. If there is insufficient NADPH, oxidized glutathione will accumulate and, if it leaks out of the cell, a reduction in the intracellular glutathione pool occurs and the cell FR defence mechanism is impaired. Glutathione peroxidase is a selenium-containing enzyme. A deficiency of this element could result in a decrease in the capacity of the tissue to deal with oxidative stress. Glutathione is also present in fairly high concentrations in cells such as the myocyte. Its rapid depletion under oxidative stress and slow regeneration may be another way by which excessive oxygen radical production can overwhelm anti-oxidant defence in the tissues such as the heart (Lesnefsky et al 1989). Thiols such as glutathione have also been shown to be decreased in vascular disease (Belch et al 1989).

The transition metals, copper and iron, are both important as they can catalyse free radical formation. It is therefore unsurprising that the body keeps the majority of its iron and copper tightly bound to haemoglobin, myoglobin and proteins such as ferritin, transferrin, lactaferrin, caeruloplasmin and albumin (Aust & White 1985). Indeed the presence of free radicals or iron near to endothelial cells potentiates damage mediated by PMNs in vitro probably by the formation of $OH^{\bullet}$ (Balla et al 1991). In a case controlled study of 84 patients with MI, ferritin levels were significantly higher in the patient group immediately post-MI and 6 weeks later (van der Schouw et al 1990). There may also be an association between the size of infarct and the rise in serum ferritin (Griffiths et al 1985) though this has not been confirmed by all authors. Iron chelators such as desferrioxamine appear to reduce infarct size in experimental animals though again this has not been validated in humans (Halliwell 1989). In contrast, zinc has a clear anti-oxidant role probably through the protection of sulphydryl groups against oxidation and by preventing $OH^{\bullet}$ and $O_2^{\bullet -}$ production by transition metals (Bray & Bettger 1990).

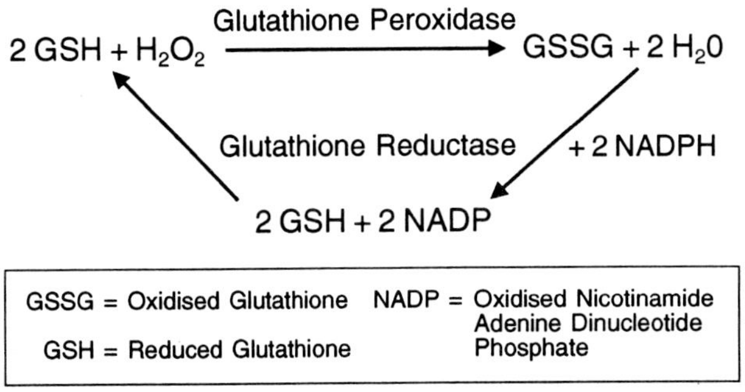

Fig. 47.9 The glutathione cycle.

Secondary defence mechanisms

Cell membranes and LDL circulating in plasma contain α-tocopherol which functions as a chain-breaking anti-oxidant. FRs initiate chain reactions by reacting with non-radical species. However, if two FRs interact this leads to the production of a non-radical and termination of the chain reaction (chain-breaking). α-Tocopherol is a lipid soluble molecule with an OH group whose hydrogen atom is very easy to remove. Thus when the hydroxyl and lipid peroxy radicals are generated they combine preferentially with the anti-oxidant instead of with an adjacent FA. This terminates the chain reaction hence the name chain-breaking anti-oxidant. α-Tocopherol is of course transferred into a new radical tocopherol-$O^{\bullet}$ but this is poorly reactive being unable to attack adjacent sidechains. The tocopherol radical can migrate to the membrane surface and be converted back to α-tocopherol by reacting with vitamin C. It should be noted that the terms α-tocopherol and vitamin E are often used synonymously. This is not quite correct. Vitamin E is defined nutritionally as a factor needed in the diet of pregnant female rats to prevent re-absorption of the fetus and compounds other than α-tocopherol (e.g. β, γ and δ-tocopherol) have similar affects in this assay. However, α-tocopherol is the most important lipid soluble chain-breaking anti-oxidant in vivo in humans (Halliwell 1990). Vitamin C, in contrast, is hydrophilic and actually exists in a relatively non-reactive FR form. It can react with $O_2^{\bullet -}$ and $OH^{\bullet}$ radicals preventing further propagation of chain reactions.

EVIDENCE FOR ROS INVOLVEMENT IN VASCULAR DISEASE

Recent work in a number of areas supports the hypothesis that ROS are involved in the mediation of vascular damage and thrombosis. Due to their very reactive nature, direct measurement of FRs is difficult though animal work using electron spin resonance spectroscopy (ESR) is of interest. ESR spectroscopy relies on a 'trapping' technique in which FRs react with reagents to produce longer-lived products which can then be detected by their ESR. Increased FR generation has been reported in animal tissues such as heart and brain when subjected to reperfusion (Schmidley 1990). Obviously such tests cannot be applied to living tissue although the technique of magnetic resonance imaging shows some promise in this area. In the meantime indirect assessments are utilized to assess the involvement of ROS in vascular disease. These take a number of forms:

1. Animal work involving the use of endogenous and exogenous FR scavengers and anti-oxidants
2. Measurement of scavenging and anti-oxidant behaviour in ischaemic states
3. Measurement of oxidative products such as MDA and diene-conjugates in thrombotic vascular disease.

Scavengers and anti-oxidants in animal models of ischaemia

The most convincing evidence in support of the concept of FR involvement in ischaemia-reperfusion injury comes from observations showing that FR scavengers have a protective action in animal models in which myocardial infarct size, contractility and reperfusion arrhythmias have been measured. In isolated perfused rabbit hearts subjected to 2 hours of global ischaemia the presence of SOD and catalase in the perfusion fluid greatly enhanced left ventricular function recovery after reperfusion (Shlafer et al 1982a). In a second study Shlafer et al (1982b) investigated isolated cat hearts which were subjected to the same ischaemic insult. One group acted as a control whereas the second group received a cardioplegic solution supplemented with SOD and catalase. Again, recovery was best seen in the scavenger-treated group. Since then a number of other workers have confirmed these findings in other species (Gardner et al 1983, Werns et al 1985). Scavengers other than SOD and catalase have been investigated. Zinc decreases reperfusion arrhythmias in an isolated perfused rat heart model (Powell et al 1990). Allopurinol, a xanthine oxidase inhibitor, and mannitol have also been studied in isolated heart models and found to preserve myocardial function (McCord 1985). The same protection was afforded by these various scavengers in intact animals during the investigation of models of myocardial ischaemia and stroke (Engler & Gilpin 1989). The main criticism of these studies, however, is that all involve pre-treatment with pharmacological doses of the scavenger. Although these experiments may point the finger at FRs as mediators of reperfusion damage, they do not reflect the true in vivo situation.

Scavengers and anti-oxidants in human thrombotic vascular disease

It has been suggested that both over-production of FRs or under-protection by scavengers and anti-oxidants can lead to FR-mediated damage. The elevation of lipid peroxide levels in the above vascular diseases suggests that one or other of these systems is operating. Patients with vascular disease, both PAD and CAD, have low levels of SOD activity and plasma thiols in RBCs. Similar findings were reported in congestive heart failure (McMurray et al 1990) and following myocardial infarction (Belch et al 1988).

The anti-oxidant vitamins are probably also important. Riemersma et al (1991) investigated the vitamin status of 555 subjects. The 125 cases of angina detected had lower levels of vitamin C and vitamin E compared to controls although the relationship of angina with low levels of vitamin C was lessened after accounting for smoking habit.

Oxidative products in ischaemic/thrombotic disease

The majority of work in living tissue has been carried out by measuring the by-products of lipid peroxidation such as MDA or conjugated dienes. The MDA assay has several shortcomings, not least being its lack of specificity for FR-mediated injury. However, newer assay techniques, using HPLC, are now becoming available and some interesting work has already been published.

A number of risk factors for arterial disease/thrombotic events have been recognised. One of these is time of day with most thrombotic events occurring in the early morning. As with WBC aggregation there is also a circadian rhythm in the level of lipid peroxides (Bridges et al

1992a). In normal subjects, a decrease in lipid peroxidation is seen in the early mornings. In contrast, in patients with ischaemic heart disease this morning dip is lost suggesting a mechanism for the additional risk of infarct at that time of day (Bridges et al 1992b). Smoking also increases lipid peroxide levels (Bridges et al 1993b) as does hyperlipidaemia (Stringer et al 1989).

Diabetes is a disease in which there is premature macro- and microvascular disease. Diene conjugates and MDA levels are increased in diabetes (Jennings et al 1987) and this elevation is most marked in those patients already having evidence of microangiopathy. Increased FR activity as measured by lipid peroxide levels has also been documented in atherosclerotic vascular disease. Stringer et al (1989) evaluated 100 patients with angiographically proven occlusive arterial disease, 50 had CAD, 50 had PAD. They compared the patients MDA levels with those of 75 controls. Significant increases in lipid peroxide levels were found in both disease groups, although, to date, the elevated lipid peroxide levels have not been shown to correlate with angiographic measurement of the extent of the vascular disease (Bridges et al 1992c). In contrast, in congestive heart failure secondary to ischaemic heart disease, not only are the lipid peroxides increased (McMurray et al 1990) but this elevation correlates with the severity of the disease as measured by left ventricular ejection fraction. (Belch et al 1991b).

The above studies were carried out in stable disease situations, however, if a further insult is added then a worsening situation develops. For example, during cardiac pacing to angina a further elevation in lipid peroxide levels occurs in patients with ischaemic heart disease (Oldroyd et al 1990). The advent of myocardial infarction onto established CAD further elevates lipid peroxidation as measured by high breath pentane concentrations (Weitz et al 1991). Pentane is generated by lipid peroxydation mediated by ROS and can be measured on breath samples by gas chromatography. Diabetics undergoing laser photocoagulation for retinopathy also further increase their oxidized lipid levels (Jennings et al 1991), as do patients with vasospastic disease following cold exposure (Lau et al 1992). Reperfusion following ischaemia is probably an important source of FR mediated damage in vascular disease and a number of such reperfusion states have been studied. Levels of lipid peroxides are elevated following both peripheral and coronary artery balloon angioplasty (Lau et al 1991, Roberts et al 1990). Patients receiving successful thrombolytic therapy for acute MI show increased lipid peroxide levels (Davies et al 1990). However, although thrombolysis can successfully restore coronary patency, a degree of left ventricular dysfunction often remains. This may be mediated partly through free radical damage and interventions aimed at scavenging free radicals at this time point may be useful.

THERAPEUTIC CONSIDERATIONS

White cells are able to inhibit flow in the microcirculation through both rheological and secretory changes in the cell. Thus, therapies which inhibit WBC activation or neutralize the WBC release products in the early stages of ischaemia/thrombosis may be beneficial. Artificially induced neutropenia prior to the ischaemic insult prevents widespread tissue damage in animals but this has limited therapeutic implications in man. There are, however, a number of compounds whose use appears feasible in humans, thus it may be possible to give pharmacological doses of physiological scavengers and anti-oxidants, or chelate transitional ions. Furthermore, compounds already in use might exert some of their beneficial antithrombotic effects through a mechanism involving attenuation of FR-induced damage. In addition, certain drugs used in other clinical situations apart from thrombosis/ischaemia may also have FR modulating activity and find an alternative usage in this area.

Physiological scavengers as therapeutic agents

Nearly all published work in this area relates to in vitro or animal studies though the development of compounds suitable for human use is currently being undertaken. SOD continues to be available in health food stores in an oral tablet form despite the irrationality of such a preparation as indicated by animal studies (Giri & Misra 1984). The medical use of SOD will depend on local installation, controlled parenteral delivery and/or the development of conjugates with enhanced survival features. Polyethylene glycol-conjugation will lengthen SOD's half life as will making the protein cationic. This is also true for catalase (Greenwald 1990). Genetic engineering has modified the SOD molecule, again prolonging its half life and work is in progress evaluating SOD-pyran polymers. In humans, no good trial has studied SOD and/or catalase in thrombotic vascular disease although many animal studies suggest protection by both these compounds from ischaemia-reperfusion injury. Adjunct treatment to both thrombolysis and angioplasty is an attractive area for study of these compounds as the safety data are favourable. SOD has been administered safely to human neonates with no evidence of local allergic hypersensitivity or toxicity (Rosenfield et al 1982). One aspect yet to be determined is that of the dosage schedule. The dose response curve for SOD in patients may be bell shaped with a loss of effect at high doses (Omar & McCord 1990).

As neither $O_2^{\bullet -}$ nor H_2O_2 cause oxidative change in the absence of iron, it has been proposed that tissue damage following reperfusion can be ameliorated by iron chelation (Aust & White 1985). Again, however, a bell shaped curve for the dose response may limit the use of agents such as desferrioxamine (Halliwell 1989). Zinc has been shown to have anti-oxidant effects. Animal work using pharmacological doses of zinc have, however, been contradictory (Bray & Bettger 1990) though most workers agree that zinc has a protective effect against liver-specific pro-oxidants. Such a use of pharmacological doses of zinc may ultimately prove to be a valuable tool in elucidating the mechanisms of anti-oxidant behaviour.

Adenosine is an endogenous arteriolar vasodilator present in relatively high concentrations at the time of reperfusion (Berne 1980). It is a metabolic by-product of ATP with numerous properties that may attenuate the reperfusion injury including inhibition of $O_2^{\bullet -}$ and proteolytic enzyme release by neutrophils (Cronstein et al 1985). Intravenous administration of this agent during early reperfusion is associated with a permanent enhancement of myocardial salvage (Pitarys et al 1991). Again, however, the work has been carried out only in animals.

Physiological anti-oxidants as therapeutic agents

The concept that vitamin E may be a useful therapeutic agent is suggested by four main lines of evidence. Chronic vitamin E deficiency in animals produces atherosclerotic-like lesions which in turn can be reduced by vitamin E supplementation (Nafstad 1974), dietary vitamin E can ameliorate atherosclerosis induced prematurely by hyperlipidaemia in animal models of vascular disease (Szczeklik et al 1985), vitamin E reduces hyperlipidaemia in animals (Muckle & Nazir 1989) and plasma vitamin E is inversely correlated with mortality from CAD (Gey & Puska 1989). It is also of interest that vitamin E supplementation inhibits the oxidized LDL modification induced by that major risk factor for vascular disease, cigarette smoking (Scheffler et al 1990). Vitamin E may thus be a necessary anti-oxidant for the prevention of disease but little evidence exists to suggest a use for vitamin E after the development of ischaemia. The patient must have a high blood level before the ischaemia occurs which is difficult to obtain if the ischaemia is unexpected. Furthermore, the concentration at the site of the damage must be high, which requires taking large, sometimes intolerable, amounts of the vitamin (Zylke 1988).

Other anti-oxidants such as vitamin C have been less well studied but may also have protective rather than therapeutic potential (Paterson & O'Rourke 1987). Carotenoids serve as our major dietary source of retinol. They have pro-vitamin A activity and can function directly as anti-oxidants (Krinsky 1989), however their therapeutic use has yet to be assessed despite the fact that they are used routinely as anti-oxidants in food. Flavinoids are a group of naturally occurring benzo-gamma-pyrone derivatives of low molecular weight. They are widespread in the plant kingdom and have been used in China for centuries as a treatment for vascular diseases. The group includes such compounds as quercetin and rutin. These are known $OH^{\bullet}$ scavengers and metal ion chelators (Yuting et al 1990). As with vitamins E and C they may have physiological/nutritional roles but evidence to support their use therapeutically is, at present, lacking.

'Conventional' drugs with free radical modulating effects

Some drugs used conventionally as anti-thrombotics can have additional anti-white cell 'effects'. This may be a further mechanism whereby they exert their benefit. Heparin inhibits both white cell aggregation and degranulation and warfarin has FR scavenging properties (Laghi-Pasim et al 1984). Aspirin and other cyclo-oxygenase inhibitors decrease the production of FRs by the neutrophil and may inhibit WBC aggregation (Abramson & Edelson 1984). PGI_2 and its analogues are also used in the treatment of vascular disease and their anti-white cell effects are well-documented (Belch et al 1983). Modification of other areas of AA metabolism can also affect FR production. Agents which inhibit 5-lipoxygenase limit myocardial neutrophil accumulation and infarct size, though this work has been limited to animal models (Mullane & Moncada 1983).

Other pharmaceutical agents used in the field of cardiovascular medicine may, by the nature of their structure, be expected to scavenge FRs. Captopril is used to treat heart failure, a disease in which FR pathology occurs. Captopril has a thiol group within its molecule and is a potent scavenger of FRs (Chopra et al 1989). This may explain some of its beneficial effects at other sites such as the kidney where it attenuates albuminuria in early diabetic microvascular disease (Parving et al 1988). Probucol is a lipid-lowering agent which also has anti-oxidant properties independent of its cholesterol lowering properties (Bridges et al 1991). Gliclazide, a hypoglycaemic agent, has been shown to improve platelet behaviour in maturity-onset diabetes mellitus. The mechanism for such an improvement in platelet behaviour may be through FR scavenging properties (Scott et al 1991). Allopurinol, used in acute gout, has already been discussed as being a xanthine oxidase inhibitor which attenuates reperfusion injury in animals. Ciuffeti et al (1989) have investigated this compound in patients with PAD showing attenuation of the FR-induced RBC rigidity seen after provocation of ischaemia.

Thus there is the potential for exciting new therapies for both the prevention of vascular disease and the preservation of tissue during ischaemia-reperfusion. However, unequivocal evidence supporting FR generation in ischaemia has only recently emerged and proof that their removal will be advantageous in vascular disease is still lacking in human studies.

CONCLUSION

In addition to the traditional role in combating infection and scavenging dead tissue, neutrophils may have a key role in mediating vascular damage. Studies of activation and degranulation of WBCs in ischaemia illustrate this novel role of the WBC as does study of the formation and extent of FR injury induced in animals. Evidence is now accumulating to support the extension of this hypothesis to human disease, although convincing data relating to therapy are still awaited.

It should also be remembered that neutrophils play an important role in the removal and repair of infarcted/ ischaemic tissue. Clearly the inflammatory response is necessary for the ultimate replacement of necrotic tissue with a fibrous scar of the required tensile strength. These considerations reveal a drawback in attempts to protect ischaemic tissue by attenuating the inflammatory response. High doses of methyl prednisolone, which inhibit the inflammatory response to myocardial injury, slow the removal of necrotic myocytes and healing in an experimental model of MI (Kloner et al 1978), although this deleterious effect might be more directly related to the inhibitory effects of glucocorticoids on protein synthesis and wound healing, events that are independent of neutrophil function. Caution should be exercised in the use of aggressive scavenging regimes. The gene for copper-zinc SOD is located on human chromosome number 21 and, therefore, in individuals with trisomy 21 there is 50% more intracellular SOD. This may contribute to the frequency of infection seen in these subjects (del Maestro 1980). Patients suffering from psychiatric diseases such as schizophrenia and paranoid psychosis also have increased SOD levels. Thus superoxide radical participates in essential intracellular chemical reactions and its complete scavenging may be detrimental. Therapies that modulate WBC funtion must not impair behaviour essential to health.

REFERENCES

Abramson S, Edelson H 1984 Inhibition of neutrophil activation by non-steroidal anti-inflammatory drugs. American Journal of Medicine 77: 3–6

Ameisen J C, Capron A, Joseph M et al 1985 Aspirin-sensitive asthma: Abnormal platelet response to drugs inducing asthmatic attacks. International Archives of Allergy and Applied Immunology 78: 438–448

Aust S D, White B C 1985 Iron chelation prevents tissue injury following ischaemia. Advances in Free Radical Biology and Medicine 1: 1–17

Azizova O A, Panasenko O M, Vol'Nova T V, Vladimirov Y A 1989 Free radical lipid oxidation affects cholesterol transfer between lipoproteins and erythrocytes. Free Radical Biology and Medicine 7: 251–257

Balla G, Vercellotti G M, Muller-Eberhard U, Eaton J, Jacob H S 1991 Exposure of endothelial cells to free heme potentiates damage mediated by granulocytes and toxic oxyen species. Laboratory Investigation 65(5): 648–655

Barrowcliffe T W, Gray E, Kerry P J, Gutteridge J M C 1985 Lipid peroxides, lipoproteins and thrombosis. Life Chemical Reproduction 3: 174–188

Bar-Shavit R, Kahn A, Wilner G D, Fenton J W 1983 Monocyte chemotaxis: stimulation by specific exosite region in thrombin. Science 220: 728–731

Belch J J F 1988 The role of eicosanoids in inflammation. In: Goodacre J, Dick W C (eds) Immunopathogenic mechanisms of arthritis. MTP Press, Lancaster, p 26–50

Belch J J F 1990 The role of the white blood cell in arterial disease. Blood Coagulation and Fibrinolysis 1: 183–192

Belch J J F 1992 Platelets and oxyen free radicals. Platelets 3: 1–6

Belch J J F, McKay A, McArdle B et al 1983 A double blind study of the effect of prostacyclin infusion in severe peripheral vascular disease. Lancet 8320: 315–317

Belch J J F, Saniabadi A, Forbes C D 1986 The effect of ZK36374 (Iloprost) on white cell behaviour. In: Schror K, Gryglewski R J (eds) Prostacyclin and its stable analogue illoprost. Springer, Berlin, p 97–102

Belch J J F, Chopra M, Tweddel A, Hutton I, Cobbe S, Smith W E 1988 Changes in redox status of blood in patients with acute myocardial infarction. In: Rice-Evans C, Dormandy T (eds) Free radicals: chemistry, pathology and medicine. Richelieu, London, p 321–332

Belch J J F , Chopra M, Hutchinson S, Lorimer R, Sturrock R D, Forbes C D, Smith E 1989 Free radical pathology in chronic arterial disease. Free Radical Biology and Medicine 27: 369–378

Belch J J F, Bridges A B, Scott N, Chopra M 1991a Oxygen free radicals and congestive heart failure. British Heart Journal 65: 245–8

Belch J J F, Lau C S, Shaw W, McLaren M 1991b Oxygen free radical generation following angioplasty for peripheral arterial disease. In: Palombo D, Brustia P (eds) La chirurgia vascolare nella Communita Economica Europea. Domenio Palombo, Valle D'Aosta, p 127–128

Bell D, Jackson M, Nicoll J J, Millar A, Dawes J, Muir A L 1990 Inflammatory response, neutrophil activation, and free radical production after acute myocardial infarction: effect of thrombolytic treatment. British Heart Journal 63: 82–87

Berne R M 1980 The role of adenosine in the regulation of coronary blood flow. Circulation Research 47: 807–813

Bevilacqua M P, Pober J S, Majeau G R, Cotran R S, Gimrone M A 1984 Interleukin 1 induces biosynthesis and cell surface expression of procoagulant activity in human vascular endothelial cells. Journal of Experimental Medicine 160: 618–621

Boxer L A, Allen J M, Schmidt M, Yoder M, Baehner R L 1980 Inhibition of polymorphonuclear leukocyte adherence by prostacyclin. Journal of Laboratory and Clinical Medicine 95: 672–678

Braide M, Blixt A, Bagge U 1992 Leukocyte effects on the vascular resistance and glomerular filtration of the isolated rat kidney at normal and low flow states. Circulatory Shock (in press)

Bray T M, Bettger W J 1990 The physiological role of zinc as an antioxidant. Free Radical Biology and Medicine 8: 281–291

Bridges A B, Scott N A, Belch J J F 1991 Probucol, a superoxide free radical scavenger in vitro. Atherosclerosis 89: 263–265

Bridges A B, Fisher T C, Scott N A, McLaren M, Belch J J F 1992a Circadian rhythm of white blood cell aggregation and free radical status in healthy volunteers. Free Radical Research Communication 16: 89–97

Bridges A B, McLaren M, Scott N A, Pringle T H, McNeill G P, Belch J J F 1992b Circadian variation in white cell aggregation and free radical markers in men with stable ischaemic heart disease. European Heart Journal 19: 1632–1636

Bridges A B, Scott N A, Pringle T H, McNeill G P, Belch J J F 1992c Relationship between the extent of coronary artery disease and indicators of free radical activity. Clinical Cardiology 15: 169–174

Bridges A B, Hill A, Mackay I, Belch J J F 1993a The effect of cigarette smoking on white blood cell aggregation. Journal of the Royal Society of Medicine 86: 139–140

Bridges A B, Scott N A, Parry G J, Belch J J F 1993b The effect of age, sex and smoking on indices of free radical activity in healthy humans. European Journal of Medicine 2: 205–208
Bykowska K, Kaczanowska J, Karpowicz M, Lopaciuk S, Kopec M 1985 Alterations of blood platelet function induced by neutral proteases from human leukocytes. Thrombosis Research 38: 535–546
Chopra M, Scott N, Smith W E, Belch J J F 1989 Captopril: a free radical scavenger. British Journal of Pharmacology 27: 396–399
Ciuffetti G, Mercuri M, Lombardini R, Maragoni G, Santambrogio L, Mannarino E 1989 Leucocyte behaviour in controlled ischaemia of the calves. Journal of Clinical Pathology 42: 1083–1087
Cronstein B N, Kramer S B, Weissmann G, Hirschhorn R 1983 Adenosine: A physiological modulator of superoxide anion generation by human neutrophils. Journal of Experimental Medicine 158: 1160–1177
Cronstein B N, Levine R I, Belanoff J, Weissmann G, Hirschhorn R 1985 A new function of adenosine: Protection of vascular endothelial cells against neutrophil-mediated injury. Clinical Research 33: 517
Cross A R 1990 Inhibitors of the leukocyte superoxide generating oxidase: Mechanisms of action and methods for their elucidation. Free Radical Biology and Medicine 8: 71–93
Dallegri F, Ballestreo A, Ottonellol Patrone F 1989 Platelets, as scavengers of neutrophil-derived oxidants: A possible defense mechanism at sites of vascular injury. Thrombosis and Haemostasis 61: 415–418
Davies S W, Ranjadayalan K, Wickens D G, Dormand T L, Timmis A D 1990 Lipid peroxidation associated wwith successful thrombolysis. Lancet 335: 741–743
Dean R T, Prydz H 1983 Inflammatory particles stimulate thromboplastin production by human monocytes. Thrombosis Research 30: 357–367
del Maestro R F 1980 An approach to free radicals in medicine and biology. Acta Physiologica Scandinavica 492 (suppl): 153–168
Dikskit M, Srivastava R, Scrimal R C 1989 Role of free radicals in pulmonary thromboembolism in mice 55: 549–557
Dormandy J, Nash G, Thomas P, Loosemore T 1988 White blood cells and ischaemia. Acta Chirurgica Scandinavica 546S: 33a
Engler R, Gilpin E 1989 Can superoxide dismutase alter myocardial infarct size? Circulation 79: 1137–1142
Engler R L, Dahlgren M D, Morris D D, Peterson M A, Schmid-Schonbein G W 1986 Role of leukocytes in response to acute myocardial ischaemia and reflow in dogs. American Journal of Physiology 251(20): 314–322
Esterbauer H, Zollner H, Schaur R J. Hydroxyalkenals: cytotoxic products of lipid peroxidation. ISI Atlas Science and Biochemistry 1: 311–315
Fisher T C, Belch J J F, Barbenel J C, Fisher A C 1989 In vitro human whole blood granulocyte aggregation. Clinical Science 76: 183–187
Fridovich I 1989 Superoxide dismutases. An adaptation to a paramagnetic gas. Journal of Biological Chemistry 264: 7761–7764
Friedman G D, Klatsky A L, Siegelaub A B 1974 The leukocyte count as a predictor of myocardial infarction. New England Journal of Medicine 290: 1275–1278
Gardner T J, Stewart J F, Casale A S, Downey J M, Chambers D E 1983 Reduction of myocardial ischemic injury with oxyen-derived free radical scavengers. Surgery 94(3): 423–427
Garlick P B, Davies M J, Hearse D J, Slater T F 1987 Direct detection of free radicals in the reperfused rat heart using electron spin resonance spectroscopy. Circulatory Research 61: 757–760
Gey K F, Puska P 1989 Plasma vitamins E and A inversely correlated to mortality from ischemic heart disease in cross-cultural epidemiology. Annals of the New York Academy of Sciences 570: 268–282
Gill D S, Barradas M A, Fonseca V A, Gracey L, Dandona P 1988 Increased histamine content in leukocytes and platelets of patients with peripheral vascular disease. American Journal of Clinical Practice 89(5): 622–626
Giri S N, Misra H P 1984 Fate of superoxide dismutase in mice following oral route administration. Molecular Biology 62: 258–289
Gray E, Barrowcliffe T 1983 Decreased antithrombin III activity by lipid peroxides. Thrombosis and Haemostasis 50: 162
Greenwald R A 1990 Superoxide dismutase and catalase as therapeutic agents for human disease. A critical review. Free Radical Biology and Medicine 8: 201–209
Griffiths J D, Campbell L J, Woodruff I W et al 1985 Acute changes in iron metabolism following myocardial infarction. American Journal of Clinical Pathology 84: 649–654
Grimm R H, Cohen J D, Smith W M, Falvo-Gerard L, Neaton J D 1985 Hypertension management in the Multiple Risk Factor Intervention Trial (MRFIT). Six-year intervention results for men in special intervention and normal care groups. Archives of Internal Medicine 145: 1191–1199
Gryglewski R J, Dembinska-Kiec A, Zmuda A, Gryglewski T 1978 Prostacyclin and thromboxane A_2 biosynthesis capacities of heart, arteries and platelets at various stages of experimental atherosclerosis in rabbits. Atherosclerosis 31: 385–394
Gryglewski R J, Palmer R M J, Moncada S 1987 Superoxide anion is involved in the breakdown of endothelium-derived vascular relaxing factor. Nature 320: 454–456
Haines A P, Howard D, North W R et al 1983 Haemostatic variables and the outcome of myocardial infarction. Thrombosis and Haemostasis 50: 800–803
Halliwell B 1989 Protection against tissue damage in vivo by desferrioxamine: What is its mechanism of action? Free Radical Biology and Medicine 7: 645–651
Halliwell B 1990 How to characterize a biological antioxidant. Free Radical Research and Communication 9: 1–32
Halliwell B, Gutteridge J M C 1984 Oxygen toxicity, oxygen radicals, transition metals and disease. Journal of Biochemistry 219: 1–14
Hammerschmidt D E, Greenberg C S, Yamada O, Craddock P R, Jacob H S 1981 Cholesterol and atheroma lipids activate, complement and stimulate granulocytes. A possible mechanism for amplification of ischaemic injury in atherosclerotic states. Journal of Laboratory and Clinical Medicine 98: 68–77
Jen C J, McIntire L V 1984 Characteristics of shear-induced aggregation in whole blood. Journal of Laboratory and Clinical Medicine 103: 115–124
Jennings P E, Jones A F, Florkowski C M, Lunec J, Barnett A H 1987 Increased diene conjugate in diabetic subjects with microangiopathy. Diabetic Medicine 4: 452–456
Jennings P E, MacEwen C J, Fallow T J, Scott N, Haining W M, Belch J J F 1991 Oxidative effects of laser photocoagulation. Free Radical Biology and Medicine 11: 327–330
Karlsson K, Marklund S L 1987 Heparin-induced release of extracellular superoxide dismutase to human blood plasma. Journal of Biochemistry 242: 55–59
Karpen C W, Merola A J, Trewyn R W,Cornwell D G, Panganamala R V 1981 Modulation of platelets thromboxane A_2 and arterial prostacyclin by dietary vitamin E. Prostaglandins 22: 651–661
Kloner R, Fishbein M, Len H, Maroko P, Braunwald E 1978 Mummification of the infarcted myocardium by high dose corticosteroids. Circulation 57: 56–61
Kosaka H, Hozumi M, Tyumi I 1989 The interaction between nitrogen oxides and hemoglobin and endothelium-derived relaxing factor. Free Radical Biology and Medicine 7: 653–658
Kostis J B, Turkevich D, Sharp J 1984 Association between leukocyte count and the presence and extent of coronary atherosclerosis as determined by coronary ateriography. American Journal of Cardiology 53: 997–999
Krinsky N I 1989 Antioxidant functions of carotenoids. Free Radical Biology and Medicine 7: 617–635
Kuzuya T, Hoshida S, Suzuki K et al 1988 Polymorphonuclear leukocyte activity and ventricular arrhythmia in acute myocardial infarction. The American Journal of Cardiology 62: 868–872
Lackie J M 1982 Aspects of the behaviour of neutrophil leucocytes. In: Curtis A, Dunn G (eds) Cell behaviour. Cambridge University Press, Cambridge p 319–348
Laghi-Pasim F, Pasqui A L, Ceccatelli L, Capecchi P L, Orrico A, DiPerri T 1984 Heparin inhibition of polymorphonuclear leukocyte activation in vitro. A possible pharmacological approach to granulocyte-mediated vascular damage. Thrombosis Reseach 35: 527–537
Lau C S, Scott N, Brown J E, Shaw W, Belch J J G 1991 Increased activity of oxygen free radicals during eperfusion in patients

undergoing percutaneous peripheral artery balloon angioplasty. International Angioplasty 10(4): 744–746
Lau C S, O'Dowd A, Belch J J F 1992 White blood cell activation in Raynaud's phenomenon of systemic sclerosis and vibration induced white finger syndrome. Annals of Rheumatic Diseases 51: 249–252
Lesnefsky E, Repine J E, Horwitz L D 1989 Oxidation and release of glutathione from myocardium during early reperfusion. Free Radical Biology and Medicine 7: 31–35
Lowe G D, Machado S G, Krol W F, Barton B A, Forbes C D 1985 White blood cell count and haematocrit as predictors of coronary recurrence after myocardium infarction. Thrombosis and Haemostasis 54: 700–703
Lyberg T, Prydz H 1982 Thromboplastin (factor III) activity in human monocytes induced by immune complexes. European Journal of Clinical Investigation 12: 229–234
McCord J M 1985 Oxygen-derived free radicals in postischemic tissue injury. The New England Journal of Medicine 312(3): 159–163
McMurray J, McLay J, Chopra M, Bridges A, Belch J J F 1990 Evidence for enhanced free radical activity in chronic congestive heart failure secondary to coronary artery disease. The American Journal of Cardiology 65: 1261–1262
Maisel A S, Gilpin E A, Le Winter M, Heming H, Ross J, Engler R 1985 Initial leukocyte count during acute myocardial infarction independently predicts early ventricular fibrillations.Circulation 72: 411–414
Malech H L, Gallin J I 1987 Neutrophils in human diseases. New England Journal of Medicine 317: 687–694
Marklund S L, Holme E, Hellner L 1982 Superoxide dismutase in extracellular fluids. Clinica Chimica Acta 126: 41–51
May G R, Cook P, Moore P K, Page C P 1990 In-vitro inhibition of platelet adhesion by EDRF. British Journal of Pharmacology 6: 273–274
Mehta J L, Nichols W W, Mehta P 1988 Neutrophils as potential participants in acute myocardial ischaemia: relevance to reperfusion. Journal of the American College of Cardiology 11: 1309–1316
Mehta J, Dinerman J, Mehta P et al 1989 Neutrophil function in ischaemic heart disease. Circulation 79: 549–556
Mercuri M, Ciuffetti G, Robinson M, Toole J 1989 Blood cell rheology in acute cerebral infarction. Stroke 20(7): 959–962
Mitchinson M J, Ball R Y 1987 Macrophages and atherogenesis. Lancet (July): 1146–1148
Moncada S, Gryglewski R J, Bunting S, Vane J R 1976 A lipid peroxide inhibits the enzyme in blood vessel microsomes that generate from prostaglandin enderoperoxides the substance (prostaglandin X) which prevents platelet aggregation. Prostaglandins 12: 715–737
Muckle T J, Nazir D J 1989 Variation in human blood high density lipoprotein response to oral vitamin E megadosage. American Journal of Clinical Pathology 91: 165–171
Mullane K M, Moncada S 1983 The salvage of ischaemic myocardium by BW755C in anaesthetized dogs. Prostaglandins 24: 255–266
Muxfelat M, Schaper W 1987 The activity of xanthine oxidase in hearts of pigs, guinea pigs, rabbits, rats and humans. Basic Research in Cardiology 82: 486–492
Nafstad I 1974 Endothelial damage and platelet thrombosis associated with PUFA-rich vitamin E-deficient diet fed to pigs. Thrombosis Research 5: 251–258
Nash G B, Christopher B, Morris A J R, Dormandy J A 1989 Changes in the flow properties of white blood cells after acute myocardial infarction. British Heart Journal 62: 329–34
Nawroth P P, Stern D M 1986 Modulation of endothelial cell haemostatic properties by tumour necrosis factor. Journal of Experimental Medicine 163: 740–745
Oldroyd K G, Chopra M, Rankin A C, Belch J J F, Cobbe S M 1990 Lipid peroxidation during pacing-induced myocardial ischaemia. British Heart Journal 63: 88–92
Omar B A, McCord J M 1990 The cardioprotective effect of Mn-superoxide dismutase is lost at high doses in the post-ischaemic isolated rabbit heart. Free Radical Biology and Medicine 9: 473–478
Palmer R M J, Ferrige A G, Moncada S 1987 Nitric oxide release accounts for the biological activity of endothelium-derived relaxing factor. Nature 327: 524–526
Parving H H, Hommel E, Smidt U M 1988 Protection of kidney function and clearance in albuminuria by captopril in insulin-dependent diabetics with nephropathy. British Medical Journal 297: 1086–1089
Paterson C A, O'Rourke M C 1987 Vitamin C levels in human tears. Archives of Ophthalmology 105: 376–377
Pfafferott C, Meiselman H J, Hochstein P 1982 The effect of malonyldiadehyde on erythrocyte deformability. Blood 59: 12–15
Pitarys C J, Renu-Virmani, Vildibill H D Jr, Jackson E K, Forman M B 1991 Reduction of myocardial reperfusion injury by intravenous adenosine administered during the early reperfusion period. Circulation 83: 237–247
Powell S, Saltman P, Uretzky G, Chevion M 1990 The effect of zinc on reperfusion arrythmias in the isolated perfused rat heart. Free Radical Biology and Medicine 8: 33–46
Prentice R L, Shimizu Y, Lin C H, Peterson A V, Kato H, Mason M W, Szatrowski T P 1982 Leukocyte counts and coronary heart disease in a Japanese cohort. American Journal of Epidemiology 116: 496–506
Riemersma R A, Wood D A, MacIntyre C C A, Elton R A, Gey K F, Oliver M F 1991 Risk of angina pectoris and plasma concentrations of vitamins A, C and E and carotene. Lancet 337: 1–5
Roberts M J D, Young I S, Trouton T G 1990 Transient release of lipid peroxides after coronary artery balloon angioplasty. Lancet 336: 143–145
Romson J L, Hook B G, Kunkel S L, Abrams G D, Schork M A, Lucchesi B R 1983 Reduction of the extent of ischaemic myocardial injury by neutrophil depletion in the dog. Circulation 67: 1016–1023
Rosenfeld W, Evans H, Jhaveri R et al 1982 Safety and plasma concentrations of bovine superoxide dismutase administered to human premature infants. Developmental Pharmacology and Therapeutics 5: 151–161
Salvemini D, De Nucci G, Gryglewski R J, Vane J R 1989 EDRF inhibits polymorphonuclear cell adhesion. Proceedings of the National Academy of Sciences, USA 86: 6328–6332
Saniabadi A, Lowe G D O, Barbenel J C, Forbes C D 1984 Haematocrit, bleeding time and platelet aggregation. Lancet 1: 1409–1410
Scheffler E, Huber L, Fruhbis J, Schulz I, Ziegler R, Dresel H A 1990 Alteration of plasma low density lipoprotein from smokers. Atherosclerosis 82: 261–265
Schlant R C, Forman S, Stamler V, Canner P L 1982 The natural history of coronary heart disease: prognostic factors after recovery from myocardial infarction in 2789 men. Circulation 66: 401–408
Schmidley J W 1990 Free radicals in central nervous system ischaemia. Stroke 21(7): 1086–1090
Schmid-Schönbein G W, Engler R L 1986 Granulocytes as active participants in acute myocardial ischaemia and infarction. American Journal of Cardiovascular Pathology 1(1): 15–29
Schmutz-Schumman M, De Souza V, Menz G et al 1989 Reduced production of oxygen-free radicals of platelets in aspirin-induced-asthma. Intrinsic Asthma 28: 195–203
Scott N, Jennings P E, Brown J, Belch J J F Gliclazide: a general free radical scavenger. European Journal of Clinical Pharmacology 208: 175–177
Shainkin-Kestenbaum R, Adler A J, Berlyne G M, Caruso C 1989 Effect of aluminium on superoxide dismutase. Clinical Science 77: 463–466
Shapiro D, Belch J J F, Sturrock R D, Shenkin A 1986 Effects of drugs altering arichidonic acid metabolism on interleukin-1 release from monocyte-like cells. In: Marker proteins in inflammation. de Gryter, Berlin, Vol 3: 43–45
Shlafer M, Kane P F, Kirsch M M 1982a Superoxide dismutase plus catalase enhance the efficacy of hypothermia cardioplegia to protect the globally ischaemic, reperfused heart. Journal of Thoracic Cardiovascular Surgery 83: 830–839
Shlafer M, Kane P F, Wiggens V Y, Kirsch M M 1982b Possible role for cytotoxic oxygen metabolites in the pathogenesis of cardiac ischaemic injury. Circulation 66: 85–92
Shoenfeld Y, Pinkhas J 1981 Leukopenia and low incidence of myocardical infarction. New England Journal of Medicine 305: 1606
Singal P K, Beamish R E, Dhalla N S 1983 Potential oxidative pathways of catecholamines in the formation of lipid peroxides and genesis of heart disease. Advances in Experimental Medicine and Biology 161: 391–401

Stringer M D, Gorog P G, Freeman A, Kakkar V V 1989 Lipid peroxides and atherosclerosis. British Medical Journal 298: 281–284
Szczeklik A, Gryglewski R J, Domagala B, Dworski R, Basista M 1985 Dietary supplementation with vitamin E in hyperlipoproteinemias: effects on plasma peroxides, antioxidant activity, prostacyclin generation and platelet aggregability. Thrombosis and Haemostasis 54: 425–430
Tate R M, Morris H G, Schroeder W R, Repine J E 1984 Oxygen metabolites stimulate thromboxane production and vasoconstriction in isolated saline perfused rabbit lung. Journal of Clinical Investigations 74: 608–613
van der Schouw Y T, van der Veeken P M W C, Kok F J, Koster J F, Schouten E G, Hofman A 1990 Iron status in the acute phase and six weeks after myocardial infarction. Free Radical Biology and Medicine 8: 47–53
Vermes I, Strik F 1988 Altered leukocyte rheology in patients with chronic cerebrovascular disease. Stroke 19: 631–633
Wang J, Zhen E, Zhanzheng G, Yongeai L 1989 Effect of hyperlipidaemic serum on lipid peroxidation, synthesis of prostaglandin and thromboxane by cultured endothelial cells: protective effect of anti-oxidants. Free Radical Biology and Medicine 7: 243–249
Wargovich T, Mehta J L, Nichols W W, Pepine C J, Conti C R 1985 Reduction in blood flow in normal and narrowed coronary arteries of dogs by leukotriene C4. Journal of the American College of Cardiology 6: 1047–1051
Weitz Z W, Birnbaum A J, Sobotka P A, Zarling E J, Skosey J L 1991 High breath pentane concentrations during acute myocardial infarction. Lancet 337: 933–935
Werns S W, Shea M J, Driscoll E M et al 1985 The independent effects of oxygen radical scavengers on canine infarct size. Circulation Research 56(6): 895–897
Wolbarsht M L, Fridovich I 1989 Hyperoxia during reperfusion is a factor in reperfusion injury. Free Radical Biology and Medicine 6(1): 61–62
Wolff S P, Dean R T 1986 Fragmentation of proteins by free radicals and its effect on their susceptibility to enzymic hydrolysis. Biochemical Journal 234: 399–403
Worthen G S, Seccombe J F, Clay K L, Guthrie L A, Johnson R B 1988 The priming of neutrophils by lipopolysaccharides for production of intracellular platelet plus activating factor: potential role in mediation of enhanced superoxide secretion. Journal of Immunology 140: 3553–3559
Yuting C, Rongliang Z, Zhongjian J, Yong J 1990 Flavinoids as superoxide scavengers and anti-oxidants. Free Radical Biology and Medicine 9: 19–21
Zalokar J B, Richard J L, Claude J R 1981 Leukocyte count, smoking and myocardial infarction. New England Journal of Medicine 304: 465–468
Zylke J 1988 Studying oxygen's life-and-death roles if taken from or reintroduced into tissue. Journal of the American Medical Association 259: 960–961

48. Mechanisms of atherogenesis and thrombosis

Marian A. Packham Raelene L. Kinlough-Rathbone

Atherogenesis is the formation and development of atherosclerotic lesions on the surface of arteries. It begins early in life and is the major cause of death in the Western world. Risk factors for atherosclerosis and/or its clinical complications include plasma total cholesterol levels over 200 mg/Dl (>5.2 mmol/l), low density lipoprotein (LDL) over 130 mg/Dl, and high density lipoprotein (HDL) less than 35 mg/Dl; high plasma levels of lipoprotein(a) (Lp(a)); male sex; history of myocardial infarction or sudden death before the age of 55 in a parent or sibling; cigarette smoking; hypertension; diabetes mellitus; severe obesity; high plasma levels of fibrinogen or factor VII; homocysteinaemia (Meade 1987, Roberts 1989, Malinow 1990, Scanu 1990). However, the risk factors for the initiation of atherosclerotic lesions and their progression are not identical to the risk factors for the thromboembolic clinical complications, although this distinction is seldom made.

Over the years there have been two main theories about the initiation of atherosclerotic lesions, but many investigators now believe that atherogenesis is such a complex process that both theories probably have validity. The marked variation in the composition of atherosclerotic lesions may reflect differences in factors that contribute to their development. One of the principal theories is that dietary lipids, particularly cholesterol and saturated fats, are the main cause of atherosclerotic lesions. The second theory, of injury-induced initiation, arose partly from the following findings.

1. Platelets and white blood cells interact with vessel walls in the regions of disturbed blood flow that correspond to sites where the focal lesions of atherosclerosis develop (Packham & Mustard 1986, Glagov et al 1988, Turitto 1988).
2. Atherosclerotic lesions can be induced by repeated vessel injury in experimental animals given diets that have not been enriched with cholesterol or saturated fat (Moore 1981).
3. Platelets release platelet-derived growth factor (PDGF) which causes migration and proliferation of smooth muscle cells, the most abundant cell in atherosclerotic lesions (Ross 1986).

A thrombus is a deposit formed from blood constituents on the surface of the lining of the heart or a blood vessel. Thrombi may occur anywhere in the circulation: in the arteries, veins, capillaries, or chambers of the heart. They usually, but not necessarily, are attached to the surface of the vessel or the lining of the heart. An occlusive thrombus occupies the entire lumen of the vessel and prevents blood flow, whereas a mural thrombus adheres to only one side of the vessel and blood continues to flow past it. It is unusual for an occlusive thrombus to form in a large artery; occlusive thrombi tend to form in medium-sized stenosed arteries or in smaller vessels in the microcirculation. Occlusive thrombi can form more readily in veins, although mural thrombi also occur. In 1856, Virchow proposed that three major factors determine the site and extent of a thrombus.

1. Mechanical effects in which blood flow is predominant
2. The constituents of the blood
3. The vessel wall.

It is the interactions among these three factors that determine the kind of thrombus that forms. For example, vessel injury in a vein with slowed or arrested flow will usually lead to a thrombus that is rich in fibrin and red blood cells. Conversely, a thrombus that forms at an injury site in the arterial circulation where blood flow is relatively undisturbed will consist mainly of aggregated platelets with some fibrin and will not be extensive. The role of the endothelium, no longer considered merely as an inert lining of the blood vessels, is under intensive investigation. The importance of coagulation in thrombosis was identified in the last century and is now attracting more and more attention in relation to both venous and arterial thrombi. Deficiencies of inhibitors of coagulation (antithrombin III, protein C, protein S) and deficiencies in the fibrinolytic mechanism have been recognized to contribute to an increased susceptibility to thrombosis. Since other chapters are devoted to venous thrombosis (see Chs 59–63) this chapter will be limited to considerations of arterial thrombi.

Atherogenesis and arterial thrombosis are closely linked and each contributes to the other. Although the role of platelet and leukocyte adhesion at sites of vessel injury in the initiation of atherosclerotic lesions is controversial, the progression of lesions by the organization of platelet-rich thrombi into vessel walls to produce intimal thickening has been recognized since the time of von Rokitansky (1841) and later, Duguid (1946) (see review by Schwartz et al 1988). When atherosclerotic lesions have reached advanced stages, the platelet-fibrin thrombi that form on ruptured plaques and at stenotic lesions are responsible for many of the clinical complications of atherosclerotic vessel disease such as unstable angina, myocardial infarction, and sudden death.

ATHEROGENESIS

Atherosclerotic lesions can be induced to form in two ways: by enriching the diet with cholesterol (or saturated fats) (Armstrong & Heistad, 1990) or by repeated injury of the wall of an artery of normocholesterolaemic animals or man (Tyson et al 1976, Moore 1981). Injury-induced atherosclerosis is exacerbated by lipid-enriched diets (Minick 1981). It has even been suggested that, in man, none of the ten well-recognized risk factors for atherosclerosis leads to the development of lesions unless the plasma cholesterol level is above 150 mg/Dl (3.9 mmol/l) (Roberts 1989). However, it has also been suggested that it is the progression of lesions, rather than their initiation, that is related to hyperlipidaemia (Moore 1989).

The early lesions of atherosclerosis are focal and occur at vessel orifices and branches, undoubtedly under the influence of haemodynamic factors. Any theory about the initiation of atherosclerosis must take this localization into account. In humans and experimental animals, these are sites where there is increased permeability of the vessel wall to plasma proteins and LDL, endothelial cell alterations, and the deposition of platelets and white blood cells (Packham & Mustard 1986, Schwartz et al 1989). If one subscribes to the injury theory of the initiation of atherosclerosis, then the question arises of identifying the materials and conditions that are injurious.

Even the nature of the earliest lesions of atherosclerosis is controversial. Whether the fatty dots or fatty streaks that occur on the walls of arteries early in life are composed of lipid-filled macrophages, or lipid-filled smooth muscle cells, is an unsettled question (Moore 1989, Davies et al 1991). As Davies et al (1991) have pointed out, the lipid content of plaques can range from negligible to over 50%, and it is not known whether these different types of plaque are initiated in different ways or give rise to each other. Consequently, not all investigators believe that lipid-rich lesions are the only type of early lesion (Moore 1989), in part because in some species, the multiplication of smooth muscle cells in the intima precedes the deposition of lipid (Scott et al 1986). In addition, the theory has been advanced that atherosclerosis may begin during development in the form of focal intimal cell masses (Schwartz et al 1986).

From observations that 80% of atherosclerotic plaques are of a single phenotype in females who are heterozygous for two polymorphic forms of glucose-6-phosphate dehydrogenase, Benditt (1977, 1988) suggested that the majority of atherosclerotic plaques originate, like benign tumours, as monoclonal growths, initiated by a mutational event. This theory has gained support from the application of more recently developed techniques (Parkes et al 1991). A wide variety of potential mutagenic agents has been suggested by Penn (1990). However, Schwartz et al (1986) have pointed out that if adult lesions originate in preexisting clones of intimal cells, such lesions would also appear to be monoclonal in nature.

In animals given hypercholesterolaemic diets to produce high plasma cholesterol levels (15 mmol/l) similar to those found in individuals who are homozygous for the receptor defect in familial hypercholesterolaemia, the suggested sequence of events is that monocytes adhere to the endothelium, migrate into the intima, and become macrophages which take up lipid. Before uptake by macrophages, LDL is oxidized, either in or adjacent to endothelial cells, or when it is bound to proteoglycans in the intima, and oxidized LDL is a chemoattractant for monocytes (Steinberg 1991). Eventually, the endothelium is disrupted over the lipid-laden macrophages (foam cells), and at this stage, platelets adhere and are induced to secrete growth factors, such as PDGF, which stimulate the migration and proliferation of smooth muscle cells (Faggiotto & Ross 1984, Masuda & Ross 1990). Other sources of growth factors are the macrophages, endothelial cells and the smooth muscle cells themselves (Gordon et al 1989, Ross et al 1989, Clowes 1991). As the lesions develop, many different constituents can be identified in addition to macrophages, platelets, and smooth muscle cells. The smooth muscle cells that are involved produce connective tissue matrix proteins such as collagen and proteoglycans; cholesterol, cholesteryl esters and Lp(a) accumulate; T lymphocytes are present; components of the complement system have been detected; fibrin gives rise to 'fibrous intimal thickening' (Seifert & Kazatchkine 1988, Rath et al 1989, Wight 1989, Libby & Hansson 1991). Eventually, calcification of advanced lesions may occur. The growth of lesions, however, is episodic rather than gradual, because platelet-fibrin thrombi that form intermittently on fissured plaques are organized into fibrofatty structures that contribute markedly to the size of the plaques (Schwartz et al 1988, Davies et al 1991). Some investigators have suggested that organization of thrombi is the major way in which advanced atherosclerotic lesions progress (Fuster et al 1991).

The almost overwhelming acceptance of the cholesterol

theory for the initiation of atherosclerotic lesions is based on evidence from:

1. Experimental animals in which extremely high plasma cholesterol levels (in the order of 15 mmol/l) have been induced.
2. Epidemiological studies involving patients (predominantly male) between 30 and 55 years of age.
3. Patients who are homozygous or heterozygous for familial hypercholesterolaemia.

As Stehbens (1990) has pointed out, the complications of coronary heart disease do not usually occur until middle age and beyond, whereas atherosclerosis begins as early as 3 years of age. He questions the validity of extrapolating from the risk factors for the clinical complications that are manifest in middle age to the causes of atherosclerosis which begins in infancy.

Although there is uncertainty concerning the question of whether atherosclerotic lesions that occur normally over many years are initiated by the high levels of cholesterol in the diet of most individuals in the Western world, or whether they result from injury to the endothelium produced in a wide variety of ways, there is no doubt that when the endothelium is removed or extensively damaged, platelets adhere to subendothelial structures and release their granule contents and, if blood flow is disturbed, thrombi may form. This response of platelets to extensive and severe vessel wall injury was under investigation in experimental animals for many years before it took on more importance because of the introduction of procedures such as bypass surgery, angioplasty and endarterectomy which disrupt or remove the endothelium and injure cells that are deeper in the blood vessel wall. Reocclusion of vessels and accelerated development of atherosclerotic lesions after these procedures is now recognized as a major problem to which platelets and the substances they release make a large contribution.

VESSEL WALL

The endothelium

The normal endothelium acts as a natural barrier, preventing thrombus formation on the vessel wall. However, the reasons for the non-thrombogenic nature of the endothelium have not been fully elucidated. The original suggestion of Moncada & Vane (1978) that prostaglandin I_2 (PGI_2, prostacyclin) produced by the cells of the vessel wall prevents platelet adherence is not tenable for several reasons.

1. Platelets do not adhere to endothelial cells when PGI_2 production is inhibited with aspirin (Curwen et al 1980, Dejana et al 1980)
2. Unstimulated endothelial cells do not produce PGI_2.

However, locally at a site of injury, PGI_2 produced by injured cells may limit platelet reactions. Endothelium-derived relaxing factor (EDRF), now identified as nitric oxide, also inhibits platelet reactions (Moncada et al 1987, Furchgott & Vanhoutte 1989, Vane et al 1990). The ectonucleotidase(s) of endothelial cells may limit the contribution of ADP to platelet aggregation (Marcus 1990). Normal, undamaged endothelial cells do not activate the coagulation systems. Indeed, they exhibit anticoagulant properties in at least two ways. They synthesize heparan sulphate which acts with antithrombin III to inhibit the action of factor Xa and thrombin (Rosenberg & Rosenberg 1984), and they express thrombomodulin which binds thrombin. The resulting complex of thrombin/thrombomodulin activates protein C which, in the presence of protein S, inactivates factors Va and VIIIa (Esmon 1989).

Endothelial cells can be activated by a number of diverse agents. Activation by thrombin, histamine or bradykinin causes an immediate response involving stimulation of the formation of PGI_2 and platelet-activating factor (PAF, 1-*O*-alkyl-2-acetyl-sn-glyceryl-3-phosphorylcholine) (Zavoico et al 1990), release of von Willebrand factor (vWf), and the translocation of P-selectin (GMP-140, PADGEM) from the Weibel–Palade bodies to the surface of the endothelium where it can bind polymorphonuclear leukocytes and monocytes (McEver 1991a). In contrast, cytokines such as interleukin-1 and tumour necrosis factor cause a delayed expression of adhesion molecules for leukocytes on the surface of endothelial cells which peaks between 4 and 6 hours (Pober & Cotran 1990, 1991) (see p. 1122).

Stimulated endothelial cells can release tissue plasminogen activator, and assemble a fibrinolytic system on their surface (Nachman & Hajjar 1991). The release of transforming growth factor-β (TGF-β) from platelets can stimulate endothelial cells to synthesize type 1 plasminogen activator inhibitor (PAI-1) (Slivka & Loskutoff 1991) (see Chs 24 and 25).

Interaction of leukocytes with the vessel wall

Changes in the endothelial cell surface brought about by exposure to cytokines such as interleukin-1, tumour necrosis factor, lymphotoxin and bacterial endotoxin (Nathan & Sporn 1991), result in the development of adhesive properties that involve the expression of inducible endothelial-leukocyte adhesion molecules (ELAMs) (Pober & Cotran 1990, 1991). Some of these adhesion molecules are specific for polymorphonuclear leukocytes (ELAM-1 and ICAM-1), and some are specific for monocytes. During the development of atherosclerotic lesions, monocytes adhere to the arterial endothelium and migrate into the intima where they accumulate. Cybulsky & Gimbrone (1991) have designated the adhesive molecules with which monocytes react as ATHERO-ELAMS. They have identified such a molecule in the endothelial cells overlying developing atherosclerotic plaques in rabbits, and have evidence that it may be a homologue of human VCAM-1. In the intima, the monocytes take up lipids and become foam cells (macrophages), and these cells secrete cytokines and growth factors (Monro & Cotran 1988, Hansson et al 1989).

Pober and Cotran (1990, 1991) have emphasized the role of cytokines in inflammation, particularly in the interaction of neutrophils with the endothelium in post-capillary venules, and Smith et al (1991) have suggested that the adhesion of neutrophils contributes to the injury that occurs after ischaemia and reperfusion. Increased adhesiveness of endothelial cells in culture for polymorphonuclear leukocytes was shown to be due to an inducible glycoprotein (ELAM-1) on the surface of endothelial cells (Bevilacqua et al 1987, 1989). Lymphocytes and monocytes do not appear to recognize ELAM-1, but an adhesive molecule (ICAM) that is induced more slowly on endothelial cells, can bind neutrophils and B lymphocytes (Pober & Cotran 1990). ICAM on endothelial cells is a ligand for the leukocyte adhesion molecules, lymphocyte function-associated antigen (LFA-1), also named CD11a/CD18, and Mac-1 (CD11b/CD18), which are quickly induced on neutrophils by chemotactic factors such as C5a (a fragment of the fifth component of complement), interleukin-8, PAF, and leukotriene B_4 (Smith et al 1989, 1991).

A recently characterized glycoprotein of 130 kDa (PECAM-1, endoCAM, CD31) has been identified that is common to endothelial cells, monocytes, granulocytes, and activated platelets (Albelda et al 1990, Newman et al 1990, Metzelaar et al 1991). On endothelial cells, it is localized to the intercellular junctions (Metzelaar et al 1991), and the suggestion has been made that it may be involved in cell–cell interactions. In addition, it has been speculated that exposure of PECAM-1 at sites of vascular injury could lead to platelet adhesion and aggregation, as well as being involved in the interaction of leukocytes with the endothelium (Albelda et al 1990, Newman et al 1990), although an antibody to this glycoprotein did not affect platelet adhesion to the subendothelial matrix or collagen (Metzelaar et al 1991).

Leukocytes are inflammatory cells and can injure the endothelium when they adhere to it. Any attempts to understand atherogenesis and thrombosis that are initiated by vessel wall injury have to be focused on the ways in which the endothelium can be altered or removed. Some of the other conditions or agents that injure the endothelium have been recognized and are reviewed in later sections (p. 1117–1123).

RESPONSES OF PLATELETS AND THE COAGULATION SYSTEMS TO INJURY OF AN ARTERIAL WALL

Injury to either a normal or an atherosclerotic vessel wall leads to the interaction of platelets with exposed constituents of the subendothelium or the atherosclerotic plaque, and activation of the extrinsic and intrinsic blood coagulation pathways (Coller 1992).

Platelet responses to vessel wall injury

When the subendothelium of a normal vessel is exposed, platelets adhere to the microfibrils, basement membrane, and collagen (Baumgartner et al 1976), change shape, and spread on the surface. They also bind to vWf and fibronectin in the subendothelium (Sixma et al 1991). Adhesion of platelets at high shear rates is dependent on vWf (Weiss et al 1978); the plasma and the vessel wall appear to make equal contributions to the vWf that takes part in platelet adhesion under these conditions (Sixma et al 1991). However, an involvement of vWf at low shear rates has also been suggested (Badimon et al 1989). Glycoprotein Ib on the platelet surface binds to vWf (Roth 1991), but vWf can also bind to the glycoprotein IIb/IIIa complex (GPIIb/IIIa, integrin $\alpha_{IIb}\beta_3$) and take part in aggregation under some conditions (Fujimoto & Hawiger 1982, De Marco et al 1986, Harfenist et al 1987, Weiss et al 1989). The receptor on platelets for collagen has been identified as the glycoprotein Ia/IIa complex (Nieuwenhuis et al 1985, Kehrel et al 1988), but binding to glycoprotein IV has also been demonstrated (Tandon et al 1989). Platelets are not strongly stimulated by collagen that is in the subendothelium (types IV and V), but they are strongly stimulated by collagen that is deeper in vessel walls (types I and III), and by the collagen in atherosclerotic plaques (type III) (Packham & Mustard 1984). The platelets adherent to collagen are stimulated to release the contents of their dense granules and α granules, and to mobilize arachidonic acid from membrane phospholipids to form thromboxane A_2 (TXA_2). TXA_2, and released ADP and serotonin, act synergistically to cause other platelets in the vicinity to change shape and aggregate on the platelets that are adherent to the injury site. The release of granule contents from platelets adherent to collagen, however, does not require the formation of TXA_2, since it is not inhibited by non-steroidal anti-inflammatory drugs, such as aspirin, that inhibit the cyclo-oxygenase enzyme involved in the formation of TXA_2 (Kinlough-Rathbone et al 1980). On the outer membrane of platelets that have released their granule contents, phosphatidylserine becomes available as a surface on which two steps of the intrinsic pathway of coagulation are accelerated, leading to the generation of thrombin (Bevers et al 1987, Mann et al 1990). In addition, exposed tissue factor at an injury site, acting with factor VII of the extrinsic coagulation pathway, contributes to thrombin formation (Rapaport 1991). The thrombin that forms in and around a mass of aggregating platelets has two effects. It is a strong aggregating agent that causes further release of granule contents and formation of TXA_2, although it can cause aggregation by a mechanism that is independent of the release of ADP and formation of TXA_2 (Charo et al 1977, Kinlough-Rathbone et al 1977). The unique mechanism of action of the thrombin receptor has been elucidated recently (Vu et al 1991). Thrombin also converts fibrinogen to fibrin which stabilizes the platelet aggregate.

The physiologic stimuli that induce platelet aggregation act through receptors and G-proteins (guanine nucleotide-binding regulatory proteins) (Manning & Brass 1991) to alter GPIIb/IIIa on the platelet membrane so that it becomes able to bind fibrinogen which, as a divalent molecule, forms links between adjacent platelets (Kroll & Schafer 1989, Siess 1989, Hourani & Cusack 1991). Under some circumstances, other adhesive proteins, most notably vWf, can bind to GPIIb/IIIa on the surface of activated platelets and take part in platelet-to-platelet adhesion (Weiss et al 1989).

The release of granule contents, induced by stimuli such as thrombin, collagen and TXA_2, involves transduction of a signal from a receptor, through G-proteins, to phospholipase C which catalyses the hydrolysis of phosphatidylinositol bisphosphate, forming the second messengers inositol 1,4,5-trisphosphate and 1,2-diacylglycerol. Inositol trisphosphate mobilizes internal Ca^{2+} from the endoplasmic reticulum or dense tubular system, resulting in an increase in cytosolic Ca^{2+} which is required for several platelet functions including the activities of a Ca^{2+}/calmodulin-dependent protein kinase, Ca^{2+}-dependent proteases, phospholipases C and A_2, and protein kinase C (Kroll and Schafer 1989, Siess 1989, Rink & Sage 1990, Hourani & Cusack 1991). Myosin light chain (kDa 20) is the main substrate of the Ca^{2+}/calmodulin-dependent protein kinase and its phosphorylation is associated with platelet shape change and contraction (Daniel et al 1984, Gerrard et al 1989, Kroll & Schafer 1989, Hourani & Cusack 1991).

Cleavage of actin-binding protein, talin, spectrin and several other proteins by calpain, a Ca^{2+}-dependent protease, was at one time thought to be involved in platelet aggregation and the release of granule contents, but this now appears unlikely (Fox et al 1990a). However, calpain may be responsible for the agonist-induced expression of procoagulant activity on platelets (Fox et al 1990a,b).

An increase in cytosolic Ca^{2+} is also required for the activation of phospholipase A_2 which mobilizes arachidonic acid for TXA_2 formation. The activity of protein kinase C is also dependent on Ca^{2+}, although it is active at basal levels of internal Ca^{2+} (Rink & Sage 1990). Influx of Ca^{2+} from the external medium is stimulated by some aggregating agents (Hallam & Rink 1985, Rink & Sage 1990).

Diacylglycerol (with phosphatidylserine at the inner surface of the platelet membrane) activates protein kinase C which phosphorylates a 47 kDa protein (pleckstrin) in association with aggregation, release of granule contents, and mobilization of arachidonic acid (Gerrard et al 1989, Kroll & Schafer 1989).

Some aggregating agents, notably ADP and low concentrations of PAF, cause aggregation without stimulation of phospholipase C or A_2, providing the concentration of Ca^{2+} in the extracellular medium is in the physiological range (Packham et al 1989, Packham 1991). Signal transduction mechanisms have not been as thoroughly explored with these agonists as those involved in stimulation of platelets with thrombin. These weaker agonists, however, do cause a rise in internal Ca^{2+} with influx from the external medium forming a large component of this change (Kroll & Schafer 1989). Adrenaline has little effect by itself except in a low Ca^{2+} medium such as citrated platelet-rich plasma (Lalau Keraly et al 1988, Lanza et al 1988), but it strongly potentiates the aggregating and release-inducing effects of other agonists (Kinlough-Rathbone & Mustard 1986, Hourani & Cusack 1991). Serotonin also exerts synergistic effects with other aggregating agents, in addition to affecting vessel wall tone and contributing to vasospasm under some conditions (Vanhoutte 1988, De Clerck 1991).

The constituents released from the amine storage (dense) granules of platelets include ADP and serotonin. In addition, proteins released from the α granules (fibrinogen, fibronectin, vWf, thrombospondin) are involved in platelet adhesion to, and spreading on, the subendothelium and the formation of stable aggregates. Both factor V released from platelets and factor V in plasma are activated and contribute to the formation of the prothrombinase complex on the platelet surface (Mann et al 1990). PDGF and TGF-β, released from the α granules, stimulate smooth muscle cell migration into the intima and proliferation of these cells (Assoian & Sporn 1986, Ross 1989).

The α granule membrane protein, P-selectin (GMP-140), is translocated to the surface of platelets that have released their granule contents and takes part in platelet–leukocyte adhesion (Larsen et al 1989, McEver 1991a,b). Other granule membrane proteins also appear on the surface of platelets when the release reaction occurs, but their roles in platelet reactions are as yet unknown (Nieuwenhuis et al 1987, Gerrard et al 1991).

Platelets release PAI-1 and α_2-antiplasmin, but as Coller (1990) has pointed out, both profibrinolytic and antifibrinolytic effects have been described as the result of in vitro testing, probably because platelets also can bind plasminogen to their surface directly or by means of thrombospondin. Both fibrinolysis of clots and activation of plasminogen by tissue plasminogen activator are enhanced by platelets (Coller 1990).

Blood coagulation

Platelet aggregation and blood coagulation are closely

linked in a number of ways. The generation of thrombin through activation of coagulation makes a major contribution to the formation of arterial thrombi since thrombin causes both platelet aggregation and formation of fibrin which stabilizes thrombi. Details of the intrinsic and extrinsic pathways of coagulation are described in other chapters (see Section 4) and have been reviewed elsewhere (Mann et al 1990, Davie et al 1991). There are few (if any) clotting factors on the surface of unstimulated platelets, but when platelets have been stimulated to release their granule contents, negatively charged phospholipids (phosphatidylserine and phosphatidylinositol) that are normally on the cytoplasmic side of the membrane become available and provide a surface on which the 'tenase' and prothrombinase complexes are assembled (Bevers et al 1987). Microparticles from activated platelets also exhibit this procoagulant activity (George et al 1986, Sims et al 1988, Fox et al 1990b).

The normal, undamaged vessel wall does not stimulate coagulation, but tissue factor antigen is present on the subendothelium of arteries and on fibroblasts and pericytes in the wall of blood vessels (Drake et al 1989, Fleck et al 1990). Thus, when the endothelium is disrupted, factor VII/tissue factor complexes can be formed to initiate the extrinsic coagulation pathway. Tissue factor is also recognized as one of the constituents of atherosclerotic plaques, and stimulated monocytes can express tissue factor activity (Wilcox et al 1989).

The blood coagulation systems are described in detail in other chapters (see Chs 12–23). The natural anticoagulants antithrombin III, thrombomodulin, protein C and protein S are described in the chapters on inhibitors of blood coagulation (see Chs 28–30). They serve to limit the extent of thrombus formation by inhibiting the generation of thrombin and its effects on platelets and fibrinogen. Fibrinolytic agents, which generate plasmin that acts on both fibrin and platelets, disrupt thrombi, whereas the natural inhibitors of fibrinolysis such as PAI-1, promote thrombus formation. Detailed treatment of these subjects can be found in other chapters (see Chs 24 and 25).

Fibrinogen and fibrin and their degradation products have been reported to affect the endothelium, although most of the studies appear to have been done with cultured endothelial cells. Fibrin induces the release of vWf from endothelial cells (Ribes et al 1987); cleavage of fibrinopeptide B is required for this effect (Ribes et al 1989). Fibrin also increases the synthesis of PGI_2 and tissue plasminogen activator by endothelial cells (Kaplan et al 1989) and has been reported to cause disorganization of endothelial cell monolayers (Weimar & Delvos 1986). However, Okadome & Tanaka (1986) showed in vivo in rats that endothelial cells are heterogeneous in their reactivity to fibrin.

Although fibrinogen itself has not been shown to induce morphological changes in endothelial cells (Watanabe & Tanaka 1983), the findings with fibrinogen degradation products have been somewhat conflicting. Dang et al (1985) reported that fragment D causes disorganization of cultured endothelial cell monolayers, whereas Watanabe & Tanaka (1983) showed no effect of either fragment D or E on cultured porcine aortic endothelial cells, although lower molecular weight degradation products did injure these cells. Elevated levels of degradation products of fibrinogen and fibrin, including fragment D, are characteristic of a number of syndromes such as adult respiratory distress syndrome, thrombotic thrombocytopenic purpura and disseminated intravascular coagulation, in which severe endothelial cell damage occurs.

Changes in the vessel wall following injury

There is now intense interest in the problems of intimal hyperplasia and restenosis after bypass surgery, angioplasty, and other forms of arterial reconstruction in which the vessel wall is injured (Clowes 1991). The principal cell in the lesions that form is the smooth muscle cell. However, before these techniques were in use in patients, a number of investigators were using rats and rabbits to study the response of vessel walls to removal of the endothelium with a balloon catheter (Baumgartner 1972, Stemerman & Ross 1972, Groves et al 1979, Clowes 1991). This procedure, however, may also injure the smooth muscle cells, and in addition, the ensuing changes may not be representative of those that occur when a diseased vessel wall is damaged. When the subendothelium of a normal rabbit aorta is exposed by removal of the endothelium, platelets rapidly cover most of the damaged surface but, unless blood flow conditions promote thrombus formation, the initial layer of platelets almost immediately becomes nonreactive to circulating platelets and fibrin does not form on the surface (Groves et al 1979). Experiments in which the carotid arteries of rats have been injured by passage of a balloon catheter have shown that the smooth muscle cells do not begin to divide until 24 hours after the injury (Clowes et al 1983), and several days later they begin to migrate from the media to the intima and synthesize and secrete matrix molecules (Clowes 1991). In rabbits and rats, the smooth muscle cells that form the neointima are relatively inert as far as platelet adherence and activation of coagulation are concerned (Groves et al 1979, Clowes et al 1986, Reidy 1988). If this neointima is damaged, the site of injury is more thrombogenic than the original subendothelium, and platelet-fibrin thrombi form in some areas, particularly at vessel orifices (Groves et al 1982). Endothelial cells grow over the damaged areas as a continuous sheet, beginning from sites where the endothelium has not been removed (Reidy et al 1983). However, re-endothelialization is often incomplete in experimental animals (Clowes 1991) and man (Berger et al 1972).

BLOOD FLOW

Patterns of blood flow determine the sites where atherosclerotic lesions develop, influence the interaction of platelets with surfaces, and affect the size and structure of thrombi (Glagov et al 1988, Turitto 1988) (See Ch. 51). Early investigators pointed out that when flow is slowed, more platelets come in contact with the vessel wall (Eberth & Schimmelbusch 1888) and eddies form at sites of rapid changes of flow (von Recklinghausen 1883). Using arteriovenous shunts containing models of various vessel configurations, many investigators have observed that deposits of blood materials tend to occur in areas of disturbed flow (Rowntree & Shionoya 1927, Mustard et al 1962, Goldsmith & Karino 1979, Karino et al 1982). In regions where flow separation with vortex formation occurs, increased numbers of platelets are transported to the wall along radially directed streamlines; platelet aggregates are formed and are trapped in the vortex (Goldsmith & Karino 1982, Leonard 1987). In addition, activated coagulation factors and mediators of platelet aggregation can accumulate in a vortex, increasing the likelihood of thrombus formation (Folie & McIntire 1989). In regions where vortices promote platelet adhesion and the development of platelet aggregates, atherosclerotic plaques are localized on the lateral and outer walls. Disturbed flow also allows the accumulation of injurious agents which can damage the endothelium. Atherosclerotic plaques tend to form in regions of flow separation, low flow velocity, and low shear stress, rather than in regions of high velocity and increased shear stress (Zarins et al 1983, Glagov et al 1988).

Responses of endothelial cells to shear stress have been outlined by Eskin & McIntire (1988). Under shear stress, endothelial cells in culture are elongated and aligned, with prominent stress fibres, and PGI_2 production and pinocytosis are increased. Arachidonic acid metabolism and production of tissue plasminogen activator are stimulated at arterial shear stresses (Diamond et al 1989, Nollert et al 1989). Since some of these effects would be expected to limit the deposition of platelets and fibrin, Diamond et al (1989) have suggested that they may contribute to the nonthrombogenic nature of the endothelium. However, endocytosis of LDL by cultured endothelial cells is increased by shear stress (Schwartz et al 1989). Turbulent shear stress induces endothelial cell turnover, as demonstrated by increased incorporation of tritiated thymidine into cultured cells (Davies et al 1986).

Very high shear can cause endothelial cell injury (Fry 1976). In large arteries with marked stenosis, the shear at the stenosis may be sufficiently great to dislodge the endothelium (Gertz et al 1981, Joris et al 1982), particularly in a diseased vessel where the adherence of the endothelium to the wall may be weak. Shear stress has been shown to cause platelet aggregation in vitro; ADP from red blood cells and platelets, and large vWf multimers have been implicated (Moritz et al 1983, Moake et al 1988). In pigs with von Willebrand's disease, platelet aggregates do not form in stenosed coronary arteries although in normal pigs, platelet aggregates do form under these conditions (Nichols et al 1986). The work of Folts and his colleagues (1990) has demonstrated a role for TXA_2 in shear-induced platelet aggregation, since the platelet-thrombi that form in tightly narrowed, injured coronary vessels of dogs are readily inhibited by aspirin and other non-steroidal anti-inflammatory drugs.

The physical effect of the red cells in flowing blood has a major influence on the interaction of platelets with surfaces (Turitto 1988) (see p. 1123).

It is generally accepted that vWf is involved in platelet adhesion to the subendothelium only at high shear rates (de Groot & Sixma 1987), but Badimon et al (1989) have presented evidence that vWf may also be involved under low shear conditions. If blood flow is laminar, only a thin carpet of platelets adheres to an injured surface and the surface becomes relatively non-thrombogenic long before it is re-endothelialized (Kinlough-Rathbone et al 1983). Restoration of laminar flow after angioplasty reduces the risk of acute reocclusion, even though platelets adhere to the freshly exposed surface. In contrast, when an occlusive thrombus is disrupted by fibrinolysis, but the stenotic lesion is not removed and blood flow patterns remain disturbed, thrombosis is likely to recur if the vessel wall is still thrombogenic (Mustard et al 1990).

For occlusive thrombi to form in medium-sized arteries, such as the coronary artery, marked narrowing of the vessel lumen with a major disturbance of blood flow has to have occurred. (See section on thrombus formation at stenotic lesions, p. 1114). The size of a mural thrombus is limited by blood flow which can rapidly dilute and remove aggregating stimuli and coagulation factors. In addition, platelets on the surface of a thrombus may be dislodged by the shear effects of flow. In some circumstances, increased blood viscosity may contribute to thrombosis (Smith & La Celle 1982).

ARTERIAL THROMBI

Stabilization of thrombi

Arterial thrombi are stabilized by adhesive proteins from plasma and from the α granules of platelets that have released their granule contents, by ADP from platelet dense granules or from red blood cells, and by fibrin formed under the influence of thrombin. The strength of the aggregating agents and the time over which they act influence stability. In addition, clot retraction mediated by platelet actomyosin consolidates a thrombus and makes it less susceptible to fibrinolysis (Fitzgerald 1991).

Although fibrinogen is generally accepted as having a

major role in binding activated platelets together, several lines of evidence indicate that it is not always involved. Direct visualization of fibrinogen using an immunogold-labelling technique shows many points where aggregated platelets are in contact with each other without any fibrinogen visible between them (Suzuki et al 1988, Heilmann et al 1991). Experiments with platelets from afibrinogenaemic patients showed that these platelets, which lack fibrinogen in their granules, are not more readily deaggregated than normal platelets after aggregation with thrombin (Cattaneo et al 1987). It appears that substances other than fibrinogen that are released from platelet granules can stabilize platelet aggregates; one of these substances has been identified as ADP by studies with platelets from patients with dense granule storage pool deficiency and a patient with a selective impairment of ADP-induced fibrinogen binding and aggregation (Cattaneo et al 1990). The ability of GPIIb/IIIa to bind adhesive proteins is lost within a few minutes after stimulation of platelets with weak agonists such as ADP or PAF, but after stimulation with thrombin, the complex remains indefinitely in a configuration that can bind these proteins (van Willigen & Akkerman 1992).

Other adhesive proteins that have been implicated in platelet aggregation and the stability of aggregates are vWf, which binds to both glycoprotein Ib and GPIIb/IIIa, and thrombospondin, released from the α granules of platelets, which has been suggested to stabilize the binding of fibrinogen to platelets (Silverstein et al 1987). Thrombospondin is a lectin-like molecule whose receptor on the platelet surface was thought to be glycoprotein IV (IIIb) (Asch et al 1987, McGregor et al 1989), but studies with an antibody to glycoprotein IV are open to other interpretations (Aiken et al 1990), and patients whose platelets lack this receptor bind thrombospondin in normal amounts (Tandon et al 1991).

Fibrin, which binds to platelets through GPIIb/IIIa (Hantgan 1988), is the most important stabilizing agent of thrombi that form in vivo.

Control of extension of thrombi

The growth of thrombi in vivo is limited in a number of ways. Blood flow may remove aggregating agents that would contribute to thrombus extension, and also sweep away platelets and emboli on the surface of a thrombus if their attachment is destabilized. The natural anticoagulants, antithrombin III, thrombomodulin and activated protein C, may inactivate thrombin or limit its production. Tissue plasminogen activator may cause the formation of plasmin which lyses fibrin and other protein links between platelets. PGI_2 and EDRF from stimulated endothelial cells in the vicinity of the thrombus may limit platelet adhesion to an injury site and inhibit further platelet aggregation.

Fate of thrombi

Thrombi are often unstable structures (Chesebro et al 1991, Falk 1991a). Their constituents may turn over, or the thrombi may break up under the influence of natural fibrinolytic agents and the force of flowing blood. The emboli from mural thrombi may obstruct the microcirculation downstream and have been implicated in sudden coronary death (Forrester 1991, Verheugt & Brugada 1991). Some thrombi, however, may progress to the point where they occlude the vessel. Thrombi that persist are organized and incorporated into the vessel wall, and in this way contribute to intimal thickening.

Studies of thrombus formation in the microcirculation have shown that, when the vessel wall is injured, a platelet-rich thrombus forms rapidly and undergoes episodes of dissolution and reformation until the damaged site becomes inactive (Fulton et al 1953, Berman 1961, Honour & Russell 1962). Experimental studies in dogs have shown that radioactive fibrinogen can be incorporated into large thrombi even if it is injected several hours after they have formed (Coleman et al 1975, Salimi et al 1977). Fulton & Sumner (1977) have demonstrated that fibrin continues to be laid down in coronary artery thrombi in man for several hours after initiation of a thrombus. The surface of thrombi in arterial aneurysms in humans tends to remain thrombogenic and platelets and fibrin accumulate and embolize (Francis et al 1984). Both the platelet and fibrin components of arterial thrombi can be lost and replaced; the platelets that are lost can persist in the circulation, but their survival may be shortened if they have been exposed to high local concentrations of plasmin which cleaves membrane glycoproteins (Greenberg et al 1979). Platelets that have been exposed to ADP, TXA_2 or thrombin can survive normally in vivo (Reimers et al 1976, Packham et al 1980), and it is possible to detect platelets in the circulation that have been exposed to aggregating and release-inducing agents (Cieslar et al 1979, van Oost et al 1983, Abrams & Shattil 1991).

Thrombi that persist can be organized and incorporated into the vessel wall (Jørgensen et al 1967b, Davies et al 1975, Fuster et al 1991). If a thrombus persists, smooth muscle cells migrate into it along with macrophages that phagocytose the thrombotic material. Eventually the lesion becomes covered with endothelium. During organization, occlusive arterial thrombi may be recanalized (Crawford 1977, Forrester 1991). The episodic growth of atherosclerotic lesions has been attributed to the organization and incorporation of thrombi that form on ruptured plaques (Schwartz et al 1988, Davies et al 1991, Forrester 1991, Fuster et al 1991).

Thrombus formation at stenotic lesions and on ruptured atherosclerotic plaques

Platelet-fibrin thrombi form mainly in regions of disturbed blood flow, such as around vessel orifices and bifurcations and at tight stenoses. Thrombi in coronary vessels are frequently associated with ruptured atherosclerotic plaques which provide sites that are strongly thrombogenic (Chesebro et al 1991, Falk 1991a).

It has been observed in man that rupture of an atherosclerotic plaque at a site with less than 75% narrowing is not associated with the formation of occlusive thrombi, whereas as narrowing becomes greater, ruptured plaques more and more frequently have occlusive thrombi associated with them (Falk 1983, 1991a). Many other investigators have made similar observation (Forrester 1991, Qiao & Fishbein 1991). The dynamics of thrombus growth has been studied with ^{111}In-labelled platelets in pigs with various extents of stenosis of damaged vessels (Lassila et al 1990). The highest level of platelet deposition occurred at the apex of the 80% stenosis, with embolization detectable after 30 minutes of perfusion. Chesebro et al (1991) point out that in their experiments the greatest concentration of platelets occurs within the smallest luminal diameter of the stenosis and a more fibrin-rich or reddish (red cell-rich) thrombus usually forms more distal to the stenosis. Angiographic evidence indicates that most nonocclusive thrombi are located post-stenotically, where flow separation, recirculation, and turbulence provide ideal conditions for thrombus growth (Falk 1991a). Thrombus formation on stenosed, injured vessels of dogs has been used extensively to study the effects of various inhibitors of thrombus formation (Folts 1990).

Although thrombosis that occurs as a result of fissuring of an atherosclerotic plaque is often clinically silent (Davies et al 1991), the rupture of an atherosclerotic plaque in a coronary vessel may precipitate the formation of thrombi that are responsible for the clinically recognizable complications of chronic coronary disease: unstable angina, acute myocardial infarction, and sudden death. Soft, lipid-rich plaques are most likely to rupture (Davies & Thomas 1985, Fuster et al 1990). Platelets adhere to the constituents of the plaque, and platelet aggregation and the formation of thrombin occur rapidly. The thrombogenic plaque constituents that are exposed may be influenced by the depth of the fissure in the plaque (Chesebro et al 1991). They include types I and III collagen, lipid gruel, tissue thromboplastin, and thrombin bound to extracellular matrix. The use of inhibitors of thrombin (heparin, hirudin, and synthetic thrombin inhibitors) has established that thrombin is the most important stimulus for thrombus formation under these circumstances (Jang et al 1990, Chesebro & Fuster 1991, Falk 1991a), most probably because it both affects platelets and causes fibrin formation. ADP from haemolysed red blood cells, and ADP and serotonin released from platelets, as well as TXA_2, contribute to thrombus formation. In addition, TXA_2 and serotonin may cause vessel spasm that contributes to ischaemia and may enhance thrombus formation (Fuster et al 1990). Spasm and thrombosis frequently occur together in many patients with unstable angina and other coronary events (Vetrovec et al 1982, Oliva 1983, Capone et al 1984, Falk 1991a). It is possible that spasm in a moderately stenosed vessel could lead to the formation of an occlusive thrombus, particularly in association with vascular injury or plaque rupture. The results of two clinical trials of aspirin therapy in unstable angina suggest the possibility of there being at least two processes, spasm and thrombosis (Lewis et al 1983, Cairns et al 1985). In both studies, aspirin therapy significantly reduced the incidence of myocardial infarction, but in the study by Lewis and his colleagues, there was no effect of aspirin on angina. This evidence is compatible with the concept that the angina was primarily due to spasm which would not be affected by aspirin, whereas thrombosis causing myocardial infarction would be prevented by aspirin. The studies of Chierchia et al (1982) have demonstrated that aspirin does not affect the spasm that is believed to cause unstable angina.

When mural thrombi embolize, the microemboli impact in the microcirculation distal to the thrombi. In experimental animals, emboli in coronary vessels have been shown to cause ventricular fibrillation and sudden death (Jørgensen et al 1967a, Moore et al 1981). In man, a number of autopsy studies after sudden coronary death have revealed microemboli distal to mural thrombi (Haerem 1978, El Maraghi & Genton 1980, Davies M J et al 1986, Falk 1991b, Forrester 1991, Verheugt & Brugada 1991).

Cerebral artery thrombosis is also believed to be initiated primarily by breaks or ruptures of atherosclerotic plaques (Constantinides 1967).

Deposition of platelets on atherosclerotic lesions contributes to the progression of peripheral vascular disease (Hess et al 1985, Sinzinger et al 1988).

Reocclusion due to thrombosis and accelerated atherosclerosis after bypass grafts, angioplasty, endarterectomy, and transplantation

Acute reocclusion due to thrombus formation at the sites of injury frequently occurs after the insertion of bypass grafts, after angioplasty or endarterectomy, or in transplanted hearts. However, even if the vessel remains patent initially, restenosis involving the proliferation of smooth muscle cells develops in 3 to 6 months in a number of patients (Clowes 1991, Schoen & Libby 1991). Following percutaneous transluminal coronary angioplasty, the percentage of patients having restenosis has been reported to be at least 25–35% (Wilcox 1991). Growth factors, such as basic fibroblast growth factor from damaged smooth muscle cells, contribute to the intimal hyperplasia, but PDGF may act principally by stimulating smooth muscle cell migration rather than proliferation (Clowes 1991, Ferns et al 1991).

Although the acute thrombotic events may be controlled to some extent by drugs that inhibit platelet responses and the action of thrombin (Klein et al 1990, Ellis et al 1991, Goldman et al 1991, Popma et al 1991), methods for the pharmacological control of smooth muscle cell proliferation have yet to be established (Ip et al 1991, Wilcox 1991). The formation of thrombi on the deeply injured arterial walls of experimental animals subjected to angioplasty procedures is more effectively inhibited by hirudin (or other specific thrombin inhibitors) than by heparin, indicating a major role for thrombin in acute reocclusion (Kaplan et al 1991, Lam al 1991, Wilcox 1991). These observations are in accord with the findings that clot-bound thrombin is protected from inhibition by heparin-antithrombin III, but is susceptible to inactivation by thrombin inhibitors that do not act through antithrombin III (Weitz et al 1990). However, both from in vivo experiments with rats and from in vitro experiments, there is evidence that heparin may have some inhibitory effect on smooth muscle cell proliferation (Clowes 1991, Hirsch & Karnovsky 1991).

Detection of thromboembolic processes

Activation of platelets results in detectable changes of the platelet membrane and the appearance of platelet constituents in the plasma (Abrams & Shattil 1991). Activation of coagulation and fibrinolysis leads to changes in a number of plasma proteins. In addition, detection of hypersensitive platelets by in vitro tests (Packham 1978), and detection of increased levels of some clotting factors in plasma may indicate an increased risk of thromboembolism.

When platelets have been stimulated to release their granule contents, β-thromboglobulin and platelet factor 4 appear in the plasma, as well as thromboxane B_2 (TXB_2), the product of TXA_2 which is formed in response to release-inducing agonists. These substances are detectable by radioimmunoassays. Increased levels of β-thromboglobulin, platelet factor 4, and TXB_2 have been found in the plasma of some individuals during thromboembolic episodes (Kaplan & Owen 1981, Hoet et al 1990), but not in individuals with stable, chronic atherosclerotic vessel disease (Files et al 1981). Urinary analysis of the metabolites of TXA_2 provides a noninvasive method of quantifying its endogenous production (FitzGerald et al 1983, Reilly et al 1986).

Monoclonal antibodies have been developed that react with antigens that appear on the surface of platelets from which granule contents have been released; these antibodies permit the detection of these activated platelets in whole blood by flow cytometry (Abrams & Shattil 1991). Several granule membrane proteins become exposed on the surface of platelets that have released their granule contents. These include P-selectin (GMP-140) and GMP-33 from the membrane of the α granules (Berman et al 1986, McEver 1991a, Metzelaar et al 1992); the lysosomal granule membrane proteins LAMP-1, LAMP-2 (Febbraio & Silverstein 1990, Silverstein & Febbraio 1990) and CD63 (Metzelaar et al 1990); and a 40 kDa dense granule membrane protein (Gerrard et al 1991).

Antibodies have been developed to the form of GPIIb/IIIa which enables it to bind adhesive proteins after platelet activation (Shattil et al 1985, Niiya et al 1987, Frelinger et al 1988); antibodies are available that recognize bound fibrinogen (Abrams et al 1990, Warkentin et al 1990, Zamarron et al 1990) and thrombospondin (George et al 1986); and there are antibodies to epitopes on GPIIb/IIIa that are expressed as a result of binding of a ligand containing an RGD sequence (Ginsberg et al 1990). Theoretically, these antibodies should be capable of detecting platelets that have been activated without the release of granule contents (e.g. by ADP or low concentrations of PAF) as well as platelets that have been exposed to release-inducing stimuli. Platelet-derived microparticles can be detected by flow cytometry when platelets have been activated in vivo during cardiopulmonary bypass, by thrombin plus collagen, or by the complement proteins, C5b-9 (George et al 1986, Sims et al 1988, Abrams et al 1990).

Decreased platelet survival is associated with clinical manifestations of arterial disease (Harker 1978, Kinlough-Rathbone et al 1983), but the reactions responsible for shortened platelet survival have not been established. Platelets that have adhered to injury sites on vessels walls or been incorporated into thrombi can re-enter the circulation if their attachments to the constituents of the vessel wall, to fibrin, and to each other are broken. If local activation of the fibrinolytic system occurs, and plasmin is generated, it would cleave both platelet membrane glycoproteins and fibrin and free platelets from these attachments. Since cleavage of membrane glycoproteins shortens platelet survival (Greenberg et al 1979), the shortened platelet survival observed during repeated vessel wall injury may be the result of the action of plasmin and other proteolytic enzymes on platelets. In keeping with this suggestion is the observation that inhibition of fibrinolysis with epsilon aminocaproic acid prolongs experimentally-shortened platelet survival in rats subjected to chronic vessel wall injury by indwelling aortic catheters (Winocour et al 1983).

Activation of coagulation can be detected by radioimmunoassays for fibrinopeptides A or B, cleaved from fibrinogen by the action of thrombin (Nossel 1976). Fibrinopeptide A has been found in plasma of patients with symptomatic venous thromboembolism, acute myocardial infarction, sudden coronary death, and severe coronary artery disease (Nossel 1976, Meade et al 1984, Gallino et al 1985).

Degradation products of fibrinogen and fibrin formed by activation of plasminogen have been found in the plasma of patients with clinical evidence of thromboembolic processes (Fletcher & Alkjaersig 1977, Lane et al 1982). A radioimmunoassay has been developed for the fibrinogen-derived peptide Bβ1-42 which is cleaved from fibrin I or fibrinogen by plasmin; when combined with measurement of fibrinopeptide B (residues 1–14 of the Bβ peptide, cleaved by thrombin), it is possible to examine the balance between the action of thrombin and plasmin (Weitz et al 1986).

Visualization of thrombi and stenotic lesions in vivo by various methods has been described in both humans and experimental animals by many investigators. Radiolabelled fibrinogen, platelets labelled with ^{111}Indium, or ^{111}In-labelled, platelet-specific antibodies are detected by external gamma camera imaging (Lassila et al 1990, Berridge et al 1991). Angiography or percutaneous coronary angioscopy (de Feyter et al 1991, White et al 1991), and pulsed Doppler velocity probes (Katritsis et al 1991) show vessel narrowing, but do not distinguish between atherosclerotic lesions and platelet-fibrin thrombi.

RISK FACTORS FOR ATHEROSCLEROSIS OR ITS THROMBOEMBOLIC COMPLICATIONS

Any agent that damages or removes the endothelium can initiate or exacerbate atherosclerotic lesions, particularly when cholesterol levels are high. Injurious agents may synergize with each other. Some of the agents that have been shown to damage vessel walls also increase the sensitivity of platelets to aggregating agents, or activate the coagulation mechanisms, leading to the formation of thrombi.

Hypercholesterolaemia and dietary fatty acids

Plasma cholesterol levels above 200 mg/Dl (5.2 mmol/l) are considered to promote the development of advanced atherosclerotic lesions (Grundy et al 1988, Roberts 1989, Shekelle & Stamler 1989, Oliver 1990). (See p. 1108 and Ch. 50).

High cholesterol levels have also been reported to result in platelet hypersensitivity to aggregating agents in man (Carvalho et al 1974, Colman 1978, Shattil & Cooper 1978, Corash et al 1981, Aviram & Brook 1982, Bradlow et al 1982, DiMinno et al 1986). In rats given cholesterol-enriched diets, or with genetically determined hypercholesterolaemia, platelet hypersensitivity to aggregation induced by thrombin has been noted (Winocour et al 1987, 1989). Platelets from cholesterol-fed rabbits show enhanced responses to collagen, to the thromboxane mimetic U46619, and to thrombin; these enhancements occur through both TXA_2-dependent and TXA_2-independent mechanisms (Gross et al 1991a). In contrast, platelets from Watanabe heritable hyperlipidaemic (WHHL) rabbits showed no difference from controls in their sensitivity to thrombin, but showed decreased responses to collagen and U46619, although their plasma cholesterol levels of 13.9 mmol/l were similar to those of the rabbits with diet-induced hypercholesterolaemia (15 mmol/l) (Gross et al 1991b). The lipoprotein patterns differ in these two forms of hypercholesterolaemia in rabbits, and in rats with genetically-determined hypercholesterolaemia, and it may be that it is the lipoprotein profiles, not hypercholesterolaemia per se, that influence platelet responsiveness to various aggregating agents.

Diets that are rich in saturated fatty acids of chain length 12 to 16 carbons not only raise plasma cholesterol levels (Ulbricht & Southgate 1991), but have been shown to be thrombogenic in rats and in man, whereas polyunsaturated fatty acids are antithrombotic (Hornstra 1980, 1989, Nordøy & Goodnight 1990). In early studies, Renaud and his co-workers (1970) showed that rats fed diets rich in saturated fat, particularly butter fat, had an increased susceptibility to endotoxin-induced thrombosis and that the platelets from these animals showed a hypersensitivity to thrombin-induced aggregation, but not to aggregation induced by ADP or collagen. The platelets from these animals had a membrane property that potentiated coagulation (Renaud & Gautheron 1975). It has been pointed out that the ratio of polyunsaturated to saturated fatty acids (P/S ratio) in the diet also influences platelet function in man (Renaud 1990) and in monkeys (Lewis & Taylor 1989). There is a greater response of platelets to both ADP and thrombin when the intake of saturated fatty acids is high. Diets in which the ω-6 polyunsaturated fat, linoleic acid, is enriched, to give a P/S ratio of approximately 1, cause a decrease in thrombin-induced aggregation, but enhance ADP-induced aggregation. Renaud (1990) notes that a dietary P/S ratio of 0.7 is characteristic of the Japanese in whom the clinical complications of atherosclerosis are reduced. Enrichment of diets with ω-6 polyunsaturated fatty acids has been shown to depress HDL, as well as lowering LDL (Ulbricht & Southgate 1991).

Trans polyunsaturated fatty acids (produced during the hydrogenation of liquid vegetable oils), in contrast to *cis* polyunsaturated fatty acids, have been found to raise LDL cholesterol levels and lower HDL cholesterol levels in man (Mensink & Katan 1990), and hence are considered to be atherogenic. There is a report that they enhance thrombin-induced platelet aggregation (Wahle 1989). However, in rats, *trans* fatty acids have been found to be either no different in their thrombogenicity (Hornstra 1980) or to reduce platelet sensitivity to collagen-induced aggregation (Chiang et al 1991).

Extensive investigations are underway of the effects on platelet function of enrichment of the diet with ω-3 unsaturated fatty acids (eicosapentaenoic acid (EPA) and docosahexaenoic acid (DHA) that are found in cold water fish. When EPA replaces arachidonic acid in platelet membrane phospholipids, TXA_3 instead of TXA_2 is formed when the platelets are stimulated, and PGI_3 is formed instead of PGI_2 by the endothelial cells. TXA_3 is not an effective platelet aggregating agent, whereas PGI_3 retains the inhibitory effects of PGI_2 (Ulbricht & Southgate 1991, Coller 1992). Inhibitory effects on platelet function and thrombosis of enriching the diet with ω-3 fatty acids are relatively modest.

The question of whether elevated levels of plasma triglycerides are a risk factor for coronary heart disease is unsettled (Oliver 1990, Austin 1991, Criqui 1991, Wilson et al 1991). Lp(a) levels above 0.3 g/l appear to be a major determinant of coronary heart disease; this lipoprotein has both thrombotic and atherosclerotic properties (Loscalzo 1990, Scott 1991).

Smoking

Smoking is recognized as a major risk factor for both men and women in the initiation of atherosclerotic lesions, in their progression, and in the thromboembolic complications of arterial disease (Hennekens et al 1984). Synergistic effects with other risk factors are evident, and in populations with low serum cholesterol levels, cigarette smoking is not associated with atherosclerotic disease (Keys 1980). The dietary habits of smokers may influence their susceptibility to cardiovascular events, since smokers in the United Kingdom were found to eat less polyunsaturated fat (mainly linoleic acid), less fibre, and less fish than nonsmokers (Oliver 1989). Smoking appears to have a number of effects on the cardiovascular system, including injury of the endothelium, stimulation of platelet function, increases in plasma fibrinogen and viscosity, higher haematocrit, and reduced HDL levels. There is apparently no increased risk of venous thrombosis and pulmonary embolism in smokers (Handley & Teather 1974), possibly because of stimulation of fibrinolysis by cigarette smoke (Janzon & Nilsson 1975).

Mild injury of endothelial cells has been observed in several studies of the effects of cigarette smoke or nicotine in experimental animals and on endothelial cells in culture (Pittilo et al 1982, 1990, Boutet et al 1980, Booyse et al 1981a,b). Desquamation of the endothelium has been found after exposure of rats to cigarette smoke (Sieffert et al 1981). Asmussen & Kjeldsen (1975) noted degenerative changes of the endothelium of the umbilical arteries of newborns of smoking mothers. Cigarette smoking shortens platelet survival (Mustard & Murphy 1963, Fuster et al 1981), and this may be mediated through an effect on the endothelium or on intravascular activation of platelets. The number of endothelial cells in blood is increased acutely when nonsmokers smoke cigarettes (Davis et al 1985). Early reports showed that exposure of rats to cigarette smoke led to areas of blebbing and microvillus-like projections on the luminal surface of rat aortae with adherent platelet microthrombi proximal to intercostal branches, but without endothelial cell detachment; PGI_2 production in vitro was reduced and platelets aggregated more readily (Pittilo et al 1982, Woolf et al 1983). However, the same investigators have reported more recently that nicotine, at concentrations similar to those in the plasma of smokers (10^{-9} to 10^{-6} mol/l), does not alter the morphology of endothelial cells in culture nor cause changes in the release of endothelial prostaglandins (Bull et al 1988). These in vitro results seem to indicate that nicotine is not the constituent of cigarette smoke that injures the endothelium, although oral consumption of nicotine has been shown to damage the endothelium of the aorta of rabbits (Booyse et al 1981a) and to increase endothelial cell turnover in mice (Zimmerman & McGeachie 1985, 1987). Inhalation of nicotine induces the release of catecholamines which increase heart rate, blood pressure, cardiac output and oxygen demand, with resultant ischaemia if atherosclerotic lesions restrict the normal increase in blood flow (Hennekens et al 1984).

Carbon monoxide was suggested at one time as the agent in cigarette smoke that was responsible for endothelial cell damage, but in later investigations it was not found to be injurious (Hugod et al 1978). Although the concentration of carbon monoxide in cigarette smoke is high, and it decreases the supply of oxygen available to the myocardium, there is no direct evidence that it is the main component of smoke that is harmful (Hennekens et al 1984). In fact, some studies indicate that carbon monoxide inhibits platelet aggregation and the release of granule contents in response to some agonists (Mansouri & Perry 1984, Brüne & Ullrich 1987).

It seems unlikely that direct effects of nicotine on platelets account for changes in platelet reactivity that are related to smoking (Becker et al 1988, Pfueller et al 1988). The urinary excretion by smokers of the TXA_2 metabolite 2,3-dinor-thromboxane B_2 is higher than in nonsmokers, indicating platelet activation (Rångemark & Wennmalm 1991, Uedelhoven et al 1991). Nowak et al (1987) have used the time of recovery of platelets from inhibition of cyclo-oxygenase by aspirin to show that platelets are the source of the TXA_2 metabolite in the urine. These investigators noted depressed platelet responses ex vivo to ADP and adrenaline with chronic smoking, and suggested that the effects of smoking on platelet function in vivo may result from vascular damage and the interaction of platelets with the injury sites, rather than from a direct effect of smoking on platelets. Refractoriness of platelets that have been stimulated in vivo may account for the decreased platelet aggregation after smoking that has been observed by several groups of investigators (Chao et al 1982, László et al 1983, van der Giessen et al 1983, Meade et al 1985, Nowak et al 1987, Foo et al 1991).

Other investigators have reported an enhancement of platelet responses immediately after smoking (Hawkins 1972, Levine 1973, Bierenbaum et al 1978, Renaud et al 1984, Schmidt & Rasmussen 1984, Davis et al 1989). Beswick et al (1991) have noted that these seemingly contradictory results may be related to their observation of hyposensitivity of the platelets of abstaining habitual smokers, and an acute potentiation of platelet activity upon smoking. A male/female difference has also been noted with female smokers tending to have an enhanced aggregation response to ADP, and male smokers having a depressed response (Zatta & Prosdocimi 1990). In dogs with mechanically stenosed, injured coronary arteries, cigarette smoke increased the rate and frequency of blood flow reductions resulting from the formation of platelet-rich thrombi (Keller & Folts 1988). In this model, smoke from a non-tobacco-burning cigarette also exacerbated acute thrombus formation (Gering & Folts 1990).

From the studies of the 'Pathobiological Determinants of Atherosclerosis in Youth (PDAY) Research Group' (McGill 1990) in which information is being collected about atherosclerotic lesions in the aortae, right coronary arteries, and blood of American males 15 to 34 years of age who die of violent causes, it is apparent from measurements of the postmortem serum thiocyanate concentration (a marker of smoking) that smoking is strongly associated with prevalence of raised lesions, particularly in the abdominal aorta. In the 390 young males in this study, the effect of smoking was not explained by lipoprotein levels. However, attempts to demonstrate an effect of smoking on atherosclerosis in experimental animals have been largely unsuccessful, leading McGill (1988) to raise the possibility that the human response to smoking is unique.

Compared with nonsmokers, smokers have lower levels of HDL cholesterol, higher levels of plasma fibrinogen, greater plasma viscosity and a higher haematocrit (Pooling Project Research Group 1978, Meade 1987, Feher et al 1990). Feher et al (1990) have demonstrated changes toward more normal values as early as 2 weeks after complete cessation of smoking, and point out that these factors are important in both atherogenesis and thrombogenesis. A number of studies have shown that smokers who cease smoking after a myocardial infarction have a reduced risk of death, compared with those who continue to smoke (Åberg et al 1983, Mulcahy 1983, Hermanson et al 1988). Results from the Coronary Artery Surgery Study (CASS) have shown that smoking cessation lessens the risk of death or myocardial infarction in older as well as younger persons with coronary artery disease (Hermanson et al 1988). In the Framingham Heart Study of 4255 men and women, stroke risk decreased significantly by 2 years and was at the level of nonsmokers by 5 years after cessation of smoking (Wolf et al 1988). It seems unlikely that smoking cessation would induce significant regression of atherosclerotic lesions in a few years, although their progression may be slowed. Therefore, since at least some of the effects of smoking appear to be acute rather than cumulative, the main consequence of the cessation of smoking is probably a lessening of the formation of thrombi that are responsible for many of the clinical complications of atherosclerosis.

Barry et al (1989) have carried out an investigation of the effect of smoking on the activity of ischaemic heart disease in patients with stable angina pectoris and positive exercise tolerance tests. The patients wore a Holter monitor so that 'silent' ischaemic events were recorded during everyday activities. Quantification of the amount of ischaemic ST segment depression showed that the smokers had three times the frequency of episodes of ischaemia and that the duration of ischaemia was 12 times longer in smokers than in nonsmokers. Although Cohn (1989) has suggested that these findings could be due to vasoconstriction, they may also indicate fewer thromboembolic events in nonsmokers.

For many years, the relationship between cigarette smoking and stroke was not clear, but recently, several different approaches have indicated that smoking is an independent risk factor. By arteriography, both intracranial and extracranial atherosclerosis and stenosis of carotid arteries have been found to be greater in smokers than in nonsmokers (Homer et al 1991, Ingall et al 1991). In a study of identical twins who were discordant for smoking, carotid atherosclerosis was greater in the smokers (Haapanen et al 1989). In these studies, the effect of smoking was evident even after taking into account the influence of other risk factors for stroke such as hypertension, age, and concentration of LDL cholesterol. Meta-analysis of 32 separate studies also showed an excess risk of stroke for smokers (Shinton & Beevers 1989).

Diabetes

Both insulin-dependent (type I) and non-insulin-dependent (type II) diabetes mellitus accelerate the development of microvascular and macrovascular disease and lead to a high risk of the clinical complications of atherosclerosis (Colwell 1988). The diabetic state influences the cardiovascular system in a number of ways:

- The endothelium is damaged
- Components of the vessel wall such as collagen are non-enzymatically glycosylated
- Platelet responses to some aggregating agents are enhanced
- The concentrations of fibrinogen, vWf and immune complexes in plasma are elevated
- Plasma lipids, particularly cholesterol, are increased (Colwell 1988).

Evidence for damage to the endothelium by high levels

of blood glucose is both direct and indirect. Abnormally high levels of vWf are found in the plasma of patients with diabetic microangiopathy (Porta 1988) and in diabetic patients without clinical complications (Colwell 1988). Since vWf is stored in the Weibel–Palade bodies of endothelial cells and is released upon stimulation of endothelial cells, elevated levels in plasma are indicative of alteration of the endothelium. On the surface of endothelial cells that have released vWf, the adhesive protein, P-selectin (GMP-140) is detectable (McEver 1991a). This P-selectin is on the inner membrane of the Weibel–Palade bodies and becomes part of the plasma membrane of the endothelial cells when the contents of these bodies are released. P-selectin serves as a receptor for leukocytes which may further damage the endothelium (McEver 1991b).

Other indirect evidence for damage to endothelial cells in the diabetic state are the reports of their decreased ability to synthesize PGI_2 in both experimental animals and in the umbilical vessels of infants of diabetic mothers (Setty & Stuart 1986, Colwell et al 1988). This decreased synthetic ability may be secondary to repeated stimulation or injury of the endothelium; however, PGI_2 synthesis by endothelial cells in culture is inhibited by serum from diabetic patients (Paton et al 1982, Aanderud et al 1985) so there may be other effects as well. Decreased production of plasminogen activator has also been reported, although contradictory observations have been made (Colwell 1988).

Direct evidence for non-denuding endothelial cell injury comes from examination of intimal changes in rabbit aortae after the induction of diabetes by injection of alloxan (Hadcock et al 1991). By 2 weeks, white blood cells, platelets, and fibrin-like material were observed on the surface of the endothelium. Increased endothelial cell replication was demonstrated by the uptake of tritiated thymidine, and proliferation of smooth muscle cells was evident at later times.

Damage to endothelial cells would result in earlier and more rapid development of atherosclerotic lesions and their progression would be potentiated by the abnormal lipid composition of the plasma. A role for endothelial injury is likely because the severity of atherosclerosis in diabetic patients is greater than would be predicted if the abnormalities of lipoproteins were solely responsible.

If the endothelium is disrupted so that subendothelial constituents are exposed, the glycosylated collagen in the vessel wall of diabetic patients may enhance platelet adhesion and aggregation on the denuded surface since platelets interact more strongly with glycosylated collagen than with non-glycosylated collagen (Le Papé et al 1983a,b). The increased plasma levels of vWf also promote platelet adhesion to the subendothelium.

Platelets from diabetic patients and experimental animals are hypersensitive in vitro to aggregation and release of granule contents induced by a number of agonists. Many studies have shown that these platelets synthesize more TXA_2 than platelets from normal individuals (Colwell 1988), but this increased TXA_2 formation is not responsible for all of the hypersensitivity since platelet responses to thrombin are abnormally strong even when the formation of TXA_2 has been blocked with aspirin (Winocour et al 1986). An elevated basal level of intracellular Ca^{2+} has been reported in platelets from diabetic patients (Tschöpe et al 1991), and could account for some of their enhanced responses. There are also reports of depressed responses of platelets from diabetic subjects to the inhibitory effects of PGI_2 and other inhibitors that increase the concentration of cyclic AMP in platelets (Betteridge et al 1982, Onodera et al 1982, Livingstone et al 1991).

In vivo, increased activation of platelets in diabetic patients is apparent from elevated plasma levels of β-thromboglobulin and platelet factor 4; these are platelet-specific proteins that are secreted from the α granules upon the interaction of platelets with release-inducing agents (Colwell 1988 and Ch. 6). The accompanying secretion of growth factors for smooth muscle cells from these granules may play a part in lesion development. Platelet survival is shortened in diabetic subjects and experimental animals (Ferguson et al 1975, Paton 1979, Tindall et al 1981) which may indicate increased interactions of platelets with damaged vessel walls.

Enhancement of platelet function in diabetic patients probably has more effect on the increased incidence of the thromboembolic complications of vascular disease than on its development. However, if more and larger thrombi form because of platelet hypersensitivity, when the thrombi are incorporated into the vessel wall they would have a greater effect on vessel wall thickening and narrowing of the lumen.

Treatment of insulin-dependent diabetic patients with insulin has been shown to control many of the abnormalities of platelet function, reduce the concentrations of plasma vWf and fibrinogen, and restore PGI_2 formation toward normal (Colwell 1988). Diabetic control as measured by glycosylated haemoglobin A_{1c} shows a significant correlation with microvascular disease (e.g. retinopathy) (Klein et al 1988), but not with macrovascular disease in type II diabetic subjects (Nielsen & Ditzel 1985).

The hyperinsulinaemia that occurs in some non-insulin-dependent diabetic patients also appears to accelerate the development of atherosclerosis, possibly by stimulating smooth muscle cell replication (Stolar 1988, Haffner et al 1989).

Hypertension

Hypertension is considered to be a risk factor for the clinical complications of atherosclerosis (Kannel 1991), although Roberts (1989) has pointed out that its effect is probably to accelerate the development of lesions when cholesterol levels are above 150 mg/Dl. Hypertensive experimental animals given atherogenic diets develop more atherosclerotic lesions than normotensive animals given such diets, and hypertensive individuals have more clinical complications of atherosclerosis than normotensive individuals with similar plasma lipoprotein profiles. Injury of the endothelium appears to be the main effect of hypertension. Chobanian et al (1984) observed that white cells, but not platelets, adhere to altered endothelial cells in rats in which chronic hypertension has been induced. If the arterial circulation is connected to the pulmonary circulation, thus subjecting it to arterial pressure, severe damage occurs and thrombi form (Downing et al 1963). Hypertension has been implicated in shear-related injury of arteries (Dzau 1990, Jones et al 1990). In addition, endothelium-mediated vasodilation is impaired in patients with hypertension (Panza et al 1990).

Platelets of hypertensive patients have elevated levels of cytosolic calcium (Erne et al 1984, Resink et al 1988, Schiffl 1989), and enhanced sensitivity to some activators (Erne et al 1985).

Stress and catecholamines

There has been considerable speculation that stress, or type A personality, is important in the development of arterial disease and its thromboembolic complications (Siltanen 1987, Dimsdale 1988). The controversy concerning whether or not type A personality is a risk factor may be attributable to imprecise definitions of the characteristics leading to this designation. The effects of emotional stress are less controversial (Siltanen 1987). It appears that psychosocial stress in atherosclerotic monkeys does lead to changes in endothelial cells, and exacerbated coronary artery atherosclerosis, and that these effects can be prevented by β-adrenergic blockers (Kaplan et al 1987, Strawn et al 1991). In rats, stressful stimuli cause structural changes in the arterial intima (Gordon et al 1981). Adrenaline and noradrenaline released during stress may have several effects: these include strong potentiation of platelet aggregation in response to all aggregating agents (Kinlough-Rathbone & Mustard 1986, Hourani & Cusack 1991), vessel wall damage (Hoff & Gottlob 1967, Constantinides & Robinson 1969), and coronary artery spasm (Joris & Majno 1981). Direct effects in vivo were demonstrated by studies in pigs with extracorporeal shunts in which infusion of adrenaline enhanced thrombosis in the shunts (Rowsell et al 1966). Thus increased catecholamine levels associated with stress may potentiate spasm, vessel injury, and the formation of platelet-rich thrombi.

In man, evidence of platelet activation has been observed when subjects have been placed in stressful situations (Rostrup et al 1990, Grignani et al 1991). Stress associated with the threat of unemployment has been shown to increase serum cholesterol levels in men (Mattiasson et al 1990).

Homocysteinaemia

Homocysteinaemia, caused by a deficiency of the enzyme cystathionine β-synthase, is an autosomal recessive trait. Homozygous individuals exhibit premature atherosclerotic disease in coronary, cerebral and peripheral vessels, and also venous thrombosis (McCully 1990). Heterozygotes have a milder form of the disease and may constitute 1–2% of the population (Clarke et al 1991). Less commonly, disorders of homocysteine remethylation, or deficiencies of vitamin B_{12}, folic acid or pyridoxine may be responsible for homocysteinaemia (Wilcken & Dudman 1989, Malinow 1990). Homocysteinaemia is recognized as an independent risk factor for vascular disease (McCully 1990, Clarke et al 1991). It is believed that the elevated serum levels of homocysteine damage the endothelium and thus accelerate the formation of atherosclerotic lesions and induce injury sites that serve as foci to initiate thromboembolic events (Harker et al 1976).

Viruses

The effects of viruses on platelets and on arterial walls are not well understood. Several viruses cause platelet aggregation and the release of granule contents (Terada et al 1966, Sottnek et al 1975, Larke et al 1977, Bik et al 1982), and thrombocytopenia has been noted as a complication of mumps (Graham et al 1974) and as a feature of hog cholera in which both platelets and the endothelium are damaged (Weiss et al 1973).

Burch (1974) has suggested that viral infections could be an important initiating cause of vascular lesions in both children and adults. It has been established that infection of normocholesterolaemic chickens with Marek's disease virus, a herpes virus, leads to extensive atherosclerosis (Fabricant et al 1983). Cholesterol and cholesteryl ester accumulation has been observed in the aortae of virus-infected chickens and in cultured arterial smooth muscle cells (Fabricant et al 1981, Hajjar et al 1986). These findings led to the recent interest in the role of viruses in the initiation or acceleration of atherosclerotic lesions which has centred around cytomegalovirus (CMV), a member of the herpes virus group, and herpes simplex virus (Yamashiroya et al 1988, Hendrix et al 1989, Melnick et al 1990, Bruggeman & van Dam-Mieras 1991). By in situ DNA hybridization and the avidin-biotin complex immunoperoxidase method, these viruses were detected in association with areas exhibiting early or advanced atherosclerosis in the coronary arteries and with lesion-free as well as lesion areas in the thoracic aorta of young trauma victims (Yamashiroya et al 1988). Altered cholesterol metabolism and accumulation of cholesterol in human arterial smooth muscle cells in culture has been found to be induced by herpes virus (Hajjar & Grant 1986) High levels of CMV antibody have been found in patients with atherosclerosis requiring vascular surgery (Adam et al 1987).

Experiments in which endothelial cells in culture were infected with herpes simplex virus have demonstrated that their nonthrombogenic nature is altered in several ways (van Dam-Mieras et al 1987, Visser et al 1988, Key et al 1990). Formation of the prothrombinase complex on the surface of the cells was enhanced, leading to thrombin generation and platelet attachment; PGI_2 production in response to thrombin was greatly diminished; surface thrombomodulin activity was decreased; and tissue factor synthesis was increased. All of these changes would be expected to result in the deposition of thrombi. Infection of endothelial cell monolayers with herpes viruses also causes an increased adherence of leukocytes, both monocytes and polymorphonuclear leukocytes, which may be an early event in damage of endothelial cells (Span et al 1991).

The immune system and atherogenesis

Early results from the PDAY study (Wissler 1991) indicate that atherogenesis in some young people in whom circulating immune complexes are detectable is likely to be accelerated, even when few or no classic risk factors are present. Although the involvement of the immune system in human atherogenesis is undergoing intensive investigation, it is not known whether it has a primary role, or whether the antigenic stimulus arises secondarily and contributes only to lesion progression (Libby & Hansson 1991). An immune mechanism, however, may cause the accelerated atherosclerosis that develops in the coronary arteries of transplanted hearts (Hansson et al 1989, Libby et al 1989).

Activated T-lymphocytes of different types have been found in human atheromata (Jonasson et al 1986, Libby & Hansson 1991), as well as γ-interferon (IFN-γ), a product of their activation (Hansson et al 1989). As Libby & Hansson (1991) point out, the finding of activated T cells implies antigenic stimulation, but the nature of the antigen or antigens has not been determined; a number of suggestions have been made. The focal nature of the accumulation of leukocytes at sites where atherosclerosis develops also requires an explanation. The complement system also appears to be activated locally within atherosclerotic plaques (Vlaicu et al 1985, Seifert & Hansson 1989), and products of this pathway may cause chemotaxis of leukocytes and their adherence to endothelial cells. Endothelial-leukocyte adhesion molecules (ELAMs), as well as interleukin-1, tissue necrosis factor and IFN-γ appear to be involved in the regulation of leukocyte adhesion (Libby & Hansson 1991).

The interaction of interleukin-1 and tissue necrosis factor with endothelial cells may also have accelerating effects on coagulation (Bevilacqua et al 1984, Stern et al 1985).

Oestrogen and oral contraceptives

The obvious difference between men and women in the occurrence of the clinical complications of atherosclerosis, up to the age of 45, has been attributed to a protective effect of oestrogen in premenopausal women (Bush et al 1988, Barrett-Conner & Bush 1991). This difference appears to be related to a slower rate of progression of atherosclerotic lesions in these women (Witteman et al 1989) rather than to differences in vessel wall injury, platelet reactivity, or coagulation. Emphasis has been placed on the decrease in HDL cholesterol and increase in LDL cholesterol that accompany menopause (Matthews et al 1989) and the reverse effects that result from the administration of oestrogen to postmenopausal women (Bush et al 1988, Knopp 1988). Administration of oestrogen to cholesterol-fed rabbits has been shown to increase HDL cholesterol and to inhibit the development of atherosclerotic lesions (Henriksson et al 1989). A further beneficial effect of oestrogen replacement therapy has been shown in ovariectomized cynomolgus monkeys in which the constrictor responses of atherosclerotic coronary arteries were observed to be modulated (Williams et al 1990). In women with coronary artery disease documented by angiography, oestrogen replacement after menopause has been reported to prolong survival (Sullivan et al 1990). A Mayo Clinic population-based, case-control study showed that oestrogen use reduced myocardial infarction and sudden death of women 40 to 59 years of age (Beard et al 1989). The 10-year follow-up of the Nurses' Health Study showed a reduction in the incidence of coronary heart disease and mortality from cardiovascular disease, but no change in the risk of stroke, with current oestrogen use (Stampfer et al 1991).

The oral contraceptive formulations in the 1960s and 1970s had relatively high doses of synthetic oestrogens, combined with progestins, and were associated with an increased risk of venous thromboembolism, acute myocardial infarction, and stroke (Bush et al 1988). However, even the current formulations which contain much less oestrogen are reported to adversely affect lipids and lipoproteins because of the content of progestins (Bush et al 1988). Nevertheless, past use of oral contraceptives does not appear to increase the risk of subsequent complications of cardiovascular disease (Stampfer et al 1988), as would be expected if the progression of atherosclerosis had been enhanced by the decrease in HDL cholesterol and the increase in LDL cholesterol. In experiments with female cynomolgus macaques with diet-induced atherosclerosis, Adams et al (1990) observed that although

HDL cholesterol was lowered, atherosclerosis was not increased by the oral contraceptive they administered. They concluded that ethinyloestradiol neutralized the atherogenic effect of the progestin component of the oral contraceptive.

The greater risk of venous thromboembolism seems to occur only during the use of oral contraceptives (Vessey et al 1986), probably indicating effects on the coagulation system. Analysis of plasma from women taking oral contraceptives shows higher than normal amounts of fibrinogen and fibrinopeptide A, decreased antithrombin III, and an altered fibrinolytic system (Inauen et al 1987, Leuven et al 1987). Increased formation of platelet-fibrin thrombi from flowing blood of oral contraceptive users has been demonstrated ex vivo (Inauen et al 1987); both enhanced platelet reactivity and increased formation of fibrin can be inferred from these observations. Synergistic effects of oral contraceptive use with other risk factors, such as smoking, that also affect platelets and coagulation have been well documented, but the risk of myocardial infarction appears to be limited to women who smoke (Mishell 1988, Thorneycroft 1990). The cause of myocardial infarction in these women is thrombotic, rather than atherosclerotic.

THROMBOEMBOLISM AND DISTURBANCES OF THE MICROCIRCULATION

A number of agents and conditions cause the formation of intravascular platelet-fibrin thrombi, or thrombi attached to sites of vascular injury. Mural thrombi may embolize into the microcirculation, or thrombi may be formed in it. In either case, obstruction of blood flow causes ischaemia and tissue damage. In addition, materials released from platelets can injure the endothelium.

Emboli

A well-documented example of embolic phenomena affecting the microcirculation involves mural thrombi in diseased carotid arteries which release embolic fragments of platelet aggregates or platelet-fibrin thrombi into the microcirculation of the eye and brain. These can be seen passing through the microcirculation of the retina, associated with transient disturbances of vision (Fisher 1959, Russell 1961, Gunning et al 1964). Such aggregates in the microcirculation of the brain are considered to be responsible for transient attacks of cerebral ischaemia (TIAs) (Barnett 1976). Since the frequency of these TIAs can be reduced by aspirin (Dutch TIA Trial Study Group 1991), it is considered that TXA_2 from the platelets may constrict microcirculatory vessels and promote the accumulation of emboli in the microcirculation (see Ch. 55).

Platelet emboli in the microcirculation have been implicated in some cases of sudden death in humans with advanced coronary artery atherosclerosis (Frink et al 1978, Haerem 1978, El Maraghi & Genton 1980, Forrester 1991, Verheugt & Brugada 1991). Early studies in pigs and dogs showed that embolization of the microcirculation of the heart is associated with sudden death, and areas of myocarditis and atrophy similar to the lesions in humans who die suddenly from an acute coronary artery episode (Jørgensen et al 1967b, Moore et al 1981).

Postmortem studies have indicated that some chronic nephrosclerosis in older humans could be caused by embolic material passing into the renal circulation from mural thrombi in the aorta proximal to the renal arteries (Moore & Mersereau 1968).

Emboli or microthrombi are often found in the pulmonary microcirculation. Some of these may originate from thrombi in the leg veins. During bypass operations, small thrombi may form in blood circulating extracorporeally and impact in the lung. In experimental animals, intravenous injection of platelet aggregating agents such as arachidonate, thrombin or collagen causes acute respiratory distress and death as the aggregates block the microcirculation of the lung (Kohler et al 1976, Honey et al 1986). In man also, platelet aggregates in the pulmonary circulation have been implicated as a cause of death (Pirkle & Carstens 1974).

Embolization of the arterial circulation of the lower limbs from proximal atherosclerotic lesions occurs. The emboli can be derived from thrombi or cholesterol-rich debris from ulcerated atherosclerotic plaques (Kempczinski 1979).

Red blood cells and haemolysis

Red blood cells can promote thrombosis in at least four ways.

1. Physical effects on platelets that force them toward the vessel wall (Goldsmith & Karino 1982, Aarts et al 1988, Turitto 1988, Bell et al 1990).
2. Haemolysis that results in loss of ADP, causing platelet aggregation (Born & Wehmeier 1979, Brown & Harrison 1988).
3. Haemolysis that makes negatively charged phospholipids available on the surface of the cells, thus accelerating the intrinsic pathway of coagulation.
4. Increases in cyclo-oxygenase and lipoxygenase metabolites upon stimulation of platelet-red cell mixtures with collagen or thrombin (Santos et al 1991).

Intravascular haemolysis can be produced in a variety of ways. It has been noted in association with incompatible blood transfusion, paroxysmal nocturnal haemoglobinuria, haemolytic anaemias, and sickle cell disease. High shear can also damage red blood cells sufficiently to cause the loss of ADP (Schmid-Schönbein et al 1981, Reimers et al 1984).

Microangiopathic haemolytic anaemia. The formation of fibrin in the microcirculation leads to microangiopathic haemolytic anaemia (Brain 1972). This form of anaemia is not uncommon in conjunction with disseminated intravascular coagulation, and is often associated with thrombotic thrombocytopenic purpura, the haemolytic uraemic syndrome, and polyarteritis nodosa. Red blood cells passing through fibrin strands are fragmented by the strands, resulting in haemolysis (Bull & Brain 1968).

Haemolytic-uraemic syndrome. Haemolytic anaemia, thrombocytopenia, and acute renal failure are characteristic of the haemolytic-uraemic syndrome (HUS). Although the aetiology is not known, and different diseases may lead to the syndrome, HUS has similarities to the Shwartzman reaction and to thrombotic thrombocytopenic purpura (Ruggenenti & Remuzzi 1990). Damage to the kidneys is a direct consequence of intravascular coagulation. Drummond (1985) points out the central importance of endothelial cell damage, and calls attention to the clear association between some cases of HUS and *Escherichia coli* that produce verotoxin and *Shigella dysenteriae* that produce shiga toxin (Karmali et al 1983). The disappearance of the largest vWf multimers from plasma has been observed concurrently with thrombocytopenia in about 50% of patients during severe episodes of HUS, and this finding has led to the suggestion that platelet aggregation mediated by large vWf multimers occurs in the renal vessels (Moake 1988).

Sickle cell disease. Vascular occlusion in sickle cell disease is usually attributed to sickled erythrocytes, but other mechanisms may also operate (Francis & Johnson 1991). Intimal hyperplasia and thrombosis have been noted, particularly in the cerebral arterial vasculature, and have been recognized as important factors in stroke in patients with sickle cell disease. Pulmonary thrombosis and thromboembolism have also been reported. Changes in the coagulation system, and in natural inhibitors of coagulation, increase thrombin generation and fibrin formation in this disease, and platelet activation is indicated by increased plasma levels of β-thromboglobulin and TXB_2 (Francis & Johnson 1991).

Thrombotic thrombocytopenic purpura

Thrombotic thrombocytopenic purpura (TTP) is a rare condition in which platelet-rich thrombi are found in the microcirculation of virtually all organs of the body (Lian 1988, Schmidt 1989, Ruggenenti & Remuzzi 1990). The causes are unknown and may be diverse; associations have been observed with infections, pregnancy, toxins, drugs, cancer, organ transplantation, and collagen vascular disorders. It is not known whether vascular damage is the initiating event or results from intravascular platelet agglutination or aggregation. The involvement of plasma factors is indicated by the dramatic benefit of plasma infusion or plasma exchange (Schmidt 1989). Sera from TTP patients were reported to mediate immune destruction of human endothelial cells in culture (Burns & Zucker-Franklin 1982), but Lian (1988) points out that the evidence for immune-mediated vascular injury in TTP is weak. Damage to the endothelium may be caused in other ways.

There may be several pathogenetic mechanisms. A 37 kDa platelet-agglutinating protein has been purified from the plasma of a subset of patients with TTP and shown to cause platelet agglutination through binding to glycoprotein IV (Lian et al 1991). However, vWf, particularly unusually large multimers (ULvWf), has also been implicated in the formation of the platelet thrombi. ULvWf multimers are present, during remission, in the platelet-poor plasma of the rare patients who have the chronic relapsing type of TTP (Moake 1988). These ULvWf multimers, in the presence of ADP (or presumably with other agonists that make GPIIb/IIIa able to bind adhesive proteins), can cause platelet aggregation when fluid shear forces are high, as they are in the microcirculation (Moake et al 1988). A failure of 'ULvWf processing activity' to produce vWf multimers of the sizes normally present in plasma has been suggested in these patients with chronic relapsing TTP (Moake 1988). In addition, an inciting vWf cofactor for platelet aggregation, present intermittently, has been postulated as present in the plasma of patients with this type of TTP, in which relapses often occur in association with infection or injury (Moake 1988).

In acute, nonrelapsing TTP, extensive damage of the endothelium is indicated by the brief appearance of ULvWf multimers in plasma soon after the onset of TTP. These multimers disappear as thrombi form, and the thrombi stain strongly for vWf, but only weakly for fibrinogen (Asada et al 1985). (This observation differs from the finding of fibrin-rich platelet thrombi in disseminated intravascular coagulation.) However, other explanations for the decrease in large vWf multimers in acute TTP have been suggested (Lian 1988), and TTP plasma that has been depleted of vWf is capable of agglutinating platelets. The platelet-rich thrombi that are formed in TTP are resistant to fibrinolysis, possibly because of the platelet content of inhibitors of plasminogen activator and plasmin (Kwaan 1987). In addition, damage of the endothelium may result in localized absence of fibrinolysis.

Moore et al (1990) have detected abnormally high levels of calpain in the serum of patients with TTP and have proposed that calpain proteolysis of vWf enhances its binding to GPIIb/IIIa, but this suggestion is difficult to reconcile with that of Moake (1988).

Adult respiratory distress syndrome

In the adult respiratory distress syndrome (ARDS), the

endothelial cells of the lung are injured and the coagulation system is activated (Hasleton 1983). Activated platelets have been detected in the circulation (George et al 1986). Complement activation and elevated levels of plasma C5a are considered to be involved in the formation of mixed aggregates of platelets and polymorphonuclear leukocytes (Hammerschmidt et al 1980, Ferrer-Lopez et al 1990, Damerau et al 1991) and tissue damage by the neutrophils appears to play a role.

Systemic lupus erythematosus

Systemic lupus erythematosus (SLE) is associated with recurrent thrombocytopenia and both venous and arterial thrombosis (Hamsten & Norberg 1989). Circulating antibodies to negatively charged phospholipids (lupus anticoagulant and anticardiolipin antibodies) occur in patients with this condition, but the correlation with an increase in the occurrence of arterial thrombosis is weak (Hamsten & Norberg 1989, Jouhikainen et al 1990). Spontaneous platelet aggregation has been observed (Wiener et al 1991). The early suggestion of an imbalance of TXA_2/PGI_2 synthesis as a cause of thrombosis in SLE has not been substantiated by more recent studies (Hasselaar et al 1988, Lellouche et al 1991). It is not clear that the antiphospholipid antibodies are responsible for platelet activation because antibodies against a platelet protein have also been reported to be associated with a higher risk of thrombosis in SLE patients (Jouhikainen et al 1990) and Bevers et al (1991) have observed that lupus anticoagulant antibodies are not directed to phospholipids alone, but appear to recognize a complex of lipid-bound prothrombin.

Bacteria, endotoxin and disseminated intravascular coagulation (DIC)

Activation of coagulation, leukopenia and thrombocytopenia, which may or may not be associated with thrombi in the microcirculation, are seen with some bacterial infections, particularly with Gram-negative bacteria (Guckian 1975, Rowe et al 1978, Wilson et al 1982), although platelets can also interact with Gram-positive bacteria (Beachey & Stollerman 1971, Clawson & White 1971). Many bacteria have the ability to induce platelet aggregation and the release of granule contents in vitro and in vivo (Herzberg et al 1983, 1990, Timmons et al 1986, Sullam et al 1988, Kessler et al 1991). In a study of strains of *Staphylococcus aureus* by Kessler et al (1987), the degree and rapidity of platelet aggregation in vitro was shown to correlate with the clinical occurrence of DIC and subacute bacterial endocarditis.

The α-toxin of *Staph. aureus* causes the assembly of the prothrombinase complex on platelets, resulting in the generation of thrombin (Bhakdi et al 1988, Arvand et al 1990). Interleukin-1 is released by monocytes that are exposed to α-toxin (Bhakdi et al 1989).

The endotoxin (lipopolysaccharide) formed from Gram-negative bacteria can cause DIC, obstruction of the microcirculation, and fibrin accumulation in the renal glomeruli (Müller-Berghaus 1978, Wilson et al 1982). There are a number of reports that endotoxin can injure the endothelium (Pesonen et al 1981, Harlan et al 1983, Meyrick & Brigham 1983, Reidy & Schwartz 1983). Bacterial endotoxin, like the cytokines interleukin-1, tumour necrosis factor and lymphotoxin, causes endothelial cells to synthesize and express leukocyte adhesion molecules (E-LAMS) (Bevilacqua et al 1987, Cybulsky & Gimbrone 1991) (p. 1109). Other actions of endotoxin include suppression of thrombomodulin expression on endothelial cells (Moore et al 1987), generation of tissue thromboplastin activity (Brox et al 1984) by increasing the cell surface activity of tissue factor (Colucci et al 1983), induction of the synthesis and release of plasminogen activator inhibitor (Colucci et al 1985), release of vWf in vivo (Gralnick et al 1989), and stimulation of the production of PGI_2 by cultured endothelial cells (Nawroth et al 1984, Watanabe et al 1989).

In the Shwartzman reaction, fibrin is localized in the kidneys. Experimentally, the classical Shwartzman reaction occurs following one endotoxin injection when the reticuloendothelial system has been depressed; it also occurs when two injections of endotoxin are given fairly close to each other in time (Mustard & Packham 1979).

DIC is discussed in Chapter 42.

Serum sickness and immune complexes

Vascular injury occurs in association with the immune complexes that form in serum sickness (Cochrane 1971, Minick et al 1978, Stills et al 1983). Deposition of IgG-containing immune complexes in vessel walls results in the activation of complement and attachment of monocytes and neutrophils, leading to tissue injury (Gilliland 1984). In addition, immune complexes can cause platelet aggregation (Henson & Ginsberg 1981, Pfueller 1985). It has been proposed that platelets contribute to the vascular injury by releasing serotonin and permeability factors and facilitating immune complex deposition (Kniker & Cochrane 1968, Hayslett 1984, Barnes et al 1990). However, many of the studies of serum sickness in experimental animals have involved the injection of albumin preparations that were contaminated with endotoxin which causes damage to endothelial cells. When endotoxin-free albumin was used, although immune complexes formed, interacted with platelets and shortened platelet survival, morphological evidence of vascular injury was not detectable (Parbtani et al 1990). There may also be species differences since, in the studies of Massmann et al (1987), injections of foreign serum induced immune vasculitis and accelerated the development of atherosclerotic lesions in rabbits, but injections of the same foreign serum into swine failed to produce these effects.

Myeloproliferative disorders and tumour cells

Thrombosis (and bleeding) have been described in the myeloproliferative disorders, e.g. polycythaemia vera, essential thrombocythaemia (Schafer 1984, Wehmeier et al 1991).

Most tumour cell lines and tumour tissues activate platelets and cause their aggregation, although the sensitivity of the platelets varies from donor to donor (Jamieson et al 1987). Several mechanisms have been reported for tumour cell-induced aggregation, including thrombin generated through tumour cell procoagulant activity, ADP released from tumour cells, a trypsin-sensitive surface protein on tumour cells, and a reaction requiring complement, a plasma factor, divalent cation, and a sialo-lipoprotein vesicular component of the tumour cell membrane (Lerner et al 1983, Jamieson et al 1987, Katagiri et al 1991). Since both the coagulation system and platelets can be activated by tumour cells, it is not surprising that DIC and thrombosis are associated with some forms of malignancy (Rickles & Edwards 1983, Dvorak 1987). A number of studies have implicated platelets in tumour cell metastasis (Jamieson et al 1987, Menter et al 1987, Karpatkin et al 1988, Katagiri et al 1991).

Thermal injury

According to Alkjaersig and colleagues (1980), thrombosis is an invariable reaction to a severe burn and thromboembolism frequently occurs later: microthrombi are found in the lungs and kidneys. Both vessel wall injury (Lazarus & Hutto 1982, Xuewei & Wanrhong 1983) and chronic activation of coagulation contribute to thrombus formation. DIC is often observed (Eurenius et al 1974, Wells et al 1984). Vascular injury is also a consequence of frostbite (Lazarus & Hutto 1982) and DIC may occur during rewarming following hypothermia (Mahajan et al 1981).

In heat stroke, endothelial cell damage and DIC contribute to the high mortality (Hart et al 1980, Chao et al 1981). Platelet responses to ADP in platelet-rich plasma from heat stroke patients ranged from being hypersensitive to being depressed in the study of Gader et al (1990). Decreased responsiveness in vitro may be attributable to a refractory state of platelets that have been stimulated in vivo.

Artificial surfaces and thrombosis

The development of a variety of prosthetic devices that are exposed to blood has stimulated studies of the effect of artificial surfaces on thrombus formation (Packham 1988, see also Ch. 58). Thrombus formation is a major complication of artificial heart valves, vascular catheters, cardiopulmonary oxygenators, dialysis membranes, left ventricular devices, vascular grafts, and charcoal columns used in haemoperfusion.

Contrast agents

Both ionic and non-ionic contrast agents used in angiography can cause the formation of thrombi (Grabowski & De Caterina 1991, Wiesel et al 1991).

DRUGS AND THROMBOSIS

Many chemicals, constituents of foods, and drugs affect platelet function (Packham & Mustard 1983, George & Shattil 1991, also Ch. 8). Among these are the anticoagulants that inhibit the formation of thrombin or its activity. These anticoagulants are noteworthy because they inhibit both thrombin-induced platelet aggregation and the formation of fibrin.

CONCLUSIONS

The risk factors for atherogenesis are not identical to the risk factors for the thromboembolic complications of atherosclerosis. Focal lesions of atherosclerosis show a distribution related to blood flow patterns and lesions can develop as a result of repeated vessel wall injury as well as high levels of cholesterol and saturated fat. Arterial thrombi are largely made up of platelet aggregates, stabilized by fibrin, and tend to form on ruptured atherosclerotic plaques and at sites of disturbed flow and severe stenosis. The importance of thrombin in the formation of arterial thrombi is receiving more and more attention, although the thrombogenic constituents of the subendothelium and ruptured plaques, as well as ADP, TXA_2, adrenaline and possibly serotonin also contribute. Organization of thrombi on atherosclerotic plaques is responsible for their episodic growth. The reasons for the non-thrombogenic nature of the unstimulated endothelium are not fully understood, but the endothelium is no longer regarded as a passive barrier and its responses to activation and the materials it synthesizes are being recognized. Agents and conditions that stimulate or injure the endothelium and promote thrombosis include hypercholesterolaemia, smoking, diabetes, hypertension, stress, homocysteinaemia, viruses, immune mechanisms and cytokines. The responses of platelets and the coagulation system to severe vessel wall injury are attracting intense interest because of the reocclusion problems associated with bypass surgery, angioplasty and endarterectomy. Details of the platelet reactions that result in the formation of TXA_2, release of granule contents and acceleration of the intrinsic coagulation pathway, as well as methods for detection of thromboembolic processes involving assays for activated platelets and products of the coagulation system are under active investigation. In vivo, stabilization of thrombi, control of their extension by natural anticoagulants, PGI_2, EDRF and fibrinolytic agents, and the effects of blood flow are relevant to whether thrombi persist or break up and embolize into the microcirculation. A number of pathological conditions can cause the formation of thrombi in the microcirculation.

REFERENCES

Aanderud S, Krane H, Nordøy A 1985 Influence of glucose, insulin and sera from diabetic patients on the prostacyclin synthesis in vitro in cultured human endothelial cells. Diabetologia 28: 641–644

Aarts P A M M, van den Broek S A T, Prins G W, Kuiken G D C, Sixma J J, Heethaar R M 1988 Blood platelets are concentrated near the wall and red blood cells, in the center in flowing blood. Arteriosclerosis 8: 819–824

Åberg A, Bergstrand R, Johansson S et al 1983 Cessation of smoking after myocardial infarction. Effects on mortality after 10 years. British Heart Journal 49: 416–422

Abrams C S, Ellison N, Budzynski A Z, Shattil S J 1990 Direct detection of activated platelets and platelet-derived microparticles in humans. Blood 75: 128–138

Abrams C, Shattil S J 1991 Immunological detection of activated platelets in clinical disorders. Thrombosis and Haemostasis 65: 467–473

Adam E, Melnick J L, Probtsfield J L et al 1987 High levels of cytomegalovirus antibody in patients requiring vascular surgery for atherosclerosis. Lancet ii: 291–293

Adams M R, Clarkson T B, Shively C A, Parks J S, Kaplan J R 1990 Oral contraceptives, lipoproteins, and atherosclerosis. American Journal of Obstetrics and Gynecology 163: 1388–1393

Aiken M L, Ginsberg M H, Byers-Ward V, Plow E F 1990 Effects of OKM5, a monoclonal antibody to glycoprotein IV, on platelet aggregation and thrombospondin surface expression. Blood 76: 2501–2509

Albelda S M, Oliver P D, Romer L H, Buck C A 1990 EndoCAM: a novel endothelial cell-cell adhesion molecule. Journal of Cell Biology 110: 1227–1237

Alkjaersig N, Fletcher A P, Peden J C Jr, Monafo W W 1980 Fibrinogen catabolism in burned patients. Journal of Trauma 20: 154–159

Armstrong M L, Heistad D D 1990 Animal models of atherosclerosis. Atherosclerosis 85: 15–23

Arvand M, Bhakdi S, Dahlbäck B, Preissner K T 1990 Staphylococcus aureus α-toxin attack on human platelets promotes assembly of the prothrombinase complex. Journal of Biological Chemistry 265: 14377–14381

Asada Y, Sumiyoshi A, Hayashi T, Suzumiya J, Kaketani K 1985 Immunohistochemistry of vascular lesion in thrombotic thrombocytopenic purpura, with special reference to factor VIII related antigen. Thrombosis Research 38: 469–479

Asch A S, Barnwell J, Silverstein R L, Nachman R L 1987 Isolation of the thrombospondin membrane receptor. Journal of Clinical Investigation 79: 1054–1061

Asmussen I, Kjeldsen K 1975 Intimal ultrastructure of human umbilical arteries. Observations on arteries from newborn children of smoking and nonsmoking mothers. Circulation Research 36: 579–589

Assoian R K, Sporn M B 1986 Type β transforming growth factor in human platelets: release during platelet degranulation and action on vascular smooth muscle cells. Journal of Cell Biology 102: 1217–1223

Austin M A 1991 Plasma triglyceride and coronary heart disease. Arteriosclerosis and Thrombosis 11: 2–14

Aviram M, Brook G J 1982 The effect of human plasma on platelet function in familial hypercholesterolemia. Thrombosis Research 26: 101–109

Badimon L, Badimon J J, Turitto V T, Fuster V 1989 Role of von Willebrand factor in mediating platelet-vessel wall interaction at low shear rate; the importance of perfusion conditions. Blood 73: 961–967

Barnes J L, Camussi G, Tetta C, Venkatachalam M A 1990 Glomerular localization of platelet cationic proteins after immune complex-induced platelet activation. Laboratory Investigation 63: 755–761

Barnett H J M 1976 Pathogenesis of transient ischemic attacks. In: Scheinberg P (ed) Cerebrovascular diseases. Raven Press, New York, p 1–21

Barrett-Connor E, Bush T L 1991 Estrogen and coronary heart disease in women. Journal of American Medical Association 265: 1861–1867

Barry J, Mead K, Nabel E G et al 1989 Effect of smoking on the activity of ischemic heart disease. Journal of American Medical Association 261: 398–402

Baumgartner H R 1972 Platelet interaction with vascular structures. Thrombosis et Diathesis Haemorrhagica (suppl 51) 161–176

Baumgartner H R, Muggli R, Tschopp T B, Turitto V T 1976 Platelet adhesion, release and aggregation in flowing blood: effect of surface properties and platelet function. Thrombosis and Haemostasis 35: 124–138

Beachey E H, Stollerman G H 1971 Toxic effects of streptococcal M protein on platelets and polymorphonuclear leukocytes in human blood. Journal of Experimental Medicine 134: 351–365

Beard C M, Kottke T E, Annegers J F, Ballard D J 1989 The Rochester Coronary Heart Disease Project: effect of cigarette smoking, hypertension, diabetes, and steroidal estrogen use on coronary heart disease among 40- to 59-year old women, 1960 through 1982. Mayo Clinic Proceedings 64: 1471–1480

Becker B F, Terres W, Kratzer M, Gerlach E 1988 Blood platelet function after chronic treatment of rats and guinea pigs with nicotine. Klinische Wochenschrift 66 (suppl XI): 28–36

Bell D N, Spain S, Goldsmith H L 1990 The effect of red blood cells on the ADP-induced aggregation of human platelets in flow through tubes. Thrombosis and Haemostasis 63: 112–121

Benditt E P 1977 Implications of the monoclonal character of human atherosclerotic plaques. American Journal of Pathology 86: 693–702

Benditt E P 1988 Origins of human atherosclerotic plaques. The role of altered gene expression. Archives of Pathology and Laboratory Medicine 112: 997–1001

Berger K, Sauvage L R, Rao A M, Wood S J 1972 Healing of arterial prostheses in man: its incompleteness. Annals of Surgery 175: 118–127

Berman C L, Yeo E L, Wencel-Drake J D, Furie B C, Ginsberg M H, Furie B 1986 A platelet alpha granule membrane protein that is associated with the plasma membrane after activation. Characterization and subcellular localization of platelet activation-dependent granule-external membrane protein. Journal of Clinical Investigation 78: 130–137

Berman H J 1961 Anticoagulant-induced alterations in hemostasis, platelet thrombosis, and vascular fragility in the peripheral vessels of the hamster cheek pouch. In: MacMillan R L, Mustard J F (eds) Anticoagulants and fibrinolysins. MacMillan, Canada, p 95–107

Berridge D C, Perkins A C, Frier M et al 1991 Detection and characterization of arterial thromboses using a platelet-specific monoclonal antibody (P256 Fab′). British Journal of Surgery 78: 1130–1133

Beswick A, Renaud S, Yarnell J W G, Elwood P C 1991 Platelet activity in habitual smokers. Thrombosis and Haemostasis 66: 739

Betteridge D J, El Tahir K E H, Reckless J P D, Williams K I 1982 Platelets from diabetic subjects show diminished sensitivity to prostacyclin. European Journal of Clinical Investigation 12: 395–398

Bevers E M, Rosing J, Zwaal R F A 1987 Platelets and coagulation. In: MacIntyre D E, Gordon J L (eds) Platelets in biology and pathology III. Elsevier Science (Biomedical Division), Amsterdam, p 127–160

Bevers E M, Galli M, Barbui T, Comfurius P, Zwaal R F A 1991 Lupus anticoagulant IgG's (LA) are not directed to phospholipids only, but to a complex of lipid-bound human prothrombin. Thrombosis and Haemostasis 66: 629–632

Bevilacqua M P, Pober J S, Majeau G R, Cotran R S, Gimbrone M A Jr 1984 Interleukin-1 (IL-1) induces biosynthesis and cell surface expression of procoagulant activity in human vascular endothelial cells. Journal of Experimental Medicine 160: 618–623

Bevilacqua M P, Pober J S, Mendrick D L, Cotran R S, Gimbrone M A Jr 1987 Identification of an inducible endothelial-leukocyte adhesion molecule. Proceedings of the National Academy of Sciences, United States of America 84: 9238–9242

Bevilacqua M P, Stengelin S, Gimbrone M A Jr, Seed B 1989 Endothelial leukocyte adhesion molecule 1: an inducible receptor for neutrophils related to complement regulatory proteins and lectins. Science 243: 1160–1165

Bhakdi S, Muhly M, Mannhardt U et al 1988 Staphylococcal α toxin promotes blood coagulation via attack on human platelets. Journal of Experimental Medicine 168: 527–542

Bhakdi S, Muhly M, Korom S, Hugo F 1989 Release of interleukin-1β associated with potent cytocidal action of staphylococcal alpha-toxin on human monocytes. Infection and Immunity 57: 3512–3519

Bierenbaum M L, Fleischman A I, Stier A, Somol S H, Watson P B 1978 Effect of cigarette smoking upon in vivo platelet function in man. Thrombosis Research 12: 1051–1057

Bik T, Sarov I, Livne A 1982 Interaction between vaccinia virus and human blood platelets. Blood 59: 482–487

Booyse F M, Osikowicz G, Radek J 1981a Effects of nicotine on the rabbit aortic endothelium. American Journal of Pathology 102: 229–238

Booyse F M, Osikowicz G, Radek J 1981b Effects of nicotine on cultured bovine aortic endothelial cells. Thrombosis Research 23: 169–185

Born G V R, Wehmeier A 1979 Inhibition of platelet thrombus formation by chlorpromazine acting to diminish haemolysis. Nature 282: 212–213

Boutet M, Bazin M, Turcotte H, Lagacé R 1980 Effects of cigarette smoke on rat thoracic aorta. Artery 7: 56–72

Bradlow B A, Chetty N, Birnbaum M, Baker S G, Seftel H C 1982 Platelet function in familial hypercholesterolemia in South Africa and the effect of probucol. Thrombosis Research 26: 91–99

Brain M C 1972 Microangiopathic haemolytic anaemia (MHA). British Journal of Haematology 23 (suppl): 45–52

Brown P, Harrison M J G 1988 The role of red blood cells in platelet aggregation in whole blood. Atherosclerosis 71: 261–262

Brox J H, Østerud B, Bjørklid E, Fenton J W II 1984 Production and availability of thromboplastin in endothelial cells: the effects of thrombin, endotoxin and platelets. British Journal of Haematology 57: 239–246

Bruggeman C A, van Dam-Mieras M C E 1991 The possible role of cytomegalovirus in atherogenesis. In: Melnick J L (ed) Progress in medical virology. Karger, Basel, vol 38: 1–26

Brüne B, Ullrich V 1987 Inhibition of platelet aggregation by carbon monoxide is mediated by activation of guanylate cyclase. Molecular Pharmacology 32: 497–504

Bull B S, Brain M C 1968 Experimental models of microangiopathic haemolytic anaemia. Proceedings of the Royal Society of Medicine 61: 1134–1138

Bull H A, Pittilo R M, Woolf N, Machin S J 1988 The effect of nicotine on human endothelial cell release of prostaglandins and ultrastructure. British Journal of Experimental Pathology 69: 413–421

Burch G E 1974 Viruses and arteriosclerosis. American Heart Journal 87: 407–412

Burns E R, Zucker-Franklin D 1982 Pathologic effects of plasma from patients with thrombotic thrombocytopenic purpura on platelets and cultured vascular endothelial cells. Blood 60: 1030–1037

Bush T L, Fried L P, Barrett-Connor E 1988 Cholesterol, lipoproteins, and coronary heart disease in women. Clinical Chemistry 34: B60–B70

Cairns J, Gent M, Singer J et al 1985 Aspirin, sulfinpyrazone, or both in unstable angina. Results of a Canadian multicenter trial. New England Journal of Medicine 313: 1369–1375

Capone G J, Meyer B B, Wolf N M, Meister S G 1984 Incidence of intracoronary thrombi in patients with active unstable angina pectoris. Circulation 70 (suppl II): II415

Carvalho A C A, Colman R W, Lees R S 1974 Platelet function in hyperlipoproteinemia. New England Journal of Medicine 290: 434–438

Cattaneo M, Kinlough-Rathbone R L, Lecchi A, Bevilacqua C, Packham M A, Mustard J F 1987 Fibrinogen-independent aggregation and deaggregation of human platelets: studies in two afibrinogenemic patients. Blood 70: 221–226

Cattaneo M, Canciani M T, Lecchi A et al 1990 Released adenosine diphosphate stabilizes thrombin-induced human platelet aggregates. Blood 75: 1081–1086

Chao T C, Sinniah R, Pakiam J E 1981 Acute heat stroke. Pathology 13: 145–156

Chao F C, Tullis J L, Alper C A, Glynn R J, Silbert J E 1982 Alteration in plasma proteins and platelet functions with aging and cigarette smoking in healthy men. Thrombosis and Haemostasis 47: 259–264

Charo I F, Feinman R D, Detwiler T C 1977 Interrelations of platelet aggregation and secretion. Journal of Clinical Investigation 60: 866–873

Chesebro J H, Fuster V 1991 Dynamic thrombosis and thrombolysis. Role of antithrombins. Circulation 83: 1815–1817

Chesebro J H, Zoldhelyi P, Fuster V 1991 Pathogenesis of thrombosis in unstable angina. American Journal of Cardiology 68: 2B–10B

Chiang M T, Otomo M I, Itoh H, Furukawa Y, Kimura S, Fujimoto H 1991 Effect of trans fatty acids on plasma lipids, platelet function and systolic blood pressure in stroke-prone spontaneously hypertensive rats. Lipids 26: 46–52

Chierchia S, de Caterina R, Crea F, Patrono C, Maseri A 1982 Failure of thromboxane A_2 blockade to prevent attacks of vasospastic angina. Circulation 66: 702–705

Chobanian A V, Prescott M F, Haudenschild C C 1984 Recent advances in molecular pathology. The effects of hypertension on the arterial wall. Experimental and Molecular Pathology 41: 153–169

Cieslar P, Greenberg J P, Rand M L et al 1979 Separation of thrombin-treated platelets from normal platelets by density-gradient centrifugation. Blood 53: 867–874

Clarke R, Daly L, Robinson K et al 1991 Hyperhomocysteinemia: an independent risk factor for vascular disease. New England Journal of Medicine 324: 1149–1155

Clawson C C, White J G 1971 Platelet interaction with bacteria. I. Reaction phases and effects of inhibitors. American Journal of Pathology 65: 367–380

Clowes A W 1991 Prevention and management of recurrent disease after arterial reconstruction: new prospects for pharmacological control. Thrombosis and Haemostasis 66: 62–66

Clowes A W, Reidy M A, Clowes M M 1983 Kinetics of cellular proliferation after arterial injury. I. Smooth muscle growth in the absence of endothelium. Laboratory Investigation 49: 327–333

Clowes A W, Clowes M M, Reidy M A 1986 Kinetics of cellular proliferation after arterial injury. III. Endothelial and smooth muscle growth in chronically denuded vessels. Laboratory Investigation 54: 295–303

Cochrane C G 1971 Initiating events in immune complex injury. In: Amos B (ed) Progress in immunology. Academic Press, New York, p 143–153

Cohn P F 1989 Another smoking gun linking cigarettes and heart disease. Journal of the American Medical Association 261: 438

Coleman R E, Harwig S S L, Harwig J F, Siegel B A, Welch M J 1975 Fibrinogen uptake by thrombi: effect of thrombus age. Journal of Nuclear Medicine 16: 370–373

Coller B S 1990 Platelets and thrombolytic therapy. New England Journal of Medicine 322: 33–42

Coller B S 1992 Platelets in cardiovascular thrombosis and thrombolysis. In: Fozzard H A, Haber E, Jennings R B, Katz A M, Morgan H E (eds) The heart and cardiovascular system, 2nd edn. Raven Press, New York, p 219–273

Colman R W 1978 Platelet function in hyperbetalipoproteinemia. Thrombosis and Haemostasis 39: 284–293

Colucci M, Balconi G, Lorenzet R et al 1983 Cultured human endothelial cells generate tissue factor in response to endotoxin. Journal of Clinical Investigation 71: 1893–1896

Colucci M, Paramo J A, Collen D 1985 Generation in plasma of a fast-acting inhibitor of plasminogen activator in response to endotoxin stimulation. Journal of Clinical Investigation 75: 818–824

Colwell J A 1988 Platelets, endothelium and diabetic vascular disease. Diabete & Metabolisme (Paris) 14: 512–518
Colwell J A, Lopes-Virella M F, Winocour P D, Halushka P V 1988 New concepts about the pathogenesis of atherosclerosis in diabetes mellitus. In: Levin M E, O'Neal L W (eds) The diabetic foot. C V Mosby, St. Louis, Mo, p 51–70
Constantinides P 1967 Pathogenesis of cerebral artery thrombosis in man. Archives of Pathology 83: 422–428
Constantinides P, Robinson M 1969 Ultrastructural injury of arterial endothelium. II. Effects of vasoactive amines. Archives of Pathology 88: 106–112
Corash L, Andersen J, Poindexter B J, Schaefer E J 1981 Platelet function and survival in patients with severe hypercholesterolemia. Arteriosclerosis 1: 443–448
Crawford T 1977 Pathology of ischaemic heart disease. Butterworths, London
Criqui M H 1991 Triglycerides and coronary heart disease. In: Gotto A M Jr, Paoletti R (eds) Atherosclerosis reviews, vol 22: 75–79
Curwen K D, Gimbrone M A Jr, Handin R I 1980 In vitro studies of thromboresistance: the role of prostacyclin (PGI_2) in platelet adhesion to cultured normal and virally transformed human vascular endothelial cells. Laboratory Investigation 42: 366–374
Cybulsky M I, Gimbrone M A Jr 1991 Endothelial expression of a mononuclear leukocyte adhesion molecule during atherogenesis. Science 251: 788–791
Damerau B, Meyer B, Vogt W 1991 Formation of mixed aggregates of human polymorphonuclear leukocytes and platelets by C5a-desArg. Complement and Inflammation 8: 25–32
Dang C V, Bell W R, Kaiser D, Wong A 1985 Disorganization of cultured vascular endothelial cell monolayers by fibrinogen fragment D. Science 227: 1487–1490
Daniel J L, Molish I R, Rigmaiden M, Steward G 1984 Evidence for a role of myosin phosphorylation in the initiation of the platelet shape change response. Journal of Biological Chemistry 259: 9826–9831
Davie E W, Fujikawa K, Kisiel W 1991 The coagulation cascade: initiation, maintenance, and regulation. Biochemistry 30: 10363–10370
Davies M J, Thomas A C 1985 Plaque-fissuring — the cause of acute myocardial infarction, sudden ischemic death, and crescendo angina. British Heart Journal 53: 363–373
Davies M J, Ballantine S J, Robertson W B, Woolf N 1975 The ultrastructure of organizing experimental mural thrombi in the pig aorta. Journal of Pathology 117: 75–81
Davies M J, Thomas A C, Knapman P A, Hangartner J R 1986 Intramyocardial platelet aggregation in patients with unstable angina suffering sudden ischemic cardiac death. Circulation 73: 418–427
Davies M J, Krikler D M, Katz D 1991 Atherosclerosis: inhibition or regression as therapeutic possibilities. British Heart Journal 65: 302–310
Davies P F, Remuzzi A, Gordon E J, Dewey C F Jr, Gimbrone M A Jr 1986 Turbulent fluid shear stress induces vascular endothelial cell turnover in vitro. Proceedings of the National Academy of Sciences, USA 83: 2114–2117
Davis J W, Shelton L, Eigenberg D A, Hignite C E, Watanabe I S 1985 Effects of tobacco and non-tobacco cigarette smoking on endothelium and platelets. Clinical Pharmacology and Therapeutics 37: 529–533
Davis J W, Hartman C R, Shelton L, Ruttinger H A 1989 A trial of dipyridamole and aspirin in the prevention of smoking-induced changes in platelets and endothelium in men with coronary artery disease. American Journal of Cardiology 63: 1450–1454
De Clerck F 1991 Effects of serotonin on platelets and blood vessels. Journal of Cardiovascular Pharmacology 17 (suppl 5): S1–S5
de Feyter P J, Serruys P W, Davies M J, Richardson P, Lubsen J, Oliver M F 1991 Quantitative coronary angiography to measure progression and regression of coronary atherosclerosis. Value, limitations, and implications for clinical trials. Circulation 84: 412–423
de Groot P G, Sixma J J 1987 Role of von Willebrand factor in the vessel wall. Seminars in Thrombosis and Hemostasis 13: 416–424
Dejana E, Cazenave J-P, Groves H M et al 1980 The effect of aspirin inhibition of PGI_2 production on platelet adherence to normal and damaged rabbit aortae. Thrombosis Research 17: 453–464
De Marco L, Girolami A, Zimmerman T S, Ruggeri Z M 1986 von Willebrand factor interaction with the glycoprotein IIb/IIIa complex. Its role in platelet function as demonstrated in patients with congenital afibrinogenemia. Journal of Clinical Investigation 77: 1272–1277
Diamond S L, Eskin S G, McIntire L V 1989 Fluid flow stimulates tissue plasminogen activator secretion by cultured human endothelial cells. Science 243: 1483–1485
DiMinno G, Silver M J, Cerbone A M, Rainone A, Postiglione A, Mancini M 1986 Increased fibrinogen binding to platelets from patients with familial hypercholesterolemia. Arteriosclerosis 6: 203–211
Dimsdale J E 1988 A perspective on type A behavior and coronary disease. New England Journal of Medicine 318: 110–112
Downing S E, Vidone R A, Brandt H M, Liebow A A 1963 The pathogenesis of vascular lesions in experimental hyperkinetic pulmonary hypertension. American Journal of Pathology 43: 739–765
Drake T A, Morrissey J H, Edgington T S 1989 Selective cellular expression of tissue factor in human tissues. Implications for disorders of hemostasis and thrombosis. American Journal of Pathology 134: 1087–1097
Drummond K N 1985 Hemolytic uremic syndrome — then and now. New England Journal of Medicine 312: 116–118
Duguid J B 1946 Thrombosis as a factor in the pathogenesis of coronary atherosclerosis. Journal of Pathology and Bacteriology 58: 207–212
Dutch T I A Trial Study Group 1991 A comparison of two doses of aspirin (30 mg vs 283 mg a day) in patients after a transient ischemic attack or minor ischemic stroke. New England Journal of Medicine 325: 1261–1266
Dvorak H F 1987 Thrombosis and cancer. Human Pathology 18: 275–284
Dzau V J 1990 Atherosclerosis and hypertension: mechanisms and interrelationships. Journal of Cardiovascular Pharmacology 15: (suppl 5) S59–S64
Eberth J C, Schimmelbusch C 1888 Die Thrombose nach Versuchen u. Leichenbefunden. Ferdinand Enke, Stuttgart
Ellis S G, Bates E R, Schaible T, Weisman H F, Pitt B, Topol E J 1991 Prospects for the use of antagonists to the platelet glycoprotein IIb/IIIa receptor to prevent postangioplasty restenosis and thrombosis. Journal of the American College of Cardiology 17: 89B–95B
El Maraghi N, Genton E 1980 The relevance of platelet and fibrin thromboembolism of the coronary microcirculation, with special reference to sudden cardiac death. Circulation 62: 936–944
Erne P, Bolli P, Bürgisser E, Bühler F R 1984 Correlation of platelet calcium with blood pressure. Effect of antihypertensive therapy. New England Journal of Medicine 310: 1084–1088
Erne P, Resink T J, Bürgisser E, Bühler F R 1985 Platelets and hypertension. Journal of Cardiovascular Pharmacology 7 (suppl 6): S103–S108
Eskin S G, McIntire L V 1988 Hemodynamic effects on atherosclerosis and thrombosis. Seminars in Thrombosis and Hemostasis 14: 170–174
Esmon C T 1989 The roles of protein C and thrombomodulin in the regulation of blood coagulation. Journal of Biological Chemistry 264: 4743–4746
Eurenius K, Rossi T D, McEuen D D, Arnold J, McManus W F 1974 Blood coagulation in burn injury. Proceedings of the Society for Experimental Biology and Medicine 147: 878–882
Fabricant C G, Hajjar D P, Minick C R, Fabricant J 1981 Herpesvirus infection enhances cholesterol and cholesteryl ester accumulation in cultured arterial smooth muscle cells. American Journal of Pathology 105: 176–184
Fabricant C G, Fabricant J, Minick C R, Litrenta M M 1983 Herpesvirus-induced atherosclerosis in chickens. Federation Proceedings 42: 2476–2479
Faggiotto A, Ross R 1984 Studies of hypercholesterolemia in the nonhuman primate. II. Fatty streak conversion to fibrous plaque. Arteriosclerosis 4: 341–356
Falk E 1983 Plaque rupture with severe pre-existing stenosis precipitating coronary thrombosis. Characteristics of coronary atherosclerotic plaques underlying fatal occlusive thrombi. British Heart Journal 50: 127–134

Falk E 1991a Coronary thrombosis: pathogenesis and clinical manifestations. American Journal of Cardiology 68: 28B–35B

Falk E 1991b Unstable angina with fatal outcome: dynamic coronary thrombosis leading to infarction and/or sudden death. Autopsy evidence of recurrent mural thrombosis with peripheral embolization culminating in total vascular occlusion. Circulation 71: 699–708

Febbraio M, Silverstein R L 1990 Identification and characterization of LAMP-l as an activation-dependent platelet surface glycoprotein. Journal of Biological Chemistry 256: 18531–18537

Feher M D, Rampling M W, Brown J et al 1990 Acute changes in atherogenic and thrombogenic factors with cessation of smoking. Journal of the Royal Society of Medicine 83: 146–148

Ferguson J C, MacKay N, Philip J A D, Sumner D J 1975 Determination of platelet and fibrinogen half-life with [^{75}Se]-selenomethionine: studies in normal and in diabetic subjects. Clinical Science and Molecular Medicine 49: 115–120

Ferns G A A, Raines E W, Sprugel K H, Motani A S, Reidy M A, Ross R 1991 Inhibition of neointimal smooth muscle accumulation after angioplasty by an antibody to PDGF. Science 253: 1129–1132

Ferrer-Lopez P, Renesto P, Schattner M, Bassot S, Laurent P, Chignard M 1990 Activation of human platelets by C5a-stimulated neutrophils: a role for cathepsin G. American Journal of Physiology 258: C1100–C1107

Files J C, Malpass T W, Yee E K, Ritchie J L, Harker L A 1981 Studies of human platelet α-granule release in vivo. Blood 58: 607–618

Fisher C M 1959 Observations of the fundus oculi in transient mononuclear blindness. Neurology (Minneapolis) 9: 333–347

Fitzgerald D J 1991 Platelet activation in the pathogenesis of unstable angina: importance in determining the response to plasminogen activators. American Journal of Cardiology 68: 51B–57B

FitzGerald G A, Pedersen A K, Patrono C 1983 Analysis of prostacyclin and thromboxane biosynthesis in cardiovascular disease. Circulation 67: 1174–1177

Fleck R A, Rao L V M, Rapaport S I, Varki N 1990 Localization of human tissue factor antigen by immunostaining with monospecific, polyclonal anti-human tissue factor antibody. Thrombosis Research 59: 421–437

Fletcher A P, Alkjaersig N 1977 The use and monitoring of antithrombotic drug therapy. The need for a new approach. Thrombosis and Haemostasis 38: 881–892

Folie B J, McIntire L V 1989 Mathematical analysis of mural thrombogenesis. Concentration profiles of platelet-activating agents and effects of viscous shear flow. Biophysical Journal 56: 1121–1141

Folts J D 1990 A model of experimental arterial platelet thrombosis, platelet inhibitors, and their possible clinical relevance: an update. Cardiovascular Reviews & Reports 11: 10–26

Foo L C, Roshidah I, Aimy M B 1991 Platelets of habitual smokers have reduced susceptibility to aggregating agent. Thrombosis and Haemostasis 65: 317–319

Forrester J 1991 Intimal disruption and coronary thrombosis: its role in the pathogenesis of human coronary disease. American Journal of Cardiology 68: 69B–77B

Fox J E B, Reynolds C C, Austin C D 1990a The role of calpain in stimulus-response coupling: evidence that calpain mediates agonist-induced expression of procoagulant activity in platelets. Blood 76: 2510–2519

Fox J E B, Austin C D, Boyles J K, Steffen P K 1990b Role of the membrane skeleton in preventing the shedding of procoagulant-rich microvesicles from the platelet plasma membrane. Journal of Cell Biology 111: 483–493

Francis C W, Markham R E Jr, Marder V J 1984 Demonstration of in situ fibrin degradation in pathologic thrombi. Blood 63: 1216–1224

Francis R B Jr, Johnson C S 1991 Vascular occlusion in sickle cell disease: current concepts and unanswered questions. Blood 77: 1405–1414

Frelinger A L III, Lam S C-T, Plow E F, Smith M A, Loftus J C, Ginsberg M H 1988 Occupancy of an adhesive glycoprotein receptor modulates expression of an antigenic site involved in cell adhesion. Journal of Biological Chemistry 263: 12397–12402

Frink R J, Trowbridge J O, Rooney P A Jr 1978 Nonobstructive coronary thrombosis in sudden cardiac death. American Journal of Cardiology 42: 48–51

Fry D L 1976 Hemodynamic forces in atherogenesis. In: Sheinberg P (ed) Cerebrovascular diseases, 10th Princeton Conference. Raven Press, New York, p 77–95

Fujimoto T, Hawiger J 1982 Adenosine diphosphate induces binding of von Willebrand factor to human platelets. Nature 297: 154–156

Fulton G P, Akers R P, Lutz B R 1953 White thromboemboli and vascular fragility in hamster cheek pouch after anticoagulants. Blood 8: 140–152

Fulton W F M, Sumner D J 1977 Causal role of coronary artery thrombotic occlusion in myocardial infarction: evidence of stereo-arteriography serial sections and ^{125}I-fibrinogen autoradiography. American Journal of Cardiology 39: 322

Furchgott R F, Vanhoutte P M 1989 Endothelium-derived relaxing and contracting factors. FASEB Journal 3: 2007–2018

Fuster V, Chesebro J H, Frye R L, Elveback L R 1981 Platelet survival and the development of coronary disease in the young adult: effects of cigarette smoking, strong family history and medical therapy. Circulation 63: 546–551

Fuster V, Stein B, Ambrose J A, Badimon L, Badimon J J, Chesebro J H 1990 Atherosclerotic plaque rupture and thrombosis. Evolving concepts. Circulation 82 (suppl II): II47–II59

Fuster V, Ip J H, Badimon L, Badimon J J, Stein B, Chesebro J H 1991 Importance of experimental models for the development of clinical trials on thromboatherosclerosis. Circulation 83 (suppl IV): IV15–IV25

Gader A M A, Al-Mashhadani S A, Al-Harthy S S 1990 Direct activation of platelets by heat is the possible trigger of the coagulopathy of heat stroke. British Journal of Haematology 74: 86–92

Gallino A, Haeberli A, Baur H R, Straub P W 1985 Fibrin formation and platelet aggregation in patients with severe coronary artery disease: relationship with the degree of myocardial ischemia. Circulation 72: 27–30

George J N, Shattil S J 1991 The clinical importance of acquired abnormalities of platelet function. New England Journal of Medicine 324: 27–39

George J N, Pickett E B, Saucerman S et al 1986 Platelet surface glycoproteins. Studies on resting and activated platelets and platelet membrane microparticles in normal subjects, and observations in patients during adult respiratory distress syndrome and cardiac surgery. Journal of Clinical Investigation 78: 340–348

Gering S A, Folts J D 1990 Exacerbation of acute platelet thrombus formation in stenosed dog coronary arteries with smoke from a non-tobacco-burning cigarette. Journal of Laboratory and Clinical Medicine 116: 728–736

Gerrard J M, McNicol A, Klassen D, Israels S J 1989 Protein phosphorylation and its relation to platelet function. In: Meyer P, Marche P (eds) Blood cells and arteries in hypertension and atherosclerosis. Raven Press, New York, p 93–114

Gerrard J M, Lint D, Sims P J et al 1991 Identification of a platelet dense granule membrane protein that is deficient in a patient with the Hermansky–Pudlak syndrome. Blood 77: 101–112

Gertz S D, Uretsky G, Wajnberg R S, Navot N, Gotsman M S 1981 Endothelial cell damage and thrombus formation after partial arterial constriction: relevance to the role of coronary artery spasm in the pathogenesis of myocardial infarction. Circulation 63: 476–486

Gilliland B C 1984 Serum sickness and immune complexes. New England Journal of Medicine 311: 1435–1436

Ginsberg M H, Frelinger A L, Lam S C-T et al 1990 Analysis of platelet aggregation disorders based on flow cytometric analysis of membrane glycoprotein IIb-IIIa with conformation-specific monoclonal antibodies. Blood 76: 2017–2023

Glagov S, Zarins C, Giddens D P, Ku D N 1988 Hemodynamics and atherosclerosis. Insights and perspectives gained from studies of human arteries. Archives of Pathology and Laboratory Medicine 112: 1018–1031

Goldman S, Copeland J, Moritz T et al 1991 Starting aspirin therapy after operation. Effects on early graft patency. Circulation 84: 520–526

Goldsmith H L, Karino T 1979 Mechanically induced thromboemboli. In: Hwang N H C, Gross D R, Patel D J (eds) Quantitative cardiovascular studies. Clinical and research applications of engineering principles. University Park Press, Baltimore, p 289–351

Goldsmith H L, Karino T 1982 Microrheology and clinical medicine. Unravelling some problems related to thrombosis. Clinical Hemorheology 2: 143–155
Gordon D, Guyton J R, Karnovsky M J 1981 Intimal alterations in rat aorta induced by stressful stimuli. Laboratory Investigation 45: 14–27
Gordon D, Schwartz S M, Benditt E P, Wilcox J N 1989 Growth factors and cell proliferation in human atherosclerosis. Transplantation Proceedings 21: 3692–3694
Grabowski E F, De Caterina R (guest eds) 1991 Effects of contrast media and catheters on hemostasis and thrombosis. Seminars in Hematology 28 (suppl 7): 1–80
Graham D Y, Brown C H III, Benrey J, Butel J S 1974 Thrombocytopenia. A complication of mumps. Journal of the American Medical Association 227: 1162–1164
Gralnick H R, McKeown L P, Wilson O M, Williams S B, Elin R J 1989 Von Willebrand factor release induced by endotoxin. Journal of Laboratory and Clinical Medicine 113: 118–122
Greenberg J-P, Packham M A, Guccione M A, Rand M L, Reimers H-J, Mustard J F 1979 Survival of rabbit platelets treated in vitro with chymotrypsin, plasmin, trypsin, or neuraminidase. Blood 53: 916–927
Grignani G, Soffiantino F, Zucchella M et al 1991 Platelet activation by emotional stress in patients with coronary artery disease. Circulation 83 (suppl II): II128–II136
Gross P L, Rand M L, Barrow D V, Packham M A 1991a Platelet hypersensitivity in cholesterol-fed rabbits: enhancement of thromboxane A_2-dependent and thrombin-induced, thromboxane A_2-independent platelet responses. Atherosclerosis 88: 77–86
Gross P L, Rand M L, Barrow D V, Packham M A 1991b Platelet function in Watanabe heritable hyperlipidemic rabbits. Decreased sensitivity to thromboxane A_2. Arteriosclerosis and Thrombosis 11: 610–616
Groves H M, Kinlough-Rathbone R L, Richardson M, Moore S, Mustard J F 1979 Platelet interaction with damaged rabbit aorta. Laboratory Investigation 40: 194–200
Groves H M, Kinlough-Rathbone R L, Richardson M, Jørgensen L, Moore S, Mustard J F 1982 Thrombin generation and fibrin formation following injury to rabbit neointima: studies of vessel wall reactivity and platelet survival. Laboratory Investigation 46: 605–612
Grundy S M, Barrett-Connor E, Rudel L L, Miettinen T, Spector A A 1988 Workshop on the impact of dietary cholesterol on plasma lipoproteins and atherogenesis. Arteriosclerosis 8: 95–101
Guckian J C 1975 Effect of pneumococci on blood clotting, platelets, and polymorphonuclear leukocytes. Infection and Immunity 12: 910–918
Gunning A J, Pickering G W, Robb-Smith A H T, Russell R R 1964 Mural thrombosis of the internal carotid artery and subsequent embolism. Quarterly Journal of Medicine 33: 155–195
Haapanen A, Koskenvuo M, Kaprio J, Kesäniemi Y A, Heikkilä K 1989 Carotid arteriosclerosis in identical twins discordant for cigarette smoking. Circulation 80: 10–16
Hadcock S, Richardson M, Winocour P D, Hatton M W C 1991 Intimal alterations in rabbit aortas during the first 6 months of alloxan-induced diabetes. Arteriosclerosis and Thrombosis 11: 517–529
Haerem J W 1978 Sudden, unexpected coronary death. The occurrence of platelet aggregates in the epicardial and myocardial vessels of man. Acta Pathologica Microbiologica Scandinavica 265: 1–47
Haffner S M, Stern M P, Hazuda H P, Mitchell B D, Patterson J K, Ferrannini E 1989 Parental history of diabetes is associated with increased cardiovascular risk factors. Arteriosclerosis 9: 928–933
Hajjar D P, Grant A J 1986 Human herpesvirus induces altered cholesterol metabolism and accumulation in human arterial smooth muscle cells. Circulation 74 (suppl II): II26
Hajjar D P, Fabricant C G, Minick C R, Fabricant J 1986 Virus-induced atherosclerosis. Herpesvirus infection alters aortic cholesterol metabolism and accumulation. American Journal of Pathology 122: 62–70
Hallam T J, Rink T J 1985 Agonists stimulate divalent cation channels in the plasma membrane of human platelets. FEBS Letters 186: 175–179
Hammerschmidt D E, Weaver L J, Hudson L D, Craddock P R, Jacob H S 1980 Association of complement activation and elevated plasma C5a with adult respiratory distress syndrome: pathophysiological relevance and possible prognostic value. Lancet i: 947–949
Hamsten A, Norberg R 1989 Antibodies to phospholipids in thrombotic disease. Journal of Internal Medicine 225: 363–365
Handley A J, Teather D 1974 Influence of smoking on deep vein thrombosis after myocardial infarction. British Medical Journal 3: 230–231
Hansson G K, Jonasson L, Seifert P S, Stemme S 1989 Immune mechanisms in atherosclerosis. Arteriosclerosis 9: 567–578
Hantgan R R 1988 Fibrin protofibril and fibrinogen binding to ADP-stimulated platelets: evidence for a common mechanism. Biochimica et Biophysica Acta 968: 24–35
Harfenist E J, Packham M A, Kinlough-Rathbone R L, Cattaneo M, Mustard J F 1987 Effect of calcium ion concentration on the ability of fibrinogen and von Willebrand factor to support the ADP-induced aggregation of human platelets. Blood 70: 827–831
Harker L A 1978 Platelet survival time: its measurement and use. In: Spaet T H (ed) Progress in hemostasis and thrombosis, Grune & Stratton, New York, vol 4: 321–347
Harker L A, Ross R, Slichter S J, Scott C R 1976 Homocystine-induced arteriosclerosis. The role of endothelial cell injury and platelet response in its genesis. Journal of Clinical Investigation 58: 731–741
Harlan J M, Harker L A, Reidy M A, Gajdusek C M, Schwartz S M, Striker G E 1983 Lipopolysaccharide-mediated bovine endothelial cell injury in vitro. Laboratory Investigation 48: 269–274
Hart L E, Egier B P, Shimizu A G, Tandan P J, Sutton J R 1980 Exertional heat stroke: the runner's nemesis. Journal of the Canadian Medical Association 122: 1144–1150
Hasleton P S 1983 Adult respiratory distress syndrome — a review. Histopathology 7: 307–332
Hasselaar P, Derksen R H W M, Blokzijl L, de Groot P G 1988 Thrombosis associated with antiphospholipid antibodies cannot be explained by effects on endothelial and platelet prostanoid synthesis. Thrombosis and Haemostasis 59: 80–85
Hawkins R I 1972 Smoking, platelets and thrombosis. Nature 236: 450–452
Hayslett J P 1984 Role of platelets in glomerulonephritis. New England Journal of Medicine 310: 1457–1458
Heilmann E, Hourdillé P, Pruvost A, Paponneau A, Nurden A T 1991 Thrombin-induced platelet aggregates have a dynamic structure. Time-dependent redistribution of glycoprotein IIb-IIIa complexes and secreted adhesive proteins. Arteriosclerosis and Thrombosis 11: 704–718
Hendrix M G R, Dormans P H J, Kitslaar P, Bosman F, Bruggeman C A 1989 The presence of cytomegalovirus nucleic acids in arterial walls of atherosclerotic and nonatherosclerotic patients. American Journal of Pathology 134: 1151–1157
Hennekens C H, Buring J E, Mayrent S L 1984 Smoking and aging in coronary heart disease. In: Bossé R, Rose C L (eds) Smoking and aging. Lexington Books, Lexington, MA p 95–115
Henriksson, P, Stamberger M, Eriksson M et al 1989 Oestrogen-induced changes in lipoprotein metabolism: role in prevention of atherosclerosis in the cholesterol-fed rabbit. European Journal of Clinical Investigation 19: 395–403
Henson P M, Ginsberg M H 1981 Immunological reactions of platelets. In: Gordon J L (ed) Platelets in biology and pathology –2 edn. Elsevier/North Holland, Amsterdam, p 265–308
Hermanson B, Omenn G S, Kronmal R A, Gersh B J 1988 Beneficial six-year outcome of smoking cessation in older men and women with coronary artery disease. Results from the CASS Registry. New England Journal of Medicine 319: 1365–1369
Herzberg M C, Brintzenhofe K L, Clawson C C 1983 Aggregation of human platelets and adhesion of Streptococcus sanguis. Infection and Immunity 39: 1457–1469
Herzberg M C, Erickson P R, Kane P K, Clawson D J, Clawson C C, Hoff F A 1990 Platelet-interactive products of Streptococcus sanguis protoplasts. Infection and Immunity 58: 4117–4125
Hess H, Mietaschk A, Deichsel G 1985 Drug-induced inhibition of platelet function delays progression of peripheral occlusive arterial disease. A prospective double-blind arteriographically controlled trial. Lancet i: 415–419

Hirsch G M, Karnovsky M J 1991 Inhibition of vein graft intimal proliferative lesions in the rat by heparin. American Journal of Pathology 139: 581–587

Hoet B, Arnout J, Van Geet C, Deckmyn H, Verhaeghe R, Vermylen J 1990 Ridogrel, a combined thromboxane synthase inhibitor and receptor blocker, decreases elevated plasma β-thromboglobulin levels in patients with documented peripheral arterial disease. Thrombosis and Haemostasis 64: 87–90

Hoff H F, Gottlob R 1967 A fine structure study of injury to the endothelial cells of the rabbit abdominal aorta by various stimuli. Angiology 18: 440–451

Homer D, Ingall T J, Baker H L Jr, O'Fallon W M, Kottke B A, Whisnant J P 1991 Serum lipids and lipoproteins are less powerful predictors of extracranial carotid artery atherosclerosis than are cigarette smoking and hypertension. Mayo Clinic Proceedings 66: 259–267

Honey A C, Lad N, Tuffin D P 1986 Effect of indomethacin and dazoxiben on intravascular platelet aggregation in the anaesthetized rabbit. Thrombosis and Haemostasis 56: 80–85

Honour A J, Russell R W R 1962 Experimental platelet embolism. British Journal of Experimental Pathology 43: 350–362

Hornstra G 1980 Dietary fats and arterial thrombosis. PhD thesis, University of Maastricht, Netherlands

Hornstra G 1989 Effect of dietary lipids on platelet function and thrombosis. Annals of Medicine 21: 53–57

Hourani S M O, Cusack N J 1991 Pharmacological receptors on blood platelets. Pharmacological Reviews 43: 243–298

Hugod C, Hawkins L H, Kjeldsen K et al 1978 Effect of carbon monoxide exposure on aortic and coronary intimal morphology in the rabbit: a revaluation. Atherosclerosis 30: 333–342

Inauen W, Baumgartner H R, Haeberli A, Straub P W 1987 Excessive deposition of fibrin, platelets and platelet thrombi on vascular subendothelium during contraceptive drug treatment. Thrombosis and Haemostasis 57: 306–309

Ingall T J, Homer D, Baker H L Jr, Kottke B A, O'Fallon W M, Whisnant J P 1991 Predictors of intracranial carotid artery atherosclerosis. Duration of cigarette smoking and hypertension are more powerful than serum lipid levels. Archives of Neurology 48: 687–691

Ip J H, Fuster V, Israel D, Badimon L, Badimon J, Chesebro J H 1991 The role of platelets, thrombin and hyperplasia in restenosis after coronary angioplasty. Journal of American College of Cardiology 17: 77B–88B

Jamieson G A, Bastida E, Ordinas A 1987 Interaction of platelets and tumour cells. In: MacIntyre D E, Gordon J L (eds) Platelets in biology and pathology III. Elsevier Science (Biomedical Division), Amsterdam, p 161–189

Jang I-K, Gold H K, Ziskind A A, Leinbach R C, Fallon J T, Collen D 1990 Prevention of platelet-rich arterial thrombosis by selective thrombin inhibition. Circulation 81: 219–225

Janzon L, Nilsson I M 1975 Smoking and fibrinolysis. Circulation 51: 1120–1123

Jonasson L, Holm J, Skalli O, Bondjers G, Hansson G K 1986 Regional accumulations of T cells, macrophages, and smooth muscle cells in the human atherosclerotic plaque. Arteriosclerosis 6: 131–138

Jones C J H, Singer D R J, Watkins N V, MacGregor G A, Caro C G 1990 Abnormal arterial flow pattern in untreated essential hypertension: possible link with the development of atherosclerosis. Clinical Science 78: 431–435

Jørgensen L, Rowsell H C, Hovig T, Glynn M F, Mustard J F 1967a Adenosine diphosphate-induced platelet aggregation and myocardial infarction in swine. Laboratory Investigation 17: 616–644

Jørgensen L, Rowsell H C, Hovig T, Mustard J F 1967b Resolution and organization of platelet-rich mural thrombi in carotid arteries of swine. American Journal of Pathology 51: 681–719

Joris I, Majno G 1981 Medial changes in arterial spasm induced by L-norepinephrine. American Journal of Pathology 105: 212–222

Joris I, Zand T, Majno G 1982 Hydrodynamic injury of the endothelium in acute aortic stenosis. American Journal of Pathology 106: 394–408

Jouhikainen T, Kekomäki R, Leirisalo-Repo M, Bäcklund T, Myllylä G 1990 Platelet autoantibodies detected by immunoblotting in systemic lupus erythematosus: association with the lupus anticoagulant, and with history of thrombosis and thrombocytopenia. European Journal of Haematology 44: 234–239

Kannel W B 1991 Hypertension, hypertrophy, and the occurrence of cardiovascular disease. American Journal of the Medical Sciences 302: 199–204

Kaplan A V, Leung L L-K, Leung W-H, Grant G W, McDougall I R, Fischell T A 1991 Roles of thrombin and platelet membrane glycoprotein IIb/IIIa in platelet-subendothelial deposition after angioplasty in an ex vivo whole artery model. Circulation 84: 1279–1288

Kaplan J R, Manuck S B, Adams M R, Weingand K W, Clarkson T B 1987 Inhibition of coronary atherosclerosis by propranolol in behaviorally predisposed monkeys fed an atherogenic diet. Circulation 76: 1364–1372

Kaplan K L, Owen J 1981 Plasma levels of β-thromboglobulin and platelet factor 4 as indices of platelet activation in vivo. Blood 57: 199–202

Kaplan K L, Mather T, DeMarco L, Solomon S 1989 Effect of fibrin on endothelial cell production of prostacyclin and tissue plasminogen activator. Arteriosclerosis 9: 43–49

Karino T, Motomiya M, Goldsmith H L 1982 Flow patterns in model and natural vessels. In: Stanley J C (ed) Biologic and synthetic vascular prostheses. Grune & Stratton, New York, p 153–178

Karmali M A, Petric M, Lim C, Fleming P C, Steele B T 1983 Escherichia coli cytotoxin, haemolytic-uraemic syndrome, and haemorrhagic colitis. Lancet ii: 1299–1300

Karpatkin S, Pearlstein E, Ambrogio C, Coller B S 1988 Role of adhesive proteins in platelet tumor interaction in vitro and metastasis formation in vivo. Journal of Clinical Investigation 81: 1012–1019

Katagiri Y, Hayashi Y, Baba I, Suzuki H, Tanoue K, Yamazaki H 1991 Characterization of platelet aggregation induced by the human melanoma cell line HMV-I: roles of heparin, plasma adhesive proteins, and tumor cell membrane proteins. Cancer Research 51: 1286–1293

Katritsis D, Choi M J, Webb-Peploe M M 1991 Assessment of the hemodynamic significance of coronary artery stenosis: theoretical considerations and clinical measurements. Progress in Cardiovascular Diseases 34: 69–88

Kehrel B, Balleisen L, Kokott R et al 1988 Deficiency of intact thrombospondin and membrane glycoprotein Ia in platelets with defective collagen-induced aggregation and spontaneous loss of disorder. Blood 71: 1074–1078

Keller J W, Folts J D 1988 Relative effects of cigarette smoke and ethanol on acute platelet thrombus formation in stenosed canine coronary arteries. Cardiovascular Research 22: 73–78

Kempczinski R F 1979 Lower-extremity arterial emboli from ulcerating atherosclerotic plaques. Journal of the American Medical Association 241: 807–810

Kessler C M, Nussbaum E, Tuazon C U 1987 In vitro correlation of platelet aggregation with occurrence of disseminated intravascular coagulation and subacute bacterial endocarditis. Journal of Laboratory and Clinical Medicine 109: 647–652

Kessler C M, Nussbaum E, Tuazon C U 1991 Disseminated intravascular coagulation associated with Staphylococcus aureus septicemia is mediated by peptidoglycan-induced platelet aggregation. Journal of Infectious Diseases 164: 101–107

Key N S, Vercellotti G M, Winkelmann J C et al 1990 Infection of vascular endothelial cells with herpes simplex virus enhances tissue factor activity and reduces thrombomodulin expression. Proceedings of the National Academy of Sciences, USA 87: 7095–7099

Keys A 1980 Seven countries. A multivariate analysis of death and coronary heart disease. Harvard University Press, Cambridge

Kinlough-Rathbone R L, Mustard J F 1986 Synergism of agonists. In: Holmsen H (ed) Platelet responses and metabolism. CRC Press, Boca Raton, vol 1: 193–207

Kinlough-Rathbone R L, Packham M A, Reimers H-J, Cazenave J-P, Mustard J F 1977 Mechanisms of platelet shape change, aggregation and release induced by collagen, thrombin or A23,187. Journal of Laboratory and Clinical Medicine 90: 707–716

Kinlough-Rathbone R L, Cazenave J-P, Packham M A, Mustard J F 1980 Effect of inhibitors of the arachidonate pathway on the release

of granule contents from rabbit platelets adherent to collagen. Laboratory Investigation 42: 28–34
Kinlough-Rathbone R L, Packham M A, Mustard J F 1983 Vessel injury, platelet adherence, and platelet survival. Arteriosclerosis 3: 529–546
Klein R, Klein B E K, Moss S E, Davis M D, De Mets D L 1988 Glycosylated hemoglobin predicts the incidence and progression of diabetic retinopathy. Journal of the American Medical Association 260: 2864–2871
Klein W, Eber B, Dusleag J et al 1990 Ketanserin prevents early restenosis following percutaneous transluminal coronary angioplasty. Clinical Physiology and Biochemistry 8 (suppl 3): 101–107
Kniker W T, Cochrane C G 1968 The localization of circulating immune complexes in experimental serum sickness. The role of vasoactive amines and hydrodynamic forces. Journal of Experimental Medicine 127: 119–135
Knopp R H 1988 The effects of postmenopausal estrogen therapy on the incidence of arteriosclerotic vascular disease. Obstetrics and Gynecology 72: 23S–30S
Kohler C, Wooding W and Ellenbogen L 1976 Intravenous arachidonate in the mouse: a model for the evaluation of antithrombotic drugs. Thrombosis Research 9: 67–80
Kroll M H, Schafer A I 1989 Biochemical mechanisms of platelet activation. Blood 74: 1181–1195
Kwaan H C 1987 Role of fibrinolysis in thrombotic thrombocytopenic purpura. Seminars in Hematology 24: 101–109
Lalau Keraly C, Kinlough-Rathbone R L, Packham M A, Suzuki H, Mustard J F 1988 Conditions affecting the responses of human platelets to epinephrine. Thrombosis and Haemostasis 60: 209–216
Lam J Y T, Chesebro J H, Steele P M et al 1991 Antithrombotic therapy for deep arterial injury by angioplasty. Efficacy of common platelet inhibition compared with thrombin inhibition in pigs. Circulation 84: 814–820
Lane D A, Ireland H, Wolff S, Grant R, Jennings S, Allen-Mersh T 1982 Plasma concentrations of fibrinopeptide A, fibrinogen fragment Bβ1–42 and β-thromboglobulin following total hip replacement. Thrombosis Research 26: 111–118
Lanza F, Beretz A, Stierlé A, Hanau D, Kubina M, Cazenave J-P 1988 Epinephrine potentiates human platelet activation but is not an aggregating agent. American Journal of Physiology 255: H1276–H1288
Larke R P B, Turpie A G G, Scott S, Chernesky M A 1977 Paramyxovirus-induced platelet aggregation. Requirement for neuraminic acid receptors on platelets. Laboratory Investigation 37: 150–157
Larsen E, Celi A, Gilbert G E, et al 1989 PADGEM protein: a receptor that mediates the interaction of activated platelets with neutrophils and monocytes. Cell 59: 305–312
Lassila R, Badimon J J, Vallabhajosula S, Badimon L 1990 Dynamic monitoring of platelet deposition on severely damaged vessel wall in flowing blood. Effects of different stenoses on thrombus growth. Arteriosclerosis 10: 306–315
László E, Káldi N, Kovács L 1983 Alterations in plasma proteins and platelet functions with aging and cigarette smoking in healthy men. Thrombosis and Haemostasis 49: 150
Lazarus H M, Hutto W 1982 Electric burns and frostbite: patterns of vascular injury. Journal of Trauma 22: 581–585
Lellouche F, Martinuzzo M, Said P, Maclouf J, Carreras L O 1991 Imbalance of thromboxane/prostacyclin biosynthesis in patients with lupus anticoagulant. Blood 78: 2894–2899
Leonard E F 1987 Rheology of thrombosis. In: Colman R W, Hirsh J, Marder V J, Salzman E W (eds) Hemostasis and thrombosis. Basic principles and clinical practice, 2nd edn. J B Lippincott, Philadelphia, p 1111–1122
Le Papé A, Guitton J D, Gutman N, Legrand Y, Fauvel F, Muh J P 1983a Non-enzymatic glycosylation of collagen in diabetes: incidence on increased normal platelet aggregation. Haemostasis 13: 36–41
Le Papé A, Gutman N, Guitton J D, Legrand Y, Muh J P 1983b Nonenzymatic glycosylation increases platelet aggregation potency of collagen from placenta of diabetic human beings. Biochemical and Biophysical Research Communications 111: 602–610
Lerner W A, Pearlstein E, Ambrogio C, Karpatkin S 1983 A new mechanism for tumor-induced platelet aggregation. Comparison with mechanisms shared by other tumors with possible pharmacologic strategy toward prevention of metastases. International Journal of Cancer 31: 463–469
Leuven J A G, Kluft C, Bertina R M, Hessel L W 1987 Effects of two low-dose oral contraceptives on circulating components of the coagulation and fibrinolytic systems. Journal of Laboratory and Clinical Investigation 109: 631–636
Levine P H 1973 An acute effect of cigarette smoking on platelet function. A possible link between smoking and arterial thrombosis. Circulation 48: 619–623
Lewis J C, Taylor R G 1989 Effects of varying dietary fatty acid ratios on plasma lipids and platelet function in the African green monkey. Atherosclerosis 77: 167–174
Lewis H D Jr, Davis J W, Archibald D G et al 1983 Protective effects of aspirin against acute myocardial infarction and death in men with unstable angina. Results of a Veterans Administration cooperative study. New England Journal of Medicine 309: 396–403
Lian E C-Y 1988 Thrombotic thrombocytopenic purpura. Annual Review of Medicine 39: 203–212
Lian E C-Y, Siddiqui F A, Jamieson G A, Tandon N N 1991 Platelet agglutinating protein p37 causes platelet agglutination through its binding to membrane glycoprotein IV. Thrombosis and Haemostasis 65: 102–106
Libby P, Hansson G K 1991 Biology of disease. Involvement of the immune system in human atherogenesis: current knowledge and unanswered questions. Laboratory Investigation 64: 5–15
Libby P, Salomon R N, Payne D D, Schoen F J, Pober J S 1989 Functions of vascular wall cells related to the development of transplantation-associated coronary atherosclerosis. Transplantation Proceedings 21: 3677–3684
Livingstone C, McLellan A R, McGregor M-A et al 1991 Altered G-protein expression and adenylate cyclase activity in platelets of non-insulin-dependent diabetic (NIDDM) male subjects. Biochimica et Biophysica Acta 1096: 127–133
Loscalzo J 1990 Lipoprotein(a). A unique risk factor for atherothrombotic disease. Arteriosclerosis 10: 672–679
McCully K S 1990 Atherosclerosis, serum cholesterol and the homocysteine theory: a study of 194 consecutive autopsies. American Journal of the Medical Sciences 299: 217–221
McEver R P 1991a GMP-140: A receptor for neutrophils and monocytes on activated platelets and endothelium. Journal of Cellular Biochemistry 45: 156–161
McEver R P 1991b Leukocyte interactions mediated by selectins. Thrombosis and Haemostasis 66: 80–87
McGill H C Jr 1988 The cardiovascular pathology of smoking. American Heart Journal 115: 250–257
McGill H C 1990 Relationship of atherosclerosis in young men to serum lipoprotein cholesterol concentrations and smoking. A preliminary report from the pathobiological determinants of atherosclerosis in youth (PDAY) research group. Journal of the American Medical Association 264: 3018–3024
McGregor J L, Catimel B, Parmentier S, Clezardin P, Dechavanne M, Leung L L K 1989 Rapid purification and partial characterization of human platelet glycoprotein IIIb. Interaction with thrombospondin and its role in platelet aggregation. Journal of Biological Chemistry 264: 501–506
Mahajan S L, Myers T J, Baldini M 1981 Disseminated intravascular coagulation during rewarming following hypothermia. Journal of the American Medical Association 245: 2517–2518
Malinow M R 1990 Hyperhomocyst(e)inemia. A common and easily reversible risk factor for occlusive atheroclerosis. Circulation 81: 2004–2006
Mann K G, Nesheim M E, Church W R, Haley P, Krishnaswamy S 1990 Surface-dependent reactions of the vitamin K-dependent enzyme complexes. Blood 76: 1–16
Manning D R, Brass L F 1991 The role of GTP-binding proteins in platelet activation. Thrombosis and Haemostasis 66: 393–399
Mansouri A, Perry C A 1984 Inhibition of platelet ADP and serotonin release by carbon monoxide and in cigarette smokers. Experientia 40: 515–517
Marcus A J 1990 Thrombosis and inflammation as multicellular

processes: pathophysiologic significance of transcellular metabolism. Blood 76: 1903–1907
Massmann J, Trimper B, Gebhardt G 1987 Failure of foreign serum injections to induce immune vasculitis and to accelerate spontaneous or cholesterol-induced atherosclerosis in swine. Atherosclerosis 66: 77–83
Masuda J, Ross R 1990 Atherogenesis during low level hypercholesterolemia in the nonhuman primate. I. Fatty streak formation. Arteriosclerosis 10: 164–177
Matthews K A, Meilahn E, Kuller L H, Kelsey S F, Caggiula A W, Wing R R 1989 Menopause and risk factors for coronary heart disease. New England Journal of Medicine 321: 641–646
Mattiasson I, Lindgärde F, Nilsson J Å, Theorell T 1990 Threat of unemployment and cardiovascular risk factors: longitudinal study of quality of sleep and serum cholesterol concentrations in men threatened with redundancy. British Medical Journal 301: 461–466
Meade T W 1987 The epidemiology of haemostatic and other variables in coronary artery disease. In: Verstraete M, Vermylen J, Lijnen H R, Arnout J (eds) Thrombosis and haemostasis. International society on thrombosis and haemostasis 1987 Leuven University Press, Leuven, p 37–60
Meade T W, Howarth D J, Stirling Y 1984 Fibrinopeptide A and sudden coronary death. Lancet ii: 607–609
Meade T W, Vickers M V, Thompson S G, Stirling Y, Haines A P, Miller G J 1985 Epidemiological characteristics of platelet aggregability. British Medical Journal 290: 428–432
Meade T W, Imeson J, Stirling Y 1987 Effects of changes in smoking and other characteristics on clotting factors and the risk of ischaemic heart disease. Lancet i: 986–988
Melnick J L, Adam E, DeBakey M E 1990 Possible role of cytomegalovirus in atherogenesis. Journal of the American Medical Association 263: 2204–2207
Mensink R P, Katan M B 1990 Effect of dietary trans fatty acids on high-density and low-density lipoprotein cholesterol levels in healthy subjects. New England Journal of Medicine 323: 439–445
Menter D G, Hatfield J S, Harkins C et al 1987 Tumor cell-platelet interactions in vitro and their relationship to in vivo arrest of hematogenously circulating tumor cells. Clinical and Experimental Metastasis 5: 65–78
Metzelaar M J, Sixma J J, Nieuwenhuis H K 1990 Detection of platelet activation using activation specific monoclonal antibodies. Blood Cells 16: 85–93
Metzelaar M J, Korteweg J, Sixma J J, Nieuwenhuis H K 1991 Biochemical characterization of PECAM-1 (CD31 antigen) on human platelets. Thrombosis and Haemostasis 66: 700–707
Metzelaar M J, Heijnen H F G, Sixma J J, Nieuwenhuis H K 1992 Identification of a 33-Kd protein associated with the α granule membrane (GMP-33) that is expressed on the surface of activated platelets. Blood 79: 372–379
Meyrick B, Brigham K L 1983 Acute effects of Escherichia coli endotoxin on the pulmonary microcirculation of anesthetized sheep. Structure: function relationships. Laboratory Investigation 48: 458–470
Minick C R 1981 Synergy of arterial injury and hypercholesterolemia in atherogenesis. In: Moore S (ed) Vascular injury and atherosclerosis. Marcel Dekker, New York, p 149–173
Minick C R, Alonso D R, Rankin L 1978 Role of immunologic arterial injury in atherogenesis. Thrombosis and Haemostasis 39: 304–311
Mishell D R Jr 1988 Use of oral contraceptives in women of older reproductive age. American Journal of Obstetrics and Gynecology 158: 1652–1657
Moake J L 1988 von Willebrand factor and the pathophysiology of thrombotic thrombocytopenia: from human studies to a new animal model. Laboratory Investigation 59: 415–417
Moake J L, Turner N A, Stathopoulos N A, Nolasco L, Hellums J D 1988 Shear-induced platelet aggregation can be mediated by vWF released from platelets, as well as by exogenous large or unusually large vWF multimers, requires adenosine diphosphate, and is resistant to aspirin. Blood 71: 1366–1374
Moncada S, Vane J R 1978 Pharmacology and endogenous roles of prostaglandin endoperoxides, thromboxane A_2, and prostacyclin. Pharmacological Reviews 30: 293–331
Moncada S, Palmer R M J, Higgs E A 1987 Prostacyclin and endothelium-derived relaxing factor: biological interactions and significance. In: Verstraete M, Vermylen J, Lijnen H R, Arnout J (eds) Thrombosis and haemostasis International Society on thrombosis and haemostasis 1987. Leuven University Press, Leuven p 597–618
Monro J M, Cotran R S 1988 The pathogenesis of atherosclerosis: atherogenesis and inflammation. Laboratory Investigation 58: 249–261
Moore J C, Murphy W G, Kelton J G 1990 Calpain proteolysis of von Willebrand factor enhances its binding to platelet membrane glycoprotein IIb/IIIa: an explanation for platelet aggregation in thrombotic thrombocytopenic purpura. British Journal of Haematology 74: 457–464
Moore K L, Andreoli S P, Esmon N L, Esmon C T, Bang N U 1987 Endotoxin enhances tissue factor and suppresses thrombomodulin expression of human vascular endothelium in vitro. Journal of Clinical Investigation 79: 124–130
Moore S 1981 Injury mechanisms in atherogenesis. In: Moore S (ed) Vascular injury and atherosclerosis. Marcel Dekker, New York, p 131–148
Moore S 1989 Dietary atherosclerosis and arterial wall injury. Laboratory Investigation 60: 733–736
Moore S, Mersereau W A 1968 Microembolic renal ischemia, hypertension, and nephrosclerosis. Archives of Pathology 85: 623–630
Moore S, Belbeck L W, Evans G, Pineau S 1981 Effects of complete or partial occlusion of a coronary artery. Laboratory Investigation 44: 151–157
Moritz M W, Reimers R C, Baker R K, Sutera S P, Joist J H 1983 Role of cytoplasmic and releasable ADP in platelet aggregation induced by laminar shear stress. Journal of Laboratory and Clinical Medicine 101: 537–544
Mulcahy R 1983 Influence of cigarette smoking on morbidity and mortality after myocardial infarction. British Heart Journal 49: 410–415
Müller-Berghaus G 1978 The role of platelets, leukocytes and complement in the activation of intravascular coagulation by endotoxin. In: de Gaetano G, Garattini S (eds) Platelets: A multidisciplinary approach. Raven Press, New York, p 303–320
Mustard J F, Murphy E A 1963 Effect of smoking on blood coagulation and platelet survival in man. British Medical Journal 1: 846–849
Mustard J F, Packham M A 1979 The reaction of the blood to injury. In: Movat H Z (ed) Inflammation, immunity and hypersensitivity, 2nd edn. Harper & Row, New York, p 557–664
Mustard J F, Murphy E A, Rowsell H C, Downie H G 1962 Factors influencing thrombus formation in vivo. American Journal of Medicine 33: 621–647
Mustard J F, Packham M A, Kinlough-Rathbone R L 1990 Platelets, blood flow and vessel wall. Circulation 81 (suppl I): I24–I27
Nachman R L, Hajjar K A 1991 Endothelial cell fibrinolytic activity. Annals of the New York Academy of Sciences 614: 240–249
Nathan C, Sporn M 1991 Cytokines in context. Journal of Cell Biology 113: 981–986
Nawroth P P, Stern D M, Kaplan K L, Nossel H L 1984 Prostacyclin production by perturbed bovine aortic endothelial cells in culture. Blood 64: 801–806
Newman P J, Berndt M C, Gorski J et al 1990 PECAM-1 (CD31) cloning and relation to adhesion molecules of the immunoglobulin gene superfamily. Science 247: 1219–1222
Nichols T C, Bellinger D A, Johnson T A, Lamb M A, Griggs T R 1986 von Willebrand's disease prevents occlusive thrombosis in stenosed and injured porcine coronary arteries. Circulation Research 59: 15–26
Nielsen N V, Ditzel J 1985 Prevalence of macro- and microvascular disease as related to glycosylated hemoglobin in type I and type II diabetic subjects. An epidemiologic study in Denmark. Hormone and Metabolic Research 17 (suppl): 19–22
Nieuwenhuis H K, Akkerman J W N, Houdijk W P M, Sixma J J 1985 Human blood platelets showing no response to collagen fail to express surface glycoprotein Ia. Nature 318: 470–472
Nieuwenhuis H K, van Oosterhout J J G, Rozemuller E, van Iwaarden F, Sixma J J 1987 Studies with a monoclonal antibody against activated platelets: evidence that a secreted 53 000-molecular weight

lysosome-like granule protein is exposed on the surface of activated platelets in the circulation. Blood 70: 838–845
Niiya K, Hodson E, Bader R et al 1987 Increased surface expression of the membrane glycoprotein IIb/IIIa complex induced by platelet activation. Relationship to the binding of fibrinogen and platelet aggregation. Blood 70: 475–483
Nollert M U, Hall E R, Eskin S G, McIntire L V 1989 The effect of shear stress on the uptake and metabolism of arachidonic acid by human endothelial cells. Biochimica et Biophysica Acta 1005: 72–78
Nordøy A, Goodnight S H 1990 Dietary lipids and thrombosis. Relationships to atherosclerosis. Arteriosclerosis 10: 149–163
Nossel H L 1976 Radioimmunoassay of fibrinopeptides in relation to intravascular coagulation and thrombosis. New England Journal of Medicine 295: 428–432
Nowak J, Murray J J, Oates J A, FitzGerald G A 1987 Biochemical evidence of a chronic abnormality in platelet and vascular function in healthy individuals who smoke cigarettes. Circulation 76: 6–14
Okadome K, Tanaka K 1986 Pathophysiological effects of fibrin on arterial endothelial cells in vivo: an electron microscopic study. Experimental and Molecular Pathology 44: 364–373
Oliva P B 1983 The role of coronary artery spasm in acute myocardial infarction. In: Goldberg S (ed) Coronary artery spasm and thrombosis. Davis, Philadelphia, p 45–58
Oliver M F 1989 Cigarette smoking, polyunsaturated fats, linoleic acid, and coronary heart disease. Lancet i: 1241–1242
Oliver M F 1990 Lipids and coronary disease — resolved and unresolved problems. British Medical Bulletin 46: 865–872
Onodera H, Hirata T, Sugawara H et al 1982 Platelet sensitivity to adenosine diphosphate and to prostacyclin in diabetic patients. Tohoku Journal of Experimental Medicine 137: 423–428
Packham M A 1978 Methods for detection of hypersensitive platelets. Thrombosis and Haemostasis 40: 175–195
Packham M A 1988 The behavior of platelets at foreign surfaces. Proceedings of the Society for Experimental Biology and Medicine 189: 261–274
Packham M A 1991 Platelet reactions in thrombosis. In: Gotlieb A I, Langille B L, Federoff S (eds) Atherosclerosis. Cellular and molecular interactions in the artery wall. Plenum Press, New York, p 209–225
Packham MA, Mustard J F 1983 Pharmacology of antiplatelet agents and their role in coronary disease. In: Margulies E (ed) Myocardial infarction and cardiac death. Academic Press, New York, p 93–142
Packham M A, Mustard J F 1984 Platelet adhesion. In: Spaet T H (ed) Progress in hemostasis and thrombosis. Grune & Stratton, New York, vol 7: 211–288
Packham M A, Mustard J F 1986 The role of platelets in the development and complications of atherosclerosis. Seminars in Hematology 23: 8–26
Packham M A, Guccione M A, Kinlough-Rathbone R L, Mustard J F 1980 Platelet sialic acid and platelet survival after aggregation by ADP. Blood 56: 876–880
Packham M A, Bryant N L, Guccione M A, Kinlough-Rathbone R L, Mustard J F 1989 Effect of the concentration of Ca^{2+} in the suspending medium on the responses of human and rabbit platelets to aggregating agents. Thrombosis and Haemostasis 62: 968–976
Panza J A, Quyyumi A A, Brush J E Jr, Epstein S E 1990 Abnormal endothelium-dependent vascular relaxation in patients with essential hypertension. New England Journal of Medicine 323: 22–27
Parbtani A, Kinlough-Rathbone R L, Chahil A, Richardson M, Mustard J F 1990 Survival of rabbit platelets exposed to immune complexes. Experimental and Molecular Pathology 52: 109–121
Parkes J L, Cardell R R, Hubbard F C Jr, Hubbard D, Meltzer A, Penn A 1991 Cultured human atherosclerotic plaque smooth muscle cells retain transforming potential and display enhanced expression of the myc protooncogene. American Journal of Pathology 138: 765–775
Paton R C 1979 Platelet survival in diabetes mellitus using an aspirin-labelling technique. Thrombosis Research 15: 793–802
Paton R C, Guillot R, Passa P, Canivet J 1982 Prostacyclin production by human endothelial cells cultured in diabetic serum. Diabete & Metabolisme 8: 323–328
Penn A 1990 Mutational events in the etiology of arteriosclerotic plaques. Mutation Research 239: 149–162
Pesonen E, Kaprio E, Rapola J, Soveri T, Oksanen H 1981 Endothelial cell damage in piglet coronary artery after intravenous administration of E. coli endotoxin. A scanning and transmission electron-microscopic study. Atherosclerosis 40: 65–73
Pfueller S L 1985 Immunology of the platelet surface. In: George J N, Nurden A T, Phillips D R (eds) Platelet membrane glycoproteins. Plenum Press, New York, p 327–355
Pfueller S L, Burns P, Mak K, Firkin B G 1988 Effects of nicotine on platelet function. Haemostasis 18: 163–169
Pirkle H, Carstens P 1974 Pulmonary platelet aggregates associated with sudden death in man. Science 185: 1062–1064
Pittilo R M, Mackie I J, Rowles P M, Machin S J, Woolf N 1982 Effects of cigarette smoking on the ultrastructure of rat thoracic aorta and its ability to produce prostacyclin. Thrombosis and Haemostasis 48: 173–176
Pittilo R M, Bull H A, Gulati S et al 1990 Nicotine and cigarette smoking: effects on the ultrastructure of aortic endothelium. International Journal of Experimental Pathology 71: 573–586
Pober J S, Cotran R S 1990 Cytokines and endothelial cell biology. Physiological Reviews 70: 427–451
Pober J S, Cotran R S 1991 What can be learned from the expression of endothelial adhesion molecules in tissues? Laboratory Investigation 64: 301–305
Pooling Project Research Group 1978 Relationship of blood pressure, serum cholesterol, smoking habit, relative weight and ECG abnormalities to incidence of major coronary events: final report of the Pooling Project. Journal of Chronic Diseases 31: 201–306
Popma J J, Califf R M, Topol E J 1991 Clinical trials of restenosis after coronary angioplasty. Circulation 84: 1426–1436
Porta M 1988 Von Willebrand factor as an indicator of endothelial cell dysfunction in diabetic microangiopathy: studies in vivo. Diabete e Metabolisme 14: 523–526
Qiao J-H, Fishbein M C 1991 The severity of coronary atherosclerosis at sites of plaque rupture with occlusive thrombosis. Journal of the American College of Cardiology 17: 1138–1142
Rångemark C, Wennmalm Å 1991 Cigarette smoking and urinary excretion of markers for platelet/vessel wall interaction in healthy women. Clinical Science 81: 11–15
Rapaport S I 1991 Regulation of the tissue factor pathway. Annals of the New York Academy of Sciences 614: 51–62
Rath M, Niendorf A, Reblin T, Dietel M, Krebber H-J, Beisiegel U 1989 Detection and quantification of lipoprotein(a) in the arterial wall of 107 coronary bypass patients. Arteriosclerosis 9: 579–592
Reidy M A 1988 Endothelial regeneration. VIII Interaction of smooth muscle cells with endothelial regrowth. Laboratory Investigation 59: 36–43
Reidy M A, Schwartz S M 1983 Endothelial injury and regeneration. IV. Endotoxin: a nondenuding injury to aortic endothelium. Laboratory Investigation 48: 25–34
Reidy M A, Clowes A W, Schwartz S M 1983 Endothelial regeneration. V. Inhibition of endothelial regrowth in arteries of rat and rabbit. Laboratory Investigation 49: 569–575
Reilly I A G, Doran J B, Smith B, FitzGerald G A 1986 Increased thromboxane biosynthesis in a human preparation of platelet activation: biochemical and functional consequences of selective inhibition of thromboxane synthase. Circulation 73: 1300–1309
Reimers H-J, Kinlough-Rathbone R L, Cazenave J-P et al 1976 In vitro and in vivo functions of thrombin-treated platelets. Thrombosis and Haemostasis 35: 151–166
Reimers R C, Sutera S P, Joist J H 1984 Potentiation by red blood cells of shear-induced platelet aggregation: relative importance of chemical and physical mechanisms. Blood 64: 1200–1206
Renaud S 1990 Linoleic acid, platelet aggregation and myocardial infarction. Atherosclerosis 80: 255–256
Renaud S, Gautheron P 1975 Influence of dietary fats on atherosclerosis, coagulation and platelet phospholipids in rabbits. Atherosclerosis 21: 115–124
Renaud S, Kinlough R L, Mustard J F 1970 Relationship between platelet aggregation and the thrombotic tendency in rats fed hyperlipemic diets. Laboratory Investigation 22: 339–343
Renaud S, Blache D, Dumont E, Thevenon C, Wissendanger T 1984 Platelet function after cigarette smoking in relation to nicotine and

carbon monoxide. Clinical Pharmacology and Therapeutics 36: 389–395

Resink T J, Dimitrov D, Zschauer A, Erne P, Tkachuk V A, Bühler F R 1988 Platelet calcium-linked abnormalities in essential hypertension. Annals of the New York Academy of Sciences 488: 252–265

Ribes J A, Francis C W, Wagner D D 1987 Fibrin induces release of von Willebrand factor from endothelial cells. Journal of Clinical Investigation 79: 117–123

Ribes J A, Ni F, Wagner D D, Francis C W 1989 Mediation of fibrin-induced release of von Willebrand factor from cultured endothelial cells by the fibrin β chain. Journal of Clinical Investigation 84: 435–442

Rickles F R, Edwards R L 1983 Activation of blood coagulation in cancer: Trousseau's syndrome revisited. Blood 62: 14–31

Rink T J, Sage S O 1990 Calcium signalling in human platelets. Annual Review of Physiology 52: 431–449

Roberts W C 1987 Frequency of systemic hypertension in various cardiovascular diseases. American Journal of Cardiology 60: 1E–8E

Roberts W C 1989 Atherosclerosis risk factors — are there ten or is there only one? American Journal of Cardiology 64: 552–554

Rosenberg R D, Rosenberg J S 1984 Natural anticoagulant mechanisms. Journal of Clinical Investigation 74: 1–5

Ross R 1986 The pathogenesis of atherosclerosis — an update. New England Journal of Medicine 314: 488–500

Ross R 1989 Platelet-derived growth factor. Lancet i: 1179–1182

Rostrup M, Mundal H H, Kjeldsen S E, Gjesdal K, Eide I 1990 Awareness of high blood pressure stimulates platelet release reaction. Thrombosis and Haemostasis 63: 367–370

Roth G J 1991 Developing relationships: arterial platelet adhesion, glycoprotein Ib, and leucine-rich glycoproteins. Blood 77: 5–19

Rowe MI, Marchildon MB, Arango A, Malinin T, Gans M A 1978 The mechanisms of thrombocytopenia in experimental Gram-negative septicemia. Surgery 84: 87–93

Rowntree L G, Shionoya T 1927 Studies in experimental extracorporeal thrombosis. I. A method for the direct observation of extracorporeal thrombus formation. Journal of Experimental Medicine 46: 7–12

Rowsell H C, Hegardt B, Downie H G, Mustard J F, Murphy E A 1966 Adrenaline and experimental thrombosis. British Journal of Haematology 12: 66–73

Ruggenenti P, Remuzzi G 1990 Thrombotic thrombocytopenic purpura and related disorders. Hematology/Oncology Clinics of North America 4: 219–241

Russell R W R 1961 Observations on the retinal blood vessels in monocular blindness. Lancet ii: 1422–1428

Salimi A, Oliver G C Jr, Lee J, Sherman L A 1977 Continued incorporation of circulating radiolabelled fibrinogen into preformed coronary artery thrombi. Circulation 56: 213–217

Santos M T, Valles J, Marcus A J et al 1991 Enhancement of platelet reactivity and modulation of eicosanoid production by intact erythrocytes. A new approach to platelet activation and recruitment. Journal of Clinical Investigation 87: 571–580

Scanu A M 1990 Lipoprotein(a): a genetically determined cardiovascular pathogen in search of a function. Journal of Laboratory and Clinical Medicine 116: 142–146

Schafer A I 1984 Bleeding and thrombosis in the myeloproliferative disorders. Blood 64: 1–12

Schifflh 1989 Platelet cytosolic free calcium concentration in hypertension associated with early stage kidney disease. Klinische Wochenschrift 67: 676–681

Schmid-Schönbein H, Born G V R, Richardson P D et al 1981 Rheology of thrombotic processes in flow: the interaction of erythrocytes and thrombocytes subjected to high flow forces. Biorheology 18: 415–444

Schmidt J L 1989 Thrombotic thrombocytopenic purpura: successful treatment unlocks etiologic secrets. Mayo Clinic Proceedings 64: 956–961

Schmidt K G, Rasmussen J W 1984 Acute platelet activation induced by smoking. Thrombosis and Haemostasis 51: 279–282

Schoen F J, Libby P 1991 Cardiac transplant graft arteriosclerosis. Trends in Cardiovascular Medicine 1: 216–223

Schwartz S M, Campbell G R, Campbell J H 1986 Replication of smooth muscle cells in vascular disease. Circulation Research 58: 427–444

Schwartz C J, Valente A J, Kelley J L, Sprague E A, Edwards E H 1988 Thrombosis and the development of atherosclerosis: Rokitansky revisited. Seminars in Thrombosis and Hemostasis 14: 189–195

Schwartz C J, Kelley J L, Nerem R M et al 1989 Pathophysiology of the atherogenic process. American Journal of Cardiology 64: 23G–30G

Scott J 1991 Lipoprotein(a). Thrombotic and atherogenic. British Medical Journal 303: 663–664

Scott R F, Reidy M A, Kim D N, Schmee J, Thomas W A 1986 Intimal cell mass-derived atherosclerotic lesions in the abdominal aorta of hyperlipidemic swine. Part 2. Investigation of endothelial cell changes and leukocyte adherence associated with early smooth muscle cell proliferative activity. Atherosclerosis 62: 27–38

Seifert P S, Hansson G K 1989 Complement receptors and regulatory proteins in human atherosclerotic lesions. Arteriosclerosis 9: 802–811

Seifert P S, Kazatchkine M D 1988 The complement system in atherosclerosis. Atherosclerosis 73: 91–104

Setty B N Y, Stuart M J 1986 15-Hydroxy-5,8,11,13-eicosatetraenoic acid inhibits human vascular cyclooxygenase. Potential role in diabetic vascular disease. Journal of Clinical Investigation 77: 202–211

Shattil S J, Cooper R A 1978 Role of membrane lipid composition, organization, and fluidity in human platelet function. In: Spaet T H (ed) Progress in hemostasis and thrombosis. Grune & Stratton, New York, vol 4: 59–86

Shattil S J, Hoxie J A, Cunningham MC, Brass L F 1985 Changes in the platelet membrane glycoprotein IIb-IIIa complex during platelet activation. Journal of Biological Chemistry 260: 11107–11114

Shekelle R B, Stamler J 1989 Dietary cholesterol and ischaemic heart disease. Lancet i: 1177–1178

Shinton R, Beevers G 1989 Meta-analysis of relation between cigarette smoking and stroke. British Medical Journal 298: 789–794

Sieffert G F, Keown K, Moore W S 1981 Pathologic effect of tobacco smoke inhalation on arterial intima. Surgical Forum 32: 333–335

Siess W 1989 Molecular mechanisms of platelet activation. Physiological Reviews 69: 58–177

Siltanen P 1987 Stress, coronary disease, and coronary death. Annals of Clinical Research 19: 96–103

Silverstein R L, Febbraio M 1990 LAMP-2 is an activation-dependent platelet surface protein: further evidence for platelet lysosomal membrane flow. Journal of Cell Biology 111: 66a

Silverstein R L, Leung L L K, Nachman R L 1987 Thrombospondin: A versatile multifunctional glycoprotein. Arteriosclerosis 6: 245–253

Sims P J, Faioni E M, Wiedmer T, Shattil S J 1988 Complement proteins C5b-9 cause release of membrane vesicles from the platelet surface that are enriched in the membrane receptor for coagulation factor Va and express prothrombinase activity. Journal of Biological Chemistry 263: 18205–18212

Sinzinger H, O'Grady J, Fitscha P 1988 Platelet deposition on human atherosclerotic lesions is decreased by low-dose aspirin in combination with dipyridamole. Journal of International Medical Research 16: 39–43

Sixma J J, Pronk A, Nievelstein P N E M et al 1991 Platelet adhesion to extracellular matrices of cultured cells. Annals of the New York Academy of Sciences 614: 181–192

Slivka S R, Loskutoff D J 1991 Platelets stimulate endothelial cells to synthesize type 1 plasminogen activator inhibitor. Evaluation of the role of transforming growth factor β. Blood 77: 1013–1019

Smith B D, la Celle P L 1982 Blood viscosity and thrombosis: clinical considerations. In: Spaet T H (ed) Progress in hemostasis and thrombosis. Grune & Stratton, New York, vol 6: 179–201

Smith C W, Marlin S D, Rothlein R, Toman C, Anderson D C 1989 Cooperative interactions of LEA-1 and Mac-1 with intercellular adhesion molecule-1 in facilitating adherence and transendothelial migration of human neutrophils in vitro. Journal of Clinical Investigation 83: 2008–2017

Smith C W, Anderson D C, Taylor A A, Rossen R D, Entman M L 1991 Leukocyte adhesion molecules and myocardial ischemia. Trends in Cardiovascular Medicine 1: 167–170

Sottnek H M, Cassel W A, Campbell W G Jr 1975 The pathogenesis

of vaccinia virus toxicity. I. The role of virus-platelet interaction. Laboratory Investigation 33: 514–521
Span A H M, van Dam-Mieras M C E, Mullers W, Endert J, Muller A D, Bruggeman C A 1991 The effect of virus infection on the adherence of leukocytes or platelets to endothelial cells. European Journal of Clinical Investigation 21: 331–338
Stampfer M J, Willett W C, Colditz G A, Speizer F E, Hennekens C H 1988 A prospective study of past use of oral contraceptive agents and risk of cardiovascular diseases. New England Journal of Medicine 319: 1313–1317
Stampfer M J, Colditz G A, Willett W C et al 1991 Postmenopausal estrogen therapy and cardiovascular disease. Ten-year follow-up from the Nurses' Health Study. New England Journal of Medicine 325: 756–762
Stehbens W E 1990 The epidemiological relationship of hypercholesterolemia, hypertension, diabetes mellitus and obesity to coronary heart disease and atherogenesis. Journal of Clinical Epidemiology 43: 733–741
Steinberg D 1991 Antioxidants and atherosclerosis. A current assessment. Circulation 84: 1420–1425
Stemerman M B, Ross R 1972 Experimental arteriosclerosis. I. Fibrous plaque formation in primates, an electron microscope study. Journal of Experimental Medicine 136: 769–789
Stern D, Nawroth P, Handley D, Kisiel W 1985 An endothelial cell-dependent pathway of coagulation. Proceedings of the National Academy of Sciences, USA 82: 2523–2527
Stills H F, Bullock B C, Clarkson T B 1983 Increased atherosclerosis and glomerulonephritis in cynomolgus monkeys (Macaca fascicularis) given injections of BSA over an extended period of time. American Journal of Pathology 113: 222–234
Stolar M W 1988 Atherosclerosis in diabetes: the role of hyperinsulinemia. Metabolism 37 (Suppl 1): 1–9
Strawn W B, Bondjers G, Kaplan J R et al 1991 Endothelial dysfunction in response to psychosocial stress in monkeys. Circulation Research: 68: 1270–1279
Sullam P M, Jarvis G A, Valone F H 1988 Role of immunoglobulin G in platelet aggregation by viridans group streptococci. Infection and Immunity 56: 2907–2911
Sullivan J M, Vander Zwaag R, Hughes J P et al 1990 Estrogen replacement and coronary artery disease. Effect on survival in postmenopausal women. Archives of Internal Medicine 150: 2557–2562
Suzuki H, Kinlough-Rathbone R L, Packham M A, Tanoue K, Yamazaki H, Mustard J F 1988 Immunocytochemical localization of fibrinogen during thrombin-induced aggregation of washed human platelets. Blood 71: 1310–1320
Tandon N N, Kralisz U, Jamieson G A 1989 Identification of glycoprotein IV (CD36) as a primary receptor for platelet-collagen adhesion. Journal of Biological Chemistry 264: 7576–7583
Tandon N N, Ockenhouse C F, Greco N J, Jamieson G A 1991 Adhesive functions of platelets lacking glycoprotein IV (CD36). Blood 78: 2809–2813
Terada H, Baldini M, Ebbe S, Madoff M A 1966 Interaction of influenza virus with blood platelets. Blood 28: 213–228
Thorneycroft I H 1990 Oral contraceptives and myocardial infarction. American Journal of Obstetrics and Gynecology 163: 1393–1397
Timmons S, Huzoor-Akbar, Grabarek J, Kloczewiak M, Hawiger J 1986 Mechanism of human platelet activation by endotoxic glycolipid-bearing mutant Re595 of Salmonella minnesota. Blood 68: 1015–1023
Tindall H, Paton R C, Zuzel M, McNicol G P 1981 Platelet life-span in diabetics with and without retinopathy. Thrombosis Research 21: 641–648
Tschöpe D, Rösen P, Gries F A 1991 Increase in the cytosolic concentration of calcium in platelets of diabetics type II. Thrombosis Research 62: 421–428
Turitto V T 1988 Platelet rheology. Clinical Blood Rheology 1–2: 111–128
Tyson J E, deSa D J, Moore S 1976 Thromboatheromatous complications of umbilical arterial catheterization in the newborn period. Archives of Disease in Childhood 51: 744–754
Uedelhoven W M, Rützel A, Meese C O, Weber P C 1991 Smoking alters thromboxane metabolism in man. Biochimica et Biophysica Acta 1081: 197–201
Ulbricht T L V, Southgate D A T 1991 Coronary heart disease: seven dietary factors. Lancet 338: 985–992
Van Dam-Mieras M C E, Bruggeman C A, Muller A D, Debie W H M, Zwaal R F A 1987 Induction of endothelial cell procoagulant activity by cytomegalovirus infection. Thrombosis Research 47: 69–75
van der Giessen W J, Serruys P W, Stoel I, Hugenholtz P G, Deleeuw P W, van Vliet H H D M 1983 Acute effect of cigarette smoking on cardiac prostaglandin synthesis and platelet behaviour in patients with coronary heart disease. In: Samuelsson B, Paoletti R, Ramwell P (eds) Advances in prostaglandin, thromboxane, and leukotriene research. Raven Press, New York, vol 11: 359–364
Vane J R, Änggård E E, Botting R M 1990 Regulatory functions of the vascular endothelium. New England Journal of Medicine 323: 27–36
Vanhoutte P M 1988 Platelets, endothelium and blood vessel wall. Experientia 44: 105–109
van Oost B, van Hien-Hagg I H, Timmermans A P M, Sixma J J 1983 The effect of thrombin on the density distribution of blood platelets: detection of activated platelets in the circulation. Blood 62: 433–438
van Willigen G, Akkerman J-W N 1992 Regulation of glycoprotein IIB/IIIA exposure on platelets stimulated with α-thrombin. Blood 79: 82–90
Verheugt F W A, Brugada P 1991 Sudden death after acute myocardial infarction: the forgotten thrombotic view. American Journal of Cardiology 67: 1130–1134
Vessey M, Mant D, Smith A, Yeates D 1986 Oral contraceptives and venous thromboembolism: findings in a large prospective study. British Medical Journal 292: 526
Vetrovec G W, Leinback R C, Gold H K, Cowley M J 1982 Intracoronary thrombolysis in syndromes of unstable ischemia: angiographic and clinical results. American Heart Journal 104: 946–952
Virchow R 1856 Phlogose und Thrombose im Gefassystem. Gesämmelte Abhandlungen zur Wissenchaftlichen Medicin. Staatsdruckerei, Frankfurt
Visser M R, Tracy P B, Vercellotti G M, Goodman J L, White J G, Jacob H S 1988 Enhanced thrombin generation and platelet binding on herpes simplex virus-infected endothelium. Proceedings of the National Academy of Sciences, USA 85: 8227–8230
Vlaicu R, Niculescu F, Rus H G, Cristea A 1985 Immunohistochemical localization of the terminal C5-b-9 complement complex in human aortic fibrous plaque. Atherosclerosis 57: 163–177
von Recklinghausen F 1883 Handbuch der allgemeinen Pathologie des Kreislaufs und der Ernäbrung. In: Billroth C A T, Leucke A (eds) Lief 2–3 in Deutsche Chirurgie, p xliii 521
von Rokitansky C 1841 Handbuch der pathologischen Anatomie. Braumüller, Siedel, Vienna
Vu T-K H, Hung D T, Wheaton V I, Coughlin S R 1991 Molecular cloning of a functional thrombin receptor reveals a novel proteolytic mechanism of receptor activation. Cell 64: 1057–1068
Wahle K W L 1989 Isomeric fatty acids, essential fatty acids and coronary heart disease: a perspective. Proceedings of Porim International Palm Oil Development Conference. Palm Oil Research Institute of Malaysia, p 66–70
Warkentin T E, Powling M J, Hardisty R M 1990 Measurement of fibrinogen binding to platelets in whole blood by flow cytometry: a micromethod for the detection of platelet activation. British Journal of Haematology 76: 387–394
Watanabe K, Tanaka K 1983 Influence of fibrin, fibrinogen and fibrinogen degradation products on cultured endothelial cells. Atherosclerosis 48: 57–70
Watanabe K, McCaffrey T M, Weksler B B, Jaffe E A 1989 Endotoxin stimulates the production of prostacyclin by cultured human endothelial cells. In: Samuelsson B, Wong P Y-K, Sun F F (eds) Advances in prostaglandin, thromboxane, and leukotreine research. Raven Press, New York, vol 19: 242–243
Wehmeier A, Daum I, Jamin H, Schneider W 1991 Incidence and clinical risk factors for bleeding and thrombotic complications in myeloproliferative disorders. A retrospective analysis of 260 patients. Annals of Hematology 63: 101–106
Weimar B, Delvos U 1986 The mechanism of fibrin-induced

disorganization of cultured human endothelial cell monolayers. Arteriosclerosis 6: 139–145
Weiss E, Teredesai A, Hoffmann R, Hoffmann-Fezer G 1973 Volume distribution and ultrastructure of platelets in acute hog cholera. Thrombosis et Diathesis Haemorrhagica 30: 371–380
Weiss H J, Turitto V T, Baumgartner H R 1978 Effect of shear rate on platelet interaction with subendothelium in citrated and native blood. 1. Shear rate-dependent decrease of adhesion in von Willebrand's disease and Bernard–Soulier syndrome. Journal of Laboratory and Clinical Medicine 92: 750–764
Weiss H J, Hawiger J, Ruggeri Z M, Turitto V T, Thiagarajan P, Hoffmann T 1989 Fibrinogen-independent platelet adhesion and thrombus formation on subendothelium mediated by glycoprotein IIb-IIIa complex at high shear rate. Journal of Clinical Investigation 83: 288–297
Weitz J I, Koehn J A, Canfield R E, Landman S L, Friedman R 1986 Development of a radioimmunoassay for the fibrinogen-derived peptide Bβ1–42. Blood 67: 1014–1022
Weitz J I, Hudoba M, Massel D, Maraganore J, Hirsh J 1990 Clot-bound thrombin is protected from inhibition by heparin-antithrombin III but is susceptible to inactivation by antithrombin III-independent inhibitors. Journal of Clinical Investigation 86: 385–391
Wells S, Sissons M, Hasleton P S 1984 Quantitation of pulmonary megakaryocytes and fibrin thrombi in patients dying from burns. Histopathology 8: 517–527
White C J, Ramee S R, Collins T J 1991 Percutaneous coronary angioscopy. Current status and future directions. Trends in Cardiovascular Medicine 1: 6–11
Wiener H M, Vardinon N, Yust I 1991 Platelet antibody binding and spontaneous aggregation in 21 lupus anticoagulant patients. Vox Sanguinis 61: 111–121
Wiesel M-L, Zupan M, Wolff F, Grunebaum L, Brechenmacher C, Cazenave J-P 1991 Potential thrombogenicity of angiographic contrast agents. Thrombosis Research 64: 291–294
Wight T N 1989 Cell biology of arterial proteoglycans. Arteriosclerosis 9: 1–20
Wilcken D E L, Dudman N P B 1989 Mechanisms of thrombogenesis and accelerated atherogenesis in homocysteinaemia. Haemostasis 19 (suppl 1): 14–23
Wilcox J N 1991 Thrombin and other potential mechanisms underlying restenosis. Circulation 84: 432–435
Wilcox J N, Smith K M, Schwartz S M, Gordon D 1989 Localization of tissue factor in the normal vessel wall and in the atherosclerotic plaque. Proceedings of the National Academy of Sciences, USA 86: 2839–2843
Williams J K, Adams M R, Klopfenstein H S 1990 Estrogen modulates responses of atherosclerotic coronary arteries. Circulation 81: 1680–1687
Wilson J J, Neame P B, Kelton J G 1982 Infection-induced thrombocytopenia. Seminars in Thrombosis and Hemostasis 8: 217–233
Wilson P W F, Anderson K M, Castelli W P 1991 The impact of triglycerides on coronary heart disease. The Framingham study. Gotto A M Jr, Paoletti R (eds) Atherosclerosis Reviews. Raven Press, New York, vol 22: 59–63
Winocour P D, Kinlough-Rathbone R L, Richardson M, Mustard J F 1983 Reversal of shortened platelet survival in rats by the antifibrinolytic agent, epsilon aminocaproic acid. Journal of Clinical Investigation 71: 159–164
Winocour P D, Kinlough-Rathbone R L, Mustard J F 1986 Pathways responsible for platelet hypersensitivity in rats with diabetes. I. Streptozocin-induced diabetes. Journal of Laboratory and Clinical Medicine 107: 148–153
Winocour P D, Kinlough-Rathbone R L, Morazain R, Mustard J F 1987 The effect of dietary saturated fat and cholesterol on platelet function, platelet survival and response to continuous aortic injury in rats. Atherosclerosis 65: 37–50
Winocour P D, Rand M L, Kinlough-Rathbone R L, Richardson M, Mustard J F 1989 Platelet function and survival in rats with genetically determined hypercholesterolaemia. Atherosclerosis 76: 63–70
Wissler R W 1991 Update on the pathogenesis of atherosclerosis. American Journal of Medicine 91 (suppl 1B): 3S–9S
Witteman J C M, Grobbee D E, Kok F J, Hofman A, Valkenburg H A 1989 Increased risk of atherosclerosis in women after the menopause. British Medical Journal 298: 642–644
Wolf P A, D'Agostino R B, Kannel W B, Bonita R, Belanger A J 1988 Cigarette smoking as a risk factor for stroke. The Framingham Study. Journal of the American Medical Association 259: 1025–1029
Woolf N, Pittilo R M, Machin S J 1983 Cigarette smoking and platelet adhesion. Lancet ii: 1091
Xuewei W, Wanrhong Z 1983 Vascular injuries in electrical burns — the pathological basis for mechanism of injury. Burns 9: 335–339
Yamashiroya H M, Ghosh L, Yang R, Robertson A L Jr 1988 Herpesviridae in the coronary arteries and aorta of young trauma victims. American Journal of Pathology 130: 71–79
Zamarron C, Ginsberg M H, Plow E F 1990 Monoclonal antibodies specific for a conformationally altered state of fibrinogen. Thrombosis and Haemostasis 64: 41–46
Zarins C K, Giddens D P, Bharadvaj B K, Sottiurai V S, Mabon R F, Glagov S 1983 Carotid bifurcation atherosclerosis. Quantitative correlation of plaque localization with flow velocity profiles and wall shear stresses. Circulation Research 53: 502–514
Zatta A, Prosdocimi M 1990 Platelet aggregation in male and female smokers. Thrombosis and Haemostasis 63: 140
Zavoico G B, Hrbolich J K, Gimbrone M A Jr, Schafer A I 1990 Enhancement of thrombin- and ionomycin-stimulated prostacyclin and platelet-activating factor production in cultured endothelial cells by a tumor-promoting phorbol ester. Journal of Cellular Physiology 143: 596–605
Zimmerman M, McGeachie J 1985 The effect of nicotine on aortic endothelial cell turnover. An autoradiographic study. Atherosclerosis 58: 39–47
Zimmerman M, McGeachie J 1987 The effect of nicotine on aortic endothelium. A quantitative ultrastructural study. Atherosclerosis 63: 33–41

49. Molecular and cellular mechanisms of atherogenesis: studies of human lesions linked with animal modelling

J. N. Wilcox   L. A. Harker

Atherogenesis is a complex multifactorial process which is not well understood despite extensive investigation. Progress has been limited by the lack of animal models that fully reproduce all of the important features of clinical atherosclerotic disease including: endothelial injury, smooth muscle cell (SMC) proliferation, inflammation, lipid deposition, necrosis, spontaneous lesion rupture, thrombosis, and calcification. While many aspects of the disease may be modelled individually they are not simultaneously reproduced in any single animal system. Consequently, much of our understanding of the cellular relationships in this disease must arise from direct pathological studies of human atherosclerotic plaques.

This chapter will explore how endothelial denuding and non-denuding injuries contribute to atherogenesis with special emphasis on the role of thrombus formation, organization, and healing in this process. The discussion of the molecular and cellular characteristics of human atherosclerotic lesions will be integrated with experimental findings derived from relevant animal models used to test specific hypotheses originating from the study of human lesions.

HUMAN ATHEROSCLEROTIC LESIONS

Mature human atherosclerotic plaques consist of three main regions: the fibrous cap, necrotic core, and shoulder regions. The fibrous cap overlying the necrotic core is composed predominately of SMCs and serves to hold the vessel together (Gown et al 1986, Tsukada et al 1987). Lipid deposits identified histologically as cholesterol crystal clefts are found in the centre of the necrotic core (Small 1988, Guyton & Klemp 1989). Macrophages and other inflammatory cells are found scattered throughout the necrotic core and neointima but may also be concentrated in distinct inflammatory zones within the plaque (Jonasson et al 1986, Hansson et al 1988, 1989, van der Wal 1989, Ramshaw & Parums 1990). The extent to which the human atherosclerotic plaque is covered by an intact layer of endothelial cells is disputed. Although a number of studies report a significant loss of endothelial integrity accompanying atherosclerotic disease (Gown et al 1986), it is not clear to what extent the denudation of the endothelium is attributable to tissue preparation artifacts or surgical disruption. There is a rich vascular supply to the human atheroma. Numerous small capillaries and vessels within the plaque supply this tissue with the necessary blood supply to maintain the intimal mass. These vessels appear to develop from the adventitia as an extension of the normal vasa vasorum supplying the media (Gown et al 1986).

A significant feature common to advanced atherosclerotic plaques is the presence of thrombus. Thrombus formation is initiated by rupture of the atherosclerotic plaque or from the haemorrhage of the plaque, the vasa vasorum (Drury 1954, Constantinides 1966, 1967, Chapman 1965, Friedman & van den Bovenkamp 1966, Friedman 1971) and may play a role in stimulating SMC proliferation and vascular lesion formation (Woolf 1978, Schwartz et al 1988).

There are two types of lesions considered to be precursors of atherosclerotic plaques: **fatty streaks** composed of lipid-containing macrophages; and **diffuse intimal thickening** of fibromuscular masses composed predominately of smooth muscle cells. While such lesions are often distributed at sites prone to atherosclerotic development late in life, there is no conclusive evidence that either leads directly to the mature atheroma. Fatty streaks and diffuse intimal thickenings are commonly found from birth in all individuals and may represent a normal condition of the vessel wall (Stary 1989). True pre-atherosclerotic lesions, i.e. those lesions containing lipid-filled macrophages, dispersed SMCs and extracellular lipid, are not generally found until late puberty and fully developed atherosclerotic plaques with thrombi and areas of necrosis are not found until early adulthood. These early plaques have many characteristics of the mature atheroma including a fibrous cap and the beginning of a necrotic zone surrounding a predominantly lipid core overlaid by lipid-containing macrophages.

DENUDING AND NON-DENUDING MECHANISMS OF ATHEROGENESIS

In this chapter we will discuss how vascular lesion formation is induced by denuding and non-denuding injuries to the vessel wall and describe animal models that have been used to test this hypothesis. While denuding or non-denuding injuries each initiate different molecular pathways (Fig. 49.1), both injuries ultimately lead to:

1. Proliferation of vascular SMCs and the synthesis of associated connective tissue matrix
2. Focal accumulation of monocytes/macrophages
3. Lymphocytic infiltration
4. Variable intracellular and extracellular lipid accumulation
5. Vascular lesions producing stenoses and eventual thrombotic occlusion of the vessel.

We postulate that atherosclerosis generally begins as a process of non-denuding endothelial injury generated from plasma lipoproteins diffusing into the vessel wall initiating an inflammatory lesion leading to eventual endothelial loss. Subsequent vascular lesion formation may then be accelerated by thrombin generation with platelet/fibrin thrombus formation and organization on the denuded surface.

Non-denuding injury

Vascular lesions may form in the absence of significant endothelial denudation when endothelial cells become dysfunctional due to toxic molecules arising from chemicals or lipids in the bloodstream (DiCorleto & Chisolm 1986, Freiman et al 1986, Hansson & Bondjers, 1987). Functionally normal endothelium inhibits: (1) growth of intimal SMCs; (2) contraction of SMCs; (3) infiltration of leukocytes; (4) adhesion and recruitment of platelets; and (5) the production and activity of thrombin.

At present the earliest in vivo evidence of endothelial dysfunction is impairment of its vasomotor function (Freiman et al 1986, Harrison et al 1987, Sellke et al 1990). Endothelial dependent relaxation is angiographically impaired at very early stages in the development of human coronary artery disease (Ludmer et al 1986). Vasomotor dysfunction is attributable to a loss of endothelial-derived relaxing factor (EDRF) or nitric oxide (NO) activity (Palmer et al 1987, Moncada et al 1988, Guerra et al 1989, Myers et al 1989, Bates et al 1991). This may be due to a decrease in the synthesis of nitric oxide synthase (NOS) or superoxide dismutase (SOD). NOS is the major rate limiting step in the synthesis of NO (Sessa et al 1992). Oxygen radicals break down NO but are normally degraded by SOD so that a decrease in SOD levels might decrease overall EDRF activity (Gryglewski et al 1986, Rubanyi & Vanhoutte 1986). Experimental hypercholesterolaemia in primates and pigs is associated with impairment of endothelial-dependent vasodilator function (Shimokawa & Vanhoutte 1989, Quillen et al 1991). Alteration in

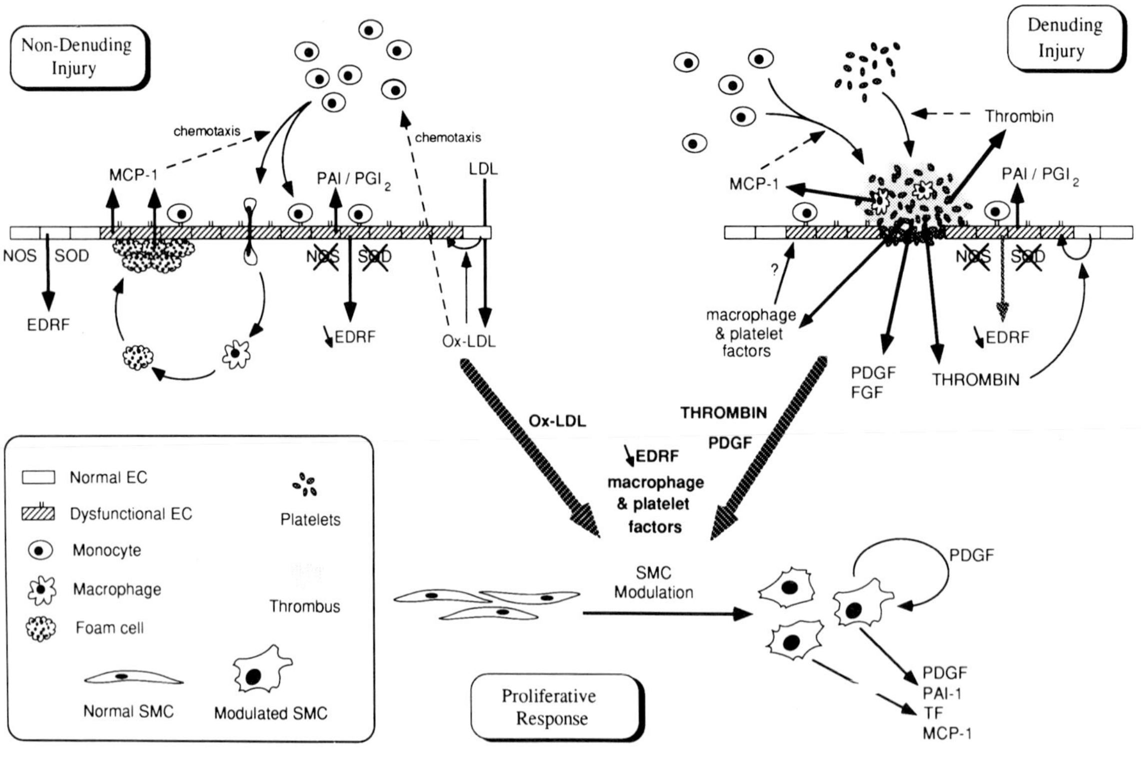

Fig. 49.1 Proposed initiating events in vascular lesion formation by both non-denuding and denuding injury to the endothelium.

endothelial-dependent relaxation is particularly evident at sites at risk of developing atherosclerosis such as at branch points in the arterial tree. These observations suggest that there is a causal relationship between site-specific defects in endothelial function and the susceptibility to atherosclerosis in these areas.

Dysfunctional endothelial cells may fail to prevent SMC proliferation either through the secretion of growth factor(s) or the absence of inhibitory factor(s). SMC proliferation under an intact endothelium may be demonstrated experimentally in animal models of hypercholesterolaemia (Faggiotto & Ross 1984, Faggiotto et al 1984), vascular grafts (Golden et al 1990, 1991), or sites of previous endothelial denuding injury. Endothelial cells overlying experimental prosthetic vascular grafts in baboons synthesize platelet-derived growth factor (PDGF) and may actively promote SMC proliferation (Golden et al 1991). Transforming growth factor β (TGF-β) is a bifunctional growth factor which under some conditions may inhibit SMC proliferation (Majack 1987, Merwin et al 1991). Altered synthesis or activity of TGF-β in dysfunctional endothelial cells may therefore promote SMC proliferation and lesion formation.

Dysfunctional endothelial cells display altered expression of leukocyte adhesion molecules (DiCorleto & Chisolm 1986, Cybulsky & Gimbrone 1991, Poston et al 1992) or monocyte chemotactic factors (Yla Herttuala et al 1991, Nelkin et al 1992). Any alteration in these factors severely impacts the binding and transmigration of inflammatory cells into nascent lesion sites as well as promoting thrombin generation and thrombus formation. Monocyte chemotactic protein-1 (MCP-l) mRNA has been detected in the endothelium overlying early atherosclerotic plaques (Yla Herttuala et al 1991, Nelken et al 1992) and its expression is increased by lipids or TGF-β in vitro (Berliner et al 1990, Cushing et al 1990, Gamble & Vadas 1991). VCAM-1 has been detected in the endothelium overlying fatty streaks in hypercholesterolaemic rabbits (Cybulsky & Gimbrone 1991) and may be found in human lesions. Normal endothelium is non-thrombogenic but dysfunctional endothelium may promote thrombosis by an upregulation of thrombogenic proteins. Synthesis of plasminogen activator inhibitor-1, tissue plasminogen activator, and tissue factor (TF) by endothelial cells is modified in vitro by cytokines which may be secreted by the inflammatory cells which first invade the lesion (Colucci et al 1983; Bevilacqua et al 1984, 1985, 1986, Nachman et al 1986, Schleef et al 1988).

Denuding injury

A denuding vascular injury, involving a loss of endothelial cells, exposes the subendothelial matrix to flowing blood. Such injuries may be produced mechanically by angioplasty or may be induced by accumulating lipids and inflammatory cells in early atherosclerotic lesions. Loss of endothelial cells from the arterial surface generally initiates platelet deposition due to the interaction of platelet glycoprotein receptors, such as GPIb exposed on the platelet membrane, or subendothelial matrix adhesion molecules such as von Willebrand factor. The binding and activation of platelets releases growth factors and other vasoactive substances from the alpha granules in the platelets. Growth factors released by platelets may stimulate the underlying SMCs to begin the proliferative process. The most important growth factor released by platelets is probably PDGF (Ross 1986).

Depending on the amount of injury to the vessel wall there may be more significant activation of the coagulation system leading to increased thrombin activity, platelet aggregation, and fibrin formation. Thrombus organization is suggested to play a role in vascular lesion formation (Duguid 1946, Schwartz et al 1988). The mechanism by which this occurs may involve thrombin which is produced during thrombus formation and may stimulate adjacent endothelial and SMCs. In vitro, thrombin acts as a mitogen for SMCs, fibroblasts, and mesangial cells (Bar Shavit et al 1990, Graham & Alexander 1990, Shultz & Raij 1990) and stimulates the release of growth factors from vascular endothelial cells and SMCs (Harlan et al 1986, Shultz et al 1989, Okazaki et al 1992). Thrombin has chemotactic activity for monocytes and thus stimulates the migration and infiltration of inflammatory cells into the site of injury (Bar Shavit & Wilner 1986, Shavit et al 1987). Organizing thrombi are sites of active inflammation and attract mononuclear and inflammatory cells. MCP-1 is found associated with macrophages and mesenchymal-appearing cells at sites of thrombus organization in human atheroma (Nelken et al 1991). Thrombin may also influence leukocyte adhesion molecule expression by surrounding endothelium which would participate in increasing leukocyte binding and transmigration into the lesion (DiCorleto & de la Motte 1989). Macrophages and T cells in the lesion may synthesize factors that also stimulate lesion development and SMC proliferation. Thrombin also induces endothelial plasminogen activator inhibitor-1 synthesis and so may modulate plasminogen activation locally (Heaton et al 1992).

Modulation of vascular smooth muscle cells

The underlying basis for vascular lesion formation ultimately depends on SMC proliferation since these cells make up the major bulk of the neointima. The onset of SMC proliferation is accompanied by morphological changes in the SMCs from a contractile quiescent state to a stellate-shaped proliferative phenotype and a loss of contractile proteins (Campbell & Campbell 1985, Mosse et al 1985). The morphological change accompanying the beginning of SMC proliferation is known as SMC modulation and the cells in this state are known as modulated or synthetic state cells. Modulated or synthetic state SMCs have low levels of α-actin expression (Gabbiani et al 1984, Barja et al 1986, Owens et al 1986, Fager et al 1989), increased numbers of intracellular organelles (Campbell & Campbell 1985, Mosse et al 1985), and are stimulated by autocrine production of PDGF and PDGF receptors (Wilcox et al 1988, Majesky et al 1990).

Experimentally it is difficult to separate out the control of SMC modulation from SMC proliferation. These may be two separate processes or one may be the natural consequence of the other. However, understanding the regulation of these processes in vascular SMCs is of paramount importance in developing strategies for the prevention of atherosclerosis and mechanical induction of vascular lesion formation after vascular surgery or angioplasty.

Both denuding and non-denuding injuries stimulate SMC modulation and proliferation through different pathways. Non-denuding injuries stimulate SMC modulation and proliferation through factors produced by the dysfunctional endothelial cells or the inflammatory cells first invading the lesion site. Alternatively, denuding injuries may stimulate SMC modulation through the action of any number of factors emanating from the thrombus including platelet- or macrophage-derived factors, PDGF, fibroblast growth factor (FGF) or thrombin.

Conversion of non-denuding into denuding injury

Non-denuding injuries and the early lesions they produce represent only the beginning of atherosclerotic plaque formation. Subsequent lesion development may proceed through some combination of denuding and non-denuding mechanisms. Continued non-denuding injuries will eventually lead to disruption of the endothelium overlying the lesion. The foamy macrophages present in these early lesions contain TF (Wilcox et al 1989). Disruption of the endothelium will therefore expose TF, initiating thrombus formation (Nemerson 1987) resulting in the release of factors from the thrombus which would stimulate SMC proliferation. Plaques appear to undergo episodic growth. The episodic progression of atherosclerotic disease may arise from periodic lesion rupture and thrombosis leading to accelerated proliferation of SMCs. This process may not be limited to only large mural thrombi; small sub-clinical (i.e. non-occlusive) thrombi forming at sites of endothelial injury may also contribute to the progression of atherosclerotic disease through effects on surrounding SMCs.

MOLECULAR MECHANISMS IN ATHEROSCLEROTIC LESION FORMATION

Growth factors and vascular lesion formation

PDGF production in human atherosclerotic plaques

PDGF is postulated to play an important part in intimal SMC proliferation in atherosclerotic plaques (Ross 1986). In vitro studies indicate that PDGF is a mitogen (Ross 1979) and chemoattractant (Grotendorst et al 1982) for SMCs. Since PDGF is secreted from activated platelets, platelet deposition and release of PDGF at sites of vascular injury might contribute to the initiation of SMC proliferation (Ross & Glomset 1976a,b). The discovery of PDGF mRNA in extracts of human atherosclerotic plaques by Northern blots (Barrett & Benditt 1987) indicates that local platelet-independent production of PDGF may also contribute to intimal SMC proliferation. However, it is unclear from the Northern blot studies which cell type(s) might be producing PDGF in the human atherosclerotic plaque since macrophages (Shimokado et al 1985, Martinet et al 1986, Mornex et al 1986), endothelial cells (Barrett et al 1984, DiCorleto 1984, Gajdusek 1984, Jaye et al 1985) and arterial SMCs (Seifert et al 1984, Nilsson et al 1985, Walker et al 1986) all synthesize PDGF in vitro.

Specific cells containing PDGF-A and -B chain mRNA are identified in human atherosclerotic plaques using in situ hybridization (Wilcox et al 1988). PDGF-A and -B chain mRNAs are predominantly found in mesenchymal-appearing intimal cells (MIC). Many MICs exhibit a stellate shape, display variable amounts of cytoplasm, and have large pale haematoxylin staining nuclei (Plate 49.1A) but do not stain well with any of the cell type-specific antibodies directed against SMCs, endothelial cells, macrophages, or T cells. Some of the PDGF-A mRNA-containing cells have the light microscope appearance of SMCs, i.e. spindle-shaped cells with long, slender nuclei (Haust 1983) and stain with alpha actin antibodies on serial sections. Endothelial cells lining subsets of the vasa vasorum vessels in the plaque are dysfunctional and synthesize PDGF-B chain mRNA (Plate 49.1B).

PDGF-β receptor mRNA is found almost exclusively in MICs (Wilcox et al 1988). Furthermore, MICs containing PDGF-β receptor mRNA are found in regions of the plaque rich in similar cells expressing PDGF-A and -B chain mRNA as well. The apparent co-localization of PDGF and PDGF receptors in the same region of the plaque and in similar cell types suggests that PDGF may be acting through autocrine and/or paracrine mechanisms to stimulate lesion formation.

The nature of the MIC is not clear. By light microscopy these cells have sometimes been referred to as intimal SMC (Ross et al 1984), stellate cells (Geer 1965), or synthetic state SMCs (Mosse et al 1985). That they do not stain with any of the cell type-specific antibodies is not surprising because immunohistochemical and ultrastructural studies of the human atherosclerotic plaque fail to identify a considerable fraction of intimal cells (Ross et al 1984, Gown et al 1986, Jonasson et al 1986). In general these cells are considered to be modified SMCs, since this cell type is believed to be the sole connective tissue cell comprising the inner tunica media from which the intimal cells are hypothesized to arise (Ross 1986). Whatever the lineage of the MIC in the human atherosclerotic plaque, this cell type comprises a large proportion of the intimal mass and appears to be responsible for a significant portion of the local PDGF production.

PDGF production in animal lesions

In experimental animal models the process of vascular lesion formation and SMC proliferation is stimulated by mechanically denuding injury to the vessel wall. Such models are used to examine the time course of growth factor expression and the control of SMC proliferation in a relatively simple system, thus contributing to our interpretation of the human studies.

Denudation, or removal of endothelial cells from the surface of an artery by balloon catheter angioplasty (BCA), stimulates SMC proliferation producing significant vascular lesions (Clowes et al 1983b, Clowes & Schwartz, 1985). This involves the passage of a balloon catheter into an artery, inflation and slow withdrawal of the inflated catheter several times to mechanically remove the endothelial cells from the surface of the vessel. SMC proliferation begins in the arterial media within 36–72 hours after balloon injury (Clowes et al 1983b). Cell proliferation continues in the media for 1 week and is followed by migration of the proliferating SMCs across the internal elastic lamina to form the neointima. Within 2 weeks after BCA of the rat common carotid artery a vascular lesion forms consisting almost exclusively of SMCs which may be one to two times the thickness of the original vessel. Cell proliferation continues in the lumenal layer of neointimal cells for several months after injury. This model is a relatively simple way to initiate SMC proliferation in vivo after a denuding injury without involving inflammatory cells or lipids.

Removal of endothelial cells from the vascular surface removes some factor(s) that inhibits the proliferation of medial SMCs. BCA of the abdominal aorta produces much smaller vascular lesions than BCA of the carotid artery. This may be explained by the presence of the intercostal arteries in the aorta which act as a source for endothelial cells restoring confluent endothelium on the injured surface. Areas of the denuded vessel which are re-endothelialized first tend to exhibit the least vascular lesion formation. In rodents there are no such side branches arising from the common carotid and re-endothelialization must proceed from the proximal and distal ends of the injured vessel. Complete re-endothelialization of the aorta frequently occurs after BCA, while even 12 weeks after BCA a central portion of the common carotid usually remains without endothelial cells (Clowes et al 1983a, Reidy et al 1983).

MICs from human atherosclerotic plaques share many characteristics with proliferating SMCs after BCA of the rat carotid artery. MICs in atherosclerotic lesions express reduced levels of smooth muscle-specific contractile proteins (Gabbiani et al 1984, Glukhova et al 1988, Wilcox et al 1988) similar to proliferating SMCs in culture (Barja et al 1986, Owens et al 1986) or after BCA of the rat carotid artery (Barja et al 1986, Clowes et al 1988). In addition proliferating SMCs in the rat carotid after BCA express PDGF mRNA (Majesky et al 1990) (Plate 49.2) another characteristic of the MIC in the human atheroma (Wilcox et al 1988).

In all experimental vascular injury models examined, SMC proliferation is accompanied by expression of PDGF-A and -β receptor mRNAs. Increased expression of PDGF-A chain mRNA can be detected in the media of the injured rat carotid as early as 6 hours after balloon denudation by Northern blots or in situ hybridization. 2 weeks after BCA, cells containing PDGF-A mRNA are localized along the lumenal surface of the vascular lesion. These cells do not express PDGF-B chain mRNA or PDGF-α receptor but strongly hybridize to the PDGF-β receptor probes. The PDGF-β receptor mRNA-containing cells extend deep into the intima and include more cells than are PDGF-A chain positive. Thymidine labelling studies indicate that the lumenal SMCs show the highest rate of proliferation in the lesion at that time (Clowes et al 1983b). PDGF-A chain and PDGF-β receptor expression have also been found in proliferating SMCs in the baboon arterial wall after BCA, surgical endarterectomy (Wilcox 1992), and during vascular lesion formation induced by implantation of prosthetic vascular grafts (Golden et al 1991). A correlation between SMC proliferation and PDGF expression suggests that PDGF is directly involved in the proliferative process, however there is no proof of this. It is equally possible that PDGF may regulate differentiation of proliferating SMCs by influencing the expression of contractile proteins in these cells (Blank et al 1988, Corjay et al 1989).

FGF during vascular lesion formation in animal models

Studies have been performed modulating the action of specific growth factors during vascular lesion formation after BCA of the rat carotid artery. The basis for these studies is the hypothesis that injection of a putative growth factor increases SMC proliferation in vivo. Conversely, inhibition of that growth factor, with an antibody for example, might inhibit SMC proliferation and/or lesion formation.

The injection of recombinant PDGF into rats after carotid BCA has little effect on the first wave of cell proliferation in the media measured 3 days after injury. Paradoxically however this treatment greatly increases the size of the neointima 2 weeks later (Jawien et al 1992). Inhibition of PDGF by injection of a neutralizing antibody to

PDGF also has little effect on SMC proliferation acutely, but slightly reduces the size of the neointima measured 7 days after injury (Ferns et al 1991). These results suggest that PDGF is not the major mitogen controlling the initiation of SMC proliferation after injury, but appears to play a more important role in regulating SMC migration to the intima.

Basic fibroblast growth factor (bFGF) is another vascular growth factor which may be an important mitogen for SMC and endothelial cells. Inhibition of bFGF, by injection of neutralizing antibodies, inhibits the first wave of SMC proliferation after balloon injury of the rat carotid artery (Lindner & Reidy 1991a,b). In addition injection of bFGF after balloon injury significantly increases SMC proliferation after balloon injury (Lindner et al 1991). These studies suggest that bFGF is an important mediator of the initial proliferative response after vascular injury. However, inhibition of bFGF for the entire period of neointimal formation has no effect upon the size of the vascular lesion and indicates that other factors are important in lesion development as well.

It has been proposed that balloon injury of the rat carotid damages medial SMCs and releases intracellular bFGF (Lindner et al 1991, Lindner & Reidy 1991a). The bFGF released from the damaged cells stimulates the remaining medial cells to begin proliferation. The first wave of SMC proliferation occurs within the media and induces transformation of a contractile SMC into the modulated phenotype producing autocrine growth factors like PDGF. These cells begin to proliferate within the media and eventually migrate to the neointima. The process of migration is as important as the first wave of SMC proliferation in determining lesion formation. At later times after injury, there is continued PDGF expression in the most lumenal cells of the neointima which co-localizes with SMC proliferation. The continued proliferation of neointimal SMCs accompanied by matrix deposition forms the vascular lesion.

Thrombin and vascular lesion formation

Procoagulant factors expressed in plaques

Atherosclerotic plaques are proliferative lesions that generate thrombin when they rupture (Falk 1983, Imparato et al 1983, Sherman et al 1986). An occlusive mural thrombus accompanies most cases of acute myocardial infarction (Davies et al 1976, Horie et al 1978, DeWood et al 1980, Buja & Willerson 1981). Plaque rupture exposes the necrotic core to the flowing blood leading to thrombus formation in both coronary (Drury 1954, Chapman 1965, Constantinides 1966, Friedman & van den Bovenkamp 1966, Friedman 1971, Falk 1983, Forrester et al 1987) and cerebral arteries (Constantinides 1967). What is it about the plaque that initiates coagulation when the plaque ruptures? While collagen and subendothelial matrix proteins are known to activate platelets (Wilner et al 1968b, Stemerman 1973, Groves et al 1979, Kinlough-Rathbone et al 1983, Parsons et al 1986) and factor XII (Niewiarowski et al 1966, Wilner et al 1968a), additional procoagulant proteins are produced locally in the atherosclerotic plaque.

Tissue factor (TF) facilitates both intrinsic and extrinsic pathways of coagulation, and is a key protein in the activation of the coagulation cascade (Nemerson 1966, Østerud & Rapaport 1977, Nemerson & Bach 1982). TF is prominent in human atherosclerotic plaques compared to normal vessels (Wilcox et al 1989) (Plate 49.3A). TF protein and mRNA are localized in macrophages adjacent to the cholesterol clefts in the necrotic core of the plaque and in foamy macrophages in the plaque intima (Plate 49.3B). It is interesting that TF is found only in those macrophages associated with lipids in the lesion. Haemosiderin-containing macrophages, activated macrophages in regions of thrombus actively ingesting fibrin and cellular debris, do not contain TF protein or mRNA. Smaller non-phagocytic macrophages in these tissues likewise do not contain TF. This association implies some link between exposure to lipids or lipid uptake by macrophages and the regulation of TF synthesis in these cells.

TF mRNA is also found in cells morphologically similar to the PDGF-producing MICs in the fibrous cap and in areas of organizing thrombi within the plaque. TF is an immediate–early gene (Hartzell et al 1989) and its synthesis may be linked to the cell cycle (Bloem et al 1989) suggesting a role in cellular growth. The finding of TF production by MICs in the human atherosclerotic plaque may therefore be in some way related to the proliferation of these cells. Whatever the function of TF in macrophages or MICs, it is likely that TF plays a significant role in the initiation of coagulation associated with plaque rupture.

PDGF expression in regions of thrombus organization in human atheroma

Fibrin deposition and thrombus organization have been suggested to play a role in plaque development (Duguid 1946, Schwartz et al 1988). The 'thrombogenic' or 'encrustation' hypothesis first proposed by von Rokitansky in 1852 suggested that plaques might develop by the incorporation of fibrin or blood products on the lumenal surface of blood vessels. Additional support for this hypothesis came with the observation by Duguid (1946) of a continuum between organizing thrombi and fibrotic intimal thickening in many atherosclerotic plaques. This was further supported by experimental studies in which the organization of chronic thrombi in rats (Poole et al 1971, van Aken et al 1980, van Aken & Emeis 1983), rabbits (Moore 1973, Sumiyoshi et al 1973), and pigs

(Jorgensen et al 1967, Woolf et al 1968) led to fibrous intimal thickenings as part of the normal healing process. MIC containing PDGF and PDGF receptor mRNAs are often found in areas of organizing thrombi within human atherosclerotic plaques (Wilcox 1991) (Plate 49.4). These cells express both PDGF isoforms as well as receptors for PDGF. The finding that organizing thrombi within human atherosclerotic plaques are often associated with smooth muscle-derived MICs that contain PDGF and PDGF receptor mRNA may begin to explain how the process of thrombus organization might lead to continued plaque development by stimulating an autocrine growth response.

We examined a model to study the organization of chronic arterial thrombi which was originally developed by Poole and co-workers (Poole et al 1971). This model consists of a single suture passed into and out of the rat aorta, combined with a gentle crush injury around the thread. A thrombus develops in the lumen on the thread and is maintained against the vessel wall for many weeks after the initial injury. Cells populating the thrombus 1 week after injury have a mesenchymal morphology similar to the MIC in the human plaque, contain PDGF-A chain mRNA but do not stain with an α-actin antibody (Wilcox et al 1990). Eventually, by 3 or 4 weeks the thrombus is fully resolved into a pseudointima that is populated by cells with a contractile morphology typical of SMCs, which stain with α-actin antibodies, while the intimal surface appears to be completely re-endothelialized. The SMCs in the pseudointima at 3 or 4 weeks however no longer hybridize with the PDGF probes.

Previously it was concluded that the thrombus developing on the thread stimulates medial SMC proliferation and migration into the thrombus which eventually develops into an intimal mass (Poole et al 1971). If the PDGF-containing mesenchymal-appearing cells in the thrombus at 1 week are the PDGF-negative SMCs present at 4 weeks, as suggested by Poole and co-workers (1971), it might be concluded that the thrombus contains cells or agents which modify SMC differentiation and/or proliferation.

Contribution of thrombin to vascular lesion formation in rats and baboons

How do thrombi stimulate vascular lesion formation? Growth factors released from platelets in thrombi may stimulate SMC proliferation. However, other components of the thrombus may be mitogenic as well. Fibrin fragments have been shown to be chemotactic for SMCs and may help stimulate a healing response in the vessel wall (Naito et al 1990, Thompson et al 1990). Macrophages are among the first cells to invade the thrombus. They synthesize PDGF and other growth factors in vitro (Shimokado et al 1985) which may affect SMC growth in vivo. In cell culture, macrophages synthesize factors which increase modulation of contractile/quiescent SMCs into the non-contractile/proliferative phenotype which might also increase lesion formation (Campbell & Campbell 1990, 1991).

Thrombin has very potent effects on vascular cells and may directly promote the proliferative response. Thrombin is chemotactic for inflammatory cells and may stimulate the migration of macrophages and T cells to the site of injury (Bar Shavit et al 1987), thus promoting the local production of macrophage-derived growth and/or differentiation factors. Importantly, thrombin may promote an autocrine growth response since it stimulates the synthesis and release of PDGF from SMC and endothelial cells (Harlan et al 1986, Shultz et al 1989, Okazaki et al 1992) and acts as a direct mitogen for SMCs and fibroblasts (Bar Shavit et al 1990, 1992, Graham & Alexander 1990, Shultz & Raij 1990). These actions of thrombin on SMCs are most likely mediated by the cellular thrombin receptor (Vu et al 1991).

Recent studies indicate that thrombin receptor synthesis is important for SMC proliferation during vascular lesion development (Wilcox et al 1992). Normal uninjured vessels do not contain thrombin receptor mRNA. However, 6 hours after BCA of the rat carotid artery there is a significant increase in PDGF-A and thrombin receptor mRNA expression in the remaining medial cells. 2 weeks after injury, thrombin receptor mRNA-containing cells are found diffusely distributed throughout the neointima while PDGF-A synthesis is confined to the most lumenal group of cells at this time.

Thrombin is involved in vascular lesion development after surgical endarterectomy of baboon carotid arteries (Wilcox et al 1992). In this model the intima and lumenal portion of the media are circumferentially removed by standard surgical techniques. Fully formed lesions develop within 30 days, consisting of SMCs, overlying endothelium and macrophages. These lesions show increased expression of thrombin receptor mRNA compared to normal control vessels (Plate 49.5). Proliferating SMCs just beneath the endothelial surface contain both PDGF-A and thrombin receptor mRNA as determined by in situ hybridization.

The co-localization of PDGF with thrombin receptor mRNA expression in the rat and primate lesions implicates thrombin in both the first wave of SMC proliferation in response to injury and in the later phases of lesion development. This conclusion is consistent with the independent observation that thrombin activity is detected at the surface of injured vessels at all stages of lesion development (Hatton et al 1989). Thrombin production is highest in the first few hours after balloon injury of the rat carotid but continues to be elevated above control levels 2 weeks later. Thus, both ligand and receptor are present in these tissues throughout neointimal development. This hypothesis is further supported by recent studies indicating that hirudin, a potent thrombin inhibitor, blocks the first wave of SMC proliferation after BCA in the baboon (Hanson et al 1992).

In vitro studies on cultured rat aortic vascular SMCs indicate that thrombin receptor synthesis is up-regulated by both bFGF and PDGF (Wilcox et al 1992). bFGF stimulates a very rapid induction of thrombin receptor mRNA within 1 hour, while PDGF has a more sustained effect and significantly increases thrombin receptor mRNA 5–10 hours after addition to the culture medium.

The association of thrombin receptor expression with proliferating SMCs at sites of vascular injury coupled with the ability of FGF to induce thrombin receptor expression and the action of hirudin to block SMC proliferation provides persuasive evidence that thrombin plays a key role during neointimal development after vascular injury. We hypothesize that FGF begins the proliferative process and stimulates thrombin receptor synthesis (Fig. 49.2). Inhibition of FGF therefore inhibits early medial SMC proliferation and prevents the early rise in thrombin receptor and PDGF expression. Subsequently, thrombin is important in maintaining the proliferative process and stimulating the autocrine production of PDGF-A chain expressed by proliferating SMCs. According to this model, FGF would have no role in the later phases of lesion development which may be driven in large part by thrombin and PDGF. This interpretation is supported by studies indicating that blockage of FGF action as late as 2 weeks after BCA of the rat carotid has no effect on ongoing cell proliferation (Lindner & Reidy 1991b, Olson et al 1992). Thus, the late phase of lesion development is largely an FGF-independent process. Further studies are needed to determine what effect the blockage of thrombin at later times might have on cell proliferation and lesion development.

Thrombin action and thrombin receptor expression may also be involved in atherogenesis and the continued development of human atherosclerotic plaques. Thrombin receptor mRNA-containing cells are present in human carotid endarterectomy specimens as determined by in situ hybridization. The majority of cells expressing thrombin receptor mRNA are morphologically similar to MICs synthesizing PDGF although macrophages and endothelial cells may express thrombin receptor mRNA as well.

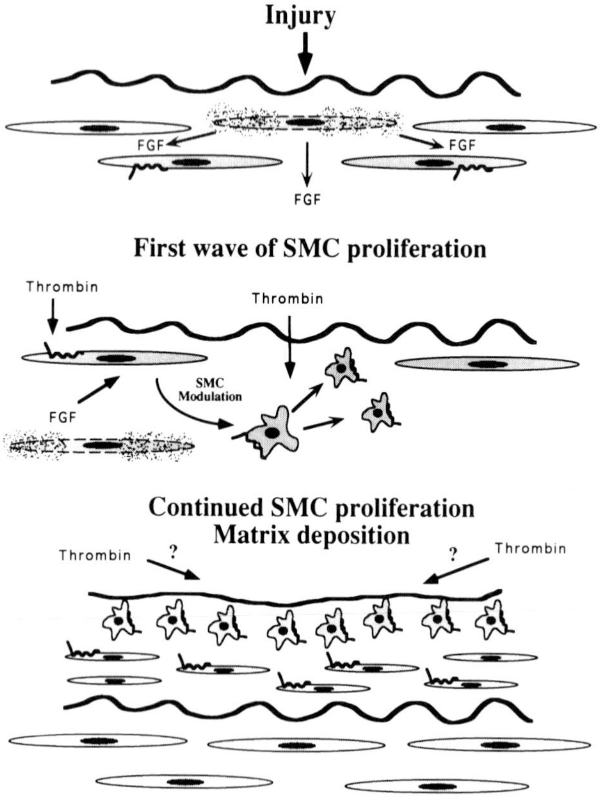

Fig. 49.2 Proposed initiating events in vascular lesion formation after balloon catheter injury. Balloon injury damages medial smooth muscle cells releasing bFGF. bFGF stimulates thrombin receptor synthesis by medial smooth muscle cells. bFGF and thrombin act to stimulate smooth muscle modulation and the first wave of medial smooth muscle proliferation. Smooth muscle cells migrate to form a neointima where they continue to proliferate on the lumenal surface possibly stimulated by continued thrombin production.

Cytokine production in human atherosclerotic lesions

Distinct inflammatory zones are found in the human atherosclerotic plaque, where significant accumulations of T cells and macrophages are found (Jonasson et al 1986). These findings have prompted investigators to propose that atherosclerotic lesion formation may involve an autoimmune process or a reaction to a viral infection of the vessel wall (Hajjar 1991). Recent studies have demonstrated local production of a group of inflammatory cytokines, members of the RANTES/SIS cytokine family, in the human lesion (Nelken et al 1991, Yla.Herttuala et al 1991). The RANTES/SIS cytokine family includes MCP-1, HIMAP, LD78, and RANTES. These are secreted molecules with potent chemotactic activity for monocytes and T cells (Schall 1991). In situ hybridization experiments indicate that there are many cells positive for these cytokine mRNAs found in atherosclerotic plaques, especially in macrophage-rich inflammatory regions. By comparison, minimal expression was noted in control arteries without atherosclerotic disease.

For example, *MCP*-1 mRNA is found in mesenchymal-appearing cells with a similar localization, morphology and staining characteristics as the PDGF-producing MIC described previously (Nelken et al 1991). *MCP*-1 is the human homologue of the mouse PDGF-inducible gene *JE* (Cochran et al 1983). The apparent co-localization of PDGF and *MCP*-1 expression in the same regions of the plaque suggests that the autocrine or paracrine stimulation of the MIC by PDGF may in turn up-regulate *MCP*-1 expression by these cells. In addition MICs and macrophages expressing *MCP*-1 can be found at sites of organizing thrombi in human atherosclerotic plaques. Thus thrombin activation and the formation of thrombus may not only contribute to SMC proliferation through an increase in PDGF expression but may also stimulate the synthesis and release of inflammatory cytokines which contribute to the ongoing inflammatory process by attracting mononuclear cells to these sites.

MCP-1 mRNA-containing cells are detected in preatherosclerotic lesions, e.g. aortic fatty streaks. *MCP*-1 is localized to macrophages and endothelial cells overlying these lesions (Yla Herttuala et al 1991, Nelken et al 1992). In vitro, minimally oxidized LDL and β VLDL upregulate *MCP*-1 mRNA and protein in human umbilical vein endothelial cells and SMCs (Territo et al 1989, Berliner et al 1990, Cushing et al 1990). Elevated lipids may play a role in initiating atherosclerotic lesion development by stimulating MCP-1 production which might initiate the inflammatory process. As monocytes and T cells begin to arrive in the lesion they too begin to synthesize additional MCP-1 and other inflammatory cytokines thereby attracting more leukocytes to the developing atherosclerotic plaque beginning the cycle of inflammation and intimal development. Alternatively, this process may begin with a diffuse fibromuscular lesion in which local production of PDGF stimulates MCP-1 synthesis by SMCs in the lesion, thus converting a predominantly smooth muscle-derived lesion into the inflammatory lesion typical of atherosclerosis.

Lipids and atherosclerosis

Clinical and epidemiological studies indicate that blood lipids or their metabolites may initiate molecular events leading to the early inflammatory lesions typical of the first stages of atherosclerosis. Fatty streaks can be found in the aortas of infants and children less than 3 years old while fibrous plaques are more commonly found beginning in the 2nd and 3rd decade of life (Stary 1989). Although evidence supporting the possible transition of fatty streaks to fibrous plaques remains inconclusive they are generally considered to be precursors of atherosclerotic lesion formation (Faggiotto & Ross 1984, Faggiotto et al 1984, Ross 1986). Fatty streaks are characterized by an accumulation of monocytes and T cells in discrete lesions under the endothelial surface. It is presumed that the monocytes, in order to reach the subendothelium, have adhered to the endothelium and migrated into the sub-endothelial space. This may involve the induction of specific adhesion molecules such as VLA-4, CD 11/18 and LECCAM on monocytes which interact with specific counter-receptors on the endothelium, e.g. VCAM-1, ICAM-1, and different selectins (E-selectin and P-selectin) for transmigration to occur (Carlos et al 1990, Springer & Lasky 1991).

Lipids alter the oxidative state of endothelial cells. Exposure of native LDL to cultured human endothelial cells results in an oxidative modification (Steinbrecher et al 1984, Parthasarathy et al 1985) that is associated with profound alterations in its biological characteristics. Oxidized LDL is taken up readily by both endothelial cells (Tanner et al 1991) and macrophages (Sparrow et al 1989) via the scavenger receptor(s), and is thought to be the major source of cholesterol in the transformation of the macrophage into a foam cell (Rosenfeld et al 1990). Intimal macrophages are also capable of oxidizing LDL and are believed to contribute to the formation of the modified lipoprotein that is entrapped in the intimal space of an atherosclerotic lesion (Steinberg et al 1989). Oxidized LDL has been demonstrated directly in atherosclerotic lesions (Rosenfeld et al 1991). LDL that is minimally modified by mild oxidation to the extent that it is not recognized by the scavenger receptor will enhance monocyte binding to the endothelium and increase production of monocyte chemoattractant factors (Berliner et al 1990). An important role of LDL oxidation in the pathogenesis of atherosclerosis is inferred by the observation that probucol, an antioxidant that inhibits LDL oxidation, retards the development of atherosclerosis in the Watanabe rabbit model of familial hypercholesterolaemia (Carew et al 1987). Although the molecular mechanisms accounting for these effects of oxidized LDL on the arterial wall are unclear, these data provide compelling evidence that the oxidative environment in the blood vessel wall is a critical factor determining susceptibility to atherosclerosis and producing endothelial dysfunctionality. Subsequently, the macrophages and foam cells in more advanced lesions could provide sufficient oxidative potential to promote progression of the lesion.

Animal models for hypercholesterolaemia

Fatty streak formation and the early phases of atherogenesis may be modelled in animals fed a high fat diet. In humans, plasma lipoproteins may be the primary source of lipid which accumulates in the arterial wall as part of the arteriosclerotic process and elevated levels of low density lipoprotein-cholesterol are thought to be a central cause of coronary artery disease. Non-human primates (Faggiotto & Ross 1984, Faggiotto et al 1984, Masuda & Ross 1990a,b), pigs (Gerrity et al 1979, Gerrity 1984) and rabbits (Rosenfeld et al 1987a,b) are susceptible to fatty streak formation when maintained on a diet consisting of high levels of cholesterol and saturated fats. These animals show many of the early vascular changes characteristic of human fatty streaks. Low level hypercholesterolaemia in non-human primates causes increased adherence of T cells and monocytes to the lumenal surface of the aorta (Masuda & Ross 1990a). Eventually, typical aortic fatty streaks are observed containing lipid-laden macrophages and T cells. Foamy macrophages are often observed on the lumenal surface over such lesions associated with large

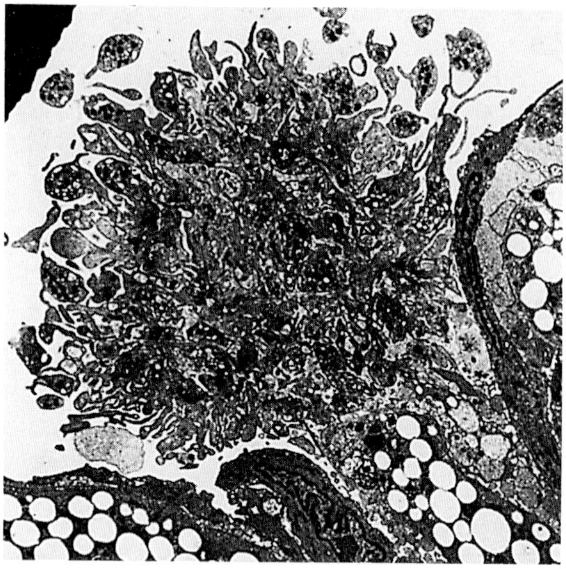

Fig. 49.3 Electron micrograph of a platelet microthrombus formed around a foamy macrophage on the surface of the aorta of a non-human primate maintained on a hypercholesterolaemic diet. Reproduced from Faggiotto and Ross 1984 with permission.

platelet microthrombi (Faggiotto & Ross 1984) (Fig. 49.3). It is likely that these macrophages contain TF (see Plate 49.3B) stimulating the formation of thrombin which may play a role in the continued development of these lesions. Long-term hypercholesterolaemia in primates results in a loss of endothelial cells stimulating further platelet deposition and mural thrombus formation (Faggiotto & Ross 1984, Faggiotto et al 1984).

SUMMARY

Denuding and non-denuding vascular injuries are postulated to initiate and sustain the development of mature clinically significant atherosclerotic plaques. The initiation of atherosclerosis may involve endothelial cell dysfunction arising from oxidative stress generated by hyperlipidaemia with the production of excessive reactive oxygen intermediates and deficient degradative enzymes such as SOD. Consequent excessive free radical formation may impair the release of functionally active NO and lead to endothelial dysfunction with altered expression of monocyte adhesion molecules and chemotactic factors. Metabolism of the fatty acids in an LDL particle increases oxidative phosphorylation with resultant increased leakage of oxidative intermediates from mitochondrial metabolism. A decreased ability to metabolize these intermediates, which might well be genetically determined, would lead ultimately to metabolic changes in endothelial cells eventually manifesting as atherosclerosis. In denuding vascular injury one of the first events following endothelial cell disruption is the formation of thrombin at the site of injury, leading to platelet activation and thrombus. Both denuding and non-denuding injuries stimulate SMC modulation and proliferation through different molecular pathways. Non-denuding injuries stimulate SMC modulation and proliferation through factors produced by the dysfunctional endothelial cells or the inflammatory cells first invading the lesion site. Alternatively, denuding injuries may stimulate SMC proliferation through the action of any number of factors emanating from the thrombus including platelet- or macrophage-derived factors, PDGF, bFGF or thrombin. Atherosclerotic plaques continue to grow for many years. The slow indolent process of non-denuding chemical injury of the endothelium and lesion formation may be periodically accelerated by thrombi forming on the lumenal surface at sites of small denuding injuries leading to progressive atherosclerotic disease.

REFERENCES

Barja F, Coughlin C, Belin D, Gabbiani G 1986 Actin isoform synthesis and mRNA levels in quiescent and proliferating rat aortic smooth muscle cells in vivo and in vitro. Laboratory Investigation 55: 226–233

Barrett T B, Gajdusek C M, Schwartz S M, McDougall J K, Benditt E P 1984 Expression of the sis gene by endothelial cells in culture and in vivo. Proceedings of the National Academy of Sciences, USA 81: 6772–6774

Barrett T B, Benditt E P 1987 Sis (platelet-derived growth factor B chain) gene transcript levels are elevated in human atherosclerotic lesions compared to normal artery. Proceedings of the National Academy of Sciences, USA 84: 1099–1103

Bar Shavit R, Wilner G D 1986 Biologic activities of nonenzymatic thrombin: elucidation of a macrophage interactive domain. Seminars in Thrombosis and Haemostasis 12: 244–249

Bar Shavit R, Hruska K A, Kahn A J, Wilner G D 1987 Thrombin chemotactic stimulation of HL-60 cells: studies on thrombin responsiveness as a function of differentiation. Journal of Cell Physiology 131: 255–261

Bar Shavit R, Benezra M, Eldor A et al 1990 Thrombin immobilized to extracellular matrix is a potent mitogen for vascular smooth muscle cells: nonenzymatic mode of action. Cell Regulation 1: 453–463

Bar Shavit R, Benezra M, Sabbah V, Bode W, Vlodavsky I 1992 Thrombin as a multifunctional protein: induction of cell adhesion and proliferation. American Journal of Respiration and Cell Molecular Biology 6: 123–130

Bates J N, Harrison D G, Myers P R, Minor R L 1991 EDRF: nitrosylated compound or authentic nitric oxide. Basic Research in Cardiology 86 (suppl 2): 17–26

Berliner J A, Territo M C, Sevanian A et al 1990 Minimally modified low density lipoprotein stimulates monocyte endothelial interactions. Journal of Clinical Investigation 85: 1260–1266

Bevilacqua M P, Pober J S, Majeau G R, Cotran R S Jr 1984 Interleukin 1 (IL-1) induces biosynthesis and cell surface expression of procoagulant activity in human vascular endothelial cells. Journal of Experimental Medicine 160: 618–623

Bevilacqua M P, Pober J S, Wheeler M E, Cotran R S Jr 1985 Interleukin-1 activation of vascular endothelium. Effects on procoagulant activity and leukocyte adhesion. American Journal of Pathology 121: 394–403

Bevilacqua M P, Schleef R R, Gimbrone M A J, Loskutoff D J 1986 Regulation of the fibrinolytic system of cultured human vascular endothelium by interleukin 1. Journal of Clinical Investigation 78: 587–591

Blank R S, Thompson M M, Owens G K 1988 Cell cycle versus density dependence of smooth muscle alpha actin expression in cultured rat aortic smooth muscle cells. Journal of Cell Biology 107: 299–306

Bloem L J, Chen L, Konigsberg W H, Bach R 1989 Serum stimulation of quiescent human fibroblasts induces the synthesis of tissue factor mRNA followed by the appearance of tissue factor antigen and procoagulant activity. Journal of Cell Physiology 139: 418–423

Buja L M, Willerson J T 1981 Clinicopathologic correlates of acute ischemic heart disease syndromes. American Journal of Cardiology 47: 343–356

Campbell G R, Campbell J H 1985 Recent advances in molecular pathology: smooth muscle phenotypic changes in arterial wall homeostasis: Implications for the pathogenesis of atherosclerosis. Experimental and Molecular Pathology 42: 139–162

Campbell G R, Campbell J H 1990 Macrophage influence on smooth muscle phenotype in atherogenesis. Advances in Experimental Medicine and Biology 273: 147–162

Campbell J H, Campbell G R 1991 The macrophage as an initiator of atherosclerosis. Clinical and Experimental Pharmacology and Physiology 18: 81–84

Carew T E, Schwenke D C, Steinberg D 1987 Antiatherogenic effect of probucol unrelated to its hypocholesterolemic effect: evidence that antioxidants in vivo can selectively inhibit low density lipoprotein degradation in macrophage-rich fatty streaks and slow the progression of atherosclerosis in the Watanabe heritable hyperlipidemic rabbit. Proceedings of the National Academy of Sciences, USA 84: 7725–7729

Carlos T M, Dobrina A, Ross R, Harlan J M 1990 Multiple receptors on human monocytes are involved in adhesion to cultured human endothelial cells. Journal of Leukocyte Biology 48: 451–456

Chapman I 1965 Morphogenesis of occluding coronary artery thrombosis. Archives in Pathology 80: 256–261

Clowes A W, Schwartz S M 1985 Significance of quiescent smooth muscle migration in the injured rat carotid artery. Circulation Research 56: 139–145

Clowes A W, Reidy M A, Clowes M M 1983a Mechanisms of stenosis after arterial injury. Laboratory Investigation 49: 208–215

Clowes A W, Reidy M A, Clowes M M 1983b Kinetics of cellular proliferation after arterial injury. I. Smooth muscle growth in the absence of endothelium. Laboratory Investigation 49: 327–333

Clowes A W, Clowes M M, Kocher O, Ropraz P, Chaponnier C, Gabbiani G 1988 Arterial smooth muscle cells in vivo: relationship between actin isoform expression and mitogenesis and their modulation by heparin. Journal of Cell Biology 107: 1939–1945

Cochran B H, Reffel A C, Stiles C D 1983 Molecular cloning of gene sequences regulated by platelet-derived growth factor. Cell 33: 939–947

Colucci M, Balconi G, Lorenzet R et al 1983 Cultured human endothelial cells generate tissue factor in response to endotoxin. Journal of Clinical Investigation 71: 1893–1896

Constantinides P 1966 Plaque fissures in human coronary thrombosis. Journal of Atherosclerosis Research 6: 1–17

Constantinides P 1967 Pathogenesis of cerebral artery thrombosis in man. Archives in Pathology 83: 422–428

Corjay M H, Thompson M M, Lynch K R, Owens G K 1989 Differential effects of platelet-derived growth factor-versus serum-induced growth on smooth muscle alpha-actin and nonmuscle beta-actin mRNA expression in cultured rat aortic smooth muscle cells. Journal of Biological Chemistry 264: 10501–10506

Cushing S D, Berliner J A, Valente A J et al 1990 Minimally modified low density lipoprotein induces monocyte chemotactic protein 1 in human endothelial cells and smooth muscle cells. Proceedings of the National Academy of Sciences, USA 87: 5134–5138

Cybulsky M I, Gimbrone M A 1991 Endothelial expression of a mononuclear leukocyte adhesion molecule during atherogenesis. Science 251: 788–791

Davies M J, Woolf N, Robertson W B 1976 Pathology of acute myocardial infarction with particular reference to occlusive coronary thrombi. British Heart Journal 38: 659–664

DeWood M A, Spores J, Notske R et al 1980 Prevalence of total coronary occlusion during the early hours of transmural myocardial infarction. New England Journal of Medicine 303: 897–902

DiCorleto P E 1984 Cultured endothelial cells produce multiple growth factors for connective tissue cells. Experimental Cell Research 153: 167–172

DiCorleto P E, Chisolm G III 1986 Participation of the endothelium in the development of the atherosclerotic plaque. Progress in Lipid Research 25: 365–374

DiCorleto P E, de la Motte C A 1989 Thrombin causes increased monocytic-cell adhesion to endothelial cells through a protein kinase C-dependent pathway. Biochemical Journal 264: 71–77

Drury R A B 1954 The role of intimal haemorrhage in coronary occlusion. Journal of Pathology and Bacteriology 67: 207–215

Duguid J B 1946 Thrombosis as a factor in the pathogenesis of coronary atherosclerosis. Journal of Pathology and Bacteriology 58: 207–212

Fager G, Hansson G K, Gown A M, Larson D M, Skalli O, Bondjers G 1989 Human arterial smooth muscle cells in culture: inverse relationship between proliferation and expression of contractile proteins. In Vitro Cell Developmental Biology 25: 511–520

Faggiotto A, Ross R 1984 Studies of hypercholesterolemia in the nonhuman primate. II. Fatty streak conversion to fibrous plaque. Arteriosclerosis 4: 341–356

Faggiotto A, Ross R, Harker L 1984 Studies of hypercholesterolemia in the nonhuman primate. I. Changes that lead to fatty streak formation. Arteriosclerosis 323: 340–1984

Falk E 1983 Plaque rupture with severe pre-existing stenosis precipitating coronary thrombosis. Characteristics of coronary atherosclerotic plaques underlying fatal occlusive thrombin. British Heart Journal 50: 127–134

Ferns G A, Raines E W, Sprugel K H, Motani A S, Reidy M A, Ross R 1991 Inhibition of neointimal smooth muscle accumulation after angioplasty by an antibody to PDGF. Science 253: 1129–1132

Forrester J S, Litvack F, Grundfest W, Hickey A 1987 A perspective of coronary disease seen through the arteries of living man. Circulation 75: 505–513

Freiman P C, Mitchell G G, Heistad D D, Armstrong M L, Harrison D G 1986 Atherosclerosis impairs endothelium-dependent vascular relaxation to acetylcholine and thrombin in primates. Circulation Research 58: 783–789

Friedman M 1971 The coronary thrombus: its origin and fate. Human Pathology 2: 81–128

Friedman M, van den Bovenkamp G J 1966 The pathogenesis of a coronary thrombus. American Journal of Pathology 48: 19–44

Gabbiani G, Kocher O, Bloom W S, Vandekerckhove J, Weber K 1984 Actin expression in smooth muscle cells of rat aortic intimal thickening, human atheromatous plaque, and cultured rat aortic media. Journal of Clinical Investigation 73: 148–152

Gajdusek C M 1984 Release of endothelial cell-derived growth factor (ECDGF) by heparin. Journal of Cell Physiology 121: 13–21

Gamble J R, Vadas M A 1991 Endothelial cell adhesiveness for human T lymphocytes is inhibited by transforming growth factor-beta 1. Journal of Immunology 146: 1149–1154

Geer J C 1965 Fine structure of human aortic intimal thickening and fatty streaks. Laboratory Investigation 14: 1764–1783

Gerrity R G 1984 Atherogenesis in the swine Evans blue model. Vasa 13: 292–297

Gerrity R G, Naito H K, Richardson M, Schwartz C J 1979 Dietary induced atherogenesis in swine. Morphology of the intima in prelesion stages. American Journal of Pathology 95: 775-792

Glukhova M A, Kabakov A E, Frid M G et al 1988 Modulation of human aorta smooth muscle cell phenotype: A study of muscle-specific variants of vinculin, caldesmon, and actin expression. Proceedings of the National Academy of Sciences, USA 85: 9542–9546

Golden M A, Hanson S R, Kirkman T R, Schneider P A, Clowes A W 1990 Healing of polytetrafluoroethylene arterial grafts is influenced by graft porosity. Journal of Vascular Surgery 11: 838–844

Golden M A, Au Y P T, Kirkman T R et al 1991 Platelet-derived growth factor activity and mRNA expression in healing vascular grafts in baboons. Association in vivo of platelet-derived growth factor mRNA and protein with cellular proliferation. Journal of Clinical Investigation 87: 406–414

Gown A M, Tsukada T, Ross R 1986 Human atherosclerosis: II.

Immunocytochemical analysis of the cellular composition of human atherosclerotic lesions. American Journal of Pathology 125: 191–207
Graham D J, Alexander J J 1990 The effects of thrombin on bovine aortic endothelial and smooth muscle cells. Journal of Vascular Surgery 11: 307–313
Grotendorst G R, Chang T, Seppa H E, Kleinman H K, Martin G R 1982 Platelet-derived growth factor is a chemoattractant for vascular smooth muscle cells. Journal of Cell Physiology 113: 261–266
Groves H M, Kinlough Rathbone R L, Richardson M, Moore S, Mustard J F 1979 Platelet interaction with damaged rabbit aorta. Laboratory Investigation 40: 194–200
Gryglewski R J, Palmer R M, Moncada S 1986 Superoxide anion is involved in the breakdown of endothelium-derived vascular relaxing factor. Nature 320: 454–456
Guerra R, Brotherton A F, Goodwin P J, Clark C R, Armstrong M L, Harrison D G 1989 Mechanisms of abnormal endothelium-dependent vascular relaxation in atherosclerosis: implications for altered autocrine and paracrine functions of EDRF. Blood Vessels 26: 300–314
Guyton J R, Klemp K F 1989 The lipid-rich core region of human atherosclerotic fibrous plaques. Prevalence of small lipid droplets and vesicles by electron microscopy. American Journal of Pathology 134: 705–717
Hajjar D P 1991 Viral pathogenesis of atherosclerosis. Impact of molecular mimicry and viral genes. American Journal of Pathology 139: 1195–1211
Hanson S R, Harker L A, Wilcox J N 1992 Unpublished observations
Hansson G K, Bondjers G 1987 Endothelial dysfunction and injury in atherosclerosis. Acta Medica Scandinavica Suppl 715: 11–17
Hansson G K, Jonasson L, Lojsthed B, Stemme S, Kocher O, Gabbiani G 1988 Localization of T lymphocytes and macrophages in fibrous and complicated human atherosclerotic plaques. Atherosclerosis 72: 135–141
Hansson G K, Holm J, Jonasson L 1989 Detection of activated T lymphocytes in the human atherosclerotic plaque. American Journal of Pathology 135: 169–175
Harlan J M, Thompson P J, Ross R R, Bowen Pope D F 1986 Alpha-thrombin induces release of platelet-derived growth factor-like molecule(s) by cultured human endothelial cells. Journal of Cell Biology 103: 1129–1133
Harrison D G Freiman P C, Armstrong M L, Marcus M L, Heistad D D 1987 Alterations of vascular reactivity in atherosclerosis. Circulation Research 61: II74–II80
Hartzell S, Ryder K, Lanahan A, Lau L F, Nathans D 1989 A growth factor-responsive gene of murine BALB/c 3T3 cells encodes a protein homologous to human tissue factor. Molecular and cell Biology 9: 2567–2573
Hatton M W, Moar S L, Richardson M 1989 Deendothelialization in vivo initiates a thrombogenic reaction at the rabbit aorta surface. Correlation of uptake of fibrinogen and antithrombin III with thrombin generation by the exposed subendothelium. American Journal of Pathology 135: 499–508
Haust D M 1983 Atherosclerosis — Lesions and Sequelae In: Silver M D (ed) Cardiovascular pathology. Churchill Livingstone, New York, vol 1: 191–315
Heaton J H, Dame M K, Gelehrter T D 1992 Thrombin induction of plasminogen activator inhibitor mRNA in human umbilical vein endothelial cells in culture. Journal of Laboratory and Clinical Medicine 120: 222–228
Horie T, Sekiguchi M, Hirosawa K 1978 Coronary thrombosis in pathogenesis of acute myocardial infarction. Histopathological study of coronary arteries in 108 necropsied cases using serial section. British Heart Journal 40: 153–161
Imparato A M, Riles T S, Mintzer R, Baumann F G 1983 The importance of hemorrhage in the relationship between gross morphologic characteristics and cerebral symptoms in 376 carotid artery plaques. Annals in Surgery 197: 195–203
Jawien A, Bowen Pope D F, Lindner V, Schwartz S M, Clowes A W 1992 Platelet-derived growth factor promotes smooth muscle migration and intimal thickening in a rat model of balloon angioplasty. Journal of Clinical Investigation 89: 507–511
Jaye M, McConathy E, Drohan W, Tong B, Deuel T, Maciag T 1985 Modulation of the sis gene transcript during endothelial cell differentiation in vitro. Science 228: 882–885
Jonasson L, Holm J, Skalli O, Bondjers G, Hansson G K 1986 Regional accumulations of T cells, macrophages, and smooth muscle cells in the human atherosclerotic plaque. Arteriosclerosis 6: 131–138
Jorgensen L, Rowsell H C, Hovig T, Mustard J F 1967 Resolution and organization of platelet-rich mural thrombi in carotid arteries of swine. American Journal of Pathology 51: 681–719
Kinlough Rathbone R L, Packham M A, Mustard J F 1983 Vessel injury, platelet adherence, and platelet survival. Arteriosclerosis 3: 529–546
Lindner V, Reidy M A 1991a Proliferation of smooth muscle cells after vascular injury is inhibited by an antibody against basic fibroblast growth factor. Proceedings of the National Academy of Sciences, USA 88: 3739–3743
Lindner V, Reidy M A 1991b Smooth muscle proliferation after vascular injury is inhibited by an antibody against basic FGF. Journal of Cellular Biochemistry 15C (suppl): 118 (abstract)
Lindner V, Lappi D A, Baird A, Majack R A, Reidy M A 1991 Role of basic fibroblast growth factor in vascular lesion formation. Circulation Research 68: 106–113
Ludmer P L, Selwyn A P, Shook T L et al 1986 Paradoxical vasoconstriction induced by acetylcholine in atherosclerotic coronary arteries. New England Journal of Medicine 315: 1046–1051
Majack R A 1987 Beta-type transforming growth factor specifies organizational behavior in vascular smooth muscle cell cultures. Journal of Cell Biology 105: 465–471
Majesky M W, Reidy M A, Bowen Pope D F, Hart C E, Wilcox J N, Schwartz S M 1990 PDGF ligand and receptor gene expression during repair of arterial injury. Journal of Cell Biology 111: 2149–2158
Martinet Y, Bitterman P B, Mornex J F, Grotendorst G R, Martin G R, Crystal R G 1986 Activated human monocytes express the c-sis proto-oncogene and release a mediator showing PDGF-like activity. Nature 319: 158–160
Masuda J, Ross R 1990a Atherogenesis during low level hypercholesterolemia in the nonhuman primate. I. Fatty streak formation. Arteriosclerosis 10: 164–177
Masuda J, Ross R 1990b Atherogenesis during low level hypercholesterolemia in the nonhuman primate. II. Fatty streak conversion to fibrous plaque. Arteriosclerosis 10: 178–187
Merwin J R, Newman W, Beall L D, Tucker A, Madri J 1991 Vascular cells respond differentially to transforming growth factors beta 1 and beta 2 in vitro. American Journal of Pathology 138: 37–51
Moncada S, Radomski M W, Palmer R M 1988 Endothelium-derived relaxing factor. Identification as nitric oxide and role in the control of vascular tone and platelet function. Biochemical Pharmacology 37: 2495–2501
Moore S 1973 Thromboatherosclerosis in normolipemic rabbits. A result of continued endothelial damage. Laboratory Investigation 29: 478–487
Mornex J F, Martinet Y, Yamauchi K et al 1986 Spontaneous expression of the c-sis gene and release of a platelet-derived growth factor-like molecule by human alveolar macrophages. Journal of Clinical Investigation 78: 61–66
Mosse P R, Campbell G R, Wang Z L, Campbell J H 1985 Smooth muscle phenotypic expression in human carotid arteries. I. Comparison of cells from diffuse intimal thickenings adjacent to atheromatous plaques with those of the media. Laboratory Investigation 53: 556–562
Myers P R, Guerra R, Harrison D G 1989 Release of NO and EDRF from cultured bovine aortic endothelial cells. American Journal of Physiology 256: H1030–H1037
Nachman R L, Hajjar H A, Silverstein R L, Dinarello C A 1986 Interleukin 1 induces endothelial cell synthesis of plasminogen activator inhibitor. Journal of Experimental Medicine 163: 1595–1600
Naito M, Hayashi T, Kuzuya M, Funaki C, Asai K, Kuzuya F 1990 Effects of fibrinogen and fibrin on the migration of vascular smooth muscle cells in vitro. Atherosclerosis 83: 9–14
Nelken N A, Coughlin S R, Gordon D, Wilcox J N 1991 Monocyte chemoattractant protein-I in human atheromatous plaques. Journal of Clinical Investigation 88: 1121–1127

Nelken N A, Wilcox J N, Coughlin S R 1992 Monocyte chemoattractant protein-1 is expressed in fatty streaks. Circulation (in press)

Nemerson Y 1966 The reaction between bovine brain tissue factor and factors VII and X. Biochemistry 5: 601–608

Nemerson Y 1987 Tissue factor and the initiation of blood coagulation. Advances in Experimental Medicine and Biology 214: 83–94

Nemerson Y 1988 Tissue factor and hemostasis. Blood 71: 1–8

Nemerson Y, Bach R 1982 Tissue factor revisited. Progress in Hemostasis and Thrombosis 6: 237–261

Niewiarowski S, Stuart R K, Thomas D P 1966 Activation of intravascular coagulation by collagen. Proceedings of the Society for Experimental Biology and Medicine 123: 196–200

Nilsson J, Sjolund M, Palmberg L, Thyberg J, Heldin C H 1985 Arterial smooth muscle cells in primary culture produce a platelet-derived growth factor-like protein. Proceedings of the National Academy of Sciences, USA 82: 4418–4422

Okazaki H, Majesky M W, Harker L A, Schwartz S M 1992 Regulation of platelet-derived growth ligand and receptor gene expressions by α-thrombin in vascular smooth muscle cells. Circulation Research 71: 1285–1293

Olson N E, Chao S, Lindner V, Reidy M A 1992 Intimal smooth muscle cell proliferation after balloon catheter injury. The role of basic fibroblast growth factor. American Journal of Pathology 140: 1017–1023

Østerud B, Rapaport S I 1977 Activation of factor IX by the reaction product of tissue factor and factor VII: additional pathway for initiating blood coagulation. Proceedings of the National Academy of Sciences, USA 74: 5260–5264

Owens G K, Loeb A, Gordon D, Thompson M M 1986 Expression of smooth muscle-specific alpha-isoactin in cultured vascular smooth muscle cells: Relationship between growth and cytodifferentiation. Journal of Cell Biology 102: 343–352

Palmer R M, Ferrige A G, Moncada S 1987 Nitric oxide release accounts for the biological activity of endothelium-derived relaxing factor. Nature 327: 524–526

Parsons T J, Haycraft D L, Hoak J C, Sage H 1986 Interaction of platelets and purified collagens in a laminar flow model. Thrombosis Research 43: 435–443

Parthasarathy S, Steinbrecher U P, Barnett J, Witztum J L, Steinberg D 1985 Essential role of phospholipase A2 activity in endothelial cell-induced modification of low density lipoprotein. Proceedings of the National Academy of Sciences, USA 82: 3000–3004

Poole J C F, Cromwell B S, Benditt E P 1971 Behavior of smooth muscle cells and formation of extracellular structures in the reaction of arterial walls to injury. American Journal of Pathology 62: 391–404

Poston R N, Haskard D O, Coucher J R, Gall N P, Johnson Tidey R R 1992 Expression of intercellular adhesion molecule-1 in atherosclerotic plaques. American Journal of Pathology 140: 665–673

Quillen J E, Sellke F W, Armstrong M L, Harrison D G 1991 Long-term cholesterol feeding alters the reactivity of primate coronary microvessels to platelet products. Arteriosclerosis and Thrombosis 11: 639–644

Ramshaw A L, Parums D V 1990 Immunohistochemical characterization of inflammatory cells associated with advanced atherosclerosis. Histopathology 17: 543–552

Reidy M A, Clowes A W, Schwartz S M 1983 Endothelial regeneration. V. Inhibition of endothelial regrowth in arteries of rat and rabbit. Laboratory Investigation 49: 569–575

Rosenfeld M E, Khoo J C, Miller E, Parthasarathy S, Palinski W, Witztum J L 1991 Macrophage-derived foam cells freshly isolated from rabbit atherosclerotic lesions degrade modified lipoproteins, promote oxidation of low-density lipoproteins, and contain oxidation-specific lipid-protein adducts. Journal of Clinical Investigation 87: 90–99

Rosenfeld M E, Tsukada T, Chait A, Bierman E L, Gown A M, Ross R 1987a Fatty streak expansion and maturation in Watanabe Heritable Hyperlipemic and comparably hypercholesterolemic fat-fed rabbits. Arteriosclerosis 7: 24–34

Rosenfeld M E, Tsukada T, Gown A M, Ross R 1987b Fatty streak initiation in Watanabe Heritable Hyperlipemic and comparably hypercholesterolemic fat-fed rabbits. Arteriosclerosis 7: 9–23

Rosenfeld M E, Palinski W, Yla Herttuala S, Carew T E 1990 Macrophages, endothelial cells, and lipoprotein oxidation in the pathogenesis of atherosclerosis. Toxicology and Pathology 18: 560–571

Ross R 1979 Platelets: cell proliferation and atherosclerosis. Metabolism 28: 410–414

Ross R 1986 The pathogenesis of atherosclerosis — an update. New England Journal of Medicine 314: 488–500

Ross R, Glomset J A 1976a The pathogenesis of atherosclerosis. New England Journal of Medicine 295: 369–377

Ross R, Glomset J A 1976b The pathogenesis of atherosclerosis (second of two parts). New England Journal of Medicine 295: 420–425

Ross R, Wight T N, Stradness E, Thiele B 1984 Human atherosclerosis. I. Cell constitution and characteristics of advanced lesions of the superficial femoral artery. American Journal of Pathology 114: 79–93

Rubanyi G M, Vanhoutte P M 1986 Superoxide anions and hyperoxia inactivate endothelium-derived relaxing factor. American Journal of Physiology 250: H822–H827

Schall T J 1991 Biology of the RANTES/SIS cytokine family. Cytokine 3: 165–183

Schleef R R, Bevilacqua M P, Sawdey M, Gimbrone M A J, Loskutoff D J 1988 Cytokine activation of vascular endothelium. Effects on tissue-type plasminogen activator and type 1 plasminogen activator inhibitor. Journal of Biological Chemistry 263: 5797–5803

Schwartz C J, Valente A J, Kelley J L, Sprague E A, Edwards E H 1988 Thrombosis and the development of atherosclerosis: Rokitansky revisited. Seminars in Thrombosis and Hemostasis 14: 189–195

Seifert R A, Schwartz S M, Bowen Pope D F 1984 Developmentally regulated production of platelet-derived growth factor-like molecules. Nature 311: 669–671

Sellke F W, Armstrong M L, Harrison D G 1990 Endothelium-dependent vascular relaxation is abnormal in the coronary microcirculation of atherosclerotic primates. Circulation 81: 1586–1593

Sessa W C, Harrison J K, Barber C M et al 1992 Molecular cloning and expression of a cDNA encoding endothelial cell nitric oxide synthase. Journal of Biological Chemistry 267: 15274–15276

Sherman C T, Litvack F, Grundfest W et al 1986 Coronary angioscopy in patients with unstable angina pectoris. New England Journal of Medicine 315: 913–919

Shimokado K, Raines E W, Madtes D K, Barrett T B, Benditt E P, Ross R 1985 A significant part of macrophage-derived growth factor consists of at least two forms of PDGF. Cell 43: 277–286

Shimokawa H, Vanhoutte P M 1989 Hypercholesterolemia causes generalized impairment of endothelium-dependent relaxation to aggregating platelets in porcine arteries. Journal of the American College of Cardiology 13: 1402–1408

Shultz P J, Raij L 1990 Inhibition of human mesangial cell proliferation by calcium channel blockers. Hypertension 15: I76–I80

Shultz P J, Knauss T C, Mene P, Abboud H E 1989 Mitogenic signals for thrombin in mesangial cells: regulation of phospholipase C and PDGF genes. American Journal of Physiology 257: F366–F374

Small D M 1988 George Lyman Duff memorial lecture. Progression and regression of atherosclerotic lesions. Insights from lipid physical biochemistry. Arteriosclerosis 8: 103–129

Sparrow C P, Parthasarathy S, Steinberg D 1989 A macrophage receptor that recognizes oxidized low density lipoprotein but not acetylated low density lipoprotein. Journal of Biological Chemistry 264: 2599–2604

Springer T A, Lasky L A 1991 Cell adhesion. Sticky sugars for selectins. Nature 349: 196–197

Stary H C 1989 Evolution and progression of atherosclerotic lesions in coronary arteries of children and young adults. Arteriosclerosis 9: I19–I32

Steinberg D, Parthasarathy S, Carew T E, Khoo J C, Witztum J L 1989 Beyond cholesterol. Modifications of low-density lipoprotein that increase its atherogenicity. New England Journal of Medicine 320: 915–924

Steinbrecher U P, Parthasarathy S, Leake D S, Witztum J L, Steinberg D 1984 Modification of low density lipoprotein by endothelial cells

involves lipid peroxidation and degradation of low density lipoprotein phospholipids. Proceedings of the National Academy of Sciences, USA 81: 3883–3887
Stemerman M B 1973 Thrombogenesis of the rabbit arterial plaque. An electron microscopic study. American Journal of Pathology 73: 7–26
Surmiyoshi A, More R H, Weigensberg B I 1973 Aortic fibrofatty type atherosclerosis from thrombus in normolipidemic rabbits. Atherosclerosis 18: 43–57
Tanner F C, Noll G, Boulanger C M, Luscher T F 1991 Oxidized low density lipoproteins inhibit relaxations of porcine coronary arteries. Role of scavenger receptor and endothelium-derived nitric oxide. Circulation 83: 2012–2020
Territo M C, Berliner J A, Almada L, Ramirez R, Fogelman A M 1989 Beta-very low density lipoprotein pretreatment of endothelial monolayers increases monocyte adhesion. Arteriosclerosis 9: 824–828
Thompson W D, Smith E B, Stirk C M, Kochhar A 1990 Atherosclerotic plaque growth: presence of stimulatory fibrin degradation products. Blood Coagulation and Fibrinolysis 1: 489–493
Tsukada T, McNutt M A, Ross R, Gown A M 1987 HHF35, a muscle actin-specific monoclonal antibody. II. Reactivity in normal, reactive, and neoplastic human tissues. American Journal of Pathology 127: 389–402
van Aken P J, Emeis J J 1983 Organization of experimentally induced arterial thrombosis in rats from two weeks until ten months: The development of an arteriosclerotic lesion and the occurrence of rethrombosis. Artery 11: 384–399
van Aken P J, Emeis J J, Lindeman J 1980 A new microsurgical method for the induction of arterial thrombosis in rats. Artery 8: 442–447
van der Wal A C, Das P K, Bentz van de Berg D, van der Loos C M, Becker A E 1989 Atherosclerotic lesions in humans. In situ immunophenotypic analysis suggesting an immune mediated response. Laboratory Investigation 61: 166–170
Vu T K, Hung D T, Wheaton V I, Coughlin S R 1991 Molecular cloning of a functional thrombin receptor reveals a novel proteolytic mechanism of receptor activation. Cell 64: 1057–1068
Walker L N, Bowen Pope D F, Ross R, Reidy M A 1986 Production of platelet-derived growth factor-like molecules by cultured arterial smooth muscle cells accompanies proliferation after arterial injury. Proceedings of the National Academy of Sciences, USA 83: 7311–7315
Wilcox J N 1991 Analysis of local gene expression in human atherosclerotic plaques by in situ hybridization. Trends in Cardiovascular Medicine 1: 17–24
Wilcox J N 1992 Unpublished observations
Wilcox J N, Smith K M, Williams L T, Schwartz S M, Gordon D 1988 Platelet-derived growth factor mRNA detection in human atherosclerotic plaques by in situ hybridization. Journal of Clinical Investigation 82: 1134–1143
Wilcox J N, Smith K M, Schwartz S M, Gordon D 1989 Localization of tissue factor in the normal vessel wall and in the atherosclerotic plaque. Proceedings of the National Academy of Sciences, USA 86: 2839–2843
Wilcox J N, Emerick G, Hultgren B, Hotchkiss A 1990 Organization of a chronic arterial thrombus in rats: an in vivo models for modulation of smooth muscle cells? Biology of Vascular Cells, Sixth International Symposium, Paris (August)
Wilcox J N, Hanson S R, Rodriguez J et al 1993 Thrombin receptor expression in vascular lesion formation. Journal of Clinical Investigation (in press)
Wilner G D, Nossel H L, LeRoy E C 1968a Activation of Hageman factor by collagen. Journal of Clinical Investigation 47: 2608–2615
Wilner G D, Nossel H L, LeRoy E C 1968b Aggregation of platelets by collagen. Journal of Clinical Investigation 47: 2616–2621
Woolf N 1978 Thrombosis and atherosclerosis. British Medical Bulletin 34: 137–142
Woolf N, Bradley J W P, Crawford T, Carstairs K C 1968 Experimental mural thrombi in the pig aorta. The early natural history. British Journal of Experimental Pathology 49: 257–264
Yla Herttuala S, Lipton B A, Rosenfeld M E et al 1991 Expression of monocyte chemoattractant protein 1 in macrophage-rich areas of human and rabbit atherosclerotic lesions. Proceedings of the National Academy of Sciences, USA 88: 5252–5256

50. Lipids and atherosclerosis

A. Gaw C. J. Packard J. Shepherd

The aetiology of coronary heart disease has been the subject of intense study over the last few decades and many contributing or risk factors have been identified (Isles & Hole 1991). The putative role of hyperlipidaemia in the development of atherosclerosis goes back almost 150 years to the work of Vogel in Leipzig (1845). It was he who first noted the presence of cholesterol in atheromatous tissue. The term atherosclerosis itself was coined by Marchand around 1860 (quoted by Aschoff 1924) but it was not until the early years of the 20th century that the association between dietary cholesterol and atherosclerotic lesions was confirmed experimentally. Anitschkow and his colleagues (1913) in St Petersburg fed egg yolk to rabbits and observed the development of lesions in their aortae, identical to the atherosclerotic lesions in man. As this work progressed, Anitsckow (1915) became convinced only two years later that, 'there can be no atheroma without cholesterol'.

From such beginnings an impressive edifice of epidemiological research has been built, culminating in incontrovertible evidence for the recognition of hyperlipidaemia as an important causative factor in the development of atherosclerosis. Because this hyperlipidaemia may be readily correctable in most cases by dietary and pharmacological means, and with benefit to the individual it has been the focus of much clinical attention.

The Lipid Research Clinics Coronary Primary Prevention Trial (1984a & b) and Helsinki Heart Study (Frick et al 1987), clearly showed that lowering plasma cholesterol levels brings benefit in terms of reduction of coronary morbidity. Such findings coupled with advances in therapeutics and biotechnology have detonated an explosion of interest and activity within the scientific and medical communities since the mid 1980s.

With the control of lipoprotein metabolism comes the control, at least in part, of the development of atheroma. There follows a discussion of lipoprotein metabolism and a description of the structure and function of the plasma lipoproteins.

LIPOPROTEIN METABOLISM

Lipoprotein classes

Lipids are important sources of energy, of synthetic precursors and cellular components. Because of this, a complex system has evolved to solve the problems of transporting lipids around the body in the aqueous environment of the plasma. This system depends on the packaging of neutral lipids (cholesteryl esters and triglyceride) with specific proteins and amphipathic lipids (phospholipids and cholesterol) to create multimolecular particles called lipoproteins that are readily miscible with water. The resolution of the plasma lipoproteins was made possible largely due to the use of the ultracentrifuge in the 1950s (Gofman et al 1950, Turner et al 1951). The most widely used system of nomenclature defines five main classes of lipoprotein on the basis of their hydrated density (d, in g/ml) (Mills et al 1984). These are chylomicrons d <0.94 g/ml; very low density lipoprotein (VLDL) d 0.94–1.006 g/ml; intermediate density lipoproteins (IDL) d 1.006–1.019 g/ml, low density lipoprotein (LDL) d 1.019–1.063 g/ml and high density lipoprotein (HDL) d 1.063–1.210 g/ml. Lipoproteins have also been defined by their electrophoretic mobility, particle size, apolipoprotein composition and flotation rate (Mills et al 1984). The last is commonly quoted and merits further explanation. In this system the lipoproteins are defined by their rate of flotation through a salt solution of fixed density in the analytical ultracentrifuge. For lipoproteins of density less than 1.063 g/ml the salt solution used is NaCl d 1.063 g/ml, while the high density lipoproteins are defined using a density solution of 1.210 g/ml. All densities are defined at 26°C and the units used are Svedberg units (S_f) where one S_f unit=10^{-13} cm.s.$^{-1}$ dyne.$^{-1}$ g^{-1} at 26°C. Both systems are very flexible, for while five main lipoprotein classes are traditionally defined, any lipoprotein preparation that does not fit these established windows may be characterized on the basis of its limiting densities or flotation rate interval. Each lipoprotein class exhibits a unique structure, function and metabolism.

The major organs involved in lipid metabolism are the intestine and the liver. Together these organs are responsible for the majority of lipoprotein synthesis and catabolism. Regulation of lipid transport is exerted through several agencies: apolipoproteins with specific signalling and cofactor functions, specific cell-surface lipoprotein receptors, intravascular lipolytic enzymes and transfer proteins that act in concert to maintain cholesterol and triglyceride homeostasis. Malfunction of these regulatory factors may cause or contribute to the development of dyslipidaemia and in turn atherosclerosis. An overview of lipoprotein metabolism illustrating the roles that each plays in lipid transport is illustrated in Figure 50.1.

Intestinal lipoprotein metabolism

Daily we ingest about 0.5 g of cholesterol (as free and esterified sterol) and 100 g of triglyceride. Digestive enzymes in the intestinal lumen hydrolyze the lipid esters, releasing free cholesterol, fatty acids and mono- and diglycerides. These amphipathic molecules form water-soluble micelles that carry the lipid to absorptive sites in the duodenum (Danielson & Sjovall 1975). Under normal circumstances, triglyceride absorption is virtually quantitative. However, only about 50% of the cholesterol is taken up, the remainder being lost in the faeces (Norum et al 1983). Within the enterocyte, absorbed cholesterol is rapidly re-esterified by the action of the membrane-bound cytoplasmic enzyme acyl coenzyme A: cholesterol acyltransferase (ACAT) (Norum et al 1983) and packaged with reconstituted triglyceride into large, lipid-rich chylomicron particles containing about 1% protein. These appear in abundance in the intestinal mucosal cells following a meal and are secreted into lacteals within the wall of the small bowel. The availability of a specific structural apolipoprotein known as apolipoprotein B (apoB) is a prerequisite for the production of such particles. Subjects with the inherited disorder known as abetalipoproteinaemia (Kane & Havel

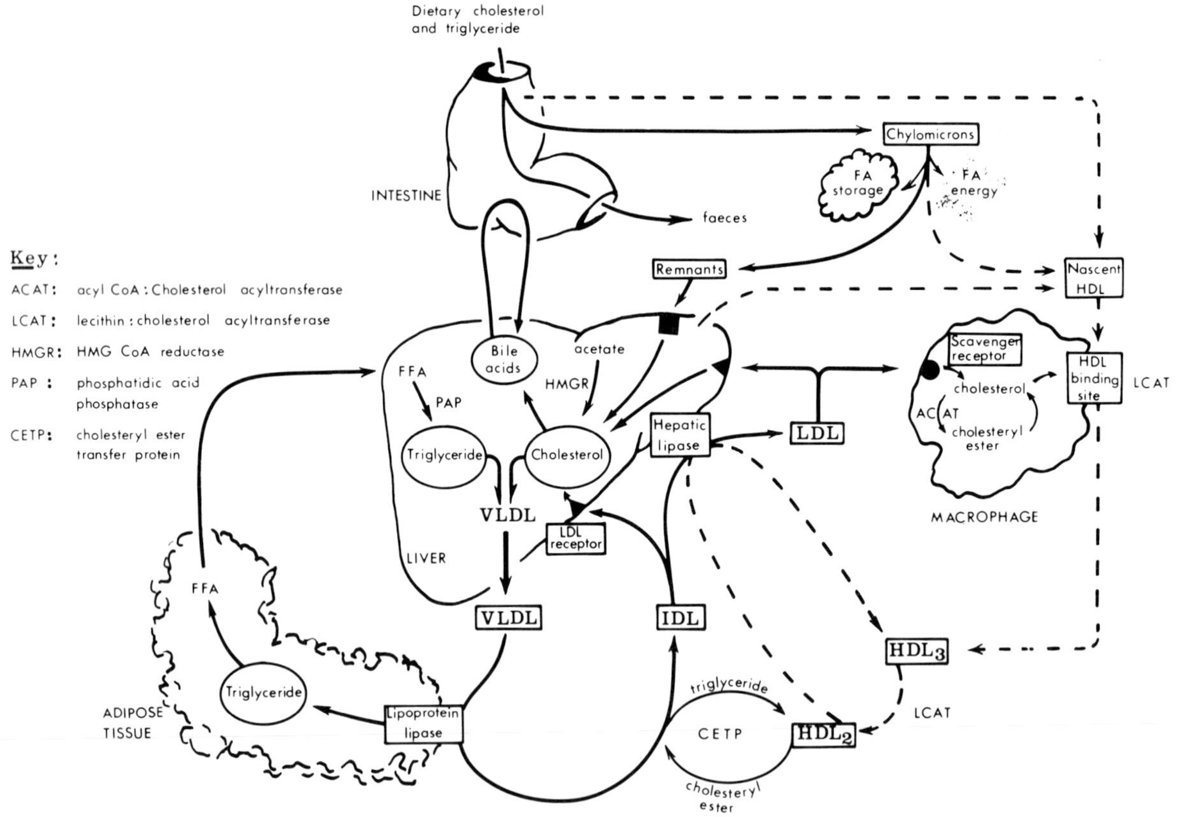

Fig. 50.1 Lipoprotein metabolism. Following its absorption, dietary fat is packaged into large, triglyceride-rich chylomicron particles within the enterocyte and secreted into the circulation. There, lipolysis reduces the particle's triglyceride core and makes redundant part of its surface coat which is shed to high density lipoprotein (HDL). The remnants produced in the process are rapidly assimilated by a receptor-mediated mechanism in the liver. In the fasting state, very low density lipoprotein (VLDL) replaces chylomicrons as the major triglyceride transporters and the liver dominates lipoprotein metabolism. Cholesterol and triglyceride elaborated in this organ, are released into the plasma where they are subject to tissue lipolysis. This degrades them to low density lipoprotein (LDL) via an intermediate species (IDL). The LDL is removed by receptors present on the liver and peripheral tissues. When these are saturated, alternative scavenger receptor pathways become dominant. Interchange of lipids between circulating lipoprotein particles is facilitated by the plasma enzyme lecithin:cholesterol acyltransferase (LCAT) and cholesteryl ester transfer protein (CETP) both of which participate in the process of reverse cholesterol transport from peripheral sites to the liver, where the sterol is excreted.

1989) fail to secrete chylomicrons from their enterocytes following a fatty meal. The condition results in failure to thrive in infancy and is associated with specific retinal and erythrocyte defects that are progressive and derive ultimately from defective absorption of fat-soluble vitamins.

ApoB found in chylomicrons is a modified, lower molecular weight form of that synthesised by the liver and secreted with VLDL. The former is termed apoB-48 and the latter apoB-100 in the nomenclature of Kane et al (1980). It has recently been noted (Levy et al 1990) that the gut also produces apoB-100 although this does not appear in chylomicrons. Other proteins are also present on the chylomicron surface. Some (apo AI, AII, AIV and possibly C) are elaborated by the gut and secreted with the chylomicron (Green & Glickman 1981) while additional peptides are acquired from high density lipoprotein (HDL) in interstitial fluid. The latter include apoC and apoE, both of which participate in subsequent processing of the particle (Imaizumi et al 1978, Green et al 1979, Green & Glickman 1981).

Several rapid changes take place in the chylomicron when it enters the plasma. Within the capillary beds of skeletal muscle and adipose tissue it is exposed to the lipolytic action of endothelium-bound lipoprotein lipase. This enzyme hydrolyses its triglyceride core, releasing free fatty acids and mono- and diglycerides for energy production or storage (Nilsson-Ehle et al 1980). Further delipidation results in the generation of so-called 'chylomicron remnants'. These particles are structurally distinct from the parent chylomicron (Mjos et al 1975), not only because they are the products of the degradation process outlined above but also because they acquire lipid, particularly cholesteryl ester, from denser lipoproteins like LDL and HDL, facilitated by cholesteryl ester transfer protein (CETP). Zilversmit (1984) demonstrated that this cholesteryl ester is exchanged for triglyceride that is transferred in the opposite direction, i.e. into LDL and HDL. Deficiency of CETP activity as described by Eto et al (1990) results in markedly elevated plasma levels of HDL. The extent of this process, which effectively enriches chylomicron remnants in cholesteryl esters, is governed by the residence time of the chylomicron in the circulation. Rapid chylomicron clearance, resulting from highly efficient lipolysis, gives the particle little opportunity to acquire cholesteryl ester. Besides these alterations in its hydrophobic core, the surface coat of the remnant shows substantial differences from that of its parent. All the apoB initially present in the particle is retained, but the relative amounts of the other proteins are altered. ApoAI and apoAII are transferred into the HDL density range (Schaefer et al 1978, Tall et al 1979) while apoAIV, upon release from the chylomicron, seems to exist free in the plasma since its affinity for other lipoproteins is low (Tall et al 1979). The C protein content initially rises as a result of transfer from HDL (Havel et al 1973). This is of particular significance with regard to apoCII since this is an obligatory cofactor for lipoprotein lipase, increasing the particle's affinity for the enzyme. The role of apoCIII, the major C peptide on the chylomicron surface, is less clear although it may be responsible for regulating the lipolysis of the particle (Ginsberg et al 1986) or delaying its hepatic clearance (Windler et al 1980). As the chylomicron progresses down the lipolytic cascade the C proteins are transferred gradually back into the reservoir within HDL. ApoE, which is acquired by the particle simultaneously with apoC, is not involved in lipolysis (Blum et al, 1982), but thereafter plays a role in triggering hepatic uptake of the remnant particle (Mahley & Innerarity 1983).

The liver is responsible for the efficient and rapid clearance of cholesteryl ester-rich chylomicron remnants from the circulation. Hepatic parenchymal cells contain, on their surfaces, receptors that recognise and bind to particular charged domains of the remnant's apoE (Brown & Goldstein 1987). This interaction results in the delivery of the particle to lysosomal degradation within the hepatocyte. The key role played by apoE in this process is evident from studies performed on individuals who express a mutant form of the E protein ($apoE_2$) in which the conformation of the receptor-binding region is altered. They exhibit delayed clearance of the remnants from the bloodstream (Gregg et al 1981). The metabolism of chylomicrons is depicted schematically in Figure 50.1, which emphasizes the bi-functionality of the process: the delivery of dietary triglyceride to skeletal muscle and adipose tissue, and of cholesterol to the liver. The activity of lipoprotein lipase in a tissue is constantly changing and is under hormonal control. Thus the enzyme has some of the properties of a membrane receptor in determining the direction of triglyceride flow.

Hepatic lipid metabolism

Although the liver has the capacity to make all the cholesterol and triglyceride that it needs, preformed components that are available either from the diet or from adipose tissue via fatty acid/albumin transport are preferred. Mobilization of depot fat in adipose tissue is under humoral control by agents such as adrenaline (Krebs & Beavo 1979). The fatty acids released from the adipocyte into the circulation are rapidly extracted by many tissues including the liver, which is able to use them for energy and as substrates for the synthesis of phospholipids and triglyceride. When the availability of these substrates is limited, the liver can generate fatty acid from small molecular weight precursors (Barter & Kelvin 1972). Similarly a cholesterol deficit can be met by endogenous synthesis, following activation of the rate-limiting enzyme 3-hydroxy 3-methylglutaryl coenzyme A reductase (HMG CoA reductase) (Goldstein & Brown 1984).

Lipids synthesized in the liver have several fates (Norum

et al 1983, Packard & Shepherd 1986). First, a significant proportion of the cholesterol and triglyceride is secreted in VLDL, the major vehicle for endogenous triglyceride transport. Secondly, lipid surplus to requirements may be stored, temporarily, as cytoplasmic oil droplets within the hepatocyte. And, thirdly, the liver cell has the unique ability (Dietschy & Wilson 1970) to eliminate cholesterol into the bile, either unchanged or following oxidation to bile acids. Gramme quantities of lipid flux through these pathways each day and so it is imperative for the hepatocellular economy that the mechanisms involved are precisely interregulated. This is achieved by the coordinated control of certain key enzymes whose activities appear in turn to be modulated by bile acids (Fig. 50.2). These compounds, produced by the liver and secreted into the gut to aid digestion, are reabsorbed in the terminal ileum and extracted from the portal blood by the liver. Their return to their site of origin in this 'enterohepatic circulation' produces several important effects (Angelin et al 1986):

1. Cholesterol 7α-hydroxylase, the rate-limiting enzyme in bile acid synthesis, is downregulated.
2. HMG CoA reductase, the enzyme that governs cholesterol production, is also suppressed, although whether this is a direct or indirect effect of bile acids is a matter of controversy.
3. Phosphatidic acid phosphatase, which stands at the fork between the pathways of triglyceride and phospholipid synthesis is inhibited, favouring production of the latter.

The net result of these regulatory events is to ensure that, as bile acids flow back to the liver, they suppress their de novo synthesis while stimulating adequate secretion of the co-emulsifier, lecithin into the bile. The enterohepatic flow of bile acids follows the cycle of dietary intake, and so strong diurnal rhythms are induced in these control mechanisms as evident from detailed studies of rats kept under conditions of controlled lighting and feeding (Dietschy & Wilson 1970, Danielson & Sjovall 1975, Myant & Mitropoulos 1977). When food is administered during the dark period, it triggers a release of bile acids from the hepatobiliary tree. This produces a peak in the synthesis of hepatic triglyceride, cholesterol and bile acids, and secretion of VLDL into the blood stream also reaches a peak (Goh & Heimberg 1979) The above phenomena are reversed in the middle of the light period when the liver is replete with recycled bile acids. However, although this scheme provides a plausible explanation for the laboratory observations, it is incomplete since even continuously fasted animals show periodicity in hepatic synthesis (Myant & Mitropoulos 1977) and in man such diurnal rhythms are less well documented, although there is some good evidence to indicate that they occur (Parker et al 1982).

It is clear from the above argument that medical and

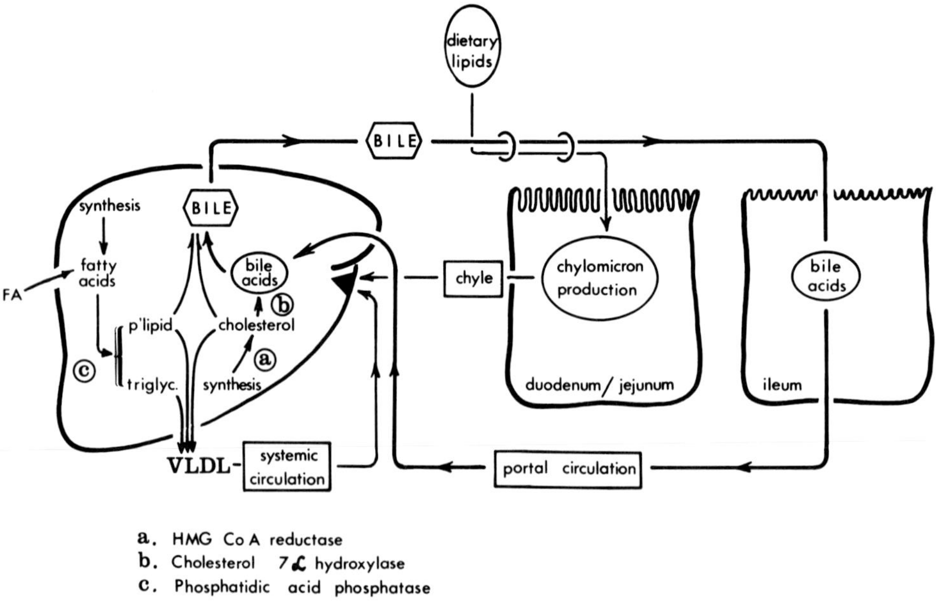

Fig. 50.2 Hepatic integration of corporeal lipid metabolism. Lipid metabolism within the liver is integrated via three key regulatory enzymes.
a. HMG CoA reductase, the pacemaker enzyme in cholesterol biosynthesis, upon demand, promotes sterol production from small molecular weight precursors like acetate. b. Cholesterol 7α-hydroxylase initiates the oxidation of cholesterol to form the bile acids required for dietary fat absorption.
c. Phosphatidic acid phosphatase stands at the branch point between production of triglyceride and phospholipid and determines the relative rates of synthesis of these two classes of lipid. All three enzymes are probably regulated in a coordinated fashion by the bile acids in the hepatocyte.

surgical interruption of the enterohepatic circulation of bile acids will have profound effects on hepatic lipid metabolism. Such therapeutic manoeuvres can therefore be used to advantage in the management of hypercholesterolaemia.

Endogenous lipoprotein metabolism

The discussion that follows outlines the pathways of endogenous lipoprotein metabolism characteristic of the post-absorptive or fasting state. The behaviour of the apolipoproteins, enzymes and cell membrane receptors involved in the process is described. This framework offers a useful basis upon which to build our understanding of these components of the system that may be anti-atherogenic, and indicates where defects may lead to hyperlipidaemia.

Metabolism of ApoB containing lipoproteins

In the post-absorptive state, VLDL replaces chylomicrons as the main vehicle of triglyceride transport in the plasma. ApoB is integral to the particle and essential for its normal secretion. ApoB in VLDL is, as noted above, the larger molecular weight apoB-100, but shares a number of antigenic sites with the gut-derived apoB-48. The B-100 protein has now been sequenced using recombinant DNA technology (Carlsson et al 1985, Chan et al 1985, Knott et al 1985). It is a huge protein of 4336 amino acid residues that has many repeat sequences. Following synthesis in the rough endoplasmic reticulum, the protein associates with a triglyceride/phospholipid droplet in its passage to the Golgi apparatus where it becomes glycosylated before being secreted (Hamilton 1983). Examination of VLDL particles isolated from purified Golgi membranes has shown that they are heterogenous, encompassing a size range from 40–70 nm. They therefore do not have a stoichiometrically definable structure (Hamilton 1983). This information accords with complementary metabolic evidence that the liver has the capacity to elaborate a range of VLDL particles whose size and lipid composition may vary in response to changes in nutritional status. Besides apoB-100, nascent VLDL particles contain a few molecules of apoC and apoE that are augmented by transfer from HDL when the lipoprotein meets the interstitial fluid.

Triglyceride-rich VLDL enter a metabolic cascade similar to that described for chylomicrons, and indeed both compete for the same lipolytic sites in skeletal muscle and adipose tissue capillary beds. Studies designed to examine the metabolism of VLDL have focussed largely on its B protein moiety. Early work with radioiodinated VLDL of density less than 1.006 kg/l (Berman et al 1978) indicated that apoB was transferred through an intermediate lipoprotein fraction, IDL to LDL. In the process the particle's core is hydrolyzed by lipoprotein lipase (Nilsson-Ehle et al 1980), a reaction that requires the participation of apoCII on the particle. Again, in parallel with chylomicron metabolism, cholesteryl esters (Eisenberg 1985) are acquired from other lipoproteins (principally HDL) by exchange, while surface coat apoC is transferred in the opposite direction (Berman et al 1978). LDL therefore represents a 'remnant' of VLDL catabolism in which the triglyceride core is virtually eliminated and apoB is the sole protein component. In most subjects, whether normolipaemic or not, the rate of synthesis of apoB into VLDL (Janus et al 1980) exceeds that into LDL. Not all VLDL particles are therefore destined to complete their journey down the delipidation cascade to LDL. This phenomenon has been examined (Packard et al 1984, Shepherd et al 1984) in detail using procedures which permit fractionation of the VLDL spectrum in order to follow the fates of particles of a narrower compositional range. The evidence that emerged indicated that lipolysis of large VLDL (S_f 60–400) generated remnants of S_f 12–60 (i.e. within the small VLDL/IDL flotation interval), most of which were removed directly from the plasma without appearing in LDL. The latter seemed to come from rapid and quantitative transformation of small VLDL particles that had been secreted directly by the liver.

Both of the major plasma lipolytic enzymes, lipoprotein lipase and hepatic lipase have been implicated in the metabolism of apoB-100-containing particles (Nicoll & Lewis 1980). It is known that the affinity of lipoprotein lipase is greater for large, triglyceride-rich particles than for smaller remnants, whereas hepatic lipase, which expresses both triglyceride lipase and phospholipase activities, seems to favour smaller VLDL and IDL particles. The complementary roles of these lipases are perhaps best exemplified in studies of patients who, for genetic reasons (Carlson et al 1986, Demant et al 1988), lack the enzymes, or in animal studies where enzyme activity has been inhibited using antibodies (Behr et al 1981, Goldberg et al 1982). Under such conditions, absence of lipoprotein lipase results in accumulation of particles of flotation rate greater than S_f 100 that contain both apoB-100 and apoB-48 (i.e. of gut and liver origin, respectively). Smaller, denser apoB-containing lipoproteins virtually disappear from the plasma. Conversely, antibody-induced inhibition of hepatic lipase in cynomolgus monkeys (Goldberg et al 1982) causes the accumulation of smaller VLDL and IDL; and LDL becomes relatively enriched in triglyceride. Similarly, individuals with hepatic lipase deficiency express high plasma concentrations of small VLDL and IDL that are accompanied by reduced circulating levels of LDL (Demant et al 1988).

Metabolism of high density lipoproteins

Besides apoB-containing particles whose metabolism is

outlined above, the plasma lipoprotein spectrum also encompasses particles whose main protein component is apoA. They lie in the density interval 1.063–1.210 g/ml and are the smallest of the lipoproteins, having a molecular weight not much different from plasma protein components such as β_2-macroglobulin. A typical HDL particle is about 7 nm in diameter and almost 3000 times smaller than the average VLDL particle in terms of volume. HDL is, therefore, the smallest of the lipoproteins yet the most numerous. This is an important fact that often escapes our attention when we consider the metabolic relationships that exist between lipoproteins. Moreover, it has profound implications relative to the structure and function of HDL particles in that each lipid and protein component found in the HDL spectrum as a whole are not represented within every constituent particle. In other words, HDL is a heterogeneous mixture of particles endowed with a diversity of metabolic properties. The recent expansion of our understanding of the functions of HDL has come largely from appreciation of its heterogeneity and from the development of techniques, e.g. immunochemical precipitation and molecular sieve electrophoresis, designed to exploit it.

HDL represents an amalgam of diverse components (Fig. 50.3) that come together following:

1. Direct secretion by the liver and intestine
2. Transfer from other lipoproteins
3. Transfer from peripheral tissues.

The major HDL proteins apoAI and apoAII are elaborated in precursor form in the liver and intestine. Estimates of the contribution from each of these organs, at least in rats, suggest that they share roughly equally in synthesis (Wu & Windmueller 1979). Certainly, intestinal apoA production is prodigious as evidenced from its copious appearance in the urine of chyluric patients (Green et al 1979). Some of the protein is secreted with chylomicrons and appears in the HDL density interval following lipolysis of these particles (Green & Glickman 1981). Consequently after a fatty meal the levels of apoAI and apoAII in the plasma rise. In addition, the intestine is capable of elaborating and secreting small apoA-containing particles directly into the HDL density interval (Green et al 1978), a process that is continuous even in the fasting state. Studies using perfused intestine preparations have shown that under conditions where lecithin:cholesterol acyltransferase (LCAT) activity is blocked, a discoidal particle is produced, rich in free cholesterol and phospholipid and with apoA arranged around its circumference. Particles with a similar structure are also isolable from lymph (Dory et al 1985), a body fluid that is naturally low in LCAT activity. Exposure of such particles to the enzymatic and transfer activities of plasma transforms them into mature spherical HDL (Dory et al 1983). The apoA proteins lost from the surface of chylomicrons during lipolysis are thought also to appear initially in bilayer disks that undergo rapid conversion in the plasma to mature HDL spheres (Tall & Small 1978). Electron micrographic studies have shown that lipolysis, by reducing the core volume of the chylomicron renders some its surface coat redundant. The monolayer responds by folding upon itself to form a frond-like bilayer that, shed into the plasma, comes under the influence of LCAT and is converted to mature HDL. The central role of LCAT in

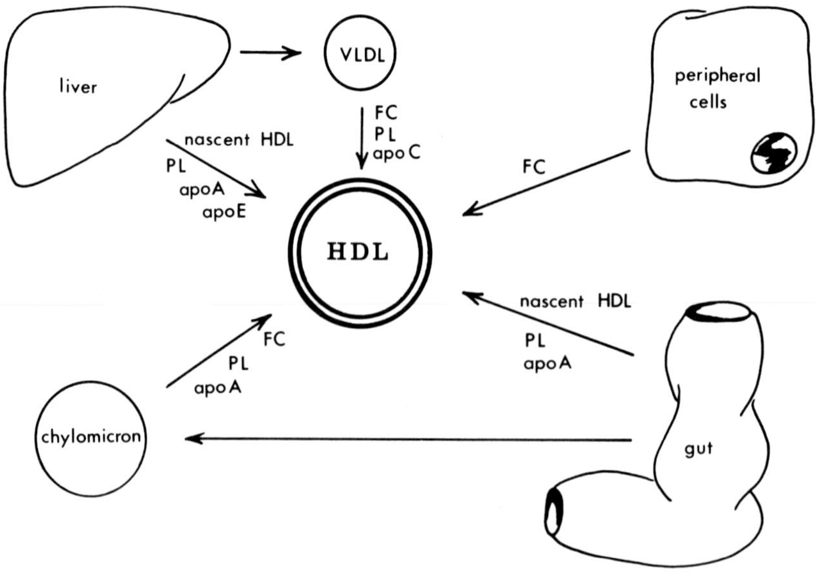

Fig. 50.3 Origins of HDL. The high density lipoprotein fraction is not only synthesised de novo by intestine and liver but also acquires components from other plasma lipoproteins and from peripheral tissues. PL, phospholipid; FC, free cholesterol.

the maturation of HDL is evident from studies of those rare patients (Norum 1984) who present with an inherited deficiency of the enzyme. Their HDL circulates as bilayer discs that readily undergo transformation in vitro to normal HDL with the addition of LCAT.

As noted above, the liver and the intestine share equally in the synthesis of HDL. Perfusion studies in rats have shown that the primary hepatic secretion product is again discoidal (Hamilton et al 1976) and rich in both apoAI and apoE. Exposure to LCAT induces its rapid conversion to HDL. In this process, apoAI is retained while E is lost to lipoproteins of lower density (Norum 1984).

The action of LCAT on discoidal HDL triggers a change in the disposition of cholesterol within the particle (Fig. 50.4). The enzyme catalyzes the transfer of a fatty acid from lecithin to the hydroxyl residue on cholesterol, leading to the generation of lysolecithin and cholesteryl ester (Norum 1984). The polarities of these products are fundamentally different from those of their precursors. Lysolecithin is more hydrophilic and dissociates readily from the lipoprotein into the aqueous environment. On the other hand, esterification of the sterol increases its hydrophobicity and causes it to partition into the nonpolar interior of the particle. The surface site vacated by the sterol is then available to accept additional cholesterol molecules either from other lipoproteins or from cell surfaces. Thus, LCAT has a dual action: it facilitates the sequestration of cholesterol within the hydrophobic core of HDL, generating in the process a chemical potential gradient which leads to continued uptake of the sterol. Even mature HDL particles have a free cholesterol/phospholipid ratio that is less than that of VLDL or LDL. Therefore it is not surprising that HDL is a good acceptor of tissue cholesterol while VLDL and LDL are not. Acquisition of cholesterol by HDL proceeds until the nascent disc is fully transformed into a pseudomicellar spherical structure. Obviously, this process would be constrained by the size of the HDL particles were it not possible for the sterol ester to undergo transfer to less dense lipoproteins facilitated by a neutral lipid transfer protein. This protein exchanges the cholesteryl ester in the core of HDL for triglyceride acquired from VLDL or chylomicrons. The triglyceride-enriched HDL then becomes more susceptible to intravascular lipolysis, which renders it smaller and denser (Deckelbaum et al 1984). Thus the size of circulating HDL depends on the balance between the opposing forces of cholesterol esterification, which increases particle size, and lipolytic digestion, which reduces it. A recent report (Cheung et al 1991) has suggested that the size of HDL particles may be clinically important. They found that smaller particle size was associated with coronary heart disease and that particle size was a much stronger predictor of disease than HDL cholesterol.

The dominant components of mature plasma HDL are

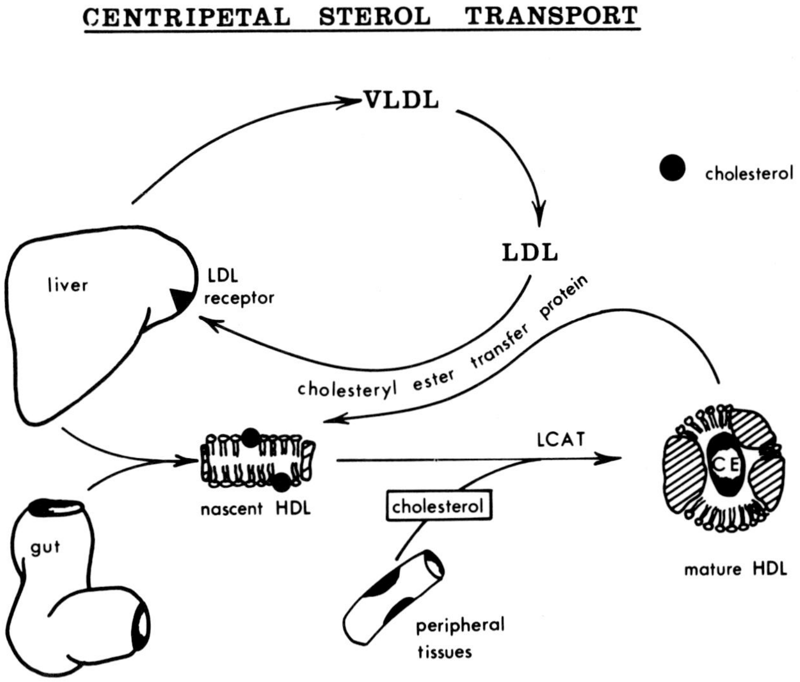

Fig. 50.4 Reverse cholesterol transport. Discoidal, nascent HDL is converted to mature spheroidal HDL by the action of lecithin:cholesterol acyltransferase (LCAT). This process allows the uptake of cholesterol from peripheral sites and other lipoproteins. The cholesteryl ester (CE) core of HDL may then be transferred, in exchange for triglyceride, into less dense lipoproteins for excretion via the liver. This process is facilitated by cholesteryl ester transfer protein (CETP).

its proteins, which constitute about 50% of its mass and cover approximately 90% of its surface. They are responsible for its interaction with enzymes (apoAI is a cofactor for LCAT) and may govern its recognition by receptors on cell membranes. Added to the structural heterogeneity within HDL is the diversity that characterizes its proteins. Of particular interest are the isoforms of apoAI and apoE, which comprise six and three major variants respectively. The apoAI polymorphism arises largely from post-translational proteolytic cleavage of the protein (Brewer et al 1983). The nascent protein first appears within the cell in a prepro-form (Law et al 1983) with a 24 amino acid extension to its amino terminus. A peptide of 18 amino acids is cleaved within the cell to release a proprotein that is secreted into the circulation. There it undergoes slower proteolytic transformation to the mature protein, with release of the six amino acid propeptide. On average, this final step takes about 6 hours. Pro-apoAI is more basic than its mature product and is distinguishable by iso-electric focusing, even although it normally only represents 1–2% of the total apoAI mass. In patients who express the HDL defect known as Tangier disease, pro-apoAI constitutes a much larger proportion of total apoAI, a finding that initially led to the proposal (Zannis et al 1982) that the disease results from defective pro-apoAI maturation. However, kinetic studies have shown (Bojanovski et al 1984) that the rates of production and clearance of the proprotein are normal in this condition. Hypercatabolism of the mature form appears to be responsible for the relative increment in the mass of pro-apoAI in the circulation. ApoAII, the other main HDL protein, is also synthesised in prepro-form. However, both pre- and pro-peptides are cleaved intracellularly, and only the mature form is found in the plasma (Gordon et al 1983). We do not yet know if there is any link between apoA maturation and the formation of nascent or mature HDL.

Although apoE represents only a minor component of HDL, its presence on some of these particles may have a profound influence on their metabolic behaviour. Particles that contain the protein can be separated from the bulk of HDL by affinity chromatography (Weisgraber & Mahley 1980). They are larger than average and bind with high affinity both to the LDL (apoB/E) receptor and to the apoE receptor on hepatocytes. Thus, the presence of apoE on HDL particles opens up the possibility that they may selectively feed into catabolic pathways controlled by the activities of these two receptors. It has already been noted that apoE exists in several isoforms, the major representatives being E2, E3 and E4. These apoE phenotypes influence the amount of apoE associated with HDL, in that individuals with the E2 phenotype transport more of the protein in that density interval than do those with E4. One of two processes may contribute to this phenomenon: either the E2-containing particles may bind less efficiently to the receptor and therefore accumulate in the plasma (Rall et al 1983), or the E2 itself may form covalent disulphide bonds with apoAII, trapping the protein in HDL in a form that is a poor ligand for the receptor (Innerarity et al 1978). Indeed, the E-AII complex has been identified by Innerarity and his colleagues (1978) as a physiological mechanism for delaying the catabolism of apoE-containing particles.

Early analytical ultracentrifugation studies made it clear that HDL was not monodisperse (de Lalla et al 1954) but rather, existed as two or more populations that were originally designated HDL_1, HDL_2 and HDL_3. It transpired that HDL_1 actually represented a mixture, the main component of which was a variant of LDL, Lp(a). Of the other two; HDL_3 (d 1.125–1.210 g/ml) was major and HDL_2 (d 1.063–1.125 g/ml) minor in mass terms, but not in clinical significance. Further work in the Donner laboratory in Berkeley, California, resolved HDL into a number of subspecies (HDL_{2a}, HDL_{2b}, HDL_{3a}, HDL_{3b}, and HDL_{3c}) using gradient gel electrophoresis (Blanche et al 1981). The importance of each fraction is now the subject of intensive investigation. The polydiversity that exists in HDL is good evidence for the existence, within the size constraints of this fraction, of a limited number of thermodynamically stable, distinct entities. Moreover, we are now beginning to relate changes in metabolism to alterations in HDL size. In hypertriglyceridaemic individuals, for example, HDL is a small, dense particle that is relatively depleted in cholesteryl ester (Deckelbaum et al 1984). As noted above, it seems to be generated by transfer of a proportion of its core cholesteryl ester into the large mass of circulating VLDL in exchange for triglyceride. The action of hepatic lipase on this particle then causes it to shrink as triglyceride and phospholipid are hydrolysed from its core and coat respectively. At the opposite end of the spectrum, patients who suffer from abetalipoproteinaemia, have extremely low plasma triglyceride levels, and large circulating HDL, which is cholesteryl ester and apoE enriched (Deckelbaum et al 1982).

Normal individuals do not remotely approach either of the above extremes, although throughout the day they do exhibit cyclical variations in plasma triglyceride that impact on the distribution of HDL and, indirectly, on coronary heart disease risk. Patsch and his colleagues (1984) have found that individuals who possess an efficient chylomicron-clearing mechanism show only minor increments in the flotation rates and negligible changes in the masses of their plasma HDL subfractions following a fatty meal. In such patients, HDL_2 and HDL_3 become enriched in phospholipid, which is gradually lost, probably through the action of hepatic lipase, as the post-prandial lipaemia resolves. HDL probably acts in this situation as a single acceptor of chylomicron coat phospholipid, shed during hydrolysis of the triglyceride-rich particle. At the other end of the normal spectrum, exist individuals whose ability to clear chylomicrons is low. They show marked and prolonged lipaemia following a fatty meal. The increased residence time of triglyceride in their plasma facilitates its transfer into HDL in exchange for cholesteryl ester. Phospholipid is also transferred from the chylomicron to HDL during the lipolytic process (Schaefer et al 1982) so that these denser particles acquire both coat and core components. This results in an increase in their susceptibility to hydrolysis by hepatic lipase that leads to a shrinkage of the particles and an increase in their density. The magnitude of this change is so great that particles, which initially appeared in the HDL_2 density interval, now isolate as HDL_3 (Patsch et al 1984). Such individuals therefore present, even in the fasting state, with a lower HDL_2/HDL_3 ratio than is found in those whose lipolytic processes are efficient. Reduced HDL levels, and in particular low HDL_2/HDL_3 ratios have been equated with increased risk of coronary heart disease (Gofman et al 1966). It is possible that this finding is not of primary importance but is merely a reflection of the status of triglyceride-rich particle metabolism. Certainly, in our laboratory (Simpson et al 1990) we have found that individuals with angiographically proven coronary heart disease not only have lower HDL_2/HDL_3 ratios in their plasma but also suffer from a defect in their ability to clear chylomicrons from their bloodstream.

Lipoprotein (a) metabolism

Lipoprotein (a) (Lp(a)) was first described by Berg (1963), and its structure has since been defined by several groups. Lp(a) is very similar to LDL in its lipid complement and like LDL contains a single copy of apoB-100. In addition it possesses a large glycoprotein called apo(a) which is thought to be linked to the apoB-100 moiety by a single disulphide bridge. Apo(a) has been shown to have striking structural homology with plasminogen (McLean et al 1987) and varies in size from approximately 400 kDa to more than 800 kDa (Utermann et al 1987). Human apo(a), like plasminogen, consists of a protease-like sequence, linked to multiple repeat domains held together by three internal disulphide bridges to produce structures called kringles because of their apparent structural similarity to pretzels. Unlike plasminogen, apo(a) is extensively glycosylated and single copy of kringle 5 is linked to a variable number of kringle 4 repeats (Gavish et al 1989).

There is much less known about the metabolism of Lp(a) than the other lipoproteins but an excellent summary of present knowledge is provided by Mbewu & Durrington (1990). Lp(a) is probably secreted directly into the circulation and is not a product of intravascular delipidation like LDL. Apo (a) is thought to be primarily of hepatic origin but its metabolic fate is unknown.

In an attempt to reveal the determinants of plasma Lp(a) levels which vary widely between subjects, the genetic basis of the apo(a) size heterogeneity has been uncovered. Genotyping of apo(a) performed by pulsed field gel electrophoresis (Lackner et al 1991) has shown that the size of the apo(a) gene correlates directly with the size of the apo(a) protein and inversely with the Lp(a) plasma concentration. Segregation analysis of the apo(a) gene also revealed that, in normals, the Lp(a) plasma level was largely determined by alleles at the apo(a) gene locus.

A number of studies have demonstrated that Lp(a) is an independent risk factor for coronary heart disease. Most recently Rosengren et al (1990) found, in a prospective study of Swedish middle-aged men, that plasma Lp(a) level is an important determinant of risk of myocardial infarction. Wiklund et al (1990) have also reported that apo(a) may be useful in the identification of those FH heterozygotes who are particularly at risk of coronary heart disease. But, how does Lp(a) contribute to such risk? Because its structure links it with both lipoprotein and thrombotic risk factors two main lines of research have been pursued in an attempt to answer this question. There is autopsy (Rath et al 1989) and biopsy (Cushing et al 1989) evidence for the presence of Lp(a) in the intima of the artery wall. Within the intima Lp(a) is thought to be immobilized by binding extracellularly to glycosaminoglycans (Bihari-Varga et al 1988). There is immunological evidence for the presence of Lp(a) in foam cells (Niendorf et al 1990), which would suggest that these lipoproteins can be taken up by macrophages and contribute to foam cell conversion. Oxidative modification of Lp(a) which has recently been described (Sattler et al 1991) may render the lipoprotein a suitable substrate for macrophage scavenger receptor-mediated uptake. Sattler et al (1991) have also discovered that Lp(a) is much more resistant to in vitro oxidation than LDL, perhaps because of its higher *N*-acetylneuraminic acid content. This relative protection from oxidation may be overcome in part by the prolonged residence of Lp(a) in the intima where it remains bound and trapped, but may also account for the apparently low intracellular levels of Lp(a).

Thrombosis is an important prodromal event in myocardial infarction. Evidence to support this statement comes not only from postmortem evidence of occlusive thrombi in coronary arteries already narrowed by atheroma, but also from the beneficial effect of post-infarction thrombolytic therapy seen in the 2nd International Study of Infarct Survival (ISIS-2 1988). The other main explanation offered for the atherogenicity of Lp(a) centres on the possible link between this lipoprotein and fibrinolysis and thrombosis. Apo(a) has a high degree of structural homology with plasminogen and has been hailed as the missing link between atherosclerosis and thrombosis. The evidence to date, while supportive of this hypothesis, in no way corfirms it. The subject is reviewed by Miles & Plow (1990) who present evidence to suggest that Lp(a) inhibits fibrinolysis by competing for plasminogen-binding sites, which in turn leads to an increased liklihood of thrombosis. Fibrinolysis may also be influenced by Lp(a)'s effect on plasminogen activator inhibitor-1 (PAI-I). Etingin et al (1991) demonstrated in cultured endothelial cells that Lp(a) regulated the expression of PAI-1, and Edelberg et al (1991) suggest that Lp(a) may regulate fibrinolysis by competing with PAI-1 and plasminogen for fibrinogen or heparin-bound tissue-type plasminogen. The effects of Lp(a) on fibronectin have also been investigated. Ehnholm et al (1990) have shown that this protein is subject to proteolytic cleavage by apo(a). The importance of each of these findings in vivo is as yet unknown but this grey area between the fields of lipoproteins and thrombosis continues to attract extensive research.

Lp(a) is an intriguing particle that has given up few of its secrets despite three decades of research. One of the most fundamental questions which remains unanswered is its physiological role. A number of hypotheses have been put forward but one of the most unusual comes from Rath & Pauling (1990) who suggest, based on evolutionary data, that Lp(a) is a surrogate for ascorbic acid.

The LDL receptor and apoB metabolism

The discovery and characterization of the LDL receptor has become the paradigm of lipoprotein research and was the result of the efforts of Brown & Goldstein (1987). This molecule is a single transmembrane glycoprotein with its 839 amino acids arranged into five functional domains. The ligand binding domain is found in the 300 amino acid N-terminal segment, which consists of seven 40 amino acid repeat units, each of which is enriched in aspartate and glutamate residues arranged in a configuration that facilitates electrostatic interaction with complementary arginine and lysine residues found on two apolipoproteins, apoB and apoE (Mahley & Innerarity 1983). The receptor therefore recognizes and interacts with particles containing these proteins, but with different affinities since the E protein binds ten times more effectively than the B. In theory then, the whole spectrum within the VLDL-LDL interval, which contains these proteins is substrate for the LDL receptor. Early metabolic studies (Bilheimer et al 1979) focused on LDL since it was the lipoprotein recognised to be markedly increased in familial hypercholesterolaemia (FH). However, as knowledge develops it is becoming clearer that the impact of receptor deficiency is felt along the length of the VLDL delipidation cascade, suggesting that the LDL receptor has a wider role in apoB metabolism than its name suggests.

Tracer kinetic analysis following administration of ^{125}I-labelled LDL to humans has shown that approximately 30–40% of the entire LDL mass in the plasma is catabolized each day. Chemical modification of the tracer with agents such as 1,2-cyclohexanedione (Shepherd et al 1979), glucose (Kesaniemi et al 1983), or 2-hydroxylacetaldehyde (Slater et al 1984), which interact with arginine or lysine residues on its apoprotein moiety, reduces its clearance by 50–70%. Since this treatment blocks binding of the lipoprotein to the receptor, clearly receptor activity must make a major contribution to LDL turnover. The role of the receptor falls by half in those subjects with heterozygous FH and is abolished in homozygous individuals (Shepherd et al 1979). In consequence, more LDL is directed into alternative catabolic mechanisms that are mediated via the macrophage scavenger receptors (Matsumoto et al 1990).

We know from extensive experiments on cultured cells that the activity of LDL receptors is regulated by variation in the intracellular sterol pool. When the requirement for cholesterol is increased, receptor synthesis is stimulated and LDL uptake promoted. Conversely, in times of surfeit, receptor expression is diminished and LDL assimilation suppressed. Extrapolation of these concepts to man has enlightened our understanding of the regulation of LDL metabolism and provided an explanation for the actions of a number of cholesterol-lowering drugs. Bile acid sequestrant resins such as cholestyramine promote faecal steroid excretion and in consequence deplete the liver of cholesterol. The organ responds both by up-regulating synthesis of the sterol from acetate and by increasing the number of LDL receptors on hepatocyte membranes. The latter of course produces the desired pharmacological action of the drug by promoting receptor-mediated clearance of LDL from the circulation (Shepherd et al 1980). A similar end result is also achieved by inhibition of cholesterologenesis in the liver using the new competitive inhibitors of HMG CoA reductase (Bilheimer et al 1983). It follows that co-administration of reductase inhibitors and sequestrant resins should have additive actions on LDL receptor activity in the liver; and indeed through this mechanism such combination therapy is capable of lowering circulating LDL by half. Moreover, these agents are so potent that they can even normalize LDL metabolism and plasma lipoprotein levels in individuals who are heterozygous for FH. They have no effect, however, on FH homozygotes who completely lack functional LDL receptors (Uauy et al 1988).

As indicated earlier, theoretical considerations suggest that we ought to expect the LDL receptor to be implicated in the metabolism of VLDL and IDL. In 1982 Soutar and her colleagues discovered that IDL clearance is retarded in FH. We have re-examined this problem in detail using cumulative flotation ultracentrifugation to follow the flux of apoB from VLDL through IDL to LDL (James et al 1989). FH homozygotes accumulate cholesterol-rich remnants within their VLDL density interval because they lack the capacity to clear them normally. IDL catabolism is also perturbed to such an extent that its pool size increases as much as that of LDL, the level of which rises 3.5 fold in the plasma. Absence of the LDL receptor therefore, has a profound impact on apoB metabolism in its entirety. But, what of its role in normolipaemic subjects? This question may be addressed by following the approach outlined earlier that relies on modification of the ligand to affect its receptor binding. Treatment of large, triglyceride-rich VLDL (Packard et al 1985) has no effect on its direct clearance from the plasma or its conversion to IDL. However, subsequent catabolism of apoB-containing particles is significantly retarded. Additional evidence supporting the view that LDL receptors participate in VLDL remnant and IDL clearance comes from clinical observation of patients with dysbetalipoproteinaemia. This condition is accompanied by high circulating levels of both these lipoprotein fractions due to their inability to bind efficiently to hepatic lipoprotein receptors. Up-regulation of the LDL receptor with an HMG CoA reductase inhibitor lowers the concentration of VLDL remnants and IDL in the plasma of these patients (Vega et al 1988).

Familial hypercholesterolaemia, the autosomal codominant trait that occurs in its heterozygous form in one in 500 of the population is associated with high levels of LDL cholesterol in the plasma and premature coronary heart disease and is known to arise because of a defect in the LDL receptor. Since its discovery more than 150 different mutations of the LDL receptor have been described (Hobbs et al 1990) which are responsible for FH. The many deletions, insertions and base pair substitutions within the LDL receptor gene can have profound effects on LDL catabolism. Recent observations suggest that similar and equally deleterious effects may result from defects in its primary ligand, apoB-100. This is most commonly seen in a condition called familial defective apoB-100 which is due to a mutation at a CG dinucleotide in residue 3500 of the apoB gene and is present again at a level of approximately 1 in 500 of the population (Innerarity et al 1990). Such changes in apoB sequence appear to be of real clinical significance and further mutations are currently being sought.

The HDL receptor and reverse cholesterol transport

From the discovery that plasma HDL levels are associated with protection from coronary heart disease (reviewed by Gordon et al 1989) came the concept that this lipoprotein acts as a vehicle to transport sterol from peripheral tissues to the liver. The necessity for such a mechanism is unquestionable since the perhydrocyclopentanophenanthrene nucleus of cholesterol cannot be catabolized to any significant extent in animals and must therefore be excreted intact via its major organ of elimination, the liver. HDL has the capacity to acquire cholesterol from cells in vitro as an initial step in the 'reverse cholesterol transport pathway' advocated by Glomset (1968).

The precise mechanism responsible for uptake is, however, currently hotly disputed. It is generally accepted that the free sterol rather than its esters participates in the transfer process. Whether this occurs during cell-lipoprotein collisions, as a result of passive diffusion, or through capture and release of HDL by cells, is not clear. The binding process would require the specificity inherent in a receptor protein, and there have been several publications claiming the detection of proteins that appear to meet this requirement. If such a mechanism exists, the binding site should be saturable and subject to regulation, on the basis, for example, of cell cholesterol content. Biesbroecke and his colleagues (1983) have evidence to suggest that the interaction of HDL with fibroblasts displays these characteristics and promotes cholesterol release from cells. Binding can be inhibited by alteration of the tyrosyl residues of the HDL protein with tetranitromethane (Tabas & Tall 1984, Chacko 1985) but is unaffected by arginine and lysine modification. The binding process seems specific for HDL proteins. LDL fails to compete, while liposomes containing apoAl, the major protein in HDL, bind with high affinity. Recently, Tozuka & Fidge (1989) have confirmed the presence of cell surface proteins that bind both HDL proteins, AI and AII. Furthermore, theme workers report that HDL_3 is the principal ligand for these receptors and that LDL was unable to compete. The removal of cholesterol from peripheral cells may also occur via an elegant internalization process involving the whole HDL particle. Postulated by Alam et al (1989), this process results in the intracellular remodelling of HDL, which increases its size and apoE content, after which the particle emerges from the cell by a process of 'retroendocytosis'. Against the receptor concept, however, is the evidence that limited proteolysis of either the lipoprotein or the cell membrane surface fails to inhibit binding. Nevertheless, data from two sources suggest that the binding process is regulated by the free cholesterol content of the cell and may be modulated by mitogens such as platelet-derived growth factor (Oppenheimer et al 1987), which was shown to decrease both HDL binding and cholesterol efflux.

A fascinating new development in this field is offered by Milda et al (1990) who offer supportive evidence for an hypothesis that the functional heterogeneity of HDL encompasses the ability of this lipoprotein to process cholesterol from peripheral cells and other plasma lipoproteins independently. This further refinement in our understanding of HDL metabolism only serves to remind us of how much we have still to learn.

The ApoE receptor and chylomicron metabolism

Dietary lipids are packaged within the enterocytes of the small intestine into large triglyceride-rich chylomicron particles that contain approximately 1–2% protein. This consists primarily of apoAI, apoAII, apoAIV and apoB-48. This shortened B protein lacks the LDL receptor-binding site, and the chylomicron must acquire an alternative receptor-binding ligand before it can be taken up by the liver (Chen et al 1987). This occurs soon after the particle enters the circulation as a result of transfer of apoE, principally from HDL. Lipolysis of the triglyceride core of the chylomicron in the capillary beds of skeletal muscle and adipose tissue generates a relatively cholesterol-enriched remnant which is purported to be atherogenic since it is able to produce cholesteryl ester deposition in macrophages. In teleological terms, there is biological benefit in clearing these remnants as quickly as possible from the bloodstream. This function is performed by the liver, which has a highly efficient uptake mechanism capable of clearing the blood of these remnants in a single pass. The LDL receptor could, in theory, participate in this process but is unlikely to do so since chylomicron remnant metabolism is not compromised in homozygous FH subjects (Rubinsztein et al 1990). The most promising putative chylomicron-remnant receptor (also called the apoE receptor) is the LDL receptor-related protein (LRP) (Herz et al 1988). LRP is a cell surface protein which is much larger than the LDL receptor but is structurally homologous, comprising the elements of four LDL receptors. LRP has been shown to be an apoE-binding protein (Beisiegel et al 1989) and to mediate the uptake of cholesteryl esters derived from apoE-enriched lipoproteins in vitro (Kowal et al 1989). One of the most intriguing aspects of this newly defined protein is the observation that it acts as a receptor for the plasma protein α_2-macroglobulin (Strickland et al 1990). If LRP does have two apparently unrelated ligands, apoE and α_2-macroglobulin, we are faced with some difficult problems. What will the primary function of this protein be in vivo, how may its expression be manipulated, and how could such a double receptor protein evolve? Some attempt to shed light on these important questions is made by Brown et al (1991) but they conclude that much more work has to be done before we will be in a position to accept the LRP as the definitive chylomicron remnant receptor which has been sought for so long.

MODIFIED LIPOPROTEINS AND ATHEROSCLEROSIS

Detailed electron microscopic studies have shown that in cholesterol-fed non-human primates the earliest prodromal sign of a developing atherosclerotic plaque is focal infiltration of the subendothelial space of the arterial wall by cells of the monocyte/macrophage series. When examined in culture, these cells are able to assimilate and deposit cholesteryl esters in intracellular lipid inclusions (Brown & Goldstein 1983). The source of this sterol has been the topic of a large body of research. Plasma LDL, the most abundant sterol transporter, does not generate these deposits. However, modified LDL particles extracted from the aorta (Hoff & Morton 1987) have this ability. They differ from the normal lipoprotein by being more electronegative, like the artificially-produced acetyl LDL which is avidly assimilated and deposited in macrophages (Goldstein et al 1979). Indeed, these cells exhibit on their membranes, proteins which facilitate the rapid unregulated uptake of acetyl LDL to the extent of generating foam cells reminiscent of those found in the atherosclerotic lesion. Because a wide variety of negatively charged compounds could compete with acetyl-LDL for these receptors they have become known as scavenger receptors (Brown et al 1980). Clearly, the physiological ligand for these receptors is not acetyl LDL, nor are they present to facilitate the production of foam cells. Steinberg et al (1989) have found that charge-modified lipoproteins in the form of oxidized LDL compete with acetyl-LDL and cause foam cell conversion. They concluded that modified lipoproteins may be the in vivo ligand for these scavenger receptors. A number of observations support the hypothesis that oxidized LDL is important in the development of atheromatous plaques. Firstly, there is immunological evidence for the presence of oxidized LDL in atheromatous lesions and even in human fatty streaks (Haberland et al 1988, Yla-Herttuala et al 1989, 1991). Secondly, LDL isolated from atherosclerotic plaques (Goldstein et al 1981, Yla-Herttuala et al 1989) is electronegative and produces foam cell transformation in vitro. Thirdly, Carew et al (1987) have attributed the protective action of the drug, probucol, to its ability to scavenge free radicals and limit the rate of LDL oxidation, rather than to its lipid-lowering properties. When the drug was administered to Watanabe rabbits, LDL uptake into atherosclerotic lesions fell by 65% while a comparative group given alternative lipid-lowering drugs showed no improvement.

The mechanism for the modification of LDL in vivo is speculative. Evidence from tissue culture work (Steinbrecher et al 1984, Henricksen et al 1987) suggests that endothelial cells or even macrophages themselves, through their ability to generate superoxide radicals, may initiate oxidative damage to the lipoprotein's lipid and protein moieties. This could obviously occur exclusively within the artery wall, accounting for the inability to detect the damaged or modified lipoproteins in the plasma.

There is evidence to suggest that multiple scavenger receptors must exist on the macrophage membrane (Sparrow et al 1989) and it is now known that these cells express at least two types of scavenger receptor protein which have been isolated and cloned (Kodama et al 1990, Rohrer et al 1990). Both human type I and type II scavenger receptors have been localized on foam cells in atheromatous plaques (Matsumoto et al 1990). The presence of macrophage scavenger receptor mRNA in atherosclerotic lesions with little associated LDL receptor mRNA (Yla-Herttuala et al 1991) further points to a key role for these scavenger receptors in the uptake of cholesterol and conversion of macrophages to foam cells.

The effects of oxidized lipoproteins on vascular tone is another important area (reviewed by Henry & Bucay 1991) where lipoproteins have been shown to have effects on the cardiovascular system additional to their long-recognized role in atherogenesis. Oxidized LDL has been found to impair arterial relaxation in vitro in response to agents that act by stimulating the release of endothelium-dependent relaxing factor (EDRF) from endothelial cells. Clinical reports (Vita et al 1990, Zeiher et al 1991) have further raised interest in this area by indicating that hypercholesterolaemia may be associated with a decreased responsiveness to endothelium-dependent vasodilators (e.g. acetylcholine). This defect, it is suggested, may seriously limit vasodilatory reserve and contribute in part to myocardial ischaemia in such patients. Such a vasomotor syndrome resulting from hypercholesterolaemia resembles the in vitro observations which have been explained by the presence of oxidized LDL. This work is still at an early stage but clearly, if confirmed, will have profound implications for clinical management.

Oxidative modification of LDL has also been postulated as one of the very first steps in the development of the fatty streak. Mild oxidation of LDL particles, resulting in so-called, minimally-modified LDL (MM-LDL), gives rise to a lipoprotein that is not chemotactic in itself but stimulates the release of monocyte chemotactic protein-1 (Berliner et al 1990, Cushing et al 1990). Moreover, MM-LDL has also been shown to promote endothelial-monocyte binding, an important step in early atherosclerotic plaque formation. A further putative link between lipoproteins and the thrombotic system has been put forward by Drake et al (1991) who showed that MM-LDL when cultured with human endothelial cells induces the expression of tissue factor (tissue thromboplastin) which may be involved in platelet adhesion.

CONCLUSIONS

Our current ability to modulate the lipoprotein levels in the plasma and influence the coronary heart disease risk of an individual is a reflection of the continued efforts in this field the past twenty-five years. Ongoing studies of lipoprotein metabolism will, it is hoped, shed new light on the underlying pathophysiology of atherosclerosis and in turn offer the clinician the potential of new therapeutic options.

Acknowledgements

Portions of this work were carried out under the tenure of British Heart Foundation Grants (Nos 87/101, 87/6, 89/107) and the Scottish Hospital Endowments Research Trust 908.

REFERENCES

Alam R, Yatsu F M, Tsui L, Alam S 1989 Receptor-mediated uptake and 'retroendocytosis' of high-density lipoproteins by cholesterol-loaded human monocyte-derived macrophages: possible role in enhancing reverse cholesterol transport. Biochimica et Biophysica Acta 1004: 292–299

Angelin B, Bjorkheim I, Einarsson K 1986 Cholesterol 7a hydroxylase and bile acid synthesis in relation to triglyceride and lipoprotein metabolism. In: Fears R, Sabine J R (eds) Cholesterol 7a hydroxylase. CRC Press, Boca Raton, Fl p 167–177

Anitschkow N N 1915 New data on the question of pathology and aetiology of atherosclerosis (arteriosclerosis) (Rus). Russian Physician 8: 184–186

Anitschkow N 1913 Uber die Veranderungen der Kaninchenaorta bei experimenteller Cholesterinsteatose. Beitrage zur pathologisten Anatomie und zur allgemeinen Pathologie 56: 379–404

Aschoff L 1924 Lectures on Pathology. Hoeber, New York

Barter P J, Nestel P J, Carroll K F 1972 Precursors of plasma triglyceride fatty acids in humans. Effect of glucose consumption, clofibrate administration and alcoholic fatty liver. Metabolism 21: 117–124

Behr S R, Patsch J R, Forte T, Bensadoun A 1981 Plasma lipoprotein changes resulting from immunologically blocked lipolysis. Journal of Lipid Research 22: 443–451

Beisiegel U, Weber W, Ihrke G, Herz J, Stanley K K 1989 The LDL-receptor related protein, LRP, is an apolipoprotein E-binding protein. Nature 341: 162–164

Berg K 1963 A new serum system in man- the Lp system. Acta Pathologica et Microbiologica Scandinavica 59: 369–382

Berliner J A, Territo M C, Sevanian A et al 1990 Minimally modified low density lipoprotein stimulates monocyte endothelial interactions. Journal of Clinical Investigation 85: 1260–1266

Berman M, Hall M, Levy R I et al 1978 Metabolism of apoB and apoC lipoproteins in man: kinetic studies in normal and hyperlipoproteinemic subjects. Journal of Lipid Research 19: 38–56

Biesbroecke R, Oram J F, Albers J J, Bierman E L 1983 Specific high affinity binding of HDL to cultured human skin fibroblasts and arterial smooth muscle cells. Journal of Clinical Investigation 71: 525–539

Bihari-Varga M, Gruber E, Rotheneder M, Zechner R, Kostner G 1988 Interaction of lipoprotein Lp (a) and low density lipoprotein with glycosaminoglycans from human aorta. Arteriosclerosis 8: 851–857

Bilheimer D W, Stone N J, Grundy S M 1979 Metabolic studies in familial hypercholesterolemia. Journal of Clinical Investigation 64: 524–533

Bilheimer, D W, Grundy S M, Brown M S, Goldstein J L 1983 Mevinolin and colestipol stimulate receptor-mediated clearance of low density lipoprotein from plasma in familial hypercholesterolemia heterozygotes. Proceedings of the National Academy of Sciences, USA 80: 4124–4128

Blanche P J, Gong E L, Forte T M, Nichols A V 1981 Characterization of human low density lipoproteins by gradient gel electrophoresis. Biochemica et Biophysica Acta 665: 408–419

Blum C B 1982 Dynamics of apolipoprotein E metabolism in humans. Journal of Lipid Research 23: 1308–1316

Bojanovski D, Gregg R E, Brewer H B 1984 In vitro conversion of pro apo $AI_{Tangier}$ to mature apo $AI_{Tangier}$. Journal of Biological Chemistry 259: 6049–6051

Brewer H B, Fairwell T, Kay L et al 1983 Human plasma pro apo AI: isolation and amino terminal sequence. Biochemical and Biophysical Research Communications 113: 626–632

Brown M S, Goldstein J L 1983 Lipoprotein metabolism in the macrophage. Annual Reviews of Biochemistry 52: 223–261
Brown M S, Goldstein J L 1987 The LDL receptor. In: Gallo L L (ed) Cardiovascular disease. Plenum Press, New York, p 87–91
Brown M S, Basu S K, Falck J R, Ho Y K, Goldstein J L 1980 The scavenger cell pathway for lipoprotein degradation: specificity of the binding site that mediates the uptake of negatively-charged LDL by macrophages. Journal of Supramolecular Structures 13: 67–81
Brown M S, Herz J, Kowal R C, Goldstein J L 1991 The low-density lipoprotein receptor-related protein: double agent or decoy? Current Opinion in Lipidology 2: 65–72
Carew T E, Schwenke D C, Steinberg D 1987 Antiatherogenic effect of probucol unrelated to its hypocholesterolemic effect: evidence that antioxidants in vivo can selectively inhibit low density lipoprotein degradation in macrophage-rich fatty streaks and slow the progression of atherosclerosis in the Watanabe heritable hyperlipidemic rabbit. Proceedings of the National Academy of Sciences, USA 84: 7725–7729
Carlsson P, Olofsson S O, Bondjers G, Darnfoss C, Wilklund O, Bjursell G 1985 Molecular cloning of human apolipoprotein B cDNA. Nucleic Acids Research 13: 8813–8826
Carlson L A, Holmqvist L, Nilsson-Ehle P 1986 Deficiency of hepatic lipase activity in post heparin plasma in familial hyperalphatriglyceridemia. Acta Medica Scandinavica 219: 435–447
Chacko G K 1985 Modification of human high density lipoprotein (HDL_3) with tetranitromethane and the effect on its binding to isolated rat liver plasma membranes. Journal of Lipid Research 26: 745–754
Chan L, van Tuinen P, Ledbetter D H, Daijer S P, Gotto A M, Chen S H 1985 The human apolipoprotein B-100 gene: a highly polymorphic gene that maps to the short arm of chromosome 2. Biochemistry and Biophysics Research Communications 133: 248–255
Chen S H, Habib G, Young C et al 1987 Apolipoprotein B48 is the product of a messenger RNA with an organ specific in-frame stop codon. Science 238: 363–366
Cheung M C, Brown B G, Wolf A C, Albers J J 1991 Altered particle size distribution of apolipoprotein A-I-containing lipoproteins in subjects with coronary artery disease. Journal of Lipid Research 32: 383–394
Cushing G L, Gaubatz J W, Nava M L et al 1989 Quantitation and localization of apolipoprotein (a) and B in coronary artery bypass vein grafts resected at re-operation. Arteriosclerosis 9: 593–603
Cushing S D, Berliner J A, Valente A J et al 1990 Minimally modified low density lipoprotein induces monocyte chemotactic protein 1 in human endothelial cells and smooth muscle cells. Proceedings of the National Academy of Sciences, USA 87: 5134–5138
Danielson H, Sjovall J 1975 Bile acid metabolism. Annual Reviews of Biochemistry 44: 233–253
Deckelbaum R J, Eisenberg S, Oschry Y, Cooper M, Blum C 1982 Abnormal high density lipoproteins of abetalipoproteinemia: relevance to normal HDL metabolism. Journal of Lipid Research 23: 1274–1282
Deckelbaum R J, Olivecrona T, Eisenberg S 1984 Plasma lipoproteins in hyperlipidemia: roles of neutral lipid exchange and lipase. In: Carlson L A, Olsson A G (eds) Treatment of hyperlipoproteinemia. Raven Press, New York, p 85–93
de Lalla O F, Elliott H A, Gofman J W 1954 Ultracentrifugal studies of high density serum lipoproteins in clinically healthy adults. American Journal of Physiology 179: 333–337
Demant T, Carlson L A, Holmquist L, Karpe F, Nilsson-Ehle P, Packard C J, Shepherd J 1988 Lipoprotein metabolism in hepatic lipase deficiency: studies on the turnover of apolipoprotein B and on the effect of hepatic lipase on high density lipoprotein. Journal of Lipid Research. 29: 1603–1611
Dietschy J M, Wilson J D 1970 Regulation of cholesterol metabolism. New England Journal of Medicine 282: 1128–1138
Dory L, Sloop C H, Boquet L M, Hamilton R L, Roheim P S 1983 Lecithin: cholesterol acyltransferase mediated modification of discoidalperipheral lymph high density lipoproteins. Proceedings of the National Academy of Sciences, USA 80: 3489–3493
Dory L, Boquet L M, Hamilton R L, Sloop C H, Roheim P S 1985 Heterogeneity of dog intestinal fluid (peripheral lymph) high density lipoproteins: implications for a role in reverse cholesterol transport. Journal of Lipid Research. 26: 519–527
Drake T A, Kannani K, Fei H, Lavi S, Berliner J A 1991 Minimally oxidized low-density lipoprotein induces tissue factor expression in cultured human endothelial cells. American Journal of Pathology 138: 601–607
Edelberg J M, Reilly C F, Pizzo S V 1991 The inhibition of tissue type plasminogen activator by plasminogen activator inhibitor-1. The effects of fibrinogen, heparin, vitronectin and lipoprotein (a). Journal of Biological Chemistry 266: 7488–7493
Ehnholm C, Jauhiainen M, Metso J 1990 Interaction of lipoprotein (a) with fibronectin and its potential role in atherogenesis. European Heart Journal 11 (suppl E): 190–195
Eisenberg S 1985 Preferential enrichment of large-sized very low density lipoprotein populations with transferred cholesteryl esters. Journal of Lipid Research 26: 487–494
Etingin O R, Hajjar D P, Hajjar K A, Harpel P C, Nachman R L 1991 Lipoprotein (a) regulates plasminogen activator inhibitor-1 expression in endothelial cells. A potential mechanism in thrombogenesis. Journal of Biological Chemistry 266: 2459–2465
Eto M, Miyata O, Noda K, Makino I 1990 A family of homozygous familial hyperalphalipoproteinemia with complete deficiency of cholesterol ester transfer activity. Artery 4: 202–212
Frick M H, Elo O, Haapa K et al 1987 Helsinki Heart Study: Primary-prevention trial with gemfibrozil in middle-aged men with dyslipidemia. New England Journal of Medicine 317: 1237–1245
Gavish D, Azrolan N, Breslow J L 1989 Plasma Lp(a) concentration is inversely correlated with ratio of kringle IV/kringle V encoding domains in the apo(a) gene. Journal of Clinical Investigation 84: 2021–2027
Ginsberg H N, Le N A, Goldberg I J R, Brown W V 1986 Apolipoprotein B metabolism in subjects with deficiency of apolipoproteins CIII and AI. Journal of Clinical Investigation 78: 1287–1295
Glomset J A 1968 The plasma lecithin: cholesterol acyltransferase reaction. Journal of Lipid Research 9: 155–164
Gofman J W, Jones H B, Lindgren F T, Lyon T P, Elliott H A, Strisower B 1950 Blood lipids and human atherosclerosis. Circulation 2: 161–177
Gofman J W, Young W, Tandy R 1966 Ischemic heart disease, atherosclerosis and longevity. Circulation 34: 679–697
Goh E H, Heimberg M 1979 Relationship between the activity of hepatic 3-hydroxyl-3-methylglutaryl coenzyme A reductase and secretion of very low density lipoprotein cholesterol in the isolated perfused liver and in the intact rat. Biochemical Journal 184: 1–6
Goldberg I J, Le N A, Paterniti J R, Ginsberg H N, Lindgren F T, Brown W V 1982 Lipoprotein metabolism during acute inhibition of hepatic triglyceride lipase in the cynomolgus monkey. Journal of Clinical Investigation 70: 1184–1192
Goldstein J L, Brown M S 1984 Progress in understanding the LDL receptor and HMG CoA reductase, two membrane proteins that regulate the plasma cholesterol. Journal of Lipid Research 25: 1450–1461
Goldstein J L, Ho Y K, Basu S K, Brown M S 1979 Binding site on macrophages that mediates uptake and degradation of acetylated low density lipoprotein, producing massive cholesterol deposition. Proceedings of the National Academy of Sciences, USA 76: 333–337
Goldstein J L, Hoff H F, Basu S K, Brown M S 1981 Stimulation of cholesteryl etser synthesis in macrophages by extracts of atherosclerotic human aortas and complexes of albumin/cholesteryl esters. Atherosclerosis 1: 210–216
Gordon J I, Budelier K A, Suus H F, Edelstein C, Scanu A M, Strauss A W 1983 Biosynthesis of human preproapolipoprotein AII. Journal of Biological Chemistry 25: 14054–14059
Gordon D J, Probstfield J L, Garrison R J et al 1989 High-density lipoprotein cholesterol and cardiovascular disease. Four prospective American studies. Circulation 79: 8–15
Green P H R, Glickman R M 1981 Intestinal lipoprotein metabolism. Journal of Lipid Research 22: 1153–1173
Green P H R, Tall A R, Glickman R M 1978 Rat intestine secretes discoidal high density lipoprotein. Journal of Clinical Investigation 61: 528–534
Green P H R, Glickman R M, Sandel C D, Blum C B, Tall A R 1979 Human intestinal lipoproteins: studies in chyluric subjects. Journal of Clinical Investigation 64: 233–242

Gregg R E, Zech L A, Schaefer E J, Brewer H B 1981 Type III hyperlipoproteinemia: defective metabolism of an abnormal apolipoprotein E. Science 221: 584–588
Haberland M E, Fong D, Cheng L 1988 Malondialdehyde-altered protein occurs in atheroma of Watanabe Heritable Hyperlipidemic rabbits. Science 241: 215–218
Hamilton R L, Williams M C, Fielding C J, Havel R J 1976 Discoidal bilayer structure of nascent high density lipoproteins from perfused rat liver. Journal of Clinical Investigation 58: 667–680
Hamilton R L 1983 Hepatic secretion of nascent plasma lipoproteins. In: Glauman H, Peters T, Redman C (eds) Plasma protein secretion by the liver. Academic Press, London, p 357–374
Havel R J, Kane J P, Kashyap M L 1973 Interchange of apolipoproteins between chylomicrons and high density lipoproteins during alimentary lipemia in man. Journal of Clinical Investigation 52: 32–38
Henricksen T, Mahoney E M, Steinberg D 1987 Enhanced macrophage delipidation of LDL previously incubated with cultured endothelial cells. Proceedings of the National Academy of Science, USA 78: 6499–6503
Henry P D, Bucay M 1991 Effects of low-density lipoproetins and hypercholesterolemia on endothelium-dependent vasodilation. Current Opinion in Lipidology 2: 306–310
Herz J, Hamann U, Rogne S, Myklebost O, Gausepohl H, Stanley K K 1988 Surface location and high affinity for calcium of a 500 kD liver membrane protein closely related to the LDL-receptor suggest a physiological role as lipoprotein receptor. European Molecular Biology Organisation Journal 7: 4119–4127
Hobbs H H, Russell D W, Brown M S, Goldstein J L 1990 The LDL receptor locus in familial hypercholesterolemia — mutational analysis of a membrane protein. Annual Review of Genetics 24: 133–170
Hoff H F, Morton R E 1987 Uptake of LDL sized particles extracted from human aortic lesions by macrophages in culture. In: Gallo L L (ed) Cardiovascular disease. Plenum Press, New York, p 87–91
Imaizumi K, Fainaru M, Havel R J 1978 Composition of proteins of mesenteric lymph chylomicrons in the rat and alterations produced upon exposure to blood serum and serum proteins. Journal of Lipid Research 19: 712–722
Innerarity T L, Mahley R W, Weisgraber K H, Bersot T P 1978 Apolipoprotein (E-AII) complex of human plasma lipoproteins. Journal of Biological Chemistry 253: 6289–6295
Innerarity T L, Mahley R W, Weisgraber K H et al 1990 Familial defective apolipoprotein B-100: a mutation of apolipoprotein B that causes hypercholesterolemia. Journal of Lipid Research 31: 1337–1349
ISIS-2 (Second International Study of Infarct of Survival) Collaborative Group 1988 Randomised trial of intravenous streptokinase, oral aspirin, both, or neither among 17 187 cases of suspected acute myocardial infarction: ISIS-2. Lancet ii: 349–360
Isles C G, Hole D J 1991 Changing trends in vascular disease: coronary heart disease risk factors today. In: Lorimer A R, Shepherd J (eds) Preventive cardiology. Blackwell Scientific, Oxford, p 1–29
James R W, Martin B, Pometta D et al 1989 Apolipoprotein B metabolism in homozygous familial hypercholesterolemia. Journal of Lipid Research 30: 159–169
Janus E D, Nicoll A M, Turner P R, Magill P, Lewis B 1980 Kinetic bases of the primary hyperlipidaemias: studies of apolipoprotein B turnover in genetically defined subjects. European Journal of Clinical Investigation 10: 161–172
Kane J P, Hardman D A, Paulus H E 1980 Heterogeneity of apolipoprotein B: isolation of a new species from human chylomicrons. Proceedings of the National Academy of Sciences, USA 77: 2465–2469
Kane J P, Havel R J 1989 Disorders of the biogenesis and secretion of lipoproteins containing the B apolipoproteins. In: Scriver et al (eds) The metabolic basis of inherited disease. McGraw-Hill, New York, vol 1: p 1139–1164
Kesaniemi Y A, Witztum J L, Steinbrecher U P 1983 Receptor mediated catabolism of LDL in man. Journal of Clinical Investigation 71: 950–959
Kodama T, Freeman M, Rohrer L, Zabrecky J, Matsudaira P, Krieger M 1990 Macrophage scavenger receptor contains a-helical and collagen-like coiled coils. Nature 343: 531–535
Kowal R C, Herz J, Goldstein J L, Esser V, Brown M S 1989 Low density lipoprotein receptor-related protein mediates uptake of cholesteryl esters derived from apoprotein E-enriched lipoproteins. Proceedings of the National Academy of Sciences, USA 86: 5810–5814
Knott T J, Rall S C, Innerarity T L et al 1985 Human apolipoprotein B: structure of carboxy-terminal domains, sites of gene expression and chromosomal localization. Science 230: 37–43
Krebs E G, Beavo J A 1979 Phosphorylation–dephosphorylation of enzymes. Annual Reviews in Biochemistry 48: 923–959
Lackner C, Boerwinkle E, Leffert C C, Rahmig T, Hobbs H H 1991 Molecular basis of apolipoprotein (a) isoform size heterogeneity as revealed by pulsed-field gel electrophoresis. Journal of Clinical Investigation 87: 2153–2161
Law S W, Gray G, Brewer H B 1983 cDNA cloning of human Apo AI: amino acid sequence of preproapo AI. Biochemical and Biophysics Research Communications 112: 257–264
Levy E, Rochette C, Londono I et al 1990 Apolipoprotein B-100: immunolocalization and synthesis in human intestinal mucosa. Journal of Lipid Research 31: 1937–1946
Lipid Research Clinics Program 1984a The Lipid Research Clinics Coronary Primary Prevention Trial results. II. Reduction in incidence of coronary heart disease. Journal of the American Medical Association 251: 351–364
Lipid Research Clinics Program 1984b The Lipid Research Clinics Coronary Primary Prevention Trial results. II. The relationship of reduction in incidence of coronary heart disease to cholesterol lowering. Journal of the American Medical Association 251: 365–374
McLean J W, Tomlinson J E, Kuang W J et al 1987 cDNA sequence of human apolipoproetin (a) is homologous to plasminogen. Nature 300: 132–137
Mahley R W, Innerarity T L 1983 Lipoprotein receptors and cholesterol homeostasis. Biochemica et Biophysica Acta 737: 197–222
Matsumoto A, Naito M, Itakura H et al 1990 Human macrophage scavenger receptors- primary structure, expression and localization in atherosclerotic lesions. Proceedings of the National Academy of Sciences, USA 87: 9133–9137
Mbewu A D, Durrington P N 1990 Lipoprotein (a): structure, properties and possible involvement in thrombogenesis and atherogenesis. Atherosclerosis 85: 1–14
Milda T, Fielding C J, Fielding P E 1990 Mechanism of transfer of LDL-derived free cholesterol to HDL subfractions in human plasma. Biochemistry 29: 10469–10474
Miles L A, Plow E F 1990 Lp(a): an interloper into the fibrinolytic system. Thrombosis and Haemostasis 63: 331–335
Mills G L, Lane P A, Weech P K 1984 The isolation and purification of plasma lipoproteins In: Burdon R H, van Knippenberg P H (eds) Laboratory techniques in biochemistry and molecular biology vol 14: A guidebook to lipoprotein technique. Elsevier, Amsterdam, p 18–116
Mjos O D, Faergeman O, Hamilton R L, Havel R J 1975 Characterization of remnants produced during the metabolism of triglyceride-rich lipoproteins of blood plasma and intestinal lymph in the rat. Journal of Clinical Investigation 56: 603–615
Myant N B, Mitropoulos K A 1977 Cholesterol 7α hydroxlase. Journal of Lipid Research 18: 135–153
Nicoll A, Lewis B 1980 Evaluation of the roles of lipoprotein lipase and hepatic lipase in lipoprotein metabolism: in vivo and in vitro studies in man. European Journal of Clinical Investigation 10: 487–495
Niendorf A, Rath M, Wolf K et al 1990 Morphological detection and quantification of lipoprotein(a) deposition in atheromatous lesions. Virchows Archiv A, Pathologie Anatomie 417: 105–111
Nilsson-Ehle P, Garfunkel A S, Schotz M C 1980 Lipolytic enzymes and plasma lipoprotein metabolism. Annual Reviews of Biochemistry 49: 667–693
Norum K R 1984 Familial lecithin: cholesterol acyltransferase deficiency. In: Miller N E, Miller G J (eds) Clinical and metabolic aspects of high density lipoproteins. Elsevier, Amsterdam, p 297–318
Norum K R, Berg T, Helgerud P, Drevon C A 1983 Transport of cholesterol. Physiological Reviews 63: 1343–1397
Oppenheimer M J, Oram J F, Bierman E L 1987 Downregulation of HDL receptor activity of cultured fibroblasts by PDGF. Arteriosclerosis 7: 325–332
Packard C J, Munro A, Lorimer A R, Gotto A M Shepherd J 1984

Metabolism of apolipoprotein B in large triglyceride-rich very low density lipoproteins of normal and hypertriglyceridemic subjects. Journal of Clinical Investigation 74: 2178–2192
Packard C J, Boag D E, Clegg R J, Bedford D, Shepherd J 1985 Effects of 1,2 cyclohexanedione modification on the metabolism of VLDL apolipoprotein B. Journal of Lipid Research 26: 1058–1067
Packard C J, Shepherd J 1986 Cholesterol 7α hydroxylase: involvement in hepatobiliary axis and regulation of plasma lipoprotein levels. In: Fears R, Sabine J R (eds) Cholesterol 7α hydroxylase. CRC Press, Boca Raton, FL, p 147–165
Parker T S, McNamara D J, Brown C et al 1982 Mevalonic acid in human plasma: relationship of concentration and circadian rhythm to cholesterol synthesis rates in man. Proceedings of the National Academy of Sciences USA 79: 3037–3041
Patsch J R, Prasad S S, Gotto A M, Bengttson-Olivecrona G 1984 Postprandial lipemia. Journal of Clinical Investigation 74: 2017–2023
Rall S C, Weisgraber K H, Innerarity T L, Mahley R W 1983 Identical structural and receptor binding defects in apolipoprotein E_2 in hypo-, normo-, and hypercholesterolemic dysbetalipoproteinemia. Journal of Clinical Investigation 71: 1023–1031
Rath M, Pauling L 1990 Hypothesis: lipoprotein (a) is a surrogate for ascorbate. Proceedings of the National Academy of Sciences, USA 16: 6204–6207
Rath M, Niendorf A, Reblin T, Dietel M, Krebber H J, Beisiegel U 1989 Detection and quantification of lipoprotein (a) in the arterial wall of 107 coronary bypass patients. Arteriosclerosis 9: 579–592
Rohrer L, Freeman M, Kodama T, Penman M, Krieger M 1990 Coiled-coil fibrous domains mediate ligand binding by macrophage scavenger type II. Nature 343: 570–572
Rosengren A, Wilhelmsen L, Eriksson E, Risberg B, Wedel H 1990 Lipoprotein (a) and coronary heart disease: a prospective case-control study in a general population sample of middle aged men. British Medical Journal 301: 1248–1251
Rubinsztein D C, Cohen J C, Berger G M, van der Westhuyzen D R, Coetzee G A 1990 Chylomicron remnant clearance from the plasma is normal in familial hypercholesterolemic homozygotes with defined receptor defects. Journal of Clinical Investigation 86: 1306–1312
Sattler W, Kostner G M, Waeg G, Esterbauer H 1991 Oxidation of lipoprotein Lp(a): a comparison with low density lipoprotein. Biochimica et Biophysica Acta 1081: 65–74
Schaefer E J, Jenkins L L, Brewer H B 1978 Human chylomicron apolipoprotein catabolism. Biochemical and Biophysics Research Communications 80: 405–412
Schaefer E J, Wetzel M G, Bengtsson G, Scow R O, Brewer H B, Olivecrona T 1982 Transfer of human lymph chylomicron constituents to other lipoprotein density fractions during in vitro lipolysis. Journal of Lipid Research 23: 1259–1273
Shepherd J, Bicker S, Lorimer A R, Packard C J 1979 Receptor-mediated low density lipoprotein catabolism in man. Journal of Lipid Research 20: 999–1006
Shepherd J, Packard C J, Bicker S, Lawrie T D V, Morgan H G 1980 Cholestyramine promotes receptor-mediated LDL catabolism. New England Journal of Medicine 302: 1219–1222
Shepherd J, Packard C J, Stewart J M et al 1984 Apolipoprotein A and B (S_f 100–400) metabolism during bezafibrate therapy in hypertriglyceridemic subjects. Journal of Clinical Investigation 74: 2164–2177
Simpson H S, Williamson C M, Olivecrona T et al 1990 Postprandial lipemia and coronary artery disease. Atherosclerosis 85: 193–202
Slater H R, McKinney L, Packard C J, Shepherd J 1984 Contribution of the receptor pathway to LDL catabolism. Arteriosclerosis 4: 604–613
Soutar A K, Myant N B, Thompson G R 1982 The metabolism of very low density and intermediate density lipoproteins in patients with familial hypercholesterolaemia. Atherosclerosis 43: 217–231
Sparrow C P, Parthasarathy S, Steinberg D 1989 A macrophage receptor that recognizes oxidized low density lipoprotein but not acetylated low density lipoprotein. Journal of Biological Chemistry 264: 2599–2604
Steinberg D, Parthasarathy S, Carew T E, Khoo J C, Witztum J L 1989 Beyond cholesterol — modifications of low-density lipoprotein that increase its atherogenicity. New England Journal of Medicine 320: 915–924
Steinbrecher U P, Parthasarathy S, Leake D S, Witztum J L, Steinberg D 1984 Modification of LDL by endothelial cells involves lipid peroxidation and degradation of LDL phospholipids. Proceedings of the National Academy of Sciences, USA 81: 3883–3887
Strickland D K, Ashcom J D, Williams S, Burgess W H, Migliorini M, Argraves W S 1990 Sequence identity between the α_2-macroglobulin receptor and low density lipoprotein receptor-related protein suggests that this molecule is a multifunctional receptor. Journal of Biological Chemistry 265: 17401–17404
Tabas I, Tall A R 1984 Mechanism of the association of HDL_3 with endothelial cells, smooth muscle cells, and fibroblasts, evidence against the role of specific ligand and receptor proteins. Journal of Biological Chemistry 259: 13897–13905
Tall A R, Small D S 1978 Plasma high density lipoproteins. New England Journal of Medicine 299: 1232–1236
Tall A R, Green P H R, Glickman R M, Riley J W 1979 Metabolic fate of chylomicron phospholipids and apoproteins in the rat. Journal of Clinical Investigation 64: 977–989
Tozuka M, Fidge N 1989 Purification and characterization of two high-density lipoprotein-binding proteins from rat and human liver. Biochemical Journal 261: 239–244
Turner R H, Snavely J R, Goldwater W H, Randolph M L, Sprague C C, Unglaub W G 1951 The study of serum lipoproteins and lipids with the aid of the quantity ultracentrifuge. Journal of Clinical Investigation. 30: 1071–1081
Uauy R, Vega G L, Grundy S M, Bilheimer D W 1988 Lovastatin therapy in receptor-negative homozygous familial hypercholesterolemia: lack of effect on low-density lipoprotein concentrations or turnover. Journal of Pediatrics 113: 387–392
Utermann G, Menzel H J, Kraft H G, Dubatt C, Kemmler H G, Seitz C 1987 Lp(a) glycoprotein phenotypes. Inheritance and relation to Lp(a)-lipoprotein concentrations in plasma. Journal of Clinical Investigation 80: 458–465
Vega G L, East C, Grundy S M 1988 Lovastatin therapy in familial dysbetalipoproteinemia: effects on kinetics of apolipoprotein B. Atherosclerosis 70: 131–143
Vita J A, Treasure C B, Nabel E G et al 1990 Coronary vasomotor response to acetylcholine relates to risk factors for coronary artery disease. Circulation 81: 491–498
Vogel J 1845 Pathologie Anatomie des menschlischen Korpers, Leipzig. The pathological anatomy of the human body. H Ballière, London, p 587
Weisgraber K H, Mahley R W 1980 Subfractionation of human high density lipoproteins by heparin-sepharose affinity chromatography. Journal of Lipid Research 21: 316–325
Wiklund O, Angelin B, Olofsson S O et al 1990 Apolipoprotein (a) and ischaemic heart disease in familial hypercholesterolaemia. Lancet 335: 1360–1363
Windler E, Chao Y, Havel R J 1980 Regeneration of the hepatic uptake of triglyceride-rich lipoproteins in the rat. Journal of Biological Chemistry 255: 8303–8307
Wu A L, Windmueller H G 1979 Relative contributions by liver and intestine to individual plasma apolipoproteins in the rat. Journal of Biological Chemistry 254: 7316–7322
Yla-Herttuala S, Palinski W, Rosenfield M E et al 1989 Evidence for the presence of oxidatively modified low density lipoprotein in atherosclerotic lesions of rabbit and man. Journal of Clinical Investigation 84: 1086–1095
Yla-Herttuala S, Rosenfeld M E, Parthasarathy S et al 1991 Gene expression in macrophage-rich human atherosclerotic lesions. 15-lipoxygenase and acetyl low density lipoprotein receptor messenger RNA colocalize with oxidation specific lipid-protein adducts. Journal of Clinical Investigation 87: 1146–1152
Zannis V I, Lees A M, Lees R S, Breslow J L 1982 Abnormal apo AI isoprotein composition in patients with Tangier disease. Journal of Biological Chemistry 257: 4978–4986
Zeiher A M, Drexler H, Wollschlager H Just H 1991 Modulation of coronary vasomotor tone in humans — progressive endothelial dysfunction with different early stages of coronary atherosclerosis. Circulation 83: 391–401
Zilversmit D B 1984 Lipid transfer proteins. Journal of Lipid Research 25: 1563–1569

51. Blood rheology, haemostasis and vascular disease

G. D. O. Lowe

Haemostasis, atherogenesis and thrombosis are each processes which occur in flowing blood. Arterial stenoses and thrombosis may cause organ damage by reducing organ blood flow (ischaemia); while venous thrombosis may embolise in flowing blood to the pulmonary arteries. Many of the potential mechanisms in haemostasis, atherogenesis, thrombosis or ischaemia have been studied in static systems, or in artificial flow conditions such as test tubes, cuvettes or microtitre plates on the laboratory bench. The role of the haemorheologist in this field is to study the flow behaviour of whole blood or plasma (macrorheology) and of its constituent cells (microrheology; Karino & Goldsmith 1987) and to apply this to the clinical problems of bleeding and vascular disorders (Dormandy 1981, Lowe 1984, 1986, 1987a,b, 1988, Goldsmith & Turitto 1986, Chien et al 1987, Karino & Goldsmith 1987).

BLOOD FLOW, SHEAR AND VISCOSITY

In the majority of blood vessels, flow is streamline or laminar (Fig. 51.1). In such flow, adjacent hypothetical fluid layers move relative to each other (shearing) because of the viscous drag exerted by the vessel wall on the flowing liquid (e.g. blood or plasma). The shear stress is the force per unit area (in units of milliPascals, mPa) which produces shearing and flow. Shear stress is related directly to flow velocity, and inversely to vessel diameter: hence it is highest for rapid flow in narrow vessels (e.g. arterial stenoses, arterioles, and capillaries). The shear rate is the velocity gradient between adjacent fluid layers (distance per second divided by distance, producing units of inverse seconds, s^{-1}).

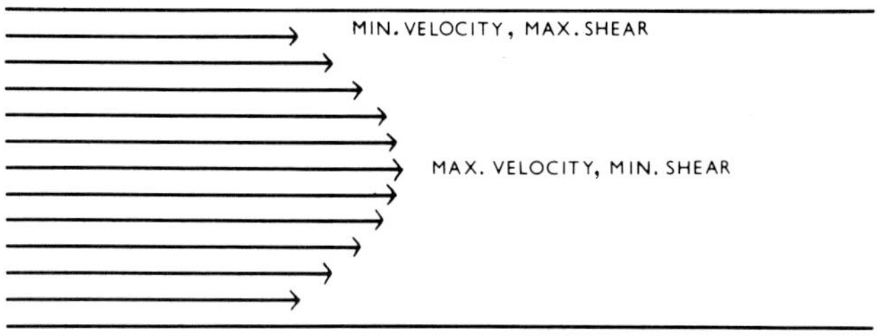

Fig. 51.1 Laminar (streamline) flow in a tube, shown in longitudinal section. The parallel fluid layers are represented by arrows. The velocity profile is parabolic, with maximal velocity at the tube axis, and minimal velocity at the tube wall. In contrast, the velocity difference (shear rate) between adjacent fluid layers is maximal at the tube wall, and minimal at the axis (from Lowe 1987a, with permission).

In streamline, nonpulsatile flow along a rigid, regular tube (Poiseuille flow), the viscous drag of the vessel wall results in a parabolic flow velocity profile, with maximal velocity at the tube axis (Fig. 51.1). In contrast, shear stresses (and shear rates) are maximal at the vessel wall. Hence blood — vessel wall interactions important in haemostasis, thrombosis and atherogenesis (platelet adhesion and aggregation; coagulation and fibrinolysis; protein and leucocyte infiltration) occur under conditions of minimal flow velocity and maximal flow force.

Non-laminar (turbulent) flow occurs in the heart chambers, in parts of the arterial tree, and in venous valves. In these areas, separation of blood flow from the mainstream may favour thrombogenesis and atherogenesis (Karino & Goldsmith 1987).

The viscosity of blood is its intrinsic resistance to flow, which arises from frictional interactions between plasma proteins and blood cells as blood flows through vessels. Viscosity is defined as the ratio of shear stress to shear rate:-

$$\text{Viscosity (mPa.s)} = \frac{\text{Shear stress (mPa)}}{\text{Shear rate (s}^{-1})}$$

The Hagen–Poiseuille Law relates the flow of a simple liquid in a straight tube to the driving pressure along the tube, the radius and length of the tube, and the viscosity of the liquid:-

$$\text{Volume flow rate} \propto \frac{\text{Pressure gradient} \times \text{Vessel radius}^4}{\text{Vessel length} \times \text{Fluid viscosity}}$$

Blood flow in vivo is pulsatile; blood vessels are neither straight nor rigid; and blood is not a simple fluid.

However if the Hagen–Poiseuille Law is taken as a first approximation, blood flow in an organ should depend on cardiac output (which produces a pressure gradient) and the resistance to blood flow within the organ, which is partly vascular resistance (the summed resistance of arteries and arterial stenoses, collateral vessels, arterioles, capillaries, venules and veins) and partly the viscous resistance of the blood:-

$$\text{Organ blood flow} \propto \frac{\text{Pressure gradient (cardiac output)}}{\underset{\text{(length/radius}^4\text{)}}{\text{Vascular resistance}} \times \underset{\text{(blood viscosity)}}{\text{Viscous resistance}}}$$

Arterial blood pressure is the product of cardiac output and total peripheral resistance, which again is partly vascular and partly viscous. Hence increases in blood viscosity may increase blood pressure, as well as decreasing blood flow.

MEASUREMENTS AND DETERMINANTS OF BLOOD RHEOLOGY

Whole-blood viscosity, the overall flow resistance of bulk blood in wide-bore vessels (e.g. arteries and veins), is determined by plasma viscosity, haematocrit (volume fraction of cells), red cell deformation, and red cell aggregation (Table 51.1). In addition to their interactive effects on whole-blood viscosity, these four rheological variables also have effects on platelet adhesion and aggregation (Ch. 11). In the microcirculation, bulk blood viscosity is not applicable: flow resistance still depends on plasma viscosity and haematocrit, but also on the deformability of individual red cells and leucocytes as they pass through the nutritive capillaries whose diameter is less than that of the resting blood cells. Due to their low concentration, leucocytes have negligible effects on bulk blood viscosity (except in rare cases of hyperleucocytic leukaemias).

Table 51.1 Determinants of blood flow behaviour

Macrovessels — whole-blood viscosity

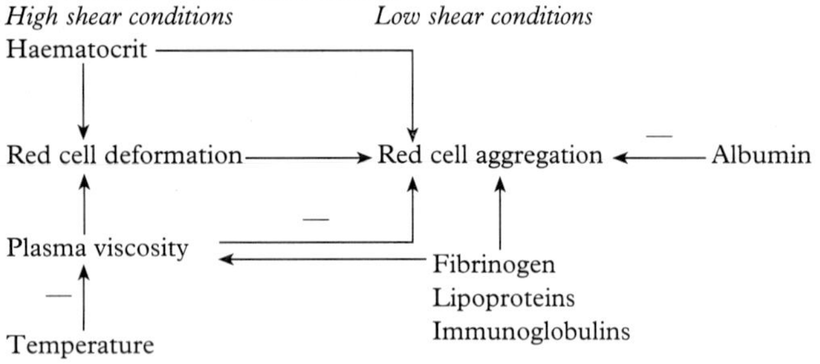

Microvessels — whole-blood filterability
Haematocrit
Plasma viscosity
Red cell aggregation
Red cell deformation (surface area: volume, membrane, haemoglobin)
Leucocyte deformation and adhesion (cell type and activation)
Platelet adhesion and aggregation

However due to their adhesiveness and low deformability they have major effects on the overall flow resistance of blood in microvessels: capillaries and venules in vivo and blood filtration in vitro (Alderman et al 1981, Chien 1988) (Table 51.1).

Plasma viscosity

Plasma viscosity is usually measured in capillary viscometers, which give accurate, precise and rapid measurements. The capillary is calibrated with standard solutions of known viscosity; the viscosity of a plasma sample is then calculated by comparing its flow rate to that of the standard solution, using the Hagen–Poiseuille equation (International Committee for Standardization in Haematology 1986). The determinants of plasma viscosity are temperature, and the plasma protein pattern. The standard temperature of measurement is 37°C: with decreases in temperature, plasma viscosity increases due to increased frictional interactions between plasma molecules (International Committee for Standardization in Haematology 1986).

The viscosity of water at 37°C is 0.69 mPa.s. The addition of small molecules has minimal effect, however the addition of plasma proteins which disturb plasma streamlines almost doubles the viscosity of plasma relative to water (mean plasma viscosity at 37°C is about 1.32 mPa.s, population range 1.15–1.50 (Lowe 1987a). The effect of individual plasma proteins on plasma viscosity increases with their concentration, molecular size and asymmetry: thus fibrinogen has a stronger effect than serum globulins (lipoproteins, immunoglobulins), which in turn have stronger effects than albumin. In acute and chronic diseases, the plasma protein pattern changes with an increase in fibrinogen and later in immunoglobulins, and a fall in albumin, and thus plasma viscosity increases. Plasma viscosity is increasingly used as a routine measure of acute and chronic phase protein reactions in disease (International Committee for Standardization in Haematology 1988).

Plasma perfuses all blood vessels in vivo, hence it is a fundamental determinant of blood flow (Schmid-Schönbein 1988). Increases in plasma viscosity within the population range are progressively associated with risk of ischaemic heart disease (Yarnell et al 1991), and above 2.0 mPa.s with the clinical plasma hyperviscosity syndrome (Somer 1987).

Haematocrit

The addition of red blood cells to plasma to form whole blood further disturbs flow streamlines and further increases viscosity. With linear increase in haematocrit, there is an exponential increase in whole-blood viscosity. However, over the population range of haematocrit (35–53%) the relationship of haematocrit to blood viscosity might equally well be linear (Lowe 1987a). The general relationship can be expressed thus (Whittington & Harkness 1982):-

$$\log \text{Whole-blood viscosity} = \text{Plasma viscosity} + \left(\text{Haematocrit} \times \text{Shear constant}\right)$$

The shear constant expresses the effects of shear-dependent red cell deformation and of shear-dependent red cell aggregation on whole-blood viscosity (Table 51.1). This equation can be used to correct whole-blood viscosity, measured at native haematocrit, to a standard haematocrit (e.g. 45%), so that the influence of other determinants of blood viscosity can be assessed (Matrai et al 1987).

In normal arterioles, red cells travel in the central, high-velocity streamlines (Fig. 51.1), resulting in dynamic reduction in haematocrit (Fåhraeus effect) and hence in blood viscosity (Fåhraeus–Lindqvist effect). Nevertheless, relationships between haematocrit and blood viscosity appear similar in the microcirculation and in the macrocirculation (Skalak & Chien 1981).

When whole-blood viscosity was measured at high shear rates (over 300 s^{-1}) at 37°C in a capillary viscometer in a large random population sample, its mean value was 3.4 mPa.s (five times the viscosity of water) at a mean haematocrit of 44% (Lowe 1987a). Over this population range of haematocrit (35–53%), the range of blood viscosity was 2.2–4.5 mPa.s. The correlation between blood viscosity and haematocrit was 0.7; hence about 50% of individual variation in blood viscosity was attributable to variation in haematocrit (Lowe 1987a). Increases in haematocrit above 38% are associated with an exponential increase in risk of thrombotic events and cardiovascular mortality (Elwood et al 1974, Pearson & Wetherley-Mein 1978, Pearson 1987) and complications of pregnancy (Lowe 1992).

Red cell deformation

Normal red blood cells are highly deformable by shear forces in flow, due to cell geometry (incomplete filling with haemoglobin resulting in an excess of surface area to volume); a flexible membrane; and a low internal viscosity (low mean cell haemoglobin concentration, MCHC; absence of nucleus or organelles). This ready deformability is responsible for not only low bulk blood viscosity in wide-bore vessels at high shear rates, but also for rapid passage of individual red cells (resting diameter 7–8 μm) through nutritive capillaries (diameter 2–6 μm) to supply oxygen to tissues.

During rapid flow in wide-bore vessels, red cells are orientated by shear forces in parallel with flow streamlines; assume ellipsoidal shapes with their long axes parallel to the direction of flow; and indeed participate in flow. The flexible red cell membrane rotates around its contents of liquid haemoglobin like the caterpillar tread of a military tank: 'tank-treading' (Schmid-Schönbein 1976). While increases in plasma viscosity and in haematocrit tend to increase high-shear whole-blood viscosity, their effects are partly minimized by increases in red cell deformation (by viscous plasma and by cell crowding respectively) (Table 51.1). Relative blood viscosity (whole-blood viscosity at a standard haematocrit of 45%, divided by plasma viscosity) is a measure of red cell rigidity (lack of deformability) in high-shear viscometric flow. Relative blood viscosity shows marked inter-individual variation, and increases when red cell geometry is altered, membrane flexibility reduced, or internal viscosity (MCHC) increased, e.g. in the sickling disorders (Lowe 1987a, Stuart & Johnson 1987).

The deformability of individual red cells in microvessels can be measured in micropipettes or by micropore filtration methods, which are much more sensitive than viscometry to the effects of rigid cells (e.g. sickle cells). The microvascular complications of the sickling disorders may partly reflect microvascular occlusion by such rigid cells (Stuart & Johnson 1987).

Red cell aggregation

With reduction in shear forces, red cells are no longer deformed, and are aggregated by plasma macromolecules into linear aggregates (rouleaux) which undergo secondary aggregation to form elastic networks within the blood. Such aggregates disturb flow streamlines and increase blood viscosity at low shear rates. For example, mean normal blood viscosity (37°C) at a shear rate of 1 s^{-1} is about 18 mPa.s, which is about five times higher than normal blood viscosity at high shear rates, i.e. above 300 s^{-1} (3.4 mPa.s). Red cell aggregation can be measured by low-shear viscometry (usually in rotational viscometers at defined, uniform shear rates or shear stresses), by photometry (as for platelet aggregation in plasma), or by sedimentation methods such as the erythrocyte sedimentation rate or ESR (International Committee for Standardization in Haematology 1986, 1988, Lowe 1987a).

As with low-shear platelet aggregation in vitro, plasma fibrinogen is the most important plasma protein which bridges cells in red cell aggregation; increases in fibrinogen from the mean normal level of 3 g/l up to 8 g/l result in large, linear increases in red cell aggregation, as measured by several methods (Lowe 1987a). However red cell aggregation is also promoted by increases in other plasma globulins such as α_2-macroglobulin, immunoglobulins and lipoproteins; and also by a decrease in plasma albumin (Table 51.1). Such changes occur in acute and chronic disease states, of which the ESR is a time-hallowed (but inferior) alternative measure to plasma viscosity (Lowe 1987a, International Committee for Standardization in Haematology 1988). Red cell aggregation also varies with plasma viscosity, haematocrit, and with aggregability of red cells (Chien 1975): the last shows marked inter-individual variation (Dormandy 1981).

Low shear rates and red cell aggregation occur at several sites in the circulation:-

1. At the axes of large vessels (Fig. 51.1), resulting in blunting of the flow velocity profile (Rampling & Challoner 1983).

2. In the arterial tree, at sites of flow separation such as bends and bifurcations where atherogenesis occurs (Motomiya & Karino 1984) (Fig. 51.2) and distal to arterial stenoses where fibrin-rich thrombi occur (Davies 1989) (Fig. 51.3).

3. In the venules (as observed, for example, in normal human conjunctivae), where red cell aggregates displace leucocytes towards the vessel wall, encouraging their adhesion and emigration in inflammatory states (the Fåhraeus–Vejlens effect), and where such processes may also perpetuate ischaemia (Schmid-Schönbein 1988).

4. In venous valve pockets, where red cell aggregation may encourage hypoxia and recirculation of activated platelets and thrombin, promoting thrombogenesis (Karino & Motomiya 1984, Lowe 1984)

In the plasma hyperviscosity syndromes, clinical symptoms may arise from the effects of immunoglobulins not only on plasma viscosity, but also on red cell aggregation in vivo (Somer 1987).

Leucocyte rheology

As previously noted, leucocytes are present at low concentration in blood and thus have minimal effects on bulk blood viscosity, except rarely in hyperleucocytic leukaemias (Lichtman et al 1987). However, the adhesiveness and poor deformability of neutrophils and monocytes (especially when activated in inflammation or ischaemia) render them important determinants of blood flow in microvessels, especially in inflammation and ischaemia (Ernst et al 1987, Lowe 1987a, Chien 1988).

Leucocytes have similar diameters to red cells (6–8 μm), but being spheres have twice their volume; moreover due to their nuclei and high-viscosity, organelle-rich cytoplasm, their cellular viscosity is higher by three orders of magnitude (Chien et al 1984, Chien 1988). Whole-blood filtration using filters with pore diameters of about 5 μm (corresponding to the mean diameter of nutritive capillaries in mammalian heart, brain and skeletal muscle) reflects pore occupation by leucocytes and red cells in

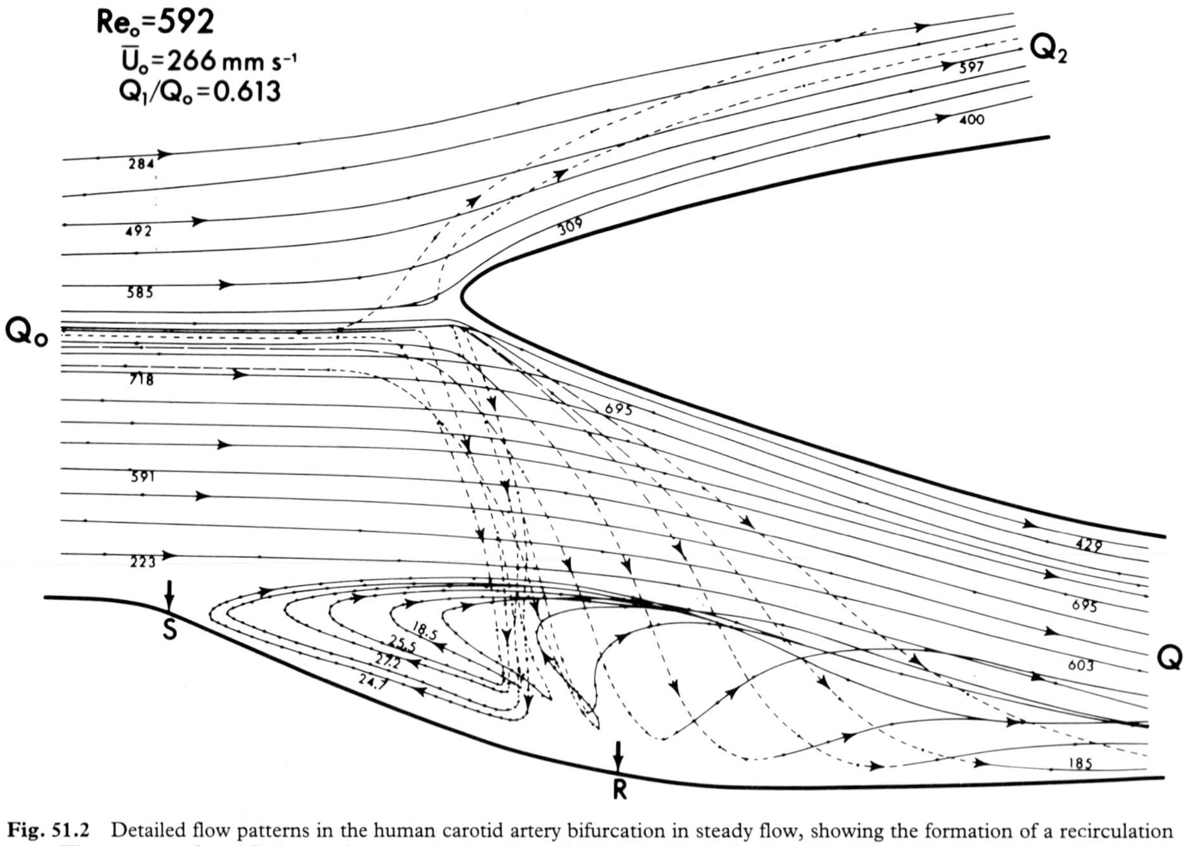

Fig. 51.2 Detailed flow patterns in the human carotid artery bifurcation in steady flow, showing the formation of a recirculation zone. The arrows at S and R denote the respective locations of the separation and stagnation points. The numbers on the streamlines (or particle paths) indicate the particle translational velocities in mm/s (after Motomiya & Karino 1984, with permission).

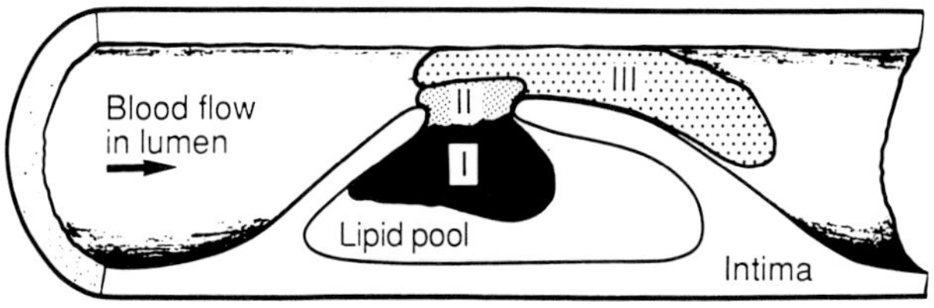

Fig. 51.3 Diagrammatic representation in a coronary artery of a reconstruction in longitudinal section of an occluding thrombus due to plaque fissuring. The thrombus within the plaque labelled I is rich in platelets; stage II contains both platelets and fibrin; while stage III thrombus which has propagated in the lumen is predominantly fibrin and red cells with a minimal platelet component. Stage I and II thrombus forms under high-shear conditions (condensation of flow streamlines through the stenosis); while stage III thrombus forms under low-shear conditions (distal to arterial occlusion) (from Davies 1989, with permission).

equal measure, because leucocytes are 700 times more likely to plug pores than red cells, although 700 times less numerous (Alderman et al 1981, Chien et al 1984, Chien 1988). The occupation of micropores by leucocytes is time-dependent, and varies with leucocyte type: monocytes and activated neutrophils have the highest flow resistance, followed by non-activated neutrophils, then by lymphocytes (Chien et al 1984, Schmalzer & Chien 1984, Nash & Meiselman 1986, Chien 1988, Lennie et al 1988). Microcirculatory studies have shown that leucocytes are also important determinants of capillary flow in vivo, especially in low-flow states (Bagge 1984, Chien 1988).

Leucocytes can also markedly affect flow in post-capillary venules, in which they are displaced towards the vessel wall by red cells, and especially by red cell aggregates in inflammatory states: the Fåhraeus–Vejlens effect (Schmid-Schönbein 1988).

These rheological effects of leucocytes probably contribute to the circulatory complications of hyperleucocytic leukaemias (Lichtman et al 1987) and of arterial disease: increases in white cell count over the population range are associated with increased risk of arterial events (Ernst et al 1987, Lowe 1987a, Yarnell et al 1991).

RHEOLOGICAL EFFECTS ON HAEMOSTASIS

Following vascular injury, haemostasis occurs as a dynamic process in flowing blood: stasis only occurs when the haemostatic plug is complete. The influence of blood flow and rheological variables on haemostasis is therefore probably important, but difficult to study in vivo apart from correlation of simple parameters with the skin bleeding time. In vitro, laminar flow systems have been employed to study the effects of flow rate, shear stress, shear rate and other rheological variables on haemostatic processes: principally platelet adhesion, aggregation and secretion; and generation of factor Xa or thrombin (Lowe 1987b, Turitto 1988, Nemerson & Turitto 1991).

Rheology and platelets

Microcirculatory studies in the rat mesentery have shown that in arterioles, the concentration of platelets near the vessel wall is twice that in the centre of the vessel; furthermore platelets align with their long axes in the flow streamlines (Tangelder et al 1982). This is probably a consequence of the axial transport of flexible red cells in high-velocity streamlines (the Fåhraeus effect) with displacement of platelets towards the vessel wall (Karino & Goldsmith 1987). Teleologically, the concentration of platelets near the vessel wall appears strategic in haemostasis. Platelets near the vessel wall are more likely to collide with the wall and with each other, and also to promote an increased concentration of platelet-secreted compounds active in haemostasis (e.g. adenosine diphosphate (ADP), serotonin, thromboxane A_2) near to the wall. In the event of vessel damage, platelets should be more likely to encounter released chemical activators (e.g. collagen) when close to the wall. Finally, platelets near the wall are exposed to the highest shear stresses (which may activate them) and have the lowest flow velocities (and hence maximal time to adhere to injured areas of the vessel wall).

Studies of the skin bleeding time have shown inverse correlations with the haematocrit (Duke 1910, Small et al 1983). The long bleeding time in anaemic patients is shortened by red cell transfusions (Hellem et al 1961, Livio et al 1982), or, in renal anaemia, by treatment with recombinant erythropoietin, due in part to increase in haematocrit and in part to correction of a platelet function defect (Zwaginga et al 1991). These effects of haematocrit on the bleeding time probably reflect the effects of increasing haematocrit on platelet adhesion (Turitto & Weiss 1980, Turitto 1988) and on platelet aggregation, at both high shear rates (Jen & McIntire 1984, Reimers et al 1984) and at low shear rates (Saniabadi et al 1984a,b, 1987, Burgess-Wilson et al 1984). Such effects of haematocrit on platelet adhesion and aggregation probably reflect both physical mechanisms (platelet diffusion) and chemical effects (release of ADP from red cells). Platelet adhesion may also be increased by red cell size, red cell rigidity, and by plasma viscosity (Aarts et al 1983, 1984, see also Ch. 11).

Platelet adhesion and aggregation are influenced not only by physical and chemical effects of red cells, but also by blood flow, shear stress and shear rate (Ch. 11). As discussed above, blood flow and the axial migration of red cells provide a continuing supply of fresh platelets near the vessel wall to replace those depleted by interaction with the vessel wall. In the Baumgartner perfusion chamber model, platelet adhesion to subendothelium, as well as thrombus growth, increase with flow rate, and specifically with wall shear rate. The shear-dependency is observed at moderate shear rates (below 600–800 s^{-1};

typical for flow in arteries and veins); and is also influenced by haematocrit (Turitto 1988). Platelet adhesion defects such as von Willebrand's disease, Bernard–Soulier syndrome, thrombasthenia and storage pool disease are associated with deficiency of shear-induced platelet deposition, indicating roles for von Willebrand factor and platelet membrane glycoproteins Ib and IIb-IIIa (Weiss et al 1986, Nemerson & Turitto 1991).

Studies of platelet aggregation in vitro have indicated the need for flow to bring platelets into contact with each other; and have shown shear-induced increases in platelet aggregation (and platelet procoagulant activity) in platelet-rich plasma (Anderson et al 1978, Moritz et al 1983, Wurzinger et al 1983) and in whole blood (Jen & McIntire 1984). While the plasma fibrinogen level is an important determinant of platelet aggregation in vitro (Lowe et al 1978a, Burgess-Wilson et al 1984, Meade et al 1985a,b), platelet adhesion and thrombus formation on subendothelium at high shear rates in the Baumgartner system appear fibrinogen-independent (Weiss et al 1989). It is possible that von Willebrand factor is the important binding protein in platelet aggregation under high-shear conditions, whereas fibrinogen may be more important under low-shear flow conditions (Nemerson & Turitto 1991).

While shear forces and haematocrit therefore promote platelet adhesion, aggregation and thrombus formation, platelet aggregates are initially unstable, friable structures which may also be dislodged and disrupted by shear forces in flowing blood, unless they are stabilized by fibrin, which greatly increases their stability against dispersion by flow (Schmid-Schönbein 1983). It is therefore important to determine rheological effects on blood coagulation and fibrin formation.

Rheology and coagulation

Shear forces and blood flow affect blood coagulation and its endpoint, fibrin formation, as well as platelet behaviour. Practical coagulationists have long appreciated that blood and plasma clotting times are affected by the frequency and technique of sample mixing in tilted clotting tubes. In rotational viscometers in which shear rates (or shear stresses) are controlled, the clotting time of blood shortens with increasing shear rates (or shear stresses) (Dintenfass 1971, Ernst et al 1984). Possible explanations include increased sample mixing (which increases the collision frequency of platelets, leucocytes and coagulation factors with each other and with the chamber surface), decreased blood viscosity after shearing (due to dispersion of red cell aggregates) which may also promote such interactions, shear-induced platelet procoagulant activity (Wurzinger et al 1983), and the effects of flow on surface-bound catalysis in the coagulation cascade (Nemerson & Turitto 1991).

Nemerson & Turitto (1991) have recently studied coagulation reactions in a flow reactor: a glass microcapillary coated internally with a continuous phospholipid bilayer incorporating tissue factor. Such a system permits study of the effects of flow on delivery of substrate and enzyme, on their reaction at the vessel wall, and on their removal; in contrast to a closed 'test-tube' system with recirculating flow. Experiments in this system showed that low factor VII concentrations delayed achievement of steady-state factor Xa production; and that the rate of formation of factor Xa increased with shear rate (Gemmell et al 1988, 1990). In the presence of factors VIII and IX, shear-induced enhancement of factor Xa production was observed (Repke et al 1990). Such studies suggest that some coagulation reactions are accelerated in the presence of high shear, and may illuminate the pathogenesis of the haemophilias. However, as with platelet thrombus formation, high shear forces may not only promote fibrin formation, but also reduce it, at least in the Baumgartner perfusion system (Weiss et al 1986). Possible explanations include increased flow removal of thrombin or fibrin monomer.

The role of plasma and blood viscosity on blood coagulation has been little studied. Theoretically, increase in plasma or blood viscosity may increase shear stresses on vascular endothelium or subendothelium and adjacent platelets, with possible consequences for coagulation on these surfaces. Plasma levels of fibrinopeptide A (a marker of ongoing thrombin activity) and of fibrin peptide $B\beta_{1-42}$ or $B\beta_{15-42}$ (markers of ongoing plasmin activity) can be used to assess the balance of coagulation and fibrinolysis (Nossel 1981). In a recent population study of middle-aged men (Lowe et al 1991), increases in plasma fibrinopeptide A (and the ratio of FpA to $B\beta_{15-42}$) were associated with several conventional cardiovascular risk factors (smoking, obesity, blood pressure, cholesterol and triglyceride) as well as with increases in fibrinogen, factor VII, and plasma viscosity which are also independent predictors of ischaemic heart disease (Meade et al 1980, 1986, Yarnell et al 1991). The strongest correlation of the FpA/$B\beta_{15-42}$ ratio was with plasma viscosity; this appeared to be independent of plasma fibrinogen levels because a similar correlation was also observed with serum viscosity (plasma viscosity less the effect of fibrinogen) (Lowe et al 1991). The effects of plasma viscosity on blood coagulation (e.g. shear effects on tissue factor-factor VIIa initiation of coagulation at the vessel wall) and on fibrinolysis (e.g. shear effects on endothelial production of tissue plasminogen activator and plasminogen activator inhibitor type 1: see p. 1175) therefore merit study. It should however be noted that extreme elevations in plasma viscosity (in the plasma hyperviscosity syndrome) are associated with a bleeding disorder, due to interference by excessive immunoglobulins with fibrin formation and polymerization as well as with platelet function (Somer 1987).

Increases in haematocrit (and hence in blood viscosity) may also promote blood coagulation. Patients with renal anaemia treated with recombinant erythropoietin to raise their haematocrit were found to develop increases in thrombin-antithrombin complexes (another marker of thrombin activity) (Taylor et al 1991) as well as increased spontaneous platelet aggregation which is known to be haematocrit-dependent (Saniabadi et al 1984a,b, 1987). Again however, extreme elevations in haematocrit (polycythaemia) have been associated with excess bleeding, possibly due to interference of excess red cells with fibrin formation, as well as to platelet dysfunction.

Rheology, endothelium and fibrinolysis

Rheological studies of cultured endothelial cells have shown that shear forces affect their morphology (elongation and orientation in the direction of flow) (Levesque & Nerem 1985) and also their function (secretion of tissue plasminogen activator and up-regulation of its messenger RNA levels) (Diamond et al 1989,1990). It is therefore likely that rheological factors may affect other antithrombotic (or prothrombotic) functions of the endothelium (or subendothelium)(Nemerson & Turitto 1991).

EPIDEMIOLOGY OF BLOOD RHEOLOGY

Recent recognition of the importance of thrombosis in vascular disease stems partly from its frequent demonstration in careful pathological studies (Davies 1989) (Fig. 51.3), partly from the efficacy of antithrombotic and thrombolytic drugs as shown in large controlled trials, and partly from epidemiological studies such as the Northwick Park Heart Study, which has shown that plasma fibrinogen, factor VII and blood fibrinolytic activity are predictors of ischaemic heart disease, as well as associated with conventional risk factors (Meade et al 1979, 1980, 1986). The epidemiology of these factors is discussed in Chapter 53. Increased plasma fibrinogen levels may promote ischaemic heart disease (and stroke) (Wilhelmsen et al 1984) by several mechanisms: infiltration of the arterial wall (Smith et al 1976, Allen et al 1988), promotion of platelet aggregation, promotion of fibrin thrombus formation, or by its rheological effects (increases in plasma viscosity, red cell aggregation, and hence in whole-blood viscosity at both high and low shear rates).

Epidemiological studies have shown that several other determinants of the flow behaviour of blood are also associated with conventional cardiovascular risk factors; are primary and/or secondary predictors of cardiovascular events; and are also associated with the presence and extent of prevalent arterial disease (Lowe 1986, Lowe et al 1993).

Age, sex, menopause and oestrogen use

The incidence of all major cardiovascular diseases (ischaemic heart disease, stroke, peripheral arterial disease and venous thromboembolism) rises exponentially with age and is higher in men than in women especially before the menopause (Shaper 1988, Anderson et al 1991, Fowkes 1991, Bamford & Warlow 1992). Men have a higher mean haematocrit than women throughout life from puberty onwards, due to the erythropoietic action of testosterone in men and possibly to menstrual blood loss and fluid retention in women. The higher haematocrit results in higher mean whole-blood viscosity in men, which may be relevant to their higher risk of atherosclerosis, thrombosis and ischaemia (Mayer 1964, Lowe et al 1980a, 1988, 1992) (Table 51.2). This hypothesis is supported by several observations:-

1. In a prospective study of women aged under 65 years (Elwood et al 1974), increase in haematocrit from mean female haematocrit of 42% to mean male haematocrit of 46% (Table 51.2) was associated with a two-fold increase in cardiovascular mortality: a substantial reduction in the sex difference.
2. In women, post-menopausal increases in haematocrit, plasma viscosity and fibrinogen reduce the sex difference in whole-blood viscosity, in parallel with reduction of the sex difference in cardiovascular disease incidence (Meade et al 1983, Campbell et al 1985, Bonithon-Kopp et al 1988, Lowe et al 1988, 1992, Lee et al 1993a) (Table 51.2).
3. Use of oestrogen-containing oral contraceptives reduces the sex differences in whole-blood viscosity (due to increases in haematocrit, plasma viscosity and fibrinogen, Lowe et al 1980a) and in cardiovascular risk.
4. Significant increases in whole-blood viscosity, haematocrit, plasma viscosity and fibrinogen were observed in a population survey in women with premature coronary heart disease, in whom the sex difference in whole-blood viscosity was again significantly reduced (Lowe et al 1989).

In men, mean levels of fibrinogen, plasma viscosity, red cell aggregation and white cell count increase with age between 25 and 64 years; however haematocrit and hence high-shear whole-blood viscosity are relatively stable (Lowe et al 1980b, 1988, 1992) (Table 51.2). In women, haematocrit as well as fibrinogen, plasma viscosity and red cell aggregation also increase with age, resulting in significant increases in high-shear whole-blood viscosity, especially after the menopause; however due to a persisting sex difference in haematocrit, mean whole-blood viscosity remains lower in postmenopausal women aged 55–64 years than in men aged 25–34 years (Table 51.2). After correction to a standard haematocrit of 45%, men still have higher blood viscosity than women; this

Table 51.2 Distributions of rheological variables by age and sex

		Age (years)				
		25–34	35–44	45–54	55–64	Total
A. First MONICA survey and scottish Heart Health Study (Lowe et al 1988)						
Number	M	44	150	266	194	654
	F	33	142	248	156	579
Whole blood viscosity (mPa.s)	M	3.41(0.40)	3.50(0.42)	3.49(0.47)	3.59(0.58)	3.52(0.49)
	F	3.03(0.27)	3.03(0.46)	3.17(0.48)	3.31(0.46)	3.17(0.48)
Haematocrit(%)	M	44.8(2.4)	46.0(3.3)	45.7(3.6)	45.5(4.0)	45.6(3.6)
	F	41.2(2.5)	41.6(3.7)	42.3(3.8)	42.9(3.3)	42.2(3.6)
Haematocrit-corrected viscosity (mPa.s)	M	3.39(0.30)	3.43(0.29)	3.44(0.29)	3.53(0.41)	3.46(0.35)
	F	3.30(0.34)	3.23(0.31)	3.33(0.38)	3.43(0.35)	3.34(0.37)
Relative viscosity	M	2.62(0.16)	2.63(0.20)	2.60(0.23)	2.62(0.26)	2.61(0.23)
	F	2.62(0.28)	2.50(0.27)	2.53(0.24)	2.56(0.23)	2.54(0.25)
Plasma viscosity (mPa.s)	M	1.30(0.08)	1.31(0.08)	1.32(0.09)	1.35(0.10)	1.33(0.09)
	F	1.26(0.06)	1.30(0.08)	1.32(0.09)	1.35(0.08)	1.32(0.09)
Fibrinogen (Clauss, g/l)	M	2.05(0.55)	2.10(0.75)	2.26(0.81)	2.36(0.95)	2.24(0.83)
	F	2.19(1.00)	2.14(0.76)	2.46(0.84)	2.69(0.92)	2.44(0.88)
Fibrinogen (Heat, ml/dl)	M	3.52(0.86)	3.90(0.92)	4.04(0.91)	4.14(1.04)	4.01(0.96)
	F	3.65(0.91)	3.77(0.69)	4.02(0.87)	4.15(1.04)	3.98(0.90)
Fibrinogen ratio (Clauss/heat)	M	0.60(0.18)	0.56 (0.21)	0.58(0.23)	0.58(0.21)	0.58(0.21)
	F	0.65(0.23)	0.58(0.22)	0.62(0.20)	0.67(0.26)	0.63(0.24)
B. Second MONICA survey (Lowe et al 1992)						
Number	M	82	119	129	147	477
	F	84	94	134	126	438
Haematocrit (%)	M	45.9(2.6)	46.4(2.9)	46.4(3.0)	46.3(3.7)	46.3(3.1)
	F	42.2(2.2)	42.3(3.4)	42.2(3.5)	43.1(2.9)	42.5(3.1)
White cells (10^9/l)	M	6.88(1.98)	7.20(2.48)	7.17(2.18)	7.16(1.82)	7.13(2.12)
	F	7.51(2.16)	7.07(1.71)	7.16(2.23)	6.92(1.99)	7.14(2.05)
Fibrinogen (Clauss, g/l)	M	1.92(0.34)	2.14(0.58)	2.41(0.59)	2.61(0.60)	2.32(0.61)
	F	2.31(0.59)	2.21(0.41)	2.46(0.56)	2.63(0.57)	2.42(0.56)
Red cell aggregation (units)[a]	M	3.05(1.04)	3.47(1.06)	3.62(1.27)	3.82(1.21)	3.54(1.19)
	F	3.41(1.19)	3.39(1.17)	3.86(1.18)	4.02(1.21)	3.71(1.22)

Data given as mean with SD in brackets from two random population samples in Glasgow, Scotland.
[a] Red cell aggregation: photometric method.

appears due to higher plasma viscosity in younger men, and lower red cell deformability (increased relative high-shear viscosity) in older men (Table 51.2).

Table 51.2 also shows several other sex differences:-

1. Women have higher levels of fibrinogen than men by the clotting-time method of Clauss (Lee et al 1990), but not by a heat precipitation method. This difference is not explained by the lower haematocrit in women and hence a greater dilution of plasma by citrate anticoagulant: it may indicate higher fibrinogen clottability in women.
2. Women have higher levels of red cell aggregation than men as measured by a photometric method; this has also been described for the ESR (Lewis 1982) and may reflect their lower haematocrit (Lowe et al 1992).
3. Women have lower levels of plasma viscosity than men before the menopause, possibly due to hormonal fluid retention.
4. Women have higher levels of white cell count than men before the menopause, and lower levels afterwards (Lewis 1982, Lowe et al 1992).

Post-menopausal hormone replacement therapy appears to protect women from ischaemic heart disease and stroke; this may be due partly to reduction in plasma fibrinogen levels (Lee et al 1993a). The effects of hormone replacement therapy on other rheological variables are not yet established.

Cigarette-smoking

Cigarette-smoking is a major, dose-dependent risk factor for ischaemic heart disease, stroke and peripheral arterial disease (Shaper 1988, Fowkes 1991, Bamford & Warlow 1992). About 50% of the increased risk of ischaemic heart disease in smokers is reversed within a year of smoking cessation; however it takes 20 years to fall to the level of risk found in those who have never smoked (Shaper 1988). Cigarette-smokers also have dose-dependent, reversible increases in plasma fibrinogen levels, and hence in plasma and whole-blood viscosity (Meade et al 1979, 1987, Lowe et al 1980, 1988, 1992, Ernst & Matrai 1987a, Kannel et al 1987a,b, Yarnell et al 1987, Feher et al 1990, Lee et al 1990) (Table 51.3). The fall in fibrinogen levels in ex-smokers parallels the reduction in risk of ischaemic heart disease (about 50% fall by a year, then a slow fall over 15–20 years to levels found in never-smokers); and increased fibrinogen level appears to account for about 50% of the effect of smoking on risk of

Table 51.3 Rheological variables in non-smokers, ex-smokers, and current cigarette-smokers

A. Edinburgh Angina Study control group (Lowe et al 1991a)

	No.	Viscosity (mPa.s) Plasma	Serum	Fibrinogen[a] (g/l)	α_2 Macroglobulin (% pool)
Men					
Non-smokers	137	1.33(0.07)	1.21(0.07)	2.04(0.46)	68.2(21.1)
Ex-smokers	103	1.34(0.09)	1.23(0.08)	2.22(0.71)	62.1(16.2)
Current smokers	119	1.37(0.10)	1.23(0.08)	2.39(0.76)	74.2(24.0)

B. Second Glasgow Monica Survey (Lowe et al 1992)

	No.	Haematocrit (%)	White cells (10^9/l)	Fibrinogen[b] (g/l)	Aggregation[c] (units)
Men					
Non-smokers	135	45.7(2.6)	6.29(1.73)	2.05(0.46)	3.66(1.12)
Ex-smokers	150	45.6(3.2)	6.60(1.77)	2.40(0.74)	3.85(1.36)
Current smokers	190	47.4(3.2)	8.09(2.21)	2.46(0.53)	3.18(0.99)
1–9 cigs/day	25	46.7(2.9)	7.31(1.72)	2.34(0.56)	3.25(1.07)
10–19	52	46.4(3.3)	7.70(1.50)	2.45(0.60)	3.28(1.09)
20–29	72	47.9(3.2)	8.46(2.27)	2.51(0.44)	3.03(0.90)
30–39	24	48.7(2.6)	8.75(3.34)	2.44(0.51)	3.25(1.06)
40+	17	47.1(3.1)	7.97(2.08)	2.45(0.61)	3.38(0.87)
Women					
Non-smokers	151	41.8(2.8)	6.58(1.97)	2.34(0.49)	3.90(1.19)
Ex-smokers	82	41.9(3.4)	6.59(2.21)	2.36(0.51)	4.02(1.25)
Current smokers	204	43.3(3.0)	7.79(1.89)	2.51(0.62)	3.44(1.18)
1–9 cigs/day	23	42.0(3.6)	7.26(1.41)	2.29(0.51)	3.68(1.24)
10–19	76	43.4(3.0)	7.88(1.89)	2.53(0.52)	3.53(1.20)
20–29	82	43.6(3.0)	7.75(1.93)	2.51(0.70)	3.32(1.18)
30–39	14	43.4(2.6)	9.09(2.05)	2.68(0.73)	3.31(1.07)
40+	9	42.0(1.8)	6.70(1.42)	2.56(0.60)	3.43(1.09)

Data from two random population samples in Scotland: mean with SD in brackets.
[a] Fibrinogen: Ellis & Stransky assay.
[b] Fibrinogen: Clauss assay.
[c] Red cell aggregation: photometric method.

ischaemic heart disease (Kannel et al 1987a, Meade et al 1987, Lee et al 1990). Smoking also damages arterial endothelium, promoting infiltration of fibrinogen into the arterial wall (Allen et al 1988); it is therefore interesting that smoking and fibrinogen levels interact in increasing the extent of peripheral arterial disease (Lowe et al 1993) and the risk of peripheral arterial graft occlusion (Wiseman et al 1989).

The reversible increase in plasma viscosity in smokers is largely due to increase in fibrinogen, because serum viscosity (plasma viscosity less the effect of fibrinogen) is only slightly increased, due to reversible increases in serum acute-phase reactant globulins such as α_2-macroglobulin (Lowe et al 1991) (Table 51.3). These reversible, dose-dependent increases in acute-phase reactant proteins are accompanied by reversible dose-dependent increases in white cell count (Lowe et al 1985, 1992) (Table 51.3), suggesting a linked response to smoking-induced tissue injury (e.g. to lung epithelium or to arterial endothelium) (Allen et al 1988). Exposure to cigarette-smoke also activates neutrophils and monocytes, reducing their deformability: this may decrease their transit time through capillaries in ischaemic tissues (promoting ischaemia) and in the lungs (promoting emphysema) (Lennie et al 1989, Drost et al 1992).

The increase in whole-blood viscosity in smokers reflects a dose-dependent, reversible increase in haematocrit, as well as in plasma viscosity (Lowe et al 1980b, 1988, 1992, Ernst & Matrai 1987a) (Table 51.3). This appears to be due to an increase in mean red cell volume rather than red cell count (Helman & Rubenstein 1975, Lowe & Forbes 1988) and hence due to a qualitative change in erythropoiesis, rather than a quantitative change or a reduction in plasma volume. Smokers increase their total haemoglobin concentration (and haematocrit) to compensate for carbon monoxide poisoning, thus maintaining the same level of functional oxyhaemoglobin as non-smokers, but at a rheological cost (Stewart et al 1974).

While the increase in fibrinogen and α_2-macroglobulin in smokers might be expected to increase red cell aggregation as well as plasma viscosity, smokers had reversible, dose-dependent *decreases* in red cell aggregation as measured by a photometric method in a population sample (Lowe et al 1992; Table 51.3). This was not explained by their higher haematocrit, and may reflect decreased red cell deformability (Lowe et al 1980c, 1992). Two other studies have confirmed that smokers do not have increased red cell aggregation, measured by low-shear viscometry (Levenson et al 1987) or by photometry (Chabanel et al 1992).

It is interesting that the dose-dependent changes in rheological variables (Table 51.3) and risk of ischaemic heart disease (Shaper 1988) are reversed in those who smoke over 40 cigarettes a day.

Blood pressure

Chronic arterial hypertension is due to increased total peripheral resistance, which consists not only of a vascular component but also a viscous component. The latter has been much neglected; however several case-control studies have suggested rheological abnormalities in essential hypertension (Letcher et al 1981) or malignant hypertension (Isles et al 1984) (for other references, see Lowe & Forbes 1988). Furthermore in two recent, large random population studies, blood pressure showed significant, independent positive correlations with high-shear whole-blood viscosity (Smith et al 1992, Fowkes et al 1993). In these studies, the effect of blood viscosity was of similar strength as traditional associations of blood pressure such as age and obesity, and a clinically significant difference in mean blood pressure (about 10 mmHg) was observed between the lowest and highest quintiles of blood viscosity.

Multivariate analysis showed that the relationship between blood viscosity and blood pressure persisted after correction for obesity and other patient characteristics; that it was not due to plasma fibrinogen levels (in contrast to a case-control study in essential hypertension — Letcher et al 1981); and that it was explained only partly by haematocrit. In the study of younger subjects (age 25–64 years but principally 40–59 years) the relationship appeared due to plasma viscosity (Smith et al 1992). Two other studies in populations of similar age have confirmed correlations between blood pressure and plasma viscosity (or serum viscosity) (Koenig et al 1989, 1991, Lowe et al 1991). In the study of older subjects (age 55–74 years) the relationship appeared due to decreased red cell deformability (increased relative high-shear viscosity) (Fowkes et al 1993). Whether this related to a possible cell sodium transport defect (Hilton 1986) is not known. Further studies are required to establish the nature of the relationship between blood viscosity and blood pressure; however it should be noted that both increased plasma viscosity and decreased red cell deformability should increase flow resistance especially in the microcirculation, where most of the increased total peripheral resistance in persons with hypertension occurs (Williams et al 1990).

By whatever mechanisms blood viscosity increases in persons with hypertension, it may play a pathogenic role:-

1. Increased viscosity *multiplies* increased vascular resistance to increase peripheral resistance and hence blood pressure.

2. Increased viscosity may increase left ventricular afterload and promote left ventricular hypertrophy, which shows a closer correlation with blood viscosity than with blood pressure or other haemodynamic variables (Devereaux et al 1984).

3. Increased viscosity may promote the ischaemic diseases (ischaemic heart disease and stroke) which account for most of the increased morbidity and mortality in hypertensive persons, and which increase with cigarette-smoking and male sex (Kannel 1991).

Figure 51.4 shows that blood pressure, cigarette-smoking and male sex have additive effects on high-shear blood viscosity in a population sample (Lowe et al 1988, Smith et al 1992). Independent effects of blood pressure and smoking on blood viscosity have also been reported by Levenson et al (1987), and are not surprising, given that smoking increases haematocrit and fibrinogen levels whereas blood pressure is associated with increases in plasma viscosity due to plasma proteins other than fibrinogen, and possibly with decreased red cell deformability.

The effects of hypotensive drugs on blood rheology in hypertensive persons are still unclear (Lowe 1988).

Blood lipids

After age, male sex, smoking and blood pressure, serum total cholesterol is the fifth conventional major risk factor for ischaemic heart disease, thrombotic stroke and peripheral arterial disease (Shaper 1988, Fowkes 1991,

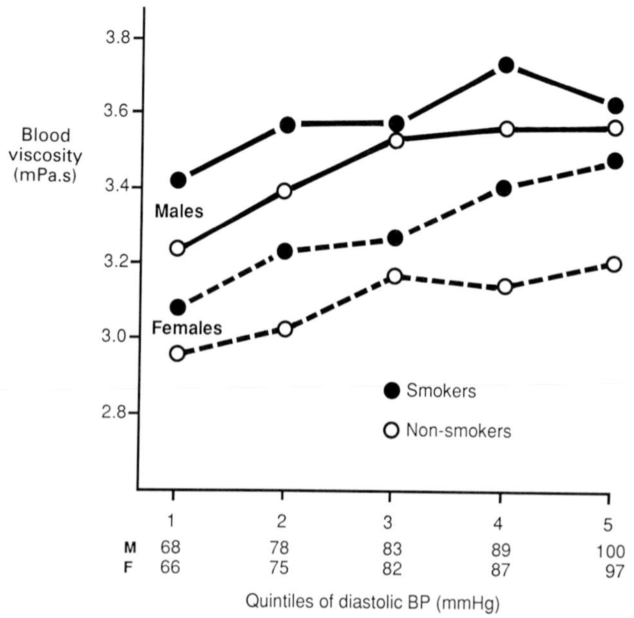

Fig. 51.4 Mean levels of high-shear whole-blood viscosity by quintiles of diastolic blood pressure, in male and female current smokers and non-smokers. Note additive effects of male sex and of cigarette smoking. Data from Glasgow MONICA Survey and Scottish Heart Health Study (Lowe et al 1988).

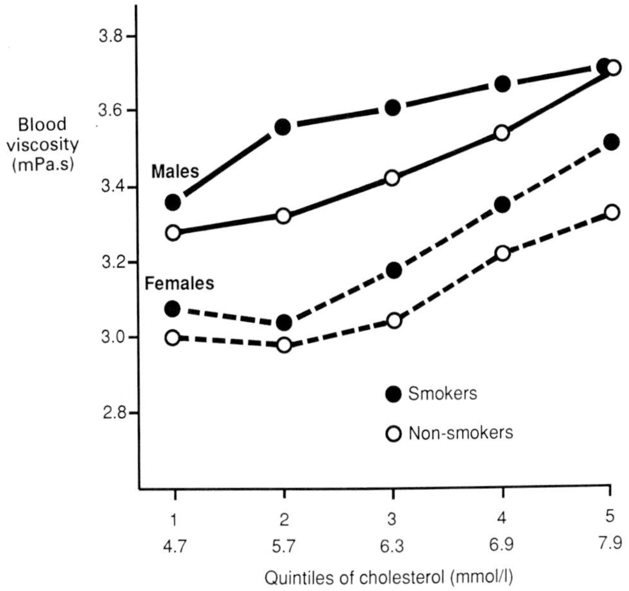

Fig. 51.5 Mean levels of high-shear whole-blood viscosity by quintiles of serum total cholesterol, in male and female current smokers and non-smokers. Note additive effects of male sex and of cigarette smoking. Data from First Glasgow MONICA Survey and Scottish Heart Health Study (Lowe et al 1988).

Bamford & Warlow 1992). Figure 51.5 shows that cholesterol, cigarette-smoking and male sex also have additive effects on high-shear blood viscosity in a population sample (Lowe et al 1988). In part, this association of cholesterol with blood viscosity is due to an association of cholesterol with haematocrit (Lowe et al 1982, 1988) and in part it is due to a direct effect of its carrier lipoproteins — low density lipoprotein (LDL) and very low density lipoprotein (VLDL) — on plasma and serum viscosity as shown by in vitro studies (Leonhardt et al 1977, Seplowitz et al 1981, Tait 1992). Five population studies have now shown independent, positive correlations of plasma viscosity with cholesterol (Lowe et al 1988, 1991, Yarnell et al 1991, Jung et al 1992, Koenig et al 1992) which are in keeping with these in vitro results and with the results of case-control studies of primary (Lowe et al 1983) and secondary (McGinley et al 1983, McRury et al 1992) hyperlipoproteinaemia. Two population studies found an inverse correlation of plasma viscosity with high density lipoprotein cholesterol (Jung et al 1992, Koenig et al 1992) which may be partly due to the inverse association of HDL cholesterol with triglyceride, which is also associated with increased plasma viscosity through its carrier protein, VLDL (Seplowitz et al 1981, Lowe et al 1991, Jung et al 1992).

High triglyceride and VLDL levels (and low HDL cholesterol levels) are also associated with increased red cell aggregation (measured by photometry) in the general population (Lowe et al 1992) and in a diabetic population (McRury et al 1993). Increased red cell aggregation has also been shown in hyperlipoproteinaemic patients, as measured by the ESR (Bottiger et al 1973) or by low-shear viscometry (Lowe et al 1982). In vitro studies have shown that VLDL and LDL directly increase red cell aggregation (Tait 1992).

Studies of lipid-lowering drugs have shown reductions in plasma viscosity, blood viscosity and red cell aggregation which are similar to those predicted from correlations in population studies; however the situation is complicated because certain fibrates (clofibrate, fenofibrate, bezafibrate) reduce plasma fibrinogen levels, gemfibrozil increases fibrinogen levels, and cholestyramine, simvastatin and pravastatin appear to have little effect on fibrinogen levels (Dormandy et al 1974, Leschke et al 1988, Jay et al 1990, Branchi et al 1992). Whether or not the different effects of these drugs on fibrinogen levels and blood rheology are important in reduction of cardiovascular risk remains to be established.

Obesity and lack of exercise

These two cardiovascular risk factors (Shaper 1988) are also associated with increased blood viscosity. In population studies, body mass index was an independent association with blood viscosity, haematocrit, fibrinogen, plasma viscosity and red cell aggregation (Lowe et al 1988, 1992, Lee et al 1990). The mechanisms for these associations are not known; weight reduction by a low-calorie diet does not appear to normalize the haemorheological abnormalities (Craveri et al 1990, 1992). These rheological abnormalities are also greater in sedentary men than in athletes (Ernst et al 1985a) and are reduced by regular exercise in volunteers (Ernst et al 1985b) and in claudicants (Ernst & Matrai 1987b).

Diabetes mellitus

In population studies, diabetes is associated with increases in plasma fibrinogen (Kannel et al 1990, Lee et al 1993b), and blood glucose with increased red cell aggregation (Lowe et al 1992). Large case-control studies of diabetics have confirmed increases in plasma viscosity and in red cell aggregation (measured by low-shear viscometry, photometry or ESR), which partly reflect increases in fibrinogen, other acute-phase proteins such as α_2-macroglobulin, and triglyceride/VLDL (McRury & Lowe 1990, McRury et al 1993). Decreased red cell deformability has been observed in some studies, but not in others, possibly due to variations in methodology and in case selection. Sensitive filtration methods have shown a small decrease in red cell deformability in diabetics, partly due to increased internal viscosity (MCHC) and partly due to change in red cell membrane composition (McRury & Lowe 1990, McRury et al 1990).

In general, the rheological abnormalities in diabetics appear to be related to both poor diabetic control and to vascular complications (McRury & Lowe 1990). Complications (both microvascular and macrovascular) are particularly common in diabetics who are hypertensive (Kannel 1991); it is therefore of interest that rheological abnormalities are greater in hypertensive diabetics than in non-hypertensive diabetics (McRury et al 1988, 1992, Rampling et al 1989).

Pregnancy

During pregnancy, an increase in plasma volume results in a fall in haematocrit, which usually outweighs progressive increases in fibrinogen, immunoglobulins and plasma viscosity, and which prevents increases in whole-blood viscosity and red cell aggregation. Failure of this normal haemodilution, and increased plasma protein changes, are associated with pregnancy hypertension and with placental insufficiency (Lowe 1992).

Diurnal and seasonal variations

The risk of myocardial infarction and stroke is highest in the early morning, at which time levels of haematocrit, fibrinogen, red cell aggregation and plasma viscosity are also highest (Lowe 1987a, Lowe et al 1992). The highest seasonal risk of cardiovascular events is in the colder winter months: increases in plasma viscosity and fibrinogen have been described at this time in elderly people (Stout & Crawford 1991), while several haemorheological changes occur in young volunteers following surface cooling (Keatinge et al 1984).

International variations

Plasma fibrinogen levels are higher in Caucasians than in the Chinese (Iso et al 1989), consistent with their higher risk of thrombotic cardiovascular disease. While there are no formal comparisons of other rheological variables, plasma viscosity appears higher in United Kingdom population samples (Lowe et al 1988, 1991, Yarnell et al 1991) than in German population samples (Jung et al 1992, Koenig et al 1992), consistent with international differences in cardiovascular risk. The lower haematocrit in persons in underdeveloped countries (due to infection, infestation and malnutrition) may also be relevant to their lower cardiovascular risk.

Primary prediction of arterial disease

Several population studies have associated increasing haematocrit (or the closely-related haemoglobin concentration) with increased risk of ischaemic heart disease, stroke, or total cardiovascular events (Heyman et al 1971, Kannel et al 1972, Elwood et al 1974, Bottiger & Carlson 1980, Kagan et al 1980, Sorlie et al 1981, Carter et al 1983, Kannel & McGhee 1984, Schatzkin et al 1984, Campbell et al 1985). In some of these studies, the effect of haematocrit (or haemoglobin level) could be accounted for by other risk factors such as smoking and blood pressure. Only the largest study (of 3-year mortality in 16 881 women aged under 65 years) displayed the data such that relative risk could be quantitated (Elwood et al 1974). Mortality was lowest (1%) at haematocrits of 38–42%, rising exponentially to relative risks of 1.5, 3.4, 4.2 and 5.8 at haematocrits of 45%, 47%, 49% and 51% respectively. In a follow-up of a cohort of 858 post-menopausal women from this study without baseline ischaemic heart disease, a haematocrit over 45% was a significant independent predictor of ischaemic heart disease mortality (Campbell et al 1985). These results are consistent with the exponential risk of thrombotic events with linear increase in haematocrit above 45% in treated patients with primary polycythaemia (Pearson & Wetherley-Mein 1978, Pearson 1987); and may reflect the exponential increases in whole-blood viscosity with linear increase in haematocrit, or increases in platelet adhesion or aggregation (Lowe 1987b, Pearson 1987).

Several other prospective studies have associated increasing white cell count with increased risk of ischaemic heart disease or stroke (Friedman et al 1974, Zalokhar et al 1981, Prentice et al 1982a,b, Grimm et al 1985, Yarnell et al 1991, Mänttäri et al 1992), which in general was not explained by a confounding effect of smoking.

Plasma fibrinogen levels are also independent predictors of ischaemic heart disease or stroke (Meade et al 1980, 1986, Wilhelmsen et al 1984, Stone & Thorp 1985, Balleisen et al 1987, Kannel et al 1987a,b, Yarnell et al 1991). In part, this may explain the predictive value of the ESR (Bottiger & Carlson 1980) or plasma viscosity (Yarnell et al 1991). However in the Caerphilly and Speedwell Studies, plasma viscosity was a rather better predictor of ischaemic heart disease than fibrinogen (Yarnell et al 1991); and other acute-phase proteins such as α_2-macroglobulin (another determinant of plasma viscosity: Lowe et al 1991, Jung et al 1992) and α_1-antitrypsin were also predictive of ischaemic heart disease (Elwood et al 1992). It is therefore possible that plasma viscosity is a more comprehensive marker than fibrinogen of a generalized protein disturbance in arterial disease (Stuart et al 1981) as well as of hyperlipoproteinaemia; and/or that increased levels of all these plasma proteins may promote ischaemic heart disease through rheological effects.

Prediction of outcome of arterial disease

Haematocrit levels do not appear to predict the outcome of acute myocardial infarction (Hershberg et al 1972), nor to predict recurrence in survivors (Schlant et al 1982,

Lowe et al 1985, Martin et al 1991). In contrast, white cell count, fibrinogen and plasma viscosity predict both acute outcome (Haines et al 1983, Maisel et al 1985) and recurrence (Schlant et al 1982, Kostis et al 1984, Lowe et al 1985, Hamsten et al 1987, Martin et al 1991).

In patients with stroke, admission levels of blood viscosity, haematocrit, fibrinogen, plasma viscosity, red cell aggregation and white cell count were associated with mortality (Lowe et al 1983, 1987a); while blood viscosity, fibrinogen, plasma viscosity and red cell aggregation were associated with recurrence (Ernst et al 1991, Resch et al 1992).

In patients with peripheral arterial disease, blood viscosity and fibrinogen levels have been associated with deterioration in walking distance (Dormandy et al 1973); white cell count with cardiovascular events (Dormandy & Murray 1991); and haematocrit and fibrinogen levels with graft occlusion (Matrai & Kollar 1987, Wiseman et al 1989).

BLOOD RHEOLOGY IN THE PATHOGENESIS OF ISCHAEMIC DISEASES

If rheological variables are associated with most cardiovascular risk factors in epidemiological studies and are also predictive of ischaemic events, their outcome and their recurrence, it is possible that they may play a role in pathogenesis of such events. This might occur through effects on atherogenesis, thrombogenesis, or on ischaemia distal to atherothrombotic stenoses (Lowe 1986). The attraction of rheological factors in pathogenesis is that they may explain the localization of these processes, which systemic risk factors do not. The late Tony Mitchell (Mitchell 1976) pointed out that 'we must avoid confusion between markers which can predict the risk of clinical events such as myocardial or cerebral infarction, and factors which actually cause vessel wall lesions. Many so-called risk factors such as smoking, hypertension and hyperlipidaemia are systemic problems, whereas the striking feature of arterial plaques is their focal distribution. The carotid sinus is a severely affected segment, yet one centimetre distally the internal carotid, perfused by the same lipid-laden, carbon monoxide containing, high pressure blood is virtually disease free.' (see Fig. 51.2).

Rheology and atherogenesis

Atherogenesis is therefore a focal disease, occurring at arterial bends and bifurcations (e.g. the carotid bifurcation) where flow separation results in areas of low-flow, low-shear recirculation of blood cells and proteins in contact with the vessel wall (Fox & Hugh 1976, Zarins et al 1983, Motomiya & Karino 1984, Ku et al 1985, Karino & Goldsmith 1987) (Fig. 51.2). Under such flow conditions, increased levels of haematocrit and fibrinogen may promote red cell aggregation and local increases in viscosity, local platelet adhesion and aggregation, local leucocyte adhesion and infiltration, and infiltration of fibrinogen and lipoproteins into the arterial wall (Lowe 1986, Lowe & Forbes 1988). Blood viscosity, haematocrit, plasma viscosity and fibrinogen levels have been correlated with the extent of coronary artery disease at angiography (Lowe et al 1980d, Kostis et al 1984, Low et al 1985), and with the extent of peripheral arterial disease (measured by ankle-brachial pressure index) in a population study (Lowe et al 1993). In another population study, fibrinogen levels correlated with the presence of carotid atherosclerosis, measured by B-mode ultrasound (Wu et al 1992).

Rheology and thrombogenesis

The effects of shear stress, haematocrit and fibrinogen on platelet adhesion and aggregation have been noted previously; as have the associations of plasma viscosity and fibrinogen with an imbalance of blood coagulation over fibrinolysis, as measured by activation markers (Lowe et al 1991). Rheological effects on thrombogenesis may be most marked at arterial stenoses, where the majority of arterial thrombi occur (Fig. 51.3). Condensation of flow streamlines through the stenosis increases local shear stresses and may initiate plaque fissuring and the formation of the initial, platelet-rich thrombus; while distal to the stenosis, flow separation results in areas of low shear stress which may favour the secondary, red-cell-rich fibrin thrombus (Schmid-Schönbein 1983, Davies 1989) (Fig. 51.3). Increased levels of haematocrit, fibrinogen and blood viscosity may favour both types of thrombus: by increasing shear stresses on cells and proteins flowing through the stenosis; and then by promoting red cell aggregation and local viscosity increases in the low-shear, post-stenotic area which might promote interactions of high-shear-activated platelets, leucocytes and coagulant enzymes. Consistent with this hypothesis, patients with acute myocardial infarction (who have occlusive arterial thrombi: Davies 1989) had significantly higher levels of blood viscosity, haematocrit, plasma viscosity and fibrinogen than patients with acute unstable angina (who have non-occlusive arterial thrombi: Davies 1989) (Lowe et al 1987b, Douglas et al 1989). Furthermore, patients with unstable angina who developed myocardial infarction had higher levels of haematocrit, plasma viscosity, fibrinogen and red cell aggregation than those who did not (Fuchs et al 1990, Neumann et al 1991).

Rheology and acute ischaemia

The predictive value of rheological variables for myocardial infarction and thrombotic stroke, their outcome, and their recurrence may reflect their effects in promoting acute ischaemia and infarction by reducing microcirculatory blood flow, as well as effects on atherogenesis or thrombogenesis. The elevations in haematocrit, white cell count, fibrinogen and plasma viscosity in patients with acute infarction may be partly consequences of infarction (haemoconcentration from catecholamine release or dehydration, acute-phase leucocytosis and protein synthesis), but may also reduce microcirculatory blood flow and promote ischaemia and infarction. Distal to atherothrombotic stenoses, fall in perfusion pressure may result in haemoconcentration, plugging of capillaries by leucocytes and rigid red cells (due to local hypoxia, acidosis and hyperosmolarity), and red cell aggregation with leucocyte margination in venules (Lowe & Forbes 1988, Schmid-Schönbein 1988).

Experimental studies of infarction have shown reduction in microcirculatory stasis, or myocardial or cerebral infarct size by haemodilution, leucocyte depletion, or inhibition of leucocyte adhesion (Lowe & Forbes 1988, Schmid-Schönbein 1988, Mori et al 1992). In clinical trials, the results of haemodilution with dextran in acute stroke have been disappointing; it should be noted that the reduction in haematocrit by dextran may be outweighed by increased plasma viscosity, as well as haemodynamic upset unless patients are haemodynamically monitored. A recent study of haemodilution in acute ischaemic stroke with albumin and crystalloids, tailored according to the individual patient's haematocrit, hydration and haemodynamic state, has shown better results than 'blind' dextran therapy (Goslinga et al 1992).

Thrombolytic therapy in acute myocardial infarction restores myocardial perfusion and reduces infarct size and mortality not only by lysing coronary thrombi, but also by acute reduction in plasma fibrinogen level and hence reduction in plasma and blood viscosity and red cell aggregation. Streptokinase causes a greater reduction in plasma and blood viscosity than does tissue plasminogen activator (t-PA) infusion, due to a greater fall in fibrinogen levels as well as generation of lower molecular weight fibrin(ogen) degradation products (Moriarty et al 1988, Douglas et al 1989, and personal unpublished observations). This rheological advantage may explain why streptokinase is as effective in reducing mortality as t-PA, despite a lower initial angiographic coronary patency rate (ISIS-3 Collaborative Group 1992). Viscosity reduction may be beneficial in acute myocardial infarction not only by increasing myocardial perfusion; but also by increasing peripheral perfusion and reducing cardiac workload (Lowe & Forbes 1988).

Rheology and chronic ischaemia

It has been suggested that intermittent claudication and angina pectoris may reflect reduction in muscle blood flow by increased blood viscosity, as well as by arterial stenoses (Dormandy et al 1973, Nicolaides et al 1977, Dormandy 1981). In the Edinburgh Artery Study, the effect of rheological variables on leg ischaemia was assessed after standardization for the degree of arterial stenoses in the lower limbs (measured by the ankle-brachial pressure index). The relative risk of claudication increased with plasma viscosity, being 3.3 for the top viscosity quintile relative to the bottom quintile (Lowe et al 1993). It is likely that this is a direct effect of viscosity on post-stenotic ischaemia. Exercise (Ernst & Matrai 1987b), stopping smoking (Ernst & Matrai 1987a) and some rheologically active drugs (Lowe 1989, 1990a,b) all reduce viscosity and increase walking distance in claudicants: effects which are quite consistent with the relationship between plasma viscosity and claudication in the older population (Lowe et al 1993). In the same study, asymptomatic leg ischaemia (post-occlusion hyperaemia) was associated with neutrophil elastase levels, suggesting a role for active leucocytes in occlusion of the nutritive microcirculation (Lowe et al 1993). Such an effect is consistent with exercise-induced leucocyte activation in claudication (Ciuffetti et al 1989, Neumann et al 1990) and with the effects of pentoxyfylline, which reduces neutrophil activation and increases walking distance in claudication (Schmalzer & Chien 1984, Lowe 1990b). Patients with critical limb ischaemia (rest pain and skin necrosis) have even higher levels of rheological abnormalities, which may be of pathogenetic importance (Lowe 1990c).

RHEOLOGY AND VENOUS THROMBOEMBOLISM

Deep vein thrombosis usually originates in venous valve pockets, where flow separation occurs resulting in recirculating vortices where low shear stress encourages cellular aggregation (Karino & Motomiya 1984) (Fig. 51.6). Such areas may act as 'in vivo aggregometers' in which interaction of systemically activated platelets, leucocytes and coagulant enzymes results in bursts of platelet aggregation, followed by conversion of red cell aggregates into red cell-fibrin masses. Progressive flow disturbance and blood activation could then result in self-propagation of thrombi in the initial layered, white/red thrombus pattern observed at necropsy, and then up the low-flow, low-shear large veins in immobile patients (Lowe 1984). These processes could be favoured by the systemic rheological disturbances associated with risk factors for venous thromboembolism such as age, male sex, oestrogen therapy, obesity, trauma, surgery, malignancy, infection, infarction and polycythaemia (Lowe 1984). A recent case-control study of 101 patients with previous (mean 8 years) spontaneous, venogram-proven deep vein thrombosis found significantly higher levels of whole-blood viscosity,

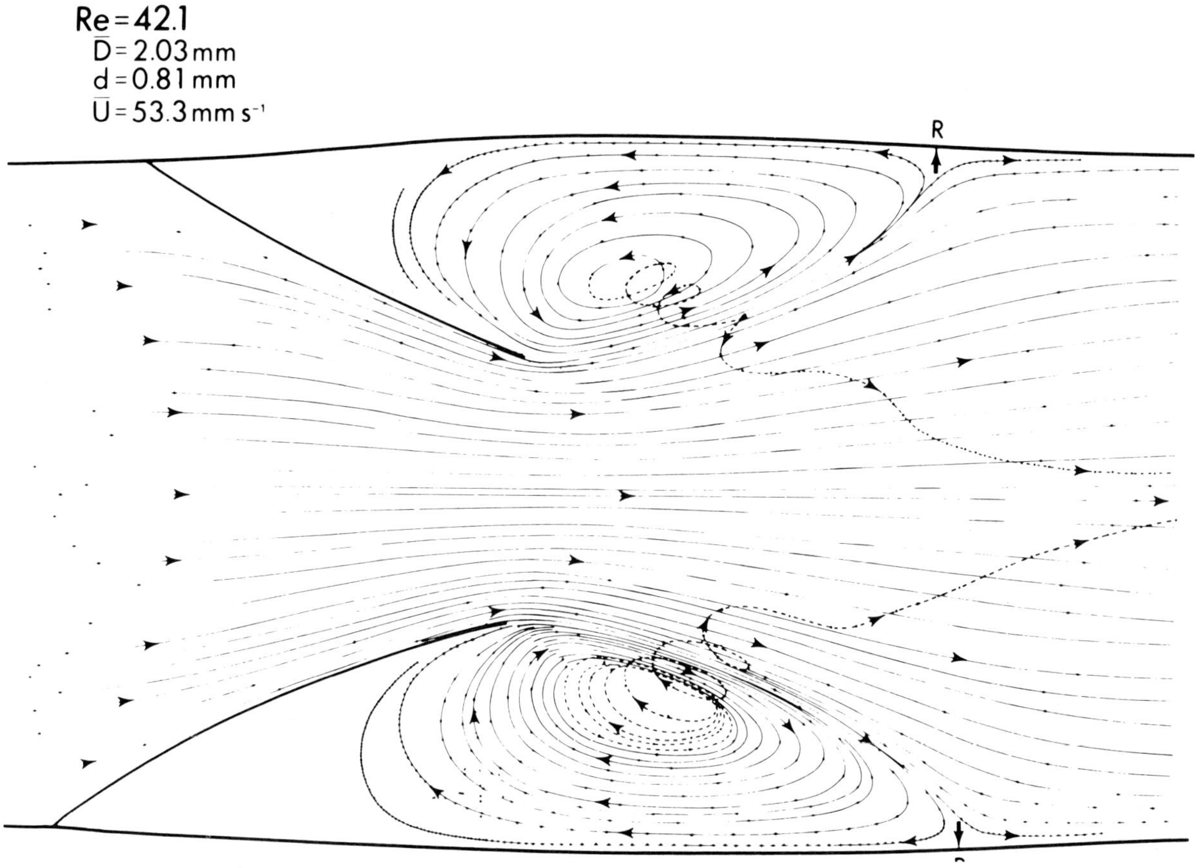

Fig. 51.6 Detailed flow patterns in the common bisector plane of the valve leaflets in a 2 mm diameter dog saphenous vein containing a bileaflet valve, showing the formation of a spiral vortex in each valve pocket. The arrows at R indicate the location of the reattachment point (after Karino & Motomiya 1984, with permission).

haematocrit, plasma viscosity, red cell aggregation and fibrinogen in the cases: multivariate analysis showed that plasma viscosity and fibrinogen remained as significant associations with thrombosis (Balendra et al 1991).

Viscosity reduction by defibrination with ancrod (Lowe et al 1978b) or by haemodilution with dextran (Vara-Thorbeck & Rosell 1988) have been shown in controlled trials to reduce significantly the incidence and extent of deep vein thrombosis in patients following hip surgery. As in acute myocardial infarction, the benefits of thrombolytic therapy in deep vein thrombosis and pulmonary embolism may reflect not only lysis of thrombi, but also reduction in fibrinogen and viscosity levels and hence increased blood flow in the legs and lungs.

Retinal blood flow disturbance is regularly observed in hyperviscosity syndromes; and increased blood viscosity has been described in patients with retinal vein thrombosis and associated with its sequel of proliferative ischaemic retinopathy. Viscosity reduction with haemodilution or stanozolol appeared to reduce the incidence of visual complications (Lowe & Foulds 1988).

RHEOLOGY AND CARDIAC THROMBOEMBOLISM

Rheological factors also appear important in pathogenesis of atrial thrombosis (which occurs in low-shear areas in dilated, fibrillating atria), valvular thrombosis (which is favoured by high-shear stresses through the valve followed by areas of flow separation), and left ventricular mural thrombosis (which occurs when endothelial damage occurs in areas of reduced contractility with flow separation) (Butchart & Bodnar 1992).

REFERENCES

Aarts P A M M, Bolhus P A, Sakariassen K S , Heethar R M, Sixma J J 1983 Red blood cell size is important for adherence of blood platelets to artery subendothelium. Blood 62: 214–217

Aarts P A M M, Heethar R M, Sixma J J 1984 Red blood cell deformability influences platelets–vessel wall interaction in flowing blood. Blood 64: 1228–1233

Alderman M J, Ridge A, Morley A A, Ryall R G, Walsh J A 1981 Effect of total leucocyte count on whole blood filterability in patients with peripheral vascular disease. Journal of Clinical Pathology 34: 163–166

Allen D R, Browse N L, Rutt D L, Butler L, Fletcher C 1988 The effect of cigarette smoke, nicotine and carbon monoxide on the permeability of the arterial wall. Journal of Vascular Surgery 7: 139–152

Anderson G H, Hellums J D, Moake J, Alfrey C P Jr 1987 Platelet response to shear stress: changes in platelet uptake, serotonin release, and ADP-induced platelet aggregation. Thrombosis Research 13: 1039–1042

Anderson F A, Wheeler H B, Goldberg R J et al 1991 A population-based perspective of the hospital incidence and case-fatality rates of deep vein thrombosis and pulmonary embolism. The Worcester DVT Study. Archives of Internal Medicine 151: 933–938

Bagge U 1984 Leukocytes and capillary perfusion in shock. In: Meiselman H J, Lichtman M A, LaCelle P L (eds) White cell mechanics: basic science and clinical aspects. Liss, New York, p 285–294

Balendra R, Rumley A, Orr M, Lennie S E, McColl P, Lowe G D O 1991 Blood lipids, coagulation, fibrinolysis and rheology in spontaneous proven deep vein thrombosis. British Journal of Haematology 77 (suppl 1): 83

Balleisen L, Schulte H, Assmann G, Epping P H, van de Loo J 1987 Coagulation factors and the progress of coronary heart disease. Lancet ii: 461

Bamford J, Warlow C P 1992 Stroke and T I A in the general population. In: Butchart E G, Bodnar E (eds) Current issues in heart valve disease: thrombosis, embolism and bleeding. I C R Publishers, London, p 3

Bonithon-Kopp C, Scarabin P Y, Malmejac A et al 1988. Menopause-related change in plasma viscosity. Clinical Hemorheology 8: 525–528

Bottiger L E, Carlson L A 1980 Risk factors for ischaemic vascular death for men in the Stockholm prospective study. Atherosclerosis 36: 389–408

Bottiger L E, Carlson L A, Ekelund L G, Olsson A C 1973 Raised E S R in asymptomatic hyperlipoproteinaemia. British Medical Journal ii: 681–684

Branchi A, Rovellini A, Gugliandolo A G, Sommariva D, Fasoli A 1992 Comparative evaluation of the effect of 3 fibrates and of 2 HMG-CoA reductase inhibitors on plasma fibrinogen in hypercholesterolemic patients. In: Ernst E, Koenig W, Lowe G D O, Meade T W (eds) Fibrinogen: a new cardiovascular risk factor. Blackwell M Z V, Vienna, p 362

Burgess-Wilson M E, Green S, Heptinstall S, Mitchell J R A 1984 Spontaneous platelet aggregation in whole blood: dependence on age and haematocrit. Lancet ii: 1213

Butchart E G, Bodnar E (eds) 1992 Current issues in heart valve disease: thrombosis, embolism and bleeding, ICR Publishers, London

Campbell M J, Elwood P C, Mackean J, Waters W E 1985 Mortality, haemoglobin level and haematocrit in women. Journal of Chronic Diseases 38: 881–889

Carter C, McGee D, Reed D, Yano K, Stemmermann G 1983 Hematocrit and the risk of coronary heart disease: the Honolulu Heart Program. American Heart Journal 105: 674–679

Chabanel A, Klaren J, Andreu G, Samama M 1992 In spite of elevated plasma fibrinogen, red blood cell aggregation is not increased in smokers. Clinical Hemorheology 12: 455–460

Chien S 1975 Biophysical behavior of red cells in suspensions. In: Surgenor D M (ed) The red blood cell. Academic Press. New York, p 1031

Chien S 1988 White blood cell rheology. In: Lowe G D O (ed) Clinical blood rheology. CRC Press, Boca Raton, vol 1: 87

Chien S, Schmid-Schönbein G W, Sung K L P, Schmalzer E A, Skalak R 1984 Viscoelastic properties of leukocytes. In: Meiselman H J, Lichtman M A, LaCelle P L (eds) White cell mechanics: basic science and clinical aspects. Liss, New York, p 19–51

Chien S, Dormandy J, Ernst E, Matrai A (eds) 1987 Clinical hemorheology. Nijhoff, Dordrecht

Ciuffetti G, Mercuri M, Mannarino E, Robinson M K, Lennie S E, Lowe G D O 1989 Peripheral vascular disease: rheologic variables during controlled ischemia. Circulation 80: 348–352

Craveri A, Tornaghi G, Paganardi L, Ranieri R, Giavardi L 1990 Weight loss does not affect the hemorheological and fibrinolytic changes in obesity. Clinical Hemorheology 10: 903–908

Craveri A, Tornaghi G, Paganardi L et al 1992 Hemorheological changes in obese children and the effect of weight loss. Clinical Hemorheology 12: 573–578

Davies M J 1989 Thrombosis and coronary atherosclerosis. In: Julian D, Kübler W, Norris R M, Swan H J C, Collen D, Verstraete M (eds) Thrombolysis in cardiovascular disease. Dekker, Basel, p 25

Devereaux R B, Drayer J I M, Chien S et al 1984 Whole blood viscosity as a determinant of cardiac hypertrophy in systemic hypertension. American Journal of Cardiology 54: 592–595

Diamond S L, Eskin S G, McIntire L V 1989 Fluid flow stimulates tissue plasminogen activator secretion by cultured human endothelial cells. Science 243: 1483–1485

Diamond S L, Sharefkin J B, Dieffenbach C, Frasier Scott K, McIntire L V, Eskin S G 1990 Tissue plasminogen activator messenger RNA levels increase in cultured human endothelial cells exposed to laminar shear stress. Journal of Cell Physiology 143: 364–371

Dintenfass L 1971 Blood microrheology — viscosity factors in blood flow, ischaemia and thrombosis. Butterworth, London

Dormandy J A 1981 Haemorheology and thrombosis. In: Bloom A L, Thomas D P (eds) Haemostasis and thrombosis, 1st edn. Churchill Livingstone, London, p 610

Dormandy J A, Murray D G 1991 The fate of the claudicant — a prospective study of 1969 claudicants. European Journal of Vascular Surgery 5: 131–133

Dormandy J A, Hoare E, Khattab A H, Arrowsmith D E, Dormandy T L 1973 Prognostic significance of rheological and biochemical findings in patients with intermittent claudication. British Medical Journal iv: 581–583

Dormandy J A, Gutteridge J M C, Hoare E, Dormandy T L 1974 Effect of clofibrate on blood viscosity in intermittent claudication. British Medical Journal iv: 259–262

Douglas J T, Lowe G D O, Hillis W S, Rao R, Hogg K J, Gemmell J D 1989 Blood and plasma hyperviscosity in acute myocardial infarction compared to unstable angina: rapid reversal by thrombolysis. Thrombosis and Haemostasis 62: 590

Drost E M, Selby C, Lannan S, Lowe G D O, McNee W 1992 Changes in neutrophil deformability following in vitro smoke exposure: mechanism and protection. American Journal of Respiratory Cell and Molecular Biology 6: 287–95

Duke W W 1910 The relation of blood platelets to hemorrhagic disease. Journal of the American Medical Association 60: 1185–86

Elwood P C, Benjamin I T, Waters W E, Sweetnam P M 1974 Mortality and anaemia in women. Lancet i: 891–894

Elwood P C, Yarnell J W G, Sweetnam P M, O'Brien J R 1992 Plasma viscosity and fibrinogen in the Caerphilly and Speedwell studies. Clinical Hemorheology 12: 545–548

Ernst E, Matrai A 1987a Abstention from chronic smoking normalizes blood rheology. Arteriosclerosis 64: 75–77

Ernst E, Matrai A 1987b Intermittent claudication, exercise and blood rheology. Circulation 76: 1110–1114

Ernst E, Matrai A, Dormandy J A 1984 Shear dependence of blood coagulation. Clinical Hemorheology 4: 395–399

Ernst E, Matrai A, Aschenbrenner E 1985a Blood rheology in athletes. Journal of Sports Medicine and Physical Fitness 25: 207–210

Ernst E, Schmid M, Matrai A 1985b Intraindividual changes of hemorheological and other variables by regular exercise. International Journal of Sports Cardiology 2: 50–54

Ernst E, Hammerschmidt D E, Bagge U, Matrai A, Dormandy J A 1987 Leukocytes and the risk of ischemic diseases. Journal of the American Medical Association 257: 2318–2324

Ernst E, Resch K L, Matrai A, Buhl M, Schlosser P, Paulsen H F 1991 Impaired blood rheology: a risk factor after stroke? Journal of Internal Medicine 229: 457–462

Feher M D, Rampling M W, Brown J et al 1990 Acute changes in atherogenic and thrombogenic factors with cessation of smoking. Journal of the Royal Society of Medicine 83: 146–148

Fowkes F G R (ed) 1991 Epidemiology of peripheral vascular disease. Springer, London
Fowkes F G R, Lowe G D O, Rumley A, Lennie S E, Smith F B, Donnan P T 1993 Relation of blood viscosity to blood pressure in a random sample of the population aged 55 to 74 years. European Heart Journal (in press)
Fox J A, Hugh A E 1976 Static zones in the internal carotid artery: correlation with boundary layer separation and stasis in model flows. British Journal of Radiology 43: 370–383
Friedman G D, Klatsky A L, Siegelaub A B 1974 The leukocyte count as a predictor of myocardial infarction. New England Journal of Medicine 290: 1275–1278
Fuchs J, Pinhas A, Davidson E, Rotenberg Z, Agmon J, Weinburger I 1990 Plasma viscosity, fibrinogen and haematocrit in the course of unstable angina. European Heart Journal 11: 1029–1032
Gemmell C H, Turitto V T, Nemerson Y 1988 Flow as a regulator of the activation of factor X by tissue factor. Blood 72: 1404–1406
Gemmell C H, Nemerson Y, Turitto V T 1990 The effects of shear rate on the enzymatic activity of the tissue factor-factor VIIa complex. Microvascular Research 40: 327–340
Goldsmith H L, Turitto V T 1986 Rheological aspects of thrombosis and haemostasis: basic principles and applications. Thrombosis and Haemostasis 55: 415–435
Goslinga H, Eijzenbach V J, Heuvelmans J H A et al 1992 Custom-tailored hemodilution with albumin and crystalloids in acute ischemic stroke. Stroke 23: 181–188
Grimm R H, Neaton J D, Ludwig W 1985 Prognostic importance of the white blood cell count for coronary, cancer and all-cause mortality. Journal of the American Medical Association 254: 1932–1937
Haines A P, Howarth D, North W R S et al 1983 Haemostatic variables and the outcome of myocardial infarction. Thrombosis and Haemostasis 50: 800–803
Hamsten A, DeFaire U, Walldius G et al 1987 Plasminogen activator inhibitor in plasma: risk factor for recurrent myocardial infarction. Lancet ii: 3–8
Hellem A J, Borchgrevink C F, Ames S B 1961 The role of red cells in haemostasis: the relation between haematocrit, bleeding time and platelet adhesiveness. British Journal of Haematology 7: 42–50
Helman N, Rubenstein L S 1975 The effects of age, sex and smoking on erythrocytes and leukocytes. American Journal of Clinical Pathology 63: 35–44
Hershberg P I, Wells R E, McGandy R B 1972 Hematocrit and prognosis in patients with acute myocardial infarction. Journal of the American Medical Association 219: 355–360
Heyman A, Karp H R, Heyden S et al 1971 Cerebrovascular disease in the biracial population of Evans County, Georgia. Archives of Internal Medicine 128: 949–955
Hilton P J 1986 Cellular sodium transport in essential hypertension. New England Journal of Medicine 314: 222–229
International Committee for Standardisation in Haematology (Expert Panel on Blood Rheology) 1986 Guidelines for measurement of blood viscosity and cell deformability. Clinical Hemorheology 6: 439–453
International Committee for Standardisation in Haematology (Expert Panel on Blood Rheology) 1988 Guidelines on selection of laboratory tests for monitoring the acute phase response. Journal of Clinical Pathology 41: 1203–1212
ISIS-3 Collaborative Group 1992 ISIS-3: a randomised comparison of streptokinase vs tissue plasminogen activator vs anistreplase and of aspirin plus heparin vs aspirin alone among 41 299 cases of suspected acute myocardial infarction. Lancet 339: 753–776
Isles C D, Lowe G D O, Rankin B M et al 1984 Abnormal haemostasis and blood viscosity in malignant hypertension. Thrombosis and Haemostasis 52: 253–255
Iso H, Folsom A R, Wu K K et al 1989 Hemostatic variables in Japanese and Caucasian men. American Journal of Epidemiology 130: 925–934
Jay R H, Rampling M W, Betteridge D J 1990 Abnormalities of blood rheology in familial hypercholesterolaemia: effects of treatment. Atherosclerosis 85: 249–256
Jen C J, McIntire L V 1984 Characteristics of shear-induced aggregation in whole blood. Journal of Laboratory and Clinical Medicine 103: 115–124
Jung F, Pindur G, Kiesewetter H 1992 Plasma viscosity dependence on proteins and lipoproteins: results of the Aachen study. Clinical Hemorheology 12: 557–571
Kagan A, Popper G S, Rhoads G G 1980 Factors related to stroke incidence in Hawaii Japanese men: the Honolulu Heart Study. Stroke 11: 14–21
Kannel W B 1991 Epidemiology of essential hypertension: the Framingham experience. Proceedings of the Royal College of Physicians of Edinburgh 21: 273–287
Kannel W B, McGhee D L 1984 Update on some epidemiological features of intermittent claudication. Journal of the American Geriatric Society 33: 13-18
Kannel W B, Gordon T, Wolf P A, McNamara P 1972 Hemoglobin and the risk of cerebral infarction: the Framingham Study. Stroke 3: 409–420
Kannel W B, D'Agostino R B, Belanger A J 1987a Fibrinogen, cigarette-smoking, and risk of cardiovascular disease: insights from the Framingham Study. American Heart Journal 113: 1006–1010
Kannel W B, Wolf P A, Castelli W P, D'Agostino R B 1987b Fibrinogen and risk of cardiovascular disease. Journal of the American Medical Association 258: 1183–1186
Kannel W B, D'Agostino R B, Wilson P W F, Belanger A J, Gagnon D R 1990 Diabetes, fibrinogen and the risk of cardiovascular disease: the Framingham experience. American Heart Journal 120: 672–676
Karino T, Goldsmith H L 1987 Rheological factors in thrombosis and haemostasis. In: Bloom A L, Thomas D P (eds) Haemostasis and thrombosis, 2nd edn. Churchill Livingstone, Edinburgh, p 739
Karino T, Motomiya M 1984 Flow through a venous valve and its implication for thrombus formation. Thrombosis Research 36: 245–257
Keatinge W R, Coleshaw S R K, Cotter F et al 1984 Increases in platelet and red cell counts, blood viscosity, and arterial pressure during mild surface cooling: factors in mortality from coronary and cerebral thrombosis in winter. British Medical Journal 289: 1405–1408
Koenig W, Sund M, Ernst E, Matrai A, Keil U, Rosenthal J 1989 Is increased plasma viscosity a risk factor for high blood pressure? Angiology 40: 153–163
Koenig W, Sund M, Ernst E, Keil U, Rosenthal J, Hombach V 1992 Association between plasma viscosity and blood pressure. Results from the MONICA-Project Augsberg. American Journal of Hypertension 4: 529–536
Koenig W, Sund M, Ernst E, Mraz W, Hombach V, Keil U 1992 Association between rheology and components of lipoproteins in human blood. Circulation 85: 2197–2204
Kostis J B, Turkevich D, Sharp J 1984 Association between leukocyte count and the presence and extent of coronary atherosclerosis as determined by coronary angiography. American Journal of Cardiology 53: 997–999
Ku D N, Giddens D P, Zarins C K, Glagov S 1985 Pulsatile flow and arteriosclerosis in the human carotid bifurcation. Positive correlation between plaque location and low and oscillating shear stress. Arteriosclerosis 5: 293–302
Lee A J, Smith W C S, Lowe G D O, Tunstall-Pedoe H D 1990 Plasma fibrinogen and coronary risk factors: the Scottish Heart Health Study. Journal of Clinical Epidemiology 43: 913–919
Lee A J, Lowe G D O, Smith W C S, Tunstall-Pedoe H D 1993a Plasma fibrinogen in women: relationships with oral contraception, the menopause and hormone replacement therapy. British Journal of Haematology 83: 616–621
Lee A J, Lowe G D O, Woodward M, Tunstall-Pedoe H D 1993b Fibrinogen in relation to personal history of prevalent hypertension, diabetes, stroke, intermittent clandication, coronary heart disease, and family history: the Scottish Heart Health Study. British Heart Journal 69: 338–342
Lennie S E, Lowe G D O, Barbenel J C, Foulds W S, Forbes C D 1988 Filterability of white blood cell subpopulations, separated by an improved method. Clinical Hemorheology 8: 811–816
Lennie S E, Lowe G D O, Lannan S, Drost E, MacNee W 1989 Decreased leucocyte filterability after exposure to cigarette smoke. Clinical Hemorheology 9: 492

Leonhardt H, Arntz H R, Klemens U H 1977 Studies of plasma viscosity in primary hyperlipoproteinaemia. Atherosclerosis 28: 29–40
Leschke M, Höffken H, Schmidtsdorff A et al 1988 Einfluss von Fenofibrat auf Fibrinogen-konzentration und Blutfluidität. Deutsche Medizinische Wochenschrift 114: 939–944
Letcher R L, Chien S, Pickering T G, Sealey J E, Laragh J H 1981 Direct relationship between blood pressure and blood viscosity in normal and hypertensive subjects. American Journal of Medicine 70: 1195–1202
Levenson J, Simon A C, Cambien F A, Beretti C 1987 Cigarette smoking and hypertension: factors independently associated with blood hyperviscosity and arterial rigidity. Atherosclerosis 7: 572–577
Levesque M J, Nerem R M 1985 The elongation and orientation of cultured endothelial cells in response to shear stress. Journal of Biochemical Engineering 107: 341–347
Lewis S M 1982 The constituents of normal blood and bone marrow. In; Hardisty R M, Weatherall D J (eds) Blood and its disorders, 2nd edn. Blackwell Scientific, Oxford, p 3
Lichtman M A, Heal J, Rowe J M 1987 Hyperleukocytic leukaemia: rheological and clinical features and management. In: Baillière's clinical haematology. Vol 1: 725–746
Livio M, Gotti E, Marchesi D, Mecca G, Remuzzi K G, de Gaetano G 1982 Uraemic bleeding: role of anaemia and beneficial effect of red cell transfusions. Lancet ii: 1013–1015
Low J, Dodds A J, McGrath M, Biggs J C 1985 Red cell deformability and other haemorheological variables in stable coronary artery disease. Thrombosis Research 38: 269–276
Lowe G D O 1984 Blood rheology and venous thrombosis. Clinical Hemorheology 4: 571–588
Lowe G D O 1986 Blood rheology in arterial disease. Clinical Science 71: 137–146
Lowe G D O (ed) 1987a Blood rheology and hyperviscosity syndromes. In: Baillière's clinical haematology 1, vol 3: 597–861
Lowe G D O 1987b Thrombosis and hemorheology. In: Chien S, Dormandy J, Ernst E, Matrai A (eds) Clinical hemorheology. Nijhoff, Dordrecht, p 195
Lowe G D O (ed) 1988 Clinical blood rheology. C R C Press, Boca Raton, Florida
Lowe G D O 1990a Drugs in cerebral and peripheral arterial disease. British Medical Journal 300: 524–528
Lowe G D O 1990b Drugs that modify red blood cell characteristics. In: Fleming J S (ed) Drugs and the delivery of oxygen to tissue. CRC Press, Boca Raton, p 253
Lowe G D O 1990c Pathophysiology of critical limb ischaemia. In: Dormandy J A, Stock G (eds) Critical limb ischaemia: its pathophysiology and management. Springer, Berlin, p 17
Lowe G D O 1992 Blood rheology in pregnancy — physiology and pathology. In: Greer I A, Turpie A G G, Forbes C D (eds) Haemostasis and thrombosis in obstetrics and gynaecology. Chapman & Hall, London, p 27
Lowe G D O, Forbes C D 1988 Rheology of cardiovascular disease. In: Lowe G D O (ed): Clinical blood rheology. CRC Press, Boca Raton, vol 2: 113
Lowe G D O, Foulds W S 1988 Rheology of retinal disorders. In: Lowe G D O (ed). Clinical blood rheology. CRC Press, Boca Raton, Florida, vol 2: 189
Lowe G D O, Reavey M M, Johnston R V, Forbes C D, Prentice C R M 1978a Increased platelet aggregates in vascular and non-vascular illness – correlation with plasma fibrinogen and effect of ancrod. Thrombosis Research 14: 377–386
Lowe G D O, Campbell A F, Meek D R, Forbes C D, Prentice C R M, Cummings S W 1978b Subcutaneous ancrod in prevention of deep-vein thrombosis after operation for fractured neck of femur. Lancet ii: 698–700
Lowe G D O, Drummond M M, Forbes C D, Barbenel J C 1980a Increased blood viscosity in young women using oral contraceptives. American Journal of Obstetrics and Gynecology 137: 840–842
Lowe G D O, Drummond M M, Forbes C D, Barbenel J C 1980b The effects of age and cigarette-smoking on blood and plasma viscosity in men. Scottish Medical Journal 25: 13–17
Lowe G D O, Drummond M M, Forbes C D, Barbenel J C, Smith S 1980c Effects of cigarette-smoking on blood rheology. In: Stoltz J F, Drouin P (eds) Hemorheology and diseases. Doin, Paris, p 349
Lowe G D O, Drummond M M, Lorimer A R et al 1980d Relationship between extent of coronary artery disease and blood viscosity. British Medical Journal i: 673–674
Lowe G D O, McArdle B M, Stromberg P et al 1982 Increased blood viscosity and fibrinolytic inhibitor in type II hyperlipoproteinaemia. Lancet i: 472–475
Lowe G D O, Jaap A J, Forbes C D 1983 Relationship of atrial fibrillation and high haematocrit to mortality in acute stroke. Lancet i: 784–786
Lowe G D O, Machado S G, Krol W F, Barton B A, Forbes C D 1985 White blood cell count and haematocrit as predictors of coronary recurrence after myocardial infarction. Thrombosis and Haemostasis 54: 700–703
Lowe G D O, Anderson J, Barbenel J C, Forbes C D 1987a Prognostic importance of blood rheology in acute stroke. In: Hartmann A, Kuschinsky W (eds) Cerebral ischemia and hemorheology. Springer, Berlin, p 496
Lowe G D O, Thomson G, Lennie S, Anderson J, Cobbe S M, Forbes C D 1987b Comparison of blood, red cell and white cell rheology in unstable angina and acute myocardial infarction. Thrombosis and Haemostasis 58: 12
Lowe G D O, Smith W C S, Tunstall-Pedoe H et al 1988 Cardiovascular risk and haemorheology: results from the Scottish Heart Health Study and the MONICA-Project, Glasgow. Clinical Hemorheology 8: 518–524
Lowe G D O, Smith W C S, Lee A J et al 1989 Blood viscosity, coronary heart disease and coronary risk factors; the Scottish Heart Health Study. Clinical Hemorheology 9: 495
Lowe G D O, Wood D A, Douglas J T et al 1991 Relationships of plasma viscosity, coagulation and fibrinolysis to coronary risk factors and angina. Thrombosis and Haemostasis 65: 339–343
Lowe G D O, Lee A J, Rumley A, Smith W C S, Tunstall-Pedoe H 1992 Epidemiology of haematocrit, white cell count, red cell aggregation and fibrinogen: the Glasgow MONICA study. Clinical Hemorheology 12: 535–544
Lowe G D O, Fowkes F G R, Dawes J, Donnan P T, Lennie S E, Housley E 1993 Blood viscosity, fibrinogen, and activation of coagulation and leukocytes in peripheral arterial disease and the normal population in the Edinburgh Artery Study. Circulation 87 (in press)
McGinley E, Lowe G D O, Boulton-Jones M, Forbes C D, Prentice C R M 1983 Blood viscosity and haemostasis in the nephrotic syndrome. Thrombosis and Haemostasis 49: 155–157
McRury S M, Lowe G D O 1990 Blood rheology in diabetes mellitus. Diabetic Medicine 7: 285–291
McRury S M, Small M, MacCuish A C, Lowe G D O 1988 Association of hypertension with blood viscosity in diabetes. Diabetic Medicine 5: 830–834
McRury S M, Small M, Anderson J, MacCuish A C, Lowe G D O 1990 Evaluation of red cell deformability by a filtration method in type 1 and type 2 diabetes with and without vascular complications. Diabetes Research 13: 61–65
McRury S M, Lennie S E, McColl P, Balendra R, MacCuish A C, Lowe G D O 1993 Increased red cell aggregation in diabetes mellitus: association with cardiovascular risk factors. Diabetic Medicine 10: 21–26
Maisel A S, Gilpin A, LeWinter M et al 1985 Initial leukocyte count during acute myocardial infarction independently predicts early ventricular fibrillation. Circulation 72 (suppl 3): 414
Mänttäri M, Manninen V, Koskinen P et al 1992 Leukocytes as a coronary risk factor in a dyslipidemic male population. American Heart Journal 123: 873–877
Martin J F, Bath P M W, Burr M L 1991 Influence of platelet size on outcome after myocardial infarction. Lancet 338: 1409–1412
Matrai A, Kollar L 1987 Importance of the preoperative hemoglobin concentration in arterial surgery. European Surgical Research 19: 1–5
Matrai A, Whittington R B, Ernst E 1987 A simple method of estimating whole blood viscosity at standardized hematocrit. Clinical Hemorheology 7: 261–265
Mayer G A 1964 Blood viscosity in healthy subjects and patients with coronary heart disease. Canadian Medical Association Journal 93: 1151–1153
Meade T W, Chakrabarti R, Haines A P, North W R S, Stirling Y

1979 Characteristics affecting fibrinolytic activity and plasma fibrinogen concentrations. British Medical Journal i: 153–156
Meade T W, North W R S, Chakrabarti R et al 1980 Haemostatic function and cardiovascular death: early results of a prospective study. Lancet i: 1050–1053
Meade T W, Haines A P, Imeson J D, Stirling Y, Thompson S G 1983 Menopausal status and haemostatic variables. Lancet i: 22–24
Meade T W, Vickers M V, Thompson S G, Stirling Y, Haines A P, Miller G J 1985a Epidemiological characteristics of platelet aggregability. British Medical Journal 290: 428–431
Meade T W, Vickers M V, Thompson S G, Seghatchian M J 1985b The effect of physiological levels of fibrinogen on platelet aggregation. Thrombosis Research 38: 527–534
Meade T W, Mellows S, Brozoviç M et al 1986 Haemostatic function and ischaemic heart disease; principal results of the Northwick Park Heart Study. Lancet ii: 533–577
Meade T W, Imeson J D, Stirling Y 1987 Effects of changes in smoking and other characteristics on clotting factors and the risk of ischaemic heart disease. Lancet ii: 986–988
Mitchell J R A 1976 Has our basic knowledge of cerebrovascular disease led to effective and rational treatment? In: Gillingham F J, Mawdsley C, Williams A E (eds) Stroke. Churchill Livingstone, Edinburgh, p 301
Mori E, del Zoppo G J, Chambers D, Copeland B R, Arfors K E 1992 Inhibition of polymorphonuclear leukocyte adherence suppresses no-reflow after focal cerebral ischemia in baboons. Stroke 23: 712–718
Moriarty A J, Highes R, Nelson S D et al 1988 Streptokinase and reduced plasma viscosity: a second benefit. European Journal of Haematology 41: 25–36
Moritz M W, Reimers R C, Baker R K, Sutera S P, Joist J H 1983 Role of cytoplasmic and releasable ADP in platelet aggregation induced by laminar shear stress. Journal of Laboratory and Clinical Medicine 101: 537–544
Motomiya M, Karino 1984 Flow patterns in the human carotid artery bifurcation. Stroke 15: 50–56
Nash G B, Meiselman H J 1986 Rheological properties of individual polymorphonuclear granulocytes and lymphocytes. Clinical Hemorheology 6: 87–97
Nemerson Y, Turitto V T 1991 The effect of flow on hemostasis and thrombosis. Thrombosis and Haemostasis 66: 272–276
Neumann F-J, Waas W, Diehm C et al 1990 Activation and decreased deformability of neutrophils after intermittent claudication. Circulation 82: 922–929
Neumann F-J, Katus H A, Hoberg E et al 1991 Increased plasma viscosity and erythrocyte aggregation: indicators of an unfavourable clinical outcome in patients with unstable angina pectoris. British Heart Journal 66: 425–430
Nicolaides A N, Bowers R, Horbourne T, Kidner P H, Besterman E M 1977 Blood-viscosity, red-cell flexibility, haematocrit and plasma fibrinogen in patients with angina. Lancet ii: 943–945
Nossel H L 1981 Relative proteolysis of the fibrinogen B β chain by thrombin and plasmin as a determinant of thrombosis. Nature 291: 165–167
Pearson T C 1987 Rheology of the absolute polycythaemias. In: Baillière's clinical haematology vol 1: 637–664
Pearson T C, Wetherley-Mein G 1978 Vascular occlusive episodes and venous haematocrit in primary proliferative polycythaemia. Lancet ii: 1219–1222
Prentice R L, Szatrowski T P, Fujikura T et al 1982a Leukocyte counts and coronary heart disease in a Japanese cohort. American Journal of Epidemiology 116: 496–509
Prentice R L, Szatrowski T P, Kato H, Mason M W 1982b Leukocyte counts and cerebrovascular disease. Journal of Chronic Diseases 35: 703–714
Rampling M W, Challoner T 1983 A theoretical analysis of the effects of varying fibrinogen concentration and haematocrit on the flow characteristics of blood in cylindrical tubes. Biorheology 20: 141–152
Rampling M W, Feher M D, Sever P S, Elkeles R S 1989 Haemorheological disturbances in non-insulin-dependent diabetes and the effects of concomitant hypertension. Clinical Hemorheology 9: 101
Reimers R C, Sutera S P, Joist J H 1984 Potentiation by red blood cells of shear-induced platelet aggregation: relative importance of chemical and physical mechanisms. Blood 64: 1200–1206
Repke D, Gemmell C H, Guha A, Turitto V T, Broze G J Jr, Nemerson Y 1990 Hemophilia as a defect of the tissue factor pathway of blood coagulation: effect of factors VIII and IX on factor X activation in a continuous flow reactor. Proceedings of the National Academy of Sciences, USA 87: 7623–7627
Resch K L, Ernst E, Matrai A, Paulsen H F 1992 Fibrinogen and viscosity as risk factors for subsequent cardiovascular events in stroke survivors. Annals of Internal Medicine 117: 371–375
Saniabadi A R, Lowe G D O, Barbenel JC, Forbes C D 1984a A comparison of spontaneous platelet aggregation in whole blood with platelet rich plasma: additional evidence for the role of ADP. Thrombosis and Haemostasis 51: 115-118
Saniabadi A R, Lowe G D O, Barbenel J C, Forbes C D 1984b Haematocrit, bleeding time, and platelet aggregation. Lancet i: 1409-1411
Saniabadi A, Lowe G D O, Madhok R et al 1987 Red blood cells mediate spontaneous aggregation of platelets in whole blood. Atherosclerosis 66: 175–180
Schatzkin A, Cupples L A , Heeren T et al 1984 The epidemiology of sudden unexpected death: risk factors for men and women in the Framingham Heart Study. American Heart Journal 107: 1300–1306
Schlant R C, Forman S, Stamler J, Canner P L 1982 The natural history of coronary heart disease: prognostic factors after recovery from myocardial infarction in 2789 men. Circulation 66: 401–414
Schmalzer E A, Chien S 1984 Filterability of subpopulations of leukocytes: effect of pentoxyfylline. Blood 64: 542-546
Schmid-Schönbein H 1976 Microrheology of erythrocytes, blood viscosity, and the distribution of blood flow in the microcirculation. International Review of Physiology 9: 1–62
Schmid-Schönbein H 1983 Haemorheology and thrombosis. In: van de Loo J, Prentice C R M, Beller F K (eds) The thromboembolic disorders. Schattauer, Stuttgart, p 45
Schmid-Schönbein H 1988 Fluid dynamics and hemorheology in vivo. In: Lowe G D O (ed) Clinical blood rheology. CRC Press, Boca Raton, vol 1: 129
Seplowitz A H, Chien S, Smith F R 1981 Effects of lipoproteins on plasma viscosity. Atherosclerosis 38: 89–95
Shaper A G 1988 Coronary heart disease. Risks and reasons. Current Medical Literature Ltd, London
Skalak R, Chien S 1981 Capillary flow: history, experiments and theory. Biorheology 18: 307–330
Small M, Lowe G D O, Cameron E, Forbes C D 1983 Contribution of the haematocrit to the bleeding time. Haemostasis 13: 379–384
Smith E B, Alexander K M, Massie I B 1976 Insoluble 'fibrin' in human aortic intima. Quantitative studies on the relationship between insoluble 'fibrin', soluble fibrinogen and low density lipoprotein. Atherosclerosis 23: 19–38
Smith W C S, Lowe G D O, Lee A J, Tunstall-Pedoe H 1992 Rheological determinants of blood pressure in a Scottish adult population. Journal of Hypertension 10: 467–472
Somer T 1987 Rheology of paraproteinaemias and the plasma hyperviscosity syndrome. In: Baillière's clinical haematology. Vol 1: 695–723
Sorlie P D, Garcia-Palmieri M R, Costas R, Havlik R 1981 Hematocrit and risk of coronary heart disease: the Puerto Rico Heart Health Program. American Heart Journal 101: 456–464
Stewart R D, Baretta E D, Platte L R et al 1974 Carboxyhemoglobin levels in American blood donors. Journal of the American Medical Association 229: 1187–1195
Stone M C, Thorp J M 1985 Plasma fibrinogen — a major coronary risk factor. Journal of the Royal College of General Practitioners 35: 565–569
Stout R W, Crawford V 1991 Seasonal variations in fibrinogen concentrations among elderly people. Lancet 338: 9–13
Stuart J, Johnson C S 1987 Rheology of the sickle cell disorders. In: Baillière's Clinical Haematology. Vol 1: 747–775
Stuart J, George A J, Davies A J, Aukland A, Hurlow R A 1981 Haematological stress syndrome in atherosclerosis. Journal of Clinical Pathology 34: 464–467
Tait G 1992 Personal communication
Tangelder G J, Slaaf D W, Teirlinck H C, Alewijnse R, Reneman R S

1982 Localization within a thin optical section of fluorescent blood platelets flowing in a microvessel. Microvascular Research 23: 214–230

Taylor J E, Henderson I S, Stewart W K, Belch J J F 1991 Erythropoietin and spontaneous platelet aggregation in haemodialysis patients. Lancet 338: 1361–1362

Turitto V T 1988 Platelet rheology. In: Lowe G D O (ed) Clinical blood rheology, Volume I. CRC Press, Boca Raton, vol 1: 111

Turitto V T, Weiss H J 1980 Red blood cells: their dual role in thrombus formation. Science 207: 541–543

Vara-Thorbeck R, Rosell J 1988 Invited commentary. World Journal of Surgery 12: 353–355

Weiss H J, Turitto V T, Baumgartner H R 1986 Role of shear rate and platelets in promoting fibrin formation on rabbit subendothelium. Studies utilizing patients with quantitative and qualitative platelet defects. Journal of Clinical Investigation 78: 1072–1082

Weiss H J, Hawiger J, Ruggeri Z M, Turitto V T, Thiagarajan P, Hoffmann T 1989 Fibrinogen-independent platelet adhesion and thrombus formation on subendothelium mediated by glycoprotein IIb-IIIa complex at high shear rate. Journal of Clinical Investigation 83: 288–297

Whittington R B, Harkness J 1982 Whole-blood viscosity, as determined by plasma viscosity, hematocrit, and shear. Biorheology 19: 175–184

Wilhelmsen L, Svardsudd K, Korsan-Bengtsen K et al 1984 Fibrinogen as a risk factor for stroke and myocardial infarction. New England Journal of Medicine 311: 501–505

Williams S A, Boolell M, McGregor G A, Smaje L H, Wasserman S M, Tooke J E 1990 Capillary hypertension and abnormal pressure dynamics in patients with essential hypertension. Clinical Science 79: 5–8

Wiseman S, Kenchington G, Dain R et al 1989 Influence of smoking and plasma factors on patency of femoro-popliteal vein grafts. British Medical Journal 299: 643–646

Wu K K, Folsom A R, Heiss G, Davis C E, Conlan M G, Barnes R 1992 Association of coagulation factors and inhibitors with carotid artery atherosclerosis. Early results of the Atherosclerosis Risk in Communities (ARIC) Study. Annals of Epidemiology 2: 471–480

Wurzinger L J, Opitz R, Blasberg P, Eschweiler H, Schmid-Schönbein H 1983 The role of hydrodynamic factors in platelet activation and thrombotic events: the effects of shear stress of short duration. In: Schettler G, Nerem R M, Schmid-Schönbein H, Mörl H, Diehm C (eds): Fluid dynamics as a localizing factor for atherosclerosis. Springer, Berlin, p 91

Yarnell J W G, Sweetnam P M, Rogers S et al 1987 Some long term effects of smoking on the haemostatic system: a report from the Caerphilly and Speedwell Collaborative Surveys. Journal of Clinical Pathology 40: 909–913

Yarnell J W G, Baker I A, Sweetnam P M et al 1991 Fibrinogen, viscosity, and white blood cell count are major risk factors for ischemic heart disease. The Caerphilly and Speedwell Collaborative Heart Disease Studies. Circulation 83: 836–844

Zalokhar J B, Richard J L, Claude J R 1981 Leukocyte count, smoking, and myocardial infarction. New England Journal of Medicine 304: 465–468

Zarins C K, Giddens D P, Bharadvaj B K, Sottiurai V S, Mabon R F, Glagov S 1983 Carotid bifurcation atherosclerosis. Quantitative correlation of plaque localisation with flow velocity profiles and wall shear stress. Circulation Research 53: 502–514

Zwaginga J J, Ijsseldijk M J W, de Groot P G et al 1991 Treatment of uremic anemia with recombinant erythropoietin also reduces the defects in platelet adhesion and aggregation caused by uremic plasma. Thrombosis and Haemostasis 66: 638–647

52. Detection of a prethrombotic state

K. A. Bauer

From a clinical standpoint, patients suspected of having a hypercoagulable state can be divided into two broad categories (Schafer 1985). The first group consists of the inherited thrombotic disorders or primary hypercoagulable states. In these instances, a specific defect in one of the three major natural anticoagulant mechanisms (namely, the heparin-antithrombin III, protein C-thrombomodulin and protein S, or plasminogen-plasminogen activator mechanisms) has been identified. Laboratory assays have been developed to screen for deficiencies of antithrombin III, protein C, and protein S, though these assays are currently able to provide diagnosis in fewer than 20% of patients with venous thromboembolism. These diagnostic tests provide relatively little assistance in the evaluation of individuals with acquired risk factors for venous thrombosis or those with arterial vascular disease. The second category consists of a heterogenous array of clinical disorders in which there is an apparent increased risk for developing thrombotic complications as compared to the general population (Table 52.1), and can be referred to as the acquired or secondary hypercoagulable states. The pathophysiological basis leading to increased coagulation system activity in most of these situations is not known with any degree of certainty. Due to their complex pathophysiology, it is unlikely that defects in merely a single component of the haemostatic mechanism will account for the thrombotic tendency in the majority of these conditions.

Table 52.1 Acquired or secondary hypercoagulable states

Diseases or syndromes	
Lupus anticoagulant	
Malignancy	
Disease-related:	includes migratory superficial thrombophlebitis (Trousseau's syndrome), nonbacterial thrombotic endocarditis, thrombosis associated with chronic disseminated intravascular coagulation
Treatment-related:	associated with the administration of various chemotherapeutic agents (L-asparaginase, mitomycin, adjuvant programmes for breast cancer)
Oestrogen administration	associated with oral contraceptives, treatment of prostate cancer with diethylstilbestrol
Infusion of prothrombin complex concentrates	
Nephrotic syndrome	
Heparin-induced thrombocytopenia	
Thrombotic thrombocytopenic purpura	
Myeloproliferative disorders	
Paroxysmal nocturnal haemoglobinuria	
Hyperlipidaemia	
Diabetes mellitus	
Homocystinuria	
Hyperviscosity	
Congestive heart failure	
Physiological factors	
Pregnancy (especially during the postpartum period)	
Postoperative state	
Immobilization	
Advancing age	
Obesity	

Prospective epidemiological studies have reported strong positive relationships between fibrinogen level and the risk of myocardial infarction (Meade et al 1980, Wilhelmsen et al 1984, Kannel et al 1987). High factor VII activity levels have also been reported to predispose patients to the onset of ischemic heart disease (Meade et al 1986). Impaired fibrinolytic activity due to high plasminogen activator inhibitor-1 levels (Hamsten et al 1987) and platelet hyperaggregability (Trip et al 1990) may also be markers that help identify individuals with an increased risk of recurrent myocardial infarction. A detailed discussion of the relationships between haemostatic factors and coronary artery disease may be found in Chapter 53.

Advances in our knowledge of the biochemistry of coagulation and fibrinolysis since the mid 1970s have facilitated the development of sensitive and specific assays that are able to detect platelet activation, the generation of coagulation enzymes, and products of intravascular fibrin formation or dissolution in the human circulation. Techniques for assessing platelet activation and fibrinolysis have been described in Chapters 6 and 26, respectively. This chapter will therefore focus on markers of coagulation activation.

Many of the protein components of the haemostatic mechanism are zymogens that are converted to serine proteases. For coagulation system enzymes to be generated at any significant rate, a zymogen, a cofactor, and a converting enzyme must form a multimolecular complex on a natural surface. These transformations are suppressed if the converting enzyme is inhibited, the protein cofactor destroyed, or the surface receptors, that are essential for the assembly of the macromolecular complex, sequestered. Previous methods for monitoring these processes in the clinic have been directed at measuring the levels of zymogens (e.g. factor X, prothrombin, protein C), inhibitors (e.g. antithrombin III), or substrates (i.e. fibrinogen) of the haemostatic system. These molecular species are present in large excess within the blood, and only a small percentage of the zymogens are converted to active enzymes under in vivo conditions. Thus, attempts to monitor thrombotic or prethrombotic states by measuring the ambient levels of zymogens, inhibitors or substrates, or by determining their catabolic rates within the circulatory system are generally of limited clinical utility. Similarly, clotting assays (e.g. activated partial thromboplastin time) that are carried out under non-physiological conditions in vitro have not proved to be particularly useful in assessing the extent of coagulation or fibrinolytic activation in vivo.

It has so far not been possible to measure directly the levels of most haemostatic enzymes in vivo. Many of the enzymes may not be available for quantification in blood as they are neutralized rapidly by naturally occurring protease inhibitors and/or bound to cellular receptors in the locale in which they are generated. Faced with these obstacles, most investigators have resorted to developing immunochemical assays for peptides that are liberated with the activation of coagulation enzymes and/or enzyme-inhibitor complexes. The assays that have been developed along with the reported in vivo half-lives for some of the species are listed in Table 52.2 and described in greater detail below. Most of these assays were initially developed in research laboratories, but some are now available commercially in kit form using either polyclonal or monoclonal antibodies.

The assay formats for these markers are generally of two types. The first is a competitive radioimmunoassay procedure. This requires an antibody population that recognizes antigenic determinants on the activation fragment or enzyme-inhibitor complex that are hidden in the parent zymogen or inhibitor. The need for highly specific antibodies to the marker of interest can sometimes be obviated by devising sample processing procedures that efficiently remove the cross-reacting species in plasma prior to assay. The second approach is the enzyme-linked immunosorbent assay (ELISA). In most instances, $F(ab')_2$ fragments directed towards epitopes on one region of the marker are bound to wells of plastic microtitre plates to 'capture' the antigen from the plasma specimens. After washing away unbound species, a second $F(ab')_2$ population recognizing epitopes in a different domain of the molecule is added to the wells. These antibody fragments are coupled to an enzyme capable of cleaving a suitable colorimetric substrate allowing the development of a titration curve.

Two coagulation enzymes, activated protein C and factor VIIa, have relatively slow in vivo inactivation mechanisms. It has therefore recently been possible to develop techniques to measure these species directly in plasma. The test for activated protein C employs an immunoenzymatic procedure (Orthner et al 1991, Gruber & Griffin 1992), while the procedure for factor VIIa employs a clotting assay using recombinant tissue factor that is C-terminally truncated (Morrissey et al 1993, Wildgoose et al 1992). This tissue factor mutant maintains cofactor activity toward factor VIIa, but does not support factor VII activation. Another novel technique first inactivates coagulation enzymes with a labelled synthetic peptide inhibitor and then employs an immunoenzymatic technique for detecting the enzyme-inhibitor complex (Mann et al 1990). This method however has

Table 52.2 Immunochemical markers of coagulation

Biochemical step	marker	$t_{1/2}$	Reference
Factor XII-factor XIIa	Factor XIIa-C1-inhibitor complex		Kaplan et al 1985, Nuijens et al 1988
Prekallikrein-kallikrein	Kallikrein-C1-inhibitor complex		Lewin et al 1983, Kaplan et al 1985
Factor IX-factor IXa	Factor IX activation peptide	15	Bauer et al 1990
	Factor IXa-antithrombin III complex	30	Takahashi et al 1991
Factor X-factor Xa	Factor X activation peptide	30	Bauer et al 1989a
	Factor Xa-antithrombin III complex		Jesty et al 1984
Prothrombin-thrombin	Prothrombin activation fragment F_{1+2}	90	Bauer et al 1985
	Thrombin-antithrombin III complex	15	Shifman & Pizzo 1982, Bauer et al 1983, Leonard et al 1983
Protein C-activated protein C	Protein C activation peptide	5	Bauer et al 1984
	Activated protein C-protein C inhibitor complex	40	Espana et al 1989, 1991
	Activated protein C-α_1-antitrypsin complex	140	Espana et al 1990, 1991
	Activated protein C-α_2-macroglobulin complex		Toh et al 1991
Fibrinogen-fibrin	Fibrinopeptide A (FPA)	3–5	Nossel et al 1971, 1974, Cronlund et al 1976
	Fibrinopeptide B (FPB)		Bilezikian et al 1975, Eckhard et al 1981

not yet demonstrated sufficient sensitivity to monitor the very low levels of many of the coagulation serine proteases that occur in blood.

The execution of clinical investigations seeking to establish a relationship between the levels of these parameters and thromboembolic disease is difficult. First, one must ensure that the selected assays are specific for the activation products of interest and possess sufficient sensitivity. Second, the tests must be properly standardized so that the assays perform in a reproducible manner. Third, care must be taken to ensure that technical factors do not introduce in vitro artifacts that can significantly alter the immunoassay results. These include the quality of the venipuncture procedures, the choice of anticoagulant cocktail for blood specimens, the sample processing procedure, and the plasma storage conditions. Fourth, objective endpoints must be used to establish a diagnosis of thrombosis, bias in patient selection should be avoided, and an appropriate control group of patients must be chosen for comparison.

ASSAYS FOR COAGULATION ACTIVATION

The blood coagulation mechanism is classically described as functionally independent extrinsic and intrinsic pathways that separately activate factor X and generate thrombin (Davie & Ratnoff 1964, MacFarlane 1964). The initiation of the intrinsic system is thought to occur with damage to the endothelium and the resulting exposure of subendothelial components such as collagen to the blood. The components of the intrinsic system include the contact factors (factor XII, prekallikrein, high molecular-weight kininogen, factor XI) as well as factors IX and VIII. The extrinsic pathway is initiated when factor VII binds to tissue factor, an integral membrane glycoprotein that is expressed constituitively by subendothelial components of the vessel wall. The factor Xa that is generated by either of the two cascades is then able to convert prothrombin to thrombin by binding to factor Va on activated platelets.

It is now appreciated that the factor VII-tissue factor mechanism is important in the physiological activation of factor IX (Biggs & Nossel 1961, Josso & Prou-Wartelle 1965). The activation of this zymogen can be monitored by measuring the levels of the factor IX activation peptide (Bauer et al 1990) or factor IXa-antithrombin III complexes (Takahashi et al 1991). These assays reflect the action of factor XIa and/or the factor VII-tissue factor complex upon factor IX (Fig. 52.1). Factor X activation mediated by the extrinsic or intrinsic pathways can be monitored by measuring the factor X activation peptide (Bauer et al 1989a).

Thrombin generation takes place at an appreciable rate under physiological conditions only in the presence of factor Xa, factor Va, calcium ions, and activated platelets. During this process, the N-terminus of the prothrombin molecule is released as the inactive F_{1+2} fragment (Figs 52.1 and 52.2). Once evolved, this serine protease

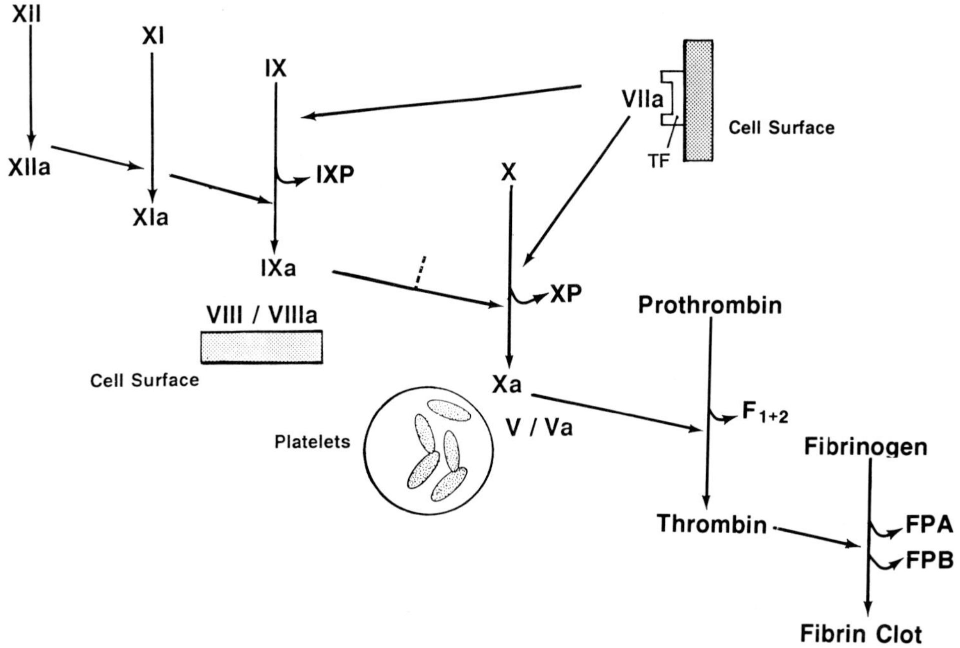

Fig. 52.1 Pathways of coagulation activation. The activation of factor IX by factor XIa or the factor VII-tissue factor (TF) mechanism liberates the factor IX activation peptide (IXP). The conversion of factor X to factor Xa by the factor IXa-factor VIII/VIIIa-cell surface complex releases the factor X activation peptide (XP). The generation of thrombin from prothrombin is mediated by factor Xa in the presence of factor Va, and activated platelets. During this process, the F_{1+2} fragment is released. Thrombin action on fibrinogen releases fibrinopeptide A (FPA) and fibrinopeptide B (FPB).

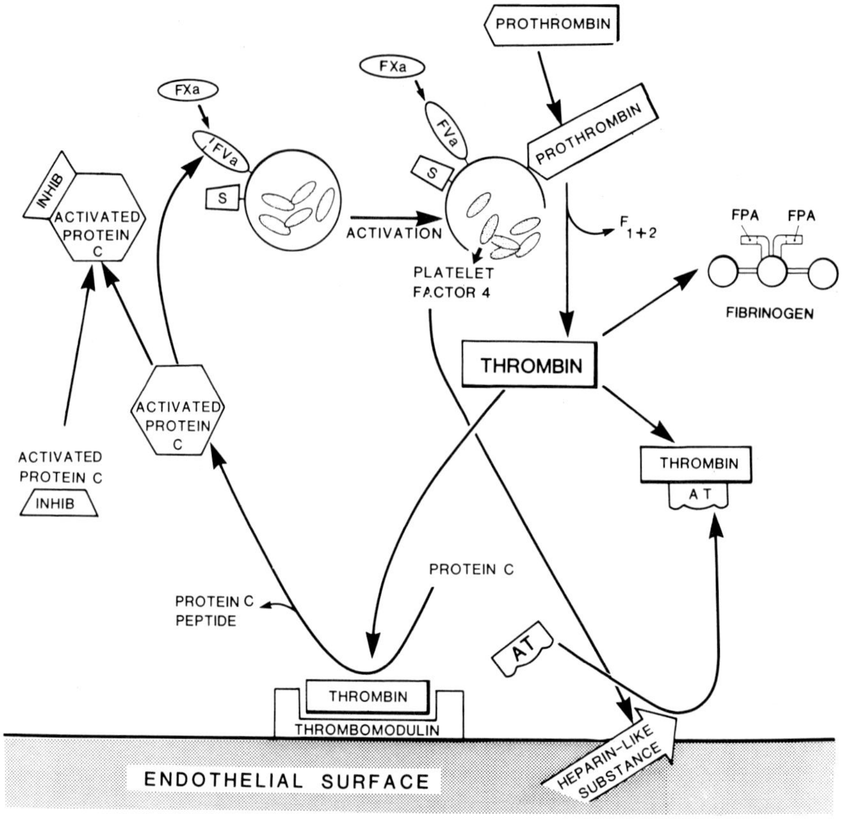

Fig. 52.2 Regulation of thrombin generation by the natural anticoagulant mechanisms of the endothelium. Factor Xa, factor Va, protein S, prothrombin activation fragment F_{1+2}, fibrinopeptide A, antithrombin, and activated protein C inhibitor(s) are designated as FXa, FVa, S, F_{1+2}, FPA, AT, and activated protein C inhibit, respectively. Thrombin may be inactivated by forming 1:1 stoichiometric complexes with its major physiological inhibitor, antithrombin III, thereby resulting in the formation of thrombin-antithrombin III complexes (thrombin-AT). Activated protein C can be neutralized by inhibitors of activated protein C (i.e. protein C inhibitor, α_1-proteinase inhibitor, and α_2-macroglobulin), which results in the generation of activated protein C inhibitor complexes.

converts fibrinogen into fibrin, releasing fibrinopeptides A and B, or it can be inhibited by the endogenous heparin sulfate-antithrombin III mechanism to form a thrombin-antithrombin III complex, a stable enzyme-inhibitor complex (Fig. 52.2). Immunoassays have been developed for the F_{1+2} fragment (Lau et al 1979, Teitel et al 1982, Hursting et al 1989, Shi et al 1989, Pelzer et al 1991) and the thrombin-antithrombin III complex (Collén & de Cock 1975, Collén et al 1977, Lau & Rosenberg 1980, Pelzer et al 1988) that can be used as indices of thrombin generation in vivo.

Alternatively, thrombin can also rapidly activate protein C by binding to thrombomodulin on vascular endothelial cells and assays have been developed to monitor this transformation (Fig. 52.2). These include measurements of the protein C activation peptide (Bauer et al 1984) and activated protein C-inhibitor complexes (Espana & Griffin 1989, Espana et al 1990, Toh et al 1991). The plasma inhibitors of activated protein C include protein C inhibitor, α_1-proteinase inhibitor, and α_2-macroglobulin.

Assays have been established for fibrinopeptide A (Nossel et al 1971, 1974, 1976, Cronlund et al 1976, Kockum & Frebelius 1980, Soria et al 1980, Woodhams & Kernoff 1981). The antibody populations employed for these assays show significant, but not absolute, specificity for fibrinopeptide A relative to fibrinogen. For this reason, it is necessary to use simple procedures that remove fibrinogen from plasma samples without altering the levels of the peptides prior to performing these assays (Nossel et al 1974, Kockum & Frebelius 1980).

APPLICATIONS

Normal levels

Normal values are usually expressed as ranges or means with standard deviations. The presence of a large number of modifying factors can result in considerable overlap in assay results between people with a pathological condition or altered physiological status and normals. While values further from the mean of the normal distribution are more likely to be abnormal, appropriate interpretation requires an appreciation of the confounding factors that can influence measurements.

The normal aging process alters coagulation activation in a predictable fashion (Bauer et al 1987, Hurstings et al 1990). With advancing age from 45–70 years, increasing numbers of patients who are otherwise normal exhibit elevated levels of prothrombin activation fragment F_{1+2}. These increased concentrations are due to increased production rather than decreased clearance of the marker as shown by direct investigation of the behaviour of radiolabelled polypeptide (Bauer et al 1987). The levels of the factor IX and factor X activation peptides also increase substantially with advancing age (Bauer et al 1990). Significant, but somewhat less striking, positive correlations have been observed between increasing age and the levels of fibrinopeptide A and protein C activation peptide (Bauer et al 1987).

It has been reported that strenuous exercise in the form of long-distance running leads to increased thrombin-antithrombin III complex levels without elevations in the levels of fibrinopeptide A (Bartsch et al 1990).

Dysfunction in normal physiological clearance mechanisms can result in substantial elevations in the levels of activation peptides. For F_{1+2}, this has been demonstrated in patients with chronic renal failure on dialysis (Weinstein et al 1985). Thus one must be cautious in interpreting an elevated level of a marker as evidence of heightened coagulation or fibrinolytic activity in disorders associated with renal (e.g. thrombotic thrombocytopenic purpura, systemic lupus erythematosus, nephrotic syndrome, renal transplant rejection) or hepatic dysfunction.

Disseminated intravascular coagulation (DIC)

A number of inciting factors can trigger DIC and increased coagulation system activation and secondary fibrinolysis are cardinal features of the disorder. The aforementioned assays should therefore be very sensitive markers of acute or chronic DIC syndromes and marked elevations in the levels of factor X activation peptide (Bauer et al 1989), protein C activation (Bauer et al 1984, Espana et al 1990), F_{1+2} (Teitel et al 1982, Bauer & Rosenberg 1984), thrombin-antithrombin III complex (Teitel et al 1982, Asakura et al 1988, Hoek et al 1988, Boisclair et al 1990), fibrinopeptide A (Nossel et al 1974, 1976, Cronlund et al 1976, Neame et al 1980, Woodhams & Kernoff 1981, Bauer & Rosenberg 1984), and fibrinopeptide B (Bilezikian et al 1975, Nossel et al 1979, Eckhardt et al 1981) have been observed in such patients. However the sensitivity and specificity of these assays as compared to other laboratory tests in populations with DIC have not been determined.

Nossel and coworkers (1979) used radioimmunoassays for fibrinopeptide A, fibrinopeptide B, and Bβ 1–42 (measured as thrombin-increasable FPB) to investigate the pathophysiology of DIC in patients receiving hypertonic saline to terminate pregnancy. Immediately after intrauterine infusion, there was a marked increase in fibrinopeptide A levels, a measure of fibrinogen proteolysis mediated by thrombin. Subsequently, a rise in the concentrations of Bβ 1–42 occurred, a measure of plasmin action on non-cross-linked fibrin I polymer. This investigation led Nossel (1981) to hypothesize that the relative rates of proteolysis of the Bβ chain of fibrinogen by thrombin and plasmin could determine the occurrence of venous thrombosis. A study by Owen et al (1983) of neurosurgical patients undergoing craniotomy found that individuals developing venous thrombosis exhibited FPA levels that were considerably greater than those of Bβ 1–42 during the 4 days preceding the onset of this disorder as compared to controls. These observations suggest that thrombosis occurs at a time when thrombin action is enhanced relative to that of plasmin.

Deep venous thrombosis (DVT)

Levels of F_{1+2} (Boneu et al 1991, Estivals et al 1991, Pelzer et al 1991), thrombin-antithrombin III complex (Hoek et al 1988, Boisclair et al 1990, Boneu et al 1991, Estivals et al 1991), fibrinopeptide A (Nossel et al 1974, 1976, Yudelman et al 1978, Yudelman & Greenberg 1982), fibrinopeptide B (Bilezikian et al 1975, Eckhardt et al 1981), and protein C activation (Espana et al 1990) are frequently elevated in symptomatic patients with venous thrombosis and/or pulmonary embolism. While these parameters are sensitive indices of haemostatic enzyme generation, the tests are not specific for intravascular thrombosis. Elevated values have been reported in nonpathological as well as pathological conditions including localized and generalized infections, neoplastic and connective tissue disease.

Fibrinopeptide A was the first coagulation activation marker to be developed and evaluated with regard to its diagnostic utility in patients with venous thromboembolism. A study by Yudelman et al (1978) found that 89% of symptomatic patients presenting with either positive venographic and/or lung scan findings had elevated fibrinopeptide A levels (> 1.3 nmol/l). The levels were generally highest in those patients presenting the shortest duration of symptoms referable to thrombosis (i.e. less than 1 day). However 15% of patients with documented thrombosis had fibrinopeptide A levels in the normal range, indicating limitations of this assay as a sole diagnostic test for venous thromboembolism. Studies using tests for F_{1+2} and thrombin-antithrombin III complex assays indicate similar limitations for these assays in the diagnosis of DVT (Hoek et al 1988, 1989, Boneu et al 1991).

Sepsis

Septicaemia frequently results in disturbances of the haemostatic mechanism. In septic shock, DIC can lead to the deposition of fibrin in the microvasculature and the failure of multiple organs. Endotoxin, a lipopolysaccharide present in the outer membrane of Gram negative bacteria, plays an important role in the development of the clinical and laboratory manifestations of septicaemia. The intravenous administration of *Escherischia coli* endotoxin to healthy volunteers under controlled conditions resulted in increased thrombin generation as monitored by the F_{1+2} and thrombin-antithrombin III complex assays that was maximal at 3–4 hours after infusion in the apparent absence of contact system activation (van Deventer et al 1990). The fibrinolytic system was also triggered by endotoxin as evidenced by increased levels of tissue plasminogen activator (tPA) and plasmin-antiplasmin complex at 2–3 hours (Suffredin et al 1989, van Deventer et al 1990). This rise in fibrinolytic activity was subsequently offset by the release of plasminogen activator inhibitor-1 (PAI-1).

Many of endotoxin's biological effects appear to be mediated by cytokines that are synthesized and released by macrophages and monocytes. High levels of the cytokine, tumour necrosis factor (TNF), have been observed within the first 2 hours after administering endotoxin to normal subjects (Michie et al 1988, van Deventer et al 1990). Bauer et al (1989b) showed that TNF has a potent procoagulant effect in vivo, monitoring coagulation activation by studying the changes in the levels of F_{1+2}, protein C activation peptide, and fibrinopeptide A following the administration of the recombinant cytokine to cancer patients. In normal volunteer studies, the early dynamics and route of coagulation activation in response to TNF administration was investigated. This resulted in the early activation of factor X, probably via the factor VII-tissue factor pathway (van der Poll et al 1990).

Coagulation factor deficiencies

The investigation of patients with hereditary coagulation factor deficiencies using the activation peptide assays has generated information regarding the pathways responsible for coagulation activation in vivo under basal conditions (i.e. the absence of thrombosis or provocative stimuli). Patients with factor VII deficiency but not factor XI deficiency, have reduced levels of factor IX activation (Bauer et al 1990, Takahashi et al 1991), whereas patients with deficiencies of factor VIII or factor IX have normal levels of factor X and prothrombin activation (Bauer et al 1989a). The infusion of relatively small doses of recombinant factor VIIa (10–20 µg/kg of body weight) in factor VII-deficient patients results in substantial elevations in the plasma concentrations of the factor IX activation peptide, factor X activation peptide, and prothrombin fragment F_{1+2} (Bauer et al 1992). Thus these data demonstrate that the factor VII-tissue factor pathway is largely responsible for the activation of factor IX as well as factor X in the basal state (Bauer et al 1989a, 1990, 1992). Using a recently developed clotting assay for factor VIIa, patients with severe factor IX deficiency were found to have circulating levels of enzyme less than 10% of that in normal individuals (Wildgoose et al 1992). These data suggest that factor IXa is the principal in vivo activator of factor VII under basal conditions.

It has also been shown that the administration of a monoclonal antibody-purified factor IX concentrate to individuals with haemophilia B causes an increase in plasma factor IX activation peptide levels that are initially greatly decreased, but does not change factor X activation peptide or F_{1+2} (Bauer et al 1992). Infusion of highly purified factor VIII concentrates into haemophilia A patients results in no significant change in the plasma concentrations of factor X activation peptide and F_{1+2} (Bauer et al 1992). These observations indicate that the factor IXa-factor VIIIa-cell surface complex is unable to activate factor X under basal conditions. In response to vascular injury or thrombotic stimuli, it is surmised that increased formation of free thrombin or factor Xa via the action of the factor VII-tissue factor pathway then generates factor VIIIa and/or a natural surface (e.g. activated platelets) on which assembly of the factor IXa-factor VIIIa complex takes place. This hypothesis is consistent with the severe bleeding tendency of most patients with factor VIII or factor IX deficiency, and the insensitivity of the factor X activation peptide and F_{1+2} assays to significant deficiencies of these two proteins.

The above mechanistic findings derived from studies of patients with coagulation factor deficiencies have significant potential implications with regard to the utility of basal coagulation system markers in diagnosing prethrombotic patients (Bauer et al 1992). It follows that the conversion of a prethrombotic state to a thrombotic event occurs due to small increases in the generation rates of haemostatic enzymes that exceed the inhibitory threshold of an individual's endogenous anticoagulant mechanisms as well as the sequestration of these proteases on specialized cell surfaces. It remains to be determined whether persons with elevated basal levels of coagulation system markers are more likely to respond in a hypersensitive fashion to environmental stimuli. Because the activity of the blood coagulation mechanism in such individuals is closer to the threshold of normal inhibitory processes, such individuals may generate slightly more thrombin via the factor VII-tissue factor mechanism via the extrinsic pathway. This thrombin could then be used to ignite the dormant intrinsic cascade, which could ultimately result in the generation of large amounts of free thrombin and the development of arterial or venous thrombosis.

Deficiencies of natural anticoagulants

Hereditary deficiencies of protein C, protein S, and antithrombin III have all been associated with hypercoagulable states, and coagulation activation has been investigated in patients with deficiencies of each of these critical anticoagulant proteins. In asymptomatic people with heterozygous deficiencies of protein C or protein S, the mean F_{1+2} concentration is significantly increased as compared to age-matched controls (Bauer et al 1988, Leroy-Matheron et al 1991, Mannucci et al 1992). Approximately one-third of patients have levels greater than the upper limit of normal controls (defined as the mean + 2 standard deviations) (Bauer et al 1988, Mannucci et al 1992). The elevated F_{1+2} concentrations are not due to diminished clearance of the fragment (Orthner et al 1991, Bauer et al 1992). Fibrinopeptide A levels were elevated in approximately 20% of subjects (Bauer et al 1988, Mannucci et al 1992).

Protein C activation as measured by the protein C activation peptide assay or an immunoenzymatic assay is reduced to about 50% of normal in asymptomatic persons with heterozygous protein C deficiency (Bauer et al 1988, Gruber & Griffin, 1992). In two adult patients with homozygous protein C deficiency, it has been shown that the levels of PCP as well as F_{1+2} can be normalized by administration of a monoclonal antibody-purified protein C concentrate (Conard et al 1991). Thus it has been shown that augmented activity of the protein C anticoagulant pathway can inhibit prothrombin activation in vivo, and that the activation of protein C by the thrombin-thrombomodulin complex is a tonically active mechanism in the regulation of coagulation system activation.

In asymptomatic patients with hereditary antithrombin III deficiency, it was initially reported that F_{1+2} levels are frequently increased as compared to age-matched unaffected siblings (Bauer et al 1985). Fibrinopeptide A measurements were similar in both groups. The plasma antithrombin III concentrations were reduced to about 50% of normal in the 22 affected people. Subsequently it was shown that the high concentrations of the fragment resulted from an in vitro effect due to the presence of low amounts of heparin (final concentration of 4 units/ml) in the anticoagulant cocktail used for sample collection, in the presence of reduced antithrombin III blood levels (Bauer et al 1991).

A recent study of 26 antithrombin III-deficient subjects from Italy did not demonstrate significant elevations in plasma F_{1+2} or fibrinopeptide A levels (Mannucci et al 1992). Another cross-sectional study of asymptomatic persons from a single large family with functional antithrombin III deficiency (antithrombin-III Hamilton, a type II mutation having diminished serine protease reactivity) found significantly higher results in affected family members (Demers et al 1992). However the mean F_{1+2} value was within the normal range and the majority had normal levels. The mean levels of TAT complex and FPA were not significantly different between the antithrombin III-deficient people and their unaffected family members (Demers et al 1992).

Coronary artery disease

Elevated levels of fibrinopeptide A have been reported early after the onset of acute transmural myocardial infarction (Johnsson et al 1979, Mombelli et al 1984, van Hulsteijn et al 1984, Eisenberg et al 1985, Rapold et al 1991) and the values then decrease over the subsequent 24 hours (Eisenberg et al 1985). The increased fibrinopeptide A levels rapidly return to normal after the administration of heparin (Mombelli et al 1984, Eisenberg et al 1985) suggesting that the generated thrombin is readily inactivated by heparin-antithrombin III complexes.

Other conditions associated with elevated levels of markers of coagulation activation

Elevated levels of markers of coagulation activation have been reported in settings in which thrombosis or DIC is not evident clinically. A list of some of these disorders is shown in Table 52.3.

Anticoagulants

In most patients with venous thromboembolism, treatment with adequate doses of heparin rapidly inhibits thrombin action upon fibrinogen and lowers elevated fibrinopeptide A levels into the normal range (Nossel et al 1974, Peuscher et al 1980a, Yudelman et al 1982). Thrombin generation as measured by the F_{1+2} and TAT assays declines gradually over the initial several days of

Table 52.3 Conditions associated with elevated levels of markers of coagulation activation (excluding thrombosis or DIC)

Condition	Marker	Reference
Systemic lupus erythematosus	FPA	Cronlund et al 1976, Hardin et al 1978
Solid tumours	F_{1+2}, FPA	Peuscher et al 1980b, Leeksma et al 1983, Bauer et al 1989b
Acute myelogenous leukaemia	F_{1+2}, FPA	Myers et al 1981, Bauer et al 1984, Gugliotta et al 1984
Sickle cell disease	F_{1+2}, FPA, D-dimer	Leichtman & Brewer 1978, Devine et al 1986, Green & Scott 1986, Francis et al 1990
Normal pregnancy	F_{1+2}	Bauer & Rosenberg 1983
Postmenopausal Oestrogen use	F_{1+2}, FPA	Caine et al 1992
Prothrombin complex concentrate administration	Factor X activation peptide, F_{1+2} FPA	Mannucci et al 1990, 1991a

heparin treatment, but often remains elevated as compared to levels in healthy controls after even a week of therapy (Estivals et al 1991). This may reflect the protection of factor Xa in the prothrombinase complex from inhibition by heparin bound to plasma antithrombin III (Teitel & Rosenberg 1983).

Therapy with oral anticoagulants such as warfarin suppresses prothrombin activation in vivo as measured by the F_{1+2} assay (Conway et al 1987, Mannucci et al 1991b). In patients with prior thrombotic histories and high F_{1+2} levels, it was demonstrated (Conway et al 1987) that stable anticoagulation at moderate intensity as reflected by International Normalized Ratios (INRs) of 2.5–3.5 produces 5–10 fold reductions in the extent of prothrombin activation. It has also been shown that the mean values of F_{1+2} decrease in parallel with the intensity of warfarin therapy. A recent study has demonstrated that a target INR range as low as 1.3–1.6 results on average in a 50% reduction in prothrombin activation from baseline levels (Millenson et al 1992). It is important to note that the findings of these studies cannot currently be translated into clinical practice as the F_{1+2} level that confers antithrombotic protection has yet to be determined.

While F_{1+2} levels are often suppressed below normal in stably anticoagulated patients on oral agents, this has not been observed for fibrinopeptide A. However it has been observed that plasma fibrinopeptide A concentrations increase above the normal range in patients with a prior history of myocardial infarction several weeks after cessation of the drug (Harenberg et al 1983).

CONCLUSION

Based on advances in our understanding of the biochemistry of the haemostatic mechanism, clinicians will have access to an expanding armamentarium of laboratory tests for evaluating the patient with a thrombotic diathesis. This chapter has described a number of sensitive methods for measuring peptides, enzyme-inhibitor complexes, and enzymes that are liberated with the activation of the coagulation system in vivo. To date, studies employing these markers indicate that a biochemical imbalance between procoagulant and anticoagulant mechanisms can be detected in the blood of humans prior to the appearance of thrombotic phenomena. However, properly designed prospective studies will be required to determine whether these assays can identify individuals who are entering a clinically relevant hypercoagulable state, as well as monitor specific therapeutic interventions designed to prevent the onset of thrombotic disease.

Acknowledgments

Supported in part by National Institutes of Health Grant Nos. HL 33014 and the Medical Research Service of the Department of Veterans Affairs.

REFERENCES

Asakura H, Saito M, Ito K, Jokaji Y, Uotani C, Kumabashiri I, Matsuda T 1988 Levels of thrombin-antithrombin III complex in plasma in cases of acute promyelocytic leukemia. Thrombosis Research 50: 895–899

Bartsch P, Haeberli A, Straub P W 1990 Blood coagulation after long distance running: antithrombin III prevents fibrin formation. Thrombosis and Haemostasis 63: 430–434

Bauer K A, Rosenberg R D 1983 Assays for thrombin generation in humans with prethrombotic states. Thrombosis and Haemosttasis 50: 159

Bauer K A, Rosenberg R D 1984 Thrombin generation in acute promyelocytic leukemia. Blood 64: 791–796

Bauer K A, Goodman T L, Rosenberg R D 1983 The rapid inhibition of thrombin and factor Xa within the circulatory system of humans. Clinical Research 31: 534a

Bauer K A, Kass B L, Beeler D L, Rosenberg R D 1984 Detection of protein C activation in humans. Journal of Clinical Investigation 74: 2033–2041

Bauer K A, Goodman T L, Kass B L Rosenberg R D 1985 Elevated factor Xa activity in the blood of asymptomatic patients with congenital antithrombin deficiency. Journal of Clinical Investigation 76: 826–836

Bauer K A, Weiss L M, Sparrow D, Vokonas P S, Rosenberg R D 1987 Aging-associated changes in indices of thrombin generation and protein C activation in humans. Normative aging study. Journal of Clinical Investigation 80: 1527–1534

Bauer K A, Broekmans A W, Bertina R M, Conard J, Horellou M-H, Samama M M, Rosenberg R D 1988 Hemostatic enzyme generation in the blood of patients with hereditary protein C deficiency. Blood 71: 1418–1426

Bauer K A, Kass B L, ten Cate H, Bednarek M A, Hawiger J J, Rosenberg R D 1989a Detection of factor X activation in humans. Blood 74: 2007–2015

Bauer K A, ten Cate H, Barzegar S, Spriggs D R, Sherman M L, Rosenberg R 1989b Tumor necrosis factor infusions have a procoagulant effect on the hemostatic mechanism of humans. Blood 74: 165–172

Bauer K A, Kass B L, ten Cate H, Hawiger J J, Rosenberg R D 1990 Factor IX is activated in vivo by the tissue factor mechanism. Blood 76: 731–736

Bauer K A, Barzegar S, Rosenberg R D 1991 Influence of anticoagulants used for blood collection on plasma prothrombin fragment F_{1+2} measurements. Thrombosis Research 63: 617–628

Bauer K A, Mannucci P M, Gringeri A, Tradati F, Barzegar S, Kass B L, ten Cate H, Kestin A S, Brettler D B, Rosenberg R D 1992 Factor IXa-factor VIIIa-cell surface complex does not contribute to the basal activation of the coagulation mechanism in vitro. Blood 79: 2039–2047

Biggs R, Nossel H L 1961 Tissue extract and the contact reaction in blood coagulation. Thrombosis et Diathesis Haemorrhagica 6: 1–4

Bilezikian S B, Nossel H L, Butler V P J, Canfield R E 1975 Radioimmunoassay of human fibrinopeptide B and kinetics of cleavage by different enzymes: Journal of Clinical Investigation 56: 438–445

Boisclair M D, Lane D A, Wilde J T, Ireland H, Preston F E, Ofosu F A 1990 A comparative evaluation of assays for markers of activated coagulation and/or fibrinolysis: thrombin-antithrombin complex, D-dimer and fibrinogen/fibrin fragment E antigen. British Journal of Haematology 74: 471–479

Boneu B, Bes G, Pelzer H, Sie P, Boccalon H 1991 D-dimers, thrombin antithrombin III complexes and prothrombin fragments 1+2: diagnostic value in clinically suspected deep vein thrombosis. Thrombosis and Haemostasis 65: 28–32

Caine Y G, Bauer K A, Barzegar S, ten Cate H, Sacks F M, Walsh

B W, Schiff I, Rosenberg R D 1992 Coagulation activation following estrogen administration to postmenopausal women. Thrombosis and Haemostasis 68: 392–395

Collen D, de Cock F A 1975 A tanned red cell hemagglutination inhibitor immunoassay (TRCHII) for the quantitative determination of thrombin-antithrombin III and plasmin-alpha$_2$ antiplasmin complexes in human plasma. Thrombosis Research 7: 235–238

Collen D, de Cock F, Verstraete M 1977 Quantitation of thrombin-antithrombin III complexes in human blood. European Journal of Clinical Investigation 7: 407–411

Conard J, Bauer K A, Schwarz H P, Horellou M H, Samama M, Rosenberg R D 1991 Normalization of markers of coagulation activation by protein C (PC) concentrate in adults with severe PC deficiency. Blood (suppl 1) 78: 186a

Conway E M, Bauer K A, Barzegar S, Rosenberg R D 1987 Suppression of hemostatic system activation by oral anticoagulants in the blood of patients with thrombotic diatheses. Journal of Clinical Investigation 80: 1535–1544

Cronlund M, Hardin J, Burton J, Lee L, Haber E, Bloch K J 1976 Fibrinopeptide A in plasma of normal subjects and patients with disseminated intravascular coagulation and systemic lupus erythematosus. Journal of Clinical Investigation 58: 142–151

Davie E, Ratnoff O D 1964 Waterfall sequence for intrinsic blood clotting. Science 145: 1310

Demers C, Ginsberg J S, Henderson P, Ofosu F A, Weitz J I, Blajchman M A 1992 Measurements of markers of activated coagulation in antithrombin III deficient subjects. Thrombosis and Haemostasis 67: 542–544

Devine D V, Kinney T R, Thomas P F, Rosse W F, Greenberg C S 1986 Fragment D-dimer levels: an objective marker of vaso-occlusive crisis and other complications of sickle cell disease. Blood 68: 317

Eckhardt T, Nossel H L, Hurlet-Jensen A, LaGamma K S, Owen J, Auerbach M 1981 Measurement of desarginine fibrinopeptide B in human blood. Journal of Clinical Investigation 67: 809–816

Eisenberg P, Sherman L A, Schechtman K, Perez J, Sobel B E, Jaffee A S 1985 Fibrinopeptide A: a marker for acute coronary thrombosis. Circulation 71: 912–918

Espana F, Griffin J H 1989 Determination of functional and antigenic protein C inhibitor and its complexes with activated protein C in plasma by ELISAs. Thrombosis Research 55: 671–682

Espana F, Vicente V, Tabernero D, Scharrer I, Griffin J H 1990 Determination of plasma protein C inhibitor and of two activated protein C-inhibitor complexes in normals and in patients with intravascular coagulation and thrombotic disease. Thrombosis Research 59: 593–608

Espana F, Gruber A, Heeb M J, Hanson S R, Harker L A, Griffin J H 1991 In vivo and in vitro complexes of activated protein C with two inhibitors in baboons. Blood 77: 1754–1760

Estivals M, Pelzer H, Sie P, Pichon J, Boccalon H, Boneu B 1991 Prothrombin fragment 1+2, thrombin-antithrombin III complexes and D-dimers in acute deep vein thrombosis: effects of heparin treatment. British Journal of Haematology 78: 421–424

Francis R, Patch J, McGehee W, Crout F 1990 Elevated prothrombin F 1.2 fragment in sickle cell disease: further evidence for activation of coagulation in the steady state. Blood 76: 61

Green D, Scott J P 1986 Is sickle cell crisis a thrombotic event? American Journal of Hematology 23: 317–321

Gruber A, Griffin J H 1992 Direct detection of activated protein C in blood from human subjects. Blood 79: 2340–2348

Gugliotta L, Vigano S, D'Angelo A, Guarini A, Tura S, Mannucci P M 1984 High fibrinopeptide A (FPA) levels in acute non-lymphocytic leukemia are reduced by heparin administration. Thrombosis Haemostasis 52: 301–304

Hamsten A, Walldius G, Szamosi A, Blombäck M, de Faire U, Dahlen G, Landou C, Wiman B 1987 Plasminogen activator inhibitor in plasma: risk factor for recurrent myocardial infarction. Lancet 2: 3–9

Hardin J A, Cronlund M, Haber E, Bloch K J 1978 Activation of blood clotting in patients with systemic lupus erythematosus. Relationship to disease activity. American Journal of Medicine 65: 430–436

Harenberg J, Haas R, Zimmermann R 1983 Plasma hypercoagulability after termination of oral anticoagulants. Thrombosis Research 29: 627–633

Hoek J A, Sturk A, ten Cate J W, Lamping R J, Berends F, Borm J J 1988 Laboratory and clinical evaluation of an assay of thrombin-antithrombin III complexes in plasma. Clinical Chemistry 34: 2058–2062

Hoek J A, Nurmohamed M T, ten Cate J W, Buller H R, Knipscheer H C, Hamelynck K J, Marti R K, Sturk A 1989 Thrombin-antithrombin III complexes in the prediction of deep vein thrombosis following total hip replacement. Thrombosis and Haemostasis 62: 1050–1052

Hursting M, Butman B, Steiner J, Moore B, Szewczvk K, Bell M, Dombrose F 1989 A quantitative ELISA for plasma prothrombin fragment 1.2 (F1.2). Blood 74: 257a

Hursting M J, Stead A, Crout F, Horvath B, Moore B 1990 Effects of age, race, sex and smoking on plasma prothrombin fragment F1.2 (F1.2) levels in a healthy population. Blood (suppl 1) 76: 423a

Jesty J, Morrison S A, Harpel P C 1984 Measurement of human activated factor X-antithrombin complex by an enzyme-linked differential-antibody immunosorbent assay. Analytical Biochemistry 139: 158–167

Johnsson H, Orinius E, Paul C 1979 Fibrinopeptide A (FpA) in patients with acute myocardial infarction. Thrombosis Research 16: 255–260

Josso F, Prou-Wartelle O 1965 Interaction of tissue factor and factor VII at the earliest phase of coagulation. Thrombosis Diathesis Haemorrhagica 17: 35–44

Kannel W, Wolf P, Castelli W, D'Agostino R 1987 Fibrinogen and risk of cardiovascular disease. Journal of the American Medical Association 258: 1183–1186

Kaplan A P, Gruber B, Harpel P C 1985 Assessment of Hageman factor activation in human plasma: Quantification of activated Hageman factor-C1 inactivator complexes by an enzyme-linked differential antibody immunosorbent assay. Blood 66: 636–641

Kockum C, Frebelius S 1980 Rapid radioimmunoassay of human fibrinopeptide A — removal of cross-reacting fibrinogen with bentonite. Thrombosis Research 19: 589–598

Lau H, Rosenberg R 1980 The isolation and characterization of a specific antibody population directed against the thrombin-antithrombin complex. Journal of Biological Chemistry 255: 5885–5893

Lau H K, Rosenberg J S, Beeler D L, Rosenberg R D 1979 The isolation and characterization of a specific antibody population directed against the prothrombin activation fragments F_2 and F_{1+2}. Journal of Biological Chemistry 254: 8751–8761

Leeksma O C, Stoepman-van Dalen E A, van Ginkel C J W, van Mourik J A, van Aken W G 1983 A reappraisal of FPA immunoreactivity in cancer patients. Thrombosis and Haemostasis 50: 400

Leichtman D, Brewer G 1978 Elevated plasma levels of fibrinopeptide A during sickle cell anemia pain crisis — evidence for intravascular coagulation. American Journal of Hematology 5: 183–190

Leonard B, Bies R, Carlson T, Reeve E B 1983 Further studies of the turnover of dog antithrombin III. Study of ^{131}I-labelled antithrombin protease complexes. Thrombosis Research 30: 165–177

Leroy-Matheron C, Gouault-Heilmann M, Levent M 1991 Prothrombin fragment 1+2 levels in patients with inherited deficiency in coagulation inhibitors. Thrombosis and Haemostasis 65: 1208

Lewin M F, Kaplan A P, Harpel P C 1983 Studies of C1 inactivator-plasma kallikrein complexes in purified systems and in plasma. Journal of Biological Chemistry 258: 6415–6421

Macfarlane R G 1964 An enzyme cascade in the blood clotting mechanism, and its function as a biochemical amplifier. Nature 202: 498–499

Mann K G, Williams E B, Krishnaswamy S, Church W, Giles A, Tracy R P 1990 Active site-specific immunoassays. Blood. 76: 755–766

Mannucci P M, Bauer K A, Gringeri A, Barzegar S, Santagostino E, Tradati F C, Rosenberg R D 1990 Thrombin generation is not increased in the blood of hemophilia B patients after the infusion of a purified factor IX concentrate. Blood 76: 2540–2545

Mannucci P M, Bauer K A, Gringeri A, Barzegar S, Santagostino E, Tradati F C, Rosenberg R D 1991a No activation of the common pathway of the coagulation cascade after a highly purified factor IX concentrate. British Journal of Haematology 79: 606–611

Mannucci P M, Bottasso B, Tripodi 1991b A. Prothrombin fragment 1+2 and intensity of treatment with oral anticoagulants. Thrombosis and Haemostasis 66: 741

Mannucci P M, Tripodi A, Bottasso B, Baudo F, Finazzi G, de

Stefano V, Palareti G, Manotti C, Mazzucconi M G, Castaman G 1992 Markers of procoagulant imbalance in patients with inherited thrombophilic syndromes. Thrombosis and Haemostasis 67: 200–202

Meade T, North W, Chakrabarti R, Stirling Y, Haines A, Thompson S 1980 Haemostatic function and cardiovascular death: early results of a prospective study. Lancet 1: 1050–1054

Meade T, Mellows S, Brozovic M, Miller G, Chakrabarti R, North W, Haines A, Stirling Y, Imeson J, Thompson S 1986 Haemostatic function and ischaemic heart disease: principal results of the Northwick Park Heart Study. Lancet 2: 533–537

Michie H R, Manogue K R, Spriggs D R, Revhaug A, O'Dwyer S, Dinarello C, Cerami, A, Wolff S M, Wilmore D W 1988 Detection of circulating tumor necrosis factor after endotoxin administration. New England Journal of Medicine 318: 1481–1486

Millenson M M, Bauer K A, Kistler J P, Barzegar S, Tulin L, Rosenberg R D 1992 Monitoring 'mini-intensity' anticoagulation with warfarin: Comparison of the prothrombin time using a sensitive thromboplastin with prothrombin fragment F1+2 levels. Blood 79: 2034–2038

Mombelli G, Im Hof V, Haeberli A et al 1984 Effect of heparin on plasma fibrinopeptide A in patients with acute myocardial infarction. Circulation 69: 684–689

Morrissey J H, Macik B G, Newenschwander P F, Comp P C 1993 Quantitation of activated factor VII levels in plasma using a tissue factor mutant selectively deficient in promoting factor VII activation. Blood 81: 734–744

Myers T J, Rickles F R, Barb C, Cronlund M 1981 Fibrinopeptide A in acute leukemia: relationship of activation of blood coagulation to disease activity. Blood 57: 518

Neame P B, Kelton J G, Walker I R, Stewart I O, Nossel H L, Hirsh J 1980 Thrombocytopenia in septicemia: the role of disseminated intravascular coagulation. Blood 56: 88–92

Nossel H L 1981 Relative proteolysis of the fibrinogen Bβ-chain as a determinant of thrombosis. Nature 291: 165–167

Nossel H, Younger L, Wilner G, Procupez T, Canfield R, Butler V Jr 1971 Radioimmunoassay of human fibrinopeptide A. Proceedings of the National Academy of Sciences, USA 68: 2350–2353

Nossel H L, Yudelman I, Canfield R E, Butler V P Jr, Spanondis K, Wilner G D, Qureshi G D 1974 Measurement of fibrinopeptide A in human blood. Journal of Clinical Investigation 54: 43–53

Nossel H L, Ti M, Kaplan K L, Spanondis K, Soland T, Butler V P Jr 1976 The generation of fibrinopeptide A in clinical blood samples: evidence for thrombin activity. Journal of Clinical Investigation 58: 1136–1144

Nossel H L, Wasser J, Kaplan K L, LaGamma K S, Yudelman I, Canfield R E 1979 Sequence of fibrinogen proteolysis and platelet release after intrauterine infusion of hypertonic saline. Journal of Clinical Investigation 64: 1371–1378

Nuijens J H, Huijbregts C C M, Eerenberg A J M, Abbink J J, Strack van Schijndel R J M, Felt-Bersma R J F, Thijs L G, Hack C E 1988 Quantification of plasma factor XIIa-C1-inhibitor and kallikrein-C1-inhibitor complexes in sepsis. Blood 72: 1841–1848

Orthner C L, Kolen B, Drohan W N 1991 A sensitive and facile assay for the measurement of activated protein C activity in vivo. Blood 78 (suppl 1): 219a

Owen J, Kvam D, Nossel H L, Kaplan K L, Kernoff P B A 1983 Thrombin and plasmin activity and platelet activation in the development of venous thrombosis. Blood 61: 476–482

Pelzer H, Schwarz A, Heimburger N 1988 Determination of human thrombin-antithrombin III complex in plasma with an enzyme-linked immunosorbent assay. Thrombosis and Haemostasis 59: 101–106

Pelzer H, Schwart A, Stuber W 1991 Determination of human prothrombin activation fragment 1+2 in plasma in plasma with an antibody against a synthetic peptide. Thrombosis and Haemostasis 65: 153–159

Peuscher F W, van Aken W G, Flier O T N, Stoepman-van Dalen E A, Cremer-Groote T M, van Mourik J A 1980a Effect of anticoagulant treatment measured by fibrinopeptide A (fpA) in patients with venous thrombo-embolism. Thrombosis Research 18: 33–43

Peuscher F W, Cleton F J, Armstrong L, Stoepman-van Dalen E A, van Mourik J A, van Aken W G 1980b Significance of plasma fibrinopeptide A (FpA) in patients with malignancy. Journal of Laboratory and Clinical Medicine 96: 5–14

Rapold J H, Grimaudo V, Declerck P J et al 1991 Plasma levels of plasminogen activator inhibitor type 1, β-thromboglobulin, and fibrinopeptide A before, during, and after treatment of acute myocardial infarction with alteplase. Blood 78: 1490

Schafer A 1985 The hypercoagulable states. Annals of Internal Medicine 102: 814–828

Shi Q, Ruiz J A, Perez L M, Denis R F, Sio R, Alvarez D, Tang S M, Mills R, Arbuthnott K, Gaur P 1989 Detection of prothrombin activation with a two-site enzyme immunoassay for the fragment F1.2. Thrombosis and Haemostasis 62: 165

Shifman M A, Pizzo S V 1982 The in vivo metabolism of antithrombin III and antithrombin III complexes. Journal of Biological Chemistry 257: 3243–3248

Soria J, Soria C, Ryckewaert J J 1980 A solid phase immuno enzymological assay for the measurement of human fibrinopeptide A. Thrombosis Research 20: 425–435

Suffredini A F, Harpel P C, Parrillo J E 1989 Promotion and subsequent inhibition of plasminogen activation after administration of intravenous endotoxin to normal subjects. New England Journal of Medicine 320: 1165–1172

Takahashi I, Kato K, Sugiura I, Takamatsu J, Kamiya T, Saito H 1991 Activated factor IX-antithrombin III complexes in human blood: Quantification by an enzyme-linked differential antibody immunoassay and determination of the in vivo half-life. Journal of Laboratory and Clinical Medicine 118: 317–325

Teitel J M, Bauer K A, Lau H K, Rosenberg R D 1982 Studies of the prothrombin activation pathway utilizing radioimmunoassays for the F_2/F_{1+2} fragment and the thrombin-antithrombin complex. Blood 59: 1086–1097

Teitel J M, Rosenberg R D 1983 Protection of factor Xa from neutralization by the heparin-antithrombin complex. Journal of Clinical Investigation 71: 1383–1391

Toh C H, Hoogendoorn H, Scully M F, Giles A R 1991 Quantification of activated protein C (APC) in complex with α_2-macroglobulin α_2-M) by ELISA in patients with disseminated intravascular coagulation (DIC). Blood 78 (suppl 1): 74a

Trip M, Manger Cats V, van Capelle F, Vreeken J 1990 Platelet hyperreactivity and prognosis in survivors of myocardial infarction. New England Journal of Medicine 322: 1549–1554

van der Poll T, Buller H R, ten Cate H, Wortel C H, Bauer K A, van Deventer S J H, Hack C E, Sauerwein H P, Rosenberg R D, ten Cate J W 1990 Coagulation activation following tumour necrosis factor administration to normal subjects. New England Journal of Medicine 322: 1622–1627

van Deventer S J H, Buller H R, ten Cate J W, Aarden L A, Hack C E, Sturk A 1990 Experimental endotoxemia in humans: analysis of cytokine release and coagulation, fibrinolytic, and complement pathways. Blood 76: 2520–2526

van Hulsteijn, H, Kolff J, Briët E, van der Laarse A, Bertina R 1984 Fibrinopeptide A and beta thromboglobulin in patients with angina pectoris and acute myocardial infarction. American Heart Journal 107: 39–45

Weinstein M J, Chute L E, Schmitt G W, Hamburger R H, Bauer K A, Troll J H, Janson P, Deykin D 1985 Abnormal factor VIII coagulant antigen in patients with renal dysfunction and in those with disseminated intravascular coagulation. Journal of Clinical Investigation 76: 1406–1411

Wildgoose P, Nemerson Y, Hansen L, Nielsen F, Glazer S, Hedner U 1992 Measurement of basal levels of factor VIIa in hemophilia A and B patients. Blood 80: 25–28

Wilhelmsen L, Svardsudd K, Korsan-Bengsten K, Welin L, Tibblin G 1984 Fibrinogen as a risk factor for stroke and myocardial infarction. New England Journal of Medicine 311: 501–505

Woodhams B J, Kernoff P B A 1981 Rapid radioimmunoassay for fibrinopeptide A in plasma. Thrombosis Research 22: 407–416

Yudelman I, Greenberg J 1982 Factors affecting fibrinopeptide-A levels in patients with venous thromboembolism during anticoagulant therapy. Blood 59: 787–792

Yudelman I M, Nossel H L, Kaplan K L, Hirsh J 1978 Plasma fibrinopeptide A levels in symptomatic venous thromboembolism. Blood 51: 1189–1195

53. The epidemiology of atheroma, thrombosis and ischaemic heart disease

T. W. Meade

It is hard to exaggerate the importance of distinguishing between the vessel wall pathology, the luminal occlusion caused by thrombosis and the clinical manifestations of ischaemic heart disease (IHD). Indeed, it can be argued that the use of umbrella terms such as 'atherosclerotic heart disease' to embrace different pathological and clinical manifestations has actually been counter-productive in delaying full appreciation of the different processes in the pathogenesis of IHD.

The term 'coronary thrombosis' was derived from clinical and pathological observations on myocardial infarction made at least 80 years ago (Herrick 1912) and perhaps even earlier (Hammer 1878). So present interest in thrombosis is a reawakening rather than a discovery. But it was probably not until the 1930s that clinically manifest IHD in the form of myocardial infarction became a familiar condition rather than the unusual occurrence or even the rarity it had hitherto been. When the growing epidemic of clinical IHD prompted an increasing and concerted research programme in the United States after the Second World War, interest largely centred on the lipid nature of the atheromatous plaque and the contributions dietary fat intake and blood cholesterol levels make to it.

Two developments in the early and mid-1970s signalled a re-emerging interest in the thrombotic component of IHD. One was the first results of randomized controlled trials of aspirin in the secondary prevention of myocardial infarction (MI) (Elwood et al 1974), along with the findings of less satisfactory but nevertheless still suggestive observational studies. Interest in aspirin had been stimulated by the demonstration of its inhibitory effects on platelet aggregation (Weiss & Aledort 1967). The other development was a debate, mainly between pathologists, as to whether thrombosis causes or is the result of MI. This question was settled, as far as it could be at that time, by a consensus view that concluded thrombosis does precede and probably causes transmural MI (Chandler et al 1974). But it was not really until 1980 — comparatively recently — that the point was finally settled when the advent of thrombolytic therapy and the need to establish the rationale for its use and effects led to angiographic studies that showed the high frequency of total coronary occlusion during MI (DeWood et al 1980). Few if any would now seriously contest the causative role of thrombosis in transmural MI and probably, though perhaps somewhat less certainly, in sub-endocardial infarction as well (Davies 1987). Even then, however, another controversy remained unresolved: the place of thrombosis in sudden coronary death. Reports in the mid-1970s of platelet thrombi and microemboli in the coronary vessels of those dying sudden vascular deaths (Haerem 1974) were often viewed with scepticism. It was not until the results of a series of particularly careful autopsy studies became available in the 1980s (for example, Davies & Thomas 1984) that the almost universal occurrence of at least a degree of thrombosis in sudden coronary death was recognised. The minority of coronary deaths in which thrombosis is not apparently associated with plaque rupture — between about 2% (Davies & Thomas 1984) and about 25% (El Fawal et al 1987) — suggests that characteristics of the circulating blood play a part in initiating some arterial thrombi as well as contributing to the consequences of plaque rupture. The reason why thrombi associated with sudden coronary death do not totally occlude the arterial lumen as often as those causing transmural MI may be the intense fibrinolytic activity accompanying sudden death, with the consequence that thrombi — initially responsible for such episodes — are at least partially lysed by the time of autopsy (Meade et al 1984, Davies 1987). Without in any way detracting from the importance of the more recent studies demonstrating the thrombotic contribution to IHD, its recognition by an earlier generation of pathologists should also be acknowledged (Duguid 1946), although it had been largely overlooked by workers in other disciplines.

EPIDEMIOLOGICAL STUDIES OF PATHOLOGY

In fact, there had also been much earlier epidemiological recognition of a thrombotic component than is generally appreciated, even though its detailed characteristics had not been identified. Thus, it was Morris who first drew attention to the involvement of a major process other than atherogenesis through his work on postmortem data (Morris 1951). Morris analysed reports on the coronary arteries of some 6000 patients aged between 50 and 69 coming to postmortem examination between 1908 and 1949 at the London hospital. Routine examination of the coronary arteries and myocardium was performed over the whole of the period in question, whatever the cause of death. 'Advanced' atheroma was used to cover lesions with calcification, ulceration, haemorrhage, stenosis or occlusion, or described merely as 'severe'. In those who died of conditions other than IHD itself (and conditions associated with it, especially hypertension) the age-standardized prevalence of advanced atheroma in 1908–13 was 30.4%. In other words, there was a high prevalence of advanced atheroma before the steep rise in the incidence of clinically manifest IHD. In 1944–49, however, the prevalence was 16.0%. The decrease was seen in all the relevant sex, age and pathological categories studied. It occurred in two phases that seemed to be connected with the two world wars. Yet over the same period, there was a seven fold increase in the number of cases of IHD in the London hospital series, complementing the country-wide increase in IHD mortality. These points are summarized in Figure 53.1. Morris concluded that 'coronary thrombosis and heart disease may not be simple and direct functions of the atheroma' and he suggested that the increase in smoking around the time of the first war might have been involved in the rise in mortality.

Soon after the findings of the London hospital autopsy series, Morris et al (1953) showed that the incidence of IHD was inversely related to the level of occupational physical activity: the lighter the work, the higher the incidence. This apparently protective effect has also been observed in terms of leisure-time activity (Morris et al 1990). It is most unlikely that it will ever be confirmed through the randomized controlled trial theoretically necessary to do so but there is now little doubt that the relationship is one of cause and effect. Furthermore, because exercise has to be current and continuing to confer protection against IHD there is growing reason to believe that it modifies the acute, thrombotic component (Morris et al 1990). This conclusion had already been suggested by the National Necropsy Survey (Morris & Crawford 1958), which dealt with the relationship between physical activity and the pathological (as distinct from clinical) manifestations of arterial disease. Pathologists in a large number of hospitals in the United Kingdom were asked to record details of the coronary arteries and myocardium according to standard criteria. Information was obtained from death certificates and other sources on levels of occupational physical activity, using the same classification as in the clinical study (Morris et al 1953). There was no relationship between the level of occupational physical activity and the extent of atheroma. On the other hand, occlusion of the coronary lumen was significantly more frequent in those who had been in light compared with heavy occupations, and large healed infarcts were some three times commoner. The findings, illustrated in Figure 53.2, were summarized by the authors as 'atheroma of coronary walls, no relationship with physical activity; occlusion or coronary lumen, some relationship; ischaemic myocardial fibrosis, much relationship'.

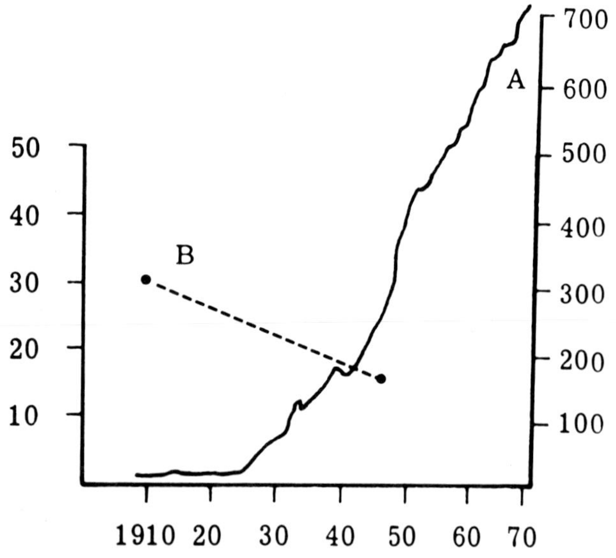

Fig. 53.1 Trends in IHD death rates and in prevalence of atheroma A (right-hand scale), male death rates per 100 000 at ages 50–69 years in England and Wales. B (left-hand scale), age-standardized prevalence, per cent, of advanced coronary atheroma in males at ages 50–69 years in 1908–13 and 1944–49 (Morris 1951).

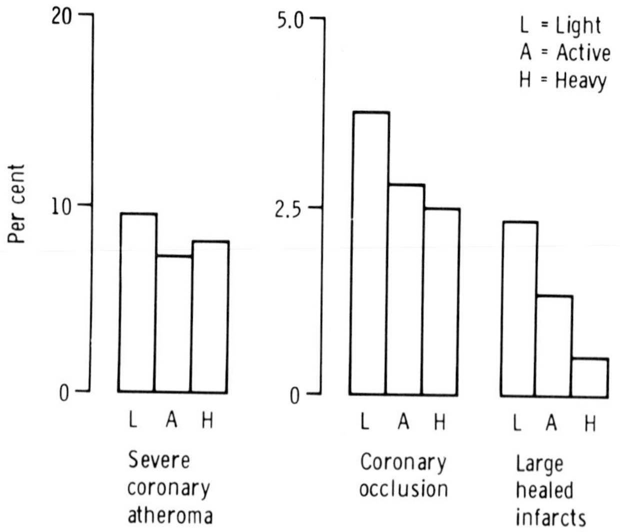

Fig. 53.2 Prevalence of different pathological manifestations of IHD according to physical activity of occupation (Morris & Crawford 1958, reproduced by permission of Update.)

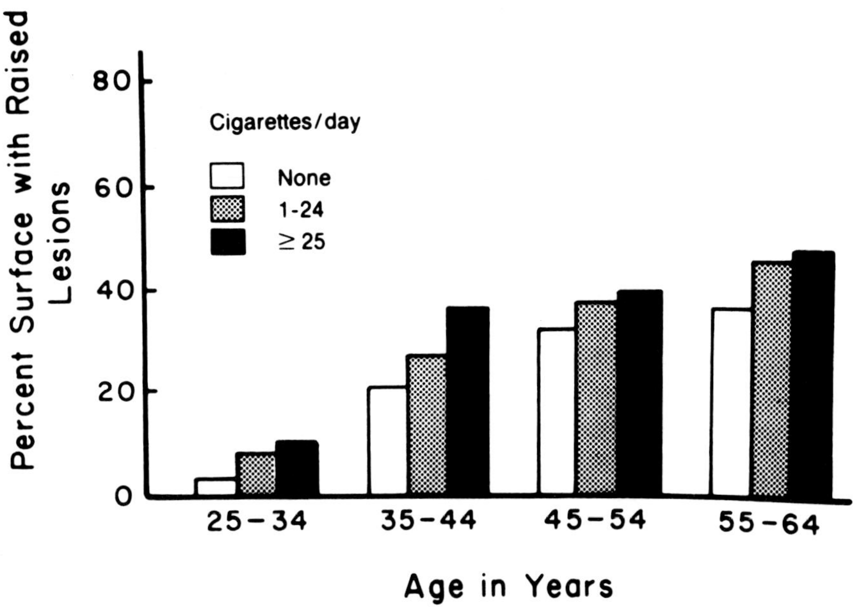

Fig. 53.3 Raised lesions (fibrous plaques and complicated lesions) in coronary arteries, by age and degree of smoking in 553 white men (McGill 1988, reproduced by permission of American Heart Journal).

The International Atherosclerosis Project (IAP) (McGill 1968) examined 25 000 aortae and sets of coronary vessels from autopsies carried out in 14 different countries with a wide range of IHD mortality rates. In summary, there was a close association between the extent of atheroma and IHD mortality. IAP also provides more direct evidence to support Morris's suggestion that smoking might have played an important part in the increasing IHD mortality from the 1920s onwards. Figure 53.3, based on IAP data (McGill 1988), shows a fairly modest effect of smoking on the extent of coronary artery atheroma. By contrast, Table 53.1 shows much larger relative risks of death from IHD in smokers compared with non-smokers. Again, therefore, the implication is that the influence of smoking on clinical disease is largely mediated through a process other than atherogenesis.

There is little to be gained from any continued polarization of views about the pathogenesis of arterial disease, although the past dominance of the lipid hypothesis in epidemiological studies justifies special consideration of other aspects. Figure 53.4 summarizes the general sequence of events by which both atheroma and thrombosis lead to clinical disease.

Table 53.1 Relative risk of ischaemic heart disease death in young male smokers compared with non-smokers

Reference source	Risk
Doll and Peto 1976	9.7
Weir and Dunn 1970	6.2
Kahn 1966	4.4
Hammond and Garfinkel 1969	2.8

THE CLINICAL SYNDROME OF IHD

The term 'ischaemic (or coronary) heart disease' is widely used to cover three main clinical manifestations. The first of these is sudden coronary death. This refers to those who collapse and die instantaneously, or within a few hours of the onset of symptoms, and accounts for a quarter or a third of first episodes of IHD (Tunstall Pedoe et al 1975) depending on the precise definition. Until 10 or 20 years

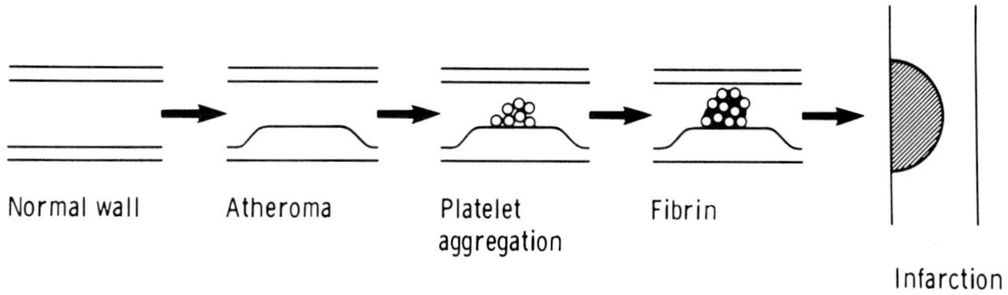

Fig. 53.4 Pathogenesis of IHD.

ago, no particular distinction was usually made between sudden death and myocardial infarction in terms of immediate precipitating causes. However, in 1975 Cobb et al (1975) reported on patients who survived sudden death as a result of an intensive community programme of instruction in cardiopulmonary resuscitation in Seattle. Only 16% of these patients went on to develop classical evidence of myocardial infarction. Those who were resuscitated were particularly prone to further episodes of sudden death and probably had a worse prognosis than those having classical episodes of non-fatal infarction. This report, which attracted considerable attention, led to a wide-spread assumption that sudden death is not a thrombotic event. There are, however, reasons for doubting this conclusion. Two other studies much less cited than the work in Seattle reported myocardial infarction developing in 39% (Liberthson et al 1974), and 44% (Goldstein et al 1981) of those resuscitated after sudden death, substantially higher than the Seattle figure. Probably the most compelling evidence comes from the autopsy study by Davies & Thomas (1984), already referred to, which made it clear that some degree of thrombosis is the rule in coronary deaths and very much the exception in sudden non-coronary deaths. Other considerations are that advanced vessel wall disease, which may itself be partly thrombotic in origin, is almost always found in sudden coronary death (Perper et al 1975).

The second main manifestation of IHD is classical myocardial infarction (MI) consisting of prolonged chest pain, characteristic electrocardiographic (ECG) changes and elevation of the level of cardiac enzymes. The high frequency — about 80% — of total coronary occlusion during the early stages of MI (DeWood et al 1980) has already been referred to.

The third main clinical manifestation is angina pectoris. By contrast with infarction, the incidence of which is higher in men than women, the incidence of angina is much the same in both sexes particularly when angina is not complicated by infarction as well (Lerner & Kannel 1986). Although IHD as a whole (death, infarction and angina) occurs more often in inactive than in active workers, angina is characterized by a higher incidence in the active than in the inactive (Morris et al 1953). In other words, when the active do develop IHD, they tend to do so in a less severe form than the inactive. Angina is rather variable in its presence or absence (Rose 1968) and is often difficult to diagnose with certainty. There is almost certainly a thrombotic component to unstable angina (Falk 1987). Sudden coronary death and myocardial infarction are referred to collectively as IHD in what follows, unless otherwise stated.

GENERAL EPIDEMIOLOGY OF IHD

This chapter is chiefly concerned with the epidemiological study of the relationships between the haemostatic system, thrombosis and IHD. A full account of all the epidemiological characteristics of IHD is therefore not attempted, only the main features being summarized.

The best known prospective study of IHD is the Framingham study, carried out in Framingham, Massachusetts. Hypercholesterolaemia, hypertension, cigarette smoking, glucose intolerance and ECG evidence of left ventricular hypertrophy have each been found to be independently associated with the subsequent risk of clinically manifest arterial disease (Gordon & Kannel 1972). Of the five variables, hypertension is particularly strongly associated with the risk of cerebrovascular disease and cigarette smoking with peripheral arterial disease. No single variable stands out so obviously on its own in the case of IHD. The Framingham results on smoking, hypertension and hypercholesterolaemia have been confirmed by many others. Morris et al (1966) reported similar findings in London busmen, and were the first to use multivariate analyses to assess the independent effects of different variables. Very extensive data from North America (Martin et al 1986) coupled with recent findings in Chinese groups (Chen et al 1991) make it clear that there is a graded relationship between cholesterol levels and IHD throughout the wide range of cholesterol levels observed in these studies. High cholesterol levels also predict recurrence of IHD (Rossouw et al 1990). There is a particularly strong and independent association between high density lipoprotein-cholesterol (HDL) and IHD, higher HDL levels being associated with a substantial degree of protection against IHD (Stampfer et al 1991). The last few years have also seen growing interest in lipoprotein (a), or Lp(a) (Editorial 1991). The association between Lp(a) and IHD is a strong one in most prevalence or case-control studies, i.e. after the onset of IHD, but since levels probably rise after clinical episodes, these associations may reflect consequence rather than cause. What prospective data there are do suggest some association (e.g. Rosengren et al 1990a) but enthusiasm for Lp(a) as a strong, independent risk factor should be tempered with caution until considerably more prospective results are available. The sequence homology of Lp(a) with plasminogen may or may not represent a significant point of contact between lipids and the haemostatic system; again, more evidence about the actual implications of the similarity in man is needed.

By comparison with Framingham, another series of studies (International Collaborative Group 1979) failed to confirm that hyperglycaemia makes an independent contribution to the onset of IHD, but evidence from the Whitehall Study (Fuller et al 1983) suggests that subjects with 2-hour glucose values above the 95th centile are at significantly increased risk. Disordered glucose metabolism manifested as insulin resistance probably explains much of the particularly high incidence of IHD in Asians (McKeigue et al 1991).

Obesity is consistently associated with an increase in risk when considered on its own but not always when included with other variables in multivariate analyses. The probable explanation is that obesity exerts its effects through mechanisms such as hyperlipidaemia and hypertension and also through the level of coagulability. Blood lipid and blood pressure levels may obscure the obesity effect in a statistical sense when several variables are considered simultaneously. In a biological sense, however, obesity almost certainly predisposes to IHD in men (Sonne-Holm et al 1983) and perhaps especially (Larsson et al 1984) in younger men, and in women (Lapidus et al 1984, Manson et al 1990), although the relationship in women is not entirely consistent (Tuomilehto et al 1987). Central obesity may be particularly relevant (Donahue et al 1987). Fluctuations in body weight may contribute to IHD, independently of obesity (Lissner et al 1991).

The risk of IHD established by the earlier prospective studies is summarized in Figure 53.5. The heights of the hatched and shaded areas represent the incidence of IHD in high and low risk groups respectively. These groups are defined according to the cholesterol and blood pressure values specified. Using this definition, 42% of the men concerned (Framingham study participants) had a 'positive test' when they were first seen. It is clear that the subsequent incidence of IHD was substantially more in this high risk group (20% in 10 years) than those without the positive test, i.e. the low risk group (7% in 10 years). But it is also clear that most of those at high risk did not experience clinical events in the next 10 years, while some of those at low risk did. In the particular context of this chapter, Figure 53.5 raises the question of whether haemostatic variables involved in thrombogenesis may explain some of the incidence in those at low risk by cholesterol/blood pressure criteria. The cut-off points for cholesterol and blood pressure in Figure 53.5 are, of course, quite arbitrary. The proportion of those at high risk who develop IHD could be increased by using much higher cut-off points, e.g. cholesterol 350 mg/ml and blood pressure 200 mmHg. But the proportion of people with such extreme values is very small. In terms of absolute numbers, most clinical events of IHD occur in those with only moderately raised values of cholesterol and blood pressure, etc.

Some further points of particular relevance to the relationship between clotting factors and IHD risk that are described in later sections should also be noted. IHD incidence and mortality increase with age and are generally higher in men than women. However, the difference between male and female rates diminishes with advancing age, one reason being the probable increase in incidence in women after the menopause (Gordon et al 1978). At any rate in men, IHD mortality is now higher among those in the lower than in the upper social classes (Marmot et al 1986, Pocock et al 1987). Mortality from IHD in the United States began to decline in the mid 1960s and it was followed by similar falls in other affluent countries such as Australia and Canada (Beaglehole 1990). Rates have now started to fall in the United Kingdom though they remain higher in Scotland and Northern Ireland than in other countries. At the same time, rates

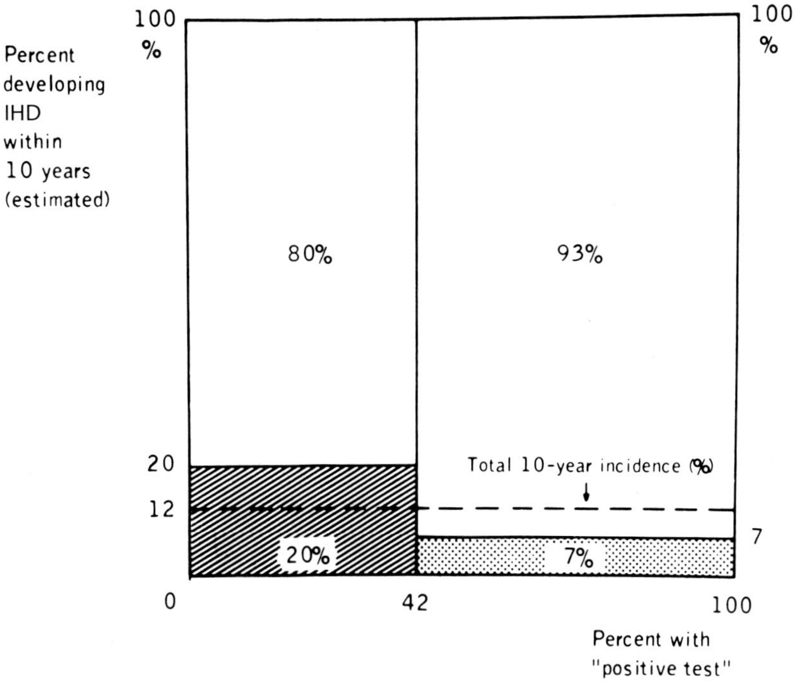

Fig. 53.5 Incidence of IHD in high (i.e. 'positive' test) and low risk groups of men aged 40–59 years. The vertical line can be moved to the right or left depending on the arbitrary definition of high and low risk groups. Here the cut offs for high risk are cholesterol ⩾ 251 mgdl^{-1} and/or systolic blood pressure ⩾ 160 mmHg. (Epstein 1969, reproduced by permission of the Natural Academy of Sciences, Washington DC.)

are increasing in many parts of the world, including some of the former eastern European countries (World Health Organization, 1989). If the risk of IHD is due to the effects of an affluent life-style superimposed on those due to adverse experiences during fetal life and during infancy (for example, poor maternal and infant nutrition) (Barker & Martyn 1992), then there may be a particularly serious impending epidemic of IHD in many third world countries as they are increasingly exposed to the harmful effects of high dietary fat consumption, smoking and other characteristics of more affluent communities. The incidence of IHD is higher between the early hours of the morning and about mid-day (Muller et al 1985, ISIS-2 Collaborative Group 1992) so that diurnal variations in haemostatic variables that might fit in with this clinical pattern may be of particular interest.

METHODOLOGICAL CONSIDERATIONS

Contemporary research on the haemostatic system in thrombotic diseases is characterized by many clinical and a growing number or epidemiological studies in which the results of clotting or platelet function tests are related to the presence or absence of disease. For obvious and understandable reasons, the value of these studies is often viewed in terms of the immediate applicability of their results. A postulated measure of 'thrombotic tendency' may successfully differentiate between groups at high and low risk of IHD and thus make a useful contribution to understanding thrombosis or atheroma in pathogenetic terms. But it does not follow that the sensitivity, specificity and predictive value of the test will be sufficiently high to justify its use to identify individuals at particular risk with a view to intervention, i.e. in prescriptive screening. In other words, the distinction between the research and clinical screening uses of epidemiology must be borne in mind.

Most measures of the haemostatic system are subject to high levels of variability: often considerably more than the variability in cholesterol, for example. Laboratory variation is part of the explanation. But it is the within-individual variation that makes it particularly difficult to characterize a person's true or habitual level. In evolutionary terms, this variability is to be expected of a system upon which changing demands may be made at quite short notice, as

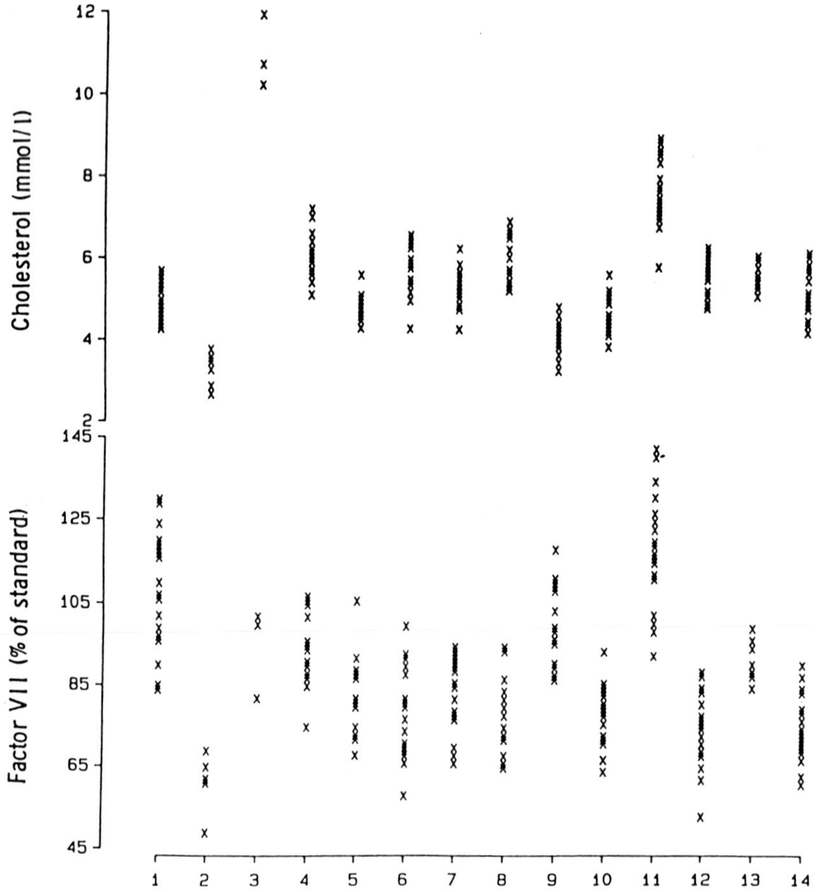

Fig. 53.6 Variability in VII_c and cholesterol in 14 volunteers over 2–3 years. The vertical axes for the two variables have been scaled so that 1 standard deviation for each is represented by the same distance. The within-person variability of the two measures can therefore be compared visually. (Reproduced by permission of the editor of Thrombosis and Haemostasis, 1987.)

requirements for haemostasis vary either physiologically or in response to circumstances that might lead to injury. Figure 53.6 compares the within-person variability in cholesterol and factor VII activity from which the greater variation in the latter can be seen (Thompson et al 1987). The main consequence of variability of this kind is that larger numbers will be required to show a relationship of factor VII with IHD than for a more stable measurement such as cholesterol. In general, the true relationship will be stronger than the observed relationship by an amount that depends on the degree of variability (the greater the variability the greater the under-estimation of the true relationship), i.e. the 'regression dilution effect' (MacMahon et al 1990).

HAEMOSTATIC VARIABLES AND IHD

Haemostasis and thrombosis are similar (though not identical) processes so the concept of thrombosis as 'haemostasis in the wrong place' (Macfarlane 1977) illustrates the general validity of considering how platelet function and the coagulation system may contribute to thrombosis and its consequences.

Coronary artery thrombi are due to platelet aggregates and to the deposition of fibrin in varying proportions. As interest in thrombosis and IHD developed, most attention was initially directed towards the contribution of platelets. Their very rapid adhesion to damaged endothelium and then to each other is central to arterial thrombosis. It is, however, fibrin which gives many developing thrombi their ultimate stability and volume. A recent biochemical (as distinct from morphological) study concluded that fibrin formation and platelet activation are probably equally important in the early hours of MI (Rapold et al 1989), providing added reason for recognising that the mechanical obstruction of the coronary artery is due to two main processes (with the possible implication that the most effective approach to antithrombotic therapy may involve platelet-active agents and anticoagulants simultaneously).

Given a major thrombotic contribution, an obvious question for the clinician or epidemiologist is the extent to which those at risk of IHD can be characterized on account of a thrombotic tendency. A major part of the answer depends on the results of studies which include measures of haemostatic function and relate these to the presence (prevalence) or subsequent onset (incidence) of IHD. So far, coagulation factor assays have generally proved more useful than platelet function tests, though this probably reflects the unsatisfactory nature of the latter rather than the importance of platelets in arterial thrombosis.

Prevalence studies

Although they are usually quicker and cheaper, prevalence studies are subject to a number of substantial drawbacks. First, an association between a clotting factor activity level and the previous occurrence of a clinical episode of IHD may be the result of the episode rather than having preceded it. This is a point of special importance in the case of fibrinogen, for example, the level of which may rise in response to a range of stimuli. Many prevalence studies have found weaker relationships than those later established in prospective studies. One reason may be the effect of a clinical episode on the measures in question, either because the episode itself has metabolic consequences on variables of potential interest or because those who have experienced them alter dietary, smoking and other habits that may affect the variables in question. More or less by definition, prevalence studies cannot include fatal episodes, the characteristics of which could differ from non-fatal episodes. Finally, many clinical cross-sectional studies have been too small or cases and controls have been inadequately matched for much confidence to be placed in their findings.

Table 53.2 summarizes the prevalence results of the Northwick Park Heart Study (NPHS) a whole population study (as distinct from a case-control study) in which cases and those so far unaffected by clinically manifest IHD were drawn from the same industrial groups and set up with the primary objective of assessing haemostatic function in the pathogenesis of IHD (Meade & North 1977). Of the two variables showing clear prospective associations with

Table 53.2 Prevalence results at entry into the Northwick Park Heart Study: mean values by presence or absence of IHD

		Myocardial infarction (N = 38)	Angina (N = 33)	All IHD (N = 71)	No IHD (N = 1350)
Factor V_c	% of standard	122.3	121.8	122.0	120.1
Factor VII_c	% of standard	106.3	108.2	107.2	102.0
Factor VIII_c	% of standard	101.1	97.3	99.4	97.6
Fibrinogen (g/l)		3.24**	3.21**	3.22**	2.91
Fibrinolytic activity (100/h)		26.3	21.5*	24.0*	28.1
Antithrombin III_c (%)		99.5	105.4*	102.3	97.9
Platelet adhesiveness (%)		46.9	41.7	44.6	42.1
Cholesterol (mmol/l)		6.29	6.40	6.34*	5.99
Systolic blood pressure (mmHg)		140.4	143.7	141.9	138.2

Numbers of cases (all IHD) by low, middle and high thirds of fibrinogen distribution (cf. Fig. 53.7) are 12, 23 and 35 (one missing value).
Compared with no IHD: * $P < 0.05$; ** $P < 0.01$.

later IHD — factor VII coagulant activity, VII_c[1] and fibrinogen (Fig. 53.7) — only fibrinogen showed a significant association in the prevalence data, though the factor VII difference was similar to that described by others. Higher levels of fibrinogen or its products in those with a past history of MI have also been reported by Yarnell et al (1985) and by Kruskal et al (1987), for example. (The findings in Table 53.2 on fibrinolytic activity and antithrombin III are considered in more detail later, in the context of prospective data.) NPHS is so far the only study to have reported prospective findings on factor VII. For the time being, therefore, confirmatory or contradictory evidence on factor VII largely depends on several case-control studies. Very consistently, these support an association between factor VII and IHD or stroke risk (Poller 1957, Carvalho de Sousa et al 1988, Hoffman et al 1989, Takano et al 1990, Suzuki et al 1991). Whether these associations reflect factor VII activity or factor VII antigen is an important question currently under detailed investigation. Work in progress (Miller 1992 personal communication) suggests that the NPHS VII_c assay is more sensitive to two-chain VIIa, than the assays used in two other studies that will eventually have prospective data (Balleisen et al 1987, Wu et al 1990).

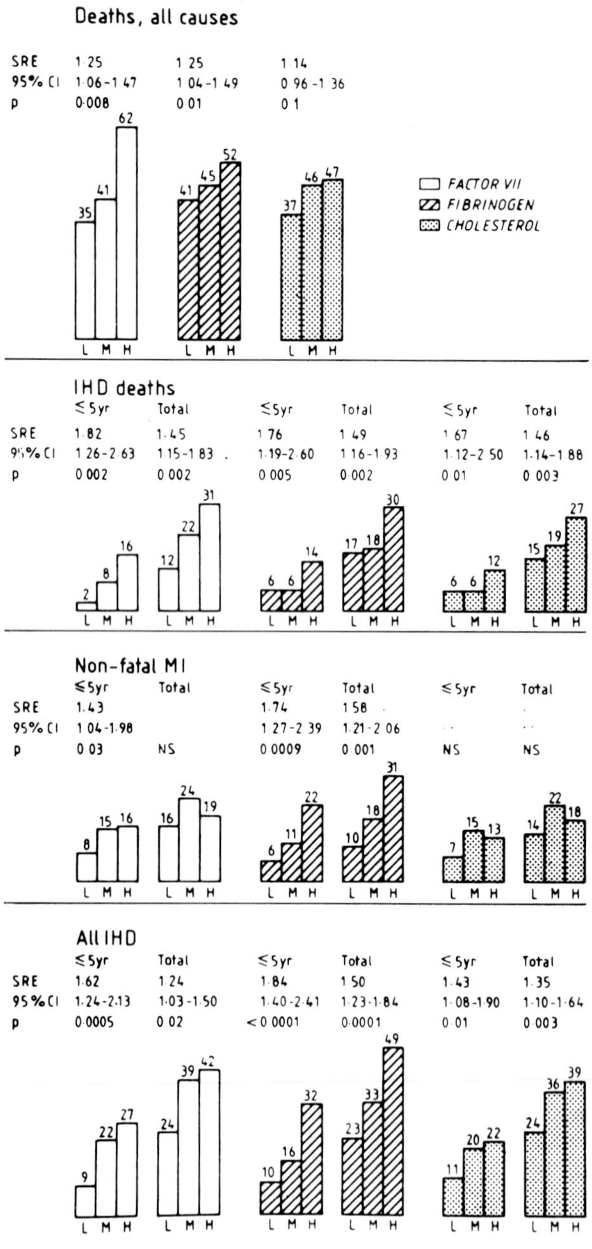

Fig. 53.7 Number of events within 5 years and for total follow-up period by low (L), middle (M) and high (H) thirds of distributions at entry into Northwick Park Heart Study. Standardized regression effects (SREs) show the increase in risk of an event for 1 standard deviation (SD) increase in the variable concerned; for example, 1 SD increase in factor VII activity increases the risk of an event within 5 years by 62%. The 95% CI shows confidence interval of SRE (Meade et al 1986, reproduced by permission of Lancet.)

Prospective studies

In the Northwick Park Heart Study (NPHS), Meade et al (1980) first showed preliminary results suggesting that high levels of VII_c and of plasma fibrinogen, and possibly also of factor VIII activity, were associated with mortality from cardiovascular disease, principally IHD. The main results of NPHS (Meade et al 1986a) are summarized in Figure 53.7. They are based on 143 deaths from all causes, of which 68 were due to IHD and on 60 non-fatal episodes of myocardial infarction. High levels of VII_c and of fibrinogen were associated with mortality from all causes. The use of deaths from all causes has the advantage that it does not depend on opinions about the cause of death. At the same time, IHD is the commonest cause in men in the age group concerned and, if high clotting factor levels are strongly associated with IHD, this should be evident in analyses based on total mortality. The relationships of VII_c and fibrinogen with the incidence of IHD itself within 5 years of recruitment were if anything stronger than for cholesterol, and were also independent of cholesterol, though the latter relationship — as expected — was also demonstrated. The association of factor VII_c with IHD was mainly due to fatal events. There were no clear relationships between VII_c or fibrinogen and the incidence of cancer, the commonest non-vascular cause of illness and death, so that the findings appear to be specific for vascular disease.

In the Gothenborg study, Wilhelmsen et al (1984) showed a relationship between high fibrinogen levels and the incidence of both IHD and, in particular, stroke in a study of 792 men born in 1913. Their findings are summarized in Table 53.3. Figure 53.8, dealing with stroke, suggests a possible interaction between fibrinogen and systolic blood pressure, men with high levels of both being

[1] The subscript c is used in this chapter for clotting factor values based on clotting (or biological) activity in NPHS and related studies.

Table 53.3 Mean plasma fibrinogen levels at entry to Gothenborg study according to subsequent outcome[a]

	IHD	Stroke	Deaths from other causes	No event
Number	92	37	60	608
Fibrinogen (g/l)	3.56*	3.70*	3.37	3.30

[a] Wilhelmsen et al 1984.
* $P < 0.01$.

at considerably greater risk than might have been expected from the sum of the two effects separately, though the small number of events on which this analysis is based needs to be taken into account.

In the Leigh study, Stone & Thorp (1985) reported an association between high fibrinogen levels and IHD incidence in a group of 297 men aged between 40 and 69 who were followed for up to 20 years. The relationship was stronger than for cholesterol, blood pressure or smoking. In this study, too, there was suggestive evidence of an interaction between fibrinogen and blood pressure. Thus, men whose systolic blood pressure and plasma fibrinogen levels fell in the top third of the respective distributions experienced 12 times the incidence of IHD compared with those in whom both levels fell in the low third.

In the Framingham Study, Kannel et al (1985) reported an association between high fibrinogen levels and the incidence of cardiovascular disease in 554 men and 761 women aged between 45 and 79 who had not previously

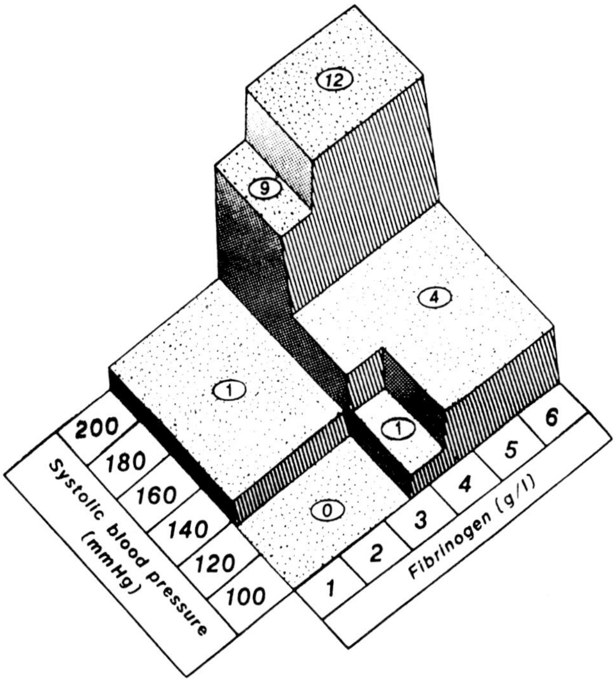

Fig. 53.8 Probability (circled percentages) of stroke in the Goteborg study according to entry blood pressure and fibrinogen levels (Wilhelemsen et al 1984, reproduced by permission of New England Journal of Medicine).

Table 53.4 Cardiovascular disease related to fibrinogen and hypertensive status: Framingham study subjects 45–79 years of age, 12-year rate per 1000[a]

	Normotensive		Mild hypertension		Definite hypertension	
Fibrinogen (g/l)	Men	Women	Men	Women	Men	Women
<2.65	2.27	1.53	4.21	1.92	5.39	3.78
2.65–3.11	2.61	1.54	5.19	2.40	4.10	2.82
>3.12	4.67	2.18	5.38	3.78	7.08	5.43

[a] Kannel 1987.

experienced a cardiovascular event, cardiovascular disease being defined as the sum of IHD, stroke, heart failure and peripheral arterial disease. Subsequent publications (Kannel et al 1987, Kannel 1987) established a clear relationship between fibrinogen and the incidence of IHD in both men and women and between fibrinogen and stroke in men but not in women (perhaps because of small numbers) and, again, also suggested (see Table 53.4) that the effects of simultaneously high levels of fibrinogen and blood pressure may be of particular importance.

In the Caerphilly study, Yarnell et al (1991) have shown a strong relationship between fibrinogen and IHD incidence that remained significant after adjusting for a variety of characteristics, including smoking habit. Viscosity was also strongly related to later IHD.

The relationship of fibrinogen to the patency of femoropopliteal vein grafts has been established (Wiseman et al 1989). In those with plasma fibrinogen concentrations below the median value, 90% of grafts were patent at 1 year compared with 57% in those with values above the median. The plasma fibrinogen level, followed by thiocyanate concentration as a measure of smoking, were the two most powerful predictors of graft status in this study. Other work also indicates the involvement of fibrinogen in the progression of peripheral arterial disease (Dormandy et al 1973, Banerjee et al 1992) and probably in its onset, too (Kannel & D'Agostino 1990).

Thus, prospective studies are very consistent in suggesting a strong relationship between the plasma fibrinogen level and the subsequent onset of clinically manifest IHD, of stroke (at least in men) and of progression in established peripheral arterial disease. The relationship between fibrinogen and stroke contrasts with the less certain association between cholesterol and stroke, thus indicating the potential value of fibrinogen as a particularly useful index of the risk of major cardiovascular disease defined as the sum of IHD and stroke.

High serum sialic acid concentrations are also associated with increased mortality from cardiovascular disease (Lindberg et al 1991, 1992a). Sialic acid occurs in fibrinogen and several other proteins. The significance of these observations needs further study.

Although considerably weaker than for VII_c and fibrinogen, there were also suggestive associations in NPHS of

Table 53.5 Dutch haemophiliacs: ratios of observed to expected deaths[a]

Disease	Observed/expected deaths
Neoplasm	2.5
Lung cancer	8.6
Accidents	2.6
Renal failure	30.0
Stroke	5.0
Ischaemic heart disease	0.2

[a] Rosendaal et al 1989.

high factor VIII_c levels and poor fibrinolytic activity with IHD incidence (Meade et al 1980, 1986b). In the case of factor VIII_c, supporting evidence comes from studies showing a lower than expected incidence of IHD in haemophiliacs exemplified by the results of a Dutch study (Rosendaal et al 1989) (Table 53.5). The higher than expected mortality from stroke and accidents is due to bleeding. The increased mortality from renal disease may partly be due to the greater prevalence of hypertension in haemophiliacs. The precise explanation for the increased mortality from malignant disease is not so far clear. By contrast, the very much lower than expected mortality from IHD is obvious. Some caution is necessary in interpreting these and other findings (Rosendaal et al 1990) since the high mortality of haemophiliacs from other causes introduces the possibility of 'competing risks' as a reason for lower mortality from IHD. However, the very considerable reduction in IHD in the Dutch study coupled with the NPHS findings and with other results (Egeberg 1962) indicate that the possible contribution of factor VIII to IHD should at least not be overlooked.

Besides the fibrinolytic system, potential defence mechanisms against thrombosis include antithrombin III and the vitamin K-dependent anticoagulatory factors, protein C and protein S. Intuitively, it is low levels that seem likely to be associated with increased risk and this is certainly true for the inherited thrombophilias leading to venous thrombosis. However, the relationships of antithrombotic factors to the risk of arterial thrombosis and thus of IHD often seem paradoxical. In the case of antithrombin III, for example, vegetarians with a lower than average risk of IHD nevertheless have significantly lower levels than non-vegetarians (Haines et al 1980). Two studies (Meilahn et al 1988, Meade et al 1990) have reported significantly higher antithrombin III levels in post-menopausal women than in pre-menopausal women of the same age, the incidence of IHD being higher in the former. Levels may also be higher in diabetics than in non-diabetics (Fuller et al 1979), the increased risk of IHD in the former being well-known. Yue et al (1976) found a gradient of rising antithrombin III values from those at low risk of IHD via those at intermediate risk or with chronic IHD to those with acute myocardial infarction. Findings at recruitment to the Northwick Park Heart Study (Table 53.2) also suggested higher rather than lower values in those who had previously experienced IHD. By contrast, others (Banerjee et al 1974, O' Brien et al 1975, Innerfield et al 1976) have reported lower levels in those with a past history of infarction or other manifestations of arterial disease. Two studies (Vigano et al 1984, O'Connor et al 1984) have reported higher rather than lower levels of protein C in those with a past history of infarction or at risk of arterial events. These apparently contradictory findings could be partly explained by postulating that antithrombin III levels, for example, tend not to be elevated in those who are at low risk of arterial disease and who do not therefore need to make an antithrombotic response. In those at high risk, on the other hand, antithrombin III levels may behave in one of two ways resulting in either low or high levels but each associated with increased risk. First, inability to increase antithrombin III levels in some may directly contribute to subsequent events in which high pro-coagulatory clotting factor levels are involved. Secondly, antithrombin III levels in others may rise as a compensatory defence mechanism. While the studies summarized are compatible with an explanation of this kind, they have so far all been cross-sectional, apart from recent preliminary prospective data from NPHS, which do now suggest that both low and high antithrombin III levels may be associated with an increased incidence of IHD (Meade et al 1991).

The associations of clotting factors with recurrence or mortality after MI are also of potential interest. Table 53.6 shows significantly higher initial fibrinogen levels in MI patients who died within the ensuing year (virtually all of IHD) compared with those who survived with similar findings for factor VIII_c (Haines et al 1983). As expected, initial values of creatine kinase were also higher in those

Table 53.6 Mean levels of haemostatic and other variables in those who died following an MI and those who survived[a]

	Number	Sex ratio M/F	Age	Creatine kinase (μ/l)	Factor VIII_c (%)	Fibrinogen (g/l)
Died within 6 weeks of MI	46	34/12	62.3	1626	176	4.68
Died between 0–6 weeks	22	19/3	64.4	1189	139	4.47
Died within 1 year (total)	68	53/15	62.9	1496**	165***	4.61**
Alive at 1 year	204	161/43	59.7	982	127	4.10

[a] Haines et al 1983.
For differences between all deaths at 1 year and survivors: ** $P < 0.01$, *** $P < 0.001$.

who died and so was the white cell count, findings which suggest that the extent of infarction and the complications of a large infarct (such as heart failure) largely determine outcome and that other influences, of which coagulability may be one, are less important than they are in influencing the onset of the initial event. However, whether the high fibrinogen levels associated with mortality after infarction also reflect infarct size or not, they may, for reasons considered elsewhere, be of pathogenetic significance nonetheless. Impaired fibrinolytic activity may also influence the recurrence of MI (Hamsten et al 1987). Among patients with unstable angina, it was those with raised fibrinogen and plasma viscosity levels who were more likely to proceed to acute MI (Fuchs et al 1990).

There is of course no doubt as to the central role of platelets in arterial thrombosis. However, in spite of the intense interest in platelet function in thrombogenesis over the last 10 or 20 years, there is still no satisfactory and generally agreed index by which to define those who may be at increased risk of IHD on account of platelet sensitivity. Renaud (1980) has established a parallel between the dietary habits of groups of farmers who contrast in their experience of IHD and a number of possible indices of platelet function, including thrombin-induced aggregability, the higher the dietary fat intake the higher the incidence of IHD and the more aggregable the platelets. In NPHS, the epidemiological characteristics of platelet aggregability using adenosine diphosphate ED_{50} (i.e. the dose of ADP at which aggregation proceeds at half its maximum velocity) are equivocal (Meade et al 1985a). Thus, aggregability increases with age, is less in black than white men and tends to be less the greater the consumption of alcohol. These findings are compatible with the increased or decreased risk of IHD in these various situations. On the other hand, aggregability is considerably greater in women than in men and is less in smokers than non-smokers. The smoking effect might be due to the in vivo aggregation of more sensitive platelets, leaving mainly the less sensitive platelets in the test system. Figure 53.9 shows that aggregability increases with increasing plasma fibrinogen concentration and the causal nature of this association, with increasing fibrinogen leading to increased aggregability, has also been established (Meade et al 1985b, Landolfi et al 1991). If platelet function is determined to any appreciable extent by external influences such as the plasma fibrinogen concentration or thrombin production, the widely held concept of aggregability as an intrinsic characteristic of the platelets themselves may be a considerable over-simplification (Lowe & Forbes 1985, Meade et al 1985a). Thus, the validity of any postulated index of platelet function must be an open question until adequate prospective data are available. A start in this direction has come from recent studies showing an association between spontaneous platelet aggregation (Trip et al 1990) or platelet volume (Martin et al 1991) and outcome after infarction

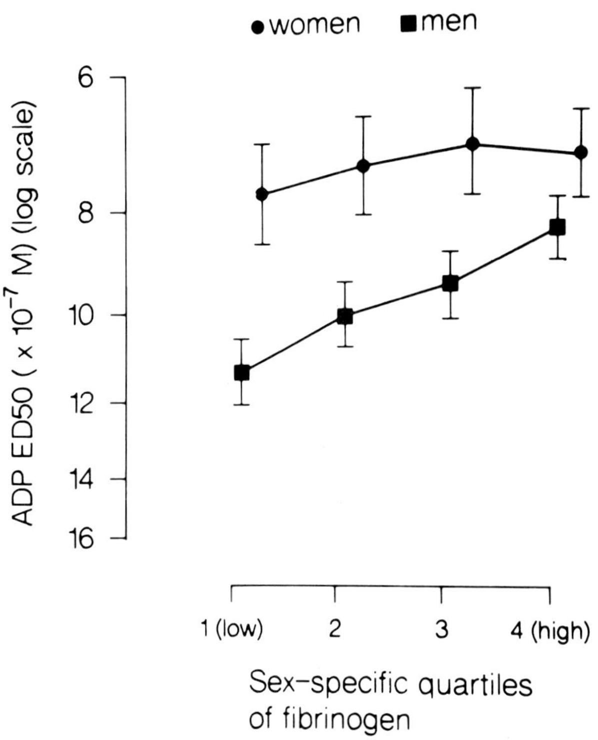

Fig. 53.9 Platelet aggregability measured by ADP ED_{50} by quartiles (1 = low) of fibrinogen concentration; means and 95% confidence intervals (Meade et al 1985a, reproduced by permission of the British Medical Journal).

but information is also needed on platelet function and first clinical episodes.

Recent reports have indicated an inverse association between serum albumin levels and mortality, including IHD mortality (Phillips et al 1989, Kuller et al 1991, Klonoff-Cohen et al 1992, Salive et al 1992), i.e. the lower the albumin the higher the mortality. The interpretation of this observation is not yet clear but the topic is an interesting one which should be kept under review.

Evidence from trials

Randomized controlled trials offer a good opportunity of studying causation (Morris & Gardner 1969) as well as establishing the clinical value of treatment and preventive measures. The purpose of referring to results of various trials here is, therefore, not so much to consider them or their clinical implications in detail (see chapters 54–56, 65–67) but to summarize their main conclusions as part of the evidence for the involvement of the haemostatic system (and of other mechanisms) in the pathogenesis of IHD.

Anticoagulants

The controversies of the 1960s and 1970s about anticoagulants are now sufficiently distant to assert (rather than have to justify in detail) the undoubted value of oral anticoagulants after myocardial infarction. Overviews of both the short-term (Chalmers et al 1977) and of the long-term trials (International Anticoagulant Review Group 1970) established a reduction in mortality of about 20% and a much larger reduction (of about 50%) in thromboembolic episodes following infarction. Interest in the anticoagulant question received a major new stimulus with the publication of the results of the trial by the Sixty Plus Reinfarction Study Research Group (1980) from the Netherlands. This trial was of the effects of taking patients off anticoagulants rather than initiating treatment and it took advantage of the lessons of the cardiovascular trials of the 1970s in terms of its design, sample size and analysis. The results are summarized in Table 53.7. Analysed on an 'intention to treat' basis (i.e including all patients as randomized, whether or not they complied fully with treatment) or on an 'on treatment' basis (i.e. including only those who adhered to the allocated treatment), there was no doubt about the substantial reduction in reinfarction conferred by anticoagulation. The 'on treatment' analysis for IHD mortality also leaves little doubt about the value of anticoagulants and the 'intention to treat' analysis strongly suggests this, too. Other findings from the Dutch trial indicated that the balance is in favour of anticoagulants so far as cerebrovascular disease is concerned. Thus, an excess of cerebral haemorrhage in those continuing on anticoagulants was more than offset by a reduction in events either certainly or probably due to thrombosis.

In 1990, the Norwegian Warfarin Reinfarction Study, WARIS, further strengthened the case for re-considering the value of oral anticoagulants (Smith et al 1990a). The trial demonstrated a significant benefit not only in reducing recurrent MI but also stroke and total mortality (Table 53.8).

Aspirin

In its overview of the secondary prevention trials (i.e. the prevention of progression or recurrence after an initial

Table 53.7 Long-term anticoagulant therapy after myocardial infarction: main results of Sixty Plus trial[a]

	Treatment		P
	Placebo N: 439	Active anticoagulation N: 439	
Intention to treat			
Death	69	51	0.071
MI	64	29	0.0005
Stroke	21	13	0.16
On treatment			
Death	49	28	0.017
MI	58	20	0.0001
Stroke	19	11	0.18

[a] Sixty Plus Research Group 1980.
Intention to treat: includes all patients as randomized, whether or not they complied with treatment. On treatment: includes only those who adhered to the allocated treatment. Intended INR 2.7–4.5. MI, myocardial infarction.

Table 53.8 The effect of warfarin anticoagulant therapy on mortality and reinfarction after myocardial infarction: main results of the WARIS trial[a]

	Treatment		P
	Placebo N: 607	Warfarin N: 607	
Intention to treat			
Death	123	94	0.03
MI	124	82	0.0007
Stroke	44	20	0.0015
On treatment			
Death	92	60	0.005
MI	122	70	0.0001
Stroke	41	16	0.0003

[a] Smith et al 1990a.
Intended INR 2.8–4.8.
'Intention to treat' and 'on treatment' – see Table 53.7.

Table 53.9 Percentage reduction in end-points attributable to aspirin according to previous history of vascular disease[a]

	Previous vascular disease at entry			
	Prior Myocardial infarction	Unstable angina	Stroke or TIA	Any vascular event
No. of trials	10	2	13	25
Non-fatal myocardial infarction	31	35	35	32
Non-fatal stroke	42	–	22	27
Vascular death	13	37	15	15
Any vascular event	22	36	22	25

[a] Hennekens et al 1989.[a]

clinical episode), the Antiplatelet Trialists Collaboration (1988) clearly demonstrated the value of aspirin. As Table 53.9 shows, benefits may vary to some extent according to the type of event initially leading to trial entry and according to later outcome (Hennekens et al 1989) but for common conditions any of these reductions are of great clinical value. In primary prevention, however, the appropriate conclusions are less clear. So far, the available data come from just two trials, one in American and the other in British doctors. The results are summarized in Figure 53.10 (Hennekens et al 1989). The American trial showed a highly significant reduction in non-fatal myocardial infarction, while the British trial showed virtually no effect. There was marginal evidence of heterogeneity between the results of the two trials, thus at least raising a question about the justification for combining their findings in an overview, particularly since the statistical test for heterogeneity is not very robust, i.e. may if anything underestimate the probability that the two trials do actually differ. There were no differences in cardiovascular or total mortality. Both trials suggested, though not significantly, that the incidence of stroke may have been greater in those taking aspirin possibly because of an increase in cerebral haemorrhage. While this might be a chance finding, the numbers of events are not trivial and the pos-

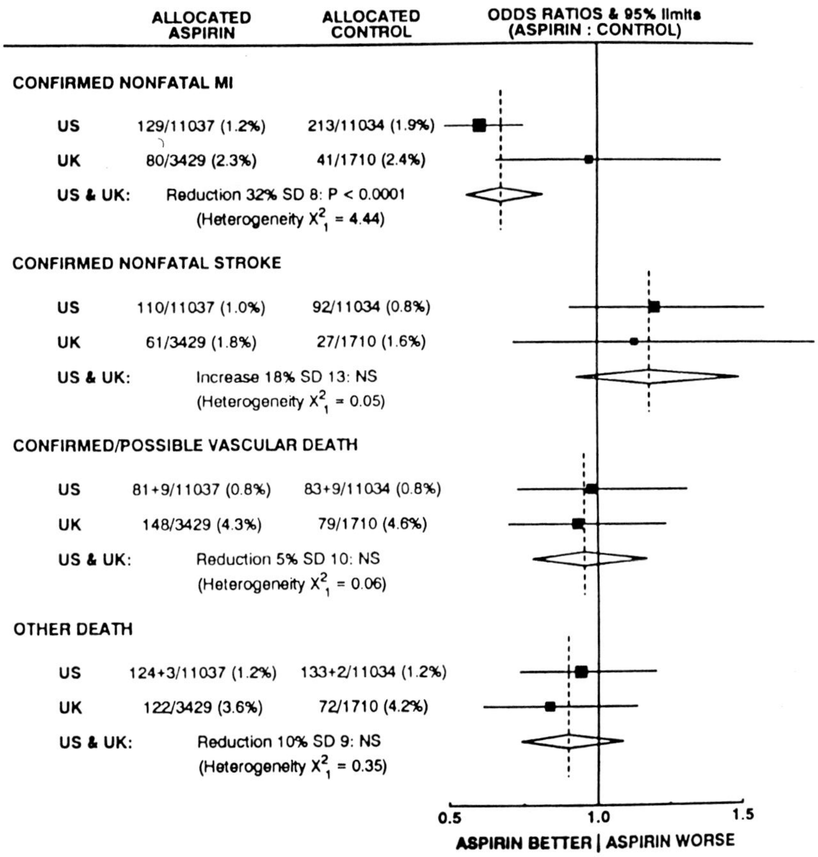

Fig. 53.10 Overview of US and UK primary prevention trial results for four end points, odds ratios (aspirin versus control), overall risk reductions, and heterogeneity tests (sum of four heterogeneity χ^2 tests = 4.9, NS). For further details, see original publication (Hennekens et al 1989). Reproduced by permission of the American Heart Association, Inc.

sibility that aspirin truly does increase the risk of stroke has been recognised (Buring et al 1990). It is therefore possible — though puzzling — that aspirin has different effects according to whether or not there is a previous history of clinically manifest disease, i.e. between the contexts of secondary and primary prevention.

The Antiplatelet Trialists Collaboration data show that aspirin has beneficial effects on deep vein thrombosis and pulmonary embolism (Meade 1992), thus overturning the conventional view that aspirin is without effect against venous thrombosis.

Since the Antiplatelet Trialists Collaboration overview (1988), the results of further aspirin trials have appeared and some of these have been concerned with lower doses of aspirin. Thus, the RISC trial (1990) in patients with unstable angina reported a reduction of about 60% in myocardial infarction or death attributable to 75 mg aspirin. The SALT trial (1991) reported an 18% reduction in major stroke or death in patients who had previously experienced transient ischaemic attacks or minor strokes. In the ISIS-2 trial (1988), the effects of 160 mg aspirin daily and of streptokinase were established in over 17 000 patients suspected of being in the early stages of myocardial infarction. While either aspirin or streptokinase singly resulted in a significant reduction in cardiovascular mortality, there was an even greater reduction in those who received both aspirin and streptokinase. In terms of pathogenesis, the clear message from this trial therefore is that modifying both platelet function and fibrin formation simultaneously is more effective than modifying either process alone. As a result of ISIS-2, the use of both aspirin and thrombolytic therapy in clinical practice for the early management of suspected myocardial infarction increased dramatically over a period of only 2 or 3 years (Collins & Julian 1991). In practical terms, it is important to consider whether oral anticoagulation may be more effective in secondary prevention than aspirin, acknowledging at the same time, that aspirin is obviously easier to use. Thus, the risk reduction in major vascular end-points attributable to aspirin in the secondary prevention of myocardial infarction is between 15 and 45% compared with between 24% and 55% in the Sixty Plus and WARIS trials (see Tables 53.7, 8 and 9). If anticoagulants do confer greater benefits than aspirin, the balance between any additional value, on the one hand, and the disadvantages of frequent blood testing and dose monitoring, on the other, may need to be considered in greater depth. At lower INRs than those achieved in conventional anticoagulation, there might not be much to chose between anticoagulants and aspirin as far as drawbacks are concerned.

Other agents

A significant recent development is recognition that anti-hypertensive treatment reduces the incidence of IHD (Collins et al 1990) as well as of stroke. It is possible that diuretics are more effective than beta-blocking agents and diuretics almost certainly confer some of their benefit through mechanisms other than the lowering of blood pressure (Medical Research Council, 1985, 1992).

There is no doubt about the value of beta-blocking agents in the secondary prevention of myocardial infarction and the implications of the trials that have established this are now expressed in clinical practice (Baber et al 1984).

The value of lipid-lowering agents in the prevention of IHD remains controversial. Overviews have concluded, on the one hand, that there is a substantial benefit (cited in Standing Medical Advisory Committee report 1990) while in another the benefit is considered only marginal (Ravnskov 1992). The uncertainty is compounded by the suggestion that lowering cholesterol levels, even if this is beneficial for IHD, increases mortality from violent causes such as accidents and suicide (Muldoon et al 1990, Lindberg et al 1992b), the hypothesis to explain this increase (if real) being changes in neurone membrane composition and neurotransmission (Engleberg 1992). The publicity accompanying the most recent results of a Finnish trial which suggested that men in the active intervention group actually fared worse than those in the comparison group (Strandberg et al 1991) paid little if any attention to the results of other trials suggesting the reverse. The individual and public health implications of this controversy are so far-reaching that a trial or trials sufficiently large to provide clear answers both to the effects of lipid lowering on IHD and on mortality from all causes must be carried out as a matter of some urgency. Similar considerations apply to the attempted prevention of IHD through life-style changes including dietary measures intended to lower cholesterol levels.

Recent years have seen the publication of several trials to slow or reverse the progression of atheroma, using dietary, pharmacological and surgical intervention and both imaging and clinical measures of outcome (Davies et al 1991). With an encouraging degree of consistency, these trials have demonstrated pathological benefits, perhaps more in terms of slowing the progression of atheroma than in achieving reversal. Some of the trials have also demonstrated clinical benefits, using 'softer' end-points such as requirements for coronary artery bypass grafting and angioplasty as well as myocardial infarction and death. How far the rather aggressive interventions used have implications for prevention in day to day clinical practice is debatable.

On balance, there is little doubt that reducing raised cholesterol levels confers a worth-while degree of protection against IHD or its recurrence. In clinical terms, it is worth bearing in mind that life-style measures intended to lower cholesterol levels will usually also lead to reductions in obesity, with benefits in terms of diabetes, arthritis and gall-bladder disease, for example, as well.

In fact, lipid-lowering agents (and perhaps diets) may exert clinical effects at least in part though different pathways than those forming the initial basis for their evaluation. Thus, the World Health Organization (WHO) primary prevention trial of clofibrate was carried out in men with high cholesterol levels and it established a reduction in the incidence of major IHD of about 20%. There may also have been an increase in mortality from non-IHD causes during the 'on treatment' phase of the trial, this effect being no longer evident, however, after treatment had stopped (Committee of Principal Investigators 1978, 1980, 1984). It is mainly for this reason that clofibrate has not been widely adopted for primary prevention. However, it has been known for some time that clofibrate also reduces plasma fibrinogen levels (Dormandy 1974), though when this effect was initially established there was little interest in the role of fibrinogen in arterial disease. A further analysis of the WHO data has now suggested that the beneficial effect of clofibrate against IHD appears to have been confined, as Table 53.10 shows, to heavy smokers who were also hypertensive (Green et al 1989). The heavy smokers will have had high fibrinogen levels. Besides suggesting that the effect of clofibrate may have been to reduce the risk of IHD through its effect on fibrinogen (as well as, or instead of, its cholesterol-lowering effect), this analysis is interesting in further supporting the possibility of an interaction between blood pressure and fibrinogen (see earlier), since it was in those at risk on both accounts in whom the benefit of treatment was mostly seen. Another fibrate, gemfibrozil, provides a further example of several pathways through which a drug may act. In the Helsinki Heart Study (Frick et al 1987), gemfibrozil reduced IHD incidence by 34%, an effect attributed to its undoubted lipid-lowering properties. However, as Table 53.11 shows, there is no doubt that gemfibrozil also reduces the thrombin level as indicated by fragment F1.2

Table 53.10 Heart attacks per 1000 per annum in WHO clofibrate trial[a]

	Non-smokers		Smokers			
			<20/day		20+/day	
	Active	Placebo	Active	Placebo	Active	Placebo
Normotensive	3.4	3.5	6.2	9.6	9.6	9.1
Hypertensive	3.9	6.0	12.1	14.3	8.7*	18.3

[a] Green et al 1989.
* $P < 0.01$.

Table 53.11 Effects of gemfibrozil: cross-over trial in 63 patients with IHD[a]

	Treatment	
	Gemfibrozil	Placebo
Cholesterol (mmol/l)**	5.46	6.21
Triglycerides (mmol/l)**	1.32	2.39
Fibrinogen (g/l)*	3.21	3.03
F1.2, (nmol/l)**	1.18	1.57

[a] Wilkes et al 1992.
* $p < 0.001$; ** $p < 0.0001$.

(Wilkes et al 1992), so that the benefit in the Helsinki trial may have been due to a short-term (lipoprotein-mediated) effect on coagulability and thrombogenic potential as well as to a longer-term influence on atheroma. As Table 53.11 also shows, gemfibrozil increases rather than reduces plasma fibrinogen. Some of the effective blood-pressure lowering agents increase plasma lipid levels (Lardinois & Neuman 1988), further emphasizing that the value of an agent must be determined by its effects on clinical events rather than the intermediate, surrogate end-points leading to their evaluation.

There is growing reason to believe that oxidized low density lipoprotein (LDL) is of particular relevance to atherogenesis (Steinberg et al 1989) and that antioxidants may be valuable in modifying it (Riemersma et al 1991).

GENERAL EPIDEMIOLOGICAL CHARACTERISTICS

Another approach to clarifying the nature of the relationship between high clotting factor levels and the incidence of IHD is to establish how far these levels vary according to personal and environmental characteristics associated with IHD. With a high degree of consistency, fibrinogen and VII_c levels tend to be high or low in association with characteristics which respectively raise or lower the risk of IHD.

Age

Both fibrinogen and VII_c levels rise with increasing age and this is illustrated by NPHS data (Meade et al 1979) in Figure 53.11. Both fibrinogen and VII_c levels tend to be higher in women than men, particularly after the age of the menopause (which accounts for the curvilinear rise in fibrinogen in women shown in Figure 53.11).

Maternal and fetal influences

There is growing evidence that adverse influences prenatally and during infancy predispose to arterial disease during adult life. This effect may well be partly mediated through fibrinogen and factor VII activity levels. Thus, as Table 53.12 shows, there is a strong relationship between low weight at 1 year of age (reflecting characteristics such as poor maternal and fetal nutrition) and high fibrinogen and VII_c levels in adult life (Barker et al 1992).

Smoking

Uniformly, all the large scale prospective studies already referred to (and several cross-sectional studies) have found the highest fibrinogen levels in smokers, intermediate levels in ex-smokers and the lowest levels in non-smokers (Meade 1987). There is a dose-response relationship between the number of cigarettes smoked and the fibrinogen level (Wilkes et al 1988). Figure 53.12 (from data at entry to NPHS) shows a rapid initial decline in fibrinogen on stopping smoking but levels remain above those for non-smokers for up to 5 and perhaps 10 years after discontinuation (Meade et al 1987a), also observed in Scottish and

Table 53.12 Mean plasma fibrinogen and factor VII_c values in men aged 59–70 years according to weight at age 1 year[a]

Weight at 1 year (1b)	N	Fibrinogen (g/l)	Factor VII_c (%)
<18	38	3.21	122
18–20	93	3.10	111
20–22	178	3.13	108
22–24	173	2.97	106
24–26	82	2.93	106
>26	33	2.93	103

[a] Barker et al 1992.
Trends: fibrinogen $p < 0.001$ VII_c $p < 0.005$.

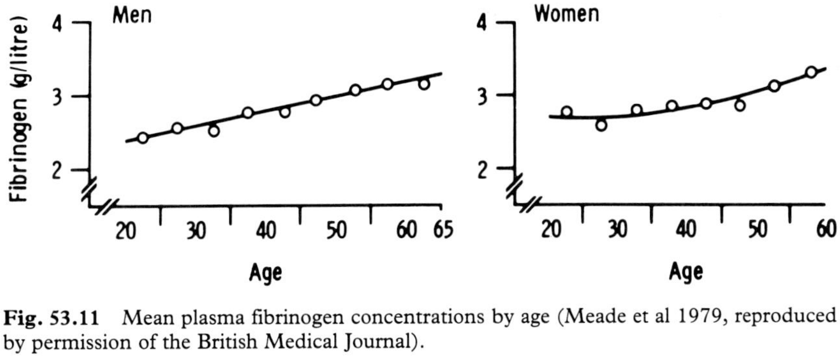

Fig. 53.11 Mean plasma fibrinogen concentrations by age (Meade et al 1979, reproduced by permission of the British Medical Journal).

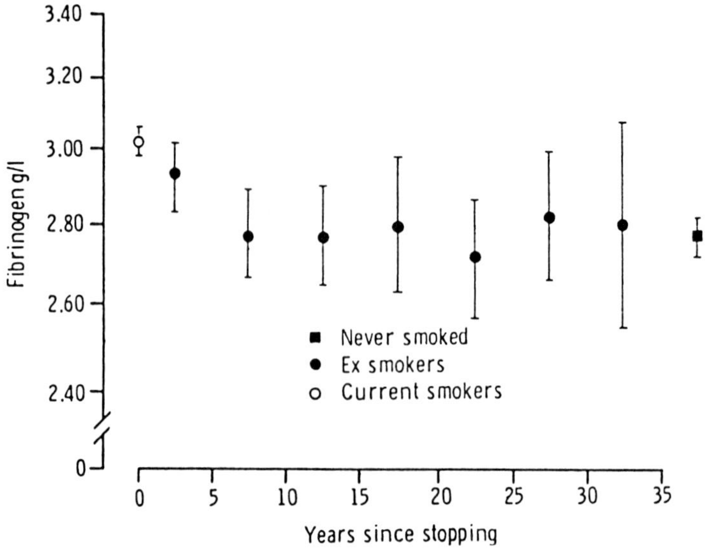

Fig. 53.12 Plasma fibrinogen (age-adjusted) by time since stopping smoking in 518 ex-smokers, in current smokers, and in non-smokers. Log scale. Bars show 95% confidence intervals (Meade et al 1987a, reproduced by permission of Lancet).

Welsh studies (Yarnell et al 1987, Lee et al 1990). The time course is similar to the decline in the risk of IHD itself after smoking cessation (Cook et al 1986, Surgeon General 1989, Dobson et al 1991). This effect has also been shown prospectively (Meade et al 1987a). Thus, over the 6-year follow-up period in NPHS, fibrinogen levels rose (over and above the increase with age) in those who started or resumed smoking while they fell in those who discontinued. The rapid initial fall in fibrinogen after discontinuation (Meade et al 1987a, Rothwell et al 1991) is one of the reasons for questioning the frequent assertion that high fibrinogen levels associated with the incidence of IHD only reflect the extent of underlying atheroma although the association would still be useful even if this were the explanation. Bearing in mind the difficulty of achieving the regression of atheroma other than by intensive methods not ordinarily used by those who are giving up smoking, it is most unlikely that the fall in fibrinogen soon after discontinuation is due to a reduction in atheroma. The extent to which fibrinogen levels are genetically determined (see p. 1218) also represents a component of high fibrinogen levels that cannot be explained as a response to atheroma. Given the strong relationship between fibrinogen levels and the risk of IHD or stroke, the fall in fibrinogen in ex-smokers is enough to account for a large part of the decline in their risk of IHD and strengthens the conclusion that much of the relationship between smoking and IHD is mediated through the fibrinogen level. It is, however, important to remember that high levels are associated with an increased risk of IHD in non-smokers (Meade et al 1986b, Yarnell et al 1991) as well as in smokers.

Diet

Excessive consumption of fat, from animal sources in particular, causes raised cholesterol levels and increases the risk of IHD. Experimental and observational studies leave no doubt as to the rapid effect of dietary fat intake on factor VII activity levels (Miller et al 1986a, 1989, 1991a). Results for an individual participant in one of the experimental studies are illustrated in Figure 53.13. At present, there is no obvious difference between the effects of saturated and polyunsaturated fatty acids on factor VII levels in the short term (Marckmann et al 1990, Miller et al 1991a), though more detailed analyses of data already collected and the results of longer-term studies may clarify this point. It may be through the effects of negatively-charged lipoproteins such as chylomicrons and very low density lipoproteins (VLDL) in activating factor XII and its activation, in turn, of factor VII that high dietary fat intake influences coagulability (Mitropoulos et al 1989). The diurnal relationship between triglycerides and VII_c, with a mid-day rise in the former followed by a rise in the latter some hours later (Miller et al 1991a), could at least partly explain the diurnal pattern in IHD onset.

The importance of data from randomized controlled comparisons as distinct from observational studies is well exemplified by work on the relationship between cereal fibre intake and the plasma fibrinogen level. Two observational (not experimental) studies did suggest an inverse relationship, i.e. lower fibrinogen levels with higher cereal fibre intakes (Fehily et al 1982, Yarnell et al 1983). However, when this topic was investigated in a randomized controlled trial (Fehily et al 1986) no relationship of fibre with fibrinogen was found. Animal studies (Pickart &

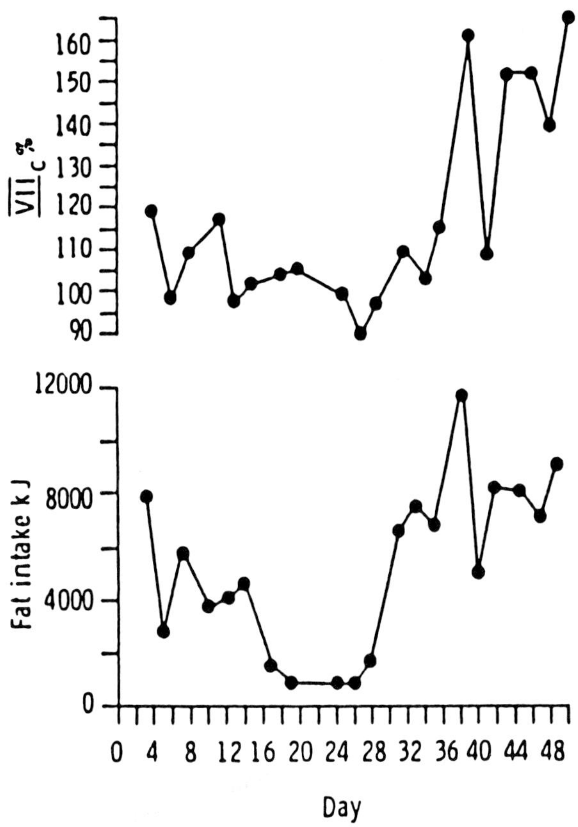

Fig. 53.13 Dietary fat intake and VII_c the following day in one individual (Miller et al 1986a, reproduced by permission of Atherosclerosis).

Thaler 1976, Pickart 1981) have shown an effect of free fatty acids on fibrinogen levels and high fibrinogen levels have been reported in hyperlipidaemia (Lowe et al 1980) but the suggestion from these observations that dietary fat might have a significant influence on fibrinogen levels has not been borne out in experimental work. Thus, in a series of studies (Simpson et al 1982, 1983, Miller et al 1986a) there were no effects of a variety of dietary measures including fat and fibre intake likely or intended to reduce the risk of vascular disease. It is possible that the duration of these studies was not sufficient to demonstrate long-term effects, though this seems unlikely even allowing for the relatively long half life of fibrinogen (3–4 days). Some trials of fish oils have shown a reduction in plasma fibrinogen levels (Hostmark et al 1988, Muller et al 1989, Radack et al 1989, Haglund et al 1990) while others have failed to do so (Rogers et al 1987, Gans et al 1988).

At best, therefore, the evidence for any marked or consistent effect of diet on the fibrinogen level in man is equivocal. If the sort of dietary modification that may be tolerable in IHD-endemic communities does indeed have little effect on the fibrinogen level, there may be a limit to which such modification can be effective through other pathways, bearing in mind the strong relationships between fibrinogen and IHD incidence. On the other hand, fish oil may be beneficial through its effects on prostaglandin metabolism (Vane & Botting 1991). The potentially harmful and beneficial effects of a range of dietary factors, including the different classes of fatty acids, have recently been reviewed (Ulbricht & Southgate 1991). Of particular interest is the potential value of linoleic and eicosapentaenoic acids through their effects on platelet composition and function (Wood et al 1987).

Regional and international comparisons

A striking part of the evidence on cholesterol in IHD has been the demonstration of regional or international differences that parallel differences in IHD mortality. This opportunity has not so far been fully exploited in the case of clotting factors. However, the results of one study (Meade et al 1986b) are summarized for VII_c and fibrinogen in Table 53.13. VII_c levels tend to rise with the incidence of IHD, particularly between those at very low risk and those at high or very high risk. In the case of fibrinogen, the highest levels are seen in rural Gambians, who experience virtually no IHD. Otherwise, with the exception of Czechoslovakia, levels increase with increasing IHD mortality and are highest in East Finland where, at the time these studies were carried out, mortality from IHD was still among the highest in the world. (Rates are now very high in Czechoslovakia.) Table 53.14 summarizes the results of another study, with generally similar results (Iso et al 1989). Thus, VII_c levels tend to be higher in those experiencing most IHD, i.e. North Americans, whether Japanese or Caucasian. Apart from the rural Japanese group, fibrinogen levels also rise with increasing IHD incidence. The high fibrinogen levels in rural groups is probably due

Table 53.13 Regional and international comparison of fibrinogen, VII_c and cholesterol (mean values)[a]

	Gambia			Czechoslovakia	England	Scotland			Finland	
Year	1977	1977	1979	1982	1979	1978	1979	1980	1979	1979
Centre	Urban	Rural	Rural	Prague	London	Glasgow	Aberdeen	South-West	Central	East
N	54	36	25	101	26	81	80	87	51	45
Age	33.4	48.8	47.7	49.6	45.4	45.5	43.9	43.4	44.2	45.2
Fibrinogen (g/l)	2.90	3.36	4.19	3.48	2.82	3.00	3.05	3.46	3.32	3.62
VII_c (% standard)	71	70	67	87	86	94	96	92	88	92
Cholesterol (mmol/l)	4.7	4.2	3.9	5.8	5.4	5.7	5.7	6.4	6.0	6.4

[a] Meade et al 1986b.

Table 53.14 Mean fibrinogen and factor VII levels in Japanese and in Caucasian and Japanese American men aged 34–55 years[a]

	Japanese		American	
	Rural	Urban	Japanese	Caucasian
N	29	34	39	35
Fibrinogen (g/l)	2.50	2.23	2.43	2.90
VII (% standard)	96	93	110	100

[a] Iso et al 1989.
Differences between groups: $P < 0.01$ for both variables.

to parasitic infestation and they indicate that high levels in the absence of other risk factors can be tolerated. This observation is not incompatible, however, with a role for fibrinogen in IHD-endemic communities with a high background prevalence of atheroma, for example. An analogous example is provided by smoking. The Japanese experience little IHD but smoke very heavily. This does not, however, argue against a strong effect of smoking in communities with other characteristics predisposing to atheroma and IHD.

Infection and inflammation

There are strong though poorly appreciated indications of an increased risk of vascular disease following infection. For example, patients admitted for acute MI had significantly higher serological indices of chronic chlamydial infection than a control group (Saikku et al 1988). In a case-control study in patients under the age of 50, there was a relative risk of no less than 9.0 for brain infarction associated with a febrile infection during the previous month (Syrjanen et al 1988). There would of course have been changes in many acute and chronic phase proteins but one of these would almost have certainly been an increase in fibrinogen. In another study, dental health was significantly worse in patients with acute MI than in controls (Mattila 1989). Again, a rise in fibrinogen levels is only one of several possible explanations but there is a strong case for further work to confirm or exclude it. Other studies linking virus infection to development of atheroma (Editorial 1978) might also be explained through effects on fibrinogen levels, at least in part. The apparently high cardiovascular mortality in patients with rheumatoid arthritis (Mutru et al 1985) and the possible involvement of fibrin deposition in Crohn's disease (Wakefield et al 1989) could also perhaps be partly explained through the effects of these diseases on fibrinogen levels. If raised fibrinogen levels do to some extent explain the fairly clear increase in risk associated with these conditions — and it must be emphasized that this is at present speculative — they illustrate the importance of not dismissing elevations in fibrinogen that may be due to relatively non-specific stimuli as biologically insignificant. It is also worth bearing in mind that high fibrinogen levels are also found in neoplastic disease and in pregnancy, both of which are also associated with an increased risk of thromboembolism. There appears to be a striking seasonal variation in plasma fibrinogen concentrations in older individuals (Stout & Crawford 1991). Levels are highest during the coldest months when mortality from both myocardial infarction and stroke are also at their highest levels. It might be that the high fibrinogen and thus mortality levels during the colder months are partly explained by respiratory and other infections which are, of course, also commonest during colder weather. However, there was no seasonal variation in white cell count in the study under consideration, which argues against this particular explanation although white cell counts may not rise as much in older as in younger patients in response to infection. The origin of high fibrinogen levels is certainly a question of considerable interest, but whatever they are — genetic, environmental or non-specific — they may lead to an increased risk of thrombosis through mechanisms discussed on p. 1219.

Menopause

The NPHS prospective findings in Table 53.15 show that fibrinogen, VII_c and cholesterol levels in those who have gone through the menopause have increased markedly compared with those who have not (Meade et al 1990). The increase in IHD incidence after the menopause is well established but it is less than might be expected as a result of the considerable effect of the menopause on VII_c and fibrinogen illustrated in Table 53.15, on the assumption that the relationship between high VII_c and fibrinogen levels is the same for women as in men. For fibrinogen, the Framingham study (Kannel et al 1987) suggests this is so. Figure 53.14, also from NPHS (Meade et al 1990), suggests what might be a partial explanation for the apparent disparity between the anticipated consequences of the effects of the menopause on VII_c and fibrinogen, on the one hand, and the increase in IHD itself. Antithrombin-III levels in pre-menopausal women are relatively low, perhaps because they do not need to mount a defence against pro-coagulatory influences that raise the

Table 53.15 Mean age-adjusted clotting factor and cholesterol levels at 6-year follow-up by menopausal status at re-examination[a]

	Continued periods (n = 136)		Menopause			
			Natural (n = 69)		Artificial (n = 28)	
	Entry	Follow-up	Entry	Follow-up	Entry	Follow-up
Factor VII_c (% standard)	102.8	101.9	107.4	121.2	99.5	106.6
Fibrinogen (g/l)	2.76	2.80	2.84	3.31	2.81	3.03
Cholesterol (mmol/l)	5.46	5.34	6.05	6.69	5.50	5.55

[a] Meade et al 1990.
All changes occurring with natural menopause: $P < 0.0001$.

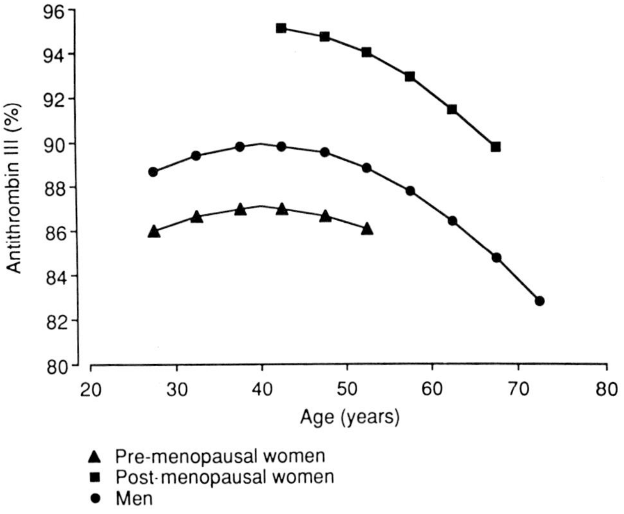

Fig. 53.14 Fitted values of antithrombin III levels in NPHS participants (Meade et al 1990, reproduced by permission of British Journal of Haematology).

risk of thrombosis. It is clear, however, that the menopause is associated with a significant increase in antithrombin-III levels, an effect also reported in another study (Meilahn et al 1988). Antithrombin-III may not have a direct effect on VII_c and does not influence fibrinogen, but increased levels after the menopause may nevertheless provide some defence against the added risk due to the general rise in coagulability. A recent prospective study in Scotland has suggested that influences other than those of widely recognized risk factors protect women against IHD (Isles et al 1992).

Obesity

Cross-sectional studies are fairly consistent in suggesting that obesity increases fibrinogen and factor VII levels (Balleisen et al 1985, Folsom et al 1991). Table 53.16 shows NPHS data. In the prospective data from NPHS, change in obesity was associated with a significant change in VII_c levels though not in fibrinogen (Meade et al 1987a). It is possible that high fibrinogen levels are also part of the syndrome characterized by obesity, insulin resistance, raised triglycerides and hypertension.

Table 53.16 Mean values of factor VII and of fibrinogen by age and with obesity as indicated by the sum of skinfold thicknesses at three sites in 1601 white NPHS men[a]

Age	Factor VII_c (% standard) Skinfold thickness (mm)			Fibrinogen (g/l) Skinfold thickness (mm)		
	<35	35–50	>50	<35	35–50	>50
18–34	85.5	93.9	99.4	2.30	2.41	2.65
35–49	88.9	99.7	105.8	2.70	2.80	2.91
50–64	98.3	106.5	106.8	3.05	3.03	3.14

[a] Meade et al 1979 and unpublished NPHS data.

Oestrogen use

Most studies suggest that the use of oral contraceptives (OC) increases fibrinogen levels (Meade et al 1977). An exception, however, is the recent Scottish Heart Health Study (Lee et al 1990), in which women with a past history of OC usage had lower fibrinogen levels than those without. This could well be due to growing awareness of characteristics (particularly smoking) that further increase the risk of thrombotic episodes in OC users and, therefore, a selective effect of OC use only in those at low risk and who are likely to have low rather than high fibrinogen levels.

Oral contraceptives raise factor VII levels in an oestrogen dose-dependent manner (Meade et al 1977). While oral contraceptives increase the risk of thromboembolism, HRT probably reduces the risk of IHD and possibly also of stroke (Meade & Berra 1992), though not to the extent often claimed. It might be – though this explanation is still largely speculative – that the higher antithrombin III levels in post- compared with pre-menopausal women (Fig. 53.14) offset the increase in clotting factors that occurs with the menopause (Meade et al 1990), thus allowing the lipid-lowering properties of oestrogens in HRT to exert their full beneficial effect. Oestrogens in the treatment of prostatic cancer raise factor VII and increase the incidence of thromboembolism (Henriksson & Edhag 1986; Henriksson et al 1986). However, they also affect other clotting factors so it is not possible to conclude with certainty that they produce their effects through factor VII though it seems likely that it is involved. Early attempts at the secondary prevention of myocardial infarction using oestrogens were discontinued when they increased rather than lowered the risk of thromboembolic episodes (Coronary Drug Project Research Group 1973). The oestrogen doses used in prostatic cancer are high and thus not necessarily indicative of the effects of the lower doses in oral contraceptives and in hormone replacement for menopausal symptoms. However, the prostatic cancer and secondary prevention findings do come from randomized controlled trials and should therefore not be overlooked in the overall assessment of oestrogens in vascular disease.

Diabetes

Fibrinogen and VII_c levels are higher in diabetics compared with non-diabetics and high levels are associated with the microvascular complications of diabetes (Fuller et al 1979). Of further interest is the apparent association between high fibrinogen levels and hypertension in non-insulin dependent diabetics (Feher et al 1988).

Social and psychological influences

There is now fairly extensive and consistent, if unexpected, evidence that adverse social or psychological circumstances lead to increased fibrinogen levels (Ernst et al 1985, Markowe et al 1985, Rosengren et al 1990b). If further studies confirm associations of this kind, they may begin more firmly to establish and explain the hitherto elusive relationship between 'stress' and IHD.

Protective characteristics: alcohol consumption and exercise

There is little doubt that moderate alcohol consumption leads to a lowering of fibrinogen levels. This conclusion is based not only on cross-sectional studies (Meade et al 1979, Lee et al 1990, Folsom et al 1991) but also on the fall in fibrinogen observed prospectively in NPHS with increased alcohol consumption (Meade et al 1987b), though a German cross-sectional study (Balleisen et al 1985) has reported no association between alcohol consumption and fibrinogen. While the magnitude of the effect of alcohol consumption on fibrinogen levels may not be large and may suggest only a modest degree of protection against IHD, it is nevertheless compatible with the evidence from studies on the relationship between alcohol consumption and IHD incidence (Marmot & Brunner 1991). Despite assertions to the contrary, several of these studies have allowed for ex-drinkers whose discontinued alcohol consumption may be the result of cardiovascular and other disease. Thus, the apparent effect of alcohol consumption on fibrinogen levels and direct studies of the relationship between alcohol consumption and IHD complement each other in suggesting that there is, indeed, some protection against IHD from moderate consumption. This conclusion is not to deny the obvious public health difficulties of explaining the relationship, though bearing in mind the potential benefit of a small effect in a common disease, it is important that it should at least be recognised.

Renaud & de Lorgeril (1992) have recently suggested that the lower incidence of IHD in France compared with Britain may be due to the effects of wine on platelet aggregability although, as already indicated, this explanation lacks the demonstration of a prospective relationship between platelet function tests and IHD whereas, this link is clear in the case of fibrinogen. Alcohol consumption also has beneficial effects on high density lipoprotein cholesterol.

Several studies are consistent in suggesting or quite firmly establishing an inverse relationship between exercise and the fibrinogen level, i.e. lower levels in those taking most exercise or in those who are physically 'fittest' (Davey-Smith et al 1989, Moller & Kirstensen 1991, Connelly et al 1992).

It is also likely that carriers of hepatitis B surface antigen, who seem to experience considerably less IHD than non-carriers, have lower fibrinogen and factor VII_c levels than the latter (Hall et al 1985, Meade et al 1987b).

Genetic contribution

At least two restriction fragment length polymorphisms (RFLPs) associated with variation in fibrinogen levels have been identified (Humphries et al 1987, Thomas et al 1991), though the finding on one of these RFLPs (Humphries et al 1987) has not been confirmed in a Scandinavian study (Berg & Kierulf 1989). Methodological differences or true variations in the association of this RFLP with fibrinogen in different populations are possible explanations. The variations at the fibrinogen locus suggested by these RFLPs account for between 3% and 15% of the variance in fibrinogen levels though, because the studies in question were based on single fibrinogen measurements, these proportions are likely to be under-estimates. Using path analysis, another study (Hamsten et al 1987b) accounted for 51% of the variance in fibrinogen in genetic terms. As the authors of this study themselves concluded, a substantial genetic determination weakens the explanation that high fibrinogen levels are only or mainly due to non-specific influences such as atheroma. Fowkes et al (1991) concluded that variation at the β fibrinogen locus is associated with an increased risk of peripheral arterial disease but that its influence is not mediated only through increased fibrinogen concentrations. They raised the possibility of a structurally variant fibrinogen, a general topic that calls for increasing attention. A genetic polymorphism associated with low VII_c levels has also been described (Green et al 1991).

CAUSALITY

Some of the reasons for believing that high clotting factor levels may be directly involved in the onset of clinically manifest IHD have already been considered but the topic is of such obvious importance that summary incorporating all the contributory evidence is worthwhile.

Considering first the epidemiological evidence, Hill (1965) suggested nine criteria by which to attempt the distinction between causation and association. The first is the *strength* of the relationship. Here, both fibrinogen and factor VII_c (the latter so far only in the Northwick Park Heart Study) are associated with the incidence of IHD at least as strongly as cholesterol and blood pressure. There is little dispute that the last two characteristics are causally involved in IHD. In the case of fibrinogen, the prospective studies are also *consistent*, i.e. the relationship has been observed in several different studies and, so far as the case-control studies on factor VII are concerned along with the prospective findings of NPHS, the same is generally true of factor VII. The associations are *specific* in the sense that they are confined to cardiovascular disease, particularly IHD but also stroke. High fibrinogen levels are not apparently related to increased risk of other diseases, though it would not be surprising if, in due course, the influence of smoking on fibrinogen levels also leads to some relationship between fibrinogen and lung cancer. (The specificity (or otherwise) of fibrinogen in the later onset of IHD should not, of course, be confused with the effects of other diseases on fibrinogen.) It is only prospective studies that can really establish *temporality*, i.e. that the putative disturbance (e.g. high fibrinogen level) precedes the clinical event and NPHS establishes this for both clotting factors. For fibrinogen, there is certainly a *biological gradient*, in that there is a graded or 'dose-response' relationship with IHD. In NPHS, the same is true for factor VII. Hill's other criteria include *experiment* and *biological plausibility*. The indications of the available trials have already been considered. The oral anticoagulant trials are clearly compatible with the possibility that high factor VII_c levels are of pathogenetic significance, though these agents also alter other vitamin-K dependent factors. Similarly, agents such as clofibrate that lower fibrinogen levels also have other potentially beneficial effects. To what extent, therefore, can the criterion of biological plausibility be considered in terms of the pathways through which high fibrinogen or high factor VII levels might operate?

Fibrinogen levels

The plasma fibrinogen level occupies a central place in the pathogenesis of IHD (and almost certainly, of stroke, too), as summarized in Figure 53.15. There are at least four ways in which high fibrinogen levels may predispose to thrombosis.

Atheroma. Several studies have now established a relationship between the fibrinogen level and the extent of atheroma, both in the coronary and carotid circulations (Schneidau et al 1989, Broadhurst et al 1990). The contribution of fibrinogen and fibrin to the atheromatous plaque throughout its evolution and development is increasingly recognised and supported by other biochemical and pathological observations (Smith et al 1990b).

Viscosity. Large, asymmetrical molecules such as fibrinogen have a marked effect on blood viscosity and there is little doubt that increasing viscosity increases the risk of thrombosis (Yarnell et al 1991, Lowe 1992).

Fibrin formation. In the rabbit, the fibrinogen concentration when coagulation is initiated influences the amount of fibrin deposited (Gurewich et al 1976, Chooi & Gallus 1989). Kinetic experiments support the same conclusion (Naski 1991). Thus, the claim on theoretical grounds that high fibrinogen levels will not influence thrombogenesis because they are in excess of those needed for haemostasis is not borne out.

Platelet aggregation. Plasma fibrinogen is a co-factor for platelet aggregation and affects aggregability throughout its physiological range. Figure 53.9 shows its effect on ADP-induced aggregation in platelet-rich plasma (Meade et al 1985a). Experimental studies show, either by defibrination with ancrod (Lowe et al 1979) or through the addition of further fibrinogen (Meade et al 1985a), that it is indeed high fibrinogen levels that influence aggregability.

Factor VII levels

Turning to factor VII, the pathogenetic significance of a constituent of the coagulation system is perhaps best judged by its potential for generating thrombin. Once again, there is a high degree of consistency between

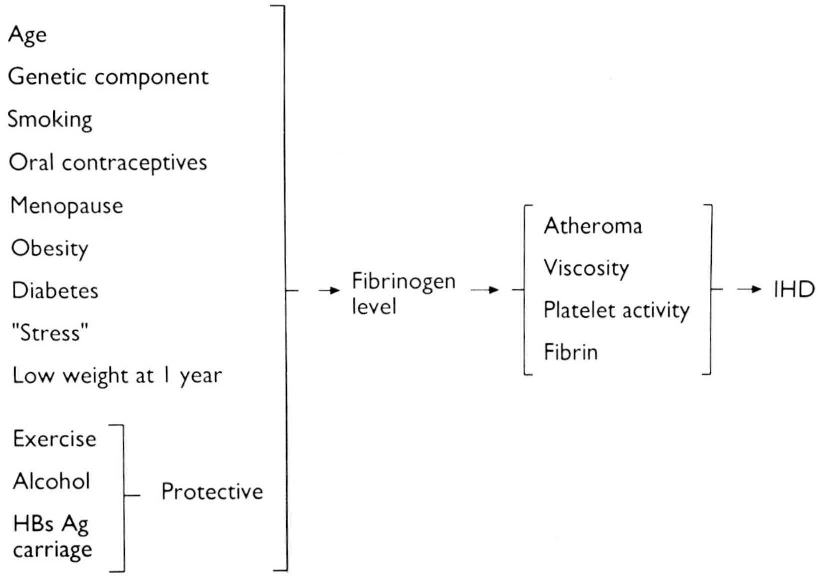

Fig. 53.15 Summary of determinants and thrombogenic pathways of fibrinogen in pathogenesis of IHD.

several studies using different approaches in demonstrating direct, significant associations between factor VII and indices of thrombin production or activity, based on fibrinopeptide A (Miller et al 1986b, Meade 1987, Lowe 1991), prothrombin activation peptide F1.2 (Miller et al 1991) or thrombin-antithrombin complexes (Carvalho de Sousa et al 1988, Suzuki et al 1991). At the very least, these findings suggest that factor VII_c is a valid index of the general level of coagulability. The clinical value of factor VII concentrates in successfully treating haemophiliacs with factor VIII antibodies is presumably mediated through increased thrombin production, providing some experimental evidence for direct involvement of factor VII in determining coagulability, although the factor VII levels following administration of concentrates greatly exceed physiological values. Factor VII concentrate may cause thrombosis (Schulman et al 1991).

CLINICAL AND RESEARCH IMPLICATIONS

What place do clotting factor assays now have in clinical and preventive practice, as far as IHD is concerned?

To return to the reasons for establishing prospective relationships between clotting factors and IHD, one purpose is to identify those at particularly high risk with the intention of intervening in that group, i.e. prescriptive screening. Whole population screening involves inviting all the middle-aged men in a general practice, for example, to undergo a series of measurements with the intention of intervening if this is indicated. Opportunistic screening is more restricted in that it involves only those who themselves decide to consult their doctors and, among those, the doctor may select only some for further investigation. The other main reason for establishing relationships between clotting factors and the later onset of IHD is to study its pathogenesis, in other words its causes and the pathways involved in its onset.

According to which of these two objectives is the main concern, there are important implications for the way in which the findings of prospective studies are analysed and considered. If the purpose is simply to predict risk, there is obviously no point in measuring redundant information, i.e. account can be taken of inter-correlations between different risk factors and attention mostly paid to those that make an independent contribution. However, not all prospective studies have identified exactly the same independent effects — for example, obesity may have an independent effect in one study but not in another – so useful information may be lost by too readily assuming that particular risk factors really are redundant.

It is, however, when the main interest is in pathogenesis that particular care about the use and interpretation of multivariate analyses is necessary. For example, triglycerides generally make no independent contribution to the risk of IHD. This is probably because of the great within-person variability in triglycerides (Austin 1989), so that they start off at a statistical disadvantage in multivariate analysis. But numerous clinical and laboratory studies over the last few years make it clear that triglycerides are centrally involved in several pathways affecting the onset of IHD, e.g. the intrinsic pathway activation of factor VII and in determining aspects of fibrinolytic activity. Indeed, over-enthusiasm for multivariate analysis may actually have delayed full recognition of the biological importance of triglycerides, though a recent study clearly showing an independent effect of triglycerides has done much to rectify this (Bainton et al 1992).

With these general principles in mind, the use to be made of the information on the two clotting factors of greatest interest, fibrinogen and factor VII, can be considered.

Dealing first with fibrinogen, the prospective studies so far published in detail all show an independent relationship between fibrinogen and IHD or stroke. Fibrinogen is significantly associated with later events in non-smokers as well as in smokers, a point that is often overlooked. So in measuring fibrinogen, new, additional information about risk is achieved. Even so, the case for whole population prescriptive screening for IHD is not strong. In opportunistic screening, however, whether in general or in hospital practice, the measurement of fibrinogen ought to become part of the routine investigation of those considered for other reasons to be at risk of thrombotic events, whether these are first events or recurrences. This raises the question of the fibrinogen level at which some kind of intervention is justified and, in this event, what the intervention ought to be. Different laboratories use different fibrinogen methods and while the relationships of various characteristics with fibrinogen itself and of fibrinogen with later IHD are very consistent from one study to another, absolute fibrinogen values vary considerably. For the time being, therefore, clinical decisions have to be based on the values and reference ranges in separate laboratories. However, the International Society on Thrombosis and Haemostasis has now established a fibrinogen standard so that this particular difficulty may soon be resolved. As to what interventions are appropriate, there are several approaches. Much the most important life-style change is the discontinuation or avoidance of smoking. But although fibrinogen levels in ex-smokers do begin to fall quite soon after discontinuation, they remain above non-smoking levels for several years, as does the risk of IHD itself. The apparently beneficial effect of strenuous exercise on fibrinogen now provides both doctors and patients with a valuable and practical incentive towards prevention, particularly where IHD risk is substantially due to raised fibrinogen levels. Another approach is to use a high fibrinogen level as a marker of risk in helping to decide, for example, whether to prescribe aspirin even though it has no effect on the fibrinogen level itself. However, the strong relationship between fibrinogen and

IHD does raise the question of specific pharmacological intervention in some circumstances. The case for clofibrate has already been considered and it may yet prove that its general abandonment after the WHO trial was premature. Bezafibrate also probably lowers fibrinogen levels (Cook & Ubben 1990). While gemfibrozil reduces the incidence of IHD, it raises rather than lowers fibrinogen levels (Wilkes et al 1992), but it reduces thrombin production the benefit of which, along with its lipid-lowering properties, evidently outweighs the fibrinogen rise. Pentoxifylline has benefical effects on blood flow (Cook & Ubben 1990) and may be particularly useful in peripheral vascular disease. Stanozolol produces a marked reduction in fibrinogen (Cook & Ubben 1990) but may adversely affect high density lipoprotein (HDL) cholesterol levels as well as having androgenic properties. Ancrod markedly lowers fibrinogen levels through its defibrinating effect but is given by infusion and is only used in rather extreme circumstances. Recently, the calcium channel-blocking agent nisoldipine has been reported to lower fibrinogen levels substantially and significantly (Salmasi et al 1991). Ticlopidine may also do so (Finelli et al 1991). But all the necessary information is not yet available and firm recommendations are not possible. It is frustrating to know, on the one hand, that high fibrinogen levels are clinically significant while, on the other hand, being uncertain as to how best to manage them: but that is the reality and it is now a challenge to all concerned to provide the further evidence needed.

Opportunistic screening for factor VII and its inclusion in clinical practice largely depend on simple and valid assay methods for two-chain VII, VII_a, and it is likely to be several years yet before this is achieved. So the value of factor VII is still very much in the research area and in studies of pathogenesis. Here, the accumulating evidence over the last few years, including the epidemiological evidence, has led to a considerable shift of emphasis to the extrinsic system as the main determinant of in vivo coagulability, with important implications for treatment and prevention. In further work, activation peptide assays seem likely to augment what has been learned from studying classical clotting factors. So growing interest in factor VII and related aspects of the extrinsic coagulation pathway still has mainly research rather than clinical implications. It has also been a major stimulus to investigating the potential value of low intensity oral anticoagulation. If this proves to be as effective in preventing thromboembolism as conventional intensity treatment, as seems likely (Meade 1992b), it will also carry with it less risk of bleeding and the need for less frequent blood tests and dose monitoring.

CONCLUSION

The involvement of thrombosis as well as atheroma in IHD is now widely recognised. Perhaps the best example of the contribution and inter-dependence of the two processes is in the role of dietary fat intake in IHD and the pathogenetic pathways this affects (Fig. 53.16). (The involvement of thrombosis in the atherogenic process itself also should not be overlooked.) It is the high mortality in those experiencing their first major episode of IHD that underlies the importance of primary prevention. If the onset and progression of significant atheroma could be forestalled, including the overwhelming consequences of plaque rupture (Richardson et al 1989), there is no reasonable doubt that epidemic IHD would pass into history. Realistically, however, the extent to which this is likely to be fully achieved in affluent communities or those in which epidemic IHD may be developing is debatable, even allowing for the welcome decline in IHD in many countries (which may have been at least partly due to reductions in thrombogenic potential as well as in atheroma). There must therefore be substantial interest in preventing the thrombotic complications of atheroma, particularly bearing in mind the implications of the pathological studies considered at the beginning of this chapter. If, as seems likely, thrombogenesis is the structural event immediately preceding and leading to myocardial infarction or sudden coronary death, this may be, as Figure 53.17 suggests, the optimal point for intervention, whether by lifestyle or pharmacological methods. This approach is entirely compatible with also trying to modify the risk factors and other pathways leading up to thrombosis.

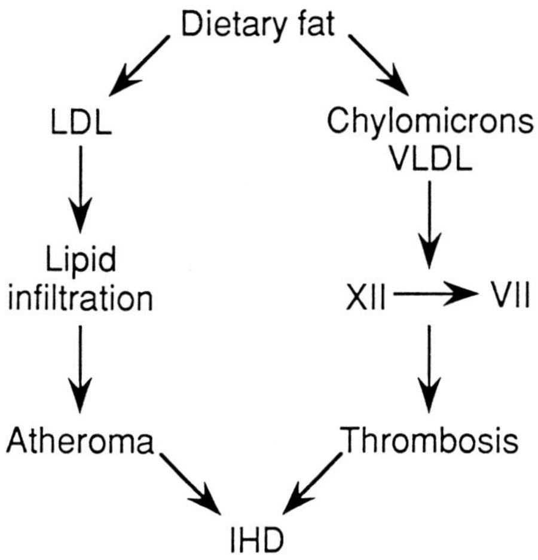

Fig. 53.16 Diet and IHD: atherogenic and thrombogenic pathways.

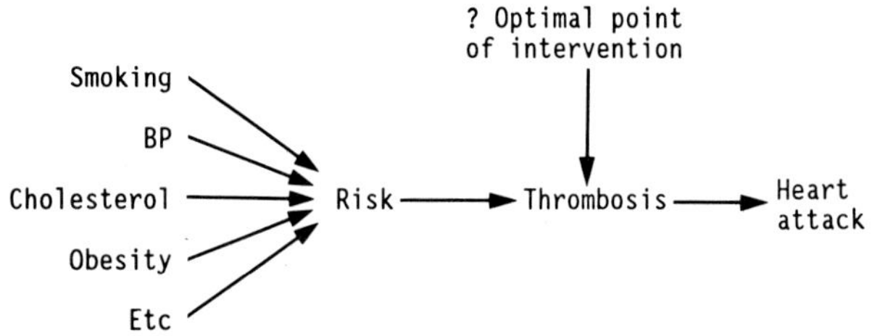

Fig. 53.17 Primary prevention of IHD: epidemiological and pathological implications.

REFERENCES

Antiplatelet Trialists' Collaboration 1988 Secondary prevention of vascular disease by prolonged antiplatelet treatment. British Medical Journal 296: 320–331

Austin M A 1989 Plasma triglyceride as a risk factor for coronary heart disease. The epidemiologic evidence and beyond. Americal Journal of Epidemiology 129: 249–259

Baber N S, Julian D G, Lewis J A, Rose G 1984 Blockers after myocardial infarction: have trials changed practice? British Medical Journal 289: 1431–1432

Bainton D, Miller N E, Bolton C H, Yarnell J W G, Sweetnam P M, Baker I A, Lewis B, Elwood P C 1992 Plasma triglyceride and high density lipoprotein cholesterol as predictors of ischaemic heart disease in British men. British Heart Journal 68: 60–66

Balleisen L, Bailey J, Epping P-H, Schulte H, van de Loo J 1985 Epidemiological study on factor VII, factor VIII and fibrinogen in an industrial population I: Baseline data on the relation to age, gender, body-weight, smoking, alcohol, pill-using, and menopause. Thrombosis and Haemostasis 54: 475–479

Balleisen L, Schulte H, Assmann G, Eppint P-H, van de Loo J 1987 Coagulation factors and the progress of coronary heart disease. Lancet 2: 461

Banerjee R, Sahni A, Kumar V, Arya M 1974 Antithrombin III deficiency in maturity onset diabetes mellitus and atherosclerosis. Thrombosis et Diathesis Haemorrhagica 31: 339–345

Banerjee A K, Pearson J, Gilliland E L, Goss D, Lewis J D, Stirling Y, Meade T W 1992 A six year prospective study of fibrinogen and other risk factors associated with mortality in stable claudicants. Thrombosis and Haemostasis (in press)

Barker D J P, Martyn C N 1992 The maternal and fetal origins of cardiovascular disease. Journal of Epidemiology and Community Health 46: 8–11

Barker D J P, Meade T W, Fall C H D, Lee A, Osmond C, Phipps K Stirling Y 1992 The relationship of fetal and infant growth to plasma fibrinogen in adult life. British Medical Journal 304: 148–152

Beaglehole R 1990 International trends in coronary heart disease mortality, morbidity, and risk factors. Epidemiologic Reviews 12: 1–15

Berg K, Kierulf P 1989 DNA polymorphisms at fibrinogen loci and plasma fibrinogen concentration. Clinical Genetics 36: 229–235

Broadhurst P, Kelleher C, Hughes L, Imeson J D, Raftery E B 1990 Fibrinogen, factor VII clotting activity and coronary artery disease severity. Atherosclerosis 85: 169–173

Buring J E, Hennekens C H, Sandercock P 1990 Aspirin and stroke. Archives Neurology 47: 1353–1354

Carvalho de Sousa J, Azevedo J, Soria C, Barros F, Ribeiro C, Parreira F, Caen J P 1988 Factor VII hyperactivity in acute myocardial thrombosis. A relation to the coagulation activation. Thrombosis Research 51: 165–173

Chalmers T C, Matta R J, Smith H, Kunzler A M 1977 Evidence favoring the use of anticoagulants in the hospital phase of acute myocardial infarction. New England Journal of Medicine 297: 1091–1096

Chandler A B, Chapman I, Erhardt L R et al 1974 Coronary thrombosis in myocardial infarction. Report of a workshop on the role of coronary thrombosis in the pathogenesis of acute myocardial infarction. America Journal of Cardiology 34: 823–833

Chen Z, Peto R, Collins R, MacMahon St, Lu J, Li W 1991 Serum cholesterol concentration and coronary heart disease in population with low cholesterol concentrations. British Medical Journal 303: 276–282

Chooi C C, Gallus A S 1989 Acute phase reaction, fibrinogen level and thrombus size. Thrombosis Research 53: 493–501

Cobb L A, Baum R S, Alvarex H, Schaffer W A 1975 Resuscitation from out-of-hospital ventricular fibrillation: 4 years follow-up. Circulation (suppl III) 51/52: 223–228

Colditz G A, Willett W C, Stampfer M J, Rosner B, Speizer F E, Hennekens C H 1987 Menopause and the risk of coronary heart disease in women. New England Journal of Medicine 316: 1105–1110

Collins R, Julian D 1991 British Heart Foundation surveys (1987 and 1989) of United Kingdom treatment policies for acute myocardial infarction. British Heart Journal 66: 250–255

Collins R, Peto R, MacMahon S, Hebert P, Fiebach N H, Eberlein K A, Godwin J, Qizilbash N, Taylor J O, Hennekens C H 1990 Blood pressure, stroke, and coronary heart disease. Lancet 355: 827–838

Committee of Principal Investigators 1978 Co-operative trial in the primary prevention of ischaemic heart disease using clofibrate. British Heart Journal 40: 1069–1118

Committee of Principal Investigators 1980 WHO cooperative trial on primary prevention of ischaemic heart disease using clofibrate to lower serum cholesterol: Mortality follow-up. Lancet 2: 379–385

Committee of Principal Investigators 1984 WHO cooperative trial on primary prevention of ischaemic heart disease with clofibrate to lower serum cholesterol: Final mortality follow-up. Lancet 2: 600–604

Connelly J B, Cooper J A, Meade T W 1992 Strenuous exercise and plasma fibrinogen. British Heart Journal 67: 351–354

Cook N S, Ubben D 1990 Fibrinogen as a major risk factor in cardiovascular disease. Trends in Pharmacological Sciences 11: 444–451

Cook D G, Shaper A G, Pocock S J, Kussick S J 1986 Giving up smoking and the risk of heart attacks. Lancet 2: 1376–1380

Coronary Drug Project 1973 Findings leading to discontinuation of the 2.5 mg/day estrogen group. Journal of the American Medical Association 226: 652–657

Davey-Smith G, Marmot M G, Etherington M, O'Brien J 1989 A work stress-fibrinogen pathway as a potential mechanism for employment grade differences in coronary heart disease rates. Abstracts, 2nd International Conference on Preventive Cardiology, Washington DC

Davies M J 1987 Thrombosis in acute myocardial infarction and sudden death: In: Mehta J L, Conti C R, Brest A N (eds) Thrombosis and platelets in myocardial ischemia. F A Divis, Philadelphia, 10: 151–159

Davies M J, Thomas A 1984 Thrombosis and acute coronary-artery lesions in sudden cardiac ischemic death. New England Journal of Medicine 310: 1137–1140

Davies M J, Krikler D M, Katz D 1991 Atherosclerosis: inhibition or regression as therapeutic possibilities. British Heart Journal 65: 302–310

DeWood M A, Spores J, Notske R, Mouser L T, Burroughs R, Golden M S, Lang H T 1980 Prevalence of total coronary occlusion during the early hours of transmural myocardial infarction. New England Journal of Medicine 303: 897–901

Dobson A J, Alexander H M, Heller R F, Lloyd D M 1991 How soon after quitting smoking does risk of heart attack decline? Journal of Clinical Epidemiology, 44: 1247–1253

Doll R, Peto R 1976 Mortality in relation to smoking 20 years' observations on male British doctors. British Medical Journal 2: 1525–1536

Donahue R P, Abbott R D, Bloom E, Reed D M, Yano K 1987 Central obesity and coronary heart disease in men. Lancet 1: 821–824

Dormandy J A, Hoare E, Khattab A H, Arrowsmith D E, Dormandy T L 1973 Prognostic significance of rheological and biochemical findings in patients with intermittent claudication. British Medical Journal 4: 581–583

Dormandy J A, Gutteridge J M C, Hoare E, Dormandy T L 1974 Effect of clofibrate on blood viscosity in intermittent claudication. British Medical Journal 4: 259–262

Duguid J B 1946 Thrombosis as a factor in the pathogenesis of coronary atherosclerosis. Journal of Pathology and Bacteriology 58: 207–212

Editorial 1978 Virus infections and atherosclerosis. Lancet 2: 821–822

Editorial 1991 Lipoprotein (a). Lancet 337: 397–398

Egeberg O 1962 Clotting factor levels in patients with coronary atherosclerosis. Scandinavian Journal of Clinical and Laboratory Investigation 14: 253–258

El Fawal M A, Berg G A, Wheatley D J, Harland W A 1987 Sudden coronary death in Glasgow: nature and frequency of acute coronary lesions. British Heart Journal 57: 329–335

Elwood P C, Cochrane A L, Burr M L et al 1974 A randomized controlled trial of acetylsalicylic acid in the secondary prevention of

mortality from myocardial infarction. British Medical Journal 1: 436–440
Engelberg H 1992 Low serum cholesterol and suicide. Lancet 339: 727–729
Epstein E H 1969 Epidemiology of coronary heart disease: risk factors and the role of thrombosis. In: Sherry S, Brinkhous K M, Genton E, Stengle J M (eds) National Academy of Sciences, Washington, DC
Ernst E, Matrai A, Bauman M 1985 Fibrinogen a possible link between social class and coronary heart disease. British Medical Journal 291: 1723
Falk E 1987 Thrombosis in unstable angina: pathologic aspects. In: Mehta J L, Conti C R, Brest A N (eds) Thrombosis and platelets in myocardial ischemia. F A Davis, Philadelphia, p 137–149
Feher M D, Rampling M W, Sever P S, Elkeles R S 1988 Diabetic hypertension — the importance of fibrinogen and blood viscosity. Journal Human Hypertension 2: 117–122
Fehily A M, Milbank J E, Yarnell J W G, Hayes T M, Kubiki A J, Eastham R D 1982 Dietary determinants of lipoproteins, total cholesterol viscosity, fibrinogen, and blood pressure. American Journal of Clinical Nutrition 36: 890–896
Fehily A M, Burr M L, Butland B K, Eastham R D 1986 A randomised controlled trial to investigate the effect of a high fibre diet on blood pressure and plasma fibrinogen. Journal Epidemiology and Community Health 40: 334–337
Finelli C, Palareti G, Poggi M et al 1991 Ticlopidine lowers plasma fibrinogen in patients with polycythaemic rubra vera and additional thrombotic risk factors. Acta Haematologie 85: 113–118
Folsom A R, Wu K K, Davis C E, Conlan M G, Sorlie P D, Syklo M 1991 Population correlates of plasma fibrinogen and factor VII, putative cardiovascular risk factors. Atherosclerosis 91: 191–205
Fowkes F G R, Connor J M, Smith F B, Wood J, Donnan P T, Lowe G D O 1992 Fibrinogen genotype and risk of peripheral atherosclerosis. Lancet 339: 696–696
Frick M H, Elo O, Haapa K et al 1987 Helsinki Heart Study: primary-prevention trial with gemfibrozil in middle-aged men with dyslipidemia. Safety of treatment, changes in risk factors, and incidence of coronary heart disease. New England Journal of Medicine 317: 1237–1245
Fuchs J, Pinhas A, Davidson E, Rotenberg Z, Agmon J, Weinberger I 1990 Plasma viscosity, fibrinogen and haematocrit in the course of unstable angina. European Heart Journal 11: 1029–1032
Fuller J H, Keen H, Jarrett R J et al 1979 Haemostatic variables associated with diabetes and its complications. British Medical Journal 2: 964–966
Fuller J H, Shipley M J, Rose G et al 1983 Mortality from coronary heart disease and stroke in relation to degree of glycaemia: the Whitehall study. British Medical Journal 287: 867–870
Gans R O B, Bilo H J G, Schouten J A, Rauwerda J A 1988 Fish oil and plasma fibrinogen. British Medical Journal 297: 978–979
Goldstein S, Landis J R, Leighton R et al 1981 Characteristics of resuscitated out-of-hospital cardiac arrest victim with coronary heart disease. Circulation 64: 977–984
Gordon T, Kannel W B 1972 Predisposition to atherosclerosis in the head, heart and legs. The Framingham Study. Journal of the American Medical Association 221: 661–666
Gordon T, Kannel W B, Hjortland M C, McNamara P M 1978 Menopause and coronary heart disease: the Framingham Study. Annals of Internal Medicine 89: 157–161
Green, K G, Heady A, Oliver M F 1989 Blood pressure, cigarette smoking and heart attack in the WHO co-operative trial of clofibrate. International Journal Epidemiology 18: 355–360
Green F R, Kelleher C K, Wilkes H C, Temple A, Meade T W, Humphries S E 1991 A common genetic polymorphism associated with lower coagulation factor VII levels in healthy individual. Arteriosclerosis and Thrombosis 11: 540–546
Gurewich V, Lipinski B, Hyde E et al 1976 The effect of the fibrinogen concentration and the leukocyte count on intravascular fibrin deposition from soluble fibrin monomer complexes. Thrombosis and Haemostasis 36: 605–614
Haerem J W 1974 Mural platelet microthrombi and major acute lesions of main epicardial arteries in sudden coronary death. Atherosclerosis 19: 529–541
Haglund O, Wallin R, Luostarinen R, Saldeen T 1990 Effects of a new fluid fish oil concentrate, ESKIMO-3, on triglycerides, cholesterol, fibrinogen and blood pressure. Journal of Internal Medicine 227: 347–353
Haines A P, Chakrabarti R, Fisher D, Meade T W, North W R S, Stirling Y 1980 Haemostatic variables in vegetarians and non-vegetarians. Thrombosis Research 19: 139–148
Haines A P, Howarth D, North W R S, Goldenberg E, Stirling Y, Meade T W, Raftery E B, Millar Craig M W 1983 Haemostatic variables and the outcome of myocardial infarction. Thrombosis and Haemostasis 50: 800–803
Hall A J, Winter P D, Wright R 1985 Mortality of hepatitis B positive blood donors in England and Wales. Lancet 1: 91–93
Hammer A 1878 Ein fall von thrombotischem verschlusse einer de Kranzarterien des herzens. Medizinische Wochenschrift 5: 97–102
Hammond E C, Garfinkel L 1969 Coronary heart disease, stroke and aortic aneuysm. Factors in the etiology. Archives of Environmental Health 19: 167–182
Hamsten A, de Faire U, Wallius G et al 1987a Plasminogen activator inhibitor in plasma: risk factor for recurrent myocardial infarction. Lancet 2: 3–9
Hamsten A, Iselius L, de Faire U, Blombäck M 1987b Genetic and Cultural inheritance of plasma fibrinogen concentration. Lancet 2: 988–990
Hennekens C H, Buring J E, Sandercock P, Collins R, Peto R 1989 Aspirin and other antiplatelet agents in the secondary and primary prevention of cardio vascular disease. Circulation 80: 749–756
Henriksson P, Edhag O 1986 Orchidectomy versus oestrogen for prostatic cancer: cardiovascular effects. British Medical Journal 2: 413–415
Henriksson P, Blombäck M, Bratt G, Edhag O, Eriksson A 1986 Activators and inhibitors of coagulation and fibrinolysis in patients with prostatic cancer treated with oestrogen or orchidectomy. Thrombosis Research 44: 783–791
Herrick J B 1912 Clinical features of sudden obstruction of the coronary arteries. Journal of the American Medical Association 23: 2015–2020
Hill A B 1965 The environment and disease: association or causation? Proceedings of Royal Society of Medicine 58: 295–300
Hoffman C J, Miller R H, Lawson W E, Hultin M B 1989 Elevation of factor VII activity and mass in young adults at risk of ischemic heart disease. Journal of American College of Cardiology 14: 941–946
Hostmark A T, Bjerkedal T, Kierulf P, Flaten H, Ulshagen K 1988 Fish oil and plasma fibrinogen. British Medical Journal 297: 180–181
Humphries S E, Cook M, Dubowitz M, Stirling Y, Meade T W 1987 Role of genetic variation at the fibrinogen locus in determination of plasma fibrinogen concentrations. Lancet 1: 1452–1455
Innerfield I, Goldfischer J, Reichter-Reiss H, Greenberg J 1976 Serum antithrombins in coronary artery disease. American Journal of Clinical Pathology 65: 64–68
International Anticoagulant Review Group 1970 Collaborative analysis of long-term anticoagulant administration after acute myocardial infarction. Lancet 1: 203–209
International Collaborative Group 1979 Joint discussion. Journal of Chronic Diseases 32: 829–837
Isles C G, Hole D J, Hawthorn V M, Lever A F 1992 Relation between coronary risk and coronary mortality in women of the Renfrew and Paisley survey: comparison with men. Lancet 339: 702–706
ISIS-2 Collaborative Group 1988 Randomised trial of intravenous streptokinase, oral aspirin, both, or neither among 17 187 cases of suspected acute myocardial infarction: ISIS-2. Lancet 2: 349–360
ISIS-2 Collaborative Group 1992 Morning peak in the incidence of myocardial infarction: experience in the ISIS-2 trial. European Heart Journal 13: 594–598
Iso H, Folsom A R, Wu K K, Finch A, Munger R G, Sato S et al 1989 Haemostatic variables in Japanese and Caucasian men. American Journal Epidemiology 130: 925–934
Kahn H A 1966 The Dorn study of smoking and mortality among US veterans: Report on eight and one-half years of observation. In: Haenzel W (ed) Epidemiological approaches to the study of cancer and other chronic diseases. National Cancer Institute Monograph No 19. US Department of Health, Education and Welfare, Public Health Service, National Institutes of Health, National Cancer Institute, p 1–125

Kannel W B 1987 Hypertension and other risk factors in coronary heart disease. American Heart Journal 114: 918–925
Kannel W B, D'Agostino R B 1990 Update of fibrinogen as a major cardiovascular risk factor: the Framingham Study. Journal of American College of Cardiology, 15: 156A
Kannel W B, Castelli W P, Meeks S L 1985 Fibrinogen and cardiovascular disease. Abstract of paper for 34th Annual Scientific Session of the American College of Cardiology, March 1985, Anaheim, California
Kannel W B, Wolf P A, Castelli W P, D'Agostino R B 1987 Fibrinogen and risk of cardiovascular disease. Journal of the American Medical Association 258: 1183–1186
Kario K, Matsuo T 1992 Coronary artery disease and factor VII hyperactivity in elderly Japanese. American Journal of Cardiology 69: 807–809
Klonoff-Cohen H, Barrett-Connor E L 1992 Albumin levels as a predictor of mortality in the healthy elderly. Journal of Clinical Epidemiology 45: 207–212
Kruskal J B, Commerford P J, Franks J J, Kirsch R E 1987 Fibrin and fibrinogen-related antigens in patients with stable and unstable coronary artery disease. New England Journal of Medicine 317: 1361–1365
Kuller L H, Eichner J E, Orchard T J, Grandits G A, McCallum L, Tracy R P 1991 The relation between serum albumin levels and risk of coronary heart disease in the multiple risk factor intervention trial. American Journal of Epidemiology 134: 1266–1277
Landolfi R, De Cristofaro R, De Candia E, Rocco B, Bizzi B 1991 Effect of fibrinogen concentration on the velocity of platelet aggregation. Blood 78: 377–381
Lapidus L, Bengtsson C, Larsson B, Pennert K, Rybo E, Sjostrom L 1984 Distribution of adipose tissue and risk of cardiovascular disease and death: A 12 year follow up of participants in the population study of women in Gothenburg, Sweden. British Medical Journal 289: 1257–1261
Lardinois C K, Neuman S L 1988 The effects of antihypertensive agents on serum lipids and lipoproteins. Archives of Internal Medicine 148: 1280–1288
Larsson B, Svardsudd K, Welin L, Wilhelmsen L, Bjorntorp P, Tibblin G 1984 Abdominal adipose tissue distribution obesity and risk of cardiovascular disease and death: 13 year follow up of participants in the study of men born in 1913. British Medical Journal 288: 1401–1404
Lee A J, Smith W C S, Lowe G D O, Tunstall-Pedoe H 1990 Plasma fibrinogen and coronary risk factors: the Scottish heart health study. Journal Clinical Epidemiology 43: 913–919
Lerner D J, Kannel W B 1986 Patterns of coronary heart disease morbidity and mortality in the sexes: A 26-year follow-up of the Framingham population. American Heart Journal 111: 383–390
Liberthson R R, Bagel E L, Hirschman J C at al 1974 Pathophysiologic observations in prehospital ventricular fibrillation and sudden cardiac death. Circulation 49: 791–798
Lindberg G, Eklund G A, Gullberg B, Rastam L 1991 Serum sialic acid concentration and cardiovascular mortality. British Medical Journal 302: 143–146
Lindberg G, Rastam L, Gullberg B, Eklund G A 1992a Serum sialic acid concentration predicts both coronary heart disease and stroke mortality: Multivariate analysis including 54 385 men and women during 20.5 years follow-up. International Journal of Epidemiology 21: 253–257
Lindberg G, Rastam L, Gullberg B, Eklund G A 1992b Low serum cholesterol concentration and short term mortality from injuries in men and women. British Medical Journal 305: 277–279
Lissner L, Odell P M, D'Agostino R B, Stokes J, Kreger B E, Belanger A J, Brownell K D 1991 Variability of body weight and health outcomes in the Framingham population. New England Journal of Medicine 324: 1839–1844
Lowe G D O 1986 Blood rheology in arterial disease. Clinical Science 71: 137–146
Lowe G D O 1991 Haemostatic changes and the hypercoagulable state. Lancet 338: 1526
Lowe G D O 1992 Blood viscosity and cardiovascular disease. Thrombosis and Haemostasis 67: 494–498
Lowe G D O, Forbes C D 1985 Platelet aggregation haematocrit and fibrinogen. Lancet 1: 395–396
Lowe G D O, Reavey M M, Johnston R V, Forbes C D, Prentice C R M 1979 Increased platelet aggregates in vascular and non-vascular illness: correlation with plasma fibrinogen and effect of ancrod. Thrombosis Research 14: 377–386
Lowe G D O, Drummond M M, Third J L H C, Bremner W F, Forbes C D, Prentice C R M, Lawrie T D V 1980 Increased plasma fibrinogen and platelet-aggregates in type II hyperlipoproteinaemia. Thrombosis and Haemostasis 42: 1503–1507
Macfarlane R G 1977 Haemostasis: Introduction. British Medical Bulletin 33: 183–185
McGill H C (ed) 1968 The geographic pathology of atherosclerosis. Laboratory Investigation 18: 463–467
McGill H C 1988 The cardiovascular pathology of smoking. American Heart Journal 115: 250–257
McKeigue P M, Shah B, Marmot M G 1991 Relation of central obesity and insulin resistance with high diabetes prevalence and cardiovascular risk in South Asians. Lancet 337: 382–386
MacMahon S, Peto R, Cutler J, Collins R, Sorlie P, Neaton J, Abbott R, Godwin J, Dyer A, Stamler J 1990 Blood pressure, stroke, and coronary heart disease. Part 1, prolonged differences in blood pressure: prospective observational studies corrected for the regression dilution bias. Lancet 335: 765–774
Manson J E, Colditz G A, Stampfer M J, Willett W C, Rosner B, Monson R R, Speizer F E, Hennekens C H 1990 A prospective study of obesity and risk of coronary heart disease in women. New England Journal of Medicine 322: 882–889
Marckmann P, Sandstrom B, Jespersen J 1990 Effects of total fat content and fatty acid composition in diet on factor VII coagulant activity and blood lipids. Atherosclerosis 80: 227–33
Markowe H L, Marmot M G, Shipley M J, Bulpitt C J, Meade T W, Stirling Y, Vickers M V, Semmence A 1985 Fibrinogen: a possible link between social class and coronary heart disease. British Medical Journal 291: 1312–1314
Marmot M, Brunner E 1991 Alcohol and cardiovascular disease: the status of the U shaped curve. British Medical Journal 303: 565–568
Marmot M G, McDowall M E 1986 Mortality decline and widening social inequalities. Lancet 2: 274–276
Martin M J, Hulley S B, Browner W S, Kuller L H, Wentworth D 1986 Serum cholesterol, blood pressure, and mortality: Implications from a cohort of 361 662 men. Lancet 2: 933–936
Martin J F, Bath P M, Burr M L 1991 Influence of platelet size on outcome after myocardial infarction. Lancet 338: 1409–1411
Mattila K J, Nieminen M S, Valtonen V V, Rasi V P, Kesaniemi A, Syrjala S L et al 1989 Association between dental health and acute myocardial infarction. British Medical Journal 298: 779–781
Meade T W 1987 The epidemiology of haemostatic and other variables in coronary artery disease. In: Verstraete M, Vermylen J, Lijnen R, Arnout J (eds) Thrombosis and haemostasis. Leuven University Press, Leuven, p 37–60
Meade T W 1992a Aspirin and myocardial infarction, an annotation on venous thrombosis. In: Vane J R, Botting R (eds) Aspirin and other salicylates. Chapman & Hall (in press)
Meade T W 1992b Low intensity oral anticoagulation. In: Thompson J, Poller L (eds) Proceedings of symposium to mark retirement of Professor Leon Poller. Churchill Livingstone (in press)
Meade T W, Berra A 1992 Hormone replacement therapy and cardiovascular disease. British Medical Bulletin 48: 276–308
Meade T W, North W R S 1977 Population-based distribution of haemostatic variables. British Medical Bulletin 33: 283–288
Meade T W, Chakrabarti R, Haines A P, Howarth D J, North W R S, Stirling Y 1977 Haemostatic, lipid and blood-pressure profiles of women on oral contraceptive containing 50 μg or 30 μg oestrogen. Lancet 2: 948–951
Meade T W, Chakrabarti R, Haines A P, North W R S, Stirling Y 1979 Characteristics affecting fibrinolytic activity and plasma fibrinogen concentrations. British Medical Journal 1: 153–156
Meade T W, North W R S, Chakrabarti R, Stirling Y, Haines A P, Thompson S G 1980 Haemostatic function and cardiovascular death: early results of a prospective study. Lancet 1: 1050–1054
Meade T W, Howarth D J, Stirling Y, Welch T P, Crompson M R

1984 Fibrinopeptide A and sudden coronary death. Lancet, 2: 607–609
Meade T W, Vickers M W, Thompson S G, Stirling Y, Haines A P, Miller G J 1985a Epidemiological characteristics of platelet aggregability. British Medical Journal 290: 428–432
Meade T W, Vickers M V, Thompson S G, Seghatchian M J 1985b The effect of physiological levels of fibrinogen on platelet aggregation. Thrombosis Research 38: 527–534
Meade T W, Mellows S, Brozovic M, Miller G J, Chakrabarti R R, North W R S, Haines A P Stirling Y, Imeson J D, Thompson S G 1986a Haemostatic function and ischaemic heart disease: principal results of the Northwick Park Heart Study. Lancet 2: 533–537
Meade T W, Stirling Y, Thompson S G, Vickers M V, Woolf L, Ajdukiewics A B, Stewart G, Davidson J F, Walker I D, Douglas A S, Richardson I M, Weir R D, Aromaa A, Impivaara O, Maatela J, Hladovec J 1986b An international and interregional comparison of haemostatic variables in the study of ischaemic heart disease. International Journal Epidemiology 15: 331–336
Meade T W, Imeson J, Stirling Y 1987a Effects of changes in smoking and other characteristics on clotting factors and the risk of ischaemic heart disease. Lancet 2: 986–988
Meade T W, Stirling Y, Thompson S G, Ajdukiewica A, Barbara J A J, Chalmers D M 1987b Carriers of hepatitis B surface antigen: possible association between low levels of clotting factors and protection against ischaemic heart disease. Thrombosis Research 45: 709–713
Meade T W, Dyer S, Howarth D J, Imeson J D, Stirling Y 1990 Antithrombin III and procoagulant activity: sex differences and effects of the menopause. British Journal of Haematology 74: 77–81
Meade T W, Cooper J, Miller G J, Howarth D, Stirling Y 1991 Antithrombin III and arterial disease. Lancet 337: 850–851
Medical Research Council Working Party 1985 MRC trial of mild hypertension: principal results. British Medical Journal 291: 97–104
Medical Research Council Working Party 1992 Medical Research Council trial of treatment of hypertension in older adults: principal results. British Medical Journal 304: 405–412
Meilahn E, Kuller L H, Kiss J E, Matthews K A, Lewis J H 1988 Coagulation parameters among pre- and post-menopausal women. American Journal of Epidemiology 128: 908
Miller G J 1992 Personal communication
Miller G J, Martin J C, Webster J, Wilkes H, Miller N E, Wilkinson W H, Meade T W 1986a Association between dietary fat intake and plasma factor VII coagulant activity – a predictor of cardiovascular mortality. Atherosclerosis 60: 269–271
Miller G J, Seghatchian M J, Walter S J, Howarth D J, Thompson S G, Esnouf M P, Meade T W 1986b An association between the factor VII coagulant activity and thrombin activity induced by surface/cold exposure of normal human plasma. British Journal of Haematology 62: 379–384
Miller G J, Cruickshank J K, Ellis L J, Thompson R L, Wilkes J H C, Stirling Y, Mitropoulos K A, Allison J V, Fox T E, Walker A O 1989 Fat consumption and factor VII coagulant activity in middle-aged men. An association between a dietary and thrombogenic coronary risk factor. Atherosclerosis 78: 19–24
Miller G J, Martin J C, Mitropoulos K A, Reeves B E A, Thompson R L, Meade T W, Cooper J A, Cruickshank J K 1991a Plasma factor VII is activated by post-prandial triglyceridaemia irrespective of dietary fat composition. Atherosclerosis 86: 163–171
Miller G J, Wilkes H C, Meade T W, Bauer K A, Barzegar S, Rosenberg R D 1990b Haemostatic changes that constitute the hypercoagulable state. Lancet 338: 1079
Mitropoulos K A, Miller G J, Reeves B E A, Wilkes H C, Cruickshank J K 1989 Factor VII coagulant activity is strongly associated with the plasma concentration of large lipoprotein particles in middle-aged men. Atherosclerosis 76: 203–208
Moller L, Kirstensen T S 1991 Plasma fibrinogen and ischaemic heart disease risk factors. Arteriosclerosis and Thrombosis 11: 344–350
Morris J N 1951 Recent history of coronary disease. Lancet 1: 1–7, 69–73
Morris J N, Crawford M D 1958 Coronary heart disease and physical activity of work. Evidence of a national necropsy survey. British Medical Journal 2: 1485–1496
Morris J N, Gardner M J 1969 Epidemiology of ischemic heart disease. American Journal of Medicine 46: 674–683
Morris J N, Head J A, Raffle P A B, Roberts C G, Parks J W 1953 Coronary heart disease and physical activity of work. Lancet 2: 1053–1057, 1111–1120
Morris J N, Kagan A, Pattison D C, Gardner M J, Raffle P A B 1966 Incidence and prediction of ischaemic heart disease in London busmen. Lancet 2: 553–559
Morris J N, Clayton D G, Everitt M G, Semmence A M, Burgess E H et al 1990 Exercise in leisure time: coronary attack and death rates. British Heart Journal 63: 325–334
Muldoon M F, Mantuck S B, Matthews K A 1990 Lowering cholesterol concentrations and mortality: a quantitative review of primary prevention trials. British Medical Journal 301: 309–314
Muller J E, Stone P H, Turi Z G, Rutherford J D, Czeisler C A, Parker C, Poole K, Passamani E, Roberts R, Robertson T, Sobel B E, Willerson J T, Braunwald E, and the MILIS study group 1985 Circadian variation in the frequency of onset of acute myocardial infarction. New England Journal of Medicine 313: 1315–1322
Muller A D, Houwelingen A C V, van Dam-Mieras M C E, Bas B M, Hornstra G 1989 Effect of a moderate fish intake on haemostatic parameters in healthy males. Thrombosis and Haemostasis 61: 468–473
Mutru O, Laakso M, Isomaki H, Koota K 1985 Ten year mortality and causes of death in patients with rheumatoid arthritis. British Medical Journal 290: 1797–1799
Naski M C, Shafer J A 1991 A kinetic model for the α-thrombin-catalyzed conversion of plasma levels of fibrinogen to fibrin in the presence of antithrombin III. Journal of Biological Chemistry 266: 13003–13010
O'Brien J, Etherington M, Jamieson S, Lawford P, Lincoln S, Alkjaersig N 1975 Blood changes in atherosclerosis and long after myocardial infarction and venous thrombosis. Thrombosis et Diathesis Haemorrhagica 34: 483–497
O'Connor N T J, Broekmans A W, Bertina R M 1984 Protein C values in coronary artery disease. British Medical Journal 289: 1192
Perper J A, Kuller L H, Cooper M 1975 Arteriosclerosis of coronary arteries in sudden unexpected deaths. Circulation (suppl III) 51/52: 27–33
Phillips A, Shaper A G, Whincup P H 1989 Association between serum albumin and mortality from cardiovascular disease, cancer, and other causes. Lancet 2: 1434–1436
Pickart L 1981 Fat metabolism the fibrinogen/fibrinolytic system and blood flow: new potentials for the pharmacological treatment of coronary heart disease. Pharmacology 23: 271–280
Pickart L R, Thaler M M 1976 Free fatty acids and albumin as mediators of thrombin-stimulated fibrinogen synthesis. American Journal of Physiology 230: 996–1002
Pocock S J, Shaper A G, Cook D G, Phillips A N, Walker M 1987 Social class differences in ischaemic heart disease in British men. Lancet 2: 197–201
Poller L 1957 Thrombosis and factor VII activity. Journal of Clinical Pathology 10: 348–350
Radack K, Deck C, Huster G 1989 Dietary supplementation with low-dose fish oils lowers fibrinogen levels: a randomized, double-blind controlled study. Annals of Internal Medicine 111: 757–758
Rapold H J, Haeberli A, Kuemmerli H, Weiss M, Baur H R Straub W P 1989 Fibrin formation and platelet activation in patients with myocardial infarction and normal coronary arteries. European Heart Journal 10: 323–333
Ravnskov U 1992 Cholesterol lowering trials in coronary heart disease: frequency of citation and outcome. British Medical Journal 305: 15–19
Regnstrom J, Nilsson J, Tornvall P, Landou C, Hamsten A 1992 Susceptibility to low-density lipoprotein oxidation and coronary atherosclerosis in man. Lancet 339: 1183–1186
Renaud S 1980 Risk factor for coronary heart disease and platelet functions. Advances in Experimental Medicine and Biology 4: 129–144
Renaud S, de Lorgeril M 1992 Wine, alcohol, platelets, and the French paradox for coronary heart disease. Lancet 339: 1523–1526
Richardson P D, Davies M J, Born G V R 1989 Influence of plaque

configuration and stress distribution on fissuring of coronary atherosclerotic plaques. Lancet 2: 941–944

Riemersma R A, Wood D A, Macintyre C C A, Elton R A, Gey K F, Oliver M F 1991 Risk of angina pectoris and plasma concentrations of vitamins A, C, and E and carotene. Lancet 337: 1–5

RISC group 1990 Risk of myocardial infarction and death during treatment with low dose aspirin and intravenous heparin in men with unstable coronary artery disease. Lancet 336: 827–830

Rogers S, James K S, Butland B K, Etherington M D, O'Brien J R, Jones J G 1987 Effects of a fish oil supplement on serum lipids, variables: a double blind randomised controlled trial in healthy volunteers. Atherosclerosis 63: 137–143

Rose G A 1968 Variability of angina. Some implications for epidemiology. British Journal of Preventive and Social Medicine 22: 12–15

Rosendaal F R, Varekamp I, Smit C et al 1989 Mortality and causes of death in Dutch haemophiliacs; 1973–86. British Journal of Haematology 71: 71–76

Rosendaal F R, Briët E, Stibb J et al 1990 Haemophilia protects against ischameic heart disease: a study of risk factors. British Journal of Haematology, 75: 525–530

Rosengren A, Wilhelmsen L, Eriksson E, Risber B, Wedel H 1990a Lipoprotein (a) and coronary heart disease: a prospective case-control study in a general population sample of middle aged men. British Medical Journal 301: 1248–1251

Rosengren A, Wilhelmsen L, Welin L, Tsipogianni, Teger-Nilsson A-C, Wedel H 1990b Social influences and cardiovascular risk factors as determinants of plasma fibrinogen concentration in a general population sample of middle aged men. British Medical Journal 300: 634–638

Rossouw J E, Lewis B, Rifkind B M 1990 The value of lowering cholesterol after myocardial infarction. New England Journal of Medicine 323: 1112–1119

Rothwell M, Rampling M W, Cholerton S, Sever P S 1991 Haemorheological changes in the very short term after abstention from tobacco by cigarette smokers. British Journal of Haematology 79: 500–503

Saikku P, Leinonen M, Mattila K, Ekman M-R, Nieminen M S, Makela P H et al 1988 Serological evidence of an association of a novel chlamydia, twar, with chronic coronary heart disease and acute myocardial infarction. Lancet 2: 983–986

Salive M E, Cornoni-Huntley J, Phillips C L, Guralnik J M, Cohen H J, Ostfeld A M, Wallace R B 1992 Serum albumin in older persons: relationship with age and health status. Journal of Clinical Epidemiology 45: 213–221

Salmasi A-M, Salmasi S, MacDonald G, Nicholaides A N 1991 Improvement of silent myocardial ischaemia and reduction of plasma fibrinogen during nisoldipine therapy in occult coronary arterial disease. International Journal of Cardiology 31: 71–80

SALT Collaborative Group 1991 Swedish aspirin low-dose trial (SALT) of 75 mg aspirin as secondary prophylaxis after cerebrovascular ischaemic events. Lancet 338: 1345–1349

Schneidau A, Harrison M J G, Hurst C, Wilkes H C, Meade T W 1989 Arterial disease risk factors and angiographic evidence of atheroma of the carotid artery. Stroke 20: 1466–1471

Schulman S, Johnsson H, Lindmarker P 1991 Thrombotic complications after substitution with a FVII concentrate. Thrombosis and Haemostasis 66: 619

Simpson H C R, Mann J I, Chakrabarti R et al 1982 Effect of high fibre diet on haemostatic variables in diabetes. British Medical Journal 284: 1608

Simpson H C R, Mann J I, Meade T W, Chakrabarti R, Stirling Y, Woolf L 1983 Hypertriglyceridaemia and hypercoagulability. Lancet 1: 786–90

Sixty-Plus Reinfarction Study Research Group 1980 A double-blind trial to assess long-term oral anticoagulant therapy in elderly patients after myocardial infarction. Lancet 2: 989–994

Smith P, Arnesen H, Holme I 1990a The effect of warfarin on mortality ad reinfarction after myocardial infarction. New England Journal of Medicine 323: 147–152

Smith E B, Keen G A, Grant A, Stirk C 1990b Fate of fibrinogen in human intima. Arteriosclerosis 10: 263–275

Sonne-Holm S, Sorensen T I A, Christensen U 1983 Risk of early death in extremely overweight young men. British Medical Journal 287: 795–797

Stampfer M J, Sacks F M, Salvini S, Willett W C, Hennekens C H 1991 A prospective study of cholesterol, apolipoproteins, and the risk of myocardial infarction. New England Journal of Medicine 325: 373–381

Standing Medical Advisory Committee 1990 Blood cholesterol testing. The cost-effectiveness of opportunistic cholesterol testing. Report to the Secretary of State for Health, May 1990

Steinberg D, Parthasarathy S, Carew T E, Khoo J C, Witztum J L 1989 Beyond cholesterol. Modifications of low-density lipoprotein that increase its atherogenecity. New England Journal of Medicine 320: 915–924

Stone M C, Thorp J M 1985 Plasma fibrinogen — a major coronary risk factor. Journal of the Royal College of General Practitioners 35: 565–569

Strandberg T E, Salomaa V V, Naukkarinen V A et al 1991 Long-term mortality after 5-year multifactorial primary prevention of cardiovascular disease in middle-aged men. Journal of the American Medical Association 266: 1225–1229

Stout R W, Crawford V 1991 Seasonal variations in fibrinogen concentrations among elderly people. Lancet 338: 9–13

Surgeon General 1989 Reducing the Health Consequences of Smoking. US Department of Health and Human Services

Suzuki T, Yamauchi K, Matsushita T, Furumichi T, Furui H, Tsuzuki J, Saito H 1991 Elevation of factor VII activity and mass in coronary artery disease of varying severity. Clinical Cardiology 14: 731–736

Syrjanen J, Valtonen V V, Ilvanainen M, Kaste M, Huttunen J K 1988 Preceding infection as an important risk factor for ischaemic brain infarction in young and middle aged patients. British Medical Journal 296: 1156–1160

Takano K, Yamaguchi T, Okada Y, Uchida K, Kisiel W, Kato H 1990 Hypercoagulability in acute ischemic stroke analysis of the extrinsic coagulation reactions in plasma by a highly sensitive automated method. Thrombosis Research 58: 481–491

Thomas A E, Green F R, Kelleher C H, Wilkes H C, Brennan P J, Humphries S E 1991 Variation in the promoter region of the B fibrinogen gene is associated with plasma fibrinogen levels in smokers and non-smokers. Thrombosis and Haemostasis 65: 487–490

Thompson S G, Martin J C, Meade T W 1987 Sources of variability in coagulation factor assays. Thrombosis and Haemostasis 58: 1073–1077

Trip M D, Cats V M, van Capelle F J L, Vreeken J 1990 Platelet hyperreactivity and prognosis in survivors of myocardial infarction. New England Journal of Medicine 322: 1549–1554

Tunstall Pedoe H, Clayton D M, Morris J N, Brigden W, McDonald L 1975 Coronary heart attacks in East London. Lancet 2: 833–838

Tuomilehto J, Salonen J T, Marti B, Jalkanen L, Puska P, Nissinen A, Wolf E 1987 Body weight and risk of myocardial infarction and death in the adult population of eastern Finland. British Medical Journal 295: 623–627

Ulbricht T L V, Southgate D A T 1991 Coronary heart disease: seven dietary factors. Lancet 338: 985–992

Vane J R, Botting R M 1991 Heart disease, aspirin, and fish oil. Circulation 84: 2588–2590

Vigano S, Mannucci P M, D'Angelo A et al 1984 Protein C antigen is not an acute phase reactant and is often high in ischemic heart disease and diabetes. Thrombosis and Haemostasis 52: 263–266

Wakefield A J, Sawyerr A M, Dhillon A P et al 1989 Pathogenesis of Crohn's disease: multifocal gastrointestinal infarction. Lancet 2: 1057–1062

Weir J M, Dunn J E 1970 Smoking and mortality a prospective study. Cancer 25: 105–112

Weiss H J, Aledort L M 1967 Impaired platelet/connective-tissue reaction in man after aspirin ingestion. Lancet 2: 495–497

Wilhelmsen L, Svardsudd K, Korsan-Bengtsen K, Welin L, Tibblin G 1984 Fibrinogen as a risk factor for stroke and myocardial infarction. New England Journal of Medicine 311: 501–505

Wilkes H C, Kelleher C, Meade T W 1988 Smoking and plasma fibrinogen. Lancet 1: 307–308

Wilkes H C, Meade T W, Barzegar S, Foley A J, Hughes L O, Bauer

K A, Rosenberg R D, Miller G J 1992 Gemfibrozil reduces plasma prothrombin fragment F1+2 concentration, a marker of coagulability, in patients with coronary heart disease. Thrombosis and Haemostasis 67: 503–506

Wiseman S, Kenchington G, Dain R et al 1989 Influence of smoking and plasma factors on patency of femoropopliteal vein grafts. British Medical Journal 299: 643–646

Wood D A, Riemersma R A, Butler S et al 1987 Linoleic and eicosapentaenoic acids in adipose tissue and platelets and risk of coronary heart disease. Lancet 1: 177–180

World Health Organization 1989 Statistics annual

Wu K K, Papp A C, Patsch W, Rock R, Eckfeldt J, Sharrett R 1990 ARIC hemostasis study — II. Organizational plan and feasibility study. Thrombosis and Haemostasis 64: 521–525

Yarnell J W G, Fehily A M, Milbank J, Kubiki A J, Eastham R, Hayes T M 1983 Derterminants of plasma lipoproteins and coagulation factors in men from Caerphilly, South Wales. Journal Epidemiology and Community Health 37: 137–140

Yarnell J W G, Sweetnam P M, Elwood P C et al 1985 Haemostatic factors and ischaemic heart disease. The Caerphilly study. British Heart Journal 53: 483–487

Yarnell J W G, Sweetnam P M, Rogers S et al 1987 Some long term effects of smoking on the haemostatic system: a report from the Caerphilly and Speedwell collaborative surveys. Journal Clinical Pathology 40: 909–913

Yarnell J W G, Baker I A, Sweetnam P M et al 1991 Fibrinogen, viscosity, and white blood cell count are major risk factors for ischemic heart disease. The Caerphilly and Speedwell Collabortive Heart Disease Studies. Circulation 83: 836–844

Yue R, Gertler M, Starr T, Koutrouby R 1976 Alterations of plasma antithrombin III levels in ischemic heart disease. Thrombosis and Haemostasis 35: 598–606

SECTION 9

Arterial disease — clinical

54. Coronary artery disease

P. J. Grant C. R. M. Prentice

The burgeoning increase in the incidence of coronary artery disease that has taken place this century has been one of the great natural disasters to affect man. The social and economic effects of the premature morbidity and mortality associated with this condition, particularly in the Western Hemisphere, are almost incalculable. These facts have combined to provide the incentive for a research effort designed to understand better the pathogenesis of this disorder, its prevention and to develop management strategies based on sound scientific principles. Great advances have taken place in the last 25 years, beginning with the routine use of cardiac catheterization and the subsequent recognition of the important role of thrombus formation on pre-existing atheroma in acute myocardial infarction. A more detailed understanding of those factors involved in the development of coronary atheroma has followed from large epidemiological studies which naturally led to intervention studies designed to enhance both primary and secondary prevention of this disorder. Finally, the management of acute myocardial infarction has been revolutionized by the large scale commercial production of plasminogen activators for clinical use. The rapid use of streptokinase, tissue plasminogen activator or urokinase has been undeniably successful in reducing the acute mortality associated with myocardial infarction.

Knowledge in all areas of ischaemic heart disease is increasing at a bewildering rate and has changed the management beyond recognition. This chapter will attempt to put into perspective some of the important advances that have recently taken place in this field.

HISTORY OF ISCHAEMIC HEART DISEASE

With the exception of one or two sporadic descriptions of a syndrome that resembled angina pectoris (Michaels 1966), this condition remained unrecognized as a clinical entity until the second half of the 18th century. In 1772, Dr William Heberden, a fellow of the Royal College of Physicians in London, published the first account of angina pectoris in a series of 20 patients (Leibowitz 1970, Fye 1985). Although it seems likely that some of his patients were not suffering from angina pectoris of ischaemic heart disease, the description of the pain in most cases was identical to that described by many patients today. Throughout the 18th and 19th centuries and up to the First World War, ischaemic heart disease, as it is now known, was considered to be a rare condition (White 1971). During the latter part of the 19th century, physicians began to study the coronary circulation and Richard Quain carried out a detailed study of what was termed fatty degeneration of the heart (Quain 1850). Following these studies, a number of physicians became convinced of the relationship between coronary thrombosis and myocardial disease (Rindfleisch 1872). The first published claim of coronary thrombosis was made in 1878, although it subsequently appears that this was in fact due to obstruction of the coronary artery by a thrombosed aortic valve vegetation (Lie 1978). During this time and up to the beginning of the 20th century it was generally believed that coronary thrombosis was a fatal event (Osler 1897). The first clinical paper delineating the clinical features of acute myocardial infarction was published in Russia in 1910 (Obrastzow & Straschesko 1910). This paper received little attention and it was the achievement of James Herrick to convince the medical community that myocardial infarction could be recognised during life (Herrick 1912). There has been considerable debate as to whether this represented the occurrence of a new disorder at around this time or if it was previously unrecognised but occurring at about the same incidence. Cogent arguments have been put forward to suggest that the former is true and that ischaemic heart disease appeared in its modern form at around the time of the Great War (Michaels 1966). During the 1920s and 1930s coronary artery disease was recognized with increasing frequency as being a problem that occurred in white affluent males in both North America and Europe. It became the leading cause of death in the United States and some other western countries at around 1940 and the incidence continued to increase throughout the 1950s. In the decade of 1960 a sudden sharp reduction in mortality from myocardial infarction was seen in the United States. Between 1968 and 1976 a 20% fall in mortality from ischaemic heart disease took place and this trend has continued up to the present time.

PATHOLOGICAL FEATURES OF CORONARY HEART DISEASE

Both autopsy and coronary arteriography studies have shown that, in patients with transmural myocardial infarction, two pathological features are nearly always present: severe atheromatous narrowing of the coronary arteries and superimposed coronary artery thrombi. The controversy over whether occlusive thrombosis was the immediate cause of myocardial infarction has been resolved in favour of thrombus occlusion over the past 30 years (Crawford 1963, Friedman & Byers 1965, Constantinides 1966, Davies et al 1976, 1979, Falk 1983). The frequency of occlusive thrombosis in transmural infarction is considerably greater than that seen in subendocardial infarction (Davies et al 1976). Again, in unstable angina pectoris the precipitating event seems to be non-occlusive, partial thrombotic obstruction of the coronary artery (Davies et al 1986, Fuster et al 1988). This information has been well documented recently by Mizuno and colleagues using direct vision angioscopy to determine the presence and degree of occlusion in the affected vessels (Mizuno et al 1991). It was found that patients with unstable angina had predominantly non-occlusive thrombus, whereas those with acute myocardial infarction had occlusive thrombus. Thus, there seems to be a progression of coronary thrombosis in which the degree of occlusion is mainly partial in unstable angina and sub-endocardial infarction, leading to complete occlusion in acute transmural myocardial infarction.

The fact that most myocardial infarctions are caused by occlusive coronary thrombus was not realised at first (Roberts & Buja 1972), because there is spontaneous resolution of thrombus in most cases with the passage of time. Thus, as the infarction ages, there is a decrease in the frequency with which occlusive thrombi are found. This was demonstrated by Mitchell and Schwartz (1965) who found that, in autopsy studies, by the time the infarction was 4 months old the incidence of occlusive thrombi had decreased significantly compared to the recent infarct. The advent of coronary arteriography was an important advance in obtaining direct information on the patency of the coronary artery. Oliva and Breckenridge (1977) and Maseri and colleagues (1978) showed that, when arteriography is carried out at the time of acute myocardial infarction, many of the apparent coronary occlusions became patent again after injection of vasodilators. Thus, reversible coronary artery spasm, usually superimposed on an atherosclerotic obstruction, could be the primary event or a secondary occurrence in the pathophysiology of acute myocardial infarction. It appears that there is a dynamic interaction between spasm, thrombus and atherosclerotic plaque preceding acute coronary artery occlusion. De Wood and colleagues (1980) showed an 87% incidence of occlusive thrombus within 4 hours of acute infarction, but this decreased to 65% over the next 24 hours. Thus, even in the era before thrombolytic therapy it was appreciated that there was a high incidence of thrombosis *causing* the infarct, but that this declined with time due to spontaneous resolution.

CLINICAL FEATURES OF CORONARY ARTERY DISEASE

The central feature of all the syndromes associated with coronary artery disease is either a reduction in or cessation of blood flow and oxygen supply to a segment of myocardium. It has been established beyond doubt that, with the exception of rare disorders such as embolism or arteritis, the underlying pathological insult leading to this is the development of coronary artery atherosclerosis. The mechanisms involved in atheroma formation are discussed in Chapters 48 and 49 and will not be dealt with in detail in this section. Atheromatous plaques are observed in their early stages in children and develop into frank obstructive lesions over many years. Factors such as regional blood flow, cholesterol levels, endothelial cell damage and local changes in haemostasis probably all have a role in determining the course that an individual plaque takes over many years. The advent of the era of coronary angiography led to the recognition of the importance of thrombosis on an established plaque in the pathogenesis of acute myocardial infarction (de Wood et al 1980). It is now recognized that there are pathological correlates for the various clinical syndromes associated with ischaemic heart disease. Although the underlying mechanisms involved in the development of coronary artery disease are common, the different courses that plaques can follow does to some extent determine the different clinical presentations within this syndrome complex.

Angina pectoris

Stable angina

The diagnosis of stable angina is made when angina has been correctly diagnosed for a number of months or years and the symptoms have become fixed. A patient with stable angina will be able to describe the precise development of the symptoms, their relationship to everyday life and exercise expenditure and after some time may regard the onset of symptoms as an 'old friend'. In general, most patients with established stable angina will complain of a crushing chest pain that develops after walking a certain distance at a certain rate. The pain might radiate into the jaw or the arms and is always relieved by rest within 2–3 minutes of cessation of exertion. Alternatively, the pain of stable angina is rapidly relieved by the use of sublingual nitrates. The symptoms of classical stable angina can be modified either by altering the rate of energy expenditure or, pharmacologically, by using sublingual nitrates prior to the onset of a degree of exercise that is known to induce the symptoms.

Unstable angina

The clinical diagnosis of unstable angina rests on the recognition that either new angina has developed or that previously stable angina has changed with respect to frequency, duration or severity. From this, three distinct clinical syndromes may be recognised, although there may be considerable overlap in clinical practice. These are: recent onset of effort angina, abrupt worsening of previously stable angina and angina at rest. Recent onset angina is defined arbitrarily as that occurring within the previous 4 weeks and in this context it is only unstable in the sense that there is a potential for rapid deterioration. Recent onset angina will either stabilize or may on occasions develop into one of the two more sinister variants of unstable angina described above. The deterioration of previously stable angina will characteristically be accompanied by a history of stable angina with relatively fixed exercise tolerance and a sudden decrease in distances that can be walked pain free. This may become progressive and culminate eventually in the development of rest pain.

Myocardial infarction

Acute myocardial infarction (AMI) can present to the clinician in different ways with quite marked differences in the patient's history. There will commonly be no prodromal phase to the illness, with onset of the characteristic chest pain the first indication that something is amiss. Alternatively, AMI may be preceeded by the onset of angina, that may initially be stable and subsequently deteriorate into unstable forms with development of rest pain. It is well recognized that the presentation of AMI will alter with increasing age, chest pain becoming less common and syncope, stroke and acute confusional states more common. The most common time of day for an AMI is early in the morning although it can occur at any time of day. The observation that the fibrinolytic system shows a diurnal variation with greatest suppression early in the morning has been used as an argument to link it causally with the development of AMI, although at the moment this remains unproven.

It is important to recognise that the older patients are more likely to present with atypical symptoms. This can be manifested by symptoms reminiscent of diseases as diverse as pulmonary embolus, biliary colic, peptic ulceration, hiatus hernia and even renal pain. The classic chest pain of AMI is identical to that of angina, except that it generally lasts for greater than 30 minutes, is not relieved by anti-anginal therapy and is unremitting. The pain is usually sited in the substernal region and radiates across the chest and commonly up into the jaw and down the left or both arms. Pain in the back is less common except in the case of a true posterior infarction, and in the circumstance of such symptoms a dissecting thoracic aortic aneurysm should be excluded. Other symptoms that commonly accompany the onset of an AMI are nausea, dyspnoea, palpitations and sweating.

Clinical signs of AMI generally confirm the impression that AMI has occurred and are not diagnostic. A patient with a small infarct who has not been haemodynamically compromised may have no signs. It is however common to hear a fourth heart sound and if there is frank heart failure, a gallop rhythm may be audible with both third and fourth heart sounds. Hypotension of varying severity may be noted and a small percentage of patients will present with cardiogenic shock which is associated with a poor prognosis. The presence of cardiac dysrhythmias such as atrial fibrillation/flutter or, more ominously, ventricular rhythm disturbances may be discovered on examination.

RISK FACTORS FOR CORONARY ARTERY DISEASE

The evaluation of a patient who presents with symptoms suggestive of myocardial ischaemia includes the detection of various risk factors. In particular, the presence of hypercholesterolaemia, hypertension, family history, cigarette smoking, diabetes mellitus or male sex are most strongly associated with coronary artery disease (Kannel & Gordon 1974, Multiple Risk Factor Intervention Trial (MRFIT) 1982, Yano et al 1984). In the MRFIT study smokers had twice the incidence of fatal myocardial infarcts compared with non-smokers. The family history is an independent risk factor for an individual's chance of developing coronary artery disease before 60 years of age. Male sex is important as coronary artery disease has tended to occur at a later age in women (Kannel & Gordon 1974, MRFIT 1982, Wei & Buckley 1982, Yano et al 1984), although this pattern may alter with changes in smoking habits. The majority of deaths from ischaemic heart disease occur in the older population (O'Rourke et al 1987, Krumholz 1989), making age itself an important risk factor for coronary artery disease.

Cholesterol, cholesterol lowering trials and coronary heart disease

There is substantial evidence that, on a national basis, there is a correlation between serum cholesterol levels and the incidence of coronary heart disease (Keys 1970) and also that the cholesterol level in a population is related to its total dietary fat intake. However, the evidence that reduction of saturated fat intake may lead to a reduced incidence of coronary heart disease is more tenuous. The problem is that although the majority of cholesterol lowering trials show a reduction in coronary heart disease, they do not show a similar drop in total mortality. It may be argued that the trials have not been sufficiently large or prolonged for the reduction in heart disease to be translated into reduced mortality and a case has been made for carrying out a large prospective trial of sufficient size to have the power to determine that a drop in total mortality does indeed take place (Collins et al 1992). In the meantime, cardiologists must make do with circumstantial evidence, or data obtained from meta-analysis of existing trials. Ravnskov has recently carried out a meta-analysis of all 22 cholesterol lowering trials, and concluded that both total and coronary heart disease specific mortality were not changed significantly (Ravnskov 1992). Of perhaps greater interest was his observation that positive trials were cited significantly more frequently in the scientific literature than the negative trials. These facts which reflect perhaps the natural human instinct for good news and also the quest for commercial success, will no doubt be disputed vigorously, and indeed, other meta-analysis studies have show a favourable effect on ischaemic heart disease of cholesterol lowering regimes (Holme 1990, Rossouw et al 1990). A further disputed point is whether cholesterol lowering agents, may, in some instances, increase mortality by promoting gall bladder disease and cancer. In some studies it has even been suggested that violent deaths, suicides and homicides have been casually related to cholesterol lowering regimes. It is more likely that these have end-points which reflect the quirk of unbalanced statistics in trials that are too small to be conclusive. Clearly, a very large trial is now required to take this controversy beyond possible doubt. It is unlikely that meta-analysis, however detailed, of many trials that vary considerably in quality, type of patient recruited, and class of drug used will clarify conclusively this controversy. Oliver has recently summarized the situation succinctly by stating that on the basis of the available evidence, the use of cholesterol lowering drugs should be confined to people at high risk of cardiovascular disease. The precise definition of high risk is flexible but in the successful Oslo heart study patients had high levels of cholesterol between 7.5–9.8 mmol/l (Hjermann et al 1981, Hjermann 1990).

Thus, there is not much evidence at present that changing the lifestyle, with the cardinal exception of stopping smoking, of people with moderate risk of cardiovascular disease will reduce morbidity or mortality. However, encouraging results from the regression trials have renewed impetus to obtain more direct clinical information on the beneficial impact of lipid lowering diets or drugs (Blankenhorn et al 1987, Brown et al 1990, Kane et al 1990).

The prethrombotic state

The haemostatic risk factors predisposing to coronary artery disease and their relationship to the prethrombotic state have been dealt with elsewhere. Nevertheless, there are special aspects in consideration of risk factors in relation to coronary heart disease that can be considered here. The fact that the mean level of some haemostatic factor was higher, or level of coagulation inhibitors lower, in people who have clinical coronary heart disease led to the concept of the hypercoagulable or prethrombotic state. The earliest studies were usually case-control studies in which patients had a variety of haemostatic factors measured which were then compared with age-matched apparently healthy people as controls.

The disadvantages of this type of study are well known to epidemiologists — the variable to be measured might be altered by the disease itself, and may reflect the degree of damage to, say, the heart after myocardial infarction rather than being its cause. The haemostatic system reacts largely as an acute phase reactant mechanism. It is better by far to carry out prospective studies, in which healthy people have measurements of the haemostatic factors carried out and are then followed up over a number of years to determine whether or not they develop clinical coronary disease. There are two main types of measurement in investigation of the prethrombotic state:

1. Measurement of abnormal levels of inactive (zymogen) coagulation or fibrinolytic factors. In these studies, the most rewarding factors identified have been fibrinogen, factor VII, factor VIII and PAI-1. It is gratifying that these factors are elevated in the 'right' direction, in that a raised fibrinogen, factor VII and factor VIII are 'prethrombotic', as well as a raised PAI-1 level.
2. Measurement of activation products of the haemostatic system. There are a variety of peptides that are liberated with the activation of haemostatic system zymogens in vivo. These can be termed 'activation markers' because they indicate that activation of the haemostatic mechanism has taken place.

Fibrinogen and factor VIII reflect, in general, the age of the patient and the extent of generalized atherosclerosis within an individual's arteries. For instance, there is a correlation between the degree of atherosclerosis in the coronary arteries, the blood viscosity and the fibrinogen level (Lowe et al 1980). In numerous studies it has been shown that the level of factor VIIIc (and von Willebrand factor, the plasma level of which is closely linked to factor VIIIc) correlates fairly well with the degree of atherosclerosis or the level of systemic disease (Jansson et al 1991). In the major prospective Northwick Park studies of healthy individuals, fibrinogen and factor VIII levels had value in predicting the occurrence of arterial vascular events such as myocardial infarction, cerebrovascular disease and vascular death (Meade et al 1986). The problem at present is that we do not have a useful drug to lower fibrinogen levels.

The use of activation markers in assessment of the prethrombotic state has been well reviewed by Bauer and Rosenberg (1987). The major markers used in clinical practice are summarized in Table 54.1. Other markers are in the course of evaluation in the clinical situation, but whether they provide any predictive factors of clinical relevance remains to be seen. The advantage of the activation markers is that they can be assayed easily and accurately by a number of immunological assays. Their half life in the circulation has been defined accurately and their stability established. All individuals have a measurable amount of all these activation markers in their circulation, confirming the original Astrup hypothesis that low grade coagulation is a continuous process in normal healthy individuals. These markers are elevated in patients with established deep vein thrombosis, pulmonary embolism and disseminated intravascular coagulation but it is unlikely that they will be sufficiently specific to act as prognostic aids for the occurrence of coronary heart disease. In patients with inherited disorders of both antithrombin III (At III), and protein C, levels of F_{1+2} are elevated, indicating increased prothrombin activation although fibrinopeptide A levels were not increased (Bauer & Rosenberg 1987). Similarly, patients (and healthy controls) on oral anticoagulants showed a reduction in F_{1+2} levels. The low grade coagulation process is accelerated in elderly individuals in that they have raised levels of F_{1+2} and fibrinopeptide A.

Measurement of activation peptides

Three of the coagulation factors, factor X, IX and prothrombin, undergo activation into active enzymes with the release into the circulation of peptides, which can be measured by immunological means. These peptides have a short half life in the circulation, from 10–90 minutes, so that their presence in the circulation means that on-going coagulation activation is taking place. Their disadvantage is that, in having a short half life, they may not reflect thrombotic or coagulation activity which is not taking place at the point of blood sampling. In a situation similar to that seen with fibrinopeptide A, there appears to be a low concentration of activation peptides in apparently normal individuals. Additionally, the coagulation system is derived teleologically from the inflammatory system, and any inflammatory stimulus will generate a rise in the acute phase reaction proteins, fibrinogen and factor VIII, as well as activation products. For instance, postoperative patients with systemic complications such as sepsis and pneumonia have as high, or higher, levels of fibrin degradation products (FDP) as those with deep vein thrombosis (Wood et al 1972). Thus a raised level of activation peptides in the circulation may not necessarily, or be likely to, indicate that thrombosis within the coronary artery is taking place.

Table 54.1 The major activation markers used in clinical practice

Parent molecule	Marker
Fibrinogen/fibrin	FDP
	D-dimer
	X linked oligomer
	Fibrinopeptide A
	Fibrinopeptide B
	Bβ 1–42 fragment
Prothrombin	F_{1+2}
	Thrombin-antithrombin complexes
Protein C	Protein C activation peptide

Any evaluation of the prethrombotic state must take into account the fact that the ageing process has an effect, not only on the plasma concentrations of clotting factors, such as fibrinogen and factor VIII, but also on the level of activation products. Bauer and colleagues (1987) studied the levels of prothrombin activation peptide (F_{1+2}), factor IX activation peptide, factor X activation peptide and fibrinopeptide A in 199 healthy males aged 42 to 80 years. There was a significant correlation between all activation peptides and the age of the patients. With increasing age, activation peptides increased in concentration, with a significant correlation between the two. Additionally, the level of βTG — a platelet release protein — indicating in vivo platelet activation rises in parallel with increasing age (Stewart et al 1983). The question may be asked why this increase in activation of platelets and coagulation occurs in elderly people. It is possible that there is an intrinsic increase in enzyme activation, mediated in part by increasing factor VIII levels seen in old age. Alternatively, the coagulation systems may be reacting to atherosclerosis or age-related changes in the vessel wall and thus merely reflecting pre-existing damage within the vessel rather than causing it. Both the factor VII-tissue factor reaction, and factor IXa-VII reactions take place in association with denuded endothelial cell surface. Any damage to endothelium will be liable to increase this area and so increase coagulation activation. So, we must be circumspect in assuming that an increase in activation products necessarily indicates on-going thrombosis or even a tendency to thrombosis. Although estimation of activation products have given us great insight into the mechanism of coagulation, they have not, as yet, provided sufficiently reliable specificity and sensitivity to be used as a clinical prognostic index. Bauer and Rosenberg (1987) have noted a close correlation in individuals between the factor IX activation peptide and factor X activation peptide suggesting that they may have increased activity of the factor VII–tissue factor pathway. These people usually have variably elevated levels of F_{1+2} and fibrinopeptide A suggesting that they have increased thrombin generation and fibrinogen to fibrin conversion. Thus, with increasing age there is a tendency to an in vivo increase in thrombin formation. These exciting findings need to be applied to long-term prospective clinical studies; there is the clear possibility that individuals at greatest risk of coronary heart disease could be detected, at time before clinical symptoms become apparent, by showing that they had elevated levels of the activation peptides.

Fibrinogen

McDonald and Edgill (1957) first discussed increased plasma fibrinogen levels in patients with angina pectoris and after myocardial infarction. Since then, an increase in fibrinogen in association with coronary artery disease has been described extensively (Mayer 1964, Bottiger & Carlson 1970, Nicolaides 1977, Wilhelmsen et al 1984, Stone & Thorp 1985, Yarnell et al 1991). The increased fibrinogen is associated with an increase in plasma viscosity which in itself may serve as a mechanism by which flow in vessels is reduced and the likelihood of thrombotic occlusion is increased (Nicolaides 1977).

Fibrinogen levels are also of predictive value for events related to coronary artery disease. Increased erthyrocyte sedimentation was associated with events in the Stockholm study (Bottiger & Carlson 1970). More recently, in the Northwick Park Heart Study it was found that men who had died from coronary artery disease had a significantly higher mean fibrinogen and factor VII levels on admission to the study than men who were still alive (Meade et al 1980, 1986).

In the prospective Goteborg study of 792 men, those who subsequently developed ischaemic heart disease had a mean fibrinogen level of 3.56 g/l which was significantly higher than those men who had no clinical event or died from a non-vascular cause (Wilhelmsen et al 1984). Similar findings were made in the Leigh study which found that the relationship between fibrinogen and incidence of ischaemic heart disease was stronger than that of smoking, cholesterol or blood pressure (Stone & Thorp 1985).

Data from the Framingham study (Kannel 1985) confirmed a positive correlation between ischaemic heart disease and fibrinogen in both men and women. The three studies just cited (Goteborg, Leigh and Framingham) showed that fibrinogen became an even stronger predictor of ischaemic events in the presence of raised blood pressure and that the two (fibrinogen and hypertension) variables in the top third of distribution acted synergistically in raising the incidence of heart disease up to 12 times greater than if these were in the lowest third. The Caerphilly study has also determined that high fibrinogen levels and plasma viscosity, which is largely determined by fibrinogen concentration, were associated with an increased incidence of coronary artery disease in their study (Yarnell et al 1991).

It has been possible to show a direct relationship between plasma viscosity, fibrinogen concentration and the degree of coronary stenosis as shown by arteriography.

Cigarette smoking

Cigarette consumption is one of the major risk factors for the development of coronary artery disease. It has been estimated that in the Western Hemisphere smoking directly causes 21% of all deaths (Department of Health and Human Services (DHHS) 1989). Cigarette smoking and coronary artery disease fit the classical requirements of epidemiological cause and effect. There is a dose–disease relationship that exists between the number of cigarettes smoked and the risk of heart disease (Doll & Peto 1976, Willett et al 1987). Most studies have demonstrated a rapid reduction in risk after cessation of smoking (Doll & Peto 1976, Rosenberg et al 1985, 1990, Willett et al 1987) to a level comparable to non-smokers after 2–3 years (Rosenburg et al 1985, 1990).

Hypertension

The relationship between elevated blood pressure and the development of coronary artery disease is strong and there is a continuous increase in the incidence of coronary artery disease with increases in both systolic and diastolic blood pressure. Diastolic measurements of 90 mmHg and above, once considered to be normotensive, are associated with a significant increase in coronary artery disease over those with lower values (Multiple Risk Factor Intervention Trial (MRFIT) 1982). Similarly, enhanced systolic pressure is associated with an increased frequency of coronary events that is related to the degree of elevation. In the MRFIT study, the absence of diabetes, smoking, hypercholesterolaemia and a diastolic pressure greater than 90 mmHg was associated with an 18 times reduction in mortality compared to those risk factors being present.

Diabetes mellitus and insulin resistance

Diabetes mellitus occurs in an estimated 1–2% of the population in the United Kingdom (Neil et al 1987). The development of vascular disease is the commonest complication associated with diabetes, macrovascular disease accounting for 75% of all deaths (Ganda 1980) whilst cardiovascular disease accounts for up to three times the mortality of non-diabetics (Garcia et al 1974). Additionally the incidence of asymptomatic ischaemic heart disease in diabetic patients has been found to be much higher than in non-diabetic subjects (Koistinen 1990). Population studies indicate that age-adjusted mortality rates for coronary heart disease are two to three times higher among diabetic men and three and seven times higher in diabetic women than in those without diabetes (Kannel & McGee

1979, Barrett-Conner & Wingard 1983, Pau et al 1986, Manson et al 1991). The deleterious effects of diabetes mellitus are related to the duration of the disease (Krolewski et al 1985) and to the presence of other risk factors (Kannel 1985, Manson et al 1991). Whilst diabetes is associated with an increased incidence in coronary artery disease, there is also an increased extent of involvement. Coronary angiography studies indicate that diabetics tend to have a greater number of vessels involved by disease (Hamby et al 1976, Dortimer et al 1978). The influence of improved diabetic control on the development of cardiovascular events is unclear. An early clinical study found no relationship between control and the prevalence of atherosclerotic heart disease (Liebow et al 1955). A more recent pathological study has confirmed these findings with no difference apparently in patients who were untreated, on diet or oral hypoglycaemic agents or insulin (Waller et al 1980). In contrast, the metabolic status immediately prior to an infarct does seem to affect outcome with mortality rates lowest in those patients with a normal glycosylated haemoglobin (Oswald et al 1984). Whilst most of the known risk factors for the development of coronary artery disease occur in excess in diabetes it has been estimated that they still only account for 25% of the excess risk (Pyörälä 1979). The presence of conventional risk factors, such as hypercholesterolaemia, is associated with a much higher coronary artery risk than in non-diabetic subjects (Pyörälä et al 1987) implying that factors unique to diabetes are playing an important role. In the diabetic milieu, three major abnormalities exist that could contribute to this state of affairs: the presence of hyperglycaemia with associated protein glycosylation, changes in lipoprotein metabolism and insulin resistance with hyperinsulinaemia. Some of the possible mechanisms involved in the pathogenesis of vascular disease in diabetes mellitus are summarized in Figure 54.1.

Glucose and glycosylation

The development of insulin in the 1920s transformed type 1 diabetes from a condition with a devastating prognosis into one dominated by the chronic existence of hyperglycaemia punctuated by episodes of ketoacidosis and hypoglycaemia. In terms of poor glycaemic control there is evidence that improvements lead to an amelioration of retinopathy (McCance et al 1989), but less evidence exists for a reduction in coronary artery disease. However, a number of potentially pathogenic effects of glucose on endothelial cells have been described to support the view that hyperglycaemia may be important in the pathogenesis of ischaemic heart disease. Glucose increases the expression of endothelial cell basement membranes and at high concentrations leads to damage to DNA (Lorenzi et al 1986, Cagliero et al 1988, 1991). Hyperglycaemia in cell culture causes enhanced tissue factor expression to thrombin (Boeri et al 1989), the release of factor VIII-related antigen (Mordes et al 1983) and an increase in the synthesis and secretion of both plasminogen activator inhibitor-1 and tissue plasminogen activator (Maiello et al 1992). These changes may indicate that, in the presence of glucose, endothelial cells become more thrombogenic thus contributing to the development of occlusive vascular disease. An alternative process whereby glucose may influence the development of vascular disease is through the production of advanced glycosylation end products (AGE). In vitro studies of AGE have provided support for this view. Glycosylation of proteins is initiated by exposure to a reducing sugar such as glucose and proceeds by an Amadori rearrangement through to a late Maillard or Browning reaction to form cross-linked pigmented and fluorescent AGE products (Monnier & Cerami 1983, Brownlee et al 1988). The rate of this reaction is dependent on time and the prevailing glucose concentration (Paulsen & Koury 1976, Brownlee et al 1984). Laboratory studies have demonstrated the presence of a specific receptor for AGE albumin on activated human monocytes. (Vlassara et al 1986, Gilcrease & Hoover 1990), the murine macrophage (RAW 264.7) cell line (Radoff et al 1990) and bovine aortic endothelial cells (Esposito et al 1989). Purification of the receptor from membranes of the macrophage cell line RAW 264.7 has revealed that it has an 83 000 dalton subunit involved in ligand binding and a 36 000 dalton subunit of unknown function (Radoff et al 1988). The receptor is reported to have an affinity constant of $1.75 \times 10^7\ M^{-1}$) with 1.5×10^5 receptors per cell on macrophages (Vlassara et al 1989a). Receptor expression is upregulated by tumour necrosis factor (Vlassara et al 1989b) and downregulated by insulin (Vlassara et al 1988a). AGE proteins themselves do not seem to affect receptor expression (Vlassara et al 1989a).

Evidence has accumulated to suggest that AGE formation alone, and the interaction of AGE with its receptor may be of importance in the pathogenesis of vascular disease. Low density lipoprotein binds to AGE collagen and it has been hypothesized that AGE formation in atherosclerotic plaques may enhance trapping of lipid molecules and promote acceleration of atheroma (Brownlee et al 1985). Cross-linkage of long-lived proteins in the vessel wall may also contribute to vascular thickening and reduced elasticity, features characteristic of early vascular disease. Important interactions have been described between AGE and the AGE receptor to indicate further involvement in the pathogenesis of vascular damage. AGE collagen has been shown to bind more avidly to activated monocytes (Gilcrease & Hoover 1992) whilst AGE albumin releases tumour necrosis factor (TNF) and interleukin-1 (IL-1) from interferon gamma activated monocytes (Vlassara et al 1988b). The release of cytokines in this way would lead to increased cellular proliferation and the induction of a procoagulant state by suppression of

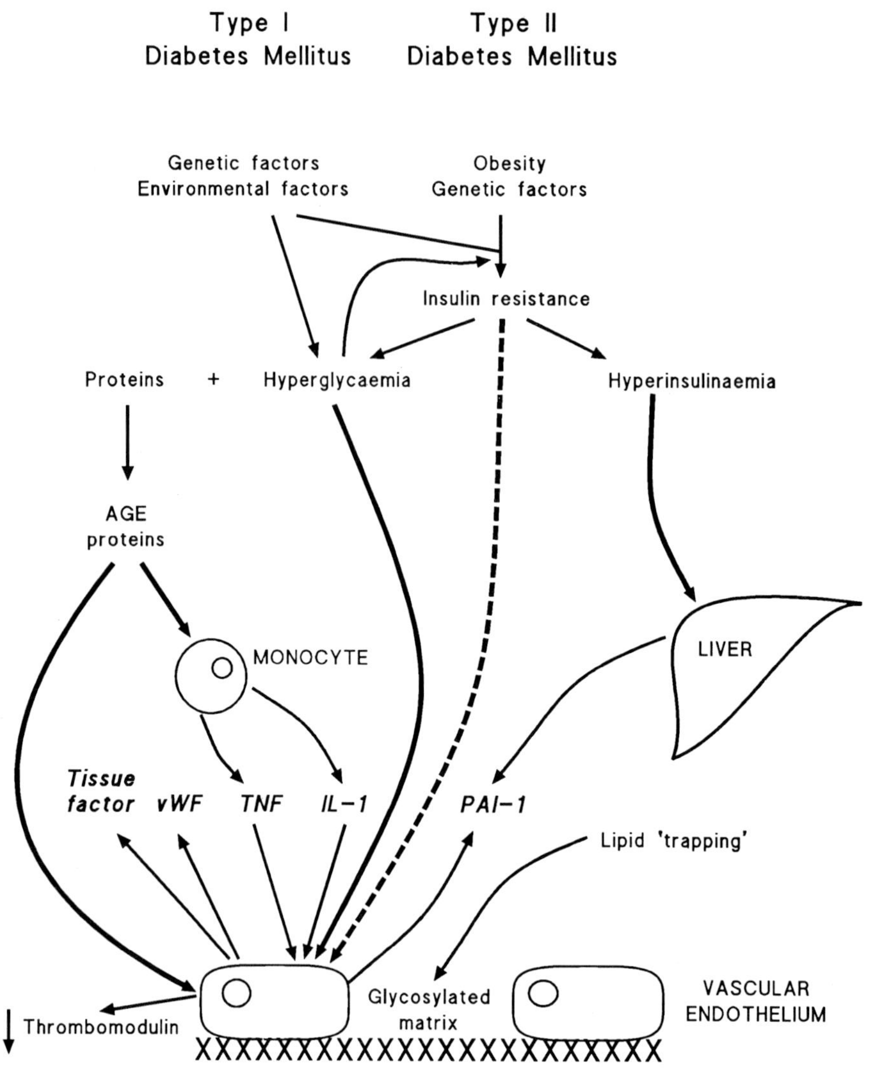

Fig. 54.1 Some possible mechanisms involved in the development of haemostatic abnormalities and the pathogenesis of macrovascular disease in diabetes mellitus. vWF, von Willebrand factor; PAI-1, plasminogen activator inhibitor-1; TNF, tumour necrosis factor; IL-1, interleukin-1; AGE, advanced glycosylation end products.

fibrinolysis (van Hinsbergh et al 1988) and release of endothelial cell tissue factor and von Willebrand factor (Bevilacqua et al 1986, Nawroth et al 1986, Breit & Green 1988, Edgington et al 1991). In the presence of AGE this would be further aggravated by the suppression by AGE albumin of endothelial cell release of thrombomodulin (Esposito et al 1989). Thrombomodulin acts to decrease the effects of an activated coagulation system in a number of ways; indirectly by activation of protein C which in turn inactivates factors V and VIII, and releases tissue plasminogen activator, and directly by binding to thrombin. The nucleophilic hydrazine, aminoguanidine hydrochloride effectively inhibits AGE formation in vivo and in vitro (Brownlee et al 1986, Nicholls & Mandel 1989). Evidence to support the role of AGE in the pathogenesis of diabetic vascular complications comes from animal work demonstrating an amelioration of both renal (Nicholls & Mandel 1989, Ellis & Bowen 1990, Hammes et al 1990) and neural lesions (Yakihashi et al 1992) after treatment with aminoguanidine. As yet, there are no clinical studies that have investigated the effects of aminoguanidine on the development of heart disease in diabetes.

Insulin resistance, coronary artery disease and hypertension

Changes in lipoprotein metabolism and insulin resistance are often placed together as risk factors for coronary artery disease as they frequently coexist. The observation that male or abdominal obesity is associated with an increased risk of adverse changes in a number of cardiovascular risk factors has a long history emanating from the original observations made by Vague (1956) and confirmed by others (Larsson et al 1984, Kaplan 1989).

The syndrome of male pattern obesity associated with insulin resistance, hypertension, lipid abnormalities and glucose intolerance has been recognized for some time (Brindley & Rolland 1989, Després et al 1990) and is known as 'Reavens syndrome' or syndrome 'X' (Reaven 1988). Whilst the role of hypertriglyceridaemia in coronary artery disease is generally under dispute, there is evidence that indicates a role in the development of diabetic heart disease (Fontbonne et al 1988, Laakso et al 1989). Low density lipoprotein when oxidized is reported to release the fibrinolytic inhibitor, PAI-1 from endothelial cells (Latron et al 1990, Stiko-Rahm et al 1990) and there is substantial evidence to implicate changes in lipoprotein metabolism in a variety of endothelial and monocyte interactions.

Insulin resistance is a common feature of both type 1 (insulin dependent) and type 2 (non-insulin dependent) diabetes mellitus (de Fronzo et al 1982a,b, Olefsky et al 1982, Nankervis et al 1984). In the presence of obesity the number of insulin receptors fall and the ability of insulin to activate the post-receptor tyrosine kinase pathway is impaired (Moller & Flier 1991). Such abnormalities tend towards normal on weight loss. The association between insulin resistance, hyperinsulinaemia and coronary artery disease is principally based on the results of large population studies which have demonstrated a relationship between insulin levels and CAD mortality (Welborn & Weame 1979, Ducimetiere et al 1980, Pyörälä et al 1985, Fontbonne et al 1988, Modan et al 1991). The explanation of these findings is unclear although there is also evidence of an association between insulin resistance, hyperinsulinaemia and hypertension (Modan et al 1985, Ferrannini et al 1987, Reaven & Hoffman 1987, Laakso et al 1989). Interestingly, this does not appear to extend to patients with insulinoma (Sawicki et al 1992) in whom hyperinsulinaemia exists without coexistent insulin resistance. However, insulin resistance seems to be a risk factor for the development of hypertension independent of obesity (Pollare et al 1990).

Insulin resistance, fibrinolysis and vascular disease

Evidence has accumulated to implicate abnormalities of both coagulation and fibrinolysis in the pathogenesis of large vessel disease. The Northwick Park study demonstrated an association between factor VII levels and the development of coronary artery disease (Meade et al 1980). Hamsten et al (1985, 1987) noted a marked decrease in t-PA activity with high levels of t-PA inhibition compared to healthy controls in young survivors of myocardial infarction. These results were consistent with the Northwick Park study which also showed depressed fibrinolysis in patients who died from cardiovascular disease (Meade et al 1980), although this association was lost on longer term follow-up. Diabetes mellitus is associated with abnormalities of both coagulation and fibrinolysis that are more frequently seen in patients with vascular complications (Bern et al 1980, Christie et al 1984). There are increases in coagulation factors VII and VIII in both type 1 and 2 diabetes, whilst in type 1 diabetes fibrinolysis is normal or increased and in type 2 diabetes it is markedly depressed due to an increase in PAI-1 concentrations (Auwerx et al 1988, Walmsley et al 1991). Laboratory studies indicate that insulin releases the fibrinolytic inhibitor PAI-1 from cells of hepatic origin (Alessi et al 1988, Kooistra et al 1989, Grant et al 1991) and population studies show an association between insulin levels and PAI-1 (Vague et al 1986, Juhan-Vague et al 1987, 1989a,b) although no study has yet shown an effect of insulin on PAI-1 concentrations in vivo (Grant et al 1990, Potter van Loon et al 1990, Landin et al 1991). Although the effects of insulin on PAI-1 in vivo have been negative, there is an interesting suggestion that patients with a particular *Hind*III polymorphism of the PAI-1 gene respond to insulin (Dawson et al 1991). If this were confirmed, this finding would help to explain some of the inconsistencies in the work on insulin and PAI-1. Over the years the sum of all these findings has led to the widely held view that insulin may be atherogenic and involved in the high mortality from CAD that occurs in diabetes (Stout & Vallance-Owen 1971, Jarrett 1988, Juhan-Vague et al 1991). There is some dispute regarding this as insulin appears not to be an independent risk factor in older men (Welin et al 1992) and Durrington cogently argues that the insulin hypothesis depends on evidence that insulin both causes and prevents atheroma (Durrington 1992). The role of insulin resistance in the aetiology of CAD is perhaps stronger and it is perhaps as an epiphenomenon to insulin resistance that hyperinsulinaemia has gained its notoriety.

PREVENTION OF CORONARY ARTERY DISEASE

Coronary heart disease remains the principal cause of death in the developed world, although there has been a decline of up to one half in the USA, Canada, Australia and New Zealand and a more recent fall of one fifth in Great Britain (Beaglehole et al 1989, Sytkowski et al 1990). Part of the decline may be attributed to a fall in smoking, especially in males, better control of hypertension, and to reduction in saturated fat in the diet. Additionally, the improvement in treatment of myocardial infarction by use of thrombolytic therapy, early aspirin therapy and beta-blockers have reduced the early mortality of myocardial infarction by over 40%, reducing the total post-infarction mortality from about 13% to 7–8%. A recent report indicates that intravenous magnesium sulphate may further lower the mortality after acute myocardial infarction. The risk of heart disease remains highest in those of low socioeconomic status in whom the risk factors remain at a higher level than in their richer compatriots.

It must be remembered that the conventional risk factors of smoking, cholesterol level, and hypertension have predictive value for less than half the attacks of coronary heart disease. While it is generally accepted that there is a rough correlation between populations of dietary fat intake, serum cholesterol level and incidence of coronary heart disease, these figures provide no predictive data for a single individual (Keys 1970). There is increasing realisation that the pathogenesis of coronary heart disease is multifactorial and that, for example, a person who smokes, has a raised cholesterol, raised fibrinogen, and hypertension would be at much higher risk than someone with only one of these risk factors. In the MRFIT study (1982), the intervention group were treated by improving all the risk factors at the same time. Despite the disappointing result that total mortality was not improved by intervention, the incidence of vascular complications was significantly improved. There are two opposing but complementary tactics by which prevention of coronary heart disease might be tackled. First, high-risk individuals can be identified and then counselled to change their lifestyle and, if necessary, given the appropriate drugs. For instance, a heavy smoking individual with raised cholesterol can be counselled to stop smoking and change to a diet low in saturated fat. If necessary, he could be treated with lipid-lowering agents such as the HMG-CoA reductase (statin) group of drugs.

The alternative approach is for a mass or population based approach to prevention (Leeder and Gliksman 1990). In this situation, widespread explanation, advertising and counselling are designed to alter a habit within the entire population (Gliksman et al 1990). The three major risk factors which can be approached in this way are smoking habit, raised cholesterol and obesity which can be changed by an altered diet. Both approaches are open to pitfalls (Hall et al 1988, McCormick at Skrabanek 1988). Rose and Day (1990) have argued cogently that the incidence of 'deviants' is directly related to the population mean, rather than there being a clear distinction between normality and deviance. In this situation, the problems of the 'deviant' minority, whether it be a heavy smoking habit, high cholesterol, obesity or hypertension cannot be managed as though they were independent of the rest of the population. The consequence is that treating 'high risk' individuals, even if they are detected, cannot be successful if the mean level of the risk factor is high in the general population. Rose and Day (1990) showed that across a wide range of societies, the average blood pressure predicts the number of hypertensive people and the average weight the number of fat people. The fact that the spread of distribution of a risk factor is not easily compressed means that it is difficult to truncate or eliminate the high tail of 'deviants'. For a strategy of prevention to succeed, the 'normal' majority must be persuaded to change in order to reduce substantially the high risk minority. Clearly the ability to formulate and carry out a mass strategy of prevention depends largely on government and political forces who will be influential by pressure of medical and public opinion on health matters. Hopefully, small changes made by the entire community may shift the mean value of risk factor prevalence so automatically reducing the high risk group. This type of approach, although superficially attractive, is beset by difficulties in a democratic society. For instance, to forbid, say, cigarette smoking and tobacco advertising may infringe the right of free action, information and communication and the population may resent the interference of government to control their behaviour. The responsibility of the doctor is to inform his patients so that they can take responsibility for maintaining their own good health. He can make each patient aware of the major risk factors for coronary heart disease. In each patient smoking habit, blood pressure and obesity are easily assessed. In high risk groups for coronary heart disease (strong family history, diabetics, previous angina or heart disease, heavy smokers, hypertensives) the serum cholesterol should also be measured.

An approach to preventive screening and practice in primary care has been formulated by the British Coronary Prevention Group and British Heart Foundation (Working Group of the Coronary Prevention Group & the British Heart Foundation 1991 based on risk assessment with the Dundee risk-disk which has been formulated by Tunstall-Pedoe and colleagues (1991). All those in clinical or family risk groups have cholesterol measurement, then receive appropriate advice concerning risk factors, or treatment. This approach involves assessment of the effect of multifactorial risk, and the final rank is based on the total of several factors. Although details in this approach have been criticized (Randall et al 1991) in that a single very high risk factor can be overlooked, this type of risk calculator provides a balanced approach to rapid detection of those at increased risk.

COAGULATION AND FIBRINOLYSIS DURING MYOCARDIAL INFARCTION

One of the major advances in the understanding and management of myocardial infarction has been the recognition that by far the commonest pathological process involves the development of thrombus on an established atherosclerotic plaque (de Wood et al 1980, Davies & Thomas 1984). Thrombus formation also has an important role in the pathogenesis of unstable angina (Davies & Thomas 1985, Falk 1985, Ambrose et al 1986, Sherman et al 1986). The implications of this observation are twofold; first it suggests that the haemostatic mechanism may have an important role in the evolution of acute myocardial infarction and that tests of haemostasis may help to predict patients at risk, and second that the development of thrombolytic agents might have a significant effect on the morbidity and mortality associated with acute myocardial infarction. The predictive value of tests of haemostasis and the clinical use of plasminogen activators are dealt with in detail elsewhere, and this section will concentrate on the changes in haemostasis that occur during and immediately after acute myocardial infarction. Changes in haemostasis that occur in relation to acute myocardial infarction are summarized in Table 54.2.

Platelets

The importance of platelets in the pathogenesis of coronary artery disease rests on two pieces of accepted wisdom; first that platelets in association with subendothelial interactions have crucial effects on haemostasis and second that the use of potent antiplatelet agents such as aspirin have beneficial effects on the clinical outcome. Evidence exists to indicate that flow disturbance in a vessel with damaged endothelium leads to attachment of platelets to the subendothelial layer. This interaction is promoted by von Willebrand factor (vWF) and clinically this has been supported by the association between increased levels of vWF and reinfarction and mortality in patients with a previous myocardial infarct (Jansson et al 1991).

Attachment of platelets would lead to the release of growth factors and platelet activation products thus further promoting the development of thrombus. Patients with unstable angina and myocardial infarction are reported to have significantly lower levels of platelet-derived growth factor (PDGF) with a general increase in beta thromboglobulin and platelet factor 4 (Tahara et al 1991).

Table 54.2 Coagulation and fibrinolysis changes during myocardial infarction

	Change	Reference
Platelets		
Platelet aggregation	↑	Gormsen et al 1977, Schwartz et al 1980
β-thromboglobulin	↑	Tahara et al 1991
Platelet factor 4	↑	Tahara et al 1991
Platelet volume	↑	Martin et al 1983a, Cameron et al 1983
Platelet survival	↓	Kutti & Weinfeld 1979
Coagulation		
Thrombin/antithrombin III	↑	Munkvad et al 1990
Antithrombin III	↓	Losito et al 1981
Fibrinopeptide A	↑	Mombelli et al 1984
Factor XII/FVII	↑	Gordon et al 1982, 1987
vWF	↑	Cucuiana et al 1980, Lonsardi et al 1981
Fibrinogen	↑	Margulis et al 1986
Factor VIII:C	→	Margulis et al 1986
Fibrinolysis		
PAI-1	↑	Almér & Ohlin 1987, Munkvad et al 1991, Goram et al 1987, Nilsson & Johnson 1987, Verheught et al 1987
Global fibrinolysis	↓	Chakrabarti et al 1968, Hume 1958, Lackner & Merskey 1960, Röjel 1959

↑, increased; ↓, decreased; →, no change.

The relationship of such observed changes to the pathogenesis of vascular disease is unclear although it has been suggested that PDGF may have a role (Nilsson 1986) and other studies have demonstrated increases in various platelet release factors in association with coronary artery disease (Handin et al 1978, Zahavi & Kakkar 1980, Levine et al 1981, Neri et al 1981, Smitherman et al 1981). In myocardial infarction the mean platelet volume is increased (Cameron et al 1983, Martin et al 1983a), larger platelets being more reactive (Martin et al 1983b). Patients with coronary heart disease have increased platelet aggregation (Gormsen et al 1977, Schwartz et al 1980, Vilen et al 1985) with reduced platelet survival (Kutti & Weinfeld 1979). Two important studies have demonstrated an association between platelet aggregation and myocardial infarction (Elwood et al 1991, Thaulow et al 1991).

Coagulation

Most evidence regarding the onset of myocardial infarction indicates that it is accompanied by the presence of a hypercoagulable state. The acute episode is associated with increased thrombin-AtIII complexes (Munkvad et al 1990), a fall in AtIII (Losito et al 1981) and increased fibrinopeptide A concentrations (Mombelli et al 1984). Activation of the natural anticoagulant, protein C, following coronary artery occlusion has been reported in an animal model (Snow et al 1991), although other inhibitors studied in man seem to be of little significance (Gram & Jespersen 1985). In addition, evidence of thrombin activation of factor XIII and the presence of cross-linked fibrin polymers in plasma indicate true activation of coagulation has occurred (Francis et al 1987). The experimental data is less clear in angina, where thrombin antithrombin-III complexes are reported to be lower than in myocardial infarction (Munkvad et al 1990) or similar (de Sousa et al 1988) although fibrinopeptide A levels are not increased (Nicols et al 1982).

In the acute event, there are strong indications that activation of both the intrinsic and extrinsic pathways of coagulation occur. Marked increases in the circulating titre of factor XII (Hageman factor) and high molecular weight kininogen with significant cold activation of factor VII have been described in survivors of myocardial infarction (Gordon et al 1987). Factor XII is reported to have a role in the enhancement of fibrinolytic activity (Gordon et al 1980), increased factor VII activity and shortening of the prothrombin time (Gordon et al 1982). It was calculated that the increase in factor XII in the post-infarction patients was responsible for 50% of the activation of factor VII and 66% of the shortening of the prothrombin time.

Other work supports some of the conclusions of this study demonstrating high levels of factor VII:C in patients with both myocardial infarction and unstable angina (de Sousa et al 1988), and the presence of factor VII-phospholipid complexes in plasma of survivors of AMI (Dalaker et al 1987). The presence of these complexes indicates that factor VII is activated and that activation of the extrinsic pathway occurs in the course of a myocardial infarction. Several studies have demonstrated an increase in von Willebrand factor (Cucuiana et al 1980, Lombardi et al 1981) and it has even been suggested as a useful diagnostic measure after 5–6 days when levels peak and cardiac enzymes have returned to normal (Margulis et al 1986). Despite the relative unanimity regarding these changes there is less certainty regarding factor VIII:C which usually rises with vWF. Margulis et al (1986) reported no change in factor VIII:C concentrations over a 14 day post-infarct period despite increases in both vWF and fibrinogen. Conversely in patients studied 3–6 months after infarction, factor VIII:C levels were raised in females (n = 32) but not in men (n = 116). Other changes noted in this study were increases in vWF and fibrinogen (Hamsten et al 1986).

Fibrinolysis

The fibrinolytic system consists of an enzyme cascade that regulates the conversion of plasminogen to plasmin. It consists of two principle activators, tissue plasminogen activator (t-PA) and urokinase (u-PA) and two inhibitors of t-PA and u-PA, plasminogen activator inhibitor-1 (PAI-1) and PAI-2. PAI-2 is present in the circulation in significant quantities during pregnancy and only about 6% of males have measurable levels in the plasma (Astedt et al 1987, Kruithof et al 1987, Lecander & Astedt 1989). As yet no work has evaluated its role in vascular disease under other circumstances. PAI-1 exists in excess over t-PA in the circulation and most interest has centred on the possible role of PAI-1 in the pathogenesis of both venous and arterial disease. A large number of studies have been carried out that consistently demonstrate a reduction in fibrinolysis in relation to coronary artery disease (Chakrabarti et al 1968, Walker et al 1977, Estellès et al 1985, Gram & Jespersen 1987, Gram et al 1987b, Mehta et al 1987, Aznar et al 1988, Francis et al 1988, Vandekerckhove et al 1988). Such studies have to be regarded with a degree of caution as there is a question mark over which comes first, suppression of fibrinolysis or coronary artery disease. In an attempt to answer this question, a small number of prospective studies have been carried out. These indicate that suppression of the fibrinolytic system in general (Meade et al 1980) and elevated PAI-1 concentrations in particular, are predictive for the occurrence of acute myocardial infarction (Hamsten et al 1985, 1987), although there is not total agreement on this issue (Jansson et al 1991). The data regarding patients with established coronary artery disease and stable angina are conflicting. In a study of 118 patients with angiographically documented coronary artery disease and 57 controls, significant increases in PAI-1 were recorded in the patients although there were no differences in global fibrinolytic activity as measured by the euglobulin clot lysis time (Paramo et al 1985). It is to be assumed that this group of patients had stable angina although this is not clarified. Of particular interest was the observation that levels of PAI-1 did not correlate with the degree of coronary lesion in the patients. A similar study carried out in patients with exercise-induced ischaemia confirmed the high PAI-1 levels that occur in this condition, but also showed a relationship between levels of PAI-1 and the severity of the coronary lesion (Sakata et al 1990). In a study of unstable angina compared to stable angina and controls, the first group had significantly higher levels of PAI-1 although there were no differences between patients with stable angina and controls (Zalewski et al 1991). To complete the confusion in this area a further study was unable to distinguish unstable angina from control subjects using either PAI-1 or D-dimer estimations (Alexopoulos et al 1991). Taken overall, the results from these studies indicate a relationship between fibrinolysis and unstable angina, but that, at best, the link is loose and not necessarily a major aetiological factor. The data regarding acute myocardial infarction are rather more convincing although even this must be regarded with a degree of caution. The original observations indicating that depressed fibrinolysis occurred following an acute myocardial infarction were made more than 30 years ago using global tests of fibrinolysis (Hume 1958, Röjel 1959, Lackner & Merskey 1960). These early studies showed that fibrinolysis is generally depressed for a few days after the event. A further study of 25 patients showed that fibrinolysis is increased after the first 5–8 hours and then reaches a nadir at 16–48 hours before returning to normal at 8–10 days (Ogston & Fullerton 1965). Since then several studies have confirmed these findings (Rawles et al 1975, Franzen et al 1983) and demonstrated that the suppression of fibrinolysis is due to an increase in levels of PAI-1 (Almér & Ohlin 1987, Gram et al 1987a, Nilsson & Johnson 1987, Verheught et al 1987, Munkvad et al 1990). A case report indicated the possible aetiological role in myocardial infarction by demonstrating high levels of PAI-1 in the plasma of a patient immediately prior to infarction (Sakata et al 1989). In a further study, patients with uncomplicated myocardial infarction were shown to have normal levels of cross-linked fibrin degradation products despite an increase in thrombin activity as inferred by fibrinopeptide A levels (Eisenberg et al 1987). This was taken to provide further evidence for an inappropriately depressed fibrinolytic system in the presence of thrombosis. These studies indicate that acute myocardial infarction is associated with depression of fibrinolysis due to high levels of the inhibitor, PAI-1. It would seem that this both contributes to the development of an intracoronary thrombus and aggravates an already serious condition by impairing lysis of the thrombus.

COMPLICATIONS OF ACUTE MYOCARDIAL INFARCTION

Although the mortality rate from acute myocardial infarction has steadily fallen over the last few years to about 10–12% the incidence of acute and chronic complications of myocardial infarction remains higher. In general, the complications of AMI are more common and more severe with a larger infarct size. Large anterior infarcts are more commonly associated with heart failure and cardiogenic shock, whilst inferior infarcts more frequently lead to the development of conduction defects such as bifascicular or complete heart block.

Acute complications

Arrhythmias

The acute occurrence of a myocardial infarction is associated with a number of life-threatening complications. Amongst these, the development of arrhythmias is common and a frequent cause of death. The origin of such conduction disturbances is most commonly in the electrically unstable region in close proximity to the infarction rather than in the conducting bundles. Such arrhythmias may be due to the release of toxic metabolites from the infarcted area or to small emboli from the thrombosed coronary artery (Davies 1987, Bashour et al 1988, Frink et al 1988). Any arrhythmia can develop after an AMI but in general those of ventricular origin (fibrillation or flutter) are a serious life-threatening event requiring immediate intervention. Atrial fibrillation and flutter may compromise cardiac output and increase the risk of embolic disease leading to the need for pharmacological intervention or cardioversion.

Cardiogenic shock

Cardiogenic shock is characterized by severe intractable hypotension secondary to loss of sufficient myocardium to sustain an adequate cardiac output. This may lead to symptoms and signs of impaired cerebrovascular and renal blood flow. Evidence exists that cardiogenic shock is amongst the commonest causes of death during the acute event (Stevenson et al 1989). Histologically, the presence of cardiogenic shock is associated with infarct extension and small areas of unrelated necrosis. The development of this condition appears to be related to a cycle of inadequate myocardial perfusion leading to poor cardiac output and further myocardial damage (Gutovitz et al 1978).

Ruptured ventricular wall

Of those patients with fatal transmural myocardial infarctions who come to autopsy, the cause of death is rupture of the left ventricular free wall in 8 to 9% (Batts et al 1990). Ruptures affect the lateral wall more commonly than the anterior or inferior walls and the midventricular level more often than the apical or basal levels (Mann & Roberts 1988, Batts et al 1990). Rupture tends to occur during the first week, when necrosis and neutrophilic infiltration have appreciably weakened the infarcted myocardium. However, up to 30% of ruptures occur within 24 hours, before necrosis and inflammation are well established (Becker & van Mantgem 1975, Batts et al 1990). The risk factors for free wall rupture include age greater than 60 years, female gender, pre-existing hypertension, absence of left ventricular hypertrophy, first myocardial infarction, and midventricular or lateral transmural infarctions (Shapira et al 1987).

Post-infarction rupture of the ventricular septum occurs less frequently, usually as a complication of transmural infarction. Septal rupture most commonly occurs during the 1st week and results in an acquired ventricular septal defect of variable size (Hutchins 1979, Edwards et al 1984). A left-to-right shunt and acute heart failure or shock are the most common manifestations. The site of the rupture tract may be a source for embolization of thrombus or necrotic myocardium. Risk factors for rupture of a large transmural septal infarction include first infarction and an occluded coronary artery with little collateral circulation (Skehan et al 1989). Mortality is higher with inferoseptal infarctions as a result of the greater likelihood of right ventricular involvement and shock.

Ruptures of the mitral papillary muscles are less frequent and occur with subendocardial as well as transmural necrosis. The underlying infarction may be small and represent the first ischaemic event. Coronary atherosclerosis is generally less extensive than in other patients with myocardial infarction. Papillary muscle rupture tends to occur during the 1st week, as do other forms of post-infarction rupture. Although mitral regurgitation is sudden in onset, its severity is variable and determined primarily by the extent of papillary muscle involvement. Rupture near the tip, with only partial involvement of a papillary muscle group, causes less severe regurgitation than disruption of the entire muscle.

Among cases of papillary muscle rupture the posteromedial muscle is the commonest site of rupture. This is probably related to the fact that its blood supply is usually from only one source, the dominant coronary artery, whereas the anterolateral muscle is supplied by branches from both the left anterior descending and the left circumflex coronary artery. Occasionally, right ventricular infarction may be associated with rupture of a tricuspid papillary muscle (Eisenberg & Suyemoto 1964).

Thrombosis in the cardiac chambers

Thrombi commonly originate in the atria, especially the left atrium, in valve disorders such as mitral stenosis, or in atrial fibrillation. In addition, mural thrombi of the left ventricle arise after myocardial infarction, on areas of ischaemic or infarcted ventricular wall and occasionally when chronic left ventricular dysfunction is present. The major and devastating complication of these thrombi is that they may become detached as emboli, travelling mainly by the carotid arteries to produce transient ischaemic attacks or a stroke.

Recent studies have shown that atrial fibrillation not only predisposes to cerebral embolism in the presence of mitral stenosis, but also when fibrillation is due to ischaemic heart disease or other causes not associated with valve disorders. In patients with cardiogenic cerebral embolism, it is estimated that there is atrial fibrillation, intermittent or sustained, in about 50%, valvular heart disease in 25% and left ventricular mural thrombi in about 30% (Cerebral Embolism Task Force 1986, 1989). In the presence of atrial fibrillation there is a risk of stroke, transient ischaemic attack or systolic embolism about five-fold greater than in patients with sinus rhythm. This risk is even greater in elderly patients over 85 years old in whom atrial fibrillation can be found in almost 50% of stroke victims. (Wolf et al 1987, Halperin & Hart 1988).

The emboli of left ventricular origin are a further source of cardiogenic cerebral emboli (Komrad et al 1984, Johannessen et al 1988). In patients dying from cerebral infarction, myocardial scarring was three times more common than in those dying from cerebral haemorrhage or cancer. Clearly, myocardial and cerebral infarction may be associated coincidentally in patients with widespread occlusive vascular disease but their concurrence may reflect the frequency with which fatal cerebral infarction complicates myocardial infarction.

In those with cerebral emboli originating from the left ventricle, 60% are associated with acute myocardial infarction and the others have ventricular thrombi associated with ventricular dysfunction from coronary heart disease, hypertension or dilated cardiomyopathy (Fuster & Halperin 1987). It is estimated that the yearly risk of stroke in survivors of myocardial infarction is as high as 5% each year. This widespread and clinically important problem becomes even larger if it is remembered that some intra-cardiac thrombi may cause 'silent' cerebral embolism which may possibly be reflected in multi-infarct dementia of the elderly (Halperin & Hart 1988).

The importance of the heart as a source of arterial emboli was emphasized by Hofmann et al (1990). They studied 153 patients admitted with arterial embolic events, of whom 84 had acute cerebral ischaemia and 19 retinal ischaemia, by both transthoracic and transoesophageal echocardiography. The first point was that transoesophageal echocardiography (TOE) was essential for proper delineation of intracardiac masses. Using both types of echocardiography, they found that 62% of the 84 patients with cerebral ischaemia had cardiac abnormalities. About one third of these had intracardiac thrombi, usually in the left atrium, one third had valvular disease and the remainder had abnormalities of wall motion or the interatrial septum. Examples of transoesophageal echocardiography showing both a normal echocardiogram and also one containing thrombus in the left and right atria are seen in Figure 54.2.

Of the 24 patients with valvular disease, an intracardiac thrombus in addition was seen in 11 patients, almost half of the total. The presence of an intracardiac mass or 'spontaneous contrast' on echocardiography was seen significantly more frequently in atrial fibrillation than in sinus rhythm. 42% of the patients with cerebral ischaemia had normal cardiac findings.

The presence of valvular disease also increases significantly the risk of arterial embolism. Potential sources of emboli include mitral and aortic valvular disease, mitral valve prolapse and mitral annulus calcification (Stafford et al 1985, Coulshed et al 1970, Jespersen & Egeblad 1987).

Transoesophageal echocardiography has revolutionized the diagnosis of intracardiac thrombi and abnormalities. Atrial thrombi missed during transthoracic examination are frequently detected from the transoesophageal approach (Aschenberg et al 1986). It is important to note that although the incidence of intracardiac masses is higher in the presence of clinical cardiac disease, Hofmann et al (1990) noted that 19% of their patients with arterial thrombi had intracardiac masses in clinically normal hearts.

Pathogenesis of intracardiac thrombi: local factors and hypercoagulability

It is clear that mechanical factors associated with poor blood flow and stasis are largely responsible for left atrial thrombi associated with atrial fibrillation or mitral stenosis. Similarly, left ventricular thrombi can be due to left ventricular dysfunction and dilation in patients with ischaemic heart disease, left ventricle aneurysm or dilated cardiomyopathy (Asinger et al 1981, Shresta et al 1983, Weinrich et al 1984). A further cause for left ventricular thrombi is the loss of protection against mural thrombosis in an infarcted area of ventricular wall compared to normal wall.

As explained in Chapter 9 vascular endothelial protection is a complex active metabolic process which may be lost in an area of infarcted tissue. Additionally, a thrombosis itself is thrombogenic, encouraging further platelet-fibrin growth on its surface (Fuster et al 1988) and this process may be accelerated in a region of endothelial or endocardial injury.

Whether conditions associated with intracardiac thrombi are characterized by a hypercoagulable state, and whether

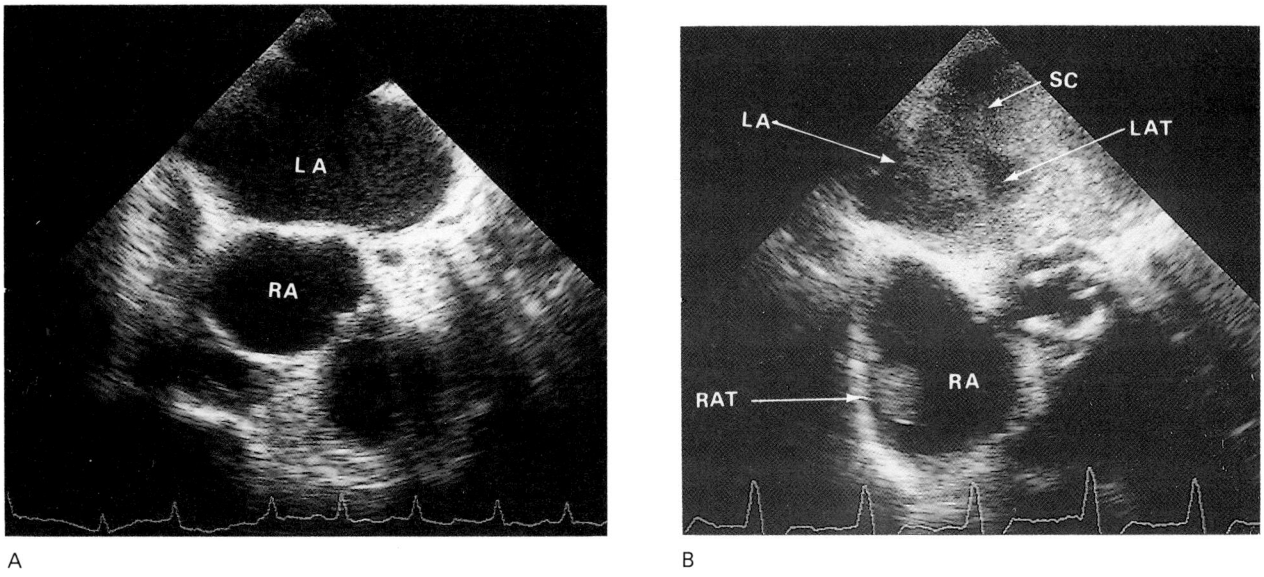

Fig. 54.2 The use of transoesophageal echocardiography to examine cardiac abnormalities. A, normal transoesophageal echocardiogram. B, echocardiogram showing a large left atrial thrombus (LAT) surrounded by spontaneous contrast (SC) and also a right atrial thrombus (RAT). The speckled appearance of spontaneous contrast is thought to indicate reflections from disturbed blood flow and may represent a risk factor for subsequent development of intracardiac thrombosis. LA, left atruim; RA, right atrium.

the patients with clinically silent thrombi can be detected by haemostatic testing is controversial. The role of high fibrinogen levels, and the related increase in plasma viscosity, has perhaps been the most rewarding area of study. Patients with high fibrinogen levels after myocardial infarction and also with chronic atrial fibrillation have a higher incidence of thromboembolism than those with lower levels (Fulton & Duckett 1990, Kumagai et al 1990). For all types of stroke, including those of embolic origin, raised plasma fibrinogen is an independent risk factor (Kannel et al 1987, Qizilbash et al 1991). The unanswered question is whether measurement of fibrinogen and possibly other haemostatic factors provides sufficient specificity to predict those patients with an initial stroke or TIA who will develop further thrombo-embolic complications. In established stroke, high haemocrit as well as high fibrinogen, fibrinopeptide A and PAI-1 are associated with increased mortality (Lowe et al 1983).

Patients with prosthetic heart valves are particularly prone to thrombo-embolic complications, the site of thrombosis being on the valve itself. Whether these patients also have evidence of a systemic hypercoagulable state is unclear. Koppensteiner et al (1991) found that patients with heart valve prostheses have increased plasma fibrinogen, plasma viscosity and red cell aggregation and these factors are more elevated in patients with mechanical valve prostheses compared to bioprostheses. It is probable that a vicious circle is set up in which prosthetic valves induce increases in fibrinogen which subsequently increase the likelihood of further thrombus formation. Similarly, in patients with mitral stenosis with intracardiac thrombosis there are increased levels of D-dimer, fibrinopeptide A and fibrin Bβ15–42 concentration compared to those without thrombi. Recent studies have shown that there are alterations of haemostasis in patients with arterial fibrillation and atrial thrombi as demonstrated by transoesophageal echocardiography (Gough et al 1992). Patients with intracardiac thrombi had elevated levels of von Willebrand factor and reduction in fibrinolytic activity measured by the euglobulin clot lysis time. In patients with spontaneous contrast in the left atrium, which is thought to represent areas of stagnant or disturbed blood flow, the haemostatic abnormalities were mid-way between those with intracardiac thrombi and those without. The onset of atrial fibrillation itself produces haemostatic abnormalities. Gustafsson et al (1990) found elevated fibrinogen, factor VIIIc, D-dimer, beta thromboglobulin and platelet factor 4 in patients with atrial fibrillation compared to those with sinus rhythm. These workers, however, did not distinguish between the patients who either had or did not have intracardiac thrombi.

Treatment of cardiac disease associated with thromboembolic risk

It is well known that mitral valve disease of rheumatic aetiology causes systemic arterial thromboembolism in a significant proportion of cases and that the problem is aggravated in the presence of atrial fibrillation (Daley et al 1951, Coulshed et al 1970). It is worth noting, however, that patients with mitral valve disease who are in sinus rhythm and give no history of paroxysmal arrhythmia can have systemic embolism. The emboli can arise not only from thrombi in the left atrial appendage but also on the surface of the damaged mitral leaflets themselves (Wooley et al 1974).

Although there is no long-term controlled clinical trial of anticoagulation in patients with mitral rheumatic valvular disease, it would now be unethical to carry this out in view of the low number of embolic events seen in these patients on anticoagulants. In a retrospective study of 500 patients, Fleming and Bailey (1971) found that the embolic complication on anticoagulants was 0.8% per patient's treatment year compared to between 4 and 8% in similar patients managed without anticoagulants (Coulshed et al 1970). Mitral valvotomy diminishes but does not abolish the risk of systemic embolism (Coulshed et al 1970). After surgery there is thus a case for continuing with anticoagulant therapy.

Atrial fibrillation

It has become apparent recently that atrial fibrillation in the absence of vascular disease causes a clinically significant risk of arterial embolism. In part this is due to the fact that atrial fibrillation is normally a result of substantial cardiac impairment. For young patients with intermittent 'lone' atrial fibrillation there seems no need for anticoagulation since they are at very low risk of stroke and their mortality rate is no greater than for patients in sinus rhythm (Kopecky et al 1985). However, in atrial fibrillation associated with older age, hypertension, thyrotoxicosis and congestive cardiac failure substantially increase the stroke risk (Staffurth et al 1977, Petersen & Hansen 1988).

Trials of antithrombotic therapy for prevention of cardiac embolism

The question of whether patients with non-valvular atrial fibrillation require anticoagulant therapy has been addressed by four major prospective trials. In the Copenhagen Atrial Fibrillation Aspirin Anticoagulant Study (AFASAK), 1007 patients were allocated to treatment with warfarin, aspirin (75 mg/day) or placebo and followed for a mean treatment period of 11 months. The primary end-points were stroke, transient ischaemic attacks and systolic embolism. Although the withdrawal rate in the warfarin group was large at 38%, the event rate, at 2.6%, was significantly less than the event rate of 5.0% in the aspirin group and 6.0% in the placebo group (Petersen et al 1989).

The Stroke Prevention in Atrial Fibrillation Study (SPAF)(1990) from the United States, has at the present time reported only preliminary results. Patients were allocated to either warfarin, aspirin (325 mg/day) or placebo unless they were not eligible for warfarin, in which case they were given aspirin or placebo. After a mean of 1.13 years, the event rate with placebo was 8.3% per year and that with active treatment (aspirin or warfarin) was 1.6%, so the placebo group was stopped. Further analysis showed that the event rate in all aspirin-treated patients was 3.2% per year, compared to 6.3% in those given placebo. Subgroup data showed that this benefit of aspirin was only apparent in patients aged 75 years or less. In older patients there was no benefit of aspirin at all, although only a relatively small proportion of the patients were in this age group.

The Boston Area Anticoagulant Trial for Atrial Fibrillation (BAATAF) (1990) randomized patients solely into warfarin and placebo groups, although aspirin was permitted in the placebo patients. The incidence of stroke over the 2.2 years of the study was much lower, at 0.41% per year in the warfarin patients than the 3.0% per year in the placebo patients, giving a risk reduction of 86%.

The most recent Canadian Atrial Fibrillation Anticoagulation study (CAFA) (Connolly 1990), terminated the placebo group early in view of the favourable treatment group outcome in the other trials. The event rate in the control group of 4.6% per year was reduced by 35% to 3.0% in the anticoagulant group.

Thus, all four trials have shown a favourable therapeutic effect, especially for oral anticoagulants. The precise role for aspirin remains unsolved. Although there is evidence from a direct comparison in the AFASAK study that anticoagulants are superior to aspirin, they are logistically more difficult to supervise and control; for this reason the treatment of choice would be a non-toxic substance that did not need laboratory control. The on-going United States SPAF study may resolve this question in that now a direct comparison of anticoagulants versus aspirin is being made.

Chronic complications of myocardial infarction

Chronic heart failure

The degree of heart failure after AMI depends on the extent of muscle loss. Because of this, persistent chronic heart failure has a poor prognosis and is indicative of end-stage ischaemic heart disease, or so-called ischaemic cardiomyopathy (Pantely & Bristow 1984).

Hearts show cardiomegaly, with moderate biventricular hypertrophy and moderate to marked four-chamber dilation. The left ventricle may be the site of one or more healed myocardial infarctions. Some patients, however, have no gross evidence of myocardial infarction (Atkinson & Virmani 1989), although all show evidence of chronic ischaemia. Mural thrombus may be present and evidence of embolization is commonly observed in other organs. The lungs exhibit chronic pulmonary hypertension, and the abdominal viscera are enlarged by chronic congestion.

Peripheral oedema and pleural or pericardial effusions are also commonly encountered.

Ventricular aneurysm

Shortly after a full thickness myocardial infarction, the force of left ventricular contraction acting on a necrotic and weakened wall commonly results in stretching and thinning of the infarcted region. This remodelling of left ventricular shape occurs most often with large infarctions (Erlebacher et al 1984) and is the precursor of aneurysm formation.

Among patients with left ventricular aneurysms, the coronary arteries are usually involved by two- or three-vessel disease. Although coronary thrombotic occlusion usually causes the underlying transmural infarction, most hearts that develop aneurysms also have little collateral blood flow (Hirai et al 1989). This suggests that once transmural infarction is established, adequate collateral blood flow may be necessary during the healing phase to prevent aneurysm formation. Left ventricular aneurysms affect men more often than women and have a poor prognosis if associated with heart failure or arrhythmias.

Rarely, post-infarction rupture of the left ventricular wall is incomplete leading to the formation of a false aneurysm, most commonly occurring along the inferior or lateral walls.

Post-infarction angina

Angina pectoris may develop after myocardial infarction and occurs more commonly with subendocardial than transmural necrosis. Chest pain is due to ischaemia either in the distribution of the infarct-related coronary artery or, paradoxically, in the distribution of a second critically narrowed artery, perhaps as a result of interrupted collateral blood flow.

Post-infarction pericarditis

Pericarditis is a potential complication of acute myocardial infarctions and usually occurs during the 1st week. It is associated with infarcts of large size (Tofler et al 1989). In some cases pericarditis is localized to the area overlying the infarction, whereas in others there is widespread involvement of the pericardial sac.

Clinically, this results in chest pain and a pericardial friction rub. Postmyocardial infarction syndrome (Dressler's syndrome) occurs weeks to months after myocardial infarction. It is characterized clinically by low-grade fever, pleuropericardial chest pain, a pericardial friction rub, and pericardial and pleural effusions that may be haemorrhagic. The cause of this syndrome is unknown, but it is thought to be related to an auto-immune mechanism or anticoagulant therapy. Although serious complications are rare, cardiac tamponade and constrictive pericarditis have been described (Blau et al 1977).

CONCLUDING REMARKS

Coronary artery disease is a condition of diverse aetiology that can present in a variety of ways with a variety of different clinical outcomes. At the centre of this syndrome is the common feature of inadequate perfusion of the myocardium. The recognition that the commonest cause of this condition is thrombus superimposed on an atheromatous plaque has led to the use of lytic agents and intensive invasive treatment that has markedly reduced the mortality and morbidity associated with this condition. In the last decade a much greater awareness has developed of the role of risk factors in the aetiology of this condition. In addition to the well known factors such as cigarette smoking, hypertension, male sex and old age, we can add cholesterol, fibrinogen, insulin resistance and a host of more or less likely candidates. It is worth noting the obvious: a relationship between something and disease does not automatically imply that reducing that something will alter disease incidence. The media in particular are guilty of jumping on each bandwagon that rolls by in this respect, although it is clearly possible that the medical profession has some role in encouraging this behaviour. Before patients can be enthusiastically encouraged to rid themselves of risk factors, it is important that evidence exists to support the value of such intervention. In the light of the largely unproven benefits of some interventions, it is worth reiterating the accelerated mortality in the MRFIT study in patients who smoked, had a diastolic pressure greater than 90 mmHg, had high cholesterol and diabetes. Most of these risk factors have the benefit of being common and reversible and should be addressed as a priority.

It is difficult to see the next major advance in the prevention or management of coronary artery disease. Perhaps the most attractive possibility is the use of gene therapy in susceptible individuals to alter levels of known risk factors. As a treatment this appears to be close in some cases and may lead to exciting advances in this important condition in the next decade.

REFERENCES

Alessi M C, Juhan-Vague I, Kooistra T, Declerck P J, Collén D 1988 Insulin stimulates the synthesis of plasminogen activator 1 by hepatocellular cell line Hep G2. Thrombosis and Haemostasis 60: 491–494

Alexopoulos D, Ambrose J A, Stump D et al 1991 Thrombosis-related markers in unstable angina pectoris. Journal of the American College of Cardiology 17: 866–871

Almér L-O, Ohlin H 1987 Elevated levels of the rapid inhibitor

of plasminogen activator. Thrombosis Research 47: 335–339
Ambrose J A, Winters S L, Arora R R et al 1986 Angiographic evolution of coronary artery morphology in unstable angina. Journal of the American College of Cardiology 5: 472–478
Aschenberg W, Schluter M, Kremer P, Schroder E, Siglow V, Bleifeld W 1986 Transesophageal two-dimensional echocardiography for the detection of left atrial appendage thrombus. Journal of the American College of Cardiology 7: 163–166
Asinger R W, Mikell F L, Elsperger J, Hodges M 1981 Incidence of left ventricular thrombosis after acute transmural myocardial infarction: serial evaluation by two-dimensional echocardiography New England Journal of Medicine 305: 297–302
Astedt B, Lecander I, Ny T 1987 The placental type plasminogen activator inhibitor PAI-2. Fibrinolysis 1: 203–208
Atkinson J B, Virmani R 1989 Congestive heart failure due to coronary artery disease without myocardial infarction: Clinicopathologic description of an unusual cardiomyopathy. Human Pathology 20: 1155–1162
Auwerx J, Bouillon R, Collen D, Geboers J 1988 Tissue-type plasminogen activator antigen and plasminogen activator inhibitor in diabetes mellitus. Arteriosclerosis 8: 68–72
Aznar J, Estellès A, Toramo G, Toramo S V, Blanch S, Es̆pana F 1988 Plasminogen activator inhibitor activity and other fibrinolytic variables in patients with coronary artery disease. British Heart Journal 59: 535–541
Barrett-Connor E, Wingard D L 1983 Sex differential in ischemic heart disease mortality in diabetics: a prospective population-based study. American Journal of Epidemiology 118: 489–496
Bashour T T, Myler R K, Andrease G E et al 1988 Current concepts in unstable myocardial ischemia. American Heart Journal 115: 850–861
Batts K P, Ackermann D M, Edwards W D 1990 Postinfarction rupture of the left ventricular free wall: Clinicopathologic correlates in 100 consectuve autopsy cases. Human Pathology 21: 520–525
Bauer K A, Rosenberg R D 1987 The pathophysiology of the prethrombotic state in humans: insights gained from studies using markers of hemostatic system activation. Blood 70: 343–350
Bauer K A, Weiss L M, Sparrow D, Vokonas P S , Rosenberg R D 1987 Aging associated changes in indices of thrombin generation and protein C activation in humans. Journal of Clinical Investigation 80: 1527–1534
Beaglehole R, Dobson A, Hobbs M S, Jackson R, Martin C A 1989 Coronary heart disease in Australia and New Zealand. International Journal of Epidemiology 18: 145–148
Becker A E, van Mantgem J-P 1975 Cardiac tamponade: A study of 50 hearts. European Journal of Cardiology 34: 349–358
Bern M M, Cassani N P, Horton J, Rand L, Davis G 1980 Changes in fibrinolysis and factor VIII coagulant antigen and ristocetin co-factor in diabetes mellitus and arteriosclerosis. Thrombosis Research 19: 831–839
Bevilacqua M P, Pober J S, Majeau G R, Fiers W, Cotran R S, Gimbrone M A Jr 1986 Recombinant tumour necrosis factor induces procoagulant activity in cultured human vascular endothelium: Characterisation and comparison with actions of interleukin 1. Proceedings of the National Academy of Sciences, USA 3: 4533–4537
Blankenhorn D H, Nessim S A, Johnson R L, Sanmarco M E, Azen S P, Cashin-Hemphill L 1987 Beneficial effects of combined cholesterol niacin therapy on coronary atherosclerosis and coronary bypass grafts. Journal of the American Medical Association 257: 3233–3240
Blau N, Shen B A, Pittman D E, Joyner C R 1977 Massive hemopericardium in a patient with postmyocardial infarction syndrome. Chest 71: 549–552
Boeri D, Almus F E, Maiello M, Cagliero E, Vijaya L, Rao M, Lorenzi M 1989 Modification of tissue-factor mRNA and protein response to thrombin and interleukin 1 by high glucose in cultured human endothelial cells. Diabetes 38: 212–218
Boston Area Anticoagulation Trial for Atrial Fibrillation Investigators 1990 The effect of low-dose warfarin on the risk of stroke in patients with nonrheumatic atrial fibrillation. New England Journal of Medicine 323: 1505–1511
Bottiger L E, Carlson L A 1970 The Stockholm Prospective Study 2. New events of coronary heart disease in men in relation to findings at initial examination. 9 year follow-up. In: Waldenstrom J, Larsson T, Ljungstedt N (eds) Early phases of coronary heart disease. The possibility of prediction. Nordiska Bokhandelns Förlag, Stockholm, p 158–179
Breit S N, Green I 1988 Modulation of endothelial cell synthesis of von Willebrand factor by mononuclear cell products. Haemostasis 18(3): 137–145
Brindley D N, Rolland Y 1989 Possible connections between stress, diabetes, obesity, hypertension and altered lipoprotein metabolism that may result in atherosclerosis. Clinical Sciences 77: 453–461
Brown G Albers J J Fisher L D Schaefer S M Lin J-T Kaplan C et al 1990 Regression of coronary artery disease as a result of intensive lipid-lowering therapy in man with high levels of apolipoprotein B. New England Journal of Medicine 322: 1289–1298
Brownlee M, Vlassara H, Cerami A 1984 Nonenzymatic glycosylation and the pathogenesis of diabetic complications. Annals of Internal Medicine 101: 527–537
Brownlee M, Vlassara H, Cerami A 1985 Nonenzymatic glycosylation products on collagen covalently trap low-density lipoprotein. Diabetes 34: 938–941
Brownlee M, Vlassara H, Kooney T, Ulrich P, Cerami A 1986 Aminoguanidine prevents diabetes-induced arterial wall protein crosslinking. Science 232: 1629–1632
Brownlee M, Cerami A, Vlassara H 1988 Advanced glycosylation end products in tissue and the biochemical basis of diabetic complications. New England Journal of Medicine 318: 1315–1321
Cagliero E, Maiello M, Boeri D, Roy S, Lorenzi M 1988 Increased expression of basement membrane components in human endothelial cells cultured in high glucose. Journal of Clinical Investigation 82: 735–738
Cagliero E, Roth T, Roy S, Lorenzi M 1991 Characteristics and mechanisms of high-glucose-induced overexpression of basement membrane components in cultured human endothelial cells. Diabetes 40: 102–110
Cameron H A, Philips R, Ibbotson R M, Carson P H M 1983 Platelet size in myocardial infarction. British Medical Journal 287: 449–451
Cerebral Embolism Task Force 1986 Cardiogenic brain embolism Archives of Neurology 43: 71–84
Cerebral Embolism Task Force 1989 Cardiogenic brain embolism: the second report of the Cerebral Embolism Task Force. Archives of Neurology 46: 727–743
Chakrabarti R, Hocking E D, Fearnley G R, Mann R D, Attwell T N, Jackson D 1968 Fibrinolytic activity and coronary artery disease. Lancet 1: 987–990
Christe M, Fritschi J, Lammie B, Tran T H, Marbet G A, Berger W, Duckert F 1984 Fifteen coagulation and fibrinolysis parameters in diabetes mellitus and in patients with vasculopathy. Thrombosis and Haemostasis 52: 138–143
Collins R, Keech A, Peto R, Sleight P et al 1992 Cholesterol and total mortality: need for larger trials. British Medical Journal: 304 1689
Connolly S J 1990 Canadian atrial fibrillation anticoagulation (CAFA) Study Circulation: 82(suppl III): 108 (abst)
Constantinides P 1966 Plaque fissure in human coronary thrombosis. Journal of Atherosclerosis 6: 1
Coulshed N, Epstein E J, McKendrick C S, Galloway R W, Walker E 1970 Systemic embolism in mitral valve disease British Heart Journal 32: 26–34
Crawford T 1963 Thrombotic occlusion and the plaque. In: Jones R J (ed) Evolution of the atherosclerotic plaque. University of Chicago Press, Chicago, p 279–300
Cucuianu M P, Missits L, Olinic N, Roman S 1980 Increased ristocetin cofactor in acute myocardial infarction: a component of the acute phase reaction. Thrombosis and Haemostasis 43: 41–44
Dalaker K, Smith P, Arnesen H, Prydz H 1987 Factor VII-phospholipid complex in male survivors of acute myocardial infarction. Acta Medica Scandinavica 222: 111–116
Daley R, Mattingley T W, Holt C H, Bland E F, White F D 1951 Systemic arterial embolism in rheumatic heart disease. American Heart Journal 42: 566–581
Davies M J 1987 Thrombosis in acute myocardial infarction and sudden death. Cardiovascular Clinics (Philadelphia) 18(1): 151–159

Davies M J, Thomas A 1984 Thrombosis and acute coronary-artery lesions in sudden cardiac ischemic death. New England Journal of Medicine 310: 1137–1140
Davies M J, Thomas A C 1985 Plaque fissuring: the cause of acute myocardial infarction, sudden ischaemic death, and crescendo angina. British Heart Journal 53: 363–373
Davies M J, Woolf N, Robertson W B 1976 Pathology of acute myocardial infarction with particular reference to occlusive coronary thrombi. British Heart Journal 38: 659
Davies M J, Fulton W F M, Robertson W B 1979 The relation of coronary thrombosis to ischaemic myocardial necrosis. Journal of Pathology 127: 99
Davies M J, Thomas A C, Knapman P, Hangartner R 1986 Intramyocardial platelet aggregation in patients with unstable angina suffering sudden ischaemic cardiac death. Circulation 73: 418–427
Dawson S, Hamsten A, Wiman B, Henney A, Humphries S 1991 Genetic variation at the plasminogen activator inhibitor-1 locus is associated with altered levels of plasma plasminogen activator inhibitor-1 activity. Arteriosclerosis and Thrombosis 11: 183–190
de Fronzo R A, Simonson D, Ferrannini E 1982a Hepatic and peripheral insulin resistance: a common feature of Type 2 (non-insulin-dependent) and Type 1 (insulin-dependent) diabetes mellitus. Diabetologia 23: 313–319
de Fronzo RA, Hendler R, Simonson D 1982b Insulin resistance is a prominent feature of insulin-dependent diabetes. Diabetes 31: 795–801
Department of Health and Human Services 1989 Reducing the health consequences of smoking: 25 years of progress: a report of the Surgeon General. Government Printing Office (DHHS publication no (CDC) 89-8411), Washington DC
de Sousa C, Azevedo J, Soria C, Barros F, Ribeiro C, Parreira F, Caen J P 1988 Factor VII hyperactivity in acute myocardial thrombosis. A relation to the coagulation activation. Thrombosis Research 51: 165–173
Després J-P, Moorjani S, Lupien P J, Tremblayh A, Nadeau A, Bouchard C 1990 Regional distribution of body fat, plasma lipoproteins, and cardiovascular disease. Arteriosclerosis 10: 497–511
de Wood M A, Spores J, Notske R, Mouser L T, Burroughs R, Golden M S, Lang M T 1980 Prevalence of total coronary occlusion during the early hours of transmural myocardial infarction. New England Journal of Medicine 303: 897–902
Doll R, Peto R 1976 Mortality in relation to smoking: 20 years' observation on male British doctors. British Medical Journal 2: 1525–1536
Dortimer A C, Shenoy P N, Shiroff R A, Leaman D M, Babb J D, Liedtke A J, Zelis R 1978 Diffuse coronary artery disease in diabetic patients: fact or fiction? Circulation 57: 133–136
Ducimetiere P, Eschwege E, Papoz L, Richard J L, Claude J R, Rosseling G 1980 Relationship of plasma insulin levels to the incidence of myocardial infarction and coronary heart disease mortality in a middle-aged population. Diabetologia 19: 205–210
Durrington P N 1992 Is insulin atherogenic? Diabetic Medicine 9: 597–600
Edgington, T S, Mackman N, Brand K, Ruf W 1991 The structural biology of expresion and function of tissue factor. Thrombosis and Haemostasis 66(1): 67–79
Edwards B S, Edwards W D, Edwards J E 1984 Ventricular septal rupture complicating acute myocardial infarction: Identification of simple and complex types in 53 autopsied hearts. American Journal of Cardiology 54: 1201–1205
Eisenberg S, Suyemoto J 1964 Rupture of a papillary muscle of the tricuspid valve following acute myocardial infarction: Report of a case. Circulation 30: 588–591
Eisenberg P R, Sherman P R, Perez J, Jaffe A S 1987 Relationship between elevated plasma levels of crosslinked fibrin degradation products (XL-FDP) and the clinical presentation of patients with myocardial infarction. Thrombosis Research 46: 109–120
Ellis E N, Bowen W 1990 Aminoguanidine ameliorates glomerular basement membrane (GBM) thickening in experimental diabetes Diabetes 39 (suppl 1): 71A (abst)
Elwood P C, Renaud S, Sharp D S, Beswick A D, O'Brien J R, Yarnell J W G 1991 Ischaemic heart disease and platelet aggregation: The Caerphilly Collaborative Heart Disease Study. Circulation 83: 38–44
Erlebacher J A, Weiss J L, Weisfedt M L, Bulkley B H 1984 Early dilation of the infarcted segment in acute transmural myocardial infarction: Role of infarct expansion in acute left ventricular enlargement. Journal of the American College of Cardiology 4: 201–208
Esposito C, Gerlach H, Bertt J, Stern D, Vlassara H 1989 Endothelial receptor-mediated binding of glucose modified albumin is associated with increased monolayer permeability and modulation of cell surface coagulant properties. Journal of Experimental Medicine 170: 1387–1407
Estellès A, Torono G, Aznar J, Espana F, Tormo V 1985 Reduced fibrinolytic activity in coronary heart disease in basal conditions and after exercise. Thrombosis Research 40: 373–383
Falk E 1983 Plaque rupture with severe pre-existing stenosis precipitating coronary thrombosis: characteristics of coronary atherosclerotic plaque underlying fatal occlusive thrombi. British Heart Journal 50: 127131
Falk E 1985 Unstable angina with fatal outcome: dynamic coronary thrombosis leading to infarction and/or sudden death. Autopsy evidence of recurrent mural thrombosis with peripheral embolization culminating in total vascular occlusion. Circulation 71: 699–708
Ferrannini E, Buzzigoli G, Bonadonna R et al 1987 Insulin resistance in essential hypertension. New England Journal of Medicine 317: 350–357
Fleming H A Bailey S M 1971 Mitral valve disease, systemic embolism and anticoagulants. Postgraduate Medical Journal 47: 599–604
Fontbonne A, Thobroutsky G, Eschwège E, Richard J L, Claude J R, Rosselin G E 1988 Coronary heart disease mortality risk: Plasma insulin level is a more sensitive marker than hypertension or abnormal glucose tolerance in overweight males. The Paris Prospective Study. International Journal of Obesity 12: 557–565
Francis C W, Connaghan D G, Scott W L, Marder V J 1987 Increased plasma concentration of cross-linked fibrin polymers in acute myocardial infarction. Circulation 75: 1170–1177
Francis R B, Kawanishi D, Baruch T, Mahrer P, Rahimtoola S, Feinstein D 1988 Impaired fibrinolysis in coronary artery disease. American Heart Journal 115: 776–780
Franzen J, Nilsson B, Johansson B W, Nilsson I M 1983 Fibrinolytic activity in men with acute myocardial infarction before 60 years of age. Acta Medica Scandinavica 214: 339–344
Friedman M, Byers S O 1965 induction of thrombi upon pre-existing arterial plaques. American Journal of Pathology 46: 567
Frink R J, Rooney P A Jr, Trowbridge J O, Rose J P 1988 Coronary thrombosis and platelet/fibrin microemboli in death associated with acute myocardial infarction. British Heart Journal 59: 196–200
Fulton R M, Duckett K 1990 Plasma-fibrinogen and thromboemboli after myocardial infarction. Lancet 2: 1161–1164
Fuster V, Halperin J L 1989 Left ventricular thrombi and cerebral embolism: an emerging approach. New England Journal of Medicine 230: 392–394
Fuster V, Badimon L, Cohen M, Ambrose J A, Badimon J J, Chesebro J H 1988 Insight into the pathogenesis of acute ischaemic syndromes Circulation 77: 1213–1220
Fye W B 1985 The delayed diagnosis of myocardial infarction: It took half a century! Circulation 72: 262–271
Ganda O P 1980 Pathogenesis of macrovascular disease in the human diabetic (review). Diabetes 29: 931–942
Garcia M J, McNamara P M, Gordon T, Kannell W B 1974 Morbidity and mortality in diabetics in the Framingham population: sixteen year follow-up study. Diabetes 23: 105–111
Gilcrease M Z, Hoover R L 1990 Activated human monocytes exhibit receptor-mediated adhesion to a non-enzymatically glycosylated protein substrate. Diabetologia 33: 329–333
Gilcrease M Z, Hoover R L 1992 Human monocyte interactions with non-enzymatically collagen. Diabetologia 35: 160–164
Gliksman M D, Dwyer T, Wlodarczyk J 1990 Differences in modifiable cardiovascular disease risk factors in Australian schoolchildren: the results of a nationwide survey. Preview Medicine 19: 291–304
Gordon E M, Ratnoff O D, Saito H, Donaldson V H, Pensky J, Jones P K 1980. Rapid fibrinolysis, augmented Hageman factor (factor XII) titers and decreased C1 esterase inhibitor titers in women taking oral contraceptives. Journal of Laboratory Clinical Medicine 96: 762–769

Gordon E M, Ratnoff O D, Jones P K 1982 Hageman factor (factor XII) titers in the cold-promoted activation of factor VII and spontaneous shortening of the prothrombin time in women using oral contraceptives. Journal of Laboratory Clinical Medicine 99: 363–369

Gordon E M, Hellerstein H K, Ratnoff O D, Arafah B M, Yamashita, T S 1987 Augmented Hageman factor and prolactin titers, enhanced cold activation of factor VII and spontaneous shortening of prothrombin time in survivors of myocardial infarction. Journal of Laboratory Clinical Medicine 109: 409–413

Gormsen J, Dalsgaard Neilsen J, Agerskov Andersen L 1977 ADP-induced platelet aggregation in vitro in patients with ischemic heart disease and peripheral thromboatherosclerosis. Acta Medica Scandinavica 201: 509–513

Gough S C L, Smyllie J, Sheldon T A, Berkin K E, Davies J A 1992 Haemostatic and fibrinolytic function in patients with atrial fibrillation and left atrial thrombi (unpublished)

Gram J, Jespersen J 1985 On the significance of Antithrombin III α_2-macroglobulin, α_2-antiplasmin, histidine-rich glycoprotein, and protein C in patients with acute myocardial infarction and deep vein thrombosis. Thrombosis and Haemostasis 54: 503–505

Gram J, Jespersen J 1987 A selective depression of tissue plasminogen activator (t-PA) activity in euglobulins characterises a risk group among survivors of acute myocardial infarction. Lancet 1: 137–139

Gram J, Jespersen J, Kluft C, Rijken D 1987a On the usefulness of fibrinolysis variables in the characterization of a risk group for myocardial reinfarction. Acta Medica Scandinavica 221: 149–153

Gram J, Kluft C, Jespersen J 1987b Depression of tissue plasminogen activator (t-PA) activity and rise of t-PA inhibition and acute phase reactants in blood from patients with acute myocardial infarction (AMI). Thrombosis and Haemostasis 58: 817–821

Grant P J, Kruithof E K O, Felley C P, Felber J B, Bachmann F 1990 Short-term infusions of insulin, triacylglycerol and glucose do not cause acute increases in plasminogen activator inhibitor-1 in man. Clinical Science 79: 513–516

Grant P J, Rüegg M, Medcalf R L 1991 Basal expression and insulin-mediated induction of PAI-1 mRNA in Hep G2 cells. Fibrinolysis 5: 81–86

Gustafsson C, Blombäck M, Britton M, Hamsten A, Svensson J 1990 Coagulation factors and the increased risk of stroke in nonvalvular atrial fibrillation. Stroke 21: 47–51

Gutovitz A L, Sobel B E, Roberts R 1978 Progressive nature of myocardial injury in selected patients with cardiogenic shock. American Journal of Cardiology 41: 469–475

Hall J, Heller R F, Dobson A J, Lloyd D M, Sanson-Fisher R W, Leeder S R 1988 A cost-effectiveness analysis of alternative strategies for the prevention of heart disease. Medical Journal of Australia 148: 273–277

Halperin J L, Hart R G 1988 Atrial fibrillation and stroke: new ideas/persisting dilemmas (editorial). Stroke 19: 937–941

Hamby R I, Sherman L, Mehta J, Aintablian A 1976 Reappraisal of the role of the diabetic state in coronary artery disease. Chest 70: 251–257

Hammes H-P, Martin S, Federlin K, Geisen K, Brownlee M 1990 Aminoguanidine treatment inhibits the development of experimental diabetic retinopathy. Diabetes 39 (suppl 1): 62A (abst)

Hamsten A, Wiman B, De Faire U, Blombäck M 1985 Increased plasma levels of a rapid inhibitor of tissue plasminogen activator in young survivors of myocardial infarction. New England Journal of Medicine 313: 1557–1563

Hamsten A, Blombäck M, Wiman B, Svensson J, Szamosi A, de Faire U, Mettinger L 1986. Haemostatic function in myocardial infarction. British Heart Journal 55: 58–66

Hamsten A, de Faire U, Waldius G, Dahlén G, Szamosi A, Landou C, Blombäck M, Wiman B 1987 Plasminogen activator inhibitor in plasma: risk factor for recurrent myocardial infarction. Lancet 2: 3–9

Handin R I, McDonough M, Lesch M 1978 Elevation of platelet factor four in acute myocardial infarction: measurement by radioimmunoassay. Journal of Laboratory and Clinical Medicine 91: 340–349

Herrick J B 1912 Certain clinical features of sudden obstruction of the coronary arteries. Journal of the American Medical Association 59: 2015–2020

Hirai T, Fujita M, Nakajima H et al 1989 Importance of collateral circulation for prevention of left ventricular aneurysm formation in acute myocardial infarction. Circulation 79: 791–796

Hjermann I 1990 The Oslo study some trial results Atherosclerosis Reviews 21: 103–108

Hjermann I, Velve Byre K, Holme I, Leren P 1981 Effect of diet and smoking intervention on the indicence of coronary heart disease: report from the Oslo study group of a randomised trial in healthy men Lancet ii: 1303–1310

Hofmann T, Kasper W, Meinertz T, Geibel A, Just H 1990 Echocardiographic evaluation of patients with clinically suspected arterial emboli Lancet 336: 1421–1424

Holme I 1990 An analysis of randomised trials evaluating the effect of cholesterol reduction on total mortality and coronary heart disease incidence. Circulation 82: 1916–1924

Hume R 1958 Fibrinolysis in myocardial infarction. British Heart Journal 20: 15–20

Hutchins G M 1979 Rupture of the interventricular septum complicating myocardial infarction: Pathological analaysis of 10 patients with clinically diagnosed perforations. American Heart Journal 97: 165–173

Jansson J-H, Nilsson T K, Johnson O 1991 von Willebrand factor in plasma: a novel risk factor for recurrent myocardial infarction and death. British Heart Journal 66: 351–355

Jarrett R J 1988 Is insulin atherogenic? Diabetologia 31: 71–75

Jespersen C M, Egeblad H 1987 Mitral annulus calcification and embolism. Acta Medica Scandinavica 222: 37–41

Johannessen K A, Nordrehaug J E, von der Lippe G,Vollset S E 1988 Risk factors for embolisation in patients with left ventricular thrombi and acute myocardial infarction. British Heart Journal 60: 104–110

Juhan-Vague I, Vague P, Alessi M C, Badier C, Valadier J, Aillaud M F 1987 Relationships between plasma insulin, triglyceride, body mass index and plasminogen activator inhibitor 1. Diabetic Medicine 13: 331–336

Juhan-Vague I, Alessi M C, Joly P, Thirion W, Vague P, Declerck P J, Serradimigni A, Collén D 1989a Plasma plasminogen activator inhibitor I in angina pectoris. Influence of plasma insulin and acute-phase response. Arteriosclerosis 9: 362–367

Juhan-Vague I, Roul C, Alessi M C, Ardissone J P, Heim M, Vague P 1989b Increased plasminogen activator inhibitor activity in non insulin dependent diabetic patients. Relationship with plasma insulin. Thrombosis and Haemostasis 61: 370–373

Juhan-Vague I, Alessi M C, Vague P 1991 Increased plasma plasminogen activator inhibitor 1 levels. A possible link between insulin resistance and atherothrombosis. Diabetologia 34: 457–462

Kane J P, Malloy M J, Ports T A, Phillips N R, Diehl J C, Havel R G 1990 Regression of coronary atherosclerosis during treatment of familial hypercholesterolemia with combined drug regimens Journal of the American Medical Association 264: 3007–3012

Kannel W B 1985 Lipids, diabetes and coronary heart disease: insights from the Framingham study. American Heart Journal 110: 1100–1107

Kannel W B 1987 Hypertension and other risk factors in coronary heart disease. American Heart Journal 114: 918–925

Kannel W B, Gordon T 1974 The Framingham Study: An Epidemiological Investigation of Cardiovascular Disease Section 30. Some Characteristics Related to the Incidence of Cardiovascular Disease and Death: The Framingham Study, 18 year follow-up. US Dept of Health Education and Welfare publication no (NIH) 74–599, Washington

Kannel WB, McGee D L 1979 Diabetes and glucose tolerance as risk factors for cardiovascular disease: the Framingham study. Diabetes Care 2: 120–126

Kannel W B, Castelli W P, Meeks S L 1985 Fibrinogen and cardiovascular disease. Abstract of paper for 34th Annual Scientific Session of the American College of Cardiology, March 1985, Anaheim, California

Kannel W B, Wolf P A, Castelli W P, D'Agostino R B 1987 Fibrinogen and the risk of cardiovascular disease: The Framingham Study. Journal of the American Medical Association 258: 1183–1186

Kaplan N M 1989 The deadly quartet: Upper-body obesity, glucose intolerance, hypertriglyceridemia, and hypertension. Archives of Internal Medicine 149: 1514–1520

Keys A 1970 Coronary heart disease in seven countries. Circulation 41: 1–211
Koistinen M J 1990 Prevalence of asymptomatic myocardial ischaemia in diabetic subjects. British Medical Journal 301: 92–95
Komrad M S, Coffey K S, McKinnis R, Massey E W, Califf R M 1984 Myocardial infarction and stroke. Neurology 34: 1403–1409
Kooistra T, Bosma P J, Tons H A M, van den Berg A P, Meyer P, Princen H M G 1989 Plasminogen activator inhibitor 1: Biosynthesis and mRNA level are increased by insulin in cultured human hepatocytes. Thrombosis and Haemostasis 62: 723–728
Kopecky S L, Gersh B J, McGoon M D et al 1985 The natural history of lone atrial fibrillation: a population-based study over three decades New England Journal of Medicine 317: 669–674
Koppensteiner R, Moritz A, Schlick W et al 1991 Blood rheology after cardiac valve replacement with mechanical prosthesis or bioprosthesis. American Journal of Cardiology 67: 79–83
Krolewski A S, Warram J H, Christlieb A R 1985 Onset, course, complications, and prognosis of diabetes mellitus. In: Marble A, Krall L P, Bradley R F, Christlieb A R, Soeldner J S (eds) Joslin's diabetes mellitus. Lea & Febiger, Philadelphia, p 251–277
Kruithof E K O, Tran-Thang C, Gudinchet A, Hauert J, Nicoloso G, Genton C, Wilti H, Bachmann F 1987 Fibrinolysis in pregnancy: a study of plasminogen activator inhibitors. Blood 69: 460–466
Krumholz H M 1989 The clinical challenges of myocardial infarction in the elderly. Western Journal of Medicine 151: 304–310
Kumagai K, Fukunami M, Ohmori M, Kitabatake A, Kamada T, Hoki N 1990 Increased intravascular clotting in patients with chronic atrial fibrillation. Journal of American College of Cardiologists 16: 377–380
Kutti J, Weinfeld A 1979 Platelet survival and platelet production in acute myocardial infarction. Acta Medica Scandinavica 205: 501–504
Laakso M, Sarlund H, Mykkänen L 1989 Essential hypertension and insulin resistance in non-insulin-dependent diabetes. European Journal of Clinical Investigation 19: 518–526
Lackner H, Merskey C 1960 Variation in fibrinolytic activity after acute myocardial infarction and after the administration of oral anticoagulant drugs and intravenous heparin. British Journal of Haematology 6: 402–413
Landin K, Tengborn L, Chmielewska J, von Schenck H, Smith U 1991 The acute effect of insulin on tissue plasminogen activator and plasminogen activator inhibitor in man. Thrombosis and Haemostasis 65: 130–133
Larsson B, Svärsudd K, Welin L, Wilhelmsen L, Björntorp P, Tibblin G 1984 Abdominal adipose tissue distribution, obesity, and risk of cardiovascular disease and death: 13 year follow-up of participants in the study of men born in 1913. British Medical Journal 288: 1401–1404
Latron Alessi M C, Anfosso F, Nalbone G, Lafont H, Juhan-Vague I 1990 Effect of low density lipoproteins on secretion of plasminogen activator inhibitor (PAI-1) by human endothelial cells and hepatoma cells. Fibrinolysis 4: 51–53
Lecander I, Astedt B 1989 Occurrence of a specific plasminogen activator inhibior of placental type, PAI-2, in men and non-pregnant women. Fibrinolysis 3: 27–30
Leeder S, Gliksman M 1990 Prospects for preventing heart disease. British Medical Journal 301: 1004–1005
Leibowitz J O 1970 The History of Coronary Heart Disease. Wellcome Institute of the History of Medicine, London
Levine S P, Lindenfeldt J, Ellis B, Raymond N M, Krentz L S 1981 Increased plasma concentrations of platelet factor 4 in coronary artery disease. Circulation 64: 626–632
Lie J T 1978 Centenary of the first correct antemortem diagnosis of coronary thrombosis by Adam Hasmmer (1818–1878). English translation of the original report. American Journal of Cardiology 42: 849–852
Liebow I M, Hellerstein H K, Miller M 1955 Arteriosclerotic heart disease in diabetes mellitus. American Journal of Medicine 18: 438–447
Lombardi R, Mannucci P M, Seghatchian M J, Vicente Gozcie V, Coppola L 1981. Alterations of Factor VIII von Willebrand Factor in clinical conditions associated with an increase in its plasma concentration. British Journal of Haematology 49: 61–68
Lorenzi M, Montisano D F, Toledo S, Barrieux A 1986 High glucose induces DNA damage in cultured human endothelial cells. Journal of Clinical Investigation 77: 322–325
Losito R, Gattiker H, Bilodeau G, Verville N, Longpré B 1981 Levels of antithrombin III, α-2-macroglobulin and alpha 1-antitrypsin in acute ischaemic heart disease. Journal of Laboratory and Clinical Medicine 97: 241–250
Lowe G D O, Drummond M M, Lorimer A R et al 1980 Relation between extent of coronary artery disease and blood viscosity British Medical Journal 1: 673–675
Lowe G D O Japp A J Forbes C D 1983 Relation of atrial fibrillation and high haematocrit in acute stroke. Lancet 1: 784–786
McCance D R, Hadden D R, Atkinson A B, Archer D B, Kennedy L 1989 Long-term glycaemic control and diabetic retinopathy. Lancet 2: 824–827
McCormick J, Skrabanek P 1988 Coronary heart disease is not preventable by population interventions. Lancet ii: 839–841
McDonald L, Edgill M 1957 Coagulability of the blood in ischaemic heart disease. Lancet ii: 457–460
Maiello M, Boeri D, Podesta F, Cagliero E, Vichi M, Odetti P, Adezati L, Lorenzi M 1992 Increased expression of tissue plasminogen activator and its inhibitor and reduced fibrinolytic potential of human endothelial cells cultured in elevated glucose. Diabetes 41: 1009–1015
Mann J M, Roberts W C 1988 Rupture of the left ventricular free wall during acute myocardial infarction: Analysis of 138 necropsy patients and comparison with 50 necropsy patients with acute myocardial infarction without rupture. American Journal of Cardiology 62: 847–859
Manson J E, Colditz G A, Stampfer M J et al 1991 A prospectlve study of maturity onset diabetes mellitus and risk of coronary heart disease and stroke in women. Archives of Internal Medicine 151: 1141–1147
Margulis T, David M, Maor N, Soff G A, Grenadier E, Palant A, Aghai E 1986 The von Willebrand factor in myocardial infarction and unstable angina: a kinetic study. Thrombosis and Haemostasis 55: 366–368
Martin J F, Plumb J, Kibley R S, Kishk Y T 1983a Changes in volume and density of platelets in myocardial infarction. British Medical Journal 287: 449–451
Martin J F, Trowbridge E A, Salmon G, Plumb J 1983b The biological significance of platelet volume: its relationship to bleeding time, platelet thromboxane B_2 production and megakaryocyte nuclear DNA concentration. Thrombosis Research 32: 443–460
Maseri A, L'Abbate A, Baroldi G et al 1978 Coronary vasospasm as a possible cause of myocardial infarction: a conclusion derived from the study of 'preinfarction' angina. New England Journal of Medicine 299: 1271–1277
Mayer G A 1964 Blood viscosity in healthy subjects and patients with coronary heart disease. Canadian Medical Association Journal 91: 951–654
Meade T W, Chakrabarti R, Haines A P, North W R S, Stirling Y, Thompson S G 1980 Haemostatic function and cardiovascular death: early results of a prospective study. Lancet 1: 1050–1053
Meade T W, Mellows S, Brozovic M et al 1986 Haemostatic function and ischaemic heart disease: principal results of the Northwick Park Heart Study. Lancet 2: 533–737
Mehta J, Mehta P, Lawson D, Saldeen T 1987 Plasma tissue plasminogen activator inhibitor levels in coronary artery disease: Correlation with age and serum triglyceride concentrations. Journal of the American College of Cardiology 9: 263–268
Michaels L 1966 Aetiology of coronary artery disease: an historical approach. British Heart Journal 28: 258–264
Mitchell J R A, Schwartz C J 1965 Arterial Disease. Blackwell, Oxford
Mizuno K, Miyamoto A, Satomura K et al 1991 Angioscopic coronary macromorphology in patients with acute coronary disorders. Lancet 337: 809–812
Modan M, Halkin L, Almog S et al 1985 Hyperinsulinaemia — A link between hypertension, obesity and glucose intolerance. Journal of Clinical Investigation 75: 805–817
Modan M, Halkin H, Or J, Karasik A, Drory Y, Fuchs Z, Lusky A, Chetrit A 1991 Hyperinsulinemia, gender and risk of atherosclerotic cardiovascular disease. Circulation 84: 1165–1175
Moller D E, Flier J S 1991 Insulin resistance — mechanisms,

syndromes and implications. New England Journal of Medicine 325: 938–948
Mombelli G, Im Hof V, Haeberli A, Straub P W 1984 Effect of heparin on plasma fibrinopeptide A in patients with acute myocardial infarction. Circulation 69: 684–689
Monnier V M, Cerami A 1983 Nonenzymatic glycosylation and browning of proteins in vivo. In: Waller G R, Feather M S (eds) The Maillard reaction in foods and nutrition. American Chemistry Society, Washington, p 431–439
Mordes D B, Lazarchick J, Colwell J A, Sens D A 1983 Elevated glucose concentrations increase factor VIIIR:Ag levels in human umbilical vein endothelial cells. Diabetes 32: 876–878
Multiple-Risk Factor Intervention Trial (MRFIT) Research Group 1982 Multiple-risk factor intervention trial: Risk factor changes in mortality results. Journal of the American Medical Association 248: 1465
Munkvad S, Jespersen J, Gram J, Kluft C 1990 Interrelationship between coagulant activity and tissue-type plasminogen activator (t-PA) system in acute ischaemic heart disease. Possible role of the endothelium. Journal of Internal Medicine 228: 361–366
Nankervis A, Proietto J, Aitken P, Alford F 1984 Impaired insulin action in newly diagnosed Type 1 (insulin-dependent) diabetes mellitus. Diabetologia 27: 497–503
Nawroth P P, Handley D A, Esmon C T, Stern D M 1986 Interleukin 1 induces endothelial cell procoagulant while suppressing cell-surface anticoagulant activity. Proceedings of the National Academy of Sciences, USA 83: 3460–3464
Neil H A W, Gatling W, Mather H M Thompson A V, Thorogood M, Fowler G H, Hill R D, Mann J 1987 The Oxford Community Diabetes Study: Evidence for an increase in the prevalence of the known diabetes in Great Britain. Diabetic Medicine 4: 539–543
Neri Serneri G G, Gensini G F, Abbate R, Mugnaini C, Favilla S, Brunelli C, Chierchia S, Parodi O 1981 Increased fibrinopeptide A formation and thromboxane A_2 production in patients with ischaemic heart disease: relationships to coronary pathoanatomy risk factors, and clinical manifestations. American Heart Journal 101: 185–194
Nicholls K, Mandel T E 1989 Advanced glycosylation end products in experimental murine diabetic nephropathy: effect of islet isografting and of aminoguanidine. Laboratory Investigation 60: 486–493
Nicolaides A N, Bowers R, Horbourne T, Kidner P H, Besterman E M 1977 Blood viscosity, red cell flexibility, haematocrit, and plasma-fibrinogen in patients with angina. Lancet ii: 943–945
Nicols A B, Owen J U, Kaplan K L, Sciacca R R, Cannon P J, Nossel H L 1982 Fibrinopeptide A, platelet factor 4 and beta thromboglobulin levels in coronary heart disease. Blood 60: 650
Nilsson J 1986 Growth factor and the pathogenesis of atherosclerosis. Atherosclerosis 62: 185–199
Nilsson T K, Johnson O 1987 The extrinsic fibrinolytic system in survivors of myocardial infarction. Thrombosis Research 48: 621–630
Obrastzow W P, Straschesko N D 1910 Zur Kenntnis der Thrombose der Koronararterien des Herzens. Zeitschrift fur Klinische Medizin 71: 116–132
Ogston D, Fullerton H W 1965 Plasma fibrinolytic activity following recent myocardial and cerebral infarction. Lancet 2: 99–101
Olefsky J M, Kolterman O G, Scarlett J A 1982 Insulin action and resistance in obesity and non-insulin-dependent type II diabetes mellitus. American Journal of Physiology 243: E15–E30
Oliva P B, Breckenridge J C 1977 Arteriographic evidence of coronary arterial spasm in acute myocardial infarction Circulation 56: 366–374
Oliver M F 1992 Doubts about preventing coronary heart disease. British Medical Journal 304: 393–394
O'Rourke R A, Chatterjee K, Wei J Y 1987 Atherosclerotic coronary heart disease in the elderly. Journal of the American College of Cardiology 10: 52A–56A
Osler W 1897 Lectures on angina pectoris and allied states. D Appleton, New York
Oswald G A, Corcoran S, Yudkin J S 1984 Prevalence and risks of hyperglycaemia and undiagnosed diabetes in patients with acute myocardial infarction. Lancet 1: 1264–1267
Pantley G A, Bristow J D 1984 Ischemic cardiomyopathy. Progress in Cardiovascular Disease 27: 95–114
Pau W H, Cedres L B, Liu K et al 1986 Relationship of clinical diabetes and asymptomatic hyperglycaemia to risk of coronary heart disease mortality In men and women. American Journal of Epidemiology 123: 504–516
Paramo J A, Colucci M, Collén D 1985 Plasminogen activator inhibitor in the blood of patients with coronary artery disease. British Medical Journal 291: 573–574
Paulsen E P, Koury M 1976 Hemoglobin $A1_C$ levels in insulin-dependent and independent diabetes mellitus. Diabetes 25 (suppl 2): 890
Petersen P, Hansen J M 1988 Stroke in thyrotoxicosis with atrial fibrillation. Stroke 19: 15–18
Petersen P, Boysen G, Godtfredsen J, Andersen E D, Andersen B 1989 Placebo controlled, randomised trial of warfarin and aspirin for prevention of thromboembolic complications in atrial fibrillation: the Copenhagen AFASAK study. Lancet 1: 175–179
Pollare T, Lithell H, Berne C 1990 Insulin resistance is a characteristic feature of primary hypertension independent of obesity. Metabolism 39: 167–174
Potter van Loon B J, de Bart A C W, Radder J K et al 1990 Acute exogenous hyperinsulinaemia does not result in elevation of plasma plasminogen activator inhibitor-1 (PAI-1) in humans. Fibrinolysis 4 (suppl 2): 93–94
Pyörälä K 1979 Relationship of glucose tolerance and plasma insulin to the incidence of coronary heart disease. Results from two population studies in Finland. Diabetes Care 2: 131–141
Pyörälä K, Savolainen E, Kaukula S, Haapakoski J 1985 Plasma insulin as coronary heart disease risk factor: Relationships to other risk factors and predictive value during 9½-year follow-up of the Helsinki Policemen Study population. Acta Medica Scandinavica 701 (suppl): 38–52
Pyörälä K, Laakso M, Uusitupa M 1987 Diabetes and atherosclerosis: An epidemiologic view. Diabetes Metabolism Reviews 3: 463–524
Qizilbash N, Jones L, Warlow C, Mann J 1991 Fibrinogen and lipid concentrations as risk factors for transient attacks and minor strokes British Medical Journal 303: 605–609
Quain R 1850 On fatty diseases of the heart. Medical Chirugica Transactions 33: 121–196
Radoff S, Vlassara H, Cerami A 1988 Characterisation of a solubilized cell-surface binding protein on macrophages specific for proteins modified non-enzymatically by advanced glycosylation end-products. Archives of Biochemistry and Biophysics 263: 418–423
Radoff S, Cerami A, Vlassara H 1990 Isolation of surface binding protein specific for advanced glycosylation end products from mouse macrophage-derived cell line RAW 264.7. Diabetes 39: 1510–1518
Randall T, Muir K, Mant D 1991 Choosing the preventive workload in general practice: practical application of the Coronary Prevention Group Guidelines and Dundee coronary risk-disk. British Medical Journal 305: 227–231
Ravnskov U 1992 Cholesterol lowering trials in coronary heart disease: frequency of citation and outcome. British Medical Journal 305: 15–19
Rawles J M, Marlow C, Ogston D 1975 Fibrinolytic capacity of arm and leg veins after femoral leg fracture and acute myocardial infarction. British Medical Journal 2: 61–62
Reaven G M 1988 Role of insulin resistance in human disease. Diabetes 37: 1595–1607
Reaven P D, Hoffman B B 1987 A role for insulin in the aetiology and course of hypertension? Lancet 2: 435–436
Rindfleisch G E 1872 Manual of pathological histology to serve as an introduction to the study of morbid anatomy, Baxter E B (trans). New Sydenham Society, London
Roberts W C, Buja L M 1972 The frequency and significance of coronary arterial thrombi and other observations in fatal acute myocardial infarction: a study of 107 necroscopy patients. American Journal of Medicine 52: 425–443
Röjel J 1959 A study of the fibrinolysin activity in thrombotic diseases. Acta Medica Scandinavica 164: 81–93
Rose G, Day S 1990 The population mean predicts the number of deviant individuals. British Medical Journal 301: 1031–1034
Rosenberg L, Kaufman D W, Helmrich S P, Shapiro S 1985 The risk of myocardial infarction after quitting smoking in men under 55 years of age. New England Journal of Medicine 313: 1511–1514
Rosenberg L, Palmer J R, Shapiro S 1990 Decline in the risk of

myocardial infarction among women who stop smoking. New England Journal of Medicine 322: 213–217
Rossouw J E, Lewis B, Rifkind B M 1990 The value of lowering cholesterol after myocardial infarction. New England Journal of Medicine 323: 1112–1119
Sakata K, Kurata C, Taguchi T et al 1989 The role of fibrinolytic system in acute myocardial infarction after normal exercise tests. European Heart Journal 10: 1118–1122
Sakata K, Kurata C, Taguchi T et al 1990 Clinical significance of plasminogen activator inhibitor activity in patients with exercise-induced ischemia. American Heart Journal 120: 831–838
Sawicki P T, Heinemann L, Starke A, Berger M 1992 Hyperinsulinaemia is not linked with blood pressure elevation in patients with insulinoma. Diabetologia 35: 649–652
Schwartz M B, Hawiger J, Timmons S, Friesinger G C 1980 Platelet aggregates in ischemic heart disease. Thrombosis and Haemostasis 43: 185–188
Shapira I, Isakov A, Burke M, Almog C H 1987 Cardiac rupture in patients with acute myocardial infarction. Chest 1987; 92: 219–223
Sherman C T, Litvack F, Grundfest W et al 1986 Coronary angioscopy in patients with unstable angina pectoris. New England Journal of Medicine 314: 913–919
Shresta N K, Moreno F L, Narciso F V, Torres L, Calleja H B 1983 Two-dimensional echocardiographic diagnosis of left atrial thrombus in rheumatic heart disease: a clinicopathologic study. Circulation 67: 341–347
Skehan J D, Carey C, Norrell M S et al 1989 Patterns of coronary artery disease in post-infarction ventricular septal rupture. British Heart Journal 62: 268–272
Smitherman T C, Milam M, Woo J, Wilerson J T, Frenkel E P 1981 Elevated beta thromboglobulin in peripheral venous blood patients with acute myocardial ischemia: direct evidence for enhanced platelet reactivity in vivo. American Journal of Cardiology 48: 395–402
Snow T R, Deal M T, Dickey D T, Esmon C T 1991 Protein C activation following coronary artery occlusion in the in situ porcine heart. Circulation 84: 293–299
Stafford W J, Petch J, Radford D J 1985 Vegetations in infective endocarditis: clinical relevance and diagnosis by cross-sectional echocardiography. British Heart Journal 53: 310–313
Staffurth J S, Gibberd M C, Tang Fui S N 1977 Arterial embolism in thyrotoxicosis with atrial fibrillation. British Medical Journal ii: 688–690
Stevenson W G, Linssen G C M, Havenith M G et al 1989 The spectrum of death after myocardial infarction: A necropsy study. American Heart Journal 118: 1182–1188
Stewart M E, Douglas J T, Lowe G D O, Prentice C R F M, Forbes C D 1983 Prognostic value of beta-thromboglobulin in patients with transient cerebral ischaemia. Lancet ii: 479–482
Stiko-Rahm A, Wiman B, Hamsten A, Nilsson J 1990 Secretion of plasminogen activator inhibitor 1 from cultured human umbilical vein endothelial cells is induced by very low density lipoprotein. Arteriosclerosis 10: 1067–1073
Stone M C, Thorp J M 1985 Plasma fibrinogen — a major coronary risk factor. Journal of the Royal College of General Practitioners 35: 565–569
Stout R W, Vallance-Owen J 1971 Insulin and atheroma. Lancet 1: 1078–1080
Stroke Prevention in Atrial Fibrillation Study Group Investigators 1990 Preliminary report of the Stroke Prevention in Atrial Fibrillation study. New England Journal of Medicine 322: 863–868
Sytkowski P A, Kannel W B, D'Agostino R B 1990 Changes in risk factors and the decline in mortality from cardiovascular disease. New England Journal of Medicine 322: 1635–1641
Tahara A, Yasuda M, Itagane H, Toda I, Teragaki M, Akioka K, Oku H, Takeuchi K, Takeda T, Bannai S, Takanashi N, Tsukada H 1991 Plasma levels of platelet-derived growth factor in normal subjects and patients with ischemic heart disease. American Heart Journal 122: 986–992
Thaulow E, Erikssen J, Sandvik L, Stormorken H, Cohn P F 1991 Blood platelet count and function are related to total and cardiovascular death in apparently health men. Circulation 84: 613–617
Tofler G H, Muller J E, Stone P H et al 1989 Pericarditis in acute myocardial infarction: Characterization and clinical significance. American Heart Journal 117: 86–92
Tunstall-Pedoe H 1991 The Dundee coronary risk-disk for management of change in risk factors. British Medical Journal 303: 744–747
Vague J 1956 The degree of masculine differentiation of obesities. A factor determining predisposition to diabetes, atherosclerosis, gout and uric calculous disease. American Journal of Clinical Nutrition 4: 20–28
Vague P, Juhan-Vague I, Aillaud M F, Badier C, Viard R, Alessi M C, Collén D 1986 Correlation between blood fibrinolytic activity, plasminogen activator inhibitor level, plasma insulin level and relative body weight in normal and obese subjects. Metabolism 2: 250–253
Vandekerckhove Y, Baele G, DePuydt H, Weyne A, Clement D 1988 Plasma tissue plasminogen activator levels in patients with coronary heart disease. Thrombosis Research 50: 449–453
van Hinsbergh V W M, Kooistra T, van de Berg E A et al 1988 Tumour necrosis factor increases the production of plasminogen activator inhibitor in human endothelial cells in vitro and in rats in vivo. Blood 72(5): 1467–1473
Verheugt F W, ten Cate J W, Sturk A et al 1987 Tissue plasminogen activator activity and inhibition in acute myocardial infarction and angiographically normal coronary arteries. American Journal of Cardiology 59: 1075–1079
Vilen L, Johansson S, Kutti J, Cronberg S, Vedin A, Wilhelmsson C 1985 ADP-induced platelet aggregation in young female survivors of acute myocardial infarction and their female controls. Acta Medica Scandinavica 217: 9–13
Vlassara H, Brownlee M, Cerami A 1986 Novel macrophage receptor for glucose-modified proteins is distinct from previously described scavenger receptors. Journal of Experimental Medicine 164: 1301–1309
Vlassara H, Brownlee M, Cerami A 1988a Specific macrophage receptor activity for advanced glycosylation end products inversely correlates with insulin levels in vivo. Diabetes 37: 456–461
Vlassara H, Brownlee M, Manogue K R, Dinarello C A, Pasagian A 1988b Cachectin/TNF and IL-1 induced by glucose-modified proteins: role in normal tissue remodelling. Science 240: 1546–1548
Vlassara H, Brownlee M, Cerami A 1989a Macrophage receptor-mediated processing and regulation of advanced glycosylation end product (AGE)-modified proteins: role in diabetes and aging. Diabetes and Nutrition 205–218
Vlassara H, Moldawer L, Chan B 1989b Macrophage/monocyte receptor for nonenzymatically glycosylated proteins is upregulated by cachectin/tumour necrosis factor. Journal of Clinical Investigation 84: 1813–1820
Walker I D, Davidson J F, Hutton I, Lawrie T D V 1977 Disordered 'fibrinolytic potential' in coronary heart disease. Thrombosis Research 10: 509–520
Waller B F, Palumbo P J, Lie J T, Roberts W C 1980 Status of the coronary arteries at necropsy in diabetes mellitus with onset after age 30 yrs. Analysis of 229 diabetic patients with and without clinical evidence of coronary heart disease and comparison to 183 control subjects. American Journal of Medicine 69: 498–506
Walmsley D, Hampton K K, Grant P J 1991 Contrasting fibrinolytic responses in Type 1 (insulin-dependent) and Type 2 (non-insulin-dependent) diabetes. Diabetic Medicine 8: 954–959
Wei J Y, Buckley B H 1982 Myocardial infarction before aged 36 years in women: Predominance of apparent nonatherosclerotic events. American Heart Journal 104: 561
Weinrich D J, Burke J F, Pauletto F J 1984 Left ventricular mural thrombi complicating acute myocardial infarction: long term follow-up with serial echocardiography. Annals of Internal Medicine 100: 789–794
Welborn T A, Weame K 1979 Coronary heart disease incidence and cardiovascular mortality in Busselton with reference to glucose and insulin concentrations. Diabetes Care 2: 154–160
Welin L, Eriksson H, Larsson B, Ohlson L-O, Svärdsudd K, Tibblin G 1992 Hyperinsulinaemia is not a major coronary risk factor in elderly men. Diabetologia 35: 766–770
White P D 1971 Perspectives. Progress in Cardiovascular Diseases 14: 250–255
Wilhelmsen L, Svärdsudd K, Korsan-Bengsten K, Welin L, Tibblin G

1984 Fibrinogen as a risk factor for stroke and myocardial infarction. New England Journal of Medicine 311: 501–505
Willett W C, Green A, Stampfer M J et al 1987 Relative and absolute excess risks of coronary heart disease among women who smoke cigarettes. New England Journal of Medicine 317: 1303–1309
Wolf P A, Abbott R D, Kannel W B 1987 Atrial fibrillation: a major contributor to stroke in the elderly: the Framingham Study. Archives of Internal Medicine 147: 1561–1564
Wood E H, Prentice C R M, McNicol G P 1972 Association of fibrinogen-fibrin related antigen (FR-antigen) with post-operative deep vein thrombosis and systemic complications. Lancet i: 166–196
Wooley C F, Baba N, Kilman J W, Ryan J M 1974 Thrombotic calcific mitral stenosis. Circulation 49: 1167–1174
Working Group of the Coronary Prevention Group and the British Heart Foundation 1991 An action plan for preventing coronary heart disease in primary care. British Medical Journal 308: 748–750
Yakihashi S, Kamijo M, Baba M, Yakihashi N, Nagai K 1992 Effect of aminoguanidine on functional and structural abnormalities in peripheral nerve of SATZ-induced diabetic rats. Diabetes 41: 47–52
Yano K, Reed S M, McGee D L 1984 Ten year incidence of coronary heart disease in the Honolulu-heart program. Relationship to biologic and lifestyle characteristics. American Journal of Epidemiology 119: 653
Yarnell J W G, Baker I A, Sweetnam P M et al 1991 Fibrinogen, viscosity, and white blood cell count are major risk factors for ischemic heart disease. The Caerphilly and Speedwell Collaborative Heart Disease Studies. Circulation 83: 836–844
Zahavi J, Kakkar V V 1980 β-Thromboglobulin — a specific marker of in vivo platelet release reaction. Thrombosis and Haemostasis 44: 23–29
Zalewski A, Shi Y, Nardone D, Bravette B, Weinstock P, Fischman D, Wilson P, Goldberg S, Levin D C, Bjornsson T D 1991 Evidence for reduced fibrinolytic activity in unstable angina at rest. Clinical, Biochemical and Angiographic correlates. Circulation 83: 1685–1691

55. Acute ischaemic stroke and transient ischaemic attacks

R. I. Lindley   C. P. Warlow

Stroke is the major cause of serious physical disability and the third most common cause of death in developed countries. Transient ischaemic attacks (TIAs) are less frequent but important to identify because appropriate medical and surgical treatment reduce the risk of subsequent stroke and coronary events. In the absence of any proven treatment for the vast majority of acute stroke patients, prevention is of particular importance. Since the early 1980s progress has been made in understanding the heterogeneous mechanisms causing the acute stroke syndrome and the qualitative similarities between minor ischaemic stroke and TIAs: anything which causes a TIA will, if prolonged cause an ischaemic stroke, whilst anything causing an ischaemic stroke will, if reversed quickly enough, cause merely a TIA.

DEFINITIONS

Research and clinical practice have been hampered by varying use of the terms 'stroke', 'transient ischaemic attack' and 'ischaemic or thrombotic stroke'. The following standardized definitions will reduce ambiguity and should be used in routine clinical practice.

Stroke. Formerly known as a cerebrovascular accident. Rapidly developing signs of focal, and at times global (applied to patients in deep coma and to those with subarachnoid haemorrhage) loss of cerebral function, with symptoms lasting more than 24 hours, or leading to death, with no apparent cause other than that of vascular origin (adapted from Hatano 1976).

Ischaemic stroke. Sometimes incorrectly called thrombotic stroke. When intracerebral haemorrhage has been excluded by a computerized tomographic (CT) scan, within 2 weeks of the onset, a stroke is presumed to be due to cerebral ischaemia causing infarction. CT is normal in the first few hours of ischaemic strokes and in some patients, e.g. many brainstem or lacunar infarcts, remains so.

Transient ischaemic attack. An acute loss of focal cerebral or monocular function with symptoms lasting less than 24 hours and which, after adequate investigation, is presumed to be due to embolic or thrombotic vascular disease (Warlow & Morris 1982).

THE CAUSES OF ISCHAEMIC STROKE AND TRANSIENT ISCHAEMIC ATTACK

Cerebral ischaemia and infarction are caused by acute occlusion of an artery supplying the brain or, less often, by low flow distal to an occluded or highly stenosed artery. Atherothromboembolism is by far the most common cause of ischaemic stroke, with haematological disorders, trauma and a variety of miscellaneous disorders the cause of the remainder.

Disorders of arteries

A large number of arterial diseases can cause stroke and these are listed in Table 55.1.

Atherothromboembolism

Thrombosis and embolism complicating atheromatous arterial disease is the most frequent cause of cerebral ischaemia. Atheroma arises at points of high levels of haemodynamic stress and turbulence, typically sites of arterial branching, tortuosity and confluence (e.g. carotid bifurcation, carotid syphon and basilar artery respectively) (Fig. 55.1). Atheromatous plaques are not static; platelet adhesion, activation and aggregation promote the formation of fibrin platelet thrombus which may propagate, embolize or resolve by fibrinolytic processes (Ross 1986). Atheromatous plaques probably become active as a result of fissuring or intraplaque haemorrhage, and then heal, at least temporarily, so atherothromboembolism can be considered as an acute-on-chronic disease. This concept would explain why TIAs tend to occur in clusters, for stroke to occur early after a TIA (and to affect the same arterial territory) (Hankey et al 1991) and for presumed artery-to-artery embolic stroke to recur early (Bamford et al 1991).

Table 55.1 Causes of arterial disease

Atheroma	
Arteritis	
	Giant cell arteritis
	Systemic lupus erythematosus
	Granulomatous angiitis
	Polyarteritis nodosa
	Wegener's granulomatosis
	Sarcoid angiitis
	Behçet's disease
	Scleroderma
	Rheumatoid disease
	Sjogren's syndrome
	Relapsing polychondritis
	Rheumatic fever
	Takayasu's disease
	Malignant atrophic papulosis (Kohlmeier-Degos disease)
Trauma	
	Penetrating injuries of the neck
	Blow to the neck
	Cervical manipulation
	Yoga
	Cervical rib
	'Whiplash' injury
	Tonsillectomy
	Strangulation
	Atlanto-axial dislocation
	Fractured clavicle
	Angiography
Dissection	
	Trauma
	Cystic medial necrosis
	Atheroma
	Marfan's syndrome
	Fibromuscular dysplasia
	Inflammatory arterial disease
	Ehlers–Danlos syndrome
	Pseudo-xanthoma elasticum
Congenital	
	Fibromuscular dysplasia
	Loops, coils, etc.
	Aneurysms
Infections	
	Tonsillitis, pharyngitis
	Cervical lymphadenitis
	Endarteritis obliterans due to:
	TB
	Syphilis
	Meningitis (bacterial or fungal)
	Herpes zoster
	Mucormycosis
Miscellaneous	
	Homocystinuria
	Neoplastic invasion of arteries
	Irradiation
	Fabry's disease
	Inflammatory bowel disease
	Mitochondrial cytopathy
	Drug abuse

Microatheroma or lipohyalinosis are terms given to a distinct small vessel arteriopathy which is thought to cause lacunar infarction, a quarter of all new cases of cerebral infarction are lacunar (Fisher 1969, 1979, Bamford & Warlow 1988). These small infarcts are found within the basal ganglia, thalamus, internal capsule and pons. The muscle and elastin in the wall of the small perforating arteries are replaced by collagen, there is subintimal hyalinization, and the vessel becomes tortuous, perhaps with the formation of microaneurysms (Charcot–Bouchard aneurysms) which may rupture. Lacunar infarction is thought to arise when this arteriopathy is complicated by in situ thrombosis. Small deep haemorrhages occur when the microaneurysms rupture, but this is much less frequent than infarction.

Trauma

The carotid arteries are vulnerable to injury, laceration and dissection. Intimal tears can lead directly to occlusion, or indirectly as a consequence of complicating thrombus with or without embolism (Pozzati et al 1989). Whilst direct blows to the neck are more likely to injure the carotid artery, rotational and hyperextension injuries are associated with vertebral artery injury (Sherman et al 1981). The increasing use of subclavian intravenous lines is an important cause of arterial trauma in hospital patients receiving chemotherapy or intensive monitoring, and can lead to stroke.

Dissection

Dissection of the neck arteries is usually due to trauma. Ischaemic stroke or ipsilateral pain (around the eye, face, neck) and Horner's syndrome, perhaps with a cervical bruit, can be the presenting features, but the dissection may be subclinical (Mokri et al 1986).

Fibromuscular dysplasia

Fibromuscular dysplasia is a rare segmental arterial disorder of unknown cause and affects small and medium sized vessels (Luscher et al 1987). It usually affects more than one artery in the same individual and is most common in the renal arteries causing hypertension. Histologically there is fibrosis and thickening of the arterial wall alternating with atrophy so that the typical angiographic appearance is likened to a 'string of beads'. The natural history is unknown and treatment with anticoagulants or arterial dilatation is entirely empirical.

Moya-moya syndrome

Moya-moya syndrome is a rare disorder almost confined to the Japanese and other Orientals. It describes a particular pattern of occlusion or stenosis of arteries at the base of the brain. In Japanese 'moya moya' means a haze, like a puff of smoke, which describes the fine anastomotic branches which develop as a consequence of the arterial occlusions (Chen et al 1988). The syndrome usually presents in infancy with recurrent cerebral ischaemia and infarction but mental retardation, headache, seizures and occasionally involuntary movements also have been re-

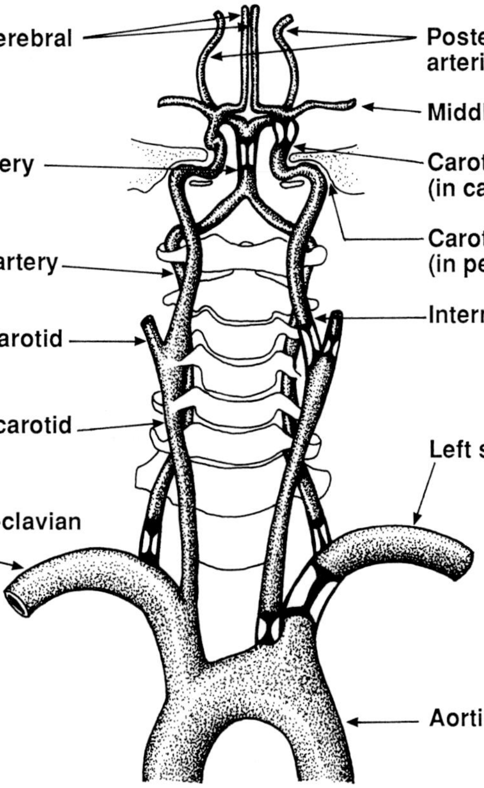

Fig. 55.1 The arterial blood supply to the brain showing sites commonly affected by atherothrombosis.

ported. In adults the presentation is more often with subarachnoid or primary intracerebral haemorrhage because of rupture of the fine collaterals which have presumably been present for many years. For most cases the cause is unknown (Bruno et al 1988) but some are congenital and others due to arterial narrowing and obstruction as a result of basal meningeal or nasopharyngeal infection, vasculitis, irradiation, trauma, fibromuscular dysplasia, tuberous sclerosis or neurofibromatosis.

Embolism from the heart (Table 55.2)

There is no doubt that emboli arising from within the heart, or passing through it from the venous system via a septal defect can reach the brain, eye and elsewhere to cause ischaemic stroke, retinal infarction and TIAs. There are a large number of potential cardiac sources of emboli (Table 55.2), most of which can be easily identified with modern non-invasive technology (see p. 1262). The real problem is deciding whether an identified *potential* embolic source is *the* source; particularly when it is common in apparently normal people (e.g. mitral valve prolapse, patent foramen ovale), or when an elderly person is affected and who might also have significant atheroma affecting the cerebral circulation (de Bono & Warlow 1981), or when the stroke is lacunar and rather unlikely to be caused by embolism from the heart or extracranial arteries. In developed countries about 20% of ischaemic stroke and

Table 55.2 Sources of embolism from the heart in anatomical sequence

Paradoxical embolism from the venous system
Pulmonary arteriovenous malformation
Atrial septal defect
Patent foramen ovale
Left atrium
Thrombus (particularly if atrial fibrillation present)
Myxoma
Sino-atrial disease
Interatrial septal aneurysm
Mitral valve
Infective endocarditis
Rheumatic endocarditis
Non-bacterial thrombotic endocarditis
Prosthetic valve
Mitral annulus calcification
Mitral leaflet prolapse
Left ventricle
Thrombosis secondary to:
Myocardial infarction
Left ventricular aneurysm
Dilating cardiomyopathy
Myxoma
Aortic valve
Infective endocarditis
Rheumatic endocarditis
Non-bacterial thrombotic endocarditis
Prosthetic valve
Sclerosis/calcification
Syphilis
Congenital cardiac disorders
Cardiac surgery
Air embolism
Platelet/fibrin embolism

TIAs are due to embolism from the heart, the most common cause being atrial fibrillation with presumed, but seldom proven, thrombus in the left atrium (Nishide et al 1983, Kittner et al 1990).

Emboli can consist of various combinations of mostly fibrin (atrial fibrillation), platelets (mitral leaflet prolapse), calcium (mitral annulus calcification), tumour (myxoma) and infected vegetations (infective endocarditis) (de Bono 1982). The emboli vary in size so they may impact in a medium sized artery to cause a substantial infarct (e.g. the origin of the middle cerebral artery) or in a small artery to cause a more restricted defect (e.g. a branch of the central retinal artery). Some emboli, like other causes of cerebral ischaemia, may be completely asymptomatic.

Atrial fibrillation carries an increased risk of embolic stroke which is substantially reduced by antithrombotic therapy (Hart 1992). The five completed randomized primary prevention trials in non-rheumatic atrial fibrillation (Petersen et al 1989, Boston Area Anticoagulation Trial for Atrial Fibrillation Investigators 1990, Connolly et al 1991, Ezekowitz et al 1991, Stroke Prevention in Atrial Fibrillation Investigators 1991) provided convincing evidence that warfarin anticoagulation reduces the risk of stroke from about 5% to 2% per year. In the trials the overall risk of serious bleeding was low (0.5–2.1% per year) for these intensively monitored group of patients. Decisions about long-term anticoagulation, therefore, should be considered if the local availability of anticoagulation monitoring is satisfactory. Aspirin also reduces stroke risk but there is still uncertainty whether it is as effective as warfarin (Hart 1992); ongoing trials are addressing this issue.

There is an increased risk of cardioembolic stroke after myocardial infarction, especially associated with left ventricular mural thrombosis complicating anterior infarction (Hart 1992). The increasing use of thrombolytic therapy does not appear to have affected the overall risk of stroke, the anticipated increase in haemorrhagic stroke being offset by the reduction in ischaemic stroke (ISIS-2 Collaborative Group 1988, Maggioni et al 1991). Aspirin treatment significantly reduces the risk of non-fatal stroke (ISIS-2 Collaborative Group 1988).

The intensity of anticoagulation remains uncertain for many of the accepted indications (e.g. for mechanical prosthetic heart valves, rheumatic valve disease). For certain cardiac abnormalities, such as atrial septal aneurysms and mitral valve prolapse, there is considerable uncertainty whether anticoagulation has any place at all in routine management (Hart 1992).

Antithrombotic treatment is not a panacea for all cardioembolic conditions, some problems are best dealt with by other means (e.g. surgery for atrial myxoma or antibiotics for infective endocarditis).

Haematological disorders (Table 55.3)

Table 55.3 Haematological causes of ischaemic stroke

Sickle cell disease
Polycythaemia
Essential thrombocythaemia
Leukaemia
Thrombotic thrombocytopenic purpura
Paroxysmal nocturnal haemoglobinuria
Disseminated intravascular coagulation
Hyperviscosity syndrome
Paraproteinaemias
'Hypercoagulability'

Polycythaemia rubra vera. This may be complicated by transient ischaemic attacks, cerebral infarction, intracranial venous thrombosis and intracranial haemorrhage (Silverstein et al 1962, Pearson & Wetherley-Mein 1978). This is because the platelet count is raised and possibly platelet activity enhanced, and because of increased whole blood viscosity. Intracranial haemorrhage is due to the defective platelet function.

Relative polycythaemia. The resultant increase in haematocrit may be a risk factor for stroke (p. 1261).

Essential thrombocythaemia. Idiopathic primary thrombocytosis, like polycythaemia rubra vera, is associated not only with thrombotic complications but intracranial haemorrhage as a result of the abnormal platelet function (Preston et al 1979, Jabaily et al 1983).

Leukaemia. Leukaemia and chemotherapy are more commonly a cause of intracranial haemorrhage (because of the haemostatic defect) than cerebral venous or arterial occlusion which can occur as a result of the increased whole blood viscosity or the complications of central intravenous line insertion.

Sickle cell disease. This may be complicated by cerebral infarction or, sometimes, intracranial haemorrhage (Wood 1978, Adams et al 1988, Pavlakis et al 1988). The patients are usually homozygous children, although sometimes a sickle cell crisis can be provoked by hypoxia in an adult heterozygote (Greenberg & Massey 1985). Stroke may also complicate haemoglobin SC disease (Fabian & Peters 1984). Small and large arteries, as well as veins, become occluded by thrombi which develop as a result of the abnormally rigid red blood cells and raised whole blood viscosity, thrombocytosis, impaired fibrinolytic activity and perhaps vessel wall changes as well.

Anaemia. Anaemia is the cause of rather non-specific neurological symptoms (such as faintness, poor concentration, tiredness and general malaise) but can cause transient ischaemic attacks if associated with severe extracranial occlusive arterial disease (Siekert et al 1960, Shahar & Sadeh 1991).

Paraproteinaemias. Neurological symptoms are caused by three mechanisms: anaemia as a result of defective erythropoiesis (see above), a haemostatic defect due to reduced platelet number, and the hyperviscosity syndrome. The hyperviscosity syndrome is characterized by headache, drowsiness, poor concentration and visual blurring (Somer 1987). Fundoscopy may reveal dilatation and tortuosity of the veins, venous occlusions, papilloedema and retinal haemorrhages. Either arterial or venous occlusion can cause cerebral infarction, and at postmortem the microcirculation is occluded with acidophilic material thought to be precipitates of the abnormal proteins. The majority of these patients can be identified with simple blood tests (see Table 55.4) because most have a raised erythrocyte sedimentation rate.

Paroxysmal nocturnal haemoglobinuria. Serious thrombotic complications can affect the brain and elsewhere. Cerebral infarction can be due to arterial or venous thrombosis. Most patients are anaemic at neurological presentation (Forman et al 1984).

Thrombotic thrombocytopenic purpura (TTP). Most commonly, this presents with a global encephalopathy on the background of systemic malaise, fever, skin purpura and proteinuria. Haemorrhagic infarcts due to platelet microthrombi occur in many organs including the brain where they can cause stroke-like episodes (Ridolfi & Bell 1981, Silverstein 1968). The differential diagnosis includes systemic lupus erythematosus, infective endocarditis, idiopathic thrombocytopenia, non-bacterial thrombotic endocarditis and disseminated intravascular coagulation.

Disseminated intravascular coagulation. Again, this is more commonly a cause of an encephalopathic illness but stroke can occur due to haemorrhagic cerebral infarction and primary intracranial haemorrhage (Schwartzman & Hill 1982). The differential diagnosis includes nonbacterial thrombotic endocarditis, cerebral hypoxia, hepatic failure and uraemia.

Hypercoagulability. This is much discussed, difficult to define, and very seldom implicated as a cause for cerebral infarction. Antithrombin III deficiency, protein S deficiency (Engesser et al 1987) and protein C deficiency (Vieregge et al 1989) are rare causes of peripheral venous thrombosis (usually recurrent and often with a family history) and even rarer causes of arterial thrombosis.

Miscellaneous causes: pregnancy and the puerperium. Stroke complicates the last trimester of pregnancy and the puerperium in no more than 30 per 100 000 deliveries in developed countries (Wiebers & Mokri 1985), rather more often in India (Srinivasan 1983). The causes and mechanisms have not been well studied but certainly include intracranial venous thrombosis: acute middle cerebral artery or other large artery occlusion, perhaps due to paradoxical embolism from the leg veins (Cross et al 1968); intracranial haemorrhage due to eclampsia (Richards et al 1988) or anticoagulants; rupture of a pre-existing aneurysm or vascular malformation; arterial dissection during labour (Wiebers & Mokri 1985); and DIC or boundary zone infarction complicating obstetric disasters. Metastases of choriocarcinoma can present with stroke-like episodes and on CT can look remarkably like primary intracerebral haemorrhages.

The risk of stroke in a future pregnancy is of crucial interest but is unknown. Presumably if no underlying cause is found for the first stroke, the risk of recurrence must be low.

EPIDEMIOLOGY

Incidence of stroke and TIA

The annual incidence of stroke in Europe and the United States is between one and two per 1000 population. Rates depend on the age of the population because of the dramatic increase in incidence with increasing age. In males there is an excess of stroke of about one third (Bamford et al 1988, Ricci et al 1991a). A major problem in stroke research and clinical practice has been the imprecise labelling of 'stroke' into ischaemic and haemorrhagic (subarachnoid haemorrhage and primary intracerebral haemorrhage) subgroups. Variations in case ascertainment and investigation in numerous epidemiological studies have led to different figures for the percentage of all strokes which are ischaemic. Varying admission and referral patterns of stroke patients can cause substantial variations in the percentage of haemorrhagic strokes in hospital-based series. Population-based surveys are more reliable; in the study from Oxfordshire, England, the proportion of first ever strokes by pathological type was: cerebral infarction 80%; primary intracerebral haemorrhage 10%; subarachnoid haemorrhage 5%; uncertain type 5% (Bamford et al 1990). Other studies are illustrated in Figure 55.2; the proportion of pathological type of stroke appears very similar, even in Japan.

The methodological problems in measuring the incidence of TIAs are greater than with stroke, due to the lack of standardized definitions in the past, the wide differential diagnosis to consider (see p. 1262), and the fact that TIAs may simply never come to medical attention. Many incidence studies have relied on retrospective hospital record review, but by excluding patients not seen in hospital, a third to a half of all TIA patients may have been missed thus underestimating the true incidence (Dennis et al 1989, Ricci et al 1991b). The community studies have explained the reason for the marked male predominance in *hospitalized* TIA patients; TIAs are nearly three times more common in men than women in middle age, and middle-aged patients are more likely to be referred to hospital than the elderly where there is little sex difference in incidence. All incidence studies, whether hospital or community based, depend on patients reporting their symptoms to a doctor, and it is unknown how many TIAs are never reported, or at least not until a stroke occurs. Thus even the community TIA incidence rate of about 0.4 per 1000 per year must be an underestimate, but at least reflects the size of the problem which presents to, and can be influenced by, medical care (Dennis et al 1989, Ricci et al 1991b).

Risk factors

Age is the strongest risk factor for TIA, cerebral infarc-

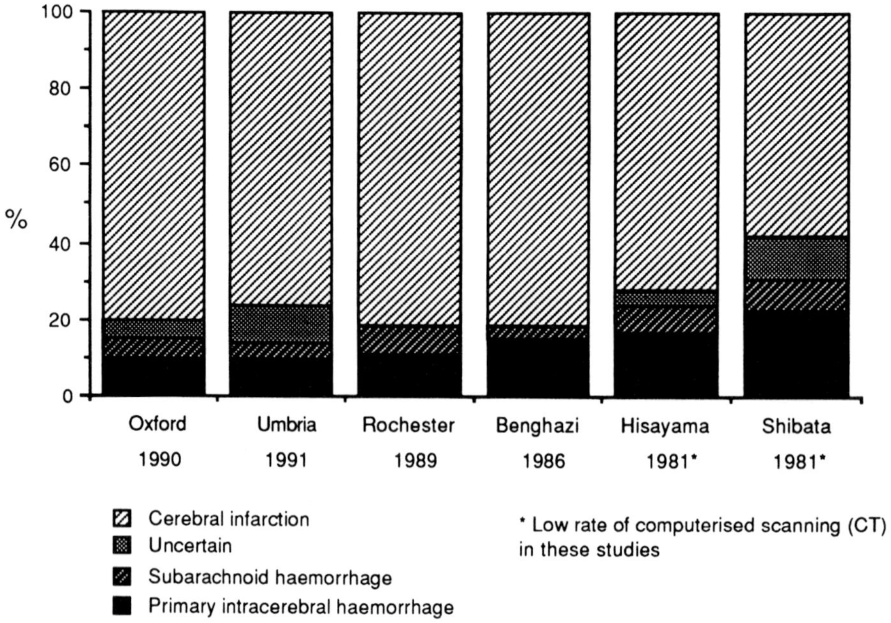

Fig. 55.2 Cause of first stroke by pathological type in community studies. Rochester included 'uncertain' strokes with cerebral haemorrhage. (Figures taken from Tanaka et al 1981, Ueda et al 1981, Ashok et al 1986, Broderick et al 1989, Bamford et al 1990, Ricci et al 1991a,b.)

tion, primary intracerebral haemorrhage and sub-arachnoid haemorrhage (Dennis et al 1989, Bamford et al 1990) and almost certainly for subtypes of cerebral infarction (e.g. lacunar infarction) (Bamford et al 1987). For example, the risk of stroke in people aged about 80 is 25 times that in people aged about 50. Like TIAs, the excess of stroke in men is most marked in middle age (but modest in size) and disappears in the elderly. This is a curious contrast to the large excess of men affected by peripheral vascular disease and coronary heart disease, also due to atheroma.

Increasing blood pressure is strongly associated with subsequent stroke risk, furthermore the concept that there is a 'threshold' of 'normal blood pressure' below which the risk of stroke remains constant has been challenged. A recent epidemiological overview has suggested that even within the diastolic blood pressure range of 70–110 mmHg, the lower the blood pressure the lower the risk of stroke. This implies that whether a patient is conventionally 'hypertensive' or 'normotensive' a lower blood pressure would eventually confer a lower risk of stroke (MacMahon et al 1990). Treatment of hypertension certainly reduces stroke risk in individuals (Collins et al 1990), but probably only contributes a small percentage to the overall reduction in stroke incidence in the community (Bonita & Beaglehole 1986). A population strategy to shift the entire blood pressure distribution curve downwards by about 5 mmHg would have a greater effect on stroke incidence than any policy based only on the treatment of high risk 'hypertensive' individuals (Rose 1981).

Coronary heart disease is clearly associated with stroke. The evidence comes from postmortem (Kagan 1976, Stemmermann et al 1984), case-control (Friedman et al 1968, Herman et al 1983, Woo et al 1991) and cohort studies (Kannel et al 1983). Rather surprisingly, data from Rochester, Minnesota, suggest that most of this association is causal (i.e. embolism from left ventricular thrombus complicating myocardial infarction) rather than due to the coincidence of atheroma in the coronary and cerebral circulation in the same (predisposed) individuals (Dexter et al 1987).

In developed countries, the most frequent *potential* cardiac source of embolism to the brain is atrial fibrillation (AF), usually 'non-rheumatic'. Both non-rheumatic, and even more so rheumatic AF, have been associated with stroke from postmortem evidence (Aberg 1969, Hinton et al 1977); case-control studies (Friedman et al 1968, Petersen et al 1987, Kempster et al 1988); and cohort studies (Wolf et al 1978, Flegel et al 1987). 'Lone' atrial fibrillation seems still to be a risk factor, albeit a weak one (Brand et al 1985). Some of the association of AF with stroke must be causal because clot undoubtedly can form in the fibrillating atrium and embolize but a coincidental association must also occur as AF can be caused by other potent risk factors for stroke (e.g. hypertension and coronary heart disease).

Smoking is a risk factor for subarachnoid haemorrhage and cerebral infarction, but there appears to be no association with primary intracerebral haemorrhage (Shinton & Beevers 1989).

Whilst lipids are an accepted risk factor for coronary heart disease, the association with stroke is less clear but almost certainly does exist (Qizilbash et al 1991, 1992). This contrast between cardiovascular and cerebrovascular disease is surprising and may be due to lipid levels being less associated with vascular events in the elderly (who are at greatest risk of stroke); lack of statistical power in cohort studies which have mostly been concerned with coronary events rather than strokes; or, perhaps, because cholesterol is negatively associated with intracranial haemorrhage which obscures any positive association with cerebral infarction in studies which have concentrated on all strokes (Tanaka et al 1982, Iso et al 1989). Other risk factors are diabetes mellitus, peripheral vascular disease, left ventricular hypertrophy, cervical bruits, and excessive alcohol intake (greater than 300 g a week).

Haematological factors

The strongest haematological variable associated with stroke is plasma fibrinogen (Wilhelmsen 1984, Kannel et al 1987, Schneidau et al 1989). This association is attenuated by cigarette smoking, hypertension and other confounding variables, but has consistently been shown to be an independent variable in multivariate analysis (Wilhelmsen 1984). It is possible that the adverse effect of smoking is mediated, at least in part, by a raised fibrinogen and thus accelerated thrombosis. However, it is not certain that raised plasma fibrinogen is causally related to stroke. Stopping smoking and treating hypertension are probably the most potent methods to reduce fibrinogen levels, at least at the present time.

Plasma factor VII coagulant activity is an independent risk factor for coronary heart disease but there are no data for stroke (Meade et al 1986). Other coagulation, fibrinolytic and platelet parameters have not consistently been associated with the risk of vascular disease.

The haematocrit is an important factor in cerebral blood flow but any effects of increasing haematocrit on the risk of stroke are weak and confounded by cigarette smoking, blood pressure and plasma fibrinogen (Kannel et al 1972).

TRANSIENT ISCHAEMIC ATTACKS

Pathophysiology

Most TIAs are presumed to be due to embolism from proximal arterial sites or from the heart, or to thrombotic occlusion of the arteries supplying the brain or eye. Angiographic studies of TIA patients suggest that embolism from atherothrombosis of the carotid bifurcation is the most common cause of symptoms, with up to 50% of patients with carotid territory attacks having significant stenosis of the symptomatic artery (Pessin et al 1977, Harrison & Marshall 1985, Bogousslavsky et al 1986). Evidence from the 'European Carotid Surgery Trial Collaborative Group' (1991) confirmed that the vast majority of later ischaemic strokes ipsilateral to the originally symptomatic internal carotid artery are the direct result of the carotid stenosis, and thus due to embolism and/or low blood flow. There are now imaging studies which suggest that some TIAs have in fact been due to small cerebral infarcts, this is not surprising since there is no qualitative difference between TIAs and ischaemic stroke (Dennis et al 1990a).

Diagnosis

As most patients are not seen during their TIA, the history obtained from the patient (and witness) is vitally important. However, even experienced neurologists can disagree about the diagnosis (Kraaijeveld et al 1984). The interobserver variability can be improved by recording the patients' symptoms in ordinary language and by using check lists of the common symptoms and standardized diagnostic criteria (Koudstaal et al 1986).

The onset of a TIA is characteristically abrupt, which helps differentiate the attack from migraine or partial seizures where there is a progression or 'march' of symptoms. It is useful to try and localize symptoms to the carotid or vertebrobasilar circulation because patients with carotid TIAs and carotid stenosis need to be considered for carotid endarterectomy (p. 1269).

Transient monocular blindness (amaurosis fugax), a carotid distribution TIA, is due to retinal ischaemia. These attacks are described as a sudden blindness in one eye, or like a shutter coming up or down obscuring the vision. They tend to be brief, lasting less than 5 minutes. If transient monocular blindness due to retinal ischaemia is witnessed, it is sometimes possible to see emboli moving in the retinal vessels. More often, asymptomatic cholesterol emboli are seen lodged in the retinal arteries after the event.

Other carotid TIAs present with various combinations of contralateral weakness of the face, arm, hand and leg. Dysphasia can occur if the dominant hemisphere is affected. Dysarthria in combination with facial weakness may also be a carotid territory TIA. Contralateral sensory disturbance may also occur but can be very difficult to distinguish from migraine or hysteria (Landi 1992). Vertebrobasilar TIAs include rotational vertigo, double vision, homonymous hemianopia, bilateral blindness, ataxia, and dysphagia. Carotid and vertebrobasilar TIAs of the brain tend to last longer than amaurosis fugax but still less than an hour in most patients.

Some patients have remarkably stereotyped TIAs and those with amaurosis fugax have usually had more attacks than those with carotid or vertebrobasilar TIAs. Up to half of TIA patients have only a single episode, multiple attacks not being necessary for diagnosis.

Differential diagnosis

One important reason for separating stroke from TIA is that the differential diagnoses differ. These differences influence the clinical assessment and the necessary investigations.

Syncope/pre-syncope. Loss of consciousness is a very rare symptom of TIA: syncope or pre-syncope should alert the clinician to the causes of global, not focal, falls in cerebral blood flow and thus cardiac arrythmias, cardiac conduction block, vaso-vagal attacks or postural hypotension need to be excluded.

Migraine. Unilateral headache preceded by pins and needles, spreading numbness or weakness, is suggestive of 'migraine with aura'. Isolated aura, 'migraine aura without headache', can occur but these patients appear to have a low risk of future vascular events and inappropriate and potentially hazardous investigations should be avoided (Dennis & Warlow 1992).

Epilepsy. Partial and generalized seizures are diagnosed by a good history, particularly if there is a witnessed account. A past history of epilepsy or previous known intracranial pathology can alert the clinician to this diagnosis.

Transient global amnesia (TGA). This is a curious but apparently benign condition in its pure form (Hodges 1991). During a TGA attack, patients characteristically lose their ability to lay down new memories. Witnesses describe the patient as vague and asking repetitive questions about their immediate environment. They know who they are and can perform normal activities (such as walking, eating and driving). There are no localizing symptoms apart from headache sometimes. The attacks generally last for a few hours with complete resolution but patients remain amnesic for the period of the attack.

Hypoglycaemia. Diabetics on oral hypoglycaemic agents or insulin are most at risk, but patients with liver failure, alcohol intoxication and insulinoma (very rarely) can suffer transient focal neurological deficits. There may be no systemic hypoglycaemic symptoms such as sweating but a useful clue is if the attacks occur at the same time each day, particularly in the morning after awakening.

Space-occupying lesions. Tumours (particularly meningiomas), subdural haematomas, vascular malformations and aneurysms can all rarely give rise to transient focal neurological deficits mimicking TIAs.

Others. Peripheral nerve lesions, paroxysmal symptoms of multiple sclerosis, drop attacks, drug reactions, cervical radiculopathy and hysteria can all occasionally be confused with transient cerebral ischaemia. Other causes of transient monocular blindness include papilloedema, glaucoma, migraine with aura, retrobulbar neuritis, retinal haemorrhage, retinal detachment, orbital tumours, macular degeneration, carotico-cavernous fistula, and intracranial arteriovenous malformations.

Investigation

There is no simple 'test' to confirm the clinical diagnosis of TIA. Investigations are performed to exclude other causes of transient focal neurological symptoms, and to document risk factors for vascular disease. It is also important to detect other likely vascular problems (e.g. cardiac or peripheral arterial disease) for relevant management (Hankey et al 1991). For most patients an ECG and chest X-ray together with haematological, biochemical and serological blood tests are indicated (Table 55.4). CT will exclude most structural lesions causing transient focal neurological deficits (e.g. a meningioma) but these are rare. If a carotid TIA patient is fit, and willing to consider surgery, it is important to investigate the degree of carotid stenosis in the safest possible manner (Hankey & Warlow 1990). As angiography carries a risk of permanent stroke of about 1%, the safest method of investigating these patients is to perform noninvasive ultrasound and Doppler scanning of the origin of the internal carotid arteries and only proceed to carotid angiography if the stenosis of the lumen is moderate to severe.

The results of these initial investigations will point the way to any further tests such as echocardiography.

Table 55.4 Investigation of TIA or stroke

Basic phase
Haemoglobin/haematocrit
Platelet count
White cell count
Erythrocyte sedimentation rate
Glucose
Cholesterol
Chest X-ray, but seldom as an emergency
Electrocardiogram
Syphilis serology
Computerized tomography scanning (see p. 1265 and Table 55.5)
Complex phase
Echocardiogram (transthoracic and/or transoesophageal)
Doppler ultrasound of the carotid arteries (Duplex scanning)
Transcranial Doppler ultrasound of the cerebral arteries
Magnetic resonance imaging (including MR angiography)
Antiphospholipid antibodies
Autoantibodies
The history, examination and results of the basic investigations will guide clinicians to the appropriate use of the more complex investigations
Risky phase
Angiography
Angiography carries a 1% risk of causing a disabling stroke. Patients must be carefully selected by appropriate use of noninvasive carotid imaging

Prognosis of TIA

TIA patients have a high risk of future vascular events (stroke, myocardial infarction and vascular death), the rates of which vary depending on the sort of patients being considered. Hospital-based series tend to have a better prognosis than community-based studies due to the bias of elderly patients not being referred. The average annual risk of stroke is about 5%, of a coronary event (myocardial infarction or sudden death) about 4% and the annual death rate is about 6% (Heyman et al 1984, Howard et al 1987, Sorensen et al 1989, Dennis et al 1990b, Hankey et al 1991). The highest risk of a stroke is in the initial weeks after presentation.

STROKE

Pathophysiology of ischaemic stroke

Approximately 80% of strokes are due to ischaemia causing cerebral infarction, but it is difficult to accurately identify the exact pathogenic mechanism in individual patients. Despite a large battery of investigations a recent multi-centre study was unable to convincingly identify the cause of stroke in 40% of cerebral infarcts (Sacco et al 1989). Even when a potential mechanism for the cause of stroke is identified it may still be uncertain that this was the actual mechanism. For example, atrial fibrillation commonly co-exists with other causes of stroke such as carotid stenosis. However, there is increasing evidence that simple *clinical* features can provide a useful indication of the likely underlying cause (Bamford et al 1991). Therefore, possible mechanisms of infarction will be discussed for each of the common clinical presentations.

Clinical features of cerebral infarction

There is huge diversity of clinical features of acute ischaemic stroke due to the many different arteries which may be involved, the size of the artery occluded, the duration of the occlusion and the collateral supply to the affected area of brain. Thus, similar lesions can produce different symptoms in different patients; a good example is that some patients can occlude their internal carotid artery without any symptoms, yet in other patients the same lesion will produce a devastating transhemispheric infarction with hemiparesis, hemianopia and dysphasia or spatial dysfunction.

The more frequently encountered syndromes are:

Lacunar stroke

Lacunar infarction is thought to be caused by thrombosis associated with microatheroma or lipohyalinosis of *a single, small perforating artery* in the brain. Embolism (cardiac or artery-to-artery) is a rare cause (Fisher 1969, Bamford et al 1987, Lodder et al 1990). The clinical syndromes associated with such single perforating artery occlusions fall into several easily identifiable sub-groups:

1. Pure motor stroke
2. Pure sensory stroke
3. Sensori-motor stroke
4. Ataxic hemiparesis.

These syndromes are usually caused by small infarcts in the internal capsule, thalamus and pons, and thus cause deficits by damage of the motor and sensory nerve tracts. Some syndromes are occasionally (<5%) due to a small primary intracerebral haemorrhage in the same place. It is an absolute requirement in the diagnosis of these syndromes that there is no evidence of higher cerebral dysfunction, such as dysphasia or sensory inattention, because this would imply damage to the cerebral cortex (see below).

Carotid territory stroke

The characteristic syndromes seen with occlusion of the internal carotid or middle cerebral artery produce the most devastating of all cerebral infarctions. These patients present with a combination of:

1. Hemiparesis
2. Homonymous hemianopia
3. Higher cerebral dysfunction (dysphasia if dominant hemisphere involved, visuospatial disorder if non-dominant hemisphere).

Bamford et al (1991) have termed the syndrome comprising *all* the above clinical features a 'total anterior circulation infarct' (TACI). This extensive deficit is due to damage to both the deep and superficial territories of the middle cerebral artery, thus involving the basal ganglia, internal capsule, motor and sensory cortex, optic radiation and language or visuospatial centres. Following demonstrated middle cerebral artery (MCA) occlusion, repeat angiography shows recanalization in a surprising number of patients (Dalal et al 1965a,b, Fieschi et al 1989). This suggests that in situ atheroma of the MCA is unusual and that the cause is embolism from the heart, or internal carotid artery.

Less extensive infarction due to occlusion of a branch of the middle cerebral artery (or perhaps complete MCA occlusion in patients with good collateral supply) causes less deficits than a TACI stroke. A partial anterior circulation infarct (PACI) consists of limited combinations of 1, 2 or 3 above, e.g. isolated dysphasia with or without motor signs. Strokes which just affect one hand, or just the leg are also likely to be peripheral cortical infarcts (as opposed to lacunes). The most striking feature of these middle cerebral artery territory distal branch occlusions is the low case fatality and high early recurrence rate compared with other subtypes of ischaemic stroke (Bamford et al 1991), perhaps because they are commonly due to embolism (from an ulcerated carotid plaque for example), and the risk of further embolism remains high until the active atheromatous lesion has healed (by re-endothelialization) or a cardiac source of embolism has resolved (e.g. fibrosis of left ventricular mural thrombus following myocardial infarction).

Vertebrobasilar territory stroke

The clinical syndromes caused by ischaemia in the vertebrobasilar territory include:

1. Ipsilateral cranial nerve palsy with contralateral motor and/or sensory deficit
2. Bilateral motor and/or sensory deficit
3. Disorders of conjugate eye movement
4. Isolated cerebellar dysfunction
5. Isolated homonymous visual field loss.

These posterior circulation infarcts (POCI) have a better prognosis than previously thought. The small proportion of POCI patients who die soon after onset presumably have involvement of vital brainstem structures, these patients are more likely to be admitted to hospital and therefore hospital series tend to be biased with the most severe cases. The significant recurrence risk of POCI strokes again suggest that embolism is an important cause in this group of patients.

Clinical features of haemorrhagic stroke

It is impossible to reliably distinguish primary intracerebral haemorrhage from cerebral infarction from just the symptoms and signs, a CT scan must be done (p. 1265). The clinical diagnosis of subarachnoid haemorrhage is more reliable although a CT scan is still required (van Gijn 1992); the characteristic features are sudden headache, loss of consciousness and the evolution of neck stiffness. A focal neurological deficit is due to associated haematoma formation (and thus there is overlap with primary intracerebral haemorrhage), or after a few days, due to arterial spasm. Certain clinical features help improve the estimate of the chances of intracranial haemorrhage (for example, apoplectic onset and impaired conscious level) (Allen 1983), but are not good enough if thrombolysis, anticoagulants (or even perhaps antiplatelet agents) are being considered (p. 1266).

Diagnosis

Has the patient had a stroke?

The clinical diagnosis of stroke can be made at the bedside or even on the telephone, in the majority of patients. There are three requirements and attention to detail will avoid errors:

1. A *focal* neurological deficit (except in subarachnoid haemorrhage)
2. A *presumed* vascular cause
3. Symptoms lasting *more than 24 hours* (or leading to death).

A convincing history of a sudden onset of focal symptoms suggests a vascular cause (as in many non-neurological vascular diseases). A rather ill-defined onset and slow progression should alert the clinician to other possibilities (e.g. tumour). By definition, those patients who satisfy the criteria in 1 and 2, but who have symptoms lasting less than 24 hours, have TIAs.

As is usually the case, a good history can be diagnostic and save costly, inappropriate and sometimes dangerous tests. This is even more important in stroke medicine, when so many patients have language problems or are drowsy or confused. One of the most useful diagnostic instruments is the telephone to obtain a clear account of the illness from relatives, carers and other witnesses. Assessment should include a full enquiry into possible risk factors for stroke, a detailed vascular history, drug history (in particular antithrombotic agents), previous functional abilities (e.g. could the patient walk prior to the stroke) and social background. Assessment of important impairments following stroke (such as swallowing, conscious level) and functional abilities (walking, use of the toilet etc.) are important but frequently omitted (or not recorded).

Differential diagnosis of stroke

Mass lesions. Metastatic tumour is the most common mass lesion with an 'acute stroke' presentation. The likelihood of tumour is increased by a rather unclear history of symptom onset and by a stuttering course (Allen 1983). The TRUST stroke trial (in which patients who had become hemiparetic in the previous 48 hours were randomized) systematically performed CT scanning in 292 patients; of these, only 4% had a primary or secondary tumour (Trust Study Group 1990). Subdural haematomas can occur without a history of obvious trauma and will be excluded by CT scanning. Occasionally cerebral abscess can present with stroke-like symptoms but the accompanying signs of infection should suggest this diagnosis.

Epilepsy. The Todd's paresis following an epileptic fit can be difficult to distinguish from a stroke (especially as a previous stroke can be the cause of the epilepsy), unless the history is clear. However it is usually accompanied by other post-ictal signs such as drowsiness, and it recovers rapidly over hours.

Migraine with prolonged aura. Migraine is more often confused with TIA (see p. 1262), but some migraine attacks can leave residual neurological deficits lasting more than 24 hours.

Hypoglycaemia. It is important to exclude hypoglycaemia as a cause of focal (or global) neurological deficits in diabetics on hypoglycaemic agents.

Confusion and acutely-ill medical patients. A confused patient gives a confused and unreliable history and it can then be very difficult to establish the onset and nature of symptoms. Hypoxia, infection and cardiac failure were the most common 'non-stroke' conditions referred to the Oxfordshire Community Stroke Project (Sandercock et al 1985). Patients with dementia are particularly difficult to assess and sometimes one has to resort to CT to help identify cerebral infarct or haemorrhage, multi-infarct disease, hydrocephalus or space-occupying lesions.

Cord and nerve root lesions. Sudden neurological deficits affecting a limb can sometimes be due to spinal cord or root lesions. Neck or radicular pain, a history of previous cervical problems, known degenerative disease of the spine together with an absence of signs attributable to a higher lesion (e.g. dysphasia or cranial nerve signs) are useful features.

Hysteria. Occasionally hysteria can mimic acute stroke. A young patient with no risk factors for stroke and without convincing signs should prompt a close enquiry into the psychological history and background of the patient.

Investigation of stroke

The investigations are similar to those described for TIA (see Table 55.4). However, these should be tempered by the patient's condition, the likelihood of recovery, and whether the results will alter the immediate or subsequent management. The aim of each stage of investigation is to identify *treatable* conditions. It is reasonable to perform the basic investigations in most patients, and thereafter reserve the complex and risky investigations for those most likely to benefit.

A CT scan (Table 55.5). Immediately after onset of symptoms, a CT scan will reliably reveal intracerebral haemorrhage as a homogeneous high density area. The haematoma gradually becomes isodense (and therefore undetectable) within a few weeks of onset. A haemorrhagic stroke can only be excluded by *early* CT, preferably within a week of onset (Hankey & Warlow 1991). It is important to note that it may take some days for cerebral infarction to become visible on a CT scan, and some infarcts remain undetected by present CT technology (especially lacunar and brainstem infarcts).

Magnetic resonance imaging. MRI is a useful addition to stroke imaging. It is less reliable than CT in differentiating haemorrhagic from ischaemic strokes, especially in the initial stages, but detects cerebral infarction earlier. Also small infarcts can be detected by MRI when CT has been normal (Hankey & Warlow 1991). Restlessness in acute stroke patients undergoing MRI and CT can cause problems. In addition, claustrophobia, pacemakers, and metal implants further restrict MRI use.

Table 55.5 Indications for CT scanning after stroke

Current (or contemplated) anticoagulant treatment
Current (or contemplated) antiplatelet treatment
Current (or contemplated) thrombolysis
Suspected cerebellar stroke
Suspected subarachnoid haemorrhage
Uncertain diagnosis
Progression of stroke after onset
Possible carotid endarterectomy later

Transcranial Doppler. TCD is a noninvasive method of measuring the velocity of blood flow in the main intracranial arteries and can detect stenosis or occlusion. It can be an alternative to angiography (especially in combination with Duplex sonography of the carotid artery in the neck) and is relatively cheap. Its disadvantages are the substantial learning curve for the operator, the inaccessibility of cranial 'windows' in about 10% of patients, the inability to identify vessels accurately and the need for patient cooperation. It is not yet a routine investigation.

Lumbar puncture. Less than 12 hours after onset of subarachnoid haemorrhage (SAH) lumbar punctures may be normal because blood may not have reached the lumbar CSF. After about 12 hours the presence of xanthochromia in blood-stained CSF suggests true subarachnoid haemorrhage rather than a traumatic tap (van Gijn 1992).

Prognosis of stroke

A fifth of stroke patients will have died by one month. There is a marked difference in the case fatality between the different stroke sub-types: whilst cerebral infarction has a 10% fatality rate at 1 month, the corresponding rates for primary intracerebral haemorrhage and subarachnoid haemorrhage are about 50%. The outcome at 1 year is illustrated in Figure 55.3.

Total anterior circulation infarction (or TACIs) have a very poor prognosis with 95% dead or severely disabled at a year. The other sub-types of cerebral infarction have a better prognosis: with about 60% attaining functional independence at 1 year (see Fig. 55.3) (Bamford et al 1991). Despite the one year mortality for lacunar infarction being the lowest at about 10%, a third of such patients are still dependent at 1 year.

MANAGEMENT OF ACUTE STROKE: SPECIFIC TREATMENT

Subarachnoid haemorrhage and primary intracerebral haemorrhage

Prompt neurological and neurosurgical assessment of patients with subarachnoid haemorrhage is essential. If appropriate, cerebral angiography should be performed with a view to surgery to prevent further aneurysmal bleeds. Nimodipine reduces the mortality and morbidity of SAH patients by the reduction of 'vasospasm' and cerebral infarction which can complicate recovery.

Patients with cerebellar haemorrhage (and those with cerebellar infarction with mass effect) can have an extremely poor prognosis due to the rapidly fatal obstructive hydrocephalus and emergency drainage of CSF may be lifesaving.

Ischaemic stroke

There is, unfortunately, no routine treatment of proven

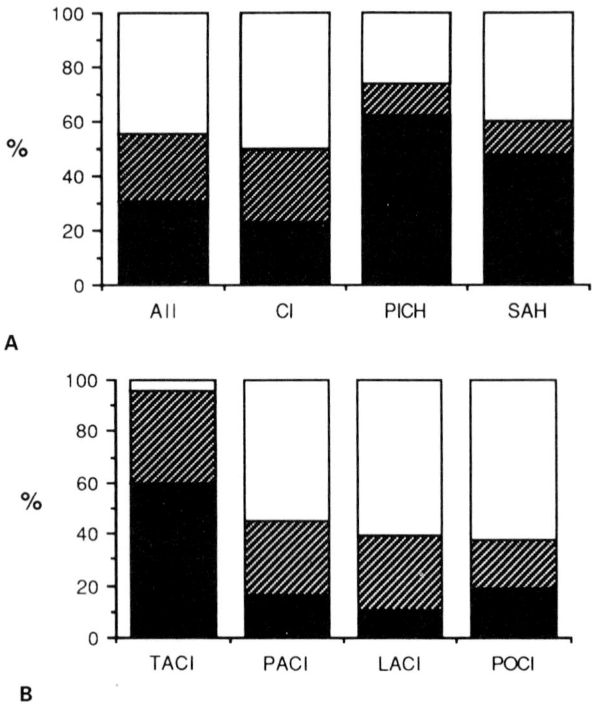

Fig. 55.3 1-year outcome after first ever stroke in Oxfordshire, UK. **A**, pathological subtypes of stroke and **B**, subtypes of ischaemic stroke. □, alive and independent; ▨, alive but dependent; ■, dead. TACI, Total anterior circulation infarct; PACI, partial anterior circulation infarct; LACI, lacunar infarct; POCI, posterior circulation infarct; All, All stroke; CI, cerebral infarction; PICH, primary intracerebral haemorrhage; SAH, subarachnoid haemorrhage (Bamford et al 1990, 1991).

benefit for acute ischaemic stroke. A lack of large appropriate clinical trials have contributed to this unhappy state of affairs, previous trials being far too small to reliably establish the risks and benefits of treatment. This contrasts markedly with acute myocardial infarction where very large multicentre trials have shown the effectiveness of beta blockade, aspirin and thrombolysis. Many physicians have a nihilistic attitude to the acute treatment of stroke, which is unfortunate; there are good reasons to believe that some simple and practical treatments might be worthwhile.

What treatments might work?

Following arterial occlusion, the amount of irreversible neuronal damage increases over time, i.e. there is some critically ischaemic tissue which could be salvaged by restoration of normal blood flow and/or by neuroprotective agents. This 'ischaemic penumbra' is electrically silent but has enough blood supply (from direct perfusion and collaterals) to maintain, temporarily, essential ion channel pumps, and thus neuronal viability (Astrup et al 1981). If the blood supply is not restored, the tissue in the ischaemic penumbra will also infarct. Thus if some of the ischaemic penumbra could be salvaged, the patient should have less neurological damage and less functional disability.

It is rather implausible that any of the many suggested treatments have a *major* beneficial effect. If they had it would have been obvious by now and the trials to date should have detected evidence of such an effect. However, as the large multicentre trials in myocardial infarction have shown, treatment with *moderate* benefits are important if applicable to large numbers of patients (Yusuf et al 1984). Beta blockers, aspirin and thrombolysis for acute myocardial infarction are all treatments with moderate benefits. It is very plausible that similar *moderate* treatment effects exist for acute ischaemic stroke, which could prevent many tens of thousands of patients from becoming disabled (or dying), but trials large enough to prove this are only just being planned.

POTENTIAL MECHANISMS AND PROMISING AGENTS FOR ACUTE STROKE MANAGEMENT

Treatments which might salvage the ischaemic penumbra and prevent the common complications of stroke can be considered under the following headings:

1. Restoring normal vascular anatomy
2. Improving blood flow
3. Protecting ischaemic neurones
4. Preventing the common complications of stroke.

1. Restoring normal vascular anatomy

Thrombolysis

Attempting to recanalize occluded cerebral arteries is an obvious approach. Thrombolysis, so successful in myocardial infarction, is unproven in acute ischaemic stroke. Unlike myocardial infarction, stroke can also be due to haemorrhage. The early unpromising randomized trials of thrombolytic therapy in acute stroke were before CT scanning and would therefore have inadvertently included some haemorrhagic stroke patients. The world literature of thrombolytic therapy in acute stroke is notable for the lack of randomized trials, thus despite many patients receiving such therapy there are no firm data on the potential risks or benefits (Wardlaw & Warlow 1992). Well-designed randomized trials now in progress in Europe and Australia will answer the important question: does thrombolytic treatment increase recanalization with reasonable safety, and does the patient benefit?

Antithrombotic treatment

Aspirin, and other antiplatelet agents, are effective *secondary* preventative treatments for patients who have survived ischaemic stroke and TIA (see p. 1268). Curiously, there have been virtually no trials published on their use for acute stroke (Sandercock et al 1993). As a result there is clinical chaos in the use of aspirin immediately after stroke with uncertain risks and benefits. Aspirin is effective in the acute phase of myocardial infarction (ISIS-2 Collaborative Group 1988) and, bearing in mind the known efficacy in secondary prevention would appear to be the most promising agent to test in acute ischaemic stroke (Lindley & Sandercock 1992). The chief concern is the risk of haemorrhagic transformation of cerebral infarcts, as some animal experiments have suggested (Clark et al 1991).

Standard and low molecular weight heparin has been tested in 1047 patients in ten randomized trials (Sandercock et al 1993). A formal overview of these studies has provided convincing evidence of the effectiveness in reducing deep venous thrombosis, but there were not enough deaths to know whether heparin causes an increase in cerebral haemorrhagic complications and thus mortality. The overview has suggested that heparin therapy may reduce mortality by about one fifth, but the confidence intervals are wide, and the results are compatible with a 15% excess of deaths with this therapy (Sandercock et al 1993).

Antithrombotic therapy appears the most promising practical therapy to test in acute ischaemic stroke. A very large multicentre collaborative study was started in pilot form in 1991 to test both aspirin and heparin (the International Stroke Trial, Sandercock et al 1993) and plans to recruit 10 000 to 20 000 patients in the early 1990s. Survival free of major disability is the major outcome of the proposed study. Until this and other studies have reported their results, the use of routine antithrombotic treatment in the *acute* phase of stroke is best restricted to randomized trials.

2. Improving cerebral blood flow

Haemodilution, to reduce the haematocrit, was thought to be promising and has been tested in several trials. The largest study included 1267 patients and failed to show any benefit (Italian Acute Stroke Study Group 1988). An overview of all the completed trials has confirmed this result (Asplund 1991). It seems unlikely that this rather complicated treatment will be evaluated any further.

Manipulation of systemic blood pressure in the acute phase of stroke could be hazardous, as yet there are no data to help advise the best policy for the control of hypertension in the immediate aftermath of acute stroke and in general this should not be treated.

3. Protecting ischaemic neurones

If neurones could be protected until spontaneous recanalization of the cerebral arteries occurs (or effective therapeutic recanalization has been achieved with thrombolysis or antithrombotic therapy) the total area of infarction might be reduced. New agents such as *N*-methyl D-aspartate (NMDA) receptor blockers appear promising in many animal experiments and are now starting clinical testing. Calcium antagonists have been the most extensively evaluated neuroprotective agents but most of the randomizied trials have been very small. The largest (the Trust Study Group 1990) randomized 1215 patients; unfortunately, even a study of this size was too small to provide reliable information on efficacy. The results suggest that if calcium antagonists are effective they have only very modest effects and a trial of 20 000 patients may be needed to provide reliable data. Interestingly, aspirin may have an additional role as a neuroprotective agent due to its effect in blocking cyclo-oxygenase, with the reduction in potent mediators of ischaemic injury (free radicals, thromboxane, prostaglandins and leukotrienes) (Lindley & Sandercock 1992).

4. Preventing the common complications of stroke

Peripheral venous thromboembolism is a common cause of morbidity in acute stroke, with about 50% of hemiplegic stroke patients developing a deep venous thrombosis (DVT). Pulmonary embolism (PE) is a frequent finding at necroscopy, 70% of the control patients who had a postmortem had evidence of pulmonary embolism compared with 29% in the heparin-treated group in one published trial (McCarthy & Turner 1986). As discussed above, the use of heparin in acute stroke is controversial due to the unknown effects on cerebral bleeding but trials are in progress.

MANAGEMENT OF MAJOR OR DISABLING ISCHAEMIC STROKE

The King's fund consensus statement provides a comprehensive guide (Consensus Conference 1988). Hospital admission may be required for the general care of the patient, but a large number of patients disabled by stroke can be and are cared for at home. Physiotherapy and occupational therapy are valuable in helping patients regain lost functional ability and avoid complications of immobility during the sometimes prolonged period of neurological recovery. Rehabilitation teams may also have to adapt the patient's home or help patients and carers find suitable accommodation if the disability prevents full independence. Most neurological recovery occurs during the first few months following stroke, thereafter recovery is slower but some patients may take up to a year to reach their maximal functional state.

Deteriorating ischaemic stroke

The separation of stroke into 'stable' or 'deteriorating'

Table 55.6 Causes of deterioration after stroke onset

General	
Hypoxia	
Hypotension	
Circulatory failure	
Pulmonary embolism	
Cardiac failure	
Arrhythmia	
Infection	
Electrolyte disturbance	
Depression	
Drugs (especially sedatives)	
Confusion in elderly demented patients admitted to hospital	
Neurological	
Propagation of intra-arterial thrombus	
Recurrent embolism from cardiac or proximal arterial source	
Haemorrhagic transformation of the infarct	
Cerebral oedema	
Seizures	
Obstructive hydrocephalus*	
Incorrect diagnosis (e.g. symptoms due to tumour)	

* Obstructive hydrocephalus due to cerebellar haemorrhage or infarction can be fatal but is potentially surgically treatable.

(stroke-in-evolution) has not been very useful. The proportion of patients with 'stroke-in-evolution' depends on how soon after the onset of symptoms the first assessment is made. There are no clinical features which can reliably determine who will deteriorate in the acute phase. Deterioration of acute ischaemic stroke can be due to general or neurological causes (see Table 55.6) and a full re-examination together with appropriate investigations (e.g. urea, electrolytes, CT scan, etc.) is required in order to correct any potentially reversible cause. The use of anticoagulation for deteriorating stroke is unproven but commonly used on an empirical basis.

Management of transient ischaemic attack and minor ischaemic stroke

Minor non-disabling ischaemic strokes should be managed in a similar manner to TIA. Once the diagnosis is made, it is important to explain to the patient the measures which will reduce future vascular events. These patients are at high risk of future stroke and vascular death and need to be assessed for suitable preventative measures. In the large UK-TIA trial one quarter of all the placebo control patients had suffered a stroke, myocardial infarction or vascular death during a mean of 4 years follow-up (UK-TIA Study Group 1991). Preventative measures to reduce the risk of vascular events are:

Modification of risk factors

Modification of risk factors can be achieved by various approaches as shown in Table 55.7 (Dunbabin & Sandercock 1990). The effect of dietary salt has been controversial for many years but recent epidemiological work has emphasized the likely causal association between salt consumption and hypertension (Frost et al 1991, Law et al 1991a, 1991b). These new studies suggest that a reduction in the incidence of stroke by a quarter is a feasible achievement by reducing the salt intake of a Western population. The implications for the clinician in advising individual patients is that a moderate reduction in dietary salt is sensible, and the effects could be as beneficial as drug treatment for hypertension.

Table 55.7 Modification of risk factors for ischaemic stroke and TIA

Dietary	Reduce salt (to reduce blood pressure)
	Reduce saturated fats (to reduce cholesterol)
	Increase fruit and vegetables
Behavioural	Stop smoking
	Regularly exercise (to reduce blood pressure and cholesterol)
	Reduce weight (to reduce blood pressure and cholesterol)
Pharmacological	Treatment of hypertension
	Treatment of hypercholesterolaemia

Despite the absence of much direct evidence, antihypertensive treatment is likely to be important for these patients in years following the acute event because there is very clear indirect evidence from statistical overviews of the *primary prevention studies* that antihypertensive treatment reduces the risk of stroke and to a lesser extent, myocardial infarction (MacMahon et al 1990, Collins et al 1990). Because TIA or minor stroke patients have a high absolute risk of stroke they may well derive a much greater absolute benefit from treatment than asymptomatic individuals with similar blood pressure.

Antiplatelet therapy

Long-term antiplatelet therapy reduces the risk of stroke by about one fifth (Antiplatelet Trialists' Collaboration 1988). If the annual risk of stroke in TIA patients is about 5%, antiplatelet therapy will reduced this to 4%. The antiplatelet effect of aspirin is well established (Vane et al 1990), and the presumed mechanism is the reduction of platelet/fibrin emboli and in situ thrombotic complications of atheromatous plaques. As aspirin is not influencing the underlying pathology, and some emboli (e.g. cholesterol) would not be influenced by aspirin therapy, it is not surprising that the effect of aspirin is modest. However, despite this, the advantage of aspirin is that it can be given routinely to virtually all TIA or minor ischaemic stroke patients. By treating 100 patients, one stroke per year is delayed or avoided (e.g. a 5% annual risk reduced to 4%). The dose of aspirin remains somewhat uncertain. There is no doubt that low dose aspirin (e.g. 30 mg daily) almost completely inhibits platelet cyclo-oxygenase and there are theoretical reasons to expect this dose to spare endothelial production of prostacyclin (which has an antiaggregation effect). In practice this thereoretical benefit has not been demonstrated. The Antiplatelet Trialists (1988) concluded that no dose of aspirin was definitely more effective than 300–325 mg daily. In the UK-TIA Study Group (1991) a daily dose of 1200 mg had the same efficacy as 300 mg but the higher dose had greater gastrointestinal side-effects. The SALT Collaborative Group from Sweden (1991) found that 75 mg of aspirin was an effective secondary preventive agent (compared with placebo). The Dutch TIA Trial Study Group (1991) found a daily dose of 30 mg as effective as 283 mg and the lower dose was less toxic. It is important that the first dose of aspirin should be at least 300 mg (as it takes a few days for platelet cyclo-oxygenase inhibition to be maximal at lower daily doses), but the maintenance dose can be as low as 30 mg. However at this very low dose the formulation of the aspirin becomes very important; the Dutch study used a pulverized carbaspirin calcium preparation. Our recommendation is that patients start with 300 mg and then the dose can be reduced to 75–150 mg using whatever formulation is convenient and available locally. The newer antiplatelet agent, ticlopidine, is a potential alternative agent for those patients who cannot tolerate aspirin, but, due to the neutropenic side-effects, this treatment has to be regularly monitored and thus is a second line option.

Carotid endarterectomy

Two large randomized trials have reported interim results on the efficacy of carotid endarterectomy to prevent stroke in symptomatic patients (European Carotid Surgery Trialists' Collaborative Group 1991, North American Symptomatic Carotid Endarterectomy Trial Collaborators 1991) (ECST and NASCET). The symptoms had to be due to cerebral (or retinal) ischaemia, non-disabling and in the carotid artery territory (e.g. TIA, amaurosis fugax, retinal infarct or minor stroke), with symptoms within the previous few months.

Those with 0–30% stenosis do not benefit from surgery: there are virtually no strokes to prevent in this category of patient, thus patients suffer the risk of surgery but derive no subsequent benefit. For patients with a 30–69% stenosis the balance of risk and benefit of carotid endarterectomy is uncertain and the two trials are continuing to randomize. Patients with 70–99% stenosis gain significant benefit from carotid endarterectomy. The ipsilateral ischaemic stroke rate is dramatically reduced after successful surgery, this reduction implying that most of these strokes must be due to atherothrombosis at the carotid bifurcation with complicating embolism and/or low blood flow. In the ECST study, removing the carotid lesion reduced the risk of ipsilateral ischaemic strokes from 17% in the control group to 3% in the surgery group in 3 years. However, endarterectomy carries a significant risk of peri-operative stroke or death (7.5% in ECST, 5.8% in NASCET). Therefore, it is imperative that the local surgical risk is known before recommending surgery for symptomatic patients with tight carotid stenosis. If the local surgical peri-operative risk of stroke or death is high (i.e. greater than 10%), surgery may not confer any absolute benefit. If the local surgical risk is lower than that in ECST and NASCET, the absolute benefits will be that much greater.

Anticoagulation

There is uncertainty about the benefit of anticoagulation in patients with TIA or minor ischaemic stroke. The lack of data causes a major therapeutic dilemma. We simply do not know if anticoagulation is a beneficial treatment for patients with TIA, whether it is more or less effective than antiplatelet agents, or whether the combination of antiplatelet and anticoagulant therapy is better than either alone. Early case reports encouraged the use of anticoagulation after TIA (Millikan et al 1955a,b) and large non-randomized series supported this (Millikan et al 1958, Whisnant et al 1973, 1978, Olsson et al 1976). The randomized trials which followed confused matters by their inconclusive results due to their small size and various design flaws (Veterans Administration 1961, Baker et al 1962, 1966, Pearce et al 1965, Bradshaw & Brennan 1975).

Secondary prevention of stroke in patients with presumed cardio-embolism

Randomized clinical trials of antiplatelet agents and anticoagulants in the *acute* phase of stroke are currently in progress (p. 1267). The value of long-term aspirin, warfarin or neither for patients in non-rheumatic atrial fibrillation is currently being evaluated in the European Atrial Fibrillation Trial. In other patients the indications for anticoagulation are still uncertain (Hart 1992).

Any benefit from anticoagulation is presumably related to the nature of the embolic source, and in practice, patients with *high* risk of embolism are anticoagulated: mitral valve disease with or without atrial fibrillation, recent myocardial infarction, prosthetic heart valve, and dilating cardiomyopathy. When to start anticoagulation after stroke in this high-risk group is controversial; too early after stroke risks haemorrhagic transformation of the infarct, too late, risks recurrent embolism. Our policy is to anticoagulate with heparin at once and then change to warfarin in a few days.

Cortical venous and/or dural sinus thrombosis

Thrombosis of the venous or dural sinuses is a rare cause of cerebral infarction. There are a variety of local and systemic predisposing conditions including haematological disorders (Table 55.8). The presentation can occasionally be with a stroke or seizures, but more commonly it is as an encephalopathy. Raised intracranial pressure can develop,

Table 55.8 Causes of cortical venous and/or dural sinus thrombosis

Local conditions affecting the veins and sinuses directly	
	Head injury
	Intracranial surgery
	Local sepsis (sinuses, ears, scalp, nasopharynx)
	Neurosyphilis
	Bacterial meningitis
	Tumour invasion of dural sinuses
	Catheterization of jugular vein, e.g. for parenteral nutrition
Systemic disorders	
	Dehydration
	Septicaemia
	Pregnancy and the puerperium
	Oral contraceptives
	Haematological disorders (Table 55.3)
	Hyperviscosity syndromes
	Inflammatory arterial disease
	Diabetes mellitus
	Congestive cardiac failure
	Inflammatory bowel disease
	Androgen therapy
	Non-metastatic effect of extracranial malignancy

mimicking 'benign intracranial hypertension'. The cerebral infarcts are commonly haemorrhagic, and an extremely important point to consider is that a CT scan can be normal despite widespread sinus thrombosis; the venous phase of cerebral angiography or magnetic resonance angiography is necessary to confirm the diagnosis (Hankey & Warlow 1991). Thrombosis of the cavernous sinus is rare but is usually secondary to venous spread of pyogenic infection from the face, sinuses or nasal space. The symptoms include orbital pain and swelling with the development of visual loss, papilloedema, with palsies of the third, fourth, fifth and sixth cranial nerves.

Treatment of sinus thrombosis has been controversial for many years; corticosteroids, anticoagulants and even thrombolysis have been used. As usual this uncertainty is due to the absence of randomized trials. However, a recent trial by Einhäupl and colleagues (1991) tested full dose heparin anticoagulation (using a dose range of 25 000 to 65 000 units/day, to maintain a PTT target range of 80–100 seconds). In this study of 20 patients, none of the heparin-treated group died, compared with three of the controls: eight heparin-treated patients completely recovered, compared with one of the controls. It is interesting to note that three of the heparin-treated patients had CT evidence of intracranial haemorrhage at the start of treatment. None of the heparin-treated group developed intracranial haemorrhage during treatment but two control patients had further intracranial haemorrhage.

REFERENCES

Aberg H 1969 Atrial fibrillation. I. A study of atrial thrombosis and systemic embolism in necropsy material. Acta Medica Scandinavica 185: 373–379

Adams R J, Nichols F T, McKie V, Milner P, Gammal T E 1988 Cerebral infarction in sickle cell anemia: Mechanism based on CT and MRI. Neurology 38: 1012–1017

Allen C M C 1983 Clinical diagnosis of the acute stroke syndrome. Quarterly Journal of Medicine 52: 515–523

Antiplatelet Trialists' Collaboration 1988 Secondary prevention of vascular disease by prolonged antiplatelet treatment. British Medical Journal 296: 320–331

Ashok P P, Radhakrishnan K, Sridharan R, El-Mangoush M A 1986 Incidence and pattern of cerebrovascular diseases in Benghazi, Libya. Journal of Neurology, Neurosurgery, and Psychiatry 49: 519–523

Asplund K 1991 Hemodilution in acute stroke. Cerebrovascular Diseases 1 (suppl 1): 129–138

Astrup J, Siesjo B K, Symon L 1981 Thresholds in cerebral ischemia – the ischemic penumbra. Stroke 12: 723–725

Baker R N, Broward J A, Fang H C et al 1962 Anticoagulant therapy in cerebral infarction. Report on co-operative study. Neurology 12: 823–829

Baker R N, Schwartz W S, Rose A S 1966 Transient ischaemic strokes. A report of a study of anticoagulant therapy. Neurology 16: 841–847

Bamford J M, Warlow C P 1988 Evolution and testing of the lacunar hypothesis. Stroke 19: 1074–1082

Bamford J M, Sandercock P, Jones L, Warlow C 1987 The natural history of lacunar infarction: The Oxfordshire Community Stroke Project. Stroke 18: 545–551

Bamford J, Sandercock P, Dennis M et al 1988 A prospective study of acute cerebrovascular disease in the community: the Oxfordshire Community Stroke Project 1981–86. 1. Methodology, demography and incident cases of first ever stroke. Journal of Neurology, Neurosurgery, and Psychiatry 51: 1373–1380

Bamford J, Sandercock P, Dennis M, Warlow C 1990 A prospective study of acute cerebrovascular disease in the community; the Oxfordshire Community Stroke Project 1981–86. 2. Incidence, case fatality rates and overall outcome at one year of cerebral infarction, primary intracerebral and subarachnoid haemorrhage. Journal of Neurology, Neurosurgery, and Psychiatry 53: 16–22

Bamford J, Sandercock P, Dennis M, Burn J, Warlow C 1991 Classification and natural history of clinically identifiable subtypes of cerebral infarction. Lancet 337: 1521–1526

Bogousslavsky J, Hachinski V C, Boughner D R, Fox A J, Vinuela F, Barnett H J M 1986 Cardiac and arterial lesions in carotid transient ischemic attacks. Archives of Neurology 43: 223–228

Bonita R, Beaglehole R 1986 Does treatment of hypertension explain the decline in mortality from stroke? British Medical Journal 292: 191–192

Boston Area Anticoagulation Trial for Atrial Fibrillation Investigators 1990 The effect of low-dose warfarin on the risk of stroke in nonrheumatic atrial fibrillation. New England Journal of Medicine 323: 1505–1511

Bradshaw P, Brennan S 1975 Trial of long-term anticoagulant therapy in the treatment of small stroke associated with a normal carotid angiogram. Journal of Neurology, Neurosurgery and Psychiatry 38: 642–647

Brand F N, Abbott R D, Kannel W B, Wolf P A 1985 Characteristics and prognosis of lone atrial fibrillation: 30-year follow-up in the Framingham Study. Journal of the American Medical Association 254: 3449–3453

Broderick J P, Phillips S J, Whisnant J P, O'Fallon W M, Bergstralh E J 1989 Incidence rates of stroke in the eighties: The end of the decline in stroke? Stroke 20: 577–582

Bruno A, Adams H P, Biller J, Rezai K, Cornell S, Aschenbrener C A 1988 Cerebral infarction due to moyamoya disease in young adults. Stroke 19: 826–833

Chen S T, Liu Y H, Hogan E L, Ryu S J 1988 Moyamoya disease in Taiwan. Stroke 19: 53–59

Clark W M, Madden K P, Lyden P D, Zivin J A 1991 Cerebral hemorrhagic risk of aspirin or heparin therapy with thrombolytic treatment in rabbits. Stroke 22: 872–876

Collins R, Peto R, MacMahon S et al 1990 Blood pressure, stroke, and coronary heart disease. Part 2, Short-term reductions in blood pressure: overview of randomised drug trials in their epidemiological context. Lancet 335: 827–838

Connolly S J, Laupaucis A, Gent M, Roberst R S, Cairns J A, Joyner C, and CAFA Study Co-investigators. 1991 Canadian Atrial Fibrillation Anticoagulation Study. Journal of the American College of Cardiology 18: 349–355

Consensus Conference 1988 Treatment of stroke. British Medical Journal 297: 126–128

Cross J N, Castro P O, Jennett W B 1968 Cerebral strokes associated with pregnancy and the puerperium. British Medical Journal 3: 214–218

Dalal P M, Shah P M, Sheth S C, Deshpande C K 1965a Cerebral embolism: Angiographic observations on spontaneous clot lysis. Lancet i: 61–64

Dalal P M, Shah P M, Aiyar R R 1965b Arteriographic study of cerebral embolism. Lancet ii: 358–361

de Bono D P, Warlow C P 1981 Potential sources of emboli in patients with presumed transient cerebral or retinal ischaemia. Lancet i: 343–345

de Bono D P 1982 Cardiac causes of transient neurologic disturbances. In: Warlow C P, Morris P S (eds) Transient ischaemic attacks. Dekker, New York 99–124

Dennis M, Warlow C 1992 Migraine aura without headache: transient ischaemic attack or not? Journal of Neurology, Neurosurgery and Psychiatry 55: 437–440

Dennis M S, Bamford J M, Sandercock P A G, Warlow C P 1989 Incidence of transient ischemic attacks in Oxfordshire, England. Stroke 20: 333–339

Dennis M, Bamford J, Sandercock P, Molyneux A, Warlow C 1990a Computed tomography in patients with transient ischaemic attacks: when is a transient ischaemic attack not a transient ischaemic attack but a stroke? Journal of Neurology 237: 257–261

Dennis M, Bamford J, Sandercock P, Warlow C 1990b The prognosis of transient ischaemic attacks in the community. The Oxfordshire Community Stroke Project. Stroke 21: 848–853

Dexter D D, Whisnant J P, Connolly D C, O'Fallon W M 1987 The association of stroke and coronary heart disease: a population study. Mayo Clinic Proceedings 62: 1077–1083

Dunbabin D W, Sandercock P A G 1990 Preventing stroke by the modification of risk factors. Stroke 21 (suppl IV): IV36–IV39

Dutch TIA Trial Study Group 1991 A comparison of two doses of aspirin (30 mg vs. 283 mg a day) in patients after a transient ischemic attack or minor ischemic stroke. New England Journal of Medicine 325: 1261–1266

Einhäupl K M, Villringer A, Meister W et al 1991 Heparin treatment in sinus venous thrombosis. Lancet 338: 597–600

Engesser L, Broekmans A W, Briet E, Brommer E J P, Bertina R M 1987 Hereditary protein S deficiency: Clinical manifestations. Annals of Internal Medicine 106: 677–682

European Carotid Surgery Trialists' Collaborative Group 1991 MRC European Carotid Surgery Trial: interim results for symptomatic patients with severe (70–99%) or with mild (0–29%) carotid stenosis. The Lancet 337: 1235–43

Ezekowitz M D, Bridgers S L, James K E, and the SPINAF Investigators 1991 Interim analysis of the VA Cooperative Study: Stroke Prevention in Nonrheumatic Atrial Fibrillation. Circulation 84 (suppl II): 450

Fabian R H, Peters B H 1984 Neurological complications of haemoglobin SC disease. Archives of Neurology 41: 289–292

Fieschi C, Argentino C, Lenzi G L, Sacchetti M L, Toni D, Bozzao L 1989 Clinical and instrumental evaluation of patients with ischemic stroke within the first six hours. Journal of the Neurological Sciences 91: 311–322

Fisher C M 1969 The arterial lesions underlying lacunes. Acta Neuropathology (Berlin) 12: 1–15

Fisher C M 1979 Capsular infarcts — the underlying vascular lesions. Archives of Neurology 36: 65–73

Flege K M, Shipley M J, Rose G 1987 Risk of stroke in non-rheumatic atrial fibrillation. Lancet i: 526–529

Forman K, Sokol R J, Hewitt S, Stamps B K 1984 Paroxysmal nocturnal haemoglobinuria. A clinicopathological study of 26 cases. Acta Haematologica 71: 217–226

Friedman G D, Loveland D B, Ehrlich S P 1968 Relationship of stroke to other cardiovascular disease. Circulation 38: 533–541

Frost C D, Law M R, Wald N J 1991 By how much does dietary salt reduction lower blood pressure? II. Analysis of observational data within populations. British Medical Journal 302: 815–818

Greenberg J, Massey E W 1985 Cerebral infarction in sickle cell trait. Annals of Neurology 18: 354–355

Hankey G J, Warlow C P 1990 Symptomatic carotid ischaemic events: safest and most cost effective way of selecting patients for angiography, before carotid endarterectomy. British Medical Journal 300: 1485–1491

Hankey G J, Warlow C P 1991 The role of imaging in the management of cerebral and ocular ischaemia. Neuroradiology 33: 381–390

Hankey G J, Slattery J M, Warlow C P 1991 The prognosis of hospital-referred transient ischaemic attacks. Journal of Neurology, Neurosurgery, and Psychiatry 54: 793–802

Harrison M J G, Marshall J 1985 Arteriographic comparison of amaurosis fugax and hemispheric transient ischaemic attacks. Stroke 16: 795–797

Hart R G 1992 Cardiogenic embolism to the brain. Lancet 339: 589–594

Hatano S 1976 Experience from a multicentre stroke register: a preliminary report. Bulletin of the World Health Organisation 54: 541–553

Herman B, Schmitz P I, Leyten A C et al 1983 Multivariate logistic analysis of risk factors for stroke in Tilburg, the Netherlands. American Journal of Epidemiology 118: 514–525

Heyman A, Wilkinson W E, Hurwitz B J et al 1984 Risk of ischaemic heart disease in patients with TIA. Neurology 34: 626–630

Hinton R C, Kistler J P, Fallon J T, Friedlich A L, Fisher C M 1977 Influence of etiology of atrial fibrillation on incidence of systemic embolism. The American Journal of Cardiology 40: 509–513

Hodges J R 1991 Transient amnesia: clinical and neuropsychological aspects. W B Saunders, London

Howard G, Toole J F, Frye-Pierson J, Hinshelwood L C 1987 Factors influencing the survival of 451 transient ischaemic attack patients. Stroke 18: 552–557

ISIS-2 Collaborative Group 1988 Randomised trial of intravenous streptokinase, oral aspirin, both, or neither among 17 187 cases of suspected acute myocardial infarction: ISIS-2. Lancet ii: 349–360

Iso H, Jacobs D R, Wentworth D, Neaton J D, Cohen J D for the MRFIT Research Group 1989 Serum cholesterol levels and six-year mortality from stroke in 350 977 men screened for the Multiple Risk Factor Intervention Trial. New England Journal of Medicine 320: 904–910

Italian Acute Stroke Study Group 1988 Haemodilution in acute stroke: Results of the Italian haemodilution trial. Lancet ii: 318–321

Jabaily J, Iland H J, Laszlo J et al 1983 Neurologic manifestations of essential thrombocythaemia. Annals of Internal Medicine 99: 513–518

Kagan A R 1976 Atherosclerosis and myocardial lesions in subjects dying from fresh cerebrovascular disease. Bulletin of the World Health Organisation 53: 597–600

Kannel W B, Gordon T, Wolf P A, McNamara P M 1972 Haemoglobin and the risk of cerebral infarction: The Framingham Study. Stroke 3: 409

Kannel W B, Wolf P A, Verter J 1983 Manifestations of coronary disease predisposing to stroke. The Framingham Study. Journal of the American Medical Association 250: 2942–2946

Kannel W B, Wolf P A, Castelli W P, D'Agostino R B 1987 Fibrinogen and risk of cardiovascular disease. Journal of the American Medical Association 258: 1183–1186

Kempster P A, Gerraty R P, Gates P C 1988 Asymptomatic cerebral infarction in patients with chronic atrial fibrillation. Stroke 19: 955–957

Kittner S J, Sharkness C M, Price T R et al 1990 Infarcts with a cardiac source of embolism in the NINCDS Stroke Data Bank: Historical features. Neurology 40: 281–284

Koudstaal P J, van Gijn J, Staal A, Duivenvoorden H J, Gerritsma J G M, Kraaijeveld C L 1986 Diagnosis of transient ischemic attacks: Improvement of interobserver agreement by a check-list in ordinary language. Stroke 17: 723–728

Kraaijeveld C L, van Gijn J, Schouten H J A, Staal A 1984 Interobserver agreement for the diagnosis of transient ischemic attacks. Stroke 15: 723–725

Landi G 1992 The clinical diagnosis of transient ischaemic attacks. Lancet 339: 402–405 la Rue L, Alter M, Lai S M et al 1987 Acute stroke, hematocrit, and blood pressure. Stroke 18: 565–569

Law M R, Frost C D, Wald N J 1991a By how much does dietary salt reduction lower blood pressure? I. Analysis of observational data among populations. British Medical Journal 302: 811–815

Law M R, Frost C D, Wald N J 1991b By how much does dietary salt reduction lower blood pressure? III. Analysis of data from trials of salt reduction. British Medical Journal 302: 819–824

Lindley R I, Sandercock P A G 1992 Why test antiplatelet therapy in acute ischaemic stroke and how can this be done? Postgraduate Medical Journal 68 (suppl 2): S14–S19

Lodder J, Bamford J M, Sandercock P A G, Jones L N, Warlow C P 1990 Are hypertension or cardiac embolism likely causes of lacunar infarction? Stroke 21: 375–381

Luscher T F, Lie J T, Stanson A W, Houser O W, Hollier L H, Sheps S G 1987 Arterial fibromuscular dysplasia. Mayo Clinic Proceedings 62: 931–952

McCarthy S T, Turner J 1986 Low-dose subcutaneous heparin in the prevention of deep-vein thrombosis and pulmonary emboli following acute stroke. Age and Ageing 15: 84–88

MacMahon S, Peto R, Cutler J et al 1990 Blood pressure, stroke, and coronary heart disease. Part 1, effects of evidence from nine prolonged differences in blood pressure: prospective observational studies corrected for the regression dilution bias. Lancet 335: 765–774

Maggioni A P, Franzosi M G, Farina M L et al 1991 Cerebrovascular events after myocardial infarction: analysis of the GISSI trial. British Medical Journal 302: 1428–1431

Meade T W, Mellows S, Brozovic M et al 1986 Haemostatic function and ischaemic heart disease: Principal results of the Northwick Park heart study. Lancet 2: 533–537

Millikan C H, Siekert R G, Shick R M 1955a Studies in cerebrovascular disease. III. The use of anticoagulant drugs in the treatment of insufficiency or thrombosis within the basilar arterial system. Staff Meetings of the Mayo Clinic 30: 116–126

Millikan C H, Siekert R G, Shick R M 1955b Studies in cerebrovascular disease. V. The use of anticoagulant drugs in the treatment of intermittent insufficiency of the internal carotid arterial system. Staff Meetings of the Mayo Clinic 30: 578–586

Millikan C H, Siekert R G, Whisnant J P 1958 Anticoagulant therapy in cerebral vascular disease – current status. Journal of the American Medical Association 166: 587–592

Mokri B, Sundt T M, Houser O W, Peipgras D G 1986 Spontaneous dissection of the cervical internal carotid artery. Annals of Neurology 19: 126–138

Nishide M, Irino T, Gotoh M, Naka M, Tsuji K 1983 Cardiac abnormalities in ischemic cerebrovascular disease studied by two-dimensional echocardiography. Stroke 14: 541–5

North American Symptomatic Carotid Endarterectomy Trial Collaborators 1991 Beneficial effect of carotid endarterectomy in symptomatic patients with high grade carotid stenosis. New England Journal of Medicine 325: 445–53

Olsson J E, Muller R, Berneli S 1976 Long-term anticoagulant therapy for transient ischaemic attacks and minor strokes with minimum residium. Stroke 7: 444–451

Pavlakis S G, Bello J, Prohovnik I et al 1988 Brain infarction in sickle cell anaemia: Magnetic resonance imaging correlates. Annals of Neurology 23: 125–130

Pearce J M S, Gubbay S S, Walton J N 1965 Long-term anticoagulant therapy in transient ischaemic attacks. Lancet i: 6–9

Pearson T C, Wetherley-Mein G 1978 Vascular occlusive episodes and venous haematocrit in primary proliferative polycythaemia. Lancet ii: 1219–1222

Pessin M S, Duncan G W, Mohr J P, Poskanzer D C 1977 Clinical and angiographic features of carotid transient ischemic attacks. The New England Journal of Medicine 296: 358–362

Petersen P, Madsen E B, Brun B, Pedersen F, Gyldensted C, Boysen G 1987 Silent cerebral infarction in chronic atrial fibrillation. Stroke 18: 1098–1100

Petersen P, Boysen G, Godtfredsen J, Anderson E D, Andersen B 1989 Placebo-controlled, randomized trial of warfarin and aspirin for prevention of thromboembolic complications in chronic atrial fibrillation: the Copenhagen AFASAK study. Lancet i: 175–179

Pozzati E, Giuliani G, Poppi M, Faenza A 1989 Blunt traumatic carotid dissection with delayed symptoms. Stroke 20: 412–416

Preston F E, Martin J F, Stewart R M, Davies-Jones G A B 1979 Thrombocytosis, circulating platelet aggregates, and neurological dysfunction. British Medical Journal 2: 1561–1563

Qizilbash N, Jones L, Warlow C, Mann J 1991 Fibrinogen and lipid concentrations as risk factors for transient ischaemic attacks and minor ischaemic strokes. British Medical Journal 303: 605–609

Qizilbash N, Duffy S W, Warlow C, Mann J 1992 Lipids are risk factors for ischaemic stroke: Overview and Review. Cerebrovascular Disease 2: 127–136

Ricci S, Celani M G, La Rosa F et al 1991a SEPIVAC: a community-based study of stroke incidence in Umbria, Italy. Journal of Neurology, Neurosurgery, and Psychiatry 54: 695–698

Ricci S, Celani M G, La Rosa F et al 1991b A community-based study of the incidence, risk factors and outcome of transient ischaemic attacks in Umbria, Italy: the SEPIVAC study. Journal of Neurology 238: 87–90

Richards A, Graham D, Bullock R 1988 Clinicopathological study of neurological complications due to hypertensive disorders of pregnancy. Journal of Neurology, Neurosurgery and Psychiatry 51: 416–421

Ridolfi R L, Bell WR 1981 Thrombotic thrombocytopenic purpura. Report of 25 cases and review of the literature. Medicine 60: 413–428

Rose G 1981 Strategy of prevention: lessons from cardiovascular disease. British Medical Journal 282: 1847–1851

Ross R 1986 The pathogenesis of atherosclerosis — an update. New England Journal of Medicine 314: 488–500

Sacco R L, Ellenberg J H, Mohr J P et al 1989 Infarcts of undetermined cause: The NINCDS stroke Data Bank. Annals of Neurology 25: 382–390

SALT Collaborative Group 1991 Swedish Aspirin Low-Dose Trial (SALT) of 75 mg aspirin as secondary prophylaxis after cerebrovascular ischaemic events. Lancet 338: 1345–1349

Sandercock P A G, Molyneux A, Warlow C 1985 Value of computed tomography in patients with stroke: Oxfordshire Community Stroke Project. British Medical Journal 290: 193–197

Sandercock P A G, van den Belt A G M, Lindley R I, Slattery J 1992 Antithrombotic therapy in acute ischaemic stroke: An overview of the completed randomised trials. Journal of Neurology, Neurosurgery and Psychiatry 56: 17–25

Schneidau A, Harrison M J G, Hurst C, Wilkes H C, Meade T W 1989 Arterial disease risk factors and angiographic evidence of atheroma of the carotid artery. Stroke: 1466–1471

Schwartzman R J, Hill J B 1982 Neurologic complications of disseminated intravascular coagulation. Neurology 32: 791–797

Shahar A, Sadeh M 1991 Severe anemia associated with transient neurological deficits. Stroke 22: 1201–1202

Sherman D G, Hart R G, Easton J D 1981 Abrupt change in head position and cerebral infarction. Stroke 12: 2–6

Shinton R, Beevers G 1989 Meta-analysis of relation between cigarette smoking and stroke. British Medical Journal 298: 789–794

Siekert R G, Whisnant J P, Millikan C H 1960 Anaemia and intermittent focal cerebral arterial insufficiency. Archives of Neurology 3: 386–390

Silverstein A, Gilbert H, Wasserman L R 1962 Neurologic complications of polycythaemia. Annals of Internal Medicine 57: 909–916

Silverstein A 1968 Thrombotic thrombocytopenic purpura. The initial neurological manifestations. Archives of Neurology 18: 358–362

Somer T 1987 Rheology of paraproteinaemias and the plasma hyperviscosity syndrome. Ballière's clinical haematology, vol 1: 695–723

Sorensen P S, Marquardsen J, Pedersen H, Heltberg A, Munck O 1989 Long-term prognosis and quality of life after reversible cerebral ischaemic attacks. Acta Neurologica Scandinavica 79: 204–213

Srinivasan K 1983 Cerebral venous and arterial thrombosis in pregnancy and puerperium. A study of 135 patients. Angiology 34: 731–746

Stemmermann G N, Hayashi T, Resch J A, Chung C S, Reed D M, Rhoads G G 1984 Risk factors related to ischaemic and hemorrhagic cerebrovascular disease at autopsy: the Honolulu Heart Study. Stroke 15: 23–28

Stroke Prevention in Atrial Fibrillation Investigators 1991 The stroke prevention in atrial fibrillation study: final results. Circulation 84: 527–539

Tanaka H, Ueda Y, Date C et al 1981 Incidence of stroke in Shibata, Japan: 1976–1978. Stroke 12: 460–466

Tanaka H, Ueda Y, Hayashi M et al 1982 Risk factors for cerebral haemorrhage and cerebral infarction in a Japanese rural community. Stroke 13: 62–73

Trust Study Group 1990 Randomised, double-blind, placebo-controlled trial of nimodipine in acute stroke. Lancet 336: 1205–1209

Ueda K, Omae T, Hirota Y et al 1981 Decreasing trend in incidence and mortality from stroke in Hisayama residents, Japan. Stroke 12: 154–160

UK-TIA Study Group 1991 The United Kingdom Transient Ischaemic Attack (UK-TIA) aspirin trial: Final results. Journal of Neurology, Neurosurgery and Psychiatry 1991 54: 1044–1054

Vane J R, Flower R J, Botting R M 1990 History of aspirin and its mechanism of action. Stroke 21 (suppl IV): IV12–IV23

van Gijn J 1992 Subarachnoid haemorrhage. Lancet 339: 653–655

Veterans Administration 1961 An evaluation of anticoagulant therapy in the treatment of cerebrovascular disease. Neurology 11: 132–138

Vieregge P, Schwieder G, Kompf D 1989 Cerebral venous thrombosis in hereditary protein C deficiency. Journal of Neurology, Neurosurgery and Pschiatry 52: 135–137

Wardlaw J M, Warlow C P 1992 Thrombolysis in acute ischaemic stroke — Does it work? Stroke 23: 1826–1839

Warlow C P, Morris P J 1982 Introduction. In: Warlow C, Morris P J (eds) Transient ischaemic attacks. Dekker, New York, p vii–xi

Whisnant J P, Matsumoto N, Elveback L R 1973 The effect of anticoagulant therapy on the progress of patients with transient cerebral ischaemic attack in a community. Rochester, Minnesota, 1955 through 1969. Mayo Clinic Proceedings 48: 844–848

Whisnant J P, Cartlidge N E F, Elveback L R 1978 Carotid and vertebral-basilar transient ischaemic attacks: effect of anticoagulants, hypertension and cardiac disorders on survival and stroke occurrence. A population study. Annals of Neurology 3: 107–115

Wiebers D O, Mokri B 1985 Internal carotid artery dissection after childbirth. Stroke 16: 956–959

Wilhelmsen L, Svardsudd K, Korsan-Bengtsen K, Larsson B, Welin L, Tibblin G 1984 Fibrinogen as a risk factor for stroke and myocardial infarction. New England Journal of Medicine 311: 501–505

Wolf P A, Dawber T R, Thomas E, Kannel W B 1978 Epidemiologic assessment of chronic atrial fibrillation and risk of stroke: The Framingham Study. Neurology 28: 973–977

Wood D H 1978 Cerebrovascular complications of sickle cell anaemia. Stroke 9: 73–75

Woo J, Lau E, Lam C W et al 1991 Hypertension, lipoprotein(a), and apolipoprotein A-1 as risk factors for stroke in the Chinese. Stroke 22: 203–208

Yusuf S, Collins R C, Peto R 1984 Why do we need some large, simple randomised trials? Statistics in Medicine 3: 409–420

56. Peripheral arterial disease

P. R. F. Bell

Peripheral arterial disease is a common condition (Dormandy & Murray 1991) caused by atherosclerosis which leads to narrowing of medium to large arteries and can progress to occlusion. The cause of atheroma remains uncertain but there are a number of contributory risk factors which include smoking (Hughson et al 1978), diabetes (Kuller et al 1985), hypercholesterolaemia (Gander 1985), hypertension (Fagrell 1990), and there is almost certainly a strong familial tendency. The process is also the normal outcome of ageing and is becoming more common as more people reach old age in relatively good health. The exact sequence of events which triggers off the development of atherosclerosis remains controversial. Endothelial damage is caused by a number of factors such as smoking, hypertension, hyperglycaemia and perhaps trauma caused by flow (Angelini et al 1991) which results in platelet aggregation and the release of various growth factors which create smooth muscle hyperplasia that later calcify to form a plaque (Plate 56.1). The usual pathological process is for an area of the vessel to become progressively narrowed by plaque formation until thrombosis suddenly occurs leading to acute or chronic ischaemia. An alternative process is the destruction of elastic tissue and collagen leading to aneurysmal dilatation of the vessel which occurs at particular sites such as the infra renal abdominal aorta. A third consequence of peripheral arterial disease is thromboembolism which needs to be covered separately.

For reasons which are not clear, plaque is laid down most commonly at particular sites, often at bifurcations, in the aorta (Fig. 56.1) and the lower limb vessels such as the iliac, femoral, popliteal and crural arteries. The aorta above the renal arteries is less commonly affected, as is the common femoral and profundafemoris arteries. The arteries of the upper limb are usually spared although the origins of the subclavian and innominate arteries can be affected. In a similar way the renal arteries can be stenosed and cause hypertension and the mesenteric vessels can similarly be involved leading to mesenteric ischaemia and sometimes necrosis of the intestines. The problem also affects the carotid, vertebral and cerebral vessels as well as the coronary circulation all of which are discussed elsewhere. Becausc of the relatively slow onset of the disease, time is usually available for a collateral circulation to develop and allow blood to bypass the area of stenosis (Fig. 56.2). In this way the circulation of the periphery is maintained for long periods of time unless the vessel is an end artery when tissue necrosis occurs. The condition is a relatively benign one as far as limb loss is concerned, a minority progressing to gangrene (Kannel & McGee 1985) (Plate 56.2). Mortality is however high due to associated disease of the cerebrovascular and coronary arterial system which will be discussed elsewhere in this book (Hoofwijk 1991).

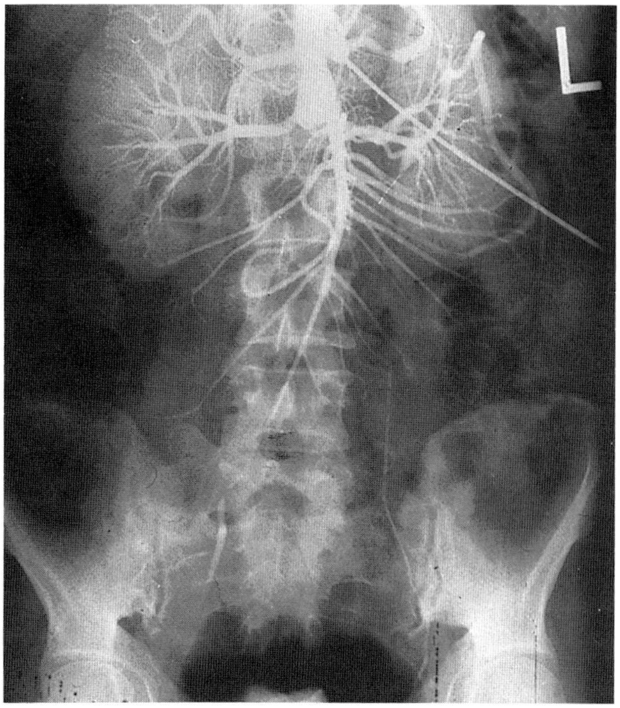

Fig. 56.1 An angiogram showing total occlusions of the aorta immediately below the renal arteries.

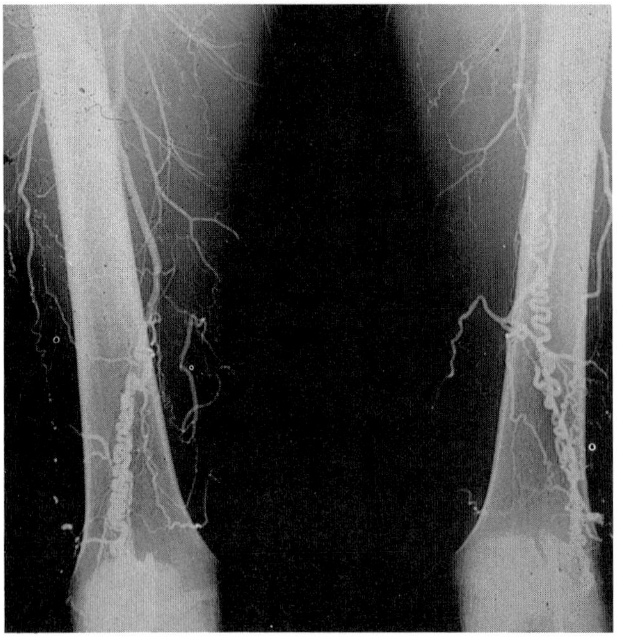

Fig. 56.2 An arteriogram showing occlusion of the femoral arteries with well developed tortuous collateral arteries carrying blood distally.

LOWER LIMB — PRESENTATION WITH CHRONIC SYMPTOMS

The majority of patients will present with chronic symptoms of limb ischaemia but a small proportion can present acutely when ischaemia can pose a serious threat to the limb. The patient will classically complain of pain after walking a certain distance which is relieved by rest and recurs on exercise (intermittent claudication). The calf is usually affected if the femoropopliteal segment is involved or the buttocks and thigh if the iliac vessels or aorta are obstructed. If the condition progresses then the claudication distance will slowly decrease until a stage is reached where the patient will be able to walk only a few yards or will develop pain at rest. The next stage is ulceration or gangrene and limb loss in a minority of patients (Kannel & McGee 1985). The stage of rest pain and gangrene or ulceration has now been defined as critical limb ischaemia with objective parameters to classify patients correctly (European Consensus Statement 1989). The progressive process towards limb loss can be arrested or slowed down if risk factors are abolished.

The history is of great importance in this condition as there are many other causes of leg pain which can, but should not, be confused with claudication. For example a slipped intravertebral disc, arthritis of the hip, various types of peripheral neuropathy, muscular pain, venous disease and spinal claudication can.all present to the vascular clinician. A careful history will however eliminate most of these, as, only if the pain occurs after walking and is absent at rest does it qualify as claudication. Examination of the patient is equally important although it must be remembered that this is taking place with the patient at rest when symptoms only occur on walking. A general examination is essential to exclude cardiac and carotid disease, the blood pressure must be taken and the pulses carefully assessed. Capillary filling at rest is not a reliable observation but elevation of the patient's legs to assess the pallor of the soles of the feet can be a useful way of assessing ischaemia. The quicker pallor occurs the more severe is the ischaemia (Plate 56.3). The presence of ulceration or early gangrene of the toes is clearly diagnostic.

Management

At the end of the examination the clinician will be in a good position to decide whether to proceed further and what to do. It is vital that the degree of disability is assessed clinically and on this will depend whether further investigations are performed. The clinician is also able to assess after palpation of the pulses whether the problem is due to aortoiliac or femoropopliteal occlusion but will not know how long the occlusion is. If patients are smoking, and they usually are, it is vital that they stop, otherwise, regardless of the treatment adopted, progression of the disease will almost certainly occur (US Surgeon General 1983). The clinician must realize that it is not sufficient merely to tell the patient to stop smoking. Help in the form of psychotherapy, acupuncture or hypnosis as well as warnings about limb loss are often needed to stop what can be a serious addiction. At the same time as stopping smoking the patient must be encouraged to exercise as there is good evidence to show that this will improve their claudication distance (Hiatt et al 1991). Walking daily through the pain will often suffice but programmed exercises are probably better. It is important that the patient is told to walk through the pain and that this will do them no harm. In general drugs do not help a patient with claudication at all (Boobis & Bell 1984). From the time of the onset of symptoms nothing should be done for a period of 3–6 months except for exercise and stopping smoking to allow maximal collateral development. If after this time the patient's condition is such that he cannot work or is inconvenienced by his problem to a significant extent, further investigation is required. If the patient's condition at the original consultation is severe, i.e. claudication of less than 50 yards, rest pain or gangrene, then investigations and treatment are urgently required. In general if a patient can walk more than 100 yards provided he walks slowly and is not having problems with work, conservative treatment is to be recommended but this will depend upon the treatment options available at each centre.

INVESTIGATION AND TREATMENT OF PATIENTS WITH SEVERE CHRONIC SYMPTOMS

If the patient is thought to be severely affected or if the condition progresses then further investigations are necessary. If there is any doubt in the clinician's mind that the symptoms are due to vascular disease, the pressures at the ankles should be measured using a simple hand held Doppler to see if there is a difference between the brachial and ankle pressures at rest. If no difference is detected, the patient should be subjected to 1 minute of exercise on a treadmill with an incline of 10° and a speed of 5 miles per hour (Laing & Greenhalgh 1980). The pressures should then be measured again and if significant vascular disease is present the pressure at the ankle will fall confirming that the pain is due to arterial insufficiency. This last test is particularly useful to distinguish claudication from other causes of leg pain. If further treatment is required it is important to reiterate that drug treatment does not usually help and the patient will have to have some form of invasive intervention, either one of the new reopening procedures or surgery, neither of which should be taken lightly. These patients have generalized arterial disease and before operative treatment in particular is undertaken they should be assessed by ECG preferably after exercise, by a duplex scan to assess the carotid arteries and a chest X-ray to exclude associated carcinoma of the lung. The haemoglobin level should also be measured as these patients are often polycythaemic. Fasting lipids are worth recording to distinguish those patients with hyperlipidaemia so measures can be taken to improve matters. Because these patients are generally in a poor condition, attempts should be made to avoid an operation if possible. Unfortunately at present there is no way of assessing the arterial tree fully without some form of angiography although advances in duplex technology using colour imaging may allow this to be done in future (Legemate et al 1989). At present some form of angiogram is required and the increasingly available intra-arterial or intravenous DSA technique is replacing conventional angiography. If DSA is not available then Seldinger angiography via the femoral or axillary artery or, as a last resort, translumbar angiography should be undertaken. It is important to remember that angiography does have some undesirable side-effects such as bleeding and embolization and should only be done prior to intervention and not merely to support the clinical findings (MacPherson et al 1980).

Treatment options

The angiogram will reveal the exact level and length of the occlusion and usually outline the vessels which are patent distal to that occlusion (Fig. 56.3). The better the run off vessels the better will be the result of intervention. In general the patients with critical ischaemia or gangrene have worse run off vessels than those with claudication and do less well whatever the treatment option undertaken.

Non-surgical procedures

Angioplasty

Angioplasty was first suggested by Dotter & Judkins (1964) and then popularized by Gruntzig & Hopff (1974) who developed a special balloon catheter which allowed the transcutaneous treatment of arterial stenosis and occlusions to become a practical possibility. The technique involves the insertion of a guidewire through a needle placed inside an artery, usually the femoral, and the advancement of a catheter with a balloon mounted at its tip over the guidewire (Fig. 56.4). Once the balloon is correctly placed across the occlusion or stenosis it is then expanded to fracture the atheromatous plaque at its weakest point and allow dilatation of the vessel (Fig. 56.5). The balloons are of a predetermined size and cannot be over distended and burst the artery unless the wrong size is used. This technique has now been available for

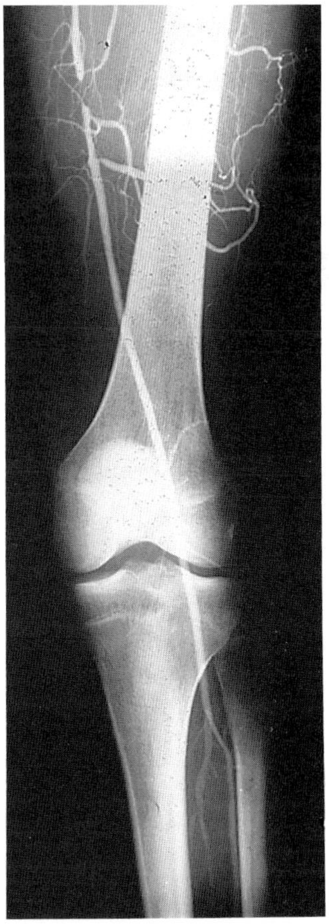

Fig. 56.3 An angiogram showing a femoral artery occlusion with good 'run off' vessels distally.

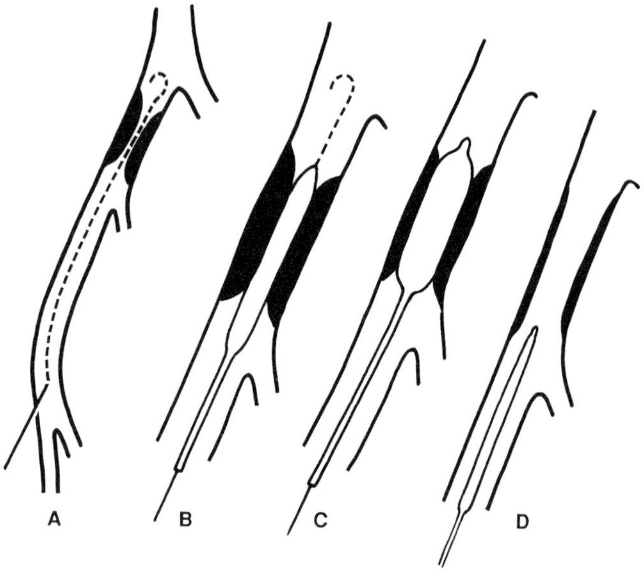

Fig. 56.4 A guide wire has been inserted via the femoral artery and passed through a stenosis of the common iliac artery (**A**). A catheter is passed over the guide wire and positioned at the stenosis (**B**). The balloon is inflated fracturing the plaque (**C**) and then deflated and withdrawn (**D**).

some years and will give good results with stenotic lesions. If however the vessels are occluded the results are less impressive (Sampson et al 1984). In general occlusion of greater than 5 cm are better treated by surgery than angioplasty and certainly lesions of greater than 10 cm in length respond relatively poorly to dilatation although this technique can work even with long occlusions (Fig. 56.6). In general patients should be offered an angioplasty as the first treatment option as symptoms can be relieved in a significant number of patients, particularly with lesions of the iliac vessels (van Ander 1985). As the disease progresses more distally the results become less acceptable and what can be treated will depend on the expertise available at each centre although very distal angioplasty can sometimes work (Fig. 56.7). Over the years, claims have been made for angioplasty but controlled trials have not been done, so even now we do not really know the place of this potentially valuable treatment in vascular occlusive disease.

It is also important to remember that complications can occur with angioplasty and it is possible for a patient to be made much worse by it, particularly if the vessel is ruptured, thromboses or embolization occurs. For these reasons it is imperative that a vascular surgeon is available to retrieve the situation if things do go wrong and angioplasty should not be carried out in centres where a vascular surgeon is not available. The patient should also be told of the possible risks of deterioration or even limb loss, even though this has a very low incidence of less than 1% (Belli et al 1990).

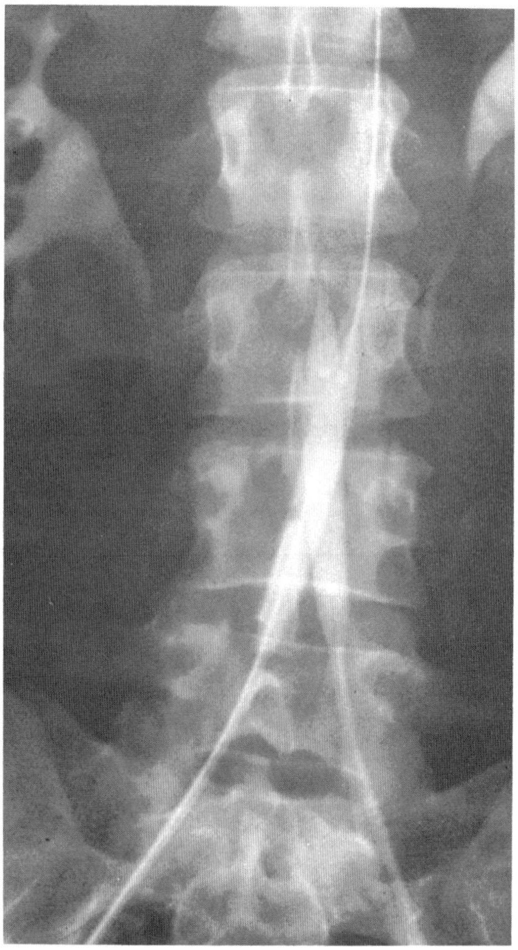

Fig. 56.5 Two balloons in place for aortic dilatation.

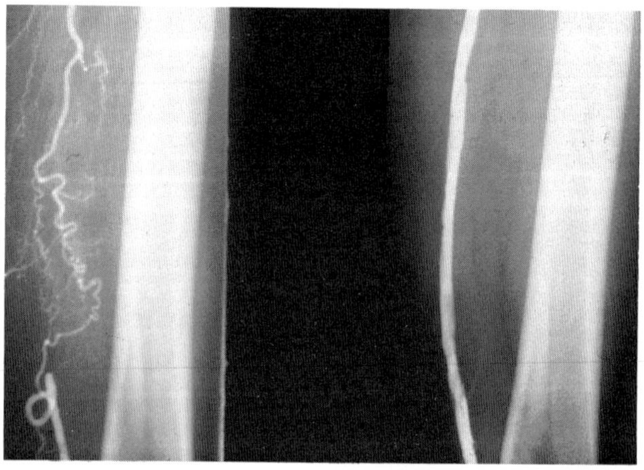

Fig. 56.6 Angiogram showing a long femoral stenosis on the left and on the right after angioplasty.

Newer procedures — laser treatment

New techniques have recently been introduced and are usually accompanied by a great deal of publicity. However trials to compare their usefulness with existing technology

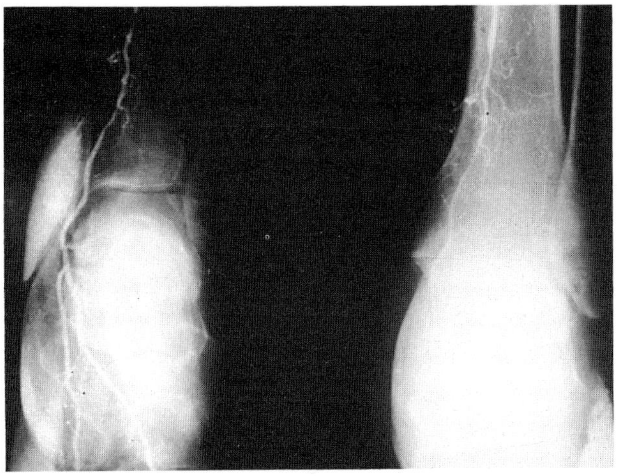

Fig. 56.7 Angioplasty of the posterior tibial artery at the ankle before on the left, and after treatment on the right.

or indeed to try and assess their place in the scheme of things remain hard to find. One example is laser technology (Murray & Cross 1991) which has been used by a number of authors to open vessels which have long occlusions of greater than 10 cm. A variety of different lasers exist, one type which has largely fallen into disrepute heats a metal tip to a high temperature allowing it to be passed through long occlusions for later dilatation. These have now been largely abandoned as the results are poor (Sanborn et al 1988). The newer generation of lasers using pulsed energy are cold or relatively so and allow vapourization of the atheroma prior to subsequent angioplasty if necessary (Murray et al 1989). The exact place of lasers in the vascular armentarium remains uncertain. A serious problem with lasers is the inability to direct the beam at the lesion rather than the arterial wall which can be perforated. Various guidance systems are evolving which include intra-arterial ultrasound or small television cameras incorporated into the catheter. The simplest system is a balloon which centres the catheter and prevents arterial perforation in most patients (Pokrovsky et al 1990). A further problem is that calcified lesions remain difficult to cross. Lasers are also very expensive, particularly the fibres, and, until comparative trials with surgery are done, their place in the treatment of vascular disease remains uncertain.

Atherectomy

Atherectomy catheters, drills and rotational devices have been used by a number of workers (Simpson et al 1988). One type is a capsule which incorporates a cutting device which can be passed down an artery to an area of stenosis and shaves off slices of atheroma in a repeatable fashion until the lesion is removed (Fig. 56.8). It is only suitable for short stenoses which generally respond well to angioplasty although eccentric or calcified lesions may do better with atherectomy (Coleman et al 1989). Again no comparative trials are available but atherectomy does tend to cause severe intimal hyperplasia (Debrosse et al 1990) which can lead to early reocclusion. The devices are also very expensive and their exact place in the treatment of arterial disease needs to be resolved.

Intravascular stents

One possible reason for the failure of atherectomy and angioplasty is that following dilatation the lesion will recur. This problem has been addressed by the use of stents which are inserted into the artery in a collapsed state following angioplasty and, when they are released from a catheter, expand to maintain the patency of the vessel (Fig. 56.9). These stents are expensive and their exact place remains uncertain. Again no trials are available to assess their efficacy and they do tend to produce intimal hyperplasia which is again counter-productive (Palmaz et al 1987). They may become much more useful when methods of preventing intimal hyperplasia are developed.

Thrombolysis

Thrombolysis using recombinant tissue plasminogen activator (rTPA) has been used successfully in myocardial

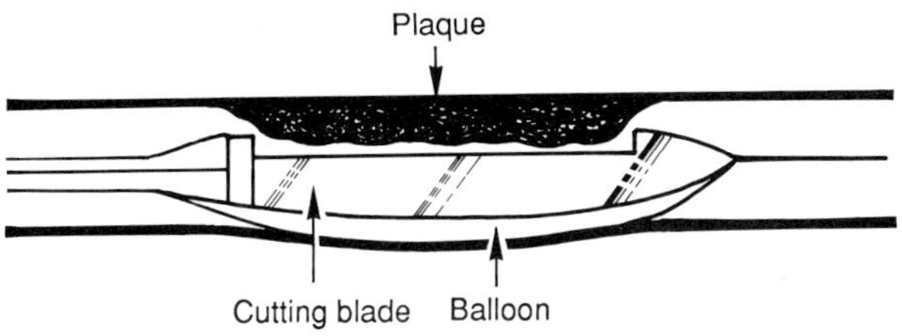

A

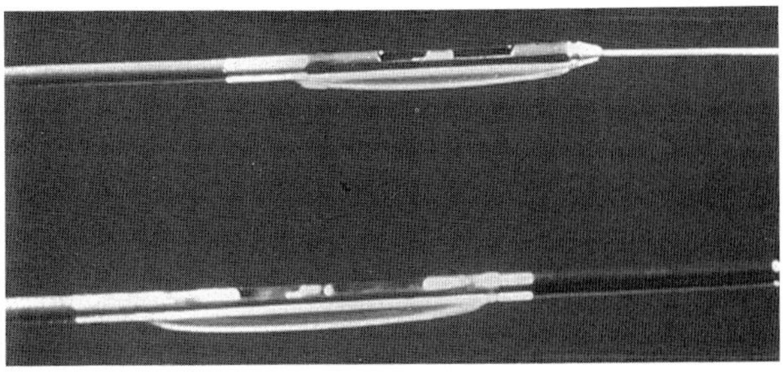

B

Fig. 56.8 An atherectomy catheter. The capsule is located in the area of the plaque and the balloon inflated. A cutting blade then passes down the length of the capsule and shaves off slices of atheroma which are trapped in the capsule and retrieved later when it is removed.

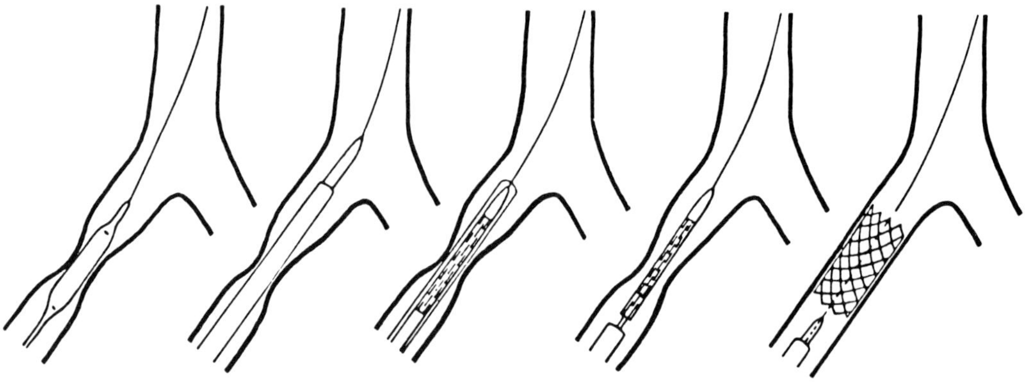

Fig. 56.9 A stent is introduced over a guide wire using a carrier. When the carrier is removed the stent expands into the stenosis holding it open.

infarction. Although rtPA has only recently been used for peripheral vascular thrombosis, even though streptokinase and urokinase have been used for some years with mixed results (Earnshaw & Shaw 1990). The usefulness of these thrombolytic agents in chronic ischaemia remains uncertain but they probably have a place in acute upon chronic or acute occlusions and this will be discussed later (p. 1284). To be effective the agent has to be given intra-arterially directly into the thrombus. Once the thrombus causing the obstruction has been removed the stenosis which caused the obstruction can then be dilated.

Surgical treatment

For some years surgery has been the only treatment available for claudication and critical ischaemia. Because there is a small but definite mortality attached to these high risk patients, surgery should generally only be used in those cases where angioplasty has failed or is impossible. Most surgical procedures are done for critical ischaemia and this can now be defined as those patients who have had rest pain for more than 3 weeks and an ankle pressure of less than 50 mmHg or a toe pressure of less an 30 mmHg or have ulceration or gangrene with similarly reduced pressures (European Consensus Statement 1989).

Aortoiliac obstruction

If the patient's aorta is blocked the obstruction can be bypassed using a bifurcated graft made of Dacron or Teflon. The graft is usually inserted between the aorta above the occlusion and into the femoral arteries in both groins (Fig. 56.10). This procedure carries a mortality of < 2% and long-term results, both in terms of limb salvage and patency, are in excess of 90% at 10 years (Nevelsteen et al 1991). The operation is to be recommended as durable and should be undertaken in those patients who are fit for the procedure. Angioplasty or other reopening methods do not usually help in this situation. The patient should of course be persuaded to stop smoking and they should also be fit for surgery. If however the patient is not fit, then the lower aorta or iliac artery can be approached retroperitoneally with good results. This approach is more difficult but less serious for the patient. (Johnson et al 1986). If the patient is unfit even for this approach then some form of extra anatomic bypass using Dacron or Teflon can be safely undertaken. For aortic obstruction the best procedure is an axillobifemoral graft with one axillary artery supplying both femorals (Plate 56.4). This operation works quite well producing limb salvage rates of 65% at 5 years in these high-risk patients (Corbett et al 1984).

If a femoral pulse is present (Fig. 56.11) on only one

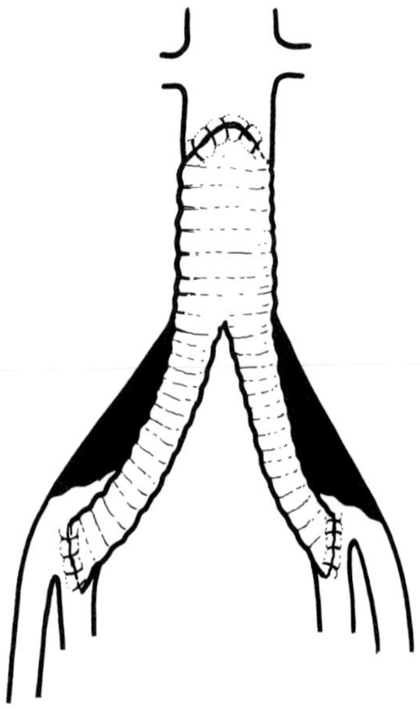

Fig. 56.10 Diagram of a bifurcated dacron graft sutured to the infra renal aorta above and the common femoral and profunda femoris artery in each groin to bypass a blocked aortoiliac segment.

side, other options are available: a crossover femorofemoral or iliofemoral graft which is a relatively atraumatic procedure can be done under local anaesthesia if necessary and allows one limb to vascularize the other. It is important to ensure that the amount of blood supplying the donor limb is adequate. This can be assessed haemodynamically by measuring the pressure of the donor femoral artery by direct puncture and comparing this with that of a radial artery. If there is a difference of more than 10 mmHg at rest there is a problem with inflow, if not the blood flow is increased by giving 20 mmHg papaverine directly into the femoral artery. If this causes a drop in pressure in the femoral artery of more than 20% there is a proximal stenosis of the donor artery making it unsuitable for a crossover graft. It can however be used if angioplasty is done prior to the operation. The results of crossover grafting are excellent with 5-year limb salvage and patency rates in excess of 80% (Fohal et al 1989).

All of these artificial grafts do have one potential complication and that is infection and it is vital that patients are given prophylactic antibiotics in order to prevent it. If a graft does however get infected it has to be removed and this inevitably causes serious problems (Perry 1985). Subsequent limb revascularization is difficult and there is a high mortality and amputation rate if this happens.

Femoropopliteal occlusion

If the patient has critical ischaemia the problem is usually due to multisegmental disease, i.e. disease affecting two vascular areas, such as the aortoiliac and femoropopliteal or crural vessels. Treatment of the proximal lesion in these cases is often enough to alleviate the critical ischaemia and convert the patient to a claudicant. If this does not work or if the popliteal occlusion is the only lesion (Fig. 56.12) it is best dealt with by a graft between the femoral artery above the occlusion and the patent vessel below it. For above knee obstructions of the popliteal artery a graft of polytetrafluorethylene [PTFE] or dacron gives good results (Quinones-Baldrich et al 1988) with limb salvage rates in critical ischaemia of 65% at 5 years. If the obstruction is lower down the leg however then the long saphenous vein should be used and will produce good limb salvage in critical ischaemia at 5 years in excess of 65% (Taylor et al 1991). The more distal the obstruction the poorer in general are the results. The vein can either be removed, reversed and used as a bypass or left in its anatomical position and the valves carefully cut by a special instrument (Fig. 56.13) which cuts the valve leaflet. This technique, termed in situ grafting, gives the best results for more distal procedures because the vessel tapers appropriately. These distal procedures are technically demanding but good limb salvage can be achieved

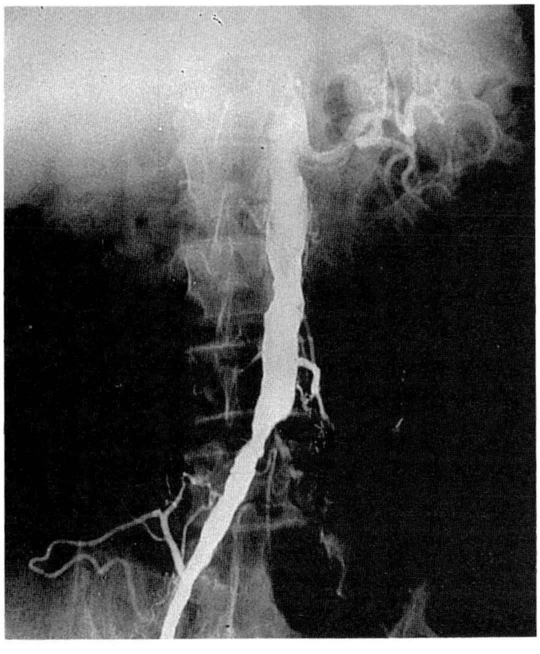

Fig. 56.11 An angiogram showing one patent femoral artery. This can be used to supply the other leg with a dacron graft which is passed under the skin suprapubically to the opposite groin.

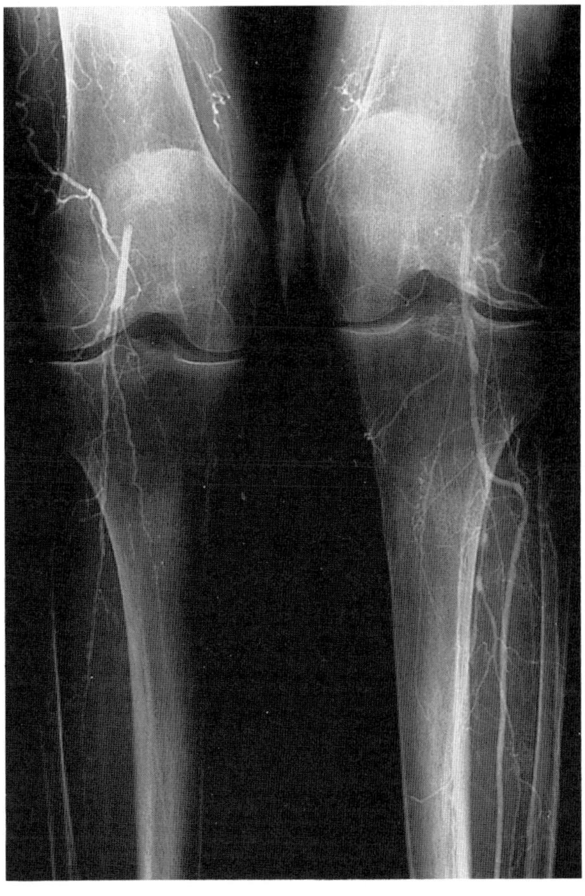

Fig. 56.12 Arteriogram showing bilateral femoropopliteal obstruction. On the left side the popliteal artery is recanalized at the knee with a good run off suitable for a bypass graft.

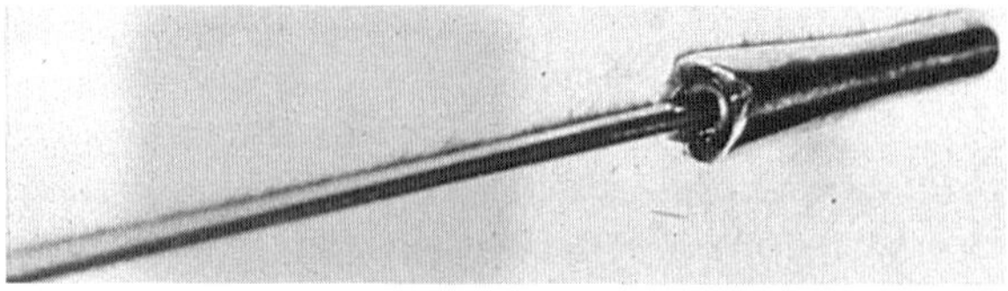

Fig. 56.13 Hall valve cutter used for in situ vein grafting.

provided great care is taken. Patient selection for these distal procedures is important so that inappropriate operations with a low success rate are not done. New techniques are emerging which can help to make these difficult decisions, for example at the time of surgery the distal vessel is isolated and the peripheral resistance measured by injecting autologous blood into it through a soft silastic cannula at 100 ml/min. The pressure generated is measured through a side arm and provides a measure of the resistance. If the resistance is high, the chances of a successful outcome are relatively poor and a primary amputation should be considered (Parvin et al 1985). After completion of the operation it is important to ensure that there are no technical problems. This can be done by doing a completion angiogram and measuring the flow through the graft using a flow meter. Flow should be between 80–100 ml/min and rise further after the injection of papaverine into the artery. Outflow resistance can again be assessed at completion if a needle is inserted into the graft (Ascer et al 1984). Enhancement of flow lasting for some hours can be achieved by the injection of a single bolus of the prostacyclin analogue, iloprost, into the graft on completion and may have a beneficial effect on outcome (Hickey et al 1991).

There is some dispute about the success rate of very distal (Fig. 56.14) procedures but provided the surgeon concerned takes enough care and is properly trained in these techniques then limb salvage rates >65% at 5 years are obtainable (Bergamini 1991) (Fig. 56.15). Recently in diabetics, where lesions are often even more distal, in situ vein grafts from a patent popliteal artery to the foot vessels have been shown to produce good results (Ricci et al 1990).

No patient should have an amputation unless a proper

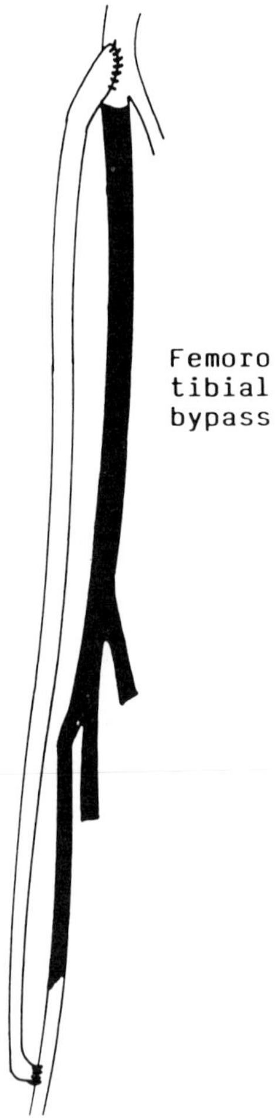

Fig. 56.14 Diagram of an in situ vein graft from the femoral to the posterior tibial artery near to the ankle.

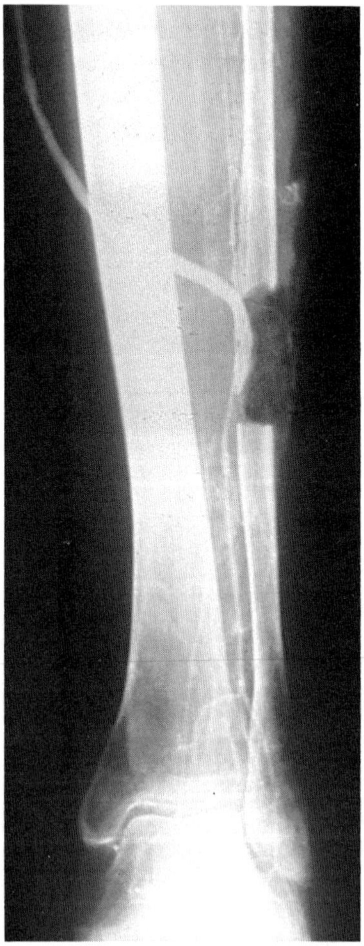

Fig. 56.15 Completion angiogram of a femorodistal peroneal in situ graft after resection of a small segment of fibula to access the distal vessel.

evaluation of the distal vessels is undertaken. In this day and age, an angiogram is not the final arbiter of operability and other tests can and should be used. Recently, for example a method called pulse generated run off (PGR) has been described as a useful method of assessing the patency of distal vessels (Beard et al 1988). In this test a cuff is placed around the calf and intermittently expanded using compressed air. The compression produces a signal in the arteries which can be heard at the ankle using doppler (Fig. 56.16). If this technique is used, the foot vessels including the pedal arch can be mapped out successfully and a vessel found for a distal anastomosis. If PGR is not available, a signal can often be heard in a pedal vessel with the leg in a dependent position, thus confirming its patency (Bell 1991). With these techniques probably less than 5% of patients are unreconstructable and with modern anaesthesia most are fit for surgery.

In recent years it has become apparent that vein grafts are, in the 1 year after implantation, prone to strictures which can develop anywhere along their length (Leopold et al 1989) (Fig. 56.17). The cause of these strictures remains obscure but a combination of hyperplasia and fibrosis occurs (Plate 56.4). After the first year they are less likely to be a problem though progression of the disease in the run off vessels can of course occur. Every patient should be followed by duplex scanning or ankle brachial pressure index measurements to detect these strictures which are otherwise asymptomatic. Duplex scanning reveals an area of increased frequency (Fig. 56.18) which should be confirmed by angiography. If, as is usually the case, a stricture is present, provided it is short it can be successfully dealt with by angioplasty. If it is a longer stricture, a vein patch needs to be applied to widen the lumen. If the vein is allowed to thrombose it is hard to salvage. Our surveillance policy has successfully abolished early vein graft failure so that patency rates of 75% at a year now approach 95% (Brennan et al 1991).

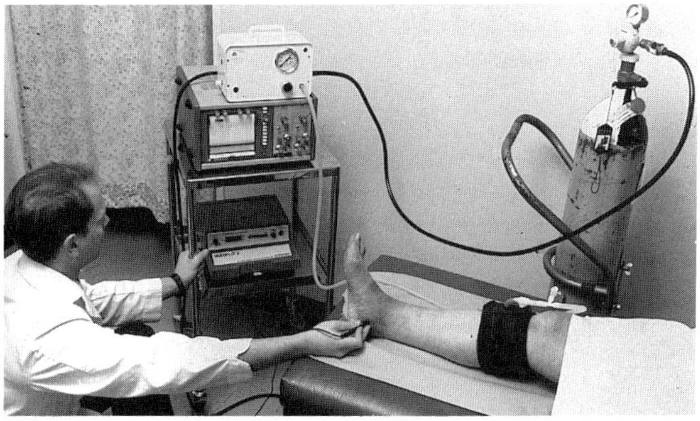

Fig. 56.16 A cuff placed around the calf vessels and intermittently compressed will produce a signal at the ankle if the distal vessels are patent.

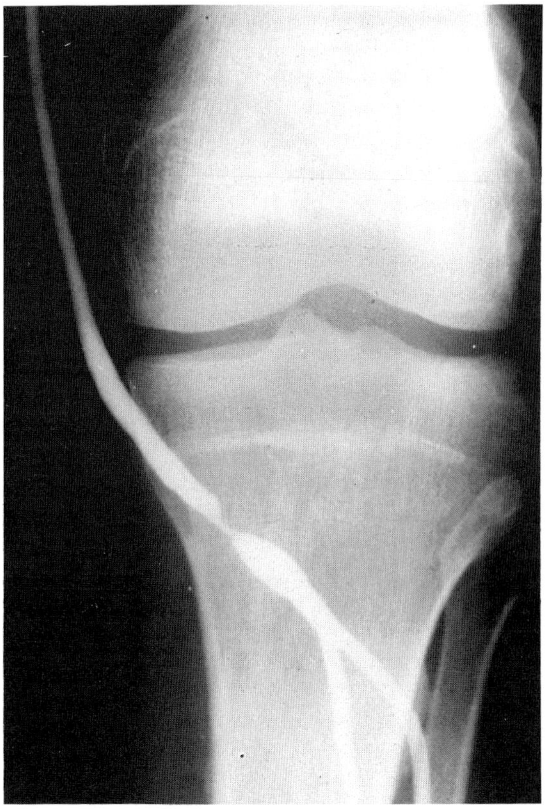

Fig. 56.17 Angiogram showing a vein graft stricture just above the knee.

Amputation

If all else fails then an amputation should be performed but this should not be the end result of a number of failed vascular procedures. As already mentioned techniques are now available which will allow the outcome to be predicted before the reconstruction is undertaken, particularly with distal procedures. If the outcome is likely to be poor (Cooper et al 1990) then a primary amputation below the knee should be considered and would be the best solution for the patient. If however there is a reasonable chance of success, which can be defined arbitrarily as limb salvage of at least 1 year in more than 25% of cases, it should be taken. Amputation is the worst solution for an elderly patient, particularly if it is above the knee and rehabilitation rates are poor under these circumstances (Gregory 1991). If possible the patient should have an amputation below the knee to allow a maximum chance of mobility, unless an above knee procedure is preferable for other reasons. There should be relatively few circumstances in which a patient with a gangrenous toe is subjected to an above knee amputation without at least an angiogram being done first and the opinion of a vascular surgeon sought about possible reconstruction. It is no longer acceptable for an arteriogram to be the arbiter of a reconstructive possibility, other tests such as simple

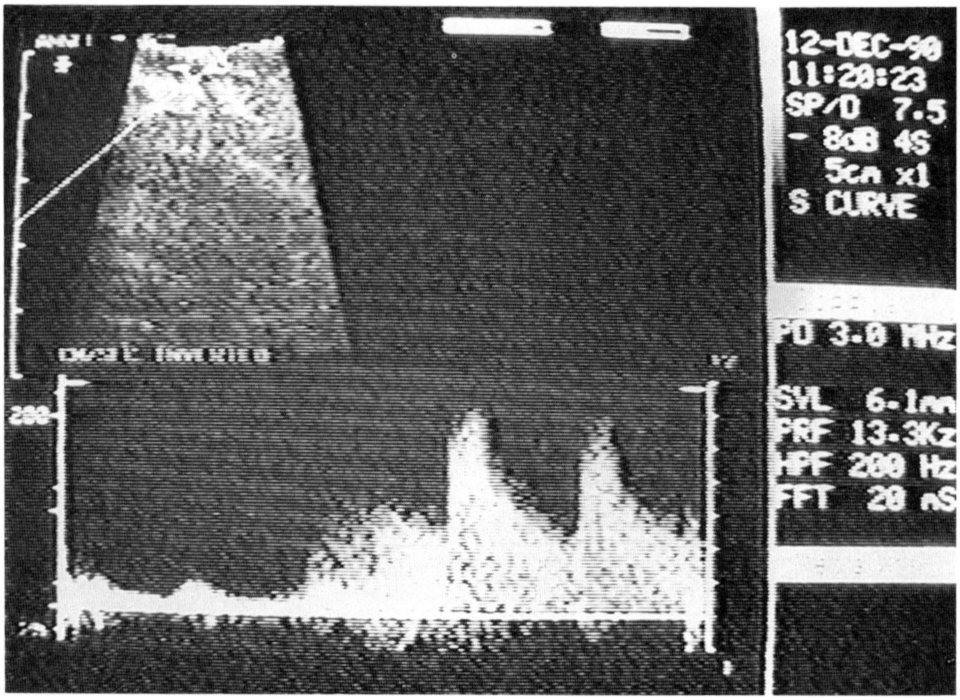

Fig. 56.18 A duplex scan of an in situ vein graft. On the left a normal frequency waveform can be seen which becomes much higher and more turbulent on the right as the probe encounters the stricture.

dependent Doppler or pulse generated run off (Beard et al 1988) are now available to demonstrate patent vessels which will allow very good results in the right hands (Bergamini et al 1991). If necessary the patient's vessels below the knee should be explored and an 'on table angiogram' carried out before the case is declared inoperable. By the same token very few patients are unfit for anaesthesia in these days of modern anaesthetic practice. Even those who are unfit can be dealt with either by spinal or local anaesthesia.

ACUTE UPON CHRONIC (SUB-ACUTE) PRESENTATION

A patient with a history of claudication due to stenosis of an appropriate vessel, as already described can at any time deteriorate particularly if smoking continues. Under these circumstances a sudden deterioration due to thrombosis or an atheromatous stenosis can lead to so-called acute upon chronic ischaemia. Under these circumstances the patient will convert from claudication to severe rest pain but will not necessarily have any neuroischaemic changes which are normally seen with acute ischaemia. Under these circumstances the physician normally has 2 or 3 days to sort out the problem and an angiogram to define the level of occlusion and look for the run off vessels should again be done. If there are good run off vessels a bypass procedure is probably the best option but an alternative is to use intra-arterial thrombolysis (Barr 1991). This technique, using low doses of either streptokinase, urokinase or tissue plasminogen activator has been used successfully on a number of occasions and will allow recanalization of the stenosed segment followed by angioplasty. Systemically administered thrombolytic agents do not work and it is essential to pass a catheter directly into the clot where the thrombolytic agents are administered in low doses and cause progressive lysis. The technique is however labour intensive and requires a good deal of supervision. As yet thrombolysis has not been compared with surgery in a randomized trial but it is a good technique to remember particularly if the run off vessels are poor (Earnshaw 1991).

Embolic disease

Under these circumstances an embolus consisting usually of thrombus moves from the heart in the left atrium or the left ventricular wall following a myocardial infarct and obstructs a major vessel which could be anywhere in the body but is often in the lower limb (Plate 56.6). When this happens the patient frequently has had no previous history of ischaemia and presents with acute ischaemia, although, occasionally, repeated emboli can cause chronic ischaemia.

Acute ischaemia

The patient will complain of severe pain in the leg with

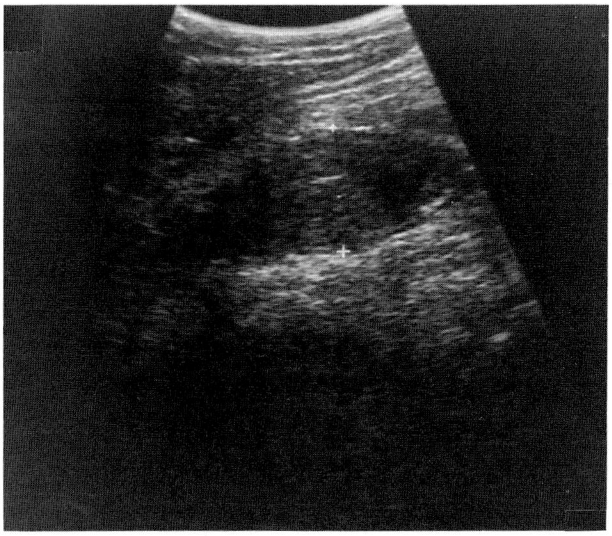

Fig. 56.19 Ultrasound scans showing a popliteal artery aneurysm.

the onset of numbness and possibly stiffness suggesting acute ischaemia is present. Under these circumstances only limited time is available, possibly less than 6 hours, before muscle death occurs. It is important that a history of myocardial infarction is excluded and the patient examined for atrial fibrillation, as these give a clue to the cause of the condition. Emboli can, of course, also come from aneurysms of the aorta or more rarely from the popliteal artery and this has to be looked for (Halliday et al 1991) (Fig. 56.19). Embolic disease can be very difficult to distinguish from thrombosis of a stenosed atheromatous segment which can also present acutely. If there is evidence of neuroischaemia with paraesthesia or blunting of sensation there is no time for thrombolysis which takes several hours and urgent surgery has to be embarked upon. As before, an angiogram should be done and if angioplasty is possible it should be carried out. If not distal vessels should be looked for using dependent doppler or pulse generated run off as already described. If the case is one of a definite embolus then the femoral artery can be exposed in the groin under local anaesthesia and an embolectomy performed using a Fogarty balloon catheter when the clot can usually be removed quite easily. Thereafter the patient should have long-term anticoagulant therapy. If however the catheter does not pass easily, the likelihood is that the case is one of acute thrombosis of a pre-existing atheromatous stenosis and the artery will need to be explored lower down and a bypass graft performed after appropriate angiography. Under these circumstances the prognosis is poor. If no run off vessels are available intra-operative thrombolysis can be carried out using streptokinase injected directly into the arteriotomy (Quinones-Baldrich et al 1989). The results of treatment for acute ischaemia are relatively poor with a high rate of limb loss. If an aortic or a popliteal aneurysm is the source of the embolus then these should be dealt with (p. 1288).

Chronic ischaemia of the hand

This is rare and is usually caused by subclavian or innominate occlusion or stenosis due to atheroma. An alternative cause is a cervical rib causing pressure on the subclavian artery leading to a post stenotic dilatation. Thrombus forms in this aneurysmal dilatation and can embolize to the hand. The symptoms are exactly the same as those seen with leg ischaemia and the patient may complain of claudication when the arm is used, particularly above the head, but gangrene is rare. An angiogram will show the lesion which may be amenable to angioplasty. If not a bypass graft from an adjacent artery such as the other subclavian artery, the carotid or aortic arch will usually solve the problem (Perry 1982) (Fig. 56.20). Distal vascular problems are unusual in the arm. If a cervical rib is present and causing difficulties, it should be removed and any obvious aneurysm of the subclavian artery resected.

Renal artery atherosclerosis

Stenosis of the origins of the renal arteries is common and is responsible for hypertension in about 10% of cases. It is also in the long term a cause of progressive and often unrecognized renal failure (Weibull et al 1990). The condition is not easily diagnosed but should be thought about because it is a remediable cause of hypertension. The difficulty is in finding a reliable and simple test to establish its presence. An IVP is still worth doing, but nowadays split renal function tests using isotope renography and renal vein sampling for renin are prob-

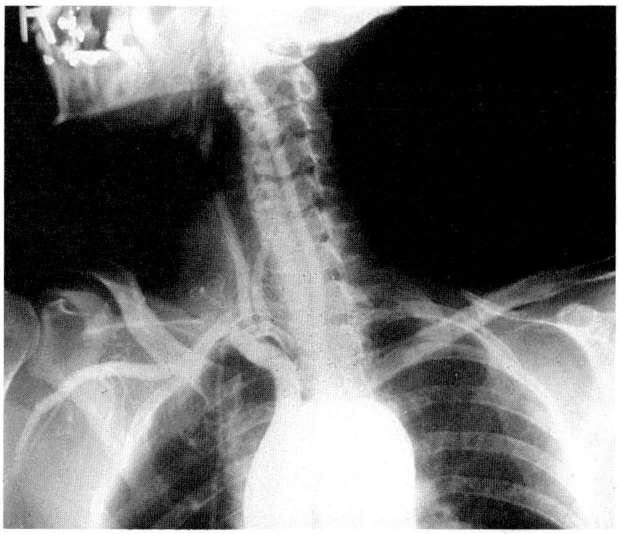

Fig. 56.20 An angiogram showing a normal right and obstructed left subclavian artery.

ably the procedures of choice. The availability of newer methods of imaging with colour duplex should also make the diagnosis of this treatable condition much easier.

As mentioned earlier the possibility of gradual renal failure must not be forgotten and the indications for treatment in this condition are uncontrolled hypertension or deteriorating renal function. This implies that a patient who is treated conservatively must be followed carefully and the renal function examined regularly. Angioplasty has made a big impact for this condition and dilatation is relatively straightforward provided the lesion is not at the aortic orifice and will give excellent long-term results. It is however potentially dangerous as giving large doses of contrast can precipitate renal failure. If angioplasty fails and should the patient's condition deteriorate as far as renal function is concerned, then surgery ought to be recommended. This can be done by using some form of bypass graft of saphenous vein, dacron or teflon from the aorta to the renal artery. A less traumatic procedure for the patient, is to connect the splenic artery on the left or the pancreaticoduodenal artery on the right to the renal artery. This is a much less onerous procedure and avoids cross clamping the aorta. The results of this type of treatment for renal artery stenosis are very good (Weibull et al 1990). If the lesions are very small and beyond the major branches of the renal artery, as can occur in fibromuscular dysplasia (Fig. 56.21), the kidney can be removed completely and, after being cooled, the lesions bypassed on the bench before the kidney is returned to the patient.

Mesenteric ischaemia

Mesenteric ischaemia is again commonly found on incidental angiography but more often than not is asymptomatic. It is said to become symptomatic if two out of the three mesenteric vessels, i.e. coeliac axis, superior mesenteric and inferior mesenteric are occluded and in this situation the patient can present with symptoms of intestinal ischaemia. Classically they will complain of severe weight loss and fear of eating because of pain. The diagnosis usually emerges after a number of possibilities have been excluded and even then is often missed. A lateral angiogram must be done to exclude the possibility as the results of bypass grafts are excellent. The colour duplex machine might make diagnosis of this condition easier.

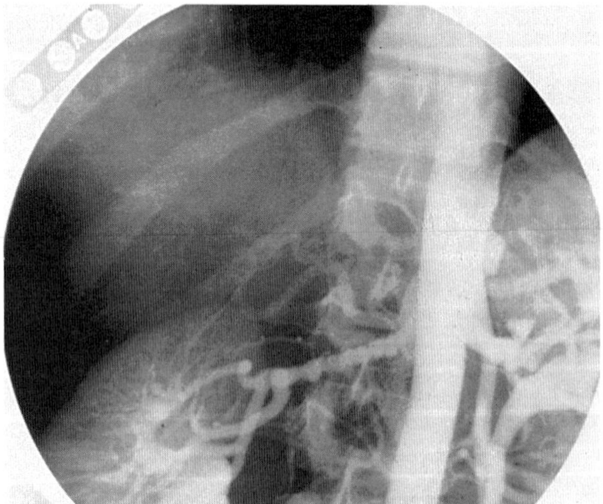

Fig. 56.21 The typical beaded appearance of fibromuscular hyperplasia affecting the right renal artery.

If the condition is not diagnosed and treated when it is in its chronic state the patient can present with acute symptoms of ischaemia and more often than not the bowel becomes gangrenous and even with surgery the outcome is very poor. There is no test at present which will discriminate acute mesenteric ischaemia from other causes of acute abdomen pain but the possibility must always be borne in mind in patients with undiagnosed abdominal pain with a leucocytosis (Baur et al 1984).

Aneurysmal disease

Abdominal aortic aneurysm

These are relatively common and present in 3–5% of males over the age of 65 as shown in recent community screening programmes (Collins 1985) looking at the aorta in an asymptomatic population. At present the natural history of this condition is unknown but when the aneurysm reaches 5.5 cm in diameter the chances of rupture within the next year are of the order of 70% (Campbell et al 1986). With smaller aneurysms there is some uncertainty but there is evidence that below 5 cm the chances of rupture are >2% (Nevitt et al 1989) which is similar to the mortality rate from surgery. Recent research has suggested that there may be an hereditary element to aortic aneurysms which are more common in the siblings of those affected (Powell et al 1991). Patients present with few symptoms and one should be aware of the possibility in anyone with vague abdominal or back pain and examine the abdomen carefully. These lesions are often found incidentally because of the widespread use of ultrasound for examining the abdomen. Quite commonly they present as a contained or intraperitoneal rupture with back pain, peritonitis and shock when the mortality can be between 50–60%. Because of its high mortality the operation should if possible be done electively, when the mortality is less than 4% (Johanson & Swedenborg 1986). If an aneurysm is suspected it can be confirmed by ultrasound (Fig. 56.22) or CAT scanning (Fig. 56.23). Prior to surgery, it is important to ensure that the aneurysm does not involve the renal arteries. This can usually be done by CAT scanning but in difficult cases an angiogram may be necessary. If the renal

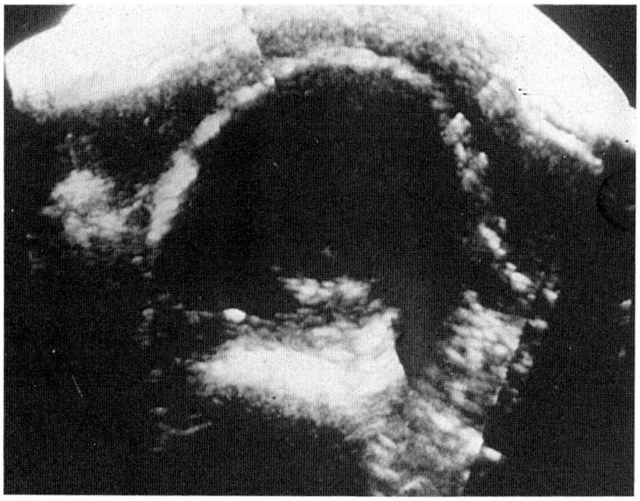

Fig. 56.22 Ultrasound scan showing a large aortic aneurysm.

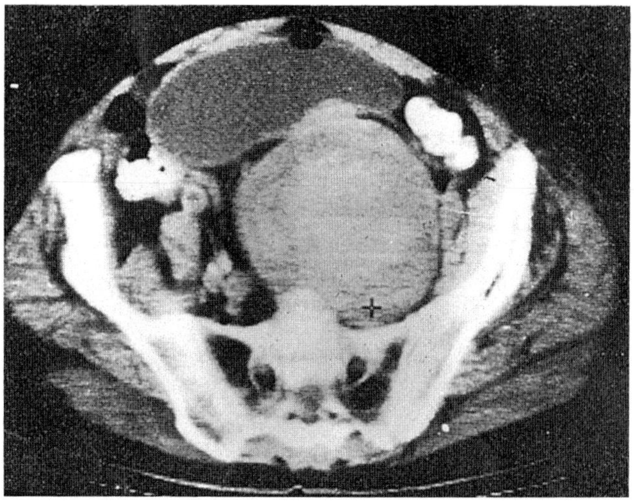

Fig. 56.23 A CAT scan showing a large aortic aneurysm.

arteries are involved the operation will be more difficult and should be planned appropriately beforehand. Unlike patients with occlusive vascular disease, if surgery is successful these patients have an almost normal life expectancy.

Patients with an aneurysm are often old but this should not be a bar to surgical treatment providing the patient can tolerate an operation, and modern anaesthesia means that most can and in fact many patients over 80 years of age do well following this procedure (Campbell et al 1986). Complications can of course occur but are relatively rare after elective surgery, they are far more common following rupture and include renal failure, coronary thrombosis and stroke. Because of the importance of this condition, screening of patients at risk, which includes those with hypertension, peripheral arterial disease and chronic obstructive airways disease, should be undertaken to offer elective surgery to those at risk.

Thoraco-abdominal aneurysms

These are relatively uncommon but can involve the descending aorta to the left of the subclavian artery down to the abdominal aorta, to involve the coeliac mesenteric and renal vessels. These aneurysms do rupture and they should be operated upon electively (Cranford & de Natale 1986) (Fig. 56.24). The operation is more difficult because all intra-abdominal branches have to be attached to the graft and there is a significant danger of paraplegia (10%) as the intercostal vessels supplying the spinal cord may be involved (Wolfe 1991). The largest of these should be attached to the graft during the procedure in order to try and avoid this problem. The most extensive aneurysm particularly those that start as high as the left subclavian artery do worse whereas those that arise in the lower thorax and upper abdomen do better and are well worth repairing. Special anaesthetic techniques are required to deal with these patients and the expertise to operate on them is only available in relatively few centres. If they are not operated on however they will rupture and in that situation are very difficult to deal with successfully.

Dissecting aneurysms

These aneurysms are common in patients who have elastic tissue disorders such as Marfan's or Ehlers–Danlos syndrome. They can also occur in patients with atheroma and usually start close to the root of the aorta but can start anywhere in the thoracic or abdominal aorta. They

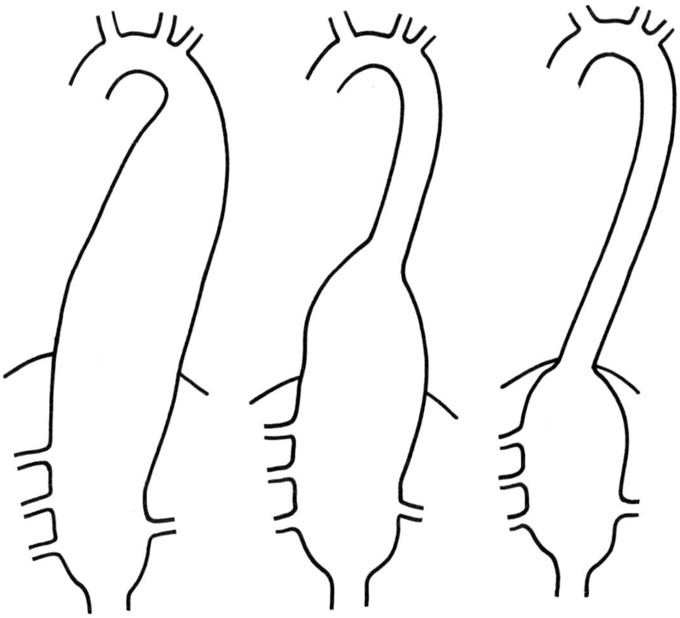

Fig. 56.24 Three types of thoraco-abdominal aortic aneurysm.

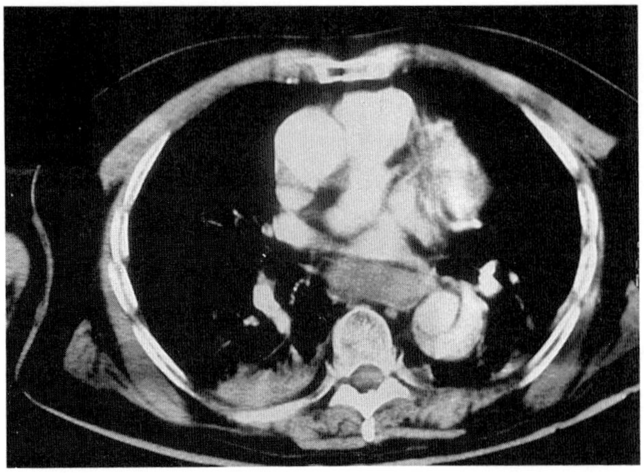

Fig. 56.25 Dissecting aneurysm of the descending thoracic aorta, the dissection can be seen clearly with two lumens visible.

classically present with severe pain starting in the chest or back which passes down towards the abdomen. The problem is due to dissection of the arterial wall to form two lumens (Fig. 56.25) and rupture or occlusion of major arterial branches is often the result. Treatment is urgent and requires replacement of the aorta with a dacron graft. The outlook, if the lesion is atheromatous, is good but in the other syndromes is relatively poor.

Femoral aneurysms

These are relatively rare and present as a swelling in the groin (Plate 56.7). Because they are often large and can rupture or thrombose they should be operated upon and replaced by a dacron prosthesis which gives good results (Graham et al 1980).

Popliteal aneurysms

Aneurysms of the popliteal artery are relatively common and often accompany aortic aneurysms (Whitehouse et al 1983). They present either as an asymptomatic swelling behind the knee or they thrombose and the patient presents with chronic or acute critical ischaemia. More rarely they can embolize and again the patient presents with acute ischaemia (Whitehouse et al 1983). Any patient presenting with acute ischaemia should be examined carefully to exclude a popliteal aneurysm. If one is present it should be dealt with after angiography. The angiogram will usually show the acutely occluded artery with a patent vessel beyond the occlusion. If this is the case the patient should be operated upon and the aneurysm bypassed using reversed vein or an artificial graft. The lesion is often bilateral and the other side should be dealt with before it too thromboses and causes acute ischaemia. If the aneurysm has not thrombosed but has embolized, the emboli are so small that limb loss is a distinct possibility. If there are no run off vessels on angiography or if the aneurysm has embolized, the most effective treatment is to attempt thrombolysis by giving small doses of streptokinase, urokinase or tissue plasminogen activator directly into the popliteal artery by the percutaneous route. Popliteal aneurysms which have thrombosed or embolized can lead to limb loss in as many as 40% of cases (Anton et al 1984). With thrombolysis and surgery where a patent distal vessel is available, good results can be obtained with long-term limb survival in excess of 70% of cases (Graham et al 1980).

Diabetes

The problems in diabetics will be discussed in Chapter 57, suffice to say that it is important to recognize that these patients can be dealt with in exactly the same way as has been described for patients with atherosclerosis without diabetes. The important thing to remember, as the reader will discover, is to distinguish between the neuropathic and neuro-ischaemic foot. The patient with neuro-ischaemic disease usually has large vessel disease of the type described earlier and the treatment is exactly the same but usually more urgent (Kolh & Lopes Virilla 1988). Pulses can usually be felt in the neuropathic foot which often has a higher than normal blood flow. There is no obstruction to major vessels (Logerfo & Coffman 1984) (Plate 56.8). In this situation infection, which can spread very rapidly, is the main problem. Urgent and radical drainage is essential if a high amputation is to be avoided. Some patients have a mixture of neuropathic and neuro-ischaemic disease.

Sympathectomy

Sympathectomy has little place in the modern treatment of peripheral vascular disease or critical ischaemia. Although it can increase skin blood flow this is at the expense of other areas. Phenol sympathectomy may be useful in some patients with severe ischaemia which is not critical and should be borne in mind for this situation.

REFERENCES

Angelini G D, Soyombo A A, Newby A C 1991 Smooth muscle proliferation in response to injury in an organ culture of human saphenous vein. European Journal of Vascular Surgery 5: 5–12

Anton G E, Hertzer N R, Beven E G et al 1986 Surgical management of popliteal aneurysms. Trends in presentation, treatment and results from 1952–1984. Journal of Vascular Surgery 3: 125–129

Ascer F, Veith F J, Morris L et al 1984 Quantitative assessment of outflow resistance in lower extremity arterial reconstructions. Journal of Surgical Research 37: 8–15

Barr H 1991 Intra arterial thrombolytic therapy in the management of

acute and chronic limb ischaemia. British Journal of Surgery 78: 284–287
Baur G M, Millay D J, Taylor L M, Porter J M 1984 Treatment of chronic visceral ischaemia. American Journal of Surgery 148: 138–144
Beard J D, Scott D J A, Evans J M, Skidmore R et al 1988 Pulse generated run off: A new method of determining calf vessel patency. British Journal of Surgery 75: 361–363
Bell P R F 1991 Arterial surgery of the lower limb. Churchill Livingstone, Edinburgh, p 7–8
Belli A M, Cumberland D C, Knox A M et al 1990 The complication rate of percutaneous peripheral balloon angioplasty. Clinical Radiology 41: 380–383
Bergamini T M 1991 Experience with in situ saphenous vein bypasses during 1981 to 1989: Determinant factors of long term patency. Journal of Vascular Surgery 13: 137–149
Boobis L, Bell P R F 1984 The place of drug therapy in peripheral arterial disease. In: Bell P R F, Tilney N L (eds) Vascular surgery. Butterworths, London, p 12–53
Brennan J A, Hartshorne T, Bell P R F 1991 The role of simple non-invasive testing in infrainguinal vein graft surveillance. European Journal of Vascular Surgery 5: 13–17
Campbell W B, Collin J, Morris P J 1986 The mortality of abdominal aortic aneurysm. Annals of the Royal College of Surgeons of England 68: 275–278
Coleman C C, Pojalaky I P, Robinson J D et al 1989 Atheroablation with the Kensey catheter: a pathological study. Radiology 170: 391–394
Collin J 1985 Screening for abdominal aortic aneurysms. British Journal of Surgery 72: 851–852
Cooper G G, Austin C, Fitzsimmons E et al 1990 Outflow resistance and early occlusion of infrainguinal bypass grafts. European Journal of Vascular Surgery 4: 279–285
Corbett R R, Taylor P R, Chilvers A et al 1984 Axillofemoral bypass grafts in poor risk patients with critical ischaemia. Annals of the Royal College of Surgeons of England 66: 170–173
Cranford E S, de Natale R W 1986 Thoracoabdominal aortic aneurysms: observations regarding natural course of disease. Journal of Vascular Surgery 3: 578–582
de Brosse D, Petit H, Torres E et al 1990 Percutaneous atherectomy with the Kensey catheter: Early and mid term results in femoropopliteal occlusions unsuitable for conventional angioplasty. Annals of Vascular Surgery 4: 550–552
Department of Health and Human Services 1983 The health consequences of smoking: Cardiovascular disease; A report of the Surgeon General. Rockville M D, Hew D (ed), p 1–11
Dormandy J A, Murray G D 1991 The fate of the claudicant — A prospective study of 1969 claudicants. European Journal of Vascular Surgery 5: 131–133
Dotter C T, Judkins M P 1964 Transluminal treatment of arteriosclerotic obstruction; Description of a new technique and a preliminary report of its application. Circulation 30: 654–670
Earnshaw J J 1991 Thrombolytic therapy in the management of acute limb ischaemia. British Journal of Surgery 78: 261–269
Earnshaw J J, Shaw J F L 1990 Survey of the use of thrombolysis for limb ischaemia in the UK and Ireland. British Journal of Surgery 72: 1041–1042
European Consensus on Critical Limb Ischaemia 1989 Lancet 1: 737–738
Fagrell B 1990 Investigations and general management of critical ischaemia. In: Dormandy J, Stock G (eds) Critical leg ischaemia. Springer Verlag, Berlin p 41–48
Fahal A H, McDonald A M, Marston A 1989 Femorofemoral bypass in unilateral iliac artery occlusion. British Journal of Surgery 76: 22–25
Gander O P 1985 Pathogenesis of macrovascular disease including the influence of lipids. In: Marble A, Kroll P, Bradley R F, Christlieb A R, Soldner J S (eds) Joclin's diabetes mellitus, 12th edn. Lea and Febiger, Philadelphia
Graham C, Zelenock G, Whitehouse W et al 1980 Clinical significance of arterio-sclerotic femoral artery aneurysms. Archives of Surgery. 115: 502–507
Gregory D A 1991 Amputations: Statistics and Trends. Annals of the Royal College of Surgeons of England 73: 137–142
Gruntzig A, Hopff H 1974 Perkutane rekanalisation chronischer casterieller verschbuese mid einen neuen dilatation skathetar: Modifikation der Dottertechnik. Deutsche Medizinische Wochenschrist 99: 2502–2511
Halliday A, Taylor P R, Wolfe J H et al 1991 The management of popliteal aneurysms: The importance of early repair. Annals of the Royal College of Surgeons of England 73: 253–257
Hiatt W R, Wolfel E E, Regensteiner J G 1991 Exercise in the treatment of intermittent claudication due to peripheral arterial disease. Vascular Medicine Review 2: 61–70
Hickey N C, Shearman C P, Crowson M C et al 1991 Iloprost improves femorodistal graft flow after a single bolus injection. European Journal of Vascular Surgery 5: 19–23
Hoofwijk A 1991 The fate of the patient with critical limb ischaemia. Critical Ischaemia 1: 15–21
Hughson W G, Marvin J I, Tibbs D J et al 1978 Intermittent claudication. Factors determining outcome. British Medical Journal 1: 1377–1379
Johanson G, Swedenborg J 1986 Ruptured abdominal aortic aneurysms: A study of incidence and mortality. British Journal of Surgery 73: 101–103
Johnson T N, McLoughlin G A, Wake P N et al 1986 Comparison of extra peritoneal and transperitoneal methods of aortoiliac reconstruction: Twenty years experience. Journal of Cardiovascular Surgery 27: 561–565
Kannel W B, McGee D L 1985 Update on some epidemiological features of intermittent claudication. Journal of the American Geriatrics Society 33: 13–18
Kolh L J H, Lopes Virilla M F 1988 A review of the development of large vessel disease in diabetes mellitus. American Journal of Medicine 85(suppl): 113–118
Kuller L H, Dorman J S, Wolf R A 1985 Cerebrovascular disease and diabetes. In: Harris M I, Hammon R F (eds) National Diabetes Data Group. Diabetes in America. NIH PAT No. 85–1468 VS Dept of Health and Human Services Public Health Service
Laing S P, Greenhalgh R M 1980 Standard exercise test to assess peripheral arterial disease. British Medical Journal 260: 13–16
Legemate D A, Teeuwen C, Hoemeveldt H et al 1989 The potential of duplex scanning to replace aortoiliac and femoropopliteal angiography. European Journal of Vascular Surgery 3: 49–55
Leopold P W, Shandalol A, Kupinski A M, Chang B B et al 1989 Use of B mode venous mapping in infra-inguinal in-situ arterial bypasses. British Journal of Surgery 76: 305–307
Logerfo F W, Coffman J D 1984 Vascular and microvascular disease of the foot in diabetes. New England Journal of Medicine 211: 1615–1619
MacPherson D S, James D C, Bell P R F 1980 Is aortography abused in lower limb ischaemia? Lancet 2: 80–81
Murray A, Cross F 1991 Laser angioplasty of peripheral arteries. Surgery 89: 2136–2139
Murray A, Mitchell D C, Grasty M et al 1989 Peripheral laser angioplasty with pulsed dye laser and ball tipped optical fibres. Lancet 2: 1471–1474
Nevelsteen A, Wontess L, Suy R 1991 Aortofemoral dacron reconstruction for aorto-iliac occlusive disease: A 25 year survey. European Journal of Vascular Surgery 5: 179–187
Nevitt M P, Ballard D J, Hallet J W 1989 Prognosis of abdominal aortic aneurysms. A population based study. New England Journal of Medicine 321: 1009–1013
Palmaz J C, Tio F O, Schatz R Z et al 1987 Self expanding endovascular prosthesis: An experimental study. Radiology 164: 709–714
Parvin S D, Evans D H, Bell P R F 1985 Peripheral resistance measurement in the assessment of severe peripheral vascular disease. British Journal of Surgery 72: 751–753
Perry M 1982 Carotid subclavian bypass. In: Greenhalgh R M (ed) Extra anatomic and secondary arterial reconstruction. Pitman Medical, London, p 295–304
Perry M D 1985 Infected aortic aneurysms. Journal of Vascular Surgery. 2: 97–99
Pokrovsky A V, Volynsky J D, Konov V I et al 1990 Recanalisation of occluded peripheral arteries by excimer laser. European Journal of Vascular Surgery 4: 575–583
Powell J T, Adamson J, Macsweeney S T et al 1991 Genetics variants

of collagen III and abdominal aortic aneurysms. European Journal of Vascular Surgery. 5: 145–149

Quinones-Baldrich W J, Baker D, Busuttil R W et al 1989 Intraoperative infusion of lytic drugs for thrombotic complications of revascularisation. Journal of Vascular Surgery 10: 408–418

Quinones-Baldrich W J, Busuttil R W, Baker J D et al 1988 Is the preferential use of polytetrafluouroethylene grafts for femoropopliteal bypass justified? Journal of Vascular Surgery 8: 219–228

Ricci M A, Graham A M, Symes J F 1990 Comparison of in situ and reversed saphenous vein grafts for infrageniculate bypass. Canadian Journal of Surgery 33: 216–220

Sampson R H, Sprayregen S, Veith F et al 1984 Management of angioplasty complications, unsuccessful procedures and early and late failures. Annals of Surgery 199: 234–40

Sanborn T A, Cumberland D C, Greenfield A F et al 1988 Initial results and one year follow up in 129 femoropopliteal lesions. Radiology 168: 121–125

Simpson J B, Selman M R, Robertson G C et al 1988 Transluminal atherectomy for occlusive peripheral vascular disease. American College of Cardiology 61: 96–101

Taylor L M Jr, Edwards J M, Porter J M 1991 Present status of reversed vein bypass grafting: Five year results of a modern series. Journal of Vascular Surgery 11: 193–206

van Ander G J, van Erp W F M, Krepel V M et al 1985 Percutaneous transluminal dilatation of the iliac artery. Radiology 156: 321–324

Weibull H G, Bergonist D, Andersson I, Choi D L, Jonsson K, Bergentz S E 1990 Symptoms and signs of thrombotic occlusion of atherosclerotic renal artery stenosis. European Journal of Vascular Surgery 4: 159–167

Whitehouse W M, Wakefield T W, Graham L M et al 1983 Limb threatening potential of arteriosclerotic popliteal artery aneurysm. Journal of Surgery 93: 694–698

Wolfe J H N 1991 Should we operate on thoraco-abdominal aneurysms. In: Barros D'Sa A, Bell P R F, Darke S G, Harris P L, (eds) Vascular surgery. Current questions. Butterworth Heinemann, Oxford, p 50–61

57. Diabetic vascular disease

D. D. Sandeman J. E. Tooke

Patients with diabetes mellitus develop a variety of vascular complications which account for most of the excess morbidity and mortality associated with the disease. Large vessel disease, or macroangiopathy which manifests as coronary artery, cerebrovascular and peripheral vascular insufficiency is not specific for diabetes, but is often more diffuse and occurs prematurely. Disease of the small vessels, microangiopathy, is more specific to diabetes and results in retinopathy, nephropathy, and possible diabetic cardiomyopathy and neuropathy.

The impact of diabetic vascular disease cannot be overstated. Indeed, Krolewski et al (1986) stated that prolonged survival with diabetes is inevitably associated with the development of clinically significant retinopathy. Morrish et al (1991) recently reported the prevalence and incidence of macrovascular disease in their London cohort of patients: The overall prevalence of macrovascular disease was 45%, ischaemic heart disease being by far the most common manifestation. Their data is in keeping with the findings of Krolewski et al (1987) who examined an American cohort of type I insulin-dependent diabetics, (IDDM) and found a cumulative incidence of ischaemic heart disease of 50% by the age of 50 years, and those of Kleinman et al (1988) in type II, non-insulin-dependent (NIDDM) subjects.

Whilst the pathogenesis of diabetic microangiopathy and accelerated macroangiopathy still eludes us, many contender mechanisms exist. The development of rational treatment is likely to arise from a greater understanding of the pathophysiology and perhaps particular attention should be directed at those potential mechanisms which offer current therapeutic potential. In this regard there is clearly a need to consider the involvement of inappropriate activation of the haemostatic system, haemodynamic factors and lipid abnormalities. Many of the factors probably have a similar role in the genesis or promotion of both micro, and macrovascular disease, with endothelial damage as a common feature (Ross 1986). However, it is arguably simpler to consider the vascular complications due to large and small vessel disease separately, and then the areas of potential overlap.

DIABETIC MICROANGIOPATHY

The term 'diabetic microangiopathy' is widely used, yet no clear and comprehensive definition exists as to what it comprises. In essence the clinical complications are a consequence of tissue ischaemia due to microvascular failure. Nevertheless, the mechanisms involved are varied and complex.

In the retina a series of degenerative changes develop which contribute to the ischaemia: along with basement membrane thickening, there is loss of pericytes, capillary closure (recognized by the finding of cellular basement membrane skeletons), capillary shunting, microaneurysm formation and increased transudation of plasma constituents (Engerman 1989). However, it is the angiogenic response to the ischaemia with resultant new vessel formation which heralds sight-threatening retinopathy particularly in type I diabetic subjects (Davis 1988).

In contrast in diabetic nephropathy the decline in glomerular filtration rate resulting in renal failure owes more to obliteration of the filtration surface area by mesangial expansion than to changes in capillary structure or function (Mauer et al 1984). Whilst these late changes (new vessel formation and mesangial expansion) are organ specific, they represent an injury response of the microcirculation to an antecedent pattern of changes both structural and functional which occurs in all microcirculatory beds as a consequence of the metabolic disturbance of diabetes. It is these early changes which represent the common process which is the basis of diabetic microangiopathy; changes in haemodynamics of the microcirculation, haemorheology, structure of the basement membrane and later modification by glycosylation have all been implicated in this process.

Microvascular haemodynamic abnormalities

Diabetes induces early functional changes in the microcirculation. These functional changes have been observed for years (Ditzel 1968) and have been the subject of much speculation culminating in three recent reviews and the proposal of the haemodynamic hypothesis of diabetic microangiopathy (Parving et al 1983, Tooke 1986, Zatz & Brenner 1986) (Fig. 57.1).

Studies in diabetic patients and in experimental diabetes reveal an early increase in microvascular flow and filtration and possibly permeability. It is argued that these changes are mediated by pre-capillary vasodilation which results in capillary hypertension. This capillary hypertension is thought to promote the capillary basement membrane thickening which characterizes diabetic microangiopathy (Williamson et al 1988).

The hypothesis has been extensively studied in the renal microcirculation in animal models. Glomerular hypertension appears to result from an imbalance in afferent and efferent arteriolar tone, and underlies the glomerular hyperfiltration that is known to occur (Hostetter et al 1981, Jensen et al 1981). These concepts are supported by studies in man (Christiansen 1985, Mogensen 1989). However, not all the animal work supports the role of glomerular hypertension (Bank et al 1987, Mauer et al 1989), and care should be taken in extrapolating from animal data to man. In our own laboratory we have found direct evidence for capillary hypertension in diabetic patients by microcannulation of the nutritive skin capillaries (Sandeman et al 1992).

Many lines of evidence support the suggestion that capillary hypertension may promote basement membrane thickening. In non-diabetic healthy man as in the giraffe, basement membrane thickening occurs at sites of relative capillary hypertension (Vracko 1970, Williamson et al 1971).

It has been suggested that the increase in wall tension, either directly or indirectly due to the increased permeation of plasma proteins (due to the pressure-induced rise in filtration), results in increased synthesis of basement membrane (Stefansson et al 1983, Williamson et al 1988). Particular attention is drawn to the possible role of the increased permeation of fibrinogen in the genesis of basement membrane thickening. Fibrinogen has been shown to induce changes in the growth and motility of vascular endothelial cells resulting in a proliferative response (Watanabe & Tanaka 1983, Rowland et al 1984, Fajdusek et al 1986). Dvorak et al (1985) reported that the fibrin content of tissues is limited by the filtration pressure suggesting a link with capillary pressure disturbance. The rate of disappearance of fibrinogen from plasma is greater in diabetics than non-diabetics which supports this possibility (Jones & Peterson 1979, 1981a,b, Bannerjee et al 1973). Whatever the precise stimulus to basement membrane thickening may be, the resultant microvascular sclerosis limits the vasodilatory reserve of the microcirculation resulting in relative ischaemia at times of high demand (Tooke 1986).

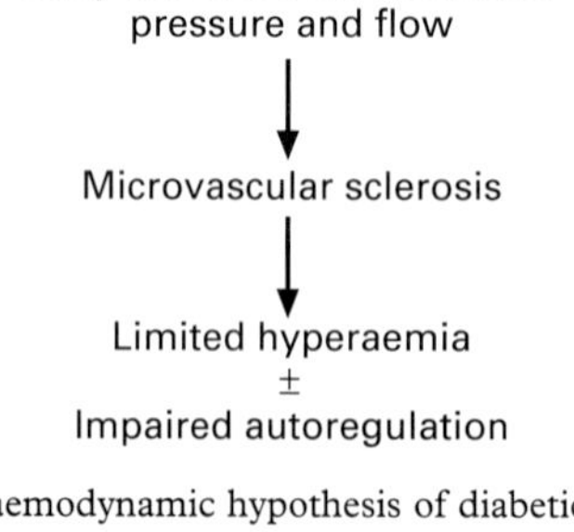

Fig. 57.1 The haemodynamic hypothesis of diabetic microangiopathy.

The haemodynamic hypothesis provides an explanation for the promoting effect of arterial hypertension upon microangiopathy (Orchard et al 1990). Capillary pressure is elevated in non-diabetic subjects with essential hypertension (Williams et al 1990): the concurrence of arterial hypertension and the pre-capillary vasodilation characteristic of poorly controlled insulin-dependent diabetes may well result in particularly high capillary pressure.

Haemorheological changes

A haemorheological model has been proposed (McMillan 1983) relating changes in red cell deformability and aggregability in diabetes to the development of diabetic microangiopathy. Such an hypothesis has immediate attraction because of the unique position of the blood to mediate widespread vascular injury. The hypothesis is made more tenable by the finding that patients who remain free of complications despite a long duration of disease exhibit less disturbance of blood rheology than those afflicted and, in keeping with the development of microvascular disease, the haemorheological changes appear to develop following puberty (McMillan et al 1981).

The mechanisms underlying reduced red cell membrane fluidity and increased aggregability are not clear. There is evidence for glycosylation of the membrane proteins responsible for shape changes and this, in addition to an alteration in the cholesterol/phospholipid ratio in the membrane, may affect fluidity (Juhan-Vague et al 1984). In addition elevated fibrinogen levels or haptoglobulin levels may contribute to the increased erythrocyte aggregation.

McMillan (1983) has suggested that during transient plugging of microvessels by red cell aggregates the wall will be briefly exposed to the entire pressure gradient of the vessel. This increased wall stress may lead to microvascular damage by the mechanisms outlined above.

An alternative and intriguing possibility links the haemodynamic and haemorheological hypotheses. It is appreciated that endothelium acts as a mechano-receptor

(Lansman 1988). Increased shear stress at the endothelium results in vasodilation, possibly mediated at the microvascular level by prostacylin (Kaley et al 1989) or other endothelium-derived relaxing factors. The rheological changes observed in diabetes would tend to increase the shear stress on the endothelial cells for any given flow rate, therapy promoting the precapillary vasodilation that is such an important component of the haemodynamic hypothesis.

Despite the attractions of these concepts it should be recalled that Branemark et al (1971) using an implanted chamber that permitted high power observation of blood cell behaviour in vivo failed to show anticipated rheological changes in diabetic patients except in the presence of ketosis.

Non enzymic glycosylation and the polyol pathway

The tissues subject to microvascular complications are those which do not require insulin for glucose uptake. Two pathways which play a part in the disposal of the excess glucose in diabetes, that is nonenzymatic glycosylation and the polyol pathway, have been implicated in the initiation and promotion of microvascular disease.

Advanced products of nonenzymic glycosylation or AGE products undoubtedly contribute to the pathogenesis of diabetic vascular disease. Their role has been extensively reviewed by Brownlee and colleagues (1988). In essence AGE products are formed irreversibly from Amadori products and accumulate throughout the life of a diabetic patient. Proteins exposed to glucose undergo nonenzymic glycosylation to form Schiff bases. These Schiff bases undergo a slow rearrangement to form the Amadori products, a reversible process which reaches equilibrium over a period of 4 weeks, whatever the lifespan of the protein (Yue et al 1983). The rate of genesis of, and therefore concentration of Amadori products is dependent on the integrated level of glucose over the period, and its formation is reversible. The level of Amadori products in turn determines the rate of accumulation of AGE products, which once formed are permanent.

AGE products probably promote vascular disease by at least two mechanisms, (1) binding of plasma constituents and (2) by changing the matrix of the vascular wall.

Microvascular sclerosis is associated with the accumulation of PAS-positive material, IgM and albumin in the vessel walls (Miller & Michael 1976, Cohn et al 1978, Michael & Brown 1981.) The plasma components are highly bound to the matrix and this binding is probably accentuated by AGE products (Brownlee et al 1983, Sensi et al 1986). Parving (1975) suggested that the continued and accelerated accumulation of plasma constituents in the vessel wall may lead to the observed narrowing of the vessels. Yet again interactions with the other mechanisms described above would be anticipated. Increased microvascular pressure would result in greater extravasation of plasma proteins, and therefore promote increased local trapping by AGE products.

Changes in the matrix of the vessel walls due to the accumulation of AGE products formed locally may have a more profound effect. The anionic proteoglycan content of the membrane has a profound effect on the permselectivity and proliferative status of the vessel wall. The basement membrane content of these substances is reduced in patients with diabetes and complications (Shimomura & Spiro 1987). This reduction may in part be explained by AGE products, the presence of which have been shown to reduce heparin binding by 80% (Brownlee et al 1987). In addition cross-linking by AGE products may prevent the normal tertiary structure of the basement membrane developing with resultant changes in its biophysical properties.

The addition of AGE products to cell cultures have caused a variety of responses in the cell culture: when bound to surface receptors, AGE products result in increased expression of coagulation factors on the endothelial cell (Eposito et al (1989) and Vlassara and co-workers (1988) demonstrated increased release of cytokines and growth factors in cell culture due to AGE products.

The polyol or sorbitol pathway is a two stage path which forms fructose from glucose. Under normal conditions the intracellular concentration of glucose is such that the activity of the pathway is low (due to the K_m of the rate limiting enzyme, aldose reductase). However, in uncontrolled diabetes, the susceptible tissues have high intracellular glucose concentrations and the pathway contributes significantly to glucose disposal. A considerable body of evidence exists in support of the concept that overactivity of this pathway may underlie diabetic vascular disease. Inhibition of the pathway by aldose reductase inhibitors, particularly in animal models has been shown to prevent the functional disturbances in the microcirculation which precede microangiopathy of the eye, kidney and nerves (Bank et al 1989a, Pugliesse et al 1990).

The mechanisms by which this pathway induces vascular injury are not clear. Imbalances in myo-inositol metabolism, changes in the ion gradients of the cell due to ATPase activity or changes in the redox potential of the cell have all been implicated and are reviewed by Pugliesse and colleagues (1991). Again potential interactions with other pathogenic mechanisms exist; for example, it is suggested that overactivity of this pathway generates the precapillary vasodilation discussed in the earlier section on microvascular haemodynamic disturbances.

Endothelial cells, platelets and prostaglandins

The topographical location of endothelial cells makes their dysfunction a prime suspect in the pathogenesis of diabetic vascular disease. Indeed as our understanding improves, the endothelial cell may turn out to be the conductor of the various pathogenetic mechanisms.

Tissue culture has revealed many abnormalities in endothelial cells and pericytes when the incubation medium contains a high glucose concentration. Delayed replication, a disturbed cell cycle, accelerated cell death and abnormal production of eicosanoids (a finding not restricted to these cells) have all been demonstrated (Kriesberg & Patel 1983, Li et al 1984, Lorenzi et al 1985, Schrier & Williams 1990).

Furthermore several markers of endothelial damage have been found to be raised in patients with diabetes-induced vascular disease. Plasma von Willebrand factor (vWF) and angiotensin-converting enzyme (ACE), are raised (Lieberman & Sastre 1980, Porta et al 1991) and levels of tissue plasminogen activator (TPA) reduced (Jensen et al 1989). Despite this suggestive data the precise impact of endothelial dysfunction upon control of the haemostatic system (Stern et al 1991) and vascular permeability (Deckert et al 1989) remain to be elucidated.

It has also been suggested that abnormalities in platelet function play a role in diabetic vascular disease (Colwell et al 1983a). Increased platelet aggregation, increased production of thromboxane, reduced endothelial production of prostacyclin and decreased platelet survival have all been demonstrated in patients and animal models of diabetes, both before and after the development of vascular disease. Indirect support for this hypothesis comes from the demonstration of protection from the development of retinopathy (as assessed by the rate of microaneurysm formation with the use of antiplatelet agents (The DAMAD Study Group 1989).

A possible role for prostanoids in the control of microvascular flow has been alluded to earlier. In support of this concept microalbuminuria, a marker of incipient nephropathy and 'malignant' angiopathy, is reduced by the thromboxane synthetase inhibitor, dazoxiben (Barnett et al 1984).

MACROANGIOPATHY

If the conventional risk factors for macrovascular disease, hypertension, hyperlipidaemia and smoking are considered, there is roughly a doubling of risk for each additional factor both in the diabetic and non-diabetic populations. Diabetes appears to confer an additional independent risk. There are many contender mechanisms to account for the promoting effect of diabetes on large vessel disease, many of which may be inferred from the account on microvascular disease; nevertheless, at the present time the mechanisms are not completely understood and the relative importance of each change is not known. It is not the intention of this section to concentrate upon general mechanisms underlying atherosclerosis in detail, which have been reviewed elsewhere (Ross & Glomset 1976, Ross 1986), but to concentrate on some mechanisms which may be particularly pertinent to the increased risk associated with diabetes.

Insulin, insulin resistance and atheroma

Stout and Vallance-Owen (1969) first suggested that insulin may contribute to the pathogenesis of macrovascular disease. Since that time the concept has evolved to include the role of insulin resistance and several proponent mechanisms have been advanced (de Fronzo & Ferrannini 1991). The stimulus for this work comes from the observation of an association between insulin resistance and hypertension, lipid disorders, obesity, non-insulin-dependent diabetes (NIDDM) and premature atherosclerotic disease. It is likely that an understanding of the mechanisms contributing to, and arising from the insulin resistance or hyperinsulinaemia will greatly advance our understanding of the pathogenesis of macrovascular disease in diabetes (and perhaps in non-diabetics as well).

It is thought that insulin resistance is an acquired defect in subjects with obesity (and in obese subjects who develop diabetes) and a primary genetic abnormality in normal weight NIDDMs (Sims et al 1973, Golay et al 1988). Moreover a close association between hyperinsulinaemia and elevated blood pressure in obese and non-obese essential hypertensive patients and NIDDM patients has been observed (de Fronzo & Ferranini 1991). Epidemiologists have demonstrated an independent role for insulin (beyond the effect on hypertension and lipids) in promoting atherosclerosis, the mechanisms of which have recently been reviewed by Stout (1990). Both these reviews discuss the evidence in detail and only the conclusions are summarized below.

Hyperinsulinaemia, or insulin resistance may have a role in the genesis of hypertension, lipid abnormalities and the promotion of the atherosclerotic plaque in diabetic and non-diabetic subjects. Hyperinsulinaemia may generate hypertension by promoting sodium retention by the kidney, by stimulating overactivity of the sympathetic nervous system directly or by increasing the flux of sodium and calcium into vascular smooth muscle cells thereby increasing their response to pressor amines, and also by stimulating a proliferative response. The characteristic lipid profile of NIDDM subjects (decreased high density lipoprotein (HDL) synthesis, increased very low density lipoprotein (VLDL) synthesis and possibly reduced low density lipoprotein (LDL) synthesis) may to a major part be secondary to increased serum insulin levels. Insulin augments VLDL synthesis in the liver, and by inhibiting lipoprotein lipase reduces VLDL clearance. It is likely that the metabolism of the raised VLDL to LDL will result in an increased flux through intermediate density lipoprotein (IDL) which is known to be highly atherogenic (Schaefer & Levy 1985). However, not all authors agree that hyperinsulinaemia stimulates VLDL over production, and insulin deficiency at the cellular level, secondary to insulin resistance (Patsch et al 1983, Gibbon 1986) may represent an alternative mechanism. There is also accumulating evidence that raised VLDL is itself associated with an increased atherogenic risk (Ginsberg 1987). Furthermore hyperinsulinaemia may also contribute to the reduced HDL levels observed in diabetes.

Insulin may act by an independent mechanism at a cellular level. Cruz and colleagues (1961) demonstrated increased atherogenesis in a femoral artery of alloxan-diabetic dogs when the artery was perfused with insulin. Insulin may promote plaque formation by enhancing LDL-receptor activity, by increasing triglyceride synthesis in arterial smooth muscle cells or by promoting proliferative changes in the muscle cells either directly or through a variety of growth factors.

Hyperlipidaemia of diabetes

Disturbances of lipoprotein synthesis and hyperlipidaemia is commonly found in diabetes and the subject has been extensively reviewed by Dunn (1990). In essence VLDL is raised in NIDDM but only raised in IDDM during poor control. HDL which is thought to be protective, is normal or raised in IDDM patients but low in NIDDMs. In addition to the changes in absolute levels of lipoproteins, qualitative differences are now appreciated which may have a significant bearing on the increased atherogenic risk.

Non-enzymic glycation of LDL has been reported to reduce peripheral receptor uptake (Witzum et al 1982, Lorenzi et al 1984), although not in all studies (Schleicher et al 1985). Reduced peripheral uptake of LDL means more is available for non-receptor mediated uptake by the large vessels particularly if there is increased endothelial permeability due to endothelial damage as discussed earlier. The effect of glycosylation of the vessel wall may tend to increase the binding of such lipoproteins (Brownlee et al 1985).

Lipid peroxidation has been shown in patients with diabetes and it is suggested that as a result these modified lipids are more atherogenic (Sato et al 1981, Baynes 1991). Increased peroxidation is associated with hypertriglyceridaemia in man and diabetic rats (and may reflect an underlying defect such as insulin resistance) (Morel & Chisolm 1989, Stringer et al 1989). The Morel and Chisolm study suggested a beneficial effect of probucol (an antoxidant as well as lipid lowering agent) despite a lack of effect upon quantitative lipid levels. Such a potential beneficial effect has not been tested in diabetic patients. The oxidative stress may be due to autoxidation reactions of sugar and sugar adducts to proteins (Hunt et al 1990) although this remains controversial (Harding & Beswick 1988). In the presence of established complications, tissue damage, cell death and metabolic stress may further increase the oxidative stress in diabetic patients (Baynes 1991).

Many other qualitative differences in lipoproteins are demonstrable in diabetes, but their functional significance is as yet not clear. The recent observation of raised lipoprotein Lp(a) in type I patients with nephropathy may contribute to their specifically increased vascular risk (Kapelrud et al 1991).

Haemostatic factors in the genesis of diabetic macrovascular disease

Platelets

It has long been speculated that platelets have a role in the promotion of macrovascular disease (Sagel et al 1975, Mustard & Packham 1984). Much work centres around the findings of reduced platelet survival and increased in vitro aggregability (reviewed by Colwell et al 1983b). It is also suggested that these changes precede the development of vascular disease and therefore may contribute to their genesis rather than progression; however, the evidence is most compelling in studies of patients with established vascular disease.

Some doubt as to the role of increased platelet activation early in the course of type I diabetes is cast by the study of Alessandrini et al 1988. In their study, patients with clinical evidence of macrovascular disease were excluded and they found no increase in the urinary excretion of the metabolites, thromboxane B_2 or 6-keto prostaglandin $F_{1\alpha}$. Such findings argue against the concept of increased platelet activity as a primary phenomenon in vivo. Using a similar protocol Davi et al (1990) examined type II subjects and revealed an increase in thromboxane metabolite excretion. Their study, whilst providing evidence for in vivo platelet hyperactivity that was related to diabetic control, included subjects who had macrovascular disease and it may be this and not the fact that they studied type II rather than type I diabetes that accounts for the difference. The observation of increased platelet volume suggests that there is increased in vivo turnover of platelets (increased synthesis of 'large' fresh platelets by the megakaryocytes) providing further although indirect evidence of in vivo platelet activation.

Tschoepe et al 1990 have provided some evidence to suggest that the factors which make platelets more thrombogenic are present when they are released from the bone marrow, and are not merely the result of interaction with established vascular disease. They demonstrated increased expression of the glycoproteins, GPIB and GPIIB/IIIA on platelets from subjects with diabetes. The presence of these glycoproteins will promote thrombogenicity and they are regulated by bone-marrow megakaryocyte thrombopoiesis and are not changed in the periphery. This finding supports the suggestion that the platelet hyperreactivity of diabetes may be a primary state. The same group have recently suggested that the megakaryocyte is altered early in diabetes by an immunologically triggered change in megakaryocyte function, and have demonstrated increased tumour necrosis factor in the bone marrow of diabetic BB rats.

Whether or not platelet dysfunction plays a primary role in diabetic vascular disease, platelet hyperactivity is likely to accelerate plaque development by a process of thrombosis and the release of platelet-derived growth factors (Colwell et al 1983). In established plaques such changes may contribute to the clinical events (Colwell et al 1983b, Trip et al 1990).

Coagulation and fibrinolysis

Diabetic blood would appear to be potentially hypercoagulable (Jones & Peterson 1981a). The prothrombotic factors, fibrinogen, factor VIIIc, von Willebrand factor, factor VII and factor XIII have all been shown to be elevated in diabetes; however, only factor VIII levels are increased in the absence of established vascular disease. Although minor perturbations of enzyme systems that inhibit the clotting cascade have been observed in diabetes they may have little clinical significance. Heterozygotes with protein C and S deficiency may have a 40–60% reduction in activity without evidence of clinically significant hypercoagulability.

Stern et al 1991 recently suggested that advanced glycosylation end products can induce suppression of thrombomodulin and expression of pro-coagulant factors by the endothelium. Changes in activity of this system related to diabetic control have been demonstrated although all the values were in the normal range.

Decreased fibrinolysis has also been described in diabetes, and may be of greater pathological significance (Auwerx et al 1988, Juhan-Vague et al 1991). Decreased fibrinolysis is due to an increased activity of plasminogen activator inhibitor-1 (PAI-1) (Wiman & Hamsted 1990). This finding is particularly noteworthy as PAI-1 levels have recently been shown to be the best predictor of disease progression in patients with coronary artery disease and glucose intolerance (Bavenholm et al 1990).

Hyperactivity of PAI-1 and resulting hypofibrinolysis may be an important component of the hyperinsulinaemia/insulin resistance phenomenon, and is possibly a major mechanism underlying accelerated atherosclerosis. In support of this contention is the observation that plasma insulin appears to be the major physiological regulator of PAI-1 activity (Vague et al 1986, Alessi et al 1988). Stimulation of increased PAI-1 could either be direct or through increased VLDL levels. In view of the increased triglyceride content of VLDL in diabetes it is of interest that triglyceride-rich VLDL appears to be a more potent stimulator of PAI-1 (Stiko-Rahm et al 1990).

IS IT POSSIBLE TO LINK SUSCEPTIBILITY TO MACRO AND MICROANGIOPATHY?

Epidemiological studies reveal both a complex interrelationship between micro- and macrovascular disease, and yet also a clear distinction. This apparent paradox is only resolved if we consider type I and type II patients separately.

Patients with impaired glucose tolerance share the increased cardiovascular disease associated with type II diabetes and the possibility that insulin resistance underlies the increased risk in both groups is discussed above.

Insulin resistance or hyperinsulinaemia cannot be an initiating factor in microvascular disease as subjects with impaired glucose tolerance do not develop the microvascular complications of diabetes. This is not to say that the microcirculation is not damaged: the impaired maximum hyperaemia seen in the feet at diagnosis of NIDDM patients might suggest that microvascular sclerosis begins prior to the diabetic state (Sandeman et al 1991). Whereas there is a wealth of data to support the policy of tight metabolic control in the prevention of microvascular complications (Hanssen et al 1986, Chase et al 1989), the pursuit of such a policy in NIDDM patients using insulin therapy, particularly if they are obese, would presumably aggravate hyperinsulinaemia and possibly worsen the macrovascular risk. The answer to this dilemma will hopefully come from the large scale prospective study of newly diagnosed NIDDM patients currently being conducted in the UK and due to report in 1994.

Considering patients with type I diabetes, a strong interrelationship between microvascular disease and macrovascular disease exists. A subgroup of type I diabetic patients develop albuminuria, and it is now accepted that this group develop renal disease. Type I patients with albuminuria also have a higher prevalence of proliferative retinopathy (Barnett et al 1985, Kofoed-Enevoldsen et al 1987) and cardiovascular mortality (Borch-Johnson et al 1985). Indeed the cardiovascular mortality as shown by this study is only marginally increased in patients without nephropathy when compared to the general population, but in those with nephropathy it is increased about 40-fold.

Deckert et al (1989) proposed that albuminuria coincided with a generalized vascular dysfunction due to increased vascular permeability. An increase in the disappearance of an intravascular mass of radiolabelled albumin is seen in type I diabetics compared to controls only when albuminuria is present. The majority of the albumin flux is through the microcirculation of the non-renal beds (Feldt-Rasmussen 1986, Bent-Hansen et al 1987). Leinonen et al (1982) demonstrated no difference in microvascular surface area in the muscle of diabetics and Deckert and colleagues (1989) therefore suggest that the increased albumin flux represents an increase in permeability, consequent on changes in the composition of the extracellular matrix. This concept is in keeping with the current injury hypothesis of atherosclerosis (Ross 1986), which suggests that increased local permeability promotes the generation of plaque. One would anticipate accelerated atherogenesis therefore in a subgroup with generalized increases in vascular permeability.

CONCLUSIONS AND THERAPEUTIC IMPLICATIONS

In summary, patients with diabetes suffer an increased morbidity and mortality from the microvascular and macrovascular complications of the disease. Although many abnormalities have been identified which may contribute to the pathogenesis of such vascular disease and plausible synergistic interactions can be forwarded, the precise significance of individual components remains to be elucidated.

Although many potential primary pathogenic mechanisms are known to be related to glycaemia, the relationship between diabetic complications and diabetic control is still a matter of debate. With respect to microvascular disease it is increasingly clear that tight control early in the course of the disease will prevent complications; once complications are established the benefit is more doubtful (Hanssen et al 1986, Ramsey et al 1988, Chose et al 1989). The role of good glycaemic control in the prevention of macrovascular disease is less clear and perhaps the method of achieving metabolic control will be as important as the glycaemic control itself. The true place of 'tight' metabolic control in the prevention of both microvascular and macrovascular disease awaits the outcome of two large trials, the Diabetes Control and Complications Trial (DCCT) in IDDM and the United Kingdom Prospective Diabetes Study (UKPDS) in NIDDM.

Not only has hypertension been shown to be a major risk factor for both macro- and microvascular disease but antihypertensive treatment has been shown to ameliorate the progression of microvascular disease (nephropathy) and probably macrovascular disease (North 1989, Parving & Hommel 1989). However, aside from this subgroup of type I patients with nephropathy there is a dearth of information on the benefit of hypotensive treatment in diabetic subjects. Extrapolation from studies in the general population may not be justified because of the many potential interactions between the therapeutic agents employed and the metabolic derangements associated with diabetes. Properly conducted long-term prospective studies are also required of drugs that modify haemostatic mechanisms, lipid metabolism and glycosylation. It is possible that we will learn as much about the mechanisms of diabetic vascular disease from such a pragmatic approach as we will from experiments conducted ex vivo.

REFERENCES

Alessi M L, Juhan-Vague I, Kooistra T et al 1988 Insulin stimulates the synthesis of plasminogen activator inhibitor 1 by the human hepatocellular line. Hep G T. Thrombosis and Haemostasis 60: 491–494

Allessandrini P, McRae J, Fenman et al 1988 Thromboxane biosynthesis and platelet function in type I Diabetes Mellitus. New England Journal of Medicine 319: 208–212

Auwerx J, Bouillon R, Collén D et al 1988 Tissue type plasminogen activator antigen and plasminogen activator inhibitor in diabetes mellitus. Arteriosclerosis 8: 68–72

Bank N, Klose R, Aynedjian H S et al 1987 Evidence against increased glomerular pressure initiating diabetic nephropathy. Kidney International 31: 898–905

Bank N, Mower P, Aynedjian H S et al 1989a Sorbinil prevents glomerular hyperperfusion in diabetic rats. American Journal of Physiology 256: F1000–F1006

Bank N, Coco M, Aynedjian H S et al 1989b Galactose feeding causes glomerular hyperperfusion: prevention by aldose reductase inhibition. American Journal of Physiology 256: F994–F999

Bannerjee R N, Sahui A L, Kumar V 1973 Fibrino-coagulopathy in maturity onset diabetes mellitus and atherosclerosis. Thrombosis et Diathesis Haemorrhagica 30: 123

Barnet A H, Dallinger K, Jennings P et al 1985 Microalbuminuria and diabetic retinopathy. Lancet i: 53–54

Barnett A H, Leatherdale B A, Polak A et al 1984 Specific thromboxane synthetase inhibition and albumin excretion rate in insulin-dependent diabetes. Lancet i: 1322–1325

Bavenholm P, Efendic S, Wiman B et al 1990 Relationship of insulin response to glucose challenge to severity and rate of progression of coronary atherosclerosis in young survivors of myocardial infarction. European Heart Journal 11 (suppl 178): 178 (abstract)

Baynes J W 1991 Role of oxidative stress in development of complications of diabetes. Diabetes 40: 405–412

Bent-Hansen L, Feldt-Rasmussen B, Kvernelund A et al 1987 Transcapillary escape rate and relative metabolic clearance of glycated and non-glycated albumin in type I (insulin dependent) diabetes mellitus. Diabetologia 30: 2–4

Borch-Johnsen K, Andersen P K, Deckert T 1985 The effect of proteinuria on relative mortality in type I (insulin-dependent) diabetes mellitus. Diabetologia 28: 390–596

Branemark P I, Rander L et al 1971 Studies in rheology of human diabetes mellitus. Diabetologia 7: 107–112

Brownlee M, Pongor S, Cerami A 1983 Covalent attachment of soluble proteins by non-enzymically glycosylated collagen: Role in the in situ formation of immune complexes. Journal of Experimental Medicine 58: 1739–1744

Brownlee M, Vlassara H, Cerami A 1985 Non-enzymic glycosylation products on collagen covalently trap low-density lipoprotein. Diabetes 34: 938–941

Brownlee M, Vlassara H, Cerami A 1987 Amino-guanidine prevents hyperglycaemia-induced defect in binding of heparin by matrix molecules. Diabetes 36: 85A

Brownlee M, Cerami A, Vlassara H 1988 Advanced products of non-enzymic glycosylation and the pathogenesis of diabetic vascular disease. Diabetes/Metabolism Reviews 4: 437–451

Chase H P, Jackson W E, Hoops S L et al 1989 Glucose control and the renal and retinal complications of insulin dependent diabetes. Journal of the American Medical Association 261: 1155–1160

Christiansen J S 1985 Glomerular hyperfiltration in diabetes mellitus. Diabetic Medicine 2: 235–244

Cohn RA, Mauer S M, Barbosa J et al 1978 Immunofluorescence studies of skeletal muscle extracellular membranes in diabetes mellitus. Laboratory Investigation 39: 13–16

Colwell J A, Winocour P D, Halushka P V 1983a Do platelets have anything to do with diabetic microvascular disease? Diabetes 32 (suppl 2): 14–19

Colwell J A, Winocour P D, Lopes-Virellu M et al 1983b New concepts about the pathogenesis of atherosclerosis in diabetes mellitus. American Journal of Medicine 75 (suppl 56): 67–80
Cruz A B, Amatuzio D S , Grande F et al 1961 Effect of intra arterial insulin on tissue cholesterol and fatty acids in alloxan-diabetic dogs. Circulation Research 9: 39–43
DAMAD Study Group 1989 Effect of aspirin alone and aspirin plus dipyridamole in early diabetic retinopathy: a multicenter randomized controlled clinical trial. Diabetes 38: 491–498
Davi G, Catalano I, Averna M et al 1990 Thromboxane biosynthesis and platelet function in type II diabetes mellitus. New England Journal of Medicine 322: 1769–1774
Davis M D 1988 Diabetic retinopathy: a clinical overview. Diabetes/Metabolism Reviews 4: 291–322
Deckert T, Feldt-Rasmussen B, Borch-Johnsen K et al 1989 Albuminuria reflects widespread vascular damage. The Steno hypothesis. Diabetologia 32: 219–226
de Fronzo R A, Ferrannini E 1991 Insulin resistance. A multifaceted syndrome responsible for NIDDM, obesity, hypertension, dyslipidaemia and atherosclerotic cardiovascular disease. Diabetes Care 14: 173–194
Ditzel J 1968 Functional microangiopathy in diabetes mellitus. Diabetes 17: 388–397
Dunn F L 1990 Hyperlipidaemia in diabetes mellitus. Diabetes/Metabolism Reviews 6: 47–61
Dvorak H F, Senger D R, Dvorak A M et al 1985 Regulation of extravascular coagulation by microvascular permeability. Science 227: 1059–1061
Engerman R L 1989 Pathogenesis of diabetic retinopathy. Diabetes 38: 1143–1155
Engerman R L, Kern T S 1984 Experimental galactosemia produces diabetic-like retinopathy. Diabetes 33: 97–100
Esposito C, Gerlach H, Brett J et al 1989 Endothelial receptor-mediated binding of glucose-modified albumin is associated with increased monolayer permeability and modulation of cell surface coagulant properties. Journal of Experimental Medicine 170: 1387–1407
Fajdusek C, Carbon S, Ross R, Nawroth P and Stern D 1986 Activation of coagulation factors releases endothelial cell mitogen. Journal of Cell Biology 103: 419–428
Feldt-Rasmussen B 1986 Increased transcapillary escape rate of albuminuria in type I (insulin dependent) diabetic patients with microalbuminuria. Diabetes Research 7: 159–164
Gabbay K H, Snider J H 1972 Nerve conduction defect in galactose-fed rats. Diabetes 21: 295–300
Gibbon G F 1986 Hyperlipidaemia of diabetes. Clinical Science 71: 477–486
Ginsberg H N 1987 Very low density lipoprotein metabolism in non insulin dependent diabetes mellitus. Diabetes/Metabolism Reviews 2: 571–589
Golay A, Felber J P, Jequier E et al 1988 Metabolic basis of obesity and non-insulin dependent diabetes mellitus. Diabetes/Metabolism Reviews 4: 727–747
Hanssen K F, Dahl-Jorgensen K, Lauritzen T et al 1986 Diabetic control and microvascular complications: the near normoglycaemic experience. Diabetologia 29: 677–684
Harding J J, Beswick H T 1988 The possible contribution of glucose autoxidation to protein modification in diabetes. Biochemical Journal 249: 618–619
Hostetter T H, Troy J L, Brenner B M 1981 Glomerular haemodynamics in experimental diabetes mellitus. Kidney International 19: 410–415
Hunt J V, Smith C C T, Wolff S P 1990 Autoxidative glycosylation and possible involvement of peroxidases and free radicals in LDL modification by glucose. Diabetes 39: 1420–1424
Jensen P K, Christiansen J S, Steven K et al 1981 Renal function in streptozotocin-diabetic rats. Diabetologia 21: 409–415
Jensen T, Byerre-Knudsen J, Feldt-Rasmussen B et al 1989 Features of endothelial dysfunction in early diabetic nephropathy. Lancet i: 461–463
Jones R L, Peterson C M 1979 Reduced fibrinogen survival in diabetes mellitus: A reversible phenomenon. Journal of Clinical Investigation 63: 485–493
Jones R L, Peterson C M 1981a Haematological alterations in diabetes mellitus. American Journal of Medicine 70: 339–352
Jones R L, Peterson C M 1981b The fluid phase of coagulation and the accelerated atherosclerosis of diabetes mellitus. Diabetes 30 (suppl 2): 33–38
Juhan-Vague I, Driss F, Roul C et al 1984 Abnormalities of erythrocyte membrane lipids in insulin-dependent diabetics are improved by short term strict control of diabetics. Clinical Haemorheology 4: 455–459
Juhan-Vague I, Alessi M C, Vague Ph 1991 Increased plasma plasminogen activator inhibitor 1 levels. A possible link between insulin resistance and atherothrombosis. Diabetologia 34: 457–462
Kaley G, Rodenburg J M, Messina E J, Wollin M S 1989 Endothelium-associated vasodilations in rat skeletal muscle microcirculation. American Journal of Physiology 256: 720–725
Kapelrud H, Bangstad H J, Dahl-Jorgensen K et al 1991 Serum Lp(a) lipoprotein concentrations in insulin dependent diabetic patients with microalbuminuria. British Medical Journal 303: 675–678
Kleinman J C, Donahue R P, Harris M I et al 1988 Morbidity among diabetics in a national sample. American Journal of Epidemiology 128: 389–401
Kofoed-Enevoldsen A, Jensen T, Borch-Johnsen K et al 1987 Incidence of retinopathy in Type I (insulin dependent) diabetes: Association with clinical nephropathy. Journal of Diabetic Complications 3: 96–99
Kriesberg J I, Patel P V 1983 The effect of insulin, glucose and diabetes on prostaglandin (PG) production by rat kidney glomeruli and cultured mesangial cells. Prostaglandins and Leukotrienes in Medicine 11: 431–442
Krolewski A S, Warram J H, Rand L I et al 1986 Risk of proliferative diabetic retinopathy in juvenile onset type I diabetes: A 40 year follow up study. Diabetes Care 9: 443–452
Krolewski A S, Kosinski E J, Warram J H et al 1987 Magnitude and determinants of coronary artery disease in juvenile onset, insulin dependent diabetes mellitus. American Journal of Cardiology 59: 750–755
Lansman J B 1988 Endothelial mechanoreceptors: Going with the flow. Nature 311: 481–482
Leinonen H, Matikainen E, Juntunen J 1982 Permeability and morphology of skeletal muscle capillaries in Type I (insulin dependent) diabetes mellitus. Diabetologia 22: 158–162
Li W, Shen S, Khatami M et al 1984 Stimulation of retinal capillary pencyte protein and collagen synthesis in culture by high-glucose concentration. Diabetes 33: 785–789
Lieberman J, Sastre A 1980 Serum angiotensin-converting enzyme: elevation in diabetes mellitus. Annals of Internal Medicine 93: 825–826
Lorenzi M, Cagliero E, Markey B et al 1984 Interaction of human endothelial cells with elevated glucose concentrations and native glycosylated low density lipoproteins. Diabetologia 26: 218–222
Lorenzi M, Cagliero E, Toledo S 1985 Glucose toxicity for human endothelial cells in culture: delayed replication, disturbed cell cycle and accelerated death. Diabetes 34: 621–627
McMillan D E 1983 The effect of diabetes on blood flow properties. Diabetes 32 (suppl 2): 56–63
McMillan D E, Ulterback N G, Walff C W 1981 Blood viscosity in young and old diabetics. Paediatric and Adolescent Endocrinology 9: 8–14
Mauer S M, Steffes M W, Ellis E N et al 1984 Structural-functional relationships in diabetic microangiopathy. Journal of Clinical Investigation 74: 1143–1155
Mauer S M, Steffes M W, Agar S et al 1989 Effects of dietary protein content in streptozotocin diabetic rats. Kidney International 35: 48–59
Michael A F, Brown D M 1981 Increased concentration of albumin in kidney basement membranes in diabetes mellitus. Diabetes 30: 843–846
Miller K, Michael A F 1976 Immunopathology of renal extracellular membranes in diabetes: Specificity of tubular basement membrane immunofluorescence. Diabetes 25: 701–708
Mogensen C 1989 Hyperfiltration, hypertension and diabetic nephropathy in IDDM patients. Diabetes Nutrition and Metabolism 2: 227–244
Morel D W, Chisolm G M 1989 Antioxidant treatment of diabetic rats

inhibits lipoprotein oxidation and cytotoxity. Journal of Lipid Research 30: 1827–1834

Morrish N J, Stevens L K, Fuller J H, Jarret R J 1991 Incidence of macrovascular disease in diabetes mellitus: The London cohort of the WHO Multinational Study of Vascular Disease in Diabetics. Diabetologia 3: 584–589

Mustard J F, Packham M A 1984 Platelets and diabetes mellitus. New England Journal of Medicine 311: 665–666

Nelson R G, Loon N, Bennet P H et al 1990 Glomerular filtration and barrier function in non-insulin dependent diabetes mellitus. Diabetes 39: 72A

North R H 1989 Diabetic nephropathy: Haemodynamic basis and implications for disease management. Annals of Internal Medicine 110: 795–813

Orchard T J, Dorman J S, Maser R E 1990 Factors associated with avoidance of severe complications after 25 years of IDDM. Diabetes Care 13: 741–747

Parving H H 1975 Microvascular permeability to plasma protein in hypertension and diabetes mellitus in man — on the pathogenesis of hypertensive and diabetic microangiopathy. Danish Medical Bulletin 22: 217–233

Parving H H, Hommel E 1989 Prognosis in diabetic nephropathy. British Medical Journal 299: 230–233

Parving H H, Viberti G C, Keen H et al 1983 Haemodynamic factors in the genesis of diabetic microangiopathy. Metabolism 32: 943–949

Patsch W, Franz S, Schonfeld G 1983 Role of insulin in lipoprotein secretion by cultured rat hepatocytes. Journal of Clinical Investigation 2: 445–453

Pickup J C, Collins A C G, Walker J D et al 1989 Patterns of hyperinsulinaemia in Type I diabetic patients with and without nephropathy. Diabetic Medicine 6: 685–691

Porta M, La Selva M, Molinghi P A 1991 von Willebrand factor and endothelial abnormalities in diabetic microangiopathy. Diabetes Care 14 (suppl 1): 167–172

Pugliese G, Tilton R G, Speedy A et al 1990 Vascular filtration function in galactose-fed versus diabetic rats: the role of polyol pathway activity. Metabolism 39: 690–697

Pugliese G, Tilton R G, Williamson J R 1991 Glucose-induced metabolic imbalances in the pathogenesis of diabetic vascular disease. Diabetes/Metabolism Reviews 7: 35–59

Ramsey R C, Goetz F C, Sutherland D E R et al 1988 Progression of diabetic retinopathy after pancreas transplantation for insulin dependent diabetes mellitus. New England Journal of Medicine 318: 208–214

Rippe B, Folkow B 1977 Capillary permeability to albumin in normotensive and spontaneously hypertensive rats. Acta Physiologia Scandinavica 101: 72–83

Ross R 1986 The pathogenesis of atherosclerosis — an update. New England Journal of Medicine 314: 488–500

Ross R, Glomset J A 1976 The pathogenesis of atherosclerosis. New England Journal of Medicine 295: 369–377

Rowland F N, Donovan M J, Picciano P T et al 1984 Fibrin mediated vascular injury: identification of fibrin peptides that mediate endothelial cell retraction. American Journal of Pathology 117: 418–428

Sagel J, Colwell J A, Crook L et al 1975 Increased platelet aggregation in early diabetes mellitus. Annals of Internal Medicine 32: 733–738

Sandeman D D, Shore A C, Tooke J E 1992 Relation of skin capillary pressure in patients with insulin dependent diabetes mellitus to complications and metabolic control. New England Journal of Medicine 327: 760–764

Sandeman D D, Shore A C, Tooke J E 1991b Pre-capillary vasodilation underlies capillary hypertension in Type I diabetes mellitus. Clinical Science 3: 13P

Sato Y, Holta N, Sakumoto N et al 1981 Lipid peroxidase level in plasma of diabetic patients. Biochemical Medicine 25: 373–378

Schaefer E J, Levy R I 1985 Pathogenesis and management of lipoprotein disorders. New England Journal of Medicine 312: 1300–1310

Schleicher E, Olgemoller B, Schon J et al 1985 Limited non-enzymic glycosylation of low density lipoprotein does not alter its catabolism in tissue culture. Biochemica et Biophysica Acta 846: 226–233

Schrier R U, Williams B 1990 High extracellular glucose concentrations (HG), increase prostaglandin (PG) production by rat mesangial cells (GMC) and vascular smooth muscle cell (VSMC). Kidney International 38: 448A

Sensi M, Tanzi P, Bruno M R et al 1986 Human glomerular basement membrane: Altered binding characteristics following in vitro non-enzymatic glycosylation. Annals of the New York Academy of Sciences 488: 549–552

Shimomura H, Spiro R G 1987 Studies on macromolecular components of human glomerular basement membrane and alterations in diabetes: Decreased levels of heparin sulphate proteoglycan and laminin. Diabetes 36: 374–381

Sims E A H, Danford E, Horton E S et al 1973 Endocrine and metabolic effects of experimental obesity in man. Recent Progress in Hormone Research 29: 457–496

Stefansson E, Landers M B M, Wolbarst M L 1983 Oxygenation and vasodilation in relation to diabetic and other proliferative retinopathies. Ophthalmic Surgery 14: 209–226

Stern D M, Esposito C, Gerlach H et al 1991 Endothelium and regulation of coagulation. Diabetes Care 14 (suppl 1): 160–166

Stiko-Rahm A, Wiman B, Hamsted N et al 1990 Secretion of plasminogen activator inhibitor from cultured human umbilical vein endothelial cells induced by very low density lipoprotein. Arteriosclerosis 10: 1067–1073

Stout R W 1990 Insulin and atheroma. 20-Yr perspective. Diabetes Care 13: 631–654

Stout R W, Vallance-Owen J 1969 Insulin and atheroma. Lancet i: 1078–1080

Stringer M D, Gorog P G, Freeman A et al 1989 Lipid peroxidases and atherosclerosis. British Medical Journal 298: 281–284

Tilton R G, Chang K, Pugliesse G et al 1989 Prevention of haemodynamic and vascular albumin filtration changes in diabetic rats by aldose reductase inhibitors. Diabetes 38: 1258–1270

Tomlinson D R, Moriarty R J, Mayer J H 1984 Prevention and reversal of defective axonal transport and motor nerve conduction velocity in rats with experimental diabetes by treatment with the aldose reductase inhibitor sorbinil. Diabetes 33: 470–476

Tooke J E 1986 Microvascular haemodynamics in diabetes mellitus. Clinical Science 80: 443–453

Trip M D, Cats V M, van Capelle F J L et al 1990 Platelet hyper-reactivity and prognosis in survivors of myocardial infarction. New England Journal of Medicine 322: 1549–1554

Tschoepe D, Roesen P, Kaufmann L et al 1990 Evidence for abnormal platelet glycoprotein expression in diabetes mellitus. European Journal of Clinical Investigation 20: P166–170

Vague Ph, Juhan-Vague I, Aillaud M F et al 1986 Correlation between blood fibrinolytic activity, plasminogen activator inhibitor level, plasma insulin level and relative body weight in normal and obese subjects. Metabolism 2: 250–253

Vlassara H, Brownlee M, Manogue K R et al 1988 Catechin/TNF and IL-4 induced by glucose-modified proteins: role in normal tissue remodelling. Science 240: 1546–1548

Vracko R 1970 Skeletal muscle capillaries in non diabetics: a quantitative analysis. Circulation 41: 285–297

Watanabe K, Tanaka K 1983 Influence of fibrin, fibrinogen and fibrinogen degradation products on cultured endothelial cells. Atherosclerosis 48: 57–70

Williams S A, MacGregor G A, Smaje L H et al 1990 Capillary hypertension and abnormal pressure dynamics in patients with essential hypertension. Clinical Science 79: 5–8

Williamson J R, Vogler N, Kilo C 1971 Regional variations in the width of the basement membrane of muscle capillaries in man and giraffe. American Journal of Pathology 63: 359–370

Williamson J R, Tilton R G, Chang K et al 1988 Basement membrane abnormalities in diabetes mellitus: relationship to clinical microangiopathy. Diabetes/Metabolism Reviews 4: 339–370

Wiman B, Hamsted A 1990 The fibrinolytic enzyme system and its role in the etiology of thrombo-embolic disease. Seminars in Thrombosis and Haemostasis 26: 207–216

Witzum J L, Mahoney E M, Branks M J et al 1982 Non-enzymic glycosylation of low-density lipoprotein alters its biological activity. Diabetes 31: 283–291

Yue D K, McLennan S, Turtle J R 1983 Non-enzymic glycosylation of tissue protein in diabetes in the rat. Diabetologia 24: 377–381

Zatz R, Brenner B M 1986 Pathogenesis of diabetic microangiopathy: the haemodynamic view. American Journal of Medicine 80: 443–453

58. Thrombosis and artificial surfaces

C. D. Forbes J. M. Courtney

BLOOD INTERACTIONS WITH ARTIFICIAL SURFACES

The investigation of thrombus formation on artificial surfaces has been promoted by the clinical utilization of synthetic materials in applications involving contact with blood, although consideration of the influence on blood coagulation of different artificial surfaces and the contrast between an artificial surface and the normal endothelium extend well beyond the present interest (Thackrah 1819, Brücke 1857, Lister 1863). Similarly, if a biomaterial is defined as a material of natural or synthetic origin, used in contact with tissue, blood or biological fluid, the application of biomaterials can be considered as covering a period of about 100 years (Williams 1987). However, recent improvements in technology and clinical procedures have led to an increase in the number of biomaterials utilized and in the range of applications. It is believed that knowledge of the blood response to artificial surfaces is essential for improved clinical performance and that this is relevant for both procedures under development, such as the artificial heart (Didisheim et al 1989, Kambic & Nosé 1991) and long-established procedures, such as the artificial kidney (Nosé 1988, Ringoir & Vanholder 1990).

There has been a consistent interest in blood–biomaterial interactions, the effect of materials on blood constituents and the events inducing thrombus formation on artificial surfaces (Feijen 1977, Forbes & Prentice 1978, Bruck 1980, Andrade et al 1981, Forbes 1981, Szycher 1983, Murabayashi & Nosé 1986, Forbes et al 1989). It is now recognized that the complexity of the blood response to an artificial surface may be increased in the clinical situation by device components and utilization, the nature of the application and patient status (Klinkmann et al 1987, Courtney et al 1993a).

It is convenient to consider blood coagulation in terms of contributions from features such as platelet activation, intrinsic, extrinsic and common coagulation pathways and the control systems participating in thrombus inhibition and fibrinolysis (Mustard & Packham 1977, Ratnoff 1977, Ratnoff & Forbes 1984). A similar approach can be adopted for consideration of the events following contact of blood with an artificial surface, if two basic differences are acknowledged (Forbes & Prentice 1978). Firstly, in the absence of special modification, artificial surfaces cannot perform an active role in thromboresistance similar to that achieved by the endothelium and cannot provide a non-attractive surface comparable to that of the endothelium (Mason et al 1977, 1979). Secondly, while the endothelium does not appear to adsorb proteins under physiological conditions, protein adsorption is a critical feature of blood–biomaterial interactions (Szycher 1983, Brash 1991).

The response of blood to an artificial surface can be viewed (Fig. 58.1) as the involvement of protein adsorption; platelet adhesion, release and aggregation; activation of the intrinsic coagulation; participation of the fibrinolytic, complement and kallikrein-kinin systems and the interaction of cellular elements (Fig. 58.2). The response is such that thrombus formation is generally inevitable, making simultaneous therapy with anticoagulants, platelet aggregation inhibitors or plasminogen activators necessary for the clinical use of artificial surfaces.

Protein adsorption on artificial surfaces

The rapid adsorption of protein onto an artificial surface is regarded as the first event to occur following blood–surface contact, with subsequent phenomena determined to a large extent by interactions of blood with the adsorbed protein layer (Brash 1991). The undoubted role of adsorbed protein on blood–biomaterial interactions is reflected in the use of the term 'conditioning layer' (Baier 1977, Brash 1983, Klinkmann 1984). However, this layer should not be considered passive (Bruck 1980). There is the possibility of transient adsorption, denaturation, or changes in conformation (Lee & Hairston 1971, Ihlenfeld & Cooper 1979), with the protein layer continuously altering in composition and physical and biological properties (Brash 1991). Information on protein adsorption

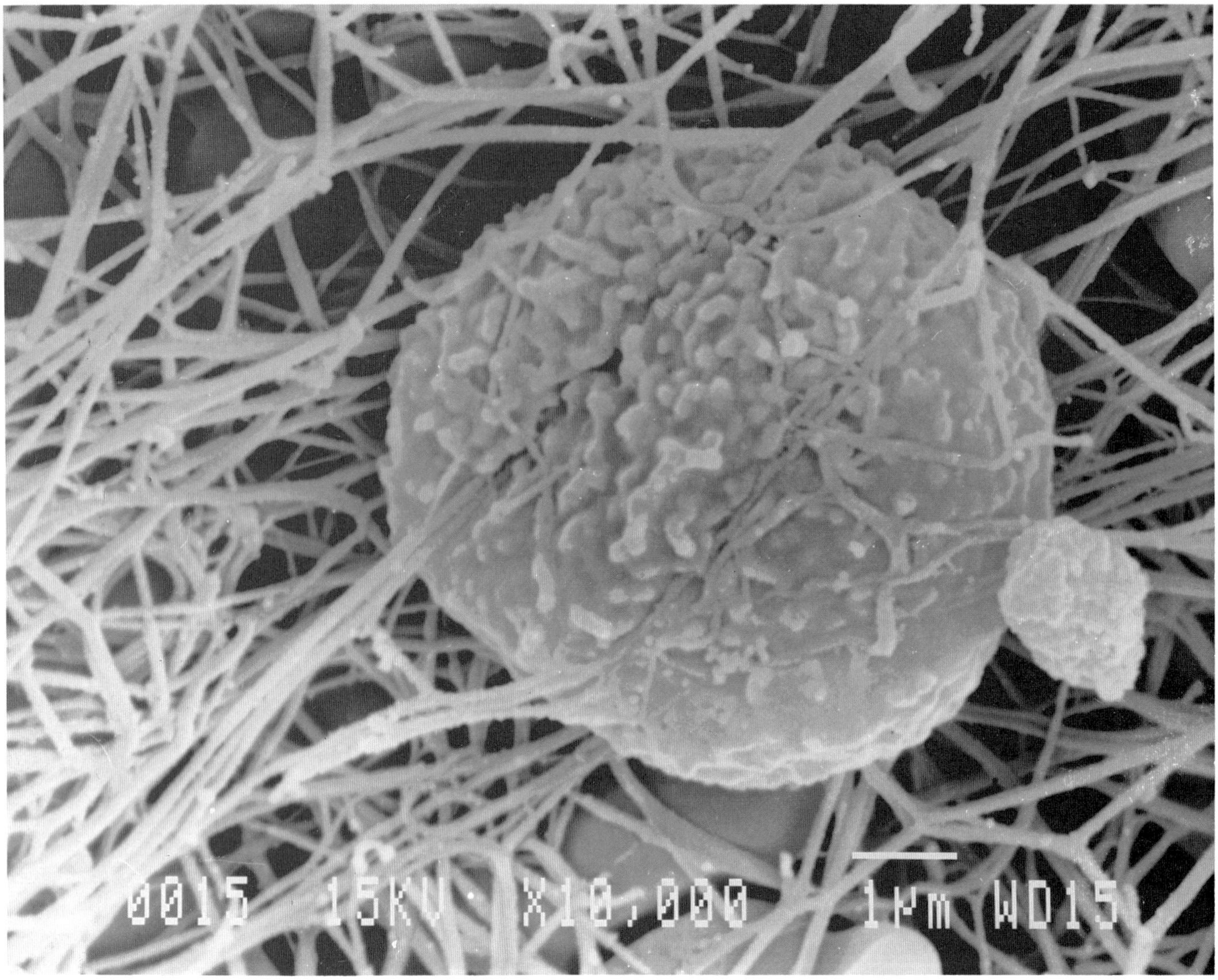

Fig. 58.1 Micrographs showing blood contact with an acrylonitrile-sodium methallyl sulphonate copolymer haemodialysis membrane (AN69S). **A**, Lymphocyte entrapped in fibrin network.

has been acquired in studies of adsorption from solution (Brash & Lyman 1969, Berger & Salzman 1974, Bagnall 1978, Chan & Brash 1981), plasma (Vroman et al 1972, 1980, Uniyal & Brash 1982, Brash & ten Hove 1984, Breemhaar et al 1984, Horbett 1984, Brash & Thibodeau 1986) or blood (Gendrau et al 1981, Chuang 1984, Owen et al 1985, Seifert & Greer 1985, Horbett 1986).

The spontaneous nature of protein adsorption onto artificial surfaces is promoted by the amphipathic (polar/nonpolar) character of protein molecules, which provides a driving force for the concentration of proteins at interfaces, and by the limited solubility of proteins due to the high molecular weight of the macromolecules (Brash 1983). Reduction in the free energy of the system can result from an enthalpy decrease when adsorption is exothermic or from an entropy increase caused by disruption of structured water near the protein or artificial surface.

The nature of an artificial surface determines the manner and extent of protein attachment. With glass surfaces, electrostatic adsorption is important (Chan & Brash 1981). With polymeric surfaces, attachment may be caused by hydrophobic interaction resulting from the interaction of non-polar protein and non-polar surface groups in the polar aqueous medium (Brash 1983). In general, protein adsorption is considered to be greater and to involve stronger binding on hydrophobic than on hydrophilic surfaces (Brash et al 1974, Hoffman 1974, Waugh et al 1975, 1978, Chuang et al 1978, Brash & Uniyal 1979, Ratner 1981), with hydrophobicity also influencing conformation changes in adsorbed protein (Absolom et al 1983). Protein adsorption is more readily and rapidly reversible on hydrophilic than on hydrophobic surfaces (Brash & Lyman 1969, Brash & Uniyal 1979). The reversibility of the chemical bond determines the state of equilibrium (Vroman et al 1972).

When blood contacts an artificial surface, plasma pro-

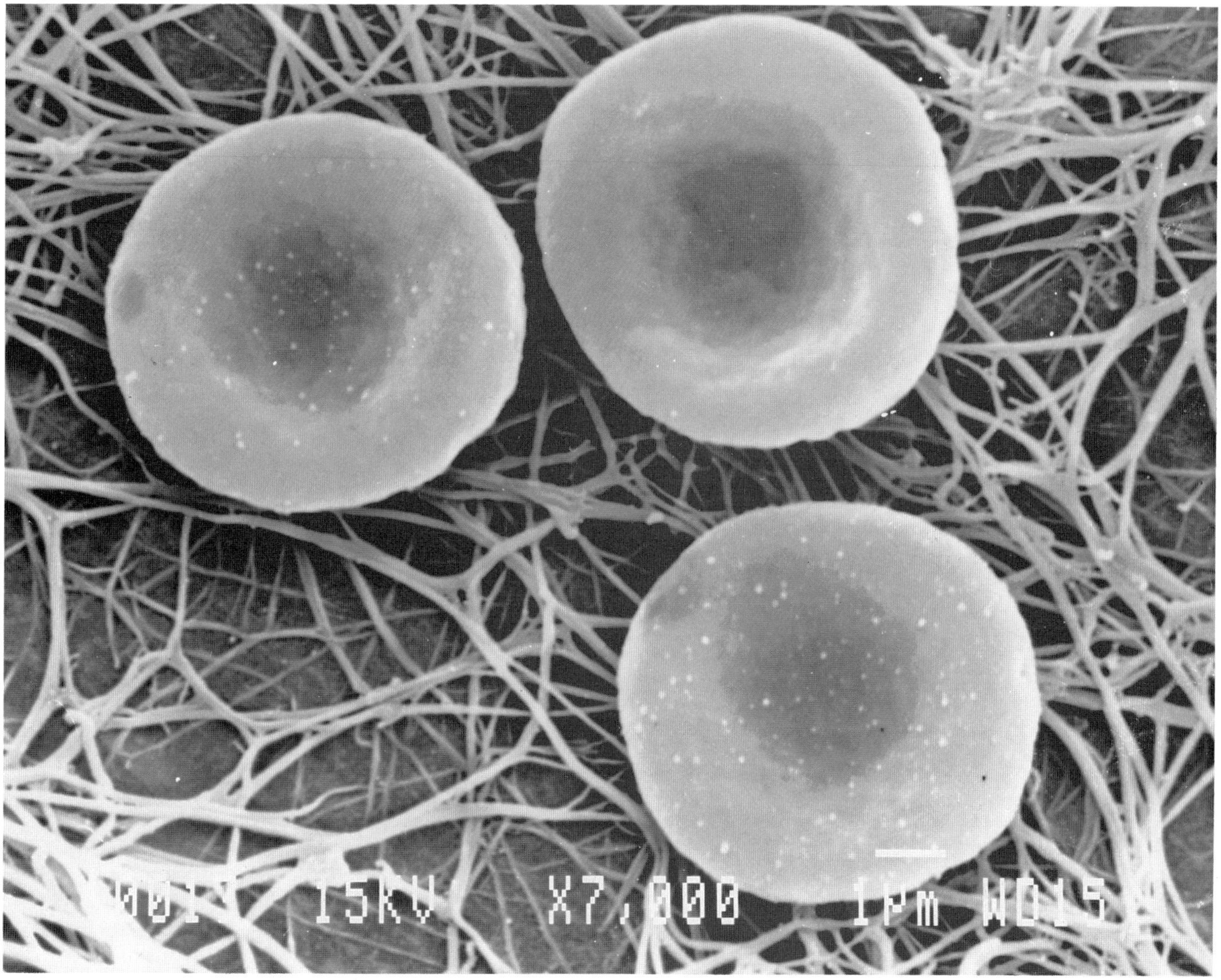

Fig. 58.1 **B**, Erythrocytes on fibrin.

teins are adsorbed onto the surface rapidly and selectively to form a protein layer about 100 nm thick, with the composition of the adsorbed protein layer exerting a controlling influence on subsequent blood–surface interactions (Baier et al 1971, Lyman et al 1974). With respect to the influence on platelets, the proteins which have been most widely studied are albumin, fibrinogen and γ-globulin (IgG). The general conclusion is that platelet adhesion to artificial surfaces is inhibited by prior adsorption of albumin and promoted by prior adsorption of fibrinogen or IgG (Packham et al 1969, Salzman et al 1969, Zucker & Vroman 1969, Lyman et al 1970, Jenkins et al 1973, Whicher & Brash 1978, Absolom et al 1979, Neumann et al 1979, Adams & Feurstein 1980).

Preferential adsorption of fibrinogen has been reported in comparison to albumin and γ-globulin (Lee et al 1974, Brash & Davidson 1976, Brash & Uniyal 1979) and to lipoproteins and coagulation factors (Vroman et al 1972). Fibrinogen strongly attracts platelets and platelet reactivity correlates with the degree of preferential fibrinogen adsorption (Brash & Uniyal 1979), although the influence of the protein diminishes after a rapid conformational change (Vroman et al, 1980). The close relationship between fibrinogen and platelets is exemplified by the fact that defibrinated or afibrinogenaemic plasma does not support platelet accumulation unless fibrinogen is added (Zucker & Vroman 1969, Mason et al 1971). Fibrinogen is required for adenosine diphosphate (ADP)-induced platelet aggregation and two classes of ADP-stimulated platelet receptors have been proposed (Plow & Marguerie 1980, Kornecki et al 1981, Di Minno et al 1983). Therefore, it is possible that the adsorption of fibrinogen on artificial surfaces is not independent of platelet deposition but is associated with specific receptors on adherent platelets (Young et al 1983).

The indication that fibrinogen adsorption is transient

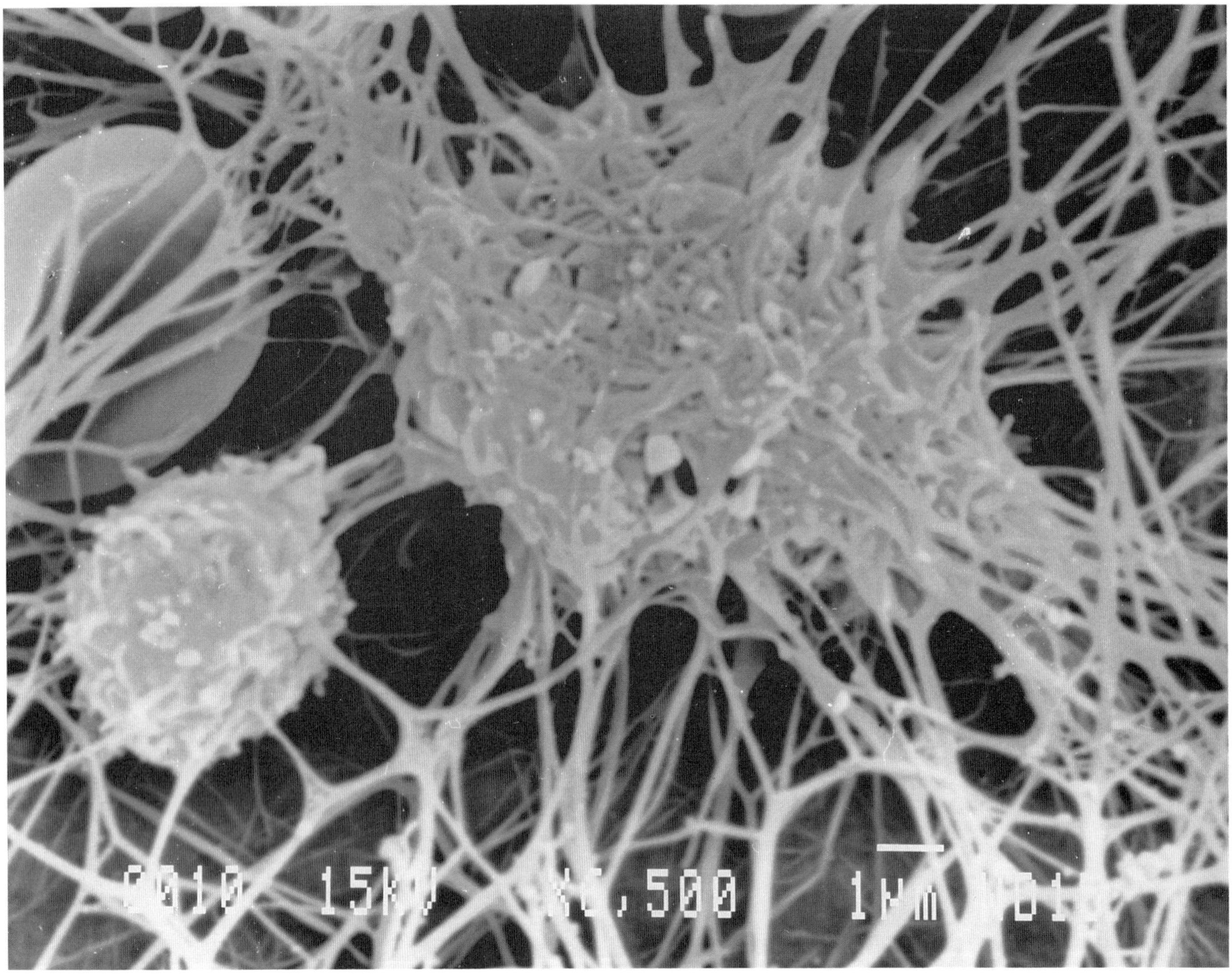

Fig. 58.1 C, Platelet aggregate with red cell in fibrin, the other cell may be a megaplatelet.

(Vroman & Adams 1969) has been confirmed (Uniyal & Brash 1982, Brash & ten Hove 1984, Breemhaar et al 1984, Horbett 1984) and the phenomenon has been designated the 'Vroman Effect' (Brash & ten Hove 1984, Horbett 1984). Of particular interest, is the demonstration that adsorbed fibrinogen is replaced by high molecular weight kininogen (Vroman et al 1980), a protein involved in the contact phase of the intrinsic coagulation. This means that with respect to artificial surfaces, a low Vroman effect with fibrinogen retention should induce less activation of the intrinsic coagulation, while a high Vroman Effect with fibrinogen displacement should induce less platelet reactivity (Brash 1991). The timing of fibrinogen adsorption and its removal from artificial surfaces may have important clinical implications (Vroman 1983) and the critical role of fibrinogen in thrombosis on artificial surfaces is further emphasized by the possible interaction of fibrinogen with leukocytes (Szycher 1983).

The adsorption of γ-globulin on artificial surfaces has been reported to promote platelet adhesion and stimulate the platelet release reaction (Evans & Mustard 1968) and γ-globulin adsorption may be followed by leukocyte adhesion (Adams et al 1978).

Albumin is rapidly adsorbed to most artificial surfaces, although it may not be a major adsorbed component (Uniyal & Brash 1982). The ability of adsorbed albumin to reduce platelet and leukocyte adhesion (Salzman et al 1969, Lyman et al 1970) and to inhibit thrombus formation (Packham et al 1969) has been utilized in the preparation of artificial surfaces with enhanced blood compatibility (Fougnot et al 1984, Engbers & Feijen 1991, Courtney et al 1993b).

While there has been an emphasis on fibrinogen, γ-globulin and albumin, the presence of other proteins in the adsorbed layer is generally accepted and the possible influence of even trace amounts of proteins supports further

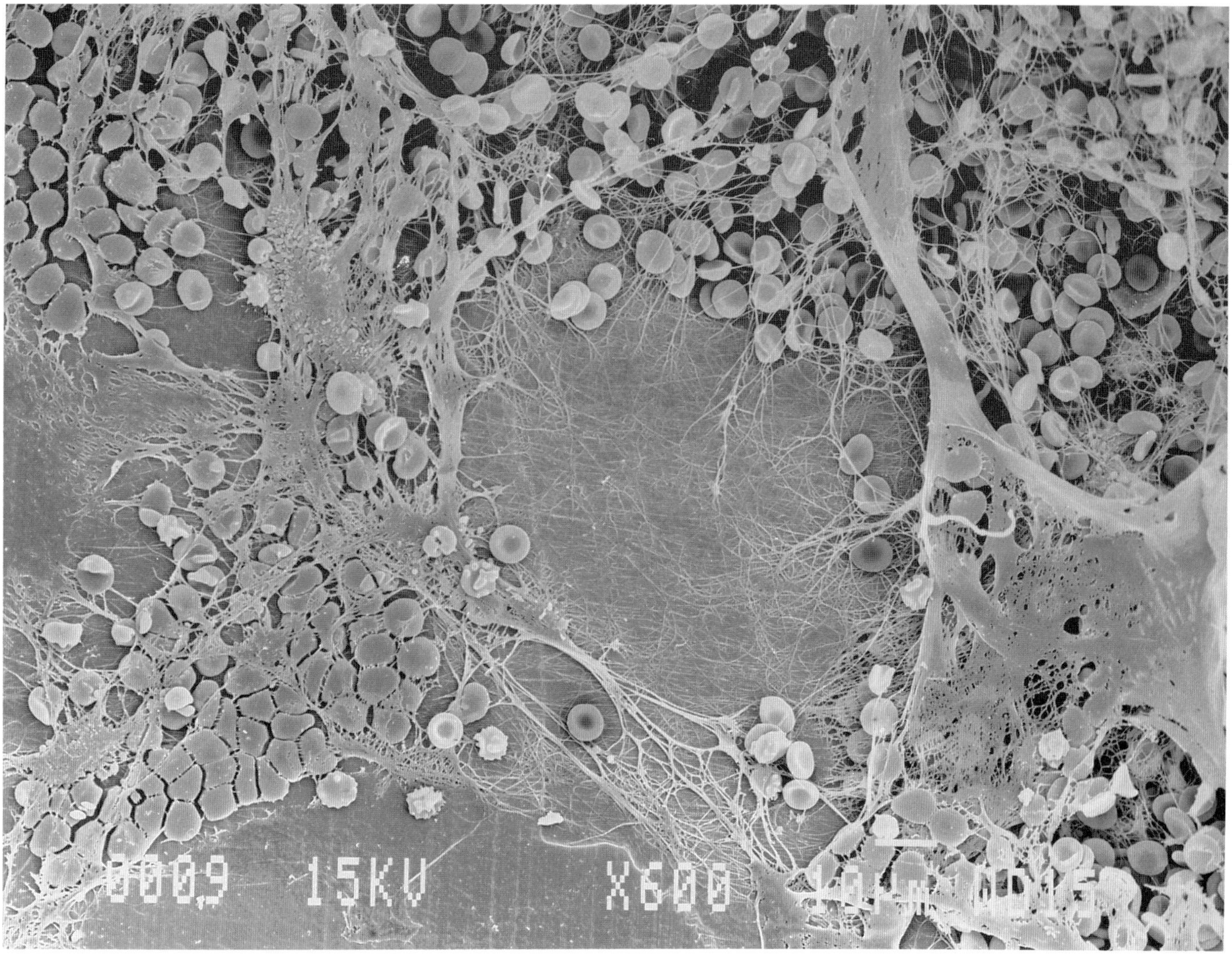

Fig. 58.1 **D**, Fibrin on the surface with a platelet aggregate, erythrocytes in the fibrin and damaged erythrocytes (pressure influence).

investigation (Brash 1983). Adsorbed proteins identified include fibronectin (Adams & Feuerstein 1981, Grinnell & Feld 1981, Grinnell & Phan 1983) with a possible role in leukocyte adhesion (Vroman 1983); lipoproteins, IgA, IgM and IgD (Limber et al 1974, Limber & Mason 1975); von Willebrand/factor VIII protein complex (Horbett & Counts 1984) with a possible link to increased platelet adhesion (Young et al 1982a); and plasminogen (Brash 1991) with a possible effect on surface-associated fibrinolytic activity.

Protein adsorption following blood exposure to an artificial surface is relevant for initiation of the intrinsic pathway by the contact activation phase, involving interaction of the contact proteins factor XII (Hageman factor), factor XI, high molecular weight kininogen (HMWK) and prekallikrein (Griffin & Cochrane 1979). A sequence of enzymatic reactions results from the adsorption of HMWK and factor XII. Bound HMWK forms a complex with prekallikrein. This complex cleaves factor XII into factor XIIa, which catalyses the conversion into kallikrein of the prekallikrein participating in the complex with HMWK. Since kallikrein activates factor XII, a cycle of reaction ensures the rapid availability of factor XII on, or near, the artificial surface. HMWK is also able to form a complex with factor XI, thus making factor XI available to factor XIIa and enabling the progression of the coagulation cascade.

Platelet reactions induced by artificial surfaces

In blood–biomaterial interactions, contact of blood with an artificial surface leads almost inevitably to the adhesion and aggregation of platelets (Mason 1972, Mason et al 1976), with the extent of platelet adhesion strongly dependent on the nature of the adsorbed protein layer. Consideration of the platelet-collagen reaction (Jamieson

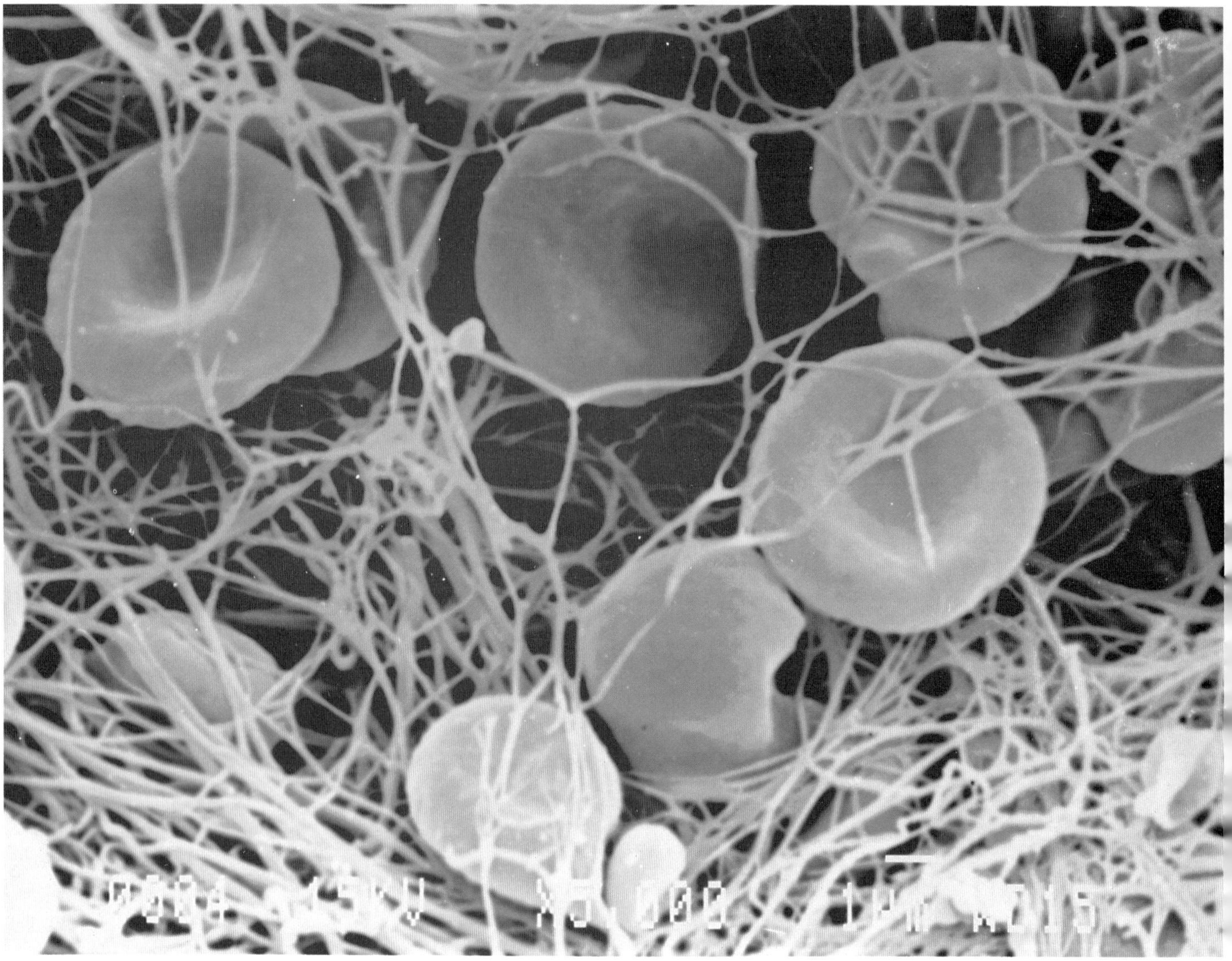

Fig. 58.1 **E**, Erythrocytes in fibrin and damaged erythrocytes.

1973) supports the view that the interaction of platelets with adsorbed fibrinogen or γ-globulin can be attributed to the formation of a complex between glycosyl transferases located in the platelet membrane and incomplete heterosaccharides of fibrinogen or γ-globulin (Evans & Mustard 1968, Kim et al 1974, Lee & Kim 1974). By this reasoning, the inhibition of platelet adhesion by adsorbed albumin might be due to the absence of saccharide chains. The adherence of circulating platelets to protein-coated surfaces leads to a change in platelet shape from anucleate discs to anucleate spheres with long filiform pseudopodia, the coalescence of platelets into an irregular monolayer and, with increasing platelet adhesion, the formation of mounds with leukocytes and erythrocytes entrapped in fibrin (Salzman et al 1977).

Following platelet adhesion to an artificial surface, it can be expected that the platelet release reaction (Holmsen et al 1969) will take place in the adherent platelets, with platelet aggregation then occurring on the surface (Baumgartner et al 1976). This has encouraged interest in the possible influence of surface properties on the release of different platelet constituents. The release of serotonin (5-hydroxytryptamine) was reported to be less dependent than platelet adhesion on surface properties and, unlike platelet adhesion, serotonin release increased with hydrophilicity (Brash & Whicher 1977). β-thromboglobulin (βTG) release is influenced by surface properties in vitro (Bowry et al 1984) and increased levels of βTG and platelet factor 4 (PF_4) have been detected after the implantation of heart valves (Davies et al 1979, Dudczak et al 1979) and during haemodialysis (Adler & Berlyne 1981, Mahiout et al 1987). Liberation of thromboxane B_2 (TXB_2) has been reported during intra-aortic balloon pumping and elevated TXB_2 levels have been observed during cardiopulmonary bypass (Davies et al 1980).

The progression of blood clotting on an artificial surface

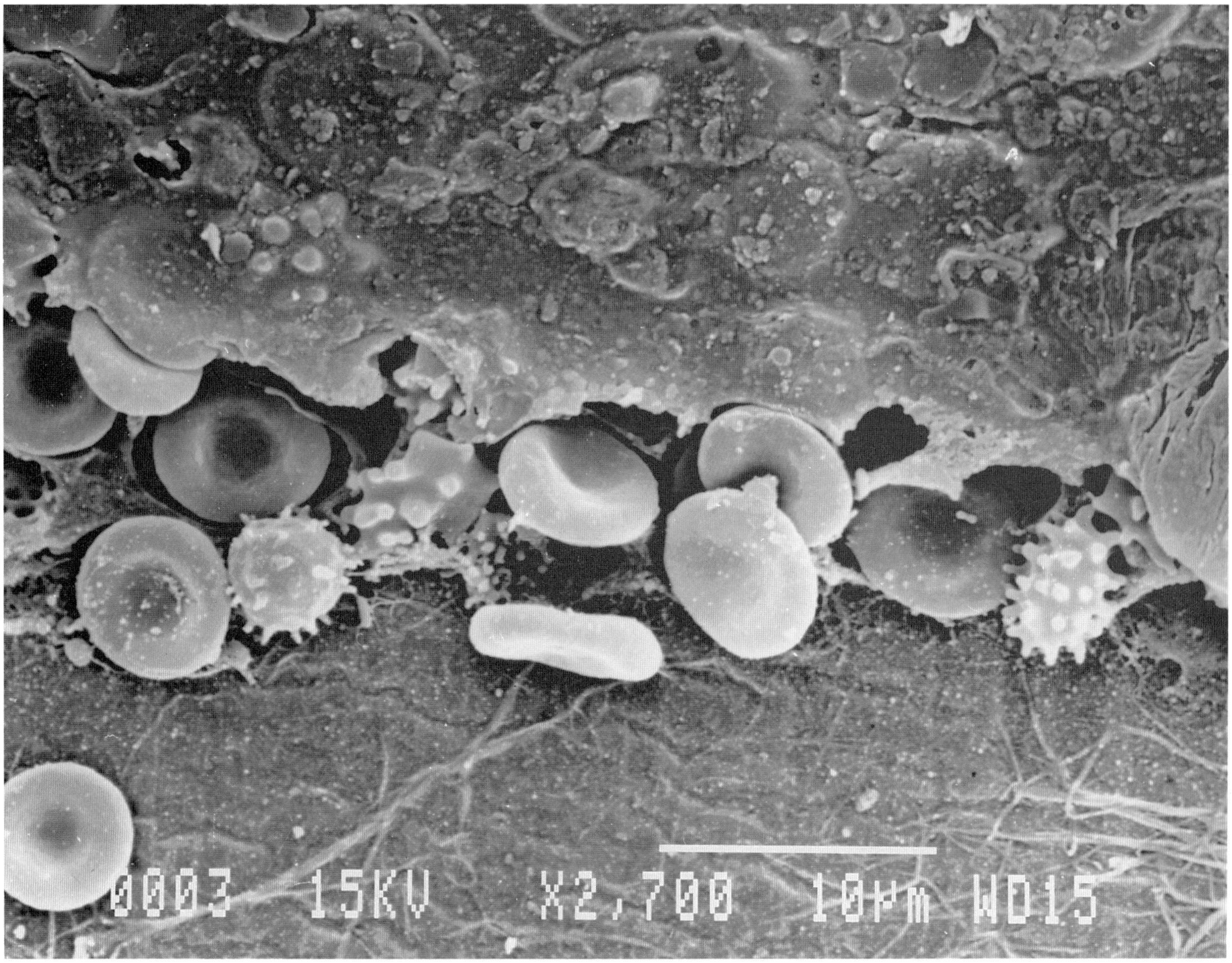

Fig. 58.1 F, From the bottom, polymer surface, protein, cells, protein.

means that an interaction between platelets and the intrinsic pathway is likely (Feijen 1977). Intrinsic coagulation may be induced by thromboplastins liberated from platelets (Needleman & Hook 1982, Walsh 1982) or by factor XII activation caused by platelets stimulated by released ADP. Thrombin formation resulting from intrinsic pathway activation leads to the rapid production of a fibrin monolayer on an artificial surface and the promotion of platelet adhesion and aggregation (Waugh & Baughman 1969, Chuang et al 1979). Thrombin generation may also induce the platelet release reaction and the secretion of PF_4, TXB_2 and thrombospondin (Patrono et al 1980, Phillips et al 1980, Shuman & Levine 1980). It is possible that thrombospondin may play an important role in mediating platelet aggregation on an artificial surface (Young et al 1982b).

The platelet response in blood–biomaterial interactions is influenced by diffusion (Feurstein et al 1975) and shear forces (Richardson et al 1977), with the shear rate and contact time critical for platelet adhesion (Rieger 1980).

Erythrocytes

In blood contact with an artificial surface, erythrocytes adhere to the adsorbed protein layer (Feijen 1977) and under certain conditions, haemolysis occurs, with the platelet release reaction induced by liberated ADP and erythrocyte ghosts (Stormorken 1971). The pattern of protein adsorption can also be influenced by erythrocytes. The addition of erythrocytes to protein solutions leads to a reduction in the amount of protein adsorbed (Brash & Uniyal 1976, Uniyal et al 1982) and this 'red cell effect' has been attributed to erythrocyte-surface contact resulting in deposition of membrane components and a new less adsorptive surface. Since similar reductions in

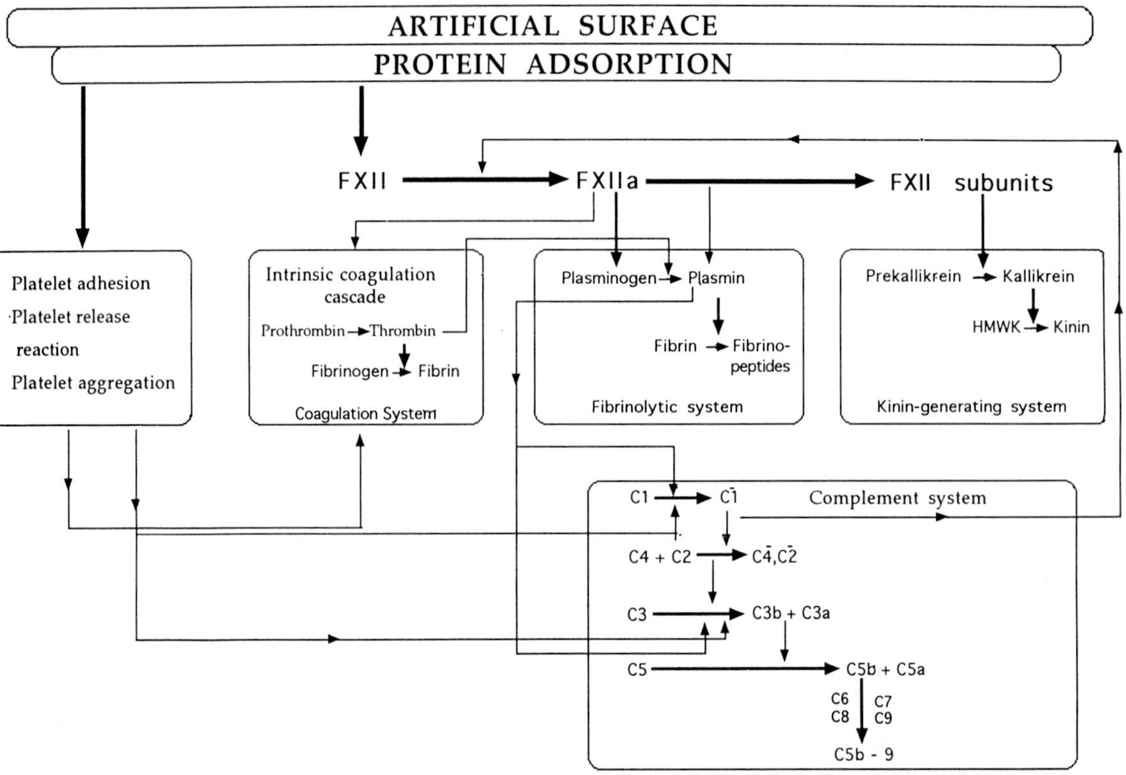

Fig. 58.2 Interactions of blood with an artificial surface. (From Courtney et al Monitoring of the blood response in blood purification. Artificial Organs 17 (4), Blackwell Scientific Publications Inc.

adsorption have been obtained with normal and ghost cells, the influence appears primarily membrane- or particle-related, although there is the possibility of some effect arising from the competitive adsorption of released haemoglobin. While erythrocytes deposit integral membrane proteins on contacting surfaces without being lysed (Borenstein & Brash 1986), evidence supports the view that whole blood flowing over an artificial surface will induce haemolysis, thus increasing the local concentration of free haemoglobin in the plasma. Since haemoglobin has a high surface activity (Horbett et al 1977, Uniyal et al 1982), the adsorption of haemoglobin is likely. This is supported by the detection of haemoglobin following clinical use of membrane blood oxygenators (Owen et al 1985) and the artificial heart (Coleman et al 1986).

In thrombus formation on artificial surfaces, platelet adhesion can be promoted by the hydrodynamic behaviour of red cells, a reduction in the adsorption of platelet-protective proteins or the deposition of an adhesive substance by the red cells (Brash 1983). Blood–surface contact can lead to significant changes in the metabolism of erythrocyte membranes. There is a possibility of shear-induced haemolysis and in coagulation under low shear forces, entrapped erythrocytes and fibrin form the red thrombus (Bruck 1980).

Leukocytes

The adhesion of leukocytes to artificial surfaces has been recognized for a considerable time (Kusserow et al 1971) and the preferential adsorption of polymorphonuclear leukocytes in preference to lymphocytes is supported by evidence from in vitro studies (Lederman et al 1978, Absolom et al 1979) and leukopheresis (Wright et al 1978). Leukocyte adhesion is influenced by the adsorbed protein layer, with enhanced adhesion reported for surfaces coated with IgG, thrombin and prothrombin (Altieri & Edgington 1989). With respect to sensitivity to mechanical trauma, leukocytes appear similar to platelets (Dewitz et al 1977). Leukocyte damage and aggregation are influenced by shear stress and the incorporation of leukocytes into platelet microaggregates has been observed (Dewitz et al 1978).

In thrombus formation on artificial surfaces, the action of leukocytes contrasts with the primarily passive role of the erythrocytes (Szycher 1983). There is attraction of leukocytes to the thrombus and in the thrombosis process, leukocytes may contribute to platelet recruitment by enzymatic release and then participate in fibrinolysis. A direct role of leukocytes in thrombus formation on artificial surfaces resulting from granulocyte adhesion and its effect on platelet aggregation (Cumming 1980) is supported by granulocyte possession of endogenous procoagulant activity (Niemetz 1972, Saba et al 1973) and proaggregatory activity (Harrison et al 1966).

The interaction of leukocytes with artificial surfaces may induce changes in cell function. White cell damage caused by blood response to an artificial surface (Kusserow et al 1971) leads to an impairment in phagocytosis and a reduced ability to combat infection. Leukocyte adhesion is often followed by activation and the stimulation of cell functions such as protein synthesis, leading to production and release of substances, including superoxide and other free radicals, leukotrienes, interleukins, tumour necrosis factor, plasminogen activator, prostaglandins, histamine and platelet activating factor (Bourne 1974, Ringoir & Vanholder 1986, Tetta et al 1987).

The investigation of the response of white cells to contact with artificial surfaces has become increasingly linked to the relationship between leukocytes and complement activation, with this relationship particularly relevant for extracorporeal applications (Farrell 1984, Ringoir & Vanholder 1986).

Complement activation by artificial surfaces

The influence of artificial surfaces on the complement system has become an important feature in the study of blood-biomaterial interactions (Herzlinger 1983, Chenoweth 1986, Kazatchkine & Carreno 1987), although such interest is recent in comparison to that relating to surface-induced complement activation in immunology (Herzlinger 1983). The focus on complement activation in blood-contacting applications has been promoted by clinical evidence obtained during haemodialysis with regenerated cellulose membranes demonstrating the occurence of complement activation and leukopenia (Farrell 1984).

A critical step in complement activation is cleavage of the C3 molecule. In the classical pathway, C3 activation follows activation of C1, C2 and C4, and in the alternative pathway, C3 activation does not involve earlier complement components. The fact that polysaccharides are known alternative pathway activators is in agreement with the view that complement activation by cellulose membranes is via the alternative pathway. There is also evidence that complement activation during cardiopulmonary bypass is initiated by the alternative pathway and for artificial surfaces generally, alternative pathway activation is considered relevant. However, leukopheresis studies have indicated that artificial surfaces may activate complement by a process similar to that of the classical pathway (Nusbacher et al 1978) and classical pathway involvement in cardiopulmonary bypass is a possibility (Jones et al 1982).

Complement components of particular interest are the anaphylatoxin molecules, C3a, C4a and C5a, which function as inflammatory mediators. Complement activation is responsible for granulocyte deviations (Craddock et al 1977a, McGillen & Phair 1979, Hammerschmidt et al 1980), with C5a playing a major role (Hammerschmidt et al 1980, Hugli & Chenoweth 1980). Evidence that neutrophil degranulation induces complement activation has focused attention on the possible relationship between complement activation and granulocyte aggregation (Falkenhagen et al 1984).

The clinical implications of complement activation and the indication that complement activation could mediate leukocyte and platelet adhesion to polymer surfaces (Herzlinger & Cumming 1980) has encouraged the development of biomaterials with a reduced influence on the complement system.

Fibrinolytic activity

The integrated nature of the action of the different systems participating in the response of blood to artificial surfaces (Murabayashi & Nosé 1986) makes it necessary to take into account fibrinolysis and fibrinolytic activity, although the role of artificial surfaces in fibrinolysis is an aspect of blood-biomaterial interactions which has not received great attention (Brash 1991). Surface-induced fibrinolytic activity can be demonstrated by measurement of the levels of fibrin degradation products and activation of the fibrinolytic system has been reported for different clinical applications, including haemodialysis (Kurz et al 1985) and cardiopulmonary bypass (Paramo et al 1991).

BLOOD COMPATIBILITY EVALUATION

While test procedures for predicting the clinical performance of artificial surfaces in blood-contacting applications are subject to limitations (Bruck 1982), the establishment of procedures capable of promoting the quality control and development of materials is an important objective (Klinkmann 1984). The basic features of blood compatibility assessment are parameter selection, the method of achieving blood–material contact and the nature of the blood used.

Parameter selection may require a compromise between the advantages of multiparameter assessment and the benefit of measuring a single parameter by a consistent methodology. Multiparameter assessment facilitates the achievement of a broad perspective and reduces potential errors in biomaterial development, e.g. detection of materials exerting little influence on platelets but inducing complement activation (Payne & Horbett 1987). Within the basic aim of trying to achieve a correlation between a characteristic of the test material and a representative parameter of the blood response, parameter selection is based on relevant features, such as protein adsorption, platelet reactions, intrinsic coagulation, fibrinolysis, leukocyte alterations and complement activation.

In vitro evaluation

Protein adsorption has been determined by the use of radiolabelling, gel electrophoresis, chromogenic substrates of an enzyme-conjugated antibody or infrared spectroscopy (Brash 1991). Platelet reactions have been monitored by platelet adhesion determined by radiolabelling (Goldman et al 1984), platelet loss which differentiates between platelets involved in adhesion and in aggregate formation (Courtney et al 1987), platelet function represented by induced platelet aggregation (Saniabadi et al 1983) and platelet release as represented by measurement of serotonin (Whicher et al 1980), βTG (Bowry et al 1984) and TXB_2 (Mantovani et al 1984). Interest in the intrinsic coagulation has focused on the contact activation phase, with measurement of a factor XII-like activity (Irvine et al 1989) and measurement of bradykinin has been reported recently (Lemke & Finke 1992). Assessment of complement activation has benefited from the availability of radioimmunoassays for specific complement components (Hugli & Chenoweth 1980, Chenoweth & Hugli 1982) to enable measurement of components such as C3a and C5a.

The selected method for assessing blood–biomaterial contact should ensure a blood response dependent on the artificial surface rather than the contact procedure and within the accuracy range of the measurement methodology. Blood–material contact has been achieved by flow through systems and by rocking (Lindsay et al 1973), rotation (Bowry et al 1982) or oscillation (Bowry et al 1984). Surfaces have been evaluated in the form of beads (Lindon et al 1978) or discs (Turitto & Leonard 1972). Test cells vary in complexity from incubation cells relevant for rapid screening (Yu et al 1991) to cells with closely controlled blood flow and wall shear rates relevant for more detailed investigation of blood–material interactions (Weng et al 1991).

Ex vivo evaluation

Single pass ex vivo systems have been utilized in the evaluation of haemodialysis membranes (Bosch et al 1987, Mahiout et al 1987). Such systems ensure control of blood flow and facilitate multiparameter assessment but may require a donation of 500 ml of blood for each test.

In animal-based systems, arteriovenous shunts have been used in the dog (Ihlenfeld et al 1978, Ihlenfeld & Cooper 1979, Young et al 1982a, 1983, Seifert & Greer 1985), sheep (Lindon et al 1980) and baboon (Hanson et al 1980, Lambrecht et al 1983, Horbett 1986). The emphasis has been on the investigation of the deposition of radiolabelled proteins and platelets. The ex vivo stagnation point flow system based on the dog (Petschek et al 1968) utilizes an artery passed through a steel tube and everted to ensure that blood does not contact any artificial surface prior to contact with the surface of the test material. This system has been used in the investigation of platelets, leukocytes and the complement system (Cumming 1980).

In vivo evaluation

The basis of in vivo procedures is the implantation of test materials for designated periods. Examples are the vena cava ring test (Gott & Furuse 1971) and the renal embolus test (Kusserow et al 1970).

Summary

There is no ideal procedure for linking an evaluation procedure for a test material to the potential clinical performance of that material. In vitro procedures enable the use of human blood but cannot take into account the interrelationships between the patient and the clinical use of the material (Lindsay et al 1980, Klinkmann et al 1987, Courtney et al 1993a) and do not normally consider the influence of the disease state (Andrade et al 1981). Ex vivo procedures using human blood are focused on the evaluation of miniature devices. Data acquired from animal experiments must be interpreted with the recognition of species-related differences for blood components (Henson 1969, Grabowski et al 1977).

MODIFICATION OF SURFACES TO IMPROVE BLOOD COMPATIBILITY

Approaches used to improve the blood compatibility of artificial surfaces may be considered in terms of the following: alteration to surface properties, increase of hydrophilicity, chemical modification, attachment of antithrombotic agents, treatment of surfaces with protein, preparation of biomembrane-mimetic surfaces (Gilchrist & Courtney 1980, Fougnot et al 1984, Engbers & Feijen 1991, Courtney et al 1993b).

Alteration to surface physical properties

Blood compatibility may be strongly influenced by the physical nature of an artificial surface. An adverse blood response can result from excessive surface roughness causing mechanical damage or producing deleterious effects on blood flow due to material shape and presentation. Therefore, achievement of a smoother surface may represent an initial simple step in enhancing blood compatibility. In contrast, blood compatibility in certain applications may be improved by the formation of a neointima induced by a porous surface. Examples of this approach include the use of expanded polymers (Baker et al 1976), textured polymers (Szycher et al 1980) and woven and knitted fabric structures (Snyder & Botzko 1982, Hood et al 1984). The relevance of the physical nature of a surface means that it is important to take surface texture into consideration with surface chemistry and to realize that surface texture plays a complex and sometimes major role.

Increase in hydrophilicity

The achievement of blood compatibility improvement by an increase in the hydrophilicity of a surface is based on the belief that protein adsorption and cellular adhesion will decrease with increasing hydrophilicity. The most hydrophilic artificial surfaces are obtained with polymeric hydrogels (Hoffman 1975, Ratner 1981), which swell extensively in aqueous media while remaining insoluble. The poor mechanical strength of hydrogels limits the applicability and procedures for increasing hydrophilicity may require coating or copolymerization.

Earlier investigations utilized hydrophilic polymers based on hydroxyethylmethacrylate (HEMA) (Kaganov et al 1976) but the present emphasis is on the utilization of poly(ethylene oxide) (PEO). While polymers containing HEMA activate complement through hydroxyl groups (Payne & Horbett 1987), PEO can reduce complement activation (Yu et al 1991). Techniques for utilizing PEO cover direct adsorption of PEO-containing surfactants onto a hydrophobic polymer (Lee et al 1989, 1990), covalent grafting of PEO onto a hydrophobic polymer substrate by photoinduction (Mori et al 1982, Nagaoka et al 1984), cross linking (Brinkman et al 1989, 1990), or direct reaction (Golander & Kiss 1988, Nojiri et al 1990, Desai & Hubbell 1991), and by copolymerization (Merrill et al 1982, Takahara et al 1985, 1991, Goodman et al 1989, Yu et al 1991).

Chemical modification

The blood response to a polymer can be altered by chemical modification, where a functional group undergoes replacement or substitution. Recent biomaterial interest has focused on the chemical modification of cellulose membranes, principally to achieve a reduction in complement activation. The hydroxyl groups of cellulose have been replaced by acetate (Ivanovich et al 1983, Chenoweth 1984, Johnson 1989, Lucchi et al 1989, Moll et al 1990), diethylaminoethyl (Cheung et al 1986, Falkenhagen et al 1987, Lucchi et al 1989) and anhydride (Johnson 1989, Johnson et al 1990). The influence of chemical modification is dependent on the nature of the substituting group and the degree of substitution, while the integrated nature of the blood response means that an improvement with respect to one parameter may be offset by an increased adverse influence on another (Courtney et al 1989).

Attachment of antithrombotic agents

As an alternative or supplement to the administration of antithrombotic agents, the blood compatibility of artificial surfaces can be improved by the attachment of anticoagulants, platelet aggregation inhibitors or plasminogen activators. Efforts have been dominated by the utilization of heparin and heparin-based procedures for enhancing blood compatibility extend back 30 years.

Utilization of heparin

Heparin has been incorporated into polymers (Salyer et al 1971) but most procedures have involved heparin attachment to the artificial surface by ionic or covalent bonding (Gilchrist & Courtney 1980, Kim et al 1983, Fougnot et al 1984, Larm et al 1989, Engbers & Feijen 1991, Courtney et al 1993b).

Since heparin has a strong anionic character, ionic bonding is readily achieved on cationic surfaces or surfaces rendered cationic by pretreatment or copolymerization. The first procedure reported (Gott et al 1963) comprised the sequential treatment of a polymer with colloidal graphite, the cationic surfactant benzalkonium chloride and heparin. This procedure is generally unsuitable for flexible materials which require elimination of the graphite layer of the coating and an alternative method of providing groups for heparin attachment. A procedure avoiding the use of graphite and applicable to a range of polymers involves contacting the polymer with a suitable cationic surfactant, followed by contact with heparin (Grode et al 1969). Heparinization of flexible and rigid polymers can be accomplished by the incorporation into the polymer of a heparin complex. Investigation has been made of complexes of heparin with benzalkonium chloride (Usdin & Fourt 1960, Fourt et al 1966), hexadecylpyridinium chloride (Hersh et al 1971), tridodecylmethylammonium chloride (Grode et al 1972, Leininger et al 1972) and cetylpyridinium chloride (Schmer et al 1976). In other methods for heparinization by incorporation, an epichlorohydrin-ethylene oxide copolymer has been incorporated into poly(vinyl chloride) and reacted with amine and heparin (Falb 1975), and different polymers have been modified by a system comprising a soluble metal salt, a solvent and heparin, with the metal salt polymerizing in the treated polymer matrix (Dyck 1972). The ionic attachment of heparin can also be achieved if artificial surfaces contain tertiary amine or quaternary ammonium groups, an approach utilized for elastomers (Falb et al 1966, Yen & Rembaum 1971) and copolymers of cellulose acetate (Martin et al 1970), acrylonitrile (Courtney et al 1976), methyl acrylate (Paik Sung et al 1976), methyl methacrylate (Courtney et al 1978) and cellulose (Holland et al 1978, Schmitt et al 1983). A characteristic of artificial surfaces modified by the ionic attachment of heparin is the removal of the anticoagulant in contact with blood or plasma (Falb et al 1967). This leaching effect has been utilized in the preparation of polymers designed to ensure a controlled release of heparin (Tanzawa et al 1973, Miyama et al 1977). In contrast, heparin removal during blood-surface contact has been reduced through cross-linking of the surface heparin by reaction with glutaraldehyde (Lagergren & Eriksson 1971, Schmitt et al 1983, Barbucci et al 1985).

Procedures for ionic binding of heparin do not permit long-term retention in contact with blood and the effectiveness of artificial surfaces modified by ionic binding may require a minimal release rate of heparin (Idezuki et al 1975). It is generally accepted that the long-term retention of heparin and the preparation of more stable surfaces can be achieved through covalent binding. Heparinization of artificial surfaces by covalent binding normally involves functionalization, to produce groups such as OH or NH_2, capable of reacting with COOH groups in the heparin molecules. Covalent binding has been used in the heparinization of silicone rubber (Grode et al 1972), poly(vinyl alcohol) (Merrill et al 1970), agarose (Schmer 1972, Danishefsky & Tzeng 1974) polyhydroxyethylmethacrylate (Miura et al 1980), styrene-butadiene copolymer (Goosen et al 1980), cellulose (Hasenfratz & Knaup 1981) and in the preparation of a copolymer of heparin and poly(methyl methacrylate) (Labarre et al 1974, 1977).

Standard techniques for covalent attachment do not always produce surfaces with improved blood compatibility (Hoffman et al 1972, Merrill et al 1970). The effectiveness of covalent binding is dependent on the possible utilization of the functional groups in the active sites of the heparin molecule during the attachment procedure and inhibition of blood-heparin contact by protein adsorption (Larm et al 1989), as well as the mobility of the heparin chain on the artificial surface. Furthermore, while artificial surfaces with covalently bound heparin are reported to form a complex with antithrombin III (Fougnot et al 1984), not all surfaces can catalyse the thrombin-inhibiting reaction. On the basis that a suitable surface must maintain the ability of heparin to bind and activate antithrombin III (Larsson et al 1980), procedures for covalent attachment have taken into account the effect of the attachment process on antithrombin III binding sites. Protection of the antithrombin III binding sites during heparin immobilization has been achieved by a technique producing end-point attachment of heparin (Larm et al 1989). In the belief that a more controlled heparin immobilization may require an appropriate spacer between the heparin molecule and the polymer matrix (Ebert & Kim 1982), poly(ethylene oxide) chains have been used as spacers for the covalent attachment of heparin to polyurethane (Park et al 1988), polysiloxane (Grainger & Kim 1988) and polystyrene (Vulic et al 1988) in triblock copolymers. Another approach to heparinization involves the covalent attachment of an albumin-heparin conjugate (Hennink et al 1983) in order to obtain the benefits of both heparin attachment and albumin adsorption.

The nature of the clinical application has a strong influence on the success of heparinized surfaces. There has been an emphasis on catheters (Heyman et al 1985, Eloy et al 1987) and extracorporeal purification procedures. In haemodialysis, there has been evaluation of systems based on ionic binding (Schmer et al 1976, 1977) and covalent binding (Lins et al 1984). While regular application in haemodialysis has not been achieved, interest remains because the systemic use of heparin has the potential disadvantages of a risk of haemorrhage (Leonard et al 1969) and an adverse effect on platelets (Lindsay et al 1977, Kelton 1986), while heparinized systems may not only inhibit platelet reactions but also reduce complement activation. In cardiopulmonary bypass, membrane oxygenators have been heparinized by ionic binding (Rea et al 1972, Hagler et al 1975) and covalent binding (Mottaghy et al 1989, von Segesser & Turin 1989, Nilsson et al 1990, Palatianos et al 1990, Tong et al 1990, Videm et al 1991), with the latter approach more likely to gain clinical utilization.

Utilization of platelet aggregation inhibitors

An improvement in blood compatibility resulting from reduced platelet adhesion and aggregation rather than inhibition of the intrinsic coagulation is the basis for the use of surface attachment of platelet aggregation inhibitors. Prostaglandin immobilization (Grode et al 1974) has been demonstrated to produce antiplatelet effects in vitro (Ebert et al 1982), while improved blood compatibility with dipyridamole bound to cellulose has been attributed to the promotion of albumin adsorption or interaction with the enzymatic components of the platelet membrane and blocking of the platelet aggregation cascade (Marconi et al 1979). The possibility of reduced platelet adhesion and aggregation by the controlled release of a platelet aggregation inhibitor has been indicated by the incorporation of prostaglandins into poly(vinyl chloride) and polyurethane (McRea & Kim 1978, McRea et al 1981) but the preferred approach to the immobilization of platelet aggregation inhibitors is that of covalent binding, with options for functionalization and selection of coupling agents (Ebert et al 1982, Bamford & Middleton 1983).

Utilization of plasminogen activators

The immobilization of plasminogen activators is intended to produce artificial surfaces which are fibrinolytically active and capable of reducing thrombus formation by dissolution. Approaches have focused on the attachment of the enzyme urokinase (Kusserow et al 1973, Ohshiro & Kosaki 1980, Sugitachi et al 1980, Watanabe et al 1981, Aoshima et al 1982, Ohshiro 1983, Senatore et al 1986). The attachment of urokinase can be by ionic binding (Aoshima et al 1982) or covalent binding (Watanabe et al

1981). A disadvantage is that plasminogen activation may be uncontrolled.

Treatment of surfaces with protein

The preparation of artificial surfaces with improved blood compatibility by deposition of protein has been strongly influenced by the fact that the adsorption of albumin leads to reduced platelet adhesion. This has been utilized in the identification of polymers capable of albumin adsorption (Lyman et al 1975) or the preparation of polymers with enhanced albumin adsorption, such as alkyl derivatized polyurethane (Munro et al 1983) and cellulose acetate (Frautschi et al 1983). A variation has been the treatment of polyurethane with an albumin-IgG complex (Mohammad & Olsen 1986). The effectiveness of albumin adsorption is dependent on the nature of the clinical application. In haemoperfusion, where the passage of blood over sorbents may induce a severe fall in platelets, success has been reported with albumin adsorption onto cellulose nitrate-coated activated carbon (Chang 1977) or polystyrene-divinylbenzene resin (Falkenhagen et al 1981) maintaining platelet counts at acceptable levels.

The term 'biolization', introduced by Nosé et al (1971), is applied to the chemical and thermal treatment of tissue components, such as proteins, either coated onto a polymer or blended with a polymer (Kambic et al 1983). On this basis, biolized materials include polymers coated with protein, polymers blended with protein, and polymer-protein blends laminated to a base polymer. Treatment of the modified surface with glutaraldehyde is a feature of biolization. Examples of biolized materials evaluated are natural rubber treated with albumin or gelatin (Imai et al 1971), polyurethane treated with gelatin (Kambic et al 1978) and a polyolefin elastomer treated with gelatin (Kiraly et al 1977).

A more recent utilization of protein is the development of a gelatin-coated vascular prosthesis designed to avoid the need for a preclotting stage (Maini 1989).

Preparation of biomembrane-mimetic surfaces

Biomembrane-mimetic surfaces are designed to mimic the biological membrane of blood cells and thereby avoid recognition by the blood as foreign. The preparation of such surfaces on polymers has been promoted by the efforts of Chapman and coworkers (Chapman & Charles 1992). A key step is the utilization on an artificial surface of the phosphorylcholine (PC) head group, a major component of erythrocyte and platelet outer membrane surfaces. Diacetylenic polymers containing PC groups have been synthesized (Durrani & Chapman 1987) and coated onto hydrophobic polymers such as poly(vinyl chloride), polyethylene, polypropylene and polystyrene, with a reported reduction in fibrinogen adsorption and platelet adhesion (Chapman & Charles 1992). Blood compatibility improvement has also been claimed by the synthesis of functionally active PC-containing compounds and the covalent attachment of these compounds to polymer surfaces containing OH, COOH or COCl groups (Durrani et al 1986, Hayward et al 1986a,b, Hall et al 1989). In another technique for the preparation of biomembrane-mimetic surfaces, a monomer containing PC, 2-methacryloyloxyethyl methacrylate (MPC) has been copolymerized with butyl methacrylate (Ishihara et al 1990) or styrene (Kojima et al 1991), with reduced protein adsorption and platelet activation reported (Ishihara et al 1991). Grafting of MPC onto cellulose has been achieved (Ishihara et al 1992) and may reduce both platelet reactions and complement activation.

CLINICAL IMPLICATIONS OF MATERIAL–BLOOD INTERACTIONS

Cardiopulmonary bypass

The major use of cardio-pulmonary bypass is in cardiac surgery to enable the heart and lungs to be bypassed by an extracorporeal circuit in which the pumping function and oxygenation of blood is replaced. Blood is removed from the vena cavae and passes through a heat exchanger which regulates the temperature. To this may be added filtered blood which has been removed by suction from the bypassed heart. The blood is then passed through an oxygenator and returned to a reservoir where it is then filtered and by means of a mechanical pump is returned at arterial pressure to the aortic arch. Numerous design advances on this basic concept have been made since the first description of a functioning machine by Gibbon (1954). One of the most important was development of membrane-based devices for oxygenation as separation of the blood and gas phases by a gas-permeable membrane which reduces trauma to cells, reduces activation of coagulation proteins and so enables the bypass process to be extended (Clowes et al 1956, Drinker 1972, Courtney et al 1993a). Major haemostatic parameter changes are not seen when membrane oxygenators are used unless there is prolongation of the bypass (Bick 1991). Also the biological responses to cardiopulmonary bypass may be altered by use of pulsatile flow (Bregman et al 1981, Taylor 1986).

To avoid thrombus formation on the various membranes of the system it is usual to use heparin as the anticoagulant (Uziel et al 1986). Some workers also use prostacyclin to reduce adhesion and consumption of platelets (Madhok et al 1985).

Despite the advances in development of the circuit, the alteration of the membranes and the more effective use of antithrombotics, activation of plasma coagulation proteins, platelets, white cells and complement still occurs and remains a clinical problem (Courtney et al 1993a).

This is a result of blood changes due to the nature of the operation itself and other physical factors such as temperature, mechanical trauma and mode of blood flow as well as surface contact (Edmunds & Stephensen 1982, Courtney et al 1993a). In addition the use of priming fluids may produce dilution of coagulation factors and compound the bleeding problems (de Leval et al 1981) and some priming fluids may contain heparin, acid-citrate-dextrose or dextrans (Edie et al 1981).

Morbidity after cardiopulmonary bypass results not only from bleeding but also from particulate material forming microemboli and entering the cerebral circulation (Solis et al 1974). Such microemboli may be composed of cell aggregates composed of platelets, white cells and red cells, denatured proteins, fat, calcium salt complexes and antifoam substances, not all of which are effectively filtered out (Pearson 1981).

Haemodialysis and related procedures

Membrane-based haemodialysis remains the commonest treatment of severe chronic renal failure. This removes solutes predominantly by diffusion with a small contribution from convective solute transfer during the removal of water by ultrafiltration. This is the most common situation in man in which blood is recurrently exposed to artificial membranes (usually regenerated cellulose) and the related vascular catheters and plastic tubing of the equipment. Despite numerous attempts to replace the cellulose membranes they still predominate due to their cheapness (Courtney et al 1984). Numerous studies have now shown the alterations of blood components on contact with cellulose especially consumption coagulopathy (Courtney et al 1993a) and neutropenia with activation of the complement cascade (Courtney et al 1990).

All membranes, whether cellulose, modified cellulose or synthetic, adsorb proteins from plasma and the site, extent and distribution are dependent on blood flow. The predominant proteins are albumin (Kuwahara et al 1989) fibrinogen (McLaughlin et al 1989) and fibronectin (Pertosa et al 1989). This protein adsorption occurs with the first pass of blood.

It has also long been recognised that soon after the start of dialysis the white cell count falls and returns to normal over a period of an hour or so (Kaplow & Goffinet 1968). The sequestered white cells are easily recognized on scanning electron microscopy of the membrane where they relate to platelets and to fibrin thrombi. There is evidence that, in addition, sequestration of both granulocytes and monocytes occurs in the lung microvasculature as a result of complement activation (Toren et al 1970, Craddock et al 1977a). It has been suggested that the pulmonary sequestration of neutrophils results from down-regulation of neutrophil receptors for C5a-des-Arg (Skubitz & Craddock 1981).

Leukocyte adherence is associated with complement activation on the membrane and the main active components are C3a and C5a, which are mediators of granulocyte chemotaxis, aggregation and activation with oxygen free radical production (Chenoweth & Hugli 1980).

Pulmonary dysfunction following haemodialysis has been variously ascribed to arterial hypoxaemia resulting from loss of hydrogen ion and carbon dioxide via the membrane (Jones et al 1980), as well as to activation of complement and leukostasis in pulmonary capillaries (Craddock et al 1977b). Such a postulate is theoretically attractive, as direct measurement now demonstrates that the potential for capillary plugging by white cells is a reflection of the white cell deformability, which is about 1000 times that of the red cell.

To reduce the incidence of clotting in the haemodialysis circuit it is conventional practice to give standard heparin in doses of approximately 30 iu/kg body weight as a bolus followed by 30 iu/kg/h. Little attempt has been made to monitor accurately the effects of dosage and, as thrombus formation occurs, the dose may be doubled or trebled with resultant bleeding after removal of the needles. Heparin action requires to be monitored and the dose altered as necessary — this is best done using an activated PTT assay, which can now be automated for use in dialysis units, and which gives the answer within a few minutes. Low molecular weight heparin may also be used for this purpose but would seem to offer no advantage (Bambauer et al 1990, von Bonsdorf et al 1990). Similarly hirudin and dermatan have been tried. There is a report of anaphylactoid reactions with ACE inhibitors when acrilonitrile membranes were used (Anon 1992).

A recurrent problem is a low incidence of thrombocytopenia due to standard heparin (Kelton 1986). This may lead to serious bleeding complications and the discontinuance of dialysis. An alternative is to replace standard heparin with a low molecular weight heparin, which has no effect on platelets. To overcome the problem of platelet activation a variety of antithrombotic agents may be used. These include aspirin and dipyridamole (Lindsay et al 1972) and triclopidine (Maeda et al 1980). None of these agents is entirely satisfactory as they all have additional side-effects which are undesirable. Prostacyclin has answered the need in this situation and has now been extensively used (Zusman et al 1981). Unfortunately, the therapeutic dose levels and the toxic levels are close, and many patients will experience nausea, flushings, and headache. There may also be a fall in blood pressure. New analogues of prostacyclin are now becoming available with long plasma half lives, and these seem to have fewer side-effects.

In patients with a high bleeding risk it is possible to perform heparin-free haemodialysis using a high blood flow with saline flushes of the blood lines (Preuschof et al 1988).

Catheters and transvenous lines

With the increasing complexity of modern medicine and the widespread use of life-support systems, it is rare for any seriously ill patient to escape having some kind of arterial or venous catheter or line inserted for infusion of fluids, parenteral hyperalimentation, long-term chemotherapy (Hickman cannula), angioplasty, angiography or parenteral feeding. Such procedures are often associated with localized thrombus deposition on the material surface exposed to flowing blood (Walters et al 1972, Nolewajka et al 1980, Pandian et al 1980, Brismar et al 1981). With the use of indwelling transfemoral lines for pacing, an incidence of femoral thrombosis of up to 30% may be found and in central venous catheterization for measurement of central venous pressure or for alimentation a similar incidence is common (Nolewajka et al 1980, Pandian et al 1980).

Three types of thrombus may be found; the commonest occurs on the catheter or line (sleeve thrombus) and the second forms on the wall of the vessel (mural thrombus), probably at points at which endothelium is damaged. The third type forms inside the catheter. Soon after insertion a monolayer of fibrin and platelets may be demonstrated on the artificial surface, the extent depending on the material used and its surface characteristic (Nachnani et al 1972, Hoar et al 1978, Libsack & Kollmeyer 1979). This sleeve of thrombus is stripped off when the catheter is removed and may then embolize to the periphery or form an occlusive thrombus at the site of vessel puncture. Fine bore silicone rubber and polyurethane polymer catheters are least likely to damage endothelium and accelerate mural thrombus (Peters et al 1984). Knotting or looping of the catheter within the vein alters blood flow and may stimulate thrombosis. Rarely does embolization present a clinical problem despite the demonstration by Siegelman et al (1968) that over 40% of patients have platelet-fibrin emboli in small peripheral arteries after arteriography.

On the venous side, a local thrombophlebitis is inevitable if a cannula is left in situ for several days (Hershey et al 1984). This may result from local thrombosis, chemical irritation or low grade infection. It is probably worthwhile changing the site of such indwelling catheters if they are required in the long term, and this will avoid complications such as thrombosis, sepsis and local tissue reactions.

Attempts have been made to reduce platelet-fibrin deposition using a wide range of antiplatelet agents, anticoagulants and fibrinolytic stimulators. Thrombus in the lumen may be avoided by priming the catheter with heparin, 1000 iu/ml. If occlusion does occur then an infusion of streptokinase or urokinase, 5000 iu/ml, will rapidly lyse the thrombus.

Artificial heart valves

Over the years the design and construction of prosthetic heart valves have undergone great change (Black et al 1983). Use of more biocompatible material has reduced the risk of thromboembolism, but this still remains, with infection, one of the greatest hazards (Bloch et al 1984) and actuarial analysis shows that thromboembolism is a continued time-related risk for any patient with heart valve replacement (Barnhorst et al 1975, Salomon et al 1977). When the earlier type of valve was used the incidence of embolism was as high as 50% (Gadboys et al 1967). However, this figure has been substantially reduced by better design and materials (Dellsperger et al 1991) and the use of anticoagulants in combination with antiplatelet agents. It is probable that the initiating factor in thrombosis is platelet deposition on the ring, flap or ball, and this may be accentuated by release of ADP from damaged red cells (Weily & Genton 1970, Turpie et al 1982). Measurement of platelet survival shows significant shortening, and scanning electron microscopy of valves removed at operation or postmortem demonstrates platelet adhesion and aggregation. Routine assessment of platelet survival and βTG levels may be used as an indicator of potential thrombogenicity (Conard et al 1984).

Tissue valves have some advantages, offering better shape and function without the need for anticoagulation. Problems include calcification in the long-term and questions about long-term function (Lee & Boughner 1991). Thromboembolic events are more likely to occur in the first 2 years with bioprostheses, whereas with mechanical prostheses thrombotic events may occur at any time (Farah et al 1984). Mitral valve replacement, however, involves a substantially higher risk than aortic valve replacement (Roux et al 1984).

Reduction of the risk of embolization from a prosthetic valve may be achieved by administration of oral anticoagulants in combination with an antiplatelet agent such as dipyridamole (Silverton et al 1984, Dalen & Hirsh 1986).

Left ventricular support and the artificial heart

Support of the failing left ventricle is theoretically an exciting concept in the case of a patient awaiting valve replacement, heart transplantation or in those with cardiogenic shock after myocardial infarction (Bolooki 1977, Ige et al 1978, Okada et al 1979). The major clinical problems remain, however, of thrombus formation and bleeding from the use of anticoagulants. Such devices are usually inserted via the left femoral artery and located in the abdominal aorta by way of a short section of vascular prosthetic graft. Inflation of the balloon occurs in diastole after the aortic valve closes and deflation is synchronized with systole. Such devices may possibly have a place in the short-term management of patients with circulatory collapse, i.e. maintaining the circulation of vital organs until drugs or pacing procedures become effective. Most of the devices consist of a flexible polyurethane bladder lined by polyester fibres on which endothelialization eventually occurs (Norman 1977). After insertion they are rapidly covered by a layer of fibrin with adherent platelets and this may form a source of emboli into the peripheral arteries (Schoen et al 1972). As a result of their action, local damage to the endothelium is common, and in up to 10% of patients, haemolysis with release of red cell ADP may promote a thrombotic tendency (Green et al 1987, Taenaka et al 1989). Local infusions of heparin and a variety of antiplatelet agents may be of value (Bick 1984).

Similar problems are present in all the different forms of the artificial hearts (total or partial). Current designs still need an external power source and valves, required to control direction of blood flow, and infection are still problems. Already artificial hearts have been used in the human with some success (the Jarvik-7 heart device keeps the recipient alive until their cardiovascular status has improved sufficiently for transplantation) (Griffith et al 1987). The vast majority of work continues in experimental animals as both mechanical and materials problems remain unsolved (DeVries et al 1984, Burns & Olsen 1989, Solen et al 1989).

Arterial grafts

Optimal criteria for arterial prostheses have been laid down by Sauvage et al (1973) and Wesolowski (1978), and these are met by many of the newer materials, such as porous woven Dacron (which is preclotted), expanded microporous polytetrafluoroethylene and glutaraldehyde-treated human femoral artery (Clyne et al 1979, Klimach & Charlesworth 1983). Many of these materials become coated with a cellular neointima and rely on this for thromboresistance. With grafts of small diameter (below 6 mm), there is a high incidence of thrombotic occlusion and only autologous veins seem to be consistently successful in this situation although it is known that platelet activation may be responsible for intimal hyperplasia of the graft wall. Thrombus deposition on grafts is best measured dynamically using ^{51}Cr-labelled platelets or imaging with ^{111}In (Goldman 1983, Goldman et al 1984). However, these tests are expensive and time-consuming, and have little use in clinical practice. Of more value are tests of platelet release products, such as βTG or PF4, or of fibrinogen activation, such as fibrinogen turnover or FPA levels (Bowry et al 1984).

Many studies have shown a clear relationship between platelet uptake and graft patency in experimental animals (Christenson et al 1981) and in the human (Goldman et al 1984). Many authors have used the above tests to devise a thrombogenicity rating for graft materials. However, laboratory tests in vitro may not correlate closely with survival of the grafts in vivo (Eikhoff et al 1983).

CONCLUSION

Biocompatibility of a material implies that when used in a clinical situation it is non-thrombogenic, non-toxic, and does not remove proteins or blood cells, does not stimulate an inflammatory response or activate any of the triggered enzyme systems in plasma (Klinkmann 1984, Forbes et al 1989).

Chemical changes in polymers and the use of new therapeutic agents to suppress platelet–surface interaction have produced rapid progress in the construction and design of medical equipment. In addition, the testing of new materials may be carried out rapidly in vitro, in vivo, and ex vivo. The major advance will be made when a material with the same properties as normal human endothelium is produced, but as yet none is available.

Acknowledgements

Scanning electron micrographs were kindly supplied by the Microscopy Group, Bioengineering Unit, University of Strathclyde. The authors acknowledge assistance provided by Sumuk Sundaram, Jing Yu and Nina Lamba, Bioengineering Unit, University of Strathclyde.

REFERENCES

Absolom D R, Neumann A W, Zingg W, van Oss C J 1979 Thermodynamic studies of cellular adhesion. Transactions of the American Society for Artificial Internal Organs 25: 152–156

Absolom D R, Zingg W, Policova Z, Neumann A W 1983 Determination of the surface tension of protein coated materials by means of the advancing solidification front technique. Transactions of the American Society for Artificial Internal Organs 29: 146–151

Adams G A, Feurstein I A 1980 Visual fluorescent and radio-isotopic evaluation of platelet accumulation and embolization. Transactions of the American Society for Artificial Internal Organs 26: 17–22

Adams G A, Feuerstein I A 1981 How much fibrinogen or fibronectin is enough for platelet adhesion? Transactions of the American Society for Artificial Internal Organs 27: 219–224

Adams A L, Fischer G C, Vroman L 1978 The complexity of blood at simple interfaces. Journal of Colloid and Interface Science 65: 468–478

Adler A J, Berlyne G M 1981 β-Thromboglobulin and platelet factor-4 levels during hemodialysis with polyacrylonitrile. American Society for Artificial Internal Organs Journal 4: 100–102

Altieri C D, Edgington T S 1989 Sequential receptor cascade for coagulation proteins on monocytes. Journal of Biological Chemistry 264: 2969–2972

Andrade J D, Coleman D L, Didisheim P, Hanson S R, Mason R, Merrill E 1981 Blood–materials interactions — 20 years of frustration. Transactions of the American Society for Artificial Internal Organs 27: 659–662

Anon 1992 Anaphylactoid reactions to high-flux polyacrylonitrile membranes in combination with ACE inhibitors. Current Problems (Committee on Safety of Medicines) No 33: 2

Aoshima R, Kand Y, Takada A, Yamashita A 1982 Sulfonated poly (vinylidene fluoride) as a biomaterial: immobilization of urokinase and biocompatibility. Journal of Biomedical Materials Research 16: 289–299
Bagnall R D 1978 Adsorption of plasma proteins on hydrophobic surfaces. II. Fibrinogen and fibrinogen-containing protein mixtures. Journal of Biomedical Materials Research 12: 203–217
Baier R E 1977 The organization of blood components near interfaces. Annals of the New York Academy of Sciences 283: 17–36
Baier R E, Loeb G I, Wallace G T 1971 Role of an artificial boundary in modifying blood proteins. Federation Proceedings 30: 1523–1538
Baker L D Jr, Johnson J M, Goldfarb D 1976 Expanded polytetrafluoroethylene (PTFE) subcutaneous arteriovenous conduit: an improved vascular access for chronic hemodialysis. Transactions of the American Society for Artificial Internal Organs 22: 382–385
Bambauer R, Rucker S, Weber U, Kohler M 1990 Comparison of low molecular weight heparin and standard heparin in hemodialysis. Transactions of the American Society of Artificial Internal Organs 36: 646–649
Bamford C H, Middleton I P 1983 Studies on functionalizing and grafting to poly (ether-urethanes). European Polymer Journal 19: 1027–1035
Barbucci R, Casini G, Ferruti P, Tempesti F 1985 Surface-grafted heparinizable materials. Polymer 26: 1349–1352
Barnhorst D A, Oxman H A, Connolly D C, Pluth J R, Danielson G K, Wallace R B, McGoon D C 1975 Long-term follow-up of isolated replacement of the aortic and mitral valve with Starr–Edwards prosthesis. American Journal of Cardiology 35: 228–231
Baumgartner H R, Muggli R, Tschopp T B, Turitto V T 1976 Platelet adhesion, release and aggregation in flowing blood: effects of surface properties and platelet function. Thrombosis and Haemostasis 35: 124–138
Berger S, Salzman E W 1974 Thromboembolic complications of prosthetic devices. Progress in Hemostasis and Thrombosis 2: 273–309
Bick R 1991 Alterations of hemostasis associated with surgery, cardiovascular surgery, prosthetic devices and transplantation. In: Ratnoff O D, Forbes C D (eds) Disorders of Hemostasis, 2nd edn. W B Saunders, Philadelphia, p 382–422
Bick R L, Schmalhorst W R, Arbegast N R 1976 Alterations of hemostasis associated with cardiopulmonary bypass. Thrombosis Research 8: 285–302
Black M M, Drury P J, Tindale W B 1983 Twenty-five years of heart-valve substitute: a review. Journal of the Royal Society of Medicine 76: 667–680
Bloch G, Vouhe P R, Menu P et al 1984 Long-term evaluation of bioprosthetic valves: 615 consecutive cases. European Heart Journal 5 (suppl): 73–80
Bolooki N 1977 Application of intra-aortic balloon pumping. Futura, New York
Borenstein N, Brash J L 1986 Red blood cells deposit membrane components on contacting surfaces. Journal of Biomedical Materials Research 20: 723–730
Bosch T, Schmidt B, Spencer P C et al 1987 Ex vivo biocompatibility evaluation of a new modified cellulose membrane. Artificial Organs 11: 144–148
Bourne H R 1974 Immunology. In: Ramwell P W (ed) The prostaglandins. Plenum, New York, vol 2: 277–291
Bowry S K, Courtney J M, Prentice C R M, Paul J P 1982 Blood compatibility of polymers: an in vitro method of assessment. In: Winter G D, Gibbons D F, Plenck H Jr (eds) Biomaterials 1980. Wiley, London, p 435–444
Bowry S K, Courtney J M, Prentice C R M, Douglas J F 1984 Utilization of the platelet release reaction in the blood compatibility assessment of polymers. Biomaterials 5: 289–292
Brash J L 1983 Protein adsorption and blood interactions. In: Szycher M (ed) Biocompatible polymers, metals, and composites. Technomic, Lancaster, PA, p 35–52
Brash J L 1991 Role of plasma protein adsorption in the response of blood to foreign surfaces. In: Sharma C P, Szycher M (eds) Blood compatible materials and devices. Technomic, Lancaster, P A, p 3–24
Brash J L, Davidson V J 1976 Adsorption on glass and polyethylene from solutions of fibrinogen and albumin. Thrombosis Research 9: 249–259
Brash J L, Lyman D J 1969 Adsorption of plasma proteins in solution to uncharged hydrophobic polymer surfaces. Journal of Biomedical Materials Research 3: 175–189
Brash J L, ten Hove P 1984 Effect of plasma dilution on adsorption of fibrinogen to solid surfaces. Thrombosis and Haemostasis 51: 326–330
Brash J L, Thibodeau J A 1986 Identification of proteins adsorbed from human plasma to glass bead columns: plasmin-induced degradation of adsorbed fibrinogen. Journal of Biomedical Materials Research 20: 1263–1275
Brash J L, Uniyal S 1976 Adsorption of albumin and fibrinogen to polyethylene in presence of red cells. Transactions of the American Society for Artificial Internal Organs 22: 253–259
Brash J L, Uniyal S 1979 Dependence of albumin-fibrinogen simple and competitive adsorption on surface properties of biomaterials. Journal of Polymer Science C66: 377–389
Brash J L, Whicher S J 1977 Interaction of platelets with surfaces: a factorial study of adhesion and associated release of serotonin. In: Kenedi R M, Courtney J M, Gaylor J D S, Gilchrist J (eds) Artificial organs. Macmillan, London, p 263–272
Brash J L, Uniyal S, Samak Q 1974 Exchange of albumin adsorbed on polymer surfaces. Transactions of the American Society for Artificial Internal Organs 20: 69–76
Breemhaar W, Brinkman E, Ellens D J, Beugeling T, Bantjes A 1984 Preferential adsorption of high density lipoprotein from blood plasma onto biomaterial surfaces. Biomaterials 5: 269–274
Bregman D, Marrin C A S, Spotnitz H M 1981 Pulsatile flow in extracorporeal circulation. In: Ionescu M I (ed) Techniques in extracorporeal circulation, 2nd edn. Butterworth, London, p 601
Brinkman E, Poot A, Beugeling T, van der Does L, Bantjes A 1989 Surface modification of copolyether-urethane catheters with poly-(ethylene oxide). International Journal of Artificial Organs 12: 390–394
Brinkman E, Poot A, van der Does L, Bantjes A 1990 Platelet deposition studies on copolyether urethanes modified with poly(ethylene oxide). Biomaterials 11: 200–205
Brismar B, Hardstedt C, Jacobsen S 1981 Diagnosis of thrombosis by catheter phlebography after prolonged central venous catheterization. Annals of Surgery 194: 779–783
Bruck S D 1980 Properties of biomaterials in the physiological environment. CRC Press, Boca Raton
Bruck S D 1982 On the evaluation of medical plastics in contact with blood. Biomaterials 3: 121–123
Brücke E 1857 Ueber die Ursache der Gerinnung des Blutes. Archiv für Pathologische Anatomie and Physiologie und für Klinische Medicin, R Virchow (ed) 12: 81–100
Burns G L, Olsen D B 1989 Immune response changes with blood pump use in calves. Transactions of the American Society for Artificial Internal Organs 35: 700–702
Chan B M C, Brash J L 1981 Adsorption of fibrinogen on glass: reversibility aspects. Journal of Colloid and Interface Science 82: 217–225
Chang T M S 1977 Protective effects of microencapsulation (coating) on platelet depletion and particulate embolism in the clinical applications of charcoal haemoperfusion. In: Kenedi R M, Courtney J M, Gaylor J D S, Gilchrist T (eds) Artificial organs. Macmillan, London, p 164–177
Chapman D, Charles S A 1992 A coat of many lipids — in the clinic. Chemistry in Britain 28: 253–256
Chenoweth D E 1984 Complement activation during hemodialysis: clinical observations, proposed mechanisms and theoretical implications. Artificial Organs 8: 281–287
Chenoweth D E 1986 Complement activation produced by biomaterials. Transactions of the American Society for Artificial Internal Organs 32: 226–232
Chenoweth D E, Hugli T E 1980 Human C5a and C5a analogs as probes of the neutrophil C5a receptor. Molecular Immunology 17: 151–161
Chenoweth D E, Hugli T E 1982 Assays for chemotactic factors and anaphylatoxins. In: Nakamura R M, Dito W R, Tucker E S III (eds)

Immunologic analysis: recent progress in diagnostic laboratory immunology. Masson, New York, p 227–237
Cheung A K, Chenoweth D E, Otsuka D, Henderson L W 1986 Compartmental distribution of complement activation products in artificial kidneys. Kidney International 30: 74–80
Christenson J T, Megerman J, Hanel K C, L'Italien G J, Strauss H W, Abbott W M 1981 Precision of early graft occlusion using indium-III labelled platelets. Journal of Cardiovascular Surgery 22: 264–270
Chuang H Y K 1984 In situ immunoradiometric assay of fibrinogen adsorbed to artificial surfaces. Journal of Biomedical Materials Research 18: 547–559
Chuang H Y K, King W F, Mason R G 1978 Interaction of plasma proteins with artificial surfaces: protein adsorption isotherms. Journal of Laboratory and Clinical Medicine 92: 483–496
Chuang H Y K, Crowther P E, Mohammad S F, Mason R G 1979 Interactions of thrombin and antithrombin III with artificial surfaces. Thrombosis Research 14: 273–282
Clowes J H A Jnr, Hopkins A L, Neville W E 1956 An artificial lung dependent upon diffusion of oxygen and carbon dioxide through plastic membranes. Journal of Thoracic and Cardiovascular Surgery 32: 630–635
Clyne C A C, McVergh J A, Fox M J, Jantet G H, Jamieson C W 1979 PTFE (Goretex) femoro-popliteal reconstruction for limb salvage. Annals of the Royal College of Surgeons (England) 61: 301–303
Coleman D L, Meuzelaar H L C, Kessler T R, McLennen W M, Richards J M, Gregonis DE 1986 Retrieval and analysis of a clinical total artificial heart. Journal of Biomedical Materials Research 20: 417–431
Conard J, Horellou M H, Baillet M et al 1984 Plasma beta-thromboglobulin in patients with valvular heart disease with or without valve replacement: relationship with thromboembolic accidents. European Heart Journal 5 (suppl): 13–18
Courtney J M, Park G B, Fairweather I A, Lindsay R M 1976 Polymer structure and blood compatibility — application of an acrylonitrile copolymer. Biomaterials, Medical Devices, and Artificial Organs 4: 263–275
Courtney J M, Park G B, Prentice C R M, Winchester J F, Forbes C D 1978 Polymer modification and blood compatibility. Journal of Bioengineering 2: 241–249
Courtney J M, Gaylor J D S, Klinkman H, Holtz M 1984 Poymer membranes. In: Hastings G W, Ducheyne P (eds) Macromolecular biomaterials. CRC Press, Boca Raton, p 143–180
Courtney J M, Travers M, Bowry S K, Prentice C R M, Lowe G D O, Forbes C D 1987 Measurement of the platelet loss in the blood compatibility assessment of biomaterials. Biomaterials 8: 231–233
Courtney J M, Robertson L M, Jones C et al 1989 Blood compatibility of biomaterials in artificial organs. In: Paul J P, Barbenel J C, Courtney J M, Kenedi R M (eds) Progress in bioengineering. Adam Hilger, Bristol, p 21–27
Courtney J M, Irvine L, Travers M 1990 Hemodialysis membranes. In: Williams D (ed) Concise encyclopedia of medical and dental materials. Pergamon, Oxford, p 212–219
Courtney J M, Sundaram S, Forbes C D 1993a Extracorporeal situations: biocompatibility aspects of the application of biomaterials. In: Forbes C D, Cushieri A (eds) Management of bleeding disorders in surgical practice. Blackwell Scientific, Oxford, p 236–276
Courtney J M, Yu J, Sundaram S 1993b Immobilisation of macromolecules for obtaining biocompatible surfaces. In: Sleytr U B, Messner P, Pum D, Sàra M (eds) Immobilised macromolecules: application potentials. Springer-Verlag, London, p 175–194
Craddock P R, Hammerschmidt D E, White J G, Dalmasso A P, Jacob H S 1977a Complement (C5a)-induced granulocyte aggregation in-vitro. A possible mechanism of complement mediated leukostasis and leukopenia. Journal of Clinical Investigation 60: 260–264
Craddock P R, Fehr J, Brigham K L, Kronenberg R S, Jacobs H S 1977b Complement and leukocyte-pulmonary dysfunction in hemodialysis. New England Journal of Medicine 296: 796–774
Cumming R D 1980 Important factors affecting initial blood–material interactions. Transactions of the American Society for Artificial Internal Organs 26: 304–308
Dalen J E, Hirsh J 1986 American College of Chest Physicians and The National Heart, Lung, Blood Institute National Conference on Antithrombotic Therapy. Archives of Internal Medicine 146: 462–472
Danishefsky I, Tzeng F 1974 Preparation of heparin-linked agarose and its interaction with plasma. Thrombosis Research 4: 237–246
Davies G C, Sobel M, Salzman E W 1979 Plasma thromboxane B_2 (TXB_2) and fibrinopeptide A (FpA) in patients with thrombosis and during contact of blood with artificial surfaces. Proceedings of the VII International Congress in Thrombosis and Haemostasis, London. Thrombosis and Haemostasis 42: 72
Davies G C, Sobel M, Salzman E W 1980 Elevated plasma fibrinopeptide A and thromboxane B_2 levels during cardiopulmonary bypass. Circulation 61: 808–814
de Leval M R, Hill J D, Mielke C H 1981 Haematological aspects of extracorporeal circulation. In: Ionescu M I (ed) Techniques in extracorporeal circulation, 2nd Edn. Butterworths, London, p 369–389
Dellsperger K C, Chandran K B 1991 Prosthetic heart valves. In: Sharma C P, Szycher M J (eds) Blood compatible materials and devices. Technomic, Lancaster PA, p 153–165
Desai N P, Hubbell J A 1991 Biological responses to polyethylene oxide modified polyethylene terephthalate surfaces. Journal of Biomedical Materials Research 25: 829–843
DeVries W G, Andersen J L, Jouce L D et al 1984 Clinical use of the total artificial heart. New England Journal of Medicine 310: 273–278
Dewitz T S, Hung T C, Martin R R, McIntire L V 1977 Mechanical trauma in leukocytes. Journal of Laboratory and Clinical Medicine 90: 728–736
Dewitz T S, Martin R R, Solis R T, Hellums H D, McIntire L V 1978 Microaggregate formation in whole blood exposed to shear stress. Microvascular Research 16: 263–271
Di Minno G, Thiagarajan P, Perussia B et al 1983 Exposure of platelet fibrinogen-binding sites by collagen, arachidonic acid, and ADP: inhibition by a monoclonal antibody to the glycoprotein IIb-IIIa complex. Blood 61: 140–148
Didisheim P, Olsen D B, Farrer D J et al 1989 Infections and thromboembolism with implantable cardiovascular devices. Transactions of the American Society for Artificial Internal Organs 35: 54–70
Drinker P A 1972 Progress in membrane oxygenator design. Anaesthesiology 37: 242–260
Dudczak R, Niessner H, Thaler E et al 1979 β-Thromboglobulin (βTG), platelet factor 4 and fibrinopeptide A (FPA) in patients with porcine (PO) and prosthetic heart valves. Proceedings of the VII International Congress in Thrombosis and Haemostasis, London. Thrombosis and Haemostasis 42: 72
Durrani A A, Chapman D 1987 Modification of polymer surfaces for biomedical applications. In: Feast W J, Munro H S (eds) Polymer surfaces and interfaces. Wiley, New York, p 189–200
Durrani A A, Hayward J A, Chapman D 1986 Biomembranes as models for polymer surfaces. II. The synthesis of reactive species for covalent coupling of phosphorylcholine to polymer surfaces. Biomaterials 7: 121–125
Dyck M F 1972 Inorganic heparin complexes for the preparation of nonthrombogenic surfaces. Journal of Biomedical Materials Research 6: 115–141
Ebert C D, Kim S W 1982 Immobilized heparin: spacer arm effects on biological interactions. Thrombosis Research 26: 43–57
Ebert C D, Lees E S, Kim S W 1982 The antiplatelet activity of immobilized prostacyclin. Journal of Biomedical Materials Research 16: 629–638
Edie R N, Haubert S M, Malm J R 1981 The use of haemodilution and non-haemic prime for cardio-pulmonary bypass. In: Ionescu M I (ed) Techniques in extracorporeal circulation, 2nd edn. Butterworths, London, p 179–198
Edmunds L H Jr, Stephensen L W 1982 Cardiopulmonary bypass for open heart surgery. In: Glen W W L, Baue A E, Linskog B S (eds) Thoracic and cardiovascular surgery. Appleton-Century-Crofts, New York, p 1091–1106
Eikhoff J H, Buchardt Hansen H J, Bromme A et al 1983 A randomised clinical trial of PTFE versus human umbilical vein for femoro-popliteal bypass surgery. Preliminary results. British Journal of Surgery 70: 85–88
Eloy R, Belleville J, Paul J et al 1987 Thromboresistance of bulk heparinized catheters in humans. Thrombosis Research 45: 223–233

Engbers G H, Feijen J 1991 Current techniques to improve the blood compatibility of biomaterial surfaces. International Journal of Artificial Organs 14: 199–215
Evans G, Mustard J F 1968 Platelet-surfaces reaction and thrombosis. Surgery 64: 273–280
Falb R D 1975 Surface-bonded heparin. In: Kronenthal R L, Oser Z, Martin E (eds) Polymers in medicine and surgery. Plenum Press, New York, p 77–86
Falb R D, Grode G A, Leininger R I 1966 Elastomers in the human body. Rubber Chemistry and Technology 39: 1288–1292
Falb R D, Takahashi M T, Grode G A, Leininger R I 1967 Studies on the stability and protein adsorption characteristics of heparinized polymer surfaces by radioisotope labelling techniques. Journal of Biomedical Materials Research 1: 239–251
Falkenhagen D, Esther G, Courtney J M, Klinkmann H 1981 Optimization of albumin coating for resins. Artificial Organs 5 (suppl): 195–199
Falkenhagen D, Böttcher M, Ramlow W et al 1984 The investigation of biomaterials by sequential plasmaperfusion. In: Paul J P, Gaylor J D S, Courtney J M, Gilchrist T (eds) Biomaterials in artificial organs. Macmillan, London, p 228–237
Falkenhagen D, Bosch T, Brown G S et al 1987 A clinical study on different cellulosic membranes. Nephrology, Dialysis, Transplantation 2: 537–545
Farah E, Enriquez-Sarano M, Vahanian A et al 1984 Thromboembolic and haemorrhagic risk in mechanical and biological aortic prostheses. European Heart Journal 5 (suppl): 43–47
Farrell P C 1984 Biocompatibility aspects of extracorporeal circulation. In: Paul J P, Gaylor J D S, Courtney J M, Gilchrist T (eds) Biomaterials in artificial organs. Macmillan, London, p 342–350
Feijen J 1977 Thrombogenesis caused by blood-foreign surface interaction. In: Kenedi R M, Courtney J M, Gaylor J D S, Gilchrist T (eds) Artificial organs. Macmillan, London, p 235–247
Feuerstein I A, Brophy J M, Brash J L 1975 Platelet transport and adhesion to reconstituted collagen and artificial surfaces. Transactions of the American Society for Artificial Internal Organs 21: 427–434
Forbes C D 1981 Thrombosis and artificial surfaces. Clinics in Haematology 10: 653–668
Forbes C D, Prentice C R M 1978 Thrombus formation and artificial surfaces. British Medical Bulletin 34: 201–207
Forbes C D, Courtney J M, Saniabadi A R, Morrice L M A 1989 Thrombus formation in artificial organs. In: Paul J P, Barbenel J C, Courtney J M, Kenedi R M (eds) Progress in bioengineering. Adam Hilger, Bristol, p 13–20
Fougnot C, Labarre D, Jozefonwicz J, Jozefowicz M 1984 Modifications to polymer surfaces to improve blood compatibility. In: Hastings G W, Ducheyne P (eds) Macromolecular biomaterials. CRC Press, Boca Raton, p 215–238
Fourt L, Schwartz A M, Quasius A, Bowman R L 1966 Heparin-bearing surfaces and liquid surfaces in relation to blood coagulation. Transactions of the American Society for Artificial Internal Organs 12: 155–162
Frautschi J R, Munro M S, Lloyd D R, Eberhart R C 1983 Alkyl derivatized cellulose acetate membranes with enhanced albumin affinity. Transactions of the American Society for Artificial Internal Organs 29: 242–244
Gadboys H L, Lirwak R S, Niemetz J, Wisch N 1967 Role of anticoagulants in preventing embolisation from prosthetic heart valves. Journal of the American Medical Association 202: 282–286
Gendrau R M, Winters S, Leininger R I, Fink D, Hassler C R, Jakobsen R J 1981 Fourier transform infrared spectroscopy of protein adsorption from whole blood: ex vivo dog studies. Applied Spectroscopy 35: 353–357
Gibbon J H (Jr) 1954 The application of a mechanical heart and lung apparatus to cardiac surgery. Minnesota Medicine 37: 171–176
Gilchrist T, Courtney J M 1980 The design of biocompatible polymers. In: Ariëns E J (ed) Drug design. Academic Press, New York, vol X: 251–275
Golander C G, Kiss E 1988 Protein adsorption on functionalized and ESCA-characterized polymer films studied by ellipsometry. Journal of Colloid and Interface Science 121: 240–253
Goldman M D 1983 Aspirin and dipyridamole reduce platelet deposition on prosthetic femoro-popliteal grafts in man. Annals of Surgery 198: 713–716
Goldman M, Hall C E, Gunson B K, Hawker R J, McCollum C N 1984 Indium labelled platelet deposition on prosthetic grafts. In: Paul J P, Gaylor J D S, Courtney J M, Gilchrist T (eds) Biomaterials in artificial organs. Macmillan, London, p 277–287
Goodman S L, Grasel T, Cooper S L, Albrecht R M 1989 Platelet shape change and cytoskeletal reorganization on polyurethaneureas. Journal of Biomedical Materials Research 23: 105–123
Goosen M F A, Sefton M V, Hatton M W C 1980 Inactivation of thrombin by antithrombin III on a heparinized biomaterial. Thrombosis Research 20: 543–554
Gott V R, Furuse A 1971 Antithrombogenic surfaces, classification and in vivo evaluation. Federation Proceedings 30: 1679–1685
Gott V L, Whitten J D, Dutton R C 1963 Heparin bonding on colloidal graphite surfaces. Science 142: 1297–1298
Grabowski E F, Didisheim P, Lewis J C, Franta J T, Stropp J Q 1977 Platelet adhesion to foreign surfaces under controlled conditions of whole blood flow: human vs rabbit, dog, calf, sheep, macaque, and baboon. Transactions of the American Society for Artificial Internal Organs 23: 141–149
Grainger D W, Kim S W 1988 Poly (dimethylsiloxane)-poly (ethylene oxide)-heparin block copolymers. 1. Synthesis and characterization. Journal of Biomedical Materials Research 22: 231–249
Green K, Liska J, Egberg N et al 1987 Hemostatic disturbances associated with implantation of an artificial heart. Thrombosis Research 48: 349–362
Griffin J H, Cochrane C G 1979 Recent advances in the understanding of contact activation reactions. Seminars in Thrombosis and Hemostasis 5: 254–273
Griffith B P, Hardesty R L, Kormos R L et al 1987 Temporary use of the Jarvik-7 total artificial heart before transplantation. New England Journal of Medicine 316: 130–134
Grinnell F, Feld M K 1981 Adsorption characteristics of plasma fibronectin in relationship to biological activity. Journal of Biomedical Materials Research 15: 363–381
Grinnell F, Phan V 1983 Deposition of fibronectin on material surfaces exposed to plasma. Journal of Cell Physiology 116: 289–296
Grode G A, Anderson S J, Grotta H M, Falb R D 1969 Nonthrombogenic surfaces via a simple coating process. Transactions of the American Society for Artificial Internal Organs 15: 1–6
Grode G A, Falb R D, Crowley J P 1972 Biocompatible materials for use in the vascular system. Journal of Biomedical Materials Research Symposium 3: 77–84
Grode G A, Pitman J, Crowley J P, Leininger R I, Falb R D 1974 Surface-immobilized prostaglandin as a platelet protective agent. Transactions of the American Society for Artificial Internal Organs 20: 38–41
Hagler H K, Powell W M, Eberle J W, Sugg W L, Platt M R, Watson J T 1975 Five-day partial bypass using a membrane oxygenator without systemic heparinization. Transactions of the American Society for Artificial Internal Organs 21: 178–185
Hall B, Bird R le R, Kojima M, Chapman D 1989 Biomembranes as models for polymer surfaces. V. Thromboelastographic studies of polymeric lipids and polyesters. Biomaterials 10: 219–224
Hammerschmidt D E, Bowers T K, Lammi-Keefe C J, Jacob H S, Craddock P R 1980 Granulocyte aggregometry: a sensitive technique for the detection of C5a and complement activation. Blood 55: 898–902
Hanson S R, Harker L A, Ratner B D, Hoffman A S 1980 In vivo evaluation of artificial surfaces with a nonhuman primate model of arterial thrombosis. Journal of Laboratory and Clinical Medicine 95: 289–304
Harrison M J, Emmons P R, Mitchell J R 1966 The effect of white cells on platelet aggregation. Thrombosis Diathesis Haemorrhagica 16: 105–121
Hasenfratz H, Knaup G 1981 Improvement of the blood compatibility of cellulosic membranes through the immobilization of heparin and measurement of biological heparin activity. Artificial Organs 5 (suppl): 507–511
Hayward J A, Durrani A A, Shelton C J, Lee D C, Chapman D 1986a Biomembranes as models for polymer surfaces. III. Characterization

of a phosphorylcholine surface covalently bound to glass. Biomaterials 7: 126–131
Hayward J A, Durrani A A, Lu Y C, Clayton C R, Chapman D 1986b Biomembranes as models for polymer surfaces. IV. ESCA analyses of a phosphorylcholine surface covalently bound to hydroxylated substrates. Biomaterials 7: 252–258
Hennink W E, Dost L, Feijen J, Kim S W 1983 Interaction of albumin-heparin conjugate preadsorbed surfaces with blood. Transactions of the American Society for Artificial Internal Organs 29: 200–205
Henson P M 1969 The adhesion of leukocytes and platelets induced by fixed IgG antibody or complement. Immunology 16: 107–121
Hersh L S, Weetall H H, Brown I W Jr 1971 Heparinized polyester fibres. Journal of Biomedical Materials Research Symposium 1: 99–104
Hershey C O, Tomford J W, McLaren C E et al 1984 The natural history of intravenous catheter-associated phlebitis. Archives of Internal Medicine 144: 1373–1375
Herzlinger G A 1983 Activation of complement by polymers in contact with blood. In: Szycher M (ed) Biocompatible polymers, metals, and composites. Technomic, Lancaster PA, p 89–101
Herzlinger G A, Cumming R D 1980 Role of complement activation in cell adhesion to polymer blood contact surfaces. Transactions of the American Society for Artificial Internal Organs 26: 165–170
Heyman P W, Cho C S, McRea J C, Olsen D B, Kim S W 1985 Heparinized polyurethanes: in vitro and in vivo studies. Journal of Biomedical Materials Research 19: 419–436
Hoar P F, Stone J G, Wicks A E, Edie R N, Scholes J V 1978 Thrombogenesis associated with Swan–Ganz catheters. Anesthesiology 48: 445–447
Hoffman A 1974 Principles governing biomolecule interactions at foreign interfaces. Journal of Biomedical Materials Research 8: 77–83
Hoffman A S 1975 Hydrogels — a broad class of biomaterials. In: Kronenthal R L, Oser Z, Martin E (eds) Polymers in medicine and surgery. Plenum Press, New York, p 33–44
Hoffman A S, Schmer G, Harris C, Kraft W G 1972 Covalent bonding of biomolecules to radiation-grafted hydrogels on inert polymer surfaces. Transactions of the American Society for Artificial Internal Organs 18: 10–17
Holland F F, Gidden H E, Mason R G, Klein E 1978 Thrombogenicity of heparin-bound DEAE cellulose hemodialysis membranes. American Society for Artificial Internal Organs Journal 1: 24–36
Holmsen H, Day H J, Stormorken J 1969 The blood platelet release reaction. Scandinavian Journal of Haematology 8 (suppl): 1–26
Hood R G, Pollock J G, Guidoin R 1984 The knitted structure and its interaction with tissue and blood. In: Paul J P, Gaylor J D S, Courtney J M, Gilchrist T (eds) Biomaterials in artificial organs. Macmillan, London, p 269–276
Horbett T A 1984 Mass action effects on the adsorption of fibrinogen from hemoglobin solutions and from plasma. Thrombosis and Haemostasis 51: 174–181
Horbett T A 1986 The kinetics of baboon fibrinogen adsorption to polymers: in vitro and in vivo studies. Journal of Biomedical Materials Research 20: 739–772
Horbett T A, Counts R B 1984 von Willebrand factor/factor III adsorption to surfaces from human plasma. Thrombosis Research 36: 599–608
Horbett T A, Weathersby P K, Hoffman A S 1977 The preferential adsorption of hemoglobulin to polyethylene. Journal of Bioengineering 1: 61–77
Hugli T, Chenoweth D E 1980 Biologically active peptides of complement: significance of C3a and C5a measurements. In: Nakamura R M, Dito W R, Tucker E S III (eds) Immunoassays: clinical laboratory techniques for the 1980s. Liss, New York, p 443–460
Idezuki Y, Watanabe H, Hagiwara M et al 1975 Mechanism of antithrombogenicity of a new heparinized hydrophilic polymer: chronic in vivo studies and clinical application. Transactions of the American Society for Artificial Internal Organs 21: 436–448
Ige S R, Hibbs C W, Trone R et al 1978 Intra-aortic balloon pumping: theory and practice. Experience with 325 patients. Artificial Organs 2: 249–256
Ihlenfeld J V, Cooper S L 1979 Transient in vivo protein adsorption onto polymeric biomaterials. Journal of Biomedical Materials Research 13: 577–591
Ihlenfeld J V, Mathis T R, Barber T A 1978 Transient in vivo thrombus deposition onto polymeric biomaterials: role of plasma fibronectin. Transactions of the American Society for Artificial Internal Organs 24: 727–734
Imai Y, Tajima K, Nosé Y 1971 Biolized materials for cardiovascular prosthesis. Transactions of the American Society for Artificial Internal Organs 17: 6–9
Irvine L, Courtney J M, Lowe G D O 1989 Polymer modification and contact activation. In: Polymers in medicine and surgery, Plastics and Rubber Institute, London, p 21/1–21/6
Ishihara K, Aragaki R, Ueda T, Watanabe A, Nakabayashi N 1990 Reduced thrombogenicity of polymers having phospholipid polar groups. Journal of Biomedical Materials Research 24: 1069–1077
Ishihara K, Ziats N P, Tierney B P, Nakabayashi N, Anderson J M 1991 Protein adsorption from human plasma is reduced on phospholipid polymers. Journal of Biomedical Materials Research 25: 1397–1407
Ishihara K, Takayama R, Nakabayashi N 1992 Improvement of blood compatibility on cellulose dialysis membrane. Biomaterials 13: 235–239
Ivanovich P, Chenoweth D E, Schmidt R et al 1983 Symptoms and activation of granulocytes and complement with two dialysis membranes. Kidney International 24: 758–763
Jamieson G A 1973 Role of glycoproteins in platelet function. In: Gerlach E, Moser K, Deutsch E, Williams W (eds) Erythrocytes, thrombocytes, leukocytes: recent advances in membrane and metabolic research. Thieme Willmans, Stuttgart, p 209–232
Jenkins C S P, Packham M A, Guccione M A, Mustard J F 1973 Modification of platelet adherence to protein-coated surfaces. Journal of Laboratory and Clinical Medicine 81: 280–290
Johnson R J 1989 The design of cellulosic based membranes that do not activate complement. Medical Progress Through Technology 15: 77–81
Johnson R J, Lelah M D, Sutliff T M, Boggs D R 1990 A modification of cellulose that facilitates the control of complement activation. Blood Purification 8: 318–328
Jones R H, Broadfield R H, Parsons V 1980 Arterial hypoxemia during hemodialysis for acute renal failure in mechanically ventilated patients: Observations and mechanisms. Clinical Nephrology 14: 18–22
Jones H M, Mathews N, Vaughan R S, Stark J M 1982 Cardiopulmonary bypass and complement activation. Involvement of classical and alternative pathways. Anaesthesia 37: 629–633
Kaganov A L, Stamberg J, Synek P 1976 Hydrophilized polyethylene catheters. Journal of Biomedical Materials Research 10: 1–7
Kambic H E, Nosé Y 1991 Biomaterials for blood pumps. In: Sharma C P, Szycher M (eds) Blood compatible materials and devices. Technomic, Lancaster PA, p 141–151
Kambic H, Barenburg S, Harasaki H, Gibbons D, Kiraly R, Nosé Y 1978 Glutaraldehyde-protein complexes as blood compatible coatings. Transactions of the American Society for Artificial Internal Organs 24: 426–437
Kambic H E, Murabayashi S, Nosé Y 1983 Biolized surfaces as chronic blood compatible interfaces. In: Szycher M (ed) Biocompatible polymers, metals, and composites. Technomic, Lancaster PA, p 179–198
Kaplow L S, Goffinet J A 1968 Profound neutropenia during the early phase of hemodialysis. Journal of the American Medical Association 203: 1135–1137
Kazatchkine M D, Carreno M P 1987 Activation of the complement system at the interface between blood and artificial surfaces. Biomaterials 9: 30–35
Kelton J C 1986 Heparin-induced thrombocytopenia. Haemostasis 16: 173–186
Kim S W, Lee R G, Oster H et al 1974 Platelet adhesion to polymer surfaces. Transactions of the American Society for Artificial Internal Organs 20: 449–455
Kim S W, Ebert C D, Lin J Y, McRea J C 1983 Nonthrombogenic polymers: pharmaceutical approaches. American Society for Artificial Internal Organs Journal 6: 76–87

Kiraly R J, Arconti R, Hillegass D, Harasaki H, Nosé Y 1977 High flex rubber for blood pump diaphragms. Transactions of the American Society for Artificial Internal Organs 23: 127–132

Klimach O, Charlesworth D 1983 Femoro-tibial bypass for limb salvage using human umbilical vein. British Journal of Surgery 70: 1–3

Klinkmann H 1984 The role of biomaterials in the application of artificial organs. In Paul J P, Gaylor J D S, Courtney J M, Gilchrist T (eds) Biomaterials in artificial organs. Macmillan, London, p 1–8

Klinkmann H, Falkenhagen D, Courtney J M 1987 Clinical relevance of biocompatibility — the material cannot be divorced from the device. In: Gurland H J (ed) Uremia therapy. Springer-Verlag, Berlin, p 125–138

Kojima M, Ishihara K, Watanabe A, Nakabayashi N 1991 Interaction between phospholipids and biocompatible polymers containing a phosphorylcholine moiety. Biomaterials 12: 121–124

Kornecki E, Niewiarowski S, Morinelli T A, Kloczewiak M 1981 Effects of chymotrypsin and adenosine diphosphate on the exposure of fibrinogen receptors on normal human and Glanzmann's thrombasthenic platelets. Journal of Biological Chemistry 256: 5696–5701

Kurz H, Lerner R G, Weseley S, Nelson J C 1985 Changes in fibrinolytic activity during the course of a single hemodialysis session. Clinical Nephrology 24: 1–4

Kusserow B, Larrow R, Nichols J 1970 Observations concerning prosthesis-induced thromboembolic phenomena made with an in vivo embolus test system. Transactions of the American Society for Artificial Internal Organs 16: 58–62

Kusserow B, Larrow R, Nichols J 1971 Perfusion- and surface-induced injury in leucocytes. Federation Proceedings 30: 1516–1520

Kusserow B K, Larrow R W, Nichols J E 1973 The surface bonded, covalently crosslinked urokinase surface. In vitro and chronic in vivo studies. Transactions of the American Society for Artificial Internal Organs 19: 8–12

Kuwahara T, Markert M, Wauters J P 1989 Proteins adsorbed on haemodialysis membranes modulate neutrophil activation. Artificial Organs 13: 427–431

Labarre D, Baffa M C, Josefowicz M 1974 Preparation and properties of heparin-poly(methyl methacrylate) copolymers. Journal of Polymer Science: Polymer Symposia 47: 131–137

Labarre D, Josefowicz M, Boffa M C 1977 Properties of heparin-poly(methyl methacrylate) copolymers II. Journal of Biomedical Materials Research 11: 283–295

Lagergren H R, Eriksson J C 1971 Plastics with a monolayer of cross-linked heparin: preparation and evaluation. Transactions of the American Society for Artificial Internal Organs 17: 10–12

Lambrecht L K, Lelah M D, Jordan C A, Pariso M E, Albrecht R M, Cooper S L 1983 Evaluation of thrombus onto polymeric biomaterials in a new subhuman primate ex vivo series shunt model. Transactions of the American Society for Artificial Internal Organs 29: 194–199

Larm O, Larsson R, Olsson P 1989 Surface-immobilized heparin. In: Lane D A, Lindahl U (eds) Heparin. Chemical and biological properties, clinical applications. Edward Arnold, London, p 597–608

Larsson R, Olsson P, Lindahl U 1980 Inhibition of thrombin on surfaces coated with immobilized heparin and heparin-like polysaccharides: a crucial non-thrombogenic principle. Thrombosis Research 19: 43–54

Lederman D M, Cumming R D, Petschek H E, Levine P H, Krinsky N I 1978 The effect of temperature on the interaction of platelets and leukocytes with materials exposed to flowing blood. Transactions of the American Society for Artificial Internal Organs 24: 557–560

Lee J M, Boughner D R 1991 Bioprosthetic heart valves: tissue mechanics and implications for design. In: Sharma C P, Szycher M (eds) Blood compatible materials and devices. Technomic, Lancaster PA, p 167–188

Lee J H, Kopecek J, Andrade J D 1989 Protein-resistant coatings prepared by PEO-containing block copolymer surfactants. Journal of Biomedical Materials Research 23: 351–368

Lee J H, Kopeckova P, Kopecek J, Andrade J D 1990 Surface properties of copolymers of alkyl methacrylates with methoxy(polyethylene oxide) methacrylates and their application as protein-resistant coatings. Biomaterials 11: 455–464

Lee R G, Kim S W 1974 The role of carbohydrate in platelet adhesion to foreign surfaces. Journal of Biomedical Materials Research 8: 393–398

Lee R G, Adamson C, Kim S W 1974 Competitive adsorption of plasma proteins onto polymer surfaces. Thrombosis Research 4: 485–490

Lee W H Jr, Hairston 1971 Structural effects on blood proteins at the gas-blood interface. Federation 'Proceedings 30: 1615–1620

Leininger R I, Crowley J P, Falb R D, Grode G A 1972 Three years' experience in vivo and in vitro with surfaces and devices treated by the heparin complex method. Transactions of the American Society for Artificial Internal Organs 18: 312–315

Lemke H-D, Finke E 1992 Generation of bradykinin in human plasma using AN69 and PAN 17DX membranes in the presence of an ACE-inhibitor in vitro. Abstracts of the Twenty Ninth Congress of the European Dialysis and Transplant Association – European Renal Association, p 163

Leonard C D, Weil E, Scribner B H 1969 Subdural haematomas in patients undergoing haemodialysis Lancet 11: 239–240

Libsack C V, Kollmeyer K R 1979 Role of catheter surface morphology on intravascular thrombosis of plastic catheters. Journal of Biomedical Materials Research 13: 459–466

Limber G K, Mason R G 1975 Studies of proteins elutable from Cuprophane exposed to human plasma. Thrombosis Research 6: 421–430

Limber G K, Glenn C H, Mason R G 1974 Studies of proteins elutable for certain artificial surfaces exposed to human plasma. Thrombosis Research 5: 735–746

Lindon J N, Rodvien R, Brier D, Greenberg R, Merrill E, Salzman E W 1978 In vitro assessment of interaction of blood with model surfaces. Journal of Laboratory and Clinical Medicine 92: 904–915

Lindon J N, Collins R E C, Coe N P, Jagoda A, Brier-Russell D, Merrill E W, Salzman E W 1980 In vivo assessment in sheep of thromboresistant materials by determination of platelet survival. Circulation Research 46: 84–90

Lindsay R M, Prentice C R M, Ferguson D, Burton J A, McNicol G P 1972 Reduction of thrombus formation on dialyser membranes by aspirin and RA233. Lancet 2: 1287–1290

Lindsay R M, Prentice C R M, Ferguson D, Muir W M, McNicol G P 1973 A method for the measurement of platelet adhesiveness by use of dialysis membranes in a test cell. British Journal of Haematology 24: 377–389

Lindsay R M, Rourke J T B, Reid B D et al 1977 The role of heparin on platelet retention by acrylonitrile copolymer dialysis membranes. Journal of Laboratory and Clinical Medicine 89: 724–734

Lindsay R M, Mason R G, Kim S W, Andrade J D, Hakim R M 1980 Blood surface interactions. Transactions of the American Society for Artificial Internal Organs 26: 603–610

Lins L E, Olsson P, Hjelte M B, Larsson R, Larm O 1984 Haemodialysis in dogs with a heparin coated hollow fiber dialyser. Proceedings of the European Dialysis and Transplant Association 21: 270–275

Lister J 1863 On the coagulation of blood. Proceedings of the Royal Society (London) 12: 580–611

Lucchi L, Bonucchi D, Acerbi M A et al 1989 Improved biocompatibility by modified cellulosic membranes: the case of Hemophan. Artificial Organs 13: 417–421

Lyman D J, Klein K G, Bash J L, Fritzinger B K 1970 The interaction of platelets with polymer surfaces. Thrombosis et Diathesis Haemorrhagica 23: 120–128

Lyman D J, Metcalf L C, Albo D Jr, Richards K F, Lamb J 1974 The effect of chemical structure and surface properties of synthetic polymers on the coagulation of blood. III. In vivo adsorption of proteins on polymer surfaces. Transactions of the American Society for Artificial Internal Organs 20: 474–478

Lyman D J, Knutson K, McNeill B, Shibatani K 1975 The effects of chemical structure and surface properties of synthetic polymers on the coagulation of blood. IV. The relation between polymer morphology and protein adsorption. Transactions of the American Society for Artificial Internal Organs 21: 49–53

McGillen J J, Phair J P 1979 Adherence, augmented adherence, and aggregation of polymorphonuclear leucocytes. Journal of Infectious Diseases 139: 69–73

McLaughlin K M, Travers M, Simpson K et al 1989 The assessment of fibrinogen and fibrinolysis during haemodialysis. International Journal of Artificial Organs 12: 587
McRea J C, Kim S W 1978 Characterization of controlled release of prostaglandin from polymer matrices for thrombus prevention. Transactions of the American Society for Artificial Internal Organs 24: 746–751
McRea J C, Ebert C D, Kim S W 1981 Prostaglandin releasing polymers — stability and efficacy. Transactions of the American Society for Artificial Internal Organs 27: 511–516
Madhok R, Forbes C D, Dawson H, Brannan J J, Taylor K M 1985 Effects of prostacyclin on platelet aggregation during cardio-pulmonary bypass. In: Hagh S, Sebening F (eds) 30 years of extracorporeal circulation. Deutches Hertzentrum, München, p 363–372
Maeda K, Usuda M, Kawaguchi S et al 1980 Effects of ticlopidine on thrombotic obstruction of A-V shunts and on dialysance of artificial kidneys. Artificial Organs 4: 30–33
Mahiout A, Meinhold H, Kessel M, Schulze H, Baurmeister U 1987 Dialyzer membranes: effect of surface area and chemical modification of cellulose on complement and platelet activation. Artificial Organs 11: 149–154
Maini R 1989 The development of a presealed Dacron vascular prosthesis. In: Paul J P, Barbenel J C, Courtney J M, Kenedi R M (eds) Progress in bioengineering. Adam Hilger, Bristol, p 37–40
Mantovani E, Marconi W, Cebo B, Togna A R, Togna G, Caprino L 1984 A native whole blood test for the evaluation of blood–surface interactions: determination of thromboxane production. International Journal of Artificial Organs 7: 147–150
Marconi W, Bartoli F, Mantovani E et al 1979 Development of new antithrombogenic surfaces by employing platelet antiaggregating agents: preparation and characterization. Transactions of the American Society for Artificial Internal Organs 25: 280–285
Martin F E, Shuey H F, Saltonstall C W Jr 1970 Improved membranes for hemodialysis. Journal of Macromolecular Science-Chemistry A4: 635–654
Mason R G 1972 The interaction of blood hemostatic elements with artificial surfaces. Progress in Hemostasis and Thrombosis 1: 141–164
Mason R G, Read M S, Brinkhous K M 1971 Effect of fibrinogen concentration on platelet adhesion to glass. Proceedings of the Society for Experimental Biology and Medicine 137: 680–682
Mason R G, Mohammad S F, Chuang H Y K, Richardson P D 1976 The adhesion of platelets to subendothelium, collagen and artificial surfaces. Seminars in Thrombosis and Hemostasis 3: 98–116
Mason R G, Sharp D, Chuang H Y K, Mohammad S F 1977 The endothelium: roles in thrombosis and hemostasis. Archives of Pathology and Laboratory Medicine 101: 61–64
Mason R G, Mohammad S F, Saba H J, Chuang H Y K, Lee E L, Balis J U 1979 Functions of endothelium. Pathobiology Annual 9: 1–48
Merrill E W, Salzman E W, Wong P S L, Ashford T P, Brown A H, Austen W G 1970 Polyvinyl alcohol-heparin hydrogel 'G'. Journal of Applied Physiology 29: 723–730
Merrill E W, Salzman E W, Wan S et al 1982 Platelet-compatible hydrophilic segmented polyurethanes from polyethylene glycols and cyclohexane diisocyanate. Transactions of the American Society for Artificial Internal Organs 28: 482–487
Miura Y, Aoyagi S, Kusada Y, Miyamoto K 1980 The characteristics of anticoagulation by covalently immobilized heparin. Journal of Biomedical Materials Research 14: 619–630
Miyama H, Harumiya N, Mori Y, Tanzawa H 1977 A new antithrombogenic heparinized polymer. Journal of Biomedical Materials Research 11: 251–265
Mohammad S F, Olsen D B 1986 Reduced platelet adhesion and activation of coagulation factors on polyurethane treated with albumin-IgG complex. Transactions of the American Society for Artificial Internal Organs 32: 323–326
Moll S, De Moerloose P, Rieber G, Schifferli G, Leski M 1990 Comparison of two hemodialysis membranes, polyacrylonitrile and cellulose acetate. International Journal of Artificial Organs 13: 273–279
Mori Y, Nagaoka S, Takiuchi H et al 1982 A new antithrombogenic material with long polyethyleneoxide chains. Transactions of the American Society for Artificial Internal Organs 28: 459–463
Mottaghy K B, Oedekoven B, Schaich-Lester P, Pöppel K, Küpper W 1989 Application of surfaces with end point attached heparin to extracorporeal circulation with membrane lungs. Transactions of the American Society for Artificial Internal Organs 35: 146–152
Munro M S, Eberhart R C, Maki N J, Brink B E, Fry W J 1983 Thromboresistant alkyl derivatized polyurethanes. American Society for Artificial Internal Organs Journal 6: 65–75
Murabayashi S, Nosé Y 1986 Biocompatibility: bioengineering aspects. Artificial Organs 10: 114–121
Mustard J F, Packham M A 1977 Normal and abnormal haemostasis. British Medical Bulletin 33: 187–192
Nachnani G H, Lessin L S, Motomiya T, Jensan W N 1972 Scanning electron microscopy of thrombogenesis on vascular catheter surfaces. New England Journal of Medicine 286: 139–140
Needleman S W, Hook J C 1982 Platelets and leukocytes. In: Colman R W, Hirsh J, Marder V J, Salzman E W (eds) Hemostasis and thrombosis: Basic principles and clinical practice. Lippincott, Philadelphia, p 716–725
Neumann A W, Moscarello M A, Zingg W, Hum O S, Chang S K 1979 Platelet adhesion from human blood to bare and protein coated polymer surfaces. Journal of Polymer Science Polymer Symposia 66: 391–398
Niemetz J 1972 Coagulant activity of leukocytes. Tissue factor activity. Journal of Clinical Investigation 51: 307–313
Nilsson L, Storm K E, Thelin S et al 1990 Heparin-coated equipment reduces complement activation during cardiopulmonary bypass in the pig. Artificial Organs 14: 46–48
Nojiri C, Okano T, Jacobs H A et al 1990 Blood compatibility of PEO grafted polyurethane and HEMA/styrene block copolymer surfaces. Journal of Biomedical Materials Research 24: 1151–1171
Nolewajka A J, Goddard M D, Brown T C 1980 Temporary transvenous pacing and femoral vein thrombosis. Circulation 62: 646–650
Norman J C 1977 Intracorporeal partial artificial hearts: initial results in ten patients. Artificial Organs 1: 41–52
Nosé Y 1988 Long term compatibility of artificial kidneys. Artificial Organs 12: 1
Nosé Y, Tajima K, Imai Y et al 1971 Artificial heart constructed with biological material. Transactions of the American Society for Artificial Internal Organs 17: 482–487
Nusbacher J, Rosenfeld S J, MacPherson J L, Thiem P A, Leddy J P 1978 Nylon fiber leukapheresis: associated complement component changes and granulocytopenia. Blood 51: 359–365
Ohshiro T 1983 Antithrombogenic characteristics of immobilized urokinase on synthetic polymers. In: Szycher M (ed) Biocompatible polymers, metals, and composites. Technomic, Lancaster PA, p 275–299
Ohshiro T, Kosaki G 1980 Urokinase immobilized on medical polymeric materials: fundamental and clinical studies. Artificial Organs 4: 58–64
Okada M, Shiozawa T, Iizuka M 1979 Experimental and clinical studies on the effect of intra-aortic balloon pumping for cardiogenic shock following acute myocardial infarction. Artificial Organs 3: 271–276
Owen D R, Chen C M, Oschner J A, Zone R M 1985 Interactions of plasma proteins with selective artificial surfaces. Transactions of the American Society for Artificial Internal Organs 31: 240–243
Packham M A, Evans G, Glynn M F, Mustard J F 1969 The effect of plasma proteins on the interaction of platelets with glass surfaces. Journal of Laboratory and Clinical Medicine 73: 686–697
Paik Sung C S, Bush J, McKie D B, Merrill E W 1976 Copolymers containing aminohexyl residues in side chains. Journal of Applied Polymer Science 20: 2603–2605
Palatianos G M, Dewanjee M K, Kapadvanjwala M, Novak S, Sfakianakis G N, Kaiser G A 1990 Cardiopulmonary bypass with a surface heparinized extracorporeal perfusion system. Transactions of the American Society for Artificial Internal Organs 36: M476–M479
Pandian N G, Kosowsky B D, Gurewich V 1980 Transfemoral temporary pacing and deep vein thrombosis. American Heart Journal 100: 847–851
Paramo J A, Rifon J, Llorend R, Casures J, Paloma A J, Rocha E 1991

Intra and postoperative fibrinolysis in patients undergoing cardiopulmonary bypass surgery. Haemostasis 21: 58–64
Park K D, Okano T, Nojiri C, Kim S W 1988 Heparin immobilization onto segmented polyurethaneurea surfaces — effect of hydrophilic spacers. Journal of Biomedical Materials Research 22: 977–992
Patrono C, Ciabattoni G, Pinca E 1980 Low dose aspirin and inhibition of thromboxane B_2 production in healthy subjects. Thrombosis Research 17: 317–327
Payne M S, Horbett T A 1987 Complement activation by hydroxyethylmethacrylate-ethylmethacrylate copolymers. Journal of Biomedical Materials Research 21: 843–859
Pearson D T 1981 Cardiotomy reservoirs and blood filters. In: Ionescu M I (ed) Techniques in Extracorporeal Circulation, 2nd edn. Butterworths, London, p 155–178
Pertosa G, Pastore A, Schena F P 1989 Influence of different dialyzer membranes on plasma fibronectin levels in hemodialyzed patients. International Journal of Artificial Organs 12: 36–40
Peters J L, Belsham P A, Taylor B A, Watt-Smith S 1984 Long-term venous access. British Journal of Hospital Medicine 32: 230–242
Petschek H, Adamis D, Kantrowitz A R 1968 Stagnation flow thrombus formation. Transactions of the American Society for Artificial Internal Organs 14: 256–263
Phillips D R, Jennings L K, Prasanna H R 1980 Ca^{2+}-mediated association of glycoprotein G (thrombin-sensitive protein, thrombospondin) with human blood. Journal of Biological Chemistry 255: 11629–11632
Plow E F, Marguerie G A 1980 Participation of ADP in the binding of fibrinogen to thrombin-stimulated platelets. Blood 56: 553–555
Preuschof L, Keller F, Seeman J, Offerman G 1988 Heparin-free hemodialysis with prophylactic change of dialyser and blood lines. International Journal of Artificial Organs 11: 255–258
Ratner B D 1981 Biomedical applications of hydrogels: review and critical appraisal. In: Williams D F (ed) Biocompatibility of clinical implant materials. CRC Press, Boca Raton, vol 2: 145–175
Ratnoff O D 1977 The surface-mediated initiation of blood coagulation and related phenomena. In: Ogston D, Bennett B (eds) Haemostasis. Biochemistry, physiology and pathology. Wiley, London, p 25–55
Ratnoff O D, Forbes C D (eds) 1984 Disorders of haemostasis. Grune and Stratton, London
Rea W J, Whitley D, Eberle J W 1972 Long-term membrane oxygenation without systemic heparinization. Transactions of the American Society for Artificial Internal Organs 18: 316–320
Richardson P D, Mohammad S F, Mason R G 1977 Flow chamber studies of platelet adhesion at controlled, spatially varied shear rates. Proceedings of the European Society for Artificial Organs 4: 175–188
Rieger H 1980 Dependency of platelet aggregation (PA) in vitro on different shear rates. Thrombosis and Haemostasis 44: 166
Ringoir S, Vanholder R 1986 An introduction to biocompatibility. Artificial Organs 10: 20–27
Ringoir S, Vanholder R 1990 New trends in dialysis. Contributions to Nephrology 82: 102–106
Roux M, Ponzio J, Brunet M, Garaix J 1984 Systemic thromboembolic accidents in the early post operative period in patients with prosthetic valves. European Heart Journal 5 (suppl): 27–31
Saba H J, Herion J C, Walker R I, Roberts H R 1973 The procoagulant activity of granulocytes. Proceedings of the Society for Experimental Biology and Medicine 142: 614–620
Salomon N W, Stinson E B, Griep R B, Shumway N E 1977 Mitral valve replacement: Long-term evaluation of prosthesis-related mortality and morbidity. Circulation 56 (suppl 11): 94–101
Salyer I O, Blardinelli A J, Ball G L III et al 1971 New blood-compatible polymers for artificial heart applications. Journal of Biomedical Materials Research Symposium 1: 105–127
Salzman E W, Merrill E W, Binder A, Wolf C R W, Ashford T P, Austen W G 1969 Protein platelet interactions on heparinized surfaces. Journal of Biomedical Materials Research 3: 69–81
Salzman E W, Lindon J, Brier D, Merrill E W 1977 Surface-induced platelet adhesion, aggregation and release. Annals of the New York Academy of Sciences 283: 114–127
Saniabadi A R, Lowe G D O, Forbes C D, Prentice C R M, Barbenel J C 1983 Platelet aggregation studies in whole human blood. Thrombosis Research 30: 625–632
Sauvage L R, Yates S G, Berger K, Nakagawa Y, Wood S J 1973 Prosthetic arteries and valves: Thrombogenicity healing and design. In: Schmer G, Strandjord J E (eds) Coagulation, current research and clinical applications. Academic Press, New York, p 189–198
Schmer G 1972 The biological activity of covalently immobilized heparin. Transactions of the American Society for Artificial Internal Organs 18: 321–323
Schmer G, Teng L N L, Cole J J et al 1976 Successful use of a totally heparin grafted hemodialysis system in sheep. Transactions of the American Society for Artificial Internal Organs 22: 654–662
Schmer G, Teng L N L, Vizzo J E, Graefe U, Milutinovich J, Cole J J, Scribner B H 1977 Clinical use of a totally heparin grafted hemodialysis system in uremic patients. Transactions of the American Society for Artificial Internal Organs 23: 177–183
Schmitt E, Holtz M, Klinkmann H, Esther G, Courtney J M 1983 Heparin binding and release properties of DEAE cellulose membranes. Biomaterials 4: 309–313
Schoen F J, DeLaria G A, Berostein B F 1972 Evaluation of intra-aortic balloon surfaces by scanning electron microscopy. Surgical Forum 23: 167–168
Seifert L M, Greer R T 1985 Evaluation of in vivo adsorption of blood elements onto hydrogel-coated silicone rubber by scanning electron microscopy and Fourier transform infrared spectroscopy. Journal of Biomedical Materials Research 19: 1043–1071
Senatore F, Bernard F, Meisner K 1986 Clinical study of urokinase-bound fibrocollagenous tubes. Journal of Biomedical Materials Research 20: 177–188
Shuman M A, Levine S P 1980 Relationship between secretion of platelet factor 4 and thrombin generation during in vitro blood clotting. Journal of Clinical Investigation 65: 307–313
Siegelman S S, Caplan L H, Annes G P 1968 Complication to catheter angiography. Study with oscillometry and pull-out angiograms. Radiology 91: 251–253
Silverton N P, Abdulali S A, Yakirevich V S, Tandon A P, Ionescu M I 1984 Embolism, thrombosis and anticoagulant haemorrhage in mitral valve disease. A prospective study of patients having valve replacement with the pericardial xenograft. European Heart Journal 5 (suppl): 19–25
Skubitz K H, Craddock P R 1981 Reversal of hemodialysis granulocytopenia and pulmonary leukostasis. A clinical manifestation of selective down-regulation of granulocyte responses to C5a-des-Arg. Journal of Clinical Investigation 676: 1383–1391
Snyder R W, Botzko K M 1982 Woven, knitted and externally supported Dacron vascular prostheses. In: Stanley J C (ed) Biologic and synthetic vascular prostheses. Grune and Stratton, New York, p 488–489
Solen K A, Mohammed S F, Reynolds L O et al 1989 Characterisation of blood microemboli associated with ex-vivo left ventricular assist devices in a bovine model. Transactions of the American Society for Artificial Internal Organs 35: 370–372
Solis R T, Noon G P, Beall A C, de Bakey M E 1974 Particulate microembolism during cardiac operation. Annals of Thoracic Surgery 17: 332–334
Stormorken 1971 Platelets, thrombosis and hemolysis. Federation Proceedings 30: 1551–1555
Sugitachi A, Tanaka M, Kawahara T, Takagi K 1980 Antithrombogenicity of UK-immobilized polymer surfaces. Transactions of the American Society for Artificial Internal Organs 26: 274–278
Szycher M 1983 Thrombosis, hemostasis, and thrombolysis at prosthetic interfaces. In: Szycher M (ed) Biocompatible polymers, metals, and composites. Technomic, Lancaster PA, p 1–33
Szycher M, Poirier V, Bernhard W F, Franzblau C, Haudenschild C C, Toselli P 1980 Integrally textured polymeric surfaces for permanently implantable cardiac assist devices. Transactions of the American Society for Artificial Internal Organs 26: 493–498
Taenaka Y, Matsuda T, Takano H et al 1989 Influences of ventricular assist device pumping on blood coagulation. Transactions of the American Society for Artificial Internal Organs 35: 396–398
Takahara A, Tashita J, Kajiyama T, Takayanagi M, MacKnight W J 1985 Microphase separated structure, surface composition and blood compatibility of segmented poly(urethaneureas) with various soft segment components. Polymer 26: 987–996

Takahara A, Okkema A Z, Wabers H, Cooper S L 1991 Effect of hydrophilic soft segment side chains on the surface properties and blood compatibility of segmented polyurethaneureas). Journal of Biomedical Materials Research 25: 1095–1118

Tanzawa H, Mori Y, Harumiya N et al 1973 Preparation and evaluation of a new athrombogenic heparinized hydrophilic polymer for use in cardiovascular system. Transactions of the American Society for Artificial Internal Organs 19: 188–194

Taylor K M 1986 Pulsatile perfusion. In: Taylor K M (ed) Cardiopulmonary bypass principles and management. Chapman and Hall, London, p 85

Tetta C, Segoloni G, Carnussi G et al 1987 In vitro complement-independent activation of human neutrophils by haemodialysis membranes. International Journal of Artificial Organs 12: 502–504

Thackrah C T 1819 An inquiry into the nature and properties of the blood, as existent in health and disease. Cox, London

Tong S-D, Rolfs M R, Hsu L-C 1990 Evaluation of Duraflo II heparin immobilized cardiopulmonary bypass circuits. Transactions of the American Society for Artificial Internal Organs 36: M654–M656

Toren M, Goffnet J A, Kaplow L S 1970 Pulmonary bed sequestration of neutrophils during hemodialysis. Blood 36: 337–340

Turitto V T, Leonard E F 1972 Platelet adhesion to a spinning surface. Transactions of the American Society for Artificial Internal Organs 18: 348–354

Turpie A G G, deBoer A C, Genton E 1982 Platelet consumption in cardiovascular disease. Seminars in Thrombosis and Hemostasis 8: 161–185

Uniyal S, Brash J L 1982 Patterns of adsorption of proteins onto foreign surfaces. Thrombosis and Haemostasis 47: 285–290

Uniyal S, Brash J L, Degterev I A 1982 Influence of red blood cells and their components on protein adsorption. American Chemical Society Advances in Chemistry 199: 277–292

Usdin V R, Fourt L 1969 Effect of proteins on elution of heparin from anticoagulant surfaces. Journal of Biomedical Materials Research 3: 107–113

Uziel L, Colombo A, Cacciabue E, Cugno M, Agostini A 1986 Extracorporeal circulation. Problems and answers. In: Dawids S, Bantjes A (eds) Blood compatible materials and their testing. Martinus Nijhoff, Hingham, p 29

Videm V, Nilsson L, Venge P, Svennevig J L 1991 Reduced granulocyte activation with a heparin-coated device in an in vitro model of cardiopulmonary bypass. Artificial Organs 15: 90–95

von Bonsdorff M, Stiekema J, Harjanne A, Alapiessa U 1990 A new low molecular weight heparinoid Org 10172 as anticoagulant in hemodialysis. International Journal of Artificial Organs 13: 103–108

von Segesser L K, Turina M 1989 Cardiopulmonary bypass without systemic heparinization. Performance of heparin-coated oxygenators in comparison with classic membrane and bubble oxygenators. Journal of Thoracic and Cardiovascular Surgery 98: 386–396

Vroman L 1983 Protein/surface interaction. In: Szycher M (ed) Biocompatible polymers, metals, and composites. Technomic, Lancaster PA, p 81–88

Vroman L, Adams A L 1969 Identification of rapid changes at plasma-solid interfaces. Journal of Biomedical Materials Research 3: 43–67

Vroman L, Adams A L, Klings M 1971 Interactions among human blood proteins at interfaces. Federation Proceedings 30: 1494–1502

Vroman L, Adams A L, Klings M, Fischer G C, Munoz P C, Solensky R P 1972 Reactions of formed elements of blood with plasma proteins at interfaces. Annals of the New York Academy of Sciences 283: 65–76

Vroman L, Adams A L, Fischer G C, Munoz P C 1980 Interaction of high molecular weight kininogen, factor XII and fibrinogen in plasma at interfaces. Blood 55: 156–159

Vulic I, Okano T, Kim S W, Feijen J 1988 Synthesis and characterization of polystyrene-poly (ethylene oxide)-heparin block copolymers. Journal of Polymer Science: Polymer Chemistry 26: 381–391

Walsh P N 1982 Platelet-coagulant protein interactions. In: Colman R W, Hirsh J, Marder V J, Salzman E W (eds) Hemostasis and thrombosis: Basic principles and clinical practice. Lippincott, Philadelphia, p 404–420

Walters M B, Stanger H A D, Rotem C E 1972 Complications with percutaneous central venous catheters. Journal of the American Medical Association 220: 1455–1457

Watanabe S, Shimuzu Y, Teramatsu T, Mirachi T, Hino T 1981 The in vitro and in vivo behaviour of urokinase immobilized onto collagen-synthetic polymer composite material. Journal of Biomedical Materials Research 15: 553–563

Waugh D F, Baughman D J 1969 Thrombin adsorption and possible relations to thrombus formation. Journal of Biomedical Materials Research 3: 145–164

Waugh D J, Anthony L J, Ng H 1975 The interactions of thrombin with borosilicate glass. Journal of Biomedical Materials Research 9: 511–536

Waugh D J, Lippe A J, Freund Y R 1978 Interactions of bovine thrombin and plasma albumin with low energy surfaces. Journal of Biomedical Materials Research 12: 599–625

Weily H S, Genton E 1970 Altered platelet function in patients with prosthetic mitral valves. Effects of sulphinpyrazone therapy. Circulation 42: 967–972

Weng D, Gaylor J D S, Courtney J M, Lowe G D O 1991 In vitro investigation of blood-biomaterials interactions. Artificial Organs 15: 307

Wesolowski S A 1978 Foundations of modern vascular grafts. In: Sawyer P N, Kaplitt M J (eds) Vascular grafts. Appleton-Century-Crofts, New York, p 27–53

Whicher S J, Brash J L 1978 Platelet–foreign surface interactions: release of granule constituents from adherent platelets. Journal of Biomedical Materials Research 12: 181–201

Whicher S J, Uniyal S, Brash J L 1980 Platelet–foreign surface interactions: the release reaction from singly adherent platelets and adherent platelet aggregates. Transactions of the American Society for Artificial Internal Organs 26: 268–273

Williams D F (ed) 1987 Definitions in biomaterials. Elsevier, Amsterdam

Wright D G, Kauffman J C, Terpstra G K, Graw R G, Deisseroth A B, Gallin J J 1978 Mobilization and exocytosis of specific (secondary) granules by human neutrophils during adherence to nylon wool infiltration leukapheresis (FL). Blood 52: 770–782

Yen S P S, Rembaum A 1971 Complexes of heparin with elastomeric positive polyelectrolytes. Journal of Biomedical Materials Research Symposium 1: 83–97

Young B R, Lambrecht L K, Cooper S L, Mosher D F 1982a Plasma proteins: their role in initiating platelet and fibrin deposition on biomaterials. American Chemical Society Advances in Chemistry 199: 317–350

Young B R, Doyle M J, Collins W E et al 1982b Effect of thrombospondin and other platelet α-granule proteins on artificial surface-induced thrombosis. Transactions of the American Society for Artificial Internal Organs 28: 498–503

Young B R, Lambrecht L K, Albrecht R M, Mosher D F, Cooper S L 1983 Platelet-protein interactions at blood–polymer interfaces in the canine test model. Transactions of the American Society for Artificial Internal Organs 29: 442–446

Yu J, Sundaram S, Weng D, Courtney J M, Moran C R, Graham N B 1991 Blood interactions with novel polyurethaneurea hydrogels. Biomaterials 12: 119–120

Zucker M B, Vroman L 1969 Platelet adhesion by fibrinogen adsorbed onto glass. Proceedings of the Society for Experimental Biology and Medicine 131: 318–320

Zusman R M, Rubin R H, Cato A E et al 1981 Hemodialysis using prostacyclin instead of heparin as the sole antithrombotic agent. New England Journal of Medicine 304: 934–939

SECTION 10

Venous thrombosis

59. Epidemiology of pulmonary embolism and deep vein thrombosis

S. Z. Goldhaber

Venous thrombosis was not reported prior to the 13th century (Dexter & Folchi 1974) and appears to be a relatively new disease, described with increasing frequency during the past 200 years. The harbingers of this condition — hypercoagulability, stasis, and vein wall trauma (known as Virchow's triad) — may be associated with Westernization of our society, as epitomized by the chair, which has permeated everyday life and symbolizes an increase in immobility, constipation, and varicose veins (Dexter, 1973).

Environmental and aetiologic factors associated with deep venous thrombosis (DVT) and pulmonary embolism (PE) have fascinated investigators for more than 50 years. One case series of 100 PE patients found no obvious cause in 70; the most commonly recognized precipitating factor was a bowel movement, identified in 15 patients (de Takats et al 1940). PEs tended to occur several days after a cold wave and were most common in winter months.

PE and DVT account for more than 250 000 hospitalizations per year in the USA (Gillum 1987) and constitute the third most common cardiovascular disease, after acute ischaemic syndromes and stroke. About two-thirds of cases are first time episodes; the remaining third arise in patients with recurrent venous thromboembolism (Anderson et al 1991) (Fig. 59.1).

Unfortunately, PE causes as many as 50 000 deaths per year in the United States and, in the past 2 decades, there has been no decline in the PE death rate when it is examined either nationally (Fig. 59.2) (Lilienfeld et al 1990a) or in specific American cities (Fig. 59.3) (Lilienfeld et al 1990b). The death rate from PE is higher in men than in women and in nonwhites than in whites (Fig. 59.2). In Canada, the PE death rate is slightly lower than in the USA (Soskolne et al 1990). However, in Canada as in the USA more men than women die of PE, and there has

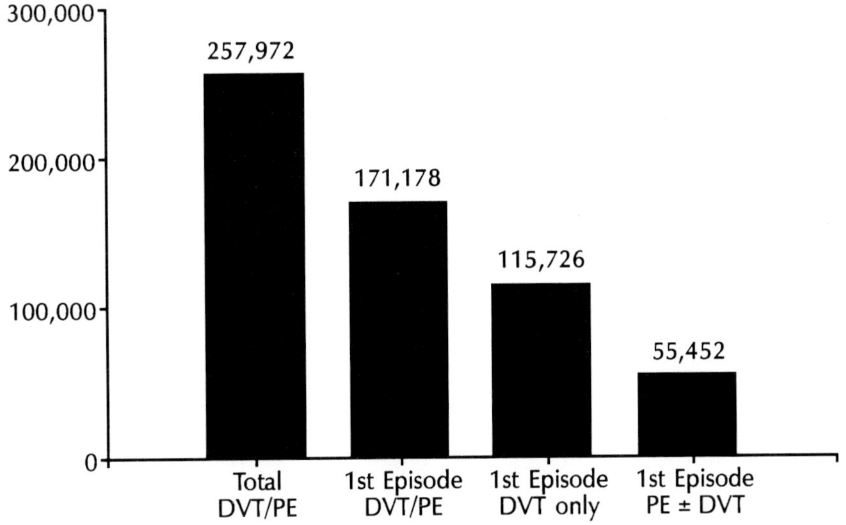

Fig. 59.1 Estimated number of cases of venous thromboembolism in the United States in 1986. The Worcester DVT study based on a 15-hospital survey in the Worcester, Massachusetts area. A population-based perspective of the incidence and case-fatality rates of venous thrombosis and pulmonary embolism: The Worcester DVT Study. (Adapted from data in Anderson F A Jr et al 1991, Archives of Internal Medicine 151: 933–938.)

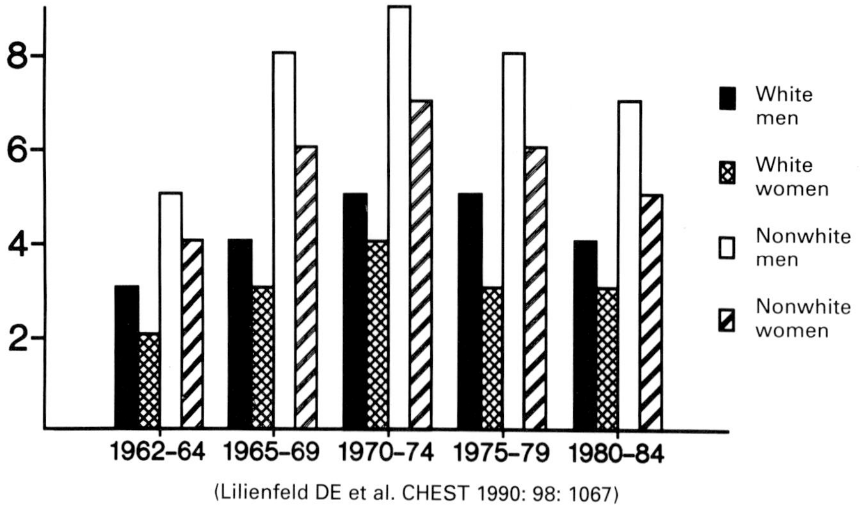

Fig. 59.2 Pulmonary embolism deaths. Average annual age-adjusted death rate per 100 000 population from pulmonary embolism in the United States from 1962–84, based on data from the National Hospital Discharge Survey. (Adapted from data in Lilienfeld D E et al 1990 Mortality from pulmonary embolism in the United States: 1962 to 1984. Chest 98: 1067–1072.)

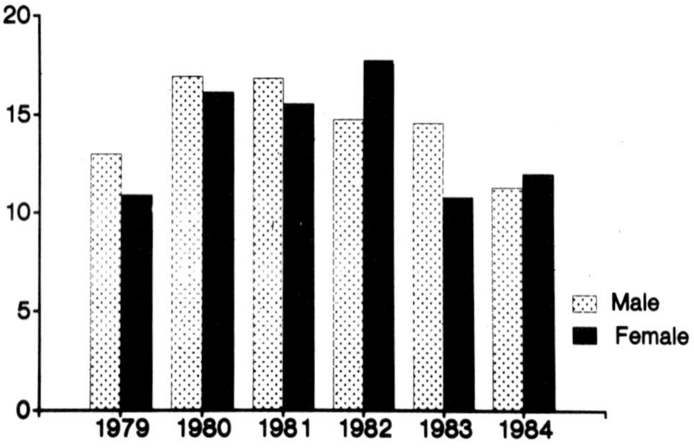

Fig. 59.3 Case fatality rate for pulmonary embolism in two cities in the USA. Annual age-adjusted case fatality rate per 100 hospital discharges for pulmonary embolism in the 'twin cities' of Minneapolis and St Paul, Minnesota, USA based on examination of hospital discharge records. From 1979 to 1984, there was no change in mortality from pulmonary embolism. (Adapted from data in Lilienfeld D E et al 1990 Hospitalization and case fatality for pulmonary embolism in the twin cities: 1979–1984. American Heart Journal 120: 392–395.)

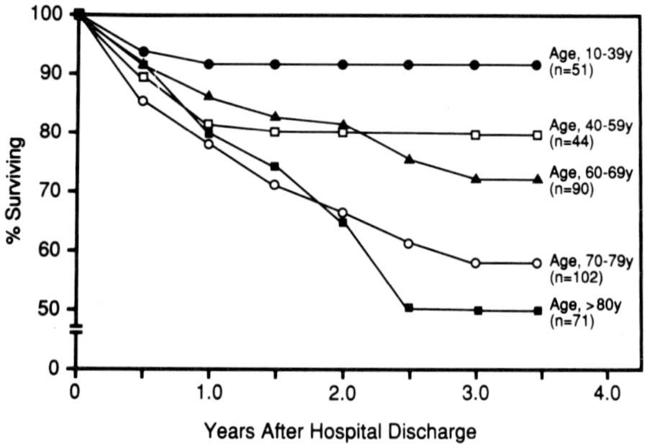

Fig. 59.4 Survival after a first episode of DVT and/or PE. Age-specific survival rates in 358 patients discharged from hospitals in the Worcester, Massachusetts area of the USA with a first episode of clinically recognized DVT and/or PE: The Worcester DVT Study. A population-based perspective of the incidence and case-fatality rates of venous thrombosis and pulmonary embolism. (From Anderson F A Jr et al 1991 Archives of Internal Medicine 151: 933–938.)

been no decline in the death rate for the past 25 years. In both the United States (Fig. 59.4) and in Canada, survival after PE declines with increasing age.

Venous thromboembolism (VTE) occurs much less often in Asian (Woo et al 1988) and African (Thomas et al 1960) populations compared with Western communities. The lower rates in other parts of the world may provide clues to aetiologic factors in the West. For example, differences in diet, exercise, and bowel habits (e.g. squatting vs. toilet) may contribute to the lower rates of PE and DVT in non-Western societies.

AUTOPSY STUDIES

The autopsy can be viewed as an epidemiologic tool for furthering our understanding of PE. Unfortunately, despite the availability of lung scanning and pulmonary angiography, PE contributing to patient death is diagnosed antemortem in only one of approximately every three cases (Goldhaber et al 1982, Rubinstein et al 1988). In one autopsy study of patients with major PE, 83% had deep venous thrombosis (DVT) at autopsy but only 19% of patients had clinically suspected DVT prior to death (Sandler & Martin 1989). These findings suggest that clinical suspicion for DVT and PE should often be intensified in order to establish the presence of venous thrombosis prior to death. Elderly institutionalized patients seem to be especially susceptible to PE (Taubman & Silverstone 1986, Gross et al 1988).

One study surveyed 2067 autopsies from 32 university and community hospitals throughout the USA (Battle et al 1987). In each case, the premortem and postmortem diagnoses were compared to determine how often the clinical and pathological diagnoses differed. Of all disease entities that were encountered, PE had the highest proportion of diagnostic discrepancies; found in 47% of 206 cases.

Susceptibility to postoperative PE continues for more than one month after surgery. In an analysis of autopsied surgical patients in Malmo, Sweden, where the autopsy rate remained high throughout the study, PE that was considered the cause or a major contributor to death occurred in 25% of PE patients between postoperative days 15 and 30, and in 15% after postoperative day 30 (Fig. 59.5) (Bergqvist & Lindblad 1985).

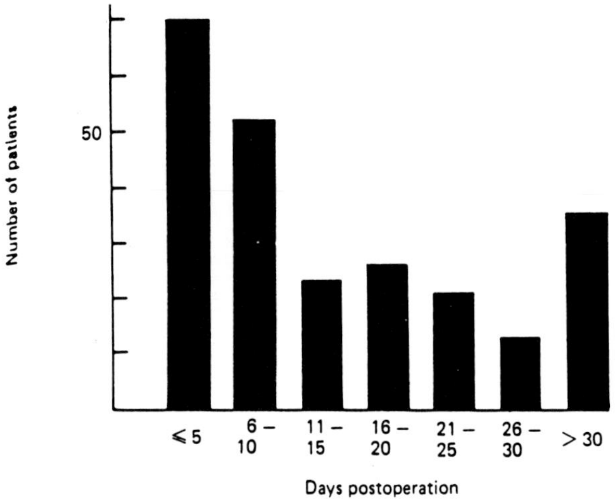

Fig. 59.5 The interval between operation and death in patients with autopsy proven fatal PE, or PE contributing to the cause of death. (From Bergqvist D, Lindblad B 1985 A 30-year survey of pulmonary embolism verified at autopsy: an analysis of 1274 surgical patients. British Journal of Surgery 72: 105–108.)

BLOOD TESTS

Seasonal variation

If one concedes that elevated fibrinogen levels predispose to intravascular thrombosis, the clinically observed increase in PE in winter months (de Takats et al 1940) might possibly be explained by a seasonal increase in fibrinogen concentration during the winter (Stout & Crawford, 1991). In a study of 100 individuals aged 75 and over, each person was visited monthly for one year. Body and environmental temperatures were recorded, and blood samples were obtained monthly. Mean core body temperature was significantly lower in the coldest 6 months, regardless of whether the subject lived in the community or was institutionalized (Fig. 59.6). There was a strong inverse correlation between fibrinogen level and temperature. Plasma fibrinogen concentrations were 23% higher in the coldest 6 months compared with summer months (Fig. 59.7).

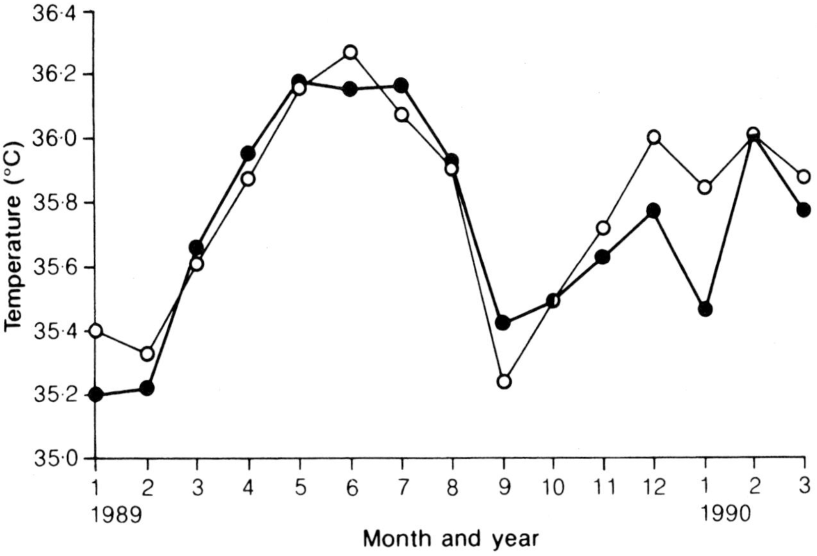

Fig. 59.6 Core body temperatures. Relationship between month and core body temperature. ○—○, community and ●—●, institution. (From Stout R V, Crawford V 1991 Seasonal variations in fibrinogen concentrations among elderly people. Lancet 2: 9–13.)

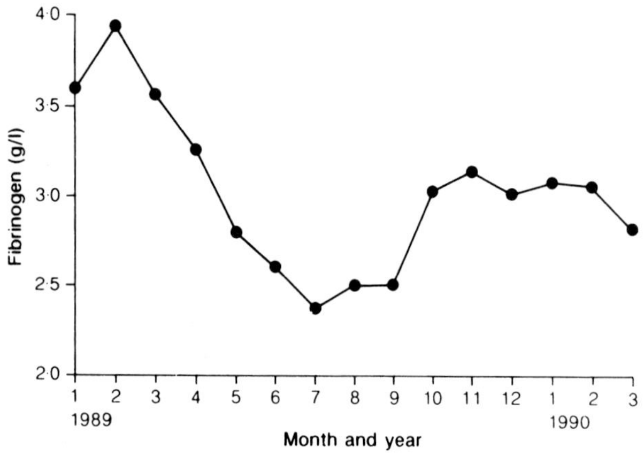

Fig. 59.7 Relationship between month and mean plasma fibrinogen concentration. (From Stout R W, Crawford V 1991 Seasonal variations in fibrinogen concentrations among elderly people. Lancet 2: 9–13.)

D-dimer as a diagnostic test

The D-dimer is a cross-linked fibrin degradation product that circulates in plasma after lysis of fibrin by plasmin. Among patients with DVT or PE, endogenous fibrinolysis occurs and leads to an increase in circulating cross-linked fibrin degradation products (D-dimer). Therefore, D-dimer has been proposed as a diagnostic screening test among populations suspected of venous thrombosis. Among 104 patients suspected of DVT who underwent venography, all patients with positive leg venograms had elevated D-dimer levels, measured by an enzyme-linked immunoassay. Plasma D-dimer levels were highest among patients with thrombosis extending proximally into pelvic veins, least in those with thrombosis restricted to distal veins, and intermediate with extension into the thigh (Rowbotham et al 1987). This observation suggests that plasma D-dimer levels may be a useful screening test among a population of patients suspected of DVT.

In a prospective series of 171 consecutive patients suspected of PE, 32% were diagnosed with this condition, and all but one had elevated D-dimer concentrations above 500 µg/l (Bounameaux et al 1991). D-dimer was measured in plasma with an enzyme-linked immunosorbent assay (STAGO). The technician who performed the assay was not aware of the final diagnosis. The sensitivy of elevated D-dimer for PE was 98% and the specificity was 39%; the positive and negative predictive values were 44% and 98%, respectively. The sensitivity of the elevated plasma D-dimer measurement remained high even 3 days (96%) and 7 days (93%) after presentation to the emergency ward. Thus, elevated plasma D-dimer levels may be an excellent screening test for PE, assuming that the proper D-dimer assay kit is chosen and utilized correctly.

ACQUIRED HYPERCOAGULABLE STATE

Primary hypercoagulable state

In an unselected population study of patients with DVT,

Table 59.1 Primary hypercoagulable states

Antithrombin III deficiency
Protein C deficiency
Protein S deficiency
Excessive plasminogen activator inhibitor

deficiencies of antithrombin III, protein C, and protein S were the most commonly identified hypercoagulable disorders and accounted for 8% of the patients (Heijboer et al 1990) (Table 59.1). In a study of 141 venous thrombosis patients less than 45 years of age, 9% had protein C or S deficiency, 3% had antithrombin III deficiency, 2% had a plasminogen abnormality, and 1% had a fibrinogen abnormality (Gladson et al 1988). In another study of 88 patients with venous thrombosis, 19% had increased levels of plasminogen activator inhibitor (Tabernero et al 1989).

'Lupus anticoagulant', an antibody that interferes with phospholipid-dependent coagulation reactions, usually prolongs the activated partial thromboplastin time but, nevertheless, is a *procoagulant* that is often present in patients without lupus. Patients with lupus anticoagulant often have elevated titres of anticardiolipin antibodies which are assayed with the negatively charged phospholipid, cardiolipin, as the antigen. Lupus anticoagulant and elevated anticardiolipin antibodies may be especially ominous in pregnant women. These markers of an acquired hypercoagulable state are associated with recurrent venous thrombosis during pregnancy as well as recurrent first or second trimester miscarriages.

THE PE-DVT RELATIONSHIP (Table 59.2)

Silent PE frequently accompanies clinically apparent DVT of the legs. Approximately half of patients with DVT proximal to the calf have asymptomatic PE (Huisman et al 1989). It is often not appreciated that between 15% (Huisman et al 1989) and 30% (Doyle et al 1987) of patients with isolated calf vein thrombosis also have asymptomatic PE. This is an important observation, because noninvasive leg examination with compression ultrasound is becoming increasingly accurate in the diagnosis of symptomatic individuals with isolated calf vein thrombosis (Yucel et al 1991). Symptomatic patients with isolated calf vein thrombosis who do not receive anticoagulation had, in one randomized controlled trial, a 29% likelihood of recurrent proximal leg DVT or PE within 3 months after the diagnosis was established (Lagerstedt et al 1985).

Table 59.2 The PE-DVT relationship: frequent sources of PE

Proximal leg DVT
Isolated calf vein thrombosis
Pelvic thrombosis
Renal vein/inferior vena caval thrombosis
Upper extremity thrombosis
Central venous catheters

Upper extremity venous thrombosis is occurring with greater frequency because of increasing intravenous drug abuse, especially cocaine (Lisse et al 1989), and because of more frequently inserted indwelling central venous catheters for hyperalimentation or for cancer chemotherapy (Anderson et al 1987, 1989). One group of investigators obtained lung scans prospectively in 20 patients with central venous catheter-related thrombosis. They found that five of the 20 patients had high probability scans for PE (Monreal et al 1991).

ACQUIRED CONDITIONS ASSOCIATED WITH PE (Table 59.3)

Certain types of surgery, such as orthopaedic surgery of the lower extremity, gynaecologic cancer, or major abdominal surgery, confer a particularly high risk for postoperative PE, which may occur as late as a month after hospital discharge (Fig. 59.5). Less well appreciated is that venous thrombosis occurs with high frequency after coronary artery bypass grafting (Josa et al 1993), renal transplantation (Allen et al 1987), and splenectomy (Pimpl et al 1989). Patients immobilized because of trauma or medical illness are also at special risk for developing PE (Gardlund 1985).

Occult cancer may be present among patients with PE (Gore et al 1982) or DVT (Goldberg et al 1987). The most frequently associated malignancies are adenocarcinomas of the lung, gastrointestinal tract, breast, and uterus. Among patients with DVT who are younger than 50 years of age, the relative risk of occult cancer was 19.0 (95% CI 2.2, 168) in one study (Goldberg et al 1987).

In women with stage II breast cancer, the adjuvant anticancer chemotherapy itself appears to contribute to the risk of venous thrombosis (Levine et al 1988). There was a 6.8% incidence of thrombosis during chemotherapy, and an incidence of 10.3% among those women over age 50 years. No thrombosis occurred during 2413 patient-months without chemotherapy. An association between venous thromboembolism and antineoplastic chemotherapy has also been reported for patients with germ cell tumours (Cantwell et al 1988) and non-Hodgkin's lymphoma (Glenn et al 1988).

Table 59.3 Acquired conditions associated with PE

Surgery:	orthopaedic
	gynaecological cancer
	major abdominal
	coronary artery bypass grafting (Josa et al 1993)
	renal transplantation
	splenectomy
Trauma	
Immobilized medical patients	
Cancer	
Pregnancy/oral contraceptives	
Obesity	
Air travel	

Cancer patients are also prone to tumour as well as thrombotic PE. Tumour PE, which has a clinical presentation similar to thrombotic PE, is more difficult to diagnose antemortem than thrombotic PE (Goldhaber et al 1987, Schriner et al 1991).

Almost all oral contraceptives (OCs) utilize low dose oestrogens which contain less than 50 μg oestrogen. The most reliable estimates of venous thromboembolism risk from OCs are derived from data in the Oxford Family Planning Association. A prospective study of its members includes over 17 000 women, of whom 56% used OCs at the time of recruitment (Vessey et al 1986). For women using OCs containing more than 50 μg oestrogen, the crude incidence of certain or probable venous thromboembolism was 0.62 per 1000 women years. In contrast, among women using OCs containing less than 50 μg oestrogen, the rate was 0.39 per 1000 woman years. In the Nurses' Health Study, current oral contraceptive use tripled the risk of PE, but use of post-menopausal oestrogens did not appear to be an important risk factor for PE (Stampfer et al 1992).

PE is also associated with pregnancy (Dixon et al 1987), particularly among women confined to bed because of preeclampsia, eclampsia, or caesarean section. The risk of PE is much greater during the first 6 weeks postpartum than during the pregnancy itself. One study demonstrated that PE is the leading medical cause of maternal mortality: four times more common among obstetrical patients than death from haemorrhage or an anaesthetic accident and twice as common as death from an ectopic pregnancy or infection (Sachs et al 1987). In a recent study commissioned by the Centers for Disease Control, PE was the leading cause of death following the delivery of a live birth (Koonin et al 1991).

Data from the Framingham Heart Study have indicated that obesity among women is a long-term risk factor for PE (Goldhaber et al 1983). In the Nurses' Health Study marked obesity more than doubled the risk of PE (Goldhaber et al 1993). Among hospitalized patients, obesity may also increase the likelihood of PE.

In otherwise apparently healthy individuals, PE can be associated with long air flights (Cruickshank et al 1988). The mechanism is presumed to be an increase in venous stasis in the legs due to immobility and dehydration.

FUTURE PERSPECTIVES (Table 59.4)

During the 1990s, the frequency of upper extremity throm-

Table 59.4 Future perspectives

Increased frequency of upper extremity thrombosis
Increased recognition of isolated calf thrombosis
Increased diagnosis of PE after hospital discharge
Increased identification of PE among the institutionalized elderly population
Increased emphasis on prevention of PE

bosis will continue to rise because of increased use of long term in-dwelling central venous catheters. As compression ultrasound becomes more widespread and as technology in noninvasive diagnosis improves, not only upper extremity thrombosis but also isolated calf vein thrombosis (Yucel et al 1991) will be recognized more often.

In the future, there will also be an increased appreciation for the surprisingly large proportion of PE that occurs after patients are discharged from the hospital (Scurr et al 1988, Huber et al 1991). Improved home health care services will have to be developed because many patients are less mobile at home than in the hospital and, therefore, more susceptible to PE. As the population ages, an increasing number of elderly individuals will be institutionalized. Their risk of PE will need to be addressed more thoroughly so that effective preventive measures can be implemented (Goldhaber 1993).

REFERENCES

Allen R D M, Michie C A, Murie J A, Morris P J 1987 Deep venous thrombosis after renal transplantation. Surgery, Gynecology Obstetrics 164: 137–142

Anderson A J, Krasnow S H, Boyer M W, Raucheisen M L, Grant C E, Gasper O R, Hoffmann J K, Cohen M H 1987 Hickman catheter clots: A common occurrence despite daily heparin flushing. Cancer Treatment Reports 71: 651–653

Anderson A J, Krasnow S H, Boyer M W, Cutler D J, Jones B D, Citron M L, Ortega L G, Cohen M H 1989 Thrombosis: The major Hickman catheter complication in patients with solid tumor. Chest 95: 71–75

Anderson F A Jr, Wheeler H B, Goldberg R J, Hosmer D W, Patwardhan N A, Jovanovic B, Forcier A, Dalen J E 1991 A population-based perspective of the incidence and case-fatality rates of venous thrombosis and pulmonary embolism: The Worcester DVT Study. Archives of Internal Medicine 151: 933–938

Battle R M, Pathak D, Humble C G, Key C R, Vanatta P R, Hill R B, Anderson R E 1987 Factors influencing discrepancies between antemortem and postmortem diagnoses. Journal of American Medical Association 258: 339–344

Bergqvist D, Lindblad B 1985, A 30-year survey of pulmonary embolism verified at autopsy: an analysis of 1274 surgical patients. British Journal of Surgery 72: 105–108

Bounameaux H, Cirafici P, de Moerloose P, Schneider P-A, Slosman D, Reber G, Unger P-F 1991 Measurement of D-dimer in plasma as diagnostic aid in suspected pulmonary embolism. Lancet 1: 196–200

Cantwell B M J, Mannix K A, Roberts J T, Ghani S E, Harris A L 1988 Thromboembolic events during combination chemotherapy for germ cell malignancy. Lancet 2: 1086–1087

Cruickshank J M, Gorlin R, Jennett B 1988 Air travel and thrombotic episodes: The economy class syndrome. Lancet 2: 497–498

de Takats G, Mayne A, Petersen W F 1940 The meteorologic factor in pulmonary embolism. Surgery 7: 819–827

Dexter L 1973 The chair and venous thrombosis. Transactions of the American Clinical and Climatological Association 84: 1–15

Dexter L, Folch-Pi W 1974 Venous thrombosis. An account of the first documented case. Journal of the American Medical Association 228: 195–196

Dixon J E 1987 Pregnancies complicated by previous thromboembolic disease. British Journal of Hospital Medicine 37: 449–452

Doyle D J, Turpie A G G, Hirsh J, Best C, Kinch D, Levine M N, Gent M 1987 Adjusted subcutaneous heparin or continuous intravenous heparin in patients with acute deep vein thrombosis: A randomized trial. Annals of Internal Medicine 107: 441–445

Gardlund B 1985 Fatal pulmonary embolism in hospitalized non-surgical patients. Acta Medica Scandinavica 218: 417–421

Gillum R F 1987 Pulmonary embolism and thrombophlebitis in the United States, 1970–1985. American Heart Journal 114: 1262–1264

Gladson C L, Scharrer I, Hach V, Beck K H, Griffin J H 1988 The frequency of type I heterozygous protein S and protein C deficiency in 141 unrelated young patients with venous thrombosis. Thrombosis and Haemostasis 59: 18–22

Glenn L D, Armitage J O, Goldsmith J C, Sorensen S, Howe D, Weisenberg D D 1988 Pulmonary emboli in patients receiving chemotherapy for non-Hodgkin's lymphoma. Chest 94: 589–594

Goldberg R J, Seneff M, Gore J M, Anderson F A, Jr, Greene H L, Wheeler H B, Dalen J E 1987 Occult malignancy in patients with deep venous thrombosis. Archives of Internal Medicine 147: 251–253

Goldhaber S Z 1993 Prevention of venous thrombosis. Marcel Dekker Inc, New York, p 60

Goldhaber S Z, Hennekens C H, Evans D A, Newton E C, Godleski J J 1982 Factors associated with correct antemortem diagnosis of major pulmonary embolism. American Journal of Medicine 73: 822–826

Goldhaber S Z, Savage D D, Garrison R J, Castelli W P, Kannel W B, McNamara P M, Gherardi G, Feinleib M 1983 Risk factors for pulmonary embolism. The Framingham Study. American Journal of Medicine 74: 1023–1028

Goldhaber S Z, Dricker E, Buring J E, Eberlein K, Godleski J J, Mayer R J, Hennekens C H 1987 Clinical suspicion of autopsy-proven thrombotic and tumor pulmonary embolism in cancer patients. American Heart Journal 114: 1432–1435

Goldhaber S Z, Stampfer M J, Manson J E, Colditz G A, Willett W C, Speizer F E, Hennekens C H 1993 Prospective study of risk factors for pulmonary embolism in women. Journal of the American College of Cardiology, 318 A (abstract)

Gore J M, Appelbaum J S, Greene H L, Dexter L, Dalen J E 1982 Occult cancer in patients with acute pulmonary embolism. Annals of Internal Medicine 96: 556–560

Gross J S, Neufeld R R, Libow L S, Gerber I, Rodstein M 1988 Autopsy study of the elderly institutionalized patient. Review of 234 autopsies. Archives of Internal Medicine 148: 173–176

Heijboer H, Brandjes D P, Büller H R, Sturk A, ten Cate J W 1990 Deficiencies of coagulation-inhibiting and fibrinolytic proteins in outpatients with deep-vein thrombosis: New England Journal of Medicine 323: 1512–1516

Huber O, Bounameaux H, Borst F, Rohner A 1991 Postoperative pulmonary embolism after hospital discharge: An underestimated risk. Archives of Surgery (in press)

Huisman M V, Buller H R, ten Cate J W, van Royen E A, Vreeken J, Kersten M-J, Bakx R 1989 Unexpected high prevalence of silent pulmonary embolism in patients with deep venous thrombosis. Chest 95: 498–502

Josa M, Siouff S Y, Silverman A B, Barsaimian E M, Khari S F, Sharma G V R K 1993 Pulmonary embolism after cardiac surgery. Journal of the American College of Cardiology 21: 990–996

Koonin L M, Atrash H K, Lawson H W, Smith J C 1991 Maternal Mortality Surveillance, United States 1979–1986. In: CDC Surveillance Summaries, MMWR (No ss–2): 1–13

Lagerstedt C I, Olsson C-G, Fagher B O, Öqvist B W, Albrechtsson U 1985 Need for long-term anticoagulant treatment in symptomatic calf-vein thrombosis. Lancet 2: 515–518

Levine M N, Gent M, Hirsh J, Arnold A, Goodyear M D, Hryniuk W, De Pauw S 1988 The thrombogenic effect of anticancer drug therapy in women with stage II breast cancer. New England Journal of Medicine 318: 404–407

Lilienfeld D E, Chan E, Ehland J, Godbold J H, Landrigan P J, Marsh G 1990a Mortality from pulmonary embolism in the United States: 1962 to 1984. Chest 98: 1067–1072

Lilienfeld D E, Godbold J H, Burke G L, Sprafka J M, Pham D L,

Baxter J 1990b Hospitalization and case fatality for pulmonary embolism in the twin cities: 1979–1984. American Heart Journal 120: 392–395
Lisse J R, Davis C P, Thurmond-Anderle M E 1989 Upper extremity deep venous thrombosis: Increased prevalence due to cocaine abuse. American Journal of Medicine 87: 457–458
Monreal M, Lafoz E, Ruiz J, Valls R, Alastrue A 1991 Upper-extremity deep venous thrombosis and pulmonary embolism. A prospective study. Chest 99: 280–283
Pimpl W, Dapunt O, Kaindl H, Thalhamer J 1989 Incidence of septic and thromboembolic-related deaths after splenectomy in adults. British Journal of Surgery 76: 517–521
Rowbotham B J, Carroll P, Whitaker A N, Bunce I H, Cobcroft R G, Elms M J, Masci P P, Bundesen P G, Rylatt D B, Webber A J 1987 Measurement of crosslinked fibrin derivatives – Use in the diagnosis of venous thrombosis. Thrombosis and Haemostasis 57: 59–61
Rubinstein I, Murray D, Hoffstein V 1988 Fatal pulmonary emboli in hospitalized patients. An autopsy study. Archives in Internal Medicine 148: 1425–1426
Sachs B P, Brown D A J, Driscoll S G, Schulman E, Acker D, Ransil B J, Jewett J F 1987 Maternal mortality in Massachusetts. Trends and prevention. New England Journal of Medicine 316: 667–672
Sandler D A, Martin J F 1989 Autopsy proven pulmonary embolism in patients: are we detecting enough deep vein thrombosis? Journal of the Royal Society of Medicine 82: 203–205
Schriner R W, Ryu J H, Edwards W D 1991 Microscopic pulmonary tumor embolism causing subacute cor pulmonale: A difficult antemortem diagnosis. Mayo Clinical Proceedings 66: 143–148
Scurr J H, Coleridge-Smith P D, Hasty J H 1988 Deep vein thrombosis: a continuing problem. British Medical Journal 297: 28
Soskolne C L, Wong A W, Lilienfeld D E 1990 Trends in pulmonary embolism death rates for Canada and the United States, 1962–87. Canada Medical Association Journal 142: 321–324
Stampfer M J, Goldhaber S Z, Manson J E, Colditz G A, Speizer F E, Willett W C, Hennekens C H 1992 A prospective study of exogenous hormones and risks of pulmonary embolism in women. Circulation 86: I–676 (abstract)
Stout R W, Crawford V 1991 Seasonal variations in fibrinogen concentrations among elderly people. Lancet 2: 9–13
Tabernero M D, Estellés A, Vicente V, Alberca I, Aznar J 1989 Incidence of increased plasminogen activator inhibitor in patients with deep venous thrombosis and/or pulmonary embolism. Thrombosis Research 56: 565–570
Taubman L B, Silverstone F A 1986 Autopsy proven pulmonary embolism among the institutionalized elderly. Journal of the American Geriatric Society 34: 752–756
Thomas W A, Davies J N P, O'Neal R M, Dimakulangan A A 1960 Incidence of myocardial infarction correlated with venous and pulmonary thrombosis and embolism. A geographic study based on autopsies in Uganda, East Africa and St. Louis, USA. American Journal of Cardiology 5: 41–47
Vessey M, Mant D, Smith A, Yeates D 1986 Oral contraceptives and venous thromboembolism: findings in a large prospective study. British Medical Journal 292: 526
Woo K S, Tse L K K, Tse C Y, Metreweli C, Vallance-Owen J 1988 The prevalence and pattern of pulmonary thromboembolism in the Chinese in Hong Kong. International Journal of Cardiology 20: 373–380
Yucel E K, Fisher J S, Egglin T K, Geller S C, Waltman A C 1991 Isolated calf venous thrombosis: Diagnosis with compression US. Radiology 179: 443–446

60. Pathogenesis of venous thrombosis

D. P. Thomas

Knowledge of current concepts of the pathogenesis of venous thrombosis is important, not only for its own sake, but also as an aid in formulating important questions that need to be considered about the disease process. For example, why do thrombi develop primarily in the deep veins of the legs, in seemingly normal vessels, and in patients confined to bed? Is the disease purely a local phenomenon or a local expression of a systemic process? How should such thrombi be prevented, and what is the rationale for treatment? The approach of a clinician to the prophylaxis and management of disease is inevitably strongly influenced by concepts of pathogenesis; this chapter therefore serves as an introduction to the field of venous thromboembolic disease.

It has been known for over 200 years that blood in isolated veins does not clot for many hours (Hewson 1771, Lister 1863). The normal non-thrombogenicity of the intact endothelium (due, for example, to local prostacyclin production (Moncada et al 1977), cell surface glycosaminoglycans (Wight 1980) and plasminogen activator (Lokskutoff & Edgington 1977), and the presence of potent circulating physiological inhibitors of clotting (such as ATIII and protein C — Abildgaard 1979, Esmon et al 1982), combine to maintain the normal fluidity of the blood. Why, then, does the blood thrombose in specific veins of some patients? Does this result from additional factor(s) in certain situations, such as the postoperative state, or is thrombosis primarily caused by a failure of normal defence mechanisms, such as fibrinolysis? It is unlikely that a single factor, or even a set of factors, can explain all causes of venous thrombosis. Any theory of pathogenesis has to reconcile the following observations:

- Deep vein thrombosis (DVT) occurs in the veins of the lower limbs and main pelvic veins, especially in the pockets of valves (Sevitt & Gallagher 1959).
- Autopsy studies have failed to demonstrate significant vessel wall damage in the venous valve pockets of patients with thrombosis (McLachlin & Paterson 1951, Hume et al 1970, Sevitt 1978).
- While deep vein thrombosis can occur in apparently healthy mobile young adults, most cases are found in patients over the age of 40 years, at rest in bed (Hume et al 1970), commonly in association with an underlying cause such as a surgical operation, a heart attack, or childbirth.
- DVT is usually preventable, either by minimizing venous stasis in the leg veins (Hills et al 1972, Scurr et al 1977), or by impairing thrombin generation by the prophylactic administration of anticoagulant drugs (Sevitt & Gallagher 1959, Kakkar 1975).

No theory of pathogenesis is likely to be acceptable if it seriously conflicts with any of these observations.

EXPERIMENTAL STUDIES

Recent experimental data point to the conclusions that local venous stasis is a necessary but not a sufficient cause of thrombosis, that endothelial damage of veins with or without superimposed stasis represents a relatively weak thrombogenic stimulus, and that the most likely additional factor that produces DVT in the presence of stasis is an ill-defined change in the blood, commonly called the hypercoagulable state.

White cell migration

The migration of white cells through the vessel wall during stasis has been suggested as a cause of endothelial damage, thereby exposing subendothelial collagen and producing platelet adhesion with subsequent thrombus formation. Stewart and colleagues suggested that, during surgical operations, blood-borne products of tissue injury increase endothelial permeability and also cause leukocyte invasion, thus producing endothelial damage (Stewart et al 1974, 1980). Another hypothesis has suggested that localized hypoxaemia from stasis produces endothelial damage and that when blood flow is restored, the damaged areas attract phagocytic blood cells which become attached to the damaged endothelium (Malone 1977).

The validity of the hypothesis that stasis-induced leukocyte migration exposes subendothelium, providing a focus for platelet adhesion and aggregation, so leading to thrombus formation, was examined by Thomas et al (1983). Control jugular venous segments of experimental animals left in situ throughout the course of the experiment had an essentially normal endothelium. Scanning electron microscopy (SEM) revealed a flat intact endothelial surface with well demarcated cell margins, numerous small blebs, and raised endothelial nuclei (Fig. 60.1). Veins containing blood, ligated for 30–60 minutes, showed a strikingly different appearance. SEM showed leukocytes on the endothelial surface and occasionally passing through the endothelium (Fig. 60.2). Some areas of the endothelium also displayed prominent surface protrusions, too numerous to be solely cell nuclei, and sometimes two protuberances were observed within the margin of one endothelial cell. Transmission electron microscopy (TEM) revealed the presence of subendothelial polymorphonuclear leukocytes and these, together with the endothelial cell nuclei, were the cause of the surface protuberances (Fig. 60.2). Thus, migration of leukocytes was induced by stasis, although the migration was patchy in distribution. Leukocytes could be seen inserted into the endothelial layer and in most instances the cell and endothelium were in close contact. Later, the cells were located beneath the endothelium but above the basal lamina. Apart from leukocyte invasion, few other changes were detected in the vessel wall during or after stasis.

It is well known that various stimuli produce the inflammatory response of leukocytes sticking to the vessel wall and their migration through intercellular junctions (Cohnheim 1889, Allison et al 1955, Florey 1970). The reactions associated with venous stasis may be regarded as comparable to inflammation. However, no evidence was found that the vessel wall changes produced by venous stasis, including the migration of leukocytes, led to platelet adherence and aggregation, or formation of a thrombus (Thomas et al 1983). Schaub et al (1984) examined the ultrastructural effects of local stasis on the jugular veins of cats. In animals in which the vein was examined after three successive 5-minute periods of stasis and reflow, large areas of the luminal surface contained adherent leukocytes, some of which were migrating through the endothelium. However, there was no evidence of platelet deposition or fibrin formation. Only when the veins had been ligated and left in situ for as long as 24 or 72 hours was there evidence of fibrin formation, together with deposition of leukocytes, platelets and erythrocytes. Most thrombi were found at side branches and valve pockets. Schaub et al also suggested that leukocytes play a primary role in the initiation of deep vein thrombosis; prolonged periods of total stasis (24 hour or more) lead to loss of endothelial continuity, as a result of leukocyte invasion, and this eventually leads to thrombus formation. Against this hypothesis is the evidence that stasis alone, even in the presence of surgical trauma, is not a sufficient thrombogenic stimulus by itself. Furthermore,

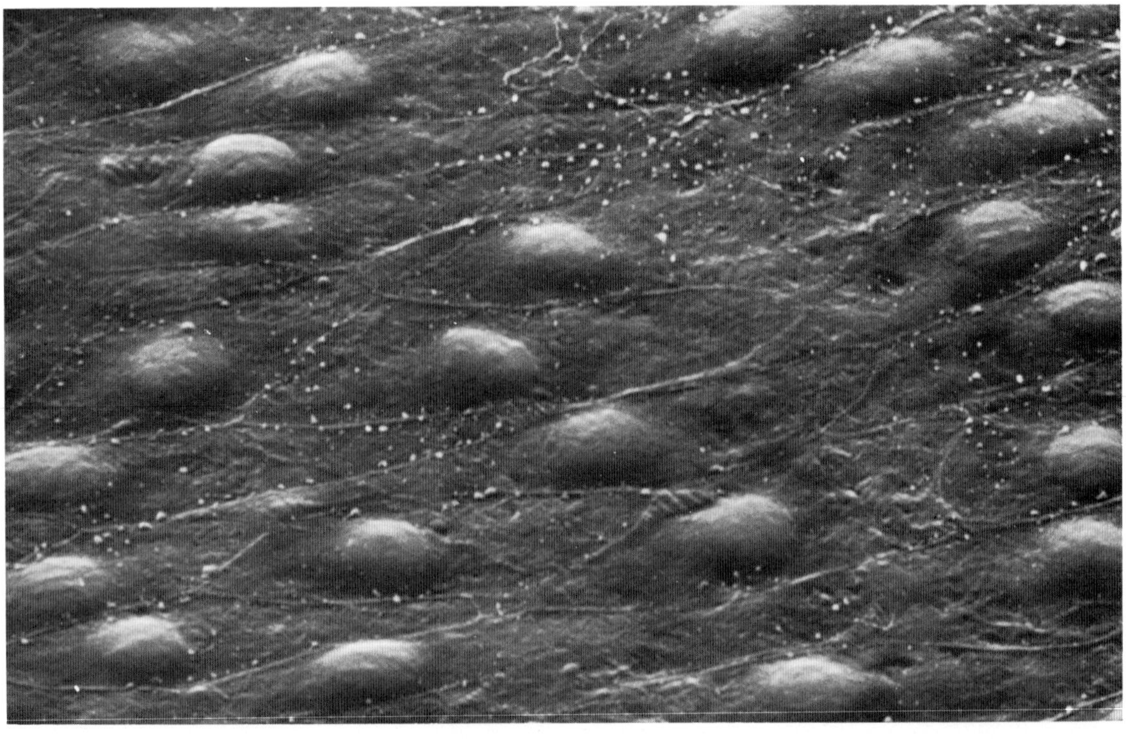

Fig. 60.1 Normal venous endothelium (rabbit). The raised nuclei and cell margins can be clearly seen (SEM × 1400).

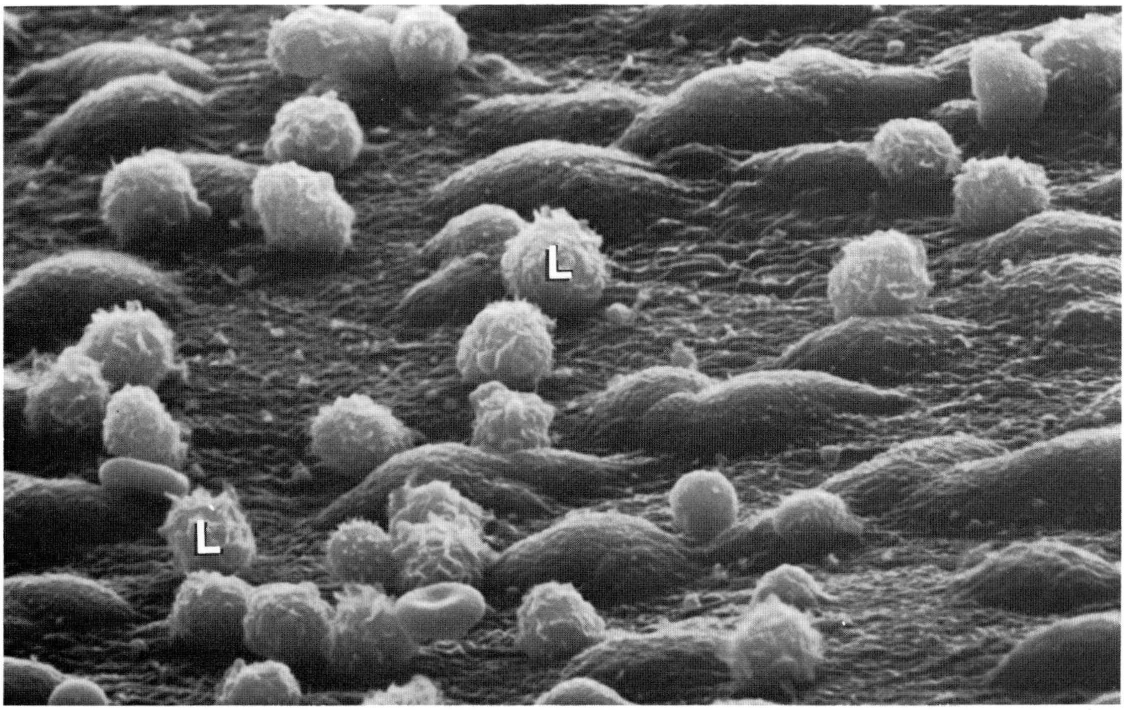

Fig. 60.2 The effect of 60 min of total venous stasis. Numerous polymorphonuclear leukocytes (L) can be seen adhering to the vessel wall. In addition to cell nuclei, some projections are produced by leukocytes that have already passed through the endothelial layer (SEM × 2500).

while stasis alone provokes leukocyte adherence and migration, without fibrin deposition, some other factor(s) must also be operative to convert an area of static blood into a localized thrombus. Leukocyte adherence to, and migration through, the endothelium appears to be a rapid and universal response to stasis, whereas thrombosis is a relatively slowly developing and exceptional phenomenon. While leukocyte migration almost certainly occurs during venous thrombogenesis, it is doubtful that the association is causative.

Hamer et al (1981) measured and compared the PO_2 of the blood in the lumen and valve pockets of veins in patients and dogs, and demonstrated that the blood within the valve pockets became rapidly hypoxic during induction of stasis. This demonstration of hypoxaemia, particularly in those sites where venous thrombi commonly originate in man, led them to suggest that hypoxic endothelial damage is a 'potential link in the chain of events which culminates as venous thrombosis'.

The failure to find platelets in the endothelial gaps produced by leukocyte migration might be explained on technical grounds associated with preparation of the vein for SEM, since no such gaps were seen in specimens examined by TEM (Thomas et al 1983). An alternative possibility is that the act of leukocyte migration causes local release of prostacyclin from the endothelium (Moncada et al 1977), sufficient to prevent platelet adherence at the site of migration, despite temporary exposure of the subendothelial collagen. If total stasis is prolonged to extreme lengths (1–3 days), it is not surprising that desquamation of the endothelium occurs, with deposition of platelets and fibrin (Schaub et al 1984). However, it seems unlikely that such extreme conditions of stasis are commonly encountered in patients.

The effect of thrombin

It has been suggested that the primary event in venous thrombogenesis is the generation of thrombin in the presence of vascular stasis (Wessler 1962, Hume et al 1970). Whether the thrombin acts only on blood platelets and fibrinogen or also acts on the endothelium is unknown, though studies with cultured endothelial cells have shown that thrombin in low concentrations leads to signs of endothelial cell injury (Barnhart & Chen 1978a,b). Rabbit veins were subjected to high local concentrations of purified thrombin, injected in vivo (Thomas et al 1982). Autologous platelets labelled with ^{III}Indium oxine were used to assess the extent of platelet adherence and the veins were also examined by TEM and SEM. No evidence of significant vessel wall damage was found in response to either high local concentrations of thrombin or the presence of venous thrombi (Fig 60.3). Less than one unit of thrombin was sufficient to clot the blood contained within the isolated segment, and no difference in radioactivity was found between control and thrombin-treated segments following the infusion of autologous indium-labelled platelets. Even when an excess of

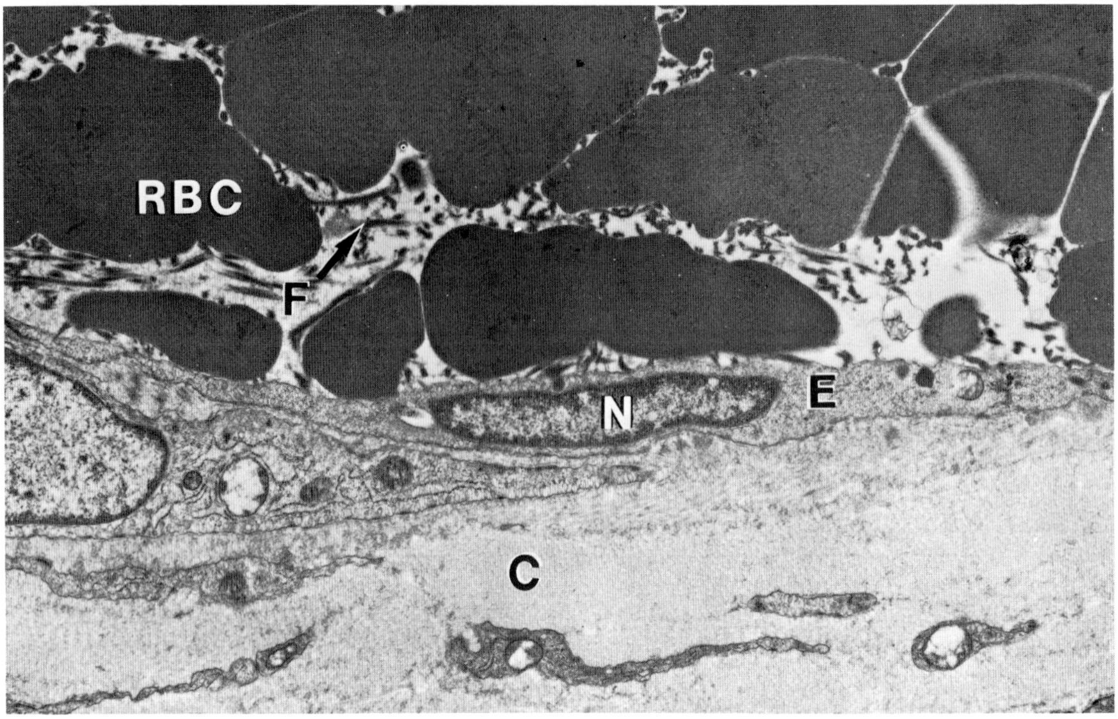

Fig. 60.3 A section of a vein containing a stasis thrombus, showing an intact endothelial cell (E) with nucleus (N), and subendothelial collagen (C). The fibrin (F) and red blood cells (RBC) of the thrombus can also be seen. (Reproduced with permission from Thomas et al 1983.) (TEM × 10 000).

purified thrombin (40 u) was injected, the radioactivity of the vein wall following restoration of blood flow was not increased significantly over the contralateral control vein. However, when thrombin was injected into the veins of animals pre-injected with aspirin, there was a significant rise in the radioactivity of the vessel wall. The infusion of prostacyclin reduced this high value back to levels not significantly different from the control. These observations suggest that platelet adherence occurs if the vessel wall prostacyclin is inhibited by aspirin-induced impairment of cyclo-oxygenase (Smith & Willis 1971).

Lough & Moore (1975) reported that the injection of thrombin into the aorta of rabbits, with re-establishment of blood flow after thrombus formation, resulted in focal separation of the endothelium from the elastica, and they suggested that injury can occur as a result of interaction between a forming thrombus and the endothelium. However, their experiments did not indicate that the endothelial cells themselves were damaged as a result of thrombin injection. Ashford & Freiman (1967) reported platelet aggregates adjacent to apparently intact endothelium after minimal mechanical injury, although Thomas et al (1982) demonstrated by SEM the relative scarcity of such platelet accumulations, even in thrombin-treated segments. It is likely that these occasional platelet aggregates develop in response to the minimal trauma that is an inevitable concomitant of surgical dissection.

It is doubtful whether the impact of thrombin on endothelial cells in the absence of blood is physiologically relevant. The normal protective mechanisms of the blood against thrombin, e.g. ATIII, adsorption of thrombin to fibrin (Liu 1981), make it unlikely that the cell wall is exposed to concentrations of thrombin sufficient to cause damage. Lollar & Owen (1980) suggested that thrombin in the circulation binds to active-site-independent, high-affinity binding sites on the endothelial cell surface, and that heparan sulphate may be responsible for this binding of thrombin and catalysis of the thrombin-ATIII reaction. Hatton et al (1980) demonstrated that thrombin binds to rabbit endothelial cells, and found approximately 5.8×10^5 molecules of thrombin associated with each cell. They also suggest that cell surface glycosaminoglycans, such as heparan sulphate, could be responsible for much of this binding. Endothelial cells grown in vitro may have less surface glycosaminoglycan available for thrombin binding, and this could explain the apparent greater susceptibility to damage by thrombin of endothelial cells grown in tissue culture. In any event, endothelial cells in vivo appear to be well adapted to tolerate local thrombin generation; even the presence of a stasis thrombus does not damage the endothelium, at least in short-term experiments (Fig. 60.3).

Role of activated clotting factors

The efficacy of activated clotting factors in producing stasis thrombi was strikingly demonstrated by Gitel et al (1977): the minimal amounts required to produce a complete thrombus after 10 minutes stasis in the jugular veins of rabbits were 1.1 nmol for thrombin, 0.12 nmol for activated factor X, and 0.02 nmol for activated factor IX. Their findings were in keeping with the hypothesis that, because of biochemical amplification during coagulation, the further removed an activated clotting factor is from fibrin formation, the fewer are the number of molecules of protease required to produce a thrombotic event. Indeed, they found that as little as 100 ng of factor IXa produced partial thrombi after 10 minute stasis in 2 kg rabbits. Activation of the intrinsic clotting system, whether it be by serum (Wessler et al 1959), endotoxin (Thomas & Wessler 1964), kaolin (Henderson & Rapaport 1962), or a highly purified clotting factor (Gitel et al 1977), when combined with local stasis, leads to rapid clotting of non-circulating blood.

The permissive role that stasis plays in venous thrombogenesis has been highlighted by work on protein C (Esmon & Esmon 1984, Stenflo 1984). As pointed out by Esmon and colleagues (1982), the surface-to-volume ratio is low in large vessels and, as a consequence, the concentration of endothelial-bound thrombomodulin is also low. When stasis occurs, the thrombin generated does not interact significantly with the endothelium because of the relatively low availability of endothelial cell surface. Activation of protein C would be slow under these circumstances, as such activation occurs mainly in the microcirculation. Esmon et al (1982) suggested that adequate blood flow from the major veins is likely to be essential for the formation of the protein C activation complex, and that failure to activate protein C may contribute to stasis-induced thrombosis. Busch & Owen (1982) commented that, because of protein C inactivation of thrombin in the microcirculation, circulating blood behaves as if it were heparinized. In contrast, non-circulating blood has lost one of its most powerful defence mechanisms against clotting. Nevertheless, as indicated earlier, this is not by itself sufficient to promote clotting in areas of stasis. It is the simultaneous combination of stasis and activated clotting factors that represents such a potent thrombogenic stimulus in experimental studies.

Vessel wall damage

Vessel wall damage has never been convincingly demonstrated as a significant aetiological factor in venous thrombosis. Postmortem studies in man failed to show any significant histological lesion in the vessel wall that could serve as a nidus for thrombus formation (Sevitt 1978). However, it has been difficult to exclude the possibility that some subtle change in the vessel wall, perhaps as a result of anoxia, has altered the normal non-thrombogenicity of the endothelium, so that platelets adhere and become the focus of an early thrombus. The suggestion that venous thrombi could form in the absence of vessel wall damage was first put forward in recent times by Wessler (1962), although much earlier Cohnheim (1889) noted that coagulation could take place even when the endothelium is 'perfectly intact and physiological'. Wessler (1962) proposed that venous thrombi developed when local stasis occurred in the presence of systemic hypercoagulability, although neither acting alone was a sufficient stimulus. This hypothesis obviated the need for vessel wall damage as an essential prerequisite for venous thrombosis. Subsequent studies have refined this concept, particularly in relation to the role of the nidi in valve pocket thrombi in man, in which platelets are relatively few or even absent (Hume et al 1970, Sevitt 1978). While the combination of stasis and hypercoagulability can readily produce venous thrombosis in experimental animals (Wessler 1962), the elusive nature of hypercoagulability in man has prevented the full acceptance of the hypothesis that these two factors are not only necessary but are also sufficient to initiate venous thrombosis. Nevertheless, there remains a view that vessel wall damage is, in some way, an essential initiating component (Day et al 1977, Kakkar & Day 1983).

Mechanical injury to veins caused by the brief application of surgical clamps demonstrated two main patterns on ultrastructural examination (Thomas et al 1985). The damaged endothelium either remained essentially intact, although obviously perturbed, or the endothelium became denuded and the subendothelial collagen exposed. Where endothelium was shed, there was considerable subendothelial oedema. The most striking feature by SEM was the relatively thin covering of activated platelets, adhering to the exposed subendothelium (Fig. 60.4). Nevertheless, no fibrin was observed, even after blood flow had been restored for 60 min, although after this time there were numerous white cells adhering to both the exposed subendothelium and the nearby relatively undamaged endothelium. Only collagen was covered by platelets, and some red blood cells, with later arrival of white cells. The absence of fibrin, even after 1 h of restored blood flow, suggests that more extensive injury was needed to promote fibrin formation in a low velocity blood flow system, perhaps because insufficient platelets were recruited at any one site to form a 'critical mass' for thrombin generation. In any event, mechanical injury, to the extent that was induced in these experiments, was an insufficient stimulus for local fibrin formation. These findings were in keeping with earlier work showing that fibrin strands were not detectable in association with adhering platelets in the balloon de-endothelialized rabbit aorta in vivo (Sheppard & French 1971, Baumgartner & Haudenschild 1972). This is in contrast to what happens when a vessel is cut, when a platelet plug with associated fibrin forms rapidly (Sixma & Wester 1977). When the vein-crushing experiments were repeated, with the addition of total stasis, the blood contained within the crushed segments remained fluid, even after 30 min of stasis. In the light of the ultrastructural studies, this is perhaps not surprising.

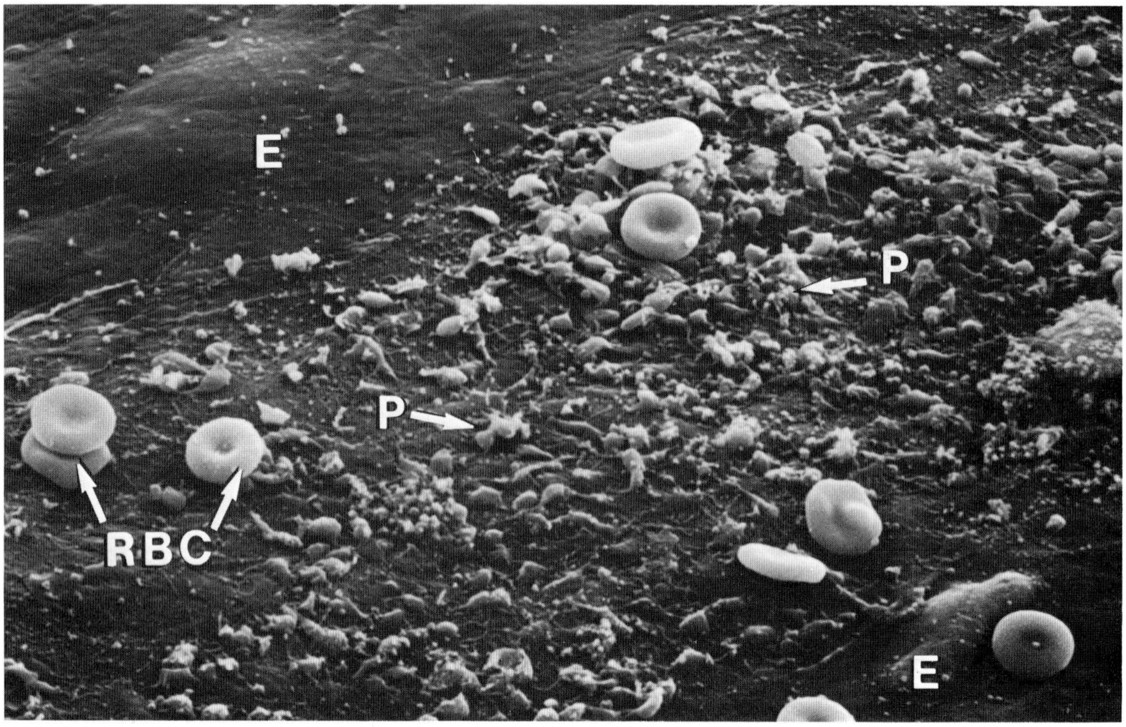

Fig. 60.4 A vein subjected to a crushing injury, with resultant loss of endothelium seen diagonally across the picture. Note the covering of activated platelets (P) where the endothelium has been removed, and the absence of fibrin. Intact endothelium (E) can be seen at the top left and bottom right of the picture, and there are scattered red blood cells (RBC) present (SEM × 2000).

If 60 minutes of blood flow after injury is insufficient to cause local fibrin deposition at the site of injury, then it is unlikely that fibrin formation would occur during subsequent stasis. However, it is possible that continued blood flow prevents the build-up of local procoagulants, that would become manifest in the presence of stasis. This proved not to be the case, at least within the time-course of the experiments (Aronson & Thomas 1985, Thomas et al 1985). They concluded that even demonstrable vessel wall damage appears to be a poor stimulus to fibrin formation at a local site of injury. A crush injury, such as might occur during a surgical operation, does not by itself (or in combination with stasis) lead to the formation of experimental venous thrombi. Perhaps even more surprising, crushing the vein with a clamp did not cause the local release of sufficient tissue factor in these experiments to produce thrombosis after 30 min of stasis. In contrast, even a trace amount of an activated clotting factor is a highly potent stimulus to fibrin formation in the presence of stasis.

It is generally agreed that the initiator of clot formation in vivo is tissue factor expressed on cell surfaces, generating the tissue factor-VIIa complex that activates factor X and IX (see Ch. 15). The blood clotting cascade then proceeds on cell-surface membranes, and the platelet membranes usually provide this essential surface. However the factors that lead to the expression of tissue factor procoagulant activity (PCA) in seemingly normal veins are still far from clear. Nawroth et al (1986) suggested that human recombinant (hr) interleukin-1 (IL-I) caused the expression of PCA on the vessel wall surface, leading to fibrin deposition. Cultured endothelial cells have also been shown to produce tissue factor-like PCA following incubation with human monocyte-derived IL-1. Merton et al (1991) studied the effect of systemic IL-1 on venous endothelium of rabbits in the presence and absence of stasis. 1 μg/kg of recombinant human IL-1β was injected intravenously and allowed to circulate for 0.5 or 5 hours, after which complete stasis was induced for 1 hour in isolated jugular vein segments. When the veins were examined by scanning electron microscopy, the endothelium was perturbed with increased surface microvilli, blebs and gaps at cell junctions, when compared with saline controls. Fibrin deposition was also observed after IL-1β, as was the adherence of essentially non-activated platelets to the endothelium (Fig. 60.5). However, no macroscopic thrombi were formed in the isolated vein segments. Thus, while IL-1 caused sufficient changes in the endothelium to produce fibrin and platelet deposition on the vessel wall, there was insufficient amplification of procoagulant activity to cause coagulation of the blood within an isolated venous segment, at least to the extent of producing an occlusive thrombus.

Schleef et al (1988) have shown that the fibrinolytic

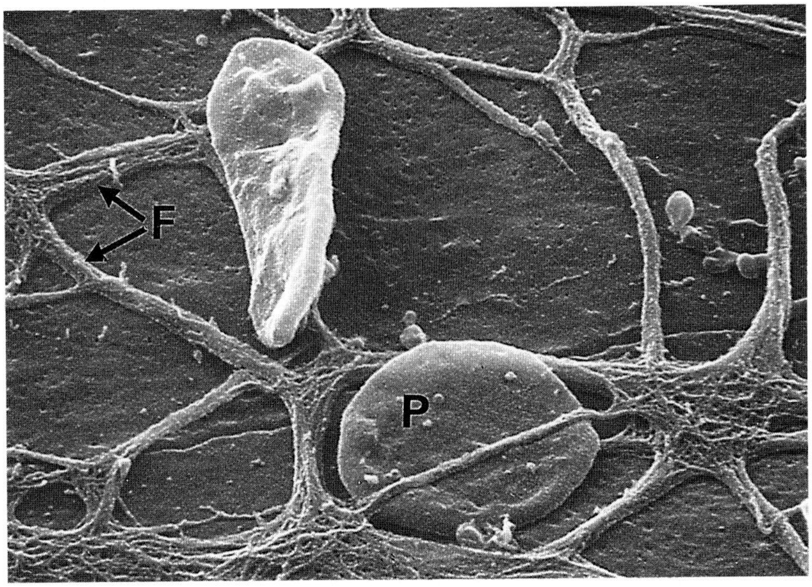

Fig. 60.5 Endothelium 4 h after IL-1 (1 μg/kg) administration and stasis (1 h), showing intact endothelial cells with adherent fibrin (F) and platelets (P) (x 20 000).

activity of endothelial cells is modulated by incubation with cytokines (IL-1 and TNF) leading to a decrease in t-PA antigen and an increase in latent and active PAI-1 activity. While this overall depression of fibrinolysis may be sufficient to favour fibrin deposition, in the presence of increased PCA, this was not sufficient to provoke macroscopic fibrin formation in blood contained within isolated vein segments in the experiments of Merton et al (1991). It is possible that repeated exposure of the vessel wall to cytokines and PCA, especially in postoperative patients, may represent a sufficient stimulus for the eventual development of occlusive thrombi. While inflammatory cytokines are potent modulators of several endothelial functions that are likely to be relevant to thrombosis (Stern et al 1988), such as IL-1 inducing rapid expression of tissue factor PCA on the surface of endothelial cells in vitro (Nawroth et al 1986), the chain of events that links trace amounts of fibrin on the vessel wall (Nawroth et al 1986, Merton et al 1991) to the development of clinically significant thrombi remains to be established. It is worth remembering that most DVT detected by ^{125}I-labelled fibrinogen undergo spontaneous lysis (Kakkar et al 1969), strongly suggesting that the development of a large thrombus from a small platelet-fibrin nidus occurs primarily in those patients in whom fibrinolysis is impaired.

PATHOLOGICAL STUDIES IN MAN

Site of origin of venous thrombi

There is disagreement on the primary site of origin of deep vein thrombi. In general, the disagreement exists (a) between those who examine leg veins at autopsy and those who examine leg veins in living patients using venographic techniques, and (b) between those who study medical and surgical patients, and those who study patients undergoing hip surgery.

a. Method of examination

Careful venous dissection at autopsy demonstrated thrombi in a variety of locations in the thigh and leg (McLachlin & Paterson 1951, Sevitt & Gallagher 1959). Thrombi in calf veins were often found to be independent of thrombi present in thigh veins. Sevitt (1978) concluded that the varied patterns of thrombosis can be explained on the basis that thrombi begin at one or more of several sites. He recognised six main primary sites of origin:

1. Iliac vein, generally above the inguinal ligament
2. Common femoral vein
3. Deep femoral vein
4. Popliteal vein
5. Posterior tibial veins
6. Intramuscular veins of the calf, particularly the soleal veins.

Sevitt also concluded that the concept of multiple independent sites of origin is supported by the occurrence of small isolated thrombi, usually in valve cusps. However, he added that thrombi in calf veins are usually the earliest and most frequent manifestation of deep vein thrombosis (DVT), and that the independent thigh vein thrombi form later in many subjects. While there is no doubt that what pathologists find at autopsy is valid, their results may not necessarily reflect the distribution of thrombi in living patients. The earliest phases of a dynamic process cannot be studied at autopsy, and pathologists tend to see venous thromboembolism in its more advanced stages.

In contrast, clinicians studying the disease in the post-operative patients tend to have a somewhat different view-point, particularly if they have employed ascending venography and labelled fibrinogen as diagnostic tools (Nicolaides et al 1971, Thomas & O'Dwyer 1977, Stamatakis et al 1978). For example, in a study of almost 1000 patients, Stamatakis et al (1978) found in a total of 535 limbs containing thrombi that 92% of thrombi were present in the calf with either no further clot, or clot in continuity with that in more proximal veins. Their study was carried out using ascending venography, mostly on postoperative, non-orthopaedic patients. However, in 8% of their patients, thrombi originated either in multiple discontinuous sites in the legs and pelvis, or in proximal major veins without concomitant calf involvement. Stamatakis and his colleagues concluded that in patients surviving an episode of DVT (and this represents the great majority), thrombi most frequently take origin from the deep veins of the calf. There is no conclusive evidence that the soleal veins are invariably the starting point of DVT, and calf vein thrombi are as likely to originate in stem veins as from soleal muscle veins (Thomas & O'Dwyer 1977). In contrast, as discussed below, ilio-femoral thrombi may be found in significant numbers of patients with pelvic disease or who have undergone hip surgery.

b. Nature of operative procedure

The disagreement regarding the sites of origin of DVT may be more apparent than real, reflecting different patient populations studied at different phases of their disease. Thrombi can certainly arise in the proximal major veins without calf involvement, and Athanasoulis (1976) found an incidence of 34% in patients undergoing total hip replacement, as compared with 6% in a group of patients without hip surgery. However, hip surgery patients form a special group, both from the viewpoint of pathogenesis and also their relative resistance to prophylaxis. (see Ch. 62).

The balance of evidence from studies in living patients points to the deep veins of the calves as the site of origin of thrombi in the great majority of patients without local trauma; at a later stage in the disease, independent thrombi may form elsewhere in the lower limbs.

Pathogenesis of DVT in patients undergoing hip surgery

These patients differ from other patients developing DVT in two important respects: they have a relatively high incidence of isolated femoral vein thrombi, and prophylaxis by a fixed dose of low-dose heparin is less effective. Additional predisposing factors to thrombosis exist in these patients, and an indication of what these factors may be has been given by Stamatakis et al (1977). Of 169 patients studied who underwent total hip replacement, 81 developed venographic evidence of thrombi in the operated leg. In 57% of patients developing thrombosis, the femoral vein was the apparent site of origin, and 75% of these thrombi arose from the wall of the femoral vein at the level of the lesser trochanter. In 8 patients, intra-operative venography revealed severe distortion of the common femoral vein, producing almost total occlusion. Stamatakis and colleagues suggested that intra-operative damage to the femoral vein results from manipulation of the leg, and that this is an important reason for the high incidence of upper femoral DVT in these patients. Local damage to the femoral vein, due to surgical manipulation, together with an unusual degree of intra-operative venous stasis, are additional thrombogenic stimuli, as is the presence of circulating tissue thromboplastin (Giercksky et al 1979).

By comparison, Maffei et al (1984), in experimental studies in dogs, found minimal ultrastructural changes in femoral veins subjected to torsion during surgical manipulation and thermal damage from locally-applied methymethacrylate. No quantitative differences were observed between control animals and the experimental groups. These observations are in keeping with those reported by Thomas et al (1985) and Aronson & Thomas (1985), where even direct mechanical trauma to the exterior of veins had relatively little effect on the endothelium, and did not lead to the formation of stasis thrombi (see p. 1340).

Various explanations can be offered for the relative inefficacy of fixed-dose heparin prophylaxis in patients undergoing hip surgery. For example, low plasma heparin levels, such as occur with subcutaneous heparin administration, did not protect against stasis thrombosis following the infusion of large amounts of tissue thromboplastin in experimental animals (Gitel & Wessler 1979). When the dose of heparin was adjusted for each patient undergoing hip surgery to yield partial thromboplastin times in the high-normal range, the incidence of postoperative DVT fell to levels comparable to those obtained following general surgery (Leyvraz et al 1983). Some of these relatively immobile patients may also have started to thrombose before operation (Heatly et al 1976); for such patients, low-dose heparin is inadequate therapy.

Valve pocket thrombi

Sevitt (1974, 1978) made a careful histological study of valve pocket thrombi, to ascertain the nature of the nidi from which they grow and their manner of growth to visible thrombi (Fig. 60.6). Most recent thrombi have a

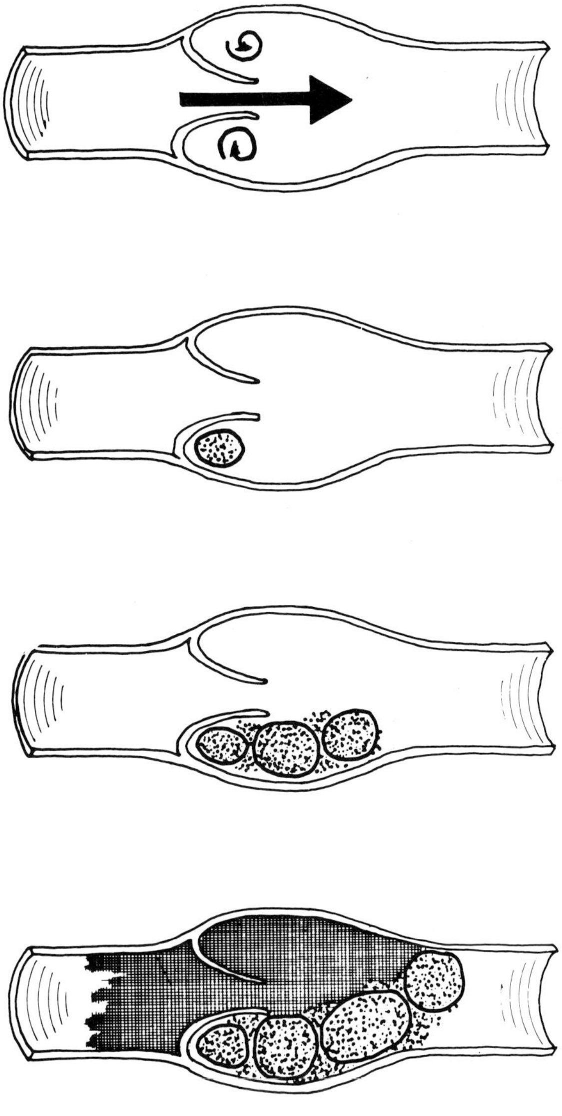

Fig. 60.6 A schematic representation of the evolution of a valve cusp thrombus. **A** This represents an area of maximum stasis in a valve pocket, with local accumulation of activated clotting factors, platelets, leukocytes and red blood cells. **B** Following thrombin generation, a platelet-fibrin nidus forms, consisting of successive alternate layers of aggregated platelets and fibrin. **C** Platelet-fibrin aggregates developing on the propagating head of the thrombus leads to thrombus growth. **D** Extension of the thrombus in a retrograde fashion occurs when the forward propagating thrombus grows to occlude the vein sufficiently.

red area restricted distally in the valve pocket and located by the vein wall, and also a larger white region which covers most of the length of the thrombus and often covers the red area. The white area is propagated growth, and includes many well-defined platelet-fibrin units. The overlying valve cusp nearly always remains free and unattached to the thrombus. While the white coagulum of a thrombus is secondary growth similar in structure to that seen in propagating thrombi, the red areas are relatively circumscribed zones located distally in the thrombus by the vein wall, and their structure is dominated by red cells with fibrin lamina. These red areas are probably the oldest and original part of the thrombus. Although there is a relative absence of platelets in these areas, platelet aggregates soon become replaced by a predominantly fibrin structure (Mustard & Packham 1977), so it is well not to underestimate the possible role of platelets in nidus formation. Sevitt concluded from his studies of valve pocket thrombi that the nidus of origin is located distally in the pocket near the vein wall, that it is laid down on normal venous endothelium and that it is formed mainly of red cells and fibrin (Sevitt 1974). Platelet collections are either absent or few in the nidus of origin, in contrast to their predominance in the growing part of thrombi.

Karino & Motomiya (1984), in an elegant study of fluid mechanics in veins, found that a truly stagnant region existed in the deepest portions of the venous valve pocket, where a secondary vortex with low red cell concentration was located. In such regions, fluid circulated with extremely low velocities, thus creating a very low shear field. They pointed out the potential of the secondary vortex to act as an automatic trap for larger cellular aggregates involved in the valve-pocket vortices, leading to a propagated reaction and thrombogenesis. It is in such sites that the earliest valve pocket thrombi have been found in human autopsy material (Sevitt 1978).

Role of fibrinolysis

The degree of local fibrinolytic activity in the blood helps to determine the extent to which fibrin will be deposited on an initial platelet nidus or whether a platelet-fibrin nidus will propagate or disappear. Clinical states which predispose to thrombosis, such as trauma and surgery, give rise to a prolonged period of reduced fibrinolysis following an initial transient activation (Hume et al 1970). The fibrinolytic activity of the vein wall, and of venous blood removed under conditions of stasis, is also lower in the legs than in the arms, and this may explain in part why thrombi have a predilection for the lower limbs. Significantly decreased levels of endothelial fibrinolytic activity have been reported in the leg veins of patients with venous thrombosis, in comparison with veins in normals (Pandolfi et al 1969, Isacson 1971). In a clinical study of patients developing postoperative DVT, Owen et al (1983) found a sustained imbalance between fibrinopeptide A levels, reflecting fibrin I formation by thrombin proteolysis of fibrinogen, and Bβ1–42 levels, reflecting fragment X formation by plasmin proteolysis of fibrin I or fibrinogen. Their data suggest that venous thrombi develop due to excess thrombin formation, and the consequent deposition of fibrin is not removed as a result of local failure of plasmin action. This impaired fibrinolysis may reflect local failure of plasminogen activator production by endothelial cells in anoxic sites, such as the valve pockets. It is known that the fibrinolytic activity of the blood after venous stasis is substantially lower in patients with thrombosis than in controls (Pandolfi et al 1967). In keeping with these observations, Melbring et al (1983) found that both preoperatively and postoperatively, the levels of plasmin–α_2-antiplasmin (PAP) complex were significantly higher in patients who did *not* subsequently develop postoperative DVT. They concluded that patients with signs of increased fibrinolytic activity, measured as PAP in plasma, have a reduced tendency to develop postoperative DVT. Another study demonstrating that at least some patients with venous thrombosis have impaired fibrinolysis is that of Bergsdorf et al (1983) who found in patients with idiopathic thrombo-embolic disease that 37% of the patients had impaired fibrolytic activity. They suggested that this was due to an increased concentration of inhibitor to tissue-type plasminogen activator (t-PA).

Wiman et al (1985) compared the fibrinolytic system in 37 patients with a recent and confirmed incidence of deep vein thrombosis, with the findings in 20 controls. 35% of the patients had t-PA activity below the lowest activity found among healthy individuals. Furthermore, the t-PA inhibitor level in the patients was significantly increased ($p < 0.01$) as compared with controls. In 13 patients with low t-PA activity in postocclusion plasma samples, the inhibitor level was 6.0 ± 4.4 u/ml (compared with 0.7 ± 0.7 u/ml in controls), while the same group of patients had a significantly lesser release of t-PA antigen (3.7 ± 2.8 μg/l), compared with controls (9.5 ± 6.0 μg/l). Wiman and colleagues concluded that the decreased fibrinolytic activity found in a third of their patients was the result of highly increased plasma levels of the fast inhibitor towards t-PA, in combination with a poor ability to release t-PA. Juhan-Vague et al (1987) also reported deficient t-PA release and elevated plasminogen activator inhibitor levels in patients with DVT.

Harbourne et al (1991) studied 156 patients 3 months after an acute DVT, confirmed by venography. In 74 patients, the DVT was idiopathic, while in 82 there were predisposing risk factors. They measured englobulin clot lysis time, global fibrinolytic activity and plasminogen activator inhibitor levels by an ELISA assay. They demonstrated abnormal fibrinolysis in about 86% of their patients with recurrent idiopathic DVT, but in only 29% of the group with secondary DVT. Thus, while low fibrinolytic activity appears to be an important factor in the aetiology of idiopathic DVT, it seems to be less so in the more common cases of DVT secondary to some predisposing cause.

Venous thrombogenesis may therefore be regarded as the product of an unstable dynamic balance between coagulation and fibrinolysis. A shift in the balance towards fibrinolysis could prevent thrombosis or quickly lyse recent thrombi, while a shift away from fibrinolysis encourages thrombus growth (see Ch. 24).

The role of hypercoagulability

It has proved difficult to define biochemically what is meant by hypercoagulability in patients. While the evidence from experimental studies is persuasive, and the observed phenomena are at least explicable on the basis that there is local generation of thrombin in the valve cusps of the lower limbs, nevertheless direct evidence of such thrombin generation in man has not been forthcoming. Similarly, while there are many studies that suggest the existence of a 'prethrombotic state' (see Ch. 52), there is no evidence directly correlating specific serine proteases with the development of postoperative DVT. It is, of course, a formidable technical task to sample blood at the appropriate time from the valve cusps and venous sinuses in the lower limbs. If hypercoagulability is a local phenomenon in most patients, and not a systemic one, then studies of blood withdrawn from, say, the antecubital vein, may be misleading. If stasis depresses the formation of local tissue plasminogen activator, and static blood is not exposed to the inhibitory action of protein C activated by the thrombin-thrombomodulin complex in the microcirculation, then the scene is set for venous thrombogenesis. However, some other factor(s) is required to complete the process, otherwise venous thrombosis would be virtually universal in immobilized patients, instead of being comparatively uncommon. It is likely that many stimuli can give rise to activation of normally inert zymogens, although their precise nature and mode of action is still unclear. Possible trigger mechanisms include circulating tissue thromboplastin (Giercksky et al 1979), endotoxin (Thomas & Wessler 1964), activation of contact factors by ulcerated atherosclerotic plaques (Hume et al 1970), and depression of fibrinolysis by cytokines (Schleef et al 1988).

Heijboer et al (1990) studied the prevalence of isolated deficiencies of antithrombin III, protein C, protein S and plasminogen in 277 consecutive patients with venographically proved acute DVT, as compared with 138 age-matched and sex-matched controls without DVT. The overall prevalence of these deficiencies was only 8.3% (CI95%: 5.4 to 12.4) in the patients, as compared to 2.2% (CI95%: 0.5 to 6.1) in the controls. The authors concluded that in the great majority of patients with DVT (91.7%), the cause of the disorder cannot be explained by an abnormality in the coagulation or fibrinolytic system, at least as measured by their assays. They also concluded that information obtained from the medical history concerning recurrent or familial venous thrombosis is not useful for the identification of patients with protein deficiencies. The possibility remains that mild abnormalities of the coagulation-inhibiting and fibrinolytic system may be found in combination, and that these could be sufficient to produce venous thrombosis despite normal screening tests (Sas et al 1991). However, it is apparent that current screening techniques are unable to explain thrombotic events in the overwhelming majority of patients with DVT.

CONCLUSIONS

The role of vascular stasis in venous thrombosis, particularly as it is seen in the deep veins of the lower limbs, has been recognized since the mid-19th century (Virchow 1860). However, the nature of the additional factors that come into play to convert a static, but still fluid, column of blood into a thrombus remains disputed. It seems reasonable to conclude that while an impaired defence mechanism lowers the threshold at which thrombosis develops, this is still an ill-understood concept and by itself represents an inadequate explanation for most cases of deep vein thrombosis.

Any hypothesis that attempts to explain the observed phenomena has to reconcile the following facts:

- Blood does not thrombose if left for many hours in the tied-off veins of experimental animals.
- Most patients immobilized in bed do not thrombose, and this is presumably the clinical counterpart of what has been demonstrated experimentally in animals.
- Therefore, any *universal* phenomenon associated with venous stasis, such as white cell migration, or low PO_2 in valve pockets, is by itself an inadequate explanation of thrombogenesis.
- Vessel wall damage is usually absent on autopsy examination of human material; furthermore, obvious endothelial damage following crush injury in experimental animals is a relatively poor thrombogenic stimulus, and does not lead to an occluding thrombus in short-term experiments. Yet venous thrombi in man develop within hours, or at most a few days, of a precipitating event, such as a surgical operation. Thus, long-term changes in the vessel wall, while crucial for an understanding of *arterial* thrombosis, are less relevant for venous thrombogenesis.

The only known additional factor that can rapidly transform static blood into a venous thrombus is the local generation of thrombin (see Ch. 20). Platelets aggregate and fibrinogen is converted to fibrin, and the basic structure of a venous thrombus emerges. The observed phenomena are most readily explained *as if* thrombin is generated in areas of retarded blood flow, with subsequent deposition of platelets and fibrin. If drugs that prevent thrombin generation were ineffective in preventing DVT, then this hypothesis would have to be discarded. In fact, there is good evidence that prophylaxis with low dose heparin and related drugs prevents most postoperative DVT (Kakkar 1975, 1982, Kiil et al 1978, Hull et al 1982, Encke & Breddin 1988, Leyvraz et al 1991). The important pragmatic conclusion to be drawn from these clinical trials is that, when thrombin generation is impaired, so is venous thrombogenesis.

REFERENCES

Abildgaard U 1979 A review of antithrombin III. In: Collen D, Wiman B, Verstraete M (eds) The physiological inhibitors of coagulation and fibrinolysis. North-Holland/Elsevier, Amsterdam, p 19

Allison F, Smith M R, Wood B 1955 Studies on the pathogenesis of acute inflammation. In: The inflammatory reaction to thermal injury as observed in a rabbit ear chamber. Journal of Experimental Medicine 102: 655

Aronson D L, Thomas D P 1985 Experimental studies on venous thrombosis: effect of coagulants, procoagulants and vessel contusion. Thrombosis and Haemostasis 54: 866–870

Ashford T P, Freiman D G 1967 The role of the endothelium in the initial phases of thrombosis. American Journal of Pathology 50: 257

Athanasoulis C A 1976 Phlebography for the diagnosis of deep leg vein thrombosis. In: Fratantoni J, Wessler S (eds) Prophylactic therapy of deep vein thrombosis and pulmonary embolism. DHEW Publication No (NIH) 76–866, p 62–76

Barnhart M I, Chen S T 1978a Platelet-vessel wall dynamics. In: Collagen-platelet interaction. Proceedings of the First Munich Symposium on Biology of Connective Tissue. Thrombosis and Haemostasis (suppl) 63: 301

Barnhart M I, Chen S T 1978b Vessel wall models for studying interaction capabilities with blood vessels. Seminars in Thrombosis and Haemostasis 5: 112

Baumgartner H R, Haudenschild C 1972 Adhesion of platelets to subendothelium. In: Weiss H J (ed) Platelets and their role in haemostasis. Annals of the New York Academy of Sciences 201: 22

Bergsdorf N, Nilsson T, Wallén P 1983 An enzyme linked immunosorbent assay for determination of tissue plasminogen activator applied to patients with thromboembolic disease. Thrombosis and Haemostasis 50: 740

Busch P C, Owen W G 1982 Interaction of thrombin with endothelium. In: Nossel H L, Vogel H J (eds) Pathobiology of the endothelial cell. Academic Press, London, p 97

Cohnheim J 1889 In: McKee A B (ed) Lectures on general pathology. New Sydenham Society, London, vol 1: 239

Czervionke R L, Hoak J C, Fry G L 1978 Effect of aspirin on thrombin-induced adherence of platelets to cultured cells from the blood vessel wall. Journal of Clinical Investigation 62: 847

Day T K, Cowper S V, Kakkar V V, Clark K G A 1977 Early venous thrombosis. A scanning electron micrscopic study. Thrombosis and Haemostasis 37: 477

Deykin D 1966 The role of the liver in serum-induced hypercoagulability. Journal of Clinical Investigation 45: 256

Encke A, Breddin K (European Fraxiparine Study Group) 1988 Comparison of a low molecular weight heparin and unfractionated heparin for the prevention of deep vein thrombosis in patients undergoing abdominal surgery. British Journal of Surgery 75: 1058–1063

Esmon C T, Esmon N L 1984 Protein C activation. Seminars in Thrombosis and Haemostasis 10: 122

Esmon C T, Esmon N L, Saugstad J, Owen W G 1982 Activation of protein C by a complex between thrombin and endothelial cell surface protein. In: Nossel H L, Vogel H J (eds) Pathobiology of the endothelial cell. Academic Press, New York, p 121

Florey H W 1970 Inflammation. In: Florey H W (ed) General pathology. Lloyd-luke, London, p 40

Giercksky K E, Bjorklid E, Prydz H, Renck H 1979 Circulating tissue thromboplastin during hip surgery. European Journal of Surgical Research 11: 296

Gitel S N, Wessler S 1979 The antithrombotic effects of warfarin and heparin following infusions of tissue thromboplastin in rabbits: clinical implications. Journal of Laboratory and Clinical Medicine 94: 481

Gitel S N, Stephenson R C, Wessler S 1977 In vitro and in vivo correlation of clotting protease activity: effect of heparin. Proceedings of the National Academy of Sciences, USA 74: 3028

Hamer J D, Malone P C, Silver I A 1981 The PO_2 in venous valve pockets: its possible bearing on thrombogenesis. British Journal of Surgery 68: 166

Harbourne T, O'Brien D, Nicolaides A N 1991 Fibrinolytic activity in patients with idiopathic and secondary deep venous thrombosis. Thrombosis Research 64: 543–550

Hatton M W C, Dejana E, Cazenave J-P, Regoeczi E, Mustard J F 1980 Heparin inhibits thrombin binding to rabbit thoracic aorta endothelium. Journal of Laboratory and Clinical Medicine 96: 861

Heatley R V, Hughes L E, Morgan A, Okwonga W 1976 Preoperative or postoperative deep vein thrombosis? Lancet 1: 437

Henderson E S, Rapaport S I 1962 The thrombotic activity of activation product. Journal of Clinical Investigation 41: 235

Heijboer H, Desiderius P M, Brandjes M D, Bülller H R, Sturk A, ten Cate J W 1990 Deficiencies of coagulation-inhibiting and fibrinolytic proteins in outpatients with deep vein thrombosis. New England Journal of Medicine 323: 1512–1516

Hewson W 1771 An Experimental Inquiry into the properties of the blood. Cadell, London, p 20

Hills N H, Pflug J J, Jeyasingh K, Boardman L, Calnan J S 1972 Prevent of deep vein thrombosis by intermittent pneumatic compression of calf. British Medical Journal 1: 131

Hull R, Delmore T, Carter C et al 1982 Adjusted subcutaneous heparin versus warfarin sodium in the long-term treatment of venous thrombosis. New England Journal of Medicine 306: 189

Hume M, Sevitt S, Thomas D P 1970 Venous thrombosis and pulmonary embolism. Harvard University Press, Cambridge MA

Isacson S 1971 Low fibrinolytic activity of blood and vein walls in venous thrombosis. Scandinavian Journal of Haematology (Suppl) 16

Juhan-Vague I, Valadier J, Allessi M C, Ailland M F, Ausaldi J, Philip-Joet C, Holvoet P, Serradimigni A, Collén D 1987 Deficient t-PA release and elevated PA inhibitor levels in patients with spontaneous or recurrent DVT. Thrombosis and Haemostasis 57: 67–72

Kakkar V V 1975 An international multicentre trial. Prevention of fatal postoperative pulmonary embolism by low doses of heparin. Lancet 2: 45

Kakkar V V, Day T K 1983 The vessel wall and venous thrombosis. In: Woolf N (ed) Biology and pathology of the vessel wall. Praeger, Eastbourne, p 229

Kakkar V V, Flanc C, Howe C T, Clarke M B 1969 Natural history of postoperative deep-vein thrombosis. Lancet 2: 230

Kakkar V V, Djazaeri B, Fox J, Fletcher M, Scully M F, Westwick J 1982 Low molecular weight heparin and prevention of postoperative deep vein thrombosis. British Medical Journal 284: 375

Karino T, Motomiya M 1984 Flow through a venous valve and its implication for thrombus formation. Thrombosis Research 36: 245

Kiil J, Axelsen F, Kiil J, Andersen D 1978 Prophylaxis against postoperative pulmonary embolism and deep vein thrombosis by low-dose heparin. Lancet 1: 1115

Leyvraz P F, Richard J, Bachmann F et al 1983 Adjusted versus fixed-dose subcutaneous heparin in the prevention of deep-vein thrombosis after total hip replacement. New England Journal of Medicine 309: 954

Leyvraz P F, Bachmann F, Hoek J, Büller H R, Postel M, Samama M, Vandenbroek M C 1991 Prevention of deep vein thrombosis after hip replacement: randomized comparison between unfractionated heparin and low molecular weight heparin. British Medical Journal 303: 543–548

Lister J 1863 On the coagulation of the blood. Proceedings of the Royal Society 12: 580

Liu C Y 1981 Mechanism of thrombin binding by fibrin. In: Walz D A, McCoy L E (eds) Contributions to hemostasis. Annals of the New York Academy of Sciences 370: 545

Lokskutoff D J, Edgington T S 1977 Synthesis of a fibrinolytic activator and inhibitor by endothelial cells. Proceedings of the National Academy of Sciences, USA 74: 3903

Lollar P, Owen W G 1980 Clearance of thrombin from circulation in rabbits by high-affinity binding sites on endothelium. Journal of Clinical Investigation 66: 1222

Lough J, Moore S 1975 Endothelial injury induced by thrombin or thrombi. Laboratory Investigation 33: 130

McLachlin J, Paterson J C 1951 Some basic observations on venous thrombosis and pulmonary embolism. Surgery, Gynaecology and Obstetrics 93: 1

Maffei F H A, Fabris V E, Gregorio E A, Valeri V 1984 Surgical trauma and venous thrombosis in total hip replacement. Thrombosis and Haemostasis 52: 368

Malone P C 1977 A hypothesis concerning the aetiology of venous thrombosis. Medical Hypotheses 3: 189

Melbring G, Dahlgren S, Reiz S, Wiman B 1983 Fibrinolytic activity in plasma and deep vein thrombosis after major abdominal surgery. Thrombosis Research 32: 575

Merton R E, Hockley D, Gray E, Poole S, Thomas D P 1991 The effect of interleukin-1 on venous endothelium – an ultrastructural study. Thrombosis and Haemostasis 66: 725–729

Moncada S, Herman A G, Higgs E A, Vane J R 1977 Differential formation of prostacyclin (PGX or PGI_2) by layers of the arterial wall. An explanation for the anti-thrombotic properties of vascular endothelium. Thrombosis Research 11: 323

Mustard J F, Packham M A 1977 Normal and abnormal haemostasis. British Medical Bulletin 33: 187

Nawroth P P, Handley D A, Esmon C T, Stern D M 1986 Interleukin 1 induces endothelial cell procoagulant while suppressing cell surface anticoagulant. Proceedings of the National Academy of Sciences, USA 83: 3460–3464

Nicolaides A N, Kakkar V V, Field E S, Renney J T G 1971 The origin of deep vein thrombosis: a venographic study. British Journal of Radiology 44: 653

Niewiarowski S, Regoeczi E, Stewart G J, Senyi A F, Mustard J F 1972 Platelet interaction with polymerizing fibrin. Journal of Clinical Investigation 51: 685

Owen J, Kvam D, Nossel H L, Kaplan K L, Kernoff P B A 1983 Thrombin and plasmin activity and platelet activation in the development of venous thrombosis. Blood 61: 476

Pandolfi M, Nilsson I-M, Robertson B, Isacson S 1967 Fibrinolytic activity of human veins. Lancet 2: 127

Pandolfi M, Isacson S, Nilsson I-M 1969 Low fibrinolytic activity in the walls of veins in patients with thrombosis. Acta Scandinavica 186: 1

Sas G, Domjan G, Pal A 1991 Coagulation inhibition in venous thrombosis. New England Journal of Medicine 324: 1288

Schaub R G, Simmons C A, Koets M H, Romano P J, Stewart G J 1984 Early events in the formation of a venous thrombus following local trauma and stasis. Laboratory Investigation 51: 218

Schleef R R, Bevilacqua M P, Sawdey M, Gimbrone M A, Loskutoff D J 1988 Cytokine activation of vascular endothelium. Journal of Biological Chemistry 263: 5797–5803

Scurr J H, Ibrahim S Z, Faber R G, Le Quesne L P 1977 The efficacy of graduated compression stockings in the prevention of deep vein thrombosis. British Journal of Surgery 64: 371

Sevitt S 1974 The structure and growth of valve-pocket thrombi in femoral veins. Journal of Clinical Pathology 27: 517

Sevitt S 1978 Pathology and pathogenesis of deep vein thrombi. In: Bergan J J, Yao J S T (eds) Venous problems. Year Book, Chicago, p 257

Sevitt S, Gallagher N G 1959 Prevention of venous thrombosis and pulmonary embolism in injured patients. A trial of anticoagulant prophylaxis with phenindione in middle-aged and elderly patients with fractured necks of femur. Lancet 2: 981

Sheppard B L, French J E 1971 Platelet adhesion in the rabbit abdominal aorta following the removal of the endothelium: a scanning and transmission electron microscopical study. Proceedings of the Royal Society London, Series B 176: 427

Sixma J J, Wester J 1977 The haemostatic plug. Seminars in Hematology 14: 265

Smith J B, Willis A L 1971 Aspirin selectively inhibits prostaglandin production in human platelets. Nature 231: 235

Stamatakis J D, Kakkar V V, Sagar S, Lawrence D, Nairn D, Bentley P G 1977 Femoral vein thrombosis and total hip replacement. British Medical Journal 2: 223
Stamatakis J D, Kakkar V V, Lawrence D, Bentley P G 1978 The origin of thrombi in the deep veins of the lower limb: a venographic study. British Journal of Surgery 65: 449
Stenflo J 1984 Structure and function of protein C. Seminars in Thrombosis and Haemostasis 10: 109
Stern D M, Kaiser E, Nawroth P P 1988 Regulation of the coagulation system by vascular endothelial cells. Haemostasis 186: 202–214
Stewart G J, Ritchie W G M, Lynch P R 1974 Venous endothelial damage produced by massive sticking and emigration of leucocytes. American Journal of Pathology 74: 507
Stewart G J, Stern H S, Lynch P R, Malmud L S, Schaub R G 1980 Responses of canine jugular veins and carotid arteries to hysterectomy: increased permeability and leucocyte adhesions and invasion. Thrombosis Research 20: 473
Stuart R K, Thomas D P 1967 Comparative effects of ADP and thrombin in producing stasis thrombi. Thrombosis et Diathesis Haemorrhagica 18: 537
Thomas D P, Wessler S 1964 Stasis thrombi induced by bacterial endotoxin. Circulation Research 14: 486
Thomas D P, Merton R E, Hiller K F, Hockley D 1982 Resistance of normal endothelium to damage by thrombin. British Journal of Haematology 51: 25
Thomas D P, Merton R E, Hockley D J 1983 The effect of stasis on the venous endothelium: an ultrastructural study. British Journal of Haematology 55: 113
Thomas D P, Merton R E, Wood R D, Hockley D J 1985 The relationship between vessel wall injury and venous thrombosis: an experimental study. British Journal of Haematology 59: 449
Thomas M Lea, O'Dwyer J A 1977 Site of origin of deep vein thrombosis in the calf. Acta Radiologica Diagnosis 18: 418
Virchow R 1860 Cellular pathology. John Churchill, London
Wessler S 1962 Thrombosis in the presence of vascular stasis. American Journal of Medicine 33: 648
Wessler S, Reimer S M, Sheps M C 1959 Biologic assay of a thrombosis-inducing activity in human serum. Journal of Applied Physiology 14: 943
Wight T N 1980 Vessel proteoglycans and thrombogenesis. Progress in Hemostasis and Thrombosis 5: 1
Wiman B, Ljungberg G, Chmielewska J, Urdén G, Blombäck M, Johnsson H 1985 The role of the fibrinolytic system in deep vein thrombosis. Journal of Laboratory and Clinical Medicine 105: 265

61. Familial venous thrombophilia

C. F. Allaart E. Briët

Prior to the discovery of blood coagulation inhibitors, the importance of familial venous thrombophilia was not widely appreciated. Consecutive editions of the major internal medicine text books have included sections on this topic only since the description of protein C and protein S deficiency in the 1980s. Apparently, the older literature (Briggs 1905, Grafe 1924, Jordan & Nandorff 1956) did not get much attention.

The prevalence of familial venous thrombophilia is unknown. Most investigators have concentrated on the deficiencies of well-defined coagulation inhibitors in selected patient groups (Briët et al 1987, Scharrer et al 1987, Gladson et al 1988, Ben Tal et al 1989, Tabernero et al 1991) while few attempts have been made to estimate the prevalence of families with a tendency to venous thrombosis, within a particular population. Heijboer et al (1990) found a positive family history in 67 out of 277 patients with well-documented deep vein thrombosis (24%), which may be considered as an indication for the prevalence of hereditary factors among unselected thrombosis patients. However, in only 11 out of these 67 patients (16%) was an isolated deficiency found that was considered to explain the thrombotic tendency. Thus, about a quarter of the 277 patients with thrombosis might possess some inherited risk factor while such risk factors were detected in only 4%. This may imply that a positive family history is not specific for true familial thrombophilia or, alternatively, that we cannot detect all the biochemical abnormalities that lead to familial thrombophilia. Heijboer as well as other investigators have assigned a positive family history to any proband who has either a first degree or second degree relative with a history of deep vein thrombosis or pulmonary embolism. Defined in this way, the specificity of the family history as an instrument to detect autosomal dominant venous thrombophilia is too low. Based on age-specific incidence rates of thrombosis in the general population we may expect at least 25% of all patients with thrombosis to have one or more symptomatic relatives of the first or second degree depending on the size of the family and the ages of the family members. Similarly, for pedigrees with protein C deficiency an index patient may have as many as five affected relatives based on the age-specific incidence rates of thrombosis in subjects with protein C deficiency and on the size of the family (Briët 1992). Consequently, future studies should be carried out with more stringent requirements for a positive family history.

A comparison of the prevalences of the major inhibitor deficiencies for different patient populations is given in Table 61.1. These data illustrate that patient populations referred to centres with a special interest in familial thrombophilia have higher prevalences for each of the deficiencies than unselected patients with deep vein thrombosis. In the groups of blood donors the prevalences are even lower.

In this chapter we shall discuss the potential causes of familial venous thrombophilia and we shall describe in some detail the clinical aspects of the syndrome with particular emphasis on the deficiencies of antithrombin III, protein C and protein S.

Table 61.1 Prevalence of antithrombin III, protein C and protein S deficiency in different patient populations

	AT III	Protein C	Protein S
Healthy donors			
Tait et al 1991	3/4200[1]	–	–
Miletich et al 1987	–	1/250	–
Tait et al 1992	–	1/1000[2]	–
DVT unselected			
Heijboer et al 1990	3/277	9/277	6/277
DVT selected			
Briët et al 1987	5/113	9/113	15/113
Scharrer et al 1987	8/158	15/158	10/158
Gladson et al 1988	–	6/141	7/141
Ben Tal et al 1989	8/107	6/107	3/107
Tabernero et al 1991	1/204	3/204	3/204

[1] Excluding type 2c; [2] Probably an underestimate due to incomplete data.

POTENTIAL CAUSES OF FAMILIAL VENOUS THROMBOPHILIA

The haemostatic mechanism is controlled by several safeguards to avoid excessive clot formation and to allow clot resolution after haemostasis has served its primary purpose (Table 61.2). Abnormalities or deficiencies of these safeguards may be expected to increase the risk of thrombosis or diffuse intravascular coagulation. Generally speaking one might anticipate any inherited condition associated with increased rates of thrombin formation as a potential cause of inherited thrombophilia. Such a condition might be due to low levels of procoagulant inhibitors or to high levels of the procoagulant components themselves. Likewise, delayed fibrinolysis due to low levels of profibrinolytic components, to high levels of fibrinolytic inhibitors or to abnormalities in fibrin might have the same effect. In this chapter, our starting point is the family with a tendency to recurrent superficial or deep venous thrombosis and pulmonary embolism and one of the questions to be answered is which of the potential causes have been shown to be true causes of this inherited syndrome. The causal relationship between an abnormality of one of the components with the inherited thrombotic syndrome cannot be accepted unless the abnormality co-segregates with the clinical manifestations in the pedigree. The cases of plasminogen deficiency and dysplasminogenaemia may serve as examples to illustrate this critical approach.

We re-analysed the data published by Shigekiyo et al (1992) concerning two families with type 1 plasminogen deficiency and summarized the findings in Table 61.3. The data do not lend support to a clinically significant association between the deficiency and thrombosis. A somewhat absurd result is found if we carry out the same analysis on the dysplasminogenaemia family published by Aoki et al (1978) (Table 61.4). The proband had an impressive history of serious thrombotic events, but none of his relatives was symptomatic. Moreover one of the relatives with dysplasminogenaemia appeared homozygous or double heterozygous for the defect and had plasminogen activity levels as low as 10% of normal. This person is now 21 years of age and has remained asymptomatic thus far (Aoki 1992). Considering these findings we feel that the case for a causal relationship between type 1 plasminogen deficiency and dysplasminogenaemia with venous thrombotic disease is weak at best. The same conclusion was reached by Dolan & Preston (1988).

Table 61.2 Regulators of blood coagulation

Component	Function
Antithrombin III Heparin cofactor II	Serine protease inhibition
TFPI	Inhibition of factor VIIa–tissue factor complex
Thrombomodulin	Inhibition of thrombin, activation of protein C
Protein C Protein S	Inhibition of factors Va and VIIIa
β_2-Glycoprotein I	Inhibition of coagulant-active phospholipids
t-PA Plasminogen Factor XII	Profibrinolytic factors
PAI HRG	Antifibrinolytic factors

TFPI, tissue factor pathway inhibitor; t-PA, tissue plasminogen activator; PAI, plasminogen activator inhibitor; HRG, histidine-rich glycoprotein.

Table 61.3 The association between plasminogen deficiency and thrombosis. Re-analysis of data from Shigekiyo et al (1992).

		History of thrombosis	
		yes	no
Plasminogen deficiency	yes	2	17
	no	0	19

Probands were excluded from the analysis. Chi-square = 2.1, $p > 0.1$.

Table 61.4 The association between dysplasminogenaemia and thrombosis (re-analysis of data from Aoki et al 1978).

		History of thrombosis	
		yes	no
Dysplasminogenaemia	yes	0	13
	no	0	4

Three families have been described (Johansson et al 1978, Jorgensen et al 1982, Stead et al 1983) with autosomal dominant thrombophilia supposedly caused by defective fibrinolytic activity. Unfortunately, protein C and S assays were not available at the time of these studies and the methodology of the assays for tissue plasminogen activator (t-PA) and its inhibitor (PAI-1) has been improved considerably since then. Other and later studies concerning the components of the fibrinolytic system, plasminogen (Aoki et al 1978, Dolan et al 1988, Shigekiyo et al 1992), histidine-rich glycoprotein (HRG) (Engesser et al 1987b) and PAI-1 (Engesser et al 1989) have not resulted in simple genetic associations between deficiencies (t-PA, plasminogen) or excessive concentrations (PAI-1, HRG) and the thrombophilic syndrome. Although a recent study (Grimaudo et al 1992) demonstrates that high levels of PAI-1 are associated with an increased risk of thrombosis, the evidence for hypofibrinolysis as a cause of dominant thrombophilia is weak.

Factor XII deficiency has been shown by several authors (Goodnough et al 1983, Mannhalter et al 1987, Lammle et al 1991) to be associated with an increased risk of thrombosis which may be explained by its role in the contact system-dependent pathway of plasminogen activation (Binnema et al 1990). However, family studies that prove factor XII deficiency to cause familial thrombophilia are not available.

In contrast, convincing evidence is available that the deficiencies of antithrombin III, protein C and protein S are associated with inherited thrombophilia. The case for dysfibrinogenaemia is less clear, but a small number of pedigrees support the notion that some forms of this disorder may be closely associated with thrombophilia. A convincing example is the pedigree of fibrinogen Vlissingen (Koopman et al 1991) which appeared to be linked to the Frankfurt IV pedigree which carries the same mutation (Briët & Haverkate 1992) (see also Ch. 22). In these families, venous as well as arterial thrombosis occurs.

Heparin cofactor II, theoretically a very attractive candidate cause of familial thrombophilia has not fulfilled this promise (Bertina et al 1987). Tissue factor pathway inhibitor (TFPI), formerly known as LACI, is the inhibitor of the factor VIIa-tissue factor complex. Since plasma concentrations of this surface-bound inhibitor may not reflect the functional state of the TFPI-gene in heterozygotes, we have sequenced the exons of this gene in 30 subjects with unexplained familial thrombophilia in order to find mutations that might explain thrombophilia; not a single mutation was found (Reitsma 1992). A similar disappointment was the result of studying the thrombomodulin gene (Reitsma 1992). Another interesting candidate cause for familial thrombophilia would be a deficiency of β_2-glycoprotein I, a putative regulator of coagulant-active phospholipid surfaces (Nimpf et al 1986). However, Bancsi et al (1992) found very similar prevalences for the deficiency in patients with unexplained familial thrombophilia and in normals. Moreover, one subject homozygous for the deficiency was still asymptomatic at age 35.

Homocystinuria is a rare, autosomal recessive disorder, usually due to cystathionine β-synthase deficiency and characterized by mental retardation, ectopia lentis, skeletal abnormalities and venous as well as arterial thrombophilia (Mudd et al 1985). At age 30, about 50% of the patients have suffered one or more thrombotic episodes, half of them venous and half arterial. The unresolved question is whether heterozygotes for the deficiency also run a higher than normal risk for thrombosis, as has been suggested by several authors (Bienvenu et al 1991, Brattstrom et al 1991, Clarke et al 1991). Since family studies have not been described in the subjects it is too early to decide whether cases of unexplained venous thrombophilia are due to this disorder.

Summarizing these data, we conclude that autosomal dominant venous thrombophilia may be caused by deficiencies of antithrombin III, protein C, protein S and by dysfibrinogenaemia. Indications that abnormalities of the other components of the system are associated with venous thrombosis are usually based on studies in unrelated patients and controls. Apparently the associated risk is not high enough to cause the familial syndrome. These findings are relevant for the choice of diagnostic tests in patients with venous thrombosis and pulmonary embolism. The search for simple genetic defects underlying autosomal dominant inherited thrombophilia remains wide open.

Antithrombin III deficiency

Thrombophilia due to antithrombin III deficiency was described first by Egeberg (1965). Since then about 200 families have been reported and several reviews are available which provide an excellent description of this autosomal dominant disorder. The most useful reviews have been published by Thaler & Lechner (1981) and by Hirsh et al (1989). Chapter 29 in this book is devoted to antithrombin III and focuses on the genetics and the biochemical aspects. In this section we shall limit ourselves to the clinical consequences of the disorder and we shall adhere to the classification of Lane et al (1991). The clinical meaning of this classification is that deficiencies of type 1, 2a and 2b are associated with thrombophilia in heterozygotes. Type 2c, characterized by abnormalities in heparin binding gives thrombophilia only in the rare homozygous patients.

As shown by Tait et al (1991), heterozygous antithrombin III deficiency (not type 2c) occurs in seven per 10 000 population and figures up to 100-fold higher are found in groups of selected patients with thrombosis (Table 61.1). Thaler & Lechner (1981) as well as Hirsh et al (1989) have calculated the cumulative risk of thrombosis from the available published family studies and arrived at strikingly similar results: the risk of a first thrombotic episode is 10% up to age 15, 50% up to age 24 and 85% up to age 50. The thrombotic tendency of antithrombin III deficiency seems to be more severe than that of the deficiencies of protein C and protein S (Table 61.5). Several authors have suggested that the deficiency is associated with significant mortality (Anonymous 1983, Cosgriff et al 1983, Michiels & van Vliet 1984). However, a formal study by Rosendaal et al (1991) on this issue did not reveal any excess mortality in comparison with the population at large.

The clinical manifestations of antithrombin III, protein C and protein S deficiency, are very similar (Table 61.6), but antithrombin III deficiency is less often associated

Table 61.5 The risk of a first thrombotic episode associated with hereditary defects

	Risk of first thrombotic episode (%)		
Deficiency of	up to 15 yr	up to 24 yr	up to 50 yr
Antithrombin III	10	50	85
Protein S	1	40	80
Protein C	1	15	50

(Based on data from Thaler & Lechner (1981), Hirsh et al (1989), Engesser et al (1987) and Allaart et al (1993).

Table 61.6 Clinical manifestations in heterozygotes for hereditary antithrombin III deficiency, protein C deficiency and protein S deficiency

Common:	Superficial vein thrombosis, often recurrent (mainly in protein C and protein S deficiency)
	Deep vein thrombosis in the legs or pelvis
	Pulmonary embolism
Also reported:	Coumarin-associated skin necrosis (mostly in protein C deficiency)
	Thrombosis in cerebral, mesenteric, portal, axillary, inferior caval, renal and retinal veins
	Arterial occlusions in coronary, femoral, splanchnic and cerebral arteries

with superficial venous thrombosis. A second difference is that pregnancy carries a higher risk of thrombotic complications in antithrombin III deficiency than in the deficiencies of protein C or protein S (Table 61.7). There are case reports of arterial thrombosis in patients with antithrombin III deficiency (Winter et al 1982a, Hossmann et al 1983, Coller et al 1987, Johnson et al 1990) and there is epidemiological evidence that low as well as high levels of antithrombin III are associated with increased risk of arterial disease (Meade et al 1991). However, the general impression is that arterial disease is not a feature of antithrombin III deficiency (Thaler & Lechner 1981, Cosgriff et al 1983, Hirsh et al 1989), with the exception of homozygous type 2c deficiency where venous as well as arterial thrombosis may occur at a very young age (Koide et al 1984, Brunel et al 1987, Ueyama et al 1990).

Protein C deficiency

Protein C, the vitamin K-dependent zymogen of a serine protease, is one of the major regulatory proteins of the coagulation cascade. Based on its anticoagulant and profibrinolytic properties, it was hypothesized that an inherited deficiency of protein C would present as a congenital tendency to develop venous thrombosis (Esmon & Owen 1981). In 1981 the first family with hereditary protein C deficiency and thrombotic disease was reported (Griffin et al 1981). Numerous others followed (Bertina et al 1982, Broekmans et al 1983b, Pabinger Fasching et al 1983, Horellou et al 1984) and since 1983 homozygotes with severe protein C deficiency have been reported also (Branson et al 1983, Marciniak et al 1983, Seligsohn et al 1984, Samama et al 1984).

Table 61.7 Pregnancy and thrombotic events in hereditary deficiencies of antithrombin III, protein C and protein S

Deficiency	No. of events/ No. of pregnancies	No of events during pregnancy/ postpartum	References
AT III	32/47	24/8	Hellgren et al 1982
AT III	27/63	9/18	Conard et al 1990
Protein S	10/44	0/10	Conard et al 1990
Protein C	33/93	5/28	Conard et al 1990
Protein C	15/87	6/9	Allaart et al 1993

Two types of hereditary protein C deficiency can be recognized based on gene product measurement: type I deficiency, where both protein C antigen and protein C activity are below the lower limit of the normal range, and type II deficiency, where the protein C antigen is within the normal range, but the protein C activity and the ratio of protein C activity over protein C antigen are below the normal range (Bertina et al 1984). However, there is an overlap between protein C levels measured in carriers of the genetic defect and in normals (Allaart et al 1993). DNA analysis now can be used to identify heterozygotes for the genetic defect underlying the deficiency. The gene for protein C is localized on chromosome 2 (Patracchini et al 1989) and it consists of nine exons (Foster et al 1985, Plutzky et al 1986). Since 1987 (Romeo et al 1987) genetic defects have been described in a large number of patients, both heterozygotes with type I or type II deficiency and homozygotes, or compound heterozygotes (Matsuda et al 1988, Grundy et al 1989, Bovill et al 1991, Gandrille et al 1991, Reitsma et al 1991a, Tsuda et al 1991).

There appear to be no differences in clinical presentation between heterozygotes who have different mutations. In symptomatic families, heterozygotes have an increased risk of developing venous thrombotic events that may occur in a wide variety of localities (Wintzen et al 1985, Green et al 1987, Orozco et al 1988, Harle et al 1989, Prat et al 1989, Allaart et al 1993) (Table 61.5). Often the thrombotic events occur 'spontaneously', at a relatively early age (Horellou et al 1984, Broekmans 1985), and recurrences are frequent (Broekmans 1985). A few cases of patients with protein C deficiency and arterial thrombotic disease have been reported (Griffin et al 1981, Horellou et al 1984, Coller et al 1987, Israels & Seshia, 1987). Whether heterozygotes in families with the deficiency and venous thrombophilia have an increased risk of developing early arterial occlusive disease is not yet clear. The data are limited. In our study of 24 families with protein C deficiency and venous thrombophilia, we found that heterozygotes appeared not to have arterial occlusions at an earlier age than their normal relatives (Allaart et al 1991).

Coumarin-induced skin necrosis has been reported in several patients (Broekmans et al 1983a,b, Klingemann et al 1984, McGehee et al 1984, Samama et al 1984, Pabinger et al 1986, Gladson et al 1987). It is thought to be caused by a discrepancy between concentrations of protein C, which has a half life of 6 hours, and other vitamin K-dependent clotting factors with longer half life times, during the starting phase of the anticoagulant therapy or during a period of increasing intensity of the therapy (Teepe et al 1986). This would explain the process of thrombosis in the subcutaneous microcirculation which leads to interstitial bleeding and necrosis of the dermis and subcutaneous fat tissue. However, coumarin-induced necrosis has also been described in patients heterozygous for protein S deficiency, even though protein S has a much longer half life of approximately 60 hours.

Clinical manifestations in children with severe protein C deficiency, who are homozygotes or compound heterozygotes, appear to be related to the level of protein C in plasma (Marlar & Neumann 1990). Infants with undetectable levels of protein C develop purpura fulminans shortly after birth (Branson et al 1983, Marciniak et al 1983, 1985, Samama et al 1984, Seligsohn et al 1984, Sills et al 1984, Auletta & Headington 1988, Peters et al 1988, Marlar et al 1989a, Marlar & Mastovich 1990). In a mechanism resembling that of coumarin-necrosis, microthrombi in the subcutaneous vessels lead to potentially lethal skin necrosis. The disorder is associated often with severe disseminated intravascular coagulation (Auletta & Headington 1988, Marlar et al 1989b, Marlar & Mastovich 1990). Cerebral and ophthalmic thrombosis may occur before birth (Marlar & Neumann 1990). If protein C levels are very low, but still detectable, skin necrosis may be absent, but life-threatening thrombosis in large vessels may develop (Seligsohn et al 1984). Recently, a number of homozygous protein C-deficient patients have been described with relatively high levels of protein C who suffered from less severe thrombotic disease which occurred at age 5 to 15 years (Estelles et al 1984, Manabe & Matsuda 1985, Sharon et al 1986, Marlar et al 1989b, Tuddenham et al 1989, Conard et al 1992).

It was hypothesized that there are two phenotypes of hereditary protein C deficiency (Bertina et al 1988). The first is the clinically dominant type where heterozygotes are symptomatic as described above. Based on the identification of such heterozygotes in selected patient groups, the prevalence in the population is estimated to be one in 16 000 (Broekmans et al 1983a), from which follows that homozygosity of this type must be rare (1:250 000 000). The other is a clinically recessive type where heterozygotes are asymptomatic and homozygotes are severely ill from birth or later in life. Based on the not so rare reports of homozygotes, and on the identification of asymptomatic heterozygotes among healthy volunteers, the prevalence in the population of the latter type is estimated to be one in 200 to 300 (Miletich et al 1987) or one in 1000 (Tait et al 1992). Surprisingly, identical genetic defects have been identified in both the clinically dominant and the clinically recessive types of protein C deficiency (Grundy et al 1989, Bovill et al 1991, Reitsma et al 1991b, Tsuda et al 1991). Consequently, it may well be that other factors, possibly also familial, play a part in the clinical expression of hereditary defects like protein C deficiency.

Protein S deficiency

Protein S is the non-enzymatic cofactor of activated protein C in the 'protein C anticoagulant pathway' (Walker 1980, 1981, Suzuki et al 1983, 1984, de Fouw et al 1986). In plasma it is present in both a free form and bound to complement factor 4b-binding protein (C4b-binding protein) (Dahlback 1983a,b). Only the free form is functionally active (Bertina et al 1985, Dahlback 1986). Since 1984 many families with venous thrombophilia and hereditary protein S deficiency have been reported (Schwarz et al 1984, Broekmans et al 1985, Young et al 1991). It is thought that the high affinity of C4b-binding protein for protein S causes free protein S to be very low when total protein S is reduced, or when acute phase reactant C4b-binding protein is increased, whereas very high levels of free protein S are found in cases were C4b-binding protein is deficient (Comp et al 1990, Griffin et al 1991, Nelson & Long 1991). Based on the measurement of both protein S and C4b-binding protein, there appear to be three different types of protein S deficiency. In type I protein S deficiency the total amount of protein S is reduced and free protein S is often very low since most will be bound to C4b-binding protein (Griffin et al 1991). In type II, the total amount of protein S as well as the equilibrium between free and bound protein S is normal, but an abnormal protein S molecule has reduced activity (Mannucci et al 1989); and in type III total protein S levels are normal, but the equilibrium between free and bound protein S is shifted towards the bound form (Comp et al 1986a). We do not favour the alternative classification by Comp et al (Comp et al 1986a), where type I deficiency describes cases with normal concentrations of complexed protein S but low concentrations of free protein S, and where type II refers to low concentrations of both free and complexed protein S, since it is not analogous with the classifications for protein C and antithrombin III deficiency, the haemophilias and von Willebrand's disease.

In the interpretation of laboratory results, one should be aware that protein S levels can be markedly decreased during pregnancy (Comp et al 1985, Comp et al 1986b) as well as during use of oestrogens in high dosage for growth retardation (Huisveld et al 1987) and to a lesser extent during the use of oral contraceptives (Boerger et al 1987). On average, protein S levels in women are slightly lower than in men (Boerger et al 1987). Protein S levels decrease during vitamin K deficiency and treatment with vitamin K-antagonists (Bertina et al 1985).

DNA-analysis can be of help in identifying heterozygotes for hereditary protein S deficiency. Two highly homologous genes for protein S are located on chromosome 3 (Ploos van Amstel et al 1987). The PSα gene consists of 15 exons and is the active gene, whereas the PSβ gene is a pseudogene which contains several splice-site, nonsense and missense mutations that make gene expression impossible (Ploos van Amstel et al 1990). Genetic abnormalities in the PSα gene, but also in the PSβ gene, have been identified in a number of families with hereditary protein S deficiency (Ploos van Amstel et al 1989a,b, Bertina et al 1990, Schmidel et al 1991).

The clinical manifestations of hereditary protein S deficiency are similar to those of antithrombin III and protein C deficiency (Table 61.5): heterozygotes in symptomatic families have an increased risk of developing venous thrombotic events at a relatively young age, often 'spontaneous' and often recurrent (Engesser et al 1987). Patients with arterial occlusions and protein S deficiency have also been reported (Mannucci et al 1986, Coller et al 1987, Israels & Seshia 1987, Schafer & von Felten 1989, Davous et al 1990, Girolami et al 1990). In a group of 37 consecutive patients who had manifestations of arterial occlusive disease before the age of 45, we found three individuals (8%) with a hereditary protein S deficiency (Allaart et al 1990). However, a study of the families of the three subjects did not show co-segregation of the arterial disease with the protein S deficiency.

There have been several reports of patients with protein S deficiency who developed skin necrosis during coumarin therapy (Friedman et al 1986, Grimaudo et al 1989, Moreb & Kitchens 1989, Goldberg et al 1991). This cannot be explained by a rapid decrease in protein S while other vitamin-K dependent factors are still relatively high, since the half life time of protein S is approximately 60 hours (Broekmans et al 1985). Therefore it is doubtful whether the theory on the development of coumarin-necrosis that was described earlier for protein C deficiency is a sufficient explanation for the phenomenon.

Severe protein S deficiency, possibly homozygous or double heterozygous, has now been reported twice (Mahasandana et al 1990, Pegelow et al 1992). The two infants developed purpura fulminans shortly after birth similar to the manifestations seen in homozygotes for protein C deficiency. Both parents of the first child were heterozygous, and healthy. The second child's father was not available for testing. There was no family history of thrombotic tendency nor was there consanguinity in either of the two families.

TREATMENT AND PROPHYLAXIS

All heterozygotes for known defects like antithrombin III, protein C and protein S deficiency, as well as members of families with unexplained thrombophilia need to be informed about the risk for thrombosis. Guidelines for treatment and prophylaxis should be given on an individual basis.

In the case of an episode of acute thrombosis, treatment with intravenous heparin and coumarins should be started simultaneously (Hull et al 1990, Brandjes et al 1992). Heparin may be discontinued when the intensity of oral anticoagulation is within the therapeutic range. In protein C-deficient patients and probably protein S-deficient patients as well, high initial doses of oral anticoagulant therapy should not be given, to avoid the development of coumarin-related necrosis. If this does develop, vitamin K_1 should be given parenterally and coumarin therapy may be temporarily suspended but need not be withdrawn (Teepe et al 1986).

Since recurrences tend to occur, long-term prophylaxis with oral anticoagulation may be considered to avoid 'spontaneous' recurrences after a first episode. Another option is to discontinue the treatment after 3 months and start prophylactic anticoagulation in situations of increased risk for venous thrombotic events, in particular after severe burns, trauma or surgery, after childbirth, during periods of immobilization, and in cases of cardiac disease or malignancy (Hirsh et al 1986). In our study of 24 families with hereditary protein C deficiency, we found that heterozygotes have a substantially greater increase in the risk for thrombosis associated with surgery or immobilization than their unaffected relatives (Table 61.8) (Allaart et al 1993). It is our opinion that in risk situations prophylactic anticoagulation is indicated for all heterozygotes, whether they have had earlier symptoms or not. Patients with recurrent thrombotic episodes should probably be receiving long-term prophylaxis with coumarin derivatives. Scientific data on the risk–benefit ratio of such a policy are unavailable, however.

As is shown in Table 61.7, pregnancy carries a considerable risk for thrombosis, particularly in antithrombin III deficiency (Winter et al 1982b, Conard et al 1990, Allaart et al 1993). Unfortunately, anticoagulant treatment during pregnancy is not without difficulties. Obviously, both treatment with heparin and with coumarins may cause bleeding complications for the mother. Oral anticoagulants, which cross the placenta, may cause fetal complications: coumarin embryopathy, which is related to exposure to coumarins in the first trimester, and central nervous system abnormalities and fetal bleeding, which may occur in any trimester. An increased rate of fetal loss has also been reported (Hall et al 1980, Iturbe-Alessio et al 1986, Briët et al 1988, Ginsberg et al 1989, Hirsh, 1991). Heparin does not cross the placenta, but may cause maternal heparin-induced osteoporosis (Wise & Hall, 1980, Howell et al 1983, Briët et al 1988). Considering

Table 61.8 Risk of thrombotic events (incidence rate ratios) associated with surgery and immobilization in normals and in heterozygous protein C deficiency (Allaart et al 1993).

	Incidence rate ratios*	
	Immobilization	Surgery
Normals	4.5	3.2
Heterozygotes	8.4	11.8

* Incidence rate ratios were calculated as the ratio of the incidence of events during years with a risk situation over the incidence of events during years without a risk situation.

the possible complications, we feel that prophylactic anticoagulation during pregnancy should not be advised as a routine for asymptomatic women who are heterozygous for protein C or protein S deficiency or who are members of families with unexplained thrombophilia. In our opinion it is justified to continue prophylactic anticoagulation in women who have been receiving it prior to pregnancy, provided the original indication was sound. In addition, the risk of thrombosis during pregnancy in previously asymptomatic antithrombin III deficiency also warrants prophylaxis. If anticoagulation is decided upon, we find the following approach convenient and safe: subcutaneous heparin, in a dosage that leads to APTTs of 1.5 times normal, is started as soon as conception is confirmed, replacing coumarins in cases of long-term anticoagulant treatment. After the 14th week of gestation coumarins with a short half life are restarted to continue up to the 36th week of pregnancy, when they are once more replaced by heparin. Coumarins with a short half life like warfarin or acenocoumarol are preferred to avoid bleeding complications for the child during parturition. On the 1st day postpartums oral anticoagulants can be started to prevent thrombotic complications of childbed both in symptomatic women and asymptomatic women with increased risk.

The use of oral contraceptives has been associated with an increased risk for venous thrombosis (Stadel 1981a,b). The effect appears to be dose-related but definitive data on the increase of the risk associated with the modern oral contraceptives are not available. Böttiger et al (1980) reported that the incidence of thrombosis among women in Scandinavia has decreased since the use of low oestrogen oral contraceptives. Gerstman et al (1991) calculated a rate of 0.42 venous thrombotic events per 1000 person-years in women who used oral contraceptives containing less than 50 μg ethinyloestradiol. A survey by the Leiden regional thrombosis service shows that the incidence of venous thrombotic events among women between 20 and 45 years of age is 0.71 per 1000 person-years, and among men of the same age range, 0.40 per 1000 person-years (Briët et al 1992). Considering that more than 50% of these women use oral contraceptives and that pregnancies and childbeds also contribute to the difference, the thrombogenic potential of the currently available oral contraceptives must be small. It is not known whether oral contraceptives add substantially to the risk of thrombosis in patients with familial thrombophilia. However, women with protein C and protein S deficiency were found not to have a higher risk for thrombotic events than men, despite the use of oral contraceptives and histories of pregnancies and childbirth (Engesser et al 1987a, Allaart et al 1993). We feel that the modern low-dose contraceptive pill can be prescribed if alternative ways of contraception are not acceptable.

As an alternative to oral anticoagulation, several groups have studied the role of anabolic steroids that raise the plasma concentrations of protein C, antithrombin III and other factors (Preston et al 1983, Kluft et al 1984, Winter et al 1984, Broekmans et al 1987). It appeared however, that prophylactic treatment with stanozolol does not prevent thrombosis in postoperative patients (Blamey et al 1984, 1985). Moreover we think that the disadvantages of long-term oral anticoagulation are less than those associated with anabolic steroids.

Homozygous and double-heterozygous protein C-deficient children who develop purpura fulminans should speedily be treated with fresh frozen plasma (FFP), 10 to 15 ml/kg every 12 hours, while other thrombotic complications should be treated symptomatically (Marlar et al 1989a). For long-term treatment of homozygous protein C deficiency, administration of protein C in the form of FFP, prothrombin complex concentrate or protein C concentrate (Vukovich et al 1988, Dreyfus et al 1991) has been successful, but the disadvantages of parenteral administration are the risk of thrombosis of the catheter, the risk of eventual loss of venous access, of local infections acquired from the catheter including septicaemia, and of transfusion-related diseases. Varying amounts of protein C in different lots of PCC may complicate stable dosage. Long-term FFP administration is not practical since it may lead to hyperproteinaemia and hypertension. To date, long-term administration of coumarins is the recommended treatment to prevent the recurrence of the symptoms although this may have adverse effects on bone development and growth in the developing child (Vermeer & Hamulyak 1991).

Antithrombin III concentrate has been used by several authors to prevent or to treat thrombosis in antithrombin III-deficient patients in the period around surgery (Mannucci et al 1982, Blanco et al 1989, Schwartz et al 1989, Menache et al 1990, Menache 1991) and around childbirth (Hellgren et al 1982, Michiels et al 1984, Samson et al 1984, Nelson et al 1985, De Stefano et al 1988, Inomoto et al 1991, Owen 1991). The reasoning behind this policy is that heparin depends on antithrombin III for its action and that it also causes antithrombin III concentrations to drop (Marciniak & Goeckerman 1977), which might lead to heparin resistance. There are indications that heparin resistance is the exception rather than the rule (Schulman & Tengborn 1992) and that childbirth can be managed with heparin alone (Vellenga et al 1983, Blondel-Hill & Mant 1992). We believe that antithrombin III concentrate can be reserved for antithrombin III-deficient patients with serious contraindications against anticoagulation and for patients in whom excessive doses of heparin are required to reach an adequate prolongation of the APTT.

REFERENCES

Allaart C F, Aronson D C, Ruys T et al 1990 Hereditary protein S deficiency in young adults with arterial occlusive disease. Thrombosis and Haemostasis 64: 206–210

Allaart C F, Poort S R, van den Velden P H, Reitsma P H, Bertina R M, Briët E 1991 Protein C deficiency is not a major risk factor for the development of arterial occlusions (abstract). Thrombosis and Haemostasis 65: 666

Allaart R C F, Poort S R, Rosendaal F R, Reitsma P H, Bertina R M, Briët E 1993 Hereditary protein C deficiency: carriers of the genetic defect have an increased risk for venous thrombotic events in symptomatic families. Lancet 341: 134–138

Anonymous 1983 Familial antithrombin III deficiency (editorial). Lancet 1: 1021–1023

Aoki N 1992 Personal communication

Aoki N, Moroi M, Sakata Y, Yoshida N, Matsuda M 1978 Abnormal plasminogen. A hereditary molecular abnormality found in a patient with recurrent thrombosis. Journal of Clinical Investigation 61: 1186–1195

Auletta M J, Headington J T 1988 Purpura fulminans. A cutaneous manifestation of severe protein C deficiency, see comments. Archives of Dermatology 124: 1387–1391

Bancsi L F J M, van der Linden I K, Bertina R M 1992 $Beta_2$-Glycoprotein I deficiency and the risk of thrombosis. Thrombosis and Haemostasis 67: 649–653

Ben Tal O, Zivelin A, Seligsohn U 1989 The relative frequency of hereditary thrombotic disorders among 107 patients with thrombophilia in Israel. Thrombosis and Haemostasis 61: 50–54

Bertina R M, Broekmans A W, van der Linden I K, Mertens K 1982 Protein C deficiency in a Dutch family with thrombotic disease. Thrombosis and Haemostasis 48: 1–5

Bertina R M, Broekmans A W, Krommenhoek van Es C, van Wijngaarden A 1984 The use of a functional and immunologic assay for plasma protein C in the study of the heterogeneity of congenital protein C deficiency. Thrombosis and Haemostasis 51: 1–5

Bertina R M, van Wijngaarden A, Reinalda Poot J, Poort S R, Bom V J 1985 Determination of plasma protein S – the protein cofactor of activated protein C. Thrombosis and Haemostasis 53: 268–272

Bertina R M, van der Linden I K, Engesser L, Muller H P, Brommer E J 1987 Hereditary heparin cofactor II deficiency and the risk of development of thrombosis. Thrombosis and Haemostasis 57: 196–200

Bertina R M, Briët E, Engesser L, Reitsma P H 1988 Protein C deficiency and the risk of venous thrombosis. New England Journal of Medicine 318: 931

Bertina R M, Ploos van Amstel H K, van Wijngaarden A et al 1990 Heerlen polymorphism of protein S, an immunologic polymorphism due to dimorphism of residue 460. Blood 76: 538–548

Bienvenu T, Ankri A, Chadefaux B, Kamoun P 1991 Plasma homocysteine assay in the exploration of thrombosis in young subjects. Presse Medicale 20: 985–988

Binnema D J, Dooijewaard G, van Iersel J J, Turion P N, Kluft C 1990 The contact system-dependent plasminogen activator from human plasma: identification and characterization. Thrombosis and Haemostasis 64: 390–397

Blamey S L, McArdie B M, Burns P, Carter D C, Lowe G D, Forbes C D 1984 A double-blind trial of intramuscular stanozolol in the prevention of postoperative deep vein thrombosis following elective abdominal surgery. Thrombosis and Haemostasis 51: 71–74

Blamey S L, Lowe G D, Bertina R M et al 1985 Protein C antigen levels in major abdominal surgery: relationships to deep vein thrombosis, malignancy and treatment with stanozolol. Thrombosis and Haemostasis 54: 622–625

Blanco A N, Meschengieser S, Penalva L B, Lazzari M A 1989 Prophylaxis during surgery in antithrombin III deficiency with low dose of concentrates. Thrombosis Research 56: 497–499

Blondel-Hill E, Mant M J 1992 The pregnant antithrombin III-deficient patient: Management without antithrombin III concentrate. Thrombosis Research 65: 193–198

Boerger L M, Morris P C, Thurnau G R, Esmon C T, Comp P C 1987 Oral contraceptives and gender affect protein S status. Blood 69: 692–694

Böttiger L E, Boman G, Eklund G, Westerholm B 1980 Oral contraceptives and thromboembolic disease: effect of lowering oestrogen content. Lancet 1: 1097–1101

Bovill E G, Tomczak J, Grant V, Pilimer E, Rainville I, Long G L 1991 Association of two novel mutations in the GLA-domain (Glu 20 to Ala and Val 34 to Met) with symptomatic type II protein C deficiency (abstract). Thrombosis and Haemostasis 65: 647

Brandjes D P M, Heijboer H, Büller H R, de Rijk M, Jagt H, ten Cate J W 1992 Acenocousmarol and heparin compared with acenocousmarol alone in the initial treatment of proximal vein thrombosis. New England Journal of Medicine 327: 1485–1489

Branson H E, Katz J, Marble R, Griffin J H 1983 Inherited protein C deficiency and coumarin-responsive chronic relapsing purpura fulminans in a newborn infant. Lancet 2: 1165–1168

Brattstrom L, Tengborn L, Lagerstedt C, Israelsson B, Hultberg B 1991 Plasma homocysteine in venous thromboembolism. Haemostasis 21: 51–57

Briët E 1992 Familial thrombotic disorders. State of the art lectures 24th ISH Congress, August 1992, London. British Journal of Haematology 81S: 74 (abstract)

Briët E, Haverkate F 1992 unpublished information

Briët E, Engesser L, Brommer E J P, Broekmans A W, Bertina R M 1987 Thrombophilia: its causes and a rough estimate of its prevalence (abstract). Thrombosis and Haemostasis 58: 39

Briët E, Broekmans A W, Engesser L 1988 Hereditary protein S deficiency. In: Bertina R M (ed) Protein C and related proteins. Churchill Livingstone, Edinburgh, p 203–212

Briggs J B 1905 Recurrent phlebitis of obscure origin. Johns Hopkins Hospital Bulletin 16: 228–233

Broekmans A W 1985 Hereditary protein C deficiency. Haemostasis 15: 233–240

Broekmans A W, Bertina R M, Loeliger E A, Hofmann V, Klingemann H G 1983a Protein C and the development of skin necrosis during anticoagulant therapy (letter). Thrombosis and Haemostasis 49: 251

Broekmans A W, van der Linden I K, Veltkamp J J, Bertina R M 1983b Prevalence of isolated protein C deficiency in patients with venous thrombotic disease and in the population (abstract). Thrombosis and Haemostasis 50: 350

Broekmans A W, Veltkamp J J, Bertina R M 1983c Congenital protein C deficiency and venous thromboembolism. A study of three Dutch families. New England Journal of Medicine 309: 340–344

Broekmans A W, Bertina R M, Reinalda Poot J et al 1985 Hereditary protein S deficiency and venous thrombo-embolism. A study in three Dutch families. Thrombosis and Haemostasis 53: 273–277

Broekmans A W, Conard J, van Weyenberg R G, Horellou M H, Kluft C, Bertina R M 1987 Treatment of hereditary protein C deficiency with stanozolol. Thrombosis and Haemostasis 57: 20–24

Brunel F, Duchange N, Fischer A M, Cohen G N, Zakin M M 1987 Antithrombin Alger: a new case of Arg 47–Cys mutation. American Journal of Hematology 25: 223–224

Clarke R, Daly L, Robinson K et al 1991 Hyperhomocysteinemia: an independent risk factor for vascular disease. New England Journal of Medicine 324: 1149–1155

Coller B S, Owen J, Jesty J et al 1987 Deficiency of plasma protein S, protein C, or antithrombin III and arterial thrombosis. Arteriosclerosis 7: 456–462

Comp P C, Vigano-D'Angelo A, Thurnau G R, Kaufmann C, Esmon C T 1985 Acquired protein S deficiency occurs in pregnancy, the nephrotic syndrome and systemic lupus erythematosus (abstract). Blood 66: 348a

Comp P C, Doray D, Patton D, Esmon C T 1986a An abnormal plasma distribution of protein S occurs in functional protein S deficiency. Blood 67: 504–508

Comp P C, Thurnau G R, Welsh J, Esmon C T 1986b Functional and immunologic protein S levels are decreased during pregnancy. Blood 68: 881–885

Comp P C, Forristall J, West C D, Trapp R G 1990 Free protein S levels are elevated in familial C4b-binding protein deficiency. Blood 76: 2527–2529

Conard J, Horellou M H, van Dreden P, Lecompte T, Samama M 1990 Thrombosis and pregnancy in congenital deficiencies in AT III, protein C or protein S: study of 78 women. Thrombosis and Haemostasis 63: 319–320

Conard J, Horellou M H, van Dreden P et al 1992 Homozygous protein C deficiency with late onset and recurrent coumarin-induced skin necrosis (letter). Lancet 339: 743–744

Cosgriff T M, Bishop D T, Hershgold E J et al 1983 Familial antithrombin III deficiency: its natural history, genetics, diagnosis and treatment. Medicine 62: 209–220

Dahlbäck B 1983a Purification of human C4b-binding protein and formation of its complex with vitamin K-dependent protein S. Biochemical Journal 209: 847–856

Dahlbäck B 1983b Purification of human vitamin K-dependent protein S and its limited proteolysis by thrombin. Biochemical Journal 209: 837–846

Dahlbäck B 1986 Inhibition of protein Ca cofactor function of human and bovine protein S by C4b-binding protein. Journal of Biological Chemistry 261: 12022–12027

Davous P, Horellou M H, Conard J, Samama M 1990 Cerebral infarction and familial protein S deficiency (letter). Stroke 21: 1760–1761

de Fouw N J, Haverkate F, Bertina R M, Koopman J, van Wijngaarden A, van Hinsbergh V W 1986 The cofactor role of protein S in the acceleration of whole blood clot lysis by activated protein C in vitro. Blood 67: 1189–1192

De Stefano V, Leone G, de Carolis S et al 1988 Management of pregnancy in women with antithrombin III congenital defect: report of four cases. Thrombosis and Haemostasis 59: 193–196

Dolan G, Preston F E 1988 Familial plasminogen deficiency and thromboembolism. Fibrinolysis 2 (suppl 2): 26–34

Dolan G, Greaves M, Cooper P, Preston F E 1988 Thrombovascular disease and familial plasminogen deficiency: a report of three kindreds. British Journal of Haematology 70: 417–421

Dreyfus M, Magny J F, Bridey F et al 1991 Treatment of homozygous protein C deficiency and neonatal purpura fulminans with a purified protein C concentrate. New England Journal of Medicine 325: 1565–1568

Egeberg O 1965 Inherited antithrombin deficiency causing thrombophilia. Thrombosis et Diathesis Haemorrhagica 13: 516–530

Engesser L, Broekmans A W, Briët E, Brommer E J, Bertina R M 1987a Hereditary protein S deficiency: clinical manifestations. Annals of Internal Medicine 106: 677–682

Engesser L, Kluft C, Briët E, Brommer E J 1987b Familial elevation of plasma histidine-rich glycoprotein in a family with thrombophilia. British Journal of Haematology 67: 355–358

Engesser L, Brommer E J, Kluft C, Briët E 1989 Elevated plasminogen activator inhibitor (PAI), a cause of thrombophilia? A study in 203 patients with familial or sporadic venous thrombophilia. Thrombosis and Haemostasis 62: 673–680

Esmon C T, Owen W G 1981 Identification of an endothelial cell cofactor for thrombin-catalyzed activation of protein C. Proceedings of the National Academy of Sciences, USA 78: 2249–2252

Estelles A, Garcia Plaza I, Dasi A et al 1984 Severe inherited 'homozygous' protein C deficiency in a newborn infant. Thrombosis and Haemostasis 52: 53–56

Foster D C, Yoshitake S, Davie E W 1985 The nucleotide sequence of the gene for human protein C. Proceedings of the National Academy of Sciences, USA 82: 4673–4677

Friedman K D, Marlar R A, Houston J G, Montgomery R R 1986 Warfarin-induced skin necrosis in a patient with protein S deficiency (abstract). Blood 68: 33A

Gandrille S, Vidaud M, Aiach M et al 1991 Six previously undescribed mutations in nine families with protein C quantitative deficiency (abstract). Thrombosis and Haemostasis 65: 646

Gerstman B B, Piper J M, Tomita D K, Ferguson W J, Stadel B V, Lundin F E 1991 Oral contraceptive estrogen dose and the risk of deep venous thromboembolic disease. American Journal of Epidemiology 133: 32–37

Ginsberg J S, Hirsh J, Turner D C, Levine M N, Burrows R 1989 Risks to the fetus of anticoagulant therapy during pregnancy. Thrombosis and Haemostasis 61: 197–203

Girolami A, Simioni P, Lazzaro A R, Pontara E, Ruzza G 1990 Heterozygous protein-S deficiency: a study of a large kindred. Acta Haematologica (Basel) 84: 162–168

Gladson C L, Groncy P, Griffin J H 1987 Coumarin necrosis, neonatal purpura fulminans, and protein C deficiency. Archives of Dermatology 123: 1701a–1706a

Gladson C L, Scharrer I, Hach V, Beck K H, Griffin J H 1988 The frequency of type I heterozygous protein S and protein C deficiency in 141 unrelated young patients with venous thrombosis. Thrombosis and Haemostasis 59: 18–22

Goldberg S L, Orthner C L, Yalisove B L, Elgart M L, Kessler C M 1991 Skin necrosis following prolonged administration of coumarin in a patient with inherited protein S deficiency. American Journal of Hematology 38: 64–66

Goodnough L T, Saito H, Ratnoff O D 1983 Thrombosis or myocardial infarction in congenital clotting factor abnormalities and chronic thrombocytopenias: A report of 21 cases and a review of 50 previously reported cases. Medicine 62: 248–255

Grafe E 1924 Zur kenntnis der kavathrombose. Munchener Medizinische Wochenschrift 1: 643–644

Green D, Ganger D R, Blei A T 1987 Protein C deficiency in splanchnic venous thrombosis. American Journal of Medicine 82: 1171–1174

Griffin J H, Evatt B, Zimmerman T S, Kleiss A J, Wideman C 1981 Deficiency of protein C in congenital thrombotic disease. Journal of Clinical Investigation 68: 1370–1373

Griffin J H, Fernandez J A, Gruber A 1991 Critical reevaluation of free protein S (PS) and C4b-binding protein (C4BP) levels and implications for thrombotic risk. Thrombosis and Haemostasis 65: 711 (abstract)

Grimaudo V, Gueissaz F, Hauert J, Sarraj A, Kruithof E K, Bachmann F 1989 Necrosis of skin induced by coumarin in a patient deficient in protein S. British Medical Journal 298: 233–234

Grimaudo V, Bachmann F, Hauert J, Christe M-A, Kruithof E K O 1992 Hypofibrinolysis in patients with a history of idiopathic deep vein thrombosis and/or pulmonary embolism. Thrombosis and Haemostasis 67: 397–401

Grundy C, Chitolic A, Talbot S, Bevan N, Kakkar V, Cooper D N 1989 Protein C London 1: recurrent mutation at Arg 169 (CGGGTGG) in the protein C gene causing thrombosis. Nucleic Acids Research 17: 10513

Hall J G, Pauli R M, Wilson K M 1980 Maternal and fetal sequelae of anticoagulation during pregnancy. American Journal of Medicine 68: 122–140

Harle J R, Aillaud M F, Quinsat D et al 1989 Cerebral thrombophlebitis disclosing functional protein C deficiency (letter). Annales de medicine Interne 140: 233–234

Heijboer H, Brandjes D P M, Buller H R, Sturk A, ten Cate J W 1990 Deficiencies of coagulation-inhibiting and fibrinolytic proteins in outpatients with deep-vein thrombosis. New England Journal of Medicine 323: 1512–1516

Hellgren M, Tengborn L, Abildgaard U 1982 Pregnancy in women with congenital antithrombin III deficiency: experience of treatment with heparin and antithrombin. Gynecologic and Obstetric Investigation 14: 127–141

Hirsh J 1991 Oral anticoagulant drugs. New England Journal of Medicine 324: 1865–1875

Hirsh J, Hull R D, Raskob G E 1986 Epidemiology and pathogenesis of venous thrombosis. Journal of the American College of Cardiology 8: 104B–113B

Hirsh J, Piovella F, Pini M 1989 Congenital antithrombin III deficiency. Incidence and clinical features. American Journal of Medicine 87: 34S–38S

Horellou M H, Conard J, Bertina R M, Samama M 1984 Congenital protein C deficiency and thrombotic disease in nine French families. British Medical Journal 289: 1285–1287

Hossmann V, Heiss W D, Bewermeyer H 1983 Antithrombin III deficiency in ischaemic stroke. Klinische Wochenschrift 61: 617–620

Howell R, Fidler J, Letsky E, de Swiet M 1983 The risks of antenatal subcutaneous heparin prophylaxis: a controlled trial. British Journal of Obstetrics and Gynaecology 90: 1124–1128

Huisveld I A, Greven E C G, Bouma B N 1987 Protein C and protein S levels in tall girls treated with ethinyloestradiol (abstract). Thrombosis and Haemostasis 58: 406

Hull R D, Raskob G E, Rosenbloom D et al 1990 Heparin for 5 days as compared with 10 days in the initial treatment of proximal venous thrombosis. New England Journal of Medicine 332: 1260–1264

Inomoto T, Takamoto M, Tamura R, Maegawa M, Kamada M, Takayanagi M 1991 Effective prophylaxis of thrombosis by antithrombin III concentrate in a pregnant woman with congenital antithrombin III deficiency: relations between plasma antithrombin III activity and the plasma levels of hemostatic molecular markers. Haemostasis 21: 147–154

Israels S J, Seshia S S 1987 Childhood stroke associated with protein C or S deficiency. Journal of Pediatrics 111: 562–564

Iturbe-Alessio I, Del Carmen Fonseca M, Mutchinik O, Santos M A, Zajarias A, Salazar E 1986 Risks of anticoagulant therapy in pregnant women with artificial heart valves. New England Journal of Medicine 315: 1390–1393

Johansson L, Hedner U, Nilsson I M 1978 A family with thromboembolic disease associated with deficient fibrinolytic activity in vessel wall. Acta Medica Scandinavica 203: 477–480

Johnson E J, Prentice C R, Parapia L A 1990 Premature arterial disease associated with familial antithrombin III deficiency. Thrombosis and Haemostasis 63: 13–15

Jordan F L J, Nandorff A 1956 The familial tendency in thrombo-embolic disease. Acta Medica Scandinavica 156: 267–275

Jorgensen M, Mortensen Z J, Madsen A G, Thorsen S, Jacobsen B 1982 A family with reduced plasminogen activator activity in blood associated with recurrent venous thrombosis. Scandinavian Journal of Haematology 29: 217–223

Klingemann H G, Broekmans A W, Bertina R M, Egbring R, Loeliger E A 1984 Protein C deficiency — a risk factor for venous thrombosis. Klinische Wochenschrift 62: 975–978

Kluft C, Bertina R M, Preston F E et al 1984 Protein C, an anticoagulant protein, is increased in healthy volunteers and surgical patients after treatment with stanozolol. Thrombosis Research 33: 297–304

Koide T, Odani S, Takahashi K, Ono T, Sakuragawa N 1984 Antithrombin III Toyama: replacement of arginine-47 by cysteine in hereditary abnormal antithrombin III that lacks heparin-binding ability. Proceedings of the National Academy of Sciences, USA 81: 289–293

Koopman J, Haverkate F, Briët E, Lord S T 1991 A congenitally abnormal fibrinogen (Vlissingen) with a 6-base deletion in the gamma-chain gene, causing defective calcium binding and impaired fibrin polymerization. Journal of Biological Chemistry 266: 13456–13461

Lammle B, Wuillemin W A, Huber I et al 1991 Thromboembolism and bleeding tendency in congenital factor XII deficiency — a study on 74 subjects from 14 Swiss families. Thrombosis and Haemostasis 65: 117–121

Lane D A, Ireland H, Olds R J, Thein S L, Perry D J, Aiach M 1991 Antithrombin III: A database of mutations. Thrombosis and Haemostasis 66: 657–661

McGehee W G, Klotz T A, Epstein D J, Rapaport S I 1984 Coumarin necrosis associated with hereditary protein C deficiency. Annals of Internal Medicine 101: 59–60

Mahasandana C, Suvatte V, Chuansumrit A et al 1990 Homozygous protein S deficiency in an infant with purpura fulminans. Journal of Pediatrics 117: 750–753

Manabe S, Matsuda M 1985 Homozygous protein C deficiency combined with heterozygous dysplasminogenemia found in a 21-year-old thrombophilic male. Thrombosis Research 39: 333–341

Mannhalter C, Fischer M, Hopmeier P, Deutsch E 1987 Factor XII activity and antigen concentrations in patients suffering from recurrent thrombosis. Fibrinolysis 1: 259–263

Mannucci P M, Boyer C, Wolf M, Tripodi A, Larrieu M J 1982 Treatment of congenital antithrombin III deficiency with concentrates. British Journal of Haematology 50: 531–535

Mannucci P M, Tripodi A, Bertina R M 1986 Protein S deficiency.associated with 'juvenile' arterial and venous thromboses (letter). Thrombosis and Haemostasis 55: 440

Mannucci P M, Valsecchi C, Krachmalnicoff A, Faioni E M, Tripodi A 1989 Familial dysfunction of protein S. Thrombosis and Haemostasis 62: 763–766

Marciniak E, Goeckerman J P 1977 Heparin-induced decrease in circulating antithrombin III. Lancet 2: 581–584

Marciniak E, Wilson H D, Marlar R A 1983 Neonatal purpura fulminans as expression of homozygosity for protein C deficiency (abstract). Blood 62: 303a

Marciniak E, Wilson H D, Marlar R A 1985 Neonatal purpura fulminans: a genetic disorder related to the absence of protein C in blood. Blood 65: 15–20

Marlar R A, Mastovich S 1990 Hereditary protein C deficiency: a review of the genetics, clinical presentation, diagnosis and treatment. Blood Coagulation and Fibrinolysis 1: 319–330

Marlar R A, Neumann A 1990 Neonatal purpura fulminans due to homozygous protein C or protein S deficiencies. Seminars in Thrombosis and Hemostaiss 16: 299–309

Marlar R A, Montgomery R R, Broekmans A W 1989a Report on the diagnosis and treatment of homozygous protein C deficiency. Report of the Working Party on Homozygous Protein C Deficiency of the ICTH Subcommittee on Protein C and Protein S. Thrombosis and Haemostasis 61: 529–531

Marlar R A, Montgomery R R, Broekmans A W 1989b Diagnosis and treatment of homozygous protein C deficiency. Report of the Working Party on Homozygous Protein C Deficiency of the ICTH Subcommittee on Protein C and Protein S. Journal of Pediatrics 114: 528–534

Matsuda M, Sugo T, Sakata Y et al 1988 A thrombotic state due to an abnormal protein C. New England Journal of Medicine 319: 1265–1268

Meade T W, Cooper J, Miller G J, Howarth D J, Stirling Y 1991 Antithrombin III and arterial disease. Lancet 338: 850–851

Menache D 1991 Replacement therapy in patients with hereditary antithrombin III deficiency. Seminars in Hematology 28: 31–38

Menache D, O'Malley J P, Schorr J B et al 1990 Evaluation of the safety, recovery, half-life, and clinical efficacy of antithrombin III (human) in patients with hereditary antithrombin III deficiency. Cooperative Study Group. Blood 75: 33–39

Michiels J J, van Vliet H H 1984 Hereditary antithrombin III deficiency and venous thrombosis. Netherlands Journal of Medicine 27: 226–232

Michiels J J, Stibbe J, Vellenga E, van Vliet H H 1984 Prophylaxis of thrombosis in antithrombin III-deficient women during pregnancy and delivery. European Journal of Obstetrics, Gynecology and Reproductive Biology 18: 149–153

Miletich J, Sherman L, Broze G Jr 1987 Absence of thrombosis in subjects with heterozygous protein C deficiency. New England Journal of Medicine 317: 991–996

Moreb J, Kitchens C S 1989 Acquired functional protein S deficiency, cerebral venous thrombosis, and coumarin skin necrosis in association with antiphospholipid syndrome: report of two cases. American Journal of Medicine 87: 207–210

Mudd S H, Skovby F, Levy H L et al 1985 The natural history of homocystinuria due to cystathionine beta-synthase deficiency. American Journal of Human Genetics 37: 1–31

Nelson R M, Long G L 1991 Solution-phase equilibrium binding interaction of human protein S with C4b-binding protein. Biochemistry 30: 2384–2390

Nelson D M, Stempel L E, Brandt J T 1985 Hereditary antithrombin III deficiency and pregnancy: report of two cases and review of the literature. Obstetrics and Gynecology 65: 848–853

Nimpf J, Bevers E M, Bomans P H H et al 1986 Prothrombinase activity of human platelets is inhibited by beta 2-glycoprotein I. Biochimica et Biophysica Acta 884: 142–149

Orozco H, Guraieb E, Takahashi T et al 1988 Deficiency of protein C in patients with portal vein thrombosis. Hepatology 8: 1110–1111

Owen J 1991 Antithrombin III replacement therapy in pregnancy. Seminars in Hematology 28: 46–52

Pabinger Fasching I, Bertina R M, Lechner K, Niessner H, Korninger C 1983 Protein C deficiency in two Austrian families. Thrombosis and Haemostasis 50: 810–813

Pabinger I, Karnik R, Lechner K, Slany J, Niessner H 1986 Coumarin induced acral skin necrosis associated with hereditary protein C deficiency. Blut 52: 365–370

Patracchini P, Aiello V, Palazzi P, Calzolari E, Bernardi F 1989 Sublocalization of the human protein C gene on chromosome 2q13-q14. Human Genetics 81: 191–192

Pegelow C H, Ledford M, Young J, Zilleruelo G 1992 Severe protein S deficiency in a newborn. Pediatrics 89: 674–676
Peters C, Casella J F, Marlar R A, Montgomery R R, Zinkham W H 1988 Homozygous protein C deficiency: observations on the nature of the molecular abnormality and the effectiveness of warfarin therapy. Pediatrics 81: 272–276
Ploos van Amstel J K, van der Zanden A L, Bakker E, Reitsma P H, Bertina R M 1987 Two genes homologous with human protein S cDNA are located on chromosome 3. Thrombosis and Haemostasis 58: 982–987
Ploos van Amstel H K, Huisman M V, Reitsma P H, Wouter ten Cate J, Bertina R M 1989a Partial protein S gene deletion in a family with hereditary thrombophilia. Blood 73: 479–483
Ploos van Amstel H K, Reitsma P H, Hamulyak K, de Die Smulders C E, Mannucci P M, Bertina R M 1989b A mutation in the protein S pseudogene is linked to protein S deficiency in a thrombophilic family. Thrombosis and Haemostasis 62: 897–901
Ploos van Amstel H K, Reitsma P H, van der Logt C P, Bertina R M 1990 Intron-exon organization of the active human protein S gene PS alpha and its pseudogene PS beta: duplication and silencing during primate evolution. Biochemistry 29: 7853–7861
Plutzky J, Hoskins J A, Long G L, Crabtree G R 1986 Evolution and organization of the human protein C gene. Proceedings of the National Academy of Sciences, USA 83: 546–550
Prat F, Ouzan D, Trecziak N, Trepo C 1989 Portal and mesenteric thrombosis revealing constitutional protein C deficiency (letter). Gut 30: 416
Preston F E, Malia R G, Greaves M, Kluft C, Bertina R M, Segal D S 1983 Effect of stanozolol on antithrombin III and protein C (letter). Lancet 2: 517–518
Reitsma P H 1992 Personal communication
Reitsma P H, Poort S R, Allaart C F, Briët E, Bertina R M 1991a The spectrum of genetic defects in a panel of 40 Dutch families with symptomatic protein C deficiency type I: heterogeneity and founder effects. Blood 78: 890–894
Reitsma P H, Poort S R, Bertina R M 1991b Genetic abnormalities in the protein C genes of homozygous and compound heterozygotes for protein C deficiency (abstract). Thrombosis and Haemostasis 65: 808
Romeo G, Hassan H J, Staempfli S et al 1987 Hereditary thrombophilia: identification of nonsense and missense mutations in the protein C gene. Proceedings of the National Academy of Sciences, USA 84: 2829–2832
Rosendaal F R, Heijboer H, Briët E et al 1991 Mortality in hereditary antithrombin-III deficiency — 1830 to 1989. Lancet 337: 260–262
Samama M, Horellou M H, Soria J, Conard J, Nicolas G 1984 Successful progressive anticoagulation in a severe protein C deficiency and previous skin necrosis at the initiation of oral anticoagulant treatment (letter). Thrombosis and Haemostasis 51: 132–133
Samson D, Stirling Y, Woolf L, Howarth D, Seghatchian M J, de Chazal R 1984 Management of planned pregnancy in a patient with congenital antithrombin III deficiency. British Journal of Haematology 56: 243–249
Schafer H P, von Felten A 1989 Protein-S deficiency in young patients with thrombotic brain infarction. Schweizerische Medizinische Wochenschrift 119: 489–492
Scharrer I, Hach-Wunderle V, Heyland H, Kuhn C 1987 Incidence of defective t-PA release in 158 unrelated young patients with venous thrombosis in comparison to PC-, PS-, AT III-, fibrinogen- and plasminogen deficiency. Thrombosis and Haemostasis 58: 72 (abstract)
Schmidel D K, Nelson R M, Broxson E H Jr, Comp P C, Marlar R A, Long G L 1991 A 5.3-kb deletion including exon XIII of the protein S alpha gene occurs in two protein S-deficient families. Blood 77: 551–559
Schulman S, Tengborn L 1992 Treatment of venous thromboembolism in patients with congenital deficiency of antithrombin III. Thrombosis and Haemostasis 68: 634–636
Schwarz H P, Fischer M, Hopmeier P, Batard M A, Griffin J H 1984 Plasma protein S deficiency in familial thrombotic disease. Blood 64: 1297–1300
Schwartz R S, Bauer K A, Rosenberg R D, Kavanaugh E J, Davies D C, Bogdanoff D A 1989 Clinical experience with antithrombin III concentrate in treatment of congenital and acquired deficiency of antithrombin. The Antithrombin III Study Group. American Journal of Medicine 87: 53S–60S
Seligsohn U, Berger A, Abend M et al 1984 Homozygous protein C deficiency manifested by massive venous thrombosis in the newborn. New England Journal of Medicine 310: 559–562
Sharon C, Tirindelli M C, Mannucci P M, Tripodi A, Mariani G 1986 Homozygous protein C deficiency with moderately severe clinical symptoms. Thrombosis Research 41: 483–488
Shigekiyo T, Uno Y, Tomonari A et al 1992 Type I congenital plasminogen deficiency is not a risk factor for thrombosis. Thrombosis and Haemostasis 67: 189–192
Sills R H, Marlar R A, Montgomery R R, Deshpande G N, Humbert J R 1984 Severe homozygous protein C deficiency. Journal of Pediatrics 105: 409-413
Stadel B V 1981a Oral contraceptives and cardiovascular disease (first of two parts). New England Journal of Medicine 305: 612–618
Stadel B V 1981b Oral contraceptives and cardiovascular disease (second of two parts). New England Journal of Medicine 305: 672–677
Stead N W, Bauer K A, Kinney T R et al 1983 Venous thrombosis in a family with defective release of vascular plasminogen activator and elevated plasma factor VIII/von Willebrand's factor. American Journal of Medicine 74: 33–39
Suzuki K, Nishioka J, Hashimoto S 1983 Regulation of activated protein C by thrombin-modified protein S. Journal of Biochemistry (Tokio) 94: 699–705
Suzuki K, Nishioka J, Matsuda M, Murayama H, Hashimoto S 1984 Protein S is essential for the activated protein C-catalyzed inactivation of platelet-associated factor Va. Journal of Biochemistry (Tokio) 96: 455–460
Tabernero M D, Tomas J F, Alberca I, Orfao A, Lopez Borrasca A, Vicente V 1991 Incidence and clinical characteristics of hereditary disorders associated with venous thrombosis. American Journal of Hematology 36: 249–254
Tait R C, Walker I D, Perry D J et al 1991 Prevalence of antithrombin III deficiency subtypes in 4000 healthy blood donors (abstract). Thrombosis and Haemostasis 65: 534
Tait R C, Walker I D, Islam S I A I et al 1992 Prevalence of protein C deficiency in the general population. 24th ISH Congress, August 1992, London. British Journal of Haematology 81S: 4 (abstract)
Teepe R G, Broekmans A W, Vermeer B J, Nienhuis A M, Loeliger E A 1986 Recurrent coumarin-induced skin necrosis in a patient with an acquired functional protein C deficiency. Archives of Dermatology 122: 1408–1412
Thaler E, Lechner K 1981 Antithrombin III deficiency and thromboembolism. Clinics in Haematology 10: 369–390
Tsuda S, Reitsma P H, Miletich J 1991 Molecular defects causing heterozygous protein C deficiency in three asymptomatic kindreds (abstract). Thrombosis and Haemostasis 65: 647
Tuddenham E G, Takase T, Thomas A E et al 1989 Homozygous protein C deficiency with delayed onset of symptoms at 7 to 10 months. Thrombosis Research 53: 475–484
Ueyama H, Murakami T, Nishiguchi S et al 1990 Antithrombin Kumamoto. Identification of a point mutation and genotype analysis of the family. Thrombosis and Haemostasis 63: 231–234
Vellenga E, van Imhoff G W, Aarnoudse J G 1983 Effective prophylaxis with oral anticoagulants and low-dose heparin during pregnancy in an antithrombin III deficient woman (letter). Lancet, 2: 224
Vermeer C, Hamulyak K 1991 Pathophysiology of vitamin K-deficiency and oral anticoagulants. Thrombosis and Haemostasis 66: 153–159
Vukovich T, Auberger K, Weil J, Engelmann H, Knobl P, Hadorn H B 1988 Replacement therapy for a homozygous protein C deficiency-state using a concentrate of human protein C and S. British Journal of Haematology 70: 435–440
Walker F J 1980 Regulation of activated protein C by a new protein. A possible function for bovine protein S. Journal of Biological Chemistry 255: 5521–5524

Walker F J 1981 Regulation of activated protein C by protein S. The role of phospholipid in factor Va inactivation. Journal of Biological Chemistry 256: 11128–11131

Winter J, Donald D, Bennet B, Douglas A S 1982a Arterial thrombosis and accelerated atheroma in a member of a family with familial antithrombin III deficiency. Postgraduate Medical Journal 58: 108–109

Winter J H, Fenech A, Mackie M, Bennett B, Douglas A S 1982b Treatment of venous thrombosis in antithrombin III deficient patients with concentrates of antithrombin III. Clinical and Laboratory Haematology 4: 101–108

Winter J H, Fenech A, Bennett B, Douglas A S 1984 Prophylactic antithrombotic therapy with stanozolol in patients with familial antithrombin III deficiency. British Journal of Haematology 57: 527–537

Wintzen A R, Broekmans A W, Bertina R M et al 1985 Cerebral haemorrhagic infarction in young patients with hereditary protein C deficiency: evidence for 'spontaneous' cerebral venous thrombosis. British Medical Journal 290: 350–352

Wise P H, Hall A J 1980 Heparin-induced osteopenia in pregnancy. British Medical Journal 2: 110–111

Young R L, Goepfert A R, Goldzieher H W 1991 Estrogen replacement therapy is not conducive of venous thromboembolism. Maturitas 13: 189–192

62. Prevention of venous thromboembolism

V. V. Kakkar

Venous thromboembolism is a frequent complication of the primary illness in hospital patients. Apart from the immediate risk to life, the late sequelae of extensive deep vein thrombosis must be considered: swelling of the legs, varicose veins, ulceration and other trophic changes. It is sometimes asked whether postoperative pulmonary embolism is preventable and, furthermore, whether it is worth preventing, since the mortality due to this complication is extremely low and all prophylactic measures require supervision and involve extra work. Data will be presented to support the argument that not only should venous thromboembolism be prevented but also that measures now available make prevention a practical proposition.

Approximately 80% of pulmonary emboli occur without premonitory signs of peripheral venous thrombosis and, consequently, treatment with heparin and oral anticoagulants to prevent embolism is often not given. To adopt a policy of treating massive pulmonary embolism or its precursor, peripheral venous thrombosis, is to expose patients to an unacceptable risk of fatal complications. The most rational approach is therefore to develop an effective method of prophylaxis, if the mortality due to pulmonary embolism and the misery due to the postphlebitic syndrome are to be significantly reduced. If such a method is to be adopted on a wide scale, it should fulfil the following criteria: it must be simple, safe and effective; it must be applicable to all types of patient at risk of developing deep vein thrombosis; and it must cover the period of risk, which in surgical patients has been shown to extend from the time of operation through the first 7–10 postoperative days.

AVAILABLE METHODS

Venous thrombi are generally regarded as an expression of blood coagulation leading to fibrin formation in the presence of venous stasis (see Ch. 60). The main attempts to prevent deep vein thrombosis can be conveniently divided into two groups: those directed towards the elimination of stasis in the deep veins of the legs and those employed to counteract changes in blood coagulability.

Elimination of stasis

Despite general agreement that stasis plays a significant role in the pathogenesis of venous thrombosis and despite increasing awareness of the hazards of bed-rest, there is conflicting evidence as to the efficacy or early ambulation and leg exercises in reducing the incidence of deep vein thrombosis (Sabri et al 1971). Earlier conclusions were based on physical signs alone, which are inadequate to diagnose the existence of venous thrombosis. Although elastic stockings have been shown to increase the rate of venous return, studies using the ^{125}I-labelled fibrinogen test (an accurate and objective method of detecting deep vein thrombosis) have failed to confirm the beneficial effects in surgical patients who wore elastic stockings throughout their hospital stay (Rosengarten et al 1970). Elevation of the lower extremities has also been claimed to increase the rate of venous return but, again, controlled studies have shown this to be ineffective in preventing venous thrombosis.

The limitations of intensive physical prophylaxis in general surgical cases were clearly demonstrated by Flanc et al (1969), using the ^{125}I-labelled fibrinogen test to detect leg vein thrombi. In this study, patients wore elastic stocking from admission to discharge, had frequent and vigorous leg exercise before and after operation, had the foot of the bed elevated, and were provided with a foot board to aid plantar flexion against resistance. Pressure on the calves during operation was avoided by the use of a sorbo-rubber stand and, after operation, the legs were kept elevated until consciousness permitted exercise and movement. Ambulation began between the 1st and 3rd postoperative days, depending on the operation. Despite all efforts, the overall results of these physical measures were disappointing: thrombosis was detected in 25% of 67 patients having intensive physiotherapy and in 35% of 65 concurrent controls. However, a significant reduction was seen in elderly patients undergoing major operations, in whom the incidence of thrombosis was 24%, compared with 61% in the controls. Different results have been reported by Tsapogas et al (1971), who found these methods to be highly effective.

More specific attempts have been made to prevent stasis during operation, and several methods for increasing venous return from the lower limbs have been investigated. One of these is electrical stimulation of the calf muscles during operation: two electrodes are applied to the calf and a low voltage current is used to contract the muscles every 2–4 seconds. The beneficial results of this method of preventing stasis and consequently of reducing thrombosis, first reported by Doran et al (1964), have now been investigated by several other workers, using the radioactive fibrinogen test for assessment.

Another method, pneumatic compression of the calves (Hills et al 1972), involves encasing the legs in an envelope of plastic material and rhythmically altering the pressure to squeeze the calf muscles and increase venous return. In practice, an electric pump inflates each legging alternatively so that compression at 40–50 mmHg for 1 minute is achieved, followed by relaxation for 1 minute. The advantage of this method is that it can be used not only during operation but also in the postoperative period. There is little doubt that these methods lessen stasis and lower the incidence of venous thrombosis, except in 'high-risk' patients undergoing operation for malignant disease. However, such physical methods present almost insuperable difficulties as a long-term solution: they must be applied to both legs and, during certain types of operation — for example, for repair of fractured neck of femur or those in which the patient is in the lithotomy position — they are either impracticable or extremely inconvenient. Some of the methods are uncomfortable for conscious patients and, most importantly, the logistical problem of applying such physical measures on a large scale would strain the resources of even the most lavishly equipped hospital.

Counteracting blood coagulability

Many attempts have also been made to prevent thrombosis by simpler methods, such as the use of chemical agents. These can be broadly classified into three main groups: drugs that alter platelet function, those that interfere with the coagulation mechanism, and drugs that act on venous endothelium to increase naturally occurring fibrinolytic activity. However, there is still a good deal of confusion, and the reason for this is that in the majority of studies clinical methods were used to assess therapeutic effectiveness. This form of assessment is well known to be unreliable for detecting the presence or absence of thrombosis.

DRUGS THAT ALTER PLATELET FUNCTION

It has been suggested that adhesion of platelets to subendothelial connective tissue at the site of presumed damage to the venous endothelium, and subsequent events leading to platelet aggregation, may account for thrombus formation. If platelet aggregation can be prevented, it is conceivable that the thrombus will not form. It is with this background that various drugs that interface with the different aspects of platelet function have been investigated; these include aspirin, dextran (usually dextran 70), dipyridamole and chloroquine.

Aspirin

Conflicting data exist regarding the antithrombotic effect of aspirin in animals. Female albino rabbits receiving a single dose of between 15 and 100 mg/kg of aspirin had a lower incidence of femoral vein thrombosis induced by sodium morrhuate than control animals (Peterson & Zucker 1970). In another study, aspirin not only failed to protect rabbits but actually facilitated thrombus formation when administered in a dose of 200 mg/kg 30 minutes before the induction of stenosis and stasis in the jugular veins (Kelton et al 1978).

The minimum effective dose of aspirin is not known. Some inactivation of platelet cyclo-oxygenase is seen 24 hours after the oral intake of only 20 mg in man, while a dose of 300–600 mg produces almost total enzyme inhibition for 24 hours (Burch et al 1978) and reduces platelet aggregation for 2–7 days. This would suggest that aspirin need be given only every 2nd or 3rd day to maintain its effect. However, since 10% of normal platelets is sufficient to normalize the bleeding time in aspirin-treated patients (Handin & Valeri 1971) or to counteract the antithrombotic effect of aspirin in the animal model (Cerkus et al 1978), it has been suggested that aspirin should be given daily.

The first clinical trial evaluating the antithrombotic potential of aspirin in venous disease was reported by Salzman et al in 1971. Since then the results of further trials have been published and they are summarized in Table 62.1. Aspirin has been shown to be ineffective in reducing the incidence of venous thrombosis after elective general surgery in two double-blind trials (Report of the Steering Committee 1972, Encke et al 1976) and had an equivocal effect in an open study (Clagett & Salzman, 1974), all using leg scanning to detect thrombosis. By contrast, Harris et al (1977) found an impressive and statistically significant decrease of venous thrombosis after elective hip replacement in men treated with aspirin, but no protective effect occurred in women. Other trials have found no prophylactic effect (Hume et al 1977, Soreff et al 1977, Stamatakis et al 1978) and the issue awaits further study (Table 62.2).

Table 62.1 Prevention of venous thromboembolism after general surgery

	Aspirin dose	Diagnosis	Control			Aspirin		
			Number	% DVT	% PE	Number	% DVT	% PE
Report of the Steering Committee (1972)	600 mg	^{125}I-fibrinogen test	150	22.0	–	153	29.0	–
Clagett & Salzman (1974)	1300 mg	^{125}I-fibrinogen	49	20.4	–	56	12.5	–
Loew et al (1974)	1500 mg	Clinical	527	5.1	3.2	570	2.0	0.8

DVT, deep vein thrombosis; PE, pulmonary embolism.

Table 62.2 Prevention of venous thromboembolism after orthopaedic surgery

	Aspirin dose	Diagnosis	Placebo			Aspirin		
			Number	% DVT	% PE	Number	% DVT	% PE
Soreff et al (1975)	2.0 g	Venogram	14	36.0	–	21	47.0	–
Zekert et al (1974)	1.5 g	Clinical and autopsy (fatal PE)	120	14.1*	11.6	120	5.8	2.5
Stamatakis et al (1978)	1.2 g	Venogram		NP		30	80	–

* Statistically significant (P < 0.05); DVT, deep vein thrombosis; PE, pulmonary embolism.

One randomized double-blind trial has also suggested that aspirin prevents pulmonary embolism after hip fracture (Zekert et al 1974). In this study, all patients who died after hip fracture had an autopsy, which showed major pulmonary embolism in one of 120 aspirin-treated patients and in eight of 120 control patients ($p < 0.05$). However, essential information relating to the site and extent of pulmonary emboli, and the criteria used for classification of fatal pulmonary embolism, were not defined.

Dextran

A commonly used agent for prevention of venous thromboembolism is dextran, which is a partially hydrolyzed glucose polymer produced from the bacteria *Leuconostoc mesenteriodes*. There are two dextran preparations suitable for clinical use, dextran 70 (average molecular weight 70 000), and dextran 40, or 'low molecular wight dextran' (average molecular weight 40 000). The two preparations are not distinct; the lower molecular weight spectrum of one overlaps the upper molecular weight spectrum of the other. The rationale for using dextran as a prophylactic agent is based on the fact that its infusion is followed by a decrease in platelet adhesiveness and a defect in the release reaction of platelets and platelet aggregation (Bygdeman et al 1966, Cronberg et al 1966). The exact mechanism of this action is unclear, although it has been suggested that dextran is adsorbed on to the surface of platelets (Rothman et al 1957), that it may increase the electrical negativity of platelets (Swank 1958), and that it makes the platelet less vulnerable, having a so-called 'stenoplastic' effect. Platelet function depends, among other things, on a normal concentration and function of von Willebrand factor. Studies have shown that although infusion of 500 ml of 6% dextran 70 has no effect on factor VIIIc, von Willebrand factor values were markedly decreased (Aberg et al 1975). The decreased thrombus stability observed after dextran may also be secondary to the effect of dextran on von Willebrand factor, probably via its effect on platelet function. There is, however, no conclusive evidence on this point as yet. The polymerization of fibrinogen by thrombin occurs more readily in the presence of dextran, and the fibrin clots have a different structure (Mazaffar et al 1976). The fibres in such clots are coarser and the tensile strength is decreased. It has been observed that these changes are accompanied by an increased clot lysability by plasmin (Tangen et al 1972). However, to achieve such an increased clot lysability (Aberg et al 1975), a high concentration of dextran is necessary (10 mg/ml plasma). In addition, by virtue of their volume-expanding properties, dextrans increase blood flow and may prevent venous stasis.

First evaluated as a prophylactic antithrombotic agent in 1962 by Kockenburg, dextran has now been examined in concurrent trials by several workers, especially in Sweden (Johnson et al 1986). They have shown that dextran (usually dextran 70) reduces the incidence of thromboembolism among general surgical patients with fractured neck of femur, and in gynaecological patients undergoing operation (Ahlberg et al 1968). Bygdeman et al (1970) listed eight surgical studies in which a total of 1321 patients were given dextran 70 prophylactically, and compared them with a similar number of control patients. There was approximately a four-fold reduction in fatal emboli in the dextran-treated patients. However, in six of these eight studies there was no significant difference between control and treated patients in the incidence of fatal emboli.

A prospective, double-blind, randomly allocated trial at

the Johns Hopkins Hospital found that the prophylactic administration of dextran 70 to 'high-risk' surgical patients reduced neither the incidence of pulmonary emboli nor the overall mortality rate (Brisman et al 1971). However, two studies involving large numbers of patients demonstrated that dextran is effective in reducing the incidence of fatal postoperative pulmonary embolism.

The first study was reported by Kline et al (1975). Of 831 patients undergoing major abdominal surgery who were randomly allocated in this trial, 435 received dextran and 396 received saline infusion. The potentially lethal event in thromboembolic disease is major pulmonary embolism. In this study there were 16 cases in all: five were detected at necropsy and 11 at assessment because of significant clinical signs. Of these 11, the diagnosis was confirmed by autopsy in two and by investigation in eight. When the cases of death from pulmonary embolism were examined, it was found that seven had occurred in the saline group and there had been only one death in the dextran group. This was found to be statistically significant when examined using a one-tail Fisher exact test. A major criticism in the design of this study related to the fact that the criteria for assessing fatal pulmonary embolism were not defined. The most essential part of any clinical trial is the compatibility between the two groups of several factors which are known to influence the occurrence of deep vein thrombosis. The published results failed to indicate what risk factors were evaluated and whether in fact randomization was achieved. In the second study (Gruber et al 1980), the value of dextran infusion was compared with low dose heparin against fatal pulmonary embolism after elective operations for general, orthopaedic, urological and gynaecological conditions. Out of 3984 patients correctly admitted to the trial, 1993 were allocated to receive dextran 70, and 1991 to receive low dose heparin. Of 75 patients who died within 30 days operation, 38 had been given dextran and 37 low dose heparin. Necropsy was performed in 33 and 32 of these cases, respectively. In six patients in each group, pulmonary embolism was the sole or a contributory cause of death. Of these, five patients in the dextran group and two in the heparin group had received a full course of prophylaxis. Complications of dextran therapy include pulmonary oedema in patients with limited cardiac reserve, occasional renal failure, mild allergenic reactions, and rare anaphylactic responses.

A survey involving 236 clinics in Sweden showed that approximately 12% of clinicians do not use dextran 70 for prophylaxis because of the risk of serious anaphylactic reactions (Bergqvist et al 1980). It has also been suggested that bleeding complication approach those of oral anticoagulants in frequency (Salzman et al 1971, Harris et al 1972). Furthermore, the drug is expensive and must be given intravenously, and its use is restricted to hospitalized patients during the acute phase of their illness. These considerations preclude the use of dextran for routine prophylaxis against venous thromboembolism in non-hospitalized patients. However, it is effective, and can be recommended in selected patients in whom other means of therapy are not appropriate, provided that certain contraindications to its use are observed.

DRUG THAT ALTER THE COAGULATION MECHANISM

The second chemical approach has involved the use of drugs that interfere with the coagulation mechanism. To block or alter the coagulation sequence, two different types of drug have been used: oral anticoagulants and heparin.

Oral anticoagulation

Oral anticoagulants, properly employed (started well before operation), are the most effective and proved method of preventing venous thrombosis. Such drugs owe their anticoagulant properties to their ability to antagonize the action of vitamin K in the liver. Vitamin K is required for the synthesis of four plasma clotting factors: prothrombin (factor II), and factors VII, IX, and X (see Ch. 65).

Oral anticoagulants represent the most extensively studied method of prophylaxis in surgical and medical patients (Storm 1968, Sevitt & Gallagher 1959, Sevitt 1962, Skinner & Salzman 1967). In controlled clinical trials the incidence of venous thrombosis was 0–36.0% (average 7.7%) in the treated groups and 1.1–56.0% (average 20.8%) among controls. Pulmonary embolism occurred in 0–2.5% (average 0.8%) of the controls. The true impact of these data can only be realized by analysis according to patient categories. Encouraging results of oral anticoagulant prophylaxis have been reported in patient undergoing orthopaedic surgery, such as reconstructive hip surgery. Among such patients, there has been a reduction of approximately 66% in the incidence of deep vein thrombosis and 80% in the incidence of pulmonary embolism as compared with the randomly allocated controls. Similar results have been reported in patients undergoing thoracic and general abdominal surgery. Embolism is quite frequent in patients with heart disease, particularly in those with congestive cardiac failure. Among such patients, oral anticoagulant therapy was effective in reducing the incidence of deep vein thrombosis by approximately 80%, as compared to untreated controls.

A major drawback of oral anticoagulant therapy is the risk of massive haemorrhage during and after operation, despite laboratory control of the dosage given. The incidence of severe haemorrhage in the various reported studies has varied between 2 and 7% and the mortality rate has been in the range of 0.08–0.1%. The risk of haemorrhage and the need for strict laboratory control have undoubtedly contributed to the relatively low level of acceptance of this form of prophylaxis among surgeons generally, at least in the United States and the United Kingdom.

Low dose heparin

A form of therapy which is both effective and devoid of the drawbacks of oral anticoagulant therapy would meet a real need. Ideally, any agent used for the prophylaxis of deep vein thrombosis should be well tolerated by the patient, have no side-effects, require no special monitoring, and produce no bleeding in a clinical situation in which the patient is subjected to major tissue trauma. One approach is the use of low dose heparin, given subcutaneously, which prevents thrombosis with minimal increase in the risk of haemorrhage.

The rationale for the use of low dose heparin prophylaxis was first put forward by de Takats, who showed that small amounts of heparin will effectively block the coagulation process if given at an early stage (de Takats 1950). The prophylactic use of heparin was introduced by Sharnoff, who found accelerated blood coagulation during and after surgery and thought this might be related to thrombus formation (Sharnoff 1966). He subsequently showed that postoperative shortening of the whole blood clotting time could be prevented by prophylactic heparin (Sharnoff and de Blasio 1970).

During intravascular coagulation, thrombin is produced from its precursor, prothrombin, by the combined action of factor V and activated factor X (factor Xa) in the presence of surface lipid and calcium ions. Thrombin thus formed initiates the development of a fibrin clot by its specific action on arginine–glycine peptide bond of fibrinogen (Blombäck & Blombäck 1965), and at the same time it is inactivated by antithrombin, a specific inhibitor present in the plasma. The anticoagulant effect of heparin has been shown to occur only in the presence of antithrombin which combines with heparin to form an active complex that accelerates, by 50–100 times, the blocking of the enzymatic action of thrombin (see Ch. 64). If 'hypercoagulability' is treated with heparin before initiation of intravascular coagulation, less drug is required than if therapy is begun after thrombin formation has occurred. Support for this hypothesis has been provided by the failure of low dose heparin in patients subjected to emergency operation for fracture of the femoral neck. In these patients, the coagulation sequence has already been activated beyond the stage of thrombin generation, before the small amounts of heparin administered could be effective.

To prevent local complications, heparin should be administered subcutaneously as described by Griffith and Boggs (1964). A concentrated aqueous solution, 25 000 IU of heparin in 1 ml, should be used. Great care must be taken to avoid damaging the skin and subcutaneous fat at the site of injection and a 26-gauge needle, half an inch (1.25 cm) in length, is used. A fold of skin is raised from the abdominal wall and the needle inserted directly at right angles to the skin. The shaft of the needle is held firmly between the thumb and index finger while the heparin is injected and withdrawn at the same angle at which it was inserted. In is important that the exact amount of heparin is administered if bleeding complications are to be avoided.

During the last few year, numerous clinical trials of low dose heparin prophylaxis in a variety of patient populations have been reported. The greatest experience has been acquired in patients undergoing general abdominal, thoracic and urological operations. The results of 17 such trials in patients undergoing abdominal surgery are shown in Table 62.3. Despite variations in the study designs and regimen of low dose heparin used, in 15 studies there was evidence of a significant reduction of the incidence of deep vein thrombosis in patients receiving heparin. In the two exceptions, there was a very low incidence in the control group, and heparin treatment did not reduce the incidence below that level to any significant extent.

Low dose heparin prophylaxis has been found to be equally effective in reducing the incidence of deep vein thrombosis in patients who are confined to bed following a myocardial infarction. One of the five studies investigating a rather small number of patients showed no significant benefit, while in others a highly significant reduction was observed in patients receiving prophylaxis (Table 62.4). Similarly, low dose heparin prophylaxis has been shown to reduce the incidence of deep vein thrombosis in patients who are confined to bed after an acute stroke. In these studies of randomly allocated patients reported by McCarthy et al (1977), the incidence in 16 acute-stroke patients in a control group was 75% and this was reduced to 12.5% in those receiving heparin ($p < 0.05$).

The experience accumulated in patients undergoing orthopaedic operations, and particularly total hip replacement, demonstrates less evidence of benefit than in other groups of surgical patients receiving heparin. The reduction from a 50% incidence of deep vein thrombosis in the control group to approximately 20% in those receiving heparin was much less impressive than the benefit observed in patients undergoing major abdominal surgery (Table 62.5). One of the reasons for the failure of prophylaxis in orthopaedic patients is that torsion of the femoral vein takes place during surgery as the hip is dislocated, and the limb internally rotated. Similar damage to the femoral vein also occurs when a posterior approach is used for hip replacement. It is likely that such distortion of the femoral vein results in extensive intimal damage, exposing the subintimal tissue, leading to platelet adhesion and aggregation. Such an interaction is not affected by low dose heparin; hence, heparin fails to prevent the development of such thrombi.

Table 62.3 Effectiveness of low dose heparin in the prevention of postoperative deep vein thrombosis

	Control group Number of DVT patients	(%)	Heparin group Number of DVT patients	(%)	Statistical significance (p value)
Kakkar et al (1971)	27	26	26	4	< 0.05
Williams (1971)	29	41	27	15	< 0.02
Kakkar et al (1972)	39	42	39	8	< 0.001
Gordon-Smith et al (1972)	50	42	48	8.3	< 0.001
Nicolaides et al (1972)	122	24	122	0.8	–
Gallus et al (1973)	118	16	108	2	< 0.001
Ballard et al (1973)	55	29	55	3.6	< 0.001
Corrigan et al (1974)	434	27.8	320	7.1	< 0.005
Multi-unit controlled trial (1974)	128	37	128	12	< 0.001
Rosenberg et al (1974)	71	42	46	6.5	< 0.001
Gallus et al (1973)	412	16	408	4.2	< 0.005
International Multicentre Trial (1975)	667	24.6	625	7.7	–
Lahnborg et al (174)	54	56	58	19	< 0.001
Rem et al (1975)		35.8		13.3	–
van Geloven 1975	80	25	79	5.9	< 0.001
Abernethy (1974)		4.8		6.3	> 0.05
Covey (1975)	52	9.6	53	7.5	> 0.05

DVT, deep vein thrombosis.

Table 62.4 Low-dose heparin prophylaxis, myocardial infarction and deep vein thrombosis

	Control group Number of patients	DVT (%)	Heparin group Number of patients	DVT (%)	Statistical significance (p value)
Handley et al (1972)	24	29	26	23	NS
Gallus et al (1973)	40	22.5	38	2.6	< 0.025
Warlow et al (1973)	64	17	63	3	< 0.025
Emerson & Marks (1977)	41	34	37	5	< 0.005
Marks & Teather (1978)	37	34	37	3.4	< 0.05

NS, not significant; DVT, deep vein thrombosis.

Table 62.5 Effectiveness of low-dose heparin in prophylaxis of deep vein thrombosis in patients undergoing total hip replacement

	Control group Number of patients	DVT (%)	Heparin group Number of patients	DVT (%)
Morris & Mitchell (1977)	32	50	27	11
Hampson et al (1974)	52	54	48	46
Venous Thrombosis Clinical Study Group (1975)	27	40	25	1
Mannucci et al (1976)	46	39	45	18
Kakkar et al (1972)	18	39	15	27
Evarts & Alfidi (1973)	–	–	25	28
Dechavanne et al (1975)	27	48	27	32
Sagar et al (1976)	32	69	25	32
Harris et al (1974)	–	–	20	55
Hume et al (1973)	19	42	18	33

Prevention of extension of deep vein thrombosis

The natural history of postoperative venous thromboembolism in non-orthopaedic surgical patients has been investigated with the ^{125}I-labelled fibrinogen test and phlebography. It has been found that the majority of thrombi form in the calf veins. If one were to investigate 1000 patients older than 40 years of age undergoing major abdominal surgery, approximately 300 would develop isotopic deep vein thrombosis in the calf veins; a surprisingly high proportion would undergo spontaneous lysis, and only in about one-third of these patients would the thrombi extend more proximally from the calf into the popliteal, femoral and iliac veins. It is not known for certain in how many of such patients with extending thrombi pulmonary emboli occur, because it is difficult to diagnose such emboli accurately; however, only a small proportion (±0.5%) prove fatal. Thus, while prevention of venous thrombosis is important, the effect of prophylaxis on the incidence of extending thrombi in the proximal veins of the lower limbs is also of considerable significance, since such thrombi are the source of most major pulmonary emboli.

The effect of low dose heparin prophylaxis on the extension of venous thrombosis has been evaluated in more than 3000 patients undergoing elective surgery (Table 62.6). Of 1631 patients in the control group, thrombi were detected in 380, and extension of thrombus occurred in 99, an incidence of 6.0%. Of 1479 in the heparin group, thrombi were detected in 55, and extension occurred in only 0.6%. Again in heparin-treated patients, there was a significant reduction in the incidence of extensive thrombi likely to produce major pulmonary embolism, not only in the aggregate of the four studies, but also in each individual trial.

Prevention of fatal and non-fatal pulmonary embolism

In the final analysis, a crucial question concerns the effect of low dose heparin in the prevention of fatal and non-fatal pulmonary embolism. This end-point has been evaluated in several studies (Table 62.7). The largest of these was a multicentre, prospective, randomized, controlled trial (International Multicentre Trial 1975) which was conducted in 28 centres, each of which had a separate list of allocations to randomize patients into control and heparin groups. The heparin-treated patients received calcium heparin 5000 U subcutaneously, 2 hours preoperatively and 8-hourly for 7 days or until they became ambulant. Patients in the control group did not receive placebo injections. The major end-point of the study was fatal pulmonary embolism diagnosed at autopsy. Fatal pulmonary embolism was defined as massive fresh emboli present in the main pulmonary trunk, main pulmonary artery, or in at least two lobar arteries, demonstrated postmortem in patients in whom no other cause of death was found. This study involved 4121 patients over the age of 40 years undergoing a variety of elective major surgical procedures; 2076 of these were in the control group and 2045 received heparin. The two groups were well matched for age, sex, weight, blood group and other factors that could predispose to the development of venous thromboembolism. During the postoperative period, 180 patients (4.4%) died, 100 in the control group and 80 in the heparin group. Necropsies were performed on 72% of the patients who died in the control group and 66% of those who died in the heparin group. 16 of the control patients and two of the heparin-treated group were found to have died from massive pulmonary embolism ($p < 0.005$). Taking all pulmonary emboli together, the findings were again significant ($p < 0.005$). The findings reported in this multicentre trial were confirmed by another large-scale study (Gruber et al 1980). There can be no doubt that low dose heparin is highly effective, not only in reducing the incidence of isotopic deep vein thrombosis, but also in preventing death due to postoperative massive embolism.

Adjusted low dose heparin

In the early 1960s, Sharnoff and co-workers utilized the concept of adjusted (rather than fixed) low dose of subcutaneous heparin, based on an individual's clotting time, to prevent deep vein thrombosis in patients with hip fracture. However, such an approach did not gain widespread acceptance, possibly because the extra laboratory work was considered to be cumbersome and, more importantly, no controlled prospective trial had shown this approach to be effective. Poller and his co-workers (1982) produced further evidence that adjusted low dose heparin provides more effective prophylaxis than a fixed dosage schedule. They investigated 55 patients undergoing hip surgery who were randomized to receive either 5000 iu of heparin subcutaneously every 8 hours or to an adjusted dose regimen

Table 62.6 Effect of low-dose heparin on the proximal extension of thrombi in the popliteal, femoral and iliac veins in patients undergoing abdominal surgery

	Control group			Heparin group		
	Total number	DVT	No. with extension	Total number	DVT	No. with extension
Corrigan et al (1974)	434	121	29	320	23	1
Nicolaides et al (1972)	122	29	9	128	11	0
Gallus et al (1973)	408	66	12	412	13	3
International Multicentre Trial (1975)	667	164	49	625	48	5
Total	1631	380	99	1485	95	9
Percentage		23.3	6		5.79	0.66

Table 62.7 Low-dose heparin and prevention of postoperative fatal pulmonary embolism

	Control group		Heparin group		
	Number of patients	Pulmonary emboli	Number of patients	Pulmonary emboli	Statistical significance (p value)
International Multicentre Trial (1975)	2074	16 (0.8%)	2045	2 (0.09%)	< 0.005
Matt et al (1977)	1631	18 (1.1%)	1610	6 (0.4%)	< 0.05
Sagar et al (1975)	236	8 (3.4%)	264	0 (0.00%)	< 0.01
Total	3941	42 (0.8%)	3919	8 (0.2%)	< 0.001

with an aim to prolong the APTT to 50 seconds (the normal range observed in their laboratory being 38–45 seconds). Six of 30 patients in the fixed dose group and three of 25 in the adjusted group developed deep vein thrombosis. Although the difference is not statistically significant, their findings suggested that the adjusted dose approach merited further study. Even more encouraging results have been published by Leyvraz et al (1983). Of 79 patients who had elective total hip replacement and were included in this trial, 41 were assigned to fixed low dose subcutaneous heparin (3500 units every 8 hours), and 38 received adjusted doses of subcutaneous heparin. Heparin prophylaxis began 2 days preoperatively. In the adjusted group, the APTT was determined 2 hours after the morning injection. Heparin dosage was increased when the 6-hours post-injection APTT was less than 31.5 seconds and was decreased when this value was more than 36 seconds. Deep vein thrombosis developed in 16 of the 41 patients who received fixed doses of heparin (39%) but in only five of the 38 who received adjusted doses (13%). The difference in the frequency of deep vein thrombosis between the two groups was statistically significant ($p < 0.01$). There were no significant differences between the two groups in total heparin dosage, blood loss, or incidence of wound haematoma. The group of patients who received the adjusted dose required increasingly larger amounts of heparin throughout the first postoperative week to maintain the APTT within the designated range. These findings suggest that hip surgery, which requires extensive tissue dissection, induces a hypercoagulable state in which increasingly larger doses of heparin are required to prevent deep vein thrombosis. However, a criticism of this study is the exclusion of 17 patients from analysis after randomization. These results have now been confirmed in a larger group of patients (Leyvraz et al 1991) indicating that adjusted subcutaneous heparin prophylaxis can be useful in these particularly high-risk patients.

Complications of low dose heparin prophylaxis

The risk of haemorrhage is the main limitation on the routine use of anticoagulants for the prevention of thromboembolic disease in surgical patients. One definite criterion for evaluating this risk is the frequency of wound haematoma formation.

Two studies in which large numbers of patients were investigated reported a significant difference between the number of patients receiving heparin and the number of their control counterparts who developed wound haematomas (Gallus et al 1973, International Multicentre Trial 1975). However, a double-blind study failed to confirm such a difference (Kiil et al 1978). The reason for this discrepancy may arise from the fact that in the international multicentre trial and the study reported by Gallus and co-workers, heparin was administered every 8 hours, whereas Kiil and colleagues gave heparin every 12 hours. Similar results have been reported by other workers (Sagar et al 1975). It seems that there is a small but definite risk of bleeding when an 8-hour regimen is used, but not when a 12-hour regimen is followed.

Practical considerations

It has been suggested that heparin utilization may vary according to age, sex, or weight of the individual. Therefore, the routine use of a standard dose of subcutaneous heparin to patients undergoing surgery without any monitoring of its coagulation effect or measurement of heparin levels in the plasma may cause postoperative bleeding. However, the published findings do not support a monitoring approach. In a study reported by Pitney and Dean (1978), plasma heparin concentrations were measured at 2-hour intervals following the subcutaneous injection of two different doses of heparin. With doses of 5000 and 1000 units, peak plasma concentrations were seen most commonly 4 hours after the injection. There was a wide range of peak values at each dose level, with considerable overlap. No correlation could be shown between plasma heparin concentration and age, sex, or weight of the individual. In recent studies, the bleeding time has been measured following administration of 5000 IU of heparin subcutaneously. In none of the patients investigated did the bleeding time differ significantly during operation as compared with the preoperative value (Kakkar et al 1982). Therefore, it is unlikely that monitoring of the dose by clotting assays or even measurement of heparin level will help in reducing the frequency of bleeding complications. These can best be minimized by careful patient selection, recognition of coexistent systemic or local abnormalities that can lead to haemorrhage, and avoidance of other concomitant drug therapy — such as aspirin or corticosteroids — that can predispose to haemorrhage. It remains to be demonstrated whether careful preoperative screening — including measurement of haematocrit, prothrombin time, partial thromboplastin time, and platelet count — recommended by the Council of Thrombosis of the American Heart Association, will reduce the frequency of bleeding complications.

Low dose heparin prophylaxis is contraindicated in patients suffering from haemorrhagic disease, endocarditis, ulcers of internal organs, damaged kidney parenchyma, or severe hypertension (blood pressure >200/120 mmHg), and in patients undergoing operation on the central system, eye operations, and operations performed with the patient under spinal (not epidural) anaesthesia.

Combination of dihydroergotamine and heparin

Changes in blood coagulation and stasis in the deep veins

of the lower limbs are both considered to be important factors in the pathogenesis of deep vein thrombosis. It is therefore logical to propose that prophylaxis might be better achieved by methods that minimize or eliminate both of these factors rather than by counteracting either factor alone.

Dihydroergotamine is a potent vasoconstrictor in humans (Aellig 1975). Its site of action seems to be the capacitance vessels of the limbs. Dihydroergotamine administered subcutaneously has been shown to increase the velocity of venous flow in the major veins of the lower limbs by constricting the capacitance vessels while exerting a negligible influence on resistance vessels and capillary filtration (Mellander & Nordenfelt 1970). A single injection of 0.5 mg of dihydroergotamine has been shown to increase the mean calf muscle flow significantly, an effect that persists for up to 5 hours (Stamatakis et al 1977). It has also been shown that dihydroergotamine enhances the synthesis of prostaglandins, and this may affect platelet function. Furthermore, administration of drugs that affect vascular motility releases plasminogen activator from the vein wall (Mannucci et al 1976). Therefore, it is possible that dihydroergotamine, by producing venoconstriction through its action on α-adrenoreceptors of the vein wall, may release plasminogen activator and thus enhance fibrinolytic activity.

Heparin-Dihydergot, a fixed combination of either 5000 or 2500 iu of heparin sodium with 0.5 mg of dihydroergotamine mesylate, is available in single dose vials as the sterile, lyophilized mixture. This preparation has been developed to overcome the physicochemical incompatibility of the available parenteral formulations of both sodium and calcium heparin with that of dihydroergotamine mesylate (Lahnborg et al 1980, Kakkar et al 1985, Sasahara et al 1986).

Four clinical trials in which deep vein thrombosis was detected by the ^{125}I-fibrinogen test and venography performed in orthopaedic patients confirmed the superiority of the antithrombotic effect of the combination of dihydroergotamine and heparin compared with heparin alone (Sagar et al 1976, Stamatakis et al 1977, Kakkar et al 1979, Brucke et al 1983). Of the patients admitted to these four trials who received heparin alone, approximately 45% developed a deep vein thrombosis compared with 20% in those receiving the combination. There was no difference in the amount of operative or postoperative blood loss in the two treatment groups, although the heparin concentration in the plasma was significantly higher in the patients receiving the combined treatment (Kakkar et al 1979). In a meta-analysis of trials of dihydroergotamine plus heparin against heparin alone in the prophylaxis of postoperative venous thromboembolism, Gent and Roberts (1986) concluded that the combination, assessed in eight randomized trials, gave a pooled estimate of a 47% reduction in the risk of developing deep vein thrombosis as compared with that found when heparin alone is used. However, the most worrisome complication associated with the administration of dihydroergotamine is vasospasm. Although low doses of this agent given subcutaneously do not seem to affect arteriolar smooth muscle in the normal individual, these low doses may affect arteriolar tone in patients with a high degree of sympathetic activity (severely traumatized patients, septic shock, severe hypovolaemia). In a review of the European experience, a total of 107 vasospastic reactions have been reported, and the calculated incidence of annual vasospastic reactions is 0.003%. Most of the patients who suffered a vasospastic complication following administration of the drug did so in a clinical setting in which the drug was contraindicated. Therefore, if used according to the recommended guidelines, the anticipated frequency of side-effects and complications should be sufficiently low to make its use very safe, which is a prerequisite for any general prophylactic agent.

Low molecular weight heparins

Low molecular weight heparins (LMWH) represent the most significant recent development in antithrombotic therapy. The impetus for their development came from the multicentre trial of low dose prophylaxis, the results of which were published in 1975 and clearly demonstrated the protective effect not only against postoperative deep vein thrombosis but also against fatal and non-fatal pulmonary embolism (Kakkar 1975). The results of the multicentre trial were subsequently supported by a meta-analysis of 70 randomized trials involving 16 000 patients (Collins et al 1988); the reduction in deaths attributed to pulmonary embolism was striking, with 19 deaths in patients receiving heparin, as compared to 55 deaths in the control group ($p < 0.001$). This reduction in mortality was not offset by any increase in deaths due to other causes, and therefore total mortality was also reduced significantly. However, there were two disadvantages of low dose heparin which had to be overcome if this form of prophylaxis was to be used on a large scale. Firstly, heparin had to be administered 8- or 12-hourly, and secondly there was a definite increased risk of bleeding, mostly in the form of wound haematoma. Low molecular weight heparins were thus developed to overcome these two main disadvantages of standard heparin prophylaxis.

The potential advantages of their use as prophylactic antithrombotic agents are based on their two to four-fold longer plasma half life following subcutaneous administration when compared to unfractionated heparin (UFH) at therapeutic doses (Bara et al 1985, 1988, Bratt et al 1986, Frydman et al 1988), thus enabling them to be administered as a single daily injection. Furthermore, for an equivalent antithrombotic effect, LMWH have been shown to cause less haemorrhage in experimental models than UFH (Holmer et al 1982, Cade et al 1984), and therefore are presumed to be associated with a reduced risk of perioperative bleeding in surgical patients.

Over the past decade, LMWH have been evaluated in a number of double-blind, randomized clinical trials. The first prospective study of the efficacy of LMWH in patients was published by Kakkar et al in 1982. In this study, 150 consecutive patients undergoing major abdominal surgery were investigated. 50 of these patients received 1250 APTT units of a heparin fraction prepared by gel permeation every 12 hours, while the remaining 100 patients received a single injection of 1850 units daily. The units of activity were measured by an APTT assay, and the LMWH had an anti-Xa/APTT ratio of four. None of the patients died from pulmonary embolism and three in each group developed deep vein thrombosis detected by the ^{125}I-fibrinogen uptake test. Prophylaxis had to be discontinued in two of the 50 patients who received LMWH every 12 hours. Global clotting assays and platelet function tests indicated that both the LMWH and UFH produced comparable effects, although intra-group comparisons revealed significant differences in anti-Xa activity, lipoprotein lipase release and plasma prekallikrein and thromboxane B_2 concentration (Kakkar et al 1982). Thus this study showed that a single daily dose of LMWH administered subcutaneously was sufficient to prevent postoperative deep vein thrombosis in 97 out of 100 patients monitored by the ^{125}I-fibrinogen uptake test for at least 10 days. In a follow-up study, Kakkar and Murray (1985) assessed the efficacy and safety of the same LMWH (Choay CY216) in the prevention of deep vein thrombosis in a double-blind, randomly allocated trial involving 400 patients; half of whom received LMWH and the other half UFH. 7.5% of patients receiving UFH and 2.5% receiving LMWH developed isotopic deep vein thrombosis; the difference in the frequency of deep vein thrombosis in the two groups being statistically significant ($p < 0.05$). No significant difference between the two groups in terms of excessive incisional or total blood loss during surgery was observed. In a further 910 patients included in an 'open' study, who again received a single daily injection of LMWH, 3.4% developed isotopic deep vein thrombosis. Thus in three separate groups of patients, all over the age of 40 and undergoing major abdominal surgery (the original 100 patients, the control study in 200 patients and the 'open' study of 900 patients, with a single daily injection of low molecular wight heparin), the incidence of postoperative deep vein thrombosis was constant at about 3%. The other important finding of Kakkar & Murray (1985) was the reported incidence of haematoma of only 1.6% in 709 patients undergoing general abdominal surgery although the incidence was higher in patients undergoing gynaecological surgery. They also concluded that a single daily injection of LMWH was likely to be more acceptable to patients and would certainly save nursing time when compared with 8- or 12-hourly administration of unfractionated heparin.

Several other randomized, double-blind trials (Table 62.8) using an almost similar design, have subsequently confirmed the original observations reported by Kakkar et al (1982). LMWH (Fragmin) was compared with UFH in two trials reported by Bergqvist et al (1986, 1988). In the first study, 432 patients were randomly allocated to receive either LMWH (Fragmin) 5000 anti-Xa units 2 hours before operation, and then 5000 IU daily or UFH 5000 U twice daily. Isotopic deep vein thrombosis was detected in 6.4% of patients in the LMWH group compared with 4.3% in the UFH group. The difference was not statistically significant. However, higher frequency of bleeding complications was observed in the patients receiving LMWH (Fragmin); 11.6% compared to 4.6% in those receiving UFH, the difference being statistically significant ($p < 0.005$). In the second study, Bergqvist et al (1988) prolonged the interval between the preoperative dose of heparin from 1 to 12 h in the belief that high concentrations of heparin during surgery were responsible for most of the operative bleeding complications observed. In this study, 1002 patients undergoing elective general abdominal surgery (64% for malignant disease) were included. Deep vein thrombosis was detected in 5.5% of the 505 patients receiving LMWH and 8.7% in 497 patients in the UFH group; the difference was not statistically significant. However, in this trial, once again there was increase in the frequency of bleeding complications in patients who received LMWH (Fragmin), 6% compared with 3% in the UFH group. In three subsequent studies (Caen et al 1988, Fricker et al 1988, Hertle et al 1990) a lower dose LMWH (Fragmin) 2500 U once a day, has been compared with 5000 U of UFH given either 8- or 12-hourly. In the study reported by Caen et al (1988), 395 patients were randomized to either 2500 IU of Fragmin once daily or 5000 IU of UFH twice daily. Deep vein thrombosis was detected in 3.1% of the LMWH group compared with 3.7% in the UFH group. No difference was detected in bleeding between the two groups. In the study reported by Hartle et al (1990), 250 patients were randomized to receive either 2500 U of LMWH (Fragmin) once a day or 5000 U of UFH twice daily. The rate of thrombosis was 8% in the LMWH and 9.8% in the UFH group. However, the patients who received the LMWH required fewer transfusions postoperative ($p < 0.01$). Fricker et al randomized 80 patients undergoing surgery for malignant disease, to either LMWH (Fragmin) or UFH. In the patients receiving LMWH (Fragmin), 2500 iu were given 2 hours before surgery and 12 hours after the first injection, and then 5000 IU daily, while those in the UFH group received 5000 U 8-hourly. None of the patients in

Table 62.8 Randomized trials of low molecular weight heparin and standard heparin for the prevention of postoperative deep vein thrombosis in general abdominal surgery

	Preparation	Dose used[1]	No of patients	Frequency DVT[2] No. (%)	Frequency Overall bleeding No. (%)
Double-blind trials					
Kakkar et al (1985)	Fraxiparin	7500 OD	196	5 (2.6)*	10 (5.1)
	UFH	5000 BID	199	15 (7.5)	7 (3.5)
Caen (1988)	Fragmin	2500 OD	195	6 (3.1)	4 (2.1)
	UFH	5000 BID	190	7 (3.7)	3 (1.6)
Hartl et al (1990)	Fragmin	2500 OD	112	9 (8.0)	4 (3.6)
	UFH	5000 BID	115	9 (7.8)	4 (3.5)
Leizorovicz et al (1991)	Logiparin	2500 OD	431	34 (7.9)	9 (2.1)
		5500 OD	430	16 (3.7)	13 (3.0)
	UFH	5000 BID	429	18 (4.2)	14 (3.3)
Open trials					
Encke & Breddin (1988)	Fraxiparin	7500 OD	960	27 (2.8)*	47 (4.9)
	UFH	5000 TID	936	42 (4.5)	42 (4.5)
Bergqvist et al (1988)	Fragmin	5000 PO 5000 OD	505	28 (5.5)	30 (6.0)
	UFH	5000 BID	497	41 (8.3)	15 (3.0)*
Fricker et al (1988)	Fragmin	2500 PO 5000 OD	40	0	4 (10.0)
	UFH	5000 TID	40	0	12 (30.0)
Samama et al (1988)	Enoxaparin	1600 OD	159	6 (3.8)	4 (2.5)
	UFH	5000 TID	158	12 (7.6)	4 (2.5)

LMWH, low molecular weight heparin; UFH, unfractionated heparin; DVT, deep vein thrombosis; OD, once daily; BID, twice daily; TID, thrice daily; PO, preoperative; * Significant difference $p < 0.05$.
[1] Dosage used: IU of UFH and anti-Xa IC units of LMWH (Fraxiparin, Fragmin, Logiparin, Enoxaparin)
[2] Frequency of DVT detected by ^{125}I-fibrinogen test.

either group developed thrombosis. Severe and moderate bleeding complications were more frequently observed in the UFH group; four patients in the LMWH (Fragmin) group compared to 12 in the UFH group ($p < 0.05$). Kakkar et al (1986) studied the effect of 2500 anti-Xa units of LMWH (Fragmin) given once daily compared with another group who received 2500 U twice daily. In the single-injection group, the incidence of thrombosis was 7.4% while in the two-injection group this fell to 2.6%. In the 200 patients studied, the difference in the deep vein thromboses did not reach statistical significance. Furthermore, there was no significant difference between the two groups in terms of the number of patients having excessive postoperative blood loss, requiring prophylaxis to be discontinued or measured postoperative drainage. The authors concluded from this study that 2500 anti-Xa units of Fragmin given once daily provides an effective prophylaxis against postoperative venous thrombosis.

In a collaborative French study, 334 patients were randomized to receive either 20 mg of LMWH (Enoxaparin) or 5000 IU of UFH 8 hours. Isotopic deep vein thrombosis was detected in 7.6% of patients in the standard heparin group and 3.8% in the LMWH group; the difference was not significant. Equal numbers of patients (four) (2.5%) developed bleeding complications (Samama et al 1988).

In one of the largest early trials on LMWH, nearly 2000 patients were randomly allocated to once daily subcutaneous injection of 7500 anti-Xa IC units of LMWH (Fraxiparine) or 500 IU of calcium heparin three times a day subcutaneously (European Fraxiparine Study; Encke & Breddin et al 1988). ^{125}I-fibrinogen uptake test was performed daily for 7 postoperative days, the results of positive scans being confirmed by phlebography. Deep vein thrombosis was detected in 2.8% of patients given LMWH and in 4.5% of those receiving UFH ($p < 0.034$). The rates of proximal vein thrombosis were 0.4% and 1.4% respectively ($p < 0.05$). The two treatment regimens were equally well tolerated and the incidence of wound haematoma, perioperative blood loss and blood transfusion was similar in both groups.

In a large multicentre Italian trial, Pezzuoli et al randomized 4498 patients to receive either 7500 anti-Xa IC units of LMWH (Fraxiparine) once daily or placebo. Eight (0.36%) deaths occurred to the LMWH (Fraxiparine) group and 18 (0.80%) in the placebo group, the difference being significant ($p < 0.05$). Autopsy was performed in 88.5% of the patients who died, and two deaths were attributed directly to pulmonary embolism in the treated group (0.09%) and four in the placebo group (0.18%). There was also a statistically significant reduction in thromboembolic mortality in favour of LMWH (0.36% to

0.09%) ($p < 0.05$). Intra- and postoperative bleeding was significantly more frequent in the LMWH group ($p < 0.01$), although such bleeding complications did not cause a significant difference in prophylaxis discontinuation. However, in comparison with the placebo group, there was a significantly higher incidence ($p < 0.01$) of wound haematoma, injection site bruising, postoperative bleeding and postoperative transfusions in patients who received LMWH (Fraxiparine).

Prophylaxis in orthopaedic surgery

In a study reported by Turpie et al (1986) 100 patients undergoing elective hip surgery were randomized to receive either LMWH (Enoxaparin) 30 mg (2400 anti-Xa units) twice daily or placebo. 5% of patients in the placebo group and 11% in the LMWH (Enoxaparin) group developed venous thrombosis, the difference being statistically significant. However, no difference was detected in bleeding complications. In the study reported by Leclerc et al (1991) 111 patients having knee surgery were randomized to receive either 30 mg (2400 anti-Xa units) of LMWH (Enoxaparin) twice daily or placebo; 65% of patients in the placebo group and 20% in the Enoxaparin group developed venous thrombosis, the differences being statistically significant ($p < 0.01$). No difference was detected in the bleeding between groups. In the third placebo-controlled trial, 196 patients having hip replacement were randomized to receive either LMWH (Lomoparin) 750 anti-Xa units twice daily or placebo (Hoek et al 1989). The rate of postoperative deep vein thrombosis was 57% in the placebo group compared with 16% in the heparin group ($p < 0.001$). Major bleeding complications occurred with equal frequency in both groups but six patients in the LMWH (Lomoparin) group developed minor wound haematoma compared to none in the placebo group.

The prophylactic effects of LMWH (Fragmin) in patients undergoing total hip replacement were also investigated by Eriksson et al (1988). Patients were allocated randomly to receive either 2500 anti-Xa units of Fragmin twice daily for 7 days with the first dose given 2 hours before surgery, or 500 ml dextran 70 twice daily during the day of operation, followed by a single infusion on the 1st and 3rd postoperative day. The ^{125}I-fibrinogen uptake test and phlebography were used to detect postoperative deep vein thrombosis, which developed in 45% of patients who received dextran and 20% of patients receiving LMWH. The authors also concluded that peri- and postoperative blood loss and transfusion requirements were significantly lower in the LMWH group, as compared to the dextran group.

In the study reported by Planes et al (1988), 237 patients undergoing elective hip replacement were randomly allocated to receive either LMWH (Enoxaparin) 40 mg (3200 anti-Xa units) once daily or UFH 5000 U three times daily; both regimens were started before surgery. A highly significant reduction in the incidence of deep vein thrombosis was observed in the patients receiving LMWH (12.5%) compared to 25% with UFH ($p = 0.01$). No difference in bleeding was detected between groups (Table 62.9).

In an even larger study, 665 patients undergoing hip replacement were randomized to receive either LMWH (Enoxaparin) 30 mg twice daily or UFH 7500 U twice daily; both regimens were started preoperatively (Levine et al 1991). In the UFH group, 23% of patients developed deep vein thrombosis compared to 19% in the LMWH (Enoxaparin) group; the difference was not statistically significant. However, clinically important bleeding occurred in 9% of patients in the UFH group and 5% of the LMWH group; the difference being statistically significant ($p < 0.05$). In a study reported by Leyvraz et al (1991), 349 patients undergoing elective hip surgery were randomized to receive either adjusted-dose LMWH (Fraxiparin) once daily or adjusted-dose UFH 8-hourly, with drugs being given preoperatively. In the Fraxiparin group, 16% of patients developed deep vein thrombosis as did 16% in the UFH group; the difference not being significant. Similarly, the difference in bleeding complications was also not significant.

Dechavanne et al (1989) randomized 124 patients undergoing hip replacement to receive either LMWH (Fragmin) 2500 anti-Xa units twice daily (group I), or twice daily for the first 48 hours after surgery and then 500 anti-Xa units daily (group II) or adjusted-dose standard heparin (group III). In each group, the first dose was administered 2 hours before surgery. Deep vein thrombosis was detected in 4.9% of patients in group I, 7.3% in group II and 10% in group III. These rates were not significantly different statistically. Similarly, there were no significant differences in the frequency of bleeding complications (Table 62.9).

Mätzsch et al (1988) investigated the efficacy of LMWH (Logiparin) in 100 patients who were randomized to receive either dextran or LMWH (Logiparin) which was administered in the dose of 35 anti-Xa units/kg body weight once daily. The overall thrombosis rate was 23% in the patients receiving LMWH (Logiparin) and 39% in those receiving dextran. No bleeding complications, deaths or pulmonary emboli were recorded in either group.

Lassen et al (1991) randomized 219 patients having total hip replacement to either LMWH (Enoxaparin) 40 mg once daily commencing preoperatively or dextran. A significantly lower incidence of deep vein thrombosis of 6.5% was detected in the LMWH group compared with 21.6% in the dextran group ($p < 0.01$). No difference was detected in bleeding between groups (Table 62.9).

In a dose-ranging study, Spiro et al (1991) investigated the efficacy of three dose regimens of LMWH (Enoxaparin): 572 patients undergoing elective hip replacement were randomized to receive either 10 mg (800 anti-Xa units) once daily (group I), 40 mg (3200 anti-Xa units) once daily

Table 62.9 Randomized trials of low molecular weight heparin, placebo, standard heparin or dextran for the prevention of postoperative deep vein thrombosis in elective hip surgery

	Preparation	Dose used[1]	No. of patients	Frequency DVT No. (%)	Bleeding frequency Points[2]	No. (%)
Double-blind trials						
Placebo control						
Turpie et al (1986)	Enoxaparin	2400 BID	37	4 (10.8)	50	2 (4.0)
	Placebo		39	20 (51.3)*	50	2 (4.0)
Hoek et al (1989)	Lomoparin	750 BID	97	15 (15.3)	97	6 (6.1)*
	Placebo		97	56 (56.6)*	99	0
UFH control						
Planes et al (1988)	Enoxaparin	3200 OD	120	15 (12.5)	124	3 (2.4)
	UFH	5000 TID	108	27 (25.0)*	112	2 (1.8)
Estoppey et al (1989)	Lomoparin	750 BID	146	25 (17.1)		
	UFH + DHE	5000 U + 0.5 mg BID	149	48 (32.2)		
Levine et al (1991)	Enoxaparin	2400 BID	258	50 (19.4)	333	17 (5.1)
	UFH	7500 BID	263	63 (23.2)	332	31 (9.3)*
Eriksson et al (1991)	Fragmin	5000 OD	63	19 (30.2)	67	1 (1.5)
	UFH	5000 TID	59	25 (49.4)	68	5 (7.4)
Adjusted dose						
Leyvaz et al (1991)	Fraxiparin	Adjusted dose	134	22 (12.6)	198	1 (0.5)
	UFH	Adjusted dose	175	28 (16)	199	3 (1.5)
Dechavanne et al (1989)	Fragmin	2500 BID	38	2 (5.3)	41	7 (17.1)
	Fragmin	2500 BID/5000 OD	39	3 (7.7)	41	4 (10.0)
	UFH	Adjusted dose	38	4 (10.5)	39	4 (10.3)
Open studies						
Lassen et al (1991)	Enoxaparin	3200 OD	108	7 (6.0)	108	15 (13.9)
	Dextran	500 ml × 5	111	24 (21.6)*	111	26 (23.4)
Spiro et al (1991)	Enoxaparin	800 OD	116	36 (31)	161	8 (5.0)
		3200 OD	149	21 (14)	199	21 (10.6)
		2400 BID	143	16 (11)	208	27 (13.0)

LMWH, low molecular weight heparin; UFH, unfractionated heparin; DHE, dihydroergotamine; OD, once daily; BID, twice daily, TID, three times daily; * significant difference $p < 0.05$

[1] Dosage used: IU of UFH and anti-Xa units of LMWH (Enoxaparin, Lomoparin, Fragmin, Fraxiparin

[2] Points are scored points for assessing severity of bleeding.

(group II) or 30 mg (2400 anti-Xa units) twice daily (group III). Treatment was initiated postoperatively within 24 hours of surgery. In group I, 30% of patients developed postoperative deep vein thrombosis compared to 14% in group II and 11% in group III. However, interestingly, there was no difference in the incidence of bleeding between the three groups.

Non-surgical patients

The efficacy of LMWH has also been assessed in patients suffering thrombotic stroke since they represent a high-risk group likely to suffer from venous thromboembolic complications. In two studies, LMWH have been compared with placebo in preventing deep vein thrombosis detected by ^{125}I-fibrinogen uptake test. In the study reported by Turpie et al (1987) 75 patients proven to be suffering from ischaemic stroke, were randomized to receive either LMWH (Lomoparin), 750 anti-Xa units, or placebo, twice daily. In the placebo group 28% of patients developed deep vein thrombosis compared with 4% who received LMWH (Lomoparin); the difference being highly significant. In a subsequent study, the same authors compared the efficacy of LMWH (Lomoparin) to low dose UFH, again in patients suffering from ischaemic stroke (Turpie et al 1991). Of the patients receiving LMWH (Lomoparin), 8.9% developed isotopic deep vein thrombosis compared to 31% in the UFH group; the difference being significant ($p < 0.02$). However, no difference was detected in the bleeding complications. In another study, 60 patients suffering from ischaemic stroke were randomized to receive either LMWH (Fragmin) 2500 anti-Xa units twice daily or placebo (Prins et al 1987). The incidence of deep vein thrombosis in the placebo group of 50% was reduced to 20% in the LMWH (Fragmin) group ($p < 0.05$). No difference was detected in the bleeding complications. In a much larger study (Dahan et al 1986), 265 medical patients were randomized to receive LMWH (Enoxaparin) 60 mg (4800 anti-Xa units) once daily or placebo. Deep vein thrombosis was detected in 9.1% in the placebo group and 3.0% in the LMWH group ($p < 0.03$). Increased bleeding frequency in the form of injection site haematoma was only observed in the LMWH (Enoxaparin) group.

Multicentre trial of low molecular weight heparin

There is no doubt that several studies have clearly shown that LMWH represents a significant development in antithrombotic therapy. They have been evaluated in a number of randomized clinical trials and have been shown to be particularly effective in preventing postoperative venous thromboembolism in patients undergoing major abdominal and orthopaedic surgery. However, to date, in all the randomized clinical trials designed to compare the safety and efficacy of LMWH and UFH, relatively limited numbers of patients have been included and, thus, it has not been possible to answer the following questions which need to be resolved before recommending their use on a large scale. Is the risk of perioperative bleeding significantly reduced when LMWH is compared to UFH for prophylaxis? Does the bleeding induced by heparin prophylaxis, particular LMWH, significantly alter the outcome of surgery? What factors, in addition to heparin prophylaxis, constitute an increased risk of bleeding? How long should prophylaxis be continued, since it has been claimed that the risk of postoperative deep vein thrombosis/pulmonary embolism persists for a considerable time following discharge from hospital? A multicentre, randomized, double-blind, comparative trial of LMWH (Fragmin) and UFH for the prevention of postoperative venous thromboembolism in patients undergoing major abdominal surgery has been recently completed (Kakkar et al 1993). Surgeons in 19 hospitals took part in this study and 3938 patients were entered into the trial. Eligible patients were randomly allocated to receive subcutaneously either 2500 U of LMWH once daily plus a placebo injection or 5000 U of UFH twice daily. Of 3809 patients included in this study, perioperative deaths occurred in 110 patients (2.8%): 63 in the LMWH group and 47 (2.5%) in the UFH group ($p = 0.13$). 92 (84%) of the deaths occurred in patients who were operated for malignant disease. Autopsy was performed in 58% of patients, but in those suspected of sudden death due to cardiovascular or respiratory disease, autopsy was performed in all cases.

Pulmonary emboli were detected in 27 patients (0.7%): 13 of these occurred in the LWMH group and 14 in the UFH group. Sudden death occurred in eight of these patients and autopsy was performed in each case; five patients (0.26%) in the LWMH group and three (0.16%) in the UFH group were considered to have died from acute massive pulmonary embolism. Deep vein thrombosis were detected in 22 patients (0.58%), 11 in each group. Six patients, three in each group, developed major deep vein thrombosis. No significant difference was found in the total frequency of deep vein thrombosis or their venographic locations.

Based on subjective assessment, excessive operative and postoperative bleeding was recorded in 110 (5.9%) and 121 (6.5%) patients respectively of the LMWH group and 109 (5.7%) and 128 (6.8%) patients of the UFH group. Of these, 94 (5%) patients in each group required transfusion during surgery. During the postoperative period, 59 (3%) of patients in both groups required transfusion. Excessive drain loss was observed in 49 (2.6%) in the LMWH group and 44 (2.3%) in the standard heparin group.

Using objective criteria, bleeding events were classified as major or minor (Table 62.10). Major bleeding was defined as follows: during surgery, when excessive bleeding required discontinuation of prophylaxis or bleeding was attributable to the trial drug (heparin-associated); during the postoperative period when excessive bleeding required discontinuation of prophylaxis or reoperation to control it, or the patient developed a wound haematoma which may have required evacuation. To assess objectively the severity of bleeding, patients were scored according to the above mentioned indices of major bleeding with one point being allocated for each event. 93 incidences of major bleeding were observed in 69 (3.6%) patients in the LMWH group and 142 incidences in 91 patients (4.8%) in the standard heparin group. Non-parametric testing revealed that this

Table 62.10 An objective assessment of the frequency and severity of peri-operative bleeding

	LMWH	%	UFH	%	Significance (p)
Major bleeding events					
Total bleeding indices (number of patients)	93 (69)		142 (91)		0.058
Prophylaxis discontinued	36	1.9	40	2.1	NS
Bleeding considered heparin-related	10	0.5	12	0.6	NS
Wound haematoma	27	1.4	52	2.7	0.007
Number of operations (patients requiring re-operation for bleeding)	20 (18)	1.0	38 (33)	1.7	0.05
Patients with severe bleeding	18	1.0	36	1.9	0.02
Minor bleeding events					
Total bleeding indices (patients)	118 (117)		155 (152)		0.04
Wound oozing	44	2.3	35	1.8	NS
Injection site bruising	74	3.9	120	6.3	0.001

LMWH, low molecular weight heparin; UFH, unfractionated heparin.

difference in the indices failed to reach conventional statistical significance (p = 0.058). During surgery, 20 indices of major bleeding occurred in 18 patients in the LMWH group, and 21 indices in 16 patients in the standard heparin group. In contrast, during the postoperative period, 73 indices in 78 (4.1%) patients occurred in the standard heparin group. Severe bleeding (a score of 2 or more indices) occurred less frequently in the LMWH group with 18 (1.0%) patients versus 36 (1.9%) patients in the UFH group (RR 0.51 (CI 0.29–0.89) p = 0.002). 27 (1.4%) patients in the LMWH group and 52 (2.7%) in the UFH group developed wound haematoma, the difference being significant (RR 0.51 (CI 0.33–0.83) p = 0.007). 20 bleeding episodes in 18 (1.0%) patients in the LMWH and 38 episodes in 33 (1.7%) patients in the UFH group required further surgery, either for the evacuation of haematoma or reoperation to control bleeding. A significant difference was seen in the proportion of patients requiring reoperation (RR 0.55 (CI 0.31–0.98) p = 0.05) (Table 62.10).

Minor bleeding events included wound oozing and excessive injection site bruising. In the LMWH group, 118 such episodes occurred in 117 (6.2%) patients compared to 155 episodes in 152 (7.9%) patients in the UFH group: this difference was significant (RR 0.78 (CI 0.62–0.98) p = 0.04). However, this significant difference was due to the observed difference in injection site bruising (greater than 2 cm) between the two groups: 74 (3.9%) in the LMWH group compared to 120 (6.3%) in the standard heparin group (RR 0.62 (CI 0.47–0.83) p = 0.001).

Non-haemorrhagic adverse effects

Details were recorded on neurological, cardio-respiratory, gastrointestinal and renal complications, as well as wound infection, wound dehiscence, anastomotic failure, and other complications which could be considered to prolong hospitalization. No difference was found in the incidence of wound infection, wound dehiscence or any other complications.

Follow-up

Patients were followed up at a minimum of 4 weeks after discharge. Of the 3809 patients, 110 died in the perioperative period, leaving 3699 evaluable patients. Complete follow-up information was available in 3358 (91%) of these. 19 patients (0.57%) had died, ten (0.60%) in the LMWH group and nine (0.53%) in the UFH group. 15 (79%) of these had malignant disease. 25 patients (0.74%) developed thromboembolic complications, 15 in the LMWH group and ten in the UFH group. Of the three patients who had fatal pulmonary emboli (confirmed at autopsy) two had received LMWH and one UFH (Table 62.11).

Table 62.11 Major events in the follow-up period of the multicentre trial[1]

	LMWH	UFH
Number of patients (total = 3358)	1661	1697
Total number of deaths*	10 (0.6%)	9 (0.53%)
Cause of death		
Pulmonary:		
Pulmonary embolism	2	1
Pneumonia	1	0
Carcinomatosis	6	7
Septicaemia	1	1
Thromboembolic events (% of total number of patients)	15 (0.9%)	10 (0.6%)
Pulmonary emboli (% of total)	9 (0.5%)	5 (0.3%)
Deep vein thromboses (% of total)	8 (0.5%)	6 (0.4%)

LMWH, low molecular weight heparin, 2500 U once daily; UFH, UFH heparin, 5000 U twice daily.
[1] Kakkar et al 1993.

Low molecular weight heparin versus standard heparin in general and orthopaedic surgery: a meta-analysis

In a recent meta-analysis study, Nurmohamed et al (1992) analyzed all comparative trials of perioperative prophylaxis against deep vein thrombosis or pulmonary embolism in patients undergoing general surgery (defined as abdominothoracic or gynaecological surgery) or orthopaedic surgery (defined as elective or traumatic hip surgery). Only studies which compared LMWH and UFH, both agents being given in the currently recommended dose, were included in the analysis. A total of 8172 patients were included in this analysis, 6878 patients were in the 17 general surgery trials and 1294 in the six orthopaedic surgery trials. For the general surgical trials ^{125}I-labelled fibrinogen leg scanning was used as the end-point for the diagnosis of deep vein thrombosis, while for orthopaedic surgery, only trials in which venography was used in all patients for establishing the presence or absence of deep vein thrombosis were included. For the rate of fatal and non-fatal pulmonary embolism, the diagnosis was accepted if one or more of the following methods or criteria were applied in both study groups: necropsy, perfusion-ventilation scanning, angiography or clinical diagnosis, total mortality and major bleeding. Major bleeding was defined as clinically overt with one or more of the following criteria: fall in haemoglobin of more than 1.2 g/l, bleeding necessitating re-operation or cessation of prophylaxis, or retroperitoneal or intracranial bleeding.

In the general surgery group, 184 patients out of 3467 patients in the LMWH group developed deep vein thrombosis compared to 230 out of 3411 in the UFH group. A relative risk of deep vein thrombosis with LMWH over UFH for all surgical trials was 0.74 (95% CI 0.65–0.86). In contrast, the relative risk for all pulmonary emboli with LMWH over UFH was 0.44 (95% CI 0.21–0.95). In the general surgery trials, the absolute mean incidence of major bleeding was 2.6% in each of the two treatment groups. In the orthopaedic group, only six out of 672 patients receiving LMWH and eight out of 622 receiving UFH developed major bleeding; a relative risk of 0.75 (95% CI 0.26–2.14).

The authors concluded that at present there is no convincing evidence that, in general surgery patients, LMWH compared with UFH generates a clinically important improvement in the benefit to risk ratio. However, LMWH may be preferable for orthopaedic surgery patients, in view of the large risk-reduction for venous thrombosis.

The difference in the results of the meta-analysis and the trial reported by Kakkar et al (1993) may possibly be due to the difference in the criteria used to define major bleeding. In the meta-analysis of Nurmohamed et al (1992), major bleeding was re-assessed retrospectively using different criteria than had been employed in the initial studies. In the Kakkar trial, major bleeding was assessed prospectively using a number of objective criteria which has been defined in advance of starting the trial. In the meta-analysis no information is provided regarding the number of patients with indices of major bleeding necessitating re-operation, cessation of prophylaxis or when it was retroperitoneal or intracranial bleeding. In contrast, in our studies (as mentioned above), clinically important, severe bleeding occurred less frequently in the LMWH group with 18 patients (1.00%) versus 36 patients (1.9%) in the UFH group [RR 0.51, (CI 0.29–0.89), $p = 0.02$]. Furthermore, significantly fewer wound haematoma were observed in the LMWH group, and a fewer number of patients required evacuation of haematoma or reoperation to control bleeding.

Adoption of low molecular weight heparin prophylaxis

The evidence that LMWH and UFH can prevent venous thromboembolism in most postoperative patients is irrefutable. A number of studies have now demonstrated that a fixed dose of LMWH administered as a single daily subcutaneous injection is at least as effective a prophylactic agent as UFH given 8- or 12-hourly. Therefore, LMWH prophylaxis has a potential advantage of better acceptance by the patients and its adoption on a large scale should save considerable nursing time. However, one of the unresolved questions in the past related to the presumed greater safety of LMWH. This important question was answered by the results of a comparative trial involving approximately 4000 patients, where serious bleeding during the perioperative period was significantly reduced with LMWH, primarily due to a reduction in the frequency of postoperative bleeding complications. Furthermore, there were significantly fewer wound haematomas in the LWMH group, as well as fewer patients requiring evacuation of haematoma or re-operation to control bleeding (Kakkar et al 1992).

Another concern about the adoption of heparin prophylaxis in the past has been whether the bleeding induced significantly alters the outcome of surgery, particularly anastomic failure in patients who have colonic or gastro-oesophageal anastomosis, wound infection and wound dehiscence. In a recent report of the National Confidential Enquiry into Peri-Operative Deaths (NCEPOD, 1992), the frequency of such complication in 1109 patients who died was analyzed. When the complication rate calculated in each of the NCEPOD surgical groups was applied to the multicentre trial data (Kakkar et al 1993), the following number of events would be expected: anastomotic failure in five, wound dehiscence in four, and wound infection in seven. In fact, in the 110 patients who died during the perioperative period in the multicentre trial, anastomotic failure occurred in eight (7.3%), wound dehiscence in one (0.26%), and wound infection in 12 (11.0%). Although an accurate comparison can only be made in a double-blind, randomized trial having a control group, the comparison with the NCEPOD data does appear to suggest that the use of heparin prophylaxis does not significantly alter the outcome of surgery.

The results of the International Multicentre Trial published in 1975 laid the foundation for the adoption of low dose heparin prophylaxis. The first postoperative study of the efficacy of LMWH in patients was published in 1982 (Kakkar et al 1983). This study paved the way for many studies that have followed, confirming the original observation that a single daily fixed dose of LMWH prevented most postoperative deep vein thrombosis and was likely to be more acceptable to patients and save nursing time. The results of the latest multicentre trial (Kakkar et al 1993) indicate that both LMWH and UFH are equally effective in preventing postoperative venous thromboembolism. However, prophylaxis with LMWH in this large study was associated with a significantly reduced incidence of serious bleeding complications. In the past, thromboprophylaxis has not been used on a large scale. Although the practice is now more widely established, many high-risk patients are still not protected. This is partly because an individual surgeon, no matter how extensive his personal practice, will never recognize the success of his prophylactic action, yet will invariably be reminded of his failures in terms of bleeding complications. However, in view of such circumstances, what should be the role of a practising clinician now that we have a safe, effective prophylactic therapy which is acceptable to patients and simple for nursing staff to use? We believe that the emphasis is now on the clinicians, who should protect all high-risk patients using LMWH prophylaxis.

REFERENCES

Aberg M, Bergentz S E, Hedner U 1975 The effect of dextran on the lysability of ex vivo thrombi. Annals of Surgery 181: 342–345

Abernethy E A 1974 Postoperative embolism. A prospective study utilising low dose heparin. American Journal of Surgery 128: 739–742

Aellig W H 1975 Lentersuchung iilear die venenkon-string ierende Wirkung von Ergotverhindungen in Menschen. Triangle 14: 39–44

Ahlberg A, Nylander G, Robertson B et al 1968 Dextran in prophylaxis of thrombosis in fractures of the hip. Acta Chirurgica Scandinavica (suppl) 387–383

Ballard R M, Bradley M, Watson P J, Johnstone F W 1973 Low doses of subcutaneous heparin in the prevention of deep vein thrombosis after gynaecological surgery. Journal of Obstetrics and Gynaecology of the British Commonwealth 80: 469–472

Bara L, Samama M M 1988 Pharmacokinetics of low molecular weight heparins. Acta Chirurgica Scandinavica 543: 65

Bara L, Billaud E, Gramond G, Kher A, Samama M 1985 Comparative pharmacokinetics of low molecular weight heparin (PK 10169) and unfractionated heparin after intravenous and subcutaneous administration. Thrombosis Research 39: 631–636

Bergqvist D, Efsing M O et al 1989 Prevention of postoperative thromboembolic complications: a prospective comparison between dextran-70 dihydroergotamine, heparin and a sulphated polysaccharide. Acta Chirurgica Scandinavica 146: 559–568

Bergqvist B, Torngren S, Wallin G 1986 Low molecular weight heparin once daily compared with conventional low dose heparin twice daily: A prospective double-blind multicentre trial on prevention of postoperative thrombosis. British Journal of Surgery 73: 204–208

Bergqvist D, Matzch T, Burmark U S et al 1988 Low molecular weight heparin given in the evening before surgery compared with conventional low-dose heparin in prevention of thrombosis. British Journal of Surgery 75: 888

Blombäck B, Blombäck M 1965 Structure of N-terminal fragments of fibrinogen and specificity of the thrombin. Nature (London) 215: 1445

Bratt G, Tornebohm E, Widlund L, Lockner D 1986 Low molecular weight heparin (KABI 2165, Fragmin): Pharmacokinetics after intravenous and subcutaneous administration in human volunteers. Thrombosis Research 42: 613–619

Brisman R, Parks L C, Haller J A Jr 1971 Dextran prophylaxis in surgery. Annals of Surgery 174: 137–141

Brucke P, Dienstl E et al 1983 Prophylaxis of postoperative thromboembolism: low dose heparin versus heparin plus dihydroergotamine. Thrombosis Research 29: 377–383

Burch J W, Stanford N, Majerus P W 1978 Inhibition of platelet prostaglandin synthetase by oral aspirin. Journal of Clinical Investigation 61: 314–319

Bygdeman S, Elisson R, Gullbring B 1966 Effect of dextran infusion on the adenosine diphosphate induced adhesiveness and the spreading capacity of human blood platelets. Thrombosis et Diathesis Haemorrhagica 15: 451

Bygdeman S, Svensjo E, Tollerz G 1970 Prevention of venous thrombosis. Lancet 2: 419

Cade J F, Buchanan M R, Boneu B, Ockelford P, Carter C J, Cerskus A L, Hirsh J 1984 A comparison of the antithrombotic and haemorrhagic effects of low molecular weight heparin fractions: The influence of the method of preparation. Thrombosis Research 35: 613–619

Caen J P 1988 A randomised double-blind study between a low-molecular weight heparin (Kabi 2165) and standard heparin in the prevention of deep vein thrombosis in general surgery – A French multicentre trial. Thrombosis Research 59(2): 216

Cerkus A L, Ali M, McDonald J W D 1978 Possible significance of functional platelets circulating between doses of aspirin. Blood 52: 160

Clagett G P, Salzman E W 1974 Prevention of venous thromboembolism in surgical patients. New England Journal of Medicine 290: 93–96

Collins R, Scrimgeour A, Yusef S, Peto R 1988 Reduction in fatal pulmonary embolism and venous thrombosis by perioperative administration of subcutaneous heparin. Overview of results of randomized trials in general, orthopaedic and urological surgery. New England Journal of Medicine 318: 1162–1173

Corrigan T P, Kakkar V V, Fossard D P 1974 Low dose subcutaneous heparin — optimal dose regimen. British Journal of Surgery 61: 320

Covey T H, Sherman L, Baue A E 1975 Low dose heparin in postoperative patients. A prospective, coded study. Archives of Surgery 110: 1021

Cronberg S, Robertson B, Nilsson I M, Milehn J E 1966 Suppresive effect of dextran on platelet adhesiveness. Thrombosis et Diathesis Haemorrhagica 16: 384

Dahan R, Houlbert D, Caulin C, Cuzin E, Viltart C, Woler M, Segrestaa J M 1986 Prevention of deep vein thrombosis in elderly medical patients by a low molecular weight heparin: A randomized double-blind trial. Haemostasis 16: 159

Dechavanne M, Ville D, Viala J J et al 1975 Controlled trial of platelet antiaggregating agents and subcutaneous heparin in prevention of postoperative deep vein thrombosis in high risk patients. Haemostasis 4: 94

Dechavanne M, Ville D, Berruyer M et al 1989 Randomized trial of low molecular weight heparin (Kabi 2165) versus adjusted dose subcutaneous standard heparin in the prophylaxis of deep vein thrombosis after elective hip surgery. Haemostasis 1: 5

de Takats G 1950 Anticoagulants in surgery. Journal of the American Medical Association 142: 527–529

Doran F S A, Drury M, Sivyer A 1964 A simple way to combat the venous stasis which occurs in the lower limbs during surgical operations. British Journal of Surgery 51: 486

Emerson P A, Marks P 1977 Preventing thromboembolism after myocardial infarction – effect of low dose heparin or smoking. British Medical Journal 1: 18–20

Encke A, Stock D, Dunke H O 1976 Doppllbindusdie zur postoperativen thrombose prophylaxe mit dipyridamol Acetylsalicyslaure. Chirurgica Scandinavia 47: 670–673

Encke A, Breddin K (European Fraxiparine Study Group) 1988 Comparison of a low molecular weight heparin and unfractionated heparin for the prevention of deep vein thrombosis in patients undergoing abdominal surgery. British Journal of Surgery 75: 1058–1063

Eriksson B I, Kalebo P, Anthmyr B A, Wadenvik I, Tengborn L, Risberg B 1991 Prevention of deep vein thrombosis and pulmonary embolism after total hip replacement. Journal of Bone and Joint Surgery 73A: 484

Estoppey D, Hochreiter J, Breyer H G, Jakubek H, Leyvraz P F, Haas S, Stiekema J C J 1989 ORG 10172 (Lomoparin) versus heparin-DHE in prevention of thromboembolism in total hip replacement — A multicentre trial. Thrombosis and Haemotasis 62 (suppl): 356

Evarts M, Alfidi S 1973 Low dose heparin prophylaxis. Journal of the American Medical Association 225: 515–516

Flanc C, Kakkar V V, Clarke M B 1969 Postoperative deep vein thrombosis: effect of intensive prophylaxis. Lancet 1: 477–478

Fricker J P, Vergnes Y, Schach R et al 1988 Low dose heparin versus low molecular weight heparin (Kabi 2165, Fragmin) in the prophylaxis of thromboembolic complications of abdominal oncological surgery. European Journal of Clinical Investigation 18: 561

Frydman A, Bara L, Leroux Y, Woler M, Chauliac F, Duchier J, Samama M 1988 The antithrombotic activity and pharmacokinetics of Enoxaparin, a low molecular weight heparin, in man given single subcutaneous doses of 20 up to 80 mg. Journal of Clinical Pharmacology 28: 608–618

Gallus A S, Hirsh J, Tuttle R J, Trebilcock R, O'Brien S E 1973 Small subcutaneous doses of heparin in the prevention of venous thrombosis. New England Journal of Medicine 288: 545–551

Gent M, Roberts S S 1986 A meta-analysis of the studies of dihydroergotamine plus heparin in the prophylaxis of deep vein thrombosis. Chest 89(suppl): 397–400

Gordon-Smith I C, Grundy D J, Lequesne L P, Newcombe J F 1972 Controlled trial of two regimens of subcutaneous heparin in the prevention of postoperative deep vein thrombosis. Lancet 1: 1133–1135

Griffith J C, Boggs R P 1964 Long-term heparin therapy. The clinical usage of heparin. American Journal of Cordiology 39: 14–26

Gruber U F, Saldeen T, Brokop T et al 1980 Incidences of fatal postoperative pulmonary embolism after prophylaxis with dextran 70 and low dose heparin: an international multicentre study. British Medical Journal 280: 69–72

Hampson W J G, Harris F C, Lucas H K et al 1974 Failure of low dose heparin to prevent deep vein thrombosis after hip replacement arthroplasty. Lancet 2: 795–797

Handin R I, Valeri C R 1971 Hemostatic effectiveness of platelets stored at 22°C. New England Journal of Medicine 285: 538–554

Handley A J, Emerson P A, Fleming P R 1972 Heparin in the prevention of deep vein thrombosis after myocardial infarction. British Medical Journal 2: 436

Harris W H, Salzman E W, DeSanctis R W et al 1972 Prevention of venous thromboembolism following total hip replacement: Warfarin vs Dextran 40. Journal of American Medical Association 220: 1319–1322

Harris W H, Salzman E A, Athanasoulis C 1974 Comparison of warfarin, low molecular weight dextran, aspirin and subcutaneous heparin in prevention of venous thromboembolism following total hip replacement. Journal of Bone and Joint Surgery 50: 1552–1562

Harris W H, Salzman E W, Athanasoulis C A, Waltman A C, DeSantis R W 1977 Aspirin prophylaxis of venous thromboembolism after total hip replacement. New England Journal of Medicine 297: 1246

Hartl P, Brucke P, Dienstl E, Vinazzer H 1990 Prophylaxis of thromboembolism in general surgery: comparison between standard heparin and Fragmin. Thrombosis Research 57: 577–584

Hills N H, Pflug J J, Jeyasingh K, Boardman L, Calman J S 1972 Prevention of deep vein thrombosis by intermittent pneumatic compression of calf. British Medical Journal 1: 131–135

Hirsh J, Levine M M 1992 Low molecular weight heparin. Blood 79: 1–17

Hoek J, Nurmohamed M T, ten Cate H, ten Cate J W, Buller H 1989 Prevention of deep vein thrombosis following total hip replacement by a low molecular weight heparinoid. Thrombosis and Haemostasis 62 (suppl): 1637

Holmer E, Matsson C, Nilsson S 1982 Anticoagulant and antithrombotic effects of low molecular weight heparin fragments in rabbits. Thrombosis Research 25: 475–479

Huber O, Bounameaux H, Borst F, Rohner A 1992 Postoperative pulmonary embolism after hospital discharge — an underestimated risk. Archives in Surgery 127: 310–313

Hume M, Kuriakose T, Xavier Z L 1973 ^{125}I-fibrinogen and the prevention of venous thrombosis. Archives of Surgery 107: 803–806

Hume M, Biermaum B, Kuriakose T X, Supenant J 1977 Prevention of postoperative thrombosis by aspirin. American Journal of Surgery 133: 410–412

International Multicentre Trial 1975 Prevention of postoperative pulmonary embolism by low doses of heparin. Lancet 2: 45–51

Johnsson S R, Bygdeman S, Eliasson R 1986 Effect of dextran on postoperative thrombosis. Acta Chirurgica Scandinavica (suppl) 387: 80–82

Kakkar V V 1975 Efficacy of low dose heparin in preventing postoperative fatal pulmonary embolism: Results of an International Multicentre Trial. DHEW Publication No. (NIH) 76N-866, p 207

Kakkar V V 1979 The logistic problems encountered in the Multicentre Trial of low dose heparin prophylaxis. The challenges of clinical trials in thrombosis. Schattauer Verlag, Stuttgart, p 105

Kakkar V V, Murray W J G 1985 Efficacy and safety of low molecular weight heparin (CY216) in preventing postoperative venous thromboembolism: a cooperative study. British Journal of Surgery 72: 786–791

Kakkar V V, Field E S, Nicolaides A N et al 1971 Low doses of heparin in prevention of deep vein thrombosis. Lancet 2: 669–671

Kakkar V V, Corrigan T P, Spindler J et al 1972 Efficacy of low doses of heparin in the prevention of deep vein thrombosis after major surgery. A double-blind, randomized trial. Lancet 1: 101–106

Kakkar V V, Djazaeri B, Fok J, Fletcher M, Scully M F, Westwick J 1982 Low molecular weight heparin and prevention of postoperative deep vein thrombosis. British Medical Journal 284: 375–379

Kakkar V V, Fox P J, Murray W J G et al 1985 Heparin and dihydroergotamine prophylaxis against thromboembolism after hip arthroplasty. Journal of Bone and Joint Surgery 67B (suppl 4): 538–542

Kakkar V V, Kakkar S, Sanderson R M, Peers C E 1986 Efficacy and safety of two regimens of low molecular weight heparin fragment (Fragmin) in preventing postoperative venous thromboembolism. Haemostasis 16 (suppl 2): 19–24

Kakkar V V, Cohen A T, Edmondson R A, Philips M J et al 1993 Low molecular weight versus standard heparin for prevention of venous thromboembolism after major abdominal surgery. Lancet 341: 259–265

Kelton J G, Hirsh, Carter C J, Buchanan M R 1978 Thrombogenic effect of high dose aspirin in rabbits. Relationship to inhibition of vessel wall synthesis of prostaglandin I_2-like activity. Journal of Clinical Investigation 62: 892–895

Kiil J, Axelsen F, Kiil J, Anderson D 1978 Prophylaxis against postoperative pulmonary embolism and deep vein thrombosis by low-dose heparin. Lancet 1: 1115–1116

Kline A, Hughes L E, Campbell H et al 1975 Dextran 70 in prophylaxis of thromboembolic disease after surgery — a clinically orientated randomised double blind trial. British Medical Journal 2: 109–112

Kockenburg L J L 1962 Experimental use of Macrodex as a prophylaxis against postoperative thromboembolism. Bulletin de la Societé Internale Chirurgie 21: 501–516

Lahnborg G 1980 Effect of low dose heparin and dihydroergotamine of frequency of postoperative deep vein thrombosis in patients undergoing post-traumatic hip surgery. Acta Chirurgica Scandinavica 146: 319–322

Lahnborg G, Friman L, Bergstrom K, Lagergren H 1974 Effect of low dose heparin in incidence of postoperative embolism detected by photoscanning. Lancet 1: 329N–331N

Lassen M R 1991 The Danish Enoxaparin Study Group: low molecular heparin (enoxaparin) vs. dextran 70: the prevention of postoperative deep vein thrombosis after total hip replacement. Archives of Internal Medicine 151: 1621

Leizorovicz A, Picolet H, Peyrieux J C, Borssel J P 1991 Prevention of perioperative deep vein thrombosis in general surgery: A multicentre double blind study comparing two doses of Logiparin and standard heparin: British Journal of Surgery 78: 412

Levine M N, Hirsh J, Gent M, Turpie A G G, Leclerc J, Powers P J, Jay R M, Neemeh J 1991 Prevention of deep vein thrombosis after elective hip surgery: A randomized trial comparing low molecular weight heparin with standard unfractionated heparin. Annals of Internal Medicine 114: 545

Leyvraz P F, Richard J, Bachmann F et al 1983 Adjusted versus fixed dose subcutaneous heparin in the prevention of deep vein thrombosis after total hip replacement. New England Journal of Medicine 309: 954–958

Leyvraz P F, Bachmann F, Hoek J, Buller H R, Postel M, Samama M, Vandenbroek M D 1991 Prevention of deep vein thrombosis after hip replacement: randomized comparison between unfractionated heparin and low molecular weight heparin. British Medical Journal 303: 543

Loew D, Wellmer H E, Baer U et al 1974 Postoperative thromboembolic prophylaxe mit acetyl-salicysaune. Deutsche Medizinische Wochenschrift 99: 565–572

McCarthy S T, Robertson D, Turner J J, Hawkey C J, Macey D J 1977 Low dose heparin as a prophylaxis against deep vein thrombosis after acute stroke. Lancet 2: 800–801

Mannucci P M, Citterio L E, Panajotapoulos N 1976 Low dose heparin and DVT after total hip replacement. Thrombosis and Haemostasis 36: 157–164

Marks P, Teather D 1978 Subcutaneous heparin. A logical prophylaxis for deep vein thrombosis after myocardial infarction. Practitioner 220: 425–427

Mätzsch T, Bergqvist D, Fredin H, Hedner U 1988 Safety and efficacy of low molecular weight heparin (Logiparin) versus dextran as prophylaxis against thrombosis after total hip replacement. Acta Chirurgica Scandinavica 543: 80–84

Mazaffar T Z, Bryce W A, Dhall D P 1976 Effect of dextran on the molecular structure and tensile behaviour of human fibrin. Thrombosis and Haemostasis 35: 737

Mellander S, Nordenfelt I 1970 Comparative effects of dihydroergotamine and noradrenaline on resistance, exchange and capacitance functions in the peripheral circulation. Clinical Science 39: 183–201

Morris G K, Mitchell J R A 1977 Preventing venous thromboembolism in elderly patients with hip fractures. Studies of low dose heparin, dipyridamole, aspirin, and flurbiprofen. British Medical Journal 1: 535–537

Multi-unit Controlled trial 1974 A multi-unit controlled trial: heparin versus dextran in the prevention of deep vein thrombosis. Lancet 2: 118–120

NCEPOD 1992 The report of the National Confidential Enquiry into Perioperative Deaths 1990. Lincoln's Inn Fields, London, p 35–43

Nicolaides A N, Dupont P A, Desai S et al 1972 Small doses of subcutaneous sodium heparin in preventing deep venous thrombosis after major surgery. Lancet 2: 890–893

Nurmohamed M T, Rosendaal F R, Buller H R, Dekker E, Hommes D W, Vandenbronche Jan P, Briët E 1992 The efficacy and safety of low molecular weight heparin versus standard heparin in general and orthopaedic surgery: A meta-analysis. Lancet 340: 152–156

Peterson J, Zucker M B 1970 The effect of adenosine monophosphate, arcaine and anti-inflammatory agents on thrombosis and platelet function in rabbits. Thrombosis et Diathesis Haemorrhagica 23: 148–158

Pezzuoli G, Neriserneri G G, Settembrini P et al 1989 Prophylaxis of fatal pulmonary embolism in general surgery using low molecular weight heparin (CY216): A multicentre, double blind, randomized controlled trial versus placebo (STEP). Internal Surgery 74: 205–210

Pitney W R, Dean S 1978 Plasma heparin concentrations during subcutaneous heparin therapy. Australia and New Zealand Journal of Medicine 6: 454

Planes A, Vochelle N, Mazas F et al 1988 Prevention of postoperative venous thrombosis: a randomized trial comparing unfractionated heparin with low molecular weight heparin in patients undergoing total hip replacement. Thrombosis and Haemostasis 60: 407–410

Poller L, Taberner D A, Sandilands D G et al 1982 An evaluation of APTT monitoring of low dose heparin in hip surgery. Thrombosis and Haemostasis 47: 50–53

Prins M H, den Ottolander G J H, Gelsema R, van Woerkom T C M, Sing A K, Heller I 1987 Deep vein thrombosis prophylaxis with a low molecular weight heparin (Kabi 2165) in stroke patients. Thrombosis and Haemostasis 58 (suppl): 117

Rem J, Duckert F, Fridrich R 1975 Subkutane kleine heparindosen zur thromboserophylaxe in der allgemeinen chirurgie und urologie. Schweizerische Medizinische Wochenschrift 105: 827

Report of the steering committee on a trial sponsored by the Medical Research Council 1972 Effect of aspirin on postoperative venous thrombosis. Lancet 2: 441–444

Rosenberg I L, Evans M, Pollock A V 1974 Prevention of postoperative leg vein thrombosis: a comparison of low dose heparin and electrical calf muscle stimulation. British Medical Journal 1: 649–651

Rosengarten D S, Laird J, Jeyasingh J, Martin P 1970 The failure of compression stockings (Tubigrip) to prevent deep venous thrombosis after operation. British Journal of Surgery 57: 296–299

Rothman S, Adelson E, Schwebel A, Lingdell R D 1957 Absorption of carbon-14-dextran to human blood platelets and red blood cells in vitro. Vox Sanguinis 2: 104–109

Sabri S, Roberts V C, Cotton L T 1971 Prevention of early postoperative deep vein thrombosis by passive exercise of leg during surgery. British Medical Journal 3: 82–83

Sagar S, Massey J, Sanderson J M 1975 Low dose heparin prophylaxis against fatal pulmonary embolism. British Medical Journal 4: 257–280

Sagar S, Stamatakis J D, Nairn D et al 1976 Efficacy of low dose heparin in prevention of extensive deep vein thrombosis in patients undergoing total hip replacement. Lancet 1: 1151–1154

Salzman E W, Harris W M, deSanctis R W 1971 Reduction in venous thrombosis by agents affecting platelet function. New England Journal of Medicine 284: 1287–1291

Samama M, Bernard P, Bonnardot J P, Combe-Tamzali S, Lanson Y, Tissot E 1988 Low molecular weight heparin compared with unfractionated heparin in prevention of postoperative thrombosis. British Journal of Surgery 75: 128

Sasahara A A, Koppenhagen K, Haring R, Welzel D, Wolf H 1986 Low molecular weight heparin plus dihydroergotamine for prophylaxis of postoperative deep vein thrombosis. British Journal of Surgery 773: 697–700

Sevitt S 1962 Venous thrombosis and pulmonary embolism: their prevention by oral anticoagulants. American Journal of Medicine 33: 703–716

Sevitt S, Gallagher N G 1959 Prevention of venous thrombosis and pulmonary embolism in injured patients: a trial of anticoagulant prophylaxis with phenindione in middle aged and elderly patients with fractured necks of femur. Lancet 2: 981–989

Sharnoff J G 1966 Results on the prophylaxis of postoperative thromboembolism. Surgery, Gynecology and Obstetrics 123: 303–307

Sharnoff J G 1973 Prevention of coronary artery thrombosis by heparin prophylaxis. Lancet 2: 1321

Sharnoff J G, de Blasio G 1970 Prevention of fatal postoperative thromboembolism by heparin prophylaxis. Lancet 2: 1006–1010

Skinner D B, Salzman E W 1967 Anticoagulant prophylaxis in surgical patients. Surgery, Gynecology and Obstetrics 125: 741

Soreff J, Johnson H, Deiner L, Goransson L 1975 Acetyl salicyclic acid in a trial to diminish thromboembolic complications after elective hip surgery. Acta Orthopaediatrica Scandinavica 46: 246–255

Spiro T E, Enoxaparin Clinical Trials Group 1991 A randomized trial of enoxaparin administered postoperatively for the prevention of deep vein thrombosis following elective hip replacement. Thrombosis and Haemostasis 65(suppl): 927

Stamatakis J D, Kakkar V V et al 1977 Synergistic effect of heparin and dihydroergotamine in the prophylaxis of postoperative deep vein thrombosis. In: Pabst H W, Maurer G (eds) Postoperative thromboembolie-Prophylaxe, S. 109. Schauttauer-Verlag, Stuttgart, p 109–118

Stamatakis J D, Kakkar V V, Lawrence D, Bentley P G, Nairn D, Ward V 1978 Failure of aspirin to prevent postoperative deep vein thrombosis in patients undergoing total hip replacement. British Medical Journal 1: 1031

Storm O 1958 Anticoagulant protection in surgery. Thrombosis et Diathesis Haemorrhagica 2: 484–491

Swank R L 1958 Suspension stability of the blood after injection of dextran. Journal of Applied Physiology 12: 125–128

Tangen O, Wik K O, Almquist I A M, Arfors K E, Hint H C 1972 Effect of dextran on the structure and plasmin-induced lysis of human fibrin. Thrombosis Research 1: 487

Tsapogas M J, Goussous H, Peabody R A et al 1971 Postoperative venous thrombosis and the effectiveness of prophylactic measures. Archives in Surgery 103: 561–567

Turpie A G G, Levine M N, Hirsh J et al 1986 A randomized controlled trial of a low molecular weight heparin (enoxaparin) to prevent deep vein thrombosis in patients undergoing elective hip surgery. New England Journal of Medicine 315: 925

Turpie A G G, Levine M N, Powers P J et al 1991 A double blind randomized trial of ORG 10172 low molecular weight heparinoid versus unfractionated heparin in the prevention of deep vein thrombosis in patients with thrombotic stroke. Thrombosis and Haemostasis 65(suppl): 753

Van Geloven F J M 1975 Personal communication

Venous Thrombosis Clinical Study Group 1975 Small doses of subcutaneous sodium heparin in the prevention of deep vein thrombosis after elective hip replacement. British Journal of Surgery 62: 348–350

Warlow C, Beattie A G, Terry G, Ogston D, Kenmura N C F, Douglas A S 1973 A double blind trial of low doses of subcutaneous heparin in the prevention of deep vein thrombosis after myocardial infarction. Lancet 2: 934–936

Williams H T 1971 Prevention of postoperative deep vein thrombosis with peri-operative subcutaneous heparin. Lancet 2: 950–952

Zekert F, Kohn P, Vormittag E, Poigenfurst J, Thien M 1974 Thromboemboliėprophylaxe mit Acetylsalicylsaure bie Operationen wegen Jufgelenksnaher Frakturen. Monatschrift der unfallheilkunde 77: 97–110.

63. Diagnosis and treatment of venous thromboembolism

M. H. Prins A. G. G. Turpie

Deep vein thrombosis and pulmonary embolism are related disorders and their separation, although useful for practical purposes, is artificial as suggested by the observations that more than 70% of patients with objectively documented pulmonary embolism have deep vein thrombosis of the legs (Samama & Horellow 1982, Hull et al 1983a) and that approximately 50% of patients with objectively documented deep vein thrombosis have asymptomatic pulmonary embolism (Huisman et al 1989a). For practical purposes, the term venous thromboembolism refers to either deep vein thrombosis or pulmonary embolism or a combination of both. Treatment of venous thromboembolism is mandatory since the rate of thromboembolic complications in untreated patients is high, approaching 50% (Barritt & Jordan 1960, Hull et al 1979, Lagerstedt et al 1985). Several therapeutic modalities are available for the treatment of venous thromboembolism. These include treatment with heparin, low molecular weight heparins or heparinoids, oral anticoagulants, thrombolytic agents, or surgical treatment by physical interruption of the inferior vena cava or by removal of the thrombus.

Since deep vein thrombosis or pulmonary embolism are present in less than 50% of patients with clinically suspected venous thromboembolism when assessed by objective tests, because a diagnosis of venous thromboembolism results in patients being labelled as thrombosis prone, and because the treatment of venous thromboembolism carries definite risks of morbidity due to bleeding, it is necessary to confirm the diagnosis objectively (Moser 1990, Raskob & Hull 1990).

This chapter will examine the merits of the tools that are available for the diagnosis of venous thromboembolism and evaluate the results obtained with the various strategies that are available for its treatment.

DIAGNOSIS

Interpretation of diagnostic studies

Rules for the development and validation of the utility of new diagnostic tests have been established (Büller et al 1991) and can be divided into three stages. These are:

1. Comparison of the results of a new test with a reference standard in an initial cohort of patients and, using discriminant functional analysis or ROC-curve analysis, optimal cut-off levels or diagnostic criteria for the test are selected.
2. The developed criteria are then tested against the reference standard in a new cohort of patients. For this phase, the results of the test and reference standard should be interpreted independently and the number of patients included should be large enough to describe the behaviour of the test (i.e. its sensitivity and specificity) with relatively small confidence intervals.
3. If it is suitable for clinical use because it has high sensitivity and specificity, the test should be assessed in a management study to describe the outcome in a cohort of patients who are followed prospectively. The number of patients included in this phase should be large enough to describe the results with small confidence intervals.

Figure 63.1 demonstrates, with examples, the steps that are taken to determine the sensitivity and specificity of a new diagnostic test and how the results may be used to determine the clinical utility of the test.

Diagnosis of deep vein thrombosis of the leg

The diagnosis of deep vein thrombosis of the leg is usually suspected in patients who present with painful swelling of the leg which is most commonly unilateral but occasionally may be bilateral. The clinical characteristics of deep vein thrombosis are shown in Table 63.1. The clinical picture of deep vein thrombosis varies from no symptoms or minimal symptoms only (often in patients at risk), minor pain in the calf and slight swelling of the ankle, to an extremely painful, grossly swollen leg. When the oedema is so severe that the arteries are compressed,

A

New Test	Reference Standard Pos.	Reference Standard Neg.
Pos.	A	C
Neg	B	D

(A+B)/(A+B+C+D) = Incidence
A/(A+B) = Sensitivity
D/(D+C) = Specificity
A/(A+C) = Pos. Pred. Value
D/(D+B) = Neg. Pred. Value

A = True-positive
B = False-negative
C = False-positive
D = True-negative

B

New Test	Reference Standard Pos.	Reference Standard Neg.
Pos.	49	1
Neg	1	49

Incidence = 50%
Sensitivity = 98%
Specificity = 98%
Pos. Pred. Value = 98%
Neg. Pred. Value = 98%

C

New Test	Reference Standard Pos.	Reference Standard Neg.
Pos.	49	25
Neg	1	25

Incidence = 50%
Sensitivity = 98%
Specificity = 50%
Pos. Pred. Value = 66%
Neg. Pred. Value = 96%

D

New Test	Reference Standard Pos.	Reference Standard Neg.
Pos.	25	1
Neg	25	49

Incidence = 50%
Sensitivity = 50%
Specificity = 98%
Pos. Pred. Value = 96%
Neg. Pred. Value = 66%

Fig. 63.1 Sensitivity, specificity, positive predictive value (PPV), Negative predictive value (NPV) of a diagnostic test. A describes the characteristics of a diagnostic test. B, C and D illustrate examples of the utility of a new diagnostic test.
A. Sensitivity and specificity are characteristics of the test and the disease severity in the population studied. Positive predictive value and negative predictive value are influenced by the incidence of the disease in the population studied. A test with a high sensitivity can be used to exclude the diagnosis when the test result is negative, a test with a high specificity to establish the diagnosis when the result is positive.
B. When both sensitivity and specificity are high, a new test can be used to replace the reference standard, if the incidence of the disease is high enough to ensure a high positive predictive value and negative predictive value.
C. If a test is sensitive but not specific, further testing is necessary in patients with a positive test result to avoid treatment of patients that do not have the disease.
D. If a test is specific but not sensitive, further testing is necessary in patients with a negative test result to avoid withholding treatment in patients who have the disease of interest.

mottled cyanosis with signs of arterial insufficiency may occur, a condition known as phlegmasia cerulea dolens. Many other disorders affecting the legs can mimic deep vein thrombosis and, therefore, the differential diagnosis is extensive. A number of the alternative diagnoses to deep vein thrombosis can be made by clinical examination (for example arthritis) and others by a combination of history and examination (traumatic muscle rupture). In most instances, however, objective investigations are needed to make a definitive diagnosis.

Several studies have shown that only 30–50% of patients who, after an initial history and physical examination, are referred for objective testing to rule in or rule out deep vein thrombosis, are shown to have deep vein thrombosis (Hull et al 1981a, Lensing et al 1989). In contrast, signs and symptoms of deep vein thrombosis occur in only 10–20% of high-risk patients who are screened systematically and are shown to have deep vein thrombosis by objective tests. (Kakkar et al 1969c).

Venography

Venography is generally accepted as the reference standard for the diagnosis of deep vein thrombosis (Williams 1973). Venography provides a direct image of the lumen of the vein by injection of radiopaque contrast medium into the venous system through a dorsal foot vein. Different techniques have been used to perform venography. Using the method of Rabinov and Paulin (1972), 80–100 ml of contrast medium is injected slowly into a dorsal vein of the foot, and using fluoroscopy to obtain optimal filling, spot pictures (anteroposterior and lateral) are obtained of the calf, popliteal and femoral veins. The long leg method, which requires more contrast medium (150 ml), involves obtaining two anteroposterior and one lateral film of the entire venous system of the leg without using fluoroscopy (Lensing et al 1990a, 1992). In both techniques, spot pictures of the external iliac vein are obtained after reclining the patient to the horizontal posi-

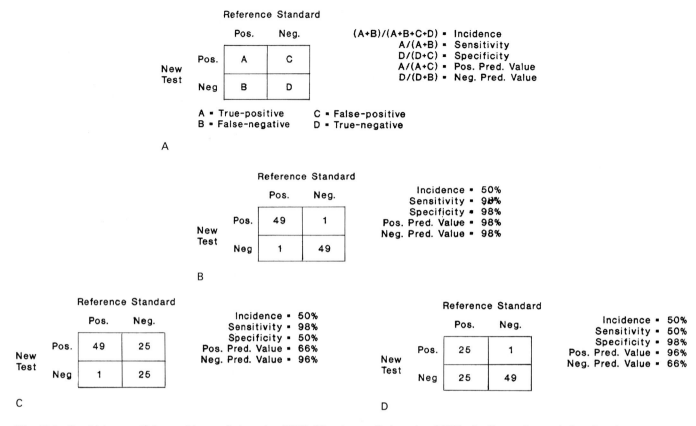

Table 63.1 Clinical characteristics of deep vein thrombosis

Underlying conditions
Immobilization (surgery or medical disorders)
Inherited deficiency of natural anticoagulants
Malignancy
Oestrogen use
Previous thrombosis
Signs and symptoms of deep vein thrombosis
Leg pain
Tenderness of the leg
Oedema below and above the knee
Palpable cord (thrombosed veins)
Increased temperature of the leg, fever
Distension of superficial veins
Discoloration, mottled cyanosis
Differential diagnosis of deep vein thrombosis
Cellulitis, arthritis, tendonitis
Lymphatic obstruction
Muscle tear or strain (exercise)
Haematoma
Ruptured Baker's cyst
External vein compression by tumour, abscess, arterial aneurysm or haematoma
Post-thrombotic syndrome
Vasomotor effects in paralysed limbs
Thromboneurosis

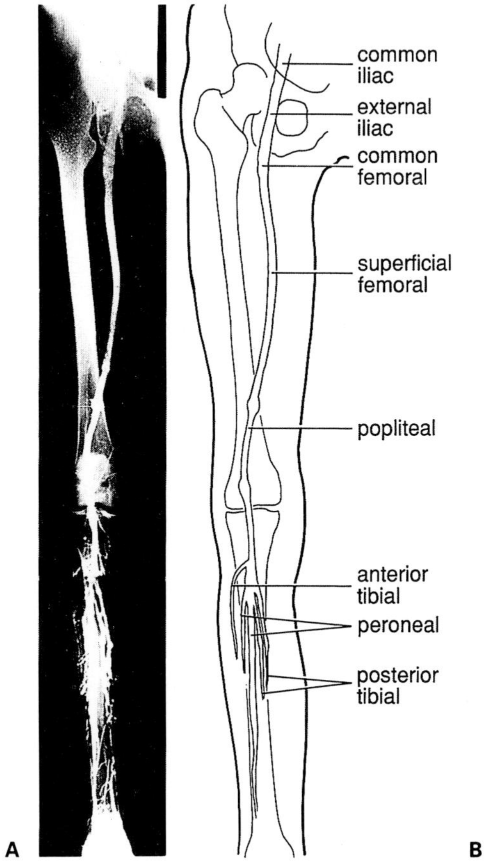

Fig. 63.2 Venograms of the leg. **A**, Example of a normal venogram obtained with the long leg technique. **B**, Schematic representation of the venogram in A with the veins labelled.

tion. Occasionally, catheterization using the Seldinger technique is required to obtain good visualization of the external iliac vein. Visualization of the internal iliac vein, common iliac vein or inferior vena cava is usually only adequately obtained with the Seldinger catheterization procedure. The use of tourniquets to enhance filling of the deep veins has been subject to debate. However, the use of a tourniquet can reduce filling of the calf veins and is, therefore, probably only useful in patients with venous insufficiency to avoid overfilling of the superficial veins (Lea Thomas 1972, Rabinov & Paulin 1972).

A long leg venogram is shown in Figure 63.2 together with a diagram of the anatomy and nomenclature of the deep venous system of the leg. Three sets of deep veins of the calf (posterior tibial, peroneal and anterior tibial veins) join to form the popliteal just below the knee. The popliteal vein becomes the superficial femoral vein approximately 5 cm above the knee, and the deep femoral vein (not commonly visualized) joins the superficial femoral vein in the upper thigh to form the common femoral vein. At the inguinal ligament, the common femoral vein becomes the external iliac vein which is joined by the internal iliac vein to form the common iliac vein in the pelvis. The deep venous system is connected to the superficial venous system by perforator veins and in the calf by a series of large muscular veins known as the soleal sinuses.

The principal criterion for the diagnosis of acute deep vein thrombosis on venography is the presence of a constant intraluminal filling defect seen in two or more views (Lea Thomas 1972, Rabinov & Paulin 1972). An intraluminal filling defect must be distinguished from artefacts such as flow from a non-opacified contributary (for example, the deep femoral or internal iliac vein) or from external compression. Non-filling of a vein is a secondary criterion for the diagnosis of deep vein thrombosis, but is regarded as less reliable and can be caused by previous deep vein thrombosis. Collaterals are commonly seen in patients with longstanding thrombotic occlusion of the deep veins.

Deep vein thrombosis is usually divided into proximal or distal thrombosis. Proximal venous thrombosis is diagnosed when a thrombus is present in the popliteal, femoral or iliac veins with or without calf vein thrombosis, while distal thrombosis is diagnosed when the thrombi are confined to the calf veins and do not reach or are not accompanied by thrombosis in the proximal veins. This differentiation into proximal and calf vein thrombosis is not only theoretical but also of practical importance, since it has been demonstrated that the likelihood of a major pulmonary embolism arising from venous thrombosis confined to the calf is very low (Kakkar et al 1969c, Moser & Lemoine 1981, Hull et al 1985a, Huisman et al 1989a). The venographic extent of thrombosis can be approximated quantitatively, a technique that is particularly applicable for clinical trials (Marder et al 1977).

There are a number of limitations of venography. 5–10%

of venograms using the Rabinov and Paulin technique are inadequate for interpretation (McLachlan et al 1979). In addition, the observer variability in the interpretation of venograms by the Rabinov and Paulin technique is considerable, with kappa values being reported to be between 0.65 and 0.85 (McLachlan et al 1979, Sauerbrei et al 1981, Picolet et al 1990). A recent study suggests that the interobserver variability (kappa 0.92) and inadequacy rate (2% or less) may be better with the long leg method (Lensing et al 1990a, 1992), but this observation has yet to be confirmed.

The diagnosis of acute recurrent deep vein thrombosis with venography poses a special problem. The most definitive diagnostic criterion is the demonstration of an intraluminal filling defect which was not present on the original venogram. However, if a previous venogram is not available, the presence of an intraluminal filling defect may be regarded as diagnostic, since previous venous thrombosis usually results in total occlusion of the veins in conjunction with the presence of collaterals (Rabinov & Paulin 1972).

The disadvantages of venography are that it is invasive and time-consuming, there is a potential for allergic reactions to the iodide-containing contrast medium, and the possibility of producing contrast-induced thrombosis which has been reported to occur in approximately 2% of patients, even when a modern non-ionic contrast medium with low osmolality is used (Rabinov & Paulin 1972). In addition, extravasation of contrast material into subcutaneous tissues is painful and may result in skin necrosis (Albrechtsson & Olsson 1976). In pregnant patients, the amount of radiation (even with lower abdominal shielding) is a limiting factor of venography.

The clinical utility of a technically adequate, negative venogram in patients suspected of venous thrombosis has been demonstrated in a management study (Hull et al 1981b) in which it has been shown that the incidence of venous thromboembolism during 3 months of follow-up among 160 patients suspected of thrombosis who had a negative venogram and who were not treated with anticoagulants was low. In the two patients in whom thrombosis occurred, it was related to the initial venography.

Clinical signs and symptoms

A number of studies have attempted to assess the sensitivity and specificity of clinical signs and symptoms of deep vein thrombosis by comparing their presence with the results of venography. A major limitation in these studies is that the signs and symptoms themselves usually lead to inclusion of deep vein thrombosis in the differential diagnosis and therefore to the performance of venography (Sandler et al 1984). The most specific sign (>90%) of deep vein thrombosis is the presence of swelling above the knee. However, only a minority of patients have extensive above-knee oedema and thus the sensitivity of this sign is low. The specificity of the other clinical signs and symptoms of deep vein thrombosis are all below 70% and therefore not useful in clinical decision making. In a retrospective study (Landefeld et al 1990) it was reported that 97% of deep vein thrombi could be detected if venography was limited to patients with suspected deep vein thrombosis who had one or more of the following features: swelling below or above the knee, recent immobility, cancer or fever. However, using these clinical features, venography would not have been done in 19 (16%) of the 119 patients in the group, and among those 19 patients there was one proximal deep vein thrombosis (95% confidence interval 0.1–26.3%). Thus, this approach of using venography only in patients with certain clinical features cannot be recommended.

Impedance plethysmography

Impedance plethysmography is one of the most extensively evaluated objective tests used as an alternative for venography in the diagnosis of deep vein thrombosis. The technique is based on the measurement of electrical resistance of the calf, which is related to the volume of blood in the calf. After standardized periods of venous occlusion applied to the thigh (45, 45, 120, 45, and 120 seconds respectively), the decrease in blood volume of the calf (assessed by electrical resistance) after release of the blood pressure cuff is slower if the proximal deep veins are occluded. To diagnose deep vein thrombosis, the increase in electrical conductance during occlusion is plotted against the decrease during the first 3 seconds after release of the occlusion and the result compared with a discriminant line based on a formal comparison of a cohort of patients who had undergone both venography and impedance plethysmography. The test result with the highest rise and fall in resistance is used for the diagnostic decision. If the highest rise and fall do not occur in the same occlusion period the test is regarded as technically inadequate and should be repeated (Hull et al 1976, 1978). Because changes in blood volume of the calf are indirectly assessed by impedance plethysmography, it can only detect proximal deep vein thrombosis; calf vein thrombosis cannot be reliably detected. Impedance plethysmography cannot discriminate between different causes of venous outflow obstruction and it is, therefore, important to consider possible causes of a false positive test (e.g. malignant obstruction of a vein, increased central venous pressure).

The test is performed with the patient in a supine position with slight external rotation of the leg and with the hip and knee flexed to an angle of 15° (Hull et al 1976). In pregnant patients the test can best be performed in the lateral recumbent position to avoid pressure of the gravid uterus on the iliac vein (Clarke-Pearson & Creasman

1981, Hull et al 1990a). For an adequate impedance plethysmography result, the cooperation of the patient is needed, since the results are also influenced by muscle contractions.

Many studies have compared the electrical impedance technique using the Codman apparatus with venography in symptomatic patients suspected of having deep vein thrombosis (Table 63.2). In all of the reported studies, the sensitivities and specificities of impedance plethysmography for proximal deep vein thrombosis were high (above 90%). Pooling the results, the sensitivity of impedance plethysmography for proximal deep vein thrombosis is 94%, and the specificity 95% (Hull et al 1976, 1977, 1978, 1981a, Flanigan et al 1978, Toy & Schrier 1978, Cooperman et al 1979, Gross & Burney 1979, Foti & Gurewich 1980, Liapis et al 1980). The significance of abnormal tests in both legs simultaneously was addressed in one study which showed that deep vein thrombosis was present in only 14 (26%) out of 53 patients suggesting that bilateral abnormal tests may be caused by mechanisms other than deep vein thrombosis, such as heart failure (Curley et al 1987).

In asymptomatic patients at risk for thrombosis, the sensitivity of impedance plethysmography for proximal deep vein thrombosis has been shown to be low (12%, 50%, and 70% respectively) in three published studies (Paiement et al 1988, Cruickshank et al 1989, Skjeldal et al 1990). Thus, impedance plethysmography alone cannot be used to exclude a diagnosis of deep vein thrombosis in prospective clinical trials assessing thrombosis prophylaxis.

The natural history of abnormal impedance has recently been defined, and in 95% of patients the test returns to normal 9–12 months after the acute event (Jay et al 1984). However, it is doubtful whether impedance plethysmography can be used to diagnose recurrent deep vein thrombosis even if the test returns to normal after treatment of the first episode of deep vein thrombosis, since in one study (Huisman et al 1988) the test was falsely positive in two of 13 (15%) patients (95% CI 0.2–36.1%). In addition, in another study the utility of impedance plethysmography in the diagnosis of recurrent thrombosis in which return of the initial test to normal was not determined, 15 out of 73 positive tests were not associated with an acute recurrent event and were, therefore, falsely positive (Hull et al 1983a).

Table 63.2 Sensitivity and specificity of plethysmographic techniques for proximal deep vein thrombosis in symptomatic patients

Study	Sensitivity (%)	Specificity (%)
Electrical impedance plethysmography		
Hull et al 1976	93 (124/133)	97 (124/133)
Hull et al 1977	98 (59/60)	95 (108/114)
Hull et al 1978	92 (155/169)	96 (304/317)
Toy & Schrier 1978	94 (15/16)	100 (9/9)
Flanigan et al 1978	96 (52/54)	95 (93/98)
Gross & Burney 1979	100 (9/9)	94 (32/34)
Cooperman et al 1979	87 (20/23)	96 (72/75)
Foti & Gurewich 1980	90 (19/21)	79 (19.24)
Liapis et al 1980	91 (43/47)	90 (219/243)
Hull et al 1981a	95 (74/78)	98 (157/160)
Computerized impedance plethysmography		
Agnelli et al 1990	97 (34/35)	87 (54/61)
Prandoni et al 1991a	86 (44/51)	95 (143/150)

Bracketed figures are the number of patients/total number of patients.

Two studies have assessed the sensitivity and specificity of a new impedance plethysmography apparatus, the Computerized Impedance Plethysmograph (CIP) which is also based on blood volume changes in the calf (used by the original Codman apparatus) to detect deep vein thrombosis but utilizes different technology to compute and register the result of the test. The reported sensitivities and specificities (Agnelli et al 1990, Prandoni et al 1991a) for proximal deep vein thrombosis in symptomatic patients are in the same range as those of the standard electrical impedance test using the Codman apparatus (Table 63.2).

Strain-gauge and air plethysmography (both tests that are also based on changes in volume of the calf), for the diagnosis of proximal deep vein thrombosis in symptomatic patients have been less extensively evaluated and many of the published studies used different criteria for a positive test. Recent prospective evaluations of their sensitivities report lower figures than those reported with electrical impedance (Barnes et al 1977, Nicholas et al 1977, Boccalon 1981, Hanel et al 1981, Bounameux et al 1982, George and Berry 1990, Holmgren et al 1990).

The use of impedance plethysmography for the management of patients suspected of deep vein thrombosis is based on two hypotheses: 1) Isolated distal vein thrombosis does not require antithrombotic treatment unless it extends into the more proximal veins and 2) in most instances, extension of calf vein thrombosis occurs in untreated patients relatively soon after the onset of symptoms and can be detected by serial testing.

Several studies have prospectively evaluated impedance plethysmography testing in the management of patients suspected of thrombosis; these are summarized (along with management studies using venography, leg scanning and ultrasound) in Table 63.3. In most studies, serial testing was done on the day of referral and repeated on day 3, 5, 7, and 10. Among the patients with repeatedly negative impedance plethysmography, the pooled incidence of non-fatal venous thromboembolism was 1.1%, with no fatal pulmonary emboli during follow-up. Thus, serial impedance plethysmography is a practical and safe alternative to venography in the management of patients with suspected deep vein thrombosis. Serial impedance plethysmography testing has also been demonstrated to be a safe alternative for the management of suspected venous thrombosis in pregnancy, since the incidence of thrombosis was zero during an approximately 6-month period of

Table 63.3 Management studies. Clinical outcome in patients suspected of deep vein thrombosis with a negative objective test that are not given anticoagulant treatment

Study	Population	Pro-/retrospective	Number	Incidence of VTE Fatal No. (%)	Total No. (%)
Venography					
Hull et al 1981b	In and out-patients	Pro	160	0 (0.0)	2 (1.3)
Impedance plethysmography					
Hull et al 1985a	In and out-patients	Pro	311	0 (0.0)	6 (1.9)
Hull et al 1990a	Pregnant patients	Pro	139	0 (0.0)	0 (0.0)
Huisman et al 1986	Out-patients	Pro	289	0 (0.0)	1 (0.2)
Huisman et al 1989b	Out-patients	Pro	131	0 (0.0)	1 (0.8)
Jonker 1991	Out-patients	Retro	1691	0 (0.0)	15 (0.9)
Jonker 1991	Out-patients	Retro	121	0 (0.0)	0 (0.0)
Huisman et al 1988	Recurrence	Pro	18	0 (0.0)	0 (0.0)
Computerized impedance plethysmography					
Prandoni et al 1991b	1st episode/out-patients	Pro	311	4 (1.3)	11 (3.2)
Jonker 1991	Out-patients	Retro	418	0 (0.0)	11 (2.6)
IPG and ^{125}I-labelled fibrinogen leg scan					
Hull et al 1981a	In and out-patients	Pro	163	0 (0.0)	2 (1.2)
Hull et al 1985a	In and out-patients	Pro	323	0 (0.0)	7 (2.2)
Hull et al 1983a	Recurrence	Pro	181	0 (0.0)	3 (1.7)
Ultrasound					
Vaccaro et al 1990	In and out-patients	Retro	1022	2 (0.2)	5 (0.5)
Heijboer et al 1991a	Out-patients	Pro	196	0 (0.0)	2 (1.1)

VTE, venous thromboembolism

follow-up of 139 pregnant patients with suspected deep vein thrombosis who had negative serial tests (Hull et al 1990a). The use of serial impedance plethysmography for the diagnosis of recurrent deep vein thrombosis has been shown to be safe (incidence 0/18; 0.0%, 95% CI 0.0–18.5%) but because of the small number of patients involved, the confidence interval of the estimated incidence of recurrent deep vein thrombosis is large.

Serial computerized impedance plethysmography has been evaluated in one prospective management study (Prandoni et al 1991b) which was interrupted because of a high incidence of fatal pulmonary embolism (4/311; 1.3%, 95% CI 0.0–2.5%) and non-fatal venous thromboembolism 1.9% (7/311). A retrospective analysis of data comparing the two electrical plethysmography techniques has confirmed the worse outcome with the CIP machine (Jonker 1992), but the reasons for the different results obtained with the two instruments is unclear.

B-mode ultrasound

The use of B-mode ultrasound to diagnose deep vein thrombosis utilizes a two-dimensional image of the anatomical structure of the venous system produced by reflected sound waves. Flow data can be added to the B-mode image by technology which detects a frequency change in a reflected sound wave that is caused by a moving object (in this case the erythrocyte). When these flow data are transformed into an audible sound the technique is called duplex scanning. Colour-coded reproduction of the data can also be added to the two-dimensional picture, a technique known as colour-coded duplex. Among the several potential criteria for the presence of a thrombus (e.g. absence of flow, visible outline in a vein compatible with a thrombus), repeated evaluations have shown that the only criterion which is reliable and necessary in order to obtain a high sensitivity and specificity for the diagnosis of deep vein thrombosis is the absence of total compressibility of the deep veins on B-mode imaging (Hill et al 1988, White et al 1989, Schindler et al 1990).

Many studies have evaluated the sensitivity and specificity of B-mode ultrasound for the diagnosis of proximal vein thrombosis in symptomatic patients (Appelman et al 1987, Cronan et al 1987, Vogel et al 1987, O'Leary et al 1988, Lensing et al 1989, Monreal et al 1989b, White et al 1989, Ezekowitz et al 1990) and are summarized in Table 63.4. Most of these studies only tested compressibility of the femoral vein near the inguinal ligament and the popliteal vein in the popliteal fossa. The pooled sensitivity of B-mode ultrasound for proximal deep vein thrombosis is 97% and the pooled specificity 98%. Duplex and colour-coded duplex scans have not been shown to improve the results observed with B-mode ultrasound (Table 63.4). There is no reported experience with B-mode ultrasound in the diagnosis of recurrent deep vein thrombosis, but it may be useful, since it was recently reported that 50% of the compression ultrasound tests reverted to normal during a 9 month period after the acute episode (Murphy & Cronan 1990).

Table 63.4 Sensitivity and specificity of ultrasound techniques for proximal deep vein thrombosis in symptomatic patients

Study	Sensitivity (%)	Specificity (%)
B-mode ultrasound		
Appelman et al 1987	96 (50/52)	97 (58/60)
Cronan et al 1987	93 (25/27)	100 (24/24)
Vogel et al 1987b	95 (19/20)	100 (33/33)
Habscheid et al 1990	97 (68/70)	100 (104/104)
O'Leary et al 1988	92 (22/24)	98 (25/26)
Lensing et al 1989	100 (66/66)	99 (142/143)
Monreal et al 1989b	95 (40/42)	95 (18/19)
Duplex		
Elias et al 1987	100 (241/241)	98 (601/613)
O'Leary et al 1988	92 (22/24)	92 (24/26)
Mantoni et al 1989	97 (34/35)	96 (48/50)
Colour-coded duplex		
Schindler et al 1990	98 (54/55)	100 (39/39)
Rose et al 1990	96 (25/26)	100 (49/49)

The results of ultrasound techniques in screening of patients at high risk for thrombosis are inconsistent, and the reported sensitivity for proximal thrombosis, even when compressibility is tested in multiple segments of the thigh, has varied between 53% and 100% (Comerota et al 1988, Borris et al 1989, Froehlich et al 1989, Ginsberg et al 1990, Woolson et al 1990). However in each of the studies, the specificity for proximal thrombosis was high (>95%), and therefore a positive test is clinically useful in high-risk patients screened for deep vein thrombosis.

Studies that have evaluated the sensitivity of ultrasound for the diagnosis of distal thrombosis by testing the compressibility of the peroneal and posterior tibial veins in multiple positions have reported sensitivities ranging from 50–93% (Habscheid et al 1990, Mussurakis et al 1990, Rose et al 1990). The addition of flow data (i.e. duplex or colour-coded duplex scanning) has not been shown to lead to better results.

A major advantage of ultrasound over impedance plethysmography is direct visualization of the veins, which probably accounts for its high specificity, and its potential to demonstrate the presence of alternative disorders leading to leg symptoms, e.g. calf muscle haematoma, Baker's cysts.

Two management studies of B-mode ultrasound in the diagnosis of deep vein thrombosis have been completed (Table 63.3). The first was a retrospective study of 1022 patients that did not include serial testing (Vaccaro et al 1990), and the second, a prospective study in 196 patients with serial testing (Heijboer et al 1991b). The incidence of venous thromboembolism (fatal and non-fatal was extremely low in patients with negative tests in both studies (0.2% and 1.2%). Ultrasound was performed on day 1, 3 and 7 in the prospective study. It is possible that, due to the high sensitivity of ultrasound for proximal deep vein thrombosis and the possibility of introducing testing of multiple segments of the proximal veins in the thigh, the number of tests in the series can be reduced to two, thus reducing the costs of serial testing.

Fibrinogen leg-scanning

Radio-labelled (^{125}Iodine) fibrinogen leg scanning is a non-invasive test that has been used extensively in the detection of deep vein thrombosis in high-risk patients and has been used to confirm the diagnosis of deep vein thrombosis in symptomatic patients (Flanc et al 1968). The principle of this test involves the detection of radio-labelled fibrinogen that is incorporated into existing or developing thrombi. 100 microcurie of ^{125}I-labelled fibrinogen is injected in an antecubital vein, and the surface radioactivity is measured using a surface counter and followed over time at points on the calf and along the course of the popliteal and superficial femoral veins of both legs. The criteria for the presence of a thrombus are a relative increase in radioactivity of more than 20% over one or more points that persist for more than 24 hours, in comparison with: 1) the same point 24 hours previously, 2) adjacent points in the same leg or 3) equivalent points in the opposite leg. The duration of scanning is limited to approximately 7 days by the half life of fibrinogen. Haematomas, surgical wounds or wounds secondary to trauma, cellulitis and localized inflammation will give rise to false positive tests.

In symptomatic patients the sensitivity of leg scanning for proximal vein thrombosis is low, but it is highly sensitive in the diagnosis of distal vein thrombosis, while its specificity for both proximal and distal thrombosis is approximately 85% (Browse et al 1971, Browse 1972, Kakkar 1972, Walker 1972, Hirsh et al 1974, Hull et al 1981a). Fibrinogen leg scanning alone is thus not suitable for the diagnosis of deep vein thrombosis in symptomatic patients, but it could, in principle, be used to detect calf vein thrombosis in patients managed with impedance plethysmography or ultrasound. Its use has been evaluated in combination with impedance plethysmography for the detection of proximal thrombosis in symptomatic patients suspected of having a first episode of thrombosis. However, this combined approach has not been shown to be clinically superior to serial impedance testing alone (Table 63.3) (Hull et al 1985b).

In patients suspected of an acute recurrent episode of thrombosis, fibrinogen leg scanning in combination with impedance plethysmography has been used to rule in or rule out recurrent thrombosis. In this situation a reference standard is lacking and therefore its use is based on description of the clinical results in patients managed by a priori criteria. In a study of 181 patients with suspected recurrent deep vein thrombosis it was found that in patients with negative impedance plethysmography and a negative fibrinogen leg scan in whom anticoagulant treatment was withheld, the incidence of recurrent venous thromboembolism was only 1.7% during a 20-month period of follow-up, while in 89 patients with a positive leg scan alone or a positive impedance test or venogram with a positive leg scan, who were treated with anticoagulants, the incidence of recurrence was 20% (Hull et al 1983b).

Fibrinogen leg scanning has been extensively used as a diagnostic tool for venous thromboembolism in clinical trials of thrombosis prophylaxis. Studies that performed confirmatory venography in patients with a positive leg scan reported that the positive predictive value varied between 70–90% (Negus et al 1968). However, in general, gynaecological and urological surgery and in medical patients, a formal prospective comparison with a reference standard has not been performed and, therefore, the sensitivity of leg scanning in these situations is unknown.

In hip surgery, fibrinogen leg scanning either alone or in combination with impedance plethysmography has been shown to have disappointingly low sensitivity and specificity (Harris et al 1975, 1976, Loudon et al 1978, Paiement et al 1988, Cruickshank et al 1989, Faunoe et al 1990), except in one study which showed a sensitivity of leg-scanning of 95% for all deep vein thrombosis in patients.

Other tests for deep vein thrombosis

Many other tests for deep vein thrombosis have been proposed, but none have been evaluated in management studies and only some have been compared to the reference standard in a sufficiently large cohort of patients.

The diagnosis of thrombosis with simple doppler ultrasonography (without B-mode imaging) depends on the detection and description of venous flow by an alteration in the reflected wave length of a beam of ultrasound, caused by moving erythrocytes, that is made audible. The normal flow in a vein is phasic which disappears on increase of abdominal pressure (Valsalva manoeuvre). Using doppler ultrasound, deep vein thrombosis is diagnosed when there is no flow, or when the flow in not phasic or does not disappear with the Valsalva manoeuvre. However, these diagnostic criteria are mainly subjective and observer dependent which is probably the reason for the wide range of sensitivities for proximal thrombosis which have been reported with this technique (Sigel et al 1972, Richards et al 1976, Dosick & Blakemore 1978, Flanigan et al 1978, Maryniak & Nicholson 1979, Bendick et al 1983, Turnbull et al 1990). A recent report (Lensing et al 1990b) proposed standardization of the criteria, by documenting the sound waves and the intra-abdominal pressure, which resulted in a high sensitivity (91%) and specificity (98%) of the technique in symptomatic outpatients. However, widespread availability of B-mode ultrasound will probably preclude the further development of this test refinement.

Of the available isotope techniques other than ^{125}I-labelled fibrinogen leg scanning, only ^{99m}Technetium-plasmin scanning has been compared to the reference standard in a sufficiently large cohort (Husted et al 1984, Lagerstedt et al 1989). The sensitivity of this technique for the diagnosis of deep vein thrombosis was reported to be 95% but its specificity was only 47%. The test could therefore be used to exclude the diagnosis of thrombosis, while patients with a positive test could be assessed with a confirmatory test. Before this approach can be recommended for widespread use, a management study to demonstrate the safety of withholding anticoagulant therapy in patients with a negative test should be performed.

Many other isotope imaging techniques have been proposed to diagnose deep vein thrombosis. These include ^{99m}Technetium-labelled albumin aggregates, red blood cells, streptokinase, urokinase, and sulphur colloid and ^{111}Indium-labelled platelets (Henkin et al 1973, Kempi et al 1974, Millar & Smith 1974, Persson & Darte 1977, Davies et al 1980, Vieras et al 1980, Singer et al 1984, Christensen et al 1987). However, these techniques have only been evaluated in relatively small studies (fewer than 100 patients) and therefore their estimated sensitivities and specificities have relatively large confidence intervals, or they were not compared with the reference standard and are, therefore, not of practical value.

In recent years magnetic resonance imaging (MRI) has been introduced as an important diagnostic modality in clinical practice (Blackmore et al 1990). This technique is based on the detection of signals, produced by the nuclei of atoms when they are destabilized by a strong magnetic pulse. These signals can be transformed into high resolution two-dimensional images of the structures studied. Initial evaluations of magnetic resonance imaging in the diagnosis of deep vein thrombosis have been carried out, but no formal comparison with recognized standards have been reported (Erdman 1990). However, due to the costs associated with this technique and the high sensitivity and specificity of the readily available, less expensive ultrasound techniques, it is unlikely that magnetic resonance imaging will be used routinely for the diagnosis of deep vein thrombosis of the legs.

Thermography, which requires specialized equipment that is expensive, is a technique based on the temperature increase in the leg associated with thrombosis. Thermography has been tested in several studies, but the range of reported specificities vary widely (48–100%) as do the sensitivities (79–100%) (Cooke & Pilcher 1974, Ritchie et al 1979, Watz & Bygdeman 1979, Aronen et al 1981, Holmgren et al 1990). Liquid crystal thermography, using simple portable equipment has been shown to be even less promising (Pochaczevsky et al 1982, Sandler & Martin 1985, Thomas et al 1989). Neither of these tests have been tested in a management study.

A variety of laboratory tests have been proposed as screening techniques for the detection of deep vein thrombosis. These include measurement of C-reactive protein, thrombin-antithrombin III complexes, fibinopeptide A, thrombin-increasable fibrinopeptide B, fibrin and fibrinogen degradation products, fibrin monomer, D-dimer, tissue-plasminogen antigen, plasminogen activator inhibitor activity, circulating platelet-aggregates, beta-thromboglobulin and platelet factor 4 (Gurewich et al 1973, Kockum 1976, Yudelman et al 1977, Smith et al 1978, deBoer et al 1981, Owen et al 1983, Hoek et al 1989, Thomas et al 1989, van Bergen et al 1989, Boisclair et al 1990, Halvorsen et al 1991). Most of these laboratory tests have only a limited sensitivity and specificity for the diagnosis of deep vein thrombosis (Declerck et al 1987, Van Bergen et al 1989, Boisclair et al 1990, Speiser et al 1990, Boneu et al 1991) or the assays require a complex laboratory procedure (Kockum 1976, Yudelman et al 1977), thus limiting their use in clinical practice.

The most promising laboratory test is based on the detection of D-dimer, a degradation product of fibrin that contains parts of cross-linked fibrin strands. Studies using enzyme linked immunoassay techniques for D-dimer have shown that, in out-patients suspected of deep vein thrombosis, D-dimer levels below 200 ng/ml virtually exclude a diagnosis of deep vein thrombosis. In in-patients, however, the cut-off level for a normal test is higher at 500 ng/ml or less (Declerck et al 1987, Heaton et al 1987, Rowbotham et al 1987, Ott et al 1988, Bounameux et al 1989, Chapman et al 1990, Speiser et al 1990, Boneu et al 1991, Kroneman et al 1991). This difference in the reference value is probably due to the presence of co-morbid conditions in hospitalized patients giving rise to higher levels of D-dimer in the absence of thrombosis. Using this test, approximately 50% of outpatients who would eventually test negative for deep vein thrombosis would be recognized. However the quantitative ELISA assay used to detect D-dimer has not been tested in a management study and may well prove to be too expensive when results are needed quickly to guide the clinical management of individual patients. Results obtained with various rapid Latex-based semi-quantitative tests are less consistent and no ideal assay for D-dimer has been developed commercially (Chapman et al 1990, Grau et al 1991).

Guidelines for the use of diagnostic tests in management of patients with suspected deep vein thrombosis

Symptomatic patients without previous thrombotic episodes

Patients with leg symptoms in whom the diagnosis of deep vein thrombosis cannot be confidently excluded after an initial history and clinical examination, should undergo objective testing for deep vein thrombosis. Generally it is not necessary to start anticoagulant treatment immediately in patients with suspected deep vein thrombosis if objective testing is readily available.

Several approaches to the management of patients with suspected deep vein thrombosis have been tested in prospective cohort (management) studies. Three diagnostic strategies have proved to be safe and effective; these are venography, impedance plethysmography or ultrasound. The advantages and disadvantages of these tests are summarized in Table 63.5. The choice of strategy to be followed will depend on the available diagnostic tools and should take into consideration the cost-effectiveness of the various approaches. There are a number of disadvantages to the use of venography. Venography will be impossible to perform or technically inadequate in approximately 10% of patients, and in these patients other objective tests should be used or the patients should be treated based on the clinical examination. In addition, some patients will develop contrast-induced thrombosis. This complication should be suspected in patients with a negative venogram who subsequently complain of an increase in leg symptoms.

If either impedance plethysmography or ultrasound are used, it is necessary to repeat the tests serially in patients with an initial negative test to exclude an extending calf vein thrombosis. In patients with positive impedance plethysmography, underlying conditions that are known to lead to a falsely positive test result should be considered and, if present, the diagnosis of deep vein thrombosis should be confirmed by ultrasound or venography.

A practical approach to the diagnosis of deep vein thrombosis is outlined in Fig. 63.3 and is based on the assumption that if a suspicion of deep vein thrombosis exists and the results of objective tests are inadequate it is better to treat the patient than to withhold treatment. A cost-effectiveness analysis has estimated that out-patient management with impedance plethysmography is more efficient (costs per correct diagnosis) than management using venography or by treating patients on the basis of clinical symptoms alone (Hull et al 1981c).

The availability of a rapid, economical test for D-dimer, that has been validated in a management study, could change the management of patients suspected of deep vein thrombosis. If the need to perform 50% fewer diag-

Table 63.5 Advantages and disadvantages of the diagnostic tools available for the diagnosis of deep vein thrombosis

Diagnostic method	Advantages	Disadvantages
Venography	Specific	10% failure Time consuming Side-effects
IPG	Rapid Economical	Repeated testing False positives
B-Mode Ultrasound	Rapid High specificity	Repeated testing
Leg scan	Sensitive to calf thrombi	Takes 24 h Combined testing Disease transmission

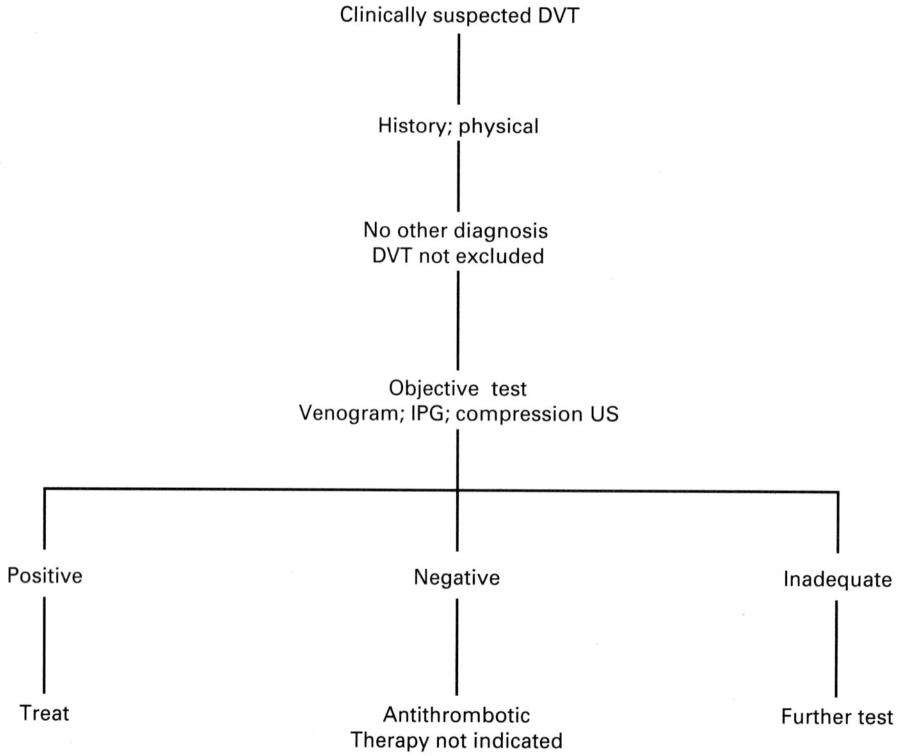

Fig. 63.3 The management of patients with suspected deep vein thrombosis.

nostic evaluations by venography, impedance plethysmography or ultrasound in patients with a negative D-dimer test could be validated, the savings in time and costs would be highly significant. Another potential development is the reduction of number of tests necessary in the management of patients suspected of deep vein thrombosis and managed with ultrasound, since the sensitivity of this technique is high and potentially screening of multiple segments of the thigh can be used in symptomatic patients.

Symptomatic patients with previous thrombotic episodes

The accurate diagnosis of acute recurrent deep vein thrombosis has important clinical implications since the patient may be labelled as being thrombophilic or may be exposed to the risk of complications associated with long-term anticoagulant treatment. Thus, an objective diagnosis of recurrent deep vein thrombosis is necessary but is difficult to obtain due to lack of a clear reference standard. There have been only two relevant studies in this patient group (Hull et al 1983b, Huisman et al 1988). One study used serial impedance plethysmography alone but only included a very small cohort of patients suspected of an acute recurrent event and therefore the safety of this approach is not proven (Huisman et al 1988). The other study used a laborious approach that included a combination of leg scanning and serial impedance plethysmography, and showed a low incidence of recurrent venous thromboembolism in patients with negative tests. This approach is summarized in Figure 63.4. Since impedance plethysmography was frequently falsely positive, venographic or leg scan confirmation of a positive impedance test is probably needed.

Future developments will include the application of compression ultrasound in the diagnosis and management of recurrent deep vein thrombosis, since this examination frequently returns to normal after the initial episode (Murphy & Cronan 1990) and possibly also the addition of D-dimer testing (Kroneman et al 1991).

Patients at risk for deep vein thrombosis

In medical patients and in general, urological, gynaecological and neurosurgical patients receiving adequate deep vein thrombosis prophylaxis, the incidence of thromboembolic complications is sufficiently low to render the need for systematic testing for deep vein thrombosis at discharge unnecessary. However, the need for continuing prophylaxis after discharge is unknown. A recent study (Scurr et al 1988) described a relatively high incidence of asymptomatic thrombosis occurring in general surgical patients after discharge from hospital and the requirement for prophylaxis post-discharge should be tested prospectively.

In patients who undergo hip surgery, the incidence of deep vein thrombosis remains significant even with current prophylactic regimens and is approximately 20% when assessed by venography (Hirsh 1991a). In this setting,

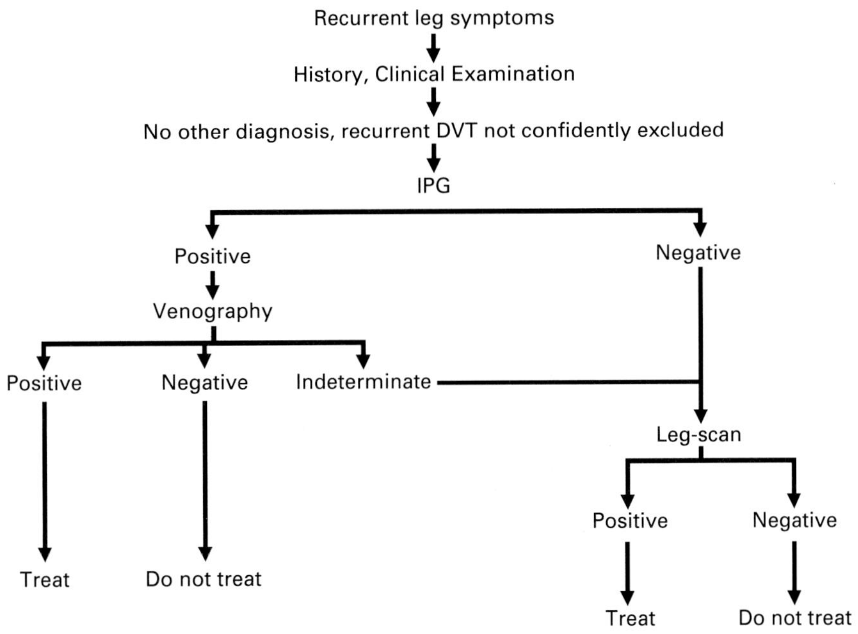

Fig. 63.4 The management of patients with suspected recurrent deep vein thrombosis (modified from Hull 1983a).

venography is the only appropriate diagnostic tool, since the sensitivity of ultrasound, impedance plethysmography and leg-scanning is sub-optimal in asymptomatic patients. Therefore two approaches can be recommended for these patients: 1) patients are not tested for the presence of deep vein thrombosis, but are continued on anticoagulation or 2) venography is performed in all patients and anticoagulation continued only in patients who have an abnormal venogram (Hirsh 1990).

Diagnosis of pulmonary embolism

Pulmonary embolism may be suspected in patients who present with sudden dyspnoea, pleuritic chest pain, haemoptysis, acute right-sided heart failure or cardiovascular collapse. The clinical features and differential diagnosis of pulmonary embolism are summarized in Table 63.6. The clinical presentation in patients with objectively documented pulmonary embolism can vary between no symptoms in patients presenting with deep vein thrombosis in whom pulmonary embolism was documented as an incidental finding, to severe dyspnea and cyanosis, or cardiovascular collapse and death in massive pulmonary embolism (large embolus obstructing the pulmonary artery trunk).

Many clinical signs and abnormal test results are associated with pulmonary embolism (tachypnoea, pleural friction rub, increased central venous pressure, low arterial pO_2, increased lactate dehydrogenase or abnormal liver enzymes, right ventricular strain or dysrhythmias on electrocardiogram, wedge-shaped infiltrates or diminished vascular pattern on chest X-ray) but none are sensitive or specific for the diagnosis of pulmonary embolism (Hull et al 1988, Kelley et al 1991, Stein et al 1991a). However, these clinical features and tests can be useful in the diagnosis of alternative diseases included in the differential diagnosis, or for therapeutic decisions (e.g. oxygen administration).

Table 63.6 The clinical characteristics of pulmonary embolism

Underlying conditions
Immobilization (surgery or disease)
Inherited deficiency of natural anticoagulants
Malignancy
Oestrogen use
Previous thrombosis
Signs and symptoms of pulmonary embolism
Sudden dyspnoea, cyanosis
Haemoptysis
Pleuritic chest pain, pleural friction rub
Hypotension, tachycardia, atrial fibrillation
Increased central venous pressure, accentuation of pulmonic component of second heart sound
Evidence of deep venous thrombosis
Fever
Differential diagnosis of pulmonary embolism
Myocardial disease (infarction, myocarditis, valve rupture)
Pericardial disease (pericarditis, cardiac tamponade)
Aortic aneurysm
Pneumonia, bronchitis, bronchiolitis
Pneumothorax, haemothorax
Tuberculosis, bronchial malignancy
Thoracic, chondral, osseous or muscle pain
Thromboneurosis

Pulmonary angiography

Pulmonary angiography results in visualization of the

lumen of the pulmonary vasculature by catheterization of the pulmonary arteries through the right heart and is accepted as the reference standard for the diagnosis of pulmonary embolism. In order to obtain high resolution images, selective catheterization of the right or left pulmonary artery or their branches is normally carried out. The criterion for the diagnosis of pulmonary embolism on angiography is the presence of a constant intraluminal filling defect or a sudden cut-off of vessels with a diameter of more than 2.5 mm (Dalen et al 1971, Bookstein & Silver 1974). Abrupt cut-offs in smaller vessels, tapering and pruning of vessels or oligaemia are not specific for pulmonary embolism as those appearances also occur in a variety of other pulmonary diseases (Dalen et al 1971).

Pulmonary angiography requires considerable technical expertise, is invasive and time consuming, all features that limit its general applicability. If digital intravenous subtraction angiography, which is much simpler to perform, could be shown to be as sensitive or specific as standard angiography, its use would be much more generally acceptable. However, the requirement for high resolution images has limited the application of intravenous digital subtraction angiography techniques for pulmonary angiography. Three relatively small studies have reported that, if adequately performed, the technique is as good as direct angiography (Goodman & Brant-Zawadzki 1982, Pond et al 1983, Bjoerk 1986). However, a direct validation of intravenous digital subtraction angiography by comparing it with standard pulmonary angiography has not been performed in a large cohort of patients, and is probably not feasible due to the large amount of contrast that would be required if both studies were to be performed within a short time.

Complications of pulmonary angiography include allergy to the contrast medium, cardiac dysrhythmias, endocardial damage and cardiac perforation. The incidence of these adverse effects is low and is reported to be approximately 1–4% (Dalen et al 1971). The frequency of these adverse effects can be reduced with the use of modern pliable pig-tail catheters (Mills et al 1980). Mortality associated with pulmonary angiography is low (0.2–0.5%) and usually only occurs in patients with severe pulmonary hypertension and cardiac enlargement with increased right ventricular end-diastolic pressure (Perlmut et al 1982, Nicod et al 1984).

The clinical validity of withholding anticoagulant treatment in patients with a negative angiogram has been shown in a management study in which the incidence of venous thromboembolism during follow-up was examined. Venous thromboembolism did not occur among 167 patients suspected of pulmonary embolism who had negative angiography (Novelline et al 1978). A management study using intravenous digital subtraction angiography has not been performed.

Isotope lung scan

Isotope lung scanning is the most commonly performed specific diagnostic test for pulmonary embolism and was introduced approximately 30 years ago. The original isotope scans were carried out by injection of ^{99m}Technetium macro-aggregated albumin particles (approximately 400 000) or ^{99m}Technetium-microspheres (approximately 100 000) into an ante-cubital vein to block approximately 0.1% of the lung capillaries to provide an image of lung perfusion. After injection of the isotope, images are taken in four to six projections (anterior, posterior, right and left postero- and antero-oblique), which are interpreted with the aid of a chart of the lung segments, to determine the presence of a perfusion defect in the same segment in different views. The use of a lung segment chart has been shown to decrease the observer variability in the interpretation of lung scans (Hoey et al 1980, Lensing et al 1991).

Initial studies have shown that a normal perfusion scan virtually excludes a diagnosis of pulmonary embolism (indicating a high sensitivity of an abnormal scan), but that the presence of perfusion defects is non-specific due to diminished blood flow in poorly ventilated areas as a result of local vasoconstrictory reflexes that occur with many other lung diseases. To enhance the usefulness of perfusion scanning, ventilation scanning was introduced on the premise that pulmonary embolism would be characterized by the presence of perfusion defects in the absence of ventilation defects (Moser et al 1971). This is in contrast with other non-vascular lung diseases in which abnormal ventilation would occur (e.g. bullae, bronchiectasis or pleural effusion). Four isotopes may be used for ventilation scanning: ^{127}Xenon, ^{133}Xenon, ^{81m}Krypton and ^{99m}Technetium-diethylene triamine penta-acetic acid (Secker-Walker & Siegel 1973, Jacobstein 1974, Alderson et al 1976, McNeil 1976, Atkins et al 1977, Goris et al 1977, Hull et al 1983b). With the xenon isotopes and with krypton, a rebreathing technique is used and with the technetium-labelled diethylene triamine penta-acetic acid, a nebulizer is used with a bacterial filter to remove the isotope from the exhaled air (Secker-Walker & Siegel 1973, Hull et al 1983b). The energy levels of the radiation produced by the isotopes, and the doses of the isotopes that are used, dictate the sequence of ventilation or perfusion (Secker-Walker & Siegel 1973). For ^{133}Xenon and ^{99m}Technetium-diethylene triamine penta-acetic acid, ventilation scanning has to be performed before the perfusion scan and for the other two isotopes, ventilation scanning (if indicated) can be performed after the perfusion scan. Xenon isotopes have a long half life and after rebreathing, poorly ventilated areas are indistinguishable from normally ventilated areas due to equilibration. Therefore, the images with xenon must be made in the initial phase of inhalation to demonstrate ventilation abnormalities. With xenon isotopes, one or two views are obtained in the position(s) that showed the most extensive perfusion defects (Atkins et al 1977). Images made in the wash-out phase with xenon demonstrate a reverse image (Atkins et al 1977, Goris et al 1977). With ^{81m}Krypton which has a short half life, and with the Technetium-labelled aerosol which is trapped by the small airways, six views comparable with the perfusion studies can be obtained with the patient breathing continuous labelled isotope in a closed system (Goris et al 1977, Hull et al 1983b). To interpret ventilation-perfusion studies, the concept of matched defects (i.e. perfusion defects that are matched by a defect in the ventilation scan or on the chest X-ray) or mismatched defects (i.e. perfusion defects in areas that are normally ventilated) is important. Studies that have compared ventilation-perfusion scanning with the results of pulmonary angiography have shown that the likelihood of pulmonary embolism was only high enough for diagnostic purposes when one or more ventilation/perfusion mismatches of at least the size of a lung segment

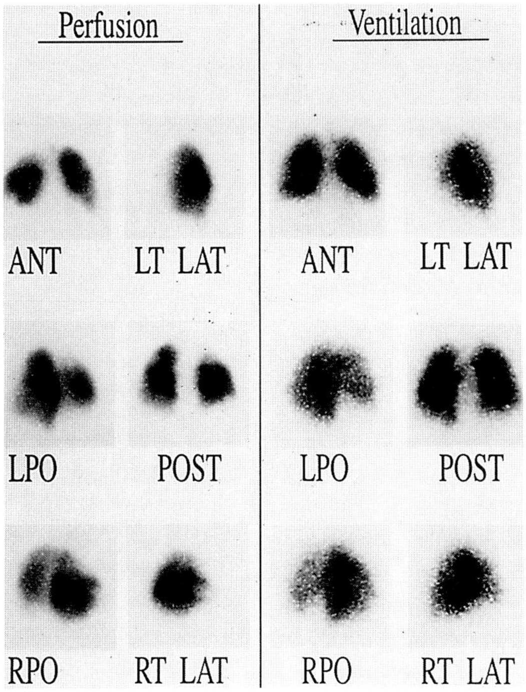

A

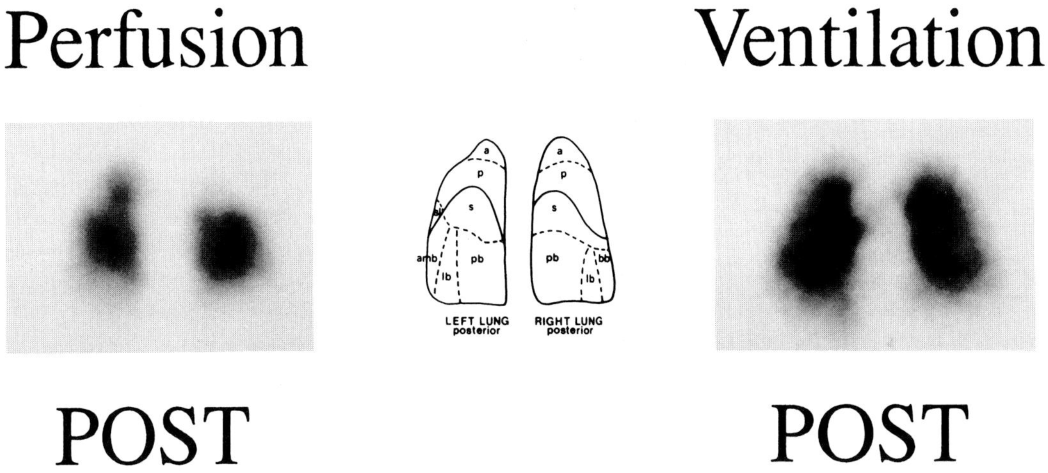

B

Fig. 63.5 Example of a high-probability ventilation-perfusion lung scan using intravenous ^{99m}TC MAA and aerosol ^{99m}TC DTPA. **A**, Six standard ventilation and perfusion images showing a segmental (right upper lobe) perfusion defect that ventilates normally. **B**, Perfusion and ventilation posterior images from the same scan along with the corresponding lung segment chart showing the right upper lobe high-probability scan.

were present. Sub-segmental mismatches or matched defects result in a probability of pulmonary embolism that is approximately equal to the initial probability and, therefore, performance of a ventilation scan when perfusion defects are subsegmental is not useful. A high probability lung scan for pulmonary embolism is shown in Figure 63.5 illustrating the lung segment chart (posterior view).

According to recent data, it seems reasonable to divide the results of perfusion/ventilation studies into three categories: negative or normal (excluding pulmonary embolism), positive or high probability (one or more ventilation/perfusion mismatches of at least segmental size, providing a 90% likelihood of pulmonary embolism), and non-diagnostic (further testing needed to rule in or rule out pulmonary embolism). The results of studies which compared ventilation-perfusion lung-scanning with pulmonary angiography are summarized in Table 63.7 (Hull et al 1983b, 1985b, Gray et al 1990, PIOPED group 1990a, Hull & Raskob 1991). Recently it was demonstrated that the diagnostic value of ventilation perfusion scans was not dependent on the presence of co-morbid pulmonary or cardiovascular disorders (Stein et al 1991b).

Studies in consecutive patients suspected of having pulmonary embolism have shown that approximately 25–30% of scans in patients suspected of pulmonary embolism are normal (negative) and 20–25% are high probability (positive) scans (Hull et al 1983b, 1985b, Gray et al 1990, PIOPED group 1990a, Webber et al 1990, Hull & Raskob 1991). In the remaining 50% of patients, the scan is non-diagnostic, and further testing to rule in or rule out pulmonary embolism is necessary. One approach would be to perform pulmonary angiography in all of these patients. However, the observation that more than 70% of patients with objectively documented pulmonary embolism have deep vein thrombosis has lead to the use of serial impedance plethysmography or venography in such patients. In management studies (Table 63.8) it has been shown that it is safe to withhold anticoagulant treatment in patients suspected of pulmonary embolism with a normal perfusion scan or a non-diagnostic scan, who have negative serial impedance tests or a normal venogram (Hull et al 1989, Kruit et al 1991).

Table 63.7 The prevalence of pulmonary embolism assessed by pulmonary angiography in relation to ventilation-perfusion scan result in patients suspected of pulmonary embolism

Study	Scan result		
	High probability %	Non-diagnostic %	Normal %
Gray et al 1990	93 (13/14)	4 (1/29)	0 (0/10)
Hull et al 1983b	91 (32/35)	42 (20/48)	–[1]
Hull et al 1985b	88 (21/24)	40 (27/68)	–[1]
Hull et al 1988	95 (19/20)	33 (15/46)	–[1]
Hull & Raskob 1991	62 (52/84)	22 (44/199)	1 (2/200)
PIOPED group[2] 1990a	87 (102/117)	26 (144/560)	10[3] (5/50)[3]

[1] For ethical reasons a pulmonary angiography was not performed in patients with a normal perfusion scan

[2] No difference in results for patients with or without co-morbid pulmonary or cardiovascular disease

[3] Only patients with a high index of clinical suspicion underwent angiography.

Table 63.8 Management studies in pulmonary embolism. Clinical outcome in patients suspected of pulmonary embolism with a negative objective test who are not given anticoagulant treatment

Study	Incidence of venous thromboembolism	
	Fatal (%)	Total (%)
Pulmonary angiography		
Novelline et al 1978	0.0 (0/167)	0.0 (0/147)
Normal ventilation perfusion lung scan		
Kipper et al 1982	0.0 (0/68)	0.0 (0/68)
Hull et al 1985b	0.0 (0/515)	0.6 (3/515)
Kruit et al 1991	0.0 (0/44)	2.3 (1/44)
Hull et al 1990b	0.0 (0/315)	1.1 (3/315)
Normal ventilation-perfusion scan or normal serial IPG		
Hull et al 1989	0.1 (1/686)	1.9 (13/686)
Normal ventilation-perfusion scan or normal venography		
Kruit et al 1991	0.0 (0/106)	1.9 (2/106)

Other diagnostic tests for pulmonary embolism

Fibrin-fibrinogen degradation products, D-dimer and fibrinopeptide A have been evaluated to a limited extent in patients suspected of pulmonary embolism (Wilson et al 1971, Rickman et al 1973, Light et al 1974, Bynum et al 1976, van Hulsteijn et al 1982, Mombelli et al 1987, Bounameux et al 1991, Tulchinsky et al 1991). Normal D-dimer or urinary fibrinopeptide A have been shown to virtually exclude pulmonary embolism of recent onset, but the applicability of these tests in management studies is hampered by the complexity of the ELISA-procedure used to obtain the test results. Rapid semi-quantitative tests for D-dimer have not yet been evaluated, and management studies have not been performed.

Platelet scintigraphy has been proposed as a diagnostic tool for pulmonary embolism, but has not been adequately evaluated (Davis et al 1980, Moser 1990). There are initial reports of the potential usefulness of magnetic resonance imaging in pulmonary embolism and infarction (Pope et al 1987, White et al 1989, Kessler et al 1991) but further evaluation of this technique is required before it can be recommended for clinical use.

Management of patients suspected of pulmonary embolism

The management of a patient with suspected pulmonary embolism will depend on the severity of the illness at presentation. In severely ill patients suspected of pulmonary embolism without evidence of major bleeding, it would be prudent to start heparin before any diagnostic test is done. If a patient is critically ill and thrombolysis or operative treatment is contemplated, an emergency pulmonary angiography should be performed. In most other cases, a perfusion scan can usually be obtained within hours, but some delay is sometimes unavoidable for a ventilation scan due to the availability of suitable isotopes. A practical approach to the management of pulmonary embolism is shown in Figure 63.6. It is likely that in the management of patients with a non-diagnostic scan, compression ultrasound will be a safe alternative to impedance plethysmography, although this has not yet been demonstrated scientifically.

TREATMENT

Interpretation of treatment studies

Criteria for the level of evidence provided by results from clinical studies on the treatment or prevention of thromboembolic diseases and the strength of the clinical recommendation based on the results of these studies have been developed (Sackett 1989). In general, strong recommendations (level I) can be based on randomized clinical trials that included a sufficient number of patients to produce a significant result or to have a small type-II error. Smaller, non-significant randomized trials (level II) can only give rise to recommendations of medium strength, while non-randomized studies, or studies lacking a control group or using historic controls can only lead to weak recommendations.

Treatment of deep vein thrombosis

The goals of treatment of deep vein thrombosis are to prevent major pulmonary embolism, to prevent extension of the thrombus, to enhance thrombolysis, and to prevent the post-thrombotic syndrome.

In clinical trials of the treatment of deep vein thrombosis, many end-points have been considered. These include lysis assessed by repeat venography, assessment of venous flow, changes in perfusion scan defects that occur in patients with clinically apparent deep vein thrombosis, the occurrence of clinically important episodes of venous thromboembolism, the incidence of the post-thrombotic syndrome and the frequency of bleeding, practically, the last three outcomes are the most important.

The importance of early effective treatment is supported by the fact that in patients with untreated or suboptimally treated deep vein thrombosis, the incidence of recurrent venous thromboembolism approximates 25–50%, and the frequency of the post-thrombotic syndrome is 90% (Hoejensgaard & Stürüp 1953, Barritt & Jordan 1960, Hull et al 1979, Lagerstedt et al 1985).

Treatment options can be divided into general measures and specific interventions (anti-coagulants, thrombolytic agents, venous interruption). General measures include immobilization to reduce pain and prevent embolization, elevation of the limb to reduce oedema and pain, avoidance of pressure on the swollen leg (blanket arch), and analgesics for pain management. The use of these

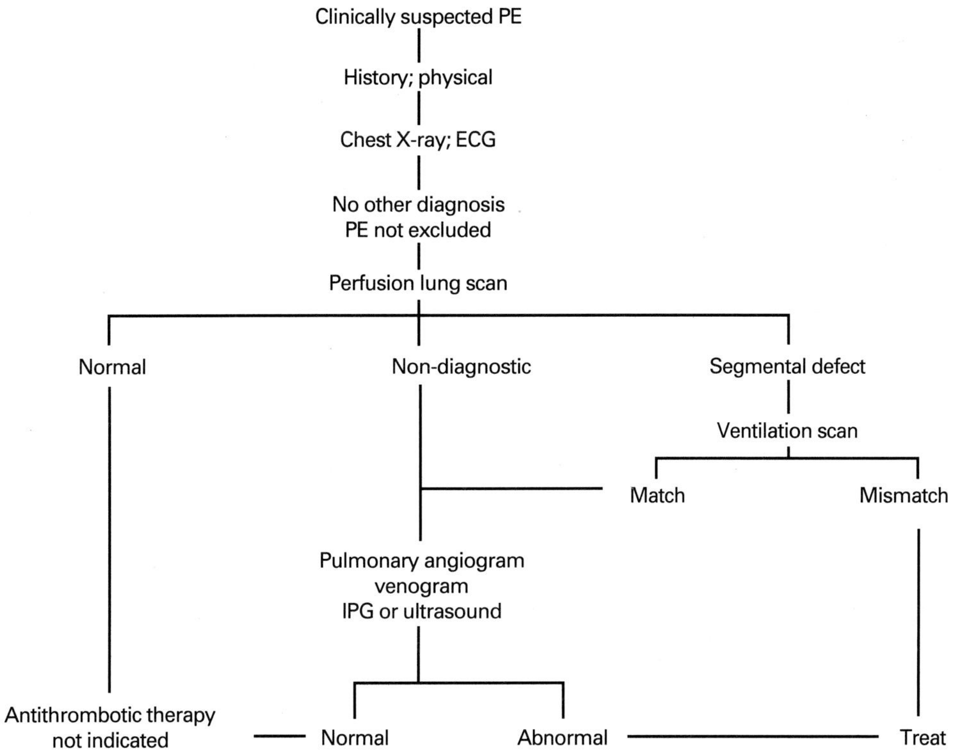

Fig. 63.6 Management of patients with suspected pulmonary embolism.

measures is based on anecdotal evidence and should be dictated by the clinical situation. Drugs for pain management include the nonsteroidal anti-inflammatory drugs, which are highly effective but probably increase the risk of bleeding especially when used in conjunction with anticoagulants.

Several specific treatments of deep vein thrombosis are available. They include:

1. Initial antithrombotic therapy with thrombolytic agents to reduce the thrombus mass and to restore venous patency, anticoagulation with unfractionated heparin, low molecular weight heparin, ancrod, or oral anticoagulants alone, or in rare cases, thrombectomy.
2. Secondary prophylaxis with oral anticoagulants or subcutaneous heparin.
3. Surgical interruption of the vena cava or insertion

Table 63.9 Results of level I and II studies on the initial treatment of deep venous thrombosis is using clinical end-points

Study	Regimen	Bleeding incidence %	VTE incidence %
Heparin: continuous intravenous vs intermittent subcutaneous			
Bentley et al 1980	Subcutaneous	4 (2/50)	–
	Intravenous	10 (5/50)	–
Andersson et al 1982	Subcutaneous	3 (2/72)	1 (1/72)
	Intravenous	6 (4/69)	1 (1/69)
Hull et al 1986	Subcutaneous	5 (3/57)	19 (11/57)
	Intravenous	7 (4/58)	5 (3/58)
Doyle et al 1987	Subcutaneous	10 (5/51)	0 (0/51)
	Intravenous	10 (5/52)	0 (0/52)
Walker et al 1987	Subcutaneous	0 (0/50)	4 (2/50)
	Intravenous	0 (0/50)	6 (3/50)
Pini et al 1990	Subcutaneous	7 (10/138)	3 (4/138)
	Intravenous	10 (13/133)	2 (2/133)
Heparin: continuous intravenous vs intermittent intravenous			
Salzman et al 1975	Intermittent	26 (37/140)	2 (2/140)
	Continuous	28 (19/69)	2 (1/69)
Glazier & Crowell 1976	Intermittent	33 (7/21)	0 (0/21)
	Continuous	0 (0/20)	5 (1/20)
Mant et al 1977	Intermittent	44 (16/36)	–
	Continuous	45 (18/40)	–
Wilson & Lampman 1979	Intermittent	37 (15/40)	–
	Continuous	12 (5/40)	–
Fagher et al 1981	Intermittent	31 (4/13)	–
	Continuous	20 (3/15)	–
Wilson et al 1981	Intermittent	44 (27/62)	6 (4/62)
	Continuous	29 (15/52)	27 (14/52)
Heparin: long vs short duration			
Gallus et al 1986	5 days	16 (22/139)	9 (5/139)
	10 days	26 (33/127)	5 (6/127)
Hull et al 1990c	5 days	9 (9/99)	7 (7/99)
	10 days	12 (12/100)	7 (7/100)
Standard heparin (iv) vs low molecular weight heparin (sc)			
Hull et al 1992	LMWH (fixed)	4 (8/213)	3 (6/213)
	UFH (adjusted)	8 (18/219)	7 (15/219)
Prandoni et al 1992	LMWH (fixed)	4 (3/85)	7 (6/85)
	UFH (adjusted)	11 (9/85)	14 (12/85)
Streptokinase vs heparin			
Robertson et al 1968	Streptokinase	25 (2/7)	–
	Heparin	13 (1/8)	–
Porter et al 1975	Streptokinase	17 (4/24)	–
	Heparin	4 (1/26)	–
Elliot et al 1979	Streptokinase	8 (2/25)	–
	Heparin	0 (0/25)	–
Recombinant tissue plasminogen activator vs heparin			
Turpie et al 1990	rt-PA	7 (3/41)	–
	Heparin	2 (1/42)	–
Goldhaber et al 1990	rt-PA	23 (12/53)	–
	Heparin	0 (0/12)	–

VTE, venous thromboembolism; iv, intravenous; sc, subcutaneous; LMWH, low molecular weight heparin, UFH, unfractionated heparin of a caval filter when contraindications to antithrombotic drugs exist or after the occurrence of pulmonary embolism during adequate anticoagulation.

Trials (level I and II) of the initial treatment options are summarized in Table 63.9, while those of long-term treatment options are summarized in Table 63.10.

Treatment of pulmonary embolism

The mortality due to recurrent pulmonary embolism in untreated patients who have survived the initial episode is estimated to be 20–70% (Barritt & Jordan 1960). The goals of treatment of pulmonary embolism are to increase survival from the acute episode, and to prevent recurrent pulmonary embolism thereby preserving respiratory reserve. Clinical trials of therapeutic interventions in pulmonary embolism have used both reduction in thrombus size on pulmonary angiography or perfusion scanning, and recurrent thromboembolic events as outcome measures.

General therapeutic measures include the administration of oxygen, intravenous fluids and vasopressor agents and other resuscitory measures depending on the clinical status of the patient. Specific therapeutic measures are similar to those for deep vein thrombosis. Comparative studies (level I and II) of different treatments in the initial treatment of pulmonary embolism are summarized in Table 63.11.

Specific treatment options

Unfractionated heparin

Unfractionated heparin (UFH) has been the mainstay of treatment for venous thromboembolism for the past few decades (Hirsh 1991b). The evidence for the use of heparin in the initial treatment of venous thromboembolism comes from two studies. The superiority of heparin over no anti-thrombotic treatment was addressed in one trial that demonstrated a better clinical outcome in patients with pulmonary embolism treated with heparin followed by oral anticoagulants compared with those who did not receive antithrombotic treatment (Barritt & Jordan 1960). Convincing evidence of the benefits of initial heparin comes from a recent study that compared oral anticoagulants alone with continuous intravenous heparin followed by oral anticoagulants which demonstrated that the clinical outcome was significantly better in the patients who

Table 63.10 Results of level I and II studies on the long-term treatment of venous thromboembolism using clinical end-points

Study	Regimen	Bleeding incidence	Duration of follow-up (mths)	VTE incidence
Lagerstedt et al 1985	Warfarin (INR 3–4.5)	0 (0/23)	3	0 (0/23)
	No treatment	0 (0/28)	3	29* (8/28)
Hull et al 1979	Warfarin (INR 3–4.5)	22* (7/33)	3	0* (0/35)
	Heparin 5000 U sc tid	0 (0/33)		26 (9/35)
Hull et al 1982a	Warfarin (INR 3–4.5)	18* (11/49)	3	2 (1/49)
	Warfarin (INR 2–3)	4 (2/47)		2 (1/47)
Hull et al 1982b	Warfarin (INR 3–4.5)	17* (9/35)	3	2 (1/53)
	Heparin adj. dose sc	2 (1/53)		4 (2/53)
Schulman et al 1985	Warfarin (1–6) mth)	28 (10/36)	12	9 (3/36)
	Warfarin (3–13 mth)	18 (8/37)		9 (3/37)
Holmgren et al 1985	Warfarin 1 mth	–	12	14 (10/69)
	Warfarin 6 mth	–		15 (10/66)
O'Sullivan 1972	Warfarin 6 wk	–	6	7 (7/94)
	Warfarin 6 mth	–		9 (9/92)

sc, subcutaneous, tid, three times a day; *$p < 0.05$.

Table 63.11 Results of Level I and II studies on the initial treatment of pulmonary embolism using clinical end-points

Study	Regimen	Bleeding incidence %	VTE incidence	Mortality %
Barritt & Jordan 1960	No treatment	0 (0/19)	55 (10/19)	27* (5/19)
	Heparin + Nicoumalone	8 (1/16)	0 (0/16)	8 (1/16)
UPET-1 1973	Heparin	27 (21/78)	17 (13/78)	10 (8/78)
	Urokinase	45 (37/82)	11 (9/82)	11 (9/82)
PIOPED Investigators 1990b	Heparin	0 (0/4)	–	0 (0/4)
	rt-PA (40–80 mg)	11 (1/9)	–	11 (1/9)
UPET-2 1974	Urokinase 12 h	25 (15/59)	2 (1/59)	10 (6/59)
	Urokinase 24 h	31 (17/54)	7 (4/54)	15 (8/54)
	Streptokinase	22 (12/54)	4 (2/54)	15 (8/54)
Goldhaber et al 1988	Urokinase	9 (2/23)	–	9 (2/23)
	rt-PA	5 (1/22)	–	9 (2/22)

* $p < 0.05$.

received heparin as the initial treatment (Brandjes et al 1992).

The mode of action of heparin and its pharmacokinetics and pharmacodynamics are discussed in Chapter 62. Heparin dosages in individual patients are usually titrated to obtain a desired level of anticoagulation, frequently referred to as the 'therapeutic range' (e.g. activated partial thromboplastin time of 1.5 to 2.5 times control). Several studies in patients with venous thrombosis, and also in patients with arterial thrombosis, have shown that the risk of (recurrent) thromboembolic events is higher (4 to 12- fold) if the anticoagulant response, assessed with a sensitive activated partial thromboplastin time, is less than 1.5 times control, i.e. the lower limit of the therapeutic range (Basu et al 1972, Hull et al 1986, Camilleri et al 1988, Turpie et al 1989, Prins & Hirsh 1991).

Heparin is usually administered by continuous intravenous infusion, but it can also be given by subcutaneous injection, provided that the initial dose is high enough (Andersson et al 1982, Doyle et al 1987, Walker et al 1987, Pini et al 1990) (Table 63.9, Fig. 63.7). Intermittent intravenous administration of heparin is another option that is probably comparable in efficacy but is associated with more bleeding than with either continuous intravenous infusion or subcutaneous injections (Salzman et al 1975, Glazier et al 1976) (Table 63.9, Fig. 63.8).

In patients with venous thromboembolism, treatment with intravenous heparin is usually started with a bolus of 5000 to 7500 units followed by a continuous infusion of 30 000 to 35 000 units per 24 hours. Approximately 6 hours after the start of the infusion an activated partial thromboplastin time should be determined and the heparin dose adjusted. Recently, a rigorous schedule of heparin-dose adjustments has been proposed to reach an optimal anticoagulant response in the majority of patients as soon as possible after the start of treatment (Cruickshank et al 1991). 6 hours after each dose adjustment the anticoagulant response should be checked and a new dose adjustment carried out. When a therapeutic anticoagulant response is obtained the interval for laboratory control can be prolonged to 24 hours. A nomogram for the control of intravenous heparin therapy (modified from Cruickshank et al 1991) is shown in Table 63.12.

The duration of heparin treatment in patients with venous thromboembolism has conventionally been 10 days in North America and shorter, 4–5 days, in many European

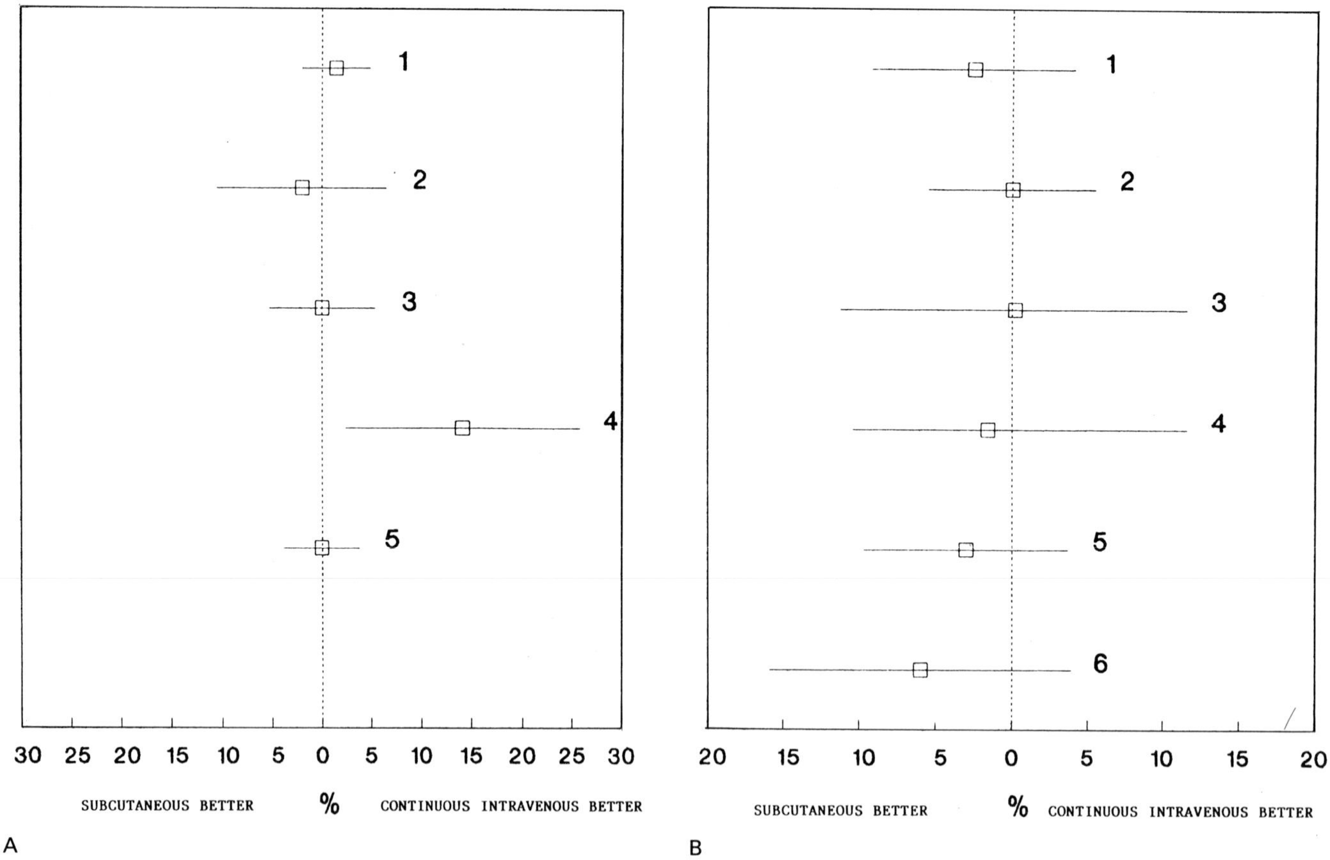

Fig. 63.7 The observed difference in incidence of recurrent venous thromboembolism (**A**) and bleeding (**B**) and their 95% confidence intervals in randomized studies comparing continuous intravenous with intermittent subcutaneous heparin in the treatment of deep vein thrombosis. 1, Pini et al 1990; 2, Walker et al 1987; 3, Doyle et al 1987; 4, Hull et al 1986; 5, Andersson et al 1982; 6, Bentley et al 1980.

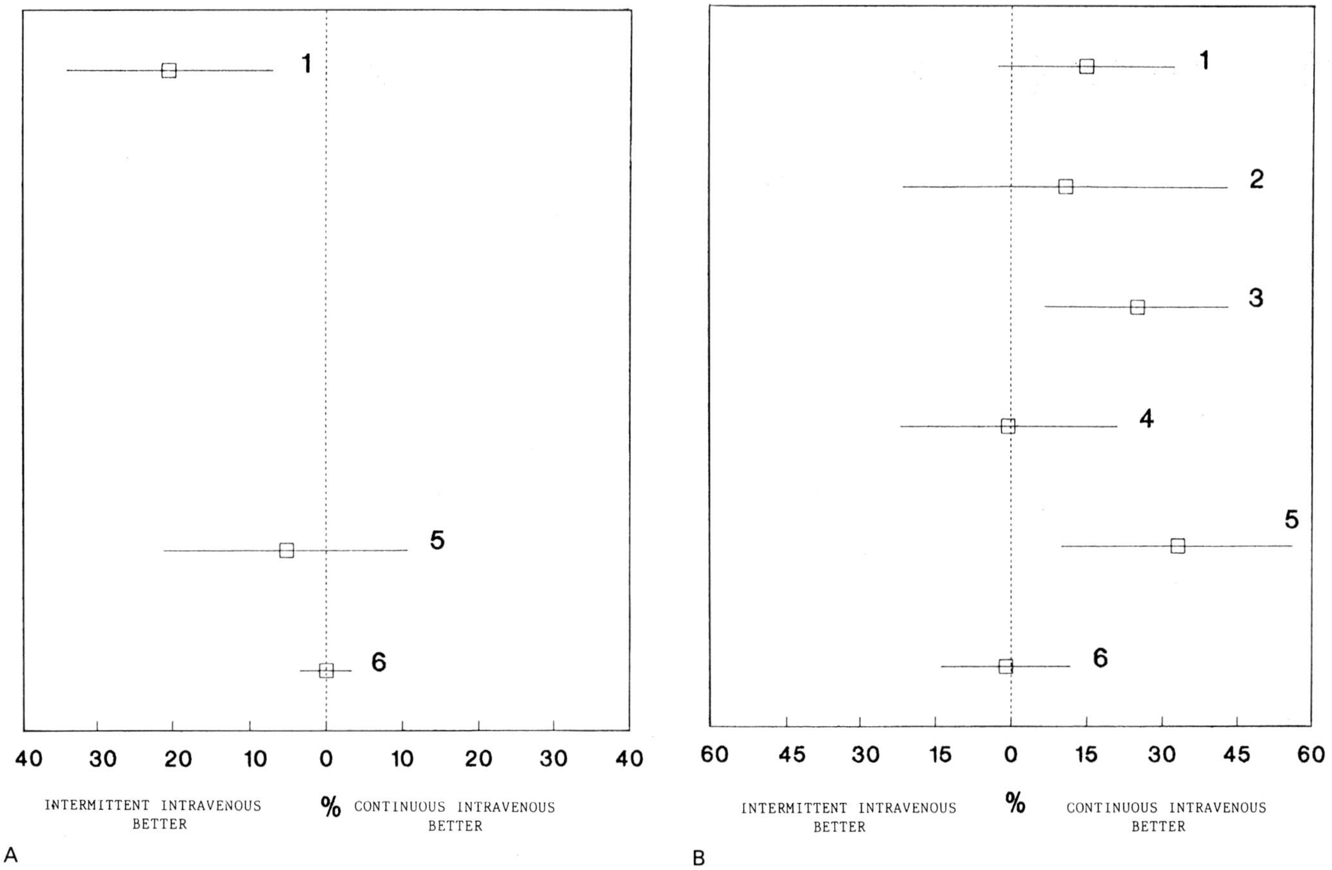

Fig. 63.8 The observed difference in incidence of recurrent venous thromboembolism (**A**) and bleeding (**B**) and their 95% confidence intervals in randomized studies comparing continuous intravenous with intermittent intravenous heparin in the treatment of deep vein thrombosis. 1, Wilson & Lampman 1979; 2, Fagher et al 1981; 3, Wilson & Lampman 1979; 4, Mant et al 1977; 5, Glazier & Crowell 1976; 6, Salzman et al 1975.

countries. Recently, the duration of heparin therapy has been the subject of two trials, one in patients with submassive venous thromboembolism (Gallus et al 1986) and another in patients with proximal deep vein thrombosis (Hull et al 1990c). The results of both studies showed that the discontinuation of heparin after 5 days of treatment is probably safe provided that oral anticoagulation started at the same time or shortly after the start of heparin therapy is in the therapeutic range for more than 24 hours before ceasing heparin (Table 63.9, Fig. 63.9).

Table 63.12 Nomogram for the adjustment of continuous intravenous heparin dosages (modified from Cruickshank et al 1991)

Start heparin treatment with a 5000 U bolus intravenously, followed by an infusion of 30 000 U/24 h. Determine the aPTT 6 h after the start of the infusion and adjust as follows

APTT (× normal)	Bolus units	Hold (min)	Dose change (units)	Repeat APTT (h)
<1.3	5000	–	+ 5000	6
1.3–1.5	–	–	+ 2500	6
1.5–2.5	–	–	–	next day
2.5–2.8	–	–	– 2500	6
>2.8	–	60	– 5000	6

For secondary prophylaxis after the initial treatment, adjusted dose subcutaneous heparin (mid-interval APTT 1.5 to 2.0 times control) is a safe alternative to oral anticoagulants (Hull et al 1982b), but low dose heparin (5000 units subcutaneously twice daily) is associated with a high risk of recurrence (Hull et al 1979).

Even with adequate treatment, however, the risk of recurrent venous thromboembolism in patients with idiopathic thrombosis is approximately 5% during the first 10 days and 10% during the 3 months after the initial event (Hull et al 1990c, Prandoni et al 1991). In patients with thrombosis secondary to a temporary risk factor, the recurrence rate is reported to be lower (Hull et al 1990c, Prandoni et al 1992).

The risk of major bleeding during heparin treatment approximates 4–7% during the initial treatment (Hull et al 1990c, Hull et al 1992, Prandoni et al 1992).

Low molecular weight heparin

Recently low molecular weight derivatives of heparin have become available for clinical use. Their pharmacology and pharmacodynamics are discussed in Chapter 62. Two

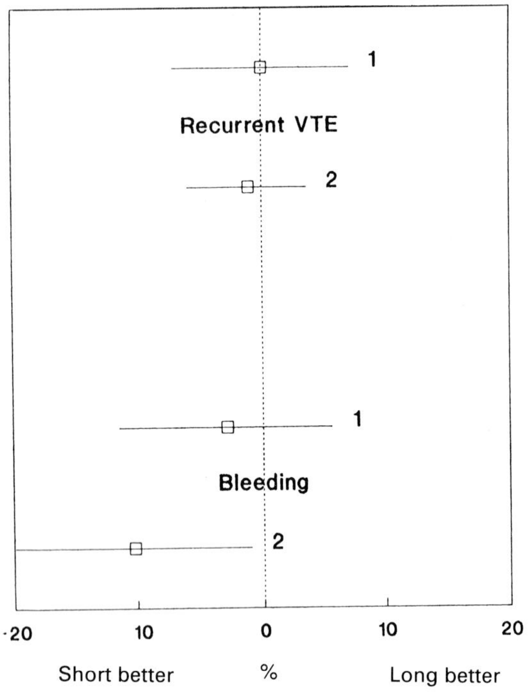

Fig. 63.9 The observed difference of recurrent venous thromboembolism and bleeding and their 95% confidence intervals in randomized studies comparing continuous intravenous heparin of long versus short duration in the treatment of venous thromboembolism. 1, Hull et al 1990c; 2, Gallus et al 1986.

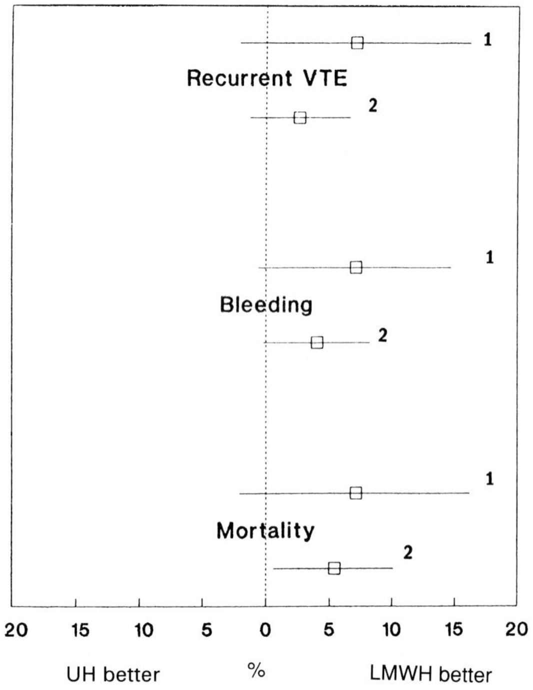

Fig. 63.10 The observed difference in incidence of recurrent venous thromboembolism, bleeding and mortality and their 95% confidence intervals in randomized studies comparing adjusted dose continuous intravenous unfractionated heparin with fixed dose subcutaneous low molecular weight heparin. 1, Prandoni et al 1992; 2, Hull et al 1992.

characteristics make these agents excellent candidates for the treatment of venous thromboembolism (Handeland et al 1990). These are: 1) their kinetics are more predictable than those of standard heparin and 2) their elimination half life is longer when compared to standard heparin. These properties make weight-adjusted fixed subcutaneous dosing of low molecular weight heparin possible in the initial treatment of venous thromboembolism.

Many randomized studies have shown that in patients with deep vein thrombosis low molecular weight heparin treatment, either intravenously with dose adjustments or subcutaneously in fixed doses, is at least as effective and probably somewhat more effective than continuous intravenous adjusted dose unfractionated heparin as observed by lysis of the thrombus on repeat venography or by the change in perfusion defects on lung-scanning (Bratt et al 1985, 1990, Holm et al 1986, Vogel & Machulik 1987, Albada et al 1989, Harenberg et al 1990, Huet et al 1990, Duroux et al 1991, Prandoni et al 1992). Recently, two large trials assessed major clinical endpoints during long-term follow-up after treatment with either unfractionated heparin or low molecular weight heparin (Hull et al 1992, Prandoni et al 1992). Both of these studies reported a lower incidence of recurrent venous thromboembolism and of major bleeding complications in patients randomized to fixed dose subcutaneous low molecular weight heparin compared to those randomized to standard unfractionated heparin treatment (Table 63.9, Fig. 63.10). The observed differences in clinical outcomes and their 95% confidence intervals reported in these two studies make it unlikely that adjusted dose intravenous unfractionated heparin treatment has a major clinical benefit over fixed dose subcutaneous low molecular weight heparin treatment. In addition, both trials reported a lower incidence of mortality due to related causes unrelated to venous thromboembolism in the patients treated with low molecular weight heparin. Whether or not this observation is causally related to the treatment is unknown. A potential development, made possible by the use of a fixed dose of subcutaneous heparin, is home treatment for patients with deep vein thrombosis who are not severely ill (Bakker et al 1988). However, before this approach is adopted for routine use, its safety and efficacy should be demonstrated in randomized trials.

Low molecular weight heparins have not been formally evaluated in treatment of patients with pulmonary embolism.

Ancrod

Ancrod is a defibrinating agent that has been evaluated in a few small trials in the treatment of deep vein thrombosis and produces a similar reduction in thrombus size compared to unfractionated heparin (Sharp et al 1968,

Kakkar et al 1969b, Pitney 1970, Davies et al 1972). Currently, its main application is in the treatment of venous thromboembolism in patients in whom unfractionated heparin results in thrombocytopenia or allergic reactions. A convenient dosage schedule is 140 units during the first 12 hours, followed by 140 units/24 hours for the next 2 to 3 days, given by continuous intravenous infusion to maintain a fibrinogen level of 50% of the initial value (Davies et al 1972). However this recommended reduction in fibrinogen is not based on scientifically proven data.

Thrombolytic agents

The role of thrombolytic agents in the treatment of venous thromboembolism is uncertain (Browse et al 1968, Goldhaber et al 1984, Marder & Sherry 1988b, Verstraete 1989, Rogers & Lutcher 1990). Currently four agents are available for clinical use: streptokinase, urokinase, recombinant tissue plasminogen activator and acylated plasminogen streptokinase activator complex (APSAC). The pharmacology and pharmacodynamics of these agents are discussed in Chapter 27. Many reports have been published on the use of thrombolytic agents in the treatment of venous thromboembolism (Table 63.13). Few of them were randomized trials that compared thrombolytic treatment to standard heparin treatment and none were large enough to demonstrate a clinical benefit in patients randomized to a thrombolytic agent.

In patients with deep vein thrombosis, the use of streptokinase is associated with a (3.7-fold) increased likelihood of achieving lysis of the thrombus than found with standard heparin treatment (Robertson et al 1968, 1970, Kakkar et al 1969b, Tsapogas et al 1973, Porter et al 1975, Elliot et al 1979, Goldhaber et al 1984). This difference is reported to persist for months to years after the acute event (Johansson et al 1979, Arnesen et al 1982). The frequency with which substantial lysis of the thrombus occurs early in the course of treatment is estimated to be between 50 to 80% (Marder and Sherry 1988b). The use of thrombolytic agents is also associated with a more rapid disappearance of clinical symptoms (Robertson 1971, Arnesen et al 1978). However the risk of major bleeding during the initial treatment is also increased (2.7-fold) compared with heparin (Robertson et al 1968, Porter et al 1975, Elliot et al 1979, Goldhaber et al 1984). Recent studies on the use of thrombolytic treatment have reported lower bleeding rates than reported in the earlier studies, largely because shorter infusions of the thrombolytic agents were used (Marder & Sherry 1988a, Levine et al 1990a,b).

Whether or not patients treated with thrombolytic agents have a lower incidence of the post-thrombotic syndrome is also an unresolved issue since the reported results are not consistent and many of the studies only analysed a small proportion of the patients initially included (Common et al 1976, Johansson et al 1979, Albrechtson et al 1981, Kakkar & Lawrence 1985).

In pulmonary embolism, the comparisons of thrombolytic agents with heparin have shown an increased lysis

Table 63.13 Dosage regimens of thrombolytic drugs used for venous thromboembolism

Study	Regimen
Pulmonary embolism	
Intravenous treatment	
UPET-I 1973	Urokinase, 4400 U/kg bolus, followed by 4400 U/kg/h for 12 h
UPET-II 1974	Urokinase as in UPET-I for 12 or 24 h Streptokinase, 250 000 U bolus, followed by 100 000 U/h for 24 h
Griguer et al 1979	Urokinase 2 700 000 U/24 h ± Lys-plasminogen (2500 U)
Goldhaber et al 1986	rt-PA, 50 mg in 2 h, then 40 mg in 4 h
Verstraete et al 1988	rt-PA, 10 mg bolus, then 40 mg in 2 h followed by 50 mg in 5 h if needed
Goldhaber et al 1988	rt-PA, 100 mg in 2 h
Levine et al 1990a, b	rt-PA, 0.6 mg/kg in 2 min
Intra-pulmonary arterial treatment	
Leeper et al 1988	Streptokinase 10 000–20 000 U/h for 9–24 h
Goldstein 1987	Streptokinase 1500 000 U in 40 min
Intra-artrial treatment	
Petitpretz et al 1984	Urokinase 15 000 U/kg bolus
Deep vein thrombosis	
Intravenous treatment	
van de Loo et al 1983	Urokinase 2200 U/kg/h, 12 h/day for 3–6 days
d'Angelo & Manucci 1984	Urokinase 1500–4000 U/kg/h for 2–7 days
Elliot et al 1979	Streptokinase 100 000 U for 3 days
Schulman et al 1984	Streptokinase 10 000 U/h for 7 days
	Streptokinase 100 000 U/h, 2 h/day for 7 days
Ruckley et al 1987	APSAC, 30 U bolus
Turpie et al 1990	rt-PA 0.5 mg/kg in 4 h (1987), in 8 h (1990) and repeated the next day (1989)
Verhaeghe et al 1989	rt-PA 100 mg in 8 h, 50 mg in 8 h the next day
Goldhaber et al 1900	rt-PA 0.05 mg/kg/h for 24 h (max 150 mg)

of the thrombus mass on repeat perfusion scan or pulmonary angiography with thrombolytic agents which results in a better haemodynamic status early (2 to 24 hours) after the acute event (UPET-I 1973, Tibbutt et al 1974, Ly et al 1978). However after several days, the difference in thrombus mass reduction, as assessed by repeat perfusion lung scan, between the two treatments was no longer apparent (UPET-I 1973, Levine et al 1990a,b).

Patients with venous thromboembolism of recent onset achieve better lysis with the use of a thrombolytic agent than patients in whom symptoms are present for a more prolonged (>3 days) period (Miller et al 1971, UPET-I 1973, UPET-II 1974, Marder & Sherry 1988a,b).

In view of the uncertainty of the clinical benefits of thrombolytic agents and the risk of bleeding associated with their use, it is reasonable to reserve their use in deep vein thrombosis for patients in whom the viability of a leg is compromised (venous gangrene) and those with extensive or painful swelling of the leg. In patients with pulmonary embolism who have refractory hypotension (i.e. hypotension that cannot be corrected with the use of vasopressor agents) or who have greater than 50% obstruction of the pulmonary vasculature, thrombolytic agents can be used to increase the likelihood of survival from the acute episode, although their superiority in this clinical setting has not been demonstrated formally. Recently, considerable effort is being invested in the development of dosage schedules of thrombolytic agents that combine safety with a major lytic effect but none of these new regimens have been evaluated sufficiently to warrant their routine use (Marder & Sherry 1988a,b, Goldhaber 1991, Levine 1991).

Oral anticoagulants

Oral anticoagulants are standard for the long-term treatment of patients with venous thromboembolism (secondary prophylaxis). Their use in patients with pulmonary embolism is associated with a better clinical outcome than no treatment (Barritt & Jordan 1960), and in patients with deep vein thrombosis the administration of oral anticoagulants has been shown to be better than no treatment (Lagerstedt et al 1985) or treatment with low dose subcutaneous heparin 5000 units twice daily (Hull et al 1979).

The pharmacology and mode of action of oral anticoagulants are described in Chapter 65. Since it takes at least 3 days before a therapeutic level of anticoagulation is achieved, the use of oral anticoagulants alone in the initial treatment of deep vein thrombosis is not recommended. This recommendation is strengthened by the results of a recent clinical trial that compared oral anticoagulants alone with the standard initial intravenous heparin. This study was interrupted early because of a disturbingly high incidence of recurrent venous thromboembolism in the group of patients treated with oral anticoagulants alone (Brandjes 1992).

The dose of oral anticoagulants should be adjusted to maintain an International Normalized Ratio at 2.0–3.0, since a higher International Normalized Ratio (3.0–4.5), though effective in preventing recurrence or extension (Hull et al 1982a), is associated with an increased risk of bleeding (Hull et al 1982a, Turpie et al 1988, Saour et al 1990, Hirsh 1991c). The best available estimate (Levine et al 1989) of the incidence of bleeding associated with a 3 month course of oral anticoagulants aimed at an International Normalized Ratio of 2.0–3.0 is 4.3% (95% CI 0.5–14.5%), while the incidence of recurrent venous thromboembolic events is reported to be 2–5% during this period (Hull et al 1982a, Schulman et al 1985, Hirsh et al 1989, Prandoni et al 1992).

Oral anticoagulants are contraindicated during pregnancy, because of teratogenicity and risk of bleeding in the foetus (Hall et al 1980, Ginsberg & Hirsh 1989, Iturbe-Alessio et al 1986). Adjusted dose subcutaneous heparin can be used for long-term treatment in this clinical setting.

Surgery

Thrombectomy for the treatment of iliofemoral thrombosis was introduced in 1948 in an attempt to reduce the incidence of pulmonary embolism and to restore normal venous flow in order to prevent the post-thrombotic syndrome (Leriche 1948, Mahorner et al 1957, Haller 1961). Early short-term evaluations of thrombectomy provided encouraging results (Haller & Abrams 1963), but the long term evaluation has not proved the beneficial effects, as demonstrated in a study in thrombectomy patients in which the symptoms of the post-phlebitic syndrome were present in 16 of 17 of the patients available for evaluation (Lansing & Davis 1968). Subsequent retrospective series of surgically-treated patients reported better results (Shionoya et al 1989). To eliminate the problem of rethrombosis in the operated vessel the use of a temporary proximal arteriovenous fistula was introduced (Plate et al 1984, Swedenborg et al 1986, Ganger et al 1989, Neglen et al 1991). This technique has been compared to medical treatment alone in a small randomized trial (Plate et al 1990) in which severe post-thrombotic sequelae after 5 years were present in six out of 22 of the medically treated patients and in three of 19 surgically treated patients. This difference is not significant, however, because of the small number of patients included in the trial and a major clinical benefit of either treatment cannot be excluded.

The weight of evidence suggests that it is prudent to reserve surgical treatment of deep vein thrombosis for patients with impending venous gangrene, for patients in whom symptoms do not respond to thrombolytic treatment, or for patients who have a contraindication for thrombolytic treatment (Lord et al 1990).

Pulmonary embolectomy can be used for the treatment of massive, life-threatening pulmonary embolism. The possibility of instituting partial femoro-femoral cardiopulmonary bypass under local anaesthesia can be life-saving in patients with severe hypotension refractory to inotropic agents, or cyanosis not improving with oxygen administration (Cross & Mowlen 1974, Alpert et al 1975, Clarke & Abrams 1986, Gray et al 1988). At present, the decision whether to use thrombolytic agents or to proceed to surgery cannot be guided by the results of randomized trials, and must be based on the clinical situation and on local practice. In patients with massive pulmonary embolism who have a contraindication to thrombolytic agents or who do not improve within a few hours after the start of thrombolytic drugs, it would be reasonable to consider pulmonary embolectomy (Glassford et al 1981, DelCampo 1985).

The results of recent series of patients who had undergone pulmonary embolectomy indicate that the procedure itself is reasonably safe in the hands of experienced teams of thoracic surgeons and anaesthetists, and that the mortality during and after the surgical procedure is mainly confined to the most severely ill patients (Gray et al 1988, Meyer et al 1991).

Venous interruption

In patients with venous thromboembolism in whom anticoagulant therapy is contraindicated or in whom pulmonary embolism occurs despite adequate anticoagulation, interruption of the great veins can be used to prevent recurrent pulmonary embolism. Formerly, the great veins were interrupted surgically by ligating the common femoral vein or ligating or plicating the inferior vena cava. However the use of these procedures was associated with high operative morbidity and mortality (6 to 23%) and a high incidence (up to 30%) of late sequelae due to venous insufficiency (Bergan & Trippel 1966, Moretz et al 1972, Coon 1974, Eberlein & Carey 1974, Couch et al 1975, Ramchandani et al 1991). Currently, insertion of filter devices in the inferior vena cava is the approach for venous interruption used most often. Since the introduction of the original stainless steel Greenfield filter, a number of other filter devices have been developed including the Bird's nest, LGM, titanium Greenfield, Simon nitinol, Guenther and Amplatz filters. These devices are designed to trap embolizing thrombi, without interruption of venous flow.

Although there are no randomized trials available, percutaneous placement seems to be associated with lower morbidity than operative placement and is regarded as the preferred way of insertion of these devices (Dorfman 1990, Hye et al 1990). Percutaneous placement is usually via the right femoral or the right internal jugular vein but if necessary the left femoral vein can be used though technically it is more difficult (Roberts et al 1987, Denny et al 1988, Pais et al 1988, Dorfman 1990). Before insertion of the device a cavogram should be obtained to ascertain the diameter of the inferior vena cava and to determine if it is patent (Dorfman 1990).

The most extensive clinical experience is with the stainless steel Greenfield filter. Surgical insertion of this device is associated with significant cost, major bleeding requiring re-exploration of the wound in 6–15% of cases and mortality, attributed to filter placement, of approximately 4% (Greenfield et al 1977, Wingerd et al 1978, Cimochowski et al 1980, Greenfield et al 1981, Greenfield et al 1988, Pais & Tobin 1989). Caval thrombosis in association with percutaneous placement of a stainless steel Greenfield filter occurs in 5% of patients, as does recurrent pulmonary embolism (Dorfman 1990).

Adverse effects associated with placement of an inferior vena caval filter, besides thrombotic obstruction of the cava and bleeding at the site of insertion, are perforation of the caval wall and sometimes penetration of other retroperitoneal organs, or migration of the device (migration to the heart usually is fatal) (Kim et al 1989, Awh et al 1991, Howerton et al 1991, Lahey et al 1991). Fortunately the incidence of these side-effects appears to be low if proper technique and positioning are used (Pais et al 1988, Dorfman 1990).

Studies with the Bird's nest filter, and the Guenther filter have produced comparable results, though in smaller numbers of patients (Fobbe et al 1988, Roehm et al 1988, Darfman 1990, Schneider et al 1990). The Amplatz and LGM filters are associated with a higher rate of caval thrombosis, while the titanium Greenfield filter was associated with a high rate of local complications and is being redesigned (Ricco et al 1988, Epstein et al 1989, Simon et al 1989, McCowan et al 1990, Greenfield et al 1990). However, the differences in reported rates of complication could be due, not only to different behaviour of the devices used, but also to differences in patient populations studied, since all the data are derived from case series or cohort studies.

The low rate of complications has prompted physicians to use placement of filter devices for more liberal indications such as primary treatment of deep vein thrombosis or pulmonary embolism in patients with cancer or other diseases who are at high risk for complications associated with anticoagulant treatment, or as an adjunct to thrombolytic treatment of deep vein thrombosis (Rohrer et al 1989, Thery et al 1990, Calligaro et al 1991, Cohen et al 1991, Fink & Jones 1991). In the few published uncontrolled studies, the results appear promising, but randomized trials are warranted in these indications (Cohen et al 1991, Calligaro et al 1991).

Management of patients with venous thromboembolism

Anticoagulant treatment should be instituted in patients in whom the diagnosis of venous thromboembolism is established and in patients who are suspected of having venous thromboembolism, but in whom the diagnosis cannot be ruled in or out within a reasonably short time interval (Hyers et al 1989). Cohort studies suggest that it is safe to withhold treatment in patients with isolated calf vein thrombosis unless extension occurs (Hull et al 1985b, Huisman et al 1986), even in the presence of a non-diagnostic ventilation-perfusion lung scan (Hull et al 1989). The necessity of treatment for patients with proximal deep vein thrombosis and isolated asymptomatic calf vein thrombosis detected by screening is not known, and will depend on the clinical status of a patient and the estimated risk of embolization.

Routine treatment should include initial heparin or low molecular weight heparin followed by secondary prophylaxis with oral anticoagulants. The duration of anticoagulant treatment is usually 3 months in patients who have a first episode of thrombosis, and longer in those who have recurrent disease or who have underlying disorders which are known to be related to a tendency for recurrent venous thromboembolism (thrombophilia). Examples of thrombophilia are the presence of malignant disease, protein C or protein S deficiency and antithrombin III deficiency. The exact duration of oral anticoagulant treatment in these circumstances is not well defined and depends on the expected benefit of continued therapy in comparison to the risks.

Thrombolytic agents should be considered in massive pulmonary embolism and impending venous gangrene or massive debilitating leg oedema (Kakkar et al 1969a). When these agents are contraindicated (Table 63.14) surgical removal of the thrombus may be considered. The insertion of a vena caval filter is indicated in patients who have a contraindication to anticoagulant treatment (Table 63.14) for the prevention of pulmonary emboli and in those in whom pulmonary embolism occurs despite anticoagulant treatment.

In patients with deep vein thrombosis it may be useful to obtain a baseline perfusion lung scan to facilitate diagnosis of pulmonary embolism if new pulmonary symptoms occur (Monreal 1989a). However, the clinical utility of this approach is not clear.

Patients with idiopathic thrombosis have an increased risk of harbouring a symptomatic or asymptomatic carcinoma (Monreal et al 1991, Prandoni et al 1992). Whether or not extensive investigations for malignancy are indicated in these patients is an unresolved issue (Prins & Hirsh 1991). All patients with objectively documented venous thromboembolism should be instructed about the need for anti-thrombotic prophylaxis in case of immobilization, because of either surgical or medical disorders.

Table 63.14 Contra-indications for full-dose anticoagulation or thrombolytic agents

Condition	Heparin/oral anticoagulants	Thrombolytic agent
Intracranial bleeding	Absolute	Absolute
Active internal bleeding	Absolute	Absolute
Active intestinal bleeding	Relative	Absolute
Recent ischaemic stroke	Relative	Absolute
Severe hypertension	Relative	Relative
Recent trauma (including cardiopulmonary resuscitation, delivery, surgery, biopsy, vessel puncture)	Relative	Relative

Venous thrombosis at other sites

Deep vein thrombosis of the lower limbs and pulmonary embolism are relatively common diseases. However, thrombosis may occur, albeit less frequently, in other parts of the venous system. Partly for this reason, and partly because of the invasiveness of the diagnostic techniques involved, only few formal comparative studies of the diagnosis and treatment of thrombosis, other than of the legs, have been performed and most knowledge is based on retrospective studies and anecdotal data.

Subclavian and axillary vein thrombosis

The diagnosis of thrombosis of the arm veins may be suspected in patients with a swollen, painful arm. However, as occurs in deep vein thrombosis of the leg, when patients at risk (e.g. those with indwelling catheters for chemotherapy) are screened prospectively, subclavian vein thrombosis is mostly found to be asymptomatic (Lokich & Becker 1983). Predisposing factors for subclavian or axillary thrombosis (Bozelli et al 1973, Hill & Berry 1990) are indwelling catheters, certain types of physical effort (e.g. baseball pitching) or local radiation for malignancy and anatomical abnormalities (e.g. thoracic outlet syndrome). Pulmonary embolism has been demonstrated in 15–30% of patients with subclavian vein thrombosis (Monreal et al 1991).

The diagnosis of subclavian vein thrombosis can be made by venography which is performed with the arm in an abducted, dependent position in order to avoid artifacts by external muscular compression (Hill & Berry 1990, Baxter et al 1991). Recently it was reported that duplex ultrasound can also be used for the diagnosis with suppression of normal phasic flow or the presence of echogenic material in the lumen of the vein used as criteria to establish the diagnosis (Kerr et al 1990, Baxter et al 1991). Treatment of subclavian vein thrombosis is the same as for deep vein thrombosis of the leg. When anatomical disorders are causative, their correction is probably indicated (Hill & Berry 1990, Nemmers et al 1990).

Cerebral venous thrombosis

Thrombosis of the cerebral veins and sinuses may be suspected in patients with signs of increased intracranial pressure, seizures or focal neurologic symptoms and signs including cranial nerve palsies (Enevoldsen & Ross Russell 1990). Predisposing causes are multiple and include trauma, sepsis, auto-immune diseases and haematologic malignancies (Enevoldsen & Ross Russell 1990).

The diagnosis of cerebral sinus thrombosis may be made by angiography of the carotid arteries, in which special attention is paid to the venous phase or by intravenous digital subtraction angiography (Barnes et al 1983). Computerized tomography scanning, even with intravenous contrast, is not sensitive for cerebral sinus thrombosis, but magnetic resonance imaging has the potential to become the diagnostic tool of choice for cerebral vein thrombosis because of its non-invasive nature (Goldberg et al 1986, Snyder et al 1986, Hulcelle et al 1989).

Whether or not anticoagulants are indicated in the treatment of cerebral sinus thrombosis has been addressed in one small clinical trial (Einhäupo et al 1991). This open trial was interrupted after inclusion of only 20 patients because of an important benefit noticed in patients treated with heparin. Because of the small number of patients included in the study, confirmatory evidence is necessary to reach a definitive conclusion regarding the benefits of heparin in this indication.

Renal vein thrombosis

Symptoms associated with renal vein thrombosis are flank pain and ipsilateral testicular pain in males. Renal vein thrombosis is mostly associated with a pre-existing nephrotic syndrome caused by membranous glomerulonephritis or membrano-proliferative glomerulonephritis. Renal vein thrombosis by itself is probably not a cause of the nephrotic syndrome (Llach et al 1980, Llach 1985). There are some reports of renal vein thrombosis associated with extensive inferior vena caval thrombosis in the absence of a nephrotic syndrome (Jackson & Thomas 1970). The diagnosis is made with cavo-renography using a catheter inserted by the Seldinger technique. Recently duplex ultrasound, colour-coded duplex ultrasound, contrast-enhanced computerized tomographic scanning and magnetic resonance imaging have been used to diagnose renal vein thrombosis.

Treatment includes heparin and thrombolytic agents, sometimes administered directly in the renal artery. Heparin treatment, followed by oral anticoagulants is reported to be associated with stabilization and even improvement of renal function (Llach 1985). Lysis of the thrombus has been reported with thrombolytic agents, but it is not known how the results with thrombolysis would compare with those with heparin alone (Vogelzang et al 1988, Kennedy et al 1991).

Mesenteric and portal vein thrombosis

The diagnosis of portal or mesenteric vein thrombosis is usually suspected in patients with abdominal pain that is frequently epigastric but can also be localized in the upper or lower quadrants of the abdomen. Leucocytosis with a shift to the left is usually present. Bloody stools are less frequently reported (Grieshop et al 1991). When ischaemia of the bowel progresses to infarction, peritoneal irritation occurs and peritoneal fluid appears (Harward et al 1989, Clavien 1990). Prior to the introduction of new diagnostic tools, the diagnosis was usually made during laparotomy or at autopsy. The diagnostic modalities that have enabled early diagnosis of mesenteric thrombosis include selective arteriography with special attention to the venous phase, splenoportal-venography, ultrasound and intravenous contrast-enhanced computer tomography (Subramanyam et al 1984, Miller & Berland 1985, Goyal et al 1989, Grieshop et al 1991).

Management of mesenteric or portal vein thrombosis includes intravenous heparin during the acute phase, and surgery if signs of peritoneal irritation or peritoneal fluid collections appear. Postoperative heparinization is recommended to prevent rethrombosis and further infarction (Umpleby 1987, Griesshop et al 1991). Usually 3 to 6 months of oral anticoagulants are given, unless a continuing risk factor (cancer, deficiency of natural anticoagulants) is present in which case life-long anticoagulants are used.

Hepatic vein thrombosis

Thrombosis of the hepatic vein and its clinical expression is frequently referred to as the Budd–Chiari syndrome. The diagnosis is suspected in patients with symptoms of portal hypertension, i.e. ascites or bleeding oesophageal varices. Most patients have abnormal liver enzymes and a prolonged prothrombin time. The diagnosis can be made directly by venography of the hepatic veins and the inferior vena cava vein by the Seldinger technique. Diagnostic alternatives include ultrasound, contrast-enhanced computer tomography and liver biopsy, the last showing centrilobular congestion and varying degrees of fibrosis (Tavill et al 1975, Wang et al 1988).

Hepatic vein thrombosis is most often found in association with myeloproliferative disorders, but can also occur in association with certain types of solid tumours, cirrhosis of the liver or it may be idiopathic (Valla et al 1985, Klein et al 1990).

Although medical management (anticoagulants with or without thrombolytic agents and diuretics) is sometimes successful, the reported 1-year survival is only 14% (McCarthy et al 1985, Klein et al 1990) which, in these studies, was limited to patients with only a partial obstruction of the hepatic veins. Current opinion is that surgical treatment is necessary for patients with a total obstruction of the hepatic veins and is associated with a 5 year survival of 60%. In patients without cirrhosis and normal liver function, a venous shunt between the portal and systemic circulation is indicated, while in patients with cirrhosis or compromised synthetic function, liver transplantation should be considered (Klein et al 1990). If venous shunting is used, a mesocaval shunt is advocated in patients without inferior caval vein obstruction and a mesoatrial shunt if inferior caval vein compression is present (Klein et al 1990).

Long-term anticoagulant treatment is usually given, although recently promising results were reported with the use of hydroxyurea and aspirin in patients that had undergone liver transplantation. This combination treatment is based on the frequent association of the Budd–Chiari syndrome with myeloproliferative disorders (Goldstein et al 1991).

Superficial vein thrombosis

The presence of a thrombus in a superficial vein is frequently called superficial thrombophlebitis if it originates in a superficial vein that is varicose. The clinical diagnosis is obvious and objective testing is usually unnecessary unless extension into the deep venous system is suspected (Rudofsky 1989).

Treatment is symptomatic and consists of local pressure, wet compresses and non-steroidal anti-inflammatory drugs, or surgical removal if extremely painful (Rudofsky 1989). For isolated superficial vein thrombosis, anticoagulant drugs are neither indicated for treatment nor for secondary prophylaxis. In iatrogenic thrombophlebitis (e.g. intravenous access, after surgery for varices) presenting with fever, the possibility of an infected thrombus mass should be considered. Blood cultures should be done and if necessary antibiotics administered (Rudofsky 1989).

REFERENCES

Agnelli G, Longetti M, Cosmi B et al 1990 Diagnostic accuracy of computerized impedance plethysmography in the diagnosis of symptomatic deep vein thrombosis: a controlled venographic study. Angiology 16: 559–564

Albada J, Nieuwenhuis H K, Sixma J J 1989 Treatment of acute venous thromboembolism with low molecular weight heparin (Fragmin). Results of a double blind randomized study. Circulation 80: 935–940

Albrechtsson U, Olsson C G 1976 Thrombotic side-effects of lower limb venography. Lancet i: 723–724

Albrechtsson U, Anderson J, Einarsson E, Eklof B, Norgren L 1981 Streptokinase treatment of deep venous thrombosis and the post-thrombotic syndrome. Archives of Surgery 116: 33–37

Alderson P O, Rujanavech N, Secker-Walker R H et al 1976 The role of ^{133}Xe ventilation studies in the scintigraphic detection of pulmonary embolism. Radiology 120: 633–640

Alpert J S, Smith R E, Ockens et al 1975 Treatment of massive embolism: the role of embolectomy. American Heart Journal 89: 413–417

Andersson G, Fagrell B, Holmgren K et al 1982 Subcutaneous administration of heparin. A randomized comparison with intravenous administration of heparin to patients with deep vein thrombosis. Thrombosis Research 27: 631–639

Appelman P T, de Jong T E, Lampmann L E 1987 Deep venous thrombosis of the leg: ultrasound findings. Radiology 163: 743–746

Arnesen H, Heilo A, Jakobsen E, Ly B, Skaga E 1978 A prospective study of streptokinase and heparin in the treatment of deep vein thrombosis. Acta Medica Scandinavica 203: 457–463

Arnesen H, Hoiseth A, Ly B 1982 Streptokinase or heparin in the treatment of deep vein thrombosis. Follow-up results of a prospective study. Acta Medica Scandinavica 211: 65–68

Aronen A J, Suorata H T, Tauvitsainen M J 1981 Thermography in deep venous thrombosis of the leg. American Journal of Radiology 137: 1179–1182

Atkins H L, Susskind H, Klopper J F et al 1977 A clinical comparison of Xe-127 and Xe-133 for ventilation studies. Journal of Nuclear Medicine 18: 653–659

Awh M H, Taylor F C, Lu C T 1991 Spontaneous fracture of a Vena-Tech inferior vena caval filter. American Journal of Roentegenology 157: 177–178

Bakker M, Dekker P J, Knot E A R, van Bergen P F M M, Jonker J J C 1988 Home treatment for deep venous thrombosis with low molecular weight heparin (letter). Lancet ii: 1142

Barnes R W, Wu K K, Howe J C J 1977 Noninvasive quantification of maximum venous outflow in acute thrombophlebitis. Surgery 82: 219–223

Barnes B D, Brant-Zadawski M, Mantzer W 1983 Digital subtraction angiography in the diagnosis of superior sinus thrombosis. Neurology 33: 508–510

Barritt D W, Jordan S C 1960 Anticoagulant drugs in the treatment of pulmonary embolism. A controlled trial. Lancet i: 1309–1312

Basu D, Gallus A, Hirsh J, Cade J 1972 A prospective study of the value of monitoring heparin treatment with the activated partial thromboplastin time. New England Journal of Medicine 287: 324–327

Baxter G M, Kincaid W, Jeffrey R F et al 1991 Comparison of colour ultrasound with venography in the diagnosis of axillary and subclavian vein thrombosis. British Journal of Radiology 64: 777–781

Bendick P J, Glover J L, Holder R W, Dilley R S 1983 Pitfalls of the Doppler examination for venous thrombosis. American Surgeon 49: 320–323

Bentley P G, Kakkar V V, Scully M F, MacGregor I R, Webb P, Chan P, Jones N 1980 An objective study of alternative methods of heparin administration. Thrombosis Research 18: 177–187

Bergan J J, Trippel O H 1966 Vena cava operations for prevention of pulmonary embolism. Surgical Clinics of North America 46: 195–207

Bjoerk L 1986 Digital angiography in pulmonary embolism. Acta Radiologica 27: 175–185

Blackmore C G, Francis C W, Bryant R G, Brenner B, Marder V J 1990 Magnetic resonance imaging of blood and clots in vitro. Investigative Radiology 25: 1316–1324

Boccalon H 1981 Venous plethysmography applied in pathologic conditions. Angiology 32: 822–829

Boisclair M D, Lane D A, Wilde J T, Ireland H, Preston F E, Ofusu F A 1990 A comparative evaluation of assays for markers of activated coagulation and/or fibrinolysis: thrombin-antithrombin complex, D-dimer and fibrinogen/fibrin fragment E antigen. British Journal of Haematology 74: 471–479

Boneu B, Bes G, Pelzer H, Sie P, Boccalon H 1991 D-dimer, thrombin antithrombin III complexes and prothrombin 1 + 2: diagnostic value in clinically suspected deep vein thrombosis. Thrombosis and Haemostasis 65: 28–32

Bookstein J J, Silver T M 1974 The angiographic differential diagnosis of acute pulmonary embolism. Radiology 110: 25–33

Borris L C, Christiansen H M, Lassen M R et al 1989 Comparison of real-time B-mode ultrasonography and bilateral ascending phlebography for detection of postoperative deep vein thrombosis following elective hip surgery. Thrombosis and Haemostasis 61: 363–365

Bounameux H, Kraehenbuehl B, Vukanovic S 1982 Diagnosis of deep vein thrombosis by combination of doppler flow examination and strain-gauge plethysmography: an alternative to venography only in particular conditions despite improved accuracy of the doppler method. Thrombosis and Haemostasis 47: 141–144

Bounameux H, Schneider P A, Reber G, de Moerloose P, Krahenbuhl B 1989 Measurement of plasma D-dimer for diagnosis of deep venous thrombosis. American Journal of Clinical Pathology 91: 82–85

Bounameux H, Cirafici P, de Moerloose P et al 1991 Measurement of D-dimer in plasma as diagnostic aid in suspected pulmonary embolism. Lancet 337: 196–200

Bozetti F, Scarpa D, Terno G et al 1983 Subclavian vein thrombosis due to indwelling catheters: a prospective study. Journal of Parenteral Nutrition 5: 240–242

Brandjes D P M, Heijboer H, Büller H R, de Rijk M, Jagt H, ten Cate J W 1992 Acenocoumarol and heparin compared with acenocoumarol alone in the initial treatment of proximal vein thrombosis. New England Journal of Medicine 327: 1485–1489

Bratt G, Tornebohn E, Granqvist S, Aberg W, Lockner D 1985 A comparison between low molecular weight heparin (KABI 2165) and standard heparin in the intravenous treatment of deep venous thrombosis. Thrombosis and Haemostasis 54(4): 813–817

Bratt G, Aberg W, Johansson M, Toernebohm E, Granqvist S, Lockner D 1990 Two daily subcutaneous injections of fragmin as compared with intravenous standard heparin in the treatment of deep venous thrombosis. Thrombosis and Haemostatis 64: 506–510

Browse N L 1972 The ^{125}I-fibrinogen uptake test. Archives of Surgery 104: 160–163

Browse N L, Lea Thomas M, Pim H P 1968 Streptokinase and deep vein thrombosis. British Medical Journal 3: 717–720

Browse N L, Chapham W F, Croft D N et al 1971 Diagnosis of established deep vein thrombosis with the ^{125}I-fibrinogen uptake test. British Medical Journal 4: 325–328

Büller H R, Lensing A W A Hirsh J, ten Cate J W 1991 Deep vein thrombosis: New non-invasive diagnostic tests. Thrombosis and Haemostasis 66: 133–137

Bynum L J, Crotty C, Wilson J E 1976 Use of fibrinogen/fibrin degradation products and soluble fibrin complexes for differentiating pulmonary embolism from non-thromboembolic lung disease. American Review of Respiratory Disease 114: 285–291

Calligaro K D, Bergen W S, Haut M J, Savarese R P, DeLaurentis D A 1991 Thromboembolic complications in patients with advanced cancer; anticoagulation versus Greenfield filter placement. Annals of Vascular Surgery 5: 186–189

Camilleri J F, Bonnet J L, Bouvier J L et al 1988 Thrombolyse intraveneuse dans l'infarctus du myocarde. Influence de la qualite de l'anticoagulation sur le taux de recidives precoces d'angor ou d'infarctus. Archives des Maladies du Coeur et Des Vaisseaux 1: 1037–1041

Chapman C S, Akhtar N, Campbell S, Miles K, O'Connor J, Mitchell V E 1990 The use of D-dimer assay by enzyme immunoassay and latex agglutination techniques in the diagnosis of deep vein thrombosis. Clinical and Laboratory Haematology 12: 37–42

Christensen W S, Wille-Jorgesen P, Kjaer L et al 1987 Contact thermography. Tc-plasmin scintimetry and Tc-plasmin scintigraphy as screening methods for deep venous thrombosis following major hip surgery. Thrombosis and Haemostasis 58: 831–833

Cimochowski G E, Evans R H, Zarins C K, Lu C T, de Meester T R 1980 Greenfield filter versus Mobin-Uddin umbrella. Journal of Thoracic and Cardiovascular Surgery 79: 358–365

Clarke D B, Abrams L D 1986 Pulmonary embolectomy: a 25 year experience. Journal of Thoracic and Vascular Surgery 92: 442–445

Clarke-Pearson D L, Creasman W T 1981 Diagnosis of deep venous thrombosis in obstetrics and gynecology by impedance plethysmography. Obstetrics and Gynecology 58: 52–56

Clavien P A 1990 Diagnosis and management of mesenteric infarction. British Journal of Surgery 77: 601–603

Cohen J R, Tenenbaum N, Citron M. 1991 Greenfield filter as primary therapy for deep venous thrombosis and/or pulmonary embolism in patients with cancer. Surgery 109: 12–15

Comerota A J, Katz M L, Grossi R J et al 1988 The comparative value of noninvasive testing for the diagnosis and surveillance of deep vein thrombosis. Journal of Vascular Surgery 7: 40–49

Common H H, Seaman A J, Roesch J, Porter J M, Dotter C T 1976 Deep vein thrombosis treated with streptokinase or heparin. Angiology 27: 645–654

Cooke E D, Pilcher M F 1974 Deep vein thrombosis. Pre-clinical diagnosis by thermography. British Journal of Surgery 61: 971–974

Coon W W 1974 Operative therapy of venous thromboembolism. Modern Concepts of Cardiovascular Diseases 43: 71–75

Cooperman M, Martin E W, Satiani B, Clark M, Evans W E 1979 Detection of deep venous thrombosis by impedance plethysmography. American Journal of Surgery 137: 252–254

Couch N P, Baldwin S S, Crane C 1975 Mortality and morbidity rates after inferior vena cava clipping. Surgery 77: 106–112

Cronan J J, Dorfman G S, Scola F H, Schepps B, Alexander J 1987 Deep venous thrombosis: Ultrasound assessment using vein compression. Radiology 162: 191–194

Cross F S, Mowlem A 1974 A survey of current status of pulmonary embolectomy for massive pulmonary embolism. Circulation 50: 236–244

Cruickshank M K, Levine M N, Hirsh J et al 1989 An evaluation of impedance plethysmography and ^{125}I-fibrinogen leg scanning in patients following hip surgery. Thrombosis and Haemostasis 62: 830–832

Cruickshank M K, Levine M N, Hirsh J, Roberts R, Siguenza M 1991 A standard heparin nomogram for the management of heparin therapy. Archives of Internal Medicine 151: 333–337

Curley F J, Pratter M R, Irwin R S et al 1987 The clinical implications of bilaterally abnormal impedance plethysmography. Archives of Internal Medicine 147: 125–129

Dalen J E, Brooks H L, Johnson L W, Meister S G, Szucs M M, Dexter L 1971 Pulmonary angiography in acute pulmonary embolism: indications, techniques and results in 367 patients. American Heart Journal 81: 175–185

D'Angelo A, Mannucci P M 1984 Outcome of treatment of deep-vein thrombosis with urokinase: relationship to dosage, duration of therapy, age of thrombus and laboratory changes. Thrombosis and Haemostasis 51: 236–239

Davies J J, Merrick M V, Sharp A A, Holt J M 1972 A controlled trial of ancrod and heparin in treatment of deep vein thrombosis of lower limb. Lancet i: 113–115

Davis H H, Siegel B A, Sherman L A et al 1980 Scintigraphy with ^{111}In-labelled autologous platelets in venous thromboembolism. Radiology 136: 203–207

deBoer A C, Han P, Turpie A G G et al 1981 Plasma and urine beta-thromboglobulin concentration in patients with deep vein thrombosis. Blood 63: 603–609

Declerck P J, Mombaerts P, Holvoet P, de Mol M, Collèn D 1987 Fibrinolytic response and fibrin fragment D-dimer levels in patients with deep vein thrombosis. Thrombosis and Haemostasis 58: 1024–1029

DelCampo C 1985 Pulmonary embolectomy: a review. Canadian Journal of Surgery 28: 111–113

Denny D F, Dorfman G S , Cronan J J et al 1988 Greenfield filter: percutaneous placement in 50 patients. American Journal of Roentgenology 150: 427–429

Dorfman G S 1990 Percutaneous inferior vena cava filters. Radiology 174: 987–992

Dosick S M, Blakemore W S 1978 The role of Doppler ultrasound in acute deep vein thrombosis. American Journal of Surgery 136: 265–268

Doyle D J, Turpie A G G, Hirsh J, Best C, Kinch D, Levine M N, Gent M 1987 Adjusted subcutaneous heparin or continuous intravenous heparin in patients with acute deep vein thrombosis. Annals of Internal Medicine 107: 441–445

Duroux P, Beclere A 1991 A randomized trial of subcutaneous low molecular weight heparin (CY-216) compared with intravenous unfractionated heparin in the treatment of deep vein thrombosis. Thrombosis and Haemostasis 65: 251–256

Eberlein T J, Carey L C 1974 Comparison of surgical managements for pulmonary emboli. Annals of Surgery 179: 836–841

Einhäupo K M, Villringer A, Meister W et al 1991 Heparin treatment in sinus venous thrombosis. Lancet 338: 597–600

Elias A, LeCorff C, Bouvier J L, Benichou M, Serradimigni A 1987 Value of real time B-mode imaging in the diagnosis of deep vein thrombosis of the lower limbs. International Angiology 6: 175–182

Elliot M S, Immelman E J, Jeffery P et al 1979 A comparative randomized trial of heparin versus streptokinase in the treatment of acute proximal venous thrombosis: an interim report of a prospective trial. British Journal of Surgery 66: 838–843

Enevoldson T P, Ross Russell R W 1990 Cerebral venous thrombosis: new causes for an old syndrome? Quarterly Journal of Medicine 77: 1255–1275

Epstein D H, Darcy M D, Hunter D W et al 1989 Experience with the Amplatz retrievable vena cava filter. Radiology 172: 105–110

Erdman W A, Jayson H T, Redman H C et al 1990 Deep venous thrombosis of extremities: role of MR imaging in the diagnosis. Radiology 174: 425–429

Ezekowitz M D, Migliaccio F, Farlow D et al 1990 Comparison of platelet scintigraphy, impedance plethysmography and color flow duplex ultrasound and venography for the diagnosis of venous thrombosis. Progress in Clinical and Biological Research 355: 23–27

Fagher B, Lundh B 1981 Heparin treatment of deep vein thrombosis. Acta Medica Scandinavica 210: 357–361

Faunoe P, Suomalainen O, Bergqvist D et al 1990 The use of fibrinogen uptake test in screening for deep vein thrombosis in patients with hip fracture. Thrombosis Research 60: 185–190

Fink J A, Jones B T 1991 The Greenfield filter as the primary means of therapy in venous thromboembolic disease. Surgery, Gynecology and Obstetrics 172: 253–256

Flanc C, Kakkar V V, Clarke M B 1968 The detection of venous thrombosis of the legs using ^{125}I-labelled fibrinogen. British Journal of Surgery 55: 742–747

Flanigan D P, Goodreau J J, Burnham S J, Bergan J J, Yao J S 1978 Vascular laboratory diagnosis of clinically suspected acute deep vein thrombosis. Lancet ii: 331–334

Fobbe F, Dietzel M, Korth R et al 1988 Guenther vena caval filter: results of long-term follow-up. American Journal of Roentgenology 151: 1031–1034

Foti M E, Gurewich V 1980 Fibrin degradation products and impedance plethysmography: measurements in the diagnosis of acute deep vein thrombosis. Archives of Internal Medicine 140: 903–908

Froehlich J A, Dorfman G S, Cronan J J et al 1989 Compression ultrasonography for the detection of deep venous thrombosis in patients who have a fracture of the hip. A prospective study. Journal of Bone and Joint Surgery 71-A: 249–256

Gallus A, Jackaman J, Tillet J, Mills W, Wycherley A 1986 Safety and efficacy of warfarin started early after submassive venous thrombosis or pulmonary embolism. Lancet ii: 1293–1296

Ganger K H, Nachbur B H, Ris H B, Zurbrugg H 1989 Surgical thrombectomy versus conservative treatment for deep venous thrombosis; functional comparison of long term results. European Journal of Vascular Surgery 3: 529–538

George J E, Berry R E 1990 Noninvasive detection of deep vein thrombosis. A critical evaluation. American Surgeon 56: 76–78

Ginsberg J S, Hirsh J 1989 Use of anti-coagulants during pregnancy. Chest 95: 156S–160S

Ginsberg J S, Brill-Edwards P, Agnelli G 1990 Deep vein thrombosis and duplex ultrasound (letter). Annals of Internal Medicine 112: 307

Glassford D M, Alford W C, Burrus G R, Stoney W S, Thomas C S 1981 Pulmonary embolectomy. Annals of Thoracic Surgery 32: 28–32

Glazier R L, Crowell E B 1976 Randomized prospective trial of continuous vs intermittent heparin therapy. Journal of the American Medical Association 236: 1365–1367

Goldberg A L, Rosenbaum A E, Wang H et al 1986 Computer assisted tomography of dural sinus thrombosis. Journal of Computer Assisted Tomography 10: 16-20

Goldhaber S Z 1991 Recent advances in the diagnosis and lytic therapy of pulmonary embolism. Chest 99: 173S–179S

Goldhaber S Z, Buring J E, Lipnick R J, Hennekens C H 1984 Pooled analysis of randomized trials of streptokinase and heparin in phlebographically documented acute deep vein thrombosis. American Journal of Medicine 76: 393–397

Goldhaber S Z, Vaughan D E, Markis J E et al 1986 Acute pulmonary embolism treated with tissue plasminogen activator. Lancet ii: 886–889

Goldhaber S Z, Kessler G M, Heit J et al 1988 Randomized controlled trial of recombinant tissue plasminogen activator versus urokinase in the treatment of acute pulmonary embolism. Lancet ii: 293–298

Goldhaber S Z, Meyerovitz M F, Green D et al 1990 Randomized controlled trial of tissue plasminogen activator in proximal deep venous thrombosis. American Journal of Medicine 88: 235–240

Goldstein M 1987 Hochdosierte kurzzeitlyse mit streptokinase bei massiver lungembolie in der fruehen postoperativen phase. Anaesthesist 36: 239–241

Goldstein R, Clark P, Klintmalm G et al 1991 Prevention of recurrent thrombosis following liver transplantation for Budd–Chiari syndrome associated with myeloproliferative disorders: treatment with hydroxyurea and aspirin. Transplantation Proceedings 23: 1559–1560

Goodman P C, Brant-Zawadski M 1982 Digital subtraction angiography. American Journal of Radiology 139: 305–309

Goris M L, Daspit S G, Walter J P et al 1977 Applications of ventilation lung imaging with ^{81m}Krypton. Radiology 122: 399–403

Goyal A K, Pokharna D S, Sharma S K, Jain T C 1989 Can sonography replace splenoportography in evaluation of patients with portal hypertension? Indian Journal of Gastroenterology 8: 157–159

Grau E, Linares M, Estany A, Martin F 1991 Utility of D dimer in the diagnosis of deep venous thrombosis in outpatients (letter). Thrombosis and Haemostasis 66: 510

Gray H H, Morgan J M, Paneth M, Miller G A H 1988 Pulmonary embolectomy for acute massive pulmonary embolism: an analysis of 71 cases. British Heart Journal 60: 196–200

Gray H W, McKillop J H, Bessent R G, Fogelman I, Smith M L, Moran F 1990 Lung scanning for pulmonary embolism: clinical and pulmonary angiographic correlations. Quarterly Journal of Medicine 77: 1135–1150

Greenfield L J, Michna B A 1988 Twelve-year clinical experience with the Greenfield vena caval filter. Surgery 104: 706–712

Greenfield L J, Zocco J, Wilk J, Schroeder T M, Elkins R C 1977 Clinical experience with the Kimray Greenfield vena cava filter. Annals of Surgery 185: 692–698

Greenfield L J, Peyton R, Crute S, Barnes R 1981 Greenfield caval filter experience. Archives of Surgery 113: 1451–1456

Greenfield L J, Cho K J, Tauscher J R 1990 Limitations of percutaneous insertion of Greenfield filters. Journal of Cardiovascular Surgery 31: 344–350

Grieshop R J, Dalsing M C, Cikrit D F, Lalka S G, Sawchuk A P 1991 Acute mesenteric venous thrombosis. Revisited in a time of diagnostic clarity. American Surgeon 57: 573–577

Griguer P, Charbonnier B, Latour F, Fauchier J P, Brochier M 1979 Plasminogen and moderate doses of urokinase in the treatment of acute pulmonary embolism. Angiology 30: 1–12

Gross W S, Burney R E 1979 Therapeutic and economic implications of emergency department evaluation for deep vein thrombosis. Journal of the American College of Emergency Physicians 8: 110–115

Gurewich V, Hume M, Patrick M 1973 The laboratory diagnosis of venous thromboembolic disease by measurement of fibrin/fibrinogen degradation products and fibrin monomer. Chest 64: 585–590

Habscheid W, Hoehman M, Wilhelm T, Epping J 1990 Real-time ultrasound in the diagnosis of acute deep venous thrombosis of the lower extremity. Angiology 16: 599–607

Hall J G, Pauli R M, Wilson K M 1980 Maternal and fetal sequelae of anticoagulation during pregnancy. American Journal of Medicine 68: 122–140

Haller J A 1961 Thrombectomy for acute iliofemoral venous thrombosis. Archives of Surgery 83: 448

Haller J R, Abrams B L 1963 Use of thrombectomy in the treatment of acute iliofemoral venous thrombosis in forty-five patients. Annals of Surgery 158: 561–566

Halvorsen S, Skjoensberg O H, Godal H C 1991 Comparison of methods of detecting soluble fibrin in plasma from patients with venous thromboembolism. Thrombosis Research 61: 341–348

Handeland G F, Abildgaard U, Holm H A, Arnesen K E 1990 Dose adjusted heparin treatment of deep venous thrombosis: a comparison of unfractionated and low molecular weight heparin. European Journal of Clinical Pharmacology 32: 107–112

Hanel K C, Abbott W M, Reidy N C et al 1981 The role of two noninvasive tests in deep venous thrombosis. Annals of Surgery 194: 725–730

Harenberg J, Huck K, Bratsch H 1990 Therapeutic application of subcutaneous low-molecular-weight heparin in acute venous thrombosis. Haemostasis 20 (suppl 1): 205–219

Harris W H, Salzman E W, Athanasoulis C et al 1975 Comparison of ^{125}I fibrinogen count scanning with phlebography for detection of venous thrombi after elective hip surgery. New England Journal of Medicine 292: 665–667

Harris W H, Athanasoulis C, Waltman A C, Salzman E W 1976 Cuff-impedance phlebography and ^{125}I fibrinogen scanning versus roentgenographic phlebography for diagnosis of thrombophlebitis following hip surgery. Journal of Bone and Joint Surgery 58-A: 939–944

Harvard T R, Green D, Bergan J J, Rizzo R J, Yao J S 1989 Mesenteric vein thrombosis. Journal of Vascular Surgery 9: 328–333

Heaton D C, Billings J D, Hickton C M 1987 Assessment of D-dimer assay for the diagnosis of deep vein thrombosis. Journal of Laboratory and Clinical Medicine 110: 588–591

Heijboer H, Brandjes D P M, Lensing A W A, Büller H R, ten Cate J W 1991a Efficacy of real-time B-mode ultrasonography versus impedance plethysmography in the diagnosis of deep vein thrombosis in symptomatic out-patients. Thrombosis and Haemostasis 65: 804 (abstract)

Heijboer H, Jongbloets L, Lensing A W A, Büller H R, ten Cate J W 1991b Detection of deep vein thrombosis with impedance plethysmography (IPG) and B-mode ultrasound (US) in hospitalized symptomatic patients. Thrombosis and Haemostasis 65: 804 (abstract)

Henkin R E, Yao J S T, Quinn J L, Bergan J J 1973 Radionuclide venography in lower extremity venous disease. Journal of Nuclear Medicine 15: 171–175

Hill S L, Berry R E 1990 Subclavian vein thrombosis: a continuing challenge. Surgery 108: 1–9

Hill S L, Martin D, McDannald E R, Donato A T 1988 Early diagnosis of iliofemoral venous thrombosis by doppler examination. American Journal of Surgery 156: 11–15

Hirsh J 1990 Prevention of venous thrombosis in patients undergoing major orthopaedic surgical procedures. Acta Chirurgica Scandinavica (suppl) 556: 30–35

Hirsh J 1991a Reliability of non-invasive tests for the diagnosis of venous thrombosis. Thrombosis and Haemostasis 65: 221–222

Hirsh J 1991b Drug therapy. Heparin. New England Journal of Medicine 324: 1565–1574

Hirsh J 1991c Drug therapy. Oral anticoagulant drugs. New England Journal of Medicine 324: 1865–1875

Hirsh J, Gallus A S, Cade J F 1974 Diagnosis of thrombosis. Evaluation of ^{125}I-fibrinogen scanning and blood tests. Thrombosis et Diathesis Haemorrhagica 32: 11–19

Hirsh J, Poller L, Deykin D, Levine M N, Dalen J E 1989 Optimal range for oral anticoagulants. Chest 95: 5S–11S

Hoejensgaard I G, Stürüp H 1953 Static and dynamic pressures in superficial and deep veins of lower extremity in man. Acta Physiologica Scandinavica 27: 49–67

Hoek J A, Nurmohamed M T, ten Cate J W et al 1989 Thrombin-antithrombin III complexes in the prediction of deep vein thrombosis following total hip replacement. Thrombosis and Haemostasis 62: 1050–1052

Hoey J R, Pfarrer P A 1980 Interobserver and intra-observer variability in lung scan reading in suspected pulmonary embolism. Clinical Nuclear Medicine 5: 508–513

Holm H A, Ly B, Handeland G F et al 1986 Subcutaneous heparin treatment of deep vein thrombosis: a comparison of unfractionated and low molecular weight heparin. Haemostasis 16: 30–37

Holmgren K, Andersson G, Fagrell B et al 1985 One month versus six-month therapy with oral anticoagulants after symptomatic deep vein thrombosis. Acta Medica Scandinavica 218: 279–284

Holmgren K, Jacobsson H, Johnsson H, Loefsjoegard-Nilsson 1990 Thermography and plethysmography, a non-invasive alternative to venography in the diagnosis of deep vein thrombosis. Journal of Internal Medicine 228: 29–33

Howerton R M, Watkins M, Feldman L 1991 Late arterial hemorrhage secondary to a Greenfield filter requiring operative intervention. Surgery 109: 265–268

Huet Y, Janvier G, Bendriss P H et al 1990 Treatment of established venous thromboembolism with enoxaparin: preliminary report. Acta Chirurgica Scandinavica (suppl) 556: 116–120

Huisman M V, Büller H R, ten Cate J W, Vreeken J 1986 Serial impedance plethysmography for suspected deep venous thrombosis in outpatients. New England Journal of Medicine 314: 823–828

Huisman M V, Büller H R, ten Cate J W 1988 Utility of impedance plethysmography in the diagnosis of recurrent deep vein thrombosis. Archives of Internal Medicine 148: 681–683

Huisman M V, Büller H R, ten Cate J W 1989a Unexpected high prevalence of silent pulmonary embolism in patients with deep vein thrombosis. Chest 95: 498–502

Huisman M V, Büller H R, ten Cate J W et al 1989b Management of clinically suspected acute venous thrombosis in outpatients with serial impedance plethysmography in a community hospital setting. Archives of Internal Medicine 149: 511–513

Hulcelle P J, Dooms G C, Mathurin P, Cornelis G 1989 MRI Assessment of unsuspected dural sinus thrombosis. Neuroradiology 31(3): 217–221

Hull R D, Raskob G E 1991 Low-probability lung scan findings: a need for change. Annals of Internal Medicine 114: 142–143

Hull R D, van Aken W G, Hirsh J et al 1976 Impedance plethysmography using the occlusive cuff technique in the diagnosis of venous thrombosis. Circulation 53: 696–700

Hull R D, Hirsh J, Sackett D L et al 1977 Combined use of leg scanning and impedance plethysmography in suspected venous thrombosis. An alternative to venography. New England Journal of Medicine 296: 1497–1500

Hull R D, Taylor D W, Hirsh J 1978 Impedance plethysmography: the relationship between venous filling and sensitivity and specificity for proximal vein thrombosis. Circulation 58: 898–902

Hull R D, Delmore T, Genton E et al 1979 Warfarin sodium versus low-dose heparin in the long-term treatment of venous thrombosis. New England Journal of Medicine 301: 855–859

Hull R D, Hirsh J, Sackett et al 1981a Replacement of venography in suspected venous thrombosis by impedance plethysmography and ^{125}I-fibrinogen leg scanning: a less invasive approach. Annals of Internal Medicine 94: 12–15

Hull R D, Hirsh J, Sackett D L et al 1981b Clinical validity of a negative venogram in patients with clinically suspected venous thrombosis. Circulation 64: 622–625

Hull R D, Hirsh J, Sackett D L et al 1981c Cost effectiveness of clinical diagnosis, venography and non-invasive testing in patients with symptomatic deep-vein thrombosis. New England Journal of Medicine 304: 1561–1567

Hull R D, Hirsh J, Jay R et al 1982a Different intensities of oral anticoagulant therapy in the treatment of proximal vein thrombosis. New England Journal of Medicine 307: 1676–1681

Hull R D, Delmore T, Carter C et al 1982b Adjusted subcutaneous heparin versus warfarin sodium in the long-term treatment of venous thrombosis. New England Journal of Medicine 306: 189–194

Hull R D, Carter C J, Jay R et al 1983a The diagnosis of acute, recurrent, deep-vein thrombosis: A diagnostic challenge. Circulation 67: 901–906

Hull R D, Hirsh J, Carter C J et al 1983b Pulmonary angiography, ventilation lung scanning, and venography for suspected pulmonary embolism with abnormal perfusion lung scan. Annals of Internal Medicine 98: 891–899

Hull R D, Hirsh J, Carter C J et al 1985a Diagnostic efficacy of impedance plethysmography for clinically suspected deep-vein thrombosis. A randomized trial. Annals of Internal Medicine 102: 21–28

Hull R D, Hirsh J, Carter C J et al 1985b Diagnostic value of ventilation-perfusion lung scanning in patients with suspected pulmonary embolism. Chest 88: 819–828

Hull R D, Raskob G E, Hirsh J et al 1986 Continuous intravenous heparin compared with intermittent subcutaneous heparin in the initial treatment of proximal vein thrombosis. New England Journal of Medicine 315: 1109–1114

Hull R D, Raskob G E, Carter C J et al 1988 Pulmonary embolism in outpatients with pleuritic chest pain. Archives of Internal Medicine 148: 838–844
Hull R D, Raskob G E, Coates G, Panju A A, Gill G J 1989 A new noninvasive management strategy for patients with suspected pulmonary embolism. Archives of Internal Medicine 149: 2549–2555
Hull R D, Raskob G E, Carter C J 1990a Serial impedance plethysmography in pregnant patients with clinically suspected deep-vein thrombosis. Clinical validity of negative findings. Annals of Internal Medicine 112: 663–667
Hull R D, Raskob C E, Coates G, Panju A A 1990b Clinical validity of a normal perfusion lung scan in patients with suspected pulmonary embolism. Chest 97: 23–26
Hull R D, Raskob G E, Rosenbloom D, Panju A A, Brill-Edwards P, Ginsberg J S, Hirsh J, Martin G J, Green D 1990c Heparin for 5 days as compared with 10 days in the initial treatment of proximal venous thrombosis. New England Journal of Medicine 322: 1260–1264
Hull R D, Raskob C E, Pineo G, Green D, Trowbridge A A, Elliot G et al 1992 Subcutaneous low-molecular weight heparin compared with continuous intravenous heparin in the treatment of proximal-vein thrombosis. New England Journal of Medicine 326: 975–982
Husted S E, Kraemmer-Nielsen H, Krüsell L et al 1984 Deep vein thrombosis detection by ^{99m}Tc-plasmin test and phlebography. British Journal of Surgery 71: 65–66
Hye R J, Mitchell A T, Dory C E, Freischlag J A, Roberts A C 1990 Analysis of the transition to percutaneous placement of Greenfield filters. Archives of Surgery 125: 1550–1553
Hyers T M, Hull R D, Weg J C 1989 Antithrombotic therapy for venous thromboembolic disease. Chest 95: 37S–51S
Iturbe-Alessio I, del Carmen Fonseca M, Mutchinik O, Santos M A, Zajarias A, Salazar E 1986 Risks of anticoagulant therapy in pregnant women with artificial heart valves. New England Journal of Medicine 315: 1390–1393
Jackson B T, Thomas M L 1970 Post thrombotic inferior vena cava obstruction: a review of 24 patients. British Medical Journal 1: 18–22
Jacobstein J G 1974 ^{133}Xe ventilation scanning immediately following the ^{99m}-Tc perfusion scan. Journal of Nuclear Medicine 15: 964–968
Jay R, Hull R, Carter C, Ockelford P, Büller H, Turpie A G G, Hirsh J 1984 outcome of abnormal impedance plethysmography results in patients with proximal vein thrombosis. Frequency of return to normal. Thrombosis Research 36: 259–263
Johansson L, Nylander G, Hedner U, Nilsson I M 1979 Comparison of streptokinase with heparin: late results in the treatment of deep venous thrombosis. Acta Medica Scandinavica 206: 93–98
Jonker J J C 1991 Computerized impedance plethysmography (letter). Thrombosis and Haemostasis 66(6): 743
Kakkar V V 1972 The diagnosis of deep vein thrombosis using the ^{125}I-fibrinogen test. Archives of Surgery 104: 152–159
Kakkar V V, Lawrence D 1985 Hemodynamic and clinical assessment after therapy for acute deep vein thrombosis. A prospective study. American Journal of Surgery 150(4A): 54–63
Kakkar V V, Flanc C, O'Shea et al 1969a Treatment of deep-vein thrombosis with streptokinase. British Journal of Surgery 56: 178–183
Kakkar V V, Flanc C, Howe C T et al 1969b Treatment of deep vein thrombosis: a trial of heparin, streptokinase and arvin. British Medical Journal 1: 806–810
Kakkar V V, Flanc C, Howe C T et al 1969c Natural history of postoperative deep vein thrombosis. Lancet ii: 230–233
Kelley M A, Carson J L, Palevsky H I, Schwartz J S 1991 Diagnosing pulmonary embolism: new facts and strategies. Annals of Internal Medicine 114: 300–306
Kempi V, van der Linden W, von Scheele C 1974 Diagnosis of deep-vein thrombosis with ^{99}Tc-streptokinase: a clinical comparison with phlebography. British Medical Journal 4: 748–749
Kennedy J S, Gerety B M, Silverman S et al 1991 Simultaneous renal arterial and venous thrombosis associated with idiopathic nephrotic syndrome: treatment with intraarterial urokinase. American Journal of Medicine 90: 125–127
Kerr T M, Lutter K S, Moeller D M et al 1990 Upper extremity thrombosis diagnosed by duplex scanning. American Journal of Surgery 160: 202–206
Kessler R, Fraisse P, Krause D, Veillon F, Vandevenn A 1991 Magnetic resonance imaging in the diagnosis of pulmonary infarction. Chest 99: 298–300
Kim D, Porter D H, Siegel J B, Simon M 1989 Perforation of the inferior vena cava with aortic and vertebral penetration by a suprarenal Greenfield filter. Radiology 172: 721–723
Kipper M S, Moser K M, Kortman K E, Ashburn W L 1982 Longterm follow-up of patients with suspected pulmonary embolism and a normal lung scan. Perfusion scans in embolic suspects. Chest 82: 411–415
Klein A S, Sitzmann J V, Coleman J, Herlong F H, Cameron J L 1990 Current management of the Budd–Chiari syndrome. Annals of Surgery 212: 144–149
Kockum C 1976 Radioimmunoassay of fibrinopeptide A: clinical applications. Thrombosis Research 8: 225–232
Kroneman H, Nieuwenhuizen W, Knot E A, van Bergen P F, de Maat, M P 1991 Correlations between plasma levels of fibrin(ogen) derivatives as quantified by different assays based on monoclonal antibodies. Thrombosis Research 61(4): 441–452
Kruit W H J, deBoer A C, Sing A K, van Roon F 1991 The significance of venography in the management of patients with clinically suspected pulmonary embolism. Journal of Internal Medicine 230 (4): 333–339
Lagerstedt C I, Olsson C G, Fagher B O, Oeqvist B W, Albrechtsson U 1985 Need for long term anticoagulant treatment in symptomatic calf vein thrombosis. Lancet ii: 515–518
Lagerstedt C, Olsson C G, Fagher B, Oeqvist B 1989 ^{99m}Tc plasmin in 394 consecutive patients with suspected deep venous thrombosis. European Journal of Nuclear Medicine 15: 771–775
Lahey S J, Meyer L P, Karchmer A W et al 1991 Misplaced caval filter and subsequent pericardial tamponade. Annals of Thoracic Surgery 51: 299–300
Landefeld C S, McGuire E, Cohen A M 1990 Clinical findings associated with acute proximal deep vein thrombosis: a basis for quantifying clinical judgment. American Journal of Medicine 88: 382–388
Lansing A M, Davis W M 1968 Five year follow-up study of iliofemoral venous thrombectomy. Annals of Surgery 168: 620–628
Lea Thomas M 1972 Phlebography. Archives of Surgery 104: 145–151
Lea Thomas M, McDonald L M 1978 Complications of ascending venography of the leg. British Medical Journal 2: 317–318
Leeper K V, Popovich J, Lesser B A et al 1988 Treatment of massive acute pulmonary embolism: the use of low doses of intrapulmonary arterial streptokinase combined with full doses of systemic heparin. Chest 93: 234–240
Lensing A W A, Prandoni P, Brandjes D et al 1989 Detection of deep-vein thrombosis by real-time B-mode ultrasonography. New England Journal of Medicine 320: 342–345
Lensing A W A, Prandoni P, Büller H R et al 1990a Lower extremity venography, with iohexol: results and complications. Radiology 177: 503–505
Lensing A W A, Levi M M, Büller H R et al 1990b Diagnosis of deep vein thrombosis using an objective Doppler method. Annals of Internal Medicine 113: 9–13
Lensing A W A, van Beekl E J R, Mingiardil A, Büller H R et al 1991 Ventilation-perfusion lung scanning and the diagnosis of pulmonary embolism: Improvement of observer agreement by the use of a lung segment reference chart. Thrombosis and Haemostasis 65(6): 1171
Lensing A W A, Büller H R, Prandoni P, Batchelor D, Molenaar A H M, Cogo A, Vigo M, Huisman P M, ten Cate J W 1992 Contrast venography, the gold standard for the diagnosis of deep vein thrombosis: improvement in observer agreement. Thrombosis and Haemostasis 67(l): 8–12
Leriche R 1948 Y-a-t-il des thromboses primitives localisees a l'embouchure de Ia vein cave? A propos de la thrombectomie dans les phlebitis: thrombose et stase. Presse Medicale 56: 825–826
Levine M N 1991 Bolus, front-loaded and accelerated thrombolytic infusions for myocardial infarction and pulmonary embolism. Chest 99: 128S–134S
Levine M N, Raskob G, Hirsh J 1989 Hemorrhagic complications of long-term anticoagulant therapy. Chest 95: 26S–36S
Levine M N, Weitz J, Turpie A G G, Andrew M, Cruickshank M, Hirsh J 1990a A new short infusion dosage regimen of recombinant

tissue plasminogen activator in patients with venous thromboembolic disease. Chest 97: 168S–171S
Levine M, Hirsh J, Weitz J et al 1990b A randomized trial of a single bolus dosage regimen of recombinant tissue plasminogen activator in patients with acute pulmonary embolism. Chest 98: 1473–1478
Liapis C D, Satiani B, Kulus M, Evans W E 1980 Value of impedance plethysmography in suspected venous disease of the lower extremity. Angiology 31: 522–525
Light R W, Bell W F 1974 LDH and fibrinogen-fibrin degradation products in pulmonary embolism. Archives of Internal Medicine 133: 372–375
Llach F 1985 Hypercoagulability, renal vein thrombosis, and other thrombotic complications of nephrotic syndrome. Kidney International 28: 429–439
Llach F, Papper S, Massry S G 1980 The clinical spectrum of renal vein thrombosis: acute and chronic. American Journal of Medicine 69: 819–827
Lokich J J, Becker B 1983 Subclavian vein thrombosis in patients treated with infusion chemotherapy for advanced malignancy. Cancer 52: 1586–1589
Lord R S, Chen F C, Devine T J, Benn I V 1990 Surgical treatment of acute deep venous thrombosis. World Journal of Surgery 14: 694–702
Loudon J R, McGarrity G, Vallance R, Baylis A C, Graham J 1978 The fibrinogen uptake test after hip surgery. British Journal of Surgery 65: 616–618
Ly B, Arnesen H, Eie H, Hol R 1978 A controlled trial of streptokinase and heparin in the treatment of major pulmonary embolism. Acta Medica Scandinavica 203: 465–470
McCarthy P M, van Heerden J A, Adson M A, Schafer L W, Wiesner R H 1985 The Budd–Chiari syndrome. Medical and surgical management of 30 patients. Archives of Surgery 120: 657–661
McCowan T C, Ferris E J, Carver D K, Baker M L 1990 Amplatz vena caval filter: clinical experience in 30 patients. American Journal of Roentgenology 155: 177–181
McLachlan M S F, Thomson J G, Taylor D W, Kelly M E, Sackett D L 1979 Observer variation in the interpretation of lower limb venograms. American Journal of Radiology 137: 227–229
McNeil B J 1976 A diagnostic strategy using ventilation-perfusion studies in patients suspect for pulmonary embolism. Journal of Nuclear Medicine 17: 613–616
Mahorner H, Castleberry J W, Coleman W O 1957 Attempts to restore function in major veins which are the site of massive thrombosis. Annals of Surgery 146: 510–522
Mant M J, O'Brien B D, Thong K L et al 1977 Haemorrhagic complications of heparin therapy. Lancet i (8022): 1133–1135
Mantoni M 1989 Diagnosis of deep venous thrombosis by duplex sonography. Acta Radiologica 30: 575–579
Marder V J, Sherry S 1988a Thrombolytic therapy: current status (first of two parts) New England Journal of Medicine 318: 1512–1520
Marder V J, Sherry S 1988b Thrombolytic therapy: current status (second of two parts) New England Journal of Medicine 318: 1585–1595
Marder V J, Soulen R L, Atchartakarn A et al 1977 Quantitative venographic assessment of deep vein thrombosis in the evaluation of streptokinase and heparin therapy. Journal of Laboratory and Clinical Medicine 89: 1018–1029
Maryniak O, Nicholson C G 1979 Doppler ultrasonography for detection of deep vein thrombosis in lower extremities. Archives of Physical Medicine and Rehabilitation 60: 277–281
Meyer G, Tamisier D, Sors H et al 1991 Pulmonary embolectomy: a 20-year experience at one center. Annals of Thoracic Surgery 51: 232–236
Millar W T, Smith J E B 1974 Localization of deep venous thrombosis using technetium^{99m}-labelled urokinase. Lancet ii: 695–696
Miller G A H, Sutton G C, Kerr I H, Gibson R V, Honey M 1971 Comparison of streptokinase and heparin in treatment of isolated acute massive pulmonary embolism. British Medical Journal 2: 681–684
Miller V E, Berland L L 1985 Pulsed doppler duplex sonography and CT of portal vein thrombosis. American Journal of Radiology 142: 91–95
Mills S R, Jackson D C, Older R A, Heaston D K, Moore A V 1980 The incidence, etiologies, and avoidance of complications of pulmonary angiography in a large series. Radiology 136: 295–299
Mombelli G, Monotti R, Haeberli A, Straub P W 1987 Relationship between fibrinopeptide A and fibrinogen/ fibrin fragment E in thromboembolism, DIC and various non-thromboembolic diseases. Thrombosis and Haemostasis 58: 758–763
Monreal M, Rey-Joly Barroso C, Ruiz Manzano J et al 1989a Asymptomatic pulmonary embolism in patients with deep vein thrombosis. Is it useful to take a lung scan to rule out this condition? Journal of Cardiovascular Surgery 30: 104–107
Monreal M, Montserrat E, Salvador R et al 1989b Real time ultrasound for the diagnosis of symptomatic thrombosis and for patients at risk: correlation with ascending conventional venography. Angiology 35: 527–533
Monreal M, Lafoz E, Ruiz J, Valls R, Alastrue A 1991 Upper extremity deep venous thrombosis and pulmonary embolism. A prospective study. Chest 99: 280–283
Moretz W H, Still J M, Griffin L H et al 1972 Partial occlusion of the inferior vena cava with a smooth teflon clip. Analysis of long term results. Surgery 71: 710–719
Moser K M 1990 State of the art. Venous thromboembolism. American Review of Respiratory Disease 141: 235–249
Moser K M, Lemoine J R 1981 Is embolic risk conditioned by location of deep venous thrombosis? Annals of Internal Medicine 94: 439–444
Moser K M, Guisan M, Cuomo A et al 1971 Differentiation of pulmonary vascular from parenchymal diseases by ventilation/ perfusion scintiphotography. Annals of Internal Medicine 75: 597–605
Murphy T P, Cronan J J 1990 Evolution of deep venous thrombosis: a prospective evaluation with US. Radiology 177: 543–548
Mussurakis S, Papaioannou S, Voros D, Vrakatselis T 1990 Compression ultrasonography as a reliable imaging monitor in deep venous thrombosis. Surgery, Gynecology and Obstetrics 171: 233–239
Neglen P, Al-Hassan Hkh, Endrys et al 1991 Iliofemoral venous thrombectomy followed by percutaneous closure of the temporary arteriovenous fistula. Surgery 110: 493–499
Negus D, Pinto D J, LeQuesne L P, Brown N, Chapman M 1968 ^{125}I-labelled fibrinogen in the diagnosis of deep-vein thrombosis and its correlation with phlebography. British Journal of Surgery 55: 835–839
Nemmers D W, Thorpe P E, Knibbe M A, Beard D W 1990 Upper extremity venous thrombosis. Case report and literature review. Orthopaedic Review 19: 164–172
Nicholas G G, Miller F J, Demuth W E, Waldhausen J A 1977 Clinical vascular laboratory diagnosis of deep venous thrombosis. Annals of Surgery 186: 213–215
Nicod P, Peterson K L, Levine M S et al 1984 Pulmonary angiography in severe chronic pulmonary hypertension. Annals of Internal Medicine 107: 565–568
Novelline R A, Baltarowich O H, Athanasoulis C A et al 1978 The clinical course of patients with suspected pulmonary embolism and a negative pulmonary arteriogram. Radiology 126: 561–567
O'Leary D H, Kane R A, Chase B M 1988 A prospective study of the efficacy of B-scan sonography in the detection of deep venous thrombosis in the lower extremities. Journal of Clinical Ultrasound 16: 1–8
O'Sullivan E F 1972 Duration of anticoagulant therapy in venous thrombo-embolism. Medical Journal of Australia 2: 1104–1107
Ott P, Astrup L, Jensen R H, Nyeland B, Pedersen B 1988 Assessment of D-dimer in plasma: diagnostic value in suspected deep venous thrombosis of the leg. Acta Medica Scandinavica 224: 263–267
Owen J, Kvam D, Nossel H L et al 1983 Thrombin and plasmin activity and platelet activation in the development of thrombosis. Blood 61: 476–482
Paiement G, Wessinger S J, Waltman A C, Harris W H 1988 Surveillance of deep vein thrombosis in asymptomatic total hip replacement patients. Impedance plethysmography and fibrinogen scanning versus roentgenographic phlebography. American Journal of Surgery 155: 400–404

Pais S O, Tobin K D 1989 Percutaneous insertion of the Greenfield filter. American Journal of Roentgenology 152: 933–938
Pais S O, Tobin K D, Austin C B, Queral L 1988 Percutaneous insertion of the Greenfield inferior vena cava filter: experience with 96 patients. Journal of Vascular Surgery 8: 460–464
Perlmutt L M, Braun S D, Newman G E et al 1982 Pulmonary arteriography in the high risk patient. Radiology 162: 187–189
Persson B R, Darte L 1977 Labelling plasmin with technetium-^{99m} for scintigraphic localization of thrombi. International Journal of Applied Radiation and Isotopes 28: 97–104
Petitpretz P, Simmoneau G, Cerrina et al 1984 Effects of a single bolus of urokinase in patients with life theatening pulmonary emboli: A descriptive trial. Circulation 70: 861–866
Picolet H, Leizorovicz A, Revel D, Chirossel P, Amiel M, Boissel J P 1990 Reliability of phlebography in the assessment of venous thrombosis in a clinical trial. Haemostasis 20: 362–367
Pini M, Pattacini C, Quintavalla R, Megha A, Tagliaferri A, Manotti C, Dettori A G 1990 Subcutaneous vs intravenous heparin in the treatment of deep venous thrombosis — A randomized clinical trial. Thrombosis and Haemostasis 64: 222–226
PIOPED Investigators 1990a Value of the ventilation/perfusion scan in acute pulmonary embolism. Results of the prospective investigation of pulmonary embolism diagnosis (PIOPED). Journal of the American Medical Association 263: 2753–2759
PIOPED Investigators 1990b Tissue plasminogen activator for the treatment of acute pulmonary embolism. Chest 97: 528–533
Pitney W R 1970 Clinical experience with arvin. Thrombosis Diathesis Hemorrhagica 38: 81–86
Plate G, Einarsson E, Ohlin P et al 1984 Thrombectomy with temporary arteriovenous fistula: the treatment of choice in acute iliofemoral venous thrombosis. Journal of Vascular Surgery 1: 867–876
Plate G, Akesson H, Einarsson E, Ohlin P, Eklof B 1990 Long-term results of venous thrombectomy combined with a temporary arterio-venous fistula. European Journal of Vascular Surgery 4: 483–489
Pochaczevsky R, Pillati G, Feldman F 1982 Liquid crystal contact thermography in deep venous thrombosis. American Journal of Roentgenology 138: 717–723
Pond G D, Ovitt T W, Capp M P 1983 Comparison of conventional angiography or pulmonary embolic disease. Radiology 147: 345–350
Pope C F, Sostman D, Carbo P, Gore J C, Holcomb W 1987 The detection of pulmonary emboli by magnetic resonance imaging: evaluation of imaging parameters. Investigative Radiology 22: 937–946
Porter J M, Seaman A J, Common H H et al 1975 Comparison of streptokinase and heparin in the treatment of venous thrombosis. American Surgeon 41: 511–519
Prandoni P, Lensing A W A, Huisman M V et al 1991a A new computerized impedance plethysmograph: Accuracy in the detection of proximal deep-vein thrombosis in symptomatic outpatients. Thrombosis and Haemostasis 65: 229–232
Prandoni P, Lensing A W A, Büller H R et al 1991b Failure of computerized impedance plethysmography in the diagnostic management of patients with clinically suspected deep vein thrombosis. Thrombosis and Haemostasis 65: 233–236
Prandoni P, Lensing A W A, Büller H et al 1992 Comparison of subcutaneous low-molecular-weight heparin with intravenous standard heparin in proximal deep-vein thrombosis. Lancet 339: 441–445
Prins M H, Hirsh J 1991 Heparin as an adjunctive treatment after thrombolytic therapy or acute myocardial infarction. American Journal of Cardiology 67: 3A–11A
Rabinov K, Paulin S 1972 Roentgen diagnosis of venous thrombosis in the leg. Archives of Surgery 104: 134–144
Ramchandani P, Zeit R M, Koolpe H A 1991 Bilateral iliac vein filtration. An effective alternative to caval filtration in patients with megacava. Archives of Surgery 126: 390–393
Raskob G E, Hull R D 1990 Diagnosis and management of pulmonary thromboembolism. Quarterly Journal of Medicine 76: 787–797
Ricco J B, Crochet D, Sebilotte P et al 1988 Percutaneous transvenous caval interruption with the 'LGM' filter: early results of a multicentre trial. Annals of Vascular Surgery 3: 242–247
Richards K L, Armstrong J D, Tikoff G et al 1976 Noninvasive diagnosis of deep venous thrombosis. Archives of Internal Medicine 136: 1091–1096
Rickman F D, Handin R, Howe J P et al 1973 Fibrin split products in acute pulmonary embolism. Annals of Internal Medicine 79: 664–668
Ritchie W G, Soulen R L, Apayowker M S 1979 Thermographic diagnosis of deep venous thrombosis. Radiology 131: 341–344
Roberts A C, Geller S C, Waltman A C, Athanasoulis C A. 1987 Kimray–Greenfield inferior vena cava filter: safety of percutaneous insertion via the femoral vein. Radiology 165: 204 (abstract)
Robertson B R 1971 On thrombosis, thrombolysis and fibrinolysis. Acta Chirurgica Scandinavica (suppl) 421: 11–21
Robertson B R, Nilsson I M, Nylander 1968 Value of streptokinase and heparin in treatment of acute deep venous thrombosis. A coded investigation. Acta Chirurgica Scandinavica 134: 203–208
Robertson B R, Nilsson I M, Nylander G M 1970 Thrombolytic effect of streptokinase as evaluated by phlebography of deep venous thrombi of the leg. Acta Chirurgica Scandinavica 136: 173–180
Roehm J O F, Johnsrude I S, Barth M H, Gianturco C 1988 The bird's nest inferior vena cava filter: progress report. Radiology 168: 745–749
Rogers L Q, Lutcher C L 1990 Streptokinase therapy for deep vein thrombosis: a comprehensive review of the English literature. American Journal of Medicine 88: 389–395
Rohrer M J, Scheidler M G, Wheeler H B, Cutler B S 1989 Extended indications for placement of an inferior vena cava filter. Journal of Vascular Surgery 10: 44–49
Rose S C, Zwiebel W J, Nelson B D et al 1990 Symptomatic lower extremity deep venous thrombosis: accuracy, limitations, and role of color duplex flow imaging in diagnosis. Radiology 175: 639–644
Rosen A, Kirobkin M, Silverman P M, Dunnick N R, Kelvin F M 1984 Mesenteric vein thrombosis: CT identification. American Journal of Radiology 143: 83–86
Rowbotham B J, Carroll P, Whitaker A N et al 1987 Measurement of cross-linked fibrin derivatives: use in the diagnosis of venous thrombosis. Thrombosis and Haemostasis 57: 59–61
Ruckley C V, Boulton F E, Redhead D 1987 The treatment of venous thrombosis of the upper and lower limbs with 'APSAC'. European Journal of Vascular Surgery 1: 107–112
Rudofsky G 1989 Pathogenese, diagnostik und therapy der thrombo-varikophlebitis. Herz 14: 283–286
Sackett D L 1989 Rules of evidence and clinical recommendations on the use of antithrombotic agents. Chest 95: 2S–4S
Samama M, Horellow M H 1982 Thrombolytic drugs and/or heparin in pulmonary embolism. Haemostasis 12: 98 (abstract)
Salzman E W, Deykin D, Mayer Shapiro R, Rosenberg R 1975 Management of heparin therapy: controlled prospective trial. New England Journal of Medicine 292: 1046–1050
Sandler D A, Martin J E 1985 Liquid crystal thermography as a screening test for deep vein thrombosis. Lancet i: 665–668
Sandler D A, Martin J F, Duncan J S et al 1984 Diagnosis of deep vein thrombosis. Comparison of clinical evaluation, ultrasound, plethysmography and venoscan with X-ray venography. Lancet ii: 716–719
Saour J N, Sieck J O, Mamo L A, Gallus A S 1990 Trial of different intensities of anticoagulation in patients with prosthetic heart valves. New England Journal of Medicine 322: 428–432
Sauerbrei E, Thomson J G, McLachlan M S F, Musial J 1981 Observer variation in lower limb venography. Journal of the Canadian Assocation of Radiology 31: 28–29
Schindler J M, Kaiser M, Gerber A et al 1990 Colour coded duplex sonography in suspected deep vein thrombosis of the leg. British Medical Journal 301: 1369–1370
Schneider P A, Geissbuhler P, Piguet J C, Bounameux H 1990 Follow-up after partial interruption of the vena cava with the Guenther filter. Cardiovascular and Interventional Radiology 13: 378–380
Schulman S, Lockner D, Granqvist S et al 1984 A randomized trial of low-dose versus high dose streptokinase in deep vein thrombosis of the thigh. Thrombosis and Haemostasis 51: 261–265
Schulman S, Lockner D, Juhlin-Dannfelt A 1985 The duration of oral anticoagulation after deep vein thrombosis. A randomized study. Acta Medica Scandinavica 217: 547–552

Scurr J H, Coleridge-Smith P D, Hasty J H 1988 Deep venous thrombosis: a continuing problem. British Medical Journal 297: 28
Secker-Walker R H, Siegel B A 1973 The use of nuclear medicine in the diagnosis of lung disease. Radiologic Clinics of North America 11: 215–241
Sharp A A, Warren B A, Raxton A M et al 1968 Anticoagulant therapy with a purified fraction of Malayan pit viper venom. Lancet i: 493–499
Shionoya S, Yamada I, Sakurai T, Ohta T, Matsubara J 1989 Thrombectomy for acute deep vein thrombosis: prevention of postthrombotic syndrome. Journal of Cardiovascular Surgery 30: 484–489
Sigel B, Felix W R, Poply G I, Ipsen J 1972 Diagnosis of lower limb venous thrombosis by Doppler ultrasound technique. Archives of Surgery 104: 174–179
Simon M, Athanasoulis C A, Kim D et al 1989 Simon nitinol inferior vena cava filter: initial clinical experience. Radiology 172: 99–103
Singer I, Royal H D, Uren R F et al 1984 Radionuclide plethysmography and Tc-99m red blood cell venography in venous thrombosis: comparison with contrast venography. Radiology 150: 213–217
Skjeldal S, Hoegevold H E, Reikeras O, Hoiseth A 1990 Plethysmographic screening for deep venous thrombosis following total hip replacement. Annales Chirurgiae et Gynaecologiae 79: 42–45
Smith R C, Duncanson J, Ruckley C V et al 1978 Beta-thromboglobulin and deep vein thrombosis. Thrombosis and Haemostasis 39: 338–342
Snyder T C, Sachder H S 1986 Magnetic resonance imaging of cerebral dural sinus thrombosis. Journal of Computer Assisted Tomography 10: 889–890
Speiser W, Mallek R, Koppensteiner R et al 1990 D-dimer and TAT measurement in patients with deep venous thrombosis: utility in diagnosis and judgement of anticoagulant treatment effectiveness. Thrombosis and Haemostasis 64: 196–201
Stein P D, Terrin M L, Hales C A et al 1991a Clinical, laboratory, roentgenographic and electrocardiographic findings in patients with acute pulmonary embolism and no pre-existing cardiac or pulmonary disease. Chest 100: 598–603
Stein P D, Coleman R E, Gottschalk E et al 1991b Diagnostic utility of ventilation/perfusion lung scans in acute pulmonary embolism is not diminished by pre-existing cardiac or pulmonoary disease. Chest 100: 604–606
Subramanyam B R, Balthazar E J, Lefleur R S, Horn S C, Hulnick D H 1984 Portal venous thrombosis: correlative analysis of sonography. American Journal of Gastroenterology 79: 773–776
Swedenborg J, Hagglof R, Jacobsson J et al 1986 Results of surgical treatment for iliofemoral thrombosis. British Journal of Surgery 73: 871–874
Tavill A S, Wood E J, Kreel L 1975 The Budd–Chiari syndrome: correlation between hepatic scintigraphy and the clinical, radiological, and pathological findings in 19 cases of hepatic venous outflow obstruction. Gastroenterology 68: 509–518
Thery C, Asseman P, Amrouni M 1990 Use of a new removable vena cava filter in order to prevent pulmonary embolism in patients submitted to thrombolysis. European Heart Journal 11: 334–341
Thomas E A, Cobby M J D, Rhys Davies E, Jeans W D, Whicher J T 1989 Liquid crystal thermography and C reactive protein in the detection of deep venous thrombosis. British Medical Journal 299: 951–952
Tibbutt D A, Davies J A, Anderson J A et al 1974 Comparison by controlled clinical trial of streptokinase and heparin in treatment of life-threatening pulmonary embolism. British Medical Journal 1: 343–347
Toy P T C Y, Schrier S L 1978 Occlusive impedance plethysmography: A noninvasive method of diagnosis of deep vein thrombosis. Western Journal of Medicine 129: 89–94
Tsapogas M J, Peabody M A, Wu K T et al 1973 Controlled study of thrombolytic therapy in deep vein thrombosis. Surgery 74: 973–984
Tulchinsky M, Zeller J A, Reba R C 1991 Urinary fibrinopeptide A in evaluation of patients wuth suspected acute pulmonary embolism. A prospective pilot study. Chest 100: 394–398
Turnbull T L, Dymowski J J, Zalut T E 1990 A prospective study of hand-held Doppler ultrasonography by emergency physicians in the evaluation of suspected deep vein thrombosis. Annals of Emergency Medicine 19: 691–695
Turpie A G G, Gunstensen J, Hirsh J, Nelson H, Gent M 1988 Randomised comparison of two intensities of oral anticoagulant therapy after tissue heart valve replacement. Lancet i: 1224–1245
Turpie A G G, Robinson J G, Doyle D J et al 1989 Comparison of high dose with low dose subcutaneous heparin to prevent left ventricular mural thrombosis in patients with acute transmural myocardial infarction. New England Journal of Medicine 320: 352–357
Turpie A G G, Levine M N, Hirsh J, Ginsberg J S, Cruickshank M, Jay R, Gent M 1990 Tissue plasminogen activator (rt-PA) vs heparin in deep vein thrombosis. Results of a randomized trial. Chest 97: 172S–175S
Umpleby H 1987 Thrombosis of the superior mesenteric vein. British Journal of Surgery 74: 694–696
UPET-I. 1973 Urokinase Pulmonary Embolism Trial: a national cooperative study. Circulation 47–2: 1–108
UPET-II 1974 Urokinase-streptokinase Embolism Trial. Phase 2 results. A cooperative study. Journal of the American Medical Association 229: 1606–1613
Vaccaro J P, Cronan J J, Dorfman G S 1990 Outcome analysis of patients with normal compression US examination, Radiology 175: 645–649
Valla D, Casadevall N, Lacombe C et al 1985 Primary myeloproliferative disorder and hepatic vein thrombosis. A prospective study of erythroid colony formation in vitro in 20 patients with Budd–Chiari syndrome. Annals of Internal Medicine 103: 329–332
van Bergen P F M M, Knot E A R, Jonker J J C, deBoer A C, de Maat M P M 1989 Can quantitative determination of fibrin(ogen) degradation products and thrombin-antithrombin III complexes predict deep venous thrombosis in outpatients? Thrombosis and Haemostasis 62: 1043–1045
van de Loo, J C W, Kriessmann A, Truebestein G et al 1983 Controlled multicentre pilot study of urokinase-heparin and streptokinase in deep vein thrombosis. Thrombosis and Haemostasis 50: 660–663
van Hulsteijn H, Briët E, Koch C, Hermans J, Bertina R 1982 Diagnostic value of fibrinopeptide A and beta-thromboglobulin in acute deep venous thrombosis and pulmonary embolism. Acta Medica Scandinavica 211: 323–330
Verstraete M 1989 Use of thrombolytic drugs in non-coronary disorders. Drugs 38: 801–821
Verstraete M, Miller G A H, Bounameaux H et al 1988 Intravenous and intrapulmonary recombinant tissue type plasminogen activator in the treatment of acute massive pulmonary embolism. Circulation 77: 353–360
Verhaeghe R, Besse P, Bounameux H, Marbet G A 1989 Multicenter pilot study of the efficacy and safety of systemic rt-PA administration in the treatment of deep vein thrombosis of the lower extremities and/or pelvis. Thrombosis Research 55: 5–12
Vieras F, Barron E L, Parker G A, Grissom M P 1980 Experimental evaluation of Tc-99m sulfur colloid as a potential imaging agent in thromboembolic disease. Journal of Nuclear Medicine 21: 723–728
Vogel C, Machulik M 1987 Efficacy and safety of low molecular weight heparin (LMW-Sandoz) in patients with deep vein thrombosis. Thrombosis and Haemostasis 57: 427 (abstract)
Vogel P, Laing F C, Jeffrey R B Jr, Wing V W 1987 Deep venous thrombosis of the lower extremity: ultrasound evaluation. Radiology 163: 747–751
Vogelzang R L, Moel D I, Cohn R L et al 1988 Acute renal vein thrombosis: successful treatment with intraarterial urokinase. Radiology 169: 681–682
Walker M G 1972 The natural history of venous thromboembolism. British Journal of Surgery 59: 753–754
Walker M C, Shaw J W, Thomson G J L, Cumming J G R, Lea Thomas M 1987 Subcutaneous calcium heparin versus intravenous sodium heparin in treatment of established acute deep vein thrombosis of the legs: a multicentre prospective randomised trial. British Medical Journal 294: 1189–1192
Wang Z, Zhu Y, Wang S et al 1989 Recognition and management of

Budd–Chiari syndrome: report of one hundred cases. Journal of Vascular Surgery 10: 149–156
Watz R, Ek I, Bygdeman S 1979 Noninvasive diagnosis of acute deep vein thrombosis. A comparison between thermography, plethysmography and phlebography. Acta Medica Scandinavica 206: 463–466
Webber M M, Comes A S, Roe D, LaFontaine R L, Hawkins R A 1990 comparison of Biello, McNeil, and PIOPED criteria for the diagnosis of pulmonary emboli on lung scans. American Journal of Roentgenology 154: 975–981
White R D, Winkler M L, Higgins C B 1987 MR imaging of pulmonary hypertension and pulmonary emboli. American Journal of Roentgenology 149: 15–21
White R H, McGahan J P, Daschbach M M, Hartling R P 1989 Diagnosis of deep-vein thrombosis using duplex ultrasound. Annals of Internal Medicine 111: 297–304
Williams W J 1973 Venography. Circulation 47: 220–221
Wilson J R, Lampman J 1979 Heparin therapy: a randomized prospective study. American Heart Journal 97: 155–158
Wilson J E, Frenkel E P, Pierce A K et al 1971 Spontaneous fibrinolysis in pulmonary embolism. Journal of Clinical Investigation 50: 474–480
Wilson J E, Bynum L J, Parkey R W 1981 Heparin therapy in venous thromboembolism. American Journal of Medicine 70: 808–816
Wingerd M, Bernhard V M, Maddison F, Towne J B 1978 Comparison of caval filters in the management of venous thromboembolism. Archives of Surgery 113: 1264–1270
Woolson S T, Alto P, McCrory D et al 1990 B-mode ultrasound scanning in the detection of proximal venous thrombosis after total hip replacement. Journal of Bone and Joint Surgery 72-A: 983–987
Yudelman I, Nossel H L, Kaplan K L et al 1977 Fibrinopeptide A levels in symptomatic thromboembolism. Archives of Internal Medicine 137: 1385–1390

SECTION 11

Antithrombotic therapy

64. Heparin and low molecular weight heparin

T. W. Barrowcliffe D. P. Thomas

Heparin is a long established antithrombotic drug, having been in successful clinical use for over 50 years. Research into its mechanism of action and many biological activities continues unabated, and significant progress has been made in recent years. An important new development has been the advent of low molecular weight (LMW) heparin, which is already in widespread clinical use. This chapter reviews the chemistry, biochemistry, and clinical use of both unfractionated and LMW heparin.

CHEMISTRY AND METHODS OF PREPARATION

Unfractionated heparin

Commercial unfractionated heparin (UFH) is derived from intestinal mucosa, mostly of pigs, though a proportion comes from cattle and sheep. Manufacturers' preparation procedures remain confidential, but are sufficiently similar that products from different manufacturers do not differ substantially. Convincing species differences have not been reported, but it should be noted that in the USA, also in Hungary and perhaps elsewhere in eastern Europe, commercial heparin is available derived from bovine lung tissue; this does show some significant chemical differences from mucosal UFH.

Heparin consists of polysaccharide chains, apparently unbranched, composed of alternating uronate and hexosamine saccharides joined by glycosidic (1–4) linkages. It is a product of biosynthetic transformation of a regular polysaccharide, in which glucuronate and *N*-acetylglucosamine alternate, by a sequence of enzymic reaction steps in which no step operates evenly or completely along the chains, resulting in a highly irregular polysaccharide in which most of the glucuronate has been epimerized to iduronate, most of the glucosamine has had its *N*-acetyl replaced by *N*-sulpho groups, and where *O*-sulpho groups occupy many of the 2- positions in the iduronates and the 6- positions in the glucosamines. Figure 64.1 shows, respectively, the invariable repeating disaccharide unit of the parent *N*-acetylheparosan (**1**), and the most frequently occurring disaccharide unit in heparin chains (**2**). This latter occurs in multi-unit sequences and on average constitutes 70% or more of each molecule. The remainder is made up from disaccharide units intermediate in structure between **1** and **2** (with perhaps a very few units of **1** surviving); the remaining glucuronate and some iduronate is unsulphated, and although most of the *N*-sulphoglucosamine is 6-sulphated as well, so is some *N*-acetyglucosamine.

Antithrombin-binding sequence

The interaction of heparin with antithrombin has been investigated by a number of groups, and it was found that only about a third of any sample of UFH would bind to the protein and activate it (Lam et al 1976, Höök et al 1976). Ultimately, a specific pentasac-charide binding sequence (**3** in Fig. 64.1) was identified as essential for this activity in UFH (Lindahl et al 1979). As indicated, some variations can be made in the substitution pattern without affecting binding or activation, but the 3-*O*-sulpho group in the centre 2,3,6-trisulphated glucosamine is essential and seems to be unique to this sequence. The presence of glucuronate next to it should also be noted. This is the only sequence so far found in heparin which has specific activity involving individual molecular species known to play a part in the coagulation cascade.

LMW heparin

LMW heparin is prepared from UFH and so shares the same basic chemical structure, but the various methods of preparation result in some minor chemical differences. Probably the most important one is that, because depolymerization creates some new low affinity chains and also to a certain extent cleaves the pentasaccharide sequence, the proportion of chains with high affinity to antithrombin III (ATIII) is lower than in UFH; around 10–20%, compared with 30–35% for UFH.

Methods of preparation

The earliest method of preparation, fractionation of UFH by enrichment of existing LMW chains, using gel filtration and/or alcohol fractionation (Johnson et al 1976, Lormeau et al 1980), was soon abandoned as being commercially uneconomic because of low yield. The products in current clinical use are prepared by one of the following four methods.

Nitrous acid. This deaminative cleavage process breaks heparin chain glycosidic linkages between the 1-

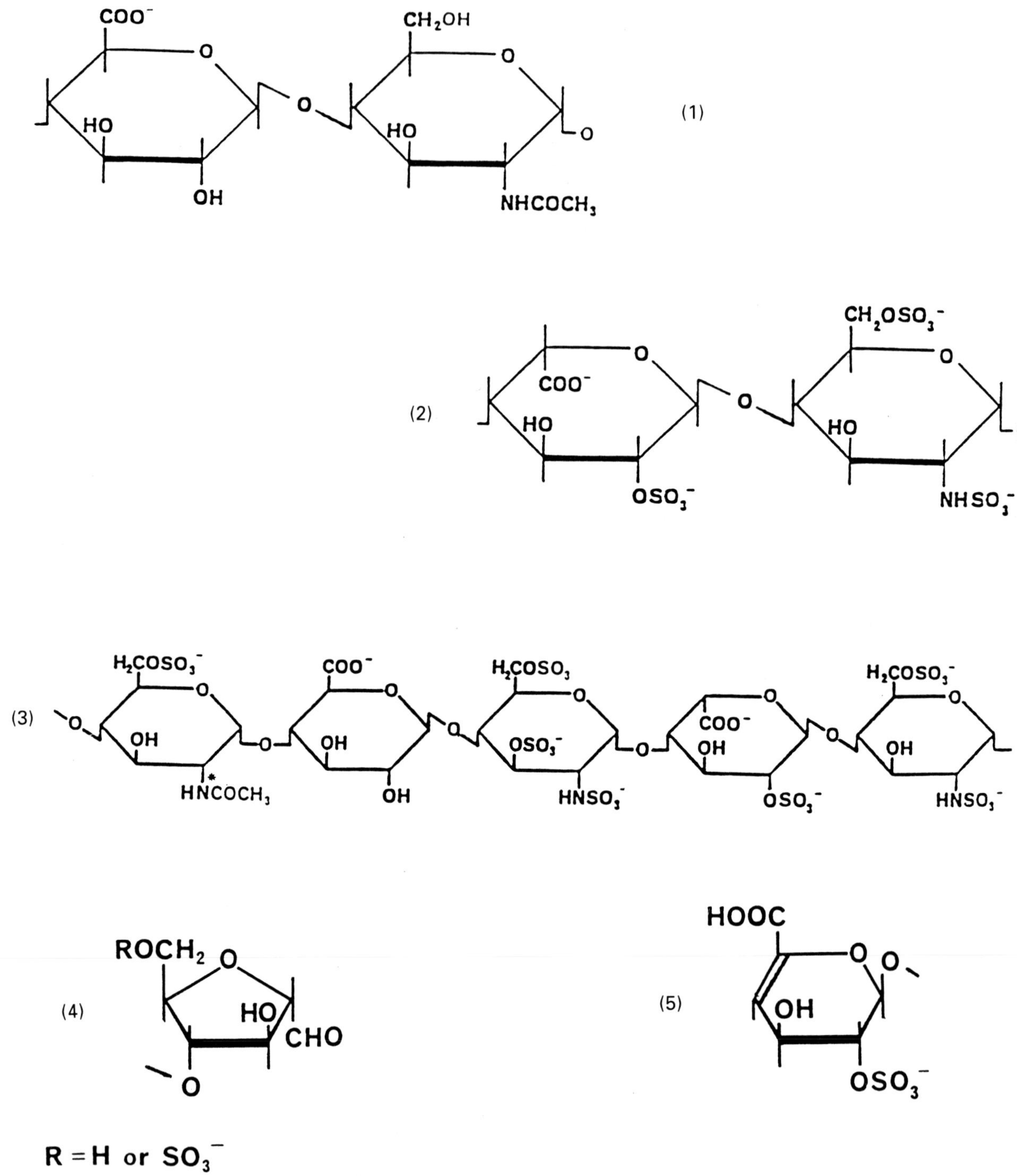

Fig. 64.1 Chemical formulae. (1) The main repeating disaccharide of the heparin precursor; (2) The main repeating disaccharide of heparin; (3) The pentasaccharide sequence with high affinity for heparin; (4) Anhydromannose, the reducing-end residue produced by degradation of heparin; (5) The sulphated uronic acid at the non-reducing end of heparin fragments produced by beta-elimination.

position of *N*-sulphated glucosamine and the 4-position of the adjacent uronate; the latter remains intact at the non-reducing end of the fragment, but the glucosamine is converted to 2,5-anhydro-D-mannose (**4** in Fig. 64.1). The sequences most vulnerable to nitrous acid are common ones not directly involved in specific activity; the 3-*O*-sulphated glucosamine in the pentasaccharide is, fortuitously, relatively resistant to nitrous acid (Casu et al 1981). Some manufacturers reduce terminal anhydromannose residues to anhydromannitol with borohydride to ensure stability, but since others leave it unchanged it is unlikely that the aldehyde group causes problems.

Heparinase. Heparinase, isolated from *Flavobacterium heparinum,* is a lyase which cleaves UFH at essentially the same positions as nitrous acid. Sulphated glucosamine remains intact at the reducing ends of the fragments, but the iduronate is dehydrogenated to yield the 4,5-unsaturated acid (**5** in Fig. 64.1) at the non-reducing ends. Control of depolymerization is conveniently effected by observing the increase in ultraviolet light absorption at 235 nm due to the formation of the unsaturated uronate (Nielsen & Østergaard 1988). The antithrombin binding sequence (**3** in Fig. 64.1) is thought to be relatively resistant to heparinase, though some cleavage does apparently occur.

β-Elimination of heparin esters. Esterification of uronate carboxyl groups in heparin greatly facilitates glycosidic cleavage by alkali, which can then occur with very little desulphation or other inactivating changes. This process of β-elimination yields fragments with the same terminal groups as those from heparinase treatment (4,5-dehydrouronate and glucosamine).

Oxidative cleavage. A variety of oxidizing agents have been used, e.g. periodate and peroxides with or without free radical catalysis. In all cases the cleavage is more random than in procedures previously described; glycosidic bonds of both uronate and glucosamine are split, so that, whereas the previous procedures yield essentially fragments with even numbers of saccharide units in their chains, oxidative cleavage yields all chain lengths.

Molecular weight distribution

The chemical differences resulting from the various preparation methods for LMW heparin are relatively minor, and probably play no part in their anticoagulant properties. Much more important potentially are differences in molecular weight distribution, since this has a considerable influence on in vivo properties, particularly pharmacokinetics. The average molecular weights of the currently used commercial preparations are similar, in the range 4000–6000, but there are detectable differences in their molecular weight profiles, which can in fact be used as a fingerprint for identification purposes. Figure 64.2 shows gel chromatograms of three of the current products. Two points should be considered when comparing these molecular weight profiles. First, a large proportion of the smallest oligosaccharide chains are likely to be inactive in relation to ATIII binding, being produced by multiple cleavage of longer chains. Unlike UFH, the proportion of high affinity chains in LMW heparin is expected to decrease with decreasing molecular weight, and indeed this has been shown to be the case (Béguin et al 1992). Secondly, the longest chains present in LMW heparin in vitro are likely to be of less importance in vivo, because absorption into the blood after subcutaneous injection

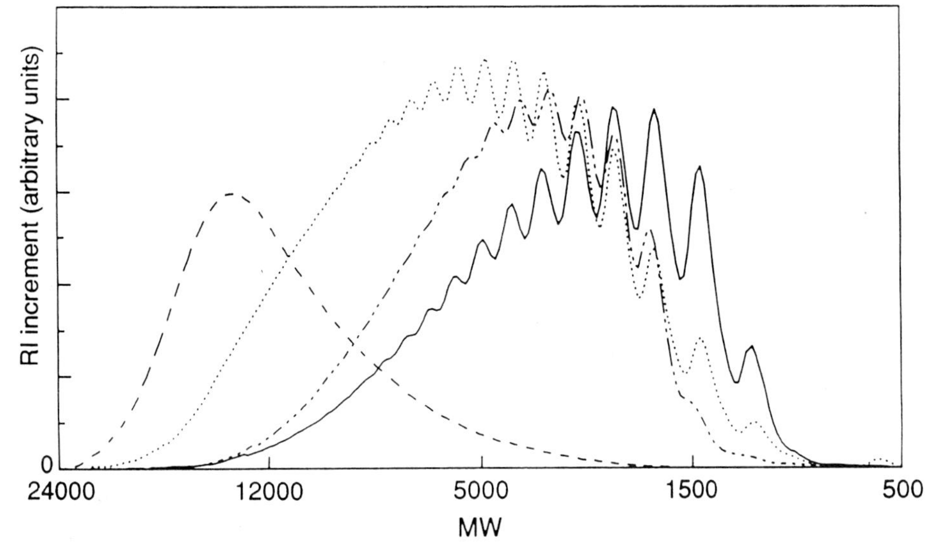

Fig. 64.2 High resolution GPC chromatograms of three commercially produced LMW heparins: Logiparim (dotted line), Fragmin (dot-dashed line) and Clexane (solid line), with unfractionated heparin (dashed-line) for comparison.

decreases with increasing molecular weight (Johnson et al 1976, Lane et al 1979, Thomas & Merton 1982). Overall, therefore, the apparently considerable differences in molecular weight distribution between products are likely to be of much less magnitude when considering active molecules present in the circulation after subcutaneous injection.

Table 64.1 summarizes the method of preparation and essential molecular weight parameters of the most commonly available LMW heparin products.

MECHANISMS OF ANTICOAGULANT ACTIVITY

Although the prime importance of binding to ATIII is well recognized, the anticoagulant activity of heparin and LMW heparin is modulated by several other types of binding, notably to coagulation proteases, heparin-neutralizing proteins, and cells. These may be particularly important for the anticoagulant properties of LMW heparin.

Binding to ATIII

There is now overwhelming evidence that the anticoagulant action of heparin in vitro is primarily due to its ability to bind tightly to ATIII, thereby accelerating the latter's rate of inhibition of all the major coagulation enzymes (Rosenberg & Damus 1973). As already indicated, binding is due to the presence in heparin chains of a specific pentasaccharide with a molecular weight of 1756 (Thunberg et al 1982, Choay et al 1983); the K_d for the interaction is 10^{-8}M. Although it is possible for chains in UFH (length 12 to over 100 saccharides) to contain more than one pentasaccharide, this is not found in practice for the majority of chains (Pejler 1988). Similarly, most of the high affinity chains in LMW heparin preparations (4 to 40 saccharides) are likely to contain only one pentasaccharide.

Molecular weight dependence of binding to ATIII

The binding of the pentasaccharide to ATIII induces a conformational change which enhances its rate of reaction with serine proteases (Einarsson & Andersson 1977, Olson & Shore 1981). Since the mechanism by which ATIII inhibits serine proteases is the same for all enzymes, it would be expected that, if ATIII binding were the only determinant of anticoagulant activity, the activity of different molecular weight fractions would be the same regardless of the enzyme or assay method used. An early indication that this was not the case came from studies in our laboratory of a series of fractions, prepared by gel filtration, ranging in molecular weight from approximately 5000 to 35 000. The APTT and anti-Xa methods gave completely different results when anticoagulant activity was plotted against molecular weight, with a sharp decrease in activity towards low molecular weight by APTT assay but an increase by anti-Xa (Andersson et al 1976). This was found for fractions prepared from both UFH and high-affinity heparin. Subsequent studies using amidolytic assays instead of clotting methods confirmed these trends (Barrowcliffe et al 1978) and it was also found that the molecular weight dependency for inhibition of thrombin was the same as for the APTT, i.e. a decrease towards lower values. Thus it became clear that the molecular weight dependence of anticoagulant activity was quite different for the two major enzymes, thrombin and factor Xa, implying some differences in mechanism of action. These in vitro results were confirmed for a variety of different heparins (Lane et al 1978, Barrowcliffe et al 1979).

Inhibition of thrombin

The mechanism of inhibition of thrombin by ATIII is reviewed in detail by Björk et al (1989). Briefly, an initial weak complex is rapidly converted to a stable 1:1 complex with very tight binding, so that the enzyme is effectively trapped. The bimolecular rate constant at 37°C has been reported as 1.4×10^4 $M.^{-1}$ s^{-1}, giving a theoretical plasma half life for thrombin of 20 seconds (Jesty 1979); the actual half life is approximately 40 seconds, probably because of the presence of fibrinogen and other thrombin substrates in plasma.

Table 64.1 Characteristics of LMW heparins in clinical use

Manufacturer	Trade name	Preparation method	Weight average molecular mass	% Polysaccharides between 2000–8000
Choay (Sanofi/Winthrop)	Fraxiparine	Nitrous acid*	4200	85
KabiPharmacia	Fragmin	Nitrous acid	5700	80
Leo	Innohep	Heparinase	6000	64
Novo/Nordisk	Logiparin	Heparinase	6000	64
Rhône-Poulenc/Rorer	Enoxaparin, Clexane, Lovenox	β-Elimination	3900	75
Sandoz	Sandoparin, Mono-Embolex NM	Nitrous acid	5100	63

* Fraxiparine may be available in two forms: one as indicated, and the other apparently a true fraction of heparin (without depolymerization).

The accelerating effect of heparin on this reaction is remarkable; an effect is demonstrable at plasma heparin concentrations as low as 0.01 IU/ml, where the plasma concentration of high affinity chains is approximately 1.3 nM, i.e. some 2000 times less than that of ATIII. At therapeutic heparin concentrations of over 1 IU/ml, the reaction is accelerated over 2000-fold, and the half life of thrombin is reduced from 40 seconds to less than 0.01 second. The ability of heparin to act at low concentrations and the fact that it is not 'consumed' during the reaction virtually define its role as a catalyst.

The activity profile of molecular weight fractions when converted to a molar basis, indicate a marked decline in the ability of each heparin molecule to catalyse thrombin inhibition as molecular weight decreases. This is seen at its most striking when fragments below molecular weight 5000 ($\approx$ 18 saccharides) are examined. In collaboration with Professor U Lindahl, three fragments with precisely defined molecular weights were studied in our laboratory; these were a decasaccharide, a 16–18 fragment, and a 20–22 fragment (Thomas et al 1982, Barrowcliffe et al 1984). As shown in Table 64.2, all three fragments had high anti-Xa activity, but the '10' and 16–18 fragments had no detectable ability to inhibit thrombin in a calcium thrombin time and very low activity by APTT. Only the 20–22 fragment displayed significant activity in these assays. These results indicate that a minimum molecular weight, occurring between 16 and 22 saccharides, is an absolute requirement for potentiation of thrombin inhibition. This requirement was defined more precisely by Lane et al (1984) using a series of homologous oligosaccharides from 8 to 20. Anti-IIa activity, i.e. ability to potentiate inhibition of thrombin does not occur until a minimum of 18 monosaccharides (molecular weight $\approx$54000) is reached, and thereafter rises sharply with increasing molecular weight. The reason for this minimum requirement was first suggested by Pomerantz and Owen (1978), who proposed a ternary complex of heparin ATIII and thrombin, with ATIII and thrombin bound to the same heparin chain. This 'template' hypothesis was further substantiated by detailed kinetic studies (Griffith 1982, Nesheim 1983) which indicated the importance of thrombin binding to heparin.

This mechanism explains the increase in anti-IIa activity with increasing molecular weight. Since the distribution of the pentasaccharide is random, a heparin fragment of, say, 20 saccharides will have a significant proportion of its chains with the pentasaccharide in the middle and insufficient chain length either side for thrombin binding. This proportion should decrease with increasing chain length, until about 32 saccharides; after this there should be sufficient space for thrombin binding wherever the pentasaccharide is located.

Another important feature of the interaction between heparin, thrombin and ATIII is that the affinity of the ATIII-thrombin complex for heparin is much lower than that of native ATIII (Carlstrom et al 1977). This can be explained by the conformational change in ATIII induced by interaction with thrombin (Peterson & Blackburn 1987). Since ATIII is always in excess of thrombin in plasma, this means that when a molecule of heparin/ATIII-thrombin complex forms, heparin will dissociate and bind preferentially to unreacted ATIII, thus being free to promote further inhibition of thrombin. It is this feature which accounts for the catalytic action of heparin, and explains why it is such an effective anticoagulant at low concentrations.

Table 64.2 In vitro anticoagulant activities of oligosaccharides with high affinity to antithrombin III

No. of saccharides	Specific activity (IU/mg)		
	Anti-Xa	APTT	TCT
10	1247	2.1	<1
16–18	1929	7.0	<1
>18	660	42	144

Inhibition of factor Xa

The inhibition of factor Xa by ATIII, in the absence of heparin, occurs by exactly the same mechanism as does the inhibition of thrombin, with initial proteolytic attack followed by formation of a stable 1:1 complex. However it is clear from the studies already mentioned that the mechanism for potentiation of factor Xa inhibition by heparin is different from that of thrombin inhibition, since oligosaccharide fragments with decreased anti-IIa activity retain their anti-Xa activity (Table 64.2). It appears that the approximation mechanism that is so necessary for inhibition of thrombin is not required for inhibition of factor Xa; the heparin-induced conformational change is sufficient. This is substantiated by the fact that binding of factor Xa to heparin is at least 100 times weaker than that of thrombin (Oosta et al 1981). There are two other aspects of the anti-Xa activity of LMW heparin which are important to understand, as they may affect the relationship between this activity and the antithrombotic action of LMW heparin.

Effect of calcium chloride ($CaCl_2$)

The effect of $CaCl_2$ on anti-Xa activity of UFH and LMW heparin was studied in our laboratory (Barrowcliffe & Le Shirley 1989), using purified human ATIII, bovine or human factor Xa, and an amidolytic method. With UFH, the addition of 3 mM $CaCl_2$ induced a marked potentiation of anti-Xa activity, almost two-fold for bovine Xa and six-fold with human Xa. This potentiation was found to be dependent on molecular weight; below 6500 there was no enhancement of activity, whereas above 6500, the potentiating effect of $CaCl_2$ increased up to a maximum at a molecular weight of between 9000 and 11 000.

These results indicate that measurements of the anti-Xa activity of LMW heparin against a UFH standard in the absence of $CaCl_2$, as is normally done, will give higher potencies than in the presence of $CaCl_2$; the latter might be thought to be more relevant to the situation in vivo.

Inhibition of factor Xa in prothrombinase

Efficient activation of prothrombin requires factor Xa to be present in a complex with Ca^{2+}, phospholipid (PL), and factor Va, commonly known as the prothrombinase complex, or simply prothrombinase. The other components of the complex enormously enhance the enzymatic action of factor Xa, and also affect its ability to be inhibited by ATIII/heparin. In vivo, activated platelets provide the phospholipid surface and also some of the factor Va. In the absence of heparin, inhibition of factor Xa by ATIII is much slower when Xa is bound to platelets (Walsh & Biggs 1972) or to Ca^{2+}/PL/FVa (Marciniak 1973, Nesheim & Mann 1983). This protective effect probably exists to ensure optimum prothrombin conversion in response to a haemostatic stimulus. A variety of studies of the effect of heparin on factor Xa inhibition in prothrombinase have shown that heparin can, to a certain extent, overcome this protective effect (Ellis et al 1986, Barrowcliffe et al 1987, Schoen et al 1989); LMW heparin appears less effective in this regard (Barrowcliffe et al 1987).

These studies all indicate that, whatever heparin is used, a higher concentration is required to inhibit factor Xa when bound in prothrombinase than when free, and that, on a molar basis LMW heparin is less effective than UFH in inhibiting prothrombinase.

Inhibition of contact system enzymes

Holmer et al (1981) found that, for factor XIa, anticoagulant activity decreased sharply with molecular weight, in a manner similar to that found for thrombin, implying the need for factor XIa to bind to the longer heparin chains, i.e. a template mechanism. For factor XIIa and kallikrein, however, high specific activities were found even down to the lowest molecular weight fractions; these enzymes therefore behave like factor Xa and can be presumed not to require enzyme binding for enhancement of activity by ATIII.

The role of UFH and ATIII in the inhibition of the contact system enzymes has been reviewed by Colman et al (1989). Although some accelerating activity of UFH can be demonstrated in purified systems, the maximum rate enhancements are far less than those observed for thrombin and factor Xa. Colman et al (1989) therefore concluded that therapeutic concentrations of heparin do not significantly enhance inactivation rates of any of the contact system enzymes. Thus the enhancement of inhibition of factor XIIa and kallikrein by LMW heparin is unlikely to contribute towards their overall anticoagulant action.

Inhibition of factor IXa

In the studies of Holmer et al (1981) the molecular weight dependence of inhibition of factor IXa by ATIII/heparin was the same as for thrombin and factor XIa, i.e. a decrease with decreasing molecular weight, and no activity below around molecular weight 5000. Thus it was assumed that factor IXa also requires enzyme binding to heparin for potentiation of ATIII inactivation, and this conclusion was reinforced by Pieters et al (1988), who found no accelerating action of the pentasaccharide on inactivation of factor IXa by purified ATIII. However in both these studies the inactivation of factor IXa was measured in the absence of Ca^{2+} ions. In a subsequent study Pieters et al (1990) measured the inhibition of factor IXa in recalcified plasma: under these conditions the rate of inhibition with UFH was enhanced, and, surprisingly, the pentasaccharide also had an inhibitory effect, albeit much less than that of UFH. About ten times more pentasacharide than UFH was needed to give a similar rate enhancement, giving an approximate potency for the pentasaccharide in this system of 15 IU/mg, compared with its anti-Xa activity of at least 300 IU/mg. The original conclusion of Holmer et al (1981) that the anti-IXa activity of LMW heparin is much lower than that of UFH is therefore still justified.

Overall effects on thrombin generation

The intended aim of any anticoagulant is to reduce, delay, or prevent the generation of thrombin. Although the inhibitory actions of heparin and LMW heparin on individual serine proteases are now fairly well characterized, the complexities of the coagulation system make it difficult to predict which reactions are most important for inhibition of thrombin generation. In addition, there is the existence of the thrombin feedback loops, whereby the first traces of thrombin produced, probably through the extrinsic pathway, activate the co-factors VIII and V, which in turn produce an enormous increase in the rate and amount of thrombin subsequently generated. In recent work by two research groups the importance of inhibition of these thrombin feedback loops by heparin and LMW heparin has been emphasized, and the contributions of inhibition of the various serine proteases to the overall inhibition of thrombin generation assessed (see Ch. 20).

In the studies of Ofosu and co-workers, the activation of prothrombin and the inhibition of the formed thrombin have been measured simultaneously in contact-activated plasma containing heparin or LMW heparin (for reviews see Ofosu et al 1989a, Ofosu 1989, Ofosu & Barrowcliffe 1990). This was done either by incorporation of ^{125}I-labelled prothrombin and subsequent gel analyses of the products, or by measurement of prothrombin and thrombin-inhibitor complexes by ELISA techniques. One of the main findings was that low concentrations of UFH could delay prothrombin activation by inhibiting the thrombin feedback loops, i.e. thrombin activation of factors VIII and V. LMW heparin at the same mass concentration was much less effective in delaying prothrombin activation because of its lower anti-IIa activity, and this accounts for the lesser effect of LMW heparin on the APTT. The anti-Xa activity of LMW heparin or UFH was considered to play little part in delaying prothrombin activation in this system.

When the concentration of LMW heparin was increased so that the anti-IIa activity was equal to that of UFH, LMW heparin was still less effective in delaying prothrombin activation (Ofosu et al 1989b). It was suggested that this was due to activation of factors VIII and V by factor Xa when thrombin activation is completely inhibited by UFH or LMW heparin. As already discussed, factor Xa in prothrombinase requires much higher concentrations of UFH for inhibition and is less readily inhibited by LMW heparin (Barrowcliffe et al 1987). More detailed studies of factor V activation have recently confirmed this hypothesis (Yang et al 1990).

Our own studies support the findings of Ofosu and colleagues. Thrombin generation in the intrinsic system was measured in plasma after surface contact activation in the presence of procoagulant phospholipids. As shown in Figure 64.3, a LMW heparin (the 1st International Standard) was a much less effective inhibitor than UFH in this system, on a weight basis, despite having similar anti-Xa activity. Further studies with high-affinity oligosaccharides showed that fragments of eight or predominantly 16 saccharides were much weaker inhibitors of thrombin generation than UFH, despite having anti-Xa activities more than five times higher, whereas an 18 saccharide fragment was almost as effective as UFH (Barrowcliffe & Thomas 1989). The 18 saccharide fragment is the smallest which is able to potentiate thrombin inhibition, and these data support the hypothesis that inhibition of thrombin itself is important for the inhibition of thrombin generation. In more recent studies the ability of several commercially available LMW heparins to inhibit thrombin generation was compared with that of UFH. As can be seen from Table 64.3, the concentrations required for 50% inhibition are much higher for the LMW heparins than for UFH, and these concentrations correlate very well with their anti-IIa activities.

In our test system it is not possible to tell whether the effect of heparin or LMW heparin is due to inhibition of the production of thrombin by the delay or prevention of prothrombin activation, or accelerated decay of the generated thrombin, or a mixture of both. Hemker and colleagues have devised a more sophisticated and reproducible form of the thrombin generation test in which

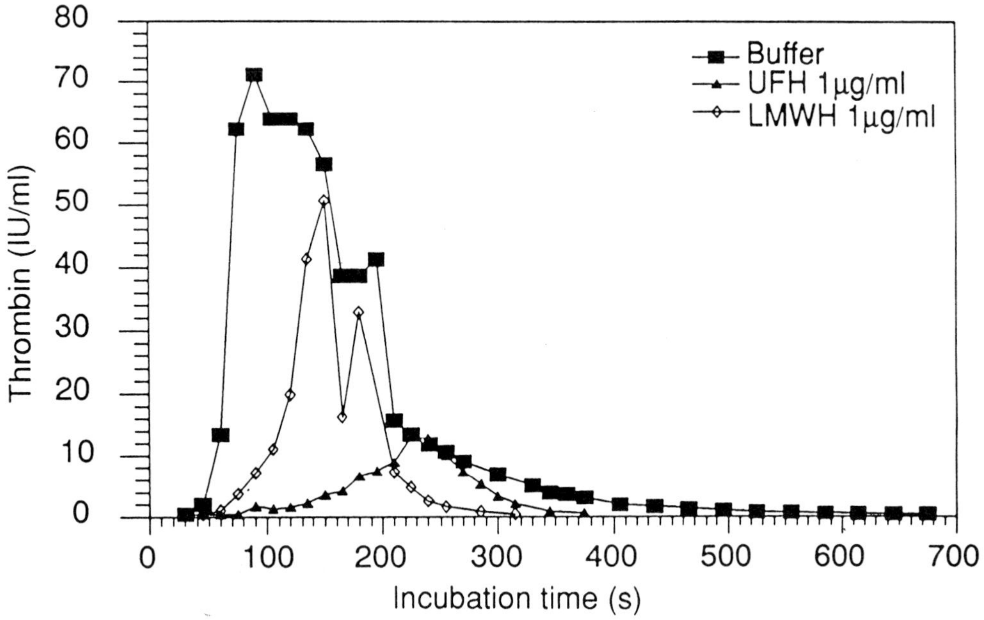

Fig. 64.3 Effects of UFH and LMW heparin on thrombin generation in plasma. Both compounds delay the appearance of thrombin, and diminish the peak and the overall amount generated. However, LMW heparin (the International Standard) is much less effective on a weight basis than UFH, despite having similar anti X-a activity.

Table 64.3 The ability of UFH and LMW heparins to inhibit intrinsic thrombin generation in human platelet-poor plasma

	EC_{50} (μg/ml)[a]
UFH (4th IS)	0.33
LMWH (1st IS)	0.60
Fragmin	0.83
Logiparin	0.92
Fraxiparine	1.37
Clexane	1.59

[a] EC_{50}: inhibition of thrombin generation expressed as the concentration required for 50% inhibition.
Data from Padilla et al 1991.

the influence of heparins on thrombin decay and prothrombin activation can be measured simultaneously (Béguin 1987, Hemker 1987, Béguin et al 1988). Effects of UFH and LMW heparin were measured using either tissue thromboplastin or kaolin plus phospholipid as the trigger. With extrinsic pathway activation (i.e. tissue thromboplastin) low concentrations of UFH (0.05 IU/ml or less) reduced thrombin generation by more than 50% without affecting prothrombinase. Only at 0.1 IU/ml was significant inhibition of prothrombinase observed.

With intrinsic pathway activation (kaolin + phospholipid), both prothrombinase and thrombin itself were inhibited. However the inhibitory action of heparin was shown to be on the formation of prothrombinase, not on prothrombinase itself, and could be explained by a twofold action; inhibition of thrombin activation of factor VIII and inactivation of factor IXa, which becomes more susceptible to heparin/ATIII inhibition when the formation of VIIIa is prevented. The anti-Xa action of heparin or LMW heparin was considered to play only a minor role in their ability to inhibit thrombin generation; activity in the extrinsic system was largely due to inhibition of thrombin activation of factor V, and in the intrinsic system to inhibition of thrombin activation of factor VIII and inactivation of factor IXa.

Studies in platelet-rich plasma showed that addition of dilute thromboplastin shortened the lag-phase for thrombin production, presumably by production of trace amounts of thrombin which activates platelets. UFH could prolong this lag phase by neutralizing the small amounts of thrombin required for platelet activation, but concentrations of up to 0.4 IU/ml did not diminish the amount of thrombin eventually formed (Béguin et al 1989a). This is in sharp contrast to the situation in platelet-poor plasma and can be explained by neutralization of the added heparin by platelet factor 4 (PF4), released after platelet activation. Since the ability of PF4 to neutralize heparin decreases with heparin molecular weight (Lane et al 1984, 1986), it might be expected that LMW heparin could be more effective than UFH as an inhibitor of thrombin generation in platelet-rich plasma; this was indeed found to be the case for Enoxaparin (Béguin et al 1989b) and Fraxiparine (Lane et al 1986).

INTERACTION WITH HEPARIN BINDING PROTEINS

The many proteins which interact with heparin can be categorized into those which enhance or inhibit anticoagulant activity, and those released from the vessel wall. Differences in the binding of UFH and LMW heparin to these proteins may be important for the therapeutic action of LMW heparin.

Heparin co-factor II (HCII)

A second heparin co-factor, distinguishable from ATIII, is a glycoprotein with a molecular weight of 65 600 (Tollefsen & Blank 1981, Tollefsen et al 1982). The concentration in normal plasma of HCII is 1.2 μM, approximately one-half that of ATIII, with which it shares similar amino acid composition (van Deerlin & Tollefsen 1991). Like ATIII, HCII inhibits thrombin by forming a stable 1:1 complex with the protease, although unlike ATIII it does not inhibit other clotting factors. While HCII is the only thrombin inhibitor in plasma that is activated by dermatan sulphate, the relative concentrations required to produce 50% inhibition of thrombin in the presence of HCII were 0.3 μg/ml of heparin and 6.4 μg/ml of dermatan sulphate, indicating that heparin is much the more active glycosaminoglycan. The physiological role of HCII remains unknown, although it seems unlikely that it has a major role in regulating intravascular coagulation (Tollefsen 1984). The potentiation of HCII activity by heparin decreases with decreasing molecular weight (Scully et al 1987), and therefore it seems unlikely that HCII plays a significant role in the anticoagulant actions of LMW heparin.

Vinazzer & Stocker (1991) reported 16 patients with heterozygous deficiency of HCII who had suffered from recurrent thromboembolic episodes. They concluded that while HCII deficiency must be considered as a possible cause of thrombophilia, such a deficiency appears to be less thrombogenic than a deficiency of other inhibitors of blood coagulation.

Platelet factor 4 (PF4)

This protein, normally present in the α granules of platelets, is potentially the most important naturally occurring heparin antagonist; it is released from platelets upon activation and if present in high enough concentration can completely neutralize the anticoagulant action of heparin. It interacts equally with high and low affinity heparin, and the presence of low affinity heparin therefore helps to 'protect' the high affinity molecules from neutralization; this may account for the potentiating effect of low affinity heparin on the antithrombotic action of high affinity molecules in animal experiments (Barrowcliffe et al 1984).

Like most heparin-binding proteins, binding affinity decreases with decreasing molecular weight; although all molecules with anti-IIa activity, i.e. down to 18 saccharides, are readily neutralized, oligosaccharides below this size become increasingly resistant to neutralization (Lane et al 1984). It has been suggested that this resistance may confer an advantage on LMW heparin, though the behaviour of the commercial LMW heparins, ranging from four to 40 saccharides is difficult to predict. Recent studies in our laboratory showed that the ability of four commercial LMW heparins to inhibit thrombin generation could be completely neutralized by PF4, though this required higher concentrations than UFH because of the larger number of molecules (Padilla et al 1992). A portion of the anti-Xa activity of these LMW heparins was resistant to neutralization by PF4 — it is not known whether this non-neutralized anti-Xa activity plays any role in vivo. Although most PF4 is found in platelets, a small proportion is present on the vascular endothelium, and can be released into the blood by heparin injection (Dawes et al 1982). The amount released by LMW heparin is less than by UFH, and calculation of the neutralizing ability of the maximum concentrations of PF4 indicate that this mechanism is unlikely to be important for either drug.

Protamine

Protamine is a highly basic protein derived from fish, and as the sulphate or chloride salt, has been used for many years as the clinical antagonist for heparin. It neutralizes all the anticoagulant activity of UFH in vitro, but around 25% of the anti-Xa activity measured after injection remains un-neutralized (Michalski et al 1978, Barrowcliffe et al 1979); this may be due to release of components with anti-Xa activity from the vessel wall (see p. 1426). As with PF4, binding affinity decreases with decreasing molecular weight, and saccharide chains below 18 units become increasingly resistant to neutralization (Holmer 1989). A significant proportion, up to 50%, of the anti-Xa activity of LMW heparin is not neutralized by protamine (Holmer & Söderström 1983, Harenberg et al 1986), either in vitro or after protamine injection. A major concern therefore is whether protamine can antagonize the haemorrhagic effect of LMW heparin in vivo. Several animal studies have shown complete neutralization of the haemorrhagic effect of LMW heparin by protamine (Diness & Østergaard 1986, van Ryn-McKenna et al 1990), but these animal models are not very sensitive, and may not accurately reflect the clinical situation. Indeed, Massonet-Castel et al (1984) found protamine of limited effectiveness in controlling bleeding induced by high doses of a LMW heparin (Enoxaparin) in extra-corporeal circulation.

Other heparin neutralizing proteins

Although histidine-rich glycoprotein (HRG) (Lijnen et al 1983) and vitronectin (Preissner et al 1985) have been shown to neutralize the anticoagulant activity of heparin in purified systems, it is uncertain whether they play a major role in circulating blood. The heparin neutralizing ability of HRG in plasma appears much less than expected from its behaviour when purified, and the same is true of vitronectin, which requires a proteolytic cleavage to expose the heparin-binding site.

The neutralization of the anticoagulant activity of heparin by HRG is a result of competition between HRG and ATIII for the binding of heparin (Lijnen et al 1983). Native HRG (M_r 75 000) occurs in plasma at a concentration of 100 ± 45 μg/l, and has been shown to interact with the main lysine-binding site of plasminogen, as well as with heparin. Lijnen et al (1984) found a significant negative correlation between the anticoagulant activity of heparin and the plasma level of HRG, and suggested that HRG modulates the anticoagulant activity of heparin in humans to an extent that may be clinically relevant. Niwa et al (1985) have suggested that HRG may also modulate in plasma the antithrombin activity of HCII in the presence of heparin or dermatan sulphate.

Proteins released by heparin

Injection of heparin leads to release of several proteins which are normally bound to vascular endothelial cells, probably via heparan sulphate molecules. The major proteins to consider are lipase enzymes, the tissue factor pathway inhibitor (TFPI), and fibrinolytic enzymes. The lipase enzymes, lipoprotein lipase (LPL) and hepatic lipase (HL), normally act in concert at the vascular endothelium to metabolize triglyceride particles and their remnants. Their release into the blood by heparin injection results in a derangement of normal lipoprotein metabolism, with an increase of plasma free fatty acids. Although this does not appear to have any acute adverse effects, prolonged use of high doses of heparin could result in depletion of lipase stores and hence decreased triglyceride clearance; such changes have been observed in patients undergoing extensive renal dialysis (Chan et al 1980). Most studies with LMW heparin have shown decreased lipase release compared to UFH (Kakkar et al 1982, Persson et al 1987), though one LMW heparin, still under development, is apparently an exception (Harenberg et al 1985).

Studies in our laboratory indicated an association between release of lipase, especially HL, and the non-neutralizable anti-Xa activity which appears in vivo after heparin injection (Barrowcliffe et al 1979); preparations of purified HL themselves displayed anti-Xa activity (Gray et al 1987). However, more recent observations suggest that TFPI (also called extrinsic pathway inhibitor, EPI, and lipoprotein-associated inhibitor, LACI) may be responsible for this 'extra' anti-Xa activity. TFPI, as well as inhibiting the tissue factor/factor VII complex, also binds to and inhibits factor Xa directly (Broze et al 1988), is released by heparin or LMW heparin injection (Sandset et al 1988, Lindahl et al 1991), and appears as a contaminant in some preparations of HL (Schmidt et al 1991). The release of TFPI could well be an important part of the antithrombotic action of heparin and LMW heparin in vivo.

A number of studies have claimed to show an enhanced fibrinolytic effect after injection of heparin or LMW heparin, possibly by release of t-PA from the vascular endothelium (Vinazzer et al 1982, Vairel et al 1983). However, most of these studies have failed to take account of the normal diurnal rhythm of the fibrinolytic system. Eriksson et al (1988) found that the changes in fibrinolytic parameters found after injection of heparin or a LMW heparin were repeated exactly when these drugs were replaced by saline, and could be explained by fluctuations in measurements during the day. There is some evidence for a genuine increase in t-PA antigen on more long-term administration of UFH (Arnesen et al 1987), but the effect is very small, and overall the effects of UFH and LMW heparin on fibrinolysis are unlikely to make a significant contribution to their antithrombotic properties.

INTERACTION WITH CELLS

Interaction of heparin and LMW heparin with platelets is considered in the section on thrombocytopenia (p. 1432). The other major cell type of importance for heparin is endothelial cells. The direct interaction of endothelial cells (EC) with heparin has been reviewed by Tobelem (1989). Binding is slow and saturable, reaching equilibrium after 4 hours. Two binding sites have been described, one with a K_d of 1.37 μM, and the other having higher affinity, K_d 0.12 μM. The binding is different according to the source of EC, the microvascular cells having highest affinity with a K_d of 0.025 μM; this is probably relevant for the pharmacokinetics of heparin and LMW heparin.

The binding is dependent on molecular weight; for any heparin, the high molecular weight molecules are preferentially selected. Several LMW heparins have been found to have much lower affinity; for CY 216 50% binding required 15 μM, and CY 222 gave a maximum of 30% binding at 100 μM. When attached to the endothelial cell surface, heparin appears to lose most of its anticoagulant activity. Furthermore, a proportion of the bound molecules are internalized on more extensive incubation, and this internalized fraction can eventually be secreted in a depolymerized form; it is possible that this phenomenon could, at least partly, account for the increase in anti-Xa/anti-IIa activity with time after subcutaneous injection. The lower affinity of LMW heparin for endothelial cells is an important factor in the improved pharmacokinetic properties of this drug, as compared to UFH.

ASSAYS AND STANDARDIZATION

Assay methods

A wide variety of assay methods has been used by manufacturer and control authorities to assess the potency of both UFH and LMW heparin, and these are reviewed in detail elsewhere (Barrowcliffe 1989, Barrowcliffe et al 1992). Broadly speaking, these assays can be divided into two types; global and specific. In the global assays, such as APTT and pharmacopoeial assays, the ability of heparin to interfere with several stages in the coagulation cascade is assessed, usually by measurement of clotting times under defined conditions. In the specific assays, i.e. anti-Xa and anti-IIa methods, potentiation of ATIII inhibition of a single enzyme is measured. Either plasma or purified ATIII can be used, and residual enzyme can be measured by its clotting activity or by a chromogenic substrate. For anti-Xa activity a variety of methods are used, but for anti-IIa activity the amidolytic assay with purified ATIII predominates, though prolongation of thrombin time is used more extensively for clinical monitoring. The majority of manufacturers of LMW heparin now use anti-Xa and anti-IIa amidolytic methods with ATIII, and these are the methods recommended by the European Pharmacopoeia (Pharmeuropa 1991).

Standards

An International Standard (IS) for UFH has existed since 1942; it has been replaced infrequently and the current standard, the 4th, was established in 1983 (Thomas et al 1984). Standardization of potency of UFH presents no major problems; when different samples are assayed against the IS by a wide variety of assay methods the results agree to within 5% (Thomas et al 1984). This is not the case with LMW heparin, however, which showed very large discrepancies between different assay methods when assayed against the IS for UFH in a number of laboratories (Barrowcliffe et al 1985). In addition to these method differences, there was also large variability between the results from different laboratories using the same method, and a pronounced tendency for the dose–response lines of the LMW heparins to be non-parallel with that of the UFH standard, rendering the assays statistically invalid.

These problems were shown to be largely resolved by establishing one preparation of LMW heparin as a reference standard against which the other preparations could be compared, and the first International Standard for LMW heparin was established in 1986 (WHO Technical Report Series 1987), after a large-scale collaborative study involving 24 laboratories in 12 countries (Barrowcliffe et al 1988).

The extent of disagreement between potencies of LMW heparin by different methods is illustrated in Table 64.4, which summarizes the potencies of the proposed LMW heparin standard when assayed against the IS for UFH. Clearly it would be impractical to issue a standard with six different potencies, and it was decided to combine all the anti-Xa results into a single figure representing the anti-Xa value of the standard, and all the 'thrombin group' assays, including APTT, into another separate figure representing the anti-IIa activity. Results from these two collaborative studies demonstrate that the use of a LMW heparin standard for assay of other LMW heparin preparations gives much closer agreement between laboratories and between methods, and this has been conformed in our laboratory by comparative assays on the various products with the manufacturers of LMW heparins.

Relevance to events in vivo

One of the major unresolved questions for LMW heparin is the relationship between its various in vitro activities and its antithrombotic action in vivo. Recent studies by the groups of Ofosu and Hemker have emphasized the importance of the anti-IIa activity of LMW heparins for their ability to inhibit thrombin generation (see p. 1422), and have suggested that their anti-Xa activity may be less relevant to their antithrombotic action in vivo. If this were true one might expect that the dosages of the different products would be more comparable when expressed as anti-IIa activity than anti-Xa activity. However this is not in fact the case; dosages of the five major clinical products for prophylaxis of DVT cover a fairly narrow range, from 2000–3500 IU (1.7-fold) when assayed for anti-Xa activity against the LMW heparin IS, whereas the range by anti-IIa assays is much wider, being more than five-fold. It is possible that modified anti-IIa methods, or thrombin generation assays, might give a better correlation with in vivo events, but in the meantime the majority of manufacturers continue to assess the dosage of their products by anti-Xa assays.

Table 64.4 Potencies of international LMW heparin standard

Method	No of laboratories	Potencies (IU/ampoule) Range	Mean	Overall means
Anti-Xa amidolytic plasma	19	1023–3197	1795	1680
Anti-Xa amidolytic ATIII	8	756–1683	1194	
Anti-Xa clotting	9	1238–4143	2209	
APTT	9	404–1000	561	
Thrombin inhibition amidolytic	10	523–1017	735	665
Thrombin time	4	532–811	714	

Data from Barrowcliffe et al 1988.
All potencies are means of at least four independent assays carried out in each laboratory against the IS for unfractionated heparin.

Because of this uncertainty about the relevance of current in vitro assays, particularly anti-Xa assays, to events in vivo, it has been suggested that comparisons between products on the basis of in vitro assays against the LMW heparin standard could be misleading (Hemker 1989).

Here the limitations of in vitro standardization must be stressed, the most important one being the difference between potency and efficacy. Potency is the biological activity determined in vitro and represents an estimate of the amount of active principle. Efficacy is the therapeutic effect in vivo and has to be determined by clinical observation. The fact that two preparations have similar activities in vitro, with a particular assay method, does not guarantee equivalency in vivo. The relationship between in vitro activities and in vivo effects must be built up over many years of accumulated clinical experience with LMW heparins, as has been the case in the past with UFH. However, in order to determine this relationship it is essential to be able to measure in vitro activities reproducibly and to compare products on a common scale. This will not be the case if different units are used for different products or if some products are prescribed only by dry weight. Standardization of LMW heparins in vitro therefore has an important contribution to make in defining the relationship between their in vitro and in vivo effects.

Monitoring

It is generally accepted that monitoring of UFH when given subcutaneously for prophylaxis of DVT is unnecessary, but high-dose intravenous therapy with UFH is usually monitored because of the danger of haemorrhage. The APTT method is used predominantly and, despite the lack of standardization of this test, a therapeutic range of 1.5–2.5 times the normal control value is widely used.

For LMW heparin, routine monitoring of prophylactic treatment is also unnecessary, but has been useful in clinical trials, particularly some of the early trials where dosages of LMW heparin were too high. For instance Levine et al (1989a) found a therapeutic range of 0.1–0.2 IU/ml when measuring activity by anti-Xa assay in blood taken 12 hours after subcutaneous injection of enoxaparin; patients whose level was below 0.1 IU/ml showed a statistically significant increase in thrombosis, whereas above 0.2 IU/ml there was a significant increase in wound haematomata. In another study, a high incidence of bleeding was associated with anti-Xa levels of around 0.4–0.5 IU/ml (Koller et al 1986), but APTT values in these patients were prolonged by only a few seconds at the most. Since prolongation of the APTT is thought to reflect primarily inhibition of the thrombin feedback loops (Ofosu & Barrowcliffe et al 1990), it appears that this mechanism may not be as important for the in vivo actions of LMW heparin as is often claimed. The same would appear to hold true for the use of LMW heparin in treatment of established DVT, where therapeutic effects have been observed with anti-Xa levels of 0.5–1.0 IU/ml and relatively little prolongation of the APTT (Bratt et al 1990). Whatever the theroretical arguments, anti-Xa assays are the only practical way of measuring the concentration of LMW heparin in the blood and appear to give useful clinical information in some circumstances.

CLINICAL USE OF HEPARIN AND LOW MOLECULAR WEIGHT HEPARIN

Heparin

Heparin is used clinically in four main ways:

1. In low dosage, by subcutaneous injection, for the prophylaxis of venous thrombosis
2. In standard dosage, intravenously, for the treatment of thrombosis in arteries and veins
3. In standard dosage, subcutaneously, for the prophylaxis and treatment of venous thromboembolism
4. As an anticoagulant for maintaining the fluidity of the blood in extracorporeal circulations, such as heart-lung machines, or in renal dialysis.

It is important to differentiate the purposes for which heparin is used therapeutically. The differing role of heparin in prophylaxis, as opposed to treatment, of disease can be best understood in relation to the central role of thrombin (see Ch. 20). When heparin is used for prophylaxis, thrombin generation is prevented. However, in acute thrombosis, there is the additional requirement of neutralizing thrombin that has already been formed, as well as of preventing further generation of thrombin. While the effective dose for preventing deep vein thrombosis (DVT) is usually 10 000 IU given subcutaneously daily in divided dosages, the dose required to control established venous thromboembolism is higher (25 000–40 000 IU) given intravenously or subcutaneously. (Table 64.5).

ATIII levels may be reduced in patients given intravenous heparin. For example, in 26 patients given 20 000–30 000 units daily for several days, Marciniak & Gockerman (1977) reported a considerable progressive reduction in antigenic protein, and suggested that ATIII depletion

Table 64.5 Clinical uses of heparin, after Hirsh 1991

Condition	Effective heparin regimen
Venous thromboembolism	
Prophylaxis of deep venous thrombosis and pulmonary embolism	5000 U subcutaneously every 8 or 12 h, or adjusted low-dose heparin*
Treatment of deep venous thrombosis	Intravenous bolus of 5000 U, followed by 30 000–35 000 U/24 h by intravenous infusion or 35 000–40 000 U/24 h subcutaneously, adjusted to maintain APTT at 1.5 to 2.5 times control value**
Coronary heart disease	
Unstable angina: after thrombolytic therapy (tPA) (patency)	Intravenous bolus of 5000 U, followed by 24 000 U/24 h by intravenous infusion, adjusted to maintain APTT at 1.5 to 2.5 times control value**
Acute myocardial infarction:	
Prevention of mural thrombosis	12 500 U, subcutaneously twice a day (fixed dose)
Prevention of death and reinfarction	Intravenous bolus of 2000 U, 12 500 U subcutaneously twice a day (fixed dose)

* 3500 U of heparin subcutaneously every 8 h, adjusted to an APTT in the upper normal range.
** Equivalent to a heparin level of 0.2–0.4 U/ml by protamine titration or 0.35–0.7 U/ml according to the level of inhibition of factor Xa.

may underline the thromboembolic complications that are sometimes encountered during heparin therapy. Kakkar et al (1980), while confirming the fall in ATIII during intravenous heparin therapy, found that the same dose of heparin given subcutaneously did not lead to ATIII depletion. In prophylaxis against DVT, and also when the acute phase of thrombosis is over, high doses of heparin may not only be unnecessary, but also undesirable in that they expose patients to the twin hazards of haemorrhage and depleted ATIII concentrations. On the other hand, Hull et al (1982) found that only when sufficient subcutaneous heparin was given to prolong the APTT to 1.5 times control levels was heparin an effective drug in the long-term prevention of recurrent thromboembolism. Under these conditions, heparin was as effective as warfarin, and associated with less bleeding.

Prophylaxis of deep vein thrombosis (DVT)

In 1988, Collins et al published an overview of results of randomized trials in general, orthopaedic, and urological surgery, and concluded that there was a reduction in fatal pulmonary embolism and venous thrombosis by perioperative administration of subcutaneous heparin (UFH). In a review of more than 70 randomized trials in 16 000 patients, they concluded that the use of subcutaneous heparin can prevent about half of all pulmonary emboli and about two thirds of all deep-vein thromboses. The reduction in deaths attributed to pulmonary embolism was striking, with 19 deaths in patients receiving heparin, as compared to 55 deaths in control patients

($P < 0.001$). This reduction in mortality was not offset by any increase in deaths due to other causes, and therefore total mortality was also reduced significantly. They concluded that a fixed dose of subcutaneous heparin administered every 12 hours will prevent about half the pulmonary emboli occurring after many types of surgery, without producing any substantial increase in serious bleeding. However, in their meta analysis, the authors noted clear and consistent evidence for an increased risk of bleeding after administration of subcutaneous heparin (overall, 419 episodes in the heparin group versus 244 in the control group) in some 13 500 patients for whom bleeding data were available. The number of fatal haemorrhages was eight in the heparin group and six in the control group.

This important meta analysis has highlighted the case for prophylaxis in patients following surgical operations. There can be no doubt that postoperative thromboembolism can be very largely prevented by prophylaxis with low-dose heparin, with only a slight increase in bleeding risk. This conclusion has led to a clear shift in perspective, so that those clinicians who do not employ some form of effective prophylaxis have now to justify their position.

Treatment of deep vein thrombosis (DVT)

The initial treatment of DVT has usually been carried out by either continuous or intermittent bolus injections of UFH by the intravenous route. In a randomized double-blind trial in 115 patients with acute proximal deep vein thrombosis (Hull et al 1986), continuous intravenous heparin was compared with intermittent subcutaneous heparin. Recurrent venous thromboembolism developed in 19.3% of patients receiving subcutaneous heparin as compared to 5.2% in patients receiving continuous intravenous heparin ($P = 0.024$). 63.2% of patients receiving subcutaneous heparin, as compared to 29.3% of patients receiving intravenous heparin, had a subtherapeutic response during the initial 24 hours or more (defined as an activated partial thromboplastin time response less than 1.5 times the control value). In both groups, recurrences were essentially confined to those patients who had an initial subtherapeutic anticoagulant response to treatment. The authors concluded that their data suggested a relation between the effectiveness of heparin and the levels of anticoagulation achieved, with this relationship explaining the observed failure of the subcutaneous regimen.

In a study by Walker et al (1987), patients receiving subcutaneous heparin showed more lysis of existing thrombi and propagation prevention than patients receiving intravenous heparin. In 49 patients receiving subcutaneous calcium heparin, two showed an increase in thrombus size, while eight showed complete lysis. In contrast, in 47 patients who received intravenous sodium heparin, thrombi increased in size in 13 while only one patient showed complete lysis ($P < 0.01$). These results differ sharply from those of Hull et al (1986), whose recurrences occurred in patients with an initial subtherapeutic anticoagulant response. Walker et al (1987) had no difficulty in maintaining their patients within the therapeutic anticoagulant range. Pini et al (1990) studied 271 patients with acute symptomatic deep vein thrombosis who were randomly assigned to receive either intermittent subcutaneous heparin or continuous heparin infusions for 6–10 days. In relation to clinical improvement, pulmonary embolism and major bleeding complications, there was no significant difference between the two groups. The authors concluded that subcutaneous intermittent therapy twice daily had a comparable efficacy to continuous intravenous heparin in the treatment of DVT.

Several studies have now shown that satisfactory results can be obtained by the subcutaneous injection of heparin twice daily with the obvious advantage of simplifying treatment and, where appropriate, permitting home treatment (Andersson et al 1982, Walker et al 1987, Pini et al 1990). In a meta-analysis of eight clinical trials comparing subcutaneous with intravenous heparin administration in patients with documented DVT, Hommes et al (1991) found the overall relative risk for efficacy (prevention of extension and recurrence) of subcutaneous versus intravenous heparin to be 0.62 (95% confidence interval (CI): 0.39–0.98). For safety (defined as major haemorrhage), the figure was 0.79 (95% CI: 0.42–1.48). Their analysis of these studies showed therefore that subcutaneously administered heparin twice daily is probably more effective and at least as safe as continuous intravenous heparin.

The vexed question of the duration of heparin treatment in patients with acute proximal venous thrombosis was examined by Hull et al (1990). In many centres, treatment of DVT is begun with a course of intravenous heparin, and continued for 10 days. Warfarin is added after some days and then continued for several months. Hull et al carried out a randomized, double-blind trial in 199 patients, comparing a 5-day course of continuous intravenous heparin (with warfarin begun on the 1st day), with a 10-day course of heparin (with warfarin begun on the 5th day). Objectively documented recurrent venous thromboembolism was 7% in both groups, while major bleeding episodes were also similar in both groups. The authors concluded that a 5-day course of heparin is as effective as a 10-day course in the treatment of DVT, with the obvious ensuing advantages for the patient. If confirmed by other studies, it would seem logical for this shorter regimen of heparin to be widely adopted in the future.

Treatment of coronary artery disease

Heparin is widely used in the treatment of coronary artery

disease, and a meta-analysis of studies carried out in patients with acute myocardial infarction who were given neither aspirin nor thrombolytic drugs found a reduction in mortality of 17% in patients given heparin, with a reduction of 22% in reinfarction (MacMahon et al 1988). More recently, there have been several studies examining the patency of the coronary arteries after thrombolytic therapy in patients also given heparin. Overall, these results suggest that heparin given in an intravenous dose of 5 000 IU, followed by 1 000 IU/hour, increases patency during the initial period after treatment, presumably by preventing rethrombosis (Table 64.5). In the European Coronary Study Group 6 trial (de Bono et al 1992), all patients were given aspirin, and patency was 80% in the group who also received heparin, whereas patency was 75% in the group who received aspirin alone ($P < 0.01$). Heparin added to a therapeutic regimen seems more effective when patients have been treated with streptokinase as opposed to tPA, which may be related to the greater anticoagulant effect produced by streptokinase combined with the action of heparin. For example, in the International Study Group (Gissi-2) trial (1990) the mortality rates were identical among those who received heparin in addition to tPA, as compared to those who did not (5.9% in both groups, after excluding patients who died before heparin was started). On the other hand, of the patients who received streptokinase and heparin the mortality rate was 7.9%, whereas it was 9.2% among the patients who received streptokinase alone. In a collaborative study comparing early intravenous heparin with oral aspirin in patients treated with tPA for coronary thrombolysis, coronary patency rates were higher with early concomitant systemic heparin treatment (88%) than with concomitant low-dose oral aspirin (52%) (Hsia et al 1990).

The precise contribution of heparin, as compared to aspirin and thrombolytic drugs, in patients with various manifestations of coronary artery disease has yet to be clearly defined. Such patients receive a cocktail of drugs, and it becomes increasingly difficult to isolate the role of a single drug, among many. However, the evidence suggests that the addition of heparin to the therapeutic regimen in patients with coronary artery disease makes a modest but significant contribution.

Low molecular weight heparin (LMW heparin)

In 1976, Johnson and colleagues first showed that a low molecular weight heparin (LMW heparin) produced by gel filtration gave higher anti-Xa blood levels following subcutaneous injection in volunteers, than did unfractionated heparin. The molecular weight of LMW heparin, which can be produced by a variety of techniques (Barrowcliffe et al 1992), varies between 3500 and 9000. LMW heparins all share the ability to enhance selectively the inhibition of certain proteases, and in particular factor Xa, while having a relatively weak effect on thrombin inhibition. Unfractionated heparins (UFH) have specific activities of 150–190 IU/mg, by whatever assay is used to assess potency. In contrast, a typical LMW heparin would have a potency by an APTT assay of around 50 IU/mg, but a potency of perhaps 120 IU/mg by an anti-Xa assay. The anti-Xa/APTT ratio for UFH is therefore always close to unity, while the ratio for a typical LMW heparin will be two or more.

Human pharmacology studies

There have been numerous studies in which the effect of LMW heparins has been studied in human volunteers (see Barrowcliffe et al 1992). Following subcutaneous injection, heparin activity as measured by anti-Xa assays is invariably higher following LMW heparins than after UFH. The pharmacokinetics of subcutaneously administered LMW heparin are quite different from UFH and, with a half life about twice that of UFH, the low molecular weight material has much greater bioavailability. However, Thomas & Merton (1982) pointed out that, while LMW heparin gave high and prolonged heparin activity by anti-Xa assay, heparin activity by sensitive APTT and calcium thrombin time assays was also at least as high as occurred following UFH, at comparable dry weight dosage. On the basis of their data, they saw no reason to anticipate a lower incidence of haemorrhagic side-effects following the use of LMW heparin.

Clinical studies

Kakkar and colleagues (Kakkar et al 1982, Kakkar & Murray 1985), in early clinical trials, found that the effect on the anti-Xa blood levels in patients given LMW heparin was sufficiently prolonged to enable only a single daily dose to be given. Further clinical use demonstrated that a single daily dose of LMW heparin is at least as effective as UFH in the prevention of postoperative DVT (Encke & Breddin 1988). The meta-analysis of Collins et al (1988) demonstrating the protective effect of low-dose subcutaneous heparin provides a useful background against which LMW heparin can be compared. If a twice-daily injection of 5000 IU of UFH is considered 'standard therapy' for the prophylaxis of postoperative DVT, how can these results be improved upon? There are three main ways in which this could happen, namely LMW heparin could be safer (less bleeding), more effective (fewer DVT and pulmonary embolism (PE)) or more convenient (less than two injections a day). In a recent important meta-analysis of LMW heparin prophylaxis in patients undergoing surgery (Nurmohamed et al 1992), the relative risk (LMW heparin versus UFH) was 0.74

(95% CI: 0.65–0.86), 0.43 (95% CI: 0.26–0.72) and 0.98 (95% CI: 0.69–1.40) for deep vein thrombosis, pulmonary embolism and major bleeding, respectively. When the analysis for the general surgery studies was limited to those of strong methodology, the benefit risk ratio was less favourable (relative risk for DVT 0.91, 95% CI: 0.68–1.23, for major bleeding 1.32, 95% CI: 0.69–2.56). However, the study also found that in orthopaedic patients the absolute benefit was greater, and LMW heparin may well be a superior drug to UFH for patients undergoing total hip replacement. This is especially true for proximal DVT, where the incidence in patients given LMW heparin is as low as 3–4%, whereas in patients treated with UFH the reported incidence varies from 13–18%. Overall, the incidence of DVT is reduced by approximately a half, as compared to conventional treatment with UFH (Leyvraz et al 1991).

In a large Canadian multicentre study (Levine et al 1991), although the improvement in patients given LMW heparin did not reach statistical significance, nevertheless the results overall favoured the use of LMW heparin. Another randomized, double-blind Canadian study (Leclerc et al 1992) was carried out in patients undergoing major knee surgery. Patients received 30 mg of Enoxaparin subcutaneously every 12 hours, and the incidence of DVT detected by venography fell from 65% in the placebo group to 19% in patients treated with LMW heparin. Bleeding complications were identical, and the authors concluded that a fixed dose regimen of Enoxaparin, started postoperatively, is an effective and safe regimen for reducing the frequency of DVT after major knee surgery. LMW heparin represents a significant therapeutic advance for the prophylaxis of DVT in orthopaedic patients, who have always been a considerable challenge for prophylaxis with UFH (Thomas 1992). The added advantage of LMW heparin is that the dose need not be monitored, and effective prophylaxis can be achieved with either a single daily dose given on a weight-adjusted basis (Leyvraz et al 1991), or a fixed dose given twice a day (Leclerc et al 1992).

Several studies have compared LMW heparin with UFH in the treatment of established venous thrombosis (Albada et al 1989, Bratt et al 1990, Duroux and Beclere 1991, Hull et al 1992). Overall, the results have been favourable, in that LMW heparins administered in a fixed or weight-adjusted dose are at least as effective as UFH, with a trend in favour of LMW heparins, particularly in relation to preventing proximal vein thrombosis. Of particular interest is the recent evidence that established deep vein thrombosis can be successfully managed by weight-adjusted doses of LMW heparin, without laboratory monitoring. For example, in a multicentre, double-blind clinical trial, Hull et al (1992) compared fixed-dose subcutaneous LMW heparin (Logiparin), given once daily with adjusted-dose intravenous heparin given by continuous infusion for the initial treatment of proximal vein thrombosis. The patients given LMW heparin received 175 anti-Xa units per kg body weight once every 24 hours. Out of a total of 432 patients, 2.8% of those who received LMW heparin and 6.9% of those who received intravenous heparin had new episodes of venous thromboembolism (P = 0.07). Only one patient on LMW heparin had major bleeding as compared to 11 patients given UFH. Hull et al (1992) concluded that LMW heparin is at least as effective and as safe as intravenous UFH, and more convenient to administer. In another recent randomized multicentre study of 149 patients, with phlebographically demonstrated proximal and/or distal DVT (Lopaciuk et al 1992), half of the patients received Fraxiparine twice a day subcutaneously (92 anti-Xa IU/kg), while the other patients received 5000 IU of calcium heparin twice a day, adjusted daily to maintain the APTT between 1.5 and 2.5 times the patient's basal value. Both types of treatment lasted 10 days, with oral anticoagulation introduced after a week, and continued for at least 3 months. The mean phlebographic score after 10 days of treatment was significantly improved in both groups as compared to baseline values, but was not significantly different between the two groups. The authors concluded that subcutaneous fixed dose LMW heparin on a weight-adjusted basis is safe and at least as effective as subcutaneous adjusted dose UFH. The important practical advantage of LMW heparin, demonstrated again by both these studies, is that laboratory monitoring is not required, thus facilitating treatment on an out-patient basis.

Heparin versus low molecular weight heparin

Unfractionated heparin (UFH) has been an essential drug for over 50 years, whereas low molecular weight heparin (LMW heparin) has only recently become generally available, and indeed is still not a licensed drug in the USA (1992). The main change in the use of UFH in recent years has been the realization that satisfactory control of some thrombotic conditions can be achieved with subcutaneous administration, and that intravenous injection of the drug is unnecessary. This greatly simplifies the management of patients with established deep vein thrombosis. While a strong case can be made for treating acute pulmonary embolism with intravenous UFH (if only to ensure that the drug enters rapidly into the circulation), once the patient has stabilized and the immediate crisis is over, then it may be appropriate to switch to subcutaneous administration and/or oral anticoagulation (see Ch. 65).

The precise indications for LMW heparin are still evolving, although it is already apparent the main advantage of this drug in the prophylaxis of venous thromboembolic disease is one of convenience, in that adequate control of the disease can be achieved with a single daily subcutaneous injection. Furthermore, laboratory monitoring is not required, although there is evidence that the drug is best administered on a weight-related basis (Leyvraz et al 1991, Hull et al 1992, Lopaciuk et al 1992). In patients undergoing total hip replacement, there is increasing evidence that LMW heparin may be more effective than UFH (Thomas 1992). However, there is no convincing evidence that LMW heparin is associated with a lower incidence of haemorrhagic complications than UFH. Indeed, the balance of evidence clearly points to the two types of heparin having closely comparable haemorrhagic complications. The precise role of LMW heparin in the treatment of other thrombotic conditions, such as acute myocardial infarction or established venous thrombosis, is still a matter for further clinical studies (Hirsh & Levine 1991).

Finally, it needs to be acknowledged that LMW heparin is currently a more expensive option for prophylaxis of DVT than is UFH. In the UK, the cost of a 5-day course of prophylaxis is approximately 2–3 times greater for LMW heparin, depending on the particular brand used (Drugs and Therapeutic Bulletin 1992). In terms of providing prophylaxis for thousands of surgical patients, this cost differential becomes a significant item in a health care budget. However, in terms of the individual patient, and the overall costs of a major surgical operation, many would take the view that the increased expenditure is trivial, and more than compensated for by the added convenience of LMW heparin for both patients and nursing staff.

Complications of heparin treatment

Haemorrhagic complications

The main adverse reaction with heparin treatment is bleeding (Hirsh 1991). This complication of treatment may be getting worse, primarily because of the increasing age of patients and the growing risk of drug interactions (Walker & Jick 1980). Although the risk of haemorrhage is real enough, it is not entirely unpredictable. For example, the various ways of giving heparin have to be separated. The risk of haemorrhage is small when heparin is given subcutaneously in low doses for prophylaxis. Apart from a slight increase in the incidence of wound haematoma in heparin-treated patients, there was no significant difference in the incidence of haemorrhagic complications between the treated and control groups in a large multicentre trial evaluating the efficacy of low-dose calcium heparin in postoperative patients (Kakkar 1975).

The position is different when heparin is given intravenously for the treatment of established disease, and the incidence of bleeding can range as high as 33% (Glazier & Crowell 1976, Mant et al 1977). Even here, however, there are certain guidelines that help to identify those patients most at risk of a haemorrhagic complication. For example, elderly women seem more liable to bleed when given heparin (Holm et al 1985) and indeed, in one series, the incidence of haemorrhagic complications was 50% in women over 60-years-old (Jick et al 1968). Walker & Jick (1980) found that bleeding was a dose-related phenomenon that occurred most commonly among women, severely ill patients, and patients who received aspirin during heparin therapy. It is of great importance whether or not haemostasis is normal at the start of treatment. In a study of 114 patients receiving heparin, Pitney et al (1970) found the incidence of haemorrhage to be 7.6% when haemostasis was normal, but it was 50% in patients with defective haemostasis. The presence of uraemia or thrombocytopenia was particularly associated with haemorrhagic complications. In the UPET study (1973), the overall incidence of haemorrhage was 27% in the heparin-treated patients, although the most common location for haemorrhage was the cutdown site.

Salzman et al (1975) also separated a high-risk category for haemorrhagic complications, defining their high-risk group as patients who had recent surgery, thrombocytopenia, uraemia, prior history of a bleeding tendency, intramuscular injections, or the concurrent administration of a platelet-suppressive drug. Of such patients who received heparin, 25% experienced major bleeding, whereas in patients with none of these associated factors the incidence of major bleeding was only 11%. In high-risk patients the danger of an adverse drug reaction must be carefully weighed against the anticipated clinical benefits.

Using four different assays, Holm et al (1985) found no significant difference in median heparin activity between patients with minor bleeding and those with no bleeding. However, with patients in whom there was major bleeding, there were significant differences in two of the assay methods (chromogenic substrate and calcium thrombin time).

Thrombocytopenia

The effect of heparin on platelets in vitro has been variously reported as enhancing, reducing or having no effect on platelet aggregation (O'Brien et al 1969, Eika 1972, 1973, Thomson et al 1973). This variation in response is likely to be a reflection of differing test systems and different heparins. Salzman et al (1980) reported that porcine intestinal mucosa heparin induced aggregation of platelets in citrated platelet-rich plasma, and enhanced platelet aggregation and serotonin secretion induced by other agents. Fractions of high molecular weight (average 20 000) were more reactive with platelets than were fractions of low molecular weight (7000). Salzman and colleagues suggested that there were two types of binding site on the heparin molecule: one that binds either to

ATIII or to platelets but has a higher affinity for the former, and a second that binds preferentially to platelets. In LMW heparin, the former binding sites appear to predominate in the high anti-thrombin affinity subfractions so that, if exposed to anti-thrombin, these molecules are unlikely to react with platelets. Thus, the formation of an antithrombin-heparin complex appears to protect platelets from aggregation by heparin. Dunn et al (1984) studied the availability of fibrinogen receptors on platelets after ADP stimulation, and found that unfractionated heparin increased the binding of fibrinogen on ADP-treated platelets. However, low molecular weight heparin fractions did not significantly increase this binding.

Clinically, thrombocytopenia is an important complication of heparin therapy. Transient thrombocytopenia following heparin has been recognized for many years (Gollub & Ulin 1962). Although the incidence of heparin-associated thrombocytopenia has been reported as high as 31% (Bell et al 1976), this figure is almost certainly too high, and a more likely figure is between <1% to 6% (Godal 1980). While thrombocytopenia may occur after either intravenous or subcutaneous injections of heparin, preparations of beef lung heparin have been reported to cause thrombocytopenia more often than porcine mucosal heparin (Bell & Royal 1980, Godal 1980, King & Kelton 1984). The declining use of beef lung heparin should lead to fewer reports of heparin-induced thrombocytopenia in the future.

Two mechanisms have been reported by which heparin-associated thrombocytopenia develops. A common but mild thrombocytopenia, as an acute transient effect, occurs in 5–30% of patients, beginning on the 2nd or 3rd day of treatment. This thrombocytopenia is of short duration and indeed may be so transient that it is not noticed clinically. This type does not produce symptoms or signs and is only detected if the clinician carries out serial platelet counts (Fratantoni et al 1975, Salzman et al 1980, Chong et al 1982). Delayed onset thrombocytopenia, occurring about a week or so after the commencement of heparin, is a more serious complication. In this syndrome, the patient's plasma contains an antibody which is believed to be heparin-dependent, and causes platelet aggregation in the presence of heparin. Once it has developed, the antibody persists for at least 6 weeks and, if heparin is administered during this period, thrombocytopenia will again develop (Ansell et al 1980, Babcock et al 1976, Silver et al 1983). Heparin administration can also be associated with complement-mediated platelet injury, with consequent thrombocytopenia (Cines et al 1980). Thrombocytopenia developing as a result of a heparin-dependent antibody has important implications, particularly if the patient develops an arterial or venous thrombosis while receiving heparin. A sudden fall in the platelet count 8 days or more after the commencement of heparin is an indication for the immediate withdrawal of the drug, and where possible the presence of antibodies should be confirmed by platelet aggregation tests (Pitney 1983).

Heparin-induced thrombocytopenia is often associated with intravascular thrombosis. This so-called 'white clot' syndrome occurs more frequently in the elderly and in patients with myeloproliferative disorders. The syndrome, which is associated with a high morbidity and mortality, is probably the result of heparin-dependent platelet membrane antibodies formed in predisposed patients (Babcock et al 1976, Rhodes et al 1977, Kapsch et al 1979). It has been suggested that platelet counts should be performed on alternate days on every patient receiving heparin (Pitney 1983).

Although the use of LMW heparin has been recommended when thrombocytopenia occurs during treatment with UFH (Huisse et al 1983), persistent heparin-induced thrombocytopenia can occur despite such treatment (Horellou et al 1984). Nevertheless, there have been several reports that patients with heparin-induced thrombocytopenia have been switched successfully to LMW heparin for further treatment. However, there have been few prospective studies in which the incidence of thrombocytopenia in a group of patients given UFH has been compared with a similar group receiving LMW heparin. One such study was that of Monreal et al (1989) who studied the incidence of thrombocytopenia in 89 consecutive patients with venous thrombosis receiving therapeutic treatment with UFH, 49 patients with hip fracture receiving prophylactic low-dose UFH and 43 patients with hip fracture who received LMW heparin. The hip fracture patients were randomly allocated to receive prophylactically either UFH or LMW heparin (Fragmin). Two patients developed thrombocytopenia while receiving UFH in high dosage but no cases of thrombocytopenia occurred in the two groups of patients on prophylactic heparinization, whether UFH or LMW heparin. The authors also reported that while elevated transaminase levels were frequently seen in patients receiving UFH, whether high-dose or low-dose, only one patient on LMW heparin developed an abnormal alanine transferase level.

In a study of eight patients with a delayed-onset thrombocytopenia induced by heparin, the platelet counts returned to normal values within 3–5 days in six patients given LMW heparin as alternate therapy, while in two patients thrombocytopenia persisted on LMW heparin therapy (Gouault-Heilmann et al 1987). Platelet aggregation tests showed a relationship between the presence or absence of a LMW heparin-dependent platelet aggregating factor in the patients' plasma and the persistence or correction of thrombocytopenia during LMW heparin therapy. The authors concluded that in vitro platelet testing may be a useful guide before substituting a LMW heparin for UFH in patients with heparin-induced thrombocytopenia.

Heparin, LMW heparin, and pregnancy

UFH is widely used for the prophylaxis and treatment of DVT and pulmonary embolism during pregnancy, primarily because UFH does not cross the placental barrier (Flessa et al 1965), and does not have any teratogenic effects (Hall et al 1980). However, UFH is not without risks to the mother and fetus (Howell et al 1983). There has been considerable interest in the use of LMW heparins in pregnancy, for much the same reason as its use in other clinical conditions, namely the convenience of a once daily injection. This is a particularly cogent argument for the use of LMW heparin in pregnancy, having in mind that treatment may be needed for weeks or even months. Of critical importance is the question of whether LMW heparin, like UFH, does not cross the placental barrier, and does not alter fetal coagulation. Several groups have addressed this question and, from both animal and human experiments, it is clear that different LMW heparins do not cross the placenta (Forestier et al 1984, 1987, Andrew et al 1985, Mätzsch 1990, Mätzsch et al 1990), at least at doses that are used clinically (see Ch. 43). The evidence therefore suggests that LMW heparin can be effective in pregnancy for the same indications as UFH, but because of the prolonged half life once daily injections are adequate for most patients.

Osteoporosis

Osteoporosis with spontaneous bone fractures of vertebrae and ribs occasionally complicates prolonged heparin treatment (Avioli 1975). Griffith et al (1965) reported that no symptoms of osteoporosis developed in 107 patients receiving 10 000 units or less of heparin daily for 1 to 5 years. However, in patients who received 15 000–30 000 units daily for 6 months or longer, six out of ten developed spontaneous fractures. De Swiet and colleagues (1983) reported a dose-related demineralization process associated with prophylactic heparin therapy in pregnancy. Prophylaxis with subcutaneous heparin (20 000 IU daily) for more than 25 weeks was particularly associated with demineralization. 12 out of 70 women given heparin during pregnancy developed osteoporosis, and two of them developed multiple fractures of the spine (Dahlman et al 1990). While most cases of osteoporosis develop after relatively prolonged use of heparin, the condition has been reported after as little as 2 months of treatment (Aarskog et al 1980).

Experimental evidence suggests that, if dosed according to similar anti-Xa activity, LMW heparin induces osteoporosis to the same extent as UFH, and in a dose-dependent manner (Mätzsch et al 1990). The pathogenesis of heparin-induced osteoporosis remains unknown, although it is likely to be a direct effect of the drug.

REFERENCES

Aarskog D, Aksues L, Lehmann V 1980 Low 1,25-dihydroxyvitamin D in heparin-induced osteopenia. Lancet 2: 650–651

Albada J, Niewenhuis H K, Sixma J J 1989 Treatment of acute venous thromboembolism with low molecular weight heparin. Circulation 80: 935–939

Anastassiades E, Lane D A, Ireland H, Flynn A, Curtis J R 1989 A low molecular weight heparin ('Fragmin') for routine hemodialysis: a crossover trial comparing three dose regimens with a standard regimen of commercial unfractionated heparin. Clinical Nephrology 32: 290–296

Andersson L-O, Barrowcliffe T W, Holmer E, Johnson E A, Sims G E C 1976 Anticoagulant properties of heparin fractionated by affinity chromatography on matrix-bound antithrombin III and by gel filtration. Thrombosis Research 9: 575–583

Andersson G, Fagrell B, Holmgren K, Johnsson H, Ljumgberg B, Nilsson E, Wilhelmsson S, Zeterquist S 1982 Subcutaneous administration of heparin. A randomized comparison with intravenous administration of heparin to patients with deep vein thrombosis. Thrombosis Research 27: 631–639

Andrew M, Boneu B, Cade J et al 1985 Placental transport of low molecular weight heparin in the pregnant sheep. British Journal of Haematology 59: 103–108

Ansell J, Slepchuk N, Kumar R, Lopez A, Southard L, Deykin D 1980 Heparin induced thrombocytopenia: a prospective study. Thrombosis and Haemostasis 43: 61–65

Arnesen H, Engebretsen L F, Ugland O M, Seljeflot J, Kierulf P 1987 Increased fibrinolytic activity after surgery induced by low dose heparin. Thrombosis Research 45: 553–559

Avioli L V 1975 Heparin-induced ostepenia: an appraisal. Advances in Experimental Medicine and Biology 52: 375–387

Babcock R B, Dumper C W, Scharfman W B 1976 Heparin-induced immune thrombocytopenia. New England Journal of Medicine 295: 237–241

Barrowcliffe T W 1989 Heparin assays and standardisation. In: Lane D A Lindahl U (eds) Heparin. Edward Arnold, London p 393–416

Barrowcliffe T W, Le Shirley Y 1989 The effect of calcium chloride on anti-Xa activity of heparin and its molecular weight fractions. Thrombosis and Haemostasis 62: 950–954

Barrowcliffe T W, Thomas D P 1989 Anticoagulant activities of heparin and fragments. In: Ofosu F A, Danishefsky I, Hirsh J (eds) Heparin and related polysaccharides. Annals of the New York Academy of Sciences 556: 132–145

Barrowcliffe T W, Johnson E A, Eggleton C A, Thomas D P 1978 Anticoagulant activities of lung and mucosal heparins. Thrombosis Research 12: 27–36

Barrowcliffe T W, Johnson E A, Eggleton C A, Kemball-Cook G, Thomas D P 1979 Anticoagulant activities of high and low molecular weight heparin fractions. British Journal of Haematology 41: 573–583

Barrowcliffe T W, Merton R E, Havercroft S J, Thunberg L, Lindahl U, Thomas D P 1984 Low-affinity heparin potentiates the action of high-affinity heparin oligosaccharides. Thrombosis Research 34: 125–133

Barrowcliffe T W, Curtis A D, Tomlinson T P, Hubbard A R, Johnson E A, Thomas D P 1985 Standardisation of low molecular weight heparins: a collaborative study. Thrombosis and Haemostasis 54: 675–679

Barrowcliffe T W, Havercroft S J, Kemball-Cook G, Lindahl U 1987 The effect of Ca^{2+} phospholipid and Factor V on the anti-(Factor Xa) activity of heparin and its high-affinity oligosaccharides. Biochemical Journal 243: 31–37

Barrowcliffe T W, Curtis A D, Johnson E A, Thomas D P 1988 An international standard for low molecular weight heparin. Thrombosis and Haemostasis 60: 1–7

Barrowcliffe T W, Johnson E A, Thomas D P 1992 Low molecular weight heparin. John Wiley, Chichester

Béguin S 1987 Thrombinoscopy — A method for the determination of

prothrombinase activity in plasma, its application to the study of different types of heparin. PhD Thesis, Maastricht
Béguin S, Lindhout T, Hemker H C 1988 The mode of action of heparin in plasma. Thrombosis and Haemostasis 60: 457–462
Béguin S, Lindhout T, Hemker H C 1989a The effect of trace amounts of tissue factor on thrombin generation in platelet rich plasma, its inhibition by heparin. Thrombosis and Haemostasis 61: 25–29
Béguin S, Mardignian J, Lindhout T, Hemker H C 1989b The mode of action of low molecular weight heparin preparation (PK 10169) and two of its major components on thrombin generation in plasma. Thrombosis and Haemostasis 61: 30–34
Béguin S, Wielders S, Lormeau J C, Hemker H C 1992 The mode of action of CY216 and CY222 in plasma. Thrombosis and Haemostasis 67: 33–41
Bell W R, Royall R M 1980 Heparin-associated thrombocytopenia: a comparison of 3 heparin preparations. New England Journal of Medicine 303: 902–907
Bell W R, Tomasulo P A, Alving B M, Duffy T P 1976 Thrombocytopenia occurring during the administration of heparin. A prospective study in 52 patients. Annals of Internal Medicine 85: 155–160
Bergqvist D, Burmark U S, Frisell J, Hallbook T, Lindblad B, Risberg B, Torngren S, Wallin G 1986 Low molecular weight heparin once daily compared with conventional low-dose heparin twice daily. A prospective double-blind multicentre trial on prevention of postoperative thrombosis. British Journal of Surgery 73: 204–208
Bergqvist D, Mätzsch T, Burmark U S, Frisell J, Guilbaud O, Hallbook T, Horn A, Lindhagen A, Ljungner H, Ljungstrom K G, Onarheim H, Risberg B, Torngren S, Ortenwall P 1988 Low molecular weight heparin given the evening before surgery compared with conventional low-dose heparin in prevention of thrombosis. British Journal of Surgery 75: 888–891
Björk I, Olson S T, Shore J D 1989 Molecular mechanisms of the accelerating effect of heparin on the reactions between antithrombin and clotting proteinases. In: Lane D A, Lindahl U (eds) Heparin. Edward Arnold, London, p 229–256
Bratt G, Aberg W, Johansson M, Tornebohm E, Granquist S, Lockner D 1990 Two daily subcutaneous injections of Fragmin as compared with intravenous standard heparin in the treatment of deep vein thrombosis (DVT). Thrombosis and Haemostasis 64: 506–510
Breddin H K 1989 Low molecular weight heparins and bleeding. Seminars in Thrombosis and Haemostasis 15: 401–404
Broze G J Jr, Warren L A, Novotny W F, Higuchi D A, Girard J J, Miletich J P 1988 The lipoprotein-associated coagulation inhibitor that inhibits the factor VII-tissue factor complex also inhibits factor Xa: insight into its possible mechanism of action. Blood 71: 335–343
Caen J P (A French Multicenter Trial) 1988 A randomized double blind study between low molecular heparin (Kabi 2165) and standard heparin in the prevention of deep vein thrombosis in general surgery. Thrombosis and Haemostasis 59: 216–220
Carlstrom A-S, Lieden K, Björk I 1977 Decreased binding of heparin to antithrombin following the interaction between antithrombin and thrombin. Thrombosis Research 11: 785–787
Casu B, Oreste P, Torri G, Zopett G, Choay J, Lormeau J C, Petitou M, Sinay P 1981 The structure of heparin oligosaccharide fragments with high anti-(factor Xa) activity containing the minimal antithrombin III binding sequence. Biochemical Journal 197: 599–609
Chan M K, Varghese Z, Persaud J W, Baillod R A, Moorhead J F. 1980 Fat clearance before and after heparin in chronic renal failure — haemodialysis reduces post-heparin fractional clearance rates of Intralipid. Clinica Chimica Acta 108: 95–101
Choay J, Petitou M, Lormeau J C, Sinay P, Casu B, Gatti G 1983 Structure-activity relationship in heparin; a synthetic pentasaccharide with high affinity for antithrombin III and eliciting high anti-factor Xa activity. Biochemical and Biophysical Research Communications 116: 492–499
Chong B H, Pitney W R, Castaldi P A 1982 Heparin-induced thrombocytopenia: association of thrombotic complications with heparin-dependent IgG antibody that induces thromboxane synthesis and platelet aggregation. Lancet 2: 1246–1248
Cines D B, Kaywin P, Bina M, Tomaski A, Schreiber A D 1980 Heparin-associated thrombocytopenia. New England Journal of Medicine 303: 788–795
Collins R, Scrimgeour A, Yusef S, Peto R 1988 Reduction in fatal pulmonary embolism and venous thrombosis by perioperative administration of subcutaneous heparin. Overview of results of randomized trials in general, orthopedic and urological surgery. New England Journal of Medicine 318: 1162–1173
Colman R W, Scott C F, Pixley R A, DeLa Cadena R A 1989 Effect of heparin on the inhibitions of the contact enzymes. Annals of the New York Academy of Sciences 556: 95–103
Dahlman T, Lindvall N, Hellgren M 1990 Osteopenia in pregnancy during long-term heparin treatment; a radiological study post partum. British Journal of Obstetrics and Gynaecology 97: 221–228
Dawes J, Pumphrey C W, McLaren K M, Prowse C V, Pepper D S 1982 The in vivo release of human platelet factor 4 by heparin. Thrombosis Research 27: 65–76
de Bono D P, Simoons M L, Tijssen J et al 1992 Effect of early intravenous heparin on coronary patency, infarct size, and bleeding complications after alteplase thrombolysis: results of a randomized double blind European Cooperative Study Group trial. British Heart Journal 67: 122–128
Dechavanne M, Ville D, Beruyer M, Trepo F, Dalery F, Clermont N, Lerat J L, Moyen B, Fischer L P, Kher A, Barbier P 1989 Randomized trial of a low molecular weight heparin (Kabi 2165) versus adjusted-dose subcutaneous standard heparin in the prophylaxis of deep-vein thrombosis after elective hip surgery. Haemostasis 1: 5–12
de Swiet M, Dorrington Ward P, Fidler J et al 1983 Prolonged heparin therapy in pregnancy causes bone demineralization. British Journal of Obstetrics and Gynaecology 90: 1129–1134
Diness V, Ostergaard P B 1986 Neutralization of a low molecular weight heparin (LHN-1) and conventional heparin by protamine sulfate in rats. Thrombosis and Haemostasis 56: 318–322
Drugs and Therapeutics Bulletin 1992 Preventing and Treating Deep Vein Thrombosis 30: 11
Dunn F W, Soria C, Thomaidis A et al 1984 Interactions of platelets with standard heparin and low molecular weight fractions. Nouvelle Revue Francais d'Hematologie 26: 249–253
Duroux P, Beclere A 1991 A randomized trial of subcutaneous low molecular weight heparin (CY216) compared with intravenous unfractionated heparin in the treatment of deep vein thrombosis. Thrombosis and Haemostasis 65: 251
Eika C 1972 On the mechanism of platelet aggregation induced by heparin, protamine and polybrene. Scandinavian Journal of Haematology 9: 248–257
Eika C 1973 Anticoagulant and platelet aggregating activities of heparin. Thrombosis Research 2: 349–360
Einarsson R, Andersson L-O 1977 Binding of heparin to human antithrombin III as studied by measurement of tryptophan fluorescence. Biochimica et Biophysica Acta 490: 104–111
Ellis V, Scully M F, Kakkar V V 1986 The acceleration of the inhibition of platelet prothrombinase complex by heparin. Biochemical Journal 233: 161–165
Encke A, Breddin K (European Fraxiparine Study Group) 1988 Comparison of a low molecular weight heparin and unfractionated heparin for the prevention of deep vein thrombosis in patients undergoing abdominal surgery. British Journal of Surgery 75: 1058–1063
Eriksson E, Wolter I M, Christenson B, Stigendal L, Risberg B 1988 Heparin and fibrinolysis — comparison of subcutaneous administration of unfractioned and low molecular weight heparin. Thrombosis and Haemostasis 59: 284–288
European Pharmacopoeia Forum 1991 Low molecular mass heparins, draft monograph. Pharmeuropa Vol 3 (No 3): 161–165
Flessa H C, Kapstrom A B, Glueck H, Will J J 1965 Placental transport of heparin. American Journal of Obstetrics and Gynecology 93: 570–573
Forestier F, Daffos F, Rainaut M, Toulemond F 1987 Low molecular weight heparin (CY 216) does not cross the placenta during the third trimester of pregnancy. Thrombosis and Haemostasis 57: 234
Forestier F, Daffos F, Capella-Pavlovsky M 1984 Low molecular weight heparin (PH 10169) does not cross the placenta during the second trimester of pregnancy. Study by direct fetal blood sapling under ultrasound. Thrombosis Research 34: 557–560

Fratantoni J C, Pollet R, Gralnick H R 1975 Heparin-induced thrombocytopenia: confirmation of diagnosis with in vitro methods. Blood 45: 395–401

Glazier R L, Crowell E B 1976 Randomized prospective trial of continuous vs intermittent heparin therapy. Journal of the American Medical Association 236: 1365–1367

Godal H C 1980 Thrombocytopenia and heparin: report of the International Committee on Haemostasis and Thrombosis. Thrombosis and Haemostasis 43: 222–224

Gollub S, Ulin A W 1962 Heparin-induced thrombocytopenia in man. Journal of Laboratory and Clinical Medicine 59: 430–435

Gouault-Heilmann M, Huet Y, Adnot S, Contant G, Bonnet F, Intrator L, Payen D, Levent M 1987 Low molecular weight heparin fractions as an alternative therapy in heparin-induced thrombocytopenia. Haemostasis 17: 134–140

Gray E, Bengtsson-Olivecrona G, Olivecrona T, Barrowcliffe T W 1987 The anti-Xa activity of human hepatic triglyceride lipase (HTGL). Journal of Laboratory and Clinical Medicine 109: 653–659

Griffith M J 1982 Kinetics of the heparin-enhanced antithrombin III/thrombin reaction. Journal of Biological Chemistry 257: 7360–7365

Griffith G C, Nichols G, Asher J D, Flanagan B 1965 Heparin osteoporosis. Journal of the American Medical Association 193: 91–94

Hall J G, Pauli R M, Wilson K M 1980 Maternal and fetal sequelae of anticoagulation during pregnancy. American Journal of Medicine 68: 122–140

Harenberg J, Gnasso A, de Vries J X, Zimmermann R, Augstin J 1985 Anticoagulant and lipolytic effects of a low molecular weight heparin fraction. Thrombosis Research 39: 683–692

Harenberg J, Giese Ch, Knodler A, Zimmermann R, Schettler G 1986 Neutralisierung von niedermolekularem Heparin Kabi 2165 mit Protaminchlorid. Klinische Wochenschrift 64: 1171–1175

Harenberg J, Kallenbach B, Martin U, Dempfle C E, Zimmermann R, Kübler W, Heene D L 1990 Randomized controlled study of heparin and low molecular weight heparin for prevention of deep-vein thrombosis in medical patients. Thrombosis Research 59: 639–650

Hemker H C 1987 The mode of action of heparin in plasma. In: Verstraete M, Vermylen J, Lijnen R, Arnout J (eds) Thrombosis and haemostasis. Leuven University Press, Leuven, p 17–36

Hemker H C 1989 A standard for low molecular weight heparin? Editorial. Haemostasis 19: 1–4

Hirsh J 1991 Heparin. New England Journal of Medicine 324: 1565–1574

Hirsh J, Levine M N 1992 Low Molecular Weight Heparin. Blood 79: 117

Holm H A, Abildgaard U, Kalvenes S 1985 Heparin assays and bleeding complications in treatment of deep venous thrombosis with particular reference to retroperitoneal bleeding. Thrombosis and Haemostasis 53: 278–281

Holmer E 1989 Low molecular weight heparin. In: Lane D A, Lindahl U (eds) Heparin. Chemical and Biological Properties; Clinical Applications. Edward Arnold, London, p 575–596

Holmer E, Söderström G 1983 Neutralisation of unfractionated heparin and a low molecular weight (LMW) heparin fragment by protamine. Thrombosis and Haemostasis 50: 103

Holmer E, Kurachi K, Söderström G 1981 The molecular-weight dependence of the rate-enhancing effect of heparin on the inhibition of thrombin, Factor Xa, Factor IXa, Factor XIa, Factor XIIa and kallikrein by antithrombin. Biochemical Journal 193: 395–400

Hommes D W, Bura A, Mazzolai L, Buller H R, ten Cate J W 1991 Subcutaneous heparin compared to continuous intravenous heparin administration in the initial treatment of deep vein thrombosis: a systemic overview and meta-analysis. Thrombosis and Haemostasis 65: 753 (abst 305)

Höök M, Björk I, Hopwood J, Lindahl U 1976 Anticoagulant activity of heparin: separation of high-activity and low-activity heparin species by affinity chromatography on immobilized antithrombin. FEBS Letters 66: 90–93

Horellou M H, Conard J, Lecrubier C et al 1984 Persistent heparin induced thrombocytopenia despite therapy with low molecular weight heparin. Thrombosis and Haemostasis 51: 134

Hoylaerts M, Owen W G, Collen D 1984 Involvement of heparin chain length in the heparin-catalyzed inhibition of thrombin by antithrombin III. Journal of Biological Chemistry 259: 5670–5677

Howell R, Fidler J, Letsky E 1983 The risks of antenatal subcutaneous heparin prophylaxis: a controlled trial. British Journal of Obstetrics and Gynaecology 90: 1124–1128

Hsia J, Hamilton W P, Keiman N, Roberts R, Chaitman B R, Ross A M 1990 A comparison between heparin and low-dose aspirin as adjunctive therapy with tissue plasminogen activator for acute myocardial infarction. New England Journal of Medicine 323: 1433–1437

Huisse M G, Huet J, Zygelman M, Guillin M C 1983 Thrombopenie induite par l'heparine standard: tentative therapeutique á l'aide d'une héparine de bas poids moléculaire. Presse Médicale 12: 643

Hull R, Delmore T, Carter C, Hirsh J, Genton E, Gent M, Turpie G, McLaughlin D 1982 Adjusted subcutaneous heparin versus warfarin sodium in the long-term treatment of venous thrombosis. New England Journal of Medicine 306: 189–194

Hull R D, Raskob G E, Hirsh J, Jay R M, LeClerc J R, Geerts W H, Rosenbloom D, Sackett D L, Anderson C, Harrison L, Gent M 1986 Continuous intravenous heparin compared with intermittent subcutaneous heparin in the initial treatment of proximal-vein thrombosis. New England Journal of Medicine 315: 1109–1114

Hull R S, Raskob G E, Rosenbloom D, Panju A A, Brill-Edwards P, Ginsberg J S, Hirsh J, Martin G J, Green D 1990 Heparin for 5 days as compared with 10 days in the initial treatment of proximal venous thrombosis. New England Journal of Medicine 322: 1260–1264

Hull R D, Raskob G E, Pineo G F et al 1992 Subcutaneous low-molecular weight heparin compared with continuous intravenous heparin in the treatment of proximal vein thrombosis. New England Journal of Medicine 326: 975–982

International Study Group (GISSI-2) 1990 In-hospital mortality and clinical course of 20 891 patients with suspected acute myocardial infarction randomized between alteplase and streptokinase with or without heparin. Lancet 336: 71–75

Ireland H, Rylance P B, Kesteven P 1989 Heparin as an anticoagulant during extracorporeal circulation. In: Lane D A, Lindahl U (eds) Heparin: chemical and biological properties, clinical applications. E A Arnold, London, p 549–574

Jesty J 1979 Dissociation of complexes and their derivatives formed during inhibition of bovine thrombin and activated factor X by antithrombin III. Journal of Biological Chemistry 254: 1044–1049

Jick H, Slone D, Borda I T, Shapiro S 1968 Efficacy and toxicity of heparin in relation to age and sex. New England Journal of Medicine 279: 284–286

Johnson E A, Kirkwood T B L, Stirling Y, Perez-Requejo J L, Ingram G I C, Bangham D R, Brozovic M 1976 Four heparin preparations: anti-Xa potentiating effect of heparin after subcutaneous injection. Thrombosis and Haemostasis 35: 586–591

Kakkar V V 1975 An international multicentre trial. Prevention of fatal postoperative pulmonary embolism by low doses of heparin. Lancet 2: 45–51

Kakkar V V, Murray W J G 1985 Efficacy and safety of low-molecular weight heparin (CY 216) in preventing postoperative venous thrombo-embolism: a co-operative study. British Journal of Surgery 72: 786–791

Kakkar V V, Bentley P G, Scully M F, MacGregor I R, Jones N A G, Wegg P J 1980 Antithrombin III and heparin. Lancet 1: 103–104

Kakkar V V, Djazaeri B, Fok J, Fletcher M, Scully M F, Westwick J 1982 Low-molecular weight heparin and prevention of postoperative deep vein thrombosis. British Medical Journal 284: 375–379

Kapsch D N, Adelstein E H, Rhodes G R, Silver D 1979 Heparin-induced thrombocytopenia, thrombosis and haemorrhage. Surgery 86: 148–155

King D J, Kelton J G 1984 Heparin-associated thrombocytopenia. Annals of Internal Medicine 100: 535–540

Koller M, Schoch U, Buchmann P, Largiader F, von Felten A, Frick P G 1986 Low molecular weight heparin (KABI 2165) as thromboprophylaxis in elective visceral surgery. A randomized double-blind study versus unfractionated heparin. Thrombosis and Haemostasis 56: 243–246

Lam L H, Silbert J E, Rosenberg R D 1976 The separation of active and inactive forms of heparin. Biochemical and Biophysical Research Communications 69: 570–577

Lane D A, Ryan K 1989 Heparin and low molecular weight heparin: is anti-factor Xa activity important? Journal of Laboratory and Clinical Medicine 114, 331–333

Lane D A, MacGregor I R, Michalski R, Kakkar V V 1978 Anticoagulant activities of four unfractionated and fractionated heparins. Thrombosis Research 12: 257–271
Lane D A, MacGregor I R, van Ross M, Cella G, Kakkar V V 1979 Molecular weight dependence of the anticoagulant properties of heparin: intravenous and subcutaneous administration of fractionated heparins to man. Thrombosis Research 16: 651–661
Lane D A, Denton J, Flynn A M, Thunberg L, Lindahl U 1984 Anticoagulant activities of heparin oligosaccharides and their neutralization by platelet factor 4. Biochemical Journal 218: 725–732
Lane D A, Pejler G, Flynnn A M, Thompson E A, Lindahl U 1986 Neutralization of heparin-related saccharides by histidine-rich glycoprotein and platelet factor 4. Journal of Biological Chemistry 261: 3980–3986
Leclerc J R, Geerts W H, Desjardius L, Jobin F, Laroche F, Delorme F, Hariernick S, Atkinson S, Bourgouin J 1992 Prevention of deep vein thrombosis after major knee surgery — a randomized double-blind trial comparing a low molecular weight heparin fragment (Enoxaparin) to placebo. Thrombosis and Haemostasis 67: 417–423
Levine M N, Planes A, Hirsh J, Goodyear M, Vochelle N, Gent M 1989 The relationship between anti-factor Xa level and clinical outcome in patients receiving enoxaparine low molecular weight heparin to prevent deep vein thrombosis after hip replacement. Thrombosis and Haemostasis 62: 940–944
Levine M N, Hirsh J, Gent M, Turpie A G, LeClerc J, Powers P J, Jay R M, Neemeh J 1991 Prevention of deep vein thrombosis after elective hip surgery. A randomized trial comparing low molecular weight heparin with standard unfractionated heparin. Annals of Internal Medicine 114: 545–551
Leyvraz P F, Richard J, Bachmann F et al 1983 Adjusted versus fixed-dose subcutaneous heparin in the prevention of deep vein thrombosis after total hip replacement. New England Journal of Medicine 309: 954–958
Leyvraz P F, Bachmann F, Hoek J, Buller H R, Postel M, Samama M, Vandenbroek M C 1991 Prevention of deep vein thrombosis after hip replacement: randomized comparison between unfractionated heparin and low molecular weight heparin. British Medical Journal 303: 543–548
Lijnen R, Hoylaerts M, Collén D 1983 Heparin binding properties of human histidine-rich glycoprotein. Mechanism and role in the neutralization of heparin in plasma. Journal of Biological Chemistry 258: 3803–3808
Lindahl U, Bäckström G, Höök M, Thunberg L, Fransson L-A, Linker A 1979 Structure of the antithrombin-binding site in heparin. Proceedings of the National Academy of Sciences, USA 76: 3198–3202
Lindahl A K, Abildgaard U, Larsen M L, Aamodt L-M, Nordfang O, Beek T C 1991 Extrinsic pathway inhibitor (EPI), and the post-heparin anticoagulant effect in tissue thromboplastin-induced coagulation. Thrombosis Research suppl XIV: 39–48
Lijnen R, Hoylaerts M, Collén D 1983 Heparin binding properties of human histidine-rich glycoprotein. Mechanism and role in the neutralization of heparin in plasma. Journal of Biological Chemistry 258: 3803–3808
Lijnen R, van Hoef B, Collén D 1984 Histidine-rich glycoprotein modulates the anticoagulant activity of heparin in human plasma. Thrombosis and Haemostasis 51: 266–268
Lopaciuk S, Meissuer A J, Filipecki S, Zawilska K, Sowier J, Cielielski L, Bielawiec M, Glowinski S, Czestochowska E et al 1992 Subcutaneous low molecular weight heparin versus subcutaneous unfractionated heparin in the treatment of deep vein thrombosis: a Polish Multicenter Trial. Thrombosis and Haemostasis 68: 14–18
Lormeau J C, Goulay J, Choay J 1980 German Patent No 2944792
MacMahon S, Collins R, Knight C, Yusef S, Peto R 1988 Reduction of major morbidity and mortality by heparin in acute myocardial infarction. Circulation 78 (suppl II): II-98
Mant M J, Thong K L, Birtwhistle R V, O'Brien B D, Hammond G W, Grace M G 1977 Haemorrhagic complications of heparin therapy. Lancet 1: 1133–1135
Marciniak E 1973 Factor Xa inactivation by antithrombin III: evidence for biological stabilisation of Factor Xa by Factor V-phospholipid complex. British Journal of Haematology 24: 391–400
Marciniak E, Gockerman J P 1977 Heparin-induced decrease in circulating antithrombin III. Lancet 2: 581–584
Massonnet-Castel S, Pelissier E, Dreyfus G, Deloche A, Abry B, Guibourt P, Terrier E, Passelecq J, Jaulmes B, Carpentier A 1984 Low molecular weight heparin in extracorporeal circulation. Lancet 1: 1182–1183
Mätzsch T 1990 Transplacental passage of an enzymatically depolymerized low molecular weight heparin as compared to standard heparin. PhD thesis, University of Lund, Lund, Sweden
Mätzsch T, Bergqvist D, Hedner U, Nilsson B, Ostergaard P 1990 Effects of low molecular weight heparin and unfragmented heparin on induction of osteoporosis in rats. Thrombosis and Haemostasis 63: 505–509
Michalski R, Lane D A, Pepper D S, Kakkar V V 1978 Neutralisation of heparin in plasma by platelet factor four and protomine sulphate. British Journal of Haematology 38: 561–571
Monreal M, Lafoz E, Salvador R, Roncales J, Navarro A 1989 Adverse effects of three different forms of heparin therapy: thrombocytopenia, increased transaminases and hyperkalaemia. European Journal of Clinical Pharmacology 37: 415–418
Nesheim M E 1983 A simple rate law that describes the kinetics of the heparin-catalysed reaction between antithrombin III and thrombin. Journal of Biological Chemistry 258: 14708–14717
Nesheim M E, Mann K G 1983 Modulation of the inhibition of factor Xa by antithrombin III upon incorporation of factor Xa into the prothrombinase complex. Blood 62 (suppl 1): 291
Nielsen J, Østergaard P 1988 Chemistry of heparin and low molecular weight heparin. Acta Chirurgica Scandinavica, (Suppl) 543: 52–56
Niwa M, Yamagishi R, Kondo S-I, Sakaragawa N, Koide T 1985 Histidine-rich glycoprotein inhibits the antithrombin activity of heparin co-factor II in the presence of heparin or dermatan sulfate. Thrombosis Research 37: 237–240
Nurmohamed M T, Rosendaal F R, Buller H R, Dekker E, Hommes D W, Vandenbroucke J P, Briët E 1992 The efficacy and safety of low molecular weight heparin versus standard heparin in general and orthopaedic surgery: a meta-analysis. Lancet 340: 152–156
O'Brien J R, Shoobridge S M, Finch W J 1969 Comparison of the effect of heparin and citrate on platelet aggregation. Journal of Clinical Pathology 22: 28–31
Ofosu F A 1989 Antithrombotic mechanisms of heparin and related compounds. In: Lane D A, Lindahl U (eds) Heparin. Edward Arnold, London, p 433–454
Ofosu F A, Barrowcliffe T W 1990 Mechanisms of action of low molecular weight heparins and heparinoids. Baillière's Clinical Haematology 3(3): 505–530
Ofosu F A, Buchanan M R, Anvari N, Smith L M, Blajchman M A 1989a Plasma anticoagulant mechanisms of heparin, heparin sulfate, and dermatan sulfate. Annals of the New York Academy of Sciences 556: 123–131
Ofosu F A, Hirsh J, Esmon C T, Modi G J, Smith L M, Anvari N, Buchanan M R, Fenton J W, Blajchman M A 1989b Unfractionated heparin inhibits the thrombin-catalyzed amplification reactions of coagulation more efficiently than those catalyzed by factor Xa. Biochemical Journal 257: 143–150
Olson S T, Shore J D 1981 Binding of high affinity heparin to antithrombin III. Characterization of the protein fluorescence enhancement. Journal of Biological Chemistry 256: 11065–11072
Oosta G M, Gardner W T, Beeler D L, Rosenberg R D 1981 Multiple functional domains of the heparin molecule. Proceedings of the National Academy of Sciences, USA 78: 829–833
Padilla A, Gray E, Pepper D S, Barrowcliffe T W 1992 Effect of platelet factor 4 (PF4) on inhibition of thrombin generation by low molecular weight (LMW) heparins. British Journal of Haematology 82: 406–413
Pejler G 1988 Why does heparin bind antithrombin? Thesis. Swedish University of Agricultural Science, Uppsala
Persson E, Nordenstrom J, Nilsson-Ehle P 1987 Plasma kinetics of liproprotein lipase and hepatic lipase activities induced by heparin and a low molecular weight heparin fragment. Scandinavian Journal of Clinical and Laboratory Investigation 47: 151–155
Peterson C B, Blackburn M N 1987 Antithrombin conformation and the catalytic role of heparin. I. Does cleavage by thrombin induce structural changes in the heparin-binding region of antithrombin? Journal of Biological Chemistry 262: 7552–7558

Pezzuoli G, Neri Serneri G G, Settembrini P, Coggi G, Olivari N, Buzzetti G, Chierichetti S, Scotti A, Scatigna M, Carnovali M 1989 Prophylaxis of fatal pulmonary embolism in general surgery using low-molecular weight heparin Cy 216: a multicentre, double-blind, randomized, controlled, clinical trial versus placebo (STEP). International Surgery 74: 205–210

Pharmeuropa, The European Pharmacopoeia Forum 1991 Low molecular mass heparins. Draft Monograph vol 3 (No 3): 161–165

Pieters J, Willems G, Hemker H C, Lindhout T 1988 Inhibition of Factor IXa and Factor Xa by antithrombin III/heparin during Factor X activation. Journal of Biological Chemistry 263: 15313–15318

Pieters J, Lindhout T, Willems G 1990 Heparin-stimulated inhibition of Factor IXa generation and Factor IXa neutralization in plasma. Blood 76(3): 549–554

Pini M, Pattacini C, Quintavalla R, Poli T, Megha A, Tagliaferri A, Manotti C, Dettori A G 1990 Subcutaneous vs intravenous heparin in the treatment of deep venous thrombosis. A randomized clinical trial. Thrombosis and Haemostasis 64: 222–226

Pitney W R 1983 How safe is heparin? Medical Journal of Australia 2(3): 11–12

Pitney W R, Pettit J E, Armstrong L 1970 Control of heparin therapy. British Medical Journal 2: 139–141

Planes A, Vochelle N, Mazas F, Mansat C, Zucman J, Landais A, Pascariello J C, Weill D, Butel J 1988 Prevention of postoperative venous thrombosis: a randomized trial comparing unfractionated heparin with low molecular weight heparin in patients undergoing total hip replacement. Thrombosis and Haemostasis 60: 407–410

Pomerantz M W, Omen W G 1978 A catalytic role for heparin. Evidence for a ternary complex of heparin cofactor thrombin and heparin. Biochemica et Biophysica Acta 535: 66–77

Preissner K T, Wassmuth R, Muller-Berghaus G 1985 Physicochemical characterisation of human S-protein and its function in the blood coagulation system. Biochemical Journal 231: 349–355

Rhodes G R, Dizon R H, Silver D 1977 Heparin-induced thrombocytopenia: eight cases with thrombotic haemmorrhagic complications. Annals of Surgery 186: 752–758

Rosenberg R D, Damus P S 1973 The purification and mechanism of action of human antithrombin-heparin cofactor. Journal of Biological Chemistry 248: 6490–6505

Salzman E W, Deykin D, Shapiro R M, Rosenberg R D 1975 Management of heparin therapy — controlled prospective trial. New England Journal of Medicine 191: 1046–1051

Salzman E W, Rosenberg R D, Smith M H, Lindon J N, Favreau L 1980 Effect of heparin and heparin fractions on platelet aggregation. Journal of Clinical Investigation 65: 64–73

Samama M, Bernard P, Bonnardot J P, Combe-Tamzali S, Lanson Y, Tissot E (GENOX multicentric trial) 1988 Low molecular weight heparin compared with unfractionated heparin in prevention of postoperative thrombosis. British Journal of Surgery 75: 128–131

Sandset M, Abildgaard U, Larsen M L 1988 Herparin induces release of extrinsic coagulation pathway inhibitor (EPI). Thrombosis Research 50: 803–813

Schmidt M, Barrowcliffe T W, Gray E, Watton J, Harenberg J 1991 Anti-Xa clotting activities in different hepatic-triglyceride lipase preparations from post-heparin plasma. Thrombosis Research 63: 503–508

Schoen P, Lindhout T, Willems G, Hemker H C 1989 Antithrombin III-dependent anti-prothrombinase activity of heparin and heparin fragments. Journal of Biological Chemistry 264: 10002–10007

Scully M J, Ellis V, Kakkar V V 1987 Comparison of the molecular mass dependency of heparin stimulation of heparin cofactor II: thrombin interaction to antithrombin III: thrombin interaction. Thrombosis Research 46: 491–502

Silver D, Kapsch D N, Tsoi E K M 1983 Heparin-induced thromboctopenia, thrombosis and haemorrhage. Annals of Surgery 198: 301–306

Tew C J, Lane D A, Thompson E, Ireland H, Curtis J R 1988 Relationship between ex vivo anti-proteinase (factor Xa and thrombin) assays and in vivo anticoagulant effect of very low molecular weight heparin, CY 222. British Journal of Haematology 70: 335–340

Thomas D P 1992 Prevention of post-operative thrombosis by low molecular weight heparin in patients undergoing hip replacement. Thrombosis and Haemostasis 67: 491–493

Thomas D P, Merton R E 1982 A low molecular weight heparin compared with unfractionated heparin. Thrombosis Research 28: 343–350

Thomas D P, Merton R E, Barrowcliffe T W, Thunberg L, Lindahl U 1982 Effects of heparin oligosaccharides with high affinity for antithrombin III in experimental venous thrombosis. Thrombosis and Haemostasis 47: 244–248

Thomas D P, Curtis A D, Barrowcliffe T W 1984 A collaborative study designed to establish the 4th International Standard for heparin. Thrombosis and Haemostasis 52: 148–153

Thomson C, Forbes C D, Prentice C R M 1973 The potentiation of platelet aggregation and adhesion by heparin in vitro and in vivo. Clinical Science and Molecular Medicine 45: 485–494

Thunberg L, Bäckström G, Lindahl U 1982 Further characterization of the antithrombin-binding sequence in heparin. Carbohydrate Research 100: 393–410

Tobelem G 1989 Endothelial cell interactions with heparin. Seminars in Thrombosis and Hemostasis 15(2): 197–199

Tollefsen D M 1984 Activation of heparin cofactor II by heparin and dermatan sulphate. Nouvelle Revue Francaise d'Hématologie 26: 211–219

Tollefsen D M 1989 Heparin cofactor II. In: Heparin. Chemical and Biological Properties; Clinical Applications. Eds D A Lane and U Lindahl. Edward Arnold, London, pp 257–274

Tollefsen D M, Blank M K 1981 Detection of a new heparin-dependent inhibitor of thrombin in human plasma. Journal of Clinical Investigation 68: 589–596

Tollefsen D M, Majerus D W, Blank M K 1982 Heparin co-factor II. Purification and properties of a heparin-dependent inhibitor of thrombin in human plasma. Journal of Biological Chemistry 257: 2162–2169

Turpie A G G, Levine M N, Hirsh J, Carter C J, Jay R M, Powers P J, Andrew M, Hull R D, Gent M 1986 A randomized controlled trial of a low-molecular weight heparin (Enoxaparin) to prevent deep-vein thrombosis in patients undergoing elective hip surgery. New England Journal of Medicine 315: 925–929

UPET (Urokinase Pulmonary Embolism Trial) 1973 A national cooperative study. Circulation 47 (suppl 2): 1–108

Vairel E G, Bouty-Boye H, Toulemonde F, Doutremepuich C, Marsh N A, Gaffney P J 1983 Heparin and a low molecular weight fraction enhances thrombolysis and by this pathway exercises aprotective effect against thrombosis. Thrombosis Research 30: 219–224

van Deerlin, V M D, Tollefsen, D M 1991 End terminal acidic domain of heparin cofactor II mediates the inhibition of thrombin in the presence of glycosaminoglycans. Journal of Biological Chemistry 266(30): 20223–20231

van Ryn-McKenna J, Cai L, Ofosu F A, Hirsh J, Buchanan M R 1990 Neutralization of Enoxaparine-induced bleeding by protamine sulfate. Thrombosis and Haemostasis 63(2): 271–274

Vinazzer H, Stocker K 1991 Heparin co-factor II: experimental approach to a new assay and clinical results. Thrombosis Research 61: 235–241

Vinazzer H, Stemberger A, Haas S, Blumel G 1982 Influence of heparin; of different heparin fractions and a low molecular weight heparin-like substance on the mechanism of fibrinolysis. Thrombosis Research 27: 341–352

Walker A M, Jick H 1980 Predictors of bleeding during heparin therapy. Journal of the American Medical Association 244: 1209–1212

Walker M G, Shaw J W, Thompson G J L, Cumming J G R, Thomas M L 1987 Subcutaneous calcium heparin versus intravenous sodium heparin in treatment of established acute deep vein thrombosis of the legs: a multicentre prospective randomized trial. British Medical Journal 294: 1189–1192

Walsh P N, Biggs R 1972 The role of platelets in intrinsic factor Xa formation. British Journal of Haematology 22: 743–760

WHO Technical Report Series, Geneva, 1987 No 760: 22

Yang X, Blajchman M A, Craven S, Smith L M, Anvari N, Ofosu F A 1990 Activation of factor V during intrinsic and extrinsic coagulation. Inhibition by heparin, hirudin and H-D-PHE-PRO-ARG-CH_2C1. Biochemical Journal 272: 399–406

65. Oral anticoagulant therapy

A. M. H. P. van den Besselaar

Oral anticoagulants are drugs interfering with the biosynthesis of vitamin K-dependent blood coagulation factors. Therefore, they are called vitamin K-antagonist drugs. Oral anticoagulants are used clinically for prophylaxis and management of venous thrombosis. They are also used prophylactically in patients with arterial disease, and with heart valve prostheses.

Bleeding is the main complication of oral anticoagulant treatment. Therefore, the therapeutic range of anticoagulant effect is extremely narrow. Standardized laboratory control is one of the essential prerequisites of oral anticoagulant treatment.

Only adequately maintained therapy is of value to a patient, and this takes considerable time and care. It requires a dedication that is not present if control is in the hands of changing staff, and, most importantly, under-anticoagulation must be treated with the same degree of urgency as over-anticoagulation. Oral anticoagulant treatment is not just prescribing a drug, but requires an organizational framework to fulfil the need of patient education, laboratory testing, and dosage regulation. Furthermore, the quality of the treatment should be assessed regularly (therapeutic quality assessment).

The first oral anticoagulant drug used clinically was 3,3′-methylene bis (4-hydroxy-2*H*-1-benzopyran-2-one), also named 'dicoumarol'. It was originally isolated from spoiled sweet clover by Link (1959). Because of poor absorption and the non-linear kinetics of dicoumarol, it is no longer used (Breckenridge 1984). Presently, there are three widely used oral anticoagulant drugs: warfarin, acenocoumarin (nicoumalone), and phenprocoumon. All three are derivatives of 4-hydroxycoumarin (Fig. 65.1). While warfarin is the most widely used coumarin in Britain and North America, in mainland Europe both acenocoumarin and phenprocoumon are extensively used in addition to warfarin.

Derivatives of indan-1,3 dione also have anticoagulant effect but for toxicological reasons these are no longer used (Breckenridge 1984).

Warfarin, acenocoumarin and phenprocoumon all contain one asymmetric carbon atom (Fig. 65.1). Each exists therefore in two enantiomeric forms. These two forms are commonly designated *R* and *S*. Chemical synthesis of these compounds results in a racemic mixture. The kinetic and dynamic properties of the enantiomers of each of the compounds differ, and a mixture of two drugs is administered when racemic warfarin, acenocoumarin or phenprocoumon is given.

VITAMIN K-DEPENDENT COAGULATION FACTOR SYNTHESIS IN THE LIVER

Vitamin K is an essential coenzyme of the post-translational carboxylation of coagulation factors II (prothrombin), VII, IX, and X, and of the physiological anticoagulants protein C and protein S. Glutamyl residues on the proteins are converted by the liver enzyme 'carboxylase' to γ-carboxyglutamyl (Gla) residues under the influence of the reduced form of vitamin K, oxygen, and carbon dioxide.

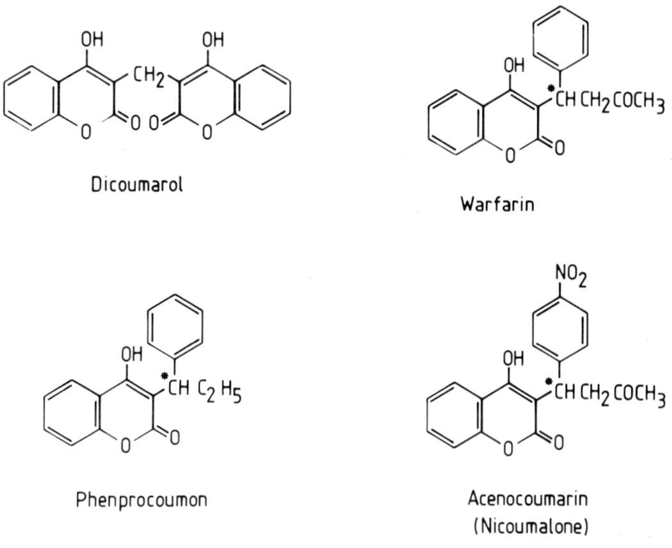

Fig. 65.1 Chemical structures of 4-hydroxycoumarin derivatives. Asymmetric carbon atoms are marked with an asterisk.

Only specific glutamyl residues are carboxylated. For example, in prothrombin, ten Gla residues are found. When the carboxylation reaction is blocked and the plasma proteins lack Gla residues, they do not interact with negatively charged phospholipids. Interaction with phospholipids is required for physiological activation of the zymogen coagulation factors. Prothrombin with no Gla residues completely lacks biological activity. The active form of vitamin K acting as coenzyme for carboxylase is the reduced (hydroquinone) form. The vitamin K-dependent carboxylase reaction produces two products, Gla residues and vitamin K 2,3-epoxide. The epoxide is recycled to the hydroquinone in two reduction steps (Fig. 65.2). In these steps, dithiol- and NAD(P)H-dependent reductases are involved. The reduction of the quinone form of vitamin K can be accomplished by two pathways, one of which is dithiol-dependent, and the other NAD(P)H-dependent. These cyclical reactions occur continuously in the liver. It was calculated that each molecule of vitamin K is recycled many hundred fold (and probably several thousand fold) before it is catabolized into inactive degradation products (Vermeer & Hamulyák 1991).

Vitamin K sources

There are two main forms of vitamin K in nature: phylloquinone (vitamin K_1) and the menaquinones (vitamin K_2). Vitamin K_1 is exclusively of plant origin, and its main sources are green vegetables like spinach, kale, cabbage and broccoli. Also cow's milk contains considerable amounts of phylloquinone. Commercially available vitamin K_1 is a synthesized compound. Menaquinone is a group name for a number of closely related products of microbial origin. Menaquinones occur in various (mainly fermented) foods like yoghurt and natta (a popular Japanese food prepared from fermented soybeans). Also the bacterial flora in the colon produce substantial amounts of menaquinones, but the extent to which they are resorbed from the colon is still a matter of investigation. The data presently available suggest that the hepatic menaquinone store predominantly originates from the diet, and not from the intestinal flora. An elaborate food analysis for menaquinone levels must be awaited to obtain more conclusive support for this hypothesis (Vermeer & Hamulyák 1991).

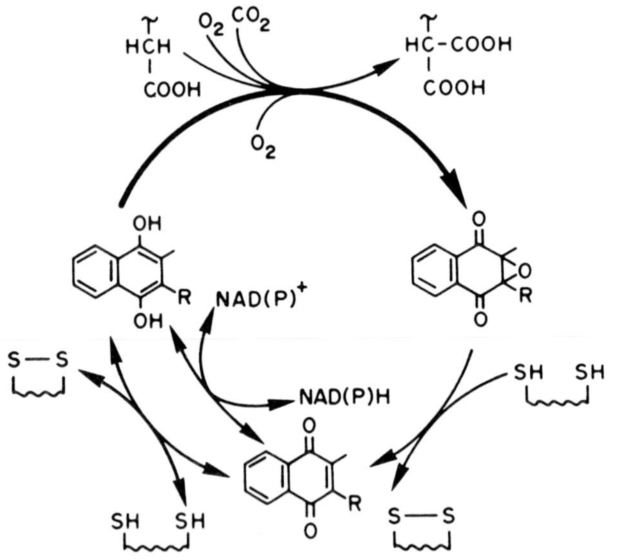

Fig. 65.2 Liver metabolism of vitamin K. The dithiol-dependent vitamin K epoxide reduction and vitamin K quinone reduction are the metabolic steps inhibited by oral anticoagulants. (From Suttie 1990, copyrighted and reprinted with the permission of Clinical Cardiology Publishing Co., Inc., and/or the Foundation for Advances in Medicine and Science.)

Vitamin K uptake from food

The uptake of phylloquinone from food is probably the most important source for vitamin K in man. The minimal daily requirement in humans is not known. Based on the data available in the literature there is a general consensus that the daily intake of 1–2 µg of phylloquinone per kg body weight is sufficient to maintain a normal haemostasis (Vermeer & Hamulyák 1991). Phylloquinone is absorbed from the ileum after solubilization in mixed micelles composed of bile salts, free fatty acids and monoglycerides. These micelles are resorbed by the intestinal mucosa, from where phylloquinone is transported via the lymph in chylomicrons to the general circulation where it is associated with lipoproteins (Shearer et al 1970). Phylloquinone accumulates mainly in the liver, but is also found in the kidney, spleen, heart, lungs and bones.

After ingestion of kale soup, the maximum phylloquinone concentration in serum is reached after 5 to 6 hours, which is about 2–3 hours later than after oral administration of solubilized phylloquinone (Langenberg 1985). This can be explained by the fact that phylloquinone in food is not readily available for absorption since the vegetable tissue has to be digested at least partly for the liberation and solubilization of phylloquinone. The systemic uptake of phylloquinone after ingestion of kale soup ranged from 14 to 42%, with a mean value of 26% (Langenberg 1985).

VITAMIN K ANTAGONISM

It is well established that 4-hydroxycoumarin anticoagulants inhibit hepatic vitamin K epoxide reductase causing the accumulation of the epoxide metabolite (Bell 1978). In this way the recycling of vitamin K is blocked, so that the supply of the hydroquinone form (the active coenzyme for carboxylase) is rapidly exhausted. This blockade causes a decrease of procoagulant activity of the vitamin K-dependent coagulation factors, resulting in a prolongation of blood coagulation time tests. However, the blockade of the vitamin K cycle may be bypassed by the administration of high doses of vitamin K because the conversion of vitamin K to the active hydroquinone form can be accomplished by two reductases, only one of which (the dithiol-dependent one) is sensitive to 4-hydroxycoumarins (Fig. 65.2).

Although the oral anticoagulants are administered as racemic mixtures, the enantiomers differ in their vitamin K-antagonist activity. *S*-warfarin is five times more potent than *R*-warfarin in terms of anticoagulant effect in man (Breckenridge et al 1974, O'Reilly 1974).

Pharmacokinetics of oral anticoagulants

Warfarin, phenprocoumon, and acenocoumarin are well and rapidly absorbed. These drugs are all extensively (>98%) bound to serum albumin. There is a wide inter-individual variation in the rate of elimination of each of the oral anticoagulants due to differences in rate of metabolism. The elimination half life of racemic warfarin ranges from 15 to 50 hours, phenprocoumon 4–9 days, and acenocoumarin 8.2–8.7 hours (Breckenridge 1984). Thus, the half life of acenocoumarin is shorter than that of warfarin which is, in turn, shorter than that of phenprocoumon. Each of the three main anticoagulants is a racemic mixture of enantiomers that are eliminated at different rates. For example, the elimination rate of *R*-warfarin is 35–45 hours whereas *S*-warfarin has a half life of 23–33 hours (Toon et al 1990). On the other hand, *S*-nicoumalone is eliminated much faster than *R*-nicoumalone (Gill et al 1988, Couet et al 1990). Because of its pharmacokinetics, *S*-nicoumalone is almost devoid of activity. The half lifetimes of *R*-phenprocoumon and *S*-phenprocoumon are identical (Heimark et al 1987).

Metabolism of oral anticoagulants

Both warfarin and phenprocoumon are metabolized by oxidative processes. The major oxidative process for both drugs is (*S*)-7-hydroxylation. However, this process is relatively more important in the elimination of warfarin. Approximately 67% of the dose of *S*-warfarin undergoes 7-hydroxylation compared with 42% of the dose of *S*-phenprocoumon. Both drugs also undergo 6-hydroxylation in a nonstereoselective manner. In contrast, 8-hydroxylation is observed for warfarin and not phenprocoumon whereas 4′-hydroxylation is observed for phenprocoumon and not warfarin. The rate of oxidative metabolism may not be the dominant factor governing the elimination rate of phenprocoumon for which conjugation appears to be an important process. Both phenprocoumon and its oxidative metabolites are conjugated extensively before excretion in the urine. The conjugate of phenprocoumon is the species that is most likely responsible for the enterohepatic recycling the drug is known to undergo. This recycling is probably a major factor governing the long elimination half life of phenprocoumon relative to warfarin.

Kinetics of vitamin K-dependent coagulation factors

The concentration of the coagulation factors in plasma is determined by a dynamic equilibrium between synthesis and degradation. The rate of synthesis in the liver is probably independent of the concentration in plasma. The rate of degradation is proportional to the plasma concentration and is characterized by its half life time. The half lives of the four vitamin K-dependent coagulation factors are very different; see Table 65.1 (Rizza & Jones 1987). The half life of protein C is relatively short, 6–9 hours (Marlar & Neumann 1990).

If the rate of synthesis of a particular coagulation factor is reduced by the administration of a coumarin derivative, a new equilibrium will be reached, and the plasma concentration of the coagulation factor will be reduced to the same extent as the rate of synthesis. In general, the level of coagulation factors in the steady state reflects the degree of inhibition of the synthesis system (Hemker & Frank 1985). Studies by Loeliger et al (1963) indicated that all four vitamin K-dependent coagulation factors were depressed to approximately the same level in steady oral anticoagulation. However, recent investigations showed that in patients stabilized on warfarin, the concentrations were not equally depressed, with factor X the lowest, factor II at intermediate value and factors VII and IX the highest (Paul et al 1987).

Bertina (1984) estimated the levels of the four vitamin K-dependent coagulation factors as a function of the intensity of steady oral anticoagulation (Fig. 65.3). The average intensity of oral anticoagulation is expressed in International Normalized Ratio (INR) units (p. 1443). The levels of all factors decrease with increasing intensity, but not at the same rate and to the same extent. The reduction of factor X from 0.22 U/ml at INR 2.70 to 0.155 U/ml at INR 4.71 is much smaller than that observed for the other factors. It should be realized that these are average values. The interindividual variation of the coagulation factors at a given prothrombin time or INR in steady anticoagulation is relatively high (Bertina & Loeliger 1980, Jones et al 1991). If it were theoretically possible to increase the synthesis rate of the coagulation

Table 65.1 Half lives of vitamin K-dependent clotting factors in man

Factor	half life
II	3 days
VII	4–6 h
IX	18–30 h
X	2 days

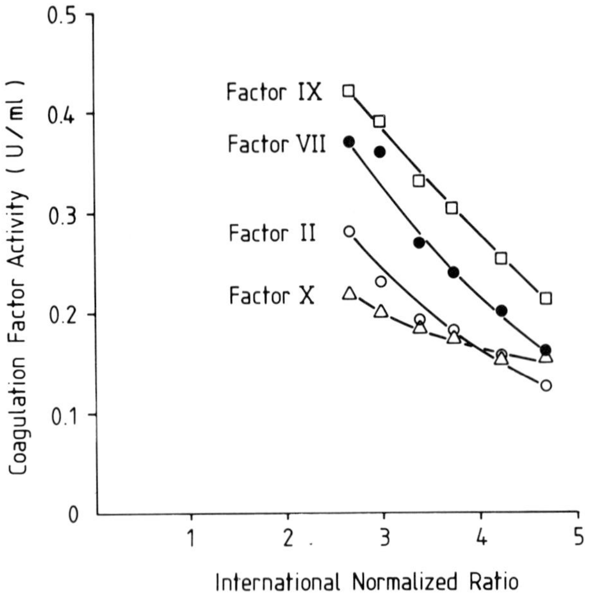

Fig. 65.3 Relationship between INR and the activities of factors II, VII, IX and X. Each data point is the mean of values from at least 17 patients (Bertina 1984).

factors in a sudden way, then the concentration of the factors in plasma would approach their new level in an exponential fashion, again determined by their half lives. Every change of synthesis rate induces a change of plasma factor level and the rate of this change is determined by the half life of the plasma factor. If the rate of synthesis is fluctuating because the oral anticoagulant is excreted rapidly, factor VII is fluctuating also because of its short half life (Thijssen et al 1988, Fiessinger et al 1989).

The kinetics of the vitamin K-dependent coagulation factors can be changed in various clinical conditions (Shetty et al 1989). The synthesis and the decay rates can be affected, which may require change in the dosage of oral anticoagulants. In liver disease, the synthesis of the coagulation factors is decreased and consequently the dosage requirement of oral anticoagulants is decreased as well. Coagulation factor degradation rates are affected by the thyroid function. Loeliger et al (1963) found evidence of increased degradation of factor VII and probably also of factors II and X in hyperthyroidism. Kellett et al (1986) observed that factor II activity is lower and the partial thromboplastin time is shorter in hyperthyroid patients than in those in the euthyroid state. Warfarin produced a greater fall in factors II and VII and a greater increase in prothrombin time ratio and partial thromboplastin time in the hyperthyroid state than in the euthyroid state. Stephens et al (1989) reported a case in which hypothyroidism necessitated a 2.75-fold increase in warfarin dosage.

Laboratory control

The prothrombin time (PT) is the primary measurement of monitoring of oral anticoagulant treatment. The prothrombin time, originally described by Quick et al (1935) is based on the tissue factor pathway of blood coagulation. The PT is sensitive to the vitamin K-dependent coagulation factors II, VII and X.

The result of the PT test is strongly dependent on the nature of the tissue extract (thromboplastin) and the method used. Many modifications of the original Quick test have been applied for monitoring of oral anticoagulant treatment. In an attempt to standardize the PT test, results were expressed as percentage prothrombin activity. However, the percentage prothrombin activity read from a curve based on dilutions of normal plasma in saline was still dependent on the tissue extract used for the PT test (Conley & Morse 1948). Similarly, the expression of the PT as a ratio (patient's PT divided by the mean normal PT) depended strongly on the modification used (Poller 1987). The multiplicity of modifications of the PT test has contributed to the confusion about the optimal therapeutic target levels of oral anticoagulation (Hirsh & Levine 1988). The confusion could only be resolved with the introduction of an international standardization system established by the World Health Organization (WHO), and recommended by the International Committee for Standardization in Haematology (ICSH) and the Scientific and Standardization Committee of the International Society on Thrombosis and Haemostasis (WHO Expert Committee on Biological Standardization 1983, Loeliger 1985).

International standardization

International standardization of the PT could be achieved by relating any given test system to an established primary standard reference method. In 1977, a research standard prepared by the International Committee on Thrombosis and Haemostasis in collaboration with the National Institute of Biological Standards and Control (NIBSC) in London, was established by the World Health Organization (WHO) as the primary international reference preparation (IRP) for thromboplastin (WHO Expert Committee on Biological Standardization 1977). This material, coded 67/40, was prepared from human brain supplemented with adsorbed bovine plasma (combined reagent), to be used according to meticulously defined instructions.

A further advance in standardization was the development of a model for the calibration of any PT test system in terms of the primary IRP, as proposed by Kirkwood (1983). In this model, a linear relationship was hypothesized between the logarithms of PTs obtained with the primary IRP method and the logarithms of PTs obtained with the test system (Fig. 65.4). Furthermore, the model required that a single relationship be valid for fresh plasma specimens of normal individuals and fresh specimens of patients on stabilized oral anticoagulant treatment:

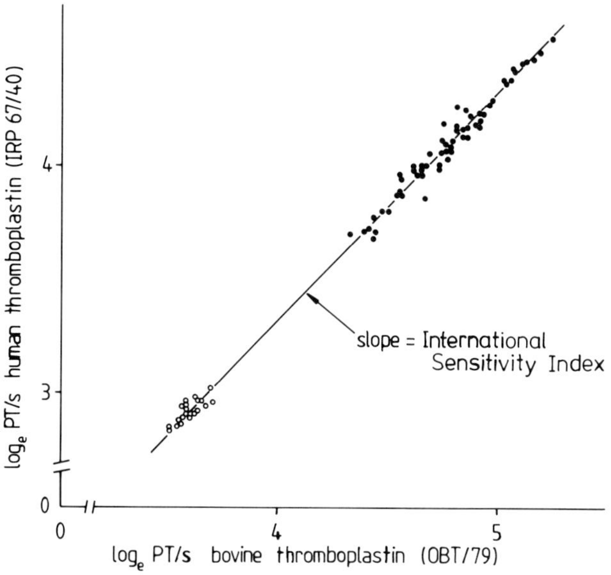

Fig. 65.4 Calibration plot of secondary reference preparation OBT/79 (thromboplastin, bovine, combined) against the primary International Reference Preparation 67/40. Healthy individuals are represented by white circles and patients on stabilized oral anticoagulant treatment by black circles (Hermans et al 1983).

$$[\log PT_{67/40} = a + c. \log PT_{test}] \qquad \text{(Equation 1)}$$

in which a and c are the intercept and slope of the calibration line, respectively. This model leads to a simple equation to transform a PT ratio (R = patient PT: mean normal PT) obtained with the working PT system into the PT ratio which would have been obtained had the primary IRP 67/40 been used:

$$[R_{67/40} = R^{ISI}] \qquad \text{(Equation 2)}$$

in which ISI is the *international sensitivity index* of the working system. The ISI is equal to the slope c. $R_{67/40}$ is usually called the international normalized ratio (INR). The INR is the universal scale to express the PT for oral anticoagulant control. This calibration model was tested successfully in an international collaborative exercise organized by the European Community Bureau of Reference (BCR) and ICSH (Hermans et al 1983). Consequently, this model was adopted by WHO (WHO Expert Committee on Biological Standardization 1983). Calibrations of other thromboplastins have been carried out in accordance with the WHO model (Thomson et al 1984, 1986, van den Besselaar et al 1986, Palareti et al 1987). However, the WHO model is empirical and for a particular combination of thromboplastins, a significant deviation from the model has been observed although a modified model could account for the experimental calibration data (Tomenson 1984, Gogstad et al 1986). Generally speaking, it is the thromboplastin manufacturer's responsibility to provide the calibration data for each batch of their material (Loeliger 1985). This can be done in several ways, i.e. by reporting of an ISI-value or providing a chart in which the relationship between PT (ratio), percentage activity and INR is given.

It should be emphasized that the INR/ISI system can only be used in oral anticoagulant control. It has no significance in other applications of the PT test.

Secondary international reference preparations for thromboplastins

The WHO model for thromboplastin calibration requires a hierarchy of standardization. Secondary reference preparations have been calibrated against the primary IRP in international collaborative exercises (Fig. 65.5). The calibration of a thromboplastin is, in general, more precise when comparisons are made between similar preparations from the same species (WHO Expert Committee on Biological Standardization 1983). The secondary reference preparations represent different species and types of reagents. It is suggested that laboratories and manufacturers use the secondary reference preparation of the same species for the calibration of their materials. The composition of the thromboplastin reagent has been shown to have considerable effect on the precision of calibration. Plain reagents (i.e. without addition of adsorbed plasma) should be calibrated against a plain secondary reference preparation; combined reagents should be calibrated against a combined reference preparation. At present only one combined reference preparation (OBT/79) is available, as the primary IRP 67/40 has been discontinued (WHO Expert Committee on Biological Standardization 1984). Secondary reference preparations are also available from the BCR (Hermans et al 1983, van den Besselaar & Bertina 1991). These reference materials are intended to be more widely available to manufacturers of commercial or noncommercial thromboplastins. The BCR reference materials have been certified in terms of the primary WHO IRP 67/40. Manufacturers of thromboplastin are being urged

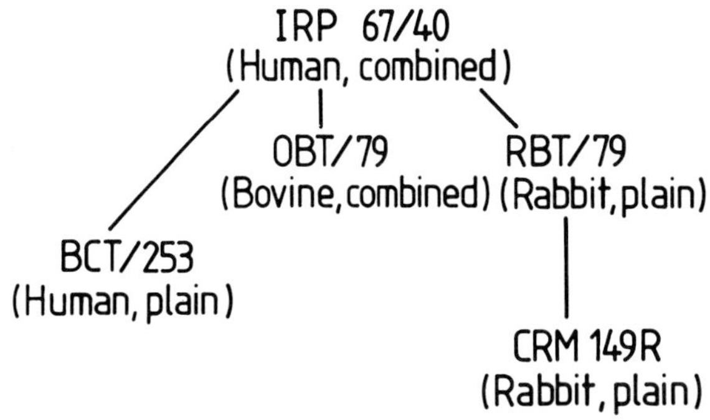

Fig. 65.5 Hierarchy of thromboplastin calibration. Secondary reference preparations were calibrated against the primary International Reference Preparation 67/40. The second reference preparation for thromboplastin, rabbit, plain (coded CRM 149R) was calibrated against its predecessor RBT/79. Each line in the diagram represents a multi-centre calibration.

to introduce a house standard or working reference preparation which is a batch of thromboplastin set aside for the calibration of individual production batches. The calibration of the house standard should be performed by comparison with a (BCR) secondary reference preparation. The calibrated house standard may then be used for lot-to-lot calibration which may be carried out with pooled plasmas (either deep-frozen or lyophilized) instead of fresh individual plasmas.

Effects of instruments

The thromboplastin reference preparations issued by WHO and BCR have been calibrated by means of manual techniques, and the ISI values of the reference preparations relate to the manual technique. However, more than 98% of larger hospital laboratories in the US rely on instruments rather than manual methods for coagulation testing and, in Europe, the proportion of laboratories using instruments is increasing. It is important to know the effect of different instruments on the PT, and more specifically, on the ISI used for oral anticoagulant control.

Several studies have shown that instruments may have a significant effect on the PT. Some studies indicated that the use of PT-ratios (patient PT: mean normal PT) would eliminate some of the bias due to differences in method (instrument) of clot detection. More recent studies indicate that instruments may have a significant effect on the PT-ratio and hence on the ISI (Ray & Smith 1990). The difference in ISI observed between two photo-optical instruments could amount to approximately 10% (Poggio et al 1989). It cannot be excluded that even greater differences in ISI between instruments exist (Hawkins et al 1989). These observations imply that the thromboplastin manufacturer should indicate the instrument(s) for which the stated ISI is valid. Preliminary results suggest that instrument-specific ISI values can allow determination of INR-equivalents with acceptable precision on lyophilized samples (van den Besselaar & Bertina 1988). Conversely, INR equivalents assigned to lyophilized plasmas might be used for local calibration of thromboplastin/instrument systems. These matters are presently under investigation.

Precision of the INR

The precision of the INR depends on the analytical precision of the ISI and PT-ratio (equation 2). Multi-centre studies have shown that the between-laboratory variation of the ISI ranges between 2 and 6% coefficient of variation (Hermans et al 1983, Thomson et al 1984, 1986, van den Besselaar & Bertina, 1991).

An important source of variation is the mean normal PT (MNPT) used for calculation of the PT-ratio. Some laboratories use the MNPT given in the thromboplastin manufacturer's chart. The MNPT determined by the local laboratory using fresh plasma from healthy volunteers may be different from the manufacturer's value (Peters et al 1989). It is recommended that the MNPT is the geometric mean of 20 fresh plasmas obtained from healthy ambulant adults, by the same technique as used for the patients' samples (Poller & Hirsh 1989). It is not practical to determine MNPT for every new batch of reagent according to the recommended procedure. The procedure may be simplified by replacing the fresh plasmas by a calibrated deep-frozen or lyophilized pooled normal plasma (Loeliger et al 1985b, Peters et al 1991).

Biological variation of the INR

Even if the ISI and PT-ratio were known without analytical error, still there would be variation of the INR, i.e. the INR would still depend to some extent on the thromboplastin/instrument used. The residual variation of the INR is the result of biological variation of the individual patient's coagulation factors and inhibitors. This can be readily appreciated from the scatter of individual patient points in a calibration plot (Fig. 65.4). The biological variation of the INR is a function of the difference between the working thromboplastin and the primary IRP 67/40. Thus, the true INR is best approximated with a thromboplastin similar to IRP 67/40. According to Loeliger (1984), calibration inaccuracy (ISI imprecision) plays only a minor role in the inter-thromboplastin variation on the INR within a single centre. Under well-controlled conditions the overall (i.e. including ISI imprecision, inter-laboratory variation of the PT ratio and biological variation) coefficient of variation of the INR is 11–13.5%, if thromboplastins with an ISI of approximately 1.0 are used (Loeliger et al 1985a).

In the induction phase of oral anticoagulant treatment, a wide divergence of INR values was observed with various thromboplastins, probably arising from the differences in responses of the thromboplastins to depression of vitamin K-dependent clotting factors (McKernan et al 1988).

INITIATION OF TREATMENT

In acute venous thrombosis or pulmonary embolism, it is common practice to initiate anticoagulation with heparin and overlap the first days of oral anticoagulant treatment with heparin, until the vitamin K-dependent factors are sufficiently depressed. However, in some areas, patients with documented deep-vein thrombosis are treated with oral anticoagulants only in a non-hospital setting. In a recent clinical trial, Brandjes et al (1991) demonstrated that this strategy for proximal deep venous thrombosis is clearly less efficacious than the combined regimen of heparin with oral anticoagulants. Gallus et al (1986) compared two anticoagulant regimens, similar except for the timing of warfarin therapy, in patients with clinically submassive venous thromboembolism. Warfarin was begun after 7 days of continuous intravenous heparin infusion or within 3 days (average 1 day) of starting heparin. The observed incidence of symptomatic recurrent venous thromboembolism during the hospital stay, the in-patient mortality and the incidence of major or minor bleeding were similar in both groups. Early warfarin treatment significantly shortened hospital stay in patients admitted solely because of submassive venous thromboembolism.

Coumarin skin necrosis

One of the rare side-effects of oral anticoagulant treatment is skin necrosis. Practically it occurs only during the induction period of treatment. There may be a causal relationship between protein C deficiency and coumarin skin necrosis. Unlike other vitamin K-dependent factors, protein C dampens the haemostatic reactions. During the initial phase of oral anticoagulant therapy there is a rapid drop not only of factor VII but also of protein C (Weiss et al 1987). Conceivably, a transient drop of protein C, occurring in the initial phase of oral anticoagulant therapy, might constitute a risk for thrombosis. This risk would be even higher in patients already suffering from hereditary protein C deficiency (Broekmans et al 1983, McGehee et al 1984, Pabinger-Fasching et al 1987). The exaggerated imbalance of procoagulant and anticoagulant factors during the initiation of oral anticoagulant treatment probably accounts for the local thrombosis of venules seen in patients with coumarin skin necrosis. Severe coumarin skin necrosis may be prevented by early administration of vitamin K when the first symptoms are detected (Brunner et al 1985, Teepe et al 1986, van Amstel et al 1978). Initiation of warfarin therapy in patients with protein C-deficiency may be achieved with a more gradual decline in protein C levels using progressively increasing warfarin doses over an extended period of time (Enzenauer et al 1990). A different strategy for anticoagulation was used by Zauber & Stark (1986), who maintained the protein C level with fresh frozen plasma infusions until complete inhibition of all functional vitamin K-dependent factors had been achieved. In that strategy, heparin infusion was continued throughout to preclude clotting, and it was continued 24 hours beyond cessation of fresh frozen plasma infusions to allow for clearance of any residual infused coagulation factors.

Recurrence of warfarin necrosis in the absence of anticoagulant therapy has been reported (Humphries et al 1991) and was most likely due to vitamin K deficiency.

A kindred with protein S deficiency have been described, in which the proposita suffered skin necrosis at the onset of treatment with oral anticoagulants (Craig et al 1990). As protein S is an important cofactor for protein C it is perhaps not surprising that protein S deficiency may also be associated with coumarin-induced skin necrosis.

Determinants of warfarin dose

Age. In the induction phase of treatment, the anticoagulant response to warfarin was found to be greater in elderly patients despite the elderly subjects being given a smaller weight-related dose (Shepherd et al 1977). There appeared to be no major age-related differences in warfarin pharmacokinetics and the increased effect of warfarin in the elderly seemed to result from increased intrinsic sensitivity to warfarin. This conclusion was confirmed by O'Malley et al (1977) in a retrospective analysis of 177 in-patients who had received warfarin. The overall trend was for the mean dose to fall, relative to age, after the 5th decade. In a review of 530 patients followed in an out-patient anticoagulation clinic, Gurwitz et al (1991) concluded that ageing does increase sensitivity to the anticoagulant effects of warfarin.

Weight. A survey of patients attending anticoagulant clinics showed the maintenance dose of warfarin to increase with weight and decrease with age (Dobrzanski et al 1983). A significant correlation was observed between age and weight considered together and the maintenance dose.

Race. There are geographical or ethnic differences in patient response to warfarin (Poller & Taberner 1982). Asian patients require nearly a 40% smaller weight-adjusted average warfarin dose than Caucasian and Hispanic patients (Weibert & Palinkas 1991).

Diet. It may be expected that the dose of oral anticoagulants required to achieve a certain intensity of anticoagulation is influenced by the vitamin K_1 content of the diet. In patients who were stabilized on phenprocoumon treatment, a decrease of the PT was caused by a change from a normal diet to a diet rich in vitamin K_1 (Langenberg 1985). In none of these patients the PT decreased to values below the lower limit of the target range (INR $\approx$ 2.5), implying that the clinical consequences of the influence of the variable vitamin K_1 content for therapy were small. However, extreme variation of dietary vitamin K_1 may result in anticoagulation instability (Kalra et al 1988).

Resistance to oral anticoagulants

Patients who require very large doses of oral anticoagulants are not uncommonly encountered in clinical practice. Such abnormal response to treatment may be due to genetic factors, excessive vitamin K intake, poor compliance, interaction with other drugs, impaired absorption, or hypothyroidism. Relative warfarin resistance may be associated also with hypercholesterolaemia (Robinson et al 1990). Hereditary warfarin resistance is a rare phenomenon in man. Only three human kindreds were described with a genetically determined resistance to warfarin (O'Reilly et al 1964, O'Reilly 1970, Alving et al 1985). The inheritance pattern in the kindreds reported by O'Reilly was compatible with the dominant expression of a single autosomal gene. It was proposed that in warfarin-resistant rats, the resistance is due to a mutation that alters the enzyme system that converts vitamin K 2,3-epoxide to reduced vitamin K (Bell 1978).

Therapeutic target ranges of oral anticoagulation

Therapeutic target ranges are narrow because under-anticoagulation gives inadequate protection against thromboembolic events, and overanticoagulation increases the bleeding risk. The required minimum anticoagulation intensity depends on the origin of the thromboembolic process. This notion led to different target ranges for various clinical states. At present, full international consensus on the target ranges of anticoagulation has not yet been achieved, though considerable progress has been made in recent years (Loeliger et al 1985b, Hirsh et al 1989, British Society for Haematology 1990).

The INR target ranges in various conditions recently suggested by the British Society for Haematology and by the Federation of Dutch Thrombosis Centres are shown in Table 65.2 and 65.3, respectively. Comparing these Tables, one can see both agreement and disagreement.

Table 65.2 Suggested INR ranges in various conditions[a]

INR	Clinical state
2.0–2.5	Prophylaxis of deep vein thrombosis including surgery on high risk patients. (2.0–3.0 for hip surgery and fractured femur operations)
2.0–3.0	Treatment of deep vein thrombosis Pulmonary embolism Systemic embolism Prevention of venous thrombo-embolism in myocardial infarction Mitral stenosis with embolism Transient ischaemic attacks Atrial fibrillation
3.0–4.5	Recurrent deep vein thrombosis and pulmonary embolism Arterial disease including myocardial infarction Mechanical prosthetic heart valves

[a] British Society for Haematology 1990.

Table 65.3 INR target ranges recommended for various indications in out-patient and home-patient therapy[a]

INR target	INR range	Indication
3.0	2.5–3.5	Primary and secondary prevention of deep vein thrombosis and pulmonary embolism Recurrent venous thromboembolism in non-anticoagulated patients Primary and secondary prevention after hip surgery
3.5	3.0–4.5	Primary and secondary prevention of arterial thromboembolism, including cardiogenic embolism Recurrent venous thromboembolism in patients treated with 3.0 INR target Tissue prosthetic heart valves
4.0	3.6–4.8	Mechanical prosthetic heart valves

[a] Federation of Dutch Thrombosis Centres 1991.

TREATMENT AND SECONDARY PREVENTION OF DEEP VENOUS THROMBOSIS

Studies by Hull et al (1982) in the treatment of deep vein thrombosis have shown that a range of 2.0–2.5 INR is effective and safe. In a retrospective study of thromboembolic recurrencies during secondary prophylaxis after deep vein thrombosis, Schulman & Lockner (1985) observed that patients without neoplastic disease never had complications if the anticoagulation intensity was ⩾2 INR.

The studies by Hull et al (1982) supported the suggested range of 2.0–3.0 INR for treatment of deep vein thrombosis (British Society for Haematology 1990). A target range of 2.0–3.5 INR was used by Gallus et al (1986), and a mean INR of 3.2 was achieved on the first day off heparin. The Federation of Dutch Thrombosis Centres recommend a target range of 2.5–3.5 INR to prevent the INR falling below the lower limit of 2.0 INR (Loeliger & Broekmans 1985). A range of 3.0–4.5 INR is suggested for recurrent deep vein thrombosis and pulmonary embolism by the British Society for Haematology, and by the Dutch Federation of Thrombosis Centres if recurrence was observed under adequately controlled low-intensity of anticoagulation, i.e. 2.5–3.5 INR.

Prophylaxis of deep vein thrombosis

The first controlled studies of prophylactic anticoagulant therapy in injured patients were performed by Sevitt & Gallagher (1959) and by Sevitt & Innes (1964). Treatment was monitored with a home-made saline extract of acetone-dried human brain. Sevitt & Innes (1964) obtained effective prophylaxis with a target range of 2–3-times prolongation of the normal prothrombin time. According to Sevitt & Innes, this target range was equivalent to 10–5% Thrombotest activity, which corresponds to 2.8–4.8 INR (Gogstad et al 1986).

A controlled study of patients undergoing upper-abdominal surgery was performed by van der Linde (1974). One group of patients were given acenocoumarol 3 days before the operation and thereafter maintained on oral anticoagulant therapy. In the other group the anticoagulant therapy was started on the 2nd postoperative day. The anticoagulant effect was controlled by the Thrombotest method. The Thrombotest level was 20–15% (1.8–2.1 INR) on the day of operation and thereafter 15–5% (2.1–4.8 INR). Thrombosis was detected in only 2% of the 97 patients who had received anticoagulants during the operation. In the other group of 104 patients, not receiving the pre-operative anticoagulants, thrombosis occurred in 30%. There was no significant difference in blood loss between the two groups. A controlled study of patients undergoing major gynaecological surgery was performed by Taberner et al (1978). Immediate preoperative anticoagulation levels of 2.0–2.5 INR and postoperative levels of 2.0–4.0 INR gave adequate protection without increased haemorrhagic risk.

In a randomized, prospective trial of patients undergoing elective total hip or knee replacement, the safety and efficacy of warfarin was studied in comparison with that of dextran 40 (Francis et al 1983). A low dose of warfarin was started 10 to 14 days pre-operatively, and the prothrombin time was regulated to between 1.5 and 3 seconds longer than control at the time of surgery (estimated INR range: 1.3–1.6). Immediately after surgery, the dose was increased to prolong the prothrombin time to 1.5 times control (estimated target level: 2.3 INR). The two-step warfarin therapy provided highly effective prophylaxis of postoperative venous thrombosis after elective hip or knee prosthetic surgery without excessive risk of perioperative bleeding.

In a Dutch consensus meeting on the prophylaxis of deep venous thrombosis, it was recommended that patients were treated for three months after hip or knee surgery aiming at 2.0–2.5 INR (van Vroonhoven 1989), but the Federation of Dutch Thrombosis Centres advised a target range of 2.5–3.5 INR, to prevent the INR falling below 2.0.

Myocardial infarction

Two recently performed studies showed that oral anticoagulants are effective in preventing death, recurrent infarction and non-haemorrhagic stroke in patients who had acute myocardial infarction. The first study involved patients aged over 60 who had been treated with anticoagulant therapy after a proven infarction at least 6 months before (the mean infarct to trial interval was 5.9 years) (Sixty-Plus Reinfarction Group 1980). The patients were then randomized either to stop or to continue therapy with a target range of 2.7–4.5 INR. The two groups were handled similarly in respect of hospital visits and blood samples, and the assessing physicians did not know the nature of the tablets being taken. This study assessed the effect of withdrawing a medication which had been used for nearly 6 years, rather than of starting treatment in routine post-infarction patients. In this selected group of elderly patients, continuation of intensive and stable oral anticoagulant therapy substantially reduced the risk of recurrent myocardial infarction and thereby of cardiac death.

The second study involved 1214 patients who had recovered from acute myocardial infarction (mean interval from the onset of symptoms to randomization, 27 days) and were randomly assigned to treatment with warfarin or placebo for an average of 37 months (Smith et al 1990). The target range of 2.8–4.8 INR was achieved by two-thirds of the warfarin-treated patients at any given time. The investigators observed a 24% reduction of mortality in the warfarin group as compared with the placebo group. Furthermore, a reduction of 34% in the number of re-infarctions and a reduction of 55% in the number of total cerebrovascular accidents was observed. Serious bleeding was noted in 0.6% of the warfarin-treated patients per year. The investigators concluded that long-term therapy with warfarin has an important beneficial effect after myocardial infarction and can be recommended in the treatment of patients who survive the acute phase. A study similar to that by Smith et al (1990) is presently being undertaken in the Netherlands under the acronym ASPECT (Anticoagulants in the Secondary Prevention of Events in Coronary Thrombosis) (Boissel 1987). ASPECT is a study designed to evaluate long-term oral anticoagulant therapy against placebo in double-blind trial. The sample size (4000) is expected to give a statistical power sufficient to detect a reasonable benefit on total mortality.

Mechanical prosthetic heart valves

Thromboembolism is the most common complication in patients with a prosthetic heart valve, although recent mechanical valves are less thrombogenic than the earlier types (Gössinger et al 1986, Butchart et al 1988). Life-long anticoagulant therapy is widely recommended for those patients.

In many clinical studies, oral anticoagulation was combined with either dipyridamole or aspirin, or both (Chesebro et al 1983, Altman et al 1991, Stein & Fuster 1991). It remains to be shown that the addition of antiplatelet drugs such as dipyridamole or aspirin reduces the incidence of thromboembolism to a degree that would justify the combination (Broekmans & Loeliger 1986). By comparing several studies in which different target levels of oral anticoagulation were used, Loeliger & Broekmans (1985) showed that the incidence of thromboembolism decreased with increasing intensity of anticoagulation. The lowest incidence of thromboembolism was 0.5–1 events per 100 patient-years, at a target intensity of 4–5 INR.

In a recent study by Saour et al (1990), two patient groups with different target intensities of anticoagulation (2.65 INR and 9.0 INR, respectively) were compared. Thromboembolism occurred with similar frequency in the two groups (4.0 and 3.7 episodes per 100 patient-years, respectively), but there was a total of 6.2 bleeding episodes per 100 patient-years in the 2.65 INR group, as compared with 12.1 episodes in the 9.0 INR group. The incidence of thromboembolism in the 2.65 INR target group agrees well with the relationship observed by Loeliger & Broekmans (1985), but the frequency in the 9.0 INR target group clearly does not! Van der Meer et al (1991) point out that this paradox can be explained by the fact that all thromboembolic events occurred at levels below the lower limit of the high intensity target range. In other words: the high intensity regimen offered complete protection as long as the target was indeed achieved. Saour et al (1990) assessed the anticoagulation intensity of their patients with use of Simplastin, a rabbit-brain thromboplastin, and an automated optical-end-point blood coagulation instrument (Coag-a-mate X2). According to these authors the ISI of their system was 2.4. This value (i.e. 2.4) was reported for Simplastin used with the manual technique (van den Besselaar et al 1986). Recent experience in the author's laboratory indicates that Simplastin used with the Schnitger & Gross coagulometer and Simplastin Automated used with the Coag-a-mate X2 is associated with an ISI of about 2.1. The anticoagulation intensity of the patients studied by Saour et al might be lower than reported as these investigators were not aware of an instrument effect on the ISI.

Intensive anticoagulation of patients with mechanical prosthetic heart valves is recommended by the American College of Chest Physicians (Hirsh et al 1989), the British Society for Haematology (1990), and the Federation of Dutch Thrombosis Centres. The Dutch recommended target range of 3.5–4.8 INR is even more intense than the American/British range of 3.0–4.5 INR.

Tissue heart valve replacement

In a recent study of oral anticoagulation after tissue heart valve replacement, one group of 102 patients was randomized to a target range of 2.0–2.25 INR, and another group of 108 patients to a target range of 2.5–4.0 INR. Treatment with warfarin was continued for 12 weeks in all patients. There were two major embolic events in the first group and four in the second. Furthermore, 11 patients in the first group and 11 patients in the second group had minor embolic events. Haemorrhagic complications were significantly more frequent with the target range of 2.5–4.0 INR than with the less intensive regimen. The conclusion that the less intensive warfarin regimen is no less effective than the 'standard' regimen (2.5–4.0 INR target range) in preventing major systemic embolism in patients with tissue valve replacement, was criticized by van der Meer et al (1991) in that both regimens were equally ineffective because of the unacceptably high incidence of thromboembolism in both groups.

Atrial fibrillation

Patients with atrial fibrillation are at increased risk of having a stroke, presumably because of emboli originating in the atria.

Some patients with atrial fibrillation — those with rheumatic mitral valve disease, previous embolism, thyrotoxicosis, and certain other cardiac conditions — are at extraordinary risk of stroke, and for these patients chronic anticoagulant prophylaxis is generally recommended (Walker 1989). Patients with atrial fibrillation unrelated to rheumatic or prosthetic valvular heart disease have a risk of ischaemic stroke about five times higher than that of persons with normal sinus rhythm. Satisfactory preventive strategies validated by adequate clinical trials have been lacking. In patients with nonrheumatic atrial fibrillation there are several large, prospective randomized clinical trials of prophylactic antithrombotic medication to reduce the frequency of stroke, systemic embolism, and other cardiovascular morbidity (Walker 1989). Three such trials are complete (Petersen et al 1989, the Boston Area Anticoagulation Trial for Atrial Fibrillation Investigators 1990, Stroke Prevention in Atrial Fibrillation Investigators 1991). The Copenhagen AFASAK study (Petersen et al 1989) of 1007 patients with chronic atrial fibrillation showed a beneficial effect of warfarin on the occurrence of thromboembolic complications, as compared with aspirin and placebo. The target intensity range in the AFASAK study was 2.8–4.2, although this was achieved for only 42% of the treatment time. The values were below 2.8 INR for 57% of the treatment time.

Low-intensity of anticoagulation (target range: 1.5–2.7 INR) was used in the Boston area anticoagulation trial for atrial fibrillation (1990) and appeared to be effective in preventing stroke in patients with nonrheumatic atrial fibrillation.

A preliminary report of the Stroke Prevention in Atrial Fibrillation Study was published in 1990. In this study, the safety and efficacy of warfarin and aspirin (as separate treatments) are tested for the primary prevention of ischaemic stroke and systemic thromboembolism in patients with nonrheumatic atrial fibrillation. The target intensity of anticoagulation was reported as 2.0–3.5 INR, but the actual target range was probably wider because of different thromboplastin reagents used in the study (Poller 1990). Final results of this study were published in 1991. During a mean follow-up of 1.3 years, the rate of primary events was reduced by 42% in the patients assigned to aspirin. In the subgroup of warfarin-eligible patients, warfarin reduced the risk of primary events by 67%. Because warfarin-eligible patients composed a subset of all aspirin-eligible patients, the magnitude of reduction in events by warfarin versus aspirin cannot be compared. The investigators concluded that patients with nonrheumatic atrial fibrillation who can safely take either aspirin or warfarin should receive prophylactic antithrombotic therapy to reduce the risk of stroke.

Although moderately intensive anticoagulation may be effective in some patients with nonrheumatic atrial fibrillation, the Federation of Dutch Thrombosis Centres recommends a target intensity of 3.5 INR, because in non-hypertensive patients the benefit outweighs the bleeding risk (Loeliger & Broekmans 1985).

Other indications

In a recent study, patients with chronic arterial occlusive

disease at the femoropopliteal level who had undergone autologous saphenous bypass surgery were randomly assigned to oral anticoagulant treatment or no treatment (Kretschmer et al 1988). The treated group had a greater probability of survival. When patients with graft occlusions were excluded from the analysis, the difference in probability of survival between the two groups remained significant. Intermittent claudication is the most common and usually the presenting symptom of chronic obstructive arterial disease of the lower limbs. Dettori et al (1989) evaluated the efficacy of pentoxifylline and acenocoumarol (target range: 2–4.5 INR) alone and in combination, in the treatment of intermittent claudication. Both pentoxifylline and acenocoumarol were significantly more effective than placebo in increasing the proportion of patients who improved their performance on the treadmill after 1 year of treatment. The combination of the two drugs did not significantly increase the benefit obtained with oral anticoagulants alone and appeared to be particularly harmful, because two fatal cerebral haemorrhages and one gastrointestinal bleeding occurred in the group treated with both active drugs. Although Dettori et al (1989) concluded that the benefits of oral anticoagulant therapy are outweighed by the risk of serious bleeding, the Federation of Dutch Thrombosis Centres recommends anticoagulation with a target range of 3.0–4.5 INR for patients with peripheral arterial disease.

Systemic arterial embolism and pulmonary embolism are well recognized complications in patients with dilated cardiomyopathy. In a study of 38 patients with dilated cardiomoypathy, Kyrle et al (1985) observed that administration of oral anticoagulants (target range: 2.1–4.8 INR) completely prevented the appearance of systemic arterial or pulmonary embolism.

CONTRAINDICATIONS TO ORAL ANTICOAGULANT

Pre-existing haemostatic defects are relative or absolute contraindications. Exceptions are the lupus inhibitors (Poller 1987).

Anticoagulants are not advised in severe hypertension, retinopathy, subacute bacterial endocarditis, uraemia, surgical disorders of the kidney, a previous cerebrovascular accident (unless embolic), trauma to the central nervous system, chronic alcoholism and the gastrointestinal disorders: peptic ulcer, hiatus hernia, hepatic disease and steatorrhoea (Poller 1987).

Breast feeding is not considered a contraindication, particularly if vitamin K_1 supplements are given to the baby (Fondevila et al 1989).

Long-term anticoagulation for out-patients or home-patients is also contraindicated if regular, standardized laboratory control is not possible or if there is a lack of patient cooperation or intelligence.

Pregnancy

Oral anticoagulants cross the placenta and may produce distinct fetal complications: a characteristic embryopathy, central nervous system abnormalities, or fetal bleeding (Harrington & Ansell 1991, Hirsh 1991). Coumarin embryopathy is a constellation of abnormalities that includes stippled epiphyses, nasal hypoplasia or punctate calcifications. Coumarin embryopathy has been reported only with exposure during the first trimester, but central nervous system abnormalities have been reported with exposure to coumarin during any trimester. Therefore, at no time during pregnancy is it truly safe for oral anticoagulant use. While heparin is likely to have no fetal side-effects (heparin does not cross the placenta), maternal complications from its use may be a limiting factor. Apart from the always-present risk of bleeding, the major concern in pregnancy is maternal heparin-induced osteoporosis.

Oral anticoagulants should not be used in the first trimester of pregnancy and if possible should be avoided throughout pregnancy. Heparin is preferred when anticoagulants are indicated in pregnant women (Ginsberg et al 1989). For all patients, oral anticoagulants must be replaced by heparin at around 36 weeks (British Society for Haematology 1990).

RESTORATION OF THE COAGULATION DEFECT

Correction of the coagulation defect may be required because of bleeding, overanticoagulation, or the need to restore good haemostasis in patients requiring surgery.

Bleeding

The method of correction depends on the severity, localization and nature of bleeding. In case of minor bleeding (e.g. haematuria and epistaxis) during the use of acenocoumarin (short half life), it may be sufficient to stop the administration of this anticoagulant temporarily. If a long-acting anticoagulant (phenprocoumon, warfarin) is used, vitamin K_1 should be administered: the maximum effect of oral vitamin K_1 is achieved only after about 24 hours (van der Meer et al 1968). Some authors maintain that vitamin K_1 should be given intravenously in case of minor bleeding (Poller 1987, British Society for Haematology 1990), but oral administration of vitamin K_1 is also adequate in most cases. Intravenous administration of vitamin K_1 should be considered in malabsorption states. A repeat course of vitamin K_1 may be necessary because the half life of vitamin K_1 is much shorter than that of warfarin and phenprocoumon.

In case of life-threatening haemorrhage, vitamin K_1 should be administered and prothrombin complex concentrate or fresh frozen plasma should be infused in order to span the time until the effect of vitamin K_1 is obtained (Poller 1987, British Society for Haematology 1990). An advantage of prothrombin complex concentrate in comparison with fresh frozen plasma is its small volume so that high concentrations of coagulation factors can be achieved rapidly. Furthermore, prothrombin complex concentrates are heat-treated for inactivation of human immunodeficiency virus (HIV). Heat treatment results also in a reduction of hepatitis non-A, non-B, but complete elimination is not achieved. Because of the risks of inducing hepatitis and HIV infection with plasma products, the application of substitution therapy should be restricted to life-threatening bleeding or bleeding resulting in disability.

Patients in shock (haemorrhagic shock or otherwise) may require infusion of coagulation factors because of insufficient liver function and poor response to vitamin K_1 administration.

Overanticoagulation

Overanticoagulation without bleeding may be corrected by stopping anticoagulant administration temporarily and/or administration of vitamin K_1, as described above. The required dose of vitamin K_1 depends on the intensity of anticoagulation. The Federation of Dutch Thrombosis Centres recommends 3–5 mg oral vitamin K_1 if the INR exceeds 8.0, and 1–2 mg for INR over 5.0. Overcorrection was observed with 2.5 mg of intravenous vitamin K_1 in patients with INR over 5 (Taberner et al 1976). Andersen & Godal (1975) studied the effect of 1 mg intravenous vitamin K_1 in patients with INR between 2.4 and 7.4, without altering the dose of warfarin. Within 24 hours, the anticoagulant intensity fell to INR values between 1.4 and 2.5. The short duration of action of vitamin K_1 during coumarin overdose has become more evident with the development of new rodenticidal coumarin anticoagulants, such as difenacoum and brodifacoum, which are more potent and persistent vitamin K_1 antagonists than warfarin (Vermeer & Hamulyák, 1991). In man, high plasma concentrations of vitamin K_1 are maintained for short periods after intravenous administration of a single (10 mg) dose, but were not achieved with an equivalent oral dose (Park et al 1984).

Surgery

Before surgery is performed in patients taking oral anticoagulants, it is common practice to reduce or stop the anticoagulant medication in order to balance the risk of thromboembolism with that of excessive bleeding. In a recent study, it was shown that tranexamic acid mouthwash after oral surgery is effective in preventing bleeding after oral surgery in patients who are being treated with anticoagulants (Sindet-Pedersen et al 1989). In another study of patients on anticoagulant therapy who underwent tooth extractions without a change in their level of anticoagulation, a biologic adhesive combined with a collagen fleece was used successfully to achieve local haemostasis at the site of the surgical wound (Martinowitz et al 1990).

In a retrospective study of patients receiving long-term warfarin therapy who underwent ocular surgery, no significant difference in haemorrhagic complications was seen between patients in whom warfarin was continued and those in whom it was discontinued. The haemorrhagic complications in the warfarin-treated patients had no long-term effect on visual acuity. One thrombotic complication was noted among the 41 patients in whom the anticoagulants were discontinued (Gainey et al 1989).

DRUG INTERACTIONS WITH ORAL ANTICOAGULANTS

Numerous drugs have been reported to interact with oral anticoagulants. However, only a small number of drug interactions that affect the pharmacokinetics or pharmacodynamics of coumarin derivatives have been well documented. Drugs can influence the pharmacokinetics of the anticoagulant by altering its metabolic clearance or its rate of absorption from the intestine. Drugs can also alter the pharmacodynamics of a coumarin derivative (without affecting its plasma levels) by altering its anticoagulant effect or the activity of other pathways of haemostasis (Hirsh 1991). Drugs may interact by more than one mechanism; for example, phenylbutazone inhibits the metabolism of S-warfarin, displaces warfarin from albumin-binding sites and may potentiate anticoagulant action by interfering with platelet function (Breckenridge 1984). A list of drugs reported as interacting with oral anticoagulants is shown in Table 65.4.

According to the Federation of Dutch Thrombosis Centres, the use of azapropazone, diflunisal, phenylbutazone, oxyphenbutazone, and high doses of aspirin (over 3 g per day) is contraindicated during oral anticoagulant therapy, because of strong potentiation of coumarin effect by these drugs and the increased risk of dangerous bleeding. According to the British Society for Haematology, the use of azapropazone and diflunisal is not contraindicated (see Table 65.4).

Pharmacokinetic drug interactions

Pharmacokinetic interactions include effects on anticoagulant absorption, distribution, protein binding, and metabolism.

Drugs affecting anticoagulant absorption

In practice, the only drug shown to influence warfarin absorption significantly is cholestyramine (Robinson et al 1971), administration of which within 3 hours after a dose of warfarin reduced the amount of warfarin absorbed.

Table 65.4 Drugs reported as interacting with oral anticoagulants

Potentiating drugs	Antagonistic drugs
Gastrointestinal tract:	
Antacids–magnesium salts	Cholestyramine
	Colestipol
Cimetidine	
Liquid paraffin and other laxatives	
Cardiovascular system:	
Amiodarone	Cholestyramine
Clofibrate	Colestipol
Dextrothyroxine	Spironolactone
Diazoxide	
Dipyridamole	
Ethacrynic acid	
Quinidine	
Sulphinpyrazone	
Respiratory system:	
	Antihistamines
Central nervous system:	
Chloral hydrate and related compounds	Barbiturates
	Carbamazepine
Chlorpromazine	Dichloralphenazone(-late)
Dextropropoxyphene	
Dichloralphenazone(-initial)	Haloperidol
Diflunisal	Phenytoin
Mefenamic acid	Primidone
Monoamine oxidase inhibitors	
Tricyclic antidepressants	
Triclofos sodium	
Infections:	
Aminoglycosides:	Griseofulvin
Amikacin	Rifampicin
Gentamicin	
Kanamycin	
Neomycin	
Streptomycin	
Tobramycin	
Co-trimoxazole	
Cephalosporins:	
Cephaloridine	
Cephazolin	
Cephamandole	
Latamoxef (Moxalactam)	
Chloramphenicol	
Cycloserine	
Erythromycin	
Isoniazid	
Ketoconazole	
Metronidazole	
Miconazole	
Nalidixic acid	
Penicillin G(-large doses, intravenous)	
Ampicillin-oral	
Quinine salts	

Potentiating drugs	Antagonistic drugs
Infections: cont'd	
Streptotriad	
Sulphonamides(-long acting)	
Tetracycline	
Endocrine system:	
Anabolic steroids	Oral contraceptives
Chlorpropamide	
Corticosteroids	
Danazol	
Glucagon	
Metoclopramide	
Propylthiouracil	
Sulphonylurea	
Thyroxine	
Tolbutamide	
Malignant disease and immunosuppression:	
Cyclophosphamide	
Mercaptopurine	
Methotrexate	
Immunosuppressant drugs	
Tamoxifen	
Musculoskeletal and joint disease:	
Allopurinol	
Aspirin and the salicylates	
Azapropazone	
Diflunisal	
Fenclofenac	
Fenoprofen	
Feprazone	
Flufenamic acid	
Flurbiprofen	
Indomethacin	
Ketoprofen	
Mefenamic acid	
Naproxen	
Paracetamol (high daily dose) with dextropropoxyphene	
Distalgesic/coproxamol)	
Piroxicam	
Sulindac	
Sulphinpyrazone	
Nutrition and blood:	
Alcohol-dose dependent potentiator	Vitamin K
	Alcohol
Ear, nose and oesophagus:	Antihistamines
	Phenazone
Skin:	
	Antihistamines
Alcoholism:	
Disulfiram (Antabuse)	

These preparations should not be regarded as contraindicated or as contraindications to warfarin administration. Their prescription may, however, cause changes in oral anticoagulant requirements. Caution is therefore advised and more frequent monitoring may be required. This list is not intended to be comprehensive. Some drugs have only been referred to in single case reports (British Society for Haematology 1990).

Cholestyramine may also interact with warfarin and phenprocoumon by interrupting enterohepatic recirculation (Meinertz et al 1977). If cholestyramine is prescribed with oral anticoagulants, cholestyramine should be administered at least 4 hours after taking the oral anticoagulant dose.

Drugs causing protein-binding displacement

While many drugs (usually highly protein-bound acidic compounds) can displace warfarin from albumin binding sites, this does not automatically produce an increased anticoagulant effect (Breckenridge 1984). In practice, protein-binding displacement alone has not been shown to produce more than a transient rise in prothrombin time (Breckenridge 1984).

Drugs that cause enzyme induction

Induction of hepatic microsomal mixed-function oxygenase activity is well recognized as a cause of interaction with oral anticoagulants. Enzyme induction increases the rate of metabolism of warfarin, decreases its plasma half life and steady state concentration and therefore reduces its anticoagulant effect. Since enzyme induction is a synthetic process, the effects of an inducing agent are not immediate. The metabolic clearance of both enantiomers of warfarin is increased by barbiturates, carbamazepine, phenytoin, griseofulvin, rifampicin. Although long-term ethanol consumption may induce drug-metabolizing enzymes, moderate ethanol intake does not appear to affect anticoagulant control (O'Reilly 1979).

Drugs that cause inhibition of metabolism

Drugs inhibiting the metabolic clearance of oral anticoagulants increase the plasma levels and potentiate the anticoagulant effect. In contrast to enzyme induction, inhibition of anticoagulant metabolism has a rapid time course. Inhibition of metabolic clearance can take place either through stereospecific or non-specific pathways. Lewis et al (1974) demonstrated that phenylbutazone inhibited the metabolism of *S*-warfarin (the more potent enantiomer) while increasing the rate of elimination of *R*-warfarin. The net effect was an increased anticoagulant response to a single dose of racemic warfarin, but no apparent change in the racemic warfarin half life.

A recent study by Kunze et al (1991) clearly demonstrated that *R*-warfarin is a potent inhibitor of the cytochrome P-450 catalyzed oxidative metabolism of *S*-warfarin to 6- and 7-hydroxywarfarin. Thus, *R*-warfarin might contribute significantly to the anticoagulant effect of the drug, not by its inherent biological activity but by inhibiting the clearance of the active *S*-enantiomer. Furthermore, the presence of other drugs which have no direct effect on the clearance of *S*-warfarin might still elicit a drug interaction by inhibiting the clearance of *R*-warfarin.

Pharmacodynamic drug interactions

Drugs can also change the pharmacodynamics of warfarin (without affecting its plasma levels). Drugs that reduce the systemic availability of vitamin K_1 should augment the response to oral anticoagulants. Mineral oils (such as liquid paraffin) and cholestyramine may reduce the absorption of vitamin K_1.

The second and third generation cephalosporins augment the anticoagulant effect by inhibiting the cyclic inter-conversion of vitamin K (Bechtold et al 1984).

Drugs that alter thyroid function (e.g. thyroxine) may affect anticoagulant control, since rates of synthesis and degradation of coagulation factors are dependent on thyroid function.

Heparin

Heparin has the potential to increase the effect of oral anticoagulants by inhibition of thrombin and other serine protease coagulation factors. However, the effect of heparin on the prothrombin time is limited.

Platelet function inhibitors

Drugs that inhibit platelet function may prolong the bleeding time and therefore have the potential to increase the risk of bleeding associated with oral anticoagulants. Aspirin produces irreversible effects on platelet function which persist for the life of the aspirin-treated platelet. Furthermore, aspirin may damage the gastric mucosa. Aspirin in very high doses may also decrease prothrombin synthesis in normal subjects. Other drugs that inhibit platelet function include nonsteroidal anti-inflammatory drugs, large doses of penicillins, and moxalactam.

In practice, the risk of serious bleeding as a result of drug interactions with oral anticoagulants can be minimized by avoiding drugs that prolong the bleeding time and anticipating other drug interactions (Hirsh 1991).

PREDICTION OF ANTICOAGULANT DOSAGE

A variety of methods have been proposed which attempt to assist the physician to predict the maintenance dose of coumarin required for therapeutic anticoagulation. The stimulus for these methods comes from two sources: firstly, the eventual dose required varies widely among apparently similar people and the consequences of either under- or over-anticoagulation are clinically important; and secondly, the time taken to initiate treatment and determine the correct maintenance dose by the traditional empirical method takes a minimum of a week and in some cases several weeks. Shortening the time needed to reach the correct maintenance dose would be important not only because the therapeutic goal is achieved more quickly but also because the cost of treatment would be reduced. A comprehensive review of prediction methods has been published by Holford (1986).

Fennerty et al (1984) developed a flexible dose induction table which derives each evening's warfarin dose during the first four treatment days from that morning's prothrombin time ratio. A randomized comparison of warfarin treatment outcomes in two groups of patients starting therapy was performed by Doecke et al (1991): in one group warfarin dosage was determined by clinical pharmacists using the dose-response protocol of Fennerty et al (1984), and in the other group dosage was prescribed empirically by resident medical staff. The mean INR for each treatment day, the mean time to reach a therapeutic level of INR, the mean maintenance dose and the mean time to reach maintenance dose were not significantly different between the protocol and empirical treatment groups. Although the mean observations of warfarin effect were similar in the two groups, there were more patients with 'excessive' warfarin effects (INR > 4.0) during empirical treatment.

In another prospective randomized trial, the accuracy of warfarin dosage-adjustment predictions using a computer program was compared with the skill of an experienced anticoagulation nurse-specialist (White & Mungall 1991). In this study, consecutive patients on long-term oral anticoagulation therapy were included who required an adjustment in the dose of warfarin. There were no significant differences between the nurse-specialist group and the computer group with respect to the mean absolute error of the prothrombin time (i.e. final PT-target PT), and the proportion of patients who had a final prothrombin time within 2 seconds of the target prothrombin time.

Dosage prediction based on a pharmacokinetic/pharmacodynamic model was evaluated in a study of in-patients, using data from the first 1–5 days of therapy (Boyle et al 1989). The results of the study confirmed previous findings that the estimation of warfarin pharmacodynamic parameters using Bayesian regression analysis cannot be based on prothrombin time data from only the first 1–3 days of therapy. Prothrombin ratios for the first 5 days of therapy were required for good predictive performance.

ORGANIZATION OF AN OUTPATIENT ANTICOAGULANT CLINIC

In the Netherlands, out-patients and home-patients treated with oral anticoagulants are controlled by special anticoagulant clinics called thrombosis centres. Each of the Dutch centres operates within a clearly defined geographical area. In each centre, all medical and patient data are stored and all activities are organized, i.e. blood sampling, laboratory monitoring, dosage prescription by the centre's physician and mailing of dosage calendars and date of next check to each patient. Immobile patients can be visited at home for blood sampling.

The indications for anticoagulant therapy are established by the treating general practioner or the specialist referring the patients to the thrombosis centre for control and guidance of this therapy. There must be good communication between the referring doctor and the thrombosis centre, also with respect to the duration of anticoagulant therapy.

Within the organization of the Dutch thrombosis centre the staff members (usually nurses) play a very important role. They must be well informed about the side-effects of anticoagulant treatment and drugs that can interact with coumarin derivatives. They must ask the patient whether anything relevant has occurred, such as bleeding, intercurrent diseases, changes in medication, etc. All relevant information is recorded and brought to the attention of the centre's physician for determination of the dose, which is also based on the laboratory results. The staff must also ensure that the patient is well informed about anticoagulant therapy and all related aspects by means of educational materials for the patients.

An increasing number of thrombosis centres are now using computers, not only for administration, but also for dosage prescription and appointment regulation (Loeliger et al 1984).

The Federation of Dutch Thrombosis Centres

Practically all out-patient clinics in the Netherlands are members of the Federation of Dutch Thrombosis Centres. Together they serve an area with a population of about 13 million individuals or 90% of the total population. In addition to the 71 centres in the Netherlands, there is also a Dutch thrombosis centre in southern Spain for Dutch patients on vacation; predominantly those who spend the winter there.

The number of patients controlled annually by the thrombosis centres is about 250 000. The number of laboratory determinations performed to check on the oral anticoagulation therapy is about 3 500 000 per year.

The goals of the Federation include:

- To provide recommendations and guidelines with respect to the desired intensity of anticoagulation
- To monitor and, when necessary, improve the quality of oral anticoagulant therapy provided by the member centres
- To provide guidelines, recommendations and educational material for the patients
- To organize refresher courses for staff, medical directors and clinical chemists of the Thrombosis Centres
- To stimulate and carry out scientific research in the field of thrombosis
- To carry out collective negotiations with the Ministry of Welfare, Public Health and Culture and those responsible for the financing.

Therapeutic quality assessment

An important part of internal quality control in the anticoagulation clinic is the assessment of therapeutic control achieved in the patients under treatment. This type of self-audit has demonstrated that the quality of oral anticoagulant therapy may require considerable improvement, particularly in short-term patients (Majumdar & Payne 1985). In some hospitals, under-anticoagulation is the main deficiency, most probably due to excessively cautious prescribing by junior staff concerned to avoid the risk of bleeding problems (Harries et al 1981). Some investigators suggested that, in out-patients, poor compliance is the major cause of unstable anticoagulation with warfarin (Kumar et al 1989).

In a study of 49 patients aged 65–89 years, a significant correlation was observed between the concomitant drug therapy and anticoagulant control, but not with the occurrence of complications and treatment failures. Poor anticoagulant control was observed particularly in those receiving drugs known to potentiate warfarin effect and in whom more changes were made to their concomitant drug therapy (Wickramasinghe et al 1988). Rospond et al (1989) evaluated some factors associated with the stability of anticoagulation therapy. The time required to become stable was not significantly related to the duration of stability. The duration of stability, however, was associated with declining probability of requiring a dosage change. Because patients who achieved 3 or more months of stable anticoagulation were less likely to require a dosage adjustment, it may be possible to monitor these individuals at less frequent intervals.

Therapeutic control of anticoagulation consists of continuous assessment of the proportion of time spent by each patient in the target INR range (van den Besselaar 1990). An overall view of an anticoagulation clinic's performance may be obtained by an assessment of the proportion of patients that is within the therapeutic range (van den Besselaar et al 1988). In the Netherlands, the Federation of Dutch Thrombosis Centres requests its members to perform such assessment of their patient populations twice a year. Until 1990, many Dutch centres used the same single target range for their patients on long-term treatment, i.e. 2.8–4.8 INR. The majority of the Dutch Centres had at least 70% of their long-term patients within the target range (Fig. 65.6). Since 1991, the Federation of Dutch Thrombosis Centres recommends differentiated target ranges for various indications (Table 65.3).

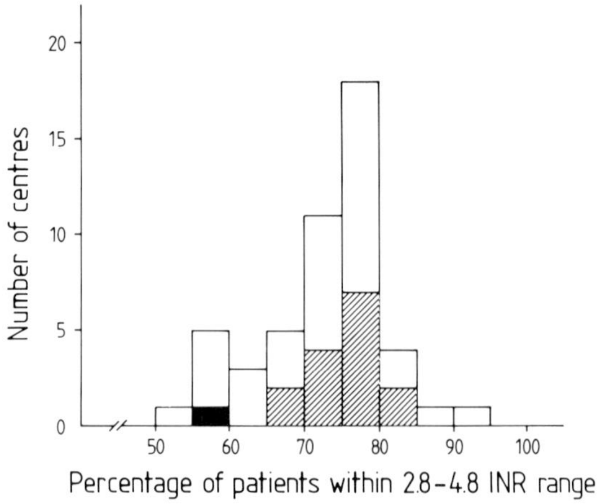

Fig. 65.6 Therapeutic control achieved by 49 Dutch thrombosis centres in 1989. White area represents centres with a single target range of 2.8–4.8 INR. Striped area represents centres with differentiated target ranges of various clinical states. The stippled area represents one centre with a single target range of 2.5–4.2 INR.

Acknowledgements

The author wishes to acknowledge the help of C. W. Gerrits-Drabbe MD for critically reading the manuscript and for providing therapeutic quality data of Dutch thrombosis centres.

Mrs M. de Mooij and Mrs M.J. Mentink prepared the typescript.

REFERENCES

Altman R, Rouvier J, Gurfinkel E, D'Ortencio O, Manzanel R, de La Fuente L, Favaloro R G 1991 Comparison of two levels of anticoagulant therapy in patients with substitute heart valves. Journal of Thoracic and Cardiovascular Surgery 101: 427–431

Alving B M, Strickler M P, Knight R D, Barr C F, Berenberg J L, Peck C C 1985 Hereditary warfarin resistance. Investigation of a rare phenomenon. Archives of Internal Medicine 145: 499–501

Andersen P, Godal H C 1975 Predictable reduction in anticoagulant activity of warfarin by small amounts of vitamin K. Acta Medica Scandinavica 198: 269–270

Bechtold H, Andrassy K, Jähnchen E, Koderisch J, Koderisch H, Weilemann L S, Sonntag H G, Ritz E 1984. Evidence for impaired hepatic vitamin K_1 metabolism in patients treated with N-methyl-thiotetrazole cephalosporins. Thrombosis and Haemostasis 51: 358–361

Bell R G 1978 Metabolism of vitamin K and prothrombin synthesis: anticoagulants and the vitamin K-epoxide cycle. Federation Proceedings 37: 2599–2604

Bertina R M 1984 The relationship between the International Normalized Ratio and the coumarin-induced coagulation defect. In: van den Besselaar A M H P, Gralnick H R, Lewis S M (eds) Thromboplastin calibration and oral anticoagulant control. Martinus Nijhoff, Boston

Bertina R M, Loeliger E A 1980 The potential use of chromogenic assays in the routine monitoring of oral anticoagulant therapy. In: Lijnen H R, Collen D, Verstraete M (eds) Synthetic substrates in clinical blood coagulation assays. Martinus Nijhoff, The Hague

Boissel J B 1987 Registry of multicenter clinical trials. Eighth report — 1986. Thrombosis and Haemostasis 57: 361–371

Boston Area Anticoagulation Trial for Atrial Fibrillation Investigators 1990 The effect of low-dose warfarin on the risk of stroke in patients with nonrheumatic atrial fibrillation. New England Journal of Medicine 323: 1505–1511

Boyle D A, Ludden T M, Carter B L, Becker A J, Taylor J W 1989 Evaluation of a Bayesian Regression program for predicting warfarin response. Therapeutic Drug Monitoring 11: 276–284

Brandjes D P M, Büller H R, Heijboer H, Jagt J, de Rijk M, ten Cate J W 1991 Comparative trial of heparin and oral anticoagulants in the initial treatment of proximal deep-vein thrombosis (DVT). Thrombosis and Haemostasis 65: 703

Breckenridge A M 1984 Clinical pharmacology of anticoagulants. In: Meade T W (ed.) Anticoagulants and myocardial infarction: a reappraisal. Wiley, Chichester

Breckenridge A, Orme M L, Wesseling H, Lewis R J, Gibbons R 1974

Pharmacokinetics and pharmacodynamics of the enantiomers of warfarin in man. Clinical Pharmacology and Therapeutics 15: 424–430
British Society for Haematology 1990 Guidelines on oral anticoagulation: 2nd edn. Journal of Clinical Pathology 43: 177–183
Broekmans A W, Loeliger E A 1986 High complication and failure rates of anticoagulant therapy are avoidable. Zeitschrift für Kadiologie 75 (suppl 2): 298–301
Broekmans A W, Bertina R M, Loeliger E A, Hofmann V, Klingemann H G 1983 Protein C and the development of skin necrosis during anticoagulant therapy. Thrombosis and Haemostasis 49: 251
Brunner W, Kuhn M, Hartmann G 1985 Die Cumarin-Nekrose. Eine seltene, schwere Komplikation der oralen Antikoagulation. Schweizerische Rundschau Medizin (PRAXIS) 74: 141–143
Butchart E G, Lewis P A, Grunkemeier G L, Kulatilake N, Breckenridge I M 1988 Low risk of thrombosis and serious embolic events despite low-intensity anticoagulation. Experience with 1004 Medtronic Hall Valves. Circulation 78 (suppl I): 166–177
Chesebro J H, Fuster V, Elveback L R, McGoon D C, Pluth J R, Puga F J, Wallace R B, Danielson G K, Orszulak T A, Piehler J M, Schaff H V 1983 Trial of combined warfarin plus dipyridamole or aspirin therapy in prosthetic heart valve replacement: danger of aspirin compared with dipyridamole. American Journal of Cardiology 51: 1537–1541
Conley C L, Morse W I 1948 Thromboplastic factors in the estimation of prothrombin concentration. American Journal of the Medical Sciences 215: 158–169
Couet W, Istin B, Decourt J P, Ingrand I, Girault J, Fourtillan J B 1990 Lack of effect of ponsinomycin on the pharmacokinetics of nicoumalone enantiomers. British Journal of Clinical Pharmacology 30: 616–620
Craig A, Taberner D A, Fisher A H, Foster D N, Mitra J 1990 Type I protein S-deficiency and skin necrosis. Postgraduate Medical Journal 66: 389–391
Dettori A G, Pini M, Moratti A, Paolicelli M, Basevi P, Quintavalla R, Manotti C, Di Lecce C 1989 Acenocoumarol and pentoxifylline in intermittent claudication. A Controlled Clinical Study. Angiology 40: 237–248
Dobrzanski S, Duncan S E, Harkiss A, Wardlaw A 1983 Age and weight as determinants of warfarin requirements. Journal of Clinical and Hospital Pharmacy 8: 75–77
Doecke C J, Cosh D G, Gallus A S 1991 Standardised initial warfarin treatment: evaluation of initial treatment response and maintenance dose prediction by randomised trial, and risk factors for an excessive warfarin response. Australian and New Zealand Journal of Medicine 21: 319–324
Enzenauer R J, Berenberg J L, Campbell J 1990 Progressive warfarin anticoagulation in protein C-deficiency: a therapeutic strategy. American Journal of Medicine 88: 697–698
Fennerty A, Dolben J, Thomas P, Backhouse G, Bentley D P, Campbell I A, Routledge P A 1984 Flexible induction dose regimen for warfarin and prediction of maintenance dose. British Medical Journal 288: 1268–1270
Fiessinger J N, Vitoux J F, Roncato M, Dellinger A, Dizien O, Aiach M 1989 Variations of prothrombin time, factor VII and protein C with a single daily dose of acenocoumarol. Haemostasis 19: 138–141
Fondevila C G, Meschengiesen S, Penalva L, Lazzari M A 1989 Effect of acenocoumarine on the breast-fed infant. Thrombosis Research 56: 29–36
Francis C W, Marder V J, Evarts C M, Yaukoolbodi S 1983 Two-step warfarin therapy. Prevention of postoperative venous thrombosis without excessive bleeding. Journal of the American Medical Association 249: 374–378
Gainey S P, Robertson D M, Fay, W, Ilstrup D 1989 Ocular surgery on patients receiving long-term warfarin therapy. American Journal of Ophthalmology 108: 142–146
Gallus A, Jackaman J, Tillett J, Mills W, Wycherley A 1986 Safety and efficacy of warfarin started early after submassive venous thrombosis or pulmonary embolism. Lancet ii: 1293–1296
Gill T S, Hopkins K J, Rowland M 1988 Stereospecific assay of nicoumalone: application to pharmacokinetic studies in man. British Journal of Clinical Pharmacology 25: 591–598
Ginsberg J S, Kowalchuk G, Hirsh J, Brill-Edwards P, Burrows R 1989 Heparin therapy during pregnancy. Risks to the fetus and mother. Archives of Internal Medicine 149: 2233–2236
Gogstad G O, Wadt J, Smith P, Brynildsrud T 1986 Utility of a modified calibration model for reliable conversion of thromboplastin times to International Normalized Ratios. Thrombosis and Haemostasis 56: 178–182
Gössinger H, Niessner H, Grubeck B, Mösslacher H, Bettelheim P, Lechner K, Mlczoch J, Domanig E 1986 Thromboembolism in patients with prosthetic heart valves. An adequately controlled intense anticoagulant therapy and its influence on the occurrence of thromboembolism in relation to valve type. Thoracic Cardiovascular Surgeon 34: 283–286
Gurwitz J H, Avorn J, Ross-Degnan D 1991 Age-related changes in warfarin pharmacodynamics. Clinical Pharmacology and Therapeutics 49: 166
Harries A D, Birtwell A J, Jones D B 1981 Anticoagulant control. Lancet i: 1320
Harrington R, Ansell J 1991 Risk-benefit assessment of anticoagulant therapy. Drug Safety 6: 54–69
Hawkins P L, Barrow D A, Maynard J R 1989 A sensitive thromboplastin reagent prepared from rabbit brain tissue factor for monitoring oral anticoagulant therapy. Thrombosis and Haemostasis 62: 530
Heimark L D, Toon S, Gibaldi M, Trager W F, O'Reilly R A, Darklis A G 1987 The effect of sulfinpyrazone on the disposition of pseudoracemic phenprocoumon in humans. Clinical Pharmacology and Therapy 42: 312–319
Hemker H C, Frank H L L 1985 The mechanism of action of oral anticoagulants and its consequences for the practice of oral anticoagulation. Haemostasis 15: 263–270
Hermans J, van den Besselaar A M H P, Loeliger E A, van der Velde E A 1983 A collaborative calibration study of reference materials for thromboplastins. Thrombosis and Haemostasis 50: 712–717
Hirsh J 1991 Oral anticoagulant drugs. New England Journal of Medicine 324: 1865–1875
Hirsh J, Levine M 1988 Confusion over the therapeutic range for monitoring oral anticoagulant therapy in North America. Thrombosis and Haemostasis 59: 129–132
Hirsh J, Poller L, Deykin D, Levin M, Dalen J E 1989 Optimal therapeutic range for oral anticoagulants. Chest 95 (suppl): 5S–11S
Holford N H G 1986 Clinical pharmacokinetics and pharmacodynamics of warfarin. Understanding the dose-effect relationship. Clinical Pharmacokinetics 11: 483–504
Hull R, Hirsh J, Jay R, Carter C, England C, Gent M, Turpie A G G, McLoughlin D, Dodd P, Thomas M, Raskob G, Ockelford P 1982 Different intensities of oral anticoagulant therapy in the treatment of proximal-vein thrombosis. New England Journal of Medicine 307: 1676–1681
Humphries J E, Gardner J H, Connelly J E 1991 Warfarin skin necrosis: recurrence in the absence of anticoagulant therapy. American Journal of Hematology 37: 197–200
Jones D W, Mackie I J, Winter M, Gallimore M, Machin S J 1991 Detection of protein C-deficiency during oral anticoagulant therapy — use of the protein C:factor VII ratio. Blood Coagulation and Fibrinolysis 2: 407–411
Kalra P A, Cooklin M, Wood G, O'Shea G M, Holmes A M 1988. Dietary modification as cause of anticoagulation instability. Lancet ii: 803
Kellett H A, Sawers J S A, Boulton F E, Cholerton S, Park B K, Toft A D 1986 Problems of anticoagulation with warfarin in hyperthyroidism. Quarterly Journal of Medicine, New Series 58(225): 43–51
Kirkwood T B L 1983 Calibration of reference thromboplastins and standardization of the prothrombin time ratio. Thrombosis and Haemostasis 49: 238–244
Kretschmer G, Wenzl E, Schemper M, Polterauer P, Ehringer H, Marcosi L, Minar E 1988 Influence of postoperative anticoagulant treatment on patient survival after femoropopliteal vein bypass surgery. Lancet i: 797–798
Kumar S, Haigh J R M, Rhodes L E, Peaker S, Davies J A, Roberts B E, Feely M P 1989 Poor compliance is a major factor in unstable

outpatient control of anticoagulant therapy. Thrombosis and Haemostasis 62: 729–732

Kunze K L, Eddy A C, Gibaldi M, Trager W F 1991 Metabolic enantiomeric interactions: the inhibition of human (S)-Warfarin-7-hydroxylase by (R)-Warfarin. Chirality 3: 24–29

Kyrle P A, Korninger C, Gössinger H, Glogar D, Lechner K, Niessner H, Pabinger I 1985 Prevention of arterial and pulmonary embolism by oral anticoagulants in patients with dilated cardiomyopathy. Thrombosis and Haemostasis 54: 521–523

Langenberg J P 1985 Bioanalysis of ultra-trace levels of K vitamins using electrofluorometric detection in HPLC. The influence of the variable vitamin K availability from normal diets on the stability of oral anticoagulant therapy. Ph.D. Thesis, University of Leiden, the Netherlands

Lewis R J, Trager W F, Chan K K, Breckenridge A, Orme M, Rowland M, Schary W 1974 Warfarin: stereochemical aspects of its metabolism and the interaction with phenylbutazone. Journal of Clinical Investigation 53: 1607–1617

Link K P 1959 The discovery of dicoumarol and its sequels. Circulation 19: 97–107

Loeliger E A 1984 Critical remarks from a clinican's point of view. In: van den Besselaar A M H P, Gralnick H R, Lewis S M (eds). Thromboplastin calibration and oral anticoagulant control. Martinus Nijhoff, Boston, p 109–116

Loeliger E A 1985 ICSH/ICTH recommendations for reporting prothrombin time in oral anticoagulant control. Thrombosis and Haemostasis 54: 155–156

Loeliger E A, Broekmans A W 1985 Optimal Therapeutic Anticoagulation. Haemostasis 15: 283–292

Loeliger E A, van der Esch B, Mattern M J, den Brabander A S A 1963a Behaviour of Factors II, VII, IX and X during long-term treatment with coumarin. Thrombosis et Diathesis Haemorrhagica 9: 74–89

Loeliger E A, van der Esch B, Mattern M J, Hemker H C 1963b The biological disappearance rate of prothrombin, factors VII, IX and X from plasma in hypothyroidism, hyperthyroidism, and during fever. Thrombosis et Diathesis Haemorrhagica 10: 267–277

Loeliger E A, van Dik-Wierda C A, van den Besselaar A M H P, Broekmans A W, Roos J 1984 Anticoagulant control and the risk of bleeding. In: Meade T W (ed) Antiocoagulants and myocardial infarction: a reappraisal. Wiley, Chichester

Loeliger E A, van den Besselaar A M H P, Lewis S M 1985a Reliability and clinical impact of the normalization of the prothrombin times in oral anticoagulant control. Thrombosis and Haemostasis 53: 148–154

Loeliger E A, Poller L, Samama M, Thomson J M, van den Besselaar A M H P, Vermylen J, Verstraete M 1985b Questions and Answers on Prothrombin Time Standardisation in Oral Anticoagulant Control. Thrombosis and Haemostasis 54: 515–517

McGehee W G, Klotz T A, Epstein D J, Rapaport S I 1984 Coumarin necrosis associated with hereditary protein C-deficiency. Annals of Internal Medicine 100: 59–60

McKernan A, Thomson J M, Poller L 1988 The reliability of international normalized ratios during short-term oral anticoagulant treatment. Clinical and Laboratory Haematology 10: 63–71

Majumdar G, Payne R W 1985 Quality of oral anticoagulant therapy. Clinical and Laboratory Haematology 7: 125–131

Marlar R A, Neumann A 1990 Neonatal purpura fulminans due to homozygous protein C- or protein S-deficiencies. Seminars in Thrombosis and Hemostasis 16: 299–309

Martinowitz U, Mazar A L, Taicher S, Varon D, Gitel S N, Ramot B, Rakocz M 1990 Dental extraction for patients on oral anticoagulant therapy. Oral Surgery, Oral Medicine, and Oral Pathology 70: 274–277

Meinentz T, Gilfrich H J, Groth U, Jonen H G, Jähnchen E 1977 Interruption of the enterohepatic circulation of phenprocoumon by cholestyramine. Clinical Pharmacology and Therapeutics 21: 731–735

Moulon R A, Neumann A 1990 Neonatal purpura fulminans due to homozygous protein C- or protein S-deficiencies. Seminars in Hemostasis and Thrombosis 16: 299–309

O'Malley K, Stevenson I H, Ward C A, Wood A J J, Crooks J 1977 Determinants of anticoagulant control in patients receiving warfarin. British Journal of Clinical Pharmacology 4: 309–314

O'Reilly R A 1970 The second reported kindred with hereditary resistance to oral anticoagulant drugs. New England Journal of Medicine 282: 1448–1451

O'Reilly R A 1974 Studies on the optical enantiomorphs of warfarin in man. Clinical Pharmacology and Therapeutics 16: 348–354

O'Reilly R A 1979 Lack of effect of mealtime wine on the hypoprothrombinemia of oral anticoagulants. American Journal of the Medical Sciences 277: 189–194

O'Reilly R A, Aggeler P M, Hoag M S, Leong L S, Kropatkin M L 1964 Hereditary transmission of exceptional resistance to coumarin anticoagulant drugs. The first reported kindred. New England Journal of Medicine 271: 809–815

Pabinger-Fasching I, Lechner K, Niessner H, Korninger C, Kyrle P A 1987 Protein C- and coagulation factor levels during the initial phase of oral anticoagulant therapy (low dose regimen) in a patient with heterozygous protein C-deficiency. Thrombosis Research 47: 705–708

Palareti G, Coccheri S, Poggi M, Bonetti M, Cervi V, Mazzuca A, Savoia M, Veri L, Fiori F, Gaspari G, Palareti A 1987 Oral anticoagulant therapy control: evidence that INR expression improves the interlaboratory comparability of results — The Bologna oral anticoagulant control exercise. Thrombosis and Haemostasis 58: 905–910

Park B K, Scott, A K, Wilson, A C, Haynes, B P, Breckenridge, A M 1984 Plasma disposition of vitamin K_1 in relation to anticoagulant poisoning. British Journal of Clinical Pharmacology 18: 655–662

Paul B, Oxley A, Brigham K, Cox T, Hamilton P J 1987 Factor II, VII, IX and X concentrations in patients receiving longterm warfarin. Journal of Clinical Pathology 40: 94–98

Peters R H M, van den Besselaar A M H P, Olthuis F M F G 1989. A multicentre study to evaluate method dependency of the International Sensitivity Index of bovine thromboplastin. Thrombosis and Haemostasis 61: 166–169

Peter R H M, van den Besselaar A M H P, Olthuis F M F G 1991 Determination of the mean normal prothrombin time for assessment of international normalized ratios — usefulness of lyophilized plasma. Thrombosis and Haemostasis 66: 442–445

Petersen P, Boysen G, Godtfredsen J, Anderson E D, Andersen B (1989) Placebo-controlled, randomized trial of warfarin and aspirin for prevention of thromboembolic complications in chronic atrial fibrillation: the Copenhagen AFASAK study. Lancet i: 175–179

Poggio M, van den Besselaar A M H P, van der Velde E A, Bertina R M 1989. The effect of some instruments for prothrombin time testing on the International Sensitivity Index (ISI) of two rabbit tissue thromboplastin reagents. Thrombosis and Haemostasis 62: 868–874

Poller L 1987 Oral anticoagulant therapy. In: Bloom A L, Thomas D P (eds) Haemostasis and thrombosis, 2nd edn. Churchill Livingstone, Edinburgh

Poller L 1990 Prevention of stroke in atrial fibrillation. New England Journal of Medicine 323: 483

Poller L, Hirsh J 1989 A simple system for the derivation of International Normalized Ratios for the reporting of prothrombin time results with North American Thromboplastin Reagents. American Journal of Clinical Pathology 92: 124–126

Poller L, Taberner D A 1982 Dosage and control of oral anticoagulants: an international collaborative study. British Journal of Haematology 51: 479–485

Quick A J, Stanley-Brown M, Bancroft F W 1935 A study of the coagulation defect in hemophilia and in jaundice. American Journal of the Medical Sciences 190: 501–511

Ray M J, Smith I R 1990 The dependence of the International Sensitivity Index on the Coagulometer used to perform the Prothrombin Time. Thrombosis and Haemostasis 63: 424–429

Rizza C R, Jones P 1987 Management of patients with inherited blood coagulation defects. In Bloom A L, Thomas D P (eds) Haemostasis and thrombosis, 2nd edn. Churchill Livingstone, Edinburgh

Robinson D S, Benjamin D M, McCormack J J 1971 Interaction of warfarin and non-systemic gastro-intestinal drugs. Clinical Pharmacology and Therapeutics 12: 491–495

Robinson A, Liau F O, Routledge P A, Backhouse G, Spragg B P, Bentley D P 1990 Lipids and warfarin requirements. Thrombosis and Haemostasis 63: 148–149

Rospond R M, Quandt C M, Clark G M, Bussey H I 1989 Evaluation of factors associated with stability of anticoagulation therapy. Pharmacotherapy 9: 207–213

Saour J N, Sieck J O, Mamo L A R, Gallus A S 1990 Trial of different intensities of anticoagulation in patients with prosthetic heart valves. New England Journal of Medicine 322: 428–432

Schulman S, Lockner D 1985 Relationship between thromboembolic complications and intensity of treatment during long-term prophylaxis with oral anticoagulants following DVT. Thrombosis and Haemostasis 53: 137–140

Sevitt N, Gallagher N G 1959 Prevention of venous thrombosis and pulmonary embolism in injured patients. Lancet ii: 981–989

Sevitt N, Innes D 1964 Prothrombin-time and Thrombotest in injured patients on prophylactic anticoagulant therapy. Lancet i: 124–129

Shearer M J, Barkhan P, Webster G R 1970 Absorption and excretion of an oral dose of tritiated vitamin K_1 in man. British Journal of Haematology 18: 297–308

Shetty H G M, Fennerty A G, Routledge P A 1989 Clinical pharmacokinetic considerations in the control of oral anticoagulant therapy. Clinical Pharmacokinetics 16: 238–253

Shepherd A M M, Hewick D S, Moreland T A, Stevenson I H 1977 Age as a determinant of sensitivity to warfarin. British Journal of Clinical Pharmacology 4: 315–320

Sindet-Pedersen S, Ramström G, Bernvil S, Blombäck M, 1989 Hemostatic effect of tranexamic acid mouthwash in anticoagulant-treated patients undergoing oral surgery. New England Journal of Medicine 320: 840–843

Sixty-Plus Reinfarction Study Research Group Report 1980 A double-blind trial to assess long-term oral anticoagulant therapy in elderly patients after myocardial infarction. Lancet ii: 989–994

Smith P, Arnesen H, Holme I 1990 The effect of warfarin on mortality and reinfarction after myocardial infarction. New England Journal of Medicine 323: 147–152

Stein B, Fuster V 1991 Invited letter concerning: anticoagulant plus platelet inhibitor therapy in patients with mechanical valve prostheses. Journal of Thoracic and Cardiovascular Surgery 101: 557–559

Stephens M A, Self T H, Lancaster D, Nash T 1989 Hypothyroidism: Effect on warfarin anticoagulation. Southern Medical Journal 82: 1585–1586

Stroke Prevention in Atrial Fibrillation Study Group Investigators 1990 Preliminary Report of the Stroke Prevention in Atrial Fibrillation Study. New England Journal of Medicine 322: 863–868

Stroke Prevention in Atrial Fibrillation Study Group Investigators 1991 Stroke prevention in Atrial Fibrillation Study. Final Results. Circulation 84: 527–539

Suttie J W 1990 Warfarin and vitamin K. Clinical Cardiology 13 (suppl 6), VI: 16–18

Taberner, D A, Thomson, J M, Poller, L 1976 Comparison of prothrombin complex concentrate and vitamin K_1 in oral anticoagulant reversal. British Medical Journal 2: 83–85

Taberner D A, Poller L, Burslem R W, Jones J B 1978 Oral anticoagulants controlled by the British comparative thromboplastin versus low-dose heparin in prophylaxis of deep vein thrombosis. British Medical Journal i: 272–274

Teepe R G C, Broekmans A W, Vermeer B J, Nienhuis A M, Loeliger E A 1986 Recurrent Coumarin-induced skin necrosis in a patient with an acquired functional protein C-deficiency. Archives of Dermatology, 122: 1408–1412

Thijssen H H W, Hamulyák K, Willigers H 1988 4-Hydroxycoumarin Oral Anticoagulants: Pharmacokinetics-Response Relationship. Thrombosis and Haemostasis 60: 35–38

Thomson J M, Tomenson J A, Poller L 1984 The calibration of the second primary international reference preparation for thromboplastin (Thromboplastin, human, plain, coded BCT/253). Thrombosis and Haemostasis 52: 336–342

Thomson J M, Darby K V, Poller L 1986 Calibration of BCT/441, the ICSH reference preparation for thromboplastin. Thrombosis and Haemostasis 55: 379–382

Tomenson J A 1984 A statistician's independent evaluation. In: van den Besselaar A M H P, Gralnick H R, Lewis S M (eds) Thromboplastin calibration and oral anticoagulant control. Boston: M Nijhoff, Boston, p 87–108

Toon S, Holt B L, Mullins F G P, Bullingham R, Aarons L, Rowland M 1990 Investigations into the potential effects of multiple dose ketorolac on the pharmacokinetics and pharmacodynamics of racemic warfarin. British Journal of Clinical Pharmacology 30: 743–750

Turpie A G G, Gustensen J, Hirsh J, Nelson H, Gent M 1988 Randomised comparison of two intensities of oral anticoagulant therapy after tissue heart valve replacement. Lancet i: 1242–1245

van Amstel W J, Boekhout-Mussert M J, Loeliger E A 1978 Successful prevention of coumarin-induced hemorrhagic skin necrosis by timely administration of vitamin K_1. Blut 36: 89–93

van den Besselaar A M H P 1990 Recommended method for reporting therapeutic control of oral anticoagulant therapy. Thrombosis and Haemostasis 63: 316–317

van den Besselaar A M H P, Bertina R M 1991 Multi-Center Calibration of the Second Reference Material for Thromboplastin, Rabbit, Plain, Coded CRM 149R. Thrombosis and Haemostasis 65: 263–267

van den Besselaar A M H P, Bertina R M 1988 Standardization and quality control in blood coagulation assays. In: Lewis S M, Verwilghen R L (eds) Quality assurance in haematology. Baillière Tindall, London, p 119–150

van den Besselaar A M H P, Hermans J, van der Velde E A, Bussemaker-Verduyn den Boer E, van Halem-Visser L P, Jansen-Grüter R, Loeliger E A 1986 The calibration of rabbit tissue thromboplastins: experience of the Dutch reference laboratory for anticoagulant control. Journal of Biological Standardization 14: 305–317

van den Besselaar A M H P, van der Meer F J M, Gerrits-Drabbe C W 1988 Therapeutic control of oral anticoagulant treatment in the Netherlands. American Journal of Clinical Pathology 90: 685–690

van der Linde D L 1974 A controlled study of the preventing of thromboembolic complications by the use of coumarin derivatives pre-operatively, during the operation, and postoperatively. In: Witkin E (ed) Venous diseases, medical and surgical management. Foundation for International Cooperation in the Medical Sciences, Montreux, Switzerland. World Meetings Registry Number B741044

van der Meer J, Hemker H C, Loeliger E A 1968 Pharmacological aspects of vitamin K_1. A clinical and experimental study in man. Thrombosis et Diathesis Haemorrhagica (suppl) 29: 46

van der Meer F J M, Rosendaal F R, Cannegieter S C, Briët E. 1992 Oral anticoagulant drugs. New England Journal of Medicine 326: 68–71

van Vroonhoven Th J M V 1989 Consensus preventie van diep veneuze trombose. Nederlands Tijdschrift voor Geneeskunde 133: 2233–2237

Vermeer C, Hamulyák K 1991 Pathophysiology of vitamin K-deficiency and oral anticoagulants. Thrombosis and Haemostasis 66: 153–159

Walker M D 1989 Atrial fibrillation and antithrombotic prophylaxis: a prospective meta-analysis. Lancet i: 325–326

Weibert R T, Palinkas L A 1991 Differences in warfarin dose requirements between Asian and Caucasian patients. Clinical Pharmacology and Therapeutics 49: 151

Weiss P, Soff G A, Halkin H, Seligsohn U 1987 Decline of proteins C and S and factors II, VII, IX and X during the initiation of warfarin therapy. Thrombosis Research 45: 783–790

White R H, Mungall D 1991 Outpatient management of warfarin therapy: comparison of computer-predicted dosage adjustment to skilled professional care. Therapeutic Drug Monitoring 13: 46–50

WHO Expert Committee on Biological Standardization 1977 Standardization in the control of anticoagulation (oral). 28th Report. Technical Report Series 610, World Health Organization, Geneva, p 45–51

WHO Expert Committee on Biological Standardizaton 1983 Requirements for thromboplastins and plasma used to control oral anticoagulant therapy. 33rd Report. Technical Report Series 687, World Health Organization, Geneva, p 81–105

WHO Expert Committee on Biological Standardization 1984 34th Report. Technical Report Series 700. World Health Organization, Geneva, p 19

Wickramasinghe L S P, Basu S K, Bansal S K 1988 Long-term oral anticoagulant therapy in elderly patients. Age and Ageing 17: 388–396

Zauber N P, Stark M W 1986 Successful warfarin anticoagulation despite protein C-deficiency and a history of warfarin necrosis. Annals of Internal Medicine 104: 659–660

66. Therapeutic uses of thrombolytic drugs

D. de Bono

Thrombolytic drugs have been used therapeutically for over forty years; in the 1980s however, the widespread acceptance of the pivotal role of thrombolytic therapy in the treatment of acute coronary thrombosis led both to an enormous expansion of knowledge and a fundamental reappraisal of many of the principles involved. This chapter aims to define and evaluate basic concepts in clinical thrombolysis, adopting where appropriate a historic approach. It then goes on to discuss the use of thrombolytic drugs in a variety of clinical conditions — including coronary thrombosis, pulmonary embolism, peripheral venous and arterial thrombosis — as evaluated in controlled clinical trials, both as an illustration of these basic concepts and as a practical guide to therapy. Finally, it will consider present directions of thrombolytic research and the advantages and limitations of present technology for studying clinical thrombolysis in practice.

BASIC CONCEPTS IN THROMBOLYTIC THERAPY

The mechanism of thrombolysis and the mode of action of thrombolytic drugs are discussed in detail elsewhere in this book (Ch. 27). Briefly, all the thrombolytic agents presently available work via a final common pathway; the conversion of plasminogen to plasmin followed by the proteolytic digestion of fibrin. It has long been recognized that while activation of fibrin-bound plasminogen in the thrombus being treated was desirable, the activation of circulating plasminogen was potentially harmful. Once the relatively meagre protection afforded by plasma α_2-antiplasmin has been saturated, continuous generation of circulating plasmin will cause systemic fibrinogenolysis. This in turn causes a haemorrhagic diathesis, partly as a consequence of fibrinogen depletion, and partly through interference with coagulation mechanisms by fibrinogen degradation products. All the strategies devised for the therapeutic use of thrombolytic drugs have aimed at maximizing the activation of fibrin-bound plasminogen, and minimizing the systemic consequences. The earliest thrombolytic agents available for clinical use, streptokinase and urokinase, activate fibrin-bound and circulating plasminogen indiscriminately. Attempts to control the rates of systemic streptokinase administration so as to preserve circulating plasma fibrinogen concentrations led to severe limitations on the ability to administer an effective therapeutic dose, and were by no means reliable in preventing haemorrhagic complications. A major insight was the realization that a more effective strategy would be to administer an initial large dose of streptokinase to convert *all* circulating plasminogen to plasmin. Since plasmin is cleared rapidly from the circulation the result is that, after an initial burst, fibrinogen degradation product concentrations return to relatively low levels and haemorrhagic complications are reduced (Sherry 1954). This concept has underlain all subsequent strategies for the therapeutic use of streptokinase or urokinase.

An advantage of being able to achieve a high plasma concentration of a thrombolytic agent is that, at least to a first approximation, plasma concentration determines the rate of entry of the fibrinolytic agent into the thrombus. Thrombi are characteristically associated with impaired local blood flow, and it may be necessary for the drug to diffuse through a stagnant column of blood to reach the thrombus. Diffusion is also the mechanism by which fibrinolytic agents reach the interior of the gel-like mass of the thrombus; albeit a path modified by fissures or cracks within the thrombus, by the mechanical effects of vascular pulsation, or by intervention with wires, catheters or balloons (Meyer et al 1982).

Local infusion of a thrombolytic drug through an indwelling vascular catheter (Boucek & Murphy 1960) is a very effective way of ensuring both a high local concentration and a route for mechanical disturbance of the thrombus. This approach has been used successfully in pulmonary embolism, coronary thrombosis, peripheral artery thrombosis and coronary vein graft thrombosis. However, the need for vascular puncture increases the risk of bleeding, and this is further enhanced if, as usually happens, sufficient thrombolytic agent leaks into the circulation to cause systemic plasminogen activation.

The necessary *duration* of thrombolytic therapy will depend partly on the mass of the thrombus, and partly on the extent to which this mass needs to be diminished in order to achieve the necessary biological effect. Thus, in acute coronary thrombosis, the initial mass of occlusive thrombus is only a fraction of a gram, though it may enlarge through prograde and retrograde extension, and even partial dissolution may restore coronary patency. Conversely, a major leg vein thrombus or pulmonary embolus may weigh 50 g or more.

It is sometimes possible to monitor the dissolution of a thrombus using serial angiography or ultrasound. This has been used to guide the duration and intensity of therapy, but it is important to realize that fibrinolytic therapy may continue in the body of the thrombus long after the fibrinolytic agent has been cleared from the bloodstream (Agnelli et al 1985, Verstraete et al 1987).

There is a strong correlation between the duration of thrombolytic therapy and the incidence of systemic bleeding complications. The relationship seems to be incremental rather than linear, and the explanation for this is unclear. The important implication is that regimes which achieve sufficient thrombolysis in a short space of time may have a favourable therapeutic safety margin even if they involve giving large doses of thrombolytic drug.

The advent of 'fibrin selective' thrombolytic agents such as recombinant human tissue type plasminogen activator (rt-PA) or anistreplase appeared initially to offer a major opportunity for combining greater efficacy with safety. Because fibrin-selectivity with currently available agents is relative rather than absolute, the most favourable circumstances for demonstrating a differential effect on thrombus-bound and circulating plasminogen would be the prolonged administration of a low dose of thrombolytic drug. If clinical circumstances demand the initial rapid administration of a large dose of thrombolytic agent, for example to secure rapid coronary patency, then some activation of circulating plasminogen is almost inevitable. This prediction has been borne out in clinical trials: the doses of rt-PA used in coronary thrombolysis are large enough to cause some systemic fibrinogenolysis, and bleeding complication rates with this agent are fairly comparable with those for streptokinase, for example, whereas in peripheral arterial thrombolysis rt-PA can be used at doses which cause little or no systemic plasminogen activation. It remains theoretically true that an agent which has a very high affinity for fibrin might still be usable under conditions which combined rapid thrombolytic efficacy with minimal systemic plasminogen activation, but such agents are not yet at the clinical trial stage.

THROMBOLYSIS IN ACUTE CORONARY THROMBOSIS

Patients with acute coronary thrombosis far outnumber all patients with other indications for thrombolytic therapy. The role of coronary thrombosis as the final precipitating factor in the majority of cases presenting as acute myocardial infarction is now well accepted (de Wood et al 1980, Davies & Thomas 1985). Thrombosis usually takes place at the site of a cracked or ruptured atheromatous plaque. The initial thrombus may be very small, and coronary occlusion intermittent. Following complete occlusion of the vessel, the thrombus may extend distally, and to some extent proximally as far as the next major sidebranch (de Bono & Bhattacharrya 1991). It is interesting to realize that although the concept of coronary thrombosis is long established (Obrastzow & Straschenko 1910, Herrick 1912), it has not been unchallenged. In the 1960s, failure to demonstrate coronary thrombus with any reliability in the vessels of patients dying after myocardial infarction led to the serious suggestion that thrombosis might be an epiphenomenon, not essential to the process of infarction. It now seems more likely that these observations were related to an underestimate of the rate of spontaneous lysis of coronary thrombi, but at the time they had a major (and largely negative) impact on early clinical trials of thrombolysis in myocardial infarction.

The first reported clinical trial of thrombolytic therapy in acute coronary thrombosis was by Fletcher and colleagues in 1959. They gave 'prolonged and massive' thrombolytic therapy, using streptokinase, to a small number of patients, and claimed a clinical improvement though not a significant mortality advantage. There followed nearly 2 decades of rather inconclusive clinical trials (Amery et al 1969, Diogardi et al 1971, European Working Party 1971, Bett et al 1973, Aber et al 1976), mostly using streptokinase given for periods of up to 48 hours. This era is perhaps best represented by the European Cooperative Study Group trial reported in 1979. This well-conducted study stratified patients into low, medium and high-risk groups, and patients in the last two were randomized to streptokinase (250 000 units loading dose followed by 100 000 units per hour for 24 hours) or placebo. There was a highly significant reduction in 1 month mortality from 31% to 16% in streptokinase-treated patients, albeit at the cost of a significantly increased risk of bleeding complications.

Three important developments which occurred while the ECSG trial was still running had an important impact on subsequent developments. First, Breddin and colleagues (1973) introduced the concept of 'high dose, short time' thrombolysis: in their trial, 750 000 units of streptokinase given over 30 minutes. Second, the work of Ruda & Chazov in the Soviet Union rekindled interest in the use of coronary catheterization both to identify occluded vessels and to administer a thrombolytic agent locally (Chazov et al 1976). Introduced into Western cardiology through the work of Rentrop and colleagues (1979) in Berlin, the major outcome of this work was the realization that a major aspect of the mechanism by which streptokinase worked was by rapidly restoring coronary patency. Angiography for the first time provided a tool for studying the process and mechanism of thrombolysis (Fig. 66.1) and for doing dose-ranging studies involving realistic numbers of patients. Finally, the development of new fibrin-specific agents such as rt-PA (Smith et al 1981, Rijken et al 1982) and anisoylated plasminogen streptokinase activator complex (APSAC, now anistreplase) introduced an element of commercial enthusiasm, urgency and finance into the field, fuelled by the hope of improving on the clinical results of the ECSG study whilst reducing the unacceptably high rate of bleeding complications.

The GISSI-1 (GISSI was an acronym for Gruppo Italiano per lo Studio della Streptochinasi nell'Infarto Miocardico; the same acronym was used in GISSI-2 but with Sopravivvenza (survival) instead of streptochinasi) was the most influential trial of the 'new era' in coronary thrombolysis (GISSI-I 1986, GISSI-I 1987). Over 30 000 patients were considered for the study, and 11 806 were recruited, of whom 5905 were allocated to receive streptokinase (1500 000 units over 1 hour) and 5901 were controls. The principal entry criteria were clinical myocardial infarction with a symptom duration of less than 12 hours and electrocardiographic evidence of myocardial ischaemia. Principal exclusions were stroke, recent surgery or trauma, and uncontrolled hypertension. The outcome measures were mortality at 3 weeks and 12 months. Overall 3-week mortality was 10.7% in the streptokinase group and 13% in the control group ($p = 0.0002$); 12-month mortality was 17.2% in the streptokinase group and 19% in controls ($p = 0.008$). When results were stratified by time from the onset of major symptoms to the administration of thrombolysis, a clear gradient emerged, with a relative risk of mortality ranging from 0.61 in patients treated within 1 hour to 0.87 in patients treated between 3 and 6 hours, and no significant benefit in patients treated later than 9 hours. Survival benefits were maintained at 1-year follow-up, and major complication rates were low; cerebral bleeding occurring in only 0.5% of streptokinase-treated patients.

The results of GISSI-1 were corroborated by another large trial, ISIS-2 (International Study of Infarct Survival) (1988). This, unlike GISSI-1, was placebo-controlled and had the additional sophistication of a 2 × 2 factorial randomization to streptokinase, aspirin, both or neither. Electrocardiographic changes were not required for entry (but were present in 98% of patients), and patients could be admitted within 24 hours of symptom onset. The principal endpoints were 5-week and 15-month survival. Streptokinase was given using the same regimen as GISSI-1, aspirin as enteric-coated tablets containing 162.5 mg acetylsalicylic acid. Both streptokinase and aspirin reduced 5-week mortality compared to placebo, and the effects seemed to be additive: 5-week mortality for combined therapy was 8.0% vs 13.2% for double placebo ($2p < 0.0001$). As in GISSI-1, there was a benefit gradient in favour of early treatment with streptokinase, but not for aspirin. Unlike the GISSI-1 trial, patients treated with active therapy still seemed to gain some benefit up to 24 hours after the start of symptoms. Bleeding requiring transfusion was uncommon (0.5% in the streptokinase group), and the overall incidence of stroke was actually lower in the streptokinase group as a small excess of cerebral haemorrhage was outweighed by a reduction in thrombotic and embolic strokes.

Between them, these two trials (and others listed in Table 66.1) have led to a general acceptance of the role of thrombolysis in acute coronary thrombosis. Remaining

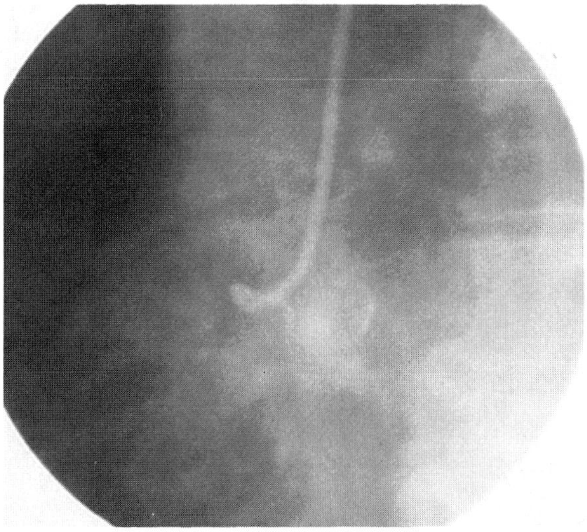

A

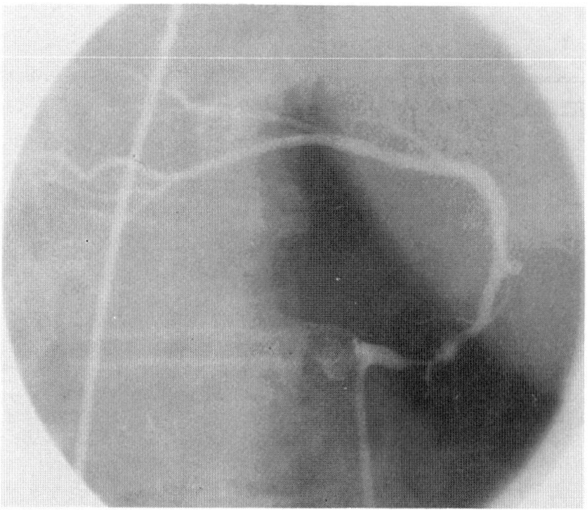

B

Fig. 66.1 Angiographic demonstration of recanalization of occluded coronary artery (using intravenous anistreplase). **A**, pretreatment showing occluded artery, **B**, showing reperfused vessel 60 minutes after intravenous injection of 30 units anistreplase.

Table 66.1 Major trials of coronary thrombolysis

Trial	No. of patients	Agent	Design	Outcome	Comment	Reference
European Cooperative Study	315	SK 250 000 U over 20 min, 100 000 U per h for 24 h	Mortality study vs control	6 month mortality: 16% SK, 31% control ($p < 0.01$)	High bleeding complication rate	European Cooperative Study Group 1979
GISSI-1	11 712	SK 150 000 U over 60 min	Mortality study vs control	21-day mortality: 10.7% SK, 13% control	Follow up medication 'ad lib'; best results with early treatment	GISSI-1 1986, 1987
ISIS-2	17 187	SK 1 500 000 U aspirin 162.5 mg	2 × 2 factorial, mortality endpoint, placebo-controlled	30-day mortality: 8% SK+ aspirin, 13% double placebo	Aspirin effect additive to SK	ISIS-2 1988
ASSET	5011	Alteplase 100 mg over 3 h, iv, heparin 24 h	Placebo-controlled mortality endpoint	28 day mortality: 7.2% alteplase, 9.8% heparin only		Wilcox et al 1988
GISSI-2/ISG	20 749	SK 1 500 000 U or alteplase 100 mg	2 × 2 factorial, open, mortality endpoint	No difference in in-hospital mortality between agents or ± heparin	Note sc heparin	GISSI-2 1990, International Study Group 1990
ISIS-3	46 092	SK 1 500 000 U or duteplase 100 mg, or anistreplase 30 U	2 × 3 factorial, placebo controlled, ± sc heparin	No difference in mortality	Heparin sc	Collins 1991

SK, streptokinase; iv, intravenous; sc, subcutaneous.

questions include the choice of the optimum therapeutic agent and regimen, the best 'follow-up' antithrombotic policy, and the role of interventions such as coronary angioplasty or bypass grafting.

CHOICE OF THROMBOLYTIC AGENT

Agents which are currently licensed for therapeutic use as thrombolytic drugs in myocardial infarction (in at least some part of the world) are streptokinase, urokinase, alteplase*, and anistreplase. Single-chain urokinase-type plasminogen activator (saruplase) has also been used in large-scale trials and is likely to be licensed shortly.

Streptokinase

Streptokinase is relatively cheap, and has been used in many more patients than any other thrombolytic agent. The regimen of 1 500 000 units of streptokinase over 60 minutes has become standardized, if not sanctified, as a result of the GISSI and ISIS trials, but in fact rests on a rather small scale dose-ranging study by Schroeder and colleagues (1983). In comparative studies against other agents using angiographic patency as the endpoint, streptokinase has been inferior to alteplase with respect to early coronary patency rates, but it has performed so far as well as alteplase and anistreplase in mortality endpoint studies. It has been argued that increasing the streptokinase dose to 2 000 000 or even 3 000 000 units would enhance early patency, but these regimens have not been subjected to large-scale trials. Bolus administration of streptokinase causes unacceptable hypotension in a large proportion of patients, but a regimen of two, slow intravenous injections of 750 000 units separated by 20 minutes has been found acceptable (Hall 1987). Following ISIS-2, streptokinase is now almost invariably combined with aspirin. Some reports indicate that streptokinase may cause a degree of platelet activation, which would make combining it with a platelet anti-aggregant even more logical (Vaughan et al 1988). The role of heparin in combination with streptokinase is discussed below (p. 1464).

Naturally-occurring antibodies to streptokinase, presumably the result of previous streptococcal infection, occur in about 20% of the adult population, but seldom seem to interfere with its thrombolytic efficacy. Therapeutic administration of streptokinase very commonly produces a substantial antibody response (Jalihal & Morris 1990) and the subsequent administration of a second dose may be associated with a reduced efficacy and an increased risk of allergic side-effects (White et al 1990). Anaphylaxis is rare, but skin rashes, fever and hypotension are common. The original recommendation was that streptokinase should not be re-used between 5 days and 3 months after first use, but these recommendations are arbitrary and based on antibody titres rather than clinical experience. If other non-cross-reactive agents such as alteplase or uroki-

* Recombinant human tissue type plasminogen activator is synthesized in cell culture as a single peptide chain which may then undergo partial proteolytic cleavage to a two-chain form. Both single and double-chain forms are biologically active, but differ somewhat in specific activity and fibrin-binding characteristics. The pharmaceutical product prepared by Genentech Inc and Boehringer Ingelheim, GmbH is predominantly single chain and has been given the approved pharmaceutical name alteplase; the predominantly double-chain form produced by Wellcome Laboratories has been given the approved name duteplase. In this chapter rt-PA is used as the class name, and alteplase or duteplase to refer to trials in which the specific agents were used.

nase are available they should be used instead of repeated therapy with streptokinase. Streptokinase is present in anistreplase, and these two agents cross-react antigenically.

Urokinase

Urokinase (low molecular weight urokinase, U-PA) has been available for almost as long as streptokinase. Although the mechanism by which it activates plasminogen is different, for practical purposes it behaves in a very similar manner to streptokinase. As a human product it is virtually non-antigenic. Its relatively long plasma half life (compared to alteplase) was initially regarded as a disadvantage, but more recently this feature has been seen as a potential method for maintaining prolonged thrombolytic activity during coronary angioplasty. A treatment regimen of 1 500 000 units intravenously as an initial bolus followed by a further 1 500 000 units over 90 minutes gave similar coronary potency rates to intravenous alteplase (Mathey et al 1985). In another study, coronary recanalization rates were proportional to intracoronary urokinase doseage up to a maximum of 960 000 units (Neuhaus et al 1988). Synergism between alteplase and urokinase was examined in the TAMI-2 trial (Topol et al 1988); coronary patency rates were similar in patients receiving 1 mg/kg alteplase and between 0.5 and 2 million units of urokinase. There was a trend towards reduced reocclusion rates in patients receiving urokinase compared with (historical) controls given only alteplase.

Alteplase

Alteplase was initially compared with streptokinase in studies with angiographic patency as end-point. These showed a trend towards better coronary patency and reperfusion rates for alteplase given in conjunction with intravenous heparin (Verstraete et al 1985, Chesebro et al 1987). Dose-ranging studies with alteplase indicated a positive relationship between dose and patency rate, but at doses above 100 mg over 3 hours the rate of cerebral haemorrhage also increased. Concern about the risk of coronary reocclusion after initial patency led to experiments with a prolonged infusion regimen, but this appears to confer no particular advantage over a 3-hour infusion (Serruys et al 1987). Placebo-controlled trials using a regimen of 100 mg alteplase (10 mg bolus, 50 mg over 1 hour, 40 mg over 2 hours) have shown a significant effect on mortality (van der Werf & Arnold 1988, Wilcox et al 1988). Recently there has been interest in 'front loaded' infusion regimens, with 100 mg infused over 90 minutes (Neuhaus et al 1989), and in single or double bolus administration. Single bolus administration appears to be less effective than infusion, but double or multiple bolus administration seems to be comparable (Khan et al 1990, Tranchesi et al 1991).

Administration of alteplase without concomitant intravenous heparin results in significantly lower coronary patency rates, especially if aspirin is omitted or given in low dosage (Bleich et al 1990, Hsai et al 1990, de Bono et al 1992). The effect of subcutaneous heparin on patency rates after alteplase has not yet been evaluated.

Despite an apparent advantage in terms of early coronary patency, trials designed to compare outcome in patients treated with streptokinase or alteplase have failed to show significant differences in either late left ventricular function (White et al 1989) or in mortality. Three large-scale mortality endpoint trials, GISSI-2 (1990), the International Study group trial (1990) and ISIS-3 (Collins 1991) have all failed to show significant survival differences between patients treated with 1 500 000 units of streptokinase and 100 mg of rt-PA (as alteplase in GISSI-2 and the International Study Group trials, duteplase in ISIS-3). In all these studies the possible interactive effect of heparin was examined by factorial randomization, and no evidence for interaction was detected. However none of the studies used intravenous heparin. Preliminary data are now (spring 1993) available on the results of the GUSTO study. 41 021 patients were randomized. 30 day mortality rates were 7.2% for streptokinase plus subcutaneous heparin, 7.4% for streptokinase plus intravenous heparin, 6.3% for alteplase (100 mg over 90 mins) plus intravenous heparin and 7.0% for streptokinase plus alteplase plus intravenous heparin. All patients received aspirin (160 mg/day). The incidence of disabling stroke was similar (0.5–0.6%) in the different groups. The mortality benefit with alteplase plus intravenous heparin was statistically significant and equivalent to about 10 extra lives saved per 1000 patients treated. An angiographic substudy in 2 400 patients showed increased early coronary patency in the alteplase group i.e there was concordance between early patency and late mortality rates.

Anistreplase

Anistreplase is the approved name given to anisoylated plasminogen streptokinase activator complex. Plasminogen temporarily inactivated by anisoylation of the enzymatic site is administered as a non-covalently bound complex with streptokinase. The complex has enhanced fibrin affinity compared with native plasminogen. In addition, it causes less hypotension when administered intravenously than equivalent amounts of streptokinase, and can therefore be given as a single slow intravenous injection rather than an infusion. Early angiographic studies comparing anistreplase with placebo gave encouraging results (Been et al 1986) and these were supported by significant reductions in mortality in clinical trials against placebo (Aims trial 1990, Swift 1991). However subsequent comparisons of coronary patency rates with intravenous anistreplase against those obtained with intravenous streptokinase have given conflicting results (Anderson et al 1989, Gemill et al 1991). Neither the ISIS-3 trial nor the recent TAPS trial (von Essen 1991) have shown a significant survival advantage to anistreplase compared with either streptokinase or rt-PA. It could be argued however that in neither case did the trial design allow for the potential advantage of anistreplase as an agent which might be rapidly administered in the community or in an emergency department.

Saruplase

Saruplase is single-chain urokinase-type plasminogen activator (also SCU-PA). It was originally investigated as a potential fibrin-specific thrombolytic agent, but clinically effective doses cause a substantial depletion of circulating fibrinogen. In angiographically-controlled trials it has been more effective than 1 500 000 units of streptokinase in producing coronary patency (PRIMI 1989) but large scale mortality endpoint trials have not yet been reported. Initial hopes for synergism between saruplase and alteplase appear to have been unfounded (Tranchesi et al 1989).

Present choice of a thrombolytic agent in myocardial infarction

Current dosage recommendations, and the advantages and disadvantages of different agents, are summarized in Table 66.2. Since no agent has been shown to be more effective than streptokinase in terms of survival, and since this agent is the least costly, it is presently the agent of choice for 'routine' thrombolytic therapy. Alteplase is probably the agent of choice in patients who have previously been exposed to streptokinase or anistreplase. Anistreplase may be favoured for emergency room or out of hospital thrombolysis because of its simple mode of administration.

Table 66.2 Comparison of current thrombolytic agents

	Alteplase	Anistreplase	Streptokinase
Source	Tissue culture expression of human gene	Bacterial + human plasminogen	Bacterial
Mode of action	All work by activating plasminogen to plasmin		
Fibrin specificity	+	(+)	–
Plasma half life (min)	5–8	≈ 90	20–30
Most common dose	100 mg over 3 h	30 U over 5 min	1 500 000 over 60 min
Potentiated by aspirin	No data	No data	Yes
Potentiated by heparin	Yes	No data	Yes?
Antibody response	Minimal	Yes	Yes

From deBono D P 1992 In: Rowlands D E (ed) Recent advances in cardiology, Churchill Livingstone, Edinburgh.

ADJUNCTIVE THERAPY IN CORONARY THROMBOLYSIS

So far, adjunctive therapy given in combination with thrombolytic agents has owed more to serendipity than to planning. A notable exception was the validation of *aspirin* in ISIS-2. The interaction of aspirin with alteplase, urokinase or anistreplase has not been formally evaluated in large-scale studies, but there seems little reason to doubt that this is a class effect which would be seen, perhaps to varying extent, with any thrombolytic agent. Consensus on aspirin dosage is converging towards an 'ISIS' type dosage of around 150 mg daily. It may be important to give a relatively large initial dose to achieve rapid suppression of platelet cyclo-oxygenase activity.

Literature on the use of heparin as an adjunct to thrombolysis is confusing in respect of the multiplicity of dose regimens, the variety of ways in which heparin dose was controlled (if at all) and the heterogeneity of outcome measures. To some extent this confusion reflects uncertainty about the object of heparin therapy: is it being used as an anti-thrombin, to prevent secondary thrombosis, or to activate endogenous fibrinolysis? As discussed above (p. 1463), intravenous heparin therapy has clearly been shown to enhance coronary patency in patients receiving alteplase thrombolysis. In the European cooperative study group trial, patients were given a standard heparin regimen of 5000 units of heparin initially followed by an infusion of 1000 units per hour. As a result, about one-third of patients were consistently well-anticoagulated (activated partial thromboplastin time >150 seconds), one third were inadequately anticoagulated (APTT <50 seconds) and the third group were intermediate between these extremes. Coronary patency rates were highest in the well-anticoagulated, and lowest in the non-anticoagulated groups (Rapold et al 1992). It is difficult in the absence of serial angiography to decide whether the benefit was due to the enhancement of thrombolysis or to the prevention of reocclusion.

Only one trial has so far formally examined the need for prolonged heparin therapy: the National Heart Institute of Australia trial (1989) randomized patients receiving alteplase thrombolysis to heparin for 24 hours followed by aspirin plus dipyridamole or to heparin for 7 days. Coronary patency and outcome were both similar at 1 week.

Most thrombolysis regimens using streptokinase or anistreplase have avoided giving early intravenous heparin for fear of bleeding complications when this was combined with the auto-anticoagulation resulting from fibrinogenolysis. The exception was the ISAM study (1986) in which 1 500 000 units of streptokinase was combined with a 5000 unit heparin bolus and 500 mg of aspirin. The incidence of 'significant' bleeding complications in this study was 5.9%, which the authors regarded as high. One small study which randomized patients receiving streptokinase to concomitant intravenous heparin or no heparin, reported enhanced reperfusion (assessed by non-invasive measures) in the heparin group (Melandri et al 1990).

Late subcutaneous heparin appears to reduce the rate of left ventricular thrombus formation (Turpie et al 1989) but had little impact on overall mortality in the GISSI-2, International Study Group or ISIS-3 trials.

Warfarin has been used in an attempt to prevent late reocclusion in a number of trials (Been et al 1986), but the recent 'APRICOT' study (Verheugt 1991) showed no difference either in later coronary patency or in the number of clinical events between patients, with a known patent coronary artery, randomized to aspirin or warfarin. A trial evaluating aspirin plus warfarin against aspirin alone is currently in progress.

Other antithrombic agents currently being evaluated as adjuncts to thrombolysis include hirudin (Ruebsamen & Eschenfelder 1991), low molecular weight hirudin analogues, and monoclonal antibodies to platelet receptors (Gold et al 1988). In experimental models these have shown promise, but results of clinical studies are awaited.

Reperfusion injury is a term invoked to explain an initial return of function after thrombolysis, followed by a decline. Several different mechanisms have been proposed, but despite much experimental work, the clinical significance of the effect remains controversial. Probably the best characterized mechanism is capillary occlusion by polymorphonuclear leukocytes, which then cause secondary tissue damage through their release of superoxide anions. The stimulus to increased polymorph adhesion is complex, and may initially involve platelet aggregating factor (PAF), with a subsequent contribution from increased expression of endothelial adhesion molecules (Mullane & Smith 1990). This effect can be counteracted by experimental neutropenia, by post-perfusion of the myocardium with a perfluorocarbon blood substitute (Kolodgie et al 1991) or (in some studies) by superoxide dismutase, but none of these appear practicable therapeutic interventions at present.

COMBINATION OF ANTITHROMBOTIC AGENTS WITH CORONARY ANGIOPLASTY

Early trials suggested a potential synergism between thrombolytic agents, which would dissolve thrombus, and coronary angioplasty, which would dispose of any residual stenotic component caused by a disrupted atheromatous plaque. These hopes have not so far been realized in clinical trials, which have shown at best, no benefit, and at worst, a disadvantage to early intervention (Simoons et al 1988, TIMI 1988, 1989). This is in part attributable to an increased rate of abrupt reocclusion in patients receiving early angioplasty . It has been suggested that a combination of alteplase with urokinase reduces this risk (Topol et al 1988) but the evidence remains meagre. Trials are also evaluating newer antithrombotic agents in the context of angioplasty.

Even if patients with abrupt reocclusion are excluded from analysis, the benefits from early angioplasty in terms of improved left ventricular function appear modest (Arnold et al 1990). Microvascular damage from dispersed thrombus is a possible but unproven explanation.

PATIENT SELECTION FOR CORONARY THROMBOLYSIS

There is now a consensus, based on the major clinical trials, that all patients with features of acute coronary thrombosis should be considered for thrombolytic therapy unless there are contraindications, or unless the expected benefit is so small as to be outweighed by the potential risk.

Clinical features. In the form of chest pain and sympathetic activation, clinical features were major selection criteria in all clinical trials. The most important differential diagnosis is from dissecting aortic aneurysm (Fig. 66.2). Other differential diagnoses, such as pericarditis, are less adversely affected by inappropriate thrombolysis.

Electrocardiographic features. In acute myocardial ischaemia, ST segment elevations were used in some trials; in others they were recorded but not used as entry criteria. There is agreement that ECG changes predict overall mortality in the order: left bundle branch block > anterior ST elevation > inferior ST elevation > normal ECG. The *proportional* survival benefit with thrombolytic therapy compared with placebo is similar for all groups: in practice this means a large absolute benefit for anterior ST elevation, a modest benefit for inferior ST elevation, and little absolute benefit for patients with normal electrocardiograms, who tend anyway to have a very good prognosis. A

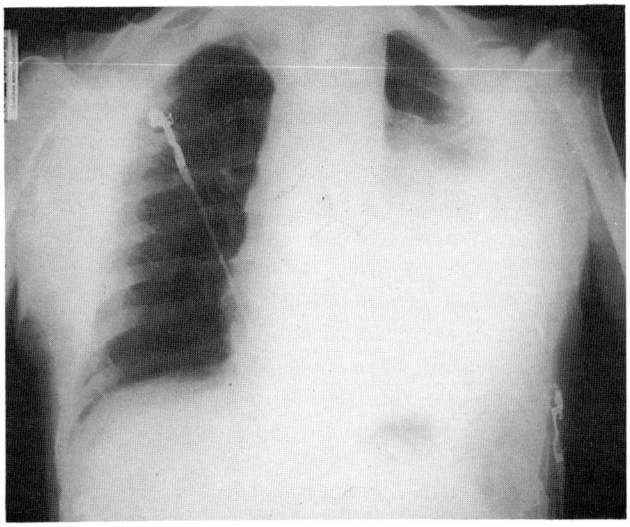

Fig. 66.2 Left haemothorax in a patient with dissecting aortic aneurysm inadvertently given streptokinase. The patient survived.

curious and unexplained exception which has been fairly consistent from trial to trial is that patients with ST depression as the only manifestation of ischaemia tend to have a high mortality with relatively little benefit from thrombolysis.

Time from onset of symptoms. This is a major determinant of benefit, in that the earlier patients are treated (ideally within 1 hour) the better the outcome, but since coronary occlusion is often intermittent, and the precise onset of symptoms hard to define, thrombolysis should not be witheld in patients with persisting chest pain or dynamic electrocardiographic changes.

Age. In itself, age is a major determinant of mortality in myocardial infarction. Many trials have applied an arbitrary age cutoff at 70 or 75, but there is no evidence of an upper age limit to the efficacy of thrombolysis, although complication rates tend to rise in the elderly.

Contraindications to thrombolysis

Contraindications have progressively contracted as the relative safety of high dose, short-term therapy has been appreciated. A previous history of cerebral haemorrhage, recent head injury, and recent (< 2 weeks) surgery — especially if vascular surgery — remain important contraindications, as are active peptic ulceration, prolonged or traumatic cardiac resuscitation, oesophageal varices, pregnancy and current menstruation. Hypertension is not in itself a contraindication, provided it can be controlled before instituting thrombolysis. Diabetic proliferative retinopathy is a theoretical contraindication, but the risk of vitreous haemorrhage must be weighed against the potentially life-saving benefits.

THROMBOLYSIS FOR ACUTE MASSIVE PULMONARY EMBOLISM

Pulmonary embolism, in early years the 'flagship' of indications for thrombolytic therapy, has been outpaced by the developments in the 1980s in coronary thrombolysis. An important and admirable reason for this is a decline in the incidence of hospital cases of pulmonary embolism as a result of effective prophylaxis. Placebo-controlled trials of thrombolysis in pulmonary embolism in the 1970s showed a trend, albeit not significant, towards mortality reduction, and a significant improvement in the angiographically-assessed rate of clearance of pulmonary thrombus (Miller et al 1971, Tibbutt et al 1974). There was also a trend towards haemodynamic improvement. It has been argued that both the requirement for the patient to have undergone (and survived) pulmonary angiography and a high crossover rate, together with a small sample size, militated against these trials showing a clear survival benefit.

Because of the difficulty of recruiting sufficient numbers of patients for mortality endpoint studies, subsequent trials have almost invariably used surrogate measures based on a 'score' calculated from the pulmonary angiogram. The Miller score (Brochier et al 1980) which takes cognisance of peripheral perfusion, is probably more discriminating than the Walsh score. Haemodynamic factors such as a rapid fall in pulmonary vascular resistance may be even more important than angiographic appearances.

Thrombolytic regimens used in pulmonary embolism have been well reviewed by Meyer and colleagues (1989). They have tended to be based on the a-priori assumption that a systemic thrombolytic state should be maintained until all thrombus has been dissolved.

Streptokinase. This has been given as a loading dose of 250 000 to 600 000 units followed by a maintenance dose of 100 000 to 250 000 units per hour for 24–72 hours. There is little evidence for the superiority of any one of these regimens over another.

Urokinase. Like streptokinase this has also been used in a variety of regimens, using either a loading dose alone, a loading dose plus a maintenance infusion, or a maintenance infusion without a loading dose. Again, in the absence of randomized trials it is difficult to identify a regimen which is clearly better than the others. It is interesting that high dose, short term 'bolus' administration of urokinase (15 000 units/kg body weight, i.e. approximately 1 000 000 to 1 500 000 units in total) appears to be as effective as prolonged administration schedules, with fewer major bleeding complications (Urokinase Pulmonary Embolism Trial 1973, Petitpretz et al 1984).

Alteplase. Alteplase has been used effectively in pulmonary embolism, but there is currently no consensus on the most appropriate dose: 100 mg over 2 hours was shown to produce more rapid angiographic clearance than urokinase 4400 units/kg as a bolus followed by 4400 units/kg/hour (Verstraete 1988), but the more interesting comparison with high dose bolus urokinase is still being investigated. Recently, a single bolus of 0.6 mg/kg has been reported as giving good results in an open study (Levine et al 1990).

Anistreplase. This has had relatively little use in pulmonary embolism, and, in the only published study, was given repeatedly in low doses, with some effect but a high incidence of bleeding complications (Vander Sande et al 1988). In our own unpublished experience, giving anistreplase as a 30 unit injection over 4 minutes (the same regimen as in acute myocardial infarction) gave very good clinical and angiographic results (Fig. 66.3) with few bleeding complications. On this basis, it might be interesting to re-examine the effects of streptokinase given in a 'myocardial infarct'-type regimen of 1 500 000 units over 60 minutes; but it should be noted that patients with massive pulmonary embolism may tolerate streptokinase-induced vasodilatation badly. There is currently a strong suspicion that the 'product licence endorsed' regimens for streptokinase or urokinase in acute massive pulmonary

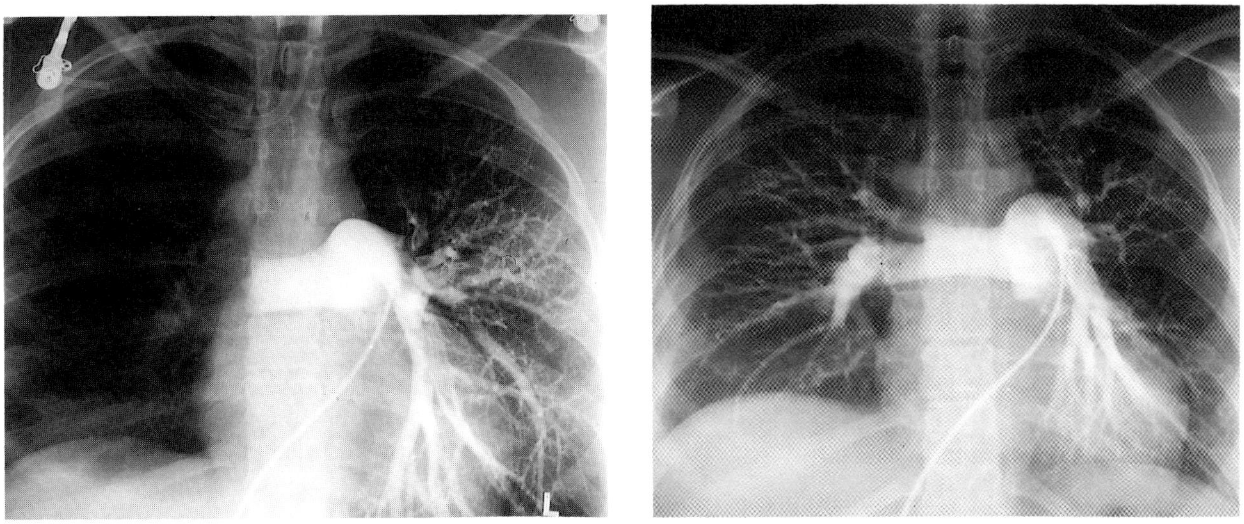

A B

Fig. 66.3 Pulmonary angiograms **A**, before and **B**, 12 hours after bolus administration of anistreplase in a 24-year-old patient with acute massive pulmonary embolism.

embolism may not be optimal either in terms of efficacy or safety, and further work on 'short-term' administration schedules would be very welcome.

THROMBOLYSIS FOR PERIPHERAL VENOUS THROMBOSIS

Peripheral venous thrombosis confined to the calf veins is common, but responds well to heparin and is seldom associated with a poor prognosis. Conversely, pulmonary embolism frequently occurs in the absence of previous overt venous thrombosis. In practice therefore thrombolytic therapy has principally been used in patients with thrombosis of the proximal leg veins (iliofemoral thrombosis). Individual studies have confirmed the ability of streptokinase to lyse angiographicaly-recognized thrombus more rapidly than heparin alone; however even with the benefit of meta-analysis, numbers have been too small and events too few, to demonstrate a convincing benefit in terms of mortality or pulmonary embolism (Goldhaber et al 1984). The effect of thrombolytic therapy on the subsequent incidence of chronic venous insufficiency has been controversial: some studies claiming and others denying benefit. All studies concur in demonstrating a higher risk of major haemorrhage in patients given thrombolytics.

Treatment regimens for deep venous thrombosis, like those for pulmonary embolism, have tended to enshrine the concept that prolonged, low-dose therapy would be more effective than short-term, high-dose therapy. Streptokinase and urokinase regimens have been similar to those used in pulmonary embolism, but usually administered for a shorter period of 12–24 hours. Alteplase has been used as an infusion of 0.5 mg/kg given over 4 or 8 hours. Both regimens were effective in producing angiographic improvement, but at the cost of a fall in plasma fibrinogen concentration, and an increased incidence of bleeding complications. Both the clinical value of thrombolytic therapy in deep vein thrombosis and the optimum treatment regimen remain to be established.

THROMBOLYSIS IN PERIPHERAL ARTERIAL OCCLUSION

Peripheral arterial occlusion presents some unique problems for thrombolytic therapy: occlusion is almost invariably complete rather than partial, and has usually been present for days if not weeks before the patient presents. Prolonged systemic administration of streptokinase to these patients was sometimes effective, but was associated with very high rates of bleeding complications. Local intra-arterial infusion of a thrombolytic agent enables a higher local concentration to be achieved (McNichol et al 1963), and this is most effectively done by using a small catheter which can actually be passed into the thrombus (Dotter et al 1974, McNamara & Fischer 1985). Urokinase or alteplase has tended to be preferred to streptokinase, possibly because they are less likely to cause febrile or allergic reactions during the somewhat prolonged infusion (Graor et al 1985). The urokinase regimen used by McNamara and Fischer (1985) was 4000 units/minute until canalization had occurred and then 1000 units/minute until complete lysis was achieved. Alteplase has been used at 0.05–0.1 mg/kg/hour. The more rapidly recanalization is achieved, the more likely is complete clearance. Late patency has been around 60%.

The major complication of thrombolysis by this technique is bleeding related to vascular puncture. This is particularly likely to occur if the artery is punctured twice, once for a diagnostic arteriogram and a second time for infusion of the thrombolytic drug. The problem can be avoided if an arterial sheath is left in situ after the initial angiogram.

Thrombolysis of thrombosed aorto-coronary bypass grafts is an essentially similar problem which can be dealt with by the same technique (Fig. 66.4). Balloon angioplasty may be needed to deal with a residual stenosis causing stasis and hence thrombosis.

THROMBOLYSIS IN STROKE

Thrombotic or embolic stroke remains a major, but as yet largely unmet, challenge for revascularization. Early studies reported some (largely unsubstantiated) benefit, but also drew attention to the increased risks of precipitating cerebral haemorrhage (see del Zoppo 1988 for review). The clinical difficulty of distinguishing between cerebral thrombosis and cerebral haemorrhage has, at least in theory, been overcome by the availability of CT scanning, and both this and acute cerebral angiography have helped to sharpen the clinical diagnosis of the syndrome of acute occlusion of the middle cerebral artery. Transcranial Doppler ultrasound provides a non-invasive means of assessing patency. Nevertheless, a major persisting problem is the tendency for reperfusion to convert a 'white' or ischaemic cerebral infarct into a red or haemorrhagic one. It appears that vascular integrity within the infarct zone is compromised by persisting ischaemia, and the immediate consequence is that the 'therapeutic time window' within which thrombolytic reperfusion may do more good than harm tends to be a narrow one: perhaps as narrow as 2 hours following occlusion. This is currently a field with intense experiental activity, albeit as yet with little clinical outcome to show for it.

COMPLICATIONS OF THROMBOLYTIC THERAPY

Haemorrhage is the major specific complication of thrombolytic therapy. Trials differ in their definition of 'major' bleeding complications, but there is agreement that the two major factors which increase bleeding risk are prolonged thrombolytic therapy and the use of procedures such as angiography or angioplasty which involve arterial or venous access. In myocardial infarction trials (short duration of thrombolysis), non-invasive studies have bleeding complication rates of 2–5%, and invasive studies 15–20%.

The incidence of *cerebral* haemorrhage in myocardial infarction trials is remarkably constant at 0.5–1% irrespective of the agent or ancillary therapy used. In trials which have distinguished cerebral haemorrhage from cerebral embolism, an increase in haemorrhage risk is often countervailed by a reduction in thrombosis/embolism. Hopes that fibrin-selective thrombolytics would cause less cerebral bleeding have not been borne out; in some studies cerebral bleeding rates have been higher with rt-PA than with streptokinase. This may simply reflect a close relationship between effective dose and body weight for rt-PA, and dose reduction is now recommended when using alteplase in patients weighing <67 kg.

Acute profuse gastrointestinal haemorrhage is usually the consequence of giving thrombolytic therapy to a patient with unsuspected active peptic ulceration. It is less common than 'coffee-ground' vomiting, which is often the result of a conjunction between thrombolysis and superficial gastric mucosal congestion and tends to follow a benign clinical course. Late (2–3 day) gastrointestinal haemorrhage may be due to stress ulceration, particularly

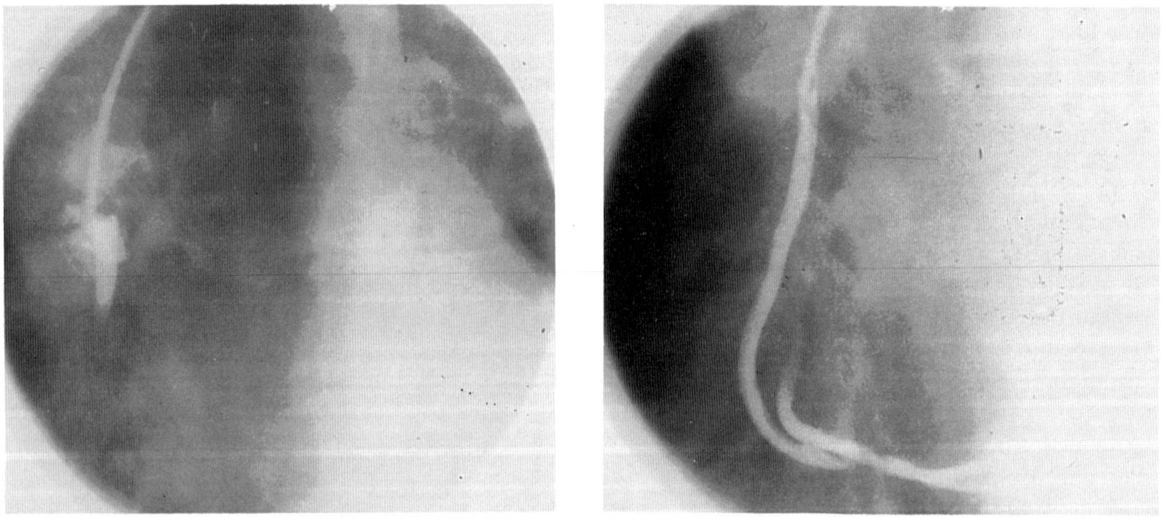

A B

Fig. 66.4 Thrombosed aorto-coronary vein graft (**A**). A 3-French gauge cannula was inserted into the thrombus via a 7 gauge guiding catheter and 250 000 streptokinase infused over 6 hours. Repeat angiography (**B**) shows patency of the graft, with a stenosis at the distal end which was subsequently angioplastied.

in gravely-ill patients; thrombolysis is probably irrelevant, but subsequent anticoagulation makes things worse.

Gingival bleeding is common, but usually benign. Microscopic haematuria is common, macroscopic haematuria is rare and may indicate an unsuspected urinary tract neoplasm.

Iatrogenic bleeding ranges from trivial to life threatening. Rupture of the heart, liver or spleen during attempted resuscitation may lead to fatal bleeding. Arterial or venous puncture should be avoided if possible; if not, a cannula should be left in situ until thrombolysis has been discontinued. If puncture of a major vein is essential for the insertion of a pacemaker electrode or Swan–Ganz catheter, an antecubital, femoral or jugular route should be preferred to the subclavian vein. Femoral artery puncture is safe provided the artery is entered cleanly and an arterial sheath left in situ. If the catheter is removed, an obturator must be left in the sheath to prevent kinking, which will cause bleeding. Bleeding around the sheath can sometimes be stopped by using a guidewire to insert the next largest size of sheath.

Reversal of thrombolysis

In practice, reversal of thrombolysis is only likely to be required in the face of severe haemorrhage from an inaccessible site, or a need for urgent surgery. The basic principles are to cease administration of the thrombolytic agent and any concomitant anticoagulants, to inhibit plasmin activity, and to replenish fibrinogen and coagulation factors. There is seldom time for elaborate laboratory tests. Continuing plasma activity of thrombolytic agents can be detected by appropriate colorimetric assays or by the euglobulin lysis time, but this is often academic. A prolonged cutaneous bleeding time is a useful bedside marker of continuing plasmin generation (Gimpel et al 1989). In experimental models plasmin inhibitors such as aprotinin and tranexamic acid have been shown to diminish haemorrhage during or following the administration of thrombolytic drugs (Gimpel et al 1989, Clozel et al 1990). Clinical experience in reversing thrombolysis is necessarily limited, but there is now extensive experience in the use of aprotinin following open-heart surgery, and it is our practice to use intravenous aprotinin 4 mg/kg, with or without additional tranexamic acid (25 mg/kg orally, 6 hourly), to inhibit plasmin activity if required.

Plasma fibrinogen concentration will almost invariably be low after streptokinase or anistreplase, but may be within the normal range after rt-PA. It does not necessaily follow, however, that all the measured fibrinogen after rt-PA is haemostatically competent. Fibrinogen replacement is advisable with fresh frozen plasma or fibrinogen concentrate, but since both of these contain plasminogen it is prudent to give a plasmin inhibitor first, or at least concurrently.

FUTURE DIRECTIONS IN THROMBOLYSIS

Myocardial infarction will continue to be the largest field for thrombolytic therapy, at least until the technical problems of thrombolytic therapy for stroke are solved. The emphasis in the development of new thrombolytic drugs seems to be moving towards ease of administration and a favourable side-effect profile rather than the out and out pursuit of thrombolytic efficacy. The large scale comparative trials of thrombolytic agents so far carried out have emphasized the difficulty and expense of proving superiority of one agent over another even when 'surrogate endpoint' studies have suggested a potential advantage. The concept of a 'fibrin selective' agent has become somewhat unfashionable, but none of the agents so far tested has really exhibited anything like absolute fibrin specificity. Angiographic endpoint trials are becoming increasingly difficult to justify ethically, because angiography can no longer simply be regarded as a prelude to angioplasty. This has emphasized the need to develop reliable non-invasive indicators of coronary reperfusion. There are likely to be major advances in our understanding of the role of adjuvant antithrombotic therapy, both with existing agents and those currently under investigation. A recent development has been a trend to investigate 'thrombolytic' drugs as antithrombotic agents in their own right, by targeting them to areas of platelet aggregation or endothelial damage (Royston et al 1987) as conjugates with platelet proteins or monoclonal antibodies.

REFERENCES

Aber C P, Bas N M, Berry C L, Carson P H M, Dobbs R J, Fox K M, Hamblin J J, Haydu S P, Howitt G, McIver J E, Portal R W, Raftery E B, Rousell R H, Stock J P P 1976 Streptokinase in acute myocardial infarction: a controlled multicentre trial in the United Kingdom, British Medical Journal ii: 1100–1105

Agnelli G, Buchanan M R, Fernandez F, Hirsh J 1985 The thrombolytic and haemorrhagic effects of tissue type plasminogen activator: influence of dosage regimens in rabbits. Thrombosis and Haemostasis 40: 764–777

Aims Trial Study group 1990 Long term effects of intravenous anistreplase in acute myocardial infarction: final report of the AIMS study. Lancet 335: 427–431

Amery A, Roeber G, Vermeulen H J, Verstraete M 1969 Single blind randomised trial comparing heparin and streptokinase treatment in recent myocardial infarction. Acta Medica Scandinavica 505 (suppl): 5–15

Anderson J L, Hackworthy R A, Sorensen S G et al 1989 Comparison of intravenous anistreplase (APSAC) and streptokinase in acute myocardial infarction: interim report of a randomised double blind patency study. Circulation 80 (suppl II): 420–422

Arnold A E R, Serruys P W, Rutsch W et al 1990 Reasons for lack of success of immediate angioplasty during recombinant tissue plasminogen activator treatment for acute myocardial infarction: a regional wall motion analysis. Journal of the American College of Cardiology 17: 11–21

Been M, de Bono D P, Muir A L, Boulton F E, Fears R, Standring R,

Ferres H 1986 Clinical effects and pharmocokinetics of intravenous APSAC — anisoylated plasminogen streptokinase activator complex (BRL26921) — in acute myocardial infarction. International Journal of Cardiology 11: 53–61

Bett J H N, Castaldi P A, Chesterman P N, Hale G S, Hirsh J, Isbister J P, McDonald I G, McLean K H, Morgan J J, O'Sullivan E F, Rosenbaum M 1973 Australian multicentre trial of streptokinase in acute myocardial infarction. Lancet i: 57–61

Bleich S D, Nichols T, Schumacher R et al 1990 Effect of heparin on coronary arterial patency after thrombolysis with tissue plasminogen activator in acute myocardial infarction. American Journal of Cardiology 66: 1412–1417

Boucek R J, Murphy W P 1960 Segmental perfusion of the coronary arteries with fibrinolysin in man following a myocardial infarction. American Journal of Cardiology 6: 525–533

Breddin K, Ehrly A M, Fechler L et al 1973 Die Kurzzeitfibrinolyse beim akuten Myokardinfarkt. Deutsche Medizinische Wochenschrift 98: 861–869

Brochier M, Raynaud P, Fauchier J P et al 1980 Comparison between lung scans and pulmonary angiograms in the evaluation of the perfusion defect in massive and submassive pulmonary embolism. In: Widimsky J (ed) Pulmonary embolism. S Karger, Basel, p 120–126

Chazov E L, Mareeva L S, Mazaev A V et al 1976 Intracoronary administration of fibrinolysin in acute myocardial infarction. Terapeuticheskii Arkhiv 48: 8–20

Chesebro J H, Knatterud G, Robert R et al 1987 Thrombolysis in myocardial infarction (TIMI) trial, phase I: a comparison between intravenous tissue plasminogen activator and intravenous streptokinase. Circulation 76: 142–154

Clozel J P, Banken L, Roux S 1990 Aprotinin: an antidote for recombinant tissue type plasminogen activator (rt-PA) active in vivo. Journal of American College of Cardiology 16: 507–510

Collins R for the ISIS-3 (Third International Study of Infarct Survival) Collaborative group 1991 Data presented at American College of Cardiology meeting, March 1991, Dallas, USA

Davies M J, Thomas A C 1985 Plaque fissuring: the cause of acute myocardial infarction, sudden ischaemic death and crescendo angina. British Heart Journal 53: 363–373

de Bono D P, Bhattacharrya A K 1991 Segmental analysis of coronary arterial stenoses in patients presenting with angina or first myocardial infarction. International Journal of Cardiology 32: 313–322

de Bono D P, Pringle S 1991 Local inhibition of thrombolysis using urokinase linked to a monoclonal antibody which recognises damaged endothelium. Thrombosis Research 61: 537–545

de Bono D P, Pringle S, Underwood I 1991 Differential effects of aprotinin and tranexamic acid on cerebral bleeding and cutaneous bleeding time during rt-PA infusion. Thrombosis Research 61: 159–163

de Bono D P, Simoons M R, Tijssen J et al 1992 Early intravenous heparin enhances coronary patency after alteplase thrombolysis: results of a randomised double blind European Cooperative Study Group trial. British Heart Journal (in press)

del Zoppo G J 1988 Thrombolytic therapy in cerebrovascular disease. Stroke 19: 1174–1179

De Wood M A, Spores J, Notske R, Mouser L T, Burroughs R, Golden M S, Lang H T 1980 Prevalence of total coronary occlusion during the early hours of myocardial infarction. New England Journal of Medicine 303: 897–902

Diogardi N, Mannucci P M, Lotto A, Rossi P, Levi G F, Lomanto B, Rota M, Mattei G, Proto C, Fiorelli G 1971 Controlled trial of streptokinase and heparin in acute myocardial infarction. Lancet ii: 891–894

Dotter C T, Rosch J, Seaman A J 1974 Selective clot lysis with low dose streptokinase. Radiology 111: 31

European Cooperative Study Group for streptokinase treatment in acute myocardial infarction 1979 Streptokinase in acute myocardial infarction. New England Journal of Medicine 310: 797–802

European Working Party 1971 Streptokinase in recent myocardial infarction: a controlled multicentre trial. British Medical Journal iii: 325–329

Fletcher A P, Alkjaersig N, Smyrniotis F E, Sherry S 1959 The treatment of patients suffering from early myocardial infarction with massive and prolonged streptokinase therapy. Transactions of the Association of American Physicians 71: 287–295

Gemill J D, Hogg K J, MacIntyre P D et al 1991 Clot specificity and coronary patency with bolus alteplase and streptokinase containing agents in myocardial infarction. European Heart Journal 12: 390 (A)

Gimpel L W, Gold H K, Leinbach R C et al 1989 Correlation between template bleeding time and spontaneous bleeding during treatment of acute myocardial infarction with recombinant tissue type plasminogen activator. Circulation 80: 581–585

GISSI-1: Gruppo Italiano per lo Studio della Streptochinasi nell'Infarto Miocardico 1986 Effectiveness of intravenous thrombolytic treatment in acute myocardial infarction. Lancet i: 397–402

GISSI-1 1987 Long term effects of intravenous thrombolysis in acute myocardial infarction. Final report of the GISSI study. Lancet i: 871–874

GISSI-2: Gruppo Italiano per lo Studio della Sopravivvenza nell'Infarto Miocardico 1990 A factorial randomised trial of alteplase versus streptokinase and heparin versus streptokinase and no heparin among 12 490 patients with acute myocardial infarction. Lancet 336: 65–71

Gold H K, Coller B S, Yasuda T et al 1988 Rapid and sustained coronary artery recanalisation with combined bolus injection of recombinant tissue type plasminogen activator and monoclonal antiplatelet GP IIb/IIIa antibody in a canine preparation. Circulation 88: 670–677

Goldhaber S Z, Buring J E, Lipnick R J, Hennekens C H 1984 Pooled analysis of randomized trials of streptokinase and heparin in phlebographically documented acute deep venous thrombosis. American Journal of Medicine 76: 393–397

Graor R A, Risius B, Denney K et al 1985 Local thrombolysis in the treatment of thrombosed arteries, bypass grafts and arteriovenous fistulae. Journal of Vascular Survery 2: 406–14

Hall G H 1987 Bolus streptokinase after myocardial infarction. Lancet 2: 96–97

Herrick J B 1912 Clinical features of sudden obstruction of the coronary arteries. Journal of the American Medical Association 59: 2015–2020

Hsia J, Hamilton W P, Kleiman N, Roberts R, Chaitman B R, Ross A M 1990 A comparison between heparin and low dose aspirin as adjunctive therapy with tissue plasminogen activator for acute myocardial infarction. New England Journal of Medicine 323: 1433–1437

International Study Group 1990 In-hospital mortality and clinical course of 20 891 patients with suspected acute myocardial infarction randomised between alteplase and streptokinase with or without heparin. Lancet 336: 71–75

ISAM Study Group 1986 A prospective study of intravenous streptokinase in acute myocardial infarction (ISAM). New England Journal of Medicine 314: 1465–1471

ISIS-2 Collaborative Group 1988 Randomised trial of intravenous streptokinase, oral aspirin, both or neither among 17 187 cases of suspected acute myocardial infarction: ISIS-2. Lancet ii: 349–360

Jalihal S, Morris G K 1990 Antistreptokinase titres after intravenous streptokinase. Lancet 335: 184–185

Khan M I, Hackett D R, Andreotti F, Davies G J, Regan T, Haider A W, McFadden E, Halson P, Maseri A 1990 Effectiveness of multiple bolus administration of tissue type plasminogen activator in acute myocardial infarction. American Journal of Cardiology 65: 1051–1056

Kolodgie F D, Virmani R, Farb A, Hart C L 1991 Limitation of no reflow injury by blood-free reperfusion with oxygenated perfluorochemical (Fluosol-DA 20%). Journal of the American College of Cardiology 18: 215–223

Levine M, Hirsh J, Weitz J et al 1990 A randomized trial of a single bolus dosage regimen of recombinant tissue plasminogen activator in patients with acute pulmonary embolism. Chest 98: 1473–79

McNamara T O, Fischer J R Thrombolysis of peripheral arterial and graft occlusions: Improved results using high dose urokinase. American Journal of Radiology 144: 769–785

McNichol G P, Reid W, Bain W H, Douglas A S 1963 Treatment of peripheral arterial occlusion by streptokinase perfusion. British Medical Journal 1: 1508

Mathey D G, Schofer J, Sheehan F H, Becker H, Tilsner V, Dodge

H T 1985 Intravenous urokinase in acute myocardial infarction. American Journal of Cardiology 55: 878–882

Melandri G, Branzi A, Semprini F, Cervi V, Galie N, Magnani B 1990 Enhanced thrombolytic efficacy and reduction of infarct size by simultaneous infusion of streptokinase and heparin. British Heart Journal 64: 118–120

Meyer J, Merx W, Doerr R, Lambertz H, Bethge C, Effert S 1982 Successful treatment of acute myocardial infarction shock by combined percutaneous transluminal coronary recanalisation and percutaneous transluminal coronary angioplasty. American Heart Journal 103: 132–134

Meyer G, Charbonnier B, Stern M, Brochier M, Sors H 1989 Thrombolysis in acute pulmonary embolism. In: Julian D G, Kubler W, Norris R M, Swan H J C, Collen D, Verstraete M (eds) Thrombolysis in cardiovascular disease. Dekker, New York, p 337–360

Miller G A H, Sutton G C, Kerr I H, Gibson R V, Honey M 1971 Comparison of streptokinase and heparin in treatment of isolated acute massive pulmonary embolism. British Medical Journal ii: 681–684

Mullane K M, Smith C W 1990 The role of leukocytes in ischaemic damage, reperfusion injury, and repair of the myocardium. In: Piper H M (ed) Pathophysiology of severe ischemic myocardial injury. Kluwer, Dordrecht, p 239–268

National Heart Foundation of Australia Coronary Thrombolysis Group 1989 A randomised comparison of oral aspirin/dipyridamole versus intravenous heparin after recombinant tissue plasminogen activator for acute myocardial infarction. Circulation 80 (suppl 2): 114 (A)

Neuhaus K L, Tebbe U, Gottwik M, Weber M A J, Feuerer W, Niederer W, Haerer W, Praetorius F, Grosser K D, Huhmann W, Hoepp H W, Alber G, Sheikhzadeh A, Schneider B 1988 Intravenous recombinant tissue plasminogen activator (rt-PA) and urokinase in acute myocardial infarction: Results of the German Activator Urokinase Study (GAUS) Journal of the American College of Cardiology 12: 581–587

Neuhaus K L, Werner F, Jeep-Tebbe S, Niederer W, Vogt A, Tebbe U 1989 Improved thrombolysis with a modified dose regimen of recombinant tissue type plasminogen activator. Journal of the American College of Cardiology 14: 1566–1569

Obrastzow W P, Straschenko N D 1910 Zur Kenntnis der Thrombose der Koronarterien des Herzens. Zeikschrift Klinische Medizinische 71: 116–125

Petitpretz P, Simmoneau G, Cerrina J et al 1984 Effects of a single bolus of urokinase in patients with life-threatening pulmonary embolism: a descriptive trial. Circulation 70: 861–866

PRIMI Trial Study Group 1989 Randomised double-blind trial of recombinant pro-urokinase against streptokinase in acute myocardial infarction. Lancet i: 863–867

Rapold H J, de Bono D P, Arnold A E R, Arnout J, de Cock F, Collen D, Verstraete M 1991 Plasma fibrinopeptide A levels in patients with acute myocardial infarction treated with alteplase: correlation with concomitant heparin, coronary artery patency, and recurrent ischaemia. Journal of the American College of Cardiology in press

Rentrop P, Blanke H, Karsch K R, Kostering K, Oster H, Leitz K 1979 Acute myocardial infarction: intracoronary application of nitroglycerine and streptokinase in combination with transluminal recanalisation, Clinical Cardiology 2: 354–363

Rijken D C, Hoylaerts M, Collén D 1982 Fibrinolytic properties of one chain and two chain human extrinsic (tissue type) plasminogen activator. Journal of Biological Chemistry 257: 2920–2925

Royston D, Bidstrup B, Taylor K M, Sapsford R N 1987 Effect of aprotinin on need for blood transfusion after open heart surgery. Lancet 2: 1289–1291

Ruebsamen K, Eschenfelder V 1991 Reocclusion after thrombolysis: a problem solved by hirudin? Blood Coagulation and Fibrinolysis 2: 97–100

Schroeder R, Biamino G, Leitner E R et al 1983 Intravenous short term infusion of streptokinase in myocardial infarction. Circulation 67: 536–548

Serruys P W, Arnold A E R, Brower R W et al 1987 Effect of continued rt-PA administration on the residual stenosis after initially successful recanalisation in acute myocardial infarction — a quantitative angiographic study of a randomised trial. European Journal of Cardiology 8: 1172–1181

Sherry S 1954 The fibrinolytic activity of streptokinase activated human plasmin. Journal of Clinical Investigation 3: 1054–1063

Simoons M L, Arnold A E R, Betriu A et al 1988 Thrombolysis with tissue plasminogen activator in acute myocardial infarction: No additional benefit from immediate percutaneous coronary angioplasty. Lancet i: 197–203

Smith R A G, Dupe R J, English P D, Green J 1981 Fibrinolysis with acyl-enzymes: a new approach to thrombolytic therapy. Nature (Lond) 290: 505–508

SWIFT (Should we intervene following thrombolysis) Trial Study group 1991 SWIFT Trial of delayed elective intervention v. conservative treatment after thrombolysis with anistreplase in acute myocardial infarction. British Medical Journal 302: 555–560

Topol E J, Califf R M, George B S et al 1988 Coronary arterial thrombolysis with combined infusion of recombinant tissue-type plasminogen activator and urokinase in patients with acute myocardial infarction. Circulation 77: 1100–1107

Tibbutt D A, Davies J A, Anderson J A et al 1974 Comparison by controlled clinical trial of streptokinase and heparin in treatment of life threatening pulmonary embolism. British Medical Journal i: 343–347

TIMI research group 1988 Immediate vs delayed catheterization and angioplasty following thrombolytic therapy for acute myocardial infarction. Journal of the American Medical Association 260: 2849–2858

TIMI research group 1989 Comparison of invasive and conservative strategies after treatment with intravenous tissue plasminogen activator in acute myocardial infarction. New England Journal of Medicine 320: 618–627

Transchesi B, Bellotti G, Chamone D F, Verstraete M 1989 Effect of combined administration of saruplase and single chain alteplase on coronary recanalisation in acute myocardial infarction. American Journal of Cardiology 64: 229–232

Tranchesi B, Chamone D F Cobbaert C, Van de Werf F, Vanhove P, Verstraete M 1991 Coronary recanalization rate after intravenous bolus of alteplase in acute myocardial infarction. American Journal of Cardiology 68: 161–165

Turpie A G G, Robinson J G, Doyle D J et al 1989 Comparison of high dose with low dose subcutaneous heparin to prevent left ventricular mural thrombosis in patients with acute transmural anterior infarction. New England Journal of Medicine 320: 352–357

Urokinase Pulmonary Embolism Trial 1973 A national cooperative study. Circulation 47 (suppl 2): 1–108

Vander Sande J, Bossaert L, Brochier M et al 1988 Thrombolytic treatment of pulmonary embolism with APSAC. European Respiration Journal 1(8): 721–726

Van de Werf F, Arnold A E R for the European Cooperative Study Group 1988 Effect of intravenous tissue plasminogen activator on infarct size, left ventricular function and survival in patients with acute myocardial infarction. British Medical Journal 297: 1374–1379

Vaughan D E, Kirshenbaum J M, Loscalzo J 1988 Streptokinase-induced antibody-mediated platelet aggregation: a potential cause of clot propagation in vivo. Journal of the American College of Cardiology 11: 1343–1348

Verheugt F 1991 The Apricot trial of anticoagulation following thrombolysis. European Cardiac Society Meeting, Amsterdam

Verstraete M, Bernard R, Bory M, Brower R W, Collen D, de Bono D P, Erbel R, Huhmann W, Lennane R J, Lubsen J, Mathey D, Meyer J, Michels H R, Rutsch W, Schartl M, Schmidt W, Uebis R, von Essen R 1985 Randomised trial of intravenous recombinant tissue type plasminogen activator versus streptokinase in acute myocardial infarction. Lancet i: 842–847

Verstraete M, Arnold A E R, Brower R W et al 1987 Acute coronary thrombolysis with recombinant human tissue type plasminogen activator: initial patency and effect of a maintenance infusion. American Journal of Cardiology 60: 231–237

Verstraete M, Miller G A H, Bounameaux H et al 1988 Intravenous and intrapulmonary recombinant tissue-type plasminogen activator in the treatment of acute massive pulmonary embolism. Circulation 77: 353–360

von Essen R for the TAPS study group 1991 Efficacy and safety of

alteplase, saruplase and anistreplase: the TAPS study. Circulation (in press)
White H D, Rivers J T, Maslowski A H et al 1989 Effect of intravenous streptokinase as compared with that of tissue type plasminogen activator on left ventricular function after first myocardial infarction. New England Journal of Medicine 320: 817–821
Wilcox R G, Von der Liffe G, Olsson C G, Jensen G, Skene A M, Hampton J R for the Asset Study Group 1988 Trial of tissue plasminogen activator for mortality reduction in acute myocardial infarction. Anglo Scandinavian Study of Early Thrombolysis (ASSET). Lancet ii: 525–530
White H D, Cross D B, William B F, Norris R M 1990 Safety and efficacy of repeat thrombolytic treatment after acute myocardial infarction. British Heart Journal 64: 177–184

67. Antiplatelet agents

V. Bertelé C. Cerletti G. de Gaetano

DEVELOPMENT OF KNOWLEDGE OF ANTIPLATELET DRUGS

The story of antiplatelet drugs started with the clinical observation of the protective effects of aspirin in the prevention of cardiovascular events when Craven reported his experience with aspirin as a 'nonspecific' prophylaxis of coronary thrombosis (Craven 1953). A few years later he was able to report that 'among 8000 men without previous symptoms of thrombosis . . . taking 5 to 10 grains (i.e. 325–650 mg) aspirin daily . . . not a single case of detectable coronary or cerebral thrombosis has occurred . . . (Craven 1956).

These observations were originally explained on the basis of the chemical similarity between salicylate and coumarin derivatives, the main anticoagulant drugs used at that time as antithrombotic prophylaxis. This observation was not related to platelets for several years until the antiplatelet effect of aspirin was discovered in 1967 (Weiss & Aledort 1967). However, it predicted the later results of randomized clinical trials and their meta-analysis.

The mechanism of action of aspirin as an antiplatelet drug (the inhibition of thromboxane A_2 production) was elucidated in the 1970s (for review see de Gaetano et al 1987). As well as its antithrombotic effect, there was significant reduction of vascular events. It is still surprising that by inhibiting the synthesis of a short half life second messenger in platelets one could reduce by a quarter the vascular events occurring in patients with previous vascular disease.

Like aspirin, which had a previous use as an analgesic and anti-inflammatory agent, sulfinpyrazone, an uricosuric drug, and dipyridamole, a coronary vasodilator, were investigated in a series of clinical trials in the 1970s aiming at assessing the benefits of the 'antiplatelet approach' in the secondary prevention of cardiovascular disease.

POTENTIAL ROLE OF ANTIPLATELET DRUGS IN PREVENTION OF THROMBOSIS

In most trials, positive trends in favour of antiplatelet drugs seldom reached statistical significance (de Gaetano et al 1982) and this disappointment provoked two reactions. The first was concern about the implications of vascular prostanoid inhibition by aspirin. As a result of the discovery of prostacyclin (Moncada et al 1976), the pharmacological action of aspirin was shown to be more complex in that besides inhibiting platelet production of the pro-aggregatory vasoconstrictor thromboxane A_2, it also inhibited vascular production of prostacyclin, a prostaglandin with biological effects opposite to thromboxane A_2 (anti-aggregation and vasodilation). This dual pharmacological activity seemed to limit its antithrombotic potential and encouraged a search for means to protect prostacyclin production while blocking thromboxane synthesis. New aspirin formulations, different dosage schedules expecially low-dose regimens, selective inhibitors of thromboxane synthase or receptor antagonists of this agonist were all proposed in the hope of finding a satisfactory pharmacological solution (de Gaetano et al 1987). Several clinical and pharmacological studies soon showed that in the thromboxane/prostacyclin balance, the former compound plays a major functional role (Pareti et al 1980) and that, though aspirin is not selective for *platelet* cyclo-oxygenase, it nevertheless blocks it more effectively than the equivalent vessel wall enzyme, whose main arachidonic acid metabolite is prostacyclin (de Gaetano et al 1987).

The second concern was regarding the pharmacological inhibition of the specific biochemical target, cyclo-oxygenase. Thromboxane synthesis is only one of the amplification pathways of platelet stimulation and parallels others such as PAF, ADP, and probably others as yet unknown whose function, left intact, might independently support a normal platelet response. Even assuming that antiplatelet treatment by aspirin was effective, it would have been a poor method of managing a complex, multifactorial condition such as thrombosis and preventing cardiovascular events, where the pathogenesis is not exclusively related to platelet response. At the beginning of the 1980s there was doubt that antiplatelet treatment could reduce cardiovascular mortality. The success of warfarin in the Sixty-Plus Reinfarction Study (SPRS Group 1980) provoked re-evaluation of the use of anticoagulants, an area which had been abandoned too quickly as being unsatisfactory 10 years before in the hope of greater efficacy with antiplatelet drugs.

Against this background of disillusionment (International Anticoagulant Review Group 1970) significantly beneficial results were obtained from the use of aspirin in patients with **unstable angina** (Lewis & Davies 1983, Cairns et al 1985) or with **aortocoronary bypass** (Chesebro et al 1982, 1984). Protection by aspirin, though considered interesting at the beginning, aroused fresh interest in its role in the prevention of cardiovascular events. The Food and Drug Administration recommended the use of aspirin for patients at risk of coronary artery disease, arguing that the advantage, though modest (20% reduction in cardiovascular events) would become worthwhile once applied to the general population (Anonymous 1985).

Proof of clinical efficacy

From a meta-analysis of the Antiplatelet Trialists' Collaboration (APT Collaboration 1988) it is expected that the use of antiplatelet drugs will prevent 25% of the expected vascular events (myocardial infarction, cerebral stroke, vascular death) in patients with previous infarction or stroke.

A more recent — still unpublished — meta-analysis from the same group (APT 1993) extends this observation to other categories of patients with different cardiovascular risks including healthy subjects in primary prevention studies. This overview confirms the previously estimated reduction of vascular events and provides evidence that the advantage is consistent across different categories of vascular conditions, in different patient groups, using different drugs and doses for different durations. Thus the efficacy of the antiplatelet approach has been eventually proven within an overall epidemiologic framework.

As far as vascular mortality is concerned (the most objective and, therefore, reliable end point), further questions should be raised. Reduction of vascular deaths by antiplatelet drugs is mostly due to the benefit observed in the coronary artery thrombosis, particularly in acute thrombotic occlusion as reported in several trials of aspirin in unstable angina and acute myocardial infarction; Veterans' Administration Cooperative Study (Lewis et al 1983), Canadian Multicenter Trial (Cairns et al 1985) and ISIS-2 (ISIS-2 1988). Much less clear is the therapeutic advantage of antiplatelet drugs in patients at risk following previous cerebrovascular accidents and even less in a healthy population for primary prevention.

What are the reasons for such different results? And what does this mean regarding clinical use of antiplatelet drugs? The potential benefit of antiplatelet agents in coronary artery disease suggests that their antithrombotic potential gives rise to their clinical efficacy. A suitable clinical trial model to prove this is represented by the ISIS-2 study. In patients with suspected acute myocardial infarction low-dose aspirin (160 mg daily) reduced the early mortality by about one-fifth, a potential benefit similar to that provided by thrombolysis with streptokinase in the same trial. The combination of the two drugs almost halved mortality in the acute phase following myocardial infarction. The results of the ISIS-2 trial should be viewed in the light of angiographic and pathological findings (de Wood et al 1980, Davies & Thomas 1985, Davies 1992), suggesting that coronary artery thrombosis is a dynamic event in the spectrum of coronary ischaemia.

Aspirin as well as streptokinase, could reduce mortality in acute myocardial infarction by interfering with the dynamic formation of a coronary thrombus still subject to opposing stimulations, i.e. thrombogenesis due to plaque fissuring and thrombolysis due to activation of endogenous fibrinolysis. The same antithrombotic mechanism may be responsible for the impressive reduction of myocardial infarction and death in another clinical situation of acute thrombogenesis, unstable angina (Lewis et al 1983, Cairns et al 1985).

The data of the still unpublished APT meta-analysis of the prevention of deep vein thrombosis deserves some additional comments (Antiplatelet Trialists' Collaboration 1993). The reduction of deep vein thrombosis in different groups of surgical and medical patients at risk is most surprising. Though of less clinical relevance in terms of absolute benefit due to the lower incidence of the events, no less surprising is the even greater avoidance of pulmonary embolism by the use of antiplatelet drugs in the same set of patients. These findings, indeed, are in contradiction to the long-held pathophysiological and therapeutical belief about the minor role of platelets and consequently of antiplatelet agents in venous thrombosis, an event which is supposed to result from primary activation of coagulation factors possibly facilitated by stasis rather than a cellular-mediated blood response to vascular lesions.

Haemorrhagic side-effects

Aspirin also acts as an antithrombotic agent in cerebrovascular disease although there is less data on this role than obtained in coronary artery disease.

In patients with atrial fibrillation who have a high risk of an embolic stroke, 325 mg aspirin daily reduced by about one half the occurrence of ischaemic stroke and systemic embolism (Stroke Prevention in Atrial Fibrillation Study 1990), a benefit not observed in a previous trial (Petersen 1989) using a lower dose of aspirin (75 mg daily). The advantage offered by antiplatelet drugs in the secondary prevention of ischaemic stroke is confirmed by meta-analysis (APT Collaboration 1993) and recent trials

(Gent et al 1989, Hass et al 1989). Antiplatelet treatment appears to reduce stroke incidence by 20% across many categories of patients and in healthy subjects in primary prevention studies.

Thus, on the basis of the available data any excess risk of haemorrhagic stroke in people given antiplatelet agents is apparently more than compensated for by the reduction of risk of strokes from other causes. While this finding is reassuring, the proportional reduction of either fatal or disabling strokes may be modest.

It is possible that the brain bleeds more easily than the heart and the results of stroke prevention studies show that, besides being antithrombotic, antiplatelet therapy may carry a significant risk of haemorrhage. No other antiplatelet drug has been shown to offer a reduced risk of haemorrhage as compared to that with aspirin (Hass et al 1989) nor are low-dose aspirin regimens of any advantage as compared with medium/high dose ones (Dutch TIA Trial Study Group 1991). Indeed, while reducing the occurrence of stroke or death after transient ischaemic attacks or minor strokes, 75 mg aspirin daily still causes a significant excess of bleeding events as compared to placebo (SALT Collaborative Group 1991).

In the Dutch TIA Trial, besides being as effective as 283 mg aspirin in prevention of vascular events, 30 mg aspirin provoked fewer episodes of minor bleeding and overall adverse events. However, there was only a trend in favour of the lower dose with regard to major bleeding complications (Dutch TIA Trial Study Group 1991). Therefore, a haemorrhagic effect seems to be unavoidably associated with the antithrombotic properties of antiplatelet drugs.

ANTIPLATELET AGENTS HAVE NO EFFECT ON ATHEROGENESIS

The most disappointing result of antiplatelet treatment concerns primary prevention of vascular events. According to the APT meta-analysis, the benefits of antiplatelet drugs on total vascular events is uncertain; their effect on vascular mortality is virtually zero. Nor could one expect any better outcome in primary prevention on the basis of the US Physicians' (SCPHSRG 1989) and the British Doctors' (Peto et al 1988) trials. In this latter study high-dose aspirin did not have any cardiovascular protection. In the US Physicians' Trial, 300 mg aspirin every other day significantly reduced both fatal and non-fatal myocardial infarction during the 5-year follow-up. However, both total and vascular mortality remained unchanged, not necessarily as a result of fatal haemorrhagic events but rather of sudden deaths generally ascribed to coronary artery thrombosis (Davies & Thomas 1984).

The limited benefit of aspirin in the US Physicians' primary prevention trial may be explained by two factors. For these low-risk subjects the proportional reduction of vascular events was lower than that estimated for the overall population considered in the APT meta-analysis. Furthermore, this proportional advantage matched a low absolute risk, due to the low incidence of all events in this particular healthy population. This resulted in a small absolute benefit, that would not increase by much even if the proportional risk reduction in primary prevention equalled that estimated for the overall population subjected to the meta-analysis. If the number of events to be prevented are few, significance is not attained. That means that if started too early before the occurrence of an acute thrombotic event, antiplatelet strategy fails. The results of primary prevention trials thus imply that antiplatelet agents while being antithrombotic, do not interfere with the atherosclerotic process. Indeed, among American doctors, aspirin protected from myocardial infarction only those over the age of 50 in whom pre-existing atherosclerotic lesions were more likely accompanied by thrombotic complications.

This is supported by the following evidence: in patients undergoing secondary prevention of vascular events after a coronary episode (i.e. those in whom atherosclerosis has developed far enough to promote local thrombosis) antiplatelet drugs prevented cerebral events as well as new coronary episodes (APT Collaboration 1988). On the other hand, in subjects in primary prevention trials in whom atherosclerotic plaques have not yet produced any clinical manifestations aspirin failed to reduce strokes, even the occlusive ones (SCPHSRG 1989).

The lack of benefit of antiplatelet therapy in the atherosclerotic process is understandable in the light of the evidence that the role of platelets in atherogenesis is not critical. Platelets seem to be involved only in the complications of severe atherosclerotic lesions with major endothelial damage. In this situation platelets adhere to the subendothelium and contribute to the proliferative lesion by releasing growth factors. In the less severe state macrophages and smooth muscle cells migrated into the intima as well as endothelial cells themselves and may provide growth factors at the site of minimal vascular injuries, thus making the platelet contribution not critical (Ross 1986).

The most convincing clinical model of the mechanism (antithrombotic rather than antiatherogenic) by which antiplatelet drugs exert vascular protection is in coronary angioplasty. In this situation of an acute vascular lesion induced by the ballooning procedure, a combination of aspirin and dipyridamole reduced the early occurrence of myocardial infarction, but failed to protect from the restenosis in the medium term. In other words antiplatelet treatment can protect from the acute thrombogenic stimulus generated by the injured vessel wall, but cannot inhibit the subsequent atherogenic-like proliferative process (Schwartz et al 1988).

Notwithstanding the above considerations, the lack of an effective strategy (pharmacological or not) to control the atherosclerotic process itself stimulates us to attempt to reduce thrombotic risk related to it and to prevent the thrombotic episodes, that can suddenly turn an asymptomatic clinical picture into acute life-threatening vascular event.

Even with this perspective, however, cardiovascular risk cannot be defined as an 'all or nothing phenomenon'. More likely its increase parallels the progress of atherosclerosis between the two extremes of the healthy physicians and the patients with life-threatening unstable angina. Thus, there must be a threshold of risk within this scale at which the advantage of preventative approaches becomes significant.

The kind of benefit provided by antiplatelet agents allows the extension of their use to categories of patients at risk in whom the advantage has never been proved directly so far. This is the case in patients with peripheral occlusive process not necessarily confined to the limbs. Indeed, coronary death rather than amputation influences the prognosis of these patients (Second Consensus Document on Critical Leg Ischaemia 1991). This document strongly recommends routine, antiplatelet prophylaxis in all patients with no contraindications and also in those undergoing invasive procedures of revascularization such as angioplasty or reconstructive surgery in whom antiplatelet treatment is indicated for its documented efficacy (Chesebro et al 1984, APT Collaboration 1988, Schwartz et al 1988).

CLINICAL PRACTICE OR BASIC RESEARCH?

Notwithstanding the evidence of a substantial clinical benefit applicable in a large variety of patient groups, the advantage offered by current antiplatelet drugs in particular clinical conditions is still questionable. Therefore, while being currently acceptable as a pragmatic strategy, the use of these drugs in the prophylaxis of vascular events must be addressed with caution in those areas in which the benefit is not definitively proved, e.g. in primary prevention of both fatal and non-fatal vascular events. Despite the therapeutic benefits so far achieved, further testing of the efficacy of antiplatelet drugs particularly in combinations is mandatory. Some of these hypotheses would be better tested in the prevention of primary vascular events. Indeed, as an intermediate approach between attempts to prevent vascular events in apparently healthy subjects and patients with previous vascular events, the test of efficacy of antiplatelet drugs in subjects with cardiovascular risk factors would be better addressed in the 'natural' environment of non-ill subjects attending their doctor for everyday problems such as high blood pressure, serum cholesterol or glucose levels, the known clinical risk associations for vascular disease.

Which antiplatelet drug to use or test?

As in most cases of meta-analysis, the APT meta-analysis considered the whole range of antiplatelet treatments. When analysed, no particular antiplatelet treatment was found to be significantly more effective than any other. The generalization of the estimated benefit to several antiplatelet drugs or combinations offers a wider range of choices according to the availability of drugs, the suitability of the dosage or formulation, the preference of the patients and the need for improving their compliance.

However, the major role of aspirin as a reference treatment for both current clinical practice and future controlled trials cannot be overlooked. Indeed, among 90 000 patients considered for the indirect comparison between different antiplatelet agents and controls, 80 000 were enrolled in trials testing aspirin efficacy. Among almost 10 000 events recorded in these trials, 8500 occurred in aspirin trials and, most important, 500 out of about 550 events avoided in the treatment groups were avoided by aspirin. Therefore, only a misleading interpretation of the APT message would suggest the conclusion that the use of any antiplatelet drug would avoid one fourth of vascular events.

Which dose of aspirin to use or test?

According to the reports of the APT Collaboration, there is no dose-dependence of the protection provided by aspirin in a large variety of categories of patients with various vascular conditions. Efficacy of a low/medium dose regimen does not appear to differ from that of a high-dose one. Moreover, however low the dose of aspirin, as long as it suppresses platelet thromboxane production it seems to prevent vascular events. Therefore, although high-dose aspirin might interfere with thrombus formation and growth by mechanisms other than thromboxane synthesis inhibition (de Gaetano et al 1986, Roncaglioni et al 1988), the lowest dose which is of proven efficacy should be recommended.

On the other hand the effects on platelet thromboxane is not the only determinant of bleeding due to aspirin (de Gaetano et al 1985, Gaspari et al 1987). It is also questionable whether a low-dose regimen actually has a lower haemorrhagic potential or whether this theoretical advantage has any clinical relevance.

Thus to the best of our present knowledge, a dose range between 50 and 300 mg daily can be recommended for the current indications of the clinical use of aspirin.

Acknowledgements

This work was supported by the National Research Council, Rome, Italy: Progetto Finalizzato FATMA, contract no. 92.00227.41. The authors thank Maria Teresa Di Prospero for her contribution in editing the manuscript.

REFERENCES

Anonymous 1985 Aspirin for heart patients. FDA Drug Bulletin 15: 34

Antiplatelet Trialists' Collaboration 1988 Secondary prevention of vascular disease by prolonged antiplatelet treatment. British Medical Journal 296: 320

Antiplatelet Trialists' Collaboration 1993: in press

Cairns J A, Gent M, Singer J et al 1985 Aspirin, sulfinpyrazone or both in unstable angina. New England Journal of Medicine 313: 1369–1375

Chesebro J H, Clements I P, Fuster V et al 1982 A platelet inhibitor drug trial in coronary-artery bypass operations: benefit of perioperative dipyridamole and aspirin therapy on early postoperative vein graft patency. New England Journal of Medicine 307: 73–80

Chesebro J H, Fuster V, Elveback L R et al 1984 Effect of dipyridamole and aspirin on the vein-graft patency after coronary bypass operations. New England Journal of Medicine 310: 209–214

Craven L L 1953 Experiences with aspirin (acetylsalicylic acid) in the non specific prophylaxis of coronary thrombosis. Mississippi Valley Medical Journal 75: 38–44

Craven L L 1956 Prevention of coronary and cerebral thrombosis. Mississippi Valley.Medical Journal 78: 213

Davies M J 1992 Anatomic features in victims of sudden coronary death. Coronary artery pathology. Circulation 85 (suppl l): 19–24

Davies M J, Thomas A C 1984 Thrombosis and acute coronary lesions in sudden cardiac ischemic death. New England Journal of Medicine 310: 1137–1140

Davies M J, Thomas A C 1985 Plaque fissuring: the cause of acute myocardial infarction, sudden ischaemic death and crescendo angina. British Heart Journal 53: 363–373

de Gaetano G, Cerletti C, Bertelé V 1982 Pharmacology of antiplatelet drugs and clinical trials on thrombosis prevention: a difficult link. Lancet ii: 974–977

de Gaetano G, Cerletti C, Dejana E, Latini R 1985 Pharmacology of platelet inhibition in humans: implications of the salicylate-aspirin interaction. Circulation 72(6): 1185–1193

de Gaetano G, Carriero M R, Cerletti C, Mussoni L 1986 Low dose aspirin does not prevent fibrinolytic response to venous occlusion. Biochemical Pharmacology 35: 3147–3150

de Gaetano G, Bertelé V, Cerletti C 1987 Pharmacology of antiplatelet drugs. In MacIntyre E, Gordon J L (eds) Platelets in biology and pathology III. Elsevier Science, London, pp 515–525

de Wood M A, Spores J, Notske R et al 1980 Prevalence of total coronary occlusion during the early hours of transmural myocardial infarction. New England Journal of Medicine 303: 897–902

Dutch T I A Trial Study Group 1991 A comparison of two doses of aspirin (30 mg vs 283 mg a day) in patients after a transient ischemic attack of minor stroke. New England Journal of Medicine 325: 1261–1266

European Working Group on Critical Leg Ischaemia 1991 Second Consensus Document on Chronic Critical Leg Ischaemia. Circulation 84 (suppl 4): 1–10

Gaspari F, Vigano' G, Orisio S, Bonati M, Livio M, Remuzzi G 1987 Aspirin prolongs bleeding time in uremia by a mechanism distinct from platelet cyclooxygenase inhibition. Journal of Clinical Investigation 79: 1788–1797

Gent M, Blakeley J A, Easton J D, CATS Group 1989 The Canadian-American ticlopidine study (CATS) in thromboembolic stroke. Lancet i: 1215–1220

Hass W K, Easton D J, Adams H P et al 1989 A randomized trial comparing ticlopidine hydrochloride with aspirin for the prevention of stroke in highrisk patients. New England Journal of Medicine 321: 501–507

International Anticoagulant Review Group 1970 Collaborative analysis of long-term anticoagulant administration after acute myocardial infarction. Lancet 1: 203–209

ISIS-2 Collaborative Group 1988 Randomised trial of intravenous streptokinase, oral aspirin, both or neither among 17,189 cases of suspected acute myocardial infarction. Lancet ii: 349–360

Lewis H D, Davies J W, Archibald D J et al 1983 Protective effect of aspirin against myocardial infarction and death in men with unstable angina: result of a Veterans Administration cooperative study. New England Journal of Medicine 309: 396–403

Moncada S, Gryglewski R, Bunting S, Vane J R 1976 An enzyme isolated from arteries transforms prostaglandin endoperoxides to an unstable substance that inhibits platelets aggregation. Nature 263: 663–665

Pareti F I, Mannucci P M, D'Angelo A, Smith J B, Sautebin L, Galli G 1980 Congenital deficiency of thromboxane and prostacyclin. Lancet i: 898–901

Petersen P, Boysen G, Godtfredsen J, Andersen E D, Andersen B 1989 Placebo-controlled randomized trial of warfarin and aspirin for prevention of thromboembolic complications in chronic atrial fibrillation: the Copenhagen AFASAK Study. Lancet i: 175–179

Peto R, Gray R, Collins R et al 1988 Randomised trial of prophylactic daily aspirin in British male doctors. British Medical Journal 296: 313–316

Roncaglioni M C, Reyers I, Cerletti C, Donati M B, de Gaetano G 1988 Moderate anticoagulation by salicylate prevents thrombosis without bleeding. Biochemical Pharmacology 37: 4743

Ross R 1986 Pathogenesis of atherosclerosis. An update. New England Journal of Medicine 314: 488–500

SALT Collaboration Group 1991 Swedish aspirin low-dose trial (SALT) of 75 mg aspirin as secondary prophylaxis after cerebrovascular ischaemic events. Lancet 338: 1345–1349

Schwartz L, Bourassa M G, Lesperance J et al 1988 Aspirin and dipyridamole in the prevention of restenosis after percutaneous transluminal coronary angioplasty. New England Journal of Medicine 318: 1714–1719

Sixty Plus Reinfarction Study Research Group 1980 A double blind trial to assess long-term oral anticoagulant therapy in elderly patients after myocardial infarction. Lancet ii: 989–993

Steering Committee of the Physicians' Health Study Research Group 1989 Final report on the aspirin component of the ongoing physicians' health study. New England Journal of Medicine 321: 129–135

Stroke Prevention in Atrial Fibrillation Study Group Investigators 1990 Preliminary report of the stroke prevention in atrial fibrillation study. New England Journal of Medicine 322: 863–868

Weiss H J, Aledort L M 1967 Impaired platelet-connective tissue interaction in men after aspirin ingestion. Lancet ii: 495–497

Index

Vol 1 pp 1–717 Vol 2 pp 719–1477